Textbook of
PULMONARY AND CRITICAL CARE MEDICINE

Textbook of PULMONARY AND CRITICAL CARE MEDICINE

Volume 1

Second Edition

Editor-in-Chief

SK Jindal

MD FAMS FNCCP FICS FCCP

Professor Emeritus

Department of Pulmonary Medicine

Postgraduate Institute of Medical Education and Research

Chandigarh, India

Medical Director, Jindal Clinics, Chandigarh

Associate Editors

Ritesh Agarwal

Ashutosh N Aggarwal

D Behera

Aditya Jindal

Suhail Raoof

PS Shankar

Section Editors

Ritesh Agarwal

Ashutosh N Aggarwal

D Behera

Sunil K Chhabra

Sahajal Dhooria

Randeep Guleria

Richard S Irwin

Aditya Jindal

SK Jindal

Sundeep Salvi

Inderpaul Singh Sehgal

Nusrat Shafiq

PS Shankar

Navneet Singh

Balamugesh T

VK Vijayan

Foreword

Sidney S Braman

JAYPEE *The Health Sciences Publisher*

New Delhi | London | Panama

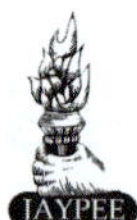

Jaypee Brothers Medical Publishers (P) Ltd.

Headquarters
Jaypee Brothers Medical Publishers (P) Ltd.
4838/24, Ansari Road, Daryaganj
New Delhi 110 002, India
Phone: +91-11-43574357
Fax: +91-11-43574314
E-mail: jaypee@jaypeebrothers.com

Overseas Offices

J.P. Medical Ltd.
83, Victoria Street, London
SW1H 0HW (UK)
Phone: +44-20 3170 8910
Fax: +44(0) 20 3008 6180
E-mail: info@jpmedpub.com

Jaypee-Highlights Medical Publishers Inc.
City of Knowledge, Building 235, 2nd Floor
Clayton, Panama City, Panama
Phone: +1 507-301-0496
Fax: +1 507-301-0499
E-mail: cservice@jphmedical.com

Jaypee Brothers Medical Publishers (P) Ltd.
17/1-B, Babar Road, Block-B
Shaymali, Mohammadpur
Dhaka-1207, Bangladesh
Mobile: +08801912003485
E-mail: jaypeedhaka@gmail.com

Jaypee Brothers Medical Publishers (P) Ltd.
Bhotahity, Kathmandu, Nepal
Phone: +977-9741283608
E-mail: kathmandu@jaypeebrothers.com

Website: www.jaypeebrothers.com
Website: www.jaypeedigital.com

Textbook of Pulmonary and Critical Care Medicine

First Edition : 2011
Second Edition : **2017**

ISBN 978-93-85999-99-4

Printed at Replika Press Pvt. Ltd.

Contributors

Amit Agarwal MD
Senior Research Fellow
Department of Pediatrics
Postgraduate Institute of Medical Education and Research
Chandigarh, India

Ritesh Agarwal MD DM
Additional Professor
Department of Pulmonary Medicine
Postgraduate Institute of Medical Education and Research
Chandigarh, India

Stuti Agarwal PhD
Senior Research Fellow
Department of Biochemistry
Postgraduate Institute of Medical Education and Research
Chandigarh, India

Ashutosh N Aggarwal MD DM
Professor
Department of Pulmonary Medicine
Postgraduate Institute of Medical Education and Research
Chandigarh, India

Deepak Aggarwal MD
Associate Professor
Department of Pulmonary Medicine
Government Medical College
Chandigarh, India

Gyanendra Agrawal MD DM
Consultant Pulmonologist
Department of Pulmonology
Jaypee Group of Hospitals
Noida, Uttar Pradesh, India

Anurag Agrawal MD PhD
Associate Professor
Academy of Scientific and Innovative Research, India and
Baylor College of Medicine, Houston, Texas, USA
Principal Scientist
Institute of Genomics and Integrative Biology
Delhi, India

Kanhaiyalal Agrawal MD
Physician
Department of Nuclear Medicine
Postgraduate Institute of Medical Education and Research
Chandigarh, India

Gautam Ahluwalia MD FAPS FICP FIACM
Professor
Department of Medicine
Dayanand Medical College and Hospital
Ludhiana, Punjab, India

Suhail Allaqaband MD FACC FCCP
Clinical Associate Professor
Cardiovascular Disease Section
Department of Medicine
University of Wisconsin School of Medicine and Public Health
Madison, Wisconsin, USA

Ashima Anand PhD
Principal Investigator
Exertional Breathlessness Studies Laboratory (DST)
Vallabhbhai Patel Chest Institute
University of Delhi, Delhi, India

Ronald Anderson PhD
Consultant
Department of Pulmonology and Internal Medicine
University of the Witwatersrand
Johannesburg, South Africa

Nidhi Anil PhD
Research Associate
Department of Pediatrics
Postgraduate Institute of Medical Education and Research
Chandigarh, India

Mark Astiz MD
Consultant
Weil Medical College
New York Methodist Hospital
Brooklyn, NY, USA

Jon G Ayres MD
Consultant
Institute of Occupational and Environmental Medicine
University of Birmingham
Birmingham, UK

Amanjit Bal MD DNB MAMS
Additional Professor
Department of Histopathology
Postgraduate Institute of Medical Education and Research
Chandigarh, India

Sandra Baldacci BSc
Project Associate
Pulmonary Environmental Epidemiology Unit
CNR Institute of Clinical Physiology
Pisa, Italy

Nargis K Bali MB
Senior Resident
Department of Clinical Microbiology
Sher-e-Kashmir Institute of Medical Sciences
Srinagar, Jammu and Kashmir, India

Daniel E Banks MD MS
Professor
Department of Medicine
Uniformed Services University of the Health Sciences
Bethesda, Maryland, USA

Ruchi Bansal MD
Consultant
Department of Medicine, Pulmonary, Critical Care and Sleep Medicine
New York Methodist Hospital
Brooklyn, New York, USA

Maj (Retd) Monica Barne MBBS
Medical Educator
Chest Research Foundation
Pune, Maharashtra, India

Peter J Barnes FRS FMedSci
Margaret Turner-Warwick Professor and Head
Department of Respiratory Medicine
Imperial College London
Airway Disease Section
National Heart and Lung Institute
London, UK

Pranab Baruwa MD
Senior Consultant
Department of Tuberculosis and Respiratory Medicine
Gauhati Medical College and Hospital
Guwahati, Assam, India

D Behera MD FCCP
Professor and Head
Department of Pulmonary Medicine
Postgraduate Institute of Medical Education and Research
Chandigarh, India

Dinkar Bhasin MD
Resident
Department of Medicine
All India Institute of Medical Sciences
New Delhi, India

Sidney S Braman MD FCCP
Professor
Department of Medicine
Icahn School of Medicine
New York, USA

Bill Brashier DTCD
Former Head
Academic Clinical and Molecular Research
Chest Research Foundation, Pune, India
Director-Scientific Operations
Novo Cellular Medicine Institute
San Fernando, Trinidad and Tobago, Caribbean

R Caroli MD
Consultant Pulmonologist
Department of Pulmonology
Fortis Hospital
Noida, Uttar Pradesh, India

Sonia Cerrai
Project Associate
Pulmonary Environment Epidemiology Unit
CNR Institute of Clinical Physiology
CNR, Pisa, Italy

VK Chadha MD
Head
Epidemiology and Research Division
National Tuberculosis Institute
Bengaluru, Karnataka, India

Arunaloke Chakrabarti MD
Professor and Head
Department of Medical Microbiology
Postgraduate Institute of Medical Education and Research
Chandigarh, India

Abha Chandra MD
Professor and Head
Department of Cardiothoracic and Vascular Surgery
Sri Venkateswara Institute of Medical Sciences
Tirupati, Andhra Pradesh, India

Dhruva Chaudhry MD DM
Professor and Head
Department of Pulmonary and Critical Care Medicine
Pt Bhagwat Dayal Sharma Post Graduate Institute of Medical Sciences
Rohtak, Haryana, India

Anil Chauhan PhD
Department of Pediatrics
Postgraduate Institute of Medical Education and Research
Chandigarh, India

Sunil K Chhabra MD
Professor and Head
Department of Cardiopulmonary Physiology
Vallabhbhai Patel Chest Institute
University of Delhi, Delhi, India

Prashant N Chhajed MD DNB
Director
Pulmonology and Centre for Sleep Disorders
Fortis Hiranandani Hospital
Navi Mumbai, Maharashtra, India

Devasahayam J Christopher MD FCCP FRCP
Professor and Head
Department of Respiratory Medicine
Christian Medical College and Hospital
Vellore, Tamil Nadu, India

Fabio Cibella
CNR Institute of Biomedicine and Molecular Immunology
Palermo, Italy

Stevens Conrad MD PhD FCCP
Professor
Department of Emergency Medicine, Pediatrics and Neurosurgery
Lousiana State University Health Sciences Centre
Shreveport, Louisiana, USA

Ashim Das MD
Professor
Department of Histopathology
Postgraduate Institute of Medical Education and Research
Chandigarh, India

Uma Devraj MD
Associate Professor
Department of Pulmonary Medicine
St John's Medical College
Bengaluru, Karnataka, India

Harakh V Dedhia MBBS
Former Professor
Department of Pulmonary and Critical Care Medicine
West Virginia University School of Medicine
Morgantown, West Virginia, USA

B Vijayalakshmi Devi MD
Additional Professor
Department of Radiodiagnosis
Sri Venkateswara Institute of Medical Sciences
Tirupati, Andhra Pradesh, India

RK Dewan MS
Consultant
Department of Thoracic Surgery
Lala Ram Sarup National Institute of Tuberculosis and Respiratory Diseases
Sri Aurobindo Marg, New Delhi, India

Lakhbir Kaur Dhaliwal MD
Former Professor and Head
Department of Obstetrics and Gynecology
Postgraduate Institute of Medical Education and Research
Chandigarh, India
Consultant Gynecologist, Mohali, Punjab, India

Rajinder Singh Dhaliwal MS MCh
Former Professor and Head
Department of Cardiothoracic and Vascular Surgery
Postgraduate Institute of Medical Education and Research
Chandigarh, India
Consultant Cardiothoracic Surgeon
Mohali, Punjab, India

Bhalinder Dhaliwal MS MCh
Resident
Department of Cardiothoracic Surgery
Postgraduate Institute of Medical Education and Research
Chandigarh, India

Raja Dhar MD MRCP MSc
Consultant
Pulmonary and Critical Care Medicine
Fortis Hospital
Kolkata, West Bengal, India

Abduljabbar Dheyab MD
Internist
Department of Pulmonary, Allergy and Critical Care Medicine
University of Massachusetts Medical School
Worcester, Massachusetts, USA

Sahajal Dhooria MD DM
Assistant Professor
Department of Pulmonary Medicine
Postgraduate Institute of Medical Education and Research
Chandigarh, India

Liesel D'silva MD DETRD
Senior Medical Advisor
Specialist in Respiratory Medicine
Mumbai, Maharashtra, India

George A D'Souza MD
Professor and Head
Department of Pulmonary Medicine
St John's Medical College
Bengaluru, Karnataka, India

Jyothy E MD DTCD
Assistant Professor
Department of Pulmonary Medicine
Government Medical College and Hospital
Kozhikode, Kerala, India

Rachael A Evans MB ChB MRCP (UK) PhD
Consultant
Department of Respiratory Medicine
West Park Healthcare Centre, University of Toronto
Toronto, Ontario, Canada

Charles Feldman MB BCh PhD DSc
Consultant
Department of Internal Medicine
University of the Witwatersrand Medical School
Johannesburg, South Africa

Kenneth R Fretwell MD
Chairman
Department of Surgery
Jamaica Hospital Medical Center
New York, USA

Joseph Friedman MD
Attending Physician
Department of Radiology
Jamaica Hospital Medical Center, New York, USA

Gajanan S Gaude MD
Professor and Head
Department of Pulmonary Medicine
Jawaharlal Nehru Medical College
Belgaum, Karnataka, India

AR Gayathri MD FCCP
Consultant
Department of Respiratory Medicine
Apollo Hospitals
Chennai, Tamil Nadu, India

Vishwsanath Gella MD DM
Senior Consultant Pulmonologist
Department of Pulmonary Medicine
Continental Hospitals
Hyderabad, Telangana, India

Liziamma George MD FCCP
Associate Professor
Department of Clinical Medicine
Weill Cornell Medical College
Director
Medical Intensive Care Unit
New York Methodist Hospital
Brooklyn, New York, USA

AG Ghoshal MD DNB FCCP
Director
National Allergy Asthma Bronchitis Institute
Kolkata, West Bengal, India

Baishakhi Ghosh PhD
Researcher
Chest Research Foundation, Pune, Maharashtra, India
Research Scholar
Symbiosis International University
Pune, Maharashtra, India

Sudheendra Ghosh C MD DTCD MPH
Ex-Professor and Head
Department of Pulmonary Medicine
Government Medical College and Hospital
Thiruvananthapuram, Kerala, India

Karthik Gnanapandithan MD
Former Senior Resident
Department of Medicine
Postgraduate Institute of Medical Education and Research
Chandigarh, India

N Goel MD
Assistant Professor
Department of Pulmonary Medicine
Vallabhbhai Patel Chest Institute
University of Delhi
Delhi, India

Roger S Goldstein MB ChB FRCP FCRP FCCP
Consultant
Department of Respiratory Medicine
West Park Healthcare Centre
Toronto, Ontario, Canada

Stephania La Grutta
Institute of Biomedicine and Molecular Immunology
Palermo, Italy

Randeep Guleria MD DM
Professor and Head
Department of Pulmonary, Critical Care and Sleep Medicine
All India Institute of Medical Sciences
Ansari Nagar, New Delhi, India

Kalpalatha K Guntupalli MD FCCP FCCM MACP
Professor
Department of Medicine
Chief, Pulmonary, Critical Care and Sleep Medicine
Baylor College of Medicine
Houston, Texas, USA

Dheeraj Gupta MD DM
Former Professor
Department of Pulmonary Medicine
Postgraduate Institute of Medical Education and Research
Chandigarh, India

KB Gupta MD
Senior Professor and Head
Department of Respiratory Medicine
Postgraduate Institute of Medical Sciences
Rohtak, Haryana, India

Mansi Gupta MBBS DM
Fellow
Department of Pulmonary Medicine
Vardhman Mahavir Medical College
Delhi, India

Nalini Gupta MD DNB
Associate Professor
Department of Cytology and Gynecologic Pathology
Postgraduate Institute of Medical Education and Research
Chandigarh, India

Nikhil Gupta MD
Assistant Professor
Department of Medicine
Era's Lucknow Medical College and Hospital
Lucknow, Uttar Pradesh, India

Prahlad R Gupta MD DM
Professor and Head
Department of Pulmonary Medicine
NIMS Medical College
Jaipur, Rajasthan, India

Richa Gupta MD
Assistant Professor
Department of Pulmonary Medicine
Christian Medical College and Hospital
Vellore, Tamil Nadu, India

Vijay Hadda MD
Assistant Professor
Department of Pulmonary, Critical Care and Sleep Medicine
All India Institute of Medical Sciences
New Delhi, India

Group Captain Ajay Handa MD DNB DM FCCP FAPS
Senior Advisor (Medicine and Pulmonary Medicine)
Professor
Department of Internal Medicine (RGUHS)
Command Hospital Air Force
Bengaluru, Karnataka, India

Shu Hashimoto MD PhD
Research Associate
Department of Internal Medicine
Nihon University
Tokyo, Japan

Miyuki Hayashi MD PhD
Research Associate
Department of Pediatrics
Nippon Medical School
Tokyo, Japan

Sean E Hesselbacher MD
Pulmonologist
Department of Pulmonary Medicine
Baylor College of Medicine
Ben Taub General Hospital
Houston, Texas, USA

Harmanjit Singh Hira MBBS MD DM FCCP
Director Professor
Department of Pulmonary Medicine
Maulana Azad Medical College and Associated Hospitals
New Delhi, India

David Honeybourne MD
Consultant Physician and Clinical Director
Honorary Clinical Reader in Respiratory Medicine and Biological Sciences
Department of Respiratory Medicine
Birmingham Heartlands Hospital
Birmingham, UK

Sunil HV MD
Head
Department of Nuclear Medicine
Postgraduate Institute of Medical Education and Research
Chandigarh, India

Christopher Kim Ming Hui MBBS MRCP
Consultant
Department of Medicine
University of Hong Kong
Queen Mary Hospital
The University of Hong Kong
Hong Kong, SAR China

Toru Igarashi MD
Research Associate
Department of Pediatrics
Nippon Medical School
Tokyo, Japan

Mary Sau Man Ip MD FRCP FHKCP FHKAM
Mok Hing Yiu Endowed Chair Professor
Head of Medicine
Chief-of-Division of Respiratory Medicine
The University of Hong Kong
Hong Kong, SAR China

Richard S Irwin MD
Professor
Department of Pulmonary, Allergy and Critical Care Medicine
University of Massachusetts Medical School
Worcester, Massachusetts, USA

Vikram Jaggi MD DNB
Medical Director
Asthma Chest and Allergy Centre
Vasant Enclave, Delhi, India

Sanjay Jain MD
Professor
Department of Internal Medicine
Postgraduate Institute of Medical Education and Research
Chandigarh, India

Ashok K Janmeja MD
Professor and Head
Department of Pulmonary Medicine
Government Medical College and Hospital
Chandigarh, India

M Fuad Jan MBBS MD
Cardiovascular Disease Fellow
Aurora Cardiovascular Services
Aurora Sinai/St. Luke's Medical Centers
Milwaukee, Wisconsin, USA

Jeba S Jenifer MD Dip Pal Med
AssociateProfessor
Palliative Care Unit
Christian Medical College
Vellore, Tamil Nadu, India

Aditya Jindal DNB DM FCCP
Consultant Interventional Pulmonology and Intensivist
Jindal Clinics
Chandigarh, India

SK Jindal MD FAMS FNCCP FICS FCCP
Professor Emeritus
Department of Pulmonary Medicine
Postgraduate Institute of Medical Education and Research
Medical Director
Jindal Clinics
Chandigarh, India

Umesh N Jindal MD
Senior Consultant and Director
Jindal IVF and Sant Memorial Hospital
Chandigarh, India

VK Jindal PhD
Honorary Professor
Department of Physics
Advanced Centre for Physics
Panjab University, Chandigarh, India

Kusum Joshi MD
Ex-Professor and Head
Department of Histopathology
Postgraduate Institute of Medical Education and Research
Chandigarh, India
Consultant Pathologist
Chandigarh, India

Mamta Kalra PhD
Senior Scientist
Immatics US Inc
Houston, Texas, USA

Madhur Kalyan MSc
Senior Research Fellow
Department of Biochemistry
Postgraduate Institute of Medical Education and Research
Chandigarh, India

F Karakontaki MD
Sismanoglio General Hospital
Athens, Greece

Surender Kashyap MD
Director
Professor and Head
Department of Pulmonary Medicine
Kalpana Chawla Government Medical College
Karnal, Haryana, India

Arvind H Kate
Institute of Pulmonology Medical Research and Development
Mumbai, Maharashtra, India

SK Katiyar MD
Former Principal and Dean
Ganesh Shankar Vidyarthi Memorial Medical College
Consultant Pulmonologist
Kanpur, Uttar Pradesh, India

S Katiyar MD
Consultant Chest Physician
Kanpur, Uttar Pradesh, India

Jean I Keddissi MD
Professor
Department of Medicine, Pulmonary Disease and Critical Care Section
University of Oklahoma Health Science Center
Oklahoma, USA

Ajmal Khan MD DM
Assistant Professor
Department of Pulmonary Medicine
Sanjay Gandhi Postgraduate Institute of Medical Education and Research
Lucknow, Uttar Pradesh, India

GC Khilnani MD
Professor
Department of Pulmonary, Critical Care and Sleep Medicine
All India Institute of Medical Sciences
New Delhi, India

Satoko Kimura MD
Research Associate
Department of Pediatrics
Nippon Medical School
Tokyo, Japan

Seth J Koenig MD FCCP
Attending Physician
Department of Pulmonary and Critical Care Medicine
Long Island Jewish Medical Center
New Hyde Park, New York, USA

Scott E Kopec MD
Department of Pulmonary Allergy and Critical Care Medicine
University of Massachusetts Medical School
Worcester, Massachusetts, USA

Parvaiz A Koul MD FACP FCCP
Professor and Head
Departments of Internal and Pulmonary Medicine
Sher-i-Kashmir Institute of Medical Sciences
Srinagar, Jammu and Kashmir, India

Sachin Kumar MD DM
Associate Professor
Department of Pulmonary Medicine
All India Institute of Medical Sciences
Raipur, Chhattisgarh, India

Suman Laal PhD
Associate Professor
Department of Pathology
New York University Langone Medical Centre
Veterans Affairs New York Harbor Healthcare System
New York, USA

Kin Bong Hubert Lam
Institute of Occupational and Environmental Medicine
University of Birmingham
Birmingham, UK

Romica Latawa PhD
Research Fellow
Department of Biochemistry
Postgraduate Institute of Medical Education and Research
Chandigarh, India

Angeline Lazarus MD MACP FCCP
Professor of Medicine
Uniformed Services University
National Naval Medical Center
Bethesda, Maryland, USA

Sneha Limaye MBBS
Research Fellow
Chest Research Foundation
Pune, Maharashtra, India

Carmen Lurashci-Monjagatta
University of Southern California
Keck School of Medicine
Los Angeles, California, USA

Macy Mei Sze Lui MBBS MRCP FHKAM FHKCP
Honorary Clinical Assistant Professor
Department of Medicine
The University of Hong Kong
Queen Mary Hospital
Hong Kong, SAR China

Karan Madan MD DM
Assistant Professor
Department of Pulmonary, Critical Care and Sleep Medicine
All India Institute of Medical Sciences
New Delhi, India

J Mark Madison MD
Professor
Department of Pulmonary, Allergy and Critical Care Medicine
University of Massachusetts Medical School
Worcester, Massachusetts, USA

Bharti Mahajan MD
Associate Professor
Department of Pharmacology
Dayanand Medical College and Hospital
Ludhiana, Punjab, India

Rajesh Mahajan MD
Professor
Department of Medicine
Dayanand Medical College and Hospital
Ludhiana, Punjab, India

Richard Mahon MD
Commander
US Navy
Naval Medical Research Center
Bethesda, Mayland, USA

Sara Maio BSc
Project Associate
Pulmonary Environmental Epidemiology Unit
CNR Institute of Clinical Physiology
Pisa, Italy

Pankaj Malhotra MD MAMS
Professor
Department of Internal Medicine
Postgraduate Institute of Medical Education and Research
Chandigarh, India

Puneet Malhotra MD DM MRCP (UK) MRCP
Special Consultant
Department of Respiratory and General Medicine
St Helens and Knowsley NHS Trust
USA

Samir Malhotra MD
Professor
Department of Pharmacology
Postgraduate Institute of Medical Education and Research
Chandigarh, India

Javaid Ahmad Malik MD DM FCCP
Additional Professor and Head
Department of Pulmonary Medicine
Sher-i-Kashmir Institute of Medical Sciences
Srinagar, Jammu and Kashmir, India

Suruchi Mandrekar MBBS FCPS
Chest Research Foundation
Pune, Maharashtra, India

William J Martin II MD
Associate Director
National Institute for Environmental Health Sciences
Director
Office of Translational Research
National Institutes of Health, North Carolina, USA

Praveen N Mathur MBBS
Professor
Department of Pulmonary, Critical Care and Occupational Medicine
Indiana University Medical Center
Indianapolis, Indiana, USA

Venkata Nagarjuna Maturu MD DM
Pulmonologist and Somnologist
Department of Pulmonology and Somnology
Yashoda Hospital
Hyderabad, Telangana, India

Dilip V Maydeo MD
Professor
Department of Tuberculosis and Respiratory Diseases
KJ Somaiya Medical College and Research Center
Mumbai, Maharashtra, India

Paul H Mayo MD FCCP
Director
Medical Intensive Care Unit
Long Island Jewish Medical Center
New Hyde Park, New York, USA
Professor
Clinical Medicine
Albert Einstein College of Medicine
Bronx, New York, USA

D Robert McCaffree MD MSHA Master FCCP
Regents' Professor
Department of Medicine, Pulmonary Disease and Critical Care Section
University of Oklahoma Health Science Center
Oklahoma, USA

Atul C Mehta MBBS FACP FCCP
Medical Director (Lung Transplantation)
Department of Pulmonary Medicine
Cleveland Clinic
Cleveland, Ohio, USA

Sanjeev Kumar Mehta MD
Senior Consultant
Lilavati Hospital
Arogya Nidhi Hospital
Mumbai, Maharashtra, India

BR Mittal MD DRM DNB MNAMS FICNM
Professor and Head
Department of Nuclear Medicine
Postgraduate Institute of Medical Education and Research
Chandigarh, India

Alladi Mohan MD
Chief
Division of Pulmonary, Critical Care and Sleep Medicine
Professor and Head
Department of Medicine
Sri Venkateswara Institute of Medical Sciences
Tirupati, Andhra Pradesh, India

Prasanta R Mohapatra MD
Professor and Head
Department of Pulmonary Medicine
All India Institute of Medical Sciences
Bhubaneswar, Odisha, India

Sachiko Mori MD
Research Associate
Department of Pediatrics
Nippon Medical School
Tokyo, Japan

Mohammad Eyman Mortada MD FACC
Electrophysiologist
Aurora Cardiovascular Services
Aurora Sinai/St Luke's Medical Centers
Milwaukee, Wisconsin, USA

Lakshmi Mudambi MD
Associate Professor
Department of Pulmonary and Critical Care Medicine
Baylor College of Medicine
Houston, Texas, USA

Jai B Mullerpattan MD
Associate Consultant
Department of Pulmonary Medicine
PD Hinduja National Hospital and Medical Research Centre
Mumbai, Maharashtra, India

Sagar Naik MD
Department of Pulmonary and Critical Care Medicine
New York Methodist Hospital
Brooklyn, New York, USA

Parmeswaran Nair MD PhD FRCP FRCPC
Professor
Department of Medicine
Division of Respirology
McMaster University
Hamilton, Ontario, Canada

R Narasimhan MD FRCP FCCP FIAB
Senior Consultant
Department of Respiratory Medicine
Apollo Hospitals
Chennai, Tamil Nadu, India

Manabu Nonaka MD
Research Associate
Department of Pediatrics
Nippon Medical School
Tokyo, Japan

Jaydeep Odhwani MD
BJ Medical College
Ahmedabad, Gujarat, India

Paulo J Oliveira MD
Assistant Professor
Department of Medicine
Division of Pulmonary, Allergy and Critical Care Medicine
University of Massachusetts Medical School
Worcester, Massachusetts, USA

Ngozi Orjioke
University of Southern California
School of Medicine
Los Angeles, California, USA

Kamlesh Pandey MBBS DNB
Chest Research Foundation
Pune, Maharashtra, India

Chandramani Panjabi MD
Head
Department of Respiratory Medicine
Mata Chanan Devi Hospital
Janakpuri, New Delhi, India

Giovanni Passalacqua MD PhD
University of Genoa
Italy

Rubal Patel MD
Tift Regional Medical Center
Tifton, Georgia, USA

Vishal K Patel MD
Department of Pulmonary and Critical Care Medicine
New York Methodist Hospital
Brooklyn, New York, USA

Ruby Pawankar MD PhD
Professor (Rhinology and Allergy)
Department of Otolaryngology
Nippon Medical School
Tokyo, Japan

Abinash Singh Paul MD DM
Consultant Pulmonologist
Department of Pulmonary Medicine
Lifeline Hospital
Dubai, United Arab Emirates

Charles Peng MD
Pulmonary, Critical Care and Sleep Medicine Fellow
Pulmonary Hypertension Center
Icahn School of Medicine at Mount Sinai
Mount Sinai Beth Israel
New York, USA

Vlasis Polychronopoulos MD PhD FCCP
Director
3rd Chest Department
Sismanoglion General Hospital
Athens, Greece

Gaurav Prakash MD DM
Assistant Professor
Bone Marrow Transplantation
Department of Internal Medicine
Postgraduate Institute of Medical Education and Research
Chandigarh, India

Rajendra Prasad MD DTCD FAMS FCCP FNCCP
Head
Department of Pulmonary Medicine
Era's Lucknow Medical College
Lucknow, Uttar Pradesh, India

Mohamed Rahman MD
Cardiovascular Disease Fellow
Aurora Cardiovascular Services
University of Wisconsin School of Medicine
Milwaukee, Wisconsin, USA

Srinivas Rajagopala MD DM
Assistant Professor (Chest Diseases)
Department of Medicine
St John's Medical College Hospital
Bengaluru, Karnataka, India

Sujeet Rajan MD
Senior Pulmonary Consultant
Bhatia Hospital
Mumbai, Maharashtra, India

Girish Raju MD
Senior Consultant
Department of Medical Oncology
St John's National Academy of Health Sciences
Bengaluru, Karnataka, India

Arvind Rajwanshi MD FRCPath
Professor and Head
Department of Cytology and Gynecologic Pathology
Postgraduate Institute of Medical Education and Research
Chandigarh, India

VR Pattabhi Raman MD
Consultant Pulmonologist
Kovai Medical Center and Hospital
Coimbatore, Tamil Nadu, India

Padmavathi Ramaswamy MD
Professor
Department of Physiology
Sri Ramachandra Medical College and Research Institute
Sri Ramachandra University
Chennai, Tamil Nadu, India

Sabiha Raoof MD FCCP
Chair
Department of Radiology
Jamaica Hospital Medical Center and Flushing Hospital
Associate Professor
Department of Medicine
Ross University, Portsmouth, Dominica, USA

Suhail Raoof MD FCCP MACP FCCM
Chief
Pulmonary Medicine
Lenox Hill Hospital, New York
Professor
Department of Medicine
Hofstra Northwell School of Medicine
New York, USA

C Ravindran MD DTCD MBA
Professor
Department of Pulmonary Medicine
Principal Medical College
Kozhikode, Kerala, India

Pallab Ray MD
Professor
Department of Medical Microbiology
Postgraduate Institute of Medical Education and Research
Chandigarh, India

Zeenat Safdar MD FACP FCCP
Associate Professor
Department of Medicine
Director
Baylor Pulmonary Hypertension Center
Pulmonary and Critical Care Medicine
Baylor College of Medicine, Houston, Texas, USA

Anthony Saleh MD FCCP
Associate Program Director
Pulmonary and Critical Care Medicine
Fellowship
New York Methodist Hospital
Brooklyn, New York, USA

Parmeet Saini MD
Pulmonary and Critical Care
New York Methodist Hospital
Brooklyn, New York, USA

Sundeep Salvi MD DNB PhD FCCP
Director
Chest Research Foundation
Pune, Maharashtra, India

Kripesh Ranjan Sarmah MD MNAMS
Assistant Professor
Department of Pulmonary Medicine
Gauhati Medical College and Hospital
Guwahati, Assam, India

Ramamurthy Sakamuri PhD
Postdoctoral Fellow
Department of Pathology
New York University Langone Medical Centre, USA

Nikhil C Sarangdhar MBBS
Assistant Professor
Department of Tuberculosis and Respiratory Diseases
KJ Somaiya Medical College
Mumbai, Maharashtra, India

Malay Sarkar MD
Associate Professor
Department of Pulmonary Medicine
Indira Gandhi Medical College
Shimla, Himachal Pradesh, India

Pralay Sarkar MD DM MRCP (UK) FCCP
Assistant Professor
Department of Pulmonary and Critical Care Medicine
Baylor College of Medicine
Houston, Texas, USA

Giuseppe Sarno
Pulmonary Environment Epidemiology Unit
Institute of Clinical Physiology
CNR, Pisa, Italy

Gwen S Skloot MD
Associate Professor
Department of Medicine
Icahn School of Medicine
Mount Sinai, New York, USA

L Keith Scott MD FCCM
Associate Professor (Medicine and Pediatrics)
Fellowship Director
Critical Care Medicine
LSU Health Sciences Center
Shreveport, Louisiana, USA

Inderpaul Singh Sehgal MD DM
Assistant Professor
Department of Pulmonary Medicine
Postgraduate Institute of Medical Education and Research
Chandigarh, India

Tavpritesh Sethi MBBS
Institute of Genomics and Integrated Biology
New Delhi, India

Nusrat Shafiq MD DM
Additional Professor
Department of Pharmacology
Postgraduate Institute of Medical Education and Research
Chandigarh, India

Ashok Shah MD
Director Professor
Department of Pulmonary Medicine
Vallabhbhai Patel Chest Institute
University of Delhi
Head
Department of Pulmonary Medicine
Faculty of Medical Sciences
University of Delhi
Delhi, India

Rakesh Shah MD
Department of Radiology
North Shore University Hospital
Manhasset, New York, USA

Walter G Shakespeare MD
Department of Pulmonary and Critical Care Medicine
Baylor College of Medicine
Houston, Texas, USA

PS Shankar MD FRCP FAMS DSc DLitt
Emeritus Professor
Department of Medicine
Rajiv Gandhi Universtiy of Health Sciences
Bengaluru, Karnataka, India
Sri Manakula Vinayagar Medical College
Puducherry, India
KBN Institute of Medical Sciences
Gulbarga, Karnataka, India

Bharat Bhushan Sharma MD
Assistant Professor
Department of Pulmonary and Allergy
Sawai Man Singh Medical College
Jaipur, Rajasthan, India

Om P Sharma MD
Former Professor (Medicine)
Keck School of Medicine
Department of Pulmonary and Critical Care Medicine
University of Southern California
Los Angeles, California, USA

Surendra K Sharma MD PhD
JC Bose National Fellow
Professor and Head
Department of Medicine
All India Institute of Medical Sciences
New Delhi, India

FD Sheski MD
Department of Pulmonary, Critical Care and
Occupational Medicine
Indiana University Medical Center
Indianapolis, Indiana, USA

Arun S Shet MD
Professor and Head
Department of Medical Oncology
St Johns National Academy of Health Sciences
Bengaluru, Karnataka, India

Hidenobu Shigemitsu MD FCCP
Professor and Chief
Department of Pulmonary and Critical Care Medicine
Fellowship Program Director
University of Nevada School of Medicine
Las Vegas, Nevada, USA

Marzia Simoni BSc
Project Associate
Pulmonary Environmental Epidemiology Unit
CNR Institute of Clinical Physiology
Pisa, Italy

Krishna K Singh PhD
Senior Technical Team Lead
Siemens Healthcare Diagnostics
Tarrytown, New York, USA

Meenu Singh MD
Professor and Incharge of Pediatric Pulmonology
Site Director
South Asian Cochrane Network
Coordinator
SAARC Telemedicine Network
Postgraduate Institute of Medical Education and Research
Chandigarh, India

Navneet Singh MD DM FACP FCCP FICS
Associate Professor
Department of Pulmonary Medicine
Postgraduate Institute of Medical Education and Research
Chandigarh, India

Virendra Singh MD
Consultant Pulmonary Physician
Asthma Bhawan
Jaipur, Rajasthan, India

Robert Smith MD
Interventional Radiologist
Department of Radiology
Jamaica Hospital Medical Center
New York, USA

Rajesh N Solanki MD FNCCP
Professor and Head
Department of Pulmonary Medicine
BJ Medical College
Ahmedabad, Gujarat, India

Andrés F Sosa MD
Fellow
Department of Pulmonary, Allergy and Critical Care Medicine
University of Massachusetts Medical School
Worcester, Massachusetts, USA

Padma Srikanth MD
Professor
Department of Microbiology
Sri Ramachandra Medical College and Research Institute
Sri Ramachandra University
Chennai, Tamil Nadu, India

Arjun Srinivasan MD DM
Consultant Pulmonologist
Department of Pulomonary and Critical Care Medicine
Kovai Medical Center and Hospital Speciality Hospital
Chennai, Tamil Nadu, India

Eleni Stagaki MD
Consultant
3rd Chest Department
Sismanoglion General Hospital
Athens, Greece

Roxana Sulica MD
Director
Pulmonary Hypertension Program
Assistant Professor of Medicine
Icahn School of Medicine
Mount Sinai, New York, USA

Balamugesh T MD DM FCCP
Professor
Department of Pulmonary Medicine
Christian Medical College
Vellore, Tamil Nadu, India

Arunabh Talwar MD FCCP
Department of Pulmonary, Critical Care and Sleep Medicine
North Shore University Hospital
Professor
Department of Medicine
New Hyde Park, New York, USA

PS Tampi MD DM
Consultant
Bombay Hospital and Medical Research Centre
Mumbai, Maharashtra, India

Vijayalakshmi Thanasekaraan MD
Consultant
Department of Pulmonary Medicine
Sri Ramachandra Medical College and Research Institute
Sri Ramachandra University
Chennai, Tamil Nadu, India

Mohankumar Thekkinkattil MD DSC AB DPPR FCCP
Head of Department and Senior Consultant Pulmonologist
Institute of Pulmonary Medicine and Research
Sri Ramakrishna Hospital
Coimbatore, Tamil Nadu, India

FE Udwadia MD
Consultant Physician
Breach Candy Hospital
Mumbai, Maharashtra, India

Zarir F Udwadia
Consultant Pulmonologist
PD Hinduja National Hospital and Medical Reasearch Centre
Mumbai, Maharashtra, India

Kumar Utsav MD
BJ Medical College
Ahmedabad, Gujarat, India

Preyas J Vaidya MD
Institute of Pulmonology, Medical Research and Development
Mumbai, Maharashtra, India

Basil Varkey MD FRCP FCCP
Professor Emeritus
Department of Medicine
Medical College of Wisconsin
Milwaukee, Wisconsin, USA

Subhash Varma MD
Professor and Head
Department of Internal Medicine
Postgraduate Institute of Medical Education and Research
Chandigarh, India

Jose Joseph Vempilly MD MRCP FCCP
Professor
Department of Clinical Medicine
Division of Pulmonary and Critical Care
UCSF Fresno, USA

Indu Verma PhD
Professor
Department of Biochemistry
Postgraduate Institute of Medical Education and Research
Chandigarh, India

Preeti Verma MD
Senior Resident
Department of Obstetrics and Gynecology
Postgraduate Institute of Medical Education and Research
Chandigarh, India

Giovanni Viegi MD
Director of Research
National Research Council (CNR)
Head
Pulmonary Environmental Epidemiology Unit
CNR Institute of Clinical Physiology
Pisa, Italy

VK Vijayan MD PhD DSc FAMS
Advisor to Director General
Indian Council of Medical Research
Bhopal Memorial Hospital and Research Centre
National Institute for Research in Environmental Health
Bhopal, Madhya Pradesh, India

Jeremy A Weingarten MD
Director
Centre for Sleep Medicine
Division of Pulmonary, Critical Care and Sleep Medicine
New York Methodist Hospital
Brooklyn, New York, USA

J Whig MD
Ex-Professor and Head
Department of Chest Diseases
Dayanand Medical College and Hospital
Consultant
Chest Physician
Ludhiana, Punjab, India

Shingo Yamanishi MD
Nippon Medical School
Tokyo, Japan

Yukiko Yokoyama MD
Nippon Medical School
Tokyo, Japan

Marc Zelter MD PhD
Former President
European Respiratory Society
Paris, France

Foreword

The 2nd edition of this *Textbook of Pulmonary and Critical Care Medicine* edited by SK Jindal, Professor Emeritus, Department of Pulmonary Medicine, Postgraduate Institute of Medical Education and Research, Chandigarh, India, again offers a thoroughly comprehensive and practical reference for the clinicians, who care for patients with respiratory diseases and critical illnesses. It is a timely follow-up to the 1st edition, given the rapid developments and advances in these fields. While this textbook will have special appeal and value to the physicians of the South-Asian continent, I can attest to the fact that it offers an authoritative addition to any practitioner's library. After receiving my copy of the 1st edition, I found myself frequently turning to the book for a refresher on topics related to the patients under my care.

I also used this textbook to supplement my lectures and seminar materials for the medical students and physicians-in-training. This new edition provides educational value for the educators, pulmonologists, intensivists, thoracic surgeons, pediatricians, postgraduate trainees, and students of medicine. It is especially unique because of the abundance of illustrations, flow charts and tables. Their clarity and, at times, simplicity, make them valuable for the novice and also very useful for the educators. The large number of radiographic and pathologic reproductions are also great teaching tools.

Once again, in this field, Professor SK Jindal has enlisted the collaboration of his colleagues from the Postgraduate Institute of Medical Education and Research in Chandigarh and of leading experts at medical schools in India and in many other countries around the globe. As a result, the textbook offers a unique exposure to special problems seen in different parts of the world. One such problem is tuberculosis (TB). Despite the fact that nearly all the cases can be cured, the WHO considers TB one of the world's biggest threats. Fifteen chapters in this book are devoted to the topics of TB, ranging from epidemiology and risk factors to the challenges in treating routine, multidrug resistant and surgically correctable disease. This section is a highlight of the book and, based on the recent WHO statistics, education about TB continues to be a high priority in highly endemic areas. For example, of the 9.6 million new cases of TB in 2014, 58% were in Southeast Asia and West Pacific Region, whereas India, Indonesia and China accounted for 23%, 10% and 10% respectively of the total globally, and more than half of the multidrug-resistant TB has occurred in India, China and the Russian Federation. The WHO report 2015 heralds an end-TB strategy to reduce TB deaths by 90% by the year 2030—a target, the readers of this book can help to achieve.

As in the previous edition of the book, there are chapters that are very helpful especially to the practicing physicians, including those who offer a systematic approach to clinical problems including, cough, dyspnea and hemoptysis, the interpretation of plain chest radiographs, the approach to chest CT scans, and the microbiologic approach to respiratory infections. An overview of the antimicrobial and immunosuppressive pharmacologic agents used to treat lung disease, is extremely useful.

What is most impressive about this edition of the book is that it continues to be comprehensive, practical, and updated. There is hardly any topic missing that might be within the scope of this book. The physicians and clinicians around the globe will benefit from Professor SK Jindal's extensive efforts.

Sidney S Braman MD FCCP
Professor
Department of Medicine
Icahn School of Medicine
New York, USA

Preface to the Second Edition

The 1st edition of this *Textbook of Pulmonary and Critical Care Medicine* received huge success all over the world. This edition, in its two volumes with over 200 authors from over 12 different countries, will serve as a reference book for the students and teachers of medicine and pulmonary sciences. There has been a constant demand for the new edition from various sections for over a year. Therefore, last year, we took the decision to revise the 1st edition.

Tremendous changes have happened in the practice of medicine including those in pulmonary medicine. Rapid advances in technology, introduction of new drugs, devices and diagnostic investigations, have made it mandatory to provide updated information to our readers. Although we have tried our best to include references to the latest publications up to the year 2016, it has not been possible in all the cases because of the longer time period required to publish such a huge text.

Electronic publications and wider availability of information on the internet seems to have relegated the printed books to the background. But textbooks remain irreplaceable. One cannot opt for shortcuts in acquisition of information and knowledge of a subject especially during training or a degree program. Internet browsing tends to promote abbreviated information, which goes against the tenets of a comprehensive program. Undoubtedly, the internet and electronic books offer great help to provide supplementary as well as complementary information. A large majority of students as well as teachers, however, continue to pose greater confidence in the print version, especially in case of the 'Text' and 'Reference' books.

There has been an enormous increase in the global burden of 'noncommunicable diseases' recognized by the UN General Assembly in one of its 'resolutions', which has made it incumbent upon all the countries to take effective steps for the control and management of these diseases. Chronic pulmonary diseases constitute one major component of this burden. Factually, the 'Third-world' countries suffer from an increasing onslaught of both communicable and noncommunicable diseases. On the other hand, the developed countries too are not immune from infectious diseases. Respiratory system is the most favored target of infectious diseases as much as of noncommunicable diseases.

We have seen a rapid expansion of pulmonary and critical care services all over the world. In India, for example, there was only one postdoctoral fellowship (DM) 'program in pulmonary and critical care medicine' in 2011, when the 1st edition of this book was published; there are at least seven such programs now in India. This has resulted in a greater visibility of the specialty as well as an increased demand for the teaching–learning material. Parallelly, there are enormous advancements made in interventional pulmonology and pulmonary critical care as well as the emergence of subspecialties such as 'sleep medicine, allergy-immunology, environmental and occupational medicine'. The increased concern about ambient and indoor air pollution as a cause of pulmonary diseases, has added an extra burden on pulmonary trainees. We have taken care to incorporate all the important areas of pulmonary medicine that might be within the scope of this book.

This current edition of the book has several new authors and topics in the text. On the other hand, some of the chapters of the earlier edition have been either pruned or deleted altogether. That has been done only to make it more interesting and reader-friendly.

SK Jindal

Preface to the First Edition

It was merely a quarter of a century ago when the specialty of pulmonary medicine was factually recognized as an important division of medicine. Until then, the lung diseases were generally dismissed as tuberculosis, or nondescriptive pneumonias and infections. Most of the nontuberculous lung diseases remained either undiagnosed or unknown. Of course, several stalwarts of the sixties and seventies had clearly identified this deficiency and made efforts to define the pulmonary problems and plan their solutions.

It was in 1989 that the first independent, postdoctoral DM Fellowship Program in Pulmonary Medicine was started at Chandigarh. Subsequently, the program was expanded to include the Critical Care as an essential component of the DM training. In addition, there were several postgraduate MD and/or diploma courses in tuberculosis and chest diseases, and/or respiratory diseases at different medical colleges. Unfortunately, most of the postgraduate programs lacked in their curricula especially for nontuberculous diseases and other systemic disorders. Moreover, the on-hand training in diagnostic and treatment modalities had been highly inadequate in the postgraduate courses. It is rather enigmatic that we still continue to lack the dedicated thoracic surgery courses and texts in various countries.

The increased importance and scope of respiratory and critical care medicine had also necessitated the need to develop the indigenous teaching and training materials including the texts with incorporation of local problems and possible solutions. Undeniably, the science is the same all over the world, but the experiences are different. Excellent text and reference materials on the subject have been available for long, which continue to guide the students, teachers and practicing physicians. In the present literature, quite a few textbooks of pulmonary medicine have been published. Ours is one more attempt in this direction to add to the existing literature on lung diseases available worldwide. This book contains contributions by approximately hundred international esteemed pulmonary medicine consultants and teachers.

There are, however, a few important additions in this present textbook. It is fairly comprehensive with contributions from several internationally eminent authors. It includes the basic principles as well as the recent advances related to different subjects. We have also attempted to incorporate allied clinical sciences relevant to the practice of the pulmonologists. A classical example is the critical care which forms an integral component of pulmonary medicine. It also incorporates tuberculosis, other pulmonary infections, environmental and occupational medicines, sleep disorders and general systemic diseases affecting the respiratory system in one or the other way. Although the critical care is relevant to most of the medical and surgical specialties, the pulmonologists have a more vested interest than that of the other specialists. Assisted respiration, which forms the core of most critical care, lies in the primary domain of pulmonologists.

We have taken care not to forget the need to push forward and meet the goals of excellence in health care. The real test of merit of a book lies in its readership by the students and adoption of its recommendations in clinical practice. Hopefully, the material in the text will benefit a diverse category of people including internists, general physicians, pulmonologists, pediatricians, intensivists, anesthesiologists and others, who need to handle patients with respiratory diseases and critical care.

SK Jindal

Acknowledgments

I thankfully acknowledge the contribution of my colleagues Dr D Behera, Dr Ashutosh N Aggarwal, Dr Ritesh Agarwal, Dr Navneet Singh, Dr Sahajal Dhooria and Dr Inderpaul Singh Sehgal, for their continued help in editing the manuscript. Unfortunately, we untimely lost our colleague Dr Dheeraj Gupta, while this edition of the textbook was still in its infancy. He had been a great source of encouragement and inspiration, the primary force in bringing out the 1st edition. Aditya, my son, has been only partially successful in bridging the gap.

I am immensely grateful to Dr Sidney S Braman, Dr Richard S Irwin, Dr Suhail Raoof, Dr PS Shankar, Dr Kalaplatha K Guntupally, Dr Ruby Pawankar and others, who have significantly contributed to this textbook. A large number of friends and eminent colleagues from across the globe have unhesitatingly spared their time as authors and coauthors with their valuable chapters and wisdom, for which, I remain obliged to them. I also greatly appreciate the help rendered by my erstwhile secretary, Ms Manju Aggarwal, for the preparation of the manuscript.

My deep appreciation is for Shri Jitendar P Vij (Group Chairman), Mr Ankit Vij (Group President), Mr Tarun Duneja (Director-Publishing), Ms Samina Khan (Executive Assistant to Director-Publishing), Mr KK Raman (Production Manager), Mr Ashutosh Srivastava (Assistant Editor), Mr Himanshu Sharma (Proofreader), Ms Yashu Kapoor (Senior Typesetter), Mr Manoj Pahuja (Senior Graphic Designer), and the other staff of M/s Jaypee Brothers Medical Publishers (P) Ltd., New Delhi, India, for taking the challenge of publication of this huge book.

Contents

VOLUME 1

Section 3: Respiratory Pharmacology
Aditya Jindal, Nusrat Shafiq

Section 4: Symptom Approach to Respiratory Disease
Richard S Irwin

Section 5: Respiratory Diagnosis

Randeep Guleria, SK Jindal

Section 6: Tuberculosis

D Behera, SK Jindal

Section 8: Asthma
SK Jindal, Inderpaul Singh Sehgal

Section 12: Occupational Disorders
PS Shankar, SK Jindal

Section 15: Pulmonary Circulatory Disorders
SK Jindal, Inderpaul Singh Sehgal

Section 16: Respiratory Sleep Disorders
Aditya Jindal

Section 17: Respiratory Critical Care
Ritesh Agarwal, Aditya Jindal

Section 21: Surgical Aspects of Respiratory Disease

SK Jindal

Section 1

History and Development

SK Jindal

1

Chapter

History of Respiratory Medicine

FE Udwadia

INTRODUCTION

The history of respiratory medicine cannot be separated from the overall history of medicine. The history of all medicines, including respiratory medicine begins with the history of man, for even primitive man realized that when a man ceases to breathe, he ceases to live. It needs also to be remembered that the history of medicine, like the history of the world is a chronicle of change. We, in the present, have built on triumphs and defeats of the past, just as those in the future will build on the successes and failures of the present.

Time present and time past
Are both perhaps present in time future,
And time future contained in time past.

Religion-ruled medicine in the ancient past; then came empiricism and then came science. Even today, medicine, including respiratory medicine, is a mixture of science and empiricism. In ancient *Ayurveda,* "phlegm" *(Kapha),* or secretions within the chest was one of the three "humors" that regulated the body, the other two being wind *(vat)* and choler *(pitta).* The Greeks paid the same importance to the humor "phlegm", but included a fourth humor "blood" and omitted "wind" from their concept of humors.

It was Hippocrates, the Father of Medicine (460–377 BC) teaching on the island of Kos, Greece, who divorced religion from medicine and who taught that disease was due to extraneous factors and influences. He introduced the importance of clinical bedside medicine, the importance of history, physical examination, and the documentation of a patient's illness. His clinical description of diseases considering the meager facilities in that age remains unsurpassed to this day and still makes fascinating reading. Among the numerous descriptions of different diseases, one also finds a description of the clinical features of tuberculosis, a disease which still plagues the developing world. Tuberculosis is an ancient disease. The earliest evidence of this disease comes from a female skeleton unearthed from a cave in Liguria, Italy dating back to around 5300 BC. Besides a description of tuberculosis in Hippocratic writings, there was awareness of the clinical features of tuberculosis in the *Rig Veda* scriptures (around 1500 BC) and in texts of *Ayurveda* (second century AD). Ancient Chinese texts as early as in the third millennium BC, the famous Egyptian George Ebers Papyrus from Thebes (1550 BC) and the Edwin Smith Papyrus (1600 BC) also give descriptions of the disease.

After Hippocrates came many contributors to medicine. The most famous of these was Claudius Galen (AD 138–201). He indeed may be considered the most influential writer of all time, as his writings in medicine became fossilized as gospel truth for almost 1500 years. Though great for his era, Galen based his deductions and theories on observations following his dissection of animals, so that among some truths that he propounded, there lay buried numerous mistakes, which hindered the progress of medicine for well over a thousand years. One of his greatest mistakes was the propagation of his belief that the blood from the right ventricle reached the left ventricle through pores (invisible small openings) within the interventricular septum. His view on the circulation of blood in humans was really a figment of imagination, yet it stood for close to 1500 years after his demise. Why should this have been so? It is because dissection of the human body was considered taboo in that day and age so that many of his hypotheses lacked the fundamentals of scientific observation, and study.

After the decline and fall of the Roman Empire (410 AD), the Western World was enveloped in the Dark Ages—war, disease and anarchy prevailed. The Dark Ages (470–1000 AD) slowly gave way to the Renaissance, a brilliant period in the history of Man.

Many medical historians are of the opinion that the history of modern medicine began with the publication in 1543 of "De Humanis Corporis Fabrica" by Andreas Vesalius, a 25-year-old young man who was professor of anatomy in the University of Padua, Italy. Vesalius dissected the human body and through meticulous observation and description illustrated the musculoskeletal framework as also the internal structure of the body in the form of exquisitely detailed anatomical plates. These were designed and executed in the studio of the great Italian artist Titian. Vesalius exploded the numerous untruths in the teaching of Galen, which had dominated medicine for well over a thousand years. He proved above all that the ventricular septum had no pores and that blood from the right ventricle could not therefore enter the left ventricle through septal pores. Vesalius described the venous system of the thorax, discovered the azygos vein and noted its entry into the superior vena cava. His numerous contraindications of the many hypotheses put forth by Galen raised a furor of opposition from the medical fraternity who believed that the teachings of Galen were sacrosanct and could not be contradicted. Vesalius disappointed, frustrated, and almost hounded by the opposition, tore up his many manuscripts and fled Padua to become physician to Charles V and then to Philip III of Spain. He never researched on anatomy again and thus was destroyed a great man in his prime—destroyed by the bigotry, jealousy and hate of lesser mortals.

The next individual who like Vesalius contradicted Galen was Michael Servetus. How was blood to reach the left ventricle from the right ventricle, if not through the pores within the septum as enunciated by Galen? Servetus had worked with Vesalius in Paris. He was Spanish, an unusual figure of the Renaissance—a humanist, a theologian and a man of medicine. In a theological treatise, Christianismi Restitutio, he briefly described the pulmonary circulation. He stated that the blood from the right ventricle had to flow through the pulmonary artery via its branches into the lungs. His theological treatise was judged to be heretical by the church, and this brave man who thought differently from the general herd of humanity was burnt at the stale for his heresy. We, however now know that Nafis, a physician from Damascus, had already described the flow of blood from the right ventricle through the lungs as early as the 13th century, 400 years ahead of Servetus. The credit for the first discovery of the pulmonary circulation should therefore go to him.

The discovery of the overall circulation of blood in man, based on meticulous observation, experimentation, and for the first time on scientific principles (akin to the principles followed by Newton and Kepler who also belonged to this Baroque age—the 17th century) is one of the greatest medical discoveries of the world. Future generations could never have contributed to cardiorespiratory medicine without this monumental discovery. The credit for this discovery goes to William Harvey. He was a physician on the staff of St Bartholomew's Hospital in London. He announced the discovery of his work in 1616. His classic work "Exercitatio anatomica de Motu Cordis et Sanguinis in Animalibus" was published rather shoddily, 12 years later in Frankfurt, in which he described circulation as we know it today. It immediately divided the world into two hostile camps—one for and one against Harvey. Truth ultimately prevailed and Harvey has the distinction of being one of the all-time greats in the field of medicine.

Though Harvey published his discovery of circulation in the 17th century, knowledge in the physiology of respiration came a century and a half later. Priestley discovered oxygen, but did not realize its importance in respiration and respiratory physiology. It was Antoine Lavoisier who named Priestley's gas oxygen and noted its characteristics and its importance in respiration. He was probably France's greatest chemist, an aristocrat by birth, who unfortunately was guillotined during the turbulent times of the French revolution.

Bernardino Ramazzini (1633–1714) pioneered the science of occupational diseases. He wrote on silicosis in stone masons and in miners working in mines. Over the next 300 years, occupational lung diseases have graduated into an important subspecialty of pulmonary medicine.

1800–2000

I shall introduce this period with none other than the great French physician René-Théophile-Hyacinthe Laennec (1781–1836) who is an immortal in the history of medicine. A pupil of Nicolas Corvisart, the first cardiologist in the Western world and also the personal physician of Napoleon Bonaparte, Laennec was a physician at Salpêtrière Hospital and the chief at the Necker Hospital in Paris in 1814. Corvisart, Laennec and others would place their ears directly to the chest to hear heart sounds. Laennec for years has been obsessed to hear sounds within the chest with greater clarity. It is said that one day when crossing the Louvre (the residential palace of the Bourbon Kings of France), he saw a boy listening with his ear to one end of a beam to scratches made by another boy with a nail at the other end of the beam. He was struck by the ease with which sound was conducted in this manner. In 1816, a young stout woman consulted him for symptoms of heart disease. Her young age and obesity did not permit him to put his ear directly to her chest (direct auscultation). He lightly rolled up a thick sheaf of paper, placing one end over the precordium and the other end over his ear. To his surprise, he could hear the heart sounds with far greater clarity than ever before, when he used to place his ear directly to the chest. He grasped the significance of this discovery and noted that the method of indirect auscultation would enable one to hear not only the beating of the heart, but likewise all movements capable of producing sound in the thoracic cavity.

Laennec in his treatise on "Mediate Auscultation" described his first monaural stethoscope, a wooden piece 9" long, 1½" in diameter. It was made in two pieces—the detachable earpiece and the chest piece, which could be screwed together. Following minor modifications, by the 19th century, rubber tubing was introduced to create a flexible monaural stethoscope. Finally, the familiar two-ear instrument with rubber tubings was devised by the American physician George P Cammann in 1852. Laennec made excellent use of his invention, studied both normal and abnormal breath sounds, described them in detail and drew conclusions from what he heard as to the nature and extent of the disease in the chest. Above all, he verified his findings with what was revealed at autopsy. He was the first man to create a diagnostic system of auscultatory findings in the diagnosis of pulmonary and cardiac disease. He described and gave the correct significance to adventitious sounds—rhonchi, râles, and through his system of mediate auscultation diagnosed pulmonary ailments such as bronchitis, pneumonia and tuberculosis.

Laennec's treatise on "Mediate Auscultation" focused particularly on pulmonary tuberculosis, which was prevalent all over the world in the 19th century. He described the early diagnosis of tuberculosis. He noted the presence of the tuberculous nodule, which was ubiquitous in every organ affected by the disease. On this basis, he postulated that tuberculosis was a single disease, which could affect many organ systems. This was indeed a remarkable observation considering that the tubercle bacillus causing the disease had not been discovered in Laennec's time. Laennec unfortunately himself suffered from and succumbed to tuberculosis—as did many of his contemporaries, including the surgical student and poet John Keats. Laennec, brilliant though he was, did arrive at some erroneous conclusions. He denied that tuberculosis was contagious when it was strongly so; he believed that it was often hereditary when it was not so. He felt that psychological factors such as grief, sorrow, and unrequited love played a role in its causation and perpetuation. Laennec's superb writings prompted Thomas Addison, the English physician to remark that Laennec contributed more to the advancement of medical art than any other single individual.

There were many great individuals during and after Laennec's time. Mention must be made of the German School of Medicine and of Rudolf Ludwig Karl Virchow who dominated medicine for more than half of the 19th century. He was unquestionably one of the greatest pathologists who ever lived and was a worthy successor to the great pathologists, Morgagni and Rokitansky. He noted that the cell was the seat of disease and described the macroscopic and microscopic changes of several diseases, including those of the lung. He was the first to show that pulmonary emboli arose from venous thrombi chiefly present in veins of the lower extremities. His work was embodied in his opus—Di cellular-pathologie. It is worth noting that none of this work would have been possible had it not been for the discovery of the microscope by the Dutch draper Anton-van Leeuwenhoek, illustrating what has been stated at the beginning of this chapter, that the history of respi-ratory medicine is inseparable from medicine as a whole.

We now go on to briefly mention just two of the many great microbe hunters in the history of medicine. Till the early part of the 19th century, disease was thought to be caused by miasmas, humors or vapors. The miasmic theory of disease was challenged by many, but ultimately shattered by Louis Pasteur, a French chemist who was born in December 1822 and who went on to study chemistry at the École Nationale in Paris. He contended through meticulous experimentation and observation that all infectious diseases were caused by microorganisms and that a specific microorganism was responsible for a specific disease. He postulated that if these microorganisms could be identified, specific vaccines could be prepared and could well prevent specific disease. This was a principle enunciated in relation to all infectious diseases, including those involving the respiratory system. It behooves the world to remember that it was a chemist and not a man trained in medicine who became one of the greatest benefactors of mankind.

Pasteur's counterpart in Germany was Robert Koch, a great microbiologist. Koch's greatest triumphs was his discovery that tuberculosis was caused by a specific organism—*Mycobacterium tuberculosis*. In 1882, Koch cultured the tubercle bacillus presenting his results in 1884 to the Berlin Physiological Society. He also presented in his paper, Koch's postulates, enunciating a specific discipline, which needs to be fulfilled, if a specific organism is to be considered responsible for a specific disease.

The history of tuberculosis now became increasingly complete. The disease could be diagnosed clinically ever since the brilliant clinical description of Laennec. The morbid anatomy had been determined by Morgagni, Rokitansky and Virchow. The possibility that tuberculosis was a communicable disease was entertained by a few prominent clinicians and pathologists. And at last, came the cause of the disease, which till the discovery of the tubercle bacillus was deemed a mystery. Yet even great minds make mistakes. In 1890, Koch announced at the Berlin International Congress that he had discovered a substance that could cure tuberculosis, a substance that could inhibit the growth of the tubercle bacillus in the test tube as also in human beings. This substance (which he kept secret for a while) was none other than a glycerin extract of the tubercle bacillus termed tuberculin. Tuberculin was administered to thousands of individuals over the next year. The treatment proved a fiasco to the embarrassment of the great Robert Koch. Yet in years to come, the preparation of tuberculin did have diagnostic use; an intradermal injection of tuberculin would often produce a strong reaction, if the patient in the past or present had been infected by tuberculosis. Even today, the tuberculin test is a worthy diagnostic aid to infection caused by the tubercle bacillus.

We must now add a post-script to the story of tuberculosis. The search of a vaccine or other means of immunization against this disease continued and continues to this day. Albert Calmette of the Pasteur Institute and Jean Marie Guérin developed a new method of preparing a vaccine. They used the live bovine strain of the tubercle bacillus and on repeated subcultures of this strain noted that the bacillus lost its virulence, but retained its protective action. The vaccine was named BCG (Bacillus Calmette-Guérin) and from 1924 was tried out on humans. Thousands of children were vaccinated.

Its efficacy was controversial. Recent work bears out its usefulness, particularly in the prevention of tuberculous meningitis, one of the worst forms of tuberculosis, which invariably caused death before the advent of antituberculosis drugs.

Mention must be made at this point of one of the unfortunate disasters in respiratory medicine. The disaster occurred in Lubeck, Germany, in 1930, when 249 babies who were supposed to be injected with BCG vaccine were inadvertently injected with a living virulent strain of *Mycobacterium tuberculosis*. About 76 babies died of progressive tuberculosis. The remaining developed mild tuberculosis, but were alive at the end of 12 years, pointing perhaps to the remarkable immunological defenses the human body is endowed with.

One of the greatest discoveries of the late 19th century was William Roentgen's discovery of X-rays in 1895—again a discovery of a physicist and not by a man trained in medicine. Radiographic examination of the chest with increasing refinements proved an invaluable asset not only in the diagnosis of pulmonary tuberculosis, but of numerous other pulmonary diseases—both infectious and noninfectious in etiology.

In 1898, Gustav Killian reported his experience with the first bronchoscopy. Technical developments over several years established bronchoscopy through a rigid bronchoscope as an important diagnostic and therapeutic modality in respiratory medicine. In 1967, Ikeda in Japan devised the flexible fiberoptic bronchoscope and this opened up new horizons following the widespread use of fiberoptic bronchoscopy in pulmonary medicine.

DISCOVERY OF CHEMOTHERAPY AND ANTIBIOTICS

The diagnosis of respiratory diseases using clinical methods, microbiology and a radiographic examination of the chest, was increasingly possible. But how was one to treat respiratory and other diseases? It was Paul Ehrlich, a disciple of Robert Koch who invented the concept of chemotherapy—the administration of a chemical substance to treat disease. In 1905, after several experiments, Paul Ehrlich discovered the first antimicrobial agent to treat syphilis. In 1925, Gerhard Dogmak invented Prontosil, the first of the sulfa drugs to be used against several microorganisms. More refined and less toxic sulfa drugs continue to be used in modern medicine. Finally, in 1929 came the great discovery of the antibiotic penicillin (a substance produced by the fungus *Penicillium notatum*), by Alexander Fleming which was available for clinical use in 1944 through the brilliant work of Chain and Florey. This discovery revolutionized the treatment of a number of incurable acute infections. Research on antibacterial effects of several fungi and moulds continued unabated. In 1942, Selman Waksman, a Russian Jew who had migrated to the USA and had become a microbiologist, discovered streptomycin from the fungus *Streptomyces griseus*. This drug was the first effective drug against the tubercle bacillus. Unfortunately, the use of this drug alone led to the multiplication of resistant strains. After that followed a quick discovery of other drugs against tuberculosis and other microorganisms. The impetus to the discovery of other drugs against tuberculosis was partly due to the fact that the tubercle bacillus quickly became resistant to the use of a single-drug regime. The discovery of para-aminosalicylic acid (PAS) was followed in 1950 by the discovery of isoniazid. Excellent clinical trials in Edinburgh by Professor John Crofton and his team showed that the combined use of streptomycin, PAS and isoniazid almost always resulted in a cure, if taken meticulously and regularly for the prescribed period of time. Poor compliance invariably resulted in resistant strains. The next few decades saw tremendous research on other drugs to counter the growing menace of tuberculosis. Numerous drugs have come into use, but other than rifampicin, none of these drugs in use can match the efficacy of streptomycin and isoniazid. The introduction of isoniazid in 1950 and rifampicin in 1965 paved the way for modern short-course chemotherapy, which was first introduced in the 1970s.

In India, initial efforts to combat tuberculosis were spearheaded by voluntary organizations and by the setting up of sanatoria in temperate hill stations. After India's independence in 1947, two pioneering institutions were established—The Tuberculosis Chemotherapy Center in Chennai and the National Tuberculosis Institute in Bengaluru under the Indian Council of Medical Research and the Government of India, respectively. These two institutes did pioneering research to help shape tuberculosis control in India and to an extent in other countries. The famous Madras chemotherapeutic trial showed that domiciliary treatment of patients with tuberculosis was successful notwithstanding poor-living conditions and a poor diet, provided there was compliance to therapy. This led to a closure of sanatoria all over the world. Several intermittent chemotherapy regimes were also devised by the Madras and Bangalore centers in collaboration with the British Research Medical Council. This indeed was excellent research in respiratory medicine the like of which has not been equaled in subsequent years in our country.

Numerous other antibiotics to counter other infections have been discovered. However, indiscriminate use of antibiotics has led to the dangerous emergence of many antibiotic-resistant bacteria. These indeed pose a great health hazard particularly in critical care units and in patients who are immunocompromised.

RESPIRATORY PHYSIOLOGY

The exchange of oxygen and carbon dioxide within the lungs was known since the beginning of the 12th century. There, however, was debate, whether oxygen was transferred from the alveoli to the capillary blood by active secretion or simple diffusion. August and Marie Krogh in a series of publications proved that the transfer of oxygen and carbon dioxide across the alveolar capillary membrane was a simple physical process of diffusion. Work on pulmonary function was carried out in several laboratories in Europe and America. Outstanding among these was the application of pulmonary function and pulmonary physiology to clinical respiratory medicine through the work of Comroe in San Francisco, America.

The knowledge on pulmonary physiology, gas exchange and pulmonary mechanics was put to clinical use in 1953 by Bjorn Ibsen who founded the first intensive care unit in the world in Copenhagen to treat patients with poliomyelitis that had caused respiratory paralysis. This was an effective counter to the epidemic of poliomyelitis that raged in that year. Ibsen's approach incorporated the use of an endotracheal tube or a tracheostomy through which, to start with, teams of medical students working in relays pumped oxygen enriched air into the lungs of paralyzed patients till such time as they could breathe spontaneously. Soon ventilators were devised first in the form of the iron lung—a contraption in which the patient was inserted (with only the head sticking out). Negative pressure induced within the machine allowed the chest to expand and the lung to inflate. Release of the negative pressure allowed the lungs to passively deflate. An improvement over the cumbersome iron lung was the invention of the ventilator, a device which could provide positive pressure ventilatory support through an endotracheal tube or a tracheostomy to a patient in respiratory failure. Over the years, the ventilator has evolved into a superb-sophisticated machine that renders mechanical ventilator support with ease and efficiency.

There is one other aspect of pulmonary medicine, which deserves an important mention. It is the epidemiological proof of the strong positive relation between cigarette and *Bidi* smoking and cancer of the lung, and of cigarette or *Bidi* smoking to chronic obstructive pulmonary disease (COPD). It was Doll and Hill who in an excellent epidemiological study in the early 50s established that the incidence of lung cancer was about 10–20 times greater in those who were heavy cigarette smokers compared to those who did not smoke. This was proven again and again by numerous other epidemiological studies. The incidence of lung cancer is shown to be reduced following the stoppage of smoking. The incidence of cancer in poor developing countries is on the rise mainly because of the increase in smoking habits in South and Southeast Asian countries.

Advances in the last half century are too numerous to be dealt with. A few of these are briefly tabled in **Table 1**.

It is impossible to discuss each of these at length in a short chapter on the History of Respiratory Medicine, but a brief mention of the history of thoracic surgery is warranted.

Table 1 Advances in the last half century

Advances
• A vast array of imaging techniques—in particular high-resolution computed tomography; CT-guided transthoracic biopsies for the evaluation of localized or peripheral lung pathologies; the discovery of positron emission tomography is chiefly used in staging lung cancer.
• The study of bronchoalveolar lavage fluid obtained through a fiberoptic bronchoscope; the widespread use of transbronchial lung biopsy and biopsy of mediastinal glands through a flexible bronchoscope.
• Advanced microbiological techniques; techniques for quicker cultures of *Mycobacterium tuberculosis* with quick drug sensitivity reports.
• A thorough physiological evaluation of lung function
• Advanced biochemical, genetic and molecular studies; unraveling of the genome of the tubercle bacillus.
• Improved pathological studies
• Powerful antibacterial drugs
• Antiviral drugs
• The development of vaccines to fight respiratory disease
• The development of intensive care
• Advanced anesthesiology and surgery, including surgery for lung transplant.

Carlo Forlanini (1847–1918) of Pavia attempted the first artificially induced pneumothorax in a patient with cavitative tuberculosis in 1888. The Carlo Forlanini Institute in Rome is a tribute to his memory. The rationale was to "relax" the cavity by partially collapsing the diseased lung. A more radical approach was the performance of thoracoplasty in 1930s, the posterior portions of the second to seventh ribs being removed enabling partial collapse of the lung on the affected side. This prompted healing of cavities in tuberculosis. The next advance in thoracic surgery was the resection of part or whole of the lung. The pioneer in this field was Evarts Graham (1883–1957) in Washington who first performed resection for lung cancer. Increasing skill and practice allowed for lobectomies, pneumonectomies and segmental resections. Thoracic surgery came in use not only in lung cancer, but also in other lung diseases, notably tuberculosis and suppurative lung disease. However neither tuberculosis nor cancer would allow an easy conquest.

The first lung transplantation (single lung transplant) was performed in 1963 by Hardy for a patient with a left lung cancer. The patient died after 18 days. Refinements in technique and postoperative care led finally to an improvement in the horrendous mortality experienced in the initial 20 years. Today double lung transplant and heart-lung transplant are successfully performed with a fairly good 3- and 5-year survival rate in a number of transplant centers in the world. Unfortunately, lung transplant surgery has not taken off in India.

Just as old problems are solved, new problems arise. The ancient problem of tuberculosis is still a menace, particularly in developing countries. The problem is confounded by the pandemic of human immunodeficiency syndrome (HIV) infection, which contributed strongly to multiple drug-resistant tuberculosis and extensive drug-resistant tuberculosis. Both tuberculosis and HIV infection literally fuel each other.

The introduction of Directly Observed Short-term Therapy (DOTS) in India has made an appreciable dent both in the detection rate and in success rates of the treatment of tuberculosis. But much more needs to be done before India and other developing countries can claim success in the control of the disease.

One can conclude by stating that though respiratory medicine has come a long way, it still has a longer way to go. It will continue to follow a trail beset with trials and tribulations, defeats and victories, interspersed with periods of great discovery and scintillating glory.

Ancient History

SK Jindal

INTRODUCTION

Breathing was perhaps the most vital physiological sign of life noticed by the ancient man. Many of the old culture including the *Aryans* (i.e. the Hindus), identified life with the number of breaths. Though there is little mention on the role of the lungs in the archaic Medicine, the anatomy of lungs was perhaps known in those periods. The oldest and best known image of the respiratory tract which dates back to 30th century BC comes from an Egyptian hieroglyph that depicts a wind pipe with a pair of lungs.[1,2] Ancient Egyptians also believed that breathing was the most vital to life. Ebers Papyrus (c.1550 BC), a detailed document on medicine of that time, written on papyri was accidently unearthed in Thebes in 1862. The papyrus, more than 20 meters long, was purchased and translated into German in 1873 by Georg Ebers.[3] Considered to be knowledge imparted by Thoth, the Egyptian God of Learning and Medicine, it mentioned about remedies for a number of diseases, including asthma.

The presence of lung diseases such as tuberculosis and asthma, were variously described in the ancient Egyptian, Greek, Indian (Vedic) and Chinese civilizations of the prebiblical periods.[4,5] The earliest mention of respiration can perhaps be traced to Erasistratus of Alexandria in Egypt who in 300 BC had postulated that it was the interplay between the air and the blood which produced the "pneuma" or the spirit essential for life. The concept of gas exchange and the role of the lungs to maintain life, however, were not known, until the 12th century of the medieval era.

MEDICAL PRACTICE

The history of medical therapy is presumably as old as the history of man. But these were largely the beliefs in magical or divine powers which underlined the practice of healing. It was only about 3000 years ago that the scientific concepts based on some logic and reason were first formulated. Medical practice in that era dealt primarily with diseases and their management in a holistic fashion. Several of the civilization in the prebiblical era started talking about the basis of human ailments. *Charaka* and *Susruta,* the two renowned Hindu physicians had extensively described about several illnesses and their management in the *Charaka* and *Susruta Samhita.*[6-9] There was little recognition of the organ system function or its malfunction. In the Ayurvedic Medicine, a disease was considered to result from an alteration of the balance between the three vital ingredients in the body, i.e. "*Vata*", "*Pitta*" and "*Kapha*".[6,8] This "*Tridosa*" (three defects) theory finds some similarity with the humoral theory of Pythagoras, Plato and Hippocrates of the Greek medicine in which the disease was believed to arise from a defect of one of the "humors" of body, of which at least one was described as the "wind" humor. The role of air to supply essential nutrients of the body was speculated in the 6th century BC.[10,11] It was Hippocrates, the Greek Physician of the 5th and 4th century BC who had laid the foundation of ancient medicine.[11] Aristotle's doctrine of four elements (earth, air, fire, water) and Hippocrate's four humors (blood, phlegm, yellow bile and black bile) continued to dominate medicine for about two millennia from 300 BC onwards. Some of these important terms used in the ancient medicine, find their linguistic relevance to the terms, we now use to describe body function and disease. For example, one can identify the "wind humor" with air, the "*Prana*" with breathing and the "*Kapha*" with the sputum. But it is not always possible to interpret the true meaning of each description and assign the due place in the context of modern respiratory medicine.

LUNGS: THE SITE OF BREATHING

Galen in the era of the Roman Empire in the 2nd century AD considered lung as a cooling device in the body to neutralize the heat produced by the heart. The Indian physicians had laid great stress on respiration, recorded the number of breaths as 22,636 times a day (i.e. 16 per minute).[12]

(The more definitive description of the site of breathing became available in the later Ayurvedic literature of 14th century in the writings of Sarangadhara who identified respiration which was implicit in the terms "Visnupadamrta" and "Ambarapiyusa" which described the course of "prana-vayu" (life air) through the interior of the lotus like heart, its exit through the throat and its re-entry to the body again to nourish the whole body.[13] The narrations of Visnupadamrta and Ambarapiyusa follow immediately after those of veins (siras) and arteries (dhamanies) which were stated to emerge from the "nalehi" and spread throughout the body. These structures under the influence of "vayu" (air) transported nutrients required by the different parts of the body for their nourishment.[13] There are further commentaries by other Indian scholars such as Adhamalla and Kasinatha Vaidya

on Sarangadhara's collection (Sarangadharasamhita) which substantiated the concepts of respiratory inhalation of Visnupadamrta (the nectar of the space) from the atmospheric air and its role in maintaining life.[14,15] *This was the transformation of basic concept "pneuma" postulated several centuries earlier by Greko-Arabian medicine. These processes could be closely identified with the overall function of respiration and of gas-exchange.)*

Lung Diseases

History of respiratory medicine is not complete without a reference to the history of tuberculosis and asthma. The saga of both tuberculosis and asthma independently runs back by 3000 years. The two are also amongst the few diseases which continue to exist in a manner that was recognized in the past.

Tuberculosis

Tuberculosis in man is known to exist since antiquity. Evidence of a wasting disease (consumption, i.e. tuberculosis) is available in one or the other form in the ancient civilizations. Some of the information of prehistoric periods are derived from the interpretation of the old cave-paintings or medical records in pictorial writing and on examination of Egyptian mummies of over 4000 years earlier. This was particularly so in case of documentation of spinal tuberculosis. Possibly, tuberculosis in the cattle preceded that in the man. The earliest likeliness of tuberculosis is derived from the Egyptian tomb portraits of hunchbacks pictured by the Egyptian artists.[16] More definitive evidence was made available in the early 20th century on examination of an Egyptian mummy (of 3400 BC) in whom the presence of vertebral destruction and an associated chronic psoas abscess was clearly demonstrated.[17] Late in the 20th century, the presence of *Mycobacterium tuberculosis* was shown in another Egyptian mummy of a child.[18] But no direct or indirect evidence of its presence is available in the subsequent periods until about 1500-2500 BC when other different civilizations had come into existence.[19] There is a more clear reference to lung fever, cough and blood spitting in the Chinese civilization of around 2600–2700 BC, as well as during the Babylonian and the Indo-Aryan periods of 1500–2000 BC.[16] There are indirect suggestions of the presence of a consumptive disease in the "*Rig Veda*" from the Indian continent, in Pen Tsao-the Chinese Materia Medica and in the Code of Hammurabi of Babylon.[16] The mention of "consumption" from around 1500 BCE was attributable to excessive fatigue, hunger, pregnancy and worries.[19] In the Vedas, the disease was known as "*yakshma*" (in Sanskrit), and since in affected the King Soma, it was described as "*rajayakshma*", i.e. the King Yakshma.[6,20-22]

Yakshma's figures in both the *Rig Veda* and the *Atharva Veda* of 1200–1500 BC at several places.[6,20-22] Sanskrit manuscript which constituted the origin of *Ayurveda*, refers to a group of diseases called "*Sosha*" with symptoms of wasting, cough and blood spitting.

> *Since, strength imparting, I hold in my hand these herbs,*
> *the life-spirit of consumption vanishes*
> *as in front of him who seizes*
> *the life soul (Yama, King of Death).*
>
> ***—Rig Veda***

> *With the word of Indra, of Mitra and of*
> *Varuna, with the voice of all the*
> *Gods, do we ward off thy Yakshma*
>
> ***—Atharva Veda***

The Laws of Manu (1000 BC) have reference to tuberculosis that persons affected by Yakshma were unclean and that the Brahmins must not marry in those families.[23]

Both *Rig Veda* and *Atharva Veda* were spiritual and philosophical texts, the reference to "*Yakshma*" was therefore generally indirect and contextual. On the other hand, the medical text of the Vedic period, *Ayurveda* which belonged to 700–800 BC era, contained direct description of "*Yakshma*"- the disease. "The physician who wants great fame cures a man attacked by consumption".[24]

Susruta-Samhita, the Ayurvedic Materia Medica of that period gives details of the origin and the symptomatology of *Yakshma*.[3,5] It was said that the disease resulted from the wrath of King *Daksha*, the God Moon who had married all the 27 daughters of the King but devoted his attention to Rohini, only one of the daughters. He later forgave the God but the disease "descended upon earth to afflict those who overstrained themselves, particularly by sexual excesses". Incidentally, the disease was commonly referred to as the King's Evil and the King fever in the later periods in Europe as well.

(The other important Indian manuscript Madhavanidana and its commentary Madhukosa written around 800–1000 CE, repeatedly refers to "consumption" or "Rajyakshma".[25]*)*

Asthma and Allergies

Unlike tuberculosis which was known for its consumptive and systemic manifestations, asthma was recognized as the "breathing disorder". In the absence of the morphological evidence of asthma, it has been difficult to trace the history farther than the availability of documented records of 1000–1500 BC. Extensive details are available in the Egyptian, Greek and Chinese literature of those periods.[26] It is said that asthma was described in the world's oldest treatise Nei Ching Su Wen, or the "Cannon of Internal Medicine", a Chinese manuscript compiled in the 26th century BC during the rule of Huang Ti (Yellow Emperor).[26,27] Shen Nong (c.2700 BC), the Father of Chinese Herbal Medicine, is believed to taste ephedra to treat asthma-like symptoms. It mentioned about a disease located in the lungs, which improved during winters. The seasonal nature and associated feature of wheezing described almost the characteristic picture of asthma.

The Egyptian Ebers Papyrus mentioned about asthma as a "disorder (WHDW) or foulness" of ducts (METU) of the lungs and other organs which could be treated with a large number of remedies.[3] It also described a special apparatus (an inhaler) for its treatment. The code of Hammurabi which belonged to the same period (1792–1750 BC) and regulated medical practice in Mesopotamia, also described about the "panting" of lungs and its treatment with the use of a breathing apparatus. Asthma in Ayurvedic literature was described as "*Tamka svasa*"—one of five types of disorders of breathing (i.e. "*svasa*"), namely *Kshudra svasa, Tamka svasa,* Pratamaka svasa, *Chinna svasa* and *Maha svasa*.[6] *Charaka Samhita*[7] gave a detailed description of clinical features of asthma—"dyspnea associated with wheezing sound. On account of the force of the paroxysm, the patient pants, coughs and becomes motionless, while thus constantly coughing, he feels faint frequently".

The concepts on the causes and treatment of the problem have considerably varied over different times. But the clinical manifestations have referred to breathlessness, coughing and panting in most descriptions. The Greek words which meant "to pant heavily" or "gasp for breath" subsequently formed the basis of the term "asthma".[28]

The other significant history relevant to the respiratory problems refers to that of a possible phenomenon of allergy reported sometimes between 3640 BC and 3300 BC.[29] King Menses of Egypt died after a wasp sting presumably because of anaphylaxis. Brittanicus, the son of Roman Emperor Claudius used to develop severe rash in the company of horses. There, however, is little to suggest a link of those phenomena with asthma or any other respiratory manifestation.

Medicine had further progressed during the period extending from about 500 BC to 3rd century AD. The Hippocratic medicine in Greece, *Susruta Samhita* in India and the Babylonian Talmud of Jews used different expressions and prescriptions for asthma. A large number of remedies had been used for treatment of asthma and other respiratory disorders in prebiblical periods. Garlic was one of the most common plant medicines used for various maladies including asthma, described in documented texts from Egypt, Greece, Rome, China and India. Ephedra, known as Ma Huang in China was used to treat asthma.[26,27] Grapes, yellow ochre and frankincense were used in Egypt to treat respiratory symptoms. Different purgatives, emetics, hot water compresses and bleeding were used in the Greco-Roman civilization. The ancient Hebrews believed in the power of God to heal different diseases. The Talmud on Hebrew laws discusses the use of "hiltith" (asafetida) to prevent and treat asthma, whooping cough and bronchitis.[30] The Talmud scholars also believed sneezing as a positive body function which pleased the God.

The disease description and the type of remedies may have varied in different eras, but all described a disease causing difficulty in breathing and/or panting which often responded to herbal or other natural treatments. As has been stated earlier, a few of the modalities included references to inhalational techniques, something which today constitutes the cornerstone of the management of asthma.

Other Respiratory Problems

It has not been possible to identify diseases which we know today, in the ancient medical texts or other historical manuscripts. It was mostly during the immediate prebiblical period before the birth of Christ when more definitive description of diseases became available. Hippocrates, the Father of Medicine, who laid the foundations of the modern medicine, had described the physical signs of "finger clubbing" and "succession splash".[31] Besides the descriptions of physical findings, epidemiology and other conditions, there are authentic references to conditions such as pneumonia, empyema and heart diseases in some of about 70 books which are attributed to him and/or his disciples.[32,33] One of the important notation in relation to lung diseases reads: "In cases where the whole lung is inflamed together with the heart... the patient is wholly paralyzed and lies cold and insensible."

Hippocrates' stress on physical examination is evident from one of his statement: "He who would make accurate forecasts as to those who will recover and those who will die and whether the disease will last whether the disease will last a greater or less number of days, must understand all the symptoms thoroughly and be able to appreciate them, estimating their powers when they are compared with one another, as I have set forth."

The developments in respiratory medicine, as in other fields in medicine as a whole had been faster in the next two millennia. Nonetheless, it remains exciting to know as to how the ancient man understood and managed the medical problems. Hidden therein are sowed the seeds of the modern medical practice.

REFERENCES

1. Nunn JF. Ancient Egyptian Medicine. Norman: University of Oklahoma Press; 1996.
2. Gardiner AH. Egyptian Grammar: Being an Introduction to the Study of Hieroglyphs, 3rd edition. Oxford: Griffith Institute, Ashmolean Museum; 1957.
3. Cohen SG. Asthma in antiquity: the Ebers papyrus. Allergy Proc. 1992;13:147-52.
4. Selwyn-Brown A. The Physician throughout the Ages. Volume I. Times Building, New York: Capehart-Brown Co Inc Publishers; 1938.
5. Lyons AS, Petrucelli RJ. Medicine: An Illustrated History. New York: HN Abrams Inc; 1987. pp. 19-41.
6. Jaggi OP. Chest diseases in ancient Hindu medicine. IJCD. 1961;3:124-8.

7. Charaka Samhita. Six vols. Jam Nagar, India: Shree Gulabkumverba Ayurvedic Soc; 1949.
8. *Susruta Samhita*. Three vols. Kolkata, India: Kavi Raj KL Bhishagratna; 1907.
9. Udwadia FE. Man and Medicine: A History. New Delhi: Oxford University Press; 2000.
10. Cournand A. Air and blood. In: Fishman AP, Richards DW (Eds). Circulation of the Blood, Men and Ideas. Bethesda, MD: American Physiological Society; 1982. pp. 3-70.
11. Fishman AP. Milestones in the history of pulmonary medicine. In: Fishman's Pulmonary Diseases and Disorders, 3rd edition. New York: McGraw-Hill; 1998.
12. Sigesrist HE. A History of Medicine. New York: Oxford University Press; 1952.
13. Dwarkanath C. The development of Indian Medicine *Sarangadhara's* contribution. New Delhi: Central Council for Research in Ayurveda and Siddha, Ministry of Health and Family Welfare, Govt. of India; 1991.
14. Pandita Sargadharacharya. The *Sarangadhara Samhita*. Pandita Parasurama Sastri, Vidyasagar (Eds). The *Sarangadhara Samhita*. Bombay: Nirmaya-Sagar Press; 1920.
15. Kutumbiah P. Ancient Indian Medicine. Mumbai: Orient Longmans; 1962.
16. Keers RY. Pulmonary tuberculosis: A Journey Down the Centuries. London: Bailliere-Tindall; 1978.
17. Cave AJE. The evidence for the incidence of tuberculosis in ancient Egypt. Br J Tuberc. 1939;33:142.
18. Zimmerman MR. Pulmonary and osseous tuberculosis in an Egyptian mummy. Bull NY Acad Med. 1979;55:604-8.
19. Herzog BH. History of tuberculosis. Respiration. 1998;65: 5-15.
20. Alladi M, Sharma SK. History. In: Sharma SK, Alladi M (Eds). Tuberculosis. New Delhi: Jaypee Brothers Medical Publishers. 2009. pp. 7-15.
21. Zimmer HR. Hindu Medicine. Baltimore: The Johns Hopkins Press; 1948.
22. Whitney. *Atharva Veda*. Lamman, Harvard Oriental Series Vol. 7 & 8; 1905.
23. Brown L. Story of Clinical Pulmonary Tuberculosis. Baltimore: Williams & Wilkins; 1936. p. 3.
24. Webb GB. Tuberculosis. New York: PB Hoeber; 1936. pp. 20-4.
25. Meulenbeld GJ. The Madhavanidana and its Chief Commentary. Leiden: EJ Brill; 1974.
26. Cserhati E. The history of bronchial asthma from the ancient times till the Middle Ages. Acta Physiol Hung. 2004;91:243-61.
27. Saavedra-Delgdo AMP, Cohen SG. Huang Ti. The Yellow Emperor and the Nei Ching: antiquities earliest reference to asthma. Allergy Proc. 1991;12:197-8.
28. McFadden ER Jr, Steven JB. History of asthma. In: Middleton E, Reed C, Ellis E (Eds). Allergy: Principles and Practice, 2nd edition. St. Louis, MO: CV Mosby; 1983. pp. 805-9.
29. Simons FER. Ancestors of Allergy. New York: Global Medical Communications Ltd; 1994.
30. Preuss J, Rosner F. Biblical and Talmudic Medicine. New York: Sanhedrin Press; 1978.
31. Jones WHS. Hippocrates. Vol I, II, and IV. London: William Heinemann; 1923-1931.
32. Katz AM. Hippocrates and the plane tree on the Island of Cos. Arch Intern Med. 1959;104:653-7.
33. Bedford DE. The ancient art of feeling the pulse. Brit Heart J. 1951;13:423-37.

SUGGESTED READING

1. Roy P. The Greatest Benefit to Mankind. New York, London: WW Norton & Co; 1997.
2. Udwadia FE. Man and Medicine, a History. New Delhi: Oxford University Press; 2002.

Anatomy and Architecture: A Clinical Perspective

SK Jindal

INTRODUCTION

The thoracic cavity bound externally by the thoracic-cage contains the lungs and the mediastinal structures between the two lungs. The thoracic cage is formed by the ribs and intercostal muscles, lined internally by the parietal pleurae. The lungs are lined on the surface by the visceral pleurae.

The respiratory systems essentially comprises of three different structural and functional units:

1. Respiratory tract (from the nose and the mouth to the alveoli), meant for air conduction.
2. Lung parenchyma (the alveoli and the surrounding interstitium, which includes the blood capillaries, lymphatics and interstitial matrix with several different kinds of cells).
3. Respiratory regulatory system.

LUNG ANATOMY AND MORPHOLOGY

Respiratory Tract or Airways

Upper Respiratory Tract

The components of the upper respiratory tract include the nose, the mouth, the pharynx and the larynx up to the level of the vocal cords. The upper respiratory tract largely lies in the domain of the otorhinolaryngologists and the oral physicians, but the diseases of different parts of the upper respiratory tract may frequently pose problems in the differential diagnosis of respiratory diseases. Several different diseases may also involve both the upper and the lower respiratory tracts. Sometimes, the diseases of the upper respiratory tract, particularly of the sinuses and the larynx, may precede or predispose to the development of diseases of the lower respiratory tract. The upper respiratory tract also performs the function of filtering, warming and humidifying the inspired air, thereby playing an important role in the pulmonary defense mechanisms.

The nasal cavity is divided into two separate parts by a median septum. The floor of the nose constitutes the hard palate and the roof of the base of the skull—maxillary, ethmoid and sphenoid bones. There are three bony projections from the lateral wall of each cavity, called superior, middle and inferior turbinates and the space between the two turbinates is the meatus. Sphenoethmoidal recess is the space above the superior turbinate. The nasal cavity is surrounded by the paranasal sinuses, which are the air containing cavities in the maxillary, frontal, ethmoid and sphenoid bones and are respectively known as the maxillary, frontal, ethmoidal and sphenoidal sinuses. The sinuses, being in continuity with the respiratory tract, bear an important clinical relationship with respiratory tract diseases.

Posteriorly, the nasal cavity continues with the nasopharynx, i.e. the part of the pharynx behind the nose. The nasopharynx contains adenoids and the lymphatic tissue. The openings of the Eustachian tubes, which connect with the middle-ear, are also located in the nasopharynx. It is through this tube that the problems of nasopharynx may directly spread to the otherwise closed, middle-ear cavity.

Nasopharynx continues inferiorly into the oropharynx—the space behind the oral cavity, up to the hyoid bone and thereafter into the hypopharynx, which extends from the hyoid bone up to the upper end of the esophagus and the larynx.

Larynx constitutes an important component of the upper respiratory tract. It is the seat of phonation and acts as sentry for the lower respiratory tract by preventing the aspiration of secretions and by regulating the flow of air. The larynx consists of several cartilages, ligaments and muscles. The laryngeal opening **(Fig. 1)** is guarded by the two vocal cords, which open with each cycle of inspiration and expiration to allow the movement of air in and out of the lungs. The vocal cords constitute both an anatomical and a functional landmark between the upper and the lower respiratory tracts. The respiratory tract below the vocal cords is normally protected from routine environmental onslaughts and is microbiologically sterile. Impaired movement or paralysis of a vocal cord compromises the respiratory defense and is also responsible for a change in the character of the voice.

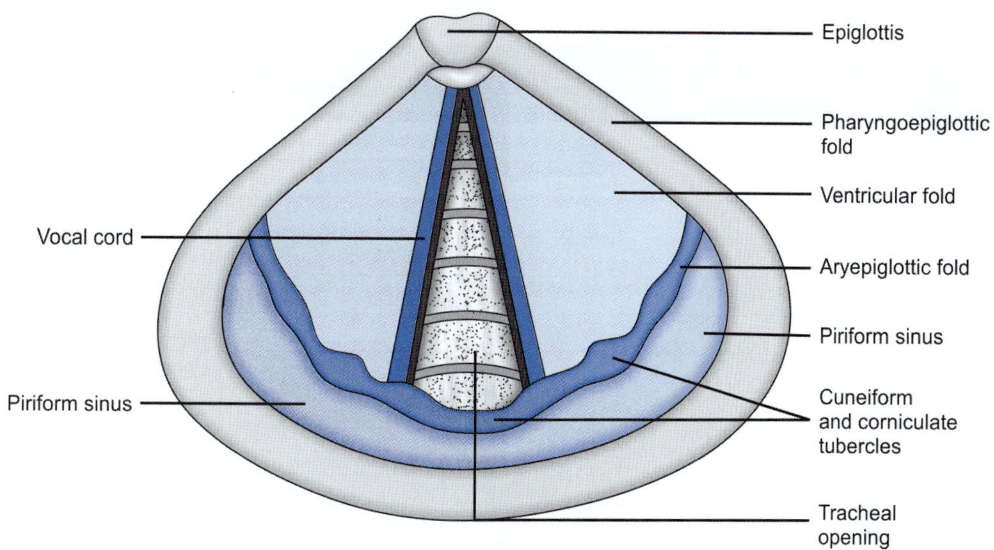

Fig. 1 Laryngeal opening as seen from above at the level of vocal cords

Lower Respiratory Tract

Starting with the trachea at the opening of the vocal cords, the lower respiratory tract consists of a branching system like that of a tree.

Trachea

The trachea extends from the level of the vocal cords above to the carina below. The extrathoracic part of the trachea begins at the level of the sixth cervical vertebra just below the cricoid cartilage and is covered anteriorly and laterally by the thyroid gland in the upper part of the neck. The lower part lies subcutaneously and enters the thoracic inlet, along with the esophagus situated behind the trachea. The intrathoracic part extends up to the fifth thoracic vertebra, corresponding anteriorly to the manubriosternal joint (Louis angle) and bifurcates at the carina into the right and left main bronchi. The tracheal wall is composed of cartilaginous rings, which do not allow the tracheal tube to collapse. The cartilaginous rings are partially incomplete posteriorly and the two posterior ends are jointed together by fibrous and elastic tissue. The tracheal lumen is somewhat oval in cross-section and remains patent throughout.

Bronchial Tree and Alveoli

The trachea divides into the two main bronchi (right and the left) which further divide into lobar, sublobar, segmental, subsegmental bronchi and the terminal bronchioles **(Fig. 2)**. The right and the left main bronchi enter the right and the left lung, respectively at the lung hila. Normally, the right main bronchus, which is in direct continuity with the trachea, is broader and shorter in length while the left main bronchus is more angulated, narrower and longer. The right bronchus is therefore the preferential site for aspiration of foreign bodies and secretions, especially in the erect position.

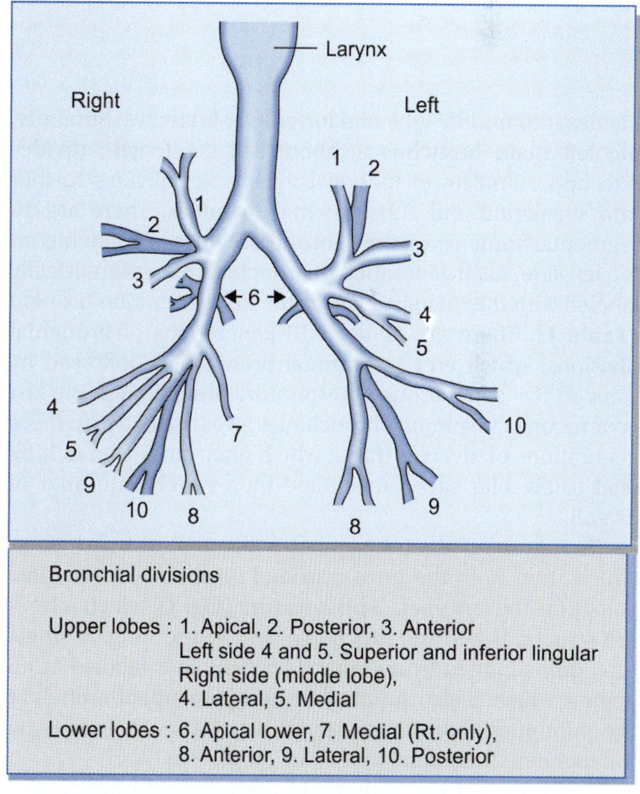

Fig. 2 Divisions of the tracheobronchial tree

The right main bronchus branches into the right upper lobe bronchus, which divides into apical, anterior and posterior branches and the intermediate bronchus, which further

Table 1 Bronchial and bronchiolar division

Structures	Generation from				
	Trachea	Bronchus	Segmental bronchiole	Terminal number	Diameter (mm)
Trachea	0			1	25
Main bronchi	1			2	11–19
Lobar bronchi	2–3			5	4.5–13.5
Segmental bronchi	3–6	0		19	4.5–6.5
Subsegmental bronchi	4–7	1		38	3–6
Bronchi		2–6		Variable	
Terminal bronchi		3–7		1,000	1.0
Bronchioles		5–14		Variable	Variable
Terminal bronchioles		6–15	0	35,000	0.65
Respiratory bronchioles			1–8	Variable	Variable
Terminal respiratory bronchioles			2–9	630,000	0.45
Alveolar ducts and sacs			4–12	14 million	0.40
Alveoli				300 million	0.25–0.3

divides into middle lobe and lower lobe branches. Similarly, the left main bronchus at about 4-5 cm length, divides into upper and lower lobe divisions, which divides further into segmental and subsegmental branches. There are 10 segmental branches on the right and 8 segmental branches on the left side. Each generation of bronchial tree is numerically labeled with the main bronchi as the first generation bronchi **(Table 1)**. There are about 8–10 generations of bronchial divisions, which end as terminal bronchioles, followed by three to five generations of respiratory bronchioles. The last generation of respiratory bronchioles gives rise to two to three generations of alveolar ducts, which after further branching lead to alveolar sacs, constituted by a variable number of alveoli.

The alveolar ducts together with the alveolar sacs, which stem from the most proximal respiratory bronchiole constitute the terminal respiratory unit **(Fig. 3)**, which is both the structural and the functional unit of the lung. A single lung unit supplied by a terminal bronchiole is labeled as an acinus, which is also supplied by an independent branch of the pulmonary blood vessels and lymphatics. Acinus is an independent functional unit of the lung.

The bronchial divisions up to the terminal bronchioles, primarily meant to conduct air to the alveoli are called the "conducting airways". They do not play any role in gas exchange during health. The respiratory tract beyond the terminal airways includes the respiratory bronchioles, alveolar ducts and the clusters of alveoli **(Fig. 3)**. This part of the respiratory tract is therefore labeled as the "gas-exchange unit" of the lung. In the two adult lungs, there are about 1,50,000 units, with about 2,000 alveoli in each unit.

The alveoli actually start appearing directly from the walls of the terminal generation of respiratory bronchioles. An alveolus is generally a polyhedral air sac with a thin and flat, single cell-layered wall.

Morphological Divisions of the Lungs

The two lungs are divided into five lobes by the presence of fissures—the right lung into three and the left into two lobes. The oblique fissure on both the sides separate the upper and the lower lobes, while the horizontal fissure on the right side divides the upper lobe into the upper and the middle lobes. The oblique fissure can be drawn on the chest wall by a line from the third dorsal vertebra opposite to the spine of scapula, sloping downward, laterally and anteriorly along the fifth rib up to the sixth costochondral junction anteriorly. The horizontal fissure on the right side may be drawn horizontally along with fourth costal cartilage to meet the oblique fissure in the mid axillary line. On the left side, the lingua, not separated by any fissure, is a part of the left upper lobe.

Each lobe is divided into segments by the presence of the septae. On the right side, the upper lobe is divided into apical, anterior and posterior segments; the middle lobe into the medial and the lateral segments; and the lower lobe into the lower apical (or superior) medial basal, lateral basal, anterior basal and posterior basal segments. On the left side, the upper lobe is divided into two, i.e. apicoposterior and anterior segments; the lingual into the superior and the inferior segments; and the lower lobe into the superior, anterior basal, posterior basal and the lateral basal segments. There is no medial basal segment on the left side. Therefore, the left

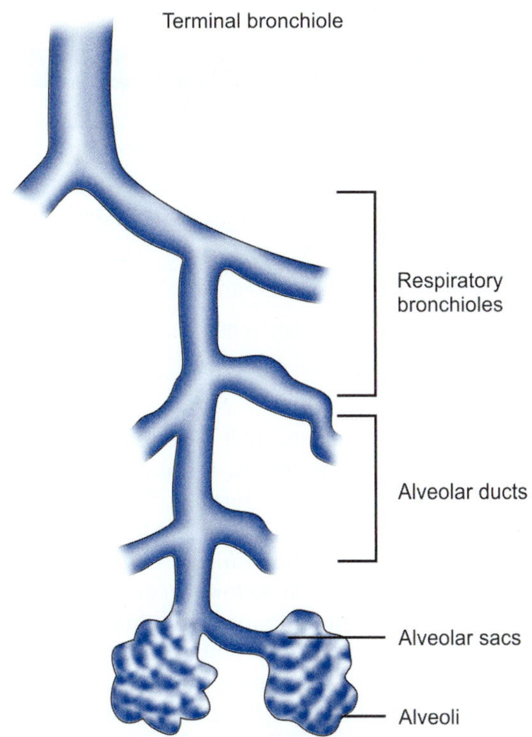

Fig. 3 Schematic structure of the terminal respiratory unit

lung contains 8 segments in comparison to 10 segments of the right lung. Each segment is further divided into subsegments and sequentially into the lobules and the acini.

Lung Hilum

The bronchus along with pulmonary vessels, lymphatics and nerves enter each lung near the center of the medial surface, called the hilum. The structures together, enclosed in a short, tabular sheet of pleura constitute the root of the lung. Inferiorly, it extends as a narrow fold called the pulmonary ligament.

ARCHITECTURE OF LUNG PARENCHYMA

The parenchyma of all the five lung lobes together consist of about 300 million alveoli, which when spread over, equal the surface area of a tennis court. The alveoli are surrounded by the lung interstitium comprising of loose-binding (extra-alveolar) connective tissue fibrils. The matrix of lung parenchyma consists of different materials, such as the collagen, elastin, glycosaminoglycan and fibronectin, which provide a framework of support of the alveolocapillary membrane that constitutes the bulk of the interstitium of the lung parenchyma. The major bulk is contributed by the collagen and the elastin, which together constitutes most of the interstitium—the glycosaminoglycan and fibronectin comprise only about 2% of the interstitium.

The basket-like arrangement of the matrix also allows the alveolar expansion in all directions. Within the lung interstitium, along the millions of alveoli, lie the divisions of the respiratory tract, i.e. the airways which supply air to the alveoli and the neurovascular bundles, which include the smaller branches of the pulmonary arteries, veins, the nerves and the lymphatics. The patency and the function of the airways, the alveoli and the vessels are maintained by the lung matrix. Any alternation in the structure and the function of the lung matrix affects the alveolar structure and function. Similarly, the pulmonary vasculature is also affected by the interstitial structure and disease.

An alveolar duct along with its peripheral structures is called a primary lobule. The smallest division of the lung parenchyma bounded by the connective tissue septae is the secondary lobule. A secondary lobule generally consists of two to five acini, i.e. two to five terminal bronchiole along with their peripheral structures.

There are small holes in the walls of the adjacent alveoli which are known as the pores of Kuhn. Communications may also exist between the terminal respiratory bronchioles and the alveoli through the canals of Lambert. These communications allow collateral ventilation, as well as the passage of alveolar cells and the microorganisms in a disease state.

Mucosal Lining and Lung Cells of the Respiratory Tract

There is a change of the mucosal epithelium from the nose to the alveoli. The nose, nasopharynx and the paranasal sinuses are lined by the ciliated columnar and the ciliated, stratified columnar epithelium. While the larynx is also lined by ciliated columnar epithelium, the vocal cords possess a squamous epithelium with no secretory functions. The entire lower respiratory tract up to the terminal bronchioles is lined by ciliated epithelium with the gradual transition of the columnar cells to the cuboidal and finally the squamous cells in the alveoli.

There are at least two epithelial cell types in the airway surface, of which nearly half are ciliated in nature. The cilia move the superficial liquid lining layer with their continuous beating. The glands in the submucosa of the airways are responsible for the production of airway secretions, which play an important role in the airway defense as well as the neurotransmission and endocrinal function.

Alveolar Walls

The alveolar wall is composed of alveolar epithelial cells, basement membrane, interstitial tissues, the capillary basement membrane and capillary endothelial cells. On the luminal side, the wall is lined by a fluid membrane—surfactant which is important to maintain the alveolar patency.

The epithelium is composed of a mosaic of lining cells, the squamous pneumocytes (Type I) and the secretory granular pneumocytes (Type II). The Type II cells are more numerous, but cover only 3% of the alveolar surface. They perform the important synthesizing and secretory functions and produce a large number of proteins including the surfactant-associated proteins and help in resorption and transepithelial exchange of fluids.

On the other hand, the Type I cells are fewer, but larger in size and cover most of the alveolar surfaces. Type I cells also express a few proteins and play some role in fluid flux. The Type I cells are complex branched cells. There are other interspersed cells such as the brush cells (Type III), mesenchymal and the endothelial cells. The brush cells have brush borders like that of the intestinal cells with possibly an absorptive function.

The alveolar macrophages are the free cells lying within the surface layers, submerged beneath the surfactant. The alveolar macrophages are capable of self renewal by mitosis. There are also Clara cells at the level of terminal bronchioles, which produce a surfactant like material. They also secrete the aqueous (or sol) layer lining of the bronchial mucosa. Kulchitsky or amine precursor uptake and decarboxylation (APUD) cells are the other important cells in the surface epithelium. They possess an endocrine function of producing serotonin. They also constitute the origin of the carcinoid tumors of lungs.

BLOOD SUPPLY OF LUNGS

The lungs receive a dual blood supply from the pulmonary and the bronchial (i.e. the systemic) circulation.

Bronchial Circulation

The bronchial circulation from the left ventricle is supplied via the bronchial arteries, which arise from the aorta or its intercostals branches. Normally, there are two main divisions (right and the left) of the bronchial artery, which follow the further bronchial divisions, but both the number and the origin of the bronchial arteries are variable and inconsistent. Terminally, the bronchial arteries are divided into bronchial arterioles and capillaries to finally anastomose with the pulmonary capillaries and constitute an extensive bronchial pulmonary vascular anastomotic bed around the terminal bronchioles and the alveoli. In healthy individuals, the bronchial circulation is small and constitutes less than 3% of the total blood supply of the lungs. It differs from the pulmonary circulation since it contains oxygenated blood from the left ventricle at systemic blood pressure levels **(Table 2)**. It is primarily nutritive in its function for the tracheobronchial tree.

Table 2 Differences between pulmonary and bronchial circulation of the lungs

	Pulmonary	*Bronchial*
Blood supply	Right ventricle	Left ventricle
Fraction of lung circulation	Most (>97%)	Less than 3%
Arterial pressure	Pulmonary	Systemic
Resistance	Low	High
Main vessels	Large-sized, elastic	Small-sized, muscular
Function	Gas exchange	Nutritive for the bronchial tree

Pulmonary Circulation

Pulmonary circulation constitutes the primary or the bulk of the blood supply of the lungs. The pulmonary artery arises from the right ventricle and divides into right and left main branches, which enter the hila of the lungs along with the right and left main bronchus, respectively and follow the airway divisions. They are further divided into medium-sized muscular arteries, arterioles and finally capillaries. The pulmonary venous system similarly consists of pulmonary vessels and veins, which follow a centripetal course and terminate into superior and inferior pulmonary veins, which drain into the left atrium, either independently or after joining together and forming a common trunk.

The pulmonary vessels lying in the alveolar walls are called alveolar vessels, while those lying in the loose binding connective tissue are called the extra-alveolar vessels. The alveolar vessels are directly affected by the changes in the alveolar pressure.

The pulmonary circulation is primarily concerned with the gas-exchange function of the lung. The extensive pulmonary capillary network around the alveoli provides a direct interface between the air in the alveoli and the blood in the capillaries, separated by a thin layer of alveolar epithelium, vascular endothelium and the lung interstitium. The pulmonary endothelial cells produce a large number of hormones and chemical mediators responsible for metabolic and endocrinal functions. The pulmonary circulation through an extensive capillary network around the alveoli has been conceptually equated to the presence of a sheet of blood all around the alveolus contained in a thin layer of capillary endothelium. The capillary network crosses several alveoli before coalescing into venules, thus providing a sufficient transit time for the blood to pass from the arterial to the venous end. This allows a free exchange of gases (oxygen and carbon dioxide) through the alveolocapillary membrane. A minor fraction of pulmonary blood flow (1–3% of total) may pass directly from the arterial to the venous side, bypassing the alveolocapillary network. This amount of nonoxygenated blood represents the shunt fraction which is present in a normal human lung.

LYMPHATIC DRAINAGE

There are considerable variations in the lymphatic drainage of the two lungs. The lymphatics of the lungs form extensive intercommunicating networks around the bronchial and the vascular divisions in the peribronchial and the perivascular spaces. These lymphatics drain into the several groups called "stations of lymph nodes", located along the bronchial tree and ultimately into the hila (right and the left along the main bronchi) and the tracheobronchial lymph nodes. The various tracheobronchial lymph nodes groups include the superior group (between the trachea and the right or the left main bronchus) para-aortic and an inferior or infracarinal (below the carina) group. The further drainage occurs into the paratracheal glands (along both sides of trachea) and the supraclavicular glands in the neck. The paratracheal lymphatics also communicate with the paraesophageal glands in the mediastinum and the retroperitoneal abdominal nodes.

The lymphatics from all the groups of tracheobronchial nodes lead into the thoracic duct on the left side and the lymphatic duct on the right side, which finally drain into the venous system, i.e. the innominate veins of the two sides. The right lung drains into the right tracheobronchial, paratracheal and supraclavicular glands, and the left lung drains into the left side glands, but there is a great degree of intercommunication between the two sides, especially of the paratracheal glands. An important exception to the same side drainage is seen for the left lower lobe lymphatics, which drain into the right-sided glands. There are also communications between the superficial and the deep lymphatic plexuses via the interlobular septal lymphatics. Thus, there is a potential for bidirectional flow of lymph.

The lymphatic drainage serves several important functions such as the removal of dust particles, toxins and microorganisms from the lungs. They also play an important role in the maintenance of lung-fluid balance. The lymph node enlargement, which occurs in several inflammatory, infective and neoplastic diseases of the lungs, may therefore provide an important clue to the differential diagnosis of these diseases. Particularly in the cases of lung cancer, the site of lymph node is important in deciding the disease-stage and treatment modality.

NERVE SUPPLY

The lungs are innervated by both the sympathetic and the parasympathetic autonomic nerve supply from the upper six thoracic sympathetic ganglia and the vagus, respectively. The innervation consists of afferent (i.e. the sensory) and the efferent (i.e. the motor pathways).

Parasympathetic (Cholinergic) Nerve Supply

The efferent fibers arise from the stretch receptors in the alveolar walls and lung interstitium and from epithelial irritant receptors of the airways. The afferents also arise from the irritant receptors of the laryngotracheal mucosa. They form a plexus around the carina and join the vagus nerve. The vagus nerves also contain the efferent fibers for the bronchial smooth muscles and the mucous glands. The efferent activation from irritant and stretch receptor stimulation causes the reflex efferent reaction causing bronchoconstriction and mucous hypersecretion.

Sympathetic (Adrenergic) Nerve Supply

The sympathetic efferent fibers from the upper thoracic sympathetic ganglia supply the pulmonary plexus around the carina and the sympathetic nerve, which innervate the bronchial smooth muscles, glands and the blood vessels. Sympathetic efferent stimulation results in bronchodilatation, vasoconstriction and diminished bronchial mucous secretion. Of the various sympathetic receptor subtypes, only the β_2 and the α-adrenergic receptors are present in the lungs. The lungs are also supplied by fibers, which are neither adrenergic nor cholinergic in action. These fibers, which are carried by the vagal nerves, may play an important role in maintaining the bronchomotor tone and in the pathogenesis of bronchospastic disorders, as in asthma.

Lung Receptors

Receptors are the nerve endings, which are sensitive to specific, sensory stimuli. As stated above, the lungs are extensively supplied by stretch and irritant receptors in the alveolar and the bronchial walls, respectively. They are present in the airway epithelium, submucous region, interalveolar septa and smooth muscles. They are also present to some extent on the pleural surface. There is no pain or thermal nerve endings. The lung interstitium also contains a large number of juxtacapillary (J) receptors around the capillary walls. These receptors, also known as Paintal's J receptors, are stimulated by the parenchymal connective tissue distortion in the presence of vascular congestion and interstitial edema. The peptidergic nerve endings present around tracheal glands have species-specific excitatory or inhibitory effect on secretary function. There is also a diffuse, neuroendocrinal system (APUD) distributed along the airway epithelium. The exact role of the APUD system is not known; it might affect the smooth muscle function.

Pleura

The membranous covering of the lung and the pleura is an important constituent of the respiratory system, both structurally and functionally. The pleura consist of a visceral layer, which lines the outer lung surface and a parietal layer, which lines the inner surface of the thoracic cage. The two pleurae together form a continuous layer joined at the hilum to constitute a potential space, the pleural cavity, which is closed on all sides and contains a small quantity of fluid to prevent friction between the two pleural layers. There occurs an excessive fluid collection in this cavity in several inflammatory, neoplastic and other diseases involving the pleura.

The visceral lining of the pleurae also extends into the oblique and the transverse fissures to form the potential pleural space between the lung lobes in the fissures. The parts of the pleurae lining, the mediastinal and the diaphragmatic surfaces, also respectively known as the mediastinal and the diaphragmatic pleura, constitute the mediastinal and the diaphragmatic pleural spaces respectively. Loculated collection of fluid may occasionally occur inside these pleural spaces in various pathological conditions.

Histologically, the pleura consists of the squamous epithelial cell lining over a connective tissue layer. The blood supply, lymphatics and nerve supply of the visceral pleura is similar to that of the lung, which it overlies. The parietal pleura is a part of the thoracic cage and derives its blood supply from the systemic circulation through the intercostals and the branches of the internal mammary arteries. Lymphatic drainage of the parietal pleura occurs to the nodes along with internal mammary artery and to the posterior mediastinal glands near the heads of the ribs. Similarly, the nerve supply of the parietal pleura is through the spinal nerves for the costal and the mediastinal pleurae and through the phrenic nerve for the diaphragmatic pleura. On the other hand, the visceral pleura is innervated by the autonomic nerves.

Thoracic Cage

The thoracic cage, which constitutes the walls of the thoracic cavity, provides a protective house for the lungs, the heart, the great vessels, the esophagus and the other mediastinal structures. It is constituted by the sternum anteriorly, the thoracic spine posteriorly and the ribs and the intercostal muscles laterally. Inferiorly, the two diaphragms on each site separate the thoracic cavity from the abdominal cavity. The contents of the neck, such as the trachea, the esophagus, the neck-vessels and the nerves, enter the thorax through the thoracic inlet at the upper end of the thoracic cavity. The thoracic inlet is constituted by the upper border of the manubrium sterni, the first rib and the first dorsal vertebra.

The thoracic cage not only contains the lungs and other thoracic structures, but also plays an important role in the process of respiration. The contraction of the inspiratory intercostals muscles, causing upward and forward movement of the ribs and the downward movement of diaphragms, results in the expansion of the thoracic cage and a fall in the intrapleural pressure, which causes the air to move into the tracheobronchial tree allowing the inspiration to occur. Expiration occurs after inspiratory muscle contraction ends and the thoracic cage returns to its original position. Expiration occurs as a passive phenomenon except in condition of respiratory distress when the expiratory muscles help the expiratory process through their active contraction.

The two lungs also provide a soft bed, the cardiac fossa for the heart. The inspiratory inflation and expiratory deflation of the lungs have an important bearing on the cardiac function. The overall mechanical cardiopulmonary interaction provides a conducive environment for an efficient circulatory function.

Respiratory Muscles

There are three groups of muscles involved in respiration:
1. The diaphragm
2. The intercostals
3. The accessory muscles of respiration.

Diaphragm: It consists of a fan-like musculotendinous structure, which consists of muscle fibers attached to the inside of the thoracic cage at the thoracic outlet, inserted into a central tendon. Based on their attachment, the muscle fibers are grouped into three parts—the sternal part attached to the xiphoid process; the costal part attached to the inner surface of the costal cartilages and anterior ends of ribs; and the lumbar part, which is attached to the medial and the lateral lumbocostal arches. Similarly, the central tendon has got the right middle and left leaflets. The diaphragm is innervated by the phrenic nerve, which arises from the cervical plexus, with fibers from third, fourth and fifth cervical segments of the spinal cord. Phrenic nerve stimulation causes the contraction of the diaphragm, which as a result of contraction, moves down and causes lung inflation due to an increase in the volume of thorax. Weakness or paralysis of the phrenic nerves results in the elevation of the diaphragm, which will also not move with the inspiratory effort.

The thoracic mediastinal structures, such as the aorta, the esophagus, the inferior vena cava, other small vessels and nerves, pass across the diaphragm to enter the abdominal cavity. There are other small recesses in the diaphragm such as the foramen of Morgagni anteriorly and the Bochdalek foramen posteriorly. Sometimes, the abdominal contents may protrude through the spaces into the thoracic cavity, i.e. the diaphragmatic or hiatus hernias. The point of esophageal entry into the abdomen serves the role of a sphincter, which allows the food to pass down into the stomach, but prevents the regurgitation of the contents into the thoracic part of esophagus. Gastroesophageal reflux, which occurs as a result of the loosening of this sphincter, plays an important role in the clinical symptomatology and etiologies of several respiratory problems.

Intercostal respiratory muscles: The intercostal muscles spread obliquely between the intercostals spaces of the ribs. The intercostals muscles directly inserted to the ribs have no tendons. There are two groups of the intercostals muscles—the internal and the external intercostals. The external intercostal muscles arise from the lower border of the upper rib and get inserted into the upper border of the lower rib of an intercostals space. They are also called the inspiratory muscles since they actively take part in the inspiratory effort by their contraction, which by raising the ribs results in the expansion of the thoracic cavity and therefore creating a rise in the negative pressure in the pleural cavity. The internal intercostals, also called the expiratory muscles, are passive during normal expiration, but assume an important role during the labored breathing in conditions causing respiratory distress when the expiration becomes an active process. The same may happen during hyperventilation, deep coughing and other similar conditions requiring a strong and active expiratory effort.

Intercostal muscles are supplied by systemic circulation through the intercostals vessels (an artery and a vein) which arise from the aorta. They are innervated by the intercostal nerves, which are derived from the inferior part of brachial plexus. The intercostal nerves along with the intercostals vessels run along the inferior borders of the ribs to supply the intercostal muscles of the respective space.

Accessory muscles of respiration: The scaleni, sterno-cleidomastoids, muscles of the alae nasi and of anterior abdominal wall (rectus abdominis, the external oblique, the internal oblique and the transverses abdominus) constitute the group of the accessory muscles of respiration since they assist respiration whenever an increased demand for augmented ventilation arises. Their role is rather limited in their overall contribution to the respiratory process. However, the presence of hyperactivity of accessory muscles is an important clinical indication of the underlying respiratory distress and/or failure.

BIBLIOGRAPHY

1. Albertine KH, Williams MC, Hyde DM. Anatomy and development of the respiratory tract. In: Mason RJ, Murray JF, Broaddus VC, et al. (Eds). Textbook of Respiratory Medicine. Elsevier Saunders; 2005. pp. 1-29.
2. Breeze RG, Wheeldon EB. The cells of the pulmonary airways. Am Rev Respir Dis. 1977;116(4):705-77.
3. Butler J. The heart is in good hands. Circulation. 1983;67(6): 1163-8.
4. Cudkowicz L, Abelmann WH, Levinson GE, Katznelson G, Jreissaty RM. Bronchial arterial blood flow. Clin Sci. 1960;19: 1-15.
5. Horsfield K, Cumming G. Functional consequences of airway morphology. J Appl Physiol. 1968;24(3):384-90.
6. Horsfield K, Cumming G. Morphology of the bronchial tree in man. J Appl Physiol. 1968;24(3):373-83.
7. Krahl VE. Anatomy of the mammalian lung. In: Fenn WO and Rahn H (Eds). Handbook of Physiology, Section 3: Respiration. Washington DC: American Physiological Society. 1964;1: 213-84.
8. Murray JF (Ed). Postnatal growth and development of the Lung. The normal lung: The basis for diagnosis and treatment of pulmonary disease. WB Saunders Company; 1976. pp. 21-57.
9. Richardson JB. Nerve supply to the lungs. Am Rev Respir Dis. 1979;1195:785-802.
10. Singhal S, Henderson R, Horsefield K, Harding K, Cumming G. Morphometry of human pulmonary arterial tree. Circ Res. 1973;33(2):190-7.
11. Turino GM. The lung parenchyma—a dynamic matrix. Am Rev Respir Dis. 1985;132:1324-34.
12. Weibel ER (Ed). Morphometry of the Human Lung. Berlin: Springer-Verlag; 1963. p. 111.
13. Weibel ER, Taylor CR. Functional design of the human lung for gas exchange. In: Fishman AP, Elias JA, Fishman JA, et al. (Eds). Pulmonary Diseases and Disorders, 3rd edition. McGraw-Hill Interamericana; 1998. pp. 21-61.

Lung Development

Meenu Singh, Nidhi Anil, Amit Agarwal

INTRODUCTION

Unlike the heart, kidneys, liver and other viscera that begin their function early in the fetal life, the lungs are nonfunctional because of the aquatic environment in utero. The lungs start function with the first breath at birth. The process of lung development involves complex morphogenesis by means of which epithelial tubules and blood vessels are formed that ultimately give rise to airways and alveoli. Lung development primarily involves two phases, i.e. prenatal and postnatal **(Table 1)**. The human lung arises from the laryngotracheal groove at around 4–6 week gestation.[1-3] During this time, the respiratory diverticulum (lung bud) appears ventrally to the caudal portion of the foregut. Location of the lung bud, along the gut tube is directed by various signals from the surrounding mesenchyme, including the growth factors.[4,5] The proximal portion of this bud gives rise to larynx and trachea, separated by the esophagus. The distal part of primitive bud gives rise to left and right main stem bronchi.

The lung development in humans follows four distinct phases, i.e. pseudoglandular stage, which lasts from 6 weeks to 16 weeks; during this period all major lung elements except alveoli, appear. This is followed by the canalicular stage (16–26 weeks) during which lumens of bronchi enlarge and become highly vascularized; by the 24-week respiratory bronchioles and alveolar buds develop. During the next phase, also known as the terminal saccular period, the blood air barrier gets established with the appearance of specialized cells of the respiratory epithelium, including the type I alveolar cells (responsible for gas exchange), and type II alveolar cells, which secrete pulmonary surfactant.[6,7] Alveolarization in humans begins after week 20 and continues up to 7 year of age, giving rise to an alveolar gas diffusion surface of 70 m^2 area and 1 µm thickness.

Table 1 Different phases of lung development

A.	*Prenatal development*: Phases		
	1. *Embryonic stage*: Day 26 to the next 7 weeks		
	2. Lung development		
	i.	Pseudoglandular	5–17 week
	ii.	Canalicular	16–26 week
	III.	Terminal saccular	24 week to until term
	iv.	Alveolar	36 week to until birth and postnatally
B.	*Postnatal*		
	Alveolar stage continues up to about 18 months of age		

DEVELOPMENT OF AIRWAY EPITHELIUM

The development of airway epithelium occurs during the embryonic stage as previously described, it relies on the epithelial-mesenchymal interactions between the components of the airway wall including surface lining fluid, submucosal gland and the basement membrane, including the basal lamina and fibroblasts.[8-10] There occurs differential growth of the epithelial tube into a mesenchymal derivative containing the cells and the matrix. This development moves from a proximal to distal pattern following the epithelial tube. Subsequent branching of the airway tree results in the development of alveolar septum.[11,12]

After the bronchial tree is established, growth occurs in two directions, either longitudinally to extend the length or circumferentially to increase its diameter. In mammals, the majority of growth occurs postnatally, thereby making the perturbations by environmental contaminants crucial.[13-16] The distal airways, located at the junction between the gas exchange area and tracheobronchial tree form the extensive transition zone of the human lung. The development of submucosal glands occurs in four phases: (1) formation of buds by projections of undifferentiated cells; (2) outgrowth and branching of the buds into cylinders; (3) differentiation of mucous cells in proximal tubules and (4) differentiation of serous cells in peripheral tubules and acini along with continuous proliferation of most distal areas.

Alveolar formation starts late, it is primarily a postnatal event. Besides the growth of the septae into the terminal

Flow chart 1 Schema of human fetal circulation

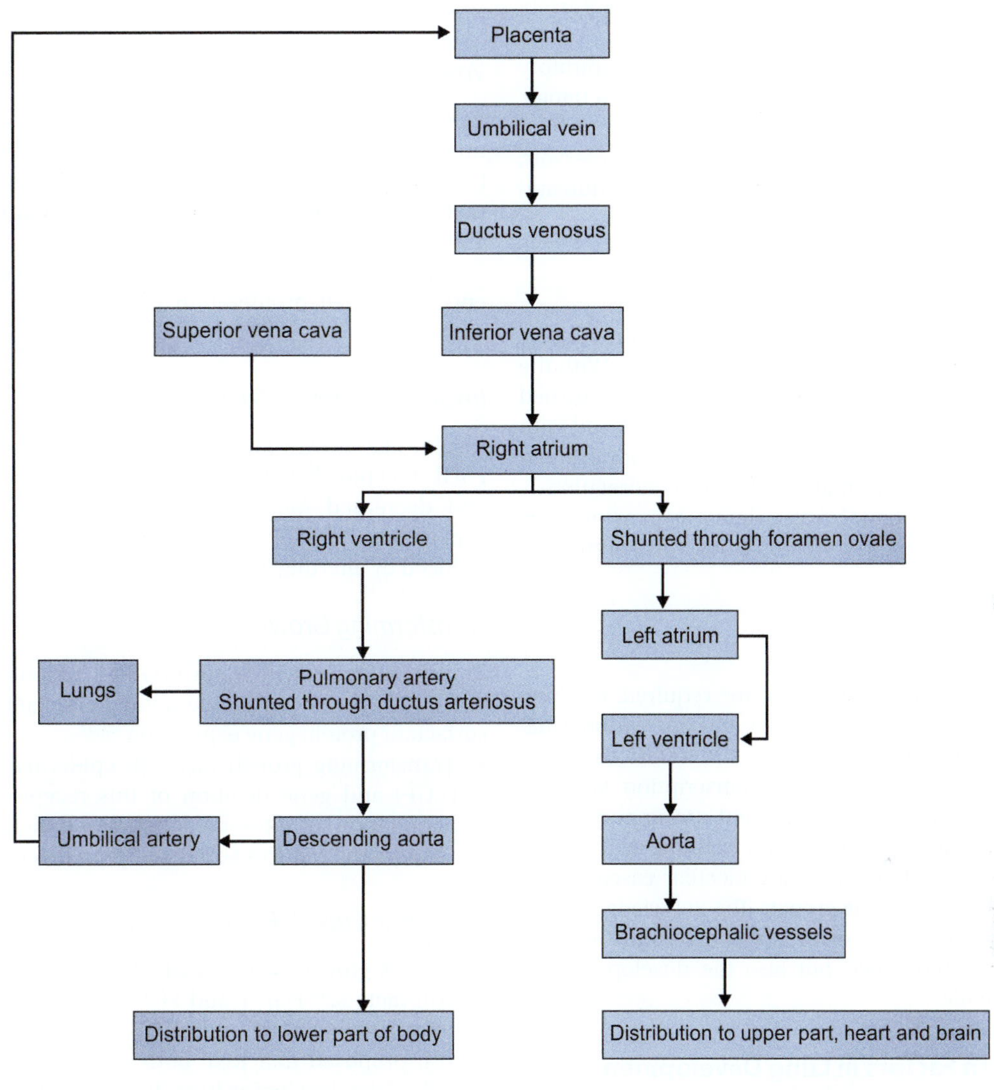

saccules, there is formation of smooth muscles, elastin and other matrix cells.

PULMONARY VASCULATURE

Primitive right and left pulmonary arteries grow caudally from the aortic sac when the lung bud is also forming. They become associated with the development of respiratory primordium. The growing pulmonary arterial system maintains this association with the development of the airway system throughout thereafter. The blood supply to the respiratory primordium drains into a venous plexus that empties into the heart through a single pulmonary vein. The venous drainage system is complete around midway through gestation and corresponds to the conducting airways and arterial system.

There is only a small proportion of blood of the total cardiac output, which flows to the lungs during fetal development. The resistance to flow in the pulmonary arteries is high. After birth, there is a sudden drop in pulmonary arterial pressure and a rise in the blood flow. This is attributed partly to the anatomical alterations and partly to local vasomotor responses.

The blood circulation during fetal life takes a somewhat different route **(Flow chart 1)**. The oxygenated blood from the placenta is returned to the fetus through the umbilical vein and flows through the ductus venosus and inferior vena cava into the right atrium, shunted through the foramen ovale into the left atrium from where it goes to the left ventricle, aorta and gets distributed preferentially to the upper part of the body, the heart and the brain, through the brachiocephalic vessels. On the other hand, the venous blood returning to the right atrium from the superior vena cava, which is poorly oxygenated passes into the pulmonary artery through the right ventricles, gets shunted into the descending aorta (through the ductus arteriosus) from where it is distributed to the lower part of the body, the placenta. The pulmonary artery blood also flows to the lungs.

The intrauterine lung performs only the nonrespiratory functions. It does not participate in gas exchange. Importantly, it is one of the important source of amniotic fluid and surfactant formation. It also serves as a blood reservoir, provides host defenses and participates in the activation and inactivation of biological substances.

BEGINNING OF POSTNATAL LIFE

The lungs take over the gas exchange function immediately after delivery, which marks the end of the fetal life. With the very first breath—the cry, the ventilatory system is "turned on". Immediately, the liquid in the lungs gets replaced with air. There occur significant changes in the pulmonary and cardiac circulation; the "normal circulation" is miraculously established with the first breath. Lung expansion gets complete during the first few breaths along with circulatory adjustments.

REGULATORY FACTORS

A number of regulatory molecules are required for lung development. Lungs are formed from anterior endodermal cells that also generate the ventral foregut. Therefore, the genes (e.g. *GATA-6, HNF-3B* and thyroid transcription factor-1) involved in ventral foregut development are important for the early lung development. Vitamin A (retinoic acid) is also essential for growth. There exists a molecular cascade that regulates and determines the growth. The knowledge of this cascade is an important area of interest to determine not only the development anomalies, but also the development of diseases, later in life.

Role of Growth Factors in Lung Development

Growth factors are known to play an important role in the development of lungs. Platelet-derived growth factor (PDGF-A and B) and their receptors PDGFR-α and β are involved in the early mid-stage of lung development. PDGE-A and B mRNA level increase[17,18] in parallel with all proliferation rates during the pseudoglandular stage of lung development; cell proliferation within lung explants is inhibited by PDGF-A and B antisense oligonucleotides, as well as PDGF neutralizing antibodies.[19,20]

- Platelet-derived growth factor-A exhibits a complete failure of alveolar septation,[18] whereas the overexpressions of PDGF-A cause marked mesenchymal cell proliferation within the lungs.
- Platelet-derived growth factor-A and B have shear stress responsive elements (SSRE) in their promoter regions suggesting their expressions levels can be influenced by the exposures of cells to physical forces. This stretch-induced cell proliferation is abolished by PDGF-B and PDGF-β antisense oligonucleotides, PDGF-BB neutralizing antibodies and a PDGFR inhibitor.[21]

Vascular Endothelial Growth Factor

Vascular endothelial growth factor (VEGF) exerts potent mitogenic effects on endothelial cells via the VEGF receptors (VEGFR2).[22] VEGF and VEGFR2 mRNA increase as the lung matures.[23,24] VEGF proteins plays a role in directing vascular growth in regions destined for gas exchange.

Vascular endothelial growth factor is responsible for the endothelial cell proliferation induced by increase in lung expansion.

Insulin-like Growth Factors

Insulin-like growth factors (IGFs) I and II act via the type I IGF receptor.[25] IGF I and II mRNA levels are increased and decreased following increase and decrease in lung expansions.[26-28] IGF may mediate changes in lung growth induced by alterting lung expansion.

Transforming Growth Factor

Transforming growth factor (TGF-β) inhibits fetal newborn and adult type II cell proliferation, surfactant synthesis and surfactant protein gene expression.[29-31]

- Transforming growth factor-β, epidermal growth factor (EGF) and gene deletion of this receptor prevents the attenuation of mesenchymal tissue between adjacent airways and reduces surfactant protein levels.

Fibroblast Growth Factor Family

Fibroblast growth factor (FGF) family consists of over 20 growth factors.[32] FGF-1 and FGF-2 differ at different stages of lung development and FGF-7 [keratino growth factor (KGF)] proposed that KGF both enhances[33-35] and inhibits growth of the developing lung. Parathyroid hormone-related protein (PTHrP) induces surfactant protein and surfactant phospholipids biosynthesis, increases PTHrP expressions and receptor binding and enhances its effects on surfactant phospholipid synthesis.[36]

Role of Environmental Factors during Lung Development

The various regulatory mechanisms are influenced by several environmental factors and results. They significantly influence the occurrence of diseases. Hypersensitivity diseases in particular, may have their roots in utero sensitization to allergens. Similarly, exposure of the fetus to tobacco smoke from a smoking mother (passive smoking) or even from other smokers in company of the pregnant mother (tertiary smoking) have been implicated in the development of allergic disorders and lung function impairment after birth.

- *Influence of in utero exposure to allergens on development*: Exposure of the fetus to allergens inhaled by the mother during pregnancy can result in its sensitization to those allergens. In one study, neonatal peripheral blood T-cells were obtained from whole blood and stimulated with several antigens or common inhaled allergens. It is well known that maternally derived T-cell would respond to commonly encountered antigens and fetal cells would respond only to the inhaled allergens.

  Maternal avoidance of allergen could influence the development of allergic reactivity in the fetus. Levels of interleukin (IL)-4, IL-5, IL-10 and γ-interferon were determined and compared with allergen data. It was observed that the cytokine levels did not correlate with allergens. It was hypothesized that T-helper (Th)-cell cytokine patterns are determined during infancy. Although the stimulation of neonatal T-cells occurs with allergen-produced cytokine profiles. It is suggested that exposure to allergens during development may be a critical factor for the development of allergenic phenotype infants and children who are genetically predisposed to allergy.

  Maternal exposure to allergens can result in a protective immunoglobulin G (IgG) response that may decrease the fetal sensitization. The degree of the production of γ interferon by stimulated T-cells has a stronger likelihood of predicting the future development of atopic disease. Th-2 phenotype during pregnancy is known to favor the prenatal development of allergy, thus the interaction between environment and genetic background during in utero life of a human infant determines the future allergic status of the child and adult.
- *Neonatal exposure to allergens:* Several infectious diseases are thought to have a role in either facilitating the development of allergic sensitization to inhaled allergens during the neonatal period or subverting the allergic response. The "hygiene hypothesis" focuses on early exposure to bacterial products that appear to have an allergy-sparing effect. In contrast, certain viral respiratory infections have been implicated in the promotion of allergen sensitization and development of asthma. Viral infections are frequently associated with wheezing in small children. The fact that many of these children progress to become asthmatic has led to the supposition that the early viral infection may either facilitate sensitization or damage airways hyperactivity.[37]

One of the major respiratory viruses that appears to have a link to asthma is respiratory syncytial virus (RSV). In the severe form, RSV causes wheezing and severe bronchiolitis and often interstitial pneumonia. It was recognized in the 1980s that children with most severe RSV, accompanied by wheezing, were often subsequently diagnosed with childhood asthma. Indeed, IgE specific for viral proteins, as well as elevated histamine concentrations in respiratory fluids, were found in severely affected children.[38]

More recently, it has been found that RSV preferentially induces a Th-2 cytokine environment in atopic children and in some animal models. Studies have shown that infection of Balb/c mice with human RSV induces a Th cell type 2 response.[39] A previous study demonstrated that some calves infected with bovine RSV[40] (a closely related bovine pathogen) develop a Th-2 cytokine response when infected with the virus. Indeed, infection of IgE is also associated with this model. Further work with the bovine model has demonstrated that the disease is exacerbated when allergen is inhaled during the virus infection[41] and that sensitization can be enhanced by exposure to allergen during the viral infection.[42]

In contrast to these observations, a recent study has demonstrated that γ-interferon is present in elevated amount in the severe cases of respiratory disease with wheezing. However, in this study, the identity of the virus causing the infection and wheezing was not elucidated.[43] Following up on these observations, Garofalo et al.[44] examined the role of Th-1 and Th-2 cytokines, as well as several chemokines in RSV disease. They found that macrophage inflammatory protein-1α was associated with severe RSV bronchiolitis. Thus, the role of cytokines in induction of clinical disease may be different to that previously thought to stimulate the subsequent development of asthma.

Role of Stem Cells in Lung Development

The vital functions of lung are in gas exchange and immune defense. These functions are fulfilled by the cellular composition and complex three-dimensional organization of the organ. In response to cellular injury by agents such as infection, toxic compounds and irradiation there is rapid proliferation and differentiation of endogenous stem and progenitor cells to repair and regenerate the damaged tissue. Normally, the cell turnover is low in the adult lung. In the mouse, different populations of epithelial progenitor cells have been identified in different regions of the respiratory system: basal cells in the proximal trachea bronchial region and submucosal glands and secretory cells in the conducting airways and bronchio alveolar duct junction. The identification of the long-term stem cells in the alveolar region is still under debate and little is known about resident stem and progenitor cells for the many mesodermal populations.

Within this framework information is provided about the origin of lung progenitor cells during development, the microenvironment in which they reside, the experimental injury and repair systems used to promote their regenerative response and some of the mechanisms regulating their behavior.[45] At least, two populations of epithelial stem/progenitor cells give rise to the lung anlage, comprising the laryngotracheal complex versus the distal lung below the first bronchial bifurcation. Residual pools of adult stem cells are hypothesized to be the source of lung regeneration and repair. These pools have been located within the basal layer of the upper airways, within or near pulmonary neuroendocrine cell rests, at the bronchoalveolar junction as well as within the alveolar epithelial surface. Rapid repair of the denuded alveolar surface after injury is clearly key to survival. Strategies to enhance endogenous alveolar epithelial repair could include protection of epithelial progenitors from injury and/or stimulation of endogenous progenitor cell function. Further work will be needed to translate stem/progenitor cell therapy for the lung.[46]

Therapeutic Role of Bone Marrow Stem Cells and Endothelial Colony Forming Cells in Children with Bronchopulmonary Dysplasia

Bronchopulmonary dysplasia (BPD) is disease resulting from impaired alveolar development and alveolar destruction. BPD continues as a major cause of neonatal morbidity and mortality. The disease is characterized by alveolar wall thickening, decreased surfactant and pulmonary hypertension due to hyperoxic condition. There are no such effective therapies to treat BPD. Recent advances in stem cell therapy have opened the pathways to counteract such type of diseases. Endothelial colony forming cells (ECFCs) and bone marrow stem cells (BMSC) has been shown to have therapeutic potential in BPD.

Endothelial colony forming cells represent a subset of circulating and resident endothelial cells capable of self-renewal and de novo vessel formation. In a recent study, it was demonstrated that cord blood derived ECFC therapy may offer new therapeutic options for lung diseases characterized by alveolar damage.[46] Another report described a population of resident pulmonary microvascular endothelial progenitor cell (EPCs) in adult rat lungs that display a high proliferative potential and capable of de novo angiogenesis in vivo.[47] These cells resemble the ECFCs previously isolated from the peripheral circulation and in human umbilical cord blood.[47] Similar cells have now been described in the mouse pulmonary circulation. It has been seen that after systemic delivery of BMSC-conditioned media in mice, inflammation and neonatal lung injury get inhibited. These effects are mediated by paracrine mechanisms through the angiogenic growth factors.

Human cord blood-derived ECFCs reverse alveolar growth arrest, preserve lung vascularity and attenuate pulmonary hypertension in hyperoxia-induced BPD in newborn rodents. There are no trials of BMSC and ECFCs in lungs of neonates with BPD, which confirms their direct role in reversing and inhibiting alveolar damage. More studies are needed in vitro and in vivo to optimize dose, timing and duration of both stem cell and cell free media treatment to delineate the mechanisms underlying BMSC and ECFCs protection in model of BPD.

SUMMARY

The respiratory system in the fetus is elegantly designed to develop from an undifferentiated epithelial tube to a complex air conducting branching system and an enormous gas-exchanging surface with a large number of differentiated cells engaged in several different functions. The immediate functional transformation and adaptation of the respiratory and circulatory systems, to the "foreign" strenuous environments after the birth is both dramatic and miraculous. Although the alveolar formation and lung development continues postnatally for some period, most of the somatic growth is complete at birth. Exogenous stem/progenitor cells can be delivered into the lung either intravenously, intratracheally, or by direct injection. Sources of exogenous stem/progenitor cells that are currently under evaluation in the context of acute lung injury and repair include embryonic stem cells, bone marrow- or fat-derived mesenchymal stem cells, circulating endothelial progenitors, and, recently, amniotic fluid stem/progenitor cells.

REFERENCES

1. Wells JM, Melton DA. Vertebrate endoderm development. Annu Rev Cell Dev Biol. 1999;15:393-410.
2. Ten Have-Opbroek AA. The development of lung in mammals: An analysis of concepts and findings. Am J Anat. 1981;162(3):201-19.
3. DeMello DE, Sawyer D, Galvin N, Reid LM. Early fetal development of lung vasculature. Am J Respir Cell Mol Biol. 1997;16(5):568-81.
4. Malpel SM, Mendelsohn C, Cardoso WV. Regulation of retinoic acid signaling during lung morphogenesis. Development. 2000;127(14):3057-67.
5. Pepicelli CV, Lewis PM, McMahon AP. Sonic hedgehog regulates branching morphogenesis in mammalian lung. Curr Biol. 1998;8(19):1083-6.
6. Warburton D, Schwarz M, Tefft D, Flores-Delgado G, Anderson KD, Cardoso WV. The molecular basis of lung morphogenesis. Mech Dev. 2000;92(1):55-81.
7. Warburton D, Bellusci S, Del Moral PM, Kaartinen V, Lee M, Tefft D, et al. Growth factor signaling in lung morphogenetic centers: automaticity, stereotypy and symmetry. Respir Res. 2003;4-5.
8. Ochs M, Nyengaard JR, Jung A, Knudsen L, Voigt M, Wahlers T, et al. The number of alveoli in human lung. Am J Respir Crit Care Med. 2004;169(1):120-4.
9. Shannon JM. Induction of alveolar type II cell differentiation in fetal tracheal epithelium by grafted distal lung mesenchyme. Dev Biol. 1994;166(2):600-14.
10. Sannes PL. Basement membrane and extracellular matrix. In: Parent RA (Ed). Comparative biology of normal lung. Boca Raton, FL: CRC Press; 1992. pp. 129-44.
11. Plopper CG, Fanucchi MV. Development of Airway epithelium. In: Harding R (Ed). The lung development aging and the environment. San Diego, CA: Elsevier; 2004. pp. 14-32.
12. Inayama Y, Hook GE, Brody AR, Cameron GS, Jetten AM, Gilmore LB, et al. The differentiation of potential of tracheal basal cells. Lab Invest. 1988;58(6):706-17.
13. Jedrychowski W, Flak E, Mróz E. The adverse effect of low levels of ambient air pollutants on lung function growth in preadolescent children. Environ Health Perspect. 1999;107(8):669-74.
14. Rosenlund M, Forastiere F, Porta D, De Sario M, Badaloni C, Perucci CA. Traffic-related air pollution in relation to respiratory symptoms, allergic sensitization and lung function in school children. Thorax. 2009;64(7):573-80.

15. Green DA, McAlpine G, Semple S, Cowie H, Seaton A. Mineral dust exposure in young Indian adults: an effect on lung growth? Occup Environ Med. 2008;65(5):306-10.
16. Islam T, Gauderman WJ, Berhane K, McConnell R, Avol E, Peters JM, et al. Relationship between air pollution, lung function and asthma in adolescents. Thorax. 2007;62(11):957-63.
17. Han RN, Mawdsley C, Souza P, Tanswell AK, Post M. Platelet-derived growth factors and growth-related genes in rat lung. III. Immunolocalization during fetal development. Pediatr Res. 1992;31(4 Pt 1):323-9.
18. Boström H, Willetts K, Pekny M, Levéen P, Lindahl P, Hedstrand H, et al. PDGF-A signalling is a critical event in lung development and alveogenesis. Cell. 1996;85(6):863-73.
19. Souza P, Sedlackova L, Kuliszewski M, Wang J, Liu J, Tseu I, et al. Antisense oligodeoxynucleotides targeting PDGF-alpha and -beta receptors in embroyonic rat lung development. Development. 1994;120(8):2163-73.
20. Souza P, Kuliszewski M, Wang J, Tseu I, Tanswell AK, Post M. PDGF-AA and its receptor influence early lung branching via an epithelial-mesenchymal interaction. Development. 1995;121(8):2559-67.
21. Liu M, Liu J, Buch S, Tanswell AK, Post M. Antisense oligonucleotides against PDGF-B and its receptor inhibit mechanical strain-induced fetal lung cell growth. Am J Physiol. 1995;269(2 Pt 1):L178-84.
22. Waltenberger J, Claesson-Welsh L, Siegbahn A, Shibuya M, Heldin CH. Different signal transduction properties of KDR and Fltl, two receptors for vascular endothelial growth factor. J Biol Chem. 1994;269(43):26988-95.
23. Bhatt AJ, Amin SB, Chess PR, Watkins RH, Maniscalco WM. Expression of vascular endothelial growth factor and Flk-1 in developing and glucocorticoid-treated mouse lung. Pediatr Res. 2000;47(5):606-13.
24. Schachtner SK, Wang Y, Scott Baldwin H. Qualitative and quantitative analysis of embryonic pulmonary vessel formation. Am J Respir Cell Mol Biol. 2000;22(2):157-65.
25. Blakesley VA, Scrimgeour A, Esposito D, Le Roith D. Signaling via the insulin-like growth factor-I receptor: does it differ from insulin receptor signaling? Cytoline Growth Factor Rev. 1996;7(2):153-9.
26. Clemmons DR. Insulin-like growth binding proteins and their role in controlling IGF actions. Cytokine Growth Factor Rev. 1997;8(1):45-62.
27. Batchelor DC, Hutchins AM, Klempt M, Skinner SJ. Developmental changes in the expression patterns of IGFs, type 1 IGF receptor and IGF-binding proteins-2 and -4 in perinatal rat lung. J Mol Endocrinol. 1995;15(2):105-15.
28. Wallen LD, Han VK. Spatial and temporal distribution of insulin-like growth factors I and II during development of rat lung. Am J Physiol. 1994;267(5 Pt 1):L531-42.
29. Torday JS, Kourembanas S. Fetal rat lung fibroblasts produce a TGF-β homolog that blocks alveolar type II cell maturation. Dev Biol. 1990;139(1):35-41.
30. Ryan RM, Mineo-Kuhn MM, Kramer CM, Finkelstein JN. Growth factors alter neonatal type II alveolar epithelial cell proliferation. Am J Physiol. 1994;266(1 Pt 1):L17-22.
31. Whitsett JA, Budden A, Hull WM, Clark JC, O'Reilly MA. Transforming growth factor-beta inhibits surfactant protein A expression in vitro. Biochim Biophys Acta. 1992;1123(3):257-62.
32. McKeehan WL, Wang F, Kan M. The heparan sulfate-fibroblast growth factor family: diversity of structure and function. Prog Nucleic Acid Res Mol Biol. 1998;59:135-76.
33. Guo L, Degenstein L, Fuchs E. Keratinocyte growth factor is required for hair development but not for wound healing. Genes Dev. 1996;10(2):165-75.
34. Post M, Souza P, Liu J, Tseu I, Wang J, Kuliszewski M, et al. Keratinocyte growth factor and its receptor are involved in regulating early lung branching. Development. 1996;122(10):3107-15.
35. Deterding RR, Jacoby CR, Shannon JM. Acidic fibroblast growth factor and keratinocyte growth factor stimulate fetal rat pulmonary epithelial growth. Am J Physiol. 1996;271(4 Pt 1):L495-505.
36. Ramierz MI, Chung UI, Williams MC. Aquaporin-5 expression, but not other peripheral lung marker genes, is reduced in PTH/PTHrP receptor null mutant fetal mice. Am J Respir Cell Mol Biol. 2000;22(3):367-72.
37. Gershwin LJ. Asthma, infection, and environment. In: Albertson M (Ed). Bronchial Asthma: Principles of Diagnosis and Treatment, Vol. 1, 4th edition. Totowa: Human Press; 2001. p. 279.
38. Welliver RC, Ogra PL. RSV, IgE, and wheezing. J Pediatr. 2001;139(6):903-5.
39. Lukacs NW, Tekkanat KK, Berlin A, Hogaboam CM, Miller A, Evanoff H, et al. Respiratory syncytial virus predisposes mice to augmented allergic airway responses via IL-13-mediated mechanisms. J Immunol. 2001;167(2):1060-5.
40. Gershwin LJ, Gunther RA, Anderson ML, Woolums AR, McArthur-Vaughan K, Randel KE, et al. Bovine respiratory syncytial virus-specific IgE is associated with interleukin-2 and -4, and interferon-gamma expression in pulmonary lymph of experimentally infected calves. Am J Vet Res. 2000;61(3):291-8.
41. Gershwin LJ, Dungworth DL, Himes SR, Friebertshauser KE. Immunoglobulin E responses and lung pathology resulting from aerosol exposure of calves to respiratory syncytial virus and Micropolyspora faeni. Int Arch Allergy Appl Immunol. 1990;92(3):293-300.
42. Gershwin LJ, Himes SR, Dungworth DL, Giri SN, Friebertshauser KE, Camacho M. Effect of bovine respiratory syncytial virus infection on hypersensitivity to inhaled Micropolyspora faeni. Int Arch Allergy Immunol. 1994;104(1):79-91.
43. Van Schaik SM, Tristram DA, Nagpal IS, Hintz KM, Welliver RC 2nd, Welliver RC. Increased production of IFN-gamma and cysteinyl leukotrienes in virus induced wheezing. J Allergy Clin Immunol. 1999;103(4):630-6.
44. Garofalo RP, Patti J, Hintz KA, Hill V, Ogra PL, Welliver RC. Macrophage inflammatory protein-1 alpha (not T helper type 2 cytokines) is associated with severe forms of respiratory syncytial virus bronchiolitis. J Infect Dis. 2001;184(4):393-9.
45. Wansleeben C, Barkauskas CE, Rock JR, Hogan BL. Stem cells of the adult lung: their development and role in homeostasis, regeneration, and disease. Wiley Interdiscip Rev Dev Biol. 2013;2(1):131-48.
46. Alphonse RS, Vadivel A, Shelley WC, Critser PJ, Ionescu L, O'Reilly M, et al. Existence, functional impairment and lung repair potential of endothelial colony forming cells in oxygen-induced arrested alveolar growth. Circulation. 2014;129(21):2144-57.
47. Alvarez DF, Huang L, King JA, ElZarrad MK, Yoder MC, Stevens T. Lung microvascular resident endothelial progenitor cells exhibit high vasculogenic capacity. Am J Physiol Lung Cell Mol Physiol. 2008;294(3):L419-30.

Genomics of Lung Diseases

L Keith Scott

INTRODUCTION

Since the discovery of Mendel's work, there have been exhaustive attempts to apply inheritance patterns to most major diseases. However, if a disease did not satisfy traditional Mendelian patterns, genetic contributions were often discounted. This led investigators to look at other contributors to a disease such as environmental factors and infectious disease-related factors. This narrow and focused research produced much of our present understanding of disease states and has generated numerous therapeutic modalities. In spite of many great successes, there were always gaps in our understanding of many diseases and traditional views did not always explain why certain diseases progressed the way they did or why there could be person to person variation of the same disease. Many felt that the variable that influenced disease individuality was exposure, timing, pathogen virulence, co-existing disease, etc. All these, we know, do influence disease states; however, traditional contributors could not always fill those gaps.

In 2001, a preliminary map of the human genome was published.[1] This provided investigators with a new way to perceive and study diseases. With advances in genomic technologies allowing high throughput analysis of a large number of genes at one time, investigators began to look at genomics in a new light and away from the traditional genetic inheritance paradigm. New tools were introduced with heavy dependence on computation with the age of bioinformatics and computational biology was born. A few years later the map of the human genome was deemed complete augmenting bioinformatic investigations further. Over the past 4–5 years, the explosion of our understanding of epigenetics and metabolomics has dramatically pushed our understanding of lung diseases specifically, and many other diseases generally.

GENOMICS AND DISEASE

Some diseases are rather easy to associate a genetic role, such as heart disease, even though they did not adhere to strict Mendelian rules. Other disease states were not as clear and the role of genetics less obvious. Questions arise and problems develop that did not make sense without some contribution of an individual's genome. For example, why would one person with an apparently normal immune system acquire pneumococcal pneumonia and barely get ill, while another, seemly equally matched person develops lethal septic shock? Was it a different bug serotype? Was that person unlucky? Only after the push to better understand the genomics of the human body, not as a function of heredity, but as a functional and dynamic process that some of these questions have answered or are beginning to be answered. After sequencing of the human genome, along with technologies that allowed high throughput genomic analysis, did our understanding take on a new level and the realization of how dynamic the genomic transcription-translation process really appears to be. This understanding, was and is, further enhanced by additional understanding of protein function and folding.

Lung diseases are an area of pathophysiology that encapsulates this process most. Few organ systems are as impacted by environmental, infectious and genomic influences as the respiratory system. This chapter will discuss the genomics of lung diseases, concentrating on major lung disease states: acute lung injury (ALI), chronic obstructive pulmonary disease (COPD)/asthma, pulmonary hypertension and interstitial lung diseases. Each disease-related section will discuss genomics related to the disease state, genomics related to therapeutic interventions and proteomics related to the disease or treatment. There will also be a brief discussion on computational biology and complexity theory and how it relates to understanding disease states.

GENOMIC NOMENCLATURE AND INVESTIGATIONAL TOOLS

To describe and present data on genomic studies, there needs to be consistent nomenclature and definitions. Below are a few definitions that will be used in this chapter.

Allele: Alleles are DNA sequences at the same physical gene locus, which may or may not result in different phenotypic traits.

Bioinformatics: The science of applying computational tools to search databases, analyze DNA sequence information, and to predict protein sequence and structure from DNA sequence data.

Epigenetics: The changes in organism behavior caused by modification of gene expression rather than alteration of the genetic code itself.

Haplotype: A set of closely-linked alleles inherited as a unit.

Homology: Genes derived from a common ancestor.

Locus (Loci): Position on a chromosome of a gene or other chromosome marker. Can also be the DNA at that position.

Metabolomics: The study of metabolic processes and by productions related to genomic and proteomic influences.

Microarrays: This is a technology that allows high throughput analysis of multiple genes from a single sample. The technology is based on probes, which are immobilized in an ordered two-dimensional pattern. Probes are either spotted cDNAs or oligonucleotides and are designed to be specific for an organism, a gene or a genetic variant.

Polymerase chain reaction (PCR): Polymerase chain reaction is a method for synthesizing millions of copies of a specific DNA sequence.

Single-nucleotide polymorphism (SNP): A single-nucleotide polymorphism is a DNA sequence where a single nucleotide in the genome differs between members of a species.

GENOMIC RESEARCH

Since the beginning of high throughput genomics, there has been a tendency to single out small number of genes and make claims as to the genes contribution to a particular disease states. This has been dubbed the reductionist approach and was more in line with the standard research paradigm.[2] It rapidly became clear that gene expression does not always translate to protein production or functionality. More recent research paradigms have focused on a system approach looking at groups of genes and evaluating these groups as a part of a system involving single or multiple pathways. This approach has been enlightening and has generated a better understanding of host-gene-protein interactions and probably more of a "real world" picture.

GENOMICS AND ACUTE LUNG INJURY

Acute lung injury (ALI) is not a homogeneous disease as once thought. Acute lung injury can be related to a primary lung insult such as aspiration or related to a process distal to the lung such as pancreatitis. This has resulted in rethinking ALI as either a primary process in which the injury is an epithelial-to-endothelial process, or a secondary process which the insult is endothelial-to-epithelial. Both disease types are phenotypically similar but may have very different morphologic response of the lung itself.[3] Although the etiology remains unclear, there does appear to be an imbalance between pro- and anti-inflammatory cytokines, oxidants and antioxidants, procoagulants and anticoagulants, neutrophil activation and neutrophil clearance, or proteases and protease inhibitors.[4] We will limit our discussion of what is felt to be the most significant proteins involved in the development of acute respiratory distress syndrome (ARDS).

Angiopoietin-2 (Ang-2) is a potent regulator of vascular permeability and inflammation in ALI and ARDS.[5] This protein aids in promoting cell-to-cell integrity and maintenance of gap junctions. Several studies have demonstrated the high levels of Ang-2 are associated with ARDS related to primary lung injury and secondary lung injury,[6,7] ventilator-induced lung injury (VILI) and hyperoxia-related ALI.[8]

Genomic studies have demonstrated differing gene expressions in animals of ALI induced by differing mechanisms. In one study, rats with ALI induced by lipopolysaccharide (LPS) and others by high volume ventilation.[9] Microarray expression analysis revealed different expressions of genes based on biologic function between the groups. Genes that showed increased expression in the LPS group were metabolism, defense response, immune cell proliferation and cell death. Those with ALI induced by volutrauma were organogenesis, morphogenesis, cell cycle and cell proliferation and differentiation. This supports the concept that ALI is really a down-stream process, or phenotype, with many different genotypic avenues leading to the injury.

These studies, however, are greatly limited by phenotypic differences, incomplete gene penetrance and gene-environmental interactions.[10] The different populations investigated and the degree of heterogeneity further complicates the data. **Table 1** lists a few of the genes that have been associated with ALI.

Polymorphisms have also been demonstrated to be a variable in the development or response to ALI. A study of European descendants with ARDS found this population to have an insertion/deletion polymorphism of the NFκB promoter. Those that were homozygous for the deletion of this promoter had higher lung injury scores but no change in outcome.[11] Similarly, the 4G/5G polymorphism of the plasminogen activator-1 gene has been shown to prolong ventilation in patients with pneumonia and ALI.[12]

Heme oxygenase-1 appears to offer cytoprotection to the development of ALI. The haplotype S-TAG of the heme oxygenase-1 gene is associated with increased ARDS risk. In a somewhat different twist, the longer the repeats of the (GT) allele of the heme oxygenase gene, the higher the heme oxygenase serum levels which resulted in reduced risk of developing ALI.[13]

The list of genomic variables will expand over the next few years with each SNP or significant gene being promoted as a target of therapy or marker of disease. It is, however, to simplistic a view that a "magic bullet" will be found using

Table 1 Numerous genes that have been reported to be associated with ALI list by gene symbol, gene name and the variant associated with the gene

Gene symbol	*Gene name*	*Associated variant*
IL-6	Interleukin 6	Gene-wide haplotypes G/C-174
TNF	Tumor necrosis factor	G/A-308
VEGF	Vascular endothelial growth factor	C/T + 938
IL-10	Interleukin-10	A/G–1,082
MIF	Macrophage inhibitory factor	Haplotypes
ACE	Angiotensin converting enzyme	I/D intron 16
NFκB	Nuclear factor κB	Ins/del ATTG-94
SFTPB	Surfactant associated protein B	T/C + 1,580 Intron 4TR
MLB2	Mannose-binding lectin	3 variant at multiple haplotypes Gly54Asp
CXCL2	Interferon gamma inducible protein	-665 TR

Table 2 Some of the major candidate genes that are differentially expressed in chronic obstructive pulmonary disease (COPD)

a1-AT Z2
Arg139
β2AR
Glu27 > Gln0.6
Haplotype-IL1RN A1/IL1B
IL8 A
IL6
MMP-1
IL4RA2
Glutathione transferases (GSTP1 *Ile105* > Val, *GSTT1* and *GSTM1*)
Heme oxygenase-1
Catalase 1 nicotine receptor *(CHRNA5)*
Abbreviations: a1-ATZ = heterozygosity for the Z allele of alpha one antitrypsin; mEH = microsomal epoxide hydrolase; β2AR = the beta 2 adrenergic receptor; *IL1RN A* = the interleukin 1 receptor antagonist; *IL8* = interleukin 8; *IL6* = interleukin 6; *MMP-1* = the matrix metalloproteinase 1; *IL4R* = the interleukin 4 receptor; glutathione transferases *(GSTP1, GSTT1* and *GSTM1)*; heme oxygenase-1; catalase; and the nicotine receptor *(CHRNA5)*

high throughput genomics. Genomics are extremely complex with gene-to-gene interactions, gene-to-environment interactions and varying penetrance all confounding the data. Although bioinformatics has come along way in accounting for these variables, the level of complexity is far beyond our current understanding. Genetics studies that investigate disease states must account for population heterogeneity. Understanding this heterogeneity will be paramount before any meaningful data can be conjectured or therapeutic interventions advanced.

GENOMICS AND CHRONIC OBSTRUCTIVE PULMONARY DISEASE/ASTHMA

Chronic obstructive pulmonary disease is a very complex disease state with both gene-environmental interactions and genetic susceptibilities. A recent study compared gene expression and SNPs in over 300 patients with COPD that had rapid decline in FEV1 to those that had a lesser degree of decline.[14] To date, these investigators have isolated over 50 genes that are differentially expressed (**Table 2** is a representative listing).

Genome wide analysis of patients with COPD was performed in 7,691 participants in the Framingham Heart Study.[15] Four SNPs on chromosome 4q were strongly associated with FEV1/FVC and one of these SNPs was also associated with FEV1/FVC in the Family Heart Study and a similar Norwegian study.[16]

Recent studies identified 200 oxidative stress-related genes that were differentially expressed in the bronchial airways between smokers with and without COPD.[17,18] Looking at genome expression of the airway epithelium demonstrates that smoking exposure produces epithelial gene expressions that are specific for this exposure[19] and are related to tobacco-related lung cancers.[20]

It is clear that the lung and epithelium of the lungs shows differing genome expressions in COPD progression and tobacco exposure. Even correlating some of these genes to eventual cancer development is an exciting advancement. However, like all genomic studies there are limitation and caution that must be observed when making broad conclusion. Even though genes may be expressed, this may not translate into protein synthesis or protein function. Therefore, proteomic studies are also needed compliment the genomic studies. With these tools in hand, investigators can shed new light in the understanding of the pathology of COPD especially on a molecular level.

A recent study by Lee et al. preformed "shotgun" protein analysis of lung tissue and epithelium of patients without COPD, smokers without COPD and COPD that had ongoing tobacco exposure.[21] They found 12 proteins that were differentially expressed. Of the 12, matrix metalloproteinase 13 [(MMP)-13] and thioredoxin-like 2 were significantly increased in the COPD patients. MP-13 was isolated mainly in the alveolar macrophages and type II pneumocytes with thioredoxin-like 2 was primarily seen in the bronchial epithelium.

There is far less data in asthma and genomic variability. Although there is obvious inheritance of allergic tendencies, less is clear about individual variation of patients with asthma, however, this is rapidly changing. One of the first steps has been improved identification of phenotypes of asthma. A recent study looking at hierarchical clustering analysis of 628 variables on 726 subjects, found five subgroups that were identified.[22] The clusters are:

- *Cluster 1*: Early onset atopic asthma with normal lung function treated with controller medications and minimal health care utilization.
- *Cluster 2*: Early onset atopic asthma and preserved lung function, but increased medication requirements and health care utilization
- *Cluster 3*: Older obese women with late onset nonatopic asthma, moderate reductions in FEV1 and frequent oral corticosteroid use to manage exacerbations.
- *Cluster 4*: Severe airflow obstruction with bronchodilator responsiveness.
- *Cluster 5*: Have severe airflow obstruction with bronchodilator responsiveness and use of oral corticosteroids.

This classification system may provide better categorization to apply genomic investigations.

Some genome comparisons have been performed but usually have identified extreme gene expression differences. As the sophistication of bioinformatics develops, less robust gene expression changes can be found and may add to the ever-increasing list of genetically determined phenotypes of asthma.[23]

In spite of the limitations to genomic studies in a disease process that affects different genetic pools, several genes have emerged consistently across diverse populations. The major genes are *TNF-α, IL4, FCERB, Adam 33,* and *GSTP1.*[24] Also, polymorphisms of the chemokine receptor-2 (CCR2) have been found to be present in asthma and may play a significant role in disease susceptibility.[25] A large cohort analysis identified a locus containing DENND1B on chromosome *1q31.3* that was associated with susceptibility to asthma.[26] This locus was found in children with both European and African descent.

More recent genomic investigations have begun to diverge from pathophysiologic variability and begun to look at therapeutic variability. Much of the attention has focused on the beta-2-adrenergic receptor *(BDRB2)*. Although there are polymorphisms identified with this gene, there is also question as to how it may affect therapy with B-agonist.[27,28] It is likely that all therapies have potential for genetic variability in responsiveness[29] which is why pharmacogenomics is such an important field in the future of asthma therapy.

GENOMICS AND INTERSTITIAL LUNG DISEASE

Interstitial lung disease is a heterogeneous group of diseases that have eluted etiologies. Diagnostic classifications have been made based on clinical course, high resolution CT scan and pathologic tissue examination. There have been high hopes that genomics would hold promise as a diagnostic tool, particularly in early disease.[30]

Sarcoidosis

This is an inflammatory lung disease that has demonstrated altered bronchoalveolar lavage (BAL) fluid with proteins that are not from leaked plasma.[31] Many of these proteins are not surprisingly related to inflammation. Many genomic studies have been able to narrow these proteins to the inhibitory nuclear factors kappa B-alpha (IκB) and nuclear factor kappa B (NFκB). Polymorphisms of the IκB promotor have been shown to be associated with sarcoidosis with the –297T allele carriage more prevalent in patients than in control groups. Three common haplotypes were found, of which haplotype 2 (GTT) was most associated with sarcoidosis. Subgroup analysis revealed that the –826T allelic carriage was most prevalent in stage II and III disease.[32] In high throughput genomic analysis, genes found to be associated with persistent disease included HLA-DRB1*1501 DQB1*0602, TNF-α, NFκB, cyclic AMP-responsive element modulator (CREM) and T-cell activation marker CD69. Those associated with self-limited disease included IL-1B, IL-8, growth-related (GRO)-beta/-gamma and CCR 2, 5, 6.[33]

Usual Interstitial Pneumonia

Usual interstitial pneumonia (UIP)/idiopathic pulmonary fibrosis is the most severe form of idiopathic interstitial pneumonia. The cellular make up is diverse and therefore the genomics of the disease is very descriptive of disease-related genomic complexity. In a study by Kelly et al.,[34] genomic expression studies were performed on differing cellular matrix of UIP lung samples. They compared fibroblast, epithelial cells and type 2 pneumocytes. Using QT-PCR, they found that tissue inhibitor of matrix metalloprotease-1 and matrix metalloprotease-2 gene expression was upregulated within the fibroblastic foci compared with the epithelium. Along with the before-mentioned mRNA, osteopontin was found to be upregulated in fibroblast, epithelial cells and type-2 pneumocytes. Also, levels of bone morphogenetic protein (BMP)-4 antagonist gremlin were found upregulated in IPF/UIP, which seems to correlate to severity of illness.[35]

Usual interstitial pneumonia again is very complex with differing states of fibrosis and repair expressing different genes and phenotypes. The phenotype of regenerative epithelium in UIP has been appeared to derive from bronchiolar basal cells and Clara cells (CC). In severe fibrotic areas, CC-10 expressing cells were more prominent, while SP-A (surfactant apoprotein) positive cells were more prominent in less fibrotic areas.[36] In a case report of a child with UIP-like histology found mutations in the adenosine triphosphate-binding-cassette-A3 gene.[37] Its implications have yet to be investigated but this further demonstrates the complexity of genomic studies, particularly applying them to disease states and, unfortunately, in translating them into therapeutics.

As for diagnostics, genomic markers may offer diagnostic differentiation among the interstitial lung diseases. For example, the TH1 cells chemo attractant monokine induced by interferon (IFN)-gamma (MIG) and IFN gamma-inducible protein of 10 kD expression were significantly higher in NSIP compared with UIP.[38]

GENOMICSANDPULMONARYHYPERTENSION

Pulmonary artery hypertension (PAH) remains an idiopathic process but there is emerging data that the disease is multi-factorial, multi-genetic and environmental. The disease is often subgrouped into idiopathic, familial and associated PAH. Heterozygous mutations in *BMPR2* can be detected in 50–70% of patients with familial PAH and 10–40% of patients with idiopathic PAH. Heterozygous or homozygous *BMPR2* (bone morphogenetic protein receptor type 2) deletion in pulmonary endothelial cells predisposes mice to develop PAH.[39] Although initially isolated in familial PAH, its presence without direct inheritance may represent a genetic milieu that promotes the development of PAH in the face of environmental factors and other inducers.[40] In children with PAH, the activin receptor-like kinase 1 gene (ALK1) has also been found in familial PAH.[41] However, its role and significance of idiopathic PAH is unknown.

Using a hypothesis generating approach to idiopathic PAH using microarray technology, have revealed a distinct expression profile in peripheral B-lymphocytes. This revealed 33 unique genes that were differentially upregulated in idiopathic PAH.

Proteomic methods of investigation have shed more light on PAH. The PAH associated with sickle cell disease cohort has been characterized by high levels of apolipoproteins A-II and B and serum amyloid A, and low levels of haptoglobin dimers and plasminogen.[42] In a cohort of idiopathic PAH, the proteins Alpha-1-antitrypsin and vitronectin were found to be downregulated compared to controls.[43]

BIOCOMPLEXITY AND COMPUTATIONAL BIOLOGY

The age of genomics is upon us and has exponentially expanded our understanding of the molecular basis of many diseases including the ones discussed above. Genomic expression studies often report a significant gene or group of genes in a disease process. Many times this is based solely on mRNA expression and is not followed through to protein translation and function. This is too simplistic as the entire landscape of genomics is changing. We are just beginning to understand that gene-to-gene interactions and gene-to-protein interactions are far more complex than previous thought. Although the basic structure of DNA is eloquently beautiful and simple, that is where simplicity ends.

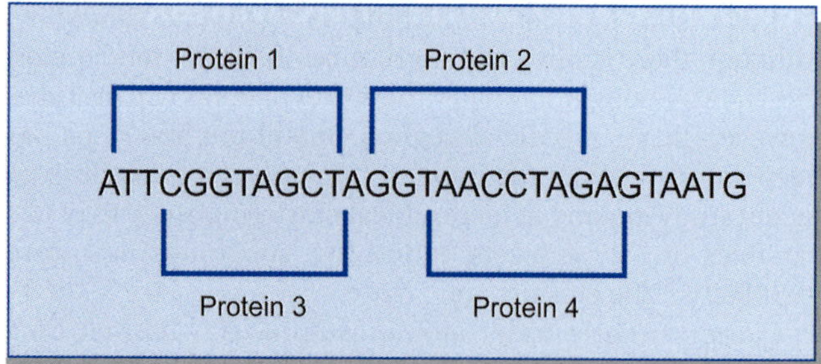

Fig. 1 Demonstrating that a specific DNA base pair sequence can represent many genes depending on the starting point and ending point of the transcription. Thus, there is cross-over among the sequence to produce many different proteins from a relatively small base pair sequence

All of us were taught the genomic paradigm of one gene-one protein and that a specific gene belongs to a specific chromosome. We know now that this is not necessarily true. Many genes and DNA sequences can cross over to transcribe different proteins on the same gene. That is to say that a long DNA sequence may transcribe albumin if started a specific DNA sequences. If, however, the DNA transcription starts one base pair away, it may transcribe a protease even though it is still within the albumin gene as shown in **Figure 1**. This means that all the DNA sequences that were once thought to be "junk" genes are a part of this shared-gene concept and this is what makes us unique as a species. Only by using bits and pieces of different genes to make a new gene so to speak, and understanding that the concept of one gene-one protein is not true, can we explain our diversity. Add that to the fact that genes seem to have the ability to change chromosomes. This is where we enter the world of complexity theory and the need to use complex computational tools to understand these complex interactions. It is likely that the only way meaningful therapeutics will emerge from this age of genomics is through these tools.

A study, which identifies a gene that shows upregulation in no way, translates to functional or phenotypic changes. Even confirming mRNA of the gene, or the presence of the translated protein, in no way assures that the protein has pathologic or physiologic function. This is one reason why there have been such disappointments in genetic therapeutics. Genomic studies need to be looked at in the context of the host, the environment and heredity to name a few confounders.[44] This interaction has prompted the new science of biocomplexity and computational biology that evaluates the biologic pathways that generate disease.

New areas of investigations are emerging all the time. For example, looking spatial relationships of a nucleosome to the gene and how this relationship may influence function.[45] However, the biggest advance recently appears to be the study of epigenetics.

EPIGENETICS

Epigenetics is a new field that is shedding new light on many diseases. Epigenetics is the evaluation of phenotypes that are unique to a cell line or species that is not directly related to the base genome sequence.[46] These phenotypes result from non-genetic influences and can persist for several generations. How this affects lung diseases is presently unknown but deserves considerable attention particularly since most lung diseases have significant environmental influences. Each of these influences can affect phenotypic expression that can not be explained by DNA sequences. This may greatly enhance our understanding of genetics and fill many questions about diseases and protein behaviors that are not easily explained by genetics alone.

Epigenetics, which includes DNA methylation, histone modifications and noncoding RNAs, affect the expression of individual genes and affect developmental patterns and tissue-specific stability. Listed below are some epigenetic data that has recently begun to shed light on several lung pathologies.

Asthma

Based on recent epigenetic research, environment and underlying genetic sequence variation influence DNA methylation, which appears to modify the risk and asthma phenotypes. Also, this DNA methylation may act as an archive of a variety of early developmental exposures that modify asthma variation further.[47]

Acute Lung Injury

The mitogen-activated protein kinase (MAPK) signaling pathway appears to have an essential role in the development of pulmonary inflammation in LPS-induced ALI/ARDS. A total of 42 methylated genes have been associated with the MAPK signaling pathway and 7 have been associated with ALI/ARDS.[48]

Chronic Obstructive Pulmonary Disease

Non-coding RNA and DNA methylation has been demonstrated in COPD and may offer a potential therapeutic target. The combination of DNA methyltransferase inhibitors and anti-inflammatory drugs provide a promising approach.[49]

Interstitial Lung Disease

The role of epigenetics in ILD is less elucidated but several epigenetic processes have been identified. One is prevention of methylation of the Thy-1 DNA and the other is evidence that the histone deacetylases inhibitor suberoylanilide hydroxamic acid may produce profound anti-inflammatory properties and lessens the fibrotic process in ILD.[50]

SUMMARY

Genomics have come of age. Genetic contributions to disease states have moved beyond inheritance. New tools such as microarrays have provided new insights into diseases, allowed new hypothesis to evolve and have thrust reductionist philosophy into the world of biocomplexity.

Lung diseases have always been difficult to study due in part to the numerous influences that foster a disease or exacerbate a disease. Genomics and epigenomics are providing new insights into these diseases that will hopefully produce better diagnostics and therapies.

REFERENCES

1. Lander ES, Linton LM, Birren B, Nusbaum C, Zody MC, Baldwin J, et al. Initial sequencing and analysis of the human genome. Nature. 2001;409(6822):860-921.
2. Kaminski N, Rosas IO. Gene expression profiling as a window into idiopathic pulmonary fibrosis pathogenesis: can we identify the right target genes? Proc Am Thorac Soc. 2006;3(4): 339-44.
3. Hoelz C, Negri EM, Lichtenfels AJ, Conceção GM, Barbas CS, Saldiva PH, et al. Morphometric differences in pulmonary lesions in primary and secondary ARDS: A preliminary study in autopsies. Pathol Res Pract. 2001;197(8):521-30.
4. Ware LB. Pathophysiology of acute lung injury and the acute respiratory distress syndrome. Semin Respir Crit Care Med. 2006;27(4):337-49.
5. van der Heijden M, van Nieuw Amerongen GP, Chedamni S, van Hinsbergh VW, Johan Groeneveld AB. The angiopoietin-Tie2 system as a therapeutic target in sepsis and acute lung injury. Expert Opin Ther Targets. 2009;13(1):39-53.
6. van der Heijden M, van Nieuw Amerongen GP, Koolwijk P, van Hinsbergh VW, Groeneveld AB. Angiopoietin-2, permeability oedema, occurrence and severity of ALI/ARDS in septic and non-septic critically ill patients. Thorax. 2008;63(10):903-9.
7. Maniatis NA, Orfanos SE. The endothelium in acute lung injury/acute respiratory distress syndrome. Curr Opin Crit Care. 2008;14(1):22-30.
8. Bhandari V, Elias JA. The role of angiopoietin 2 in hyperoxia-induced acute lung injury. Cell Cycle. 2007;6(9):1049-52.
9. dos Santos CC, Okutani D, Hu P, Han B, Crimi E, He X, et al. Differential gene profiling in acute lung injury identifies injury-specific gene expression. Crit Care Med. 2008;36(3):855-65.
10. Flores C, Ma SF, Maresso K, Ahmed O, Garcia JG. Genomics of acute lung injury. Semin Respir Crit Care Med. 2006;27(4): 389-95.
11. Adamzik M, Frey UH, Rieman K, Sixt S, Beiderlinden M, Siffert W, et al. Insertion/deletion polymorphism in the promoter of NFKB1 influences severity but not mortality of acute respiratory distress syndrome. Intensive Care Med. 2007;33(7):1199-203.
12. Sapru A, Hansen H, Ajayi T, Brown R, Garcia O, Zhuo H, et al. 4G/5G polymorphism of plasminogen activator inhibitor-1 gene is associated with mortality in intensive care unit patients with severe pneumonia. Anesthesiology. 2009;110 (5):1086-91.
13. Sheu CC, Zhai R, Wang Z, Gong MN, Tejera P, Chen F, et al. Heme oxygenase-1 microsatellite polymorphism and haplotypes are associated with the development of acute respiratory distress syndrome. Intensive Care Med. 2009;35(8):1343-51.
14. Silverman EK, Spira A, Paré PD. Genetics and genomics of chronic obstructive pulmonary disease. Proc Am Thorac Soc. 2009;6(6):539-42.
15. Wilk JB, Chen TH, Gottlieb DJ, Walter RE, Nagle MW, Brandler BJ, et al. A genome-wide association study of pulmonary

function measures in the Framingham Heart Study. PLoS Genet. 2009;5(3):e1000429.
16. Pillai SG, Ge D, Zhu G, Kong X, Shianna KV, Need AC, et al. A genome-wide association study in chronic obstructive pulmonary disease (COPD): identification of two major susceptibility loci. PLoS Genet. 2009;5(3):e1000421.
17. Hung RJ, McKay JD, Gaborieau V, Boffetta P, Hashibe M, Zaridze D, et al. A susceptibility locus for lung cancer maps to nicotinic acetylcholine receptor subunit genes on 15q25. Nature. 2008;452:633-7.
18. Pierrou S, Broberg P, O'Donnell RA, Pawlowski K, Virtala R, Lindqvist E, et al. Expression of genes involved in oxidative stress responses in airway epithelial cells of smokers with chronic obstructive pulmonary disease. Am J Respir Crit Care Med. 2007;175:577-86.
19. Spira A, Beane J, Shah V, Liu G, Schembri F, Yang X, et al. Effects of cigarette smoke on the human airway epithelial cell transcriptome. Proc Natl Acad Sci USA. 2004;101:10143-8.
20. Spira A, Beane JE, Shah V, Steiling K, Liu G, Schembri F, et al. Airway epithelial gene expression in the diagnostic evaluation of smokers with suspect lung cancer. Nat Med. 2007;13:361-6.
21. Lee EJ, In KH, Kim JH, Lee SY, Shin C, Shim JJ, et al. Proteomic analysis in lung tissue of smokers and COPD patients. Chest. 2009;135(2):344-52.
22. Moore WC, Meyers DA, Wenzel SE, Teague WG, Li H, Li X, et al. Identification of Asthma Phenotypes using Cluster Analysis in the Severe Asthma Research Program. Am J Respir Crit Care Med. 2010;181(4):315-23.
23. Agrawal A, Sinha A, Ahmad T, Aich J, Singh P, Sharma A, et al. Maladaptation of critical cellular functions in asthma: bioinformatic analysis. Physiol Genomics. 2009;40(1):1-7.
24. Weiss ST, Raby BA, Rogers A. Asthma genetics and genomics 2009. Curr Opin Genet Dev. 2009;19(3):279-82.
25. Batra J, Ghosh B. Genetic contribution of chemokine receptor 2 (CCR2) polymorphisms towards increased serum total IgE levels in Indian asthmatics. Genomics. 2009;94(3):161-8.
26. Sleiman PM, Flory J, Imielinski M, Bradfield JP, Annaiah K, Willis-Owen SA, et al. Variants of DENND1B associated with asthma in children. N Engl J Med. 2010;362(1):36-44.
27. Peters S. Part IV: Genetic variations in beta-2-adrenergic receptors: long-acting and short-acting beta-2-agonists and therapeutic response. Curr Med Res Opin. 2007;23(Suppl 3): S29-36.
28. Bleecker ER, Postma DS, Lawrance RM, Meyers DA, Ambrose HJ, Goldman M. Effect of *ADRB2* polymorphisms on response to longacting beta-2-agonist therapy: a pharmacogenetic analysis of two randomised studies. Lancet. 2007; 370(9605):2118-25.
29. Hawkins GA, Peters SP. Pharmacogenetics of asthma. Methods Mol Biol. 2008;448:359-78.
30. Agostini C, Miorin M, Semenzato G. Gene expression profile analysis by DNA microarrays: a new approach to assess functional genomics in diseases. Sarcoidosis Vasc Diffuse Lung Dis. 2002;19(1):5-9.
31. Sabounchi-Schütt F, Aström J, Hellman U, Eklund A, Grunewald J. Changes in bronchoalveolar lavage fluid proteins in sarcoidosis: a proteomics approach. Eur Respir J. 2003;21(3):414-20.
32. Abdallah A, Sato H, Grutters JC, Veeraraghavan S, Lympany PA, Ruven HJ, et al. Inhibitor kappa B-alpha (I kappa B-alpha) promoter polymorphisms in UK and Dutch sarcoidosis. Genes Immun. 2003;4(6):450-4.
33. Rutherford RM, Staedtler F, Kehren J, Chibout SD, Joos L, Tamm M, et al. Functional genomics and prognosis in sarcoidosis—the critical role of antigen presentation. Sarcoidosis Vasc Diffuse Lung Dis. 2004;21(1):10-8.
34. Kelly MM, Leigh R, Gilpin SE, Cheng E, Martin GE, Radford K, et al. Cell-specific gene expression in patients with usual interstitial pneumonia. Am J Respir Crit Care Med. 2006;174(5): 557-65.
35. Myllärniemi M, Vuorinen K, Pulkkinen V, Kankaanranta H, Aine T, Salmenkivi K, et al. Gremlin localization and expression levels partially differentiate idiopathic interstitial pneumonia severity and subtype. J Pathol. 2008;214(4):456-63.
36. Hinata N, Takemura T, Ikushima S, Yanagawa T, Ando T, Okada J, et al. Phenotype of regenerative epithelium in idiopathic interstitial pneumonias. J Med Dent Sci. 2003;50(3):213-24.
37. Young LR, Nogee LM, Barnett B, Panos RJ, Colby TV, Deutsch GH. Usual interstitial pneumonia in an adolescent with *ABCA3* mutations. Chest. 2008;134(1):192-5.
38. Honda T, Imaizumi K, Yokoi T, Hashimoto N, Hashimoto I, Kawabe T, et al. Differential Th1/Th2 chemokine expression in interstitial pneumonia. Am J Med Sci. 2010;339(1):41-8.
39. Hong KH, Lee YJ, Lee E, Park SO, Han C, Beppu H, et al. Genetic ablation of the *BMPR2* gene in pulmonary endothelium is sufficient to predispose to pulmonary arterial hypertension. Circulation. 2008;118(7):722-30.
40. Machado RD, Eickelberg O, Elliott CG, Geraci MW, Hanaoka M, Loyd JE, et al. Genetics and genomics of pulmonary arterial hypertension. J Am Coll Cardiol. 2009;54(1 Suppl):S32-42.
41. Fujiwara M, Yagi H, Matsuoka R, Akimoto K, Furutani M, Imamura S, et al. Implications of mutations of activin receptor-like kinase 1 gene *(ALK1)* in addition to bone morphogenetic protein receptor II gene *(BMPR2)* in children with pulmonary arterial hypertension. Circ J. 2008;72(1):127-33.
42. Yuditskaya S, Tumblin A, Hoehn GT, Wang G, Drake SK, Xu X, et al. Proteomic identification of altered apolipoprotein patterns in pulmonary hypertension and vasculopathy of sickle cell disease. Blood. 2009;113(5):1122-8.
43. Yu M, Wang XX, Zhang FR, Shang YP, Du YX, Chen HJ, et al. Proteomic analysis of the serum in patients with idiopathic pulmonary arterial hypertension. J Zhejiang Univ Sci B. 2007;8(4):221-7.
44. Fisher J, Piterman N. The executable pathway to biological networks. Brief Funct Genomic Proteomic. 2010;9(1):79-92.
45. Cui P, Zhang L, Lin Q, Ding F, Xin C, Fang X, et al. A novel mechanism of epigenetic regulation: nucleosome-space occupancy. Biochem Biophys Res Commun. 2010;391(1):884-9.
46. Bird A. Perceptions of epigenetics. Nature. 2007;447(7143): 396-8.
47. Wilfried K, Ziyab AH, Everson T, Holloway JW. Epigenetic Mechanisms and Models in the Origins of Asthma. Curr Opin Allergy Clin Immunol. 2013;13:63-9.
48. Zhang XQ, Lv CJ, Liu XY, Hao D, Qin J, Tian HH, et al. Genome-wide analysis of DNA methylation in rat lungs with lipopolysaccharide-induced acute lung injury. Mol Med Rep. 2013;7:417-24.
49. Schamberger AC, Mise N, Meiners S, Eickelberg O. Epigenetic Mechanisms in COPD: Implications for pathogenesis and drug discovery. Expert Opin Drug Discov. 2014;9:609-28.
50. Wang Z, Chen C, Finger SN, Kwajah S, Jung M, Schwarz H, et al. Suberoylanilide hydroxamic acid: a potential epigenetic therapeutic agent for lung fibrosis? Eur Respir J. 2009;34: 145-55.

Section 2

Respiratory Physiology

Sunil K Chhabra, Ashutosh N Aggarwal

Applied Respiratory Physics

SK Jindal, VK Jindal

INTRODUCTION

Knowledge of simple, applied physics is important to understand the movement of air in and out of the lungs, the flow of blood across the pulmonary vessels, exchange of gases and maintenance of the fluid balance. This chapter provides a brief introduction to the general physics with reference to the respiratory functioning. "More details are available in the respective chapters on individual subjects in the book".

STATE OF MATTER

Matter can exist in three different forms in nature—solid, liquid or gas; although plasma, a fourth state of matter has also been identified under the extremes of temperature and pressure. In nature, matter is either an element made from similar atoms, e.g. iron or a compound made from two or more types of atoms, e.g. water (H_2O). An element is a basic unit of matter, which retains the same properties on subdivisions by chemical or mechanical means. Oxygen and other gases, such as hydrogen, helium, chlorine and nitrogen, are elements in nature.

Atom and Element

An atom is the smallest part of an element, which acts like a "building block". On the further subdivision of an atom, the elemental properties are lost and therefore, subatomic constituents of all atoms are identical. Atoms of certain elements (e.g. hydrogen, helium) can exist in free state (H, He) and there is no difference between the atoms and molecules of these elements. Atoms of many other elements (such as oxygen) do not exist free, but combine with other atoms of the same element to form molecules (e.g. O_2, i.e. O+O). Atoms of different elements may form molecules or compounds. Hydrogen can exist in atomic or molecular form, whereas nitrogen and oxygen occurs in molecular form (N_2 and O_2).

Molecule and Compound

All substances consist of exceedingly small particles called molecules. There are about 10^{19} molecules in 1 mL of air under the normal conditions of temperature (T) and pressure (P). A molecule possesses the distinctive properties of the parent element or compound. A molecule is found to consist of two or more atoms of same kind or of different kinds.

The number of molecules comprising a macroscopic quantity of a gas is enormous typically around 10^{23} molecules. The number of molecules and their velocity determine many properties of gases.

A compound is composed of two or more elements united chemically to form a substance different from the individual elements forming that compound. For example, carbon dioxide is a compound of carbon and oxygen. On subdivisions, the compound loses its properties and may resume those of the constituent elements. Both elements and compounds exist as molecules as the smallest component.

Molecular Movement

All the molecules of matter are in a state of incessant motion. This is known as Brownian movement and forms the basis of the kinetic theory of matter. This motion results from temperature—the higher the temperature, the larger the velocity of the molecules. At absolute zero temperature, the velocity of a classical molecule goes to zero. Molecules of a gas have great mobility and travel longer distances before colliding with other molecules. It is because of this mobility that a gas has no fixed shape and mixes readily with other gases.

Atomic and Molecular Weights

The mass of an atom is concentrated at its nucleus, which contains a definite number of neutrons and protons of identical masses. The neutrons or protons are also called *nucleons*. The mass of a nucleon is ≈ 1.6×10^{-24} g [sometimes also called *atomic mass unit* (amu)]. Therefore, total number of nucleons of an atom determines the mass of an atom and is usually called *atomic weight*. This H atom has atomic weight equaling 1, whereas O atom has atomic weight equaling 16, though their actual masses are around $1 \times 1.6 \times 10^{-24}$ g and $16 \times 1.6 \times 10^{-24}$ g, respectively. Similarly, *molecular weight* is determined by summing up atomic weights of the constituent atoms forming that molecule. As an example, H_2 molecule has a molecular weight = 2, and H_2O molecule has a molecular weight = 2 + 16 = 18. For obtaining their actual weights, we multiply those weights by amu (= 1.6×10^{-24} g) to get the mass in gram.

If M is the molecular weight of given substance, then 1 molecule of that substance weighs $M \times 1.6 \times 10^{-24}$ g. This gives us that M g of the substance will have $1/1.6 \times 10^{-24}$ molecules, which is called Avogadro number, $N_0 \approx 6.02 \times 10^{23}$. It is thus clear that M g (also called 1 mole) of any substance will have N_0 molecules.

Gaseous substance (which behave like an ideal gas) follow an equation PV = nRT.

One can easily calculate the volume at NTP (normal temperature 0°C, and pressure ≡ 760 mm Hg) from n = 1 mole. It comes out to be 22.4 liters for any gas. Therefore, a quantity of any substance equaling molecular weight as g has 6.02×10^{23} molecules and as a gas, occupies 22.4 liters at NTP.

Equal volumes of gases at the same temperature and pressure contain equal number of molecules *(Avogadro's hypothesis)*.

PHYSICAL PROPERTIES OF GASES

The air we normally breathe is a mixture of gases of which oxygen and nitrogen constitute the main bulk.

Breathing of additional or supplemental gases is required in abnormal situations. The physical properties of these gases influence the mechanics of normal breathing, as well as the therapeutic strategies.

Volume

Volume is the space occupied by a gas. The volume of a cuboid-shaped vessel is determined by the multiplication of internal length, width and height of the vessel. It is expressed in cubic centimeters (cc), cubic feet or liters (L), etc. (1 L ≡ 1,000 cc or mL).

Volume = Length × Width × Height

A 10 cm cube has the volume equaling 1 L. Volume of a container of uniform cross-sectional area A and height is given by V = A h. The gas shall occupy the available volume irrespective of the amount (mass) of gas. For example, if a small vessel containing oxygen is emptied in a larger vessel, the entire volume of the larger vessel will be occupied by the same amount of gas **(Figs 1A and B)**.

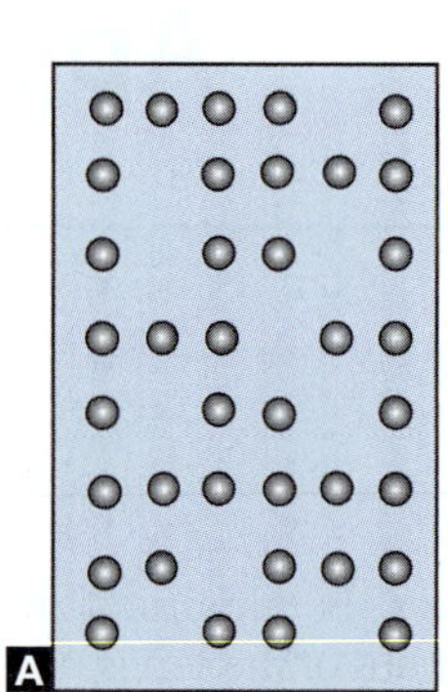

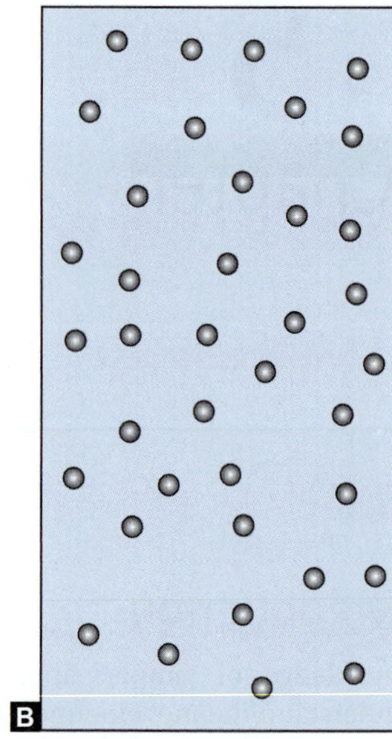

Figs 1A and B Mass of a gas such as O_2 (i.e. number of molecules) in vessels A and B is unchanged, but the volumes are different therefore, the density of the gas in vessel A is greater than that in vessel B

Mass and Weight

Mass is the bulk or the total mass of number of molecules of the gas. In the aforesaid example, the mass of the gas in two cylinders shall remain the same, although the volume has changed. The number of molecules per unit of volume in the two vessels has changed, i.e. lesser number of molecules per unit volume in the larger vessel **(Figs 1A and B)**.

Weight is often used synonymously with mass. Weight is determined by the pull of gravity on mass (i.e. m × g). Since the force of gravity on the earth is nearly constant, mass is equivalent to weight on the surface of the earth. In fact, weight is scaled to indicate mass and therefore both represent the same thing.

W ≡ gravitational force = mg

Density

Density is expressed as the weight in the grams of 1 liter of a gas. Since the weight of 22.4 liters of a gas is that of a gram molecule of that gas, 1 liter of gas shall weigh molecular weight/22.4 g. When expressed in this fashion, the density will be measured in g/liter. It is also measured in g/cc, which will equal 1/1,000 in value to that in g/liter.

Molecular weight of oxygen = 32
Density = 32/22.4
= 1.43 g/liter

The density of a gas is also expressed as relative to the density of air. Density of air shall vary depending upon its composition. For all practical purposes, it comprises of 1 volume of oxygen (about 20%) and 4 volumes of nitrogen (about 80%). At NTP, the density of air is (32 × 1/5 + 28 × 4/5)/22.4 = 1.3 g/L. Therefore, the density of oxygen relative to that of air is 1.1. When expressed this way, it becomes unimportant, if the density of individual gases was calculated in g/liter or g/cc.

Pressure (P)

The gas molecules are always in a state of motion and constantly bombard the walls of the container. The force (F) applied to (or acting upon) a unit area (A) of the wall is called the gas pressure (P = F/A). The closer the molecules, the greater the number, which strikes each unit area and therefore the greater the pressure applied. Also, larger the velocity (or temperature), larger is the impact on the walls, leading to greater pressure.

Gas pressure is generally considered as that of a stationary gas when the pressure exerted is the same at any point in a gas container. The pressure is usually expressed in the millimeters of mercury (mm Hg) or centimeters of water (cm H_2O) or pounds per square inch (psi). One millimeters of mercury means force on a unit area (1 cm^2) on which 1 mm of height of Hg is placed. The volume of height h cm on unit area is A × h = h cm^3 and the mass is hd where d is the density of the liquid. The force on unit area due to this is hdg, which is also the pressure p. Thus p due to a height h of a liquid of density d, p = hdg. The pressure due to 1 mm Hg can be calculated by putting h = 0.1 cm, d = 13.6 gm/cc and g_2 = 980 cm/S^2.

1 mm Hg ≡ 1334 CGS units or dynes/cm^2 = 133.4 Pa

(Pascal is another unit of pressure, defined as 1 Newton/ $meter^2$ = 10 dynes/cm^2).

Pressure is also measured in bars. 1 bar of pressure is 10^6 dynes/cm^2 or 10^5 Pa and is nearly 1 atm (1 atm = 1.0197 bar).

Atmospheric Pressure

Atmospheric air is pulled to the earth by gravity and generates a force upon the surface of the earth, resulting in atmospheric pressure. Atmospheric pressure is the sum of pressures of all gases (e.g. N_2, O_2 and CO_2) present in air. It is measured with the help of a glass tube filled with either mercury or water (manometer). The height of the column of mercury (or water) multiplied by its density is a measure of the atmospheric pressure. Standard pressure is measured at sea level and expressed in mm Hg (torr) or cm H_2O **(Table 1)**.

It is relevant here to mention that the lungs are subject to atmospheric pressure all the time. Since the alveoli are in direct communication with the atmosphere through the tracheobronchial tree, the alveolar pressure is the same as the atmospheric pressure. The changes in alveolar pressure during inspiratory and expiratory phases of respiration are relative to the atmospheric pressure. During inspiration when the alveolar pressure is -10 cm H_2O, it implies the presence of atmospheric pressure -10 cm H_2O (i.e. 1030-10 cm H_2O).

Table 1 Units used to express atmospheric pressure

Unit of pressure	*Equivalency*
Atmosphere (P_{atm})	1
Pascal (Pa)	1.01×10^5
cm H_2O	10^{33}
mm Hg	760
lb/in² (psi)	14.7
Bar	1.0197

Table 2 Some important pressures (mm Hg) in normal human body

Pressure	
• Alveolar	760
• *Arterial blood*	
Systolic Diastolic	100–195 60–85
• Venous blood	3–7
• *Capillaries*	
Arterial end Venous end	30 10

Similarly, when positive pressure is administered to a patient through a ventilator, the ventilator gauge pressure of 10 or 20 cm H_2O refers to a total pressure of 1040 or 1050 cm H_2O (i.e. atmospheric pressure + gauge pressure).

Partial Pressure

In a mixture of gases in a container, each gas exerts the same pressure, which it would if it alone occupied the container. There is no interference from the presence of other gas(es). The pressure exerted by each individual gas is called the partial pressure. The total pressure exerted by the mixture of gases is equal to the sum of the partial pressures of all the gases contained in the mixture (*Dalton's law*). The partial pressure is determined by the fraction of the concentration of the gas in the mixture.

The atmospheric air has a total pressure of 760 mm Hg when dry at sea level. The partial pressures of N_2 (79%) and O_2 (21%) therefore, are as follows:

P_{N_2} = 79% of P= 600.4 mm Hg

P_{O_2} = 21% of P = 159.6 mm Hg.

Other Body Pressures

The presence of air or fluid in other body cavities exerts different pressures in similar fashion as in the lungs **(Table 2)**. The interval pressures in the body are also influenced by outside environmental pressures. The total pressure is therefore the sum of the external plus the internal pressure (*gauge pressure*). For example, the internal pressures will rise in hyperbaric conditions and decrease in hypobaric conditions as at high altitudes.

Temperature and Heat

Temperature is the thermal state of a substance, which determines whether the substance will give or receive heat from another substance in contact. It is an indication of the level of molecular activity. Heat is the thermal energy of a substance, which can be given to or abstracted from it. Temperature is the measurement of heat.

Calorie is the unit of heat. It is defined as the quantity of heat required to raise the temperature of 1 g of water by 1°C. As an example, if one calorie is required to raise the temperature of 1 g of water by 1°C, 1,000 calories will be required for 1,000 g of water. The caloric value of food is expressed by a larger heat unit, i.e. the kilocalorie (cal or kcal), which is equivalent to 1,000 cal.

To raise the temperature to a given range, similar weights of different substances require different quantities of heat. The number of calories required to raise the temperature of 1 g of that substance by 1°C is the specific heat of that substance as cal/g. It could also be volume specific heat defined in cal/cc where cc is volume in cubic centimeters or mL in case of liquids and gases.

The specific heat depends on the state of the matter—solid, liquid or gas. Specific heat of water is 1 (It follows from the definition of 1 calorie).

For gases, such as O_2 and air, it is 0.0603 cal per cc, it is quite high when expressed per g.

We can calculate the total quantity of heat required to raise the temperature of a given volume by multiplying the volume with specific heat and temperature rise, i.e. volume.

(cc) × specific heat (cal per cc) × temperature rise (°C).

THE GAS LAWS

There is a definite relationship between the gasses properties described earlier. These relationships are described in different laws to understand the behavior of gases. These laws are valid for ideal gases only, where the assumption that the gas particles are very small and do not interact with each other is valid.

Boyle's Law

Pressure (P) of a gas is inversely proportional to its volume (V) provided the absolute temperature (T) of the mass of gas is kept constant. In other words, the product of pressure and volume remains constant. It follows immediately from the ideal gas equation,

$$P \propto 1/V \text{ or } P \times V = \text{constant, if T is constant.}$$

$$\text{Or } P_1 V_1 = P_2 V_2$$

The application of this law in respiratory physiology is best exemplified in the use of body plethysmography to measure total lung capacity. It is also employed in many mechanical ventilators whereby the gas is driven into patient's lungs or into the cylinder of the ventilator by the upstroke and downstroke movements of the piston.

Charles' Law

When pressure and mass of a gas are kept constant, the volume of the gas will vary directly with its absolute temperature. Again from gas equation,

$$V/T = \text{Constant (K), if P is constant}$$

It is because of this reason that volumes measured with the help of lung function equipment (at room temperature) are a little lower than those at body temperature (37°C) and need to be corrected for the same. If the temperature of a container of a gas is lowered, the volume shrinks. Therefore, more gas can be stored in the same cylinder at a lower temperature.

Gay-Lussac's Law

Temperature and pressure of a gas are directly proportional when the volume and mass are kept constant.

$$P \propto T \text{ or } P/T = K \text{ at constant V}$$

It implies an increase in pressure if the temperature is increased. For this reason safety valves are provided with devices using high pressure gases to vent high pressures in case there is an accidental heating.

The General Gas Law

Assume N ideal noninteracting molecules of a gas each of mass m are contained in a cube of volume V. They are in motion if the temperature is above 0°K (0°K = -273°C). If the temperature is T in Kelvin, the kinetic energy from each molecule is of the order of kT, where K is called Boltzmann constant ($K = 1.38 \times 10^{-16}$ CGS units). Because of this kinetic motion, the molecules of the gas keep bombarding the walls of the cube and exert pressure. The pressure increase results in extra energy (obtainable from force × distance or p × volume relation).

In this way, it is quite evident that one can equate the energy because of pressure PV as resulting from kinetic energy of N molecules, PV = NkT.

If N is expressed in N_0 (Avogadro No.), $PV = \eta N_0kT$, where $\eta = N/N_0$.

This is the gas equation valid for all ideal gases. η is the number of moles of the gas, N_0k is also called gas constant R.

$$R \simeq 6 \times 10^{23} \times 1.38 \times 10^{23} \text{ erg/deg K} \simeq 2 \text{ cal./deg K}$$

The gas equation can be used to determine how the given initial state (P_1, V_1, T_1) relates to (P_1, V_1, T_1); i.e. $P_1V_1/T_1 = P_1V_1/T_1$

It may be stated here that under the conditions of lower temperature and high pressure the gas changes its state to liquid. This is because the gas molecules get attracted to each other (van der Waals forces) rather than being repelled. The higher pressure condenses the molecules and the lower temperature reduces their activity.

The temperature at which the gas turns into liquid is the "critical temperature" of that gas. For oxygen, it is -116°C. A pressure of 50 atmospheres is required to liquefy oxygen at -116°C. To keep the oxygen in a liquid form at 1 atmosphere in a flask open to the atmosphere, the temperature is lowered to below -183°C. This principle forms the basis of the availability of oxygen in the liquid form for storage and ambulatory use.

Henry's Law

The amount of gas that enters into physical solution in a liquid is directly proportional to the partial pressure of the gas. For example, the greater the partial pressure of oxygen in the alveoli, the greater the solubility in plasma.

Graham's Law

The rate of diffusion (D) of a gas is inversely proportional to the square root of its density (d).

$$D_1d_2 = D_2d_1$$

Therefore, a light gas (such as helium) will diffuse at a faster rate than a heavier gas (such as oxygen).

Bernoulli's Principle

Flow of a gas through a partially obstructed tube can be described by Bernoulli's principle, i.e. the pressure required to produce flow is the difference in velocity at two points and the density of the gas **(Fig. 2)**.

GAS SOLUTION AND TENSION

The amount of gas dissolved in a liquid is directly proportional to the pressure of the gas (*Henry's law*). It also varies with the temperature—lesser amount is dissolved at the same pressure if temperature is increased. A state of equilibrium is reached when no further gas dissolves in the liquid. This is a state of full saturation with the gas at a given temperature and pressure. The gas in solution is said to exert the same "tension" as the partial pressure of the gas over the liquid in equilibrium with it. For example, when the partial pressure of oxygen in alveoli is 100 mm Hg, the tension of O_2 in alveolar capillaries is 100 mm Hg. At this pressure, 0.3 cc of oxygen at NTP dissolves in 100 cc of water. The weight of oxygen dissolved in 100 cc water is 1.3 × 0.3/1,000 = 0.0004 g (1.3 g/L is the density of oxygen).

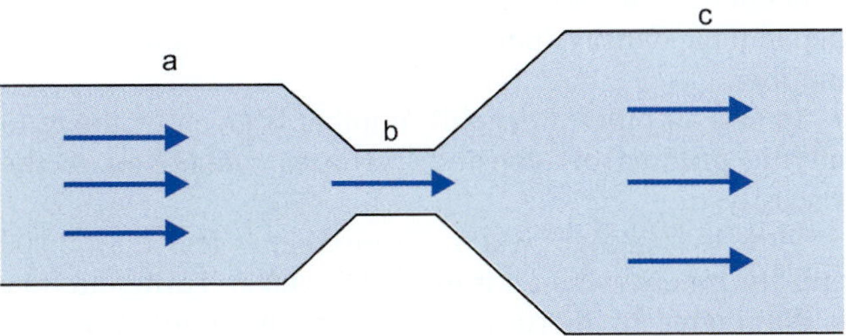

Fig. 2 Bernoulli's principle

The amount of oxygen dissolved in plasma or water is the same (0.004 g/100 mL). This is quite sufficient to supply all the oxygen necessary for the metabolism of the body.

VAPORS

Vapor is defined as the gaseous state of a substance, which at room temperature and pressure is a liquid. On the other hand a gas at room temperature exists only in the gaseous state. Like any other gas, the molecules of a vapor are continuously in violent motion and bombard the walls of the container. The force exerted on each unit area is called the pressure of the vapor (*Vapor Pressure*).

A vapor in a mixture of gases obeys the same laws as the gases. The partial pressure of the vapor in a mixture bears the same proportion to the total pressure as the volume, i.e. it depends on the percent (or fractional) concentration in the mixture. For example, the concentration of about 16% of water vapors in air at NTP, which is sufficient to saturate air with water vapors, exerts a pressure of 16% of 760 mm Hg (47 mm Hg).

The presence of water vapors in air or oxygen is referred to as *humidity*. It is largely through the process of evaporation that the molecules of water (or any other liquid) evaporate into the overlying air (or any other gas in a container).

The molecules leave the liquid substance when their kinetic energy exceeds the surface tension of the liquid. If a liquid is kept in a closed container for long, a state of equilibrium is reached when the number of molecules returning to the liquid (*condensation*) is exactly equal to the number leaving it (*evaporation*). This is called the saturation-point. This is further dependent upon temperature; if the temperature increases, the number of molecules leaving the liquid also increase and the saturation point is raised, i.e. there is a greater amount of vapors in the same amount of gas. Reverse happens with a fall in temperature.

The air we breathe is normally humid due to the presence of water vapor. The actual amount of water vapor present in air is expressed as "relative humidity", which is defined as the ratio of the amount of water vapor present in a given volume with the amount of water vapor, which the air (or the gas) is capable of holding at the given temperature, in the same volume.

The humidity of air varies with the atmospheric conditions. Once inhaled in the lungs, air gets fully saturated. The amount of water vapor required to saturate the alveolar air at body temperature and pressure is the body humidity.

The presence of water vapor in the inhaled air exerts its own partial pressure, and lowers the pressures of constituent gases of air—oxygen and nitrogen. Therefore, PN_2 or PO_2 is calculated as a proportion of the atmospheric pressure minus water vapor pressure, i.e. $P\text{-}PH_2O$.

When fully saturated, PH_2O of atmospheric air is equal to 47 mm Hg. Therefore, PO_2 = (P–PH_2O) × 21% = (760–47) × 0.21 = 150 mm Hg. The rest, i.e. 760 – (150 + 47) would be approximately the PN_2.

EXPRESSION OF GAS VOLUMES AND PRESSURES

In view of the effects of temperature, pressure and humidity on all gases, these are expressed with reference to those conditions. Some of the common expressions are:

- Standard (or normal) temperature and pressure (STP) or NTP temperature 0°C; Pressure 760 mm Hg.
- *STPD*: D indicates "dry" = complete absence of water vapor.
- Ambient temperature and pressure—dry or saturated (ATPD or ATPS). Ambient implies the room conditions.
- *Body temperature and pressure saturated (BTPS)*: Body temperature (usually 37°C), ambient pressure and water vapor pressure (47 mm Hg).

Normally, gas volume measurements are made in the ambient conditions. Conversion is required to express the volume at BTPS or STPD. STPD is used for the uniformity of expression. This is done by multiplying with conversion factors. Tables of conversion factors from ATPS to STPD, STPD to BTPS, or BTPS to ATPS are available in most laboratories. Such corrections are also required to express volume of a gas (such as O_2) produced in the laboratory. The volume is expressed at STPD, which is different than that produced at ATPS.

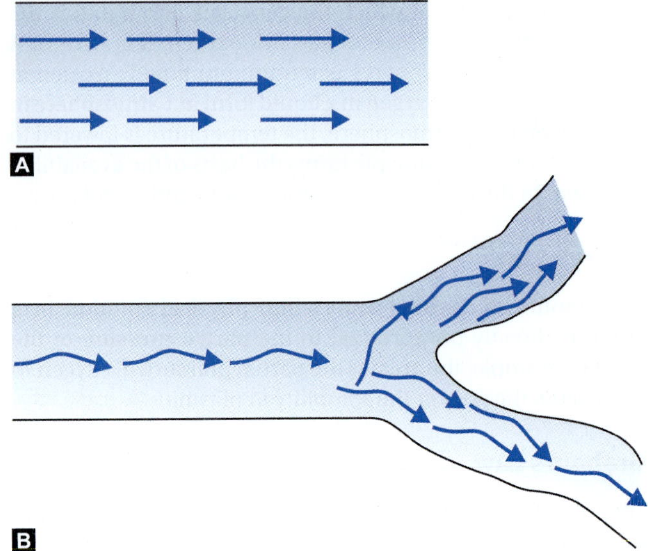

Figs 3A and B Patterns of flow: (A) Laminar flow; (B) Turbulent flow

FLOW OF GASES

Flow is the movement of particles of a liquid or a gas from higher to lower pressure. It is expressed in the terms of volume per unit time, e.g. liters per minute or per second (L/min or L/sec). The movement of air into the lungs during inspiration and out into the atmosphere during expiration is accomplished by the flow of air through tracheobronchial tree. Similarly, oxygen flows from a container cylinder to the lungs or a ventilator through connecting tubes as long as there is a pressure difference.

The flow is described as laminar, if it is smooth and gas particles move along lines parallel to the walls of the tube **(Fig. 3A)**. But it is turbulent if the lines of flow are irregular, broken up and disorderly **(Fig. 3B)**. Whether the flow is laminar or turbulent, it has to meet a certain resistance while moving from one to the other end of the tube. The laminar flow is described by the *Hagen-Poiseuille equation*, i.e. $V = \Pi \gamma^4 \Delta P/(8\,\eta l)$.

Resistance

Resistance is defined by the pressure difference under given conditions, between the entry and the exit points of a tube. The resistance is dependent on the tube length (l) and diameter. It is also directly proportional to the velocity of flow (∇) or rate in case of laminar flow. The flow is also viscosity (η) dependent and density-independent. When the flow is turbulent, the resistance rises for steeply.

In this way, the laminar flow through a straight tube of uniform size is inversely proportional to the length (l) of the tube and directly to the fourth power of radius (r).

When the flow exceeds a *"critical flow rate"*, the laminar flow is replaced by the turbulent flow throughout the length of the tube. Turbulent flow is less efficient since the ∇ P varies directly with V^2. Turbulent flow is density dependent and viscosity-independent. The critical flow varies directly with the internal diameter of the tube—the larger the diameter, the greater the flow. At a flow below the critical rate, local turbulence may occur as a result of irregularities in the pathways of the gas. During oxygen administration this may occur due to the constriction of kinking of the tubes.

Turbulence in a flowing system can also be predicted by Reynold's number. It is the ratio between inertial (density dependent, viscosity independent) and viscous (viscosity dependent, density independent) forces—a dimensionless number.

In case of pipes, Reynold's number is given by the ratio of (the product of) density × velocity × diameter to the viscosity.

Flow is "laminar" when the number is less than 2,000 and "turbulent" when it is more than 3,000. Turbulent flow is dominated by inertial forces producing random eddies and flow fluctuations. Between 2,000 and 3,000, the flow is transitional, i.e. neither fully laminar nor fully turbulent.

Flow Through Orifices

An orifice is a narrow opening of a tube. Unlike a tube, the diameter of the fluid pathway of the orifice exceeds the length. The greater the diameter compared to the length, the more does the opening approach the "ideal" orifice. The flow through an orifice depends on the diameter (or the cross-section area) of the orifice and the difference in pressures on either side of the orifice.

The intrinsic property of a liquid that influences its flow, which we earlier termed as resistance is called viscosity. It is attributed to the internal friction between different layers, which move at different speeds. While the laminar flow largely depends on viscosity, it is the density, which determines the flow when turbulent. The coefficient of viscosity is equal to the force per unit area necessary to maintain the unit difference of velocity between two parallel planes.

The flow through an orifice is at least partially turbulent. The lower the density, i.e. the lighter the gas, the greater is its volume flow for any given pressure difference on the either side of the orifice.

Wave Speed

Wave speed (c) is the speed at which a small disturbance (wave) travels in a compliant tube filled with a gas. In the airways, it depends upon the cross-sectional area of the airway, the density of the gas and the slope of the pressure area curve of the airway. Maximum flow (V_{max}) of a gas in an airway is the product of the gas velocity at wave speed and the airway area (cA). It increases as the density of the gas decreases.

Thermal Conductivity

It is a measure of a substance's capacity to conduct heat. The high thermal conductivity is likely to result in a higher skin heat loss. But respiratory heat loss depends on heat capacity not conductance.

Heliox

Heliox is a mixture of oxygen with helium (He) in varying concentrations, commonly as 20% oxygen and 80% helium. It has a lower density than that of air, i.e. oxygen (21%) with nitrogen (79%). Resistance offered to the flow of heliox is lower than that of air and of oxygen and depends on the fractional concentrations. It diffuses 1.8 times faster than oxygen. This fact is exploited in clinical practice for the treatment of acute respiratory distress of obstructive airway diseases, such as asthma, when the flow is highly turbulent. Heliox diffuses fastly than oxygen through partially obstructed airways. In view of the lower resistance offered to heliox, the breathing effort is considerably reduced and the crisis tide over.

Deposition

The particular matter inhaled in the lungs gets deposited in the tracheobronchial tree and the alveoli. The alveolar deposits have the potential to penetrate the alveolar walls and migrate to the bloodstream. The deposition is influenced by multiple factors such as the particle size, the acinus morphometry, the type of airflow, breathing patterns and lung heterogeneities.

Diffusion

The molecules in a fluid (liquid or gas) unlike in a solid, move freely in all directions. The time taken by a molecule to travel a given distance depends upon its closeness to other molecules, and the intermolecular spaces. The gas molecules do not necessarily collide with the neighboring molecules when they move around or across a membrane.

Diffusion across a membrane is determined by the difference in concentrations between the two neighboring layers of the solution. The rate of diffusion is proportional to the gradient of concentration, i.e. the change of concentration per unit length in the direction of diffusion (*Fick's law*).

Diffusion also depends on molecular movement. The rates of diffusion of gases at similar partial pressures through a porous membrane are inversely proportional to the square roots of their molecular weights (*Graham's law*). The molecular weight of oxygen and CO_2 being 32 and 44 respectively, the diffusion ratio will be 1.2.

It implies that oxygen diffuses 20% faster than CO_2 through a dry, porous membrane. It is because of the solubility of CO_2 in water of the moist alveolar membrane that the CO_2 diffusion is higher than O_2.

Solubility: Another factor, which determines diffusion across a wet film, is the solubility of the gas. The rate of diffusion is directly proportional to the solubility of the gas in the fluid.

Permeability: A membrane is permeable, if it allows the particular molecules to pass through, i.e. across the membrane. Permeability of different membranes to the molecules of different substances (solid, liquid or gases) is variable.

Osmosis: Osmosis is the migration of molecules of a solvent across a membrane. The pressure, which stops the transfer of molecules, is called the osmotic pressure of the solution. The osmotic pressure of a solution depends only on the number of dissolved particles per liter and not on the nature of the substances, which is dissolved.

The diffusion mechanisms also depend upon the pressures, volume and filtration. In respiratory system, the diffusion of gases and fluids across the alveolar membrane are critically important for normal gas-exchange functions of the lung and in the maintenance of a fluid balance.

BIBLIOGRAPHY

1. Brooks SM. Integrated Basic Science. St Louis: C.V. Mosby Company; 1966.
2. Dawson SV, Elliott EA. Wave speed limitation on expiratory flow: a unifying concept. J Appl Physiol. 1977;43(3):498-515.
3. Egan DF. Fundamentals of Respiratory Therapy. St. Louis: C.V. Mosby Company; 1966.
4. Emsley J. Nature's building blocks: An A-Z guide to the elements. New York: Oxford University Press; 2001.
5. Hess DR, Fink JB, Venkataraman ST, Kim IK, Myers TR, Tano BD. The history and physics of heliox. Respir Care. 2006;51(6):608-12.
6. Macintosh RR, Mushin WW, Epstein HG. Physics for the Anaesthetist. Philadelphia: FA Davis Company; 1970.
7. Oakes JM, Day S, Weinstein SJ, Robinson RJ. Flow field analysis in expanding healthy and emphysematous alveolar models using particle image velocimetry. J Biomech Eng. 2010;132(2):021008.
8. Riggs JH. Respiratory Facts, illustrated edition. Philadelphia; FA Davis Company; 1989.
9. West JB. Ventilation/Blood Flow and Gas Exchange. Philadelphia: FA Davis Company; 1970.
10. Young JA, Crocker D. Principles and Practice of Respiratory Therapy. Chicago: Year Book Medical Publishers Inc.

Respiratory Function and Mechanics

Dheeraj Gupta, Ritesh Agarwal, Ashutosh N Aggarwal

INTRODUCTION

Oxygen is essential for continuation of life. It is required by each human cell for its survival. It is abundantly present in atmosphere and maintains a remarkably constant concentration of 20.9% in ambient air. Oxygen is taken up by lungs through the act of inspiration and transported to cells via blood. At the cellular level, oxygen is utilized for production of energy. In this process, carbon dioxide is released and transported back via blood to lungs from where it is expired out into atmosphere. The act of exchange of oxygen and carbon dioxide is called respiration. For effective respiration, air must be drawn through the airways and distributed among approximately 400,000,000 alveolar compartments within the lung parenchyma. Although respiration is normally described as uptake of oxygen and release of carbon dioxide by the lungs, it is essentially happening at the level of lungs ("external" respiration), as well as the tissues ("internal" respiration).

The respiratory system is made up of a gas exchanging organ (the lungs) and a pump that ventilates the lungs. The pump consists of the chest wall and the respiratory muscles, which increase and decrease the size of the thoracic cavity; the areas in the brain that control the muscles; and the tracts and nerves that connect the brain to the muscles. At rest, a normal human breathes 12-15 times a minute. About 500 mL of air per breath, or 6-8 L/min, is inspired and expired. This air mixes with the gas in the alveoli, and, by simple diffusion, O_2 enters the blood in the pulmonary capillaries while CO_2 enters the alveoli. In this manner, 250 mL of O_2 enters the body per minute and 200 mL of CO_2 is excreted.

Gas exchange by human lungs is achieved with the help of four processes **(Fig. 1)**, which are also variably interdependent:

1. *Ventilation*: To and fro movement between the atmosphere and the gas exchanging units of lung.
2. *Circulation:* Supply and distribution of blood through the pulmonary capillaries.
3. *Diffusion:* The movement of O_2 and CO_2 across the air-blood barrier between alveoli and pulmonary capillaries.
4. Ventilation-perfusion relationships.

VENTILATION

Ventilation is the process of bulk movement of air from atmosphere, through the conducting airways to the terminal respiratory gas exchange units. This movement of air is made possible by force which is generated by effort of respiratory muscles (or a mechanical ventilator if the patient is being ventilated). It is also dependent on mechanical properties of the conducting airways and the lung parenchyma (i.e. the breathing units). The mechanical properties are referred to as "static" at zero (or no airflow) flow and constant volume, and "dynamic" if there is air flow.

The amount of air that moves in and out of the lungs with each inspiration and expiration respectively is called

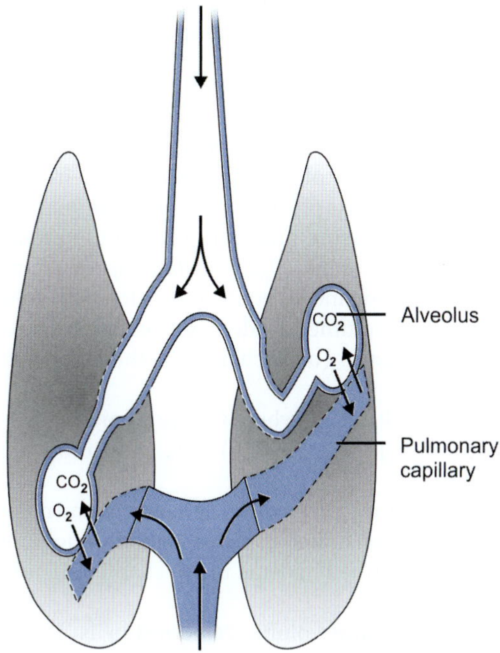

Fig. 1 Schematic diagram to represent different processes involved in respiration

the tidal volume. The air inspired over and above the tidal volume with a maximal inspiratory effort is the inspiratory reserve volume, and the volume exhaled actively after passive expiration is the expiratory reserve volume; the air left in the lungs after a maximal expiratory effort is the residual volume. The respiratory dead space is the space in the conducting zone of the airways occupied by gas that is not involved in gas exchange. The vital capacity, the largest amount of air that can be exhaled after a maximal inspiratory effort, is a frequently measured index of pulmonary function. The fraction of the vital capacity exhaled during the first-second of a forced expiration is the FEV_1. The maximal voluntary ventilation is the largest volume of gas that can be moved in to and out of the lungs in 1 minute by voluntary effort. There are several factors on which the aforementioned lung volume and the airflow depend: *Compliance* (a volume term), which is a measure of the elastic properties of lung, is an important determinant. Other elements include *resistance* (a flow term) and *inertance* (an acceleration term).

Inertance

Since the respired gases, the lungs and the chest wall all have appreciable mass and therefore inertia, they offer an impedance to change in the direction of gas flow. This component called inertance, is extremely difficult to measure, but offers impedance that increases with frequency. Hence, inertial pressure is essentially negligible for most clinical purposes and the gas flow depends primarily on the compliance and resistance characteristics of the lung parenchyma except in situations of increased respiratory frequencies like high-frequency ventilation.

Compliance

Pulmonary compliance (or distensibility) is defined as the change in the volume of lung per unit change in distending pressure, which in case of lung is the transpulmonary pressure [defined as the pressure gradient between the alveolar (P_A) and the pleural pressures (P_{pl})]. *Elastance* is the reciprocal of compliance. Compliance is equal to exhaled tidal volume (or a change in lung volume) divided by alveolar pressure minus the pleural pressure (or a change in the transpulmonary pressure).

$C = \Delta V_L / \Delta (P_A - P_{pl})$, where C = lung compliance, ΔV_L = change in lung volume, $\Delta (P_A - P_{pl})$ = change in transpulmonary pressure.

The interaction between recoil of the lungs and recoil of the chest can be demonstrated using body plethysmography. The technique is described in detail in the chapter on pulmonary function testing.

The lung pressure volume relationship is a curvilinear graph. The elastic recoil pressure of lung always tends to collapse the lung even at the residual volume. Theoretically therefore, if removed from the thoracic cage, the lungs collapse to almost an airless state.

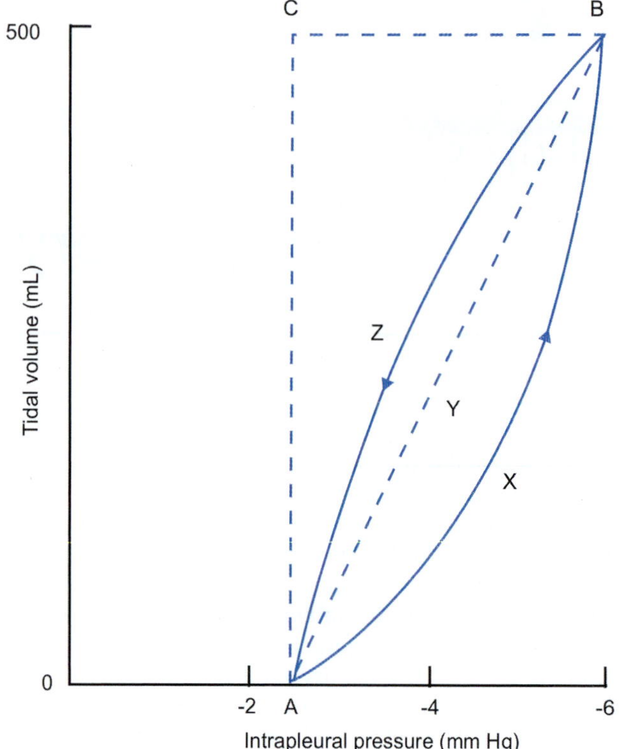

Fig. 2 Diagrammatic representation of pressure and volume changes during quiet inspiration (line AXB) and expiration (line BZA) is the compliance line

Hysteresis

The pressure-volume curve is also slightly greater when measured during deflation than when measured during inflation, a property called hysteresis **(Fig. 2)**. Hysteresis is affected by the elasticity of lung parenchyma and the surface tension of alveolar spaces. In fact, hysteresis is a universal property of all elastic materials. Pulmonary compliance is normally measured in the pressure range where the relaxation pressure curve is steepest. However, compliance depends on lung volume with highest compliance at residual lung volume and low compliance at high lung volumes.

Recruitment

This is a unique phenomenon observed in lung due to closure of some small airways at lower lung volumes. As the transpulmonary pressure rises, the closed airways open sequentially. Thus, the recruitment of additional lung units in the initial phase of inspiration starting from lower lung volumes also contributes to hysteresis. Two other important factors affecting lung compliance are the surface tension and the physical nature of lung tissues.

Surface tension exerted by air fluid interface is reduced by surfactant—a surface active compound of phospholipids produced by type II alveolar cells. Surface tension is further lowered at lower lung volumes thereby increasing the compliance and decreasing the force required during the next inflation. Also, by the Laplace law (Pressure = 2 × surface tension/radius), as the diameter of the alveoli is decreased, the pressure would increase and this would create an unstable system; this is also prevented by surfactant, which decreases surface tension with decreasing radii of alveoli, and allows gas to flow from the larger to the smaller alveolus and stability is maintained. This phenomenon is also mandatory for the maintenance of stability of alveoli at lower lung volumes.

Physical elastic properties of lung tissue per se, are due to the presence of elastic fibers in the pulmonary interstitium. Expansion in lungs is probably more due to unfolding and geometric rearrangement of elastic fibers rather than the actual lengthening. Aging alters the elastin and collagen fibers in lungs, thus increasing the compliance. Compliance is also increased in emphysema due to loss of elastic fibers of alveolar walls. It is reduced wherever there is stiffness and thickening of alveolar septae by processes such as fibrosis.

Elastic Properties of Chest Wall and Lung-chest Wall Interactions

The resting volume of thoracic cage is approximately equal to 70% of total lung capacity (TLC). It implies that if thoracic cage is opened and support of lung withdrawn, it expands from functional residual capacity (FRC) (the resting position of respiratory system at which the inward elastic recoil of the lungs is exactly balanced by the outward recoil of thoracic cage) to a volume of about 70% of TLC. At volumes less than 70% (including FRC), thoracic cage has a tendency to expand and elastic recoil pressure is opposite to that of lungs, and is directed outward.

The total compliance of the respiratory system is analogous to the electrical capacitance with the compliances of the lung and the thoracic wall arranged in series. Thus, the reciprocal of total compliance is the sum of reciprocals of the individual compliances, i.e.

1/total compliance = 1/lung compliance +1/chest wall compliance

Instead of compliance, we may consider its reciprocal, elastance and the relationship is much simpler:

Total respiratory system elastance = lung elastance + chest wall elastance.

Resistance

Resistance is the opposition to motion and in the respiratory system opposition to the flow of gas. In the lung, resistance to air flow is of two types: tissue and airway. The former, also known as elastic resistance (resistance from tissues or tissue resistance), occurs when no gas is flowing, and is due to elastic resistance of lung tissue and chest wall and the resistance imparted from surface forces at the alveolar gas/liquid interface. Approximately, 80% of the pulmonary resistance is due to airway resistance or nonelastic resistance.

Resistance to airflow is computed by the simultaneous measurements of airflow, and the driving pressure that is required to achieve the flow, i.e.

Resistance = Driving pressure/Flow = P/V

Most nonelastic resistance is provided by frictional resistance to airflow and thoracic tissue deformation, with small contributions from inertia of gas and tissue and compression of intrathoracic gas.

Airway Morphology

Airways are tubular structures designed to carry air to alveolocapillary membrane for gas exchange. The tracheobronchial tree consists of several branches, which arise by dichotomous divisions of the parent bronchus. Airway divisions from trachea to the alveoli are not uniform, may vary between 10 and 25 in different areas—divisions being less near the hilar regions and more at the bases. The diameter, angulation and course of the bronchial divisions are also different in different lung zones. For example, the air passages to alveoli at the lung bases are straighter and have large cross-sectional areas. This asymmetric pattern of branching is referred to as "irregular dichotomy". It has a bearing on the distribution of ventilation and deposition of inhaled material.

Airways are classified into two types—conducting and respiratory airways. The conducting or central airways do not participate in gas exchange. They are larger than 2 mm in diameter, have cartilaginous support, are lined by ciliated columnar epithelium and are supplied by systemic bronchial circulation. They are also able to change their diameter in response to several neurohormonal and chemical stimuli due to the presence of smooth muscles in their walls and vagal innervation. The respiratory bronchioles or terminal airways are situated beyond the conducting airways. They are less than 2 mm in diameter, lack cartilaginous support, are lined by cuboidal epithelium and supplied by pulmonary circulation. Due to their structural properties, they are susceptible to compression and closure in response to changes in intrapulmonary pressures.

The geometric features of airway divisions have a direct relationship with the partitioning of resistance and hence distribution of ventilation. There is a progressive narrowing and shortening of airways as the division progresses from trachea to the peripheral airways. Despite reduction in the diameter of daughter airways, the total cross-sectional area increases tremendously as we go peripherally. This is because the total number of airways increases geometrically with each division and the diameter of each daughter airway is more than half of the parent airway. This results in almost 2,000 fold increase in total cross-sectional area from trachea to peripheral airways.

Physical Principle of Gas Flow and Resistance

The geometric features described above are important in the distribution of resistance within the lung. The air flow decreases progressively as air moves down the bronchial tree to the peripheral zones. In the terminal bronchioles, flow is reduced to almost zero. It is the Brownian motion of the molecules, which facilitates diffusion across the alveolocapillary membrane. As the flow velocity decreases, the driving pressure and resistance also fall. It has been calculated that 80% of total measurable resistance at mouth is contributed by central or conducting airways.

The precise relationship between pressure difference and flow rate depends on the nature of flow, which may be laminar, turbulent or a mixture of the two. With *laminar flow*, gas flows along a straight unbranched tube as a series of concentric cylinders that slide over one another, with the peripheral cylinder stationary and the central cylinder moving fastest, the advancing cone forming a parabola. The advancing cone front means that some gas will reach the end of the tube despite the volume of gas entering the tube being less than the volume of the tube. This has relevance in patients being ventilated using high frequency ventilation where there is significant alveolar ventilation despite the tidal volume being less than or equal to the anatomical dead space.

In a straight unbranched tube, the *Hagen-Poiseuille equation* allows gas flow to be quantified: Flow rate = $\Delta P \times \pi \times (\text{radius})^4/8 \times \text{length} \times \text{viscosity}$, where ΔP is the pressure gradient and equals the product of flow rate and resistance: Thus, resistance = $8 \times \text{length} \times \text{viscosity}/\pi \times (\text{radius})^4$.

In this equation, the fourth power of the radius explains the critical importance of narrowing of air passages. With constant tube dimensions, viscosity is the only property of gas that is relevant under the conditions of laminar flow. Helium has a lower density, but a viscosity close to that of air, and thus will not improve gas flow if the flow is laminar.

On the other hand, *turbulent flow* occurs when gas flows at high rates through unbranched or irregular tubes, resulting in formation of eddy currents. In contrast to laminar flow, it has a square front and the volume of gas entering the tube is equal to the volume of the tube, the so called *bulk flow*. The relationship is different from the laminar flow in that the driving pressure is proportional to the square of gas flow rate and the density of gas, but independent of its viscosity and the required driving pressure is inversely proportional to the fifth power of the radius of the tubing (*Fanning's equation*).

The change in flow from laminar to turbulent characteristics is determined by a dimensionless number, the *Reynolds' number* (N_R), which is N_R = density × velocity × diameter/viscosity. The property of gas that affects N_R is the ratio of density to viscosity. Flow is laminar with N_R less than 2,000, and changes from laminar to turbulent when the N_R exceeds 4,000. Between N_R of 2,000 and 4,000, both types of flow coexist. There is also a critical length of tubing before the parabolic pattern of laminar flow is established, and thus for gases with low N_R not only will resistance be less during turbulent flow, but also laminar flow will become established more quickly after narrowed airways. In principle, turbulence occurs only in larger airways and not in smaller airways because of the large cross-sectional area, the small diameter and the slow velocity of the small airways. Heliox has a density/viscosity ratio of 0.31 compared to one for oxygen. It has a lower N_R and higher potential for laminar flow, explaining its usefulness in patients with large airway diseases.

Total and Alveolar Ventilation

The total amount of air inhaled with each inspiration gets distributed in the lungs depending upon the regional resistance and compliance of different lung units. Ventilatory requirements for adequate supply of oxygen and removal of carbon dioxide depend on metabolic demands of body. The resting ventilatory requirements are small and are met with minimal expenditure of energy. A normal individual can maintain gas exchange with a ventilation of about 80 mL/kg/minute, which is about one-tenth of the maximum ventilatory capacity. Therefore, there is a vast reserve in ventilatory capacity and problems of gas exchange would not occur, if all the inspired volume is available to the gas exchange units. Due to cyclical nature of ventilation, a significant proportion of inspired gas never reaches the alveoli—a volume known as the *dead space volume*. So, the total ventilation is contributed by the dead space ventilation (V_D) and *alveolar ventilation* (V_A), i.e. the air that reaches the alveoli to take part in gas exchange. The dead space ventilation in mL is roughly around the individual's body weight in pounds.

The volume of conducting airways, which constitute the *anatomical dead space*, is relatively fixed, i.e. about one-third of the resting tidal ventilation. Its relative proportion to the total ventilation decreases as the total ventilation increases, for example on exercise. On the other hand, a decrease in tidal volume and increase in respiratory rate (e.g. rapid shallow breathing) markedly increases the proportion of dead space ventilation thereby affecting gas exchange.

Dead space is also increased when there is presence of lung units, which are adequately perfused, but not ventilated, the so called *physiological dead space*. It is important to distinguish between the anatomic dead space (respiratory system volume exclusive of alveoli) and the physiologic dead space (volume of gas in the alveoli not equilibrating with blood, i.e. wasted ventilation). As will be discussed subsequently in this chapter, ventilation has to be matched by the perfusion of blood in the alveolar capillaries for adequate gas exchange to occur. Ventilation and perfusion are not homogeneously distributed throughout the lung, and areas which receive more ventilation relative to perfusion result in wasted ventilation and thus add to "dead space" ventilation. The sum of the dead space ventilation by these two mechanisms constitutes "**total dead space**" and is given the formula:

$$V_D/V_E = 1 - P_ECO_2/P_ACO_2,\text{ where}$$

V_D = total dead space
V_E = minute ventilation
P_ECO_2 = partial pressure of carbon dioxide in the expired air
P_ACO_2 = partial pressure of carbon dioxide in the alveolar air (which in practice is measured by the arterial PCO_2)

The relationship of total and alveolar ventilation was first described by Christian Bohr and is also known as *"Bohr dead space"*.

Distribution of Ventilation

Alveolar ventilation is distributed throughout the lungs. With each inspiration, around 500 mL of air is distributed to around 300 million alveoli such that each alveolus receives an appropriate share of the inspired gas. This fine distribution of air is essentially a function of the *"time constants"* of the regional lung units. Time constant is the product of regional compliance and resistance and thus is also called the *RC time constant*. The relative distribution of ventilation between two neighboring lung units can be understood better with the two compartment lung model. In health, the resistance and compliance of two adjacent units of lung are essentially equal and thus their RC time constant is normal with the normal distribution of ventilation. However in a diseased lung, different portions of lung may have abnormal time constants as a result of either the diseased airway lumen (increased resistance) or because of stiffness of alveolar walls (increased compliance) or both. Thus, ventilation will be maldistributed in a lung unit with abnormal RC time constant with more ventilation to areas with relatively normal time constant than other areas. A lung unit with a large time constant (i.e. greater resistance and compliance) does not completely fill by the end of inspiration and empties slowly during expiration. In contrast, a lung unit with a small-time constant (i.e. smaller resistance and compliance) fills and empties rapidly.

When a lung unit with a large-time constant is located adjacent to a lung unit with a small-time constant, the unit with the large-time constant may withdraw gas from the adjacent lung unit with a short-time constant rather than fresh inspired gas. This "to and fro" behavior is known as pendelluft, and it can occur in abnormal lungs. In addition, a lung unit with a small-time constant may receive a higher proportion of dead space gas, which reduces its alveolar ventilation. This effect is prominent in chronic obstructive lung disease, in which compliant lung units with extremely large-time constants behave essentially as dead space. The higher the respiratory rate, the greater is the discrepancy in filling and emptying between these two kinds of units, and thus greater the inhomogeneity of ventilation.

Another reason for uneven ventilation of small lung units is a gradient of gas concentration along the small airways, a condition called *stratified inhomogeneity*. Inspired gas reaches near the region of the terminal or respiratory bronchioles by convective flow, but gas flow over the rest of the distance to the alveoli is accomplished primarily by molecular diffusion within the airways. When airway calibers are altered, as in emphysema, the process of gas diffusion may be incomplete for each breath. Thus, alveoli more distal to conducting airways are less well ventilated than proximal alveoli.

Several mechanisms tend to preserve the uniform distribution of ventilation in the lung. One of these mechanisms is the pendelluft phenomenon described earlier. Another mechanism is gas exchange through collateral air channels between adjacent lung units. *Collateral ventilation* can occur between alveolo-alveolar pores of Kohn, bronchiolo-alveolar canals of Lambert, and bronchiolo-bronchiolar foramina of Martin. Another factor that tends to improve the uniformity of ventilation is the interdependence of peripheral lung units, which stems from the observation that contiguous lung units are attached integrally to each other by the connective tissue framework of the lung parenchyma. The behavior of one unit must therefore influence the behavior of its neighbors. This framework serves to offset the tendency for regional differences in compliance to make lung units larger or smaller than they should be for optimal performance.

Role of Gravity

Gravity also plays some role in the distribution of ventilation. In the upright position, ventilation per unit lung volume is greater at base of lung than at apex. This happens because at the start of inspiration, intrapleural pressure is less negative at base than at apex, and since the intrapulmonary-intrapleural pressure difference is less than at apex, the lung is less expanded. Conversely, at apex, the lung is more expanded, i.e. the percentage of maximum lung volume is greater. Because of stiffness of lung, the increase in lung volume per unit increase in pressure is smaller when the lung is initially more expanded, and ventilation is consequently greater at the base.

The ventilation differences tend to disappear in supine position, and the weight of lung makes the intrapleural pressure lower at the base in the upright position. However, the inequalities of ventilation and blood flow in humans have been found to persist to a remarkable degree in the weightlessness of space. Therefore, other as yet unknown factors apparently also play a role in producing the inequalities. It should also be noted that at very low lung volumes, such as those after forced expiration, intrapleural pressure at lung bases can actually exceed atmospheric pressure in the airways, and the small airways such as respiratory bronchioles collapse (airway closure). In older people and in those with chronic lung disease, some of the elastic recoil is lost, with a resulting decrease in intrapleural pressure. Consequently, airway closure may occur at the bases of lungs in the upright position without forced expiration, at volumes as high as the functional residual capacity.

PULMONARY CIRCULATION

The circulation of the entire cardiac output through lungs is ideally suited for rapid gas exchange. The pulmonary vascular bed resembles systemic circulation, except that the walls of pulmonary artery and its large branches are about 30% as thick as the wall of the aorta, and the small arterioles, unlike the systemic arterioles, have relatively little muscle in their walls. There is also some smooth muscle in the walls of the postcapillary venules. Also, the pulmonary capillaries are large with multiple anastomoses, so that each alveolus sits in a capillary basket. Blood from the right side of the heart flows through an intricate network of pulmonary capillaries around the alveoli.

After getting oxygenated, blood drains back into the left atrium through four pulmonary veins. The pulmonary bed is characteristically a low-pressure circuit. There is a dense network of capillaries around each alveolus. Rough estimates put the total number of capillaries at about six billion or two thousand capillaries per alveolus. Not all the capillaries are perfused under resting conditions. An increased blood flow due to an increased cardiac output (as much as 25 liters per minute during exercise in contrast to 5-6 liters during resting conditions) can be accommodated easily in pulmonary circulation without an increase in the pulmonary arterial pressure. This is made possible as a result of two major mechanisms that include *recruitment*, which is the opening of previously unperfused pulmonary capillaries in the upper lung zones, and *distension* in the entire pulmonary vasculature due to increased transmural pressure gradient. The best example of the ability of pulmonary vasculature to adapt to increased blood flow is following pneumonectomy, when the remaining lung will normally take the entire resting pulmonary blood flow without an increase in pulmonary arterial pressure.

Distribution of Perfusion

The distribution of pulmonary blood flow is nonuniform from apex to base. In upright position, upper portions of the lungs are well above the level of heart, and bases are at or below it. Consequently, there is a relatively marked pressure gradient in the pulmonary arteries from the top to the bottom of the lungs, because of effect of gravity, and a resulting linear increase in pulmonary blood flow from the apices to the bases of the lungs. The following three concepts about pressure in the pulmonary vessels are important to understanding the behavior of the pulmonary circulation.

Intravascular Pressure

This is the blood pressure inside the lumen of the vessel relative to the atmospheric pressure. The pulmonary arterial pressure (P_a) and pulmonary venous pressure (P_v) can be measured directly by placing catheters into the blood stream at specific points, and in clinical practice, capillary pressure can be estimated by wedging a catheter into a lobar branch of pulmonary artery. The "wedge" pressure measured under the conditions of "no flow" reflects the pressure downstream of the next freely communicating channels, that is, pulmonary capillaries or small pulmonary venules.

Transmural Pressure

This is the difference between the pressure inside a vessel and the pressure in the tissue around it. For example, the pressure around the pulmonary arteries and veins is approximately equal to the intrapleural pressure. The pressure around the capillaries is approximately the intra-alveolar pressure (P_A). It is this difference in transmural pressure that leads to the different behavior of alveolar and extra-alveolar vessels under conditions such as lung inflation. At the capillary level, the transmural pressure is also an important determinant of the rate of transudation of fluid across the capillary bed.

Pulmonary Driving Pressure

This is the difference in intravascular pressure between one point in the circulation and another point downstream, and is the pressure involved in overcoming the frictional resistance that impedes blood flow between two points. The driving pressure for the pulmonary circulation is the difference between the intravascular pressure in the main pulmonary artery and that immediately after the pulmonary circulation in the left atrium.

The intravascular pressures of pulmonary circulation are influenced by hydrostatic pressure created by gravity. The alveolar pressures significantly affect the intra-alveolar capillaries. As alveolar pressure is relatively independent of gravity, the relationships among pulmonary arterial, pulmonary venous and alveolar pressures must also influence the distribution of pulmonary blood flow. West subdivided the lung into four zones with differing patterns of blood flow **(Fig. 3)**. In *zone 1*, near the apex of lung, wherein the alveolar pressure exceeds both pulmonary arterial and venous pressures ($P_A > P_a > P_v$), and thus the alveolar vessels are collapsed and there is no pulmonary blood flow. In *zone 2*, the pulmonary arterial pressure exceeds the alveolar pressure, but alveolar pressure exceeds venous pressures ($P_a > P_A > P_v$). Under these conditions, the resistance to blood flow is determined by the difference between pulmonary arterial and alveolar pressures, rather than by the expected arterial-venous pressure difference. This behavior has been referred to variously as the *waterfall or sluice effect.* Also in *zone 2*, blood flow increases progressively down the lung because of the increasing hydrostatic effect on pulmonary arterial pressure, which increases the driving pressure in this region (pulmonary arterial pressure minus alveolar pressure).

In *zone 3*, the pulmonary venous pressure exceeds alveolar pressures ($P_a > P_v > P_A$), and blood flow is dependent on the pressure difference between P_a and P_v, and is maximal.

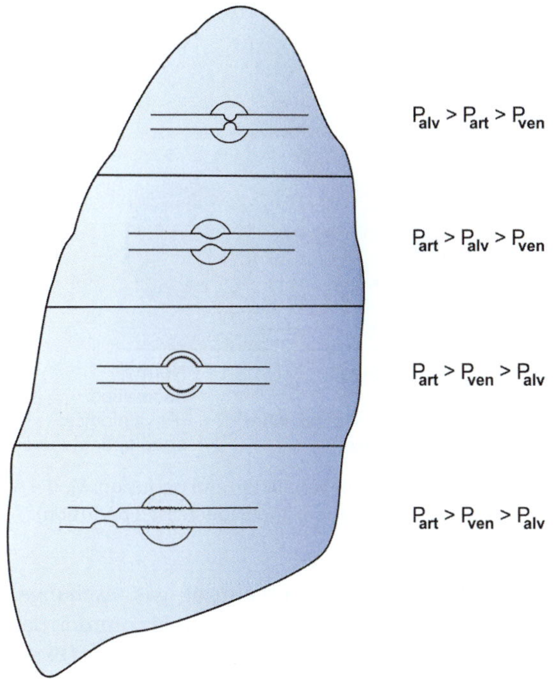

Fig. 3 West zones of perfusion

There is also a progressive increase in perfusion because of the progressive "distension" of vessels due to increase in P_a and P_v, while P_A remains constant. In *zone 4*, the relationships between intravascular and alveolar pressures are same as in *zone 3*, but the blood flow decreases slightly. *Zone 4* occurs in the lowermost region of the upright human lung and diminishes as lung volume increases. Conversely, as lung volume decreases, this region of reduced blood flow extends farther and farther up the lung, so that at FRC blood flow decreases progressively down the bottom half of the lung. At residual volume, *zone 4* extends nearly all the way up the lung, so that blood flow at the apex exceeds that at the base. This condition cannot be explained by the interactions among the pulmonary arterial, venous and alveolar pressures. Instead, the reduced blood flow in *zone 4* is probably due to the narrowing of extra-alveolar vessels at the lung base that result from lower lung inflation due to airways closing down at the "*closing volume*". The increased contribution of extra-alveolar vessels to pulmonary vascular resistance results in the presence of a zone of reduced blood flow in that region. *Zone 4* would be expected to increase in the presence of interstitial pulmonary edema, because the edematous fluid increases interstitial pressure in the vascular sheath and thereby narrows the extra-alveolar vessels. This is a plausible mechanism for the inverted distribution of blood flow (cephalization of pulmonary vasculature on chest X-ray) in pulmonary edema.

Not all the inhomogeneity of blood flow in the lung can be explained by gravitational effects. Indirect measurements of inhomogeneity (monitoring the magnitude of cardiogenic oscillations on the expired carbon dioxide tracing) of pulmonary blood flow have been made in astronauts in space shuttles, and a striking reduction in inhomogeneity of blood flow was detected during weightlessness compared with that observed in the upright posture before or after the flight. Interestingly, substantial inhomogeneity of blood flow still remained, indicating that some gravity-independent mechanism was also present. Another situation where the gravitational model fails is the situation of prone position ventilation, where the perfusion is probably more homogeneous and not dependent on gravity.

DIFFUSION

Diffusion is the rate at which oxygen from alveolus is transferred across the alveolocapillary barrier to combine with hemoglobin in the red blood cells of pulmonary capillaries **(Fig. 4)**. The situation in lungs can be visualized as a two chamber model with different partial pressures of oxygen and a liquid barrier separating the two **(Fig. 4)**. The transfer of gases from the alveoli to the capillary blood during the pulmonary transit time of 0.75 seconds depends on their reaction of the molecules with hemoglobin in the blood. For example, nitrous oxide (N_2O) does not react, and reaches equilibrium in about 0.1 seconds. In this situation, the amount of N_2O taken up is not limited by diffusion, but by the amount of blood flowing through the pulmonary capillaries, i.e. it is flow-limited.

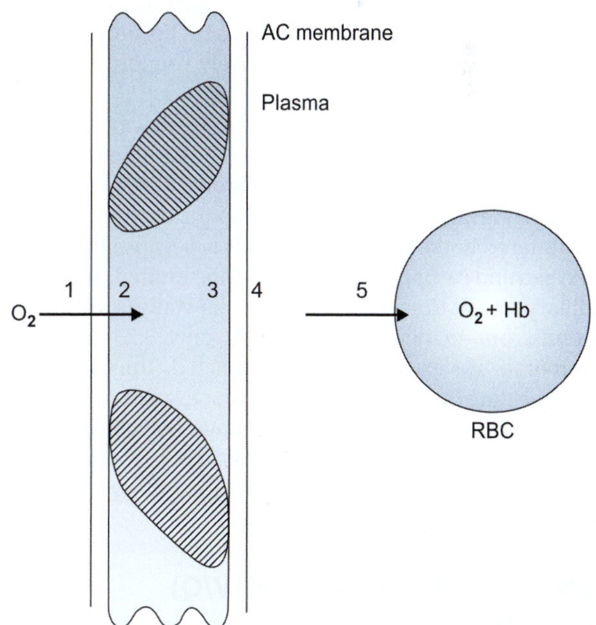

Fig. 4 Schematic diagram representing diffusion across the alveolo-capillary membrane into the red blood cell. 1 and 2 represent the inner and outer layer of the alveolar epithelium, 3 and 4 represent the inner and outer layer of the capillary endothelium, 5 represents the red blood cell (RBC) membrane

On the other hand, carbon monoxide (CO) is taken up by the hemoglobin in the red blood cells at such a high rate that the partial pressure of CO in the capillaries stays very low and equilibrium is not reached in 0.75 seconds till the blood is in the pulmonary capillaries. Therefore, the transfer of CO is not limited by perfusion at rest and instead is diffusion-limited. Oxygen is intermediate between N_2O and CO; it is taken up by hemoglobin, but much less avidly than CO, and it reaches equilibrium with capillary blood in about 0.3 seconds. Thus, its uptake is also perfusion-limited. Diffusing capacity of the lung for a given gas is directly proportionate to the surface area of the alveolocapillary membrane and inversely proportionate to its thickness. The factors that influence the movement of gas from the area of higher partial pressure (alveolus) to the area of low partial pressure (capillaries) are governed by the *Fick's law*:

V = Ad/T (P1 – P2), where
V = volume of gas diffusing per unit time (mL/minute)
A = area available for diffusion (cm^2)
P1 – P2 = pressure difference of gas on two sides (mm Hg)
d = diffusion coefficient of the barrier (cm^2/minute/mm Hg)

This *diffusion coefficient* "d" is further related to the solubility of the gas within the liquid barrier and the square root of the molecular weight of the gas. Other factors being constant, driving pressure is the most important factor determining flow of oxygen across the alveolocapillary membrane. When this pressure falls, such as travel at high altitudes, the oxygen delivery to the tissues becomes diffusion limited. Similarly, diffusion is inversely proportional to the thickness of the membrane.

Although diffusion is reduced in the presence of thickened alveolocapillary membrane (e.g. interstitial lung disease) or the loss of gas exchange areas (e.g. chronic obstructive airway disease); it is rarely the sole factor responsible for hypoxemia encountered in these conditions. This is because the transfer of oxygen and carbon dioxide is perfusion limited. The normal capillary transit time across the alveolar walls is usually 0.75 seconds, but in healthy individuals only 0.25 seconds is required for gas exchange to be completed. Thus, there is an adequate time for gas exchange to occur even in the presence of a diffusion defect. The gas exchange becomes diffusion dependent during conditions, which increase cardiac output, such as exercise, anxiety, etc. when the capillary transit time is significantly reduced.

VENTILATION-PERFUSION (V/Q) RELATIONSHIPS

The ratio of pulmonary ventilation to pulmonary blood flow for the whole lung at rest is about 0.8 to 1 (4–6 L/ minute ventilation divided by 5-6 L/minute blood flow), and this matching of distribution of ventilation and perfusion is the most important determinant of gas exchange. The ventilation-perfusion mismatch is the final common pathway to cause hypoxemia in most pulmonary diseases **(Fig. 5)**. An area of lung that is well perfused, but under ventilated acts as a right to left shunt (physiological shunt) whereas an area that is well ventilated, but under perfused acts like a dead space (physiological dead space). The spectrum of V/Q ratios in a healthy lung would vary between zero (perfused, but not ventilated) to infinity (ventilated, but not perfused).

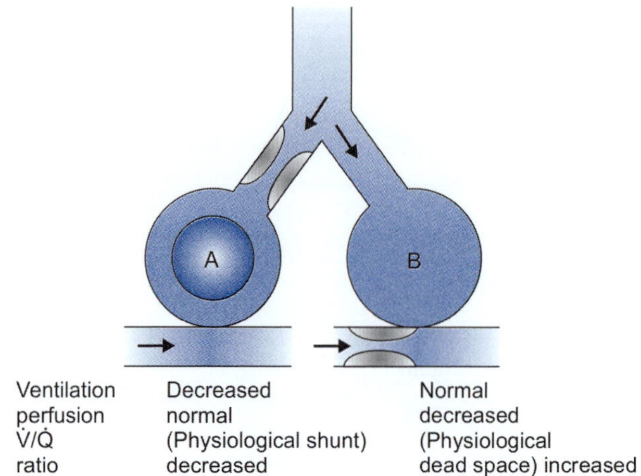

Fig. 5 Mismatching of ventilation and perfusion: Model A (diminished ventilation) and B (decreased perfusion)

The ideal V/Q ratio of one indicates perfectly matched ventilation and perfusion. Although V/Q mismatch includes both physiologic shunt and physiologic dead space, but in clinical parlance, the term generally denotes physiologic shunt as physiologic dead space is rarely, if ever, the cause of hypoxemia. In an alveolar-capillary unit with a V/Q ratio of 0 (*physiologic shunt*), the blood leaving the unit has the composition of mixed venous blood entering the pulmonary capillaries, i.e. PO_2 of 40 mm Hg and PCO_2 of 46 mm Hg whereas in an alveolar-capillary unit with a high V/Q ratio (physiologic dead space) the small amount of blood leaving the unit has partial pressures of O_2 and CO_2 are 150 mm Hg and 0 mm Hg approaching the composition of inspired gas.

Because of the sigmoid shape of the oxyhemoglobin dissociation curve, it is important to differentiate between the partial pressure and the content of oxygen in the blood. Hemoglobin is almost fully (> 90%) saturated at a PO_2 of 60 mm Hg, and little additional O_2 is carried by hemoglobin even with a substantial elevation of PO_2 above 60 mm Hg. On the other hand, significant O_2 desaturation of hemoglobin occurs once PO_2 falls below 60 mm Hg and onto the steep descending limb of the curve. As a result, blood coming from regions of the lung with a high V/Q ratio and a high PO_2 has only a small elevation in O_2 content and cannot compensate for blood coming from regions with a low V/Q ratio and a low PO_2, which has a significantly decreased O_2 content. Although V/Q mismatching can influence PCO_2, this effect is less marked and is often overcome by an increase in overall minute ventilation.

The alveolar PO_2 appears to be the most important factor involved in regulating the distribution of ventilation-perfusion within the lung. In this respect, hypoxic pulmonary vasoconstriction can be considered as part of a negative feedback loop. For example, in lung units with low V/Q ratios, there is a fall in local alveolar PO_2, and constriction of associated microcirculation reduces the local pulmonary blood flow. This tends to restore the local V/Q ratio toward its normal value. This effect can be appreciated in the residents of high altitudes, who are exposed constantly to lower ambient O_2 concentrations. Residents of high altitudes have better V/Q matching than sea level residents, as reflected by a smaller alveolar-arterial PO_2 difference.

The intensity of hypoxic pulmonary vasoconstriction varies among different lung regions, and probably depends on the smooth muscle tone in different vessels. More recently, a role for nitric oxide in regulating local ventilation-perfusion matching has been suggested as nitric oxide is a selective pulmonary vasodilator (no systemic effects), and inhibits hypoxic pulmonary vasoconstriction. Theoretically, the inhalation of nitric oxide can cause selective pulmonary vasodilation in adequately ventilated areas and improve gas exchange. The nitric oxide-mediated mechanism may also be important in patients with inflammatory lung diseases, in whom the production of nitric oxide is increased. The loss of local hypoxic vasoconstriction would worsen ventilation-perfusion mismatch.

CONTROL OF VENTILATION

The active inspiratory process facilitates expansion of the lungs. It involves contraction of intercostals muscles and diaphragm to move the chest upward and outward. By doing so the intrathoracic and alveolar pressures are lowered and the flow of the air into the lungs is facilitated. Expiration is usually a passive process. The lungs and chest collapse under their own elastic recoil and raise the intrathoracic and alveolar pressures. The air then flows out of the lungs.

Ventilation is controlled tightly through three components—sensors (or receptors), central controllers and effectors (muscles of respiration). The respiratory control mechanisms operate through both neuronal and chemical receptors. While the former are peripherally located (airway, lung, chest wall, blood vessels), the latter are both peripherally and centrally located. Control centers in the brain put together information from all these receptors, and fine-tune the neuronal drive to respiratory musculature, which in turn controls the level of ventilation.

Neuronal Receptors

The neuronal receptors vary greatly in their location and response characteristics. Some are rapidly adaptive to change in lung volume or irritation by noxious agents or inflammatory mediators. Receptor signals are mediated through the vagus nerve to the respiratory center, and have variable effects like increase in ventilation, cough and/or bronchoconstriction. Others like stretch receptors or muscle spindles in airway smooth muscles adapt slowly to lung volume changes. These get activated by lung over distension and signal the respiratory center to discontinue the stimulation of the inspiratory muscles, allowing expiration to begin. This response is called the inflation *(Herring-Breuer) reflex*. Juxtacapillary (or J) receptors located in alveolar walls sense the engorgement of the pulmonary capillaries and cause rapid shallow breathing.

Peripheral Chemoreceptors

The main location for peripheral chemoreceptors is in aortic and carotid bodies, although they may be present in other areas as well. Carotid bodies are located bilaterally at the bifurcation of common carotid arteries, and are the major receptors in adult life. They mainly respond to arterial hypoxemia, and to hypercapnia, by transmitting signals to nucleus tractus solitarius through ninth cranial nerve, resulting in hyperventilation. Other chemoreceptors in central nervous system adjust ventilation to maintain acid-base homeostasis. The more important receptors are located near ventral medullary surface and retrotrapezoid nucleus. These receptors respond to pH changes in the cerebrospinal fluid resulting from the diffusion of carbon dioxide through the blood-brain barrier.

Respiratory Center

The various positive and negative signals from all these receptors are integrated at the level of respiratory control centers in the medulla and pons, and result in appropriate modifications in frequency, depth and/or pattern of respiration. The dorsal medullary inspiratory center generates rhythmic neuronal impulses that result in contraction of inspiratory muscles. Exhalation is largely a passive process, though it can be actively controlled through ventral respiratory group of neurons in the medulla. Medullary center is controlled by pontine centers. Pneumotaxic center is located in the dorsal and superior pontine area, and is inhibitory to the medullary ventilatory drive. Apneustic area in the lower pons can stimulate respiration if the pneumotaxic center is blocked, but its function is not well understood.

Ventilatory Responses

The ventilatory response to carbon dioxide elevation in blood is largely centrally mediated and results in a proportional increase in ventilation that attempts to correct the anomaly, although normocapnia may not be achieved. Relationship between respiratory minute volume and the alveolar carbon dioxide is essentially linear. The ventilatory response to hypoxia is not so linear. Although mild hypoxemia increases discharge from the peripheral chemoreceptors, the corresponding hypocapnia from any increase in ventilation, as well as a slight alkalosis from the lesser amount of oxyhemoglobin, prevent any sustained hyperventilation. An increase in minute ventilation is only seen when arterial oxygenation falls substantially. The composite effects of hypoxemia, hypercarbia and acidosis are much more complex.

BIBLIOGRAPHY

1. Cotes JE. Lung Function. Oxford: Blackwell Scientific; 1975.
2. Cotes JE. Lung function: assessment and application in medicine. Oxford: Blackwell Publications; 1993.
3. Crystal RG, West JB. The Lung: Scientific Foundations. New York: Raven Press; 1991.
4. Fishman AP. Pulmonary circulation. In: Fishman AP, Fisher AB, Geiger SR (Eds). Handbook of Physiology, Section 3 - The respiratory system. Bethesda, MD: American Physiological Society; 1987.
5. Freedman S. Mechanics of ventilation. In: Brewers RA, Corrin B, Geddes DM, Gibson GJ, (Eds). Respiratory Medicine. London: WB Saunders; 1995.
6. Lumb AB. Nunn's Applied Respiratory Physiology, 5th edition. Edinburgh: Butterworth-Heinemann; 2000.
7. McCool FD, Hoppin FG. Respiratory mechanics. In: Baum GL, Glassroth JL, King TE, Crapo JD, Karlinsky J (Eds). Baum's Textbook of Pulmonary Diseases, 7th edition. New York: Lippincott Williams and Wilkins; 2003.
8. Milic-Emili J, Robatto FM, Bates JH. Respiratory mechanics in anesthesia. Br J Anaesth. 1990;65(1):4-12.
9. Weinberger SE, Drazen JM. Disturbances of respiratory function. In: Kasper DL, Braunwald E, Fauci AS, Hauser SL, Longo DL, Jameson JL (Eds). Harrison's Principles of Internal Medicine, 16th edition. New Delhi: McGraw Hill Medical Publishing Division; 2005. pp. 1498-505.
10. West JB. Ventilation-perfusion inequality and overall gas exchange in computer models of the lung. Respir Physiol. 1969;7(1):88-110.

Gas and Fluid Exchange in the Lung

Marc Zelter

GAS EXCHANGE

The oxygen needed by cell mitochondria for tissue respiration is extracted from atmospheric air by a succession of processes[1] including external ventilation between the lung and the air, gas distribution and gas exchange in the lung, transport of oxygen by blood and transfer to the tissues **(Fig. 1)**. Carbon dioxide, one of the two main by-products of tissue respiration, the other one being water, follows the reverse pathway. The flow process is possible because the partial pressure of oxygen decreases from one step to the next, creating the physical conditions necessary for the transfer of gas from the lung to the cell **(Fig. 2)**. The series of steps or pressure changes in oxygen from one step to the next are not even. Each of the steps involved can be characterized by what is called its conductance, defined as the maximum quantity of oxygen that can be transferred from one step to the next per unit of time and per unit of oxygen partial pressure difference. The actual mechanisms by which oxygen follows these steps may also vary from one step to the next: forced convection between atmosphere and alveoli, passive diffusion across the alveolar wall and in plasma, diffusion between plasma and intracellular red cells and then reversible chemical bondage to hemoglobin, forced convection from the lung to tissues via the systemic circulation and passive diffusion from red cells to the tissue interstitium and then by diffusion to tissue cells and mitochondria. The oxygen that has not been extracted by tissues follows the reverse pathway back to the lungs. Two of these steps require energy expenditure: ventilation and circulation.

The amount of oxygen reaching the tissues per unit of time is always superior to the oxygen consumption of these tissues so that in all circumstances there is a backflow of oxygen from the tissues to the lung. The actual oxygen consumption by the tissues is therefore the difference between the flow of oxygen from the lung to the tissues and the flow of oxygen back to the pulmonary artery from the tissues. In stable conditions, this difference is equal to the difference between the flow

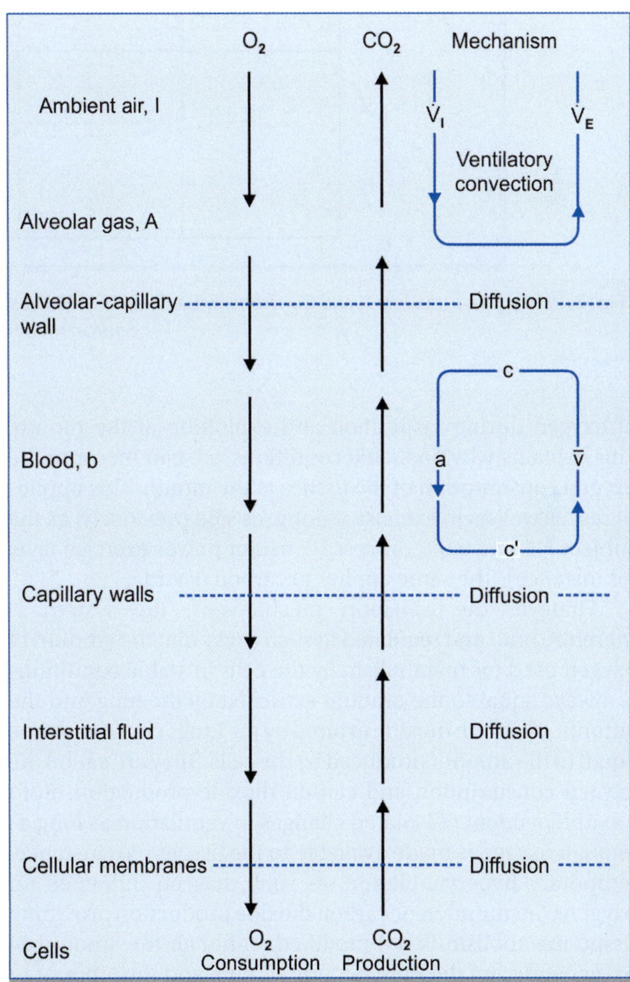

Fig. 1 Schematic representation of the steps and mechanisms of gas exchange from air to tissues

Source: Modified from Dejours[1].

Abbreviations: V_I, inspiratory flow; V_E, expiratory flow; a, arterial; c, capillary; v, mixed venous; c′ end-capillary blood

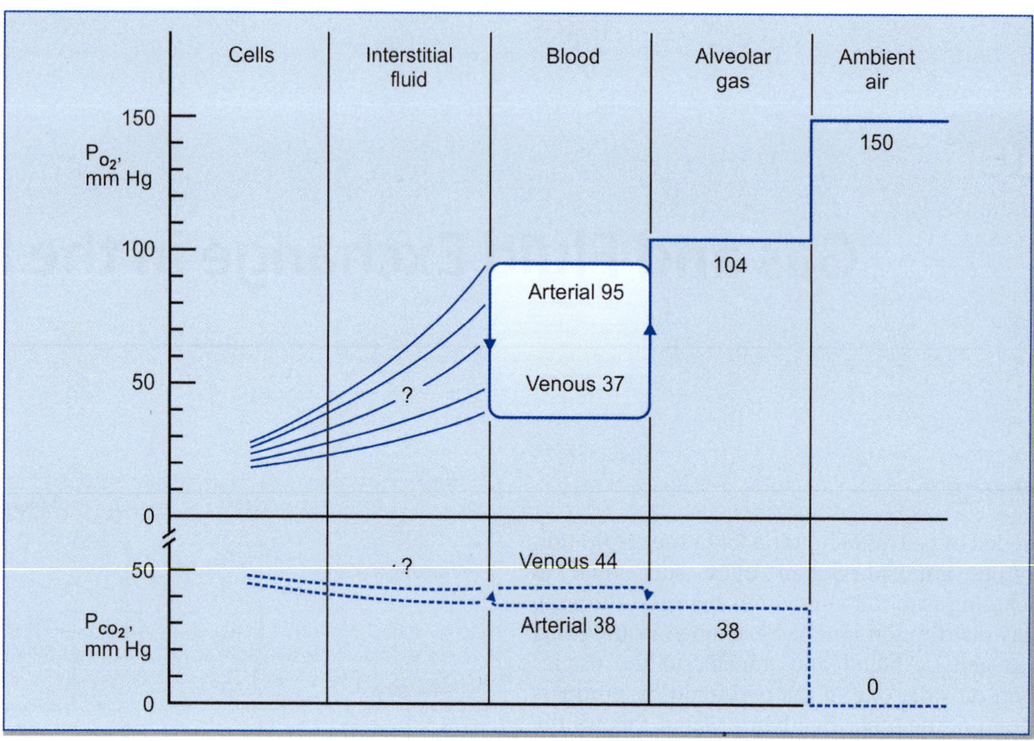

Fig. 2 Partial pressures for O_2 and CO_2 from ambient air to cells. Pressures in the interstitial fluid and in cells are still to be determined reliably *Source*: Modified from Dejours[1].

of oxygen during inspiration and expiration at the mouth. This explains why, in stable conditions, we can measure the oxygen consumption of the tissues at the mouth. This applies to rest as well as to exercise as long, as said previously, as the subject is in a stable process (constant power exercise level for instance). The same applies to carbon dioxide.

Whatever the transport mechanisms, the system is therefore built and regulated in such a way that the amount of oxygen used for metabolism by the cells in stable conditions is always equal to the amount extracted by the lung and the amount of carbon dioxide expired by the lungs per unit of time equal to the amount produced by the cells. They are called the oxygen consumption and carbon dioxide production. Both are independent of isolated changes in ventilation as long as enough oxygen is made available to the tissues. For instance, temporary hyperventilation, as such, has no influence on oxygen consumption or carbon dioxide production providing tissue metabolism is not modified, although the amount of oxygen entering the lung per unit of time and the amount of carbon dioxide leaving the lung per unit of time are higher than during normal ventilation. As suggested above, the amount of oxygen that enters the lung and is contained in the inspired air per unit time (the oxygen intake) is always larger than the amount transferred from the alveoli to the blood (the oxygen consumption). What is left is expired during the next breath. The same does not apply to carbon dioxide, as there is no carbon dioxide in the inspired air so that the amount expired per unit of time is that actually produced at tissue level, providing conditions have remained stable. The same reasoning applies to both gases in the blood: the amount of oxygen present in the blood at the output of the lung is higher than what is needed by the tissues but the tissues extract only what correspond to their consumption so that the quantity extracted from the blood by the tissues is equal to what has been extracted from the alveoli by the blood. What remains is brought back to the pulmonary artery, which is the lung input. The volume of carbon dioxide leaving the blood via the alveoli in the lung is equal to the carbon dioxide produced in the tissues, which is always less than what is transported by the pulmonary artery so that there is always carbon dioxide left in the oxygenated blood leaving the lung via the pulmonary veins. The design of the system is such that the amount of oxygen present at the output of the lung is almost always maximum in a normal individual. The concentration of oxygen in the blood leaving the lung is therefore fixed and independent of oxygen consumption. It is called the arterial blood oxygen concentration (CaO_2), as it is the concentration of oxygen reaching the systemic arteries. The amount of oxygen actually present in the arterial blood is routinely evaluated by measuring the partial pressure of oxygen (PaO_2) rather than the actual concentration because concentration cannot be measured simply; this pressure is a precious index of the ability of the lung to saturate the blood in oxygen. It is also a good index that blood can carry enough oxygen to the tissues, presuming that hemoglobin concentration in the blood and blood flow are adequate. The amount of oxygen transported by the blood cannot be assessed correctly unless we make sure the hemoglobin concentration has been measured. Saturation of blood in oxygen is defined as the ratio of oxyhemoglobin to total hemoglobin concentration. In practice, if hemoglobin concentration is normal, saturation may be computed from the oxygen pressure in blood. It is normally above 98%. If concentration is not known than saturation needs to be measured. It is imperative to state if the value has been measured or calculated. In other words we need to make sure that pressure of oxygen, saturation of hemoglobin in oxygen and hemoglobin concentration are normal before we can say that oxygen transport from the lung is normal.

INSPIRED GAS

Inspired gas is best described in terms of pressure and composition. Gas is inspired at barometric pressure P_B. At sea level pressure is about 760 mm Hg (100 kPa); it diminishes with altitude and rises during diving or during hyperbaric treatment. Inspired gas contains essentially atmospheric air, a defined chemical mixture of oxygen (21%) and nitrogen (79%) with no carbon dioxide, plus a variable amount of water vapor. Atmospheric air composition does not change with barometric pressure. Its composition remains the same at altitude and at sea level. What varies is the pressure at which it is inhaled. Composition of air may be expressed in terms of fractions of gas mixture: a fraction (F) is the percentage of one of the components in the mixture ($FO_2 = 0.21$ for oxygen). It may be expressed as partial pressure. Partial pressure is the fraction of total pressure due to each component of the gas mixture: $PO_2 = 0.21 \times P_B = 160$ mm Hg for dry air. Pressure of water vapor in the atmosphere varies with meteorological conditions. Once inspired atmospheric gas is immediately heated up to body temperature (37°C) and saturated with water vapor in the trachea. Therefore the actual inhaled gas mixture consists of dry air and water vapor. Physical laws determine the maximum amount of water vapor that can mix with air at 37°C without condensation; it depends only on temperature. The saturated water partial pressure at body temperature is 47 mm Hg. Barometric pressure being unchanged, the saturated partial pressure of water vapor being 47 mm Hg, the partial pressure of air in the inhaled mixture is P_B-47 = 713 mm Hg and consequently $P_IO_2 = 0.21 \times 713 = 150$ mm Hg.

EXPIRED GAS

After having lost oxygen to the blood and gained carbon dioxide from the blood, gas is expired from the alveoli. Because each molecule of oxygen consumed is not necessarily replaced by one molecule of carbon dioxide produced, the number of molecules expired per unit time and volume may vary with the $\dot{V}CO_2/\dot{V}O_2$ ratio, called the respiratory quotient (R). This quotient is a function of the nutriments burned by the tissues. R = 1 when the diet consists only of carbohydrates, 0.7 of lipids and 0.8 of proteins. The average value is 0.84 for a standard diet. Therefore for each mole of oxygen consumed, only 0.84 mole of carbon dioxide is produced so that fewer molecules are present in the expired gas compared to the inspired gas. This represents a change of fraction of 0.03 and is generally neglected unless focus is on metabolic exchange or oxygen consumption. Therefore although expired gas flow $\dot{V}_E$ is lower than inspired gas flow V_I they are considered equal in routine measurements.

The composition of expired gas depends on the composition of inspired gas, normally dry air and water vapor, but it may change if the subject is given oxygen therapy, or with metabolic activity ($\dot{V}O_2$), with R if diet changes, and on ventilation. Ventilation V_T is the flow produced by the action of the respiratory muscles on the thoracic cage and therefore on the lung. The flow is the product of the volume of each inspiration, also called the tidal volume V_T, by the number of expirations per unit of time, the ventilatory frequency f: $\dot{V}_T = V_T \times f$.

DEAD SPACE AND ALVEOLAR GAS

Gas exchange between inspired gas and blood occurs at the alveolar level so that gas has to be transported from the mouth to the alveoli by conducting airways. Conducting airways do not participate in gas exchange. They are part of what is called the dead space, V_D. V_D volume is around 150 mL. Functionally the lung is therefore separated in a compartment the dead space, that does not participate in gas exchange but drives gas to where exchange occurs, and a compartment that participates to gas exchange called the alveolar volume V_A. V_D and V_A are disposed in series. These definitions are physiological and do not strictly correspond to any precise anatomical volume: indeed the conducting airways are part of V_D but that is also true of part of the anatomical alveolar volume, because only a fraction of the anatomical alveoli participate to gas exchange at a given time. Consequently V_A is always smaller than the anatomical alveolar volume. The fraction of inspired gas flow that truly contributes to gas exchange is the flow that ventilates the functional part of the alveolar volume and is called alveolar ventilation ($\dot{V}_A$). It is the useful part of V_T. The inspired flow $\dot{V}_T$ is the sum of $\dot{V}_D$ and $\dot{V}_A$. The end result is that during each cycle, of the 450 mL of tidal volume 150 mL serve to ventilate dead space and only 300 mL participate in the exchange process. The composition of inspired gas does not change during inspiration. The composition of expired gas varies in time during expiration. First the volume of gas contained in the dead space is expired. It is the gas that was inspired at the end of the previous inspiration and because it has remained in the dead space

Table 1 Normal values of pressures in inspired, expired, alveolar gas and in blood (mm Hg)

	I	*E*	*A*	*a*	*v*
P_{CO_2}	0	26	39	39	44
P_{O_2}	150	118	102	91	38
P_{N_2}	563	569	572	572	572
P_{H_2O}	47	47	47	47	47
P total	760	760	760	749	701

it did not participate in gas exchange: its composition is that of inspired gas. Then a mixture of inspired gas and alveolar gas and finally pure alveolar gas are successively expired. Alveolar gas composition can be reasonably approximated in a normal subject by sampling either end tidal gas (gas at the end of a normal expiration) or better yet the end forced expiratory gas.

The normal values for inspired, expired and alveolar gas are given in **Table 1**.

Ventilation equations can be computed from what is called the mono-compartment alveolar model. The model consists in a fully functional monoalveolar lung and a single dead space.[2]

The equations are:

1. $\dot{V}_A = \{0.863 \times \dot{V}O_2 [1 - F_IO_2 (1 - R)]\}/(P_IO_2 - P_AO_2)$
2. $\dot{V}_A = (0.863 \times R \times \dot{V}CO_2)/P_ACO_2$

(The 0.863 constant results from correcting volumes and flows for pressure and temperature conditions).

Equation 2 shows that alveolar ventilation at a given metabolic rate is uniquely function of PCO_2 in normal circumstances and therefore that PCO_2 and not PO_2 is the regulating factor of ventilation.[3]

TRANSFER OF GAS ACROSS THE ALVEOLAR CAPILLARY MEMBRANE

Gases pass through the complex structure of the alveolar membrane consisting of the alveolar epithelium lined by lipoproteins, the epithelial basal membrane, the interstitium, the endothelial basal membrane and the capillary endothelium to reach plasma. Gas enter the membrane by dissolving almost instantaneously either in the lipid layer or directly in the aqueous components of the cells in proportion of its solubility which varies from very low for helium to high values for diethyl-ether which are at the extremes of the scope of gases utilized in respiratory studies. For a given partial pressure a soluble gas reaches a higher concentration at the surface within the alveolar cell than a less soluble one. The rate of diffusion will therefore be greater. The site of gas exchange within the lung is difficult to define anatomically but is confined to that part of the alveolar membrane bounded by ventilated alveoli and on the other side by microvessels that contain blood and which is believed to represent half of the alveolar membrane surface.

Other factors that contribute to gas exchange, apart from solubility and surface area, are molecular weight and thickness of the membrane and indeed the difference of partial pressures across the membrane.[4]

The overall transfer rate is:

$$Dm = k\,[(A/d \times s)/\sqrt{M}]$$

Where D is the transfer rate of the gas in volume per unit of pressure gradient per unit of time, K the diffusion coefficient in cm^2 per unit time, A the surface area, d the membrane thickness in cm, s the solubility of the gas in volume/volume per unit gas partial pressure and M the molecular weight of the gas. Dm is generally called the diffusing capacity of the gas across the membrane.

In fact, to achieve the transfer from alveoli to blood in the case of oxygen and in part for carbon dioxide, the gas after crossing the membrane and reaching the plasma must diffuse from plasma to erythrocytes and then combine chemically with hemoglobin. The gas crosses the erythrocyte membrane by facilitated diffusion due to the migration of hemoglobin molecules between the surface area and the interior of the cells. The reversible reaction by which gas combines to hemoglobin is not instantaneous and the amount of gas bound will depend on the hemoglobin concentration. The overall rate is the product of the reaction rate, the driving pressure, the volume of blood and the blood flow in the microvessels. The transfer rate for the gas from plasma to hemoglobin can be approximated from a complex equation to:

$$D' = \beta Q + \theta Vc$$

Where β is the capacitance coefficient in mmol per L of blood per unit of pressure at 37°C, θ the rate of the chemical combination, Vc the capillary volume.

Because Dm and D' have the dimension of a flow rate per unit of pressure their inverse have the dimension of a resistance so the total resistance offered against the flow of gas from the alveoli to hemoglobin is the sum of the resistance from the alveoli to plasma and from plasma to hemoglobin:

$$1/T_L = 1/Dm + 1/(\beta Q + \theta Vc)$$

T_L is called the transfer factor of the lung. The rate at which the gas leaves the plasma to combine with hemoglobin is fast compared to the rate at which it dissolves in circulating blood for carbon monoxide and nitric oxide and to a lesser extent for oxygen so that βQ can be neglected so:

$$1/T_L = 1/Dm + 1/\theta Vc$$

The transfer factor is often called the diffusing capacity but as demonstrated it incorporates resistive terms related not only to diffusion but also to chemical bonding, expressing the complexity of the transfer of oxygen from the alveoli to the blood. The speed at which the bonding of oxygen to hemoglobin occurs is relatively fast compared to the time it takes for an erythrocyte to cross the lung, so that it is not a limiting factor in the transfer of oxygen from alveoli to capillaries, at least until blood flow is very high.[5]

The physical properties of oxygen and carbon monoxide in terms of diffusion are not very different. The plasma concentration of CO remains negligible when a small quantity is breathed because of the high affinity of CO for hemoglobin so that the measurement of TLCO is easy and a good approximation of the oxygen transfer factor.[6]

GAS TRANSPORT TO AND FROM THE PERIPHERY

Oxygen Transport by the Blood

The relationship between cardiac output ($\dot{Q}$), arterial and mixed venous concentrations of oxygen in blood and oxygen consumption is:

$$\dot{V}O_2 = \dot{Q}\,(CaO_2\text{-}CvO_2).$$

The mixed venous concentration (CvO_2) is the concentration of oxygen in the pulmonary artery, just before cardiac output enters the lung, where all venous bloods from the various organs mix together. This equation states that the amount of oxygen consumed by the tissues is the difference between the total amount of oxygen brought to them by cardiac output from the lung ($\dot{Q} \times CaO_2$) and the amount that is left over and brought back to the lung by cardiac output ($\dot{Q} \times CvO_2$). As stated before, in a normal subject CaO_2 always reaches its maximum value after lung oxygenation and does not depends on the subject activity unless in extreme situations. Venous blood concentration depends on the organ activity. It varies from one organ to the other.[7,8]

Oxygen is carried in the blood in two forms, dissolved (1.5%) and combined to hemoglobin (98.5%). The amount of oxygen dissolved in the blood obeys Henry's law for dissolution of gas into liquids. It is proportional to partial pressure but the dissolution coefficient for oxygen being very low the amount of oxygen that can be transported per unit of volume of blood and per unit of time is very limited (0.3 mL/100 mL of blood). It is inadequate to cover metabolic needs. This amount rises to 2 mL/100 mL when breathing pure oxygen. The essential mechanism of oxygen transport is chemical reversible bondage to hemoglobin. The total amount of oxygen present in the blood is the sum of the dissolved and combined oxygen concentration **(Table 2)**. Dissolved oxygen is usually neglected in most calculations but dissolved oxygen is the form that allows oxygen to be transferred from erythrocytes to mitochondria in organs. It is also the physical state allowing the measure of PaO_2 by electrochemical methods.

Normal adult hemoglobin (Hemoglobin A) is a conjugated protein consisting of four polypeptide chains (globins) and of an iron porphyrin compound (heme). Oxygen binds to the heme in various successive stages, up to 4 molecules of oxygen per heme. These stages explain the sigmoid shape of the relationship between PaO_2 and oxygen concentration. A small percentage of total circulating hemoglobin is not functional because it is under the form of methemoglobin (MetHb) or because some carboxyhemoglobin has been formed in the presence of traces of carbon monoxide (HbCO). The normal concentration of hemoglobin is 9 mmol/L, equivalent to 14.6 g/100 mL, and can carry up to 20 mL of oxygen per 100 mL of blood (1.39 mL/g if only functional hemoglobin is considered, 1.36 mL if total hemoglobin is considered). The maximum volume of oxygen that can be carried by 100 mL of blood is called the total oxygen capacity. The concentration of oxygen in the blood is usually given in mL of oxygen per 100 mL of blood or in mmol/L. It is called the oxygen content. The O_2 saturation is defined as the ratio of O_2 combined with hemoglobin (oxyhemoglobin) to O_2 capacity. Normal arterial saturation is 97.5% for a PO_2 of 100 mm Hg at normal temperature and H^+ concentration. Normal mixed venous blood saturation is around 75% for a PO_2 of 40 mm Hg. Because of the sigmoid shape of the concentration and saturation curves **(Fig. 3)** there is no simple relationship between saturation, content and oxygen partial pressure; for example doubling pressure does not double saturation. The shape of the curve is beneficial to physiological functions. Because the curve is almost flat in its upper part a fairly large variation of PAO_2 will not change much the loading of oxygen. The difference in oxygen pressure between blood and alveoli will remain high all along pulmonary capillaries facilitating rapid diffusion of oxygen between alveoli and erythrocytes. Conversely because the lower part of the curve is steep a small drop in pressure will ensure a large flow of oxygen from the erythrocytes to the capillaries and then to tissues.

The affinity for oxygen of the hemoglobin molecule is modified when its stereo chemical conformation changes which happens for example when $[H^+]$ or PCO_2 changes or when another gas or molecule (carbon monoxide for example) can compete with the O_2 receptor sites.

Table 2 Normal partial pressures and concentrations of oxygen and carbon dioxide in blood

Oxygen		*a*	*v*	*(a–v)*
PO_2	mm Hg	91	38	
Dissolved	mmol/L	0.12	0.005	+0.07
HbO_2	mmol/L	8.60	6.01	+2.59
Total	mmol/L	8.72	6.01	+2.66
Carbon dioxide		*a*	*v*	*(a–v)*
PCO_2	mm Hg	39	44	
Dissolved	mmol/L	1.19	1.37	–0.18
HCO_3^-	mmol/L	19.60	20.96	–1.36
$HbCO_2$	mmol/L	1.09	1.72	–0.63
Total	mmol/L	21.88	24.05	–2.17

Abbreviations: a, arterial blood; v, mixed venous blood; (a–v), arterio–venous difference

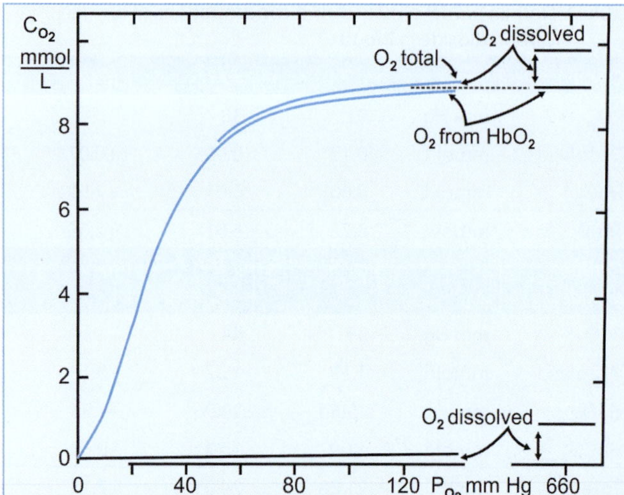

Fig. 3 Dissociation curve for oxygen and total oxygen content (CO_2): Total content of oxygen is the sum of oxygen dissolved in plasma and of oxygen combined to blood hemoglobin. Dissolved oxygen is low at atmospheric pressure breathing ambient air but can rise significantly if ambient pressure (hyperbaric condition) or oxygen fraction is raised (breathing gas with a high oxygen fraction). Content can be given in mL oxygen/100 mL of blood or mmol/L (see Table 2)

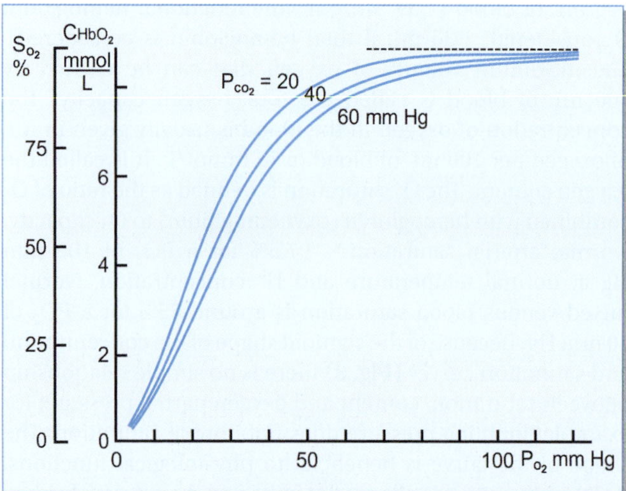

Fig. 4 Dissociation curve for oxygen for different PCO_2 in blood: Note that an increase in PCO_2 induces a shift to the right of curve. For the same PO_2 value less oxygen can be combined to hemoglobin. The process facilitates release of oxygen to the tissues as metabolism induces a rise of local PCO_2. Note that when hemoglobin concentration is known the curve is the same for saturation and content

The hemoglobin dissociation curve is shifted to the right by a rise in $[H^+]$, of temperature and of PCO_2 **(Fig. 4)**. This means that under these circumstances hemoglobin combine with less oxygen and can release more of the oxygen that was already fixed. This facilitates the release of oxygen in organs where metabolism raises temperature, PCO_2 and $[H^+]$. Organic phosphates present in the erythrocytes (2,3-diphosphoglycerate, DPG) also facilitate the release of oxygen when their concentration rises as seen in chronic hypoxia (altitude). A useful indicator of the position of the inflexion point of the dissociation curve is the value of P_{50}, the oxygen pressure at which saturation is 50%. The normal value is 26 mm Hg. It is elevated when the dissociation curve is shifted to the left, i.e. when hemoglobin can combine to more oxygen per gram and falls when it can combine to less (right shift).

Oxygen reaches mitochondria by passive convection and diffusion from the plasma. The PO_2 at tissue level and in mitochondria is very low but oxygen flow is high. Mitochondrial respiration does not stop until oxygen pressure is at extremely low levels.

The stores of oxygen in the body are very limited, in the form of combined oxygen in the blood (HbO_2) and of MbO_2 in muscles. They amount to 900 µMol/kg of body mass in a normal 70 kg man at rest. These stores allow only a few minutes of survival.

TRANSPORT OF CO_2 BY THE BLOOD

The blood transports carbon dioxide under three forms: dissolved, in bicarbonate form, in combination with proteins **(Table 2)**.

Because the solubility of CO_2 is 20 times higher that of oxygen, the amount of dissolved CO_2 is more significant in terms of transport (5% in arterial blood versus 90% for bicarbonates and 5% for proteins).

CO_2 can be transformed in bicarbonate by the following reaction:

$$CO_2 + H_2O \overset{\text{CARBONIC ANHYDRASE}}{\leftrightarrows} H_2CO_3 \leftrightarrows H^+ + HCO_3^-$$

The speed of transformation of dissolved CO_2 into carbonic acid is very slow in plasma but greatly facilitated by a specific enzyme, carbonic anhydrase, in erythrocytes. The ionization of carbonic acid occurs quickly and is spontaneously reversible. When bicarbonate concentration increases in the cell, the bicarbonate ion diffuses freely from the erythrocytes to plasma but H^+ cannot, because the membrane is little permeable to cations. Chloride ions (Cl^-) move from plasma membrane into the erythrocytes to maintain electrical neutrality in the cells, according to the Gibbs-Donnan equation.

A significant part of the free H^+ can bind to hemoglobin releasing oxygen:

$$H^+ + HbO_2 \leftrightarrows H\text{-}Hb + O_2$$

This facilitates as said previously the release of oxygen and the uptake of CO_2 in the tissue capillaries. The facilitation of CO_2 uptake by release of oxygen in the tissues is called the Haldane effect. The symmetrical facilitation of O_2 uptake by release of CO_2 in the lung is called the Bohr effect.[9]

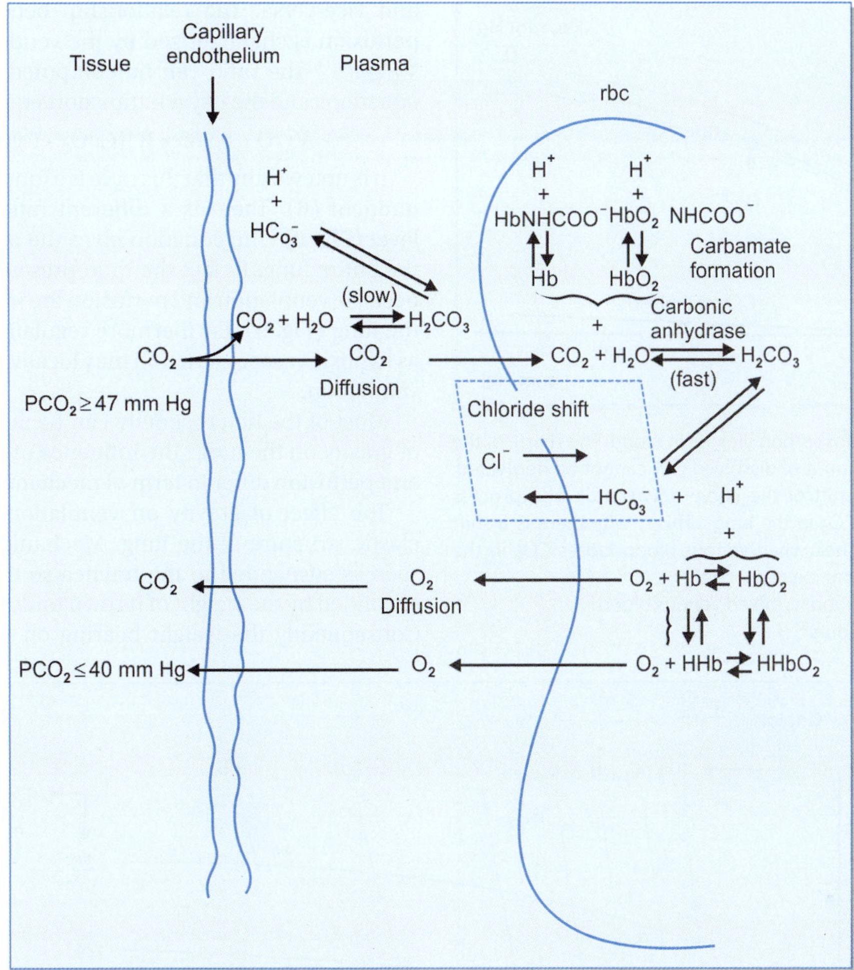

Fig. 5 Transport mechanisms for oxygen and carbon dioxide between erythrocytes and tissue (see text for explanations)

CO_2 can combine with the terminal amine groups of some blood proteins and in particular with the globins of hemoglobin forming carbamino-proteins and more specifically carbamino-hemoglobin **(Fig. 5)**. This reaction again facilitates the release of O_2 in the tissues **(Fig. 6)**.

Altogether, dissolved CO_2 constitutes 10% of the venous-arteriolar difference for CO_2 against 30% for carbamino-proteins and 60% for bicarbonate.

The dissociation curve for CO_2 differs markedly from the dissociation curves for oxygen. It is steeper than the oxygen dissociation curve for oxygen, especially in the 40–50 mm Hg range where CO_2 content varies as much as 4.7 mL/100 mL against 1.7 mL/100 mL for oxygen **(Fig. 6)**.

As stated before CO_2 content increases when the oxygen saturation of hemoglobin decreases, facilitating gas exchange at tissue level. The opposite occurs at lung level. Because of these interactions the gas contents cannot be proportional to partial pressure. This is figured when O_2 and CO_2 dissociation curves are plotted together on a PCO_2 versus PO_2 diagram (Rahn diagram)[2]: the lines of equal O_2 pressure and equal CO_2 pressure (isopleths) are neither straight nor parallel to the axes **(Fig. 7)**.

The stores of carbon dioxide in the body are very large because of the high capacitance of all tissues, including bone. CO_2 is stored mainly in the form of bicarbonates and carbamino compounds. They amount to more than 10.000 μMol/kg of body mass in a normal 70 kg man at rest. These stores change slowly except in the blood and soft tissues so that they can quickly compensate for hypo- or hypercapnia.

VENTILATION PERFUSION RATIO

The global efficacy of the lung exchanger depends strongly on the adequacy between alveolar ventilation and capillary blood flow, ensuring that ventilated zones are well perfused,

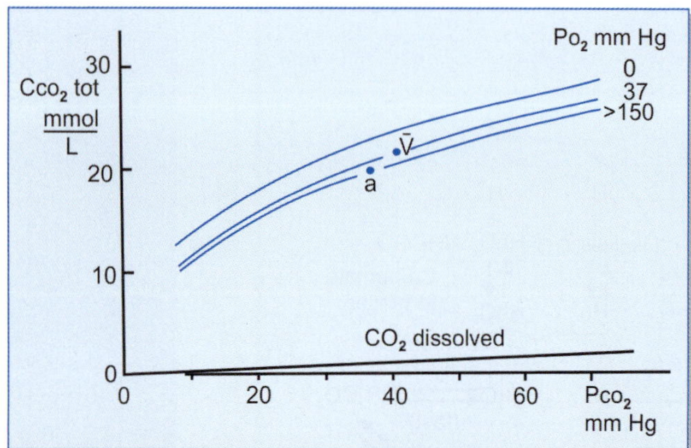

Fig. 6 Dissociation curve for carbon dioxide in blood. The shape of the curve is quite flat. The amount of dissolved CO_2 cannot be neglected. A rise in PO_2 induces a shift of the curve downwards. The process facilitates the release of CO_2 in the lungs. This is why there is a shift from one curve to the other, when venous blood looses CO_2 in the lung capillaries and takes up oxygen

Abbreviations: a, arterial blood; v, mixed venous blood.

Source: Modified from Dejours[9].

and vice-versa. The relationship between ventilation and perfusion is characterized by the ventilation-perfusion ratio $\dot{V}_A/\dot{Q}$.[10,11] The ratio can be computed from the ventilation equations and the oxygen transport equation in the blood:[12]

$$\dot{V}_A/\dot{Q} = 0.963 \times R\,[(CaO_2 - CvO_2)/P_ACO_2]$$

It is noteworthy that this ratio is a function of the respiratory quotient (R). There is a different ratio for each metabolic level **(Fig. 8)**. The equation gives the average ratio value for the entire lung. In fact the ratio presents regional variations because ventilation and perfusion are inhomogeneous within the lung **(Fig. 9)**. Furthermore regulation mechanisms such as hypoxic vasoconstriction may locally modify perfusion and ventilation.

Most of the heterogeneity can be attributed to the effects of gravity on the lung. The influence of gravity on ventilation and perfusion differ in term of mechanism and amplitude.

The effect of gravity on ventilation is secondary to the elastic structure of the lung. Mechanically the lung can be seen as suspended to the trachea so that at each level, it is expanded by the weight of its own underlying levels **(Fig. 10)**. Consequently the weight bearing on one level is inversely

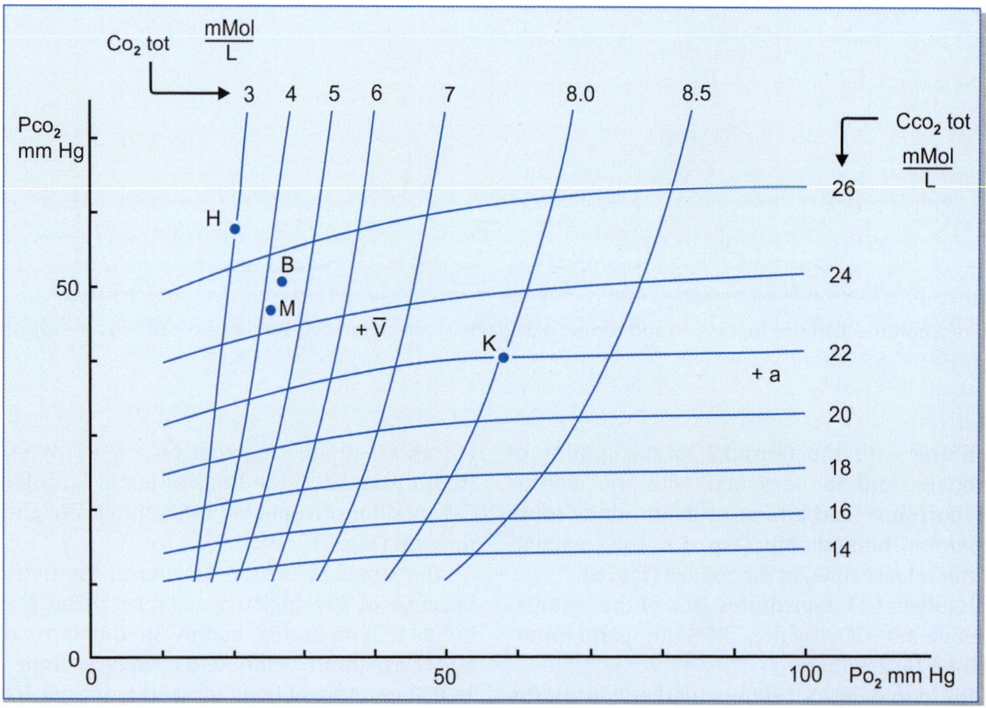

Fig. 7 The PO_2-PCO_2 diagram combines the dissociation curves for both gases. The lines represent the isopleths, the pressure curves for one gas at a given concentration of the other one. If there were no interactions between the two gases, all curves for one gas would be flat and parallel to the axis. The changes of partial pressures and of concentrations for both gases can be read on a single diagram when going from arterial to venous blood.

The difference in value between the organs venous bloods reflects the different oxygen consumption of each organ and therefore the different desaturation they produce in arterial blood to produce their corresponding venous blood, because of the various amount of oxygen teach organ extract from the same arterial blood at the input. The different venous bloods from all the different organs mix when reaching the right heart and pulmonary artery where they mix together to form mixed venous blood $\bar{v}$ which enter the lung

Source: Modified from Rahn et al[2].

Abbreviations: a; arterial blood; $\bar{v}$, mixed venous blood; H, coronary; B, brain; M, skeletal muscle; K, kidney venous bloods

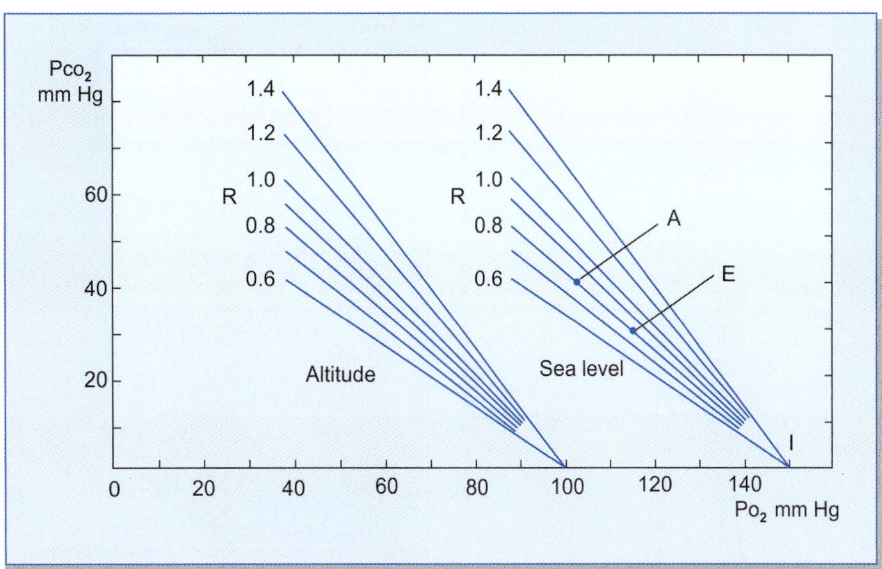

Fig. 8 Representations of R (respiratory quotient, see text for definition) lines on the PO_2-PCO_2 diagram. On the right: set of R lines at sea level (PO_2 = 150 mm Hg). On the left: set of R lines at altitude (PO_2 = 100 mm Hg). For each metabolic level represented by the ratio of CO_2 production to O_2 consumption R, possible values of PO_2 and PCO_2 are coupled and must be on the corresponding R line. For each PO_2 value there is only one possible PCO_2 value. The slope of the relationship is not modified by a change in pressure in ambient air, for example by altitude (in this example 3000 m, P_B = 526 mm Hg). R varies in physiologic conditions from 0.7 to 1 in stable conditions. When R >1 it can be inferred that the subject is in unstable or transitional condition

Abbreviations: A, alveolar; E, expiratory; I, inspiratory gas.

Source: Modified from Dejours[1].

proportional to that level and distension increases from bottom to top so that the size of alveoli increases from bottom to top. Because of the relationship between pulmonary volume and transpulmonary pressure, compliance will be lower at the apex compared to bottom so that for a given change of transpulmonary pressure during the ventilatory cycle, ventilation will be higher at the bottom compared to the apex. Alveolar ventilation increases from top to bottom.

The effect of gravity on perfusion is due to the increase in hydrostatic pressure from top to bottom within the elastic vessels of the lung that is not compensated on the external side because they are exposed on that side to the atmospheric pressure of the alveoli instead of a water column that would compensate for hydrostatic pressure at each level as this is the case in the systemic vessels. The rise in internal hydrostatic pressure results in an increase in transmural pressure so that vessel section rises and perfusion follows. Alveolar perfusion increases from top to bottom.

Although both ventilation and perfusion increase linearly from top to bottom the increase in ventilation is not proportional to that of circulation. The resulting relationship of the ratio to height is curvilinear **(Fig. 11A)**. In theory $\dot{V}_A/\dot{Q}$ may vary from zero (a perfused zone with no ventilation) to infinity (a ventilated zone with no perfusion) **(Fig. 12)**. The average lung value is 0.84.

For a given ventilation-perfusion ratio there is one and only one possible quantitative relationship between P_AO_2 and P_ACO_2 and thus between P_aO_2 and P_aCO_2. In other words for any given P_AO_2 or P_ACO_2 there is only one possible P_aCO_2 or P_aO_2. The possible paired values can be represented as a distribution curve on a PO_2-PCO_2 diagram **(Fig. 11B)**. Each level of the lung has its own $V_A/\dot{Q}$ value so that the $\dot{V}_A/\dot{Q}$ of a given level correspond to a specific paired value **(Fig. 13)**.

The range of variation of PO_2 is almost of 40 mm Hg against only 14 mm Hg for CO_2. This asymmetrical nature of the distribution curve is a consequence of the very different relationship between pressure and concentration for each gas, relatively flat for CO_2 but sigmoid for O_2 but also of the predominating role of PCO_2 in the regulation of ventilation. The largest variations of the $\dot{V}_A/\dot{Q}$ ratio are observed in the upper regions of lung. This is mostly due to the fall of local perfusion in these regions. $\dot{V}_A/\dot{Q}$ gets below its average value when going toward the bottom of the lung; the P_ACO_2-P_AO_2 diagram shows little changes in P_ACO_2 but an important drop in P_AO_2. $\dot{V}_A/\dot{Q}$ gets above 0.84 when going toward the apex; P_ACO_2 tends very quickly to very low values while PO_2 almost reaches inspired air O_2 partial pressure. Consequently the PaO_2 of blood is higher and the $PaCO_2$ lower at the apex compared to the bottom, meaning that blood oxygenation is more efficient at the apex. However because in proportion

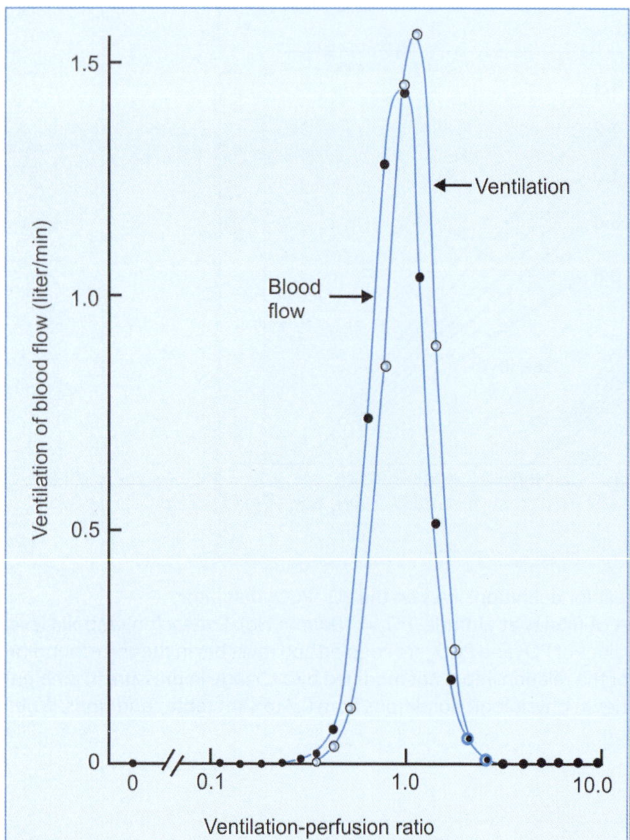

Fig. 9 Distribution of blood flow and ventilation in function of $\dot{V}_A/\dot{Q}$ in a normal young: subject: note that the horizontal scale is logarithmic. Both distributions are positioned at about a ratio close to 1 but are not superimposed

Source: Modified from Wagner et al[11].

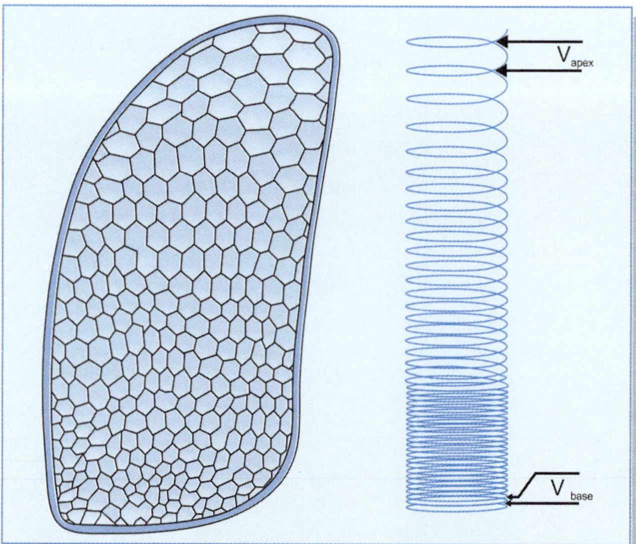

Fig. 10 Because the lung behaves like a suspended elastic structure the weight bearing on any level is that of the structure below it and therefore increases from base to apex. The resulting structure of the lung is pretty much that of a suspended spring. Distension increases from base to apex and so does the volume of the alveoli

most perfusion and ventilation take place toward the base, most of the alveolocapillary exchange is located there although it is less efficient.

GAS EXCHANGE AND [H+]

The relationship between PCO_2, HCO_3^- and $[H^+]$ implies a close relationship between these parameters and ventilation. In fact the role of ventilation on pH regulation in the organism is essential. The physiology of gas exchange cannot be fully understood unless acid-base status is known.

The end results of ventilation and blood-gas exchange can be shown on the P_AO_2-P_ACO_2 diagram on which can be super imposed the O_2 and CO_2 dissociation curves, the $\dot{V}_A/\dot{Q}$ ratio values and the R lines **(Fig. 14)**. The figure shows that when two only of these values are known all others are fixed. For example for a given R and a given inspired PO_2 there is only one possible combination of $\dot{V}_A/\dot{Q}$, P_ACO_2, P_AO_2, and R.[2]

FLUID, SOLUTES AND PROTEIN EXCHANGE IN THE LUNG

An average of 300,000 mL of blood flows per hour through the microvessels of a human lung and 299,990 reach the pulmonary venous system.[13] Although pulmonary vascular pressure is maintained at a low level, which permits high flow at low resistance, the large endothelial surface area still forms an imperfect barrier leaking water, small molecules and even proteins in all circumstances. There is therefore a permanent albeit limited outflow flux of around 10 mL per hour of fluid and proteins toward the lung interstitium **(Fig. 15)**. The lymphatic vessels due to the respiratory movements can drain this flow from the interstitium. Normally fluid is prevented to reach the alveoli from the interstitium because of the very low permeability to fluid of the alveolar barrier and because the lymphatic ducts can generally handle excess fluid, up to at least 10 times the normal value, so that fluid does not accumulate in the lung interstitium or over flood in the alveoli.[14]

The liquid and protein exchange in the lung are not confined to the alveolar wall capillaries but also occurs in the extra-alveolar lung capillaries[15] and across arterioles and venules up to two generations up or down from the capillary level **(Fig. 16)**.

The liquid draining from the alveolar wall to the extra-alveolar connective tissue space does so by a direct route via the alveolar wall junctions. The initial lymphatics are situated in the adventitia of the small extra-alveolar small

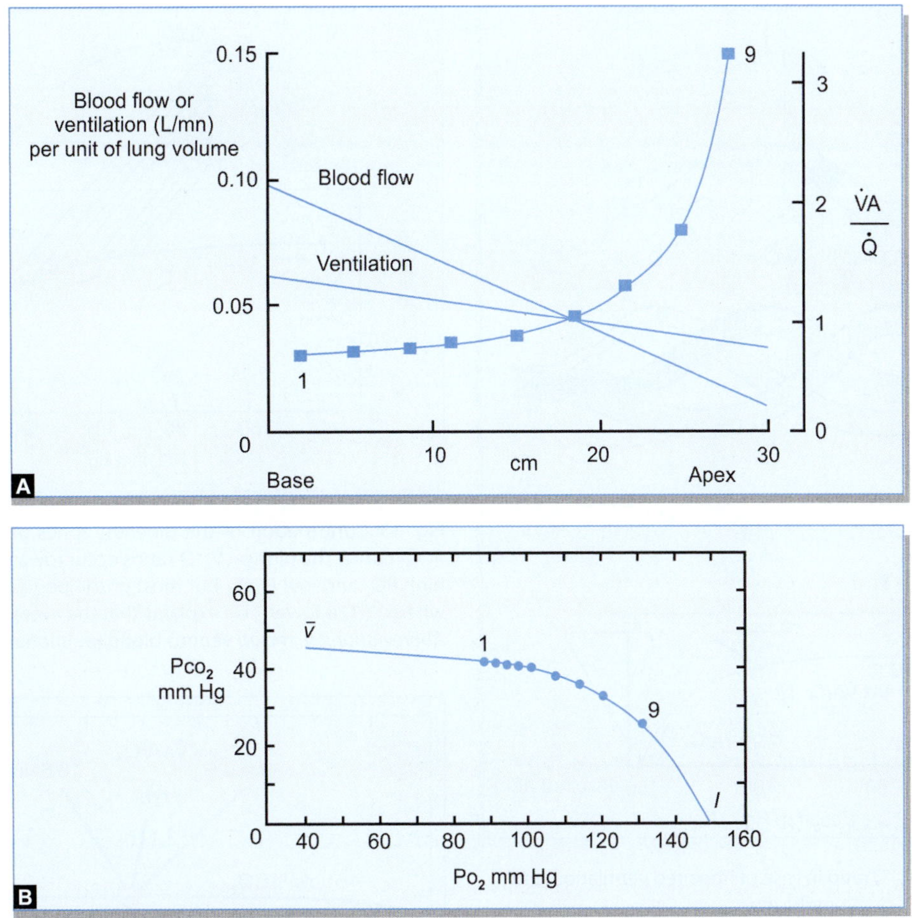

Figs 11A and B (A) Blood flow and alveolar ventilation per unit of lung volume decrease linearly from top to bottom but not with the same slope. The ratio of one to the other is therefore curvilinear. (B) For each $\dot{V}_A/\dot{Q}$ value on Figure A (1 to 9), everything being equal, there is only one possible pair of PO_2-PCO_2 values as shown on Figure B (1 to 9). The continuous line gives all the possible PO_2-PCO_2 paired values from inspired gas (I) to mixed venous blood ($\bar{v}$). Each dot on this line gives the pair corresponding to each of the $\dot{V}_A/\dot{Q}$ dots of Figure A

blood vessels,[16] within the extra-alveolar interstitium, at the junction with the alveolar space **(Fig. 17)**. The fluid is drained passively by a hydraulic pressure gradient of about 3 cm H_2O. There is no evidence of any active pumping of fluid from these initial lymphatics to the general lymphatic circulation. The lymphatic flow may increase considerably, up to 10–20 folds in correspondence with an increase of the filtration flow at the microvascular barrier.

LIQUID AND SOLUTES TRANSPORT

Transport across the microvascular endothelial barrier of the lung is qualitatively similar to that in other organs and obeys the general liquid and solute transport equations.[17] Because permeability to liquid, solutes and to proteins always vary in parallel (a change in permeability to water cannot happen without a simultaneous change in permeability to solutes and to protein) the basic Starling equation for fluid exchange, which is a simplified expression of these general equations, characterizes reasonably well exchanges through the endothelium:

$$\dot{Q}_f = K_f\,[(Pmv - Ppmv) - \sigma(\Pi mv - \Pi pmv)]$$

Where Q_f is the rate of fluid filtration, P is the fluid pressure, Π the osmotic pressure, in the microvascular (mv) and peri-microvascular interstitial fluid compartment (pmv), K_f the fluid conductance of the microvascular barrier, and σ the reflection coefficient of the membrane. K_f is the product of the permeability to fluid and small solutes per surface unit (P) by the surface of the exchange area S. σ characterizes the effective osmotic pressure of solutes, i.e. the fraction of solute concentration that cannot be balanced across the barrier because a fraction of the molecules cannot cross the barrier due to restrictive permeability because of size and structure. $\sigma = 0$ for electrolytes crossing freely and 1 for very large proteins that cannot cross at all. The value of σ in the

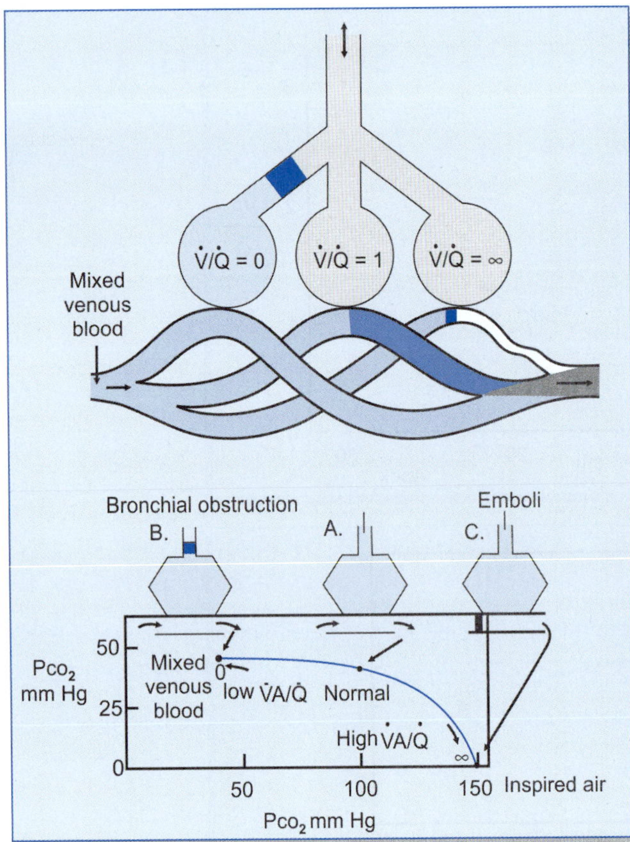

Fig. 12 Range of $\dot{V}_A/\dot{Q}$ ratio in case of impaired ventilation and perfusion

In case of bronchial obstruction, there is no ventilation but perfusion is maintained and mixed venous blood does not participate to alveolar exchange. $\dot{V}_A/\dot{Q} = 0$. In case of emboli there is no perfusion but ventilation is maintained, $\dot{V}_A/\dot{Q} = \infty$. No blood comes out of the alveoli. The blood coming out of lung is composed of oxygenated blood from perfused and ventilated alveoli and of mixed venous blood from capillaries that have not been exposed to alveolar ventilation. In normal subjects, the percentage of such capillaries is very low (less than 5%). In fact they correspond to what is called the physiologic shunt: blood flowing through capillaries that are too far from the alveolar membrane to participate to gas exchange. The physiological shunt explains why saturation cannot reach 100% in arterial blood. In pathologic situation the shunt may increase considerably and lower significantly PaO_2 because more blood flows through nonventilated area.

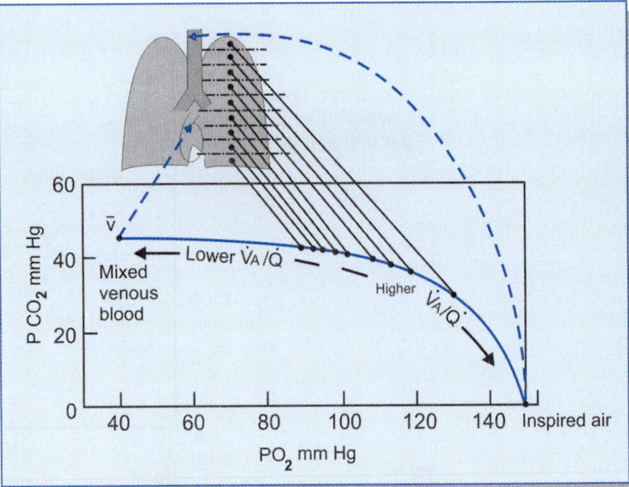

Fig. 13 Contribution of the different zones of the lung to the PO_2-PCO_2 curve: The highest $\dot{V}_A/\dot{Q}$ ratios occur toward the apex resulting in high PO_2 and low PCO_2, but most of the perfusion occurs at the base where $\dot{V}_A/\dot{Q}$ is lower. This explains that the average $\dot{V}_A/\dot{Q}$ ratio is 0.84

Abbreviations: $\bar{v}$, mixed venous blood (pulmonary artery); I, inspired air

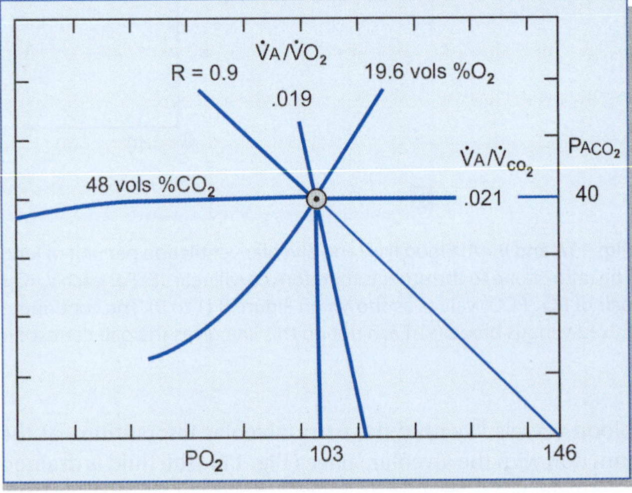

Fig. 14 The figure shows that when two values are measured, all other values are predetermined by these two measurements. This results from the fact that PO_2 and PCO_2 must be simultaneously on the PO_2-PCO_2 curve, on the R lines and on the corresponding isopleths as each should satisfy the corresponding equations. There is only one point, at the junction of all curves that satisfies these conditions. There can therefore be only one set of PO_2 and PCO_2 coupled values. It means that for a given value of one of them the other is predetermined. In a normal subject they can never vary independently one from the other

Source: Modified from Rahn et al.[2]

lung is between 0.6 and 0.8. This implies that the endothelial barrier is not fully impermeable to proteins and results in the fact that the interstitium protein concentration is about 0.8 that of plasma. It is generally believed that more than 95% of filtration fluid flows via the intercellular junctions and is therefore paracellular, and that other passive or active transcellular mechanisms are little related to bulk flow.

TYPE OF EDEMA

We can deduce from the Starling equation that two types of edema may occur: high-pressure edema, also called hemodynamic or abusively hydrostatic edema, and increased permeability edema, also called toxic edema.

In high pressure edema, the conductance of the membrane to fluid and protein remains normal. The rise in filtration flow results solely from the rise in the difference in pressure across the membrane, due exclusively to the rise of

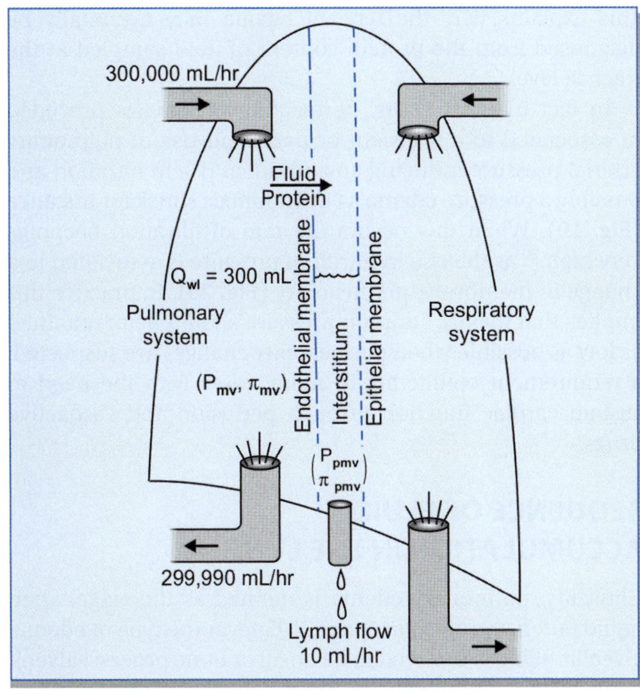

Fig. 15 The lung is composed of three compartments: vascular, interstitial and alveolar

Because the endothelial membrane is not totally impermeable to fluid and solutes, a continuous flow drains both to the interstitium according to the Starling equation. This net outward flux is drained out of the lung by the lymphatic system. The alveolar compartment remains dry due to the very low permeability of the epithelial barrier. A normal lung contains around 300 mL of water (Q_{wl}). The osmotic pressure in the interstitium is around 0.6–0.8 that of plasma

Source: Modified from Blake.[13]

Abbreviations: P, pressure; Π, osmotic pressure; mv, microvascular; pmv, peri-microvascular

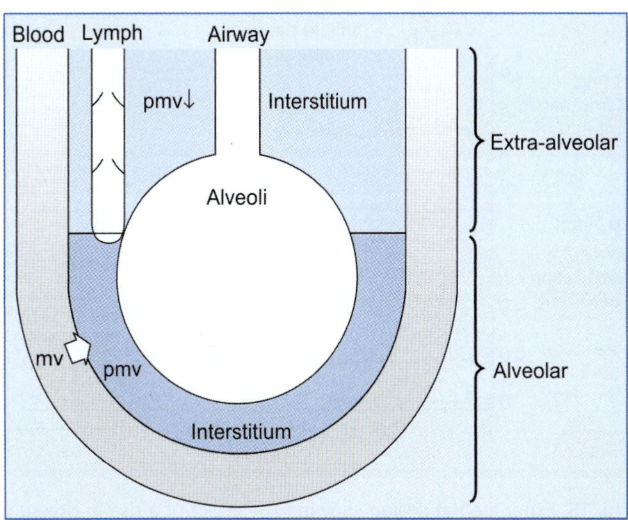

Fig. 16 Schematic representation of the alveolo-microvascular fluid exchange system in the lung.

The interstitial compartment is drained by the lymphatics. The lymphatics start at the alveolar junctions and are therefore extra-alveolar. Filtration can occur in the alveolar and in the extra-alveolar compartments. The interstitium is drained passively from the alveoli to the hilum due to the drop in pressure along the bronchoalveolar interstitium

Source: Modified from Staub.[15]

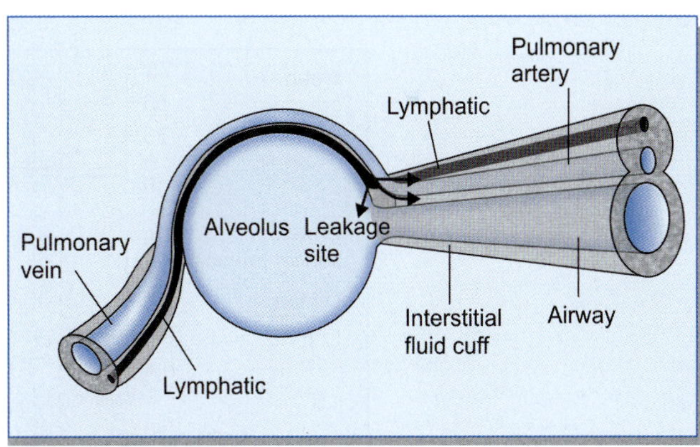

Fig. 17 Lymph drains normally via the lymphatics situated along the arterial, bronchial and venous trees. When lymphatics cannot drain anymore the excess filtration fluid, fluid accumulates first in the loose connective tissues of the bronchoarterial and venous cuffs. Then the alveoli are flooded. The most likely hypothesis explaining alveoli flooding during pressure edema is that overflow occurs in the zone that pumped out alveolar fluid at birth and that may constitute a zone of fragility

Source: Modified from Staub.[16]

the intravascular pressure. The composition of the filtration fluid remains the same as during normal filtration with a low protein concentration, which is reflected by the low protein concentration of the edema fluid.[18] This type of edema is representative of left ventricular failure, the rise of filtration pressure resulting from the rise in pressure in the left atrium **(Fig. 18)**.

In increased permeability edema, fluid and proteins conductance of the endothelium are both modified. As stated before, K_f and σ vary together but in opposite directions: K_f rises while σ decreases so that both fluid and proteins may move more freely across the barrier. The filtration flow increases even without any rise in pressure and the fluid is rich in protein, up to plasma concentration. This type of edema can be induced for instance by endotoxin, regurgitation or inhalation of toxic substances such as chlorine.

In both type of edema, as long as the fluid remains interstitial, no apparent change occurs to the epithelium. When alveolar flooding occurs the epithelium appears to become freely permeable to solutes including proteins, irrespective of the type of edema so that the composition of interstitial and alveolar fluids is identical.[19] It will be low in pressure edema and almost identical compared to plasma in permeability edema. Therefore, the concentration in protein in the alveolar edema fluid reflects that of the type of edema.

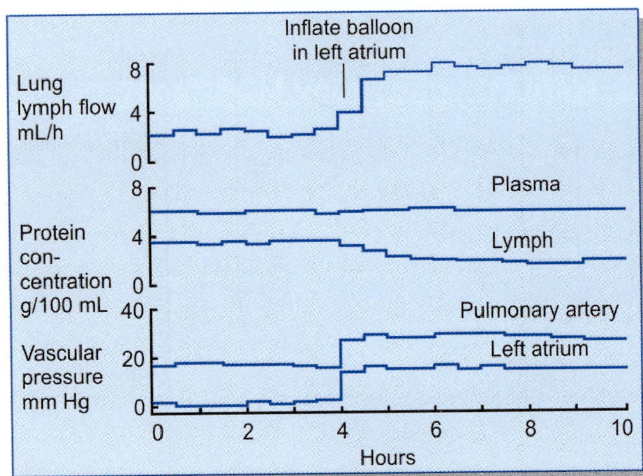

Fig. 18 Experimental design showing the effect of a rise in pressure in the right atrium by balloon inflation in a sheep: The rise in pressure in the left atrium causes almost instantaneously a rise in pressure in the pulmonary circulation. The rise of intra microvascular pressure results in a rise of fluid and small molecules filtration through the endothelial barrier, shown by the increase in lymphatic flow. Because the endothelial membrane remains intact, proteins do not cross the barrier in significant amount and a protein poor fluid filtrates to the lymph so that the ratio of lymph to plasma protein concentration drops with time. This is characteristic of pressure edema
Source: Modified from Bland et al.[18]

This explains why the type of edema may eventually be diagnosed from the protein content of fluid sampled at the trachea level.

In fact in most cases, permeability edema is preceded or associated to a transient or persistent rise of pulmonary arterial pressure inducing an additional rise in filtration and possibly a pressure edema as in endotoxic shock for instance **(Fig. 19)**. When this occurs the rate of filtration becomes very high,[20] as the rise in filtration pressure is associated to a change in membrane permeability **(Fig. 20)**. In practice this implies that ideally filtration pressure should be maintained as low as possible when permeability changes are suspected, a requirement conflicting in many cases with the need to sustain cardiac function through perfusion and vasoactive drugs.

SEQUENCE OF FLUID ACCUMULATION IN THE LUNG

Clinically, pulmonary edema is defined as the stage when liquid enters the alveolar space. Whatever the type of edema, alveolar filling is believed to be an all or none process, alveoli being filled completely at once. However much before this final and dramatic stage happens; various protective drainage mechanisms offer protection against flooding. The

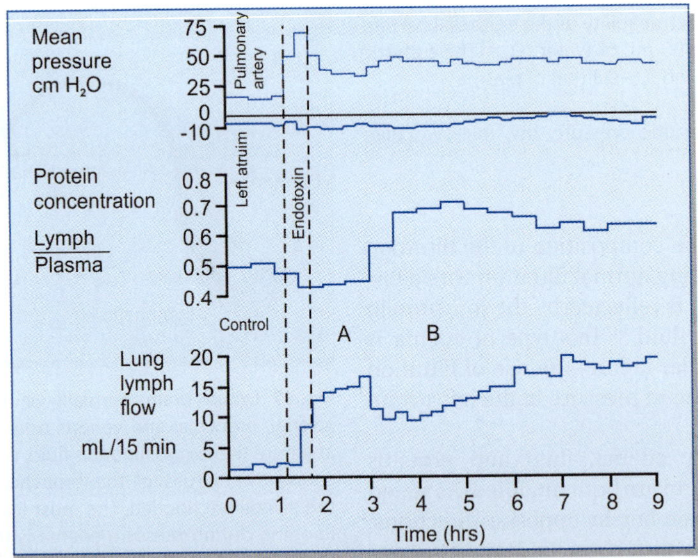

Fig. 19 Experimental design showing the succession of pressure and permeability edema in a sheep after administration of endotoxin: In the few hours following administration pressure rises in the pulmonary artery, lymph flow increases rapidly and the lymph to plasma protein concentration ratio decreases suggesting a typical pressure edema (A). However, if the animal is monitored long enough pulmonary artery pressure decreases to slightly above normal level, lung lymph flow increases slowly over several hours to reach a late high plateau although pressure has remained stable. Lymph to plasma protein ratio which has dropped initially comes back to normal slowly (B). This is interpreted as the emergence of a permeability edema characterized by a moderate pulmonary arterial pressure, a very high lymph flow and a normal lymph to plasma protein ratio suggesting the filtration of plasma and not of a protein poor fluid as in pressure edema. The slow time course is due to the necessary activation of the various biological processes leading to endothelial membrane alterations
Source: Modified from Robbins et al.[19]

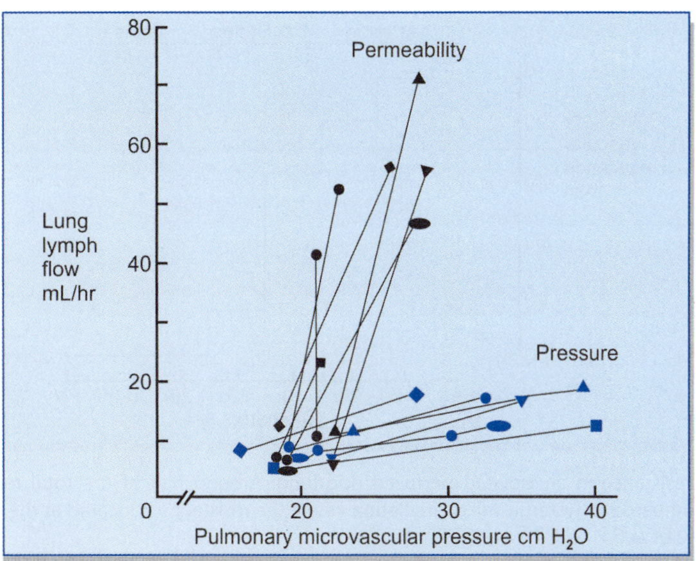

Fig. 20 Relationship between filtration flow across the endothelial barrier and membrane permeability in sheep: Black symbols show the change in lymph flow (filtration) with changes in microvascular pressure during permeability edema (endotoxin).
Open symbols show the same change during pressure edema (intact membrane).
A rise in microvascular pressure results in a dramatic increase in filtration if permeability has been altered simultaneously. A modest rise of filtration pressure in patients with toxic edema can have deleterious effects on the lung
Source: Modified from Brigham et al.[20]

first step for filtration fluid is drainage along the interstitial compartment.

Liquid and protein conductance in the interstitium do not depend on the interstitium structure although the constituting matrix structure of the interstitium may vary with pressure and volume. The interstitium does not interfere qualitatively with the fluid when flow increases. This means that the composition of pulmonary lymph is representative of filtration fluid. Interstitial edema happens only at a late stage and is quantitatively limited. The sequence of accumulation of fluid in the lung differs somewhat between hemodynamic and permeability edema. To begin with, in both types of edema, the excess fluid is drained by the lymphatic system until it is saturated, then fluid appears to collect first in the bronchoalveolar interstitial space, the so called bronchial cuffs on the venous as well as the arterial sides, then in the alveolar wall, and at the corner of the alveoli in the airspace and finally fills the airspace by a mechanism that is still poorly understood.[16]

In pressure edema it is unlikely that direct damage to the epithelium occurs except at very high pulmonary pressure (>50 mm Hg). Changes in pressure and tension across the alveolar wall cannot explain the overflow because perialveolar interstitial pressure is far too low a driving force to overcome the high epithelial hydraulic resistance. The most likely hypothesis is that overflow occurs at the junction of the alveoli with the first bronchial segments. This zone of so-called natural weakness is precisely where fluids and proteins are reabsorbed from the alveoli to the lymphatics at birth and would play an inverse passive role due to its fragility during pressure edema **(Fig. 17)**. In increased permeability edema, direct damage may occur simultaneously to the epithelial and alveolar barrier with fluid filtrating simultaneously to the cuffs and lymphatics and to the alveoli.

EFFECT OF BLOOD DISTRIBUTION IN THE LUNG

Blood flow is nonuniformly distributed in the lung on both a gravitational and a local (longitudinal) basis. There is a five-fold variation of flow over the height of the lung due to the action of gravity on distensible vessels. This results in an increasing endothelial surface area toward the bottom of the lung with an increase in filtration that is matched by a proportional increase in the lymphatic drainage structure so that there is no vertical change in fluid accumulation with height per volume unit. In the case of high-pressure edema, extravascular fluid tends to accumulate first where pressure and exchange surface per unit volume are highest. This explains the increase in water accumulation from top to bottom. In high permeability edema the repartition of extra-alveolar lung water is patchy, depending on the repartition of the lesions and at least in part independent of the vertical pressure gradient.

Filtration across the microvascular membrane is linked to the distribution of microvascular pressure and therefore of resistance along the microvessels **(Fig. 21)**. Contrary to what occurs in the systemic circulation where the drop

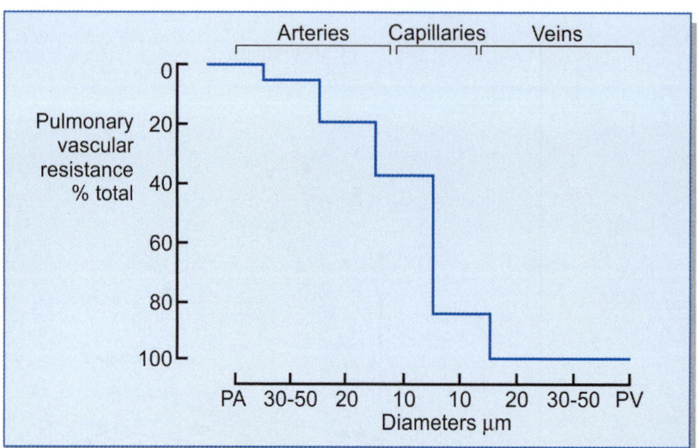

Fig. 21 Distribution of vascular resistance in an isolated perfused dog lung: Around half of the total resistance is distributed along the microvessels, a major difference compared to systemic microcirculation where the resistance is located at the arteriolar level
Source: Modified from Bhattacharya et al.[21]

in pressure and therefore resistance is localized at the arteriolar level, resistance is distributed longitudinally in pulmonary microvessels and may vary not only at the arteriolar level because of hypoxemia or hypoxia (hypoxemic vasoconstriction) but also all along the vessels[21] in response to various biological or pharmacological agents such as serotonin on the arterial side or histamine on the venules side. Consequently the filtration pressure at the filtration site is dependent on the distribution of resistance between the prefiltration and postfiltration sites **(Fig. 22)**. If the resistance is mostly on the prefiltration vessels then filtration pressure will be low compared to arteriolar pressure and well reflected by the measure of wedged capillary pressure. If resistance is mostly localized on the postfiltration side, then filtration pressure will be only slightly less than arteriolar pressure and therefore filtration rate will be high and not evaluated correctly by wedge capillary pressure. Therefore wedge capillary pressure may underestimate filtration pressure with the risk of under evaluating the outward flux especially in permeability edema.[22]

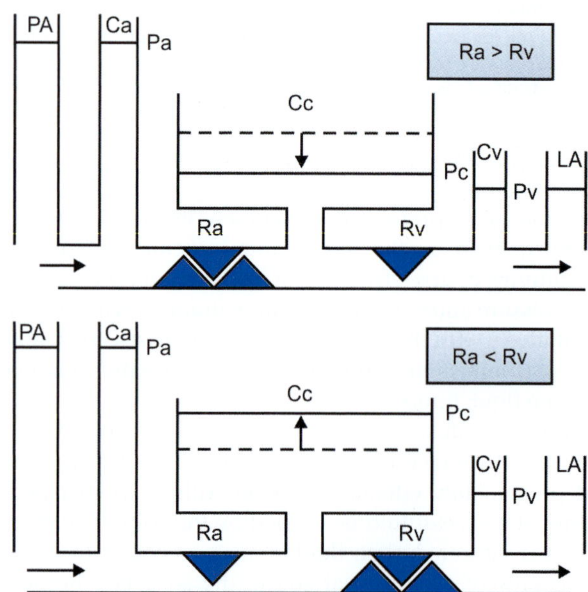

Fig. 22 Filtration pressure in the lungs depends on the longitudinal distribution of resistance along the microvessels.
When most of the resistance is located prior to the filtration site, microvascular filtration pressure and filtration are low in the filtration compartment (Ra > Rv).
When most of the resistance is located past the filtration site microvascular filtration pressure and filtration are high (Ra < Rv).
Pulmonary arterial, arteriolar, pulmonary venous and left atrial pressure are identical in both situations. Wedge capillary pressure may therefore be misleading when taken as an index of true filtration pressure during permeability edema.
Source: Modified from Grimbert et al.[22]
Abbreviations: PA, pulmonary artery; LA, left atrium; Ca, capillary arterial compartment; Cv, capillary venous compartment; Cc, pulmonary capillary compartment (filtration site)

FILTRATION THROUGH THE ENDOTHELIAL BARRIER

The role of the microvascular wall in liquid transport is not passive. Active mechanisms capable of modifying barrier properties have been identified.[23] Solutes can traverse the endothelium via the transcellular and paracellular pathways. The transcellular pathway or transcytosis is a vesicle-mediated transport of plasma proteins across the endothelium by caveolar mechanisms. The bulk of filtration of fluid and solutes occurs across a small fraction of the total microvascular surface area formed by the minute intercellular

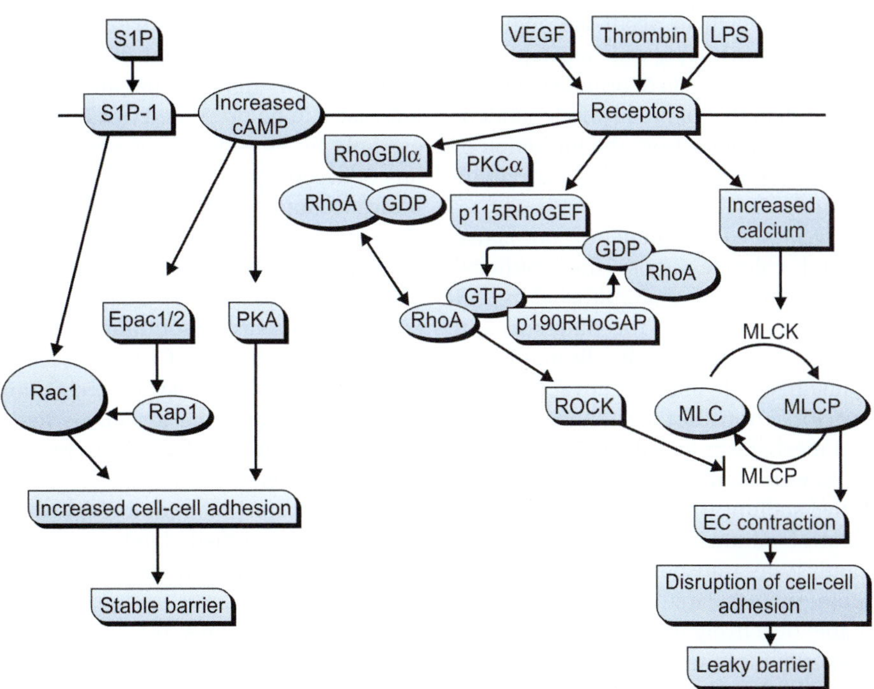

Fig. 23 Tentative representation of some of the signaling mechanisms that are involved in regulation of endothelial permeability: all mechanisms may not apply to the lung microvascular endothelium as phenotypic and genetic variations are known between endothelial cell types, depending on organs and locations in organs.
This representation makes the assumption that a common final pathway exists for various types of receptors [vascular endothelial growth factor (VEGF), thrombin, lipopolysaccharide (LPS)]. See text for details
Source: Modified from Vandenbroucke et al.[23]

spaces between cells.[24] This space primarily allows convective and diffusive transport of molecules of less than 3 nm of diameter while restricting but not totally the passage of larger molecules. The permeability of the interendothelial junction depends on the adhesive properties of the structural proteins of the tight junctions and of the adhesive junctions. These junctions are not passive and can be modified by the endothelial cells in response to specific stimuli acting on them, including sheer stress and pressure changes. The integrity of the junctions is controlled by the actin cytoskeleton through actin remodeling. Junctional permeability is modulated by inflammatory mediators, for example thrombin, tumor necrosis factor alpha (TNFα) and lipopolysaccharide (LPS) (endotoxin) **(Fig. 23)**. Mediators act through their respective endothelial surface receptors. Receptor activation increases cytosolic Ca^{++} and activates myosin light chain kinase (MCLK), GTPases RhoA, Racl and Cdc 42. Racl and Cdc 42 reinforce the junctional assemblies while Ca++ activation of MCLK and RhoA disrupt the junctions, increasing permeability. Other agents such as sphingosine-1-phosphate and cyclic adenosine monophosphate (cAMP) play a role of barrier stabilizing agents, capable of reducing increased endothelial permeability. The role on permeability of LPS, an endotoxin present on the outer membrane of Gram-negative bacteria and a major factor of acute lung injury, exemplify the relationship between the endothelial cell receptors and increased permeability. LPS binds to Toll-like receptor 4 resulting in the translocation of NF-κB to the cell nucleus initiating transcription of proinflammatory mediators, which increase permeability. LPS also promote the expression of an intercellular adhesion molecule (ICAM-1). Cross-linking of ICAM-1 activates RhoA and actin stress fiber formation; ICAM-1 also up regulates RhoA expression, resulting in on a positive feedback mechanism on permeability.

Indeed many other mechanisms may initiate the endothelial cell response such as activation of platelets, the coagulation cascade, neutrophil or macrophage activation, and others. The activation of the inflammatory cascades will be related to the initial cause of disease and takes time to proceed. This explains why the onset of permeability edema is a slow process (hours and days) compared to the onset of pressure edema that can take only minutes to develop. It is important to note that permeability edema may be secondary to the inflammation secondary to an initial mechanical or chemical aggression such as thrombi or inhalation of toxic material, which per se does not increase permeability.

RESOLUTION OF ALVEOLAR EDEMA

The first evidence that active ion transport is involved in fluid clearance from the air space was obtained in ventilated, anesthetized sheep. Fluid clearance of an instilled isomolar salt and water solution was shown to occur although the alveolar protein concentration was rising well above plasma level. It was also shown that reabsorption of protein occurred very slowly and much later than that of fluid by independent mechanisms. Further evidence comes from the inhibition of alveolar fluid clearance in various species including man by ouabaïn (90%) and amiloride (70%).

The resolution of alveolar edema depends on active transport of sodium and chloride across the epithelial barrier.[25] Regulation occurs via alveolar epithelial type I and II cells and distal airway epithelia. The differences in hydrostatic and protein osmotic pressures implicated in the Starling equation play no direct role in the removal of excess fluid or proteins. The vectorial transport of sodium, chloride and water is the central mechanism by which alveolar fluid can be cleared at birth as well as in the mature lung during pulmonary edema. Active sodium transport drives osmotic water transport. Inhibition of sodium transport by appropriate drugs reduces significantly water transport from the airspace in several species including man. Isolated epithelial cells have been shown to be capable of actively transport ions in vitro as well as in vivo. Reabsorption can occur at all levels of the distal airspaces; nonciliated cuboidal cells and Clara cells are involved in the mechanisms just as well as alveolar epithelial cells. They have all been shown to contain the required transporters. Transport by the alveolar type II cells have been extensively studied because these cells constitute 95% of the alveolar epithelium membrane and because they are fit for in vitro studies. Active sodium uptake occurs on the apical cell surface through amiloride sensitive and amiloride insensitive channels. Na, K-ATPase pumps sodium actively from the cell basolateral surface to the interstitium. An epithelial sodium channel (ENaC) has been cloned and characterized.[24] Concerning type I cell studies conducted on fresh cells have identified the expression and presence of $\alpha1$ and $\alpha2$ subunits of Na, K-ATPase on the basolateral surface of the cell as well as expression of all subunits of ENaC. The $\alpha1$ subunit of type I cells has been linked to alveolar fluid reabsorption.[22] Na uptake is sensitive to amiloride blockage. Furthermore highly selective cation channels have been identified by patch clamp and may participate in fluid clearance.

Water follows passively the sodium-induced fluid movement. The movement of liquid is generally thought to follow intercellular pathways. The identification of specialized water transporting proteins called aquaporins in the lungs has led to the hypothesis that part of the water movement might occur via transcellular channels. The predominant lung aquaporin, aquaporin 5, is expressed in the apical surface of alveolar type I cells, which have one of the highest permeability coefficient for water, leading to the hypothesis that some movement of fluid occurs across type I cells. However, experiments show that deletion of aquaporin does not seem to affect alveolar liquid clearance.

Endogenous release of catecholamine stimulates the reabsorption of fetal lung fluid from the airspaces at birth. Type I and type II cells both express and present β_2 receptors. Stimulation of these receptors in human lungs by terbutamol, salmeterol or epinephrine increases fluid clearance. This increase can be prevented by nonspecific β_2 antagonists, for example by propranolol or amiloride. This demonstrates a link between increased filtration, amiloride sensitive sodium transport, and catecholamine dependent regulation of fluid clearance.

Chloride also plays a role in the up regulation of fluid clearance across the distal lung epithelium by mediating cAMP apical uptake of sodium. Cystic fibrosis transmembrane conductance regulator (CFTR) is essential for cAMP mediated up regulation of isomolar fluid clearance from the both the distal airways and the alveoli so that CFTR might be the chloride channel involved in the process. Chloride channels are β_2 sensitive.

Various catecholamine-independent mechanisms have also been identified lately, including proinflammatory molecules such as TNF and leukotrienes D4, some growth and hormonal factors acting by transcriptional or post translational mechanisms.

CLINICAL IMPLICATIONS

Resolution of pulmonary pressure edema depends on the clearance of fluid from the alveoli, a process that requires a functional alveolar epithelium. The alveolar and distal airway epithelia are remarkably resistant to edema[17] compared to adjacent lung endothelium so that the alveolar barrier may remain functionally intact after endothelial injury. This might explain why in mild to moderate lung injury the transport of water and sodium may remain normal or even be up regulated by stress hormones.

The rate of alveoli clearance of water has been measured during major pressure (hemodynamic) edema in several species, in ex vivo human lungs and in patients. It was found to vary from 3% per hour to a maximum of 14% per hour and to be generally around maximal level providing alveolar epithelium was intact. Clearance was increased in 75% of the patients. In acute lung injury (permeability edema) alveolar clearance is impaired in 56% of the patients and there is a convincing relationship between the clearance rate, extent of epithelial injury, and patient's survival. This has encouraged strategies to increase alveolar fluid clearance essentially by means of β_2-agonist therapy but also by vasoactive agents (dobutamine, dopamine) and growth factors. However, these strategies can be meaningful only when enough of the alveolar epithelium has remained functional.[26]

MEASUREMENT OF EXTRAVASCULAR LUNG WATER

Quantification of extravascular fluid accumulation may appear a significant tool to analyze the exchange of fluids within the lung. As always in compartmental analysis, the significant approach would be to quantify the net flux of fluid and solutes across the barrier, a measurement technically very difficult to obtain, especially in a clinical setting. The measurement of extravascular lung water (EVLW) has been attempted by a variety of single pass indicator, thermal and osmotic dilution techniques based on compartmental models of water and solutes exchange or on washout procedures. All these methods have uncertain specificity and sensitivity and the normal range of EVLW has never been properly established. Major limitations are linked to the change in distribution of tracers in the lung in function of the distribution of perfusion, perfusion pressure, perfusion of extracorporeal fluids, and repartition of diseased area, all factors contributing to variations of the exchange surface area and volumes of diffusion from one time to the other. Furthermore only tracer accessible zones can be measured therefore excluding poorly perfused or ventilated areas resulting in underestimation. In fact only radiological imaging methods can detect and localize in a functionally and clinically significant manner the extent and localization of extravascular fluid accumulation although it is not quantitative.[27]

CONCLUSION

Transport of fluid and solutes through the alveolar wall is a complex process requiring the active participation of the endothelial and epithelial cells. Pressure and permeability edema have different characteristics in terms of time course and cell activation. They may occur simultaneously or successively as in Gram-negative infections. Permeability edema provokes much higher levels of filtration, compared to pressure edema, and is extremely sensitive to modest changes in filtration pressure. Filtration pressure tends to be undervalued for lack of adequate measurement technique. Treatment of pressure edema focus successfully on the mechanical change in pressure whereas permeability edema is dependent on our capacity to counter act the inflammatory mechanisms, this with limited success so far because of their complexity.

REFERENCES

1. Dejours P. Principles of comparative respiratory physiology. North Holland American Elsevier: Amsterdam; 1975.
2. Rahn H, Fenn W. A graphical analysis of the respiratory gas exchange. The American Physiological Society, 4th printing. Washington DC; 1962.
3. Berne RM, Levy MN. Physiology. Chapter 40, CV Mosby, St Louis; 1983.
4. Piiper J. Alveolar-capillary gas transfer in lungs: development of concepts and current state. Adv Exp Med Biol. 1994;345: 7-14.
5. Staub NC. Alveolar-arterial oxygen tension due to diffusion. J Appl Physiol. 1963;18:673-80.
6. Macintyre N, Crapo RO, Viegi G, Johnson DC, van der Grinten CP, Brusasco V, et al. Standardization of the single-breath determination of carbon monoxide uptake in the lung. Eur Respir J. 2005;26:720-35.
7. Roughton FJW. Transport of oxygen and carbon dioxide in Handbook of Physiology. In: Fenn WO, Rahn H (Eds). Respiration, section 3 vol 1. American Physiological Society; 1964.pp.767-826.
8. Wasserman K, Whipp BJ. Exercise physiology in health and disease. Am Rev Respir Dis. 1975;112:219-49.
9. Dejours P. Respiration. Oxford University Press; 1966.
10. Wagner PD. Ventilation-perfusion relationships. Annu Rev Physiol. 1980;42:235-47.
11. Wagner PD, Laravuso RB, Uhl RR, West JB. Continuous distributions of ventilation-perfusion ratios in normal subjects breathing air and 100 per cent O_2. J Clin Invest. 1974;54:54-68.
12. Paiva M, Engel LA. Theoretical studies of gas mixing and ventilation distribution in the lung. Physiol Rev. 1987;67:750-96.
13. Blake LH. Mathematical modelling of steady state fluid and protein exchange in lung water and solute exchange. In: Staub NC (Ed) Lung Biology in Health and Disease, volume 7. Marcel Dekker, Basel; 1978. pp. 99-128.
14. Staub NC. Pulmonary edema. Physiol Rev. 1974;54:678-811.
15. Staub NC. Lung structure and function. Basics RD. 1982;10: 1-10.
16. Staub NC. Alveolar flooding and clearance. Am Rev Respir Dis. 1983;127(5 Pt 2):S44-51.
17. Bhattacharya J. Physiological basis of pulmonary edema in pulmonary edema. In: Matthay M, Ingbar DH (Eds). Lung Biology in Health and Disease, Vol 116. Marcel Dekker New York; 1998. pp. 1-36.
18. Bland R, Hansen TA, Hazinski TA. Studies of lung fluid balance in newborn lambs. Ann N Y Acad Sci. 1982;384:126-45.
19. Robbins IM, Brigham KL, Newman JH. Increased permeability edema from sepsis/endotoxemia. In: Pulmonary Edema. Matthay M, Ingbar DH (Eds). Lung Biology in Health and Disease, volume 116. Marcel Dekker New York; 1998. pp. 203-45.
20. Brigham KL. Lung edema due to increased permeability. In: Staub NC (Ed). Lung water and solute exchange. Lung Biology in Health and Disease, volume 7. Marcel Dekker, Basel; 1978. pp. 235-76.
21. Bhattacharya J, Staub NC. Direct measurement of microvascular pressures in the isolated perfused dog lung. Science. 1980;210(4467):327-8.
22. Grimbert F, Teboul JL, Amardeil P. Pression capillaire et oedeme pulmonaire in Lemaire F, Zelter M. Oedemes pulmonaires Masson Paris. 1992.pp.61-88.
23. Vandenbroucke E, Mehta D, Minshall R, Malik AB. Regulation of endothelial junctional permeability. Ann NY Acad Sci. 2008;1123:134-45.
24. Effros RM, Parker JC. Pulmonary vascular heterogeneity and the Starling hypothesis. Microvasc Res. 2009;78:71-7.
25. Matthay MA, Robriquet L, Fang X. Alveolar epithelium: role in lung fluid balance and acute lung injury. Proc Am Thorac Soc. 2005;2(3):206-13.
26. Berthiaume Y, Matthay M. Alveolar edema clearance and acute lung injury. Respir Physiol Neurobiol. 2007;159:350-9.
27. Effros RM, Pornsuriyasak P, Porszasz J, Casaburi R. Indicator dilution measurements of extravascular lung water: basic assumptions and observations. Am J Physiol Lung Cell Mol Physiol. 2008;294:L1023-31.

Tissue Oxygenation

Puneet Malhotra, SK Jindal

Oxygen Delivery and Tissue Oxygenation

INTRODUCTION

The oxygen taken up by the blood from the alveoli is delivered to the tissues through systemic circulation [oxygen delivery (DO_2)]. The process of diffusion from the capillaries to the tissues is called internal respiration or tissue oxygenation **(Flow chart 1)**. The oxygen is consumed by the tissues for energy production.

The main determinant of tissue oxygenation is a balance between DO_2 and oxygen consumption (VO_2). An imbalance between the two results in oxygen debt.

OXYGEN DELIVERY

Oxygen delivery constitutes the total amount of oxygen delivered to the whole body. Tissue DO_2 depends on two factors: (i) arterial O_2 content (CaO_2), and (ii) cardiac output (Q), $DO_2 = Q \times CaO_2$.

The normal range for DO_2 is 520–570 mL/min/m^2 and under normal physiological conditions, DO_2 is considerably in the excess of the VO_2 (110–160 mL/min/m^2). This "spare capacity" enables the body to cope with a fall in DO_2 without initially compromising aerobic respiration.

Flow chart 1 The delivery of oxygen to tissue for cellular metabolism is a three-step process

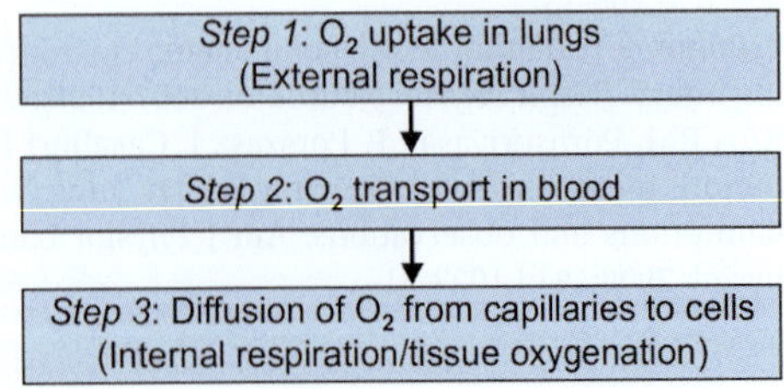

Factors Influencing Oxygen Delivery

Arterial O_2 Content (CaO_2)

It is the total amount of O_2 present in blood, i.e. combined with hemoglobin (Hb) and dissolved in plasma.

$$CaO_2 = (1.34 \times Hb \times SaO_2) + (0.0031 \times PaO_2)$$

The contribution of Hb is described by the first part of the equation. This relationship states that each gram of Hb will bind 1.34 mL of O_2, when it is fully saturated with oxygen. The SaO_2 is expressed as a fraction, not a percentage (i.e. 1.0 instead of 100%). Therefore, at a Hb level of 15 g/dL and an SaO_2 of 98%, the oxygen carried by Hb will be:

$$1.34 \times 15 \times 0.98 = 19.7 \text{ mL/100 mL}$$

From the second part of the equation one can infer that, at a PaO_2 of 100 mm Hg, the expected concentration of dissolved O_2 in blood is $0.0031 \times 100 = 0.3$ mL/100 mL. Therefore, the total concentration of O_2 in arterial blood is 19.7 + 0.3 = 20 mL/100 mL. Thus, it is clear that CaO_2 primarily depends on Hb and SaO_2 and to a lesser extent on PaO_2.

Cardiac Output

Oxygen delivery is directly related to changes in cardiac output, which is the product of heart rate and stroke volume. Any alteration in either of these two parameters alters the cardiac output. Stroke volume, the amount of blood ejected per beat is affected by the following factors:

- *Preload:* It is the load imposed on a muscle before the onset of contraction and is synonymous with the initial length (or stretch) of cardiac fibers. An increase in preload augments muscle length and leads to a more forceful cardiac contraction (Frank-Starling phenomenon). In fact, in the normal heart, the diastolic volume/preload is the principal force that governs the strength of ventricular contraction. This emphasizes the value of avoiding hypovolemia and correcting volume deficits promptly when they exist. The relationship between preload and cardiac output is, however, not linear and is also influenced by changes in ventricular compliance and geometry. Since ventricular end-diastolic volume is not easily measured at the bedside; end-diastolic pressure (EDP) and central venous pressure (CVP) are more commonly used as reflections of preload in clinical practice.

- *Afterload:* It is the sum of all forces opposing ventricular ejection. It is influenced by aortic and pulmonary arterial pressures, systemic and pulmonary vascular resistance and compliance of ventricular muscle. As the determination of these forces is complex, systolic left ventricular pressure is usually used as a reasonable measure of after load. In addition, since afterload is a transmural force, it is influenced by the pleural pressures at the surface of the heart. Positive pleural pressures can promote ventricular emptying by facilitating the inward displacement of the ventricular wall during systole and this is one of the mechanisms by which noninvasive positive pressure ventilation is beneficial in cardiogenic pulmonary edema.
- *Contractility:* It refers to the intrinsic contractile property of cardiac myocytes and is influenced by catecholamine levels, as well as extracellular calcium concentration. Cardiac contractility is measured indirectly by impedance cardiography and Doppler echocardiography.

Steps Involved in Oxygen Delivery

The delivery of O_2 to the cells, i.e. the cellular O_2 supply is not equal to all cells although all arteries in the body carry virtually identical concentrations of O_2. This is because of the following factors:

- *Differences in regional blood flow:* The gatekeeper of blood supply to a capillary network is the local arteriole. Arterioles may dilate or constrict in response to various local and central regulatory factors. Local factors causing dilatation include hypoxia, increased CO_2, increased temperature and decreased pH. The release of catecholamines is a central mechanism that attempts to preferentially distribute blood to vital organs when DO_2 is compromised. When the body is confronted with a declining DO_2, both central and local mechanisms are stimulated. In the short-term, central effects predominate while if the O_2 shortage persists, local effects override and generalized vasodilatation occurs.
- *Differences in capillary architecture:* Some cells are simply closer to capillaries than others. Because movement of O_2 depends on pressure gradients, the cells farthest away from capillaries are most vulnerable to hypoxia. In addition, many capillaries are normally closed and open only when perfusion to that particular region increases. For example, an actively contracting muscle may have 10 times more open capillaries than a resting muscle.

OXYGEN CONSUMPTION

Calculation of Oxygen Consumption

Oxygen consumption refers to the rate of uptake of O_2 by tissues from the microcirculation. It is a product of the cardiac output and the difference in oxygen content between arterial and venous blood.

$VO_2 = Q \times (CaO_2 - CVO_2)$ $VO_2 = Q \times 1.34 \times Hb \times (SaO_2 - SvO_2)$

The normal range for VO_2 is 110–160 mL/min/m^2 and it can be measured in three ways:

1. Using Fick's equation given above, requires the placement of a pulmonary artery catheter.
2. By measurement of inspired and expired minute ventilation (Vi and Ve) and of fractional concentrations of O_2 (FiO_2 and FeO_2) in the two samples. This is a noninvasive method, but is relatively unreliable in mechanically ventilated patients on high FiO_2.
$$VO_2 = (Vi \times FiO_2) - (Ve \times FeO_2)$$
3. Oxygen consumption can also be measured directly with the help of a rebreathing spirometer system filled with oxygen; the expired CO_2 is absorbed from the system and any change in the volume of gas in the spirometer reflects the VO_2.

Cellular O_2 utilization: Metabolic utilization of O_2 in cells occurs by the oxidation of pyruvic acid in the Krebs cycle **(Flow chart 2)**. This series of reactions takes place in mitochondria and results in the production of 38 molecules of ATP. The availability of O_2 is crucial in the production of ATP from adenosine diphosphate (ADP) in the Krebs' cycle. The actual process of ATP formation is called oxidative phosphorylation as phosphate is added to ADP by using the energy from oxidation. In the absence of O_2, metabolism is less efficient and only 2 molecules of ATP are generated by the metabolism of glucose (anaerobic glycolysis). Furthermore, anaerobic metabolism results in the production of lactic acid, which may lead to systemic metabolic acidosis.

More than 90% of the body's VO_2 is utilized by a single enzyme, cytochrome oxidase during the process of oxidative phosphorylation, which generates ATP. This is the most efficient means of producing ATP, since a total of 38 molecules of ATP are generated per molecule of glucose. Aerobic cellular respiration depends on the efficient supply of oxygen to the mitochondria, which is a function of the coordinated

Flow chart 2 Aerobic metabolism via oxidative phosphorylation in the mitochondria produces 19 times more energy adenosine triphosphate (ATP) than anaerobic glycolysis

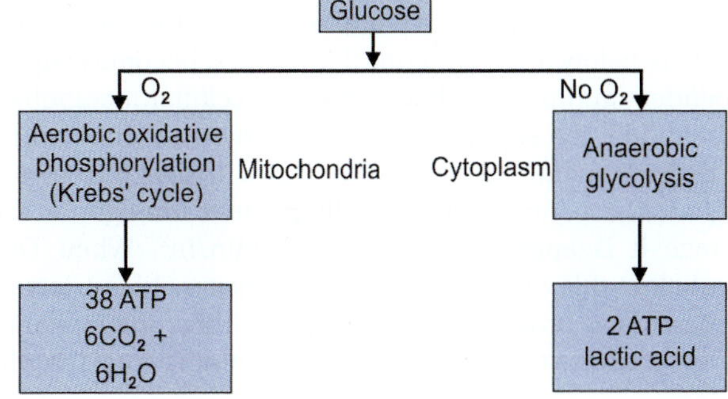

interaction between the respiratory and circulatory systems. When oxygen supply is inadequate, anaerobic metabolism sets in and generates only 2 molecules of ATP per molecule of glucose **(Flow chart 2)**. In addition H^+ ions are formed, which can lead to a systemic metabolic acidosis. Tissue oxygenation is often impaired in critically ill patients, who have poor cardiopulmonary reserve and optimizing DO_2 to meet oxygen demand, has the potential to improve outcomes in these patients.

Calculated Versus Measured Oxygen Consumption

The VO_2 is usually derived from Fick's equation and not directly measured. The derivation is based on four measured variables: Cardiac output (Q), hemoglobin concentration (Hb), arterial O_2 saturation (SaO_2) and mixed venous O_2 saturation (SvO_2). Each of these measurements varies and their summed contribution can lead to considerable variability in the final calculated VO_2. Therefore, to be considered a physiologically significant change, the calculated VO_2 should change by at least 15%.

O_2 Extraction Ratio

It is the ratio of oxygen uptake to oxygen delivery (VO_2/DO_2) and reflects the fraction of O_2 delivered to the microcirculation that is taken up by the tissues. The O_2 extraction ratio (O_2ER) varies between different organs. For example, the brain has an O_2ER of 34% while exercising muscle can remove all O_2 from its microcirculation and thus have an O_2ER approaching 100%. Overall, the normal O_2ER is 20–30%. Thus, only a small fraction of the available O_2 delivered to the capillaries is taken up into the tissues. Oxygen extraction is adjustable and in conditions where O_2 delivery is impaired, the O_2ER can increase up to 50–60%.

Oxygen Delivery: Oxygen Consumption Curve

The relationship between O_2 delivery and O_2 uptake is described by the curve in **Figure 1**. As DO_2 decreases below normal, the O_2ER increases proportionally to keep VO_2 constant. When O_2ER reaches its maximum level (50–60%), further decreases in DO_2 result in proportional decreases in VO_2. Since under normal physiological conditions, DO_2 is considerably in excess of the VO_2, tissue oxygenation to a large extent is supply-independent. However, when DO_2 falls below a certain critical level, VO_2 becomes supply dependent and this condition, in which cellular metabolism is limited by the supply of O_2 is called dysoxia. This critical O_2 delivery point (critical DO_2) varies between 150 and 1,000 mL/min/m^2 in critically ill patients though on an average it is approximately 300 mL/min/m^2. When DO_2 falls below this level, tissue hypoxia ensues, blood lactate increases and prognosis becomes poor. Thus, maintenance of DO_2 in excess of the critical delivery point is crucial in the management of critically ill patients. This is particularly true when positive end-expiratory pressure (PEEP) is being used because PEEP may be associated with a fall in DO_2 despite improvements in PaO_2 because of its effect on cardiac output.

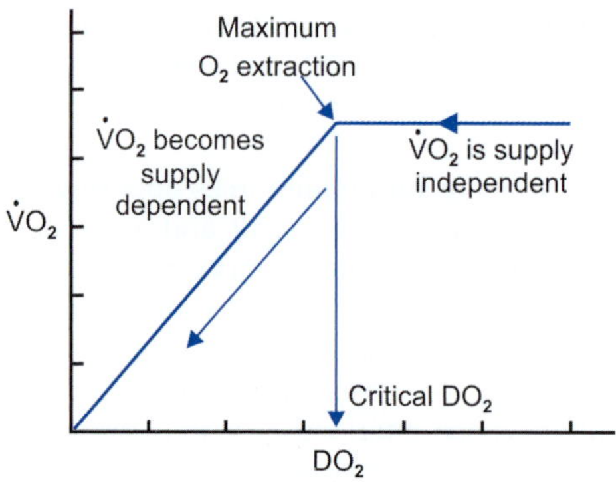

Fig. 1 Graph describing the relationship between delivery (DO_2) and O_2 uptake (VO_2). As DO_2 decreases below normal, O_2 extraction increases proportionally to keep $\dot{V}O_2$ constant and therefore, "supply independent". When DO_2 falls below a critical level, $\dot{V}O_2$ becomes "supply dependent"

Factors Influencing Oxygen Consumption

Causes of Decreased Oxygen Consumption

Decreased blood supply to tissues: Shock (cardiogenic/hypovolemic).

Cytotoxicity: An intrinsic defect in O_2 utilization at the cellular level is seen in carbon monoxide (CO) and cyanide poisoning, as well as in sepsis.

Increased O_2 demand: This is seen in most critically ill patient with increased metabolic rates, e.g. acute pancreatitis, burns, etc. It is noteworthy that tissue hypoxia in sepsis involves all the three mechanisms mentioned above: (i) decreased blood supply as a result of redistribution of blood flow due to pathologic capillary dilatation and arteriovenous shunting, as well as microvascular occlusion due to platelet and fibrin microthrombi, (ii) disruption of cellular metabolism by cytokines and free radicals and (iii) increased O_2 demand.

Causes of Increased Oxygen Consumption

Whenever stress or tissue injury occurs, there is an increase in metabolic rate and VO_2. In normal subjects, exercise increases VO_2, almost simultaneously with the onset of work. Most of this increase is accounted for by increase in cardiac output. A relative hemoconcentration and therefore increased O_2 content may also occur with the high levels of exercise. The VO_2 may increase 10- to 15-folds during exercise. In addition, O_2 extraction (see above) may also increase to as much as 80% of VO_2 in order to meet the additional O_2 requirement.

This is made possible by capillary dilatation and recruitment in exercising muscles.

Causes of increased VO_2 in sick patients include fever, tachypnea, shivering and seizures. In a very ill patient, even innocuous activities, such as chest physiotherapy, getting up or turning in bed and tracheal suctioning can increase VO_2 and tilt the already precarious O_2 balance.

Oxygen Debt (Oxygen Consumption Deficit)

Oxygen debt or VO_2 deficit is the difference between the metabolic demand for O_2 and the actual VO_2. As demand increases, VO_2 must increase to preserve aerobic metabolism. This is met with by increasing DO_2 either by physiological compensation, e.g. an increase in cardiac output or O_2ER or by therapeutic interventions such as intravenous fluids or inotropes. If this increase in DO_2 is delayed, O_2 debt continues to grow and a stage is reached from where recovery is not possible. Studies of the O_2 debt after resuscitation from hemorrhagic shock and in postoperative patients show a direct relationship between the magnitude of O_2 debt and the risk of multiorgan failure and death. This indicates that the early correction of VO_2 deficits is warranted to limit the severity of tissue ischemia.

ASSESSMENT OF TISSUE OXYGENATION

Unlike hypoxemia, which denotes a low PaO_2 and has standard normal and abnormal values, there are no normal values for tissue PO_2 and it cannot be routinely measured at the bedside. Tissue hypoxia is defined as abnormal O_2 utilization by cells and should be distinguished from other terms, such as hypoxic, anemic, histotoxic and stagnant hypoxia, which can lead to but are not synonymous with tissue hypoxia. There are three ways to detect tissue hypoxia.

Clinical Assessment

Clinical examination should be the first step in assessing tissue oxygenation. A number of well-known signs (mental obtundation, oliguria, abnormal vital signs and delayed capillary refill) often indicate specific organ dysfunction as a sequel of tissue hypoxia. However, clinical signs are often insensitive as they occur late during the course of tissue hypoxia. Direct or indirect measurements of local tissue oxygenation of an organ suspected to suffer from hypoxia will facilitate the assessment. Local tissue oxygen probes have been used in critical care areas in some instances (e.g. brain).

Physiological Parameters

Mixed Venous O_2 Saturation

Mixed venous blood represents blood returning from all the venous beds of the body, "mixed" together in the right ventricle. It is obtained from the distal end of the pulmonary artery with the help of a specialized pulmonary artery catheter, the tip of which emits infrared light and records light reflected back from Hb in circulating erythrocytes. This technique is called "reflectance spectrophotometry" (whereas pulse oximeters use transmission spectrophotometry). SvO_2 can also be measured intermittently by withdrawing blood from the catheter. In the proximal part of the pulmonary artery, blood from the two vena cavae and coronary sinus is not fully blended and, therefore, does not represent total body venous gas values. SvO_2 is a marker of the balance between whole body DO_2 and O_2 demand and is normally between 65% and 75%, i.e. O_2 demand is usually about 25–35% that of O_2 delivery.

Causes of Decreased Mixed Venous O_2 Saturation

Decrease in DO_2: This may occur due to hypovolemia, decreased cardiac output, low Hb, low PaO_2 and SaO_2.

Increase in O_2 demand: Critical illness, sepsis, thyrotoxicosis, etc.

Causes of Increased Mixed Venous O_2 Saturation

Increased DO_2: Increased cardiac output (e.g. exercise, use of inotropes), increased Hb (hypertransfusion).

Decrease in O_2 demand: Deep sedation and paralysis in ventilated patients.

Decreased tissue O_2 utilization: Cyanide and CO poisoning, sepsis.

Left-to-right shunts: These can usually be diagnosed by an abnormal "step-up" of SvO_2 at the level of the defect as the pulmonary artery catheter is passed into the right atrium or ventricle.

A limitation of SvO_2 as a parameter for assessing tissue oxygenation is that normal or increased values do not always mean that tissue oxygenation is adequate. For example, in sepsis and CO poisoning, impaired tissue O_2 utilization results in a normal or high SvO_2. In addition, pathologic vasodilatation and increased cardiac output in sepsis also tend to increase SvO_2 even though tissue hypoxia is ongoing.

Dual Oximetry

By simultaneously measuring SaO_2 by pulse oximetry, one can get a continuous measurement of whole body O_2 extraction, i.e. SaO_2–SvO_2. This method is known as dual oximetry and its normal value is 20–30%.

Oxygen Delivery/Oxygen Consumption Measurements

The measurement of changes in VO_2 in response to changes in DO_2 has been suggested as a sensitive method of determining whether tissue hypoxia exists. However, it entails multiple

Table 1 Normal values and equations of tissue oxygenation parameters

Parameter arterial O_2 content (CaO_2)	*Equation $CaO_2 = (1.34 \times Hb \times SaO_2) + (0.0031 \times PaO_2)$*	*Normal range 20 mL/dL*
Cardiac output (Q)	Q = hr × sv	4–8 L/min
Cardiac index (CI)	CI = Q/BSA	2.4–4.0 $L/min/m^2$
Oxygen delivery (DO_2)	$Q \times 1.34 \times Hb \times SaO_2$	900–1,000 mL/min
Oxygen delivery index (DO_2 index)	DO_2/BSA	520–570 $mL/min/m^2$
Oxygen uptake (VO_2)	$Q \times 1.34 \times Hb \times (SaO_2 - SvO_2)$	180–280 $mL/min/m^2$
Oxygen uptake index (VO_2 index)	$V.O_2/BSA$	110–160 $mL/min/m^2$
Oxygen extraction ratio (O_2ER)	$(SaO_2 - SvO_2/SaO_2) \times 100$	20–30%

Abbreviations: BSA, body surface area; Hb, hemoglobin; hr: heart rate; PaO_2, partial pressure of O_2 in arterial blood; SaO_2, arterial O_2 saturation; SvO_2, mixed venous O_2 saturation; sv, stroke volume

measurements at baseline and after various interventions carried out to increase DO_2 (such as the administration of fluids and inotropes) and is therefore impractical.

Biochemical Parameters

Blood Lactate Level

Blood lactate levels increase when tissue hypoperfusion results in anaerobic metabolism. This is known as Type A lactic acidosis and is different from Type B or nonhypoxic causes of lactic acidosis, e.g. delayed clearance of lactate due to liver disease, thiamine deficiency (blocks pyruvate metabolism) and metabolic alkalosis (stimulates glycolysis). A blood lactate value higher than 4 mmoL/L is generally taken as abnormal. It is easy to measure and can be followed sequentially to assess prognosis, as well as response to therapy. Recent studies indicate that blood lactate concentrations are a better prognostic indicator than oxygen-derived physiological variables.

Gastric Tonometry

Physiological variables of oxygen transport detailed above and lactate are the indices of global tissue oxygenation and cannot identify oxygen deficits in individual organs. This leads to the development of gastric tonometry to measure regional perfusion in the gut that employs a balloon in the stomach to measure intramucosal pH (pHi). Despite its complexity, tonometry is a reasonably good prognostic indicator in critically ill patients.

Sublingual Capnography

Recently capnography in the sublingual area, a technique that is less invasive and easier to use has been shown to yield tissue PCO_2 measurements that correlate with those obtained by gastric tonometry.

Nuclear Magnetic Resonance Spectrometry

This laboratory technique, not applicable at the bedside, can measure biochemical processes at the cellular level, e.g. levels of ATP, NADH and cytochrome oxidase.

Radionuclide imaging, such as positron emission tomography (PET) scanning has emerged as an important tool to characterize tumor oxygenation to optimize and individualize therapy for cancers.

Most of the different parameters of in vivo oxygen measurements measure different things and differ in their sensitivity, accuracy and repeatability. It has been proposed that a proper model that relates the various measurements to each other can serve as a powerful tool to assess tissue oxygenation. Unfortunately, such a functional model is not available as yet **(Table 1)**, whereas the measurement of SvO_2 requires the placement of a pulmonary arterial catheter.

BIBLIOGRAPHY

1. Dantzker DR, Macintyre NR, Bakow ED. Comprehensive Respiratory Care. Philadelphia: W.B. Saunders Company; 1995.
2. Dickens JJ. Central venous oxygenation saturation monitoring: A role for critical care? Curr Anaesth Crit Care. 2004;15:378-82.
3. Hollenberg SM, Ahrens TS, Annane D, Astiz ME, Chalfin DB, Dasta JF, et al. Practice parameters for hemodynamic support of sepsis in adult patients: 2004 update. Crit Care Med. 2004;32(9):1928-48.
4. Krause BJ, Beck R, Souvatzoglou M, Piert M. PET and PET/CT studies of tumor tissue oxygenation. Q J Nucl Med Mol Imaging. 2006;50(1):28-43.
5. Leach RM, Treacher DF. The pulmonary physician in critical care * 2: oxygen delivery and consumption in the critically ill. Thorax. 2002;57(2):170-7.
6. Malley WJ. Oxygen transport and internal respiration. In: Malley WJ (Ed). Clinical blood gases, 1st edition. Philadelphia: WB Saunders Company; 1990. pp. 85-101.
7. Marino P. Tissue oxygenation. In: Marino P (Ed). The ICU book, 2nd edition. Baltimore: Williams and Wilkins; 1998. pp. 187-203.

8. Nathan AT, Singer M. The oxygen trail: tissue oxygenation. Br Med Bull. 1999;55(1):96-108.
9. Ng I, Lee KK, Wong J. Brain tissue oxygenation monitoring in acute brain injury. Acta Neurochir Suppl. 2005;95:447-51.
10. Pierce LN. Guide to Mechanical Ventilation and Intensive Respiratory Care. Philadelphia: WB Saunders Company; 1995.
11. Reinhart K, Kuhn HJ, Hartog C, Bredle DL. Continuous central venous and pulmonary artery oxygen saturation monitoring in the critically ill. Intensive Care Med. 2004;30(8):1572-8.
12. Rivers E, Nguyen B, Havstad S, Ressler J, Muzzin A, Knoblich B, et al. Early goal-directed therapy in the treatment of severe sepsis and septic shock. N Engl J Med. 2001;345(19):1368-77.
13. Swartz HM, Dunn J. The difficulties in comparing in vivo oxygen measurements: turning the problems into virtues. Adv Exp Med Biol. 2005;566:295-301.
14. Tissue hypoxia: how to detect, how to correct, how to prevent? Third European Consensus Conference in Intensive Care Medicine. Organized by the Société de Réanimation de Langue Française, Cosponsored by the American Thoracic Society and the European Society of Intensive Care Medicine. J Crit Care. 1997;12(1):39-47.
15. Weibel ER. Oxygen and the History of Life. In: Weibel ER (Ed). The Pathways for Oxygen. Cambridge MA: Harvard University Press; 1984. pp. 1-30.

Respiratory Physiology in Specific Physiological States

Sunil K Chhabra, Mansi Gupta

INTRODUCTION

The respiratory system performs the essential function of gas exchange and plays its assigned role in the maintenance of the acid-base homeostasis to perfection with its basic mechanisms of the control of breathing, lung mechanics, gas diffusion and transport, and regulation of pulmonary circulation in a coordinated and integrated manner under a wide range of environmental conditions and physiological states of the body. Together with cardiovascular system and aided by an appropriate response from other systems, the human body can adapt to these variations from the normal state without any adverse consequences. These adaptations may sometimes resemble changes in pathological conditions and hence the knowledge of physiological changes in these specific states is necessary to avoid an erroneous interpretation of symptoms and signs. However, adaptations have a limit in the time course over which they develop and in the range of deviations from the normal resting state at the sea level. Due to these limits, the adaptations may fail and manifest as pathological conditions. The following sections are devoted to changes in respiratory physiology and allied systems in specific physiological states such as exercise, pregnancy, high altitude and deep diving.

EXERCISE[1-14]

While exercising, the muscles are required to perform greater work and thus require more energy. This is provided by increased aerobic metabolism and thus increased oxygen consumption. The oxygen consumption in the muscles increases with the rising intensity of exercise. An integrated response of cardiovascular and respiratory systems is required to meet the increased demand for oxygen by the muscles and to eliminate the excessive amount of CO_2. This response requires an increase in heart rate, cardiac output, regional blood flow in the exercising muscles, oxygen extraction by the tissues and ventilation to washout extra CO_2. It is coordinated and related to the workload and meets the requirements of the exercising muscles. The acute respiratory and cardiovascular responses to exercise are complimented by changes and responses in the muscles, as well as neurological and endocrinal systems in an effort to survive through a wide range of severity of exercise without adverse consequences. The physiological changes occurring in the cardiorespiratory systems on exercise are summarized in **Table 1**.

Table 1 Physiological changes in the cardiorespiratory systems on exercise

- Increased rate of oxygen consumption
- Increased CO_2 excretion
- Increased alveolocapillary gradient for oxygen
- Increased diffusion capacity
- Increased blood flow and pulmonary artery pressure
- Recruitment of underperfused pulmonary capillary beds
- Increased ventilation
- Decreased airway resistance
- Decreased ratio of Dead Space (V_D) to tidal volume (V_T)
- Rightward shift of the oxygen-hemoglobin dissociation curve
- Increased extraction of oxygen in the muscles
- Dilatation and recruitment of the capillary bed of the muscles
- Increased blood flow to muscles
- Increased arterial blood pressure
- Increased stroke volume
- Increased heart rate
- Increased venous return
- Increased cardiac output

Respiratory System

Increased extraction of oxygen in the exercising tissues results in a fall in the mixed venous PO_2 of blood reaching the right side of the heart, from a normal of 40 mm Hg to 25 mm Hg or even less. This increases the alveolocapillary gradient, even though the alveolar PO_2 is not changed. As a result, the amount of oxygen entering the blood in the lungs is increased. The increased alveolocapillary gradient for oxygen is aided by an increase in the diffusion capacity that may be up to three-fold on exercise. This results from the recruitment of underperfused pulmonary capillary beds due to increased blood flow and pulmonary artery pressures, thus providing a greater surface area across which oxygen can diffuse into the blood. The pulmonary blood flow increases from a normal of 5.5 L/minute to as much as 20–35 L/minute.

Those athletes who require greater amount of oxygen per minute have higher diffusion capacities. It is not clear how much of this increase is genetic and how much is acquired through training. Normally, there is a mild degree of ventilation-perfusion inequality due to relative under-perfusion in the upper zones of the lung. During moderate exercise, this is reduced because of the more uniform distribution of blood flow in upper zones, providing another adaptation to facilitate oxygen uptake. On the other hand, in athletes performing strenuous exercise, a mild degree of interstitial pulmonary edema related to increased pulmonary artery pressures may develop leading to mild ventilation-perfusion inequality.

The total amount of oxygen entering the blood increases from 250 mL/minute at rest to values as high as 3,000–4,000 mL/minute. In a marathon runner, it may exceed 5,000 mL/minute, a 20-fold increase. The rate of oxygen usage under maximal aerobic metabolism is written as VO_2 max. The VO_2 max of a marathoner may thus be 40–50% greater than that of an untrained person. Training does increase the VO_2 max, but only to a limited extent of about 10% over 2–3 months. However, longer periods of training may increase the VO_2 max further, and it is also probably genetically determined. The oxygen saturation, PaO_2 and the oxygen content of the blood (CaO_2) leaving the lungs remain the same as at rest. This is dictated by the oxygen hemoglobin dissociation curve, as well as the hemoglobin levels. The CO_2 excretion also increases from 200 mL/minute to as much as 8,000 mL/minute.

Oxygen consumption and total pulmonary ventilation at different levels of exercise increase with a linear relationship depending on the intensity of the exercise up to a limit. Above this limit, the aerobic metabolism in the muscles is unable to synthesize energy stores at a pace matching their utilization, and thus anaerobic metabolism sets in (anaerobic threshold). The oxygen consumption levels off, an oxygen debt is incurred and the blood lactate level rises. Ventilation increases abruptly and sharply with the onset of exercise followed by a further, more gradual increase. The initial rise in ventilation occurs primarily because of an increase in the tidal volume. Though the limit for tidal volume is the vital capacity, it plateaus off at around 50–60% of the vital capacity. The tidal volume encroaches into the inspiratory reserve volume (IRV) and, to a smaller extent, into the expiratory reserve volume (ERV). During light and moderate exercise, the contribution of an increase in the respiratory rate to minute ventilation is minimal and gradual. Ventilation decreases abruptly when exercise ceases, and is followed after a brief pause by a more gradual decline to pre-exercise values.

The increase in ventilation is proportional to the increase in oxygen consumption. It is likely that multiple mechanisms are involved in the stimulation of ventilation. The initial sharp increase at the start of an exercise is presumably due to cerebral input to the respiratory center in the anticipation of the increased needs depending on the past experiences and afferent impulses from proprioceptors in muscles, tendons and joints. The subsequent more gradual increase is probably humoral in origin. However, the arterial pH, PCO_2, and PO_2 remain constant during moderate exercise. The increase in body temperature may also play a role. Stimulation of the peripheral chemoreceptors by exercise-induced temperature rise, the plasma K^+ level, increased sensitivity of the neurons controlling the response to CO_2 and increased respiratory fluctuations in arterial PCO_2 (even though the mean arterial PCO_2 does not rise) are some of the proposed mechanisms. Oxygen may also play some role, despite the lack of a decrease in arterial PO_2, since during the performance of a given amount of work, the increase in ventilation while breathing 100% oxygen is 10–20% less than the increase while breathing air.

When exercise becomes more intense, there is liberation of CO_2 due to the buffering of the increased amount of lactic acid that is produced in the muscles. This further increases ventilation. With increased production of acid, the increase in ventilation and CO_2 production remain proportional, and thus the change in alveolar and arterial CO_2 is relatively little (isocapnic buffering). The increase in ventilation produced by the acidosis is due to the stimulation of carotid bodies. The alveolar PO_2 increases because of hyperventilation. With the further accumulation of lactic acid, the increase in ventilation becomes out of proportion to the CO_2 production, alveolar PCO_2 and arterial PCO_2 fall. The decline in arterial PCO_2 is a respiratory compensation for the metabolic acidosis produced by the additional lactic acid.

While the level of maximum ventilation achieved is dependent on the intensity of exercise, it is seldom beyond 20 times the resting level, i.e. up to 100–110 L. The maximum breathing capacity is about 150–170 L in an average person. Thus, even on intense exercise, only about 50–60% of the reserve is used. There is still sufficient reserve available for extreme circumstances such as exercise at high altitudes and in extreme environments. Further, as oxygen supply from the lungs under normal circumstances is always sufficient, respiratory system response is never the limiting factor for exercise.

The recovery of the respiratory rate after exercise to basal level is delayed until the oxygen debt is repaid. This may take as long as 90 minutes. The stimulus to ventilation after exercise is the elevated arterial H^+ concentration due to the lactic academia. The arterial PCO_2, which is normal or low, or the arterial PO_2, which is normal or high, play no role. The magnitude of the oxygen debt is the amount by which its consumption exceeds basal consumption from the end of exertion until it has returned to pre-exercise basal levels. During the repayment of the oxygen debt, its concentration in muscle myoglobin rises slightly. ATP and phosphoryl-creatinine are resynthesized, and lactic acid is removed. Eighty percent of the lactic acid is converted to glycogen and 20% is metabolized to CO_2 and H_2O. Buffering of lactic acid during strenuous exercise increases the CO_2 liberation and therefore, respiratory exchange ratio (R: the ratio of CO_2 production to oxygen consumption) rises, reaching 1.5–2.0. After exertion, while the oxygen debt is being repaid, the R falls to 0.5 or less. Typically, the R rises from about 0.8 at rest to 1.0 on aerobic exercise. This increase reflects a greater reliance on carbohydrate rather than fat to produce the required energy.

Airway resistance decreases owing to bronchodilation as soon as exercise begins. Likewise, the ratio of dead space (V_D) to tidal volume (V_T) decreases. The drop in V_D/V_T is moderate at low-to-moderate exercise intensities. The V_D itself changes minimally with bronchodilation, the change in ratio being largely due to the increased V_T. This is advantageous, as it results in greater alveolar ventilation for given minute ventilation.

Changes in the Muscle

The rate at which oxygen is transported to the mitochondria in the exercising muscle is a limiting factor for the maximum oxygen uptake. As pointed out above, the lungs are never the limiting factor for oxygen uptake in health. During exercise, because of greater oxygen extraction, the tissue and the venous PO_2 drop sharply. There is a dilatation and recruitment of the capillary bed of the contracting muscle, facilitating the delivery of oxygen from blood to cells. The blood flow to muscles during exercise increases markedly, about 25-fold during the most strenuous exercise. This results from intramuscular vasodilatation caused by the direct effects of increased muscle metabolism, and also a moderate increase in the arterial blood pressure on exercise. Muscle contractions temporarily decrease the muscle blood flow by the compression of the intramuscular blood vessels; therefore, strong tonic muscle contractions can cause rapid muscle fatigue because of the lack of delivery of enough oxygen and other nutrients during the continuous contraction.

The oxygen-hemoglobin dissociation curve is steep in the PO_2 range below 60 mm Hg, and a relatively large amount of oxygen is supplied per mm Hg fall in PO_2. Oxygen off loading is further facilitated by the rightward shift of the curve due to the accumulation of CO_2, the rise in temperature and a rise in red blood cell 2,3-diphosphoglycerate (2,3-DPG). The net effect is a three-fold increase in oxygen extraction from each unit of blood. As the local redistribution and increased cardiac output result in a 30-fold or greater increase in blood flow, it permits the metabolic rate of muscle to rise by as much as 100-fold during exercise.

Cardiovascular System

The work output, oxygen consumption, and cardiac output during exercise are directly related to each other, linearly. The increased blood flow to the muscles to meet the demand for increased oxygen consumption increases the venous return and hence the cardiac output. Normally, in an untrained person, the cardiac output can increase a little over four-fold, and in the well-trained athlete, about six-fold. Marathoners can achieve maximal cardiac outputs that are about 40% greater than those achieved by untrained persons. This occurs because of a nearly 40% increase in the cardiac muscle mass, as well as in the size of the chambers, and is observed only in the endurance types, not in the sprint types, of athletic training. At rest, a marathoner with a large heart has the same cardiac output as that of an average person. However, given the increased stroke volume, he can maintain the required cardiac output with a slower heart rate. At rest, a nonathlete person has an average stroke volume of 70–75 mL pumped at around 70 beats/minute while a marathoner has a stroke volume of around 100 mL and thus requires only 50 beats/minute to achieve the same cardiac output.

The increase in stroke volume is also greater on exercise in the marathoner and may reach 150–160 mL (about 50% increases over the resting value). At a maximal heart rate of around 180 beats/minute (up from the resting of 50 beats/minute, an almost 250% change), he will have a much greater cardiac output than a non-athlete in whom the stroke volume increases moderately to around 100–110 mL on exercise. Thus, a marathoner can increase the cardiac output to about 27–30 L/minute while a nonathlete can increase it to around 18–20 L/minute. The increase in the cardiac output till about halfway is largely accounted for by the increase in stroke volume and subsequently by the increase in heart rate as the stroke volume gets limited earlier.

During maximal exercise, the cardiac output can reach 90% of its maximum possible value, whereas as noted above, the maximum ventilation achieved is only 50–60% of the maximum capacity. Therefore, cardiovascular system is normally much more limiting on VO_2 max than is the respiratory system, because oxygen utilization by the body can only be up to the rate at which the cardiovascular system can transport oxygen to the tissues.

PREGNANCY[15-27]

Pregnancy induces major physiological changes affecting all systems of the body. These occur early in the pregnancy and continue throughout gestation, with complete reversal after delivery. Several of these changes would be considered pathological if these were to occur in the nonpregnant state and may even cause symptoms. However, in pregnancy, these changes are considered physiological because they serve to ensure a successful gestation. An understanding of these changes is necessary since inappropriate diagnosis and interventions may occur in the absence of this knowledge. Considering the scope of this chapter, the following discussion is limited to changes in the respiratory system and related cardiological and hematological aspects. These changes are summarized in **Table 2**.

Table 2 Physiological changes in cardiorespiratory and hematological systems during pregnancy

- Bronchial smooth muscle relaxation
- Reduced TLC, FRC, RV, ERV
- Increased IC
- Increased dead space ventilation
- Increased tidal volume
- Increased respiratory rate
- Increased minute ventilation
- Increase in the oxygen consumption
- Increased blood volume
- Increased red blood cell mass
- Increased left atrial size
- Increased left ventricular end-diastolic dimension
- Increased left ventricular wall thickness
- Increased left ventricular mass
- Increased cardiac output
- Decreased systemic vascular resistance
- Decreased systemic blood pressure
- Increased pulse rate

Respiratory System

Hormonal changes in pregnancy, the increased estrogen, cause edema, capillary congestion and hyperplasia of the mucus glands. It affects the mucosa of the upper respiratory tract, including the larynx, producing hyperemia, mucosal edema, hypersecretion and increased mucosal friability. This causes the voice to change along with nasal congestion. It leads to the worsening of pre-existing rhinitis. The mucosal changes in the larynx also make endotracheal intubation more difficult, should the need arise. Respiratory infections and pre-eclampsia aggravate these symptoms. As the uterus enlarges, the diaphragm is elevated by as much as 4 cm, the rib cage is displaced upwards and widens, increasing the lower thoracic diameter by 2 cm and the thoracic circumference by up to 6 cm. The abdominal muscles have a decreased tone and are less active during the pregnancy, causing respiration to be more thoracic and less diaphragmatic. The subcostal angle increases from 60–70° to around 100–110°.

Pregnancy causes significant changes in the pulmonary mechanics. The dead space volume increases due to the relaxation of the musculature of the trachea and the bronchi by progesterone. The bronchial smooth muscle relaxation may decrease asthma symptoms in some patients. A state of hyperventilation occurs and the tidal volume (V_T) increases gradually (by 35–50%) as the pregnancy progresses. The total lung capacity (TLC) is reduced slightly (4–5%) by the elevation of the diaphragm. Due to anatomical changes in the thoracic cage, the functional residual capacity (FRC), residual volume (RV), and expiratory reserve volume (ERV), all decrease by about 10–20%. The increased tidal volume and the smaller residual volume cause an increase in the alveolar ventilation (up to about 65%) during pregnancy.

Inspiratory capacity (IC) increases by 5–10%. Although there is no change in the lung compliance, there is an overall decrease in the chest wall and total respiratory compliance. The forced vital capacity (FVC) is largely unaltered till later in pregnancy as the widened chest diameters counter the effects of the raised diaphragm. Airway function is not affected and FEV_1 remains at the same level as the prepregnancy state. The FEV_1/FVC ratio is usually not affected. Therefore, the dyspnea of normal pregnancy is not responsive to bronchodilators.

There are other stimuli that increase the ventilation, including increased metabolic carbon dioxide production, as well as the high serum progesterone that has a direct effect on the respiratory center. The respiratory changes include a slight increase in the respiratory rate, and a progressive increase in the oxygen consumption of up to 15–20% above the prepregnant levels by term (due to increased maternal BMR and increased fetal energy demands). With the increase in respiratory tidal volume associated with a normal or increased respiratory rate, there is an increase in respiratory minute volume of approximately 26%. As the respiratory minute volume increases, "hyperventilation of pregnancy" occurs, causing a decrease in the alveolar CO_2. The $PaCO_2$ decreases to around 30 mm Hg in late pregnancy and the renal loss of bicarbonate compensates to maintain the pH in the normal range. This maternal hyperventilation is considered a protective measure that prevents the fetus from exposure to the excessive levels of CO_2.

At the time of labor, the functional residual capacity (FRC) decreases further. The ventilation increases, which is also driven by pain and anxiety resulting in marked hypocapnia and respiratory alkalosis. This may have adverse consequences for the fetus oxygenation by reducing the uterine blood flow. On the other hand, severe pain and anxiety can lead to rapid shallow breathing with alveolar hypoventilation, atelectasis, and mild hypoxemia in some patients. Preoxygenation is less effective and desaturation is likely to occur much faster than in the nonpregnant patient. A preoxygenation period of 3–5 minutes is advisable.

Hematological and Cardiovascular Systems

The most striking maternal physiologic alteration that occurs during pregnancy is the increase in the blood volume that varies according to the body mass of the woman, the parity, and the number of fetuses. This occurs due to the effect of progesterone and estrogen on the kidneys, leading to the activation of the renin-aldosterone-angiotensin pathway resulting in renal sodium retention and an increase in the total body water. The increase in blood volume is progressive, starting from the 6th week. The average increase in volume is 45–50% by 30–32 weeks; the level being static thereafter till term. The increased volume serves to maintain adequate fetomaternal tissue perfusion, as well as preparing the body to compensate for maternal blood loss during delivery.

The increase in plasma volume parallels the increase in the whole blood volume, the maximum extent being 50%. The red blood cell mass also increases by about 20–30%, stimulated by the rise in erythropoietin levels. There is a mild increase in the total leukocyte and platelet count. Simultaneously, platelet consumption is also increased. As plasma volume increases early in pregnancy and at a faster rate than the red blood cell volume, the hematocrit falls until the end of the second trimester, after which the increase in the red blood cells matches the increase in the plasma volume. This hemodilution results in the "physiological anemia of pregnancy". The hematocrit then stabilizes or may even increase slightly near the term. The initial hemodilution is advantageous as the reduced blood viscosity ensures adequate gaseous exchange to the fetus. The increased blood volume also delays the onset of symptoms of hypovolemia in the case of excessive bleeding during delivery. By 2 weeks postpartum, the hematological changes revert to prepregnancy status.

During pregnancy, as the uterus enlarges and the diaphragm becomes elevated, the heart is displaced upwards and somewhat to the left with rotation on its long axis, so that the apex beat is moved laterally. The cardiac capacity increases by 70-80 mL; this may be due to increased volume or hypertrophy of the cardiac muscle. The overall size of the heart appears to increase by about 12%. The left atrial size increases and correlates with the change in blood volume. The left ventricular end-diastolic dimension increases while the left ventricular end-systolic size might decrease somewhat as a result of the changes in the cardiac contractility. The left ventricular wall thickness increases by 28%, and the left ventricular mass increases by 52%.

A systolic murmur may be audible in the aortic or the pulmonary areas due to hemodilution and torsion of the great vessels. The cardiac output also starts to rise from the 5th week and increases approximately by 30-40% at 20-24 weeks gestation, reaches a maximal value of 10-30% above baseline values by 32 weeks and continues at this level until term. The cardiac output is lowest in the sitting and supine position and highest in the right or left lateral or the knee-chest position. In the supine position, the gravid uterus may compress the inferior vena cava reducing the venous return to the heart leading to a fall in the cardiac output, maternal blood pressure and placental perfusion. The descending aorta can also be compressed by the uterus causing a reduction in the uterine blood flow. Aortocaval compression is a cause of maternal hypotension from the end of the first trimester onwards, though usually it occurs after 20 weeks of gestation.

The systemic vascular resistance decreases by around 20% due to the effect of progesterone, nitric oxide, prostaglandins and atrial natriuretic peptide. The systemic blood pressure declines slightly during pregnancy. The diastolic pressure is reduced by approximately 5-10 mm Hg from about 12-26 weeks and increases thereafter to prepregnancy levels by about 36 weeks. There is an increase in the pulse rate of about 15-25%, a reflex due to reduced blood pressure and extrasystoles may occur. The pulmonary vascular resistance also decreases by 20-30%.

During labor, uterine contractions cause a 7-25% increase in the maternal cardiac output, a 7-15% decrease in the heart rate, and a resultant 7-33% increase in the stroke volume. The central venous pressure increases in parallel with the intensity of uterine contractions and increases the intra-abdominal pressure. Additionally, cardiopulmonary blood volume increases by 300-500 mL during contractions.

HIGH ALTITUDE[28-44]

Ascent to high altitude represents a physiological stress on the body. The concept of high altitude is arbitrary. Above 1,500 m, physiological changes due to hypobaric hypoxia are detectable. With ascent, the barometric pressure falls leading to a lower atmospheric partial pressure of oxygen (PO_2), that in turn leads to a lower alveolar PO_2, although the composition of air remains the same. The pressure at 5,800 m (19,000 ft) is only one-half of the normal 760 mm Hg and the PO_2 of moist inspired gas is 70 mm Hg. On the peak of Mount Everest (altitude 8,848 m, or 29,028 ft), the inspired PO_2 is only 43 mm Hg. At 19,200 m (63,000 ft), the barometric pressure is 47 mm Hg, so the inspired PO_2 is zero. Yet, more than 150 million people live at altitudes over 2,500 m (8,000 ft), and even higher than 4,900 m (16,000 ft) in the Andes.

Climbers have lived for several days at altitudes that would cause unconsciousness within a few seconds if the human body did not have the capacity for acclimatization. Respiratory changes and adaptations follow ascent, and are associated with changes in other systems of the body, especially hematological and cardiovascular that allow survival. **Table 3** summarizes the acute and chronic physiological adaptations on ascent to high altitude. It should be appreciated that these adaptations have regional, ethnic and gender variations. The physiological changes occurring in the body can be classified into acute and chronic, depending on the duration of exposure and stay at high altitude.

Acute Effects of Hypoxia

Respiratory

The minute ventilation increases to minimize the fall in alveolar PO_2 as the barometric pressure decreases. The ventilatory response increases initially on ascent as the PaO_2 falls below 60 mm Hg due to carotid chemoreceptor stimulation, then stabilizes over hours and weeks, and finally declines with deacclimatization on descent. The neural discharge from the whole carotid sinus nerve is related hyperbolically to decreasing PaO_2. Immediately following acute exposure to a very low PO_2, and lasting for perhaps half an hour, a transient "roll off" phenomenon or a hypoxic ventilatory decline may be there. Later, hypoxic stimulation of the peripheral chemoreceptors increases the alveolar ventilation to a maximum of about 1.65 times the normal.

Table 3 Physiological changes at high altitude

Acute changes
• Increase in the minute ventilation
• Increase in diffusion capacity of lungs
• Respiratory alkalosis and fall in PCO_2
• Increased pulmonary vascular resistance and perfusion
• Increased heart rate
• Increased cardiac output
• Increase in the regional blood flow by vasodilatation
• Decrease in circulating volume due to water diuresis
• Increase in the number of erythrocytes
• Leftward shift in the dissociation curve
Chronic effects
• Ventilation diminishes, but still more than at sea level
• Resting $PaCO_2$ increases towards normal, but still low
• Increased vital capacity
• Increased pulmonary vascular resistance and perfusion
• Decreased heart rate
• Increased stroke volume
• Decreased blood pressure
• Cardiac output tends to decrease back to normal
• Increased recruitment of the systemic capillary units
• Increase in the hematocrit values (polycythemia)
• Leftward shift in the dissociation curve

The increased ventilation allows alveolar CO_2 to be lowered and thus for a given FiO_2, a higher alveolar PO_2 can be achieved, as dictated by the alveolar gas equation. In extreme cases, ventilation may increase five-fold lowering alveolar CO_2 to as low as 8 mm Hg though usually in high altitude residents at 15,000 ft, it is around 33 mm Hg.

The acute increase in ventilation is inhibited by the resulting respiratory alkalosis and the fall in PCO_2 at the medullary and peripheral chemoreceptors. After a day or so, the cerebrospinal fluid (CSF) pH is brought partly back towards normal by the movement of bicarbonate out of the CSF, and after 2 or 3 days, the pH of the arterial blood is returned to near normal by the renal excretion of bicarbonate. The inhibition of ventilation is then reduced, allowing it to increase. In addition, there is evidence that the sensitivity of the carotid bodies to hypoxia increases during acclimatization. Over the next 2–5 days, the chemoreceptors increase the ventilation gradually to over five times the normal. However, the measurement of blood pH has revealed that alkalosis persists as ventilation increases. On the other hand, the cerebrospinal fluid pH may return to normal or even be relatively acidotic, causing sustained hyperventilation. The interstitial fluid around central chemoreceptors has also been found to be acidic in spite of the alkalinity of the CSF. It is possible that some mediator(s), other than H^+, may sustain the hyperventilation during the stay at high altitude.

High-altitude inhabitants exhibit a different long-term response that results in lower ventilation at any given altitude as compared to people experiencing similar altitudes for the first time suggesting that they have a diminished ventilatory response to hypoxia. The vital capacity decreases in the first 24 hours, with an increase in the residual volume and in the slope of the alveolar plateau of the single-breath nitrogen test. These changes are compatible with an increased interstitial fluid volume, resulting in airway narrowing, gas trapping, and delayed emptying of some lung units.

Cardiovascular

The initial increase in ventilation during acute hypoxia is accompanied by an increase in the cardiac output (as much as 30%) and pulmonary perfusion. This helps to sustain oxygen delivery in spite of the decreased arterial oxygen content. The increase in cardiac output is largely a result of an increased heart rate with little change in the stroke volume. This is mediated by an increase in the release of, and sensitivity to, catecholamines that override the augmented parasympathetic tone. Over the next few days at high altitude, the cardiac output decreases, primarily as a result of a decrease in the stroke volume as decreasing plasma volume reduces preload.

The hypoxic pulmonary vasoconstriction causes pulmonary hypertension. The increase in the pulmonary artery pressure starts as the alveolar PO_2 drops below 70 mm Hg, and then sharply below that. This is advantageous as it improves ventilation-perfusion matching by the redistribution of blood flow to areas of the lung that are usually poorly perfused. The increased pulmonary perfusion also improves the diffusion of oxygen.

Hematological

Hemoglobin concentration increases within 1 or 2 days of ascent and continues to rise for a number of weeks. The initial rise is due to hemoconcentration following the diuresis that occurs on initial ascent. Later, erythropoietin increases rapidly within 24–48 hours to stimulate the red blood cell production and then starts to decline within 3 weeks as acclimatization progresses. This increase allows the oxygen content to increase even though PaO_2 and saturation are diminished. The erythropoiesis, however, carries a disadvantage as it also increases the viscosity. There is a rightward shift of the O_2 dissociation curve due to an increase in the concentration of 2,3-diphosphoglycerate following respiratory alkalosis at moderate altitudes, that aids in unloading of O_2 in tissues at a given PO_2. At higher altitudes, there is a leftward shift in the dissociation curve caused by the respiratory alkalosis, and this assists in the loading of O_2 in the pulmonary capillaries.

Chronic Effects of Hypoxia or Acclimatization

Compensatory mechanisms come into play on ascent to high altitudes and allow a person to sustain and work without the deleterious effects of hypoxia on the body. This process is called "acclimatization". Ventilation continues to increase for a few weeks. A number of factors, such as regulation of brain pH, metabolic rate and turnover of neurotransmitters, might contribute to this hyperventilation. However, with residence at high altitude, ventilation diminishes, and the resting $PaCO_2$ settles at a higher level, though still lower than at sea-level. This blunting is associated with hypertrophy of the carotid bodies. The decreased energy expenditure of the lower ventilation is an advantage as it reduces the overall oxygen consumption making it easier to sustain at the lower alveolar PO_2.

Chronic exposure causes the vital capacity to increase in high-altitude natives. The increase in vital capacity is dependent on the age at which the subjects start living at high altitude. Natives born at these heights develop larger vital capacities than those who move to high altitude later in life. This is understandable as the lung growth occurs mostly till the age of 8 years. With long-term residence at high altitude, diffusion capacity of the lung increases. This may be due to increased surface area consequent upon higher lung volume and the increase in pulmonary arterial pressure, promoting more blood flow through the alveolar capillaries.

On a prolonged stay at high altitude, the parasympathetic tone plays a role in the decreased heart rate. Down regulation of α-receptors in the myocardium results in lower heart rate on exercise even though norepinephrine levels rise. This does not compromise oxygen delivery as the stroke volume is also increased. The blood pressure is generally lower in high-altitude natives that may be secondary to a primary vasodilatory effect of hypoxia on systemic arterial wall muscle, as well as its negative inotropic effect on the cardiac muscles. With a more gradual increase in the hematocrit values, lower resting heart rate and higher stroke volume, the cardiac output tends to decrease back to normal. Another hemodynamic change that occurs is the increased recruitment of the systemic capillary units in the nonpulmonary tissues that increases the tissue blood flow and hence the oxygen delivery.

Chronic exposure to high altitude results in an increase in the pulmonary vascular resistance and pulmonary hypertension (primarily at the site of pulmonary arterioles) that may be compounded by polycythemia and hypoxic pulmonary vasoconstriction which may be severe. The continued increase in hemoglobin results from increased red blood cell production (erythropoiesis) as part of acclimatization; this adaptation helps to sustain oxygen delivery in the presence of decreased arterial oxygen. In a fully acclimatized individual, the hematocrit may reach 60, with hemoglobin concentration as high as 20 g/dL. The blood volume also increases by 20–30%, resulting in a total increase of around 50% in the circulating hemoglobin. This is a slow process and takes many months to complete. These changes increase arterial oxygen content and tissue oxygen delivery.

At high altitude, adaptations occur in the oxygen-hemoglobin dissociation curve that may help to facilitate oxygen transfer. Increased 2,3-DPG concentrations have been reported that should result in a right shift in the curve. However, the persistent respiratory alkalosis more than counterbalances the 2,3-DPG effect, shifting the curve back to normal or even slightly to the left. At very high altitudes, a rightward shift of the oxygen-hemoglobin dissociation curve could be a disadvantage for oxygen transport. While favoring the unloading of oxygen from the tissues, the same would also hinder the loading of oxygen in the lungs. A left-shifted curve at extreme altitude would result in enhanced oxygen loading in the lungs and higher arterial oxygen content.

DEEP DIVING[42-56]

Deep diving is done for professional and occupational purposes and increasingly for recreation. The environment on diving changes and has effects on the body systems that can vary from trivial to profound and may sometimes be even fatal if the diver is not careful. In relation to respiration, physiological alterations occur in the breathing cycle and blood gases. There are indirect effects related to alterations in the pressure of blood gases. There occur direct pressure-related problems on descent (including effects on ears, sinuses, thorax, stomach and intestines), and on ascent (air embolism, pneumothorax, mediastinal and subcutaneous emphysema). The effects of the pressure occur especially on compressible fluids, i.e. gas compartments. Pressure has no direct effects on noncompressible tissues and fluids. In addition, there are effects of temperature stimuli. Immersion causes a central redistribution of blood volume, which is increased if cold water triggers vasoconstriction. This reduces antidiuretic hormone (ADH) release and results in a diuresis, increasing the risk of hypovolemia on surfacing. The high-risk of dehydration is further increased by the breathing of dry gas. Dehydration increases the susceptibility to diving related illnesses. Another challenge is that of temperature regulation. Water has a high thermal conductivity and capacity and the cold water predisposes the diver to, the risk of hypothermia.

Physical Principles in Deep Diving

It would be useful to review some basic laws of physical sciences to understand the diving physiology and associated abnormalities. The effect of diving deep into the sea stems from the tremendous increase in the hydrostatic pressure on the body. The human body is normally exposed to a pressure of 1 atmospheres absolute (ATA) at sea level. Water being far denser than air, for every descent of 33 feet, an additional pressure of 1 ATA is added. This is equivalent to 1.013 bar, 760 mm Hg or 14.7 psi. Thus, at 33 feet, the body is exposed to a pressure of 2 ATA, 1 ATA of pressure caused by the weight of the air above the water and the second by the weight of the water itself.

The increase in pressure causes a decrease in the volume of body cavities containing gases in accordance with the Boyle's law, i.e. the volume of gas is inversely proportional to the pressure it is subjected to, with the temperature remaining constant. Thus, compression (i.e. increased pressure) on descent will decrease the volume. If volume of a compartment is expressed as 100% at 1 ATA, it would be 50% at 2 ATA and 33% at 3 ATA and so on. Thus, proportional reduction is greatest in shallow water, i.e. the volume halves at 33 feet. The compression of the air pockets can be extremely dangerous and the lungs are especially vulnerable. An actual volume of 1 liter at a depth of 300 feet is the same quantity of air at a sea-level volume of 10 liters. Deeper a subject goes under the sea, the greater is the compression. To keep the lungs from collapsing, air must be supplied at very high pressure to keep them inflated. This exposes the blood in the lungs also to extremely high alveolar gas pressure, a condition called "hyperbarism". Beyond certain limits, these high pressures can cause tremendous alterations in body physiology, and can be lethal.

The individual gases to which a diver is exposed when breathing air are nitrogen, oxygen, and carbon dioxide; each of them at times can cause significant physiological effects at high pressures. Even gases, such as carbon monoxide that normally are in negligible concentrations, can pose hazards when their alveolar pressures are increased. Dalton's law states that the total pressure exerted by a mixture of gases is equal to the sum of the pressures of each of its constituent gases, i.e. partial pressures of each gas added up make the total pressure of the mixture. Thus, if the total pressure increases with descent, pressures of body gases in their compartments will also increase proportionately without any change in their concentrations. Henry's law states that at a constant temperature, the amount of gas that will dissolve in a liquid is directly proportional to the partial pressure of that gas at its surface. The amount also depends on the solubility coefficient of the gas. Thus, gases will increasingly dissolve in body fluids on descent depending on their solubility and, on ascent, these will bubble out as the pressure decreases. This is the physical principle underlying decompression sickness (DCS), described later.

Increased pressure, on descent, reduces the volume and increases the density of gases in the airways. This, combined with immersion, reduces pulmonary compliance, increases airways resistance and also results in increased V/Q mismatch, and an increase in the work of breathing. This increase in the work of breathing is one of the factors, which limits maximum diving depth and along with breath-holding (apnea) is responsible for dyspnea.[57] The combination of resistive and elastic loads is also responsible for the reduction in ventilation. Further, there is a density-related increase in dead space/tidal volume ratio (Vd/Vt), possibly due to the impairment of intrapulmonary gas phase diffusion and distribution of ventilation. The net result of relative hypoventilation and increased Vd/Vt is hypercapnia. Professional divers, therefore, breathe helium-oxygen mixtures that are much less dense and have reduced viscosity compared with air. The concentrations of oxygen and CO_2 do not change except when the breathing apparatus is faulty or of poor design causing CO_2 rebreathing.

Depth and Nitrogen Narcosis

About 80% of the air is nitrogen. At sea-level pressure, the nitrogen has no significant physiological effects. However, at high pressures it can affect the functioning of the central nervous system, an effect called "nitrogen narcosis".[58] The relation of depth to narcosis is sometimes informally known as "Martini law" as the symptoms of nitrogen narcosis resemble those of alcohol intoxication, developing roughly after 66 feet at the rate of the effect of one martini after every 33 feet. When the diver remains beneath the sea for an hour or more and breathes compressed air, the depth at which the first symptoms of mild narcosis appear is about 100–120 feet. Rarely, the effects may be seen with shallow dives. Individuals vary in their susceptibility. However, the problem is universal and related to the depth reached. Tolerance does not develop. The condition is entirely reversible on careful ascent.

Physiological Basis of Oxygen Toxicity

Oxygen is transported in blood largely bound to the heme portion of hemoglobin and to a much smaller extent dissolved in the blood, 0.0031 mL per mm PaO_2. Normally, at a PaO_2 of 100 mm, only 0.3 mL oxygen is dissolved in the blood, physically. When the PaO_2 in the blood rises above 100 mm Hg, the amount of oxygen dissolved in the water of the blood increases several folds. While the amount bound to hemoglobin is limited due to the saturation of the binding sites, the increase in oxygen content is largely due to an increase in the dissolved oxygen. At an alveolar PO_2 of 3,000 mm Hg (4 ATA), each 100 mL of blood contains 29 mL oxygen, 20 mL bound with hemoglobin and 9 mL dissolved in the blood water. The tissues take up their normal requirement of 5 mL leaving 24 mL of oxygen still in the blood. At this point, the PO_2 is approximately 1,200 mm Hg, which means that oxygen is delivered to the tissues at this extremely high pressure instead of at the normal value of 40 mm Hg. The normal, safe range is between 20 mm Hg and 60 mm Hg.

Pathogenesis of Decompression Sickness (Caisson Disease, Dysbarism)

An increase in the alveolar PN_2 increases the dissolved nitrogen in the capillary bed, resulting in the same level of tissue PN_2. As nitrogen is not metabolized by the body, it remains dissolved in all the body tissues. However, when the alveolar pressures return to normal, the excess nitrogen is removed by the reverse process from the tissues. This removal often takes hours to occur and is responsible for a constellation of symptoms called "decompression sickness".

At the sea level, almost exactly 1 liter of nitrogen is dissolved in the entire body, slightly more than one half of this is dissolved in the body fat, and the remaining in water, nitrogen is five times as soluble in fat as in water. After complete saturation, there is an increase of 1 L equivalent of sea-level volume of nitrogen dissolved in the body for every 33 feet depth. Equilibration of the pressure of nitrogen in all the body tissues with that in the alveoli occurs slowly as several cycles of blood flow are required and the nitrogen diffuses slowly. The equilibrium is complete in less than 1 hour, but takes much longer in fat tissue because of poor blood supply. For this reason, longer stay will allow more nitrogen to enter tissues at the same depth than a shorter stay. However, if large amount is dissolved due to a long stay, and the diver ascends quickly to surface, due to sudden fall in the pressures to 1 ATA, nitrogen (and to a small extent, other gases) move out of the liquid phase quickly and these cannot be transported to lungs fast enough to be exhaled out. Significant quantities of nitrogen bubbles can develop in the body fluids either intracellularly or extracellularly and can cause minor or serious damage in almost any area of the body, depending on the number and sizes of bubbles formed; this is the mechanism for DCS and follows the Henry's law described above.

Direct Effects of Pressure: Barotrauma

Sinuses and Middle Ear

Noncommunicating spaces are susceptible to the effects of pressure with damage occurring during compression (squeeze) or due to gas expansion on ascent. In the paranasal sinuses with blocked ostia or middle ears with blocked Eustachian tubes, descent of as little as 1-2 m is enough to cause pain, edema and even hemorrhage. Though common, middle ear barotrauma is usually minor and self-limiting. More serious injuries such as tympanic membrane rupture can occur. Differential ear equalization can result in alternobaric vertigo that is usually transient.

Pulmonary Barotrauma and Arterial Gas Embolism

Pulmonary volumes remain nearly normal while diving with breathing apparatus, but during ascent, the compressed gas in the lungs expands with the falling ambient pressure. Excessive transpulmonary pressures result if intrapulmonary gas is prevented from escaping as a result of a closed glottis, bronchospasm or gas trapping. If the rate of gas efflux from the lungs is slower than the rate of gas volume change, it will precipitate pulmonary overexpansion, and can happen in uncontrolled ascent from scuba diving at the depth of 3 feet or more.[59] Because of the heterogeneity of compliance, there are differences in the expansion of adjacent lung units causing focal shearing between vessels and airways, and rupture of small airways and/or alveoli. This may result in pneumothorax, mediastinum and subcutaneous emphysema and pneumopericardium. When the air enters pulmonary venules, it reaches the left heart resulting in arterial gas embolism.

REFERENCES

1. Grimby G. Respiration in exercise. Medicine and Science in Sports. 1969;1:9–14.
2. Davies CT, Di Prampero PE, Cerretelli P. Kinetics of cardiac output and respiratory gas exchange during exercise and recovery. J Appl Physiol. 1972;32:618–25.
3. Rowell LB. Human cardiovascular adjustments to exercise and thermal stress. Physiological Rev. 1974; 54:75–159.
4. Wasserman K, Whipp BJ. Exercise physiology in health and disease. Am Rev Respir Dis. 1975;112:219-45.
5. Wasserman K. Breathing during exercise. N Engl J Med. 1978;298:780–5.
6. Lintu N, Viitasalo A, Tompuri T, Veijalainen A, Hakulinen M, Laitinen T, et al. Cardiorespiratory fitness, respiratory function and hemodynamic responses to maximal cycle ergometer exercise test in girls and boys aged 9-11 years: the PANIC Study. Eur J Appl Physiol. 2015;115(2):235-43.
7. Johansson H, Norlander K, Hedenstrom H, Janson C, Nordang L, Nordvall L, et al. Exercise-induced dyspnea is a problem among the general adolescent population. Respir Med. 2014;108(6):852-8.
8. Younes M, Kivinen G. Respiratory mechanics and breathing pattern during and following maximal exercise. J Appl Physiol. 1984;57:1773-82.
9. Wasserman K, Whipp BJ, Casaburi R. Respiratory control during exercise. In: Fishman AP (Ed). Handbook of Physiology. Section 3: The Respiratory System, Vol II, Part 2. Bethesda, MD: American Physiological Society; 1986.
10. Leff AR, Schumacker PT. Respiratory Physiology: Basics and Applications. Philadelphia: WB Saunders; 1993.
11. Plowman SA, Smith DL. Respiratory exercise response, training adaptations, and special considerations. In: Plowman SA, Smith DL (Eds). Exercise Physiology for Health, Fitness, and Performance, 2nd edition. San Francisco: Pearson Education, Inc.; 2003. pp. 285-319.
12. Plowman SA, Smith DL. Cardiovascular Responses to Exercise. In: Plowman SA, Smith DL (Eds). Exercise Physiology for Health, Fitness, and Performance, 2nd edition. San Francisco: Pearson Education, Inc.; 2003. pp. 351-82.
13. Donley DA, Fournier SB, Reger BL, Devallance E, Bonner DE, Olfert IM, et al. Aerobic exercise training reduces arterial stiffness in metabolic syndrome. J Appl Physiol. 2014;116: 1396-404.
14. West JB. Respiratory system under stress. How gas exchange is accomplished during exercise, at low and high pressures, and at birth. In: West JB (Ed). Respiratory Physiology: The Essentials, 8th edition. US: Lippincott Williams and Wilkins; 2008. pp. 139-56.
15. Gazioglu K, Kaltreider NL, Rosen M, Yu PN. Pulmonary function during pregnancy in normal women and in patients with cardiopulmonary disease. Thorax. 1970;25:445-50.
16. Hirnle L, Lysenko L, Gerber H, Lesnik P, Baranowska A, Rachwalik M, et al. Respiratory function in pregnant women. Adv Exp Med Biol. 2013;788:153-60.
17. Contreras G, Gutiérrez M, Beroíza T, Fantín A, Oddó H, Villarroel L, et al. Ventilatory drive and respiratory muscle function in pregnancy. Am Rev Respir Dis. 1991;144:837-41.

18. Lee W. Cardiorespiratory alterations during normal pregnancy. Crit Care Clin. 1991;7:763-75.
19. Elkus R, Popovich J. Respiratory physiology in pregnancy. Clin Chest Med. 1992;13:555-65.
20. García-Rio F, Pino JM, Gómez L, Alvarez-Sala R, Villasante C, Villamor J. Regulation of breathing and perception of dyspnea in healthy pregnant women. Chest. 1996;110:446-53.
21. Crapo RO. Normal cardiopulmonary physiology during pregnancy. Clin Obstet Gynecol. 1996;39:3-16.
22. O'Day MP. Cardiorespiratory physiological adaptation of pregnancy. Semin Perinatol. 1997;21:268-75.
23. Ganong WF. Review of Medical Physiology, 22nd edition. New York: McGraw Hill; 2005.
24. Dean LS, D'Angelo R. Anatomic and Physiologic changes of pregnancy. In: Palmer CM, D'Angelo R, Paech MJ (Eds). Handbook of Obstetric Anaesthesia. Oxford: Bios Scientific Publishers Ltd.; 2002.
25. Dutta DC. Textbook Book of Obstetrics, 6th edition. 2004.
26. Renee B. Pulmonary Physiology in Pregnancy. Clin Obstet Gynecol. 2010;53:285-300.
27. Tan EB, Tan EL. Alterations in physiology and anatomy during pregnancy. Best Pract Res Clin Obstet Gynaecol. 2013;27: 791-802.
28. Rahn H, Otis AB. Man's respiratory response during and after acclimatization to high altitude. Am J Physiol. 1949;157:445-62.
29. Guleria JS, Pande JN, Sethi PK, Roy SB. Pulmonary diffusing capacity at high altitude. J Appl Physiol. 1971;31:536-43.
30. Winslow RM, Monge CC, Statham NJ, Gibson CG, Charache S, Whittembury J, et al. Variability of oxygen affinity of blood: human subjects native to high altitude. J Appl Physiol. 1981;51:1411-6.
31. West JB, Hackett PH, Maret KH, Milledge JS, Peters RM Jr, Pizzo CJ, et al. Pulmonary gas exchange on the summit of Mount Everest. J Appl Physiol Respir Environ Exerc Physiol. 1983;55:678-87.
32. West JB. Rate of ventilatory acclimatization to extreme altitude. Respir Physiol. 1988;74:323-33.
33. Goldberg SV, Schoene RB, Haynor D, Trimble B, Swenson ER, Morrison JB, et al. Brain tissue pH and ventilatory acclimatization to high altitude. J Appl Physiol. 1992;72:58-63.
34. Schmidt W, Spielvogel H, Eckardt KU, Quintela A, Peñaloza R. Effects of chronic hypoxia and exercise on plasma erythropoietin in high-altitude residents. J Appl Physiol (1985). 1993;74:1874-8.
35. Smith CA, Saupe KW, Henderson KS, Dempsey JA. Ventilatory effects of specific carotid body hypocapnia in dogs during wakefulness and sleep. J Appl Physiol. 1995;79:689-99.
36. West JB. Highlife: A History of High Altitude Physiology and Medicine. Oxford: Oxford University Press; 1998.
37. Hornbein TF, Schoene RB. High Altitude: An Exploration of Human Adaptation (Lung Biology in Health and Disease, Vol. 161), New York: Marcel Dekker; 2001.
38. Reeves JT, Stenmark KR. The pulmonary circulation at high altitude. In: Hornbein TF, Schoene RB (Eds). High Altitude: An Exploration of Human Adaptation (Lung Biology in Health and Disease, Vol. 161). New York: Marcel Dekker; 2001. pp. 293-342.
39. Wolfel EE, Levine BD. The cardiovascular system at high altitude: Heart and systemic circulation. In: Hornbein TF, Schoene RB (Eds). High Altitude: An Exploration of Human Adaptation (Lung Biology in Health and Disease, Vol. 161), New York: Marcel Dekker; 2001. pp. 235-92.
40. Ge R, Witkowski S, Zhang Y, Alfrey C, Sivieri M, Karlsen T, et al. Determinants of erythropoietin release in response to short-term hypobaric hypoxia. J Appl Physiol. 2002;92: 2361-7.
41. Wilson DF, Roy A, Lahiri S. Immediate and long-term responses of the carotid body to high altitude. High Altitude Med Biol. 2005;6:97-111.
42. Schoene RB, Swenson ER. High Altitude. In: Mason RJ, Murray JF, Broaddus VC (Eds). Textbook of Respiratory Medicine, 4th edition. Philadelphia, Pa: Saunders Elsevier; 2005: Chap. 65.
43. Ainslie PN, Lucas SJ, Burgess KR. Breathing and sleep at high altitude. Respir Physiol Neurobiol. 2013;15:188:233-56.
44. Agostoni P, Swenson ER, Fumagalli R, Salvioni E, Cattadori G, Farina S, et al. Acute high-altitude exposure reduces lung diffusion: data from the HIGHCARE Alps project. Respir Physiol Neurobiol. 2013;188:223-8.
45. Spencer MP, Campbell SD, Sealey JL, Henry FC, Lindbergh J. Experiments on decompression bubbles in the circulation using ultrasonic and electromagnetic flowmeters. J Occup Med. 1969;11:238-44.
46. Edmonds C, Thomas RL. Medical aspects of diving. 4. Med J Aust. 1972;2:1367-70.
47. Kizer KW. Diving medicine. Emerg Med Clin North Am. 1984;2:513-30.
48. Haller C, Sercombe R, Verrecchia C, Fritsch H, Seylaz J, Kuschinsky W. Effect of the muscarinic agonist carbachol on pial arteries *in vivo* after endothelial damage by air embolism. J Cereb Blood Flow Metab. 1987;7:605-11.
49. Hills BA, James PB. Microbubble damage to the blood-brain barrier: relevance to decompression sickness. Undersea Biomed Res. 1991;18:111-6.
50. Boussuges A, Blanc P, Molenat F, Bergmann E, Sainty JM. Hemoconcentration in neurological decompression illness. Int J Sports Med. 1996;17:351-5.
51. Hardy KR. Diving-related emergencies. Emerg Med Clin North Am. 1997;15:223-40.
52. Reinertsen RE, Flook V, Koteng S, Brubakk AO. Effect of oxygen tension and rate of pressure reduction during decompression on central gas bubbles. J Appl Physiol. 1998;84:351-6.
53. Wilmshurst P, Bryson P. Relationship between the clinical features of neurological decompression illness and its causes. Clin Sci (Lond). 2000;99:65-75.
54. Lippmann J, Mitchell SJ. "Nitrogen narcosis". In: Deeper into Diving, 2nd edition. Victoria, Australia: J L Publications; 2005. p. 103.
55. Rostain JC, Balon N. Recent neurochemical basis of inert gas narcosis and pressure effects. Undersea Hyperb Med. 2006;33:197-204.
56. Levett DZ, Millar IL. Bubble trouble: a review of diving physiology and disease. Postgrad Med J. 2008;84:571-8.
57. US. Navy Supervisor of Diving. US Navy Diving Manual. SS521AG-PRO-010, revision 6. US Naval Sea Systems Command. 2008.
58. Hobbs M. Subjective and behavioural responses to nitrogen narcosis and alcohol. Undersea Hyperb Med. 2008;35:175-8.
59. Moon RE, Cherry AD, Stolp BW, Camporesi EM. Pulmonary gas exchange in diving. J Appl Physiol. 2009;106:668-77.

Mechanisms of Dyspnea in Respiratory Diseases

Sunil K Chhabra, Ashima Anand

INTRODUCTION

Respiration is an automatic process that, however, can be modulated voluntarily. The respiratory drive originates in the respiratory center in the brainstem with inputs from the periphery, as well as the cerebral cortex. Normally, the sensation to breathe and the effort of breathing do not reach a person's consciousness. However, in certain physiological conditions and in pathological states, a person may become aware of his breathing activity.

The term "Dyspnea" is used to imply an uncomfortable and unpleasant awareness of an increased effort to breathe. It is a symptom, not a sign. Due to its subjective nature, dyspnea will only have a modest or no relationship with an objective measure of the functional disability of a patient. Therefore, there are no objective surrogates for dyspnea and the patient is the prime source of information. The symptom of exertional fatigue must be distinguished from dyspnea.

DEFINITIONS

The American Thoracic Society has defined dyspnea as "a term used to characterize a subjective experience of breathing discomfort that consists of qualitatively distinct sensations that vary in intensity. The experience derives from interactions among multiple physiological, psychological, social and environmental factors, and may induce secondary physiological and behavioral responses".[1]

Certain other terms used to describe alterations in respiratory rate, depth and rhythm may be associated with dyspnea. These have different clinical connotations and are not synonymous. "Tachypnea" is a rapid respiratory rate, greater than the normal frequency of 12–18 breathes per minute. It may be present with or without dyspnea. Conversely, a dyspneic patient usually has tachypnea on physical examination. "Hyperventilation" is minute ventilation that is greater than what is required to maintain a normal arterial CO_2. Thus the subject will have hypocapnia, but may not be dyspneic. "Orthopnea" or shortness of breath on assuming the supine position, results from an increase in the venous return and pulmonary blood flow that in patients with heart failure causes an increase in the left atrial and left ventricular filling pressures, leading to pulmonary vascular congestion and interstitial or alveolar edema. This is also referred to as "cardiac dyspnea." "Platypnea" is the shortness of breath when the patient is in the upright position and is a rare symptom associated with orthodeoxia (hypoxemia on standing) occurring in pulmonary or intracardiac shunts. "Trepopnea" is the shortness of breath when the patient lies on his or her side and can be relieved by moving to the opposite lateral position. "Paroxysmal nocturnal dyspnea" is waking up from sleep due to dyspnea and is usually a symptom of heart failure. As with orthopnea, the recumbent position is important, but this symptom differs in that breathlessness does not occur soon after lying down. The mechanism and the clinical implications are, however, similar with the increase in intrathoracic intravascular volume occurring due to a slow mobilization of tissue fluid such as peripheral edema. Patients with asthma and even chronic obstructive pulmonary disease (COPD) may also have disruption of sleep due to dyspnea. However, the mechanisms are different from those in heart failure.

PERCEPTION: THE SUBJECTIVE ELEMENT IN DYSPNEA

Dyspnea being a sensation, areas in the cerebral cortex concerned with perception must come into play. Indeed, the definition of dyspnea translates into a perceived unpleasant difficulty with breathing. In contrast to the physical stimuli, such as touch, pressure or temperature that are sensed by the peripheral nervous system and perceived as such by the cerebral cortex, the sensation of dyspnea is a central translation in the cerebral cortex of inputs of different nature from several peripheral sites to the respiratory center. The central cortical processing of the information from the respiratory center is modulated by psychological, behavioral and cultural factors that determine a person's ability to sense the stimulus and respond to it. This ability to sense constitutes "perception," a complex behavioral phenomenon that imparts to dyspnea, its subjective quality.[1]

The appropriate qualitative and quantitative feeling or perception of breathlessness in response to a stimulus of a particular strength and nature is impossible to define. A patient of asthma with severe airways obstruction may be asymptomatic, failing to sense the stimulus arising out of severe bronchospasm while another patient with a milder degree of airways obstruction may be very dyspneic, responding to the milder stimulus in an exaggerated manner. The former situation carries the risk of undertreatment, and the latter, overtreatment. The standards of patient care today recognize that monitoring of patients using objective outcomes, such as lung function has limitations, and, patient-reported outcomes that reflect the impact of disease on the person and on daily activities are equally, and perhaps, more important. Dyspnea is a major determinant of the person's response to his ailment, activities of daily living, functional capacity, and hence, the quality of life.

Dyspnea may occur in a variety of respiratory and cardiac conditions, both acute and chronic, as well as in other pathological states, such as anemia, thyrotoxicosis and psychiatric illness, and also in certain physiological states. Differences are expected among patients with regard to the intensity of the stimulus that will cause dyspnea, the language used to describe the sensation, as well as the psychological and physiological response to it. It is necessary for the physicians to appreciate that there are qualitative and quantitative differences in dyspnea in patients with different diseases. The underlying pathophysiological factors responsible for the sensation of dyspnea differ. Therefore, a uniform approach to treating dyspnea cannot be adopted.

Management based on an understanding of the underlying mechanisms is more scientific. While animal studies can provide information about the ventilatory responses under experimental conditions simulating physiological abnormalities encountered in different disease states, such as increased resistive or elastic loads, altered hemodynamics and blood gases, the subjective nature of dyspnea can be studied only in humans. The mechanisms have been investigated in patients with different diseases, as well as in normal subjects under the conditions of mechanical loading or altered oxygenation and acid-base milieu. Instruments have been developed and validated for the quantification of dyspnea. In recent years, there has been a further refinement of methodologies for assessment and quantification of dyspnea and understanding the neurophysiologic mechanisms that may contribute to its genesis. The availability of techniques, such as positron emission tomography (PET) and functional magnetic resonance imaging (MRI) have provided a means to study the central neuronal activity. Yet, the complex nature of the sensation of dyspnea and interplay of several neural pathways in concert makes it extremely difficult to design studies and provide definitive proofs of the responsible mechanisms. The information in literature is, therefore, often contradictory, controversial and, sometimes, even speculative.

NEURAL PATHWAYS OF DYSPNEA

The neural pathways regulating respiratory activity have been studied extensively and a vast amount of literature is available in this area.[2] The respiratory drive originates from the neurons in the medulla, called the respiratory center. The motor output travels to the diaphragm and the inspiratory muscles leading to their contraction, and, inflation of the chest wall and the lungs. The gas exchange and transport of oxygen and carbon dioxide are intimately involved in the regulation of acid-base balance. Changes in oxygen and carbon dioxide tensions in blood are sensed by central chemoreceptors in the medulla and peripheral chemoreceptors in the carotid and aortic bodies. Signals from these chemoreceptors are transmitted back to the brainstem respiratory centers that adjust breathing to maintain blood-gas and acid-base homeostasis. Mechanoreceptors in the airways, lungs and chest wall provide sensory inputs to the respiratory center on the changes in lung volumes and tissue displacement. Muscle spindles are abundant in the intercostals muscles and the diaphragm contains tendon organs that signal muscle tension and exert inhibitory influence on central respiratory activity. These provide feedback information about changes in the length and force of contraction of the respiratory muscles in response to the motor output. Afferent impulses from vagal receptors in the airways and lungs convey information on several aspects of lung physiology. These include impulses from pulmonary stretch receptors (lung expansion), irritant receptors around the epithelial cells of the bronchial walls (activated by irritants, high rates of air flow, and increases in bronchial smooth muscle tone) and C-fibers, found in the interstitium of the lung in proximity to the alveoli and pulmonary capillaries (stimulated by increases in pulmonary interstitial and capillary pressure).

Corollary Discharge to Sensory Cortex

Additionally, there is evidence that corollary signals or efferent copies of brainstem respiratory center motor output, i.e. similar parallel outputs, are also transmitted to higher brain centers in the sensory cortex and may play an important role in the perception of dyspnea. This creates a conscious awareness of the outgoing respiratory motor output to the ventilatory muscles.[3] So far, specific receptors and pathways for this parallel relay have not been identified. However, rostral projections from brainstem respiratory motor neurons to the midbrain and thalamus have recently been described in the cat.[4] Studies have shown that in conditions, such as decreasing muscle length, muscle fatigue or respiratory muscle weakness, where a greater motor command is required to achieve a given tension in the muscle, there is an increased appreciation or perception of respiratory effort.[5,6]

Further, the perception of the respiratory effort increases with increase in central respiratory motor output and is proportional to the ratio of the pressures generated by the respiratory muscles to the maximum pressure-generating capacity of those muscles.[7]

Chest Wall Receptors

There is evidence that afferent signals from mechanoreceptors in the joints, tendons, and muscles of the chest may play a role in modulating respiratory sensations. In a study using evoked-potential techniques to determine whether low-threshold muscle afferents from the chest wall project to cortical levels in conscious human subjects, evidence for a short-latency projection was provided.[8] It has been suggested that an uncomfortable sensation of breathlessness may be induced by muscle spindles in the intercostal muscles being activated out-of-phase with the respiratory cycle.[9] On the other hand, in-phase chest wall vibration (inspiratory intercostal muscles vibrated during inspiration and expiratory intercostal muscles vibrated during expiration) has been shown to decrease pathologic dyspnea in patients with chronic respiratory disease at rest and on exercise.[10-12]

Dyspnea increases with the level of respiratory chemical drive during hypercapnia, but intensity of the sensation was found to be greater when the consequent increase in ventilation was constrained. Voluntary hypoventilation produces an intense sensation of breathlessness even when blood gases are maintained constant that correlates closely with the degree to which the tidal volume is reduced.[13] In conscious patients on mechanical ventilator receiving the low levels of ventilation, dyspnea may be troublesome requiring heavy sedation.

Lung Receptors

Studies have shown that vagal influences, independent of ventilatory and blood gas changes may modulate the sensation of dyspnea. Mechanically, ventilated patients with high cervical spinal cord transaction who are thus unable to transmit impulses from chest wall receptors experience a sensation of air hunger when their ventilation is reduced.[14,15] Further, vagal blockade or vagotomy has been shown to reduce dyspnea during exercise, breath-holding and after pulmonary venous obstruction.[16-18]

The three types of sensory receptors in the lungs that have been considered as the site of origin of dyspnea are:

1. The bronchial C-fiber receptors
2. The pulmonary stretch receptors, i.e. the slowly adapting receptors (SARs) and rapidly adapting receptors (RARs) and
3. The juxtapulmonary (J) receptors also referred to as pulmonary C-fiber receptors.

The bronchial C-fiber receptors were first described by Coleridge and Coleridge.[19] These are located mainly in the wall of the large airways, both extrapulmonary and intrapulmonary, and are characteristically accessible to chemicals injected only into the bronchial circulation. Their exact anatomical location in the airway wall or in relation to the capillaries of the bronchial circulation is not known. While their natural stimulus is as yet unknown, it is hypothesized that these are likely to contribute to bronchoconstriction and mucous secretion as the chemicals that they are sensitive to, include various inflammatory mediators.[20] That they do not contribute to an acceleration of respiration was shown by Anand[21] in cats where an impressive activity produced in them by injecting phenylbiguanide into the bronchial circulation was accompanied by an inhibitory influence on respiration. Capsaicin, on the other hand, injected by a similar route is accompanied by a marked stimulation of respiration that persists after bilateral vagotomy thereby showing that the increase in respiration did not originate by their stimulation.

Located in the mucosa and smooth muscle of the extrapulmonary and intrapulmonary airways, the slowly and rapidly adapting pulmonary stretch receptors sense lung volume and are stimulated by lung inflation, and the latter, also by lung deflation.[22] These conduct their impulses in myelinated vagal afferents. According to Widdicombe,[23,24] who changed their name briefly to "irritant receptors" because these receptors could trigger cough and reactions to noxious agents, and as also reviewed recently by Ravi and Kappagoda,[25] the stimulation of RARs produces dyspnea. However, in man, a rapid voluntary hyperventilation, which would produce a high-frequency neural discharge in RARs does not give rise to dyspnea or to any kind of unpleasant sensations.[26-28] Further, these receptors produce relief from dyspnea or breathlessness under circumstances when they would be maximally stimulated.[29] After breath-holding at total lung capacity, there is immediate relief with rapid expiration, i.e. a physiological stimulus for maximizing neural output from RARs.[30] This relief is similar to the relief felt on breathing in, after holding the breath at functional residual capacity that would be attributed to the stimulation of the SARs.[29] There are no correlative studies available between humans and mammalian species on RARs and their likely role in generating dyspnea are an extrapolation of findings from the latter. So far, no human studies of dyspnegenic effects of RAR activation have been carried out. Their role in producing dyspnea on exercise is not clear. However, there is evidence in animals that RARs play a role in the respiratory responses in acute pulmonary congestion due to heart failure. Activation of RARs causes a reflex increase in respiratory rate, tracheal tone and mucus secretion in the airways. A rise in left atrial pressure (LAP) by 5 mm Hg in dogs, which is sufficient to stimulate RARs[31] may occur on exercise. This is not accompanied by dyspnea. However, sustained application of LAP of 10 mm Hg for 15 minutes produces a sustained activation of RARs along with some activity in bronchial C-fibers and very little in pulmonary C-fibers. At this level, the increase in extravascular compartment in the lung is largely in the proximal airways. Thus, it has been suggested that the RARs may come into play in the early stages of acute heart failure.[25] Pulmonary edema requires an elevation of LAP to 20 mm Hg. At this level, RARs, bronchial C-fibers and pulmonary C-fibers, all show strong activation and are likely to modulate respiratory responses in frank pulmonary edema. Interestingly, the response of the RARs to pulmonary congestion is nonadapting unlike the response to maintained inflation where rapid adaptation occurs.

The J capillary receptors, or type J-receptors, so named because they lie in close proximity to the pulmonary capillaries in the interstitium of the lung, were discovered by Paintal.[32] These are stimulated in animals by pulmonary congestion and by intravenously injected chemicals to give rise reflexly to tachypnea.[33-36] These are also called pulmonary C-fiber receptors. Majority (80%) of these are nonmyelinated C-fiber endings and 20% are A-delta fiber endings. Their natural stimulus is an increase in pulmonary blood flow leading to a rise in pulmonary capillary pressure (PCP). Doubling of pulmonary blood flow (i.e. doubling cardiac output), which will result in increasing the PCP, increases their activity from nearly 0 impulses/sec to 0.7 impulses/sec,[35] a stimulation which in earlier studies has been shown to stimulate respiration.[33,34] A correlative study of animals and human subjects demonstrated that small doses of lobeline intravenously (10–15 μg/kg) gave rise to respiratory reflexes and distinct sensations in the throat or upper chest by stimulation of J (pulmonary C-fiber) receptors.[36] The sensations felt on J-receptor stimulation resemble those reported in dyspnea,[36-40] including those perceived by patients in left ventricular failure,[40] patients of mitral stenosis on exercise,[39] and those reported by subjects with high altitude pulmonary edema,[28] suggesting a common origin of these. Thus, dyspneic sensations are produced under conditions in which the J (pulmonary C-fiber) receptors are stimulated, and, conversely no or reduced dyspnea is observed under circumstances when they are not being stimulated or their stimulation is reduced. Valvulotomy relieves dyspnea in mitral stenosis[39] even without changes in skeletal muscle peak exercise oxygen consumption[41] muscle structure or biochemistry[42] and lung-function abnormalities,[43] suggesting that J-receptors are involved in the sensation of breathlessness on exercise in these patients as surgery relieves pulmonary congestion. Paintal[26-28] has provided evidence that an increase in interstitial fluid volume resulting from elevated pulmonary arterial and capillary pressures contributes to the breathless sensation after moderate and severe exercise. In acute heart failure, their activation follows that of RARs.[25] That vagal afferents are involved in the origin of the sensation of dyspnea, is strongly supported by the observation that intravenous lobeline does not produce sensations described above in patients who have undergone bilateral lung transplantation.[44]

Chemoreceptors

Changes in arterial blood gases, hypoxia with or without hypercapnia, are commonly observed in respiratory conditions causing dyspnea and are sensed by central and peripheral chemoreceptors. Their contribution to the sensation of dyspnea becomes difficult to evaluate as changes in lung and chest wall mechanics are associated with, and usually precede the alterations in blood gases in the pathophysiology of these conditions. However, certain models and interventions allow the evaluation of dyspnea due to chemically-induced increases in respiratory motor activity, independent of changes in chest wall and lung mechanics. Both ventilator-dependent quadriplegics with high cervical spinal cord transection and normal subjects paralyzed with neuromuscular blocking agents experience the sensations of air hunger when $PaCO_2$ is increased.[45,46] Moreover, hypercapnia produces greater dyspnea than exercise and voluntary hyperventilation at similar levels of ventilation.[47] In normal subjects paralyzed with a neuromuscular blocker and receiving adequate mechanical ventilation, acute hypercapnia and hypoxia cause respiratory distress. Importantly, the changes in dyspnea ratings precede changes in ventilation.[48] It has also been shown that the administration of oxygen during exercise produces a small reduction in ventilation, but a larger and consistent decrease in dyspnea suggesting that hypoxemia itself may be a stimulus for dyspnea independent of ventilatory changes.[49]

PATHOPHYSIOLOGICAL MECHANISMS OF DYSPNEA

Dyspnea may be produced by diseases and disorders affecting the respiratory center, the ventilatory apparatus, including the airways and the lung parenchyma, gas exchange and oxygenation, and cardiopulmonary hemodynamics. As the activity of the respiratory center, the ventilatory response in the terms of changes in lung volumes, pressures and airflows, changes in blood gas tensions and alterations of cardiopulmonary hemodynamics in physiological states and diseases are integrated and influence each other. Dyspnea is likely to be precipitated and modulated by multiple factors and mechanisms in different diseases and disorders of the cardiorespiratory systems. It is also likely that dyspnea experienced by patients represents more than one sensation. The choice of phrases used by patients with a variety of conditions causing dyspnea are distinctly different.[50,51] The pathophysiological mechanisms that operate in the common causes of dyspnea are discussed in the following sections.

In obstructive airways diseases, such as COPD and asthma, the functional abnormalities that may underlie the origin of dyspnea include **(Table 1)**:

- Increased work of breathing due to increased resistive loading and functional weakness of the ventilatory muscles

- Hypoxia and hypercapnia leading to chemoreceptor activation
- Restriction of lung expansion in a hyperinflated chest and functional abnormalities in lung mechanics worsening on exertion (dynamic hyperinflation)
- Airway inflammation altering vagal afferent activity
- Afferent signals from mechanoreceptors in the joints, tendons and muscles of the chest
- Altered pulmonary circulation hemodynamics
- Associated cardiac dysfunction
- Any combination of the above.

In interstitial lung diseases (ILDs), the following abnormalities may contribute to dyspnea **(Table 2)**:

- Increased work of breathing due to increased elastic loading and functional weakness of the ventilatory muscles
- Physical restriction of thoracic expansion and functional abnormalities in lung mechanics
- Hypoxia leading to chemoreceptor activation
- Lung interstitial inflammation and fluid changes altering vagal afferent activity
- Afferent signals from mechanoreceptors in the joints, tendons and muscles of the chest
- Altered pulmonary circulation hemodynamics
- Associated cardiac dysfunction
- Any combination of the above.

With such diverse pathophysiological alterations, clearly a single mechanism or pathway cannot explain the origin of the sensation of dyspnea at rest and on exercise in these conditions.

Among the several proposed mechanisms, a popular theory that has been put forth is that dyspnea results from a disassociation or a mismatch between central respiratory motor output and incoming afferent information from the receptors in the airways, lungs and chest wall structures, i.e. the motor response is sensed as being "not matched" with the afferent inputs. The afferent feedback from the peripheral sensory receptors informs the center that the mechanical response of the lungs and chest wall (changes in volumes, pressures and airflows) are not appropriate for outgoing motor output (tension of the inspiratory muscles) leading to the sensation of dyspnea. In simple terms, the ventilatory response of the lungs and the chest wall is inappropriate for the effort. This is the crux of Campbell and Howell hypothesis of "length tension inappropriateness".[52-54] and is also termed as "neuromechanical"[55] or "efferent-reafferent dissociation".[46] In terms of this hypothesis, if the inspiratory muscles contract less than usual for the tension generated because of a noncompliant chest wall, or if the airflow generated is less than expected for a given inspiratory effort or if the volume of inspiration is less than expected for the degree of activation of the muscles, the intensity of respiratory discomfort gets intensified. This dissociation between the efferent and afferent information may occur in patients with a resistive (obstructive diseases) or elastic (restrictive diseases) mechanical load on the respiratory system, or respiratory muscle abnormalities. This mechanism may explain dyspnea associated with breath-holding, increased airways resistance, decreased lung and chest wall compliance, voluntary hypoventilation, as well as that experienced by patients on mechanical ventilation with small tidal volumes and low inspiratory flow rates. However, as discussed above, quadriplegics and normal subjects paralyzed with neuromuscular blocking agents also experience air hunger to a hypercapnic or hypoxemic stimulus and dyspnea precedes changes in ventilation.[13-15,45-47] The hypothesis also does not explain the dyspnea occurring due to changes in pulmonary hemodynamics on exertion in pulmonary and cardiac diseases.

In the absence of a single hypothesis that integrates all mechanisms of dyspnea, it is convenient to discuss origin of dyspnea in the terms of major pathophysiological alterations that occur in different diseases.

Increased Ventilatory Demand and Activity

Increased output from the brain is the primary manifestation of dyspnea in which the respiratory center may play a role in certain disorders and conditions. While it is possible to voluntarily increase ventilation, it is subjectively not an unpleasant sensation. Patients with psychiatric morbidity may hyperventilate and the corollary discharge from the respiratory center to cortical areas may also bring the increased ventilatory drive to consciousness. The dyspnea commonly seen in the first trimester of pregnancy is likely due to the stimulatory effect of progesterone on the respiratory center in the medulla. However, in most of the diseases causing dyspnea, the increased output of the respiratory center is a response to the increased ventilatory requirements sensed and communicated by the afferent inputs to the center through the neural mechanisms discussed above, rather than a primary abnormality. Abnormalities in gas exchange along with the stimulation of pulmonary receptors, as evidenced by the hyperventilation seen in patients with asthma and pulmonary embolism, may contribute to heightened activity in the center. Patients with a noncompliant wall, increased airway resistance, weakened muscles, or thickened pleura have problems with the ventilatory pump in achieving normal ventilation and derangements of the gas exchange occurring in several diseases leading to hypoxemia, with or without hypercapnia, have increased ventilatory drive to meet the increased ventilatory demand.

The intensity of dyspnea increases progressively with increase in the workload during exercise. However, halving the intensity and doubling the duration of activity reduces the maximal intensity of dyspnea to less than a third.[56,57] This is likely to be due to the increase in respiratory motor output to meet the increased ventilatory demand and a corresponding increase in the sense of effort. The cortex also takes into account the context in which the ventilation has increased in its interpretation. Increased ventilation at rest is likely to cause more dyspnea compared to an activity that gives rise to similar levels of ventilation. This is because higher ventilation at rest is seen as excessive or out-of proportion to normal requirements at rest while it is considered as more appropriate for the activity. This has been reported in COPD.[58]

Diseases of airways (COPD), lung parenchyma (ILDs) and pulmonary vasculature (pulmonary embolism) that increase dead space and other conditions causing wasted ventilation due to V/Q mismatch require an increase in the minute ventilation to achieve normal gas exchange. Hypoxemia at high altitude and in patients with respiratory disease, stimulates arterial chemoreceptors and increases respiratory motor activity. The increased ventilatory demand leads to an increased motor command under these conditions, contributing to dyspnea.

Another stimulus for excessive ventilation is a consequence of deconditioning because of prolonged inactivity imposed by cardiorespiratory diseases. Patients with COPD have an early and accelerated rise in blood lactate production by skeletal muscles during exercise and the consequent metabolic acidosis is an additional respiratory stimulus leading to excessive increase in the ventilation for a given level of exercise, and this increases dyspnea.[59] This would limit exercise capacity leading to a vicious cycle of greater inactivity and consequent deconditioning and greater dyspnea.

While the level of ventilation often correlates well with the intensity of dyspnea, increased motor output is unlikely to be solely responsible for dyspnea. Even with conditions causing increased ventilation, the subjective sensations experienced by subjects are different. As pointed out above, at similar level of ventilation, hypercapnia produces greater dyspnea than voluntary hyperventilation and exercise[47] and the relief in dyspnea with exercise in hypoxic subjects afforded by supplemental oxygen is out of proportion to the reduction in ventilation.[49] Increased ventilatory drive is unlikely to produce an uncomfortable awareness of breathing as long as the response of the chest wall and lungs is commensurate with the requirements and the effort expended in ventilation is sensed as "normal". This requires a normal lung mechanics and an efficient musculature. However, when the other alterations as discussed in the following sections occur, the increased ventilatory drive becomes the driving factor for dyspnea.

Mechanical Inefficiency of Ventilatory Pump

A weakness or mechanical inefficiency of the respiratory muscles results in a mismatch between the central respiratory motor output and achieved ventilation. Some conditions that predispose to ventilatory failure increase the work of breathing due to altered lung mechanics (COPD, asthma, ILDs, obesity, kyphoscoliosis), whereas others cause severe respiratory muscle weakness. Specific reasons for muscle weakness include critical illness (electrolyte imbalance, acidosis, shock, severe sepsis), chronic illness (poor nutrition, cachexia), and neuromuscular diseases and dysfunction (steroid myopathy). In order to generate the inspiratory pressures required to initiate inspiration, greater effort is required by the inefficient muscles and even then, the maximal inspiratory pressures may be decreased.[60] Thus, there is an increased gap in the pressures achieved and pressures required leading to an inefficient ventilatory pump and dyspnea progressively worsens.[61]

The abnormalities of lung mechanics at rest and on exercise have been studied extensively in COPD.[62] Besides a partially reversible airflow limitation, COPD is characterized by a redistribution of lung volumes at rest and on exercise. The airflow limitation results in a requirement of a longer expiratory time to exhale a given volume of air. Associated emphysema leads to a loss of elastic recoil and hence the driving pressure for expiratory airflow, causing further reduction in flow rates along with an increased size of the alveoli and larger volume to be exhaled. The increased airflow limitation (resistance) and loss of elastic recoil (reduced compliance) lead to reduced time constants of the lung units and this impedes emptying within the available expiratory time.

The result is an incomplete emptying and hyperinflation at the end of expiration [increased end-expiratory lung volume (EELV)]. As the next inspiration begins before the previous expiration has been completed, the airways pressures are still positive relative to the atmosphere [auto positive end-expiratory pressure (PEEP)]. This increases the inspiratory threshold, i.e. inspiration can begin only after this pressure is overcome. The increased inspiratory threshold thus increases the work of breathing and is also the cause of inspiratory dyspnea. On exercise, the increase in ventilation further increases the volume to be exhaled while the increase in respiratory frequency further reduces the expiratory time resulting in a progressive increase in the EELV due to the stacking of incomplete expirations and worsening of dyspnea. This phenomenon is called "dynamic hyperinflation" and occurs on even mild exertion in patients with severe COPD. The hyperinflation also causes breathing to take place on the stiffer upper portion of the pressure-volume curve, resulting in an added elastic load that further increases the inspiratory threshold load. The hyperinflation also imposes a "restriction" on the extent to which the tidal volume can be increased on exercise thus compromising ventilation. The increased resistive and elastic loads lead to increased work of breathing. Further, the low and flattened diaphragm is an inefficient muscle of inspiration. Finally, inspiratory muscle shortening with hyperinflation reduces the mechanical efficiency. In the face of the added resistive and elastic loads and mechanical disadvantages of a hyperinflated chest, to achieve a given level of ventilation requires substantial additional effort and if the ventilatory pump is able to achieve the required level of ventilation, it does so at the cost of increased work of breathing and if it is not, respiratory failure occurs. Either way, a mismatch is sensed between the respiratory drive and the achieved ventilation.

Evidence for the above concepts has been provided. On exercise, patients with mild COPD were found to have higher dyspnea ratings for a given work rate and ventilation compared to normal subjects. Changes in EELV were greater and dyspnea intensity increased as inspiratory reserve volume decreased, indicating dynamic hyperinflation. Thus, dyspnea in COPD arises out of the combined deleterious effects of higher ventilatory demand and abnormal dynamic ventilatory mechanics.[63] Bronchodilators may relieve dyspnea partly by reducing hyperinflation and restoring the lungs and the chest wall to a more mechanically advantaged position. It has been shown that more patients with COPD respond to bronchodilators by increasing the forced vital capacity, reflecting a reduced residual volume, than by an increase in expiratory flow rates and the forced expiratory volume in the first second (FEV_1).[64] An increase in the inspiratory capacity following bronchodilators also captures the same effect.[65] This is a "pharmacological lung volume reduction." The beneficial effects of lung volume reduction surgery are also attributable to reduced volumes of the chest wall and restoration of the muscle length to a more favorable and efficient position. Reduction in hyperinflation due to the prolongation of expiration favoring lung emptying is also the likely mechanism by which breathing exercises, such as pursed lip breathing, that form part of pulmonary rehabilitation programs, reduce dyspnea and improve exercise capacity.[66] The strategy of smaller tidal volumes and slower frequency with greater inspiratory-to-expiratory time ratios during mechanical ventilation of these patients also has the same physiological basis.

Changes in lung mechanics in acute exacerbations of asthma are similar with the important difference that these are largely reversible. However, asthmatic airways that have undergone substantial remodeling have a largely irreversible airway narrowing, thus increasing the work of breathing persistently and suffer from the same consequences of hyperinflation as outlined above in patients with COPD.

In ILDs, inspiratory pressures are increased due to lower lung compliance, which also reduces the tidal volume. The increased work of breathing is related to the increased elastic load, the resistive load being largely normal or low. The demand for increased ventilation is met by increasing the respiratory rate particularly during exertion. Thus, such patients typically have a rapid and shallow breathing. Reduced tidal volume also increases the proportion of wasted ventilation due to increased dead space or alveolar ventilation the center. This drives ventilation further in order to have sufficient alveolar ventilation. Tachypnea reduces expiratory time more than the inspiratory time, thus increasing the inspiratory duty cycle. The result is an increased ventilatory effort in ILD. Again, as in patients with COPD, this requires an adequately responsive ventilatory apparatus that may achieve the required ventilation, but at the cost of increased work of breathing and if it cannot, respiratory failure will follow.

Thus, in both, COPD and ILDs, the level of central respiratory motor output required to achieve the desired ventilation increases. Given the functional abnormalities in lung mechanics in these diseases discussed above, the mechanical response of the lungs is achieved at the cost of increased effort of breathing that is likely sensed as uncomfortable. In both diseases, dyspnea intensity is increased at any given ventilation compared with age-matched healthy individuals.[67] Addition of external resistive and elastic loads leads to a progressive rise in the intensity of dyspnea as the applied load increases.[68]

Harty et al.[69] applied external thoracic restriction in healthy subjects and observed that during exercise, this produced a shallow and rapid breathing pattern and was associated with greater dyspnea, with descriptors of dyspnea used by subjects (inspiratory difficulty, tightness and increased effort) similar to those reported by ILD patients. A contribution of pulmonary and chest wall mechanoreceptors in the sensation of dyspnea was suggested. O'Donnell et al.[70,71] using a combination of external chest wall restriction and added dead space in normal subjects to create a closer approximation of the physiologic disturbances caused by ILD, and, on direct studies in patients with ILD has provided evidence that the inability to expand tidal volume appropriately in the face of an increased drive to breathe contributes to the intensity and quality of dyspnea in ILD.

As the natural history of COPD and most interstitial and diffuse parenchymal lung diseases is one of progressively worsening pathology and hence the load on breathing, progressively increasing dyspnea on exertion is the classical presentation of both the types of diseases.

While the above mechanisms operating in COPD and ILDs may support Campbell and Howarth's hypothesis of "length-tension inappropriateness"[52-54] or neuromechanical dissociation, it is also difficult to prove because comprehensive measurements of efferent and afferent signals are not currently possible. Further, the pathophysiology in these states that may be responsible for dyspnea extends beyond the alterations in lung mechanics **(Tables 1 and 2)**. There are associated changes in cardiopulmonary hemodynamics on exertion along with alterations in arterial blood gases. These are sensed independent of the changes in ventilation by different pathways as described above. Thus, other mechanisms are likely to operate as well.

Afferent Pulmonary Vagal Receptors Stimulation

As discussed above, sensory receptors in the lungs are innervated by the vagus nerves and consist of three types: Pulmonary stretch receptors (SARs and RARs) and bronchial C-fiber endings in the large airways, and pulmonary C-fibers (type J-receptors).[72] While the irritant receptors appear to modify the intensity of dyspnea associated with induced

Table 1 Mechanisms of dyspnea in chronic obstructive pulmonary disease

Increased ventilatory demand
• Increased ventilation/perfusion inequality • Increased physiological dead space • Hypoxemia and hypercapnia • Early lactic acidosis due to muscle deconditioning
Inefficient ventilatory pump
• Altered lung mechanics (increased airway resistance, hyper-inflation, including dynamic, leading to increased resistive and elastic loads) • Poor nutrition • Muscle fatigue due to the sustained increased work of breathing, mechanical disadvantage and systemic inflammation
Stimulation of vagal afferents
• Airway inflammation • Increased pulmonary blood flow and congestion on exercise
Signals from mechanoreceptors in the joints, tendons and muscles of the chest
Coexistent cardiac failure (diastolic/systolic)
Psychiatric morbidity

Table 2 Mechanisms of dyspnea in interstitial lung diseases

Increased ventilatory demand
• Increased ventilation/perfusion inequality • Increased physiological dead space • Hypoxemia and hypercapnia (later stages) • Early lactic acidosis due to muscle deconditioning
Inefficient ventilatory pump
• Altered lung mechanics (deflation and decreased lung comp-liance leading to increased elastic load) • Poor nutrition • Muscle fatigue due to sustained increase in work of breathing
Stimulation of vagal afferents
• Interstitial inflammation and edema • Increased pulmonary blood flow and congestion on exercise
Signals from mechanoreceptors in the joints, tendons, and muscles of the chest
Coexistent cardiac failure (diastolic/systolic)
Psychiatric morbidity

bronchoconstriction,[73] and the airway stretch receptors appear to modify breathlessnessby altering ventilatory pattern, neither of these receptors has been shown to be specifically dyspnegenic. On the other hand, in addition to being short of breath, the sensations felt by the subjects on the stimulation of type J-receptors were found similar to the manifestation of dyspnea[36-40] and also resemble the cluster of "breathlessness-indicating sensations" of left ventricular failure patients,[39] as well as those felt by the patients of high-altitude pulmonary edema.[28]

In two recent investigations, a significant similarity was found between the nature of respiratory sensations evoked in response to intravenous lobeline and modest treadmill exercise in cardiac disease patients,[38] and with a 6-minute walk in mitral stenosis patients.[39] The latter were found to have an increase in the dose of lobeline required to produce the threshold levels of respiratory sensations after valvulotomy reduced the pulmonary wedge pressure, thus suggesting a reduction in the intensity of the natural stimulus, i.e. pulmonary congestion. This was accompanied by an increase in the symptom-free 6-minute walk distance further substantiating their role in subserving the sensation of dyspnea on the exertion and limitation of exercise. This mechanism of relief is supported by the fact that neither the skeletal muscle peak exercise oxygen consumption[41] nor muscle structure or biochemistry change[42] and lung-function abnormalities still persist.[43] The evidence points to a major role for the J-receptors in the origin of dyspnea in acute heart failure.

However, acute increases in extravascular fluid volume in the airways also activate the RARs and with larger increases, both the RAR and the C-fiber receptors in the airways and the alveoli are activated. Activation of RAR causes a reflex increase in respiratory rate, tracheal tone and mucus secretion in the airways. It has also been suggested that the RARs play a significant role mediating the respiratory reflexes associated with acute heart failure.[25] However, direct evidence in humans is lacking.

Thus, whereas the role of vagal afferents in the genesis of the sensation of dyspnea in acute heart failure is fairly well established, there is uncertainness on their contribution to dyspnea in COPD and ILDs. The level of exercise that can precipitate dyspnea in these conditions is much less than that required to alter cardiopulmonary hemodynamics and produce stimulation of these afferents and exercise limitation in normal subjects. However, these may play a facilitator role as pulmonary blood flow does increase on exercise and in addition, coexistent cardiac failure is common in these conditions. Further, inflammatory changes in the airways and the interstitium may lower the thresholds for their stimulation, as discussed later. The stimulation of J-receptors on experimental aortic occlusion in cats was more closely related to the fall in lung compliance than the increase in pulmonary artery pressure associated with congestion.[74] Interestingly, the rapid shallow breathing that is characteristic of ILDs resembles the reflex response to the stimulation of pulmonary J-receptors. Therefore, J-receptors may be responsible for the dyspnea related to interstitial edema. Direct observations on the role of J-receptors in ILDs are, however, limited and do not support the suggestion that vagal stimulation is the principle mechanism for dyspnea on exercise in ILD.[75]

Inflammation is the most prominent pathological feature of both COPD (and asthma) and ILDs. The responses of lung receptors may be altered in these conditions and may be different from those observed in normal animals, as well as human volunteers. Recent studies have revealed that the sensitivity of bronchopulmonary C-fibers can be markedly elevated in acute and chronic airway inflammatory diseases, probably caused by a sensitizing effect of certain endogenously released inflammatory mediators. Normal physiological actions, such as an increase in tidal volume (e.g. during mild exercise) can then activate these C-fiber afferents, and consequently may contribute, in part, to unpleasant breathing efforts in diseases with inflammation in the airways and parenchyma.[76] Inhaled PGE2 is known to stimulate vagal afferent receptors in the lung in particular C-fiber endings, without a significant increase in airway resistance. It significantly increases the magnitude of the dyspneic sensation when compared with inhaled saline at the same levels of workload, ventilation, and oxygen consumption on exercise and thus may modulate receptor responsiveness by lowering the thresholds for stimulation.[77] Only a small percentage (< 10%) of the bronchopulmonary C-fibers exhibit CO_2 sensitivity under control conditions, but alveolar hypercapnia exerts a consistent and pronounced stimulatory effect on the C-fiber endings during airway inflammation produced by acute exposure to ozone, infusion of inflammatory mediators, such as adenosine or prostaglandin E_2 (PGE2) and airway exposure to poly-L-lysine, a cationic protein known to induce mucosal injury.[78] Several other autacoids (e.g. bradykinin, neurotrophic factors, certain lipoxygenase metabolites, etc.) can also sensitize pulmonary C-fibers. These mediators may also contribute to the heightened respiratory discomfort found in patients with airway inflammatory diseases.[79]

Increases in pulmonary arterial and capillary pressures occur due to pulmonary vasoconstriction in healthy individuals exposed to the hypoxic environment at high altitude. Dry cough and choking sensations felt in the throat and upper chest of subjects with high altitude pulmonary edema are likely caused by the activation of pulmonary C-fibers and the same may also be the mechanism for similar respiratory sensations that occur after moderate or severe exercise at sea level.[80]

More evidence for the involvement of vagal afferents in the sensation of dyspnea has been obtained in studies employing local nerve blocks with anesthetic agents in normal subjects, as well as observations in patients who underwent vagotomy for some indications. Exercise studies in a patient who developed severe exertional dyspnea after a failed surgery that resulted in unilateral pulmonary venous obstruction demonstrated a markedly abnormal ventilatory pattern consistent with excess vagal stimuli to the respiratory center. Temporary and then permanent vagal interruption markedly altered the respiratory pattern and improved her functional status.[18] In normal human subjects, bilateral local anesthetic block of the vagus nerves at the base of the skull was found to diminish breath-holding sensation, and prolong breath-holding.[17] On the other hand, results of vagotomy in patients have been inconsistent in relieving dyspnea, although the pattern of breathing may be altered with deeper breathing.[16,81] In normal subjects, alveolar deposition of lignocaine to block unmyelinated pulmonary afferent nerves did not reduce dyspnea on exercise.[82] However, anesthesia of central airways in normal subjects was shown to produce slower and deeper breathing and reduced breathlessness on exercise.[83] In contrast, in patients with interstitial lung disease, anesthesia of the central airways did not modify the perception of dyspnea.[75] Intravenous adenosine in normal subjects does not cause bronchospasm, yet causes dyspnea, most likely by an effect on vagal C-fibers in the lungs.[84] The same effect was also seen in asthmatics.[85]

Blood-Gas Abnormalities

Blood-gas abnormalities occur frequently in acute emergencies in several respiratory diseases and also develop in due course in the natural history of several progressive chronic diseases, including COPD and ILDs. Intuitively, one may expect these to contribute to the sensation of dyspnea. However, these correlate poorly with the magnitude of dyspnea in individual patients. As both hypoxemia and hypercapnia also increase the central respiratory motor output acting through peripheral and central chemoreceptors,[86] the increased ventilation confounds any independent effect these may have on the respiratory sensations. Increased ventilation is not necessarily "unpleasant" and therefore, the contribution of changes in blood gas abnormalities to the origin of the sensation of dyspnea is difficult to evaluate.

However, dyspnea is aggravated by hypercapnia at the similar levels of ventilation on exercise and voluntary hyperventilation suggesting a direct effect on the intensity of dyspnea.[47] The effect of $PaCO_2$ on ventilation is effected through changes in hydrogen ion concentration at the medullary chemoreceptors. While this may operate during acutely developing hypercapnia, in patients with chronic hypercapnia, metabolic compensation neutralizes changes in hydrogen ion concentration and consequently limits ventilatory responses and changes in respiratory sensation. Acute changes in hydrogen ion concentration may explain the dyspnea of diabetic ketoacidosis and renal insufficiency.

Yet, a complementary role of hypoxemia in the sensation of dyspnea cannot be denied. Certainly, the administration of oxygen reduces dyspnea in both acute and chronic respiratory failure, even in the absence of any changes in ventilation.[49] Bye et al.[87] noted that exercise duration was increased with the addition of supplemental oxygen in patients with ILD. It also clearly lowered ventilation measured at a given timepoint during exercise. Marciniuk et al.[88] observed that in patients with ILD, exercise was limited primarily by dyspnea in some and by leg fatigue in others. The former had greater ventilation and demonstrated the evidence of expiratory flow limitation during exercise. However, the average arterial oxygen saturation at peak exercise was equal in both groups. This suggests that hypoxia may not be the primary mechanism causing dyspnea in ILDs. Moreover, relief in dyspnea on oxygen therapy may result from other beneficial effects, including improved ventilatory and peripheral skeletal muscle performance, as well as improved cardiac performance. It may also modify central processing of other stimuli causing dyspnea and thus influence respiratory sensation. It is also like to have a strong psychological effect, as it is synonymous with life.

Psychological Origins of Dyspnea

Considering the inherent element of perception and the subjective nature of the sensation of dyspnea, psychological factors undoubtedly play an important role in its origin. Not only factors related to personality are important as the major determinants of perception, psychiatric morbidity complicates chronic disabling diseases and thus confounds the symptoms. The communications between cortical areas concerned with the perception of dyspnea and the respiratory control center are two-way pathways. Interpretation of incoming corollary discharge to the cortical centers as being "unpleasant" is modulated by psychological, behavioral and cultural factors. However, emotional upsets may themselves lead to an increase in ventilation and a worsening of dyspnea. This is classically observed in hyperventilation states, such as acute anxiety and also contributes to dyspnea in acute exacerbations of asthma, COPD and other acute emergencies.

Associations were found between respiratory symptoms, including dyspnea and psychological scales incorporating anxiety, anger, depression, and cognitive disturbance with the perception of respiratory symptoms increasing with a rise in psychological scores.[89] The prevalence of anxiety and depression among patients with COPD is significantly higher than that in the general population and has been linked to increased mortality, decreased functional status and decreased quality of life.[90] Sarcoidosis is associated with a high rate of psychiatric comorbidity, including major depressive disorders and may contribute to a poorer quality of life.[91] A more fundamental association between psychiatric morbidity and respiratory illness has also been proposed, suggesting that a subset of patients may be more prone to develop both. In anxiety states, such as panic disorders, the respiratory abnormality most often reported is increased CO_2 sensitivity.[92]

Psychiatric morbidity and respiratory diseases may be involved in a vicious cycle, the former leading to a greater perception of symptoms of the latter, and, the latter giving rise to the former as a complication. A psychotherapeutic approach, managing both may thus be more associated with improved outcomes.[93]

SUMMARY

Dyspnea is a complex symptom of several diseases and disorders of the respiratory, cardiovascular and other systems. The subjective and complex nature of the symptoms of dyspnea makes it difficult to develop an appropriate model to study its origin. All such models have limitations and hence there are large gaps in the state of knowledge about its underlying mechanisms. It is unlikely that a common mechanism and pathway may explain its genesis. The origin of dyspnea is likely to be multifactorial and qualitative and quantitative differences exist in the perceived sensation of breathlessness in these different conditions. Increased central ventilatory drive, inefficient ventilatory pump, and stimulation of vagal afferents by inflammatory and cardiopulmonary hemodynamic changes, as well as alterations in lung mechanics, sensations from mechanoreceptors in joints, tendons and muscles of the thorax, abnormalities of arterial blood gases, and acid-base balance acting through peripheral and central chemoreceptors, and psychological factors are the multiple factors involved. Management of patients based on an understanding of the pathophysiological mechanisms of dyspnea will be more rewarding both for the patient and the physician.

REFERENCES

1. Dyspnea. Mechanisms, assessment, and management: a consensus statement. American Thoracic Society. Am J Respir Crit Care Med. 1999;159:321-40.
2. Corne S, Bshouty Z. Basic principles of control of breathing. Respir Care Clin N Am. 2005;11:147-72.
3. Chen Z, Eldridge FL, Wagner PG. Respiratory-associated rhythmic firing of midbrain neurones in cats: relation to level of respiratory drive. J Physiol. 1991;437:305-25.
4. Chen Z, Eldridge FL, Wagner PG. Respiratory-associated thalamic activity is related to level of respiratory drive. Respir Physiol. 1992;90:99-113.
5. Campbell EJ, Gandevia SC, Killian KJ, Mahutte CK, Rigg JR. Changes in the perception of inspiratory resistive loads during partial curarization. J Physiol. 1980;309:93-100.
6. Supinski GS, Clary SJ, Bark H, Kelsen SG. Effect of inspiratory muscle fatigue on perception of effort during loaded breathing. J Appl Physiol (1985). 1987;62:300-7.
7. el-Manshawi A, Killian KJ, Summers E, Jones NL. Breathlessness during exercise with and without resistive loading. J Appl Physiol (1985). 1986;61:896-905.
8. Gandevia SC, Macefield G. Projection of low-threshold afferents from human intercostal muscles to the cerebral cortex. Respir Physiol. 1989;77:203-14.
9. Homma I, Obata T, Sibuya M, Uchida M. Gate mechanism in breathlessness caused by chest wall vibration in humans. J Appl Physiol Respir Environ Exerc Physiol. 1984;56:8-11.
10. Sibuya M, Yamada M, Kanamaura A, Tanaka K, Suzuki H, Noguchi E, et al. Effect of chest wall vibration on dyspnea in patients with chronic respiratory disease. Am J Respir Crit Care Med. 1994;149:1235-40.

11. Fujie T, Tojo N, Inase N, Nara N, Homma I, Yoshizawa Y. Effect of chest wall vibration on dyspnea during exercise in chronic obstructive pulmonary disease. Respir Physiol Neurobiol. 2002;130:305-16.
12. Altose MD, Syed I, Shoos L. Effects of chest wall vibration on the intensity of dyspnoea during constrained breathing. Proc Int Union Physiol Sci. 1989;17:288.
13. Chonan T, Mulholland MB, Cherniack NS, Altose MD. Effects of voluntary constraining of thoracic displacement during hypercapnia. J Appl Physiol (1985). 1987;63:1822-8.
14. Banzett RB, Lansing RW, Brown R. High-level quadriplegics perceive lung volume change. J Appl Physiol (1985). 1987;62: 567-73.
15. Manning HL, Shea SA, Schwartzstein RM, Lansing RW, Brown R, Banzett RB. Reduced tidal volume increases 'air hunger' at fixed PCO2 in ventilated quadriplegics. Respir Physiol. 1992;90:19-30.
16. Guz A, Noble MIM, Eisele JH, Trenchard D. Experimental results of vagal blockade in cardiopulmonary disease. In: Porter R (Ed). Breathing: Hering-Breuer Centenary Symposium. Chichester: John Wiley & Sons, Ltd; 1970. pp. 315-29.
17. Noble MIM, Eisele JH, Trenchard D, Guz A. Effect of selective peripheral nerve blocks on respiratory sensations. In: Porter R (Ed). Breathing: Hering-Breuer Centenary. Chichester: John Wiley & Sons, Ltd; 1970.pp. 233-46.
18. Davies SF, McQuaid KR, Iber C, McArthur CD, Path MJ, Beebe DS, et al. Extreme dyspnea from unilateral pulmonary venous obstruction. Demonstration of a vagal mechanism and relief by right vagotomy. Am Rev Respir Dis. 1987;136:184-8.
19. Coleridge JC, Coleridge HM. Two types of afferent vagal C-fibres in the dog lung: their stimulation by pulmonary congestion. Fed Proceed. 1975;34:372.
20. Coleridge JCG, Coleridge HM. Reflexes evoked from the tracheobronchial tree and lungs. In: Cherniack NS, Widdicombe JG (Eds). Handbook of physiology, 3. The respiratory system, Vol II. Control of Breathing. Bethesda: American Physiological Society; 1986. pp. 395-429.
21. Anand A. Influence of bronchial C-fibre receptors on respiration in cats: possible role in humans. Respir Physiol. 2000; 123:1-12.
22. Knowlton GC, Larrabee MG. A unitary analysis of pulmonary volume receptors. Am J Physiol. 1946;147:100-14.
23. Widdicombe JG. Breathing and breathlessness in lung diseases. Sci Basis Med Annu Rev. 1971.pp.148-60.
24. Widdicombe JG. Nervous receptors in the respiratory tract and lungs. In: Hornbein TF (Ed). Lung Biology in Health and Disease. Regulation of Breathing, Part I. 17. New York: Marcel Dekker; 1981. pp. 429-72.
25. Ravi K, Kappagoda T. Rapidly adapting receptors in acute heart failure and their impact on dyspnea. Respir Physiol Neurobiol. 2009;167:107-15.
26. Paintal AS. Thoracic receptors connected with sensations. Br Med Bull. 1977;33:169-74.
27. Paintal AS. The nature and effects of sensory inputs into the respiratory centres. Fed Proc. 1977;36:2428-32.
28. Paintal AS. The visceral sensations—some basic mechanisms. Prog Brain Res. 1986;67:3-19.
29. Fowler WS. Breaking point of breath-holding. J Appl Physiol. 1954;6:539-45.
30. Flume PA, Eldridge FL, Edwards LJ, Houser LM. The Fowler breathholding study revisited: continuous rating of respiratory sensation. Respir Physiol. 1994;95:53-66.
31. Kappagoda CT, Man GC, Teo KK. Behaviour of canine pulmonary vagal afferent receptors during sustained acute pulmonary venous pressure elevation. J Physiol. 1987;394:249-65.
32. Paintal AS. Impulses in vagal afferent fibres form specific pulmonary deflation receptors. The response of these receptors to phenyl diguanide, potato starch, 5-hydroxytryptamine and nicotine, and their role in respiratory and cardiovascular reflexes. Quarter J Exp Physiol. 1955;40:89-111.
33. Coleridge HM, Coleridge JCG. Afferent vagal C-fibres in the dog lung: their discharge during spontaneous breathing, and their stimulation by alloxan and pulmonary congestion. In: Paintal AS, Gill-Kumar P (Eds). Krogh Centenary Symposium on Respiratory Adaptations, Capillary Exchange and Reflex Mechanisms. New Delhi: Vallabhbhai Patel Chest Institute; 1978. pp. 396-406.
34. Paintal AS. Some recent advances in studies on J receptors. Adv Exp Med Biol. 1995;381:15-25.
35. Anand A, Paintal AS. Reflex effects following selective stimulation of J receptors in the cat. J Physiol. 1980;299:553-72.
36. Raj H, Singh VK, Anand A, Paintal AS. Sensory origin of lobeline-induced sensations: a correlative study in man and cat. J Physiol. 1995;482(Pt 1):235-46.
37. Gandevia SC, Butler JE, Taylor JL, Crawford MR. Absence of viscerosomatic inhibition with injections of lobeline designed to activate human pulmonary C-fibres. J Physiol. 1998;511(Pt 1):289-300.
38. Dehghani GA, Parvizi MB, Sharief-Kazemi MB, Raj H, Anand A, Paintal AS. Presence of lobeline-like sensations in exercising patients with left ventricular dysfunction. Respir Physiol Neurobiol. 2004;143:9-20.
39. Anand A, Roy A, Bhargava B, et al. Early symptom-relief after valvulotomy in mitral stenosis indicates role of lobeline-sensitive intrapulmonary receptors. Respir Physiol Neurobiol. 2009;169:297-302.
40. Simon PG, Schwartzstein RM, Weiss JW, Lahive K, Fencl V, Teghtsoonian M, et al. Distinguishable sensations of breathlessness induced in normal volunteers. Am Rev Respir Dis. 1989;140:1021-7.
41. Marzo KP, Hermann HC, Mancini DM. Effect of balloon mitral valvuloplasty on exercise capacity, ventilation and skeletal muscle oxygenation. J Am Coll Cardiol. 1993;21:856-65.
42. Barlow CW, Long, JE, Brown G, Manga P, Meyer TE, Robbins PA. Exercise capacity and skeletal muscle structure and function before and after balloon mitral valvuloplasty. Am J Cardiol. 1995;76:684-8.
43. Gómez-Hospital JA, Cequier A, Romero PV, Cañete C, Ugartemendia C, Iràculis E, et al. Persistence of lung function abnormalities despite sustained success of percutaneous mitral valvotomy: the need for an early indication. Chest. 2005;127:40-6.
44. Butler JE, Anand A, Crawford MR, Glanville AR, McKenzie DK, Paintal AS, et al. Changes in respiratory sensations induced by lobeline after human bilateral lung transplantation. J Physiol. 2001;534(Pt 2):583-93.
45. Banzett RB, Lansing RW, Reid MB, Adams L, Brown R. 'Air hunger' arising from increased PCO2 in mechanically ventilated quadriplegics. Respir Physiol. 1989;76:53-67.
46. Banzett RB, Lansing RW, Brown R, Topulos GP, Yager D, Steele SM, et al. 'Air hunger' from increased PCO2 persists after complete neuromuscular block in humans. Respir Physiol. 1990;81:1-17.

47. Chonan T, Mulholland MB, Leitne J, Altose MD, Cherniack NS. Sensation of dyspnea during hypercapnia, exercise, and voluntary hyperventilation. J Appl Physiol (1985). 1990;68: 2100-6.
48. Chronos N, Adams L, Guz A. Effect of hyperoxia and hypoxia on exercise-induced breathlessness in normal subjects. Clin Sci (Lond). 1988;74:531-7.
49. Lane R, Cockcroft A, Adams L, Guz A. Arterial oxygen saturation and breathlessness in patients with chronic obstructive airways disease. Clin Sci (Lond). 1987;72:693-8.
50. Simon PM, Schwartzstein RM, Weiss JW, Fencl V, Teghtsoonian M, Weinberger SE. Distinguishable types of dyspnea in patients with shortness of breath. Am Rev Respir Dis. 1990;142:1009-14.
51. Elliott MW, Adams L, Cockcroft A, MacRae KD, Murphy K, Guz A. The language of breathlessness. Use of verbal descriptors by patients with cardiopulmonary disease. Am Rev Respir Dis. 1991;144:826-32.
52. Campbell EJ, Howell JB. The sensation of breathlessness. Br Med Bull. 1963;19:36-40.
53. Campbell EJ, Freedman S, Clark TJ, Robson JG, Norman J. The effect of muscular paralysis induced by tubocurarine on the duration and sensation of breath-holding. Clin Sci. 1967;32:425-32.
54. Campbell EJ, Godfrey S, Clark TJ, Freedman S, Norman J. The effect of muscular paralysis induced by tubocurarine on the duration and sensation of breath-holding during hypercapnia. Clin Sci. 1969;36:323-8.
55. O'Donnell DE, Webb KA. Exertional breathlessness in patients with chronic airflow limitation. The role of lung hyperinflation. Am Rev Respir Dis. 1993;148:1351-7.
56. Kearon MC, Summers E, Jones NL, Campbell EJ, Killian KJ. Effort and dyspnoea during work of varying intensity and duration. Eur Respir J. 1991;4:917-25.
57. Killian KJ, Summers E, Jones NL, Campbell EJ. Dyspnea and leg effort during incremental cycle ergometry. Am Rev Respir Dis. 1992;145:1339-45.
58. Burns BH, Howell JB. Disproportionately severe breathlessness in chronic bronchitis. Q J Med. 1969;38:277-94.
59. Sue DY, Wasserman K, Moricca RB, Casaburi R. Metabolic acidosis during exercise in patients with chronic obstructive pulmonary disease. Use of the V-slope method for anaerobic threshold determination. Chest. 1988;94:931-8.
60. Rochester DF. Respiratory muscles and ventilatory failure: 1993 perspective. Am J Med Sci. 1993;305:394-402.
61. Killian KJ, Jones NL. Respiratory muscles and dyspnea. Clin Chest Med. 1988;9:237-48.
62. O'Donnell DE, Banzett RB, Carrieri-Kohlman V, Casaburi R, Davenport PW, Gandevia SC, et al. Pathophysiology of dyspnea in chronic obstructive pulmonary disease: a roundtable. Proc Am Thorac Soc. 2007;4:145-68.
63. Ofir D, Laveneziana P, Webb KA, Lam YM, O'Donnell DE. Mechanisms of dyspnea during cycle exercise in symptomatic patients with GOLD stage I chronic obstructive pulmonary disease. Am J Respir Crit Care Med. 2008;177:622-9.
64. Chhabra SK, Bhatnagar S. Comparison of bronchodilator responsiveness in asthma and chronic obstructive pulmonary disease. Indian J Chest Dis Allied Sci. 2002;44:91-7.
65. Celli B, ZuWallack R, Wang S, Kesten S. Improvement in resting inspiratory capacity and hyperinflation with tiotropium in COPD patients with increased static lung volumes. Chest. 2003;124:1743-8.
66. Thoman RL, Stoker GL, Ross JC. The efficacy of purse-lips breathing in patients with chronic obstructive pulmonary disease. Am Rev Respir Dis 1966;93:100-6.
67. O'Donnell DE, Ora J, Webb KA, Laveneziana P, Jensen D. Mechanisms of activity-related dyspnea in pulmonary diseases. Respir Physiol Neurobiol. 2009;167:116-32.
68. Altose MD, Cherniack NS. Respiratory sensation and respiratory muscle activity. Adv Physiol Sci. 1981;10:111-9.
69. Harty HR, Corfield DR, Schwartzstein RM, Adams L. External thoracic restriction, respiratory sensation, and ventilation during exercise in men. J Appl Physiol (1985). 1999;86:1142-50.
70. O'Donnell DE, Chau LK, Webb KA. Qualitative aspects of exertional dyspnoea in patients with interstitial lung disease. J Appl Physiol (1985). 1998;84:2000-9.
71. O'Donnell DE, Hong HH, Webb KA. Respiratory sensation during chest wall restriction and dead space loading in exercising men. J Appl Physiol (1985). 2000;88:1859-69.
72. Coleridge JC, Coleridge HM. Afferent vagal C-fibre innervation of the lungs and airways and its functional significance. Rev Physiol Biochem Pharmacol. 1984;99:1-110.
73. Taguchi O, Kikuchi Y, Hida W, Iwase N, Satoh M, Chonan T, et al. Effects of bronchoconstriction and external resistive loading on the sensation of dyspnea. J Appl Physiol (1985). 1991;71:2183-90.
74. Paintal AS. Mechanism of stimulation of type J pulmonary receptors. J Physiol. 1969;203:511-32.
75. Winning AJ, Hamilton RD, Guz A. Ventilation and breathlessness on maximal exercise in patients with interstitial lung disease after local anaesthetic aerosol inhalation. Clin Sci (Lond). 1988;74:275-81.
76. Lee LY. Respiratory sensations evoked by activation of bronchopulmonary C-fibers. Respir Physiol Neurobiol. 2009;167:26-35.
77. Taguchi O, Kikuchi Y, Hida W, Iwase N, Okabe S, Chonan T, et al. Prostaglandin E2 inhalation increases the sensation of dyspnea during exercise. Am Rev Respir Dis. 1992;145:1346-9.
78. Lin RL, Gu Q, Lin YS, Lee LY. Stimulatory effect of CO_2 on vagal bronchopulmonary C-fiber afferents during airway inflammation. J Appl Physiol. 2005;99:1704-11.
79. Lee LY, Undem BJ. Brochopulmonary vagal sensory nerves. In: Undem BJ, Weinreich D (Eds). Advances in Vagal Afferent Neurobiology. Boca Raton: CRC Press; 2005. pp. 279-313.
80. Paintal AS. Sensation from J receptors. News in Physiological Sciences. 1995;10:238-43.
81. Bradley GW, Hale T, Pimble J, Rowlandson R, Noble MI. Effect of vagotomy on the breathing pattern and exercise ability in emphysematous patients. Clin Sci (Lond). 1982;62:311-9.
82. Stark RD, O'Neill PA, Russell NJ, Heapy CG, Stretton TB. Effects of small-particle aerosols of local anaesthetic on dyspnoea in patients with respiratory disease. Clin Sci (Lond). 1985;69:29-36.
83. Winning AJ, Hamilton RD, Shea SA, Knott C, Guz A. The effect of airway anaesthesia on the control of breathing and the sensation of breathlessness in man. Clin Sci (Lond). 1985;68: 215-25.
84. Burki NK, Dale WJ, Lee LY. Intravenous adenosine and dyspnea in humans. J Appl Physiol (1985). 2005;98:180-5.
85. Burki NK, Alam M, Lee LY. The pulmonary effects of intravenous adenosine in asthmatic subjects. Respir Res. 2006;7:139.
86. O'Donnell DE, Bain DJ, Webb KA. Factors contributing to relief of exertional breathlessness during hyperoxia in chronic airflow limitation. Am J Respir Crit Care Med. 1997;155:530-5.

87. Bye PT, Anderson SD, Woolcock AJ, Young IH, Alison JA. Bicycle endurance performance of patients with interstitial lung disease breathing air and oxygen. Am Rev Respir Dis. 1992;126:1005-12.
88. Marciniuk DD, Sridhar G, Clemens RE, Zintel TA, Gallagher CG. Lung volumes and expiratory flow limitation during exercise in interstitial lung disease. J Appl Physiol (1985). 1994;77:963-73.
89. Dales RE, Spitzer WO, Schechter MT, Suissa S. The influence of psychological status on respiratory symptom reporting. Am Rev Respir Dis. 1989;139:1459-63.
90. Putman-Casdorph H, McCrone S. Chronic obstructive pulmonary disease, anxiety, and depression: state of the science. Heart Lung. 2009;38:34-47.
91. Goracci A, Fagiolini A, Martinucci M, Calossi S, Rossi S, Santomauro T, et al. Quality of life, anxiety and depression in sarcoidosis. Gen Hosp Psychiatry. 2008;30:441-5.
92. Sardinha A, Freire RC, Zin WA, Nardi AE. Respiratory manifestations of panic disorder: causes, consequences and therapeutic implications. J Bras Pneumol. 2009;35:698-708.
93. Rosser R, Denford J, Heslop A, Kinston W, Macklin D, Minty K, et al. Breathlessness and psychiatric morbidity in chronic bronchitis and emphysema: a study of psychotherapeutic management. Psychol Med. 1983;13:93-110.

11 Chapter

Surfactant

Gyanendra Agrawal, SK Jindal

INTRODUCTION

Pulmonary surfactant is a complex mixture of phospholipids (PLs) and proteins that reduces surface tension at the air-liquid interface of the alveolus, thus preventing its collapse during end-exhalation. This chapter outlines the complexity of the surfactant system and describes its basic biophysics, physiology and biochemistry. The physiological basis for the pathology and the treatment of salient respiratory diseases due to altered surfactant metabolism in children and adults, are also reviewed briefly.

COMPOSITION OF LUNG SURFACTANT

Lung surfactant is produced by type II alveolar epithelial cells, also called pneumocytes and consists of a mixture of PLs and proteins.[1] Lung surfactant recovered from bronchoalveolar lavage (BAL) fluid, is composed of approximately 80–85% PLs, mainly dipalmitoylphosphatidylcholine (DPPC), 5–10% proteins, and 5–10% other lipids **(Table 1)**.[2]

Phospholipid Composition

Phospholipids are the main components that confer surfactant its ability to lower surface tension. The most abundant form of alveolar phospholipid (PL) is the tubular myelin, which are large relatively dense aggregates (termed large aggregate surfactant) composed of PLs and surfactant proteins (SPs). Small less dense particles (small aggregates) are also present in the alveolar space, which represent the remnants or catabolic forms of surfactant. These are taken up, reutilized or catabolized by type II pneumocytes or alveolar macrophages.

Lung surfactant contains several major PL classes—phosphatidylcholine (PC), phosphatidylglycerol (PG), phosphatidylethanolamine (PE), phosphatidylinositol (PI), phosphatidylserine (PS), sphingomyelin (SPM) and lysophospholipid (LPL) **(Table 1)**. DPPC accounts for at least 50% of PC molecular species, which is a critically important component for achieving the maximum reduction of surface tension. Surfactant is secreted into the amniotic fluid, levels of certain PLs like total PL, DPPC and lecithin to sphingomyelin ratio are used to predict the pulmonary maturity prior to the birth of preterm infants. Phosphatidylethanolamine, phosphatidylserine and lysophosphatidylcholine (LPC or PC) are present in relatively low concentrations in lung surfactant, an increase in concentration can indicate ongoing inflammation and cellular injury.[2,3]

Table 1 Composition of lung surfactants

• *Phospholipids*	*80–85%*
– Phosphatidylcholine (PC)	75% (50% DPPC)
– Phosphatidylglycerol (PG)	12%
Others	
• *Proteins*	*5–10%*
– SP-A	50–70%
– SP-B, SP-C and SP-D	30–50%
• *Neutral lipids*	*5–10%*
– Cholesterol	90–95%

Abbreviations: DPPC, dipalmitoylphosphatidylcholine; SP, surfactant protein

Protein Components

Four SPs, called SP-A, SP-B, SP-C and SP-D, named in the order of discovery, are unique to the lung and intimately associated with surfactant lipids, each playing specific roles in surfactant homeostasis or host defense. Two classes of proteins have been distinguished on the basis of their structures. The small hydrophobic SP-B and -C enhance the spreading, adsorption and stability of surfactant lipids required for the reduction of surface tension in the alveolus. They are essential for lung function and pulmonary homeostasis after birth, and are important protein components of the animal-derived surfactant replacement preparations used for the treatment of infantile respiratory distress syndrome (RDS). The two collectins, SP-A and SP-D, are relatively abundant hydrophilic proteins. They contribute to innate immunity and perhaps to the extracellular trafficking of pulmonary surfactant rather than to its surface activity.

- *Surfactant protein-A (SP-A):* SP-A is the major SP in regard to relative abundance in the surfactant complex. It is a 26–38-kDa oligomeric glycoprotein that is expressed by the Clara cells and alveolar type II cells of the distal respiratory epithelium. The deduced primary structure and amino terminal sequencing of rat SP-A reveal five discrete structural domains—(1) amino terminal domain (Asn^1-Ala^7); (2) collagen-like sequence of Gly-X-Y repeats (Gly^8-Pro^{80}); (3) hydrophobic neck region (Gly^{78}-Val^{114}); (4) Carbohydrate recognition domain (CRD) (Gly^{115}-Phe^{228}), especially mannose binding protein (MBP); and (5) two differentially occupied consensus sites for asparagine-linked glycosylation.[4] SP-A is composed of a series of discrete structural domains. Monomers of SP-A form trimers by triple-helix formation in the collagen-like domains. The fully assembled molecule is an octadecamer, stabilized by intertrimeric and intratrimeric disulfide bonds at the amino terminus. The human SP-A gene locus consists of two functional genes, SP-A1 and SP-A2, which have four coding exons located on the long arm of human chromosome 10.

  Deletion of the SP-A gene in mice does not alter survival or lung function after birth. However, they are highly susceptible to lung infection by bacterial, viral and fungal pathogens, indicating the primary role of SP-A in innate host defense of the lung. SP-A has been shown to bind to the lipid A moiety of endotoxin and to a variety of pulmonary pathogens, including *Haemophilus influenza* type A, *Streptococcus pneumoniae, Mycobacterium tuberculosis, Pneumocystis jiroveci* and influenza A virus.

  Surfactant protein-A also binds to alveolar macrophages and stimulates chemotaxis and phagocytosis.[4] SP-A also function as an alveolar opsonin to defend hosts without specific antibody or for immediate protection against remotely encountered pathogens that require the clonal expansion of lymphocytes for adequate response. It also acts an antiinflammatory agent by inhibiting certain cytokines like interleukin-1 and tumor necrosis factor-α (TNF-α). SP-A increases the association of lipids with type II cells, but does not appear to increase the internalization of lipid.

  The expression of SP-A in amniotic fluid increases in late gestation, and is a marker for determining fetal lung maturity. The levels of SP-A in BAL fluid are elevated in many diseases like sarcoidosis,[5] hypersensitivity pneumonitis,[5] idiopathic pulmonary fibrosis (IPF),[6] alveolar proteinosis[7] and asbestosis.[8] Thus, elevated SP-A levels in BAL fluids are not specific or diagnostic of a specific disease, however, may reflect acute alveolar inflammation.

- *Surfactant protein-B (SP-B):* SP-B is a relatively small, 79 amino acid, amphipathic peptide produced by type II epithelial cells lining the alveoli. It is encoded by a single gene located on chromosome 2, which is expressed in the lung by type II cells and Clara cells. SP-B is tightly associated with surfactant PLs, and forms tubular myelin in the presence of SP-A, PLs and calcium. It is then secreted into the alveoli, where it interacts at the surface of surfactant lipids, forming stable monolayers and bilayers that reduce surface tension. The dimeric structure of SP-B may account for its ability to cross-link different lipid membranes. It plays a critical role in surfactant homeostasis by promoting the adsorption of lipid molecules into the expanding surface film by a factor of greater than 150;[2] and enhancing their stability during the compression and expansion that occur during the respiratory cycle. This effect is further accelerated by the presence of calcium ions such that mixtures of PLs and SP-B display almost the same biophysical properties as the whole lung surfactant.

  Surfactant protein-B is critical for lamellar body formation and its deficiency results in the abnormal processing of SP-C due to abnormal lamellar body formation. Its transcription is regulated by transcription termination factor-1 (TTF-1).[9] The concentration of SP-B increases with advancing gestation, as does SP-A. SP-B is absolutely essential for breathing and SP-B(-/-) mice, and infants with mutations in SP-B gene die of respiratory distress after birth.[10] SP-B reconstitutes most of the surface activity of natural lung surfactant, in combination with lipids. The sequence region 64–79 of SP-B contains peptides with two or more basic residues that include arginine or lysine. This sequence has been shown to be most effective in lowering surface tension.[11]

- *Surfactant protein-C (SP-C):* SP-C is the only SP, which is expressed exclusively by type II cells in the mature lung. The human gene is found on chromosome 8 and SP-C, too, is translated as a larger preprotein and processed intracellularly. SP-C precursor protein is routed with SP-B precursor protein to multivesicular bodies, where both are processed and packaged into lamellar bodies for secretion into the air space along with PLs. Insertion of the SP-C peptide into PL membranes disrupts the packing of lipids, thereby enhancing the movement of lipid molecules between the sheets of membrane and vesicles. The main function of SP-C is to maintain the biophysical surface activity of the lipids. This occurs through an acceleration of the rate of adsorption at the air-water interface, as well as through an increase in the resistance of surfactant to inhibition by serum proteins or by edema fluid. SP-C stabilizes the surface activity of the surfactant film during the expansion and compression involved in breathing.

  Its transcription is regulated by TTF-1. SP-C (-/-) Swiss black mice does not demonstrate abnormalities in lung structure at birth.[12] In a congenic 129/Sv strain, SP-C deficient mice developed severe, progressive pulmonary disease associated with emphysema, α-smooth muscle actin staining, monocytic infiltrates, and epithelial cell dysplasia in conducting and peripheral airways.[13] SP-C is also an active component of various mammalian surfactant preparations that are used to treat RDS in preterm infants.

- *Surfactant protein-D (SP-D):* SP-D is the second hydrophilic SP and also a collectin. The molecular weight of the SP-D monomer is approximately 43 kDa that is structurally similar to SP-A and other C-type lectins. The collagenous domain of SP-D is much larger than that of SP-A, is attached directly, without a connecting region to the CRD domain. About 12 SP-D monomers are present in the lungs, three of which join to form trimers. These four trimers form a crisscross-like structure that may bind to bacterial lipopolysaccharide (LPS) and to cell surfaces, forming larger networks of cells or bacteria. The interaction of SP-D microbial pathogens is Ca^{++} and carbohydrate dependent. SP-D is produced in type II cells and in Clara cells, the gene being located on long arm of chromosome 10. The SP-D gene consists of 8 exons spanning greater than 11 kb of DNA. The majority (70%) of SP-D is found dissolved in the watery surfactant residue, whereas SP-A, SP-B and SP-C are almost entirely found in an association with lipids. Levels of SP-D and SP-A are potential markers for lung maturation because the studies of amniotic fluid and lung tissue have demonstrated the increasing levels of SP-D with increasing gestational age.

  For SP-D, there are no known functions that are related to the biophysical activity of surfactant. The molecule may be of great importance for the nonadaptive defense system of the lung. SP-D has specific binding sites on alveolar macrophages,[14] can induce a "respiratory burst", and stimulates their phagocytotic activity. SP-D also binds to polymorphonuclear granulocytes, LPS, *Escherichia coli, Pseudomonas aeruginosa,* influenza A virus and *P. jiroveci.*[2]

Other Lipids

Surfactant contains a small percentage of neutral lipids that are generally comprised of cholesterol, cholesterol esters, diglycerides, triglycerides and free fatty acids (FA). The roles of these components for surfactant function have not been fully characterized.

FUNCTIONS OF LUNG SURFACTANT (TABLE 2)

The best documented function of surfactant is its ability to reduce surface tension. Surface tension arises from the difference between the attractive forces on molecules at an air-liquid interface. As a result of this, there is a force or tension in the surface film that resists expansion of the bubble and consequently acts to contract surface area. This force is surface tension and has a value of 70 mN/m or 70 dynes/cm of water at 37°C.[9] The amphipathic properties of lung surfactant allow its alignment at the air-liquid interface. Surfactant intermolecular repulsive forces act by opposing attractive forces between molecules at the liquid surface. The presence of lung surfactant in the alveoli, therefore, reduces surface tension preventing collapse of alveoli. Natural surfactant generally lowers surface tension to less than 6 dynes/cm.[15]

Table 2 Functions of lung surfactant

• *Biophysical functions* – Reduces surface tension and prevents collapse of alveoli during expiration – Increases lung compliance and decreases work of breathing – Maintains gas exchange area of lung – Counteracts edema formation by balancing hydrostatic filtration forces – Improves mucociliary clearance – Reduces bronchoconstriction – Smooth muscle relaxant.
• *Host defense functions* – Opsonization of bacteria, viruses, fungi and allergens – Facilitate phagocytosis of pathogens – Modulate production of inflammatory mediators – Direct microbicidal activity – Promote phagocytosis of apoptotic cells.

The law of LaPlace states that the pressure difference (ΔP) across a spherical surface (e.g. alveoli) depends on the ratio between surface tension (σ) and the radius (r) of the sphere.[1,2]

$$\Delta P = \frac{2\sigma}{r}$$

A constant surface tension in conjunction with a small radius would lead to a high pressure difference across the sphere. So, there is an increased tendency for the collapse of smaller alveoli during expiration. The lowering of surface tension by the lung surfactant allows pressure differences across the alveolus to remain constant throughout the respiratory cycle; and thus, preventing collapse of alveoli and small airways. The surfactant also increases lung compliance, and reduces the work of breathing. It counteracts edema formation by balancing hydrostatic forces. Surfactant forms a nonspecific barrier against the adhesion and invasion of microorganisms into the lung.[16] Furthermore, airway surfactant was shown to improve mucociliary clearance,[17] and to reduce bronchoconstriction in response to inhaled allergens.[16] A recent study suggested the role of surfactant as a smooth muscle relaxant.[18]

Host defense functions of surfactant are primarily assured by SP-A and SP-D. Nevertheless, surfactant PLs also influences pulmonary immune function. SP-A and SP-D facilitate phagocytosis of pathogens by at least three different mechanisms—opsonization of pathogens, ligand-activation of immune cells and upregulation of cell receptors involved in microbial recognition.[19] Collectins also have a direct microbicidal activity against bacteria or fungi without the presence of immune effector cells.[19,20] The mechanisms leading to microbial killing have not been fully characterized. SP-A and SP-D promote the uptake of apoptotic cells by alveolar macrophages.[21] It also slows the release of proinflammatory mediators and inhibit the activation of nuclear factor-κB and the L-selectin-induced signal transduction.[22] The PL components in large abundance under normal conditions have been shown to suppress various lymphocyte and macrophage immune function. They suppress the proliferation, immunoglobulin production and cytotoxicity of lymphocytes; and also inhibit endotoxin-stimulated cytokine [TNF, interleukin (IL)-1, and IL-6] release from macrophages.[2]

SURFACTANT METABOLISM AND SURFACTANT FILM FORMATION (FIG. 1)

The size of the surfactant pool is tightly regulated by mechanisms controlling the synthesis, recycling and catabolism of surfactant.[23] Both during development and postnatally, the synthesis of pulmonary surfactant is subjected to precise regulatory controls. It increases markedly in late gestation and is enhanced by a variety of hormones, including the glucocorticoids. In fact, glucocorticoids are routinely used to induce lung maturity in infants at risk for preterm delivery. Thyroxine accelerates type II cell differentiation while acting synergistically with glucocorticoids to enhance the distensibility of the lung and DPPC synthesis. β-agonists and purines, such as adenosine triphosphate are also potent stimulators of surfactant secretion. Mechanical stretches, such as lung distension and hyperventilation have also been found to be involved in stimulating surfactant secretion. Certain cytokines like TNF-α and transforming growth factor beta (TGF-β) and insulin inhibit surfactant production depending on experimental conditions.

Surfactant PLs and proteins are synthesized in the endoplasmic reticulum of type II alveolar cells. In addition, SP-A, SP-B and SP-D are produced by Clara cells and submucosal

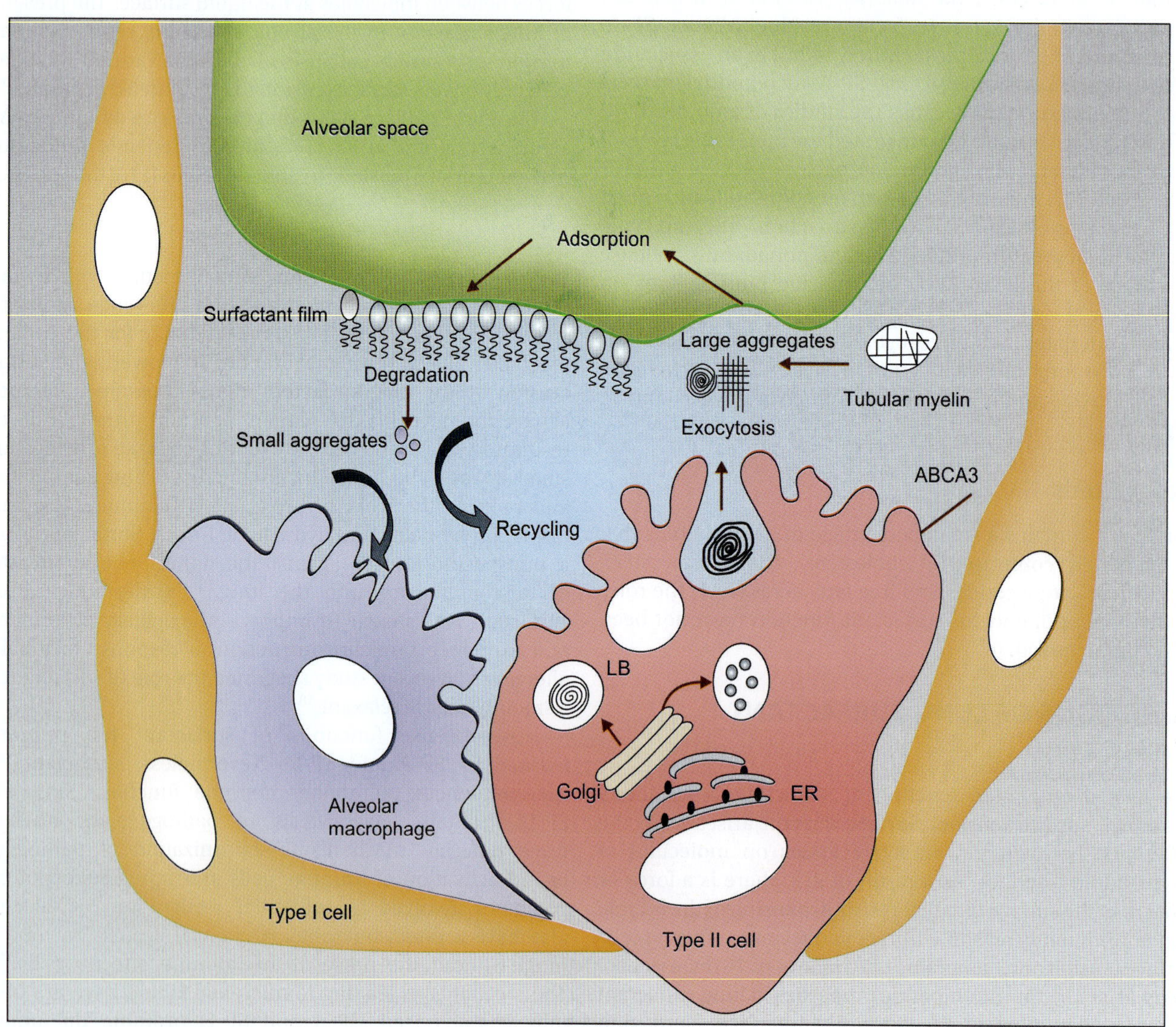

Fig. 1 Schematic representation of surfactant metabolism and surfactant film formation (see text for details)
Abbreviations: ER, endoplasmic reticulum; LB, lamellar bodies

cells. PLs and SPs are processed through the Golgi apparatus and packaged into lamellar bodies (intracellular storage organelles). ATP-binding cassette transporter A3 (ABCA3) is present in the limiting membrane of the lamellar bodies, where it is likely to regulate lipid transport at the air-liquid interface. Surfactant is exocytosed from these structures into the alveolar hypophase (a liquid layer between air and lung epithelium) where it exists in the form of heterogeneous PL-rich aggregates, including tubular myelin. Tubular myelin is the most abundant form of alveolar PL and consists of large dense aggregates. "Large aggregates" have been demonstrated to have a strong ability to lower surface tension (highly active surface) and to contain the hydrophobic SPs along with SP-A and specialized PL structures (i.e. lamellar bodies and tubular myelin). PLs from extracellular surfactant structures form continuous monolayers and multilayers of PLs that line the alveolar spaces and airways, with their polar heads oriented toward the liquid and their acyl chains toward the air.

During breathing the surfactant film at the air-liquid interface is subjected to "compression" and "expansion." The following concept has been proposed for surfactant film behavior—at the end of expiration, the surfactant film is enriched in DPPC as the PLs with unsaturated FA chains are squeezed out of the surfactant film (compression). DPPC films can be tightly compressed, which allows the achievement of very low-surface tensions at the end of expiration and thus prevents alveolar collapse. Although the ability to maximally lower surface tension is attributable to the presence of DPPC in surfactant films, proper surfactant function, which is highly dynamic in vivo, could not be achieved without the action of other lipids and SPs. The surfactant components, which are expelled during expiration, are reincorporated into the surface-active film during inspiration (expansion). This leads to enhanced surfactant spreading. PLs with unsaturated or shorter FA chains introduce fluidity into surfactant films, and allow fast surfactant adsorption and respreading at the air-liquid interface. Anionic PLs (PG and PI) enhance surfactant film adsorption and film stabilization during the respiratory cycle.[24] Surfactant proteins (SP-B, SP-C and SP-A) are essential for the packaging of surfactant PL in lamellar bodies, organization of tubular myelin, and ultimately formation of an efficient surfactant film at the air-liquid interface.

Normally, surfactant is inactivated by mechanical and biologic processes and converted into small, surface-inactive aggregates. "Small aggregates" typically represent surfactant, which is being removed from the air-liquid interface for recycling, or has been injured during inflammation. Approximately, 70–80% of the "small aggregates" are taken up by alveolar type II cells, transported to phagolysosomes, and reused or catabolized. Alveolar macrophages internalize and catabolize the remaining surfactant pool, a process critically dependent on granulocyte-macrophage colony-stimulating factor (GM-CSF).[25] Although less than 10–15% of surfactant is cleared by catabolism by the alveolar macrophages, this pathway is critical in controlling steady state surfactant concentrations in vivo. GM-CSF acts within the lung by stimulating the terminal differentiation of alveolar macrophages, principally by raising the levels of transcription factor PU.1.[7] It has been shown in experimental studies that GM-CSF and GM-CSF receptor-deficient mice are not capable of clearing SPs and PLs, causing alveolar proteinosis.[26] GM-CSF signaling also enhances the function of peroxisome-proliferator-activated receptor γ (PPARγ), another transcription factor that regulates many cellular functions, including intracellular lipid metabolism.[26] These findings explain how inhibiting the binding of GM-CSF to its receptor causes the decreased clearance of surfactant from the alveolar spaces.

DISORDERS OF SURFACTANT METABOLISM

Surfactant alterations have been implicated in the pathophysiology of a number of alveolar and airway diseases. This occurs either due to decreased production or due to accelerated breakdown by oxidation, proteolytic degradation, inhibition or inherited defects of surfactant metabolism **(Table 3)**. Decreased clearance of surfactant by alveolar cells, causing the excess deposition of surfactant in the lungs can also cause respiratory failure. Surfactant alterations have been described in a much larger number of respiratory diseases **(Table 4)**.[2] It is beyond the scope of this chapter to address all of these. Some of the important diseases linked to the altered surfactant metabolism have been briefly discussed as under.

Table 3 Mechanisms of lung surfactant abnormalities[3]

• Deficient surfactant formation (synthesis/storage/release) – Immaturity of type II pneumocytes – Injury to type II pneumocytes
• Inhibition of surfactant function (surfactant inhibitors) – Meconium – Plasma proteins – Cellular lipids – Hemoglobin
• Degradation of surfactant – Free radical injury – Proteases – Phospholipases

Infantile Respiratory Distress Syndrome

Respiratory distress syndrome is one of the most common causes of morbidity in preterm neonates, the risk increases as the gestational age decreases. The preterm infant who has RDS has low amount of surfactant that contains a lower percent of disaturated PC species, less PG, and less of all the SPs than surfactant from a mature lung. Minimal surface tensions are also higher for surfactant from preterm than term infants. Decreased alveolar surfactant activity associated with pulmonary immaturity causes atelectasis, alveolar collapse and hypoxemia. Radiological findings include a diffuse

Table 4 Disorders of surfactant metabolism

• *Decreased surfactant:* – Quantitative defect - Infantile respiratory distress syndrome – Qualitative defect - Hereditary SP-B deficiency - Hereditary SP-C deficiency - ABCA3 transporter gene mutation – Both (decreased production and inhibition of surfactant activity) - ARDS - Meconium aspiration syndrome - Pulmonary hemorrhage.
• *Excess surfactant:* Alveolar proteinosis
Abbreviations: SP, surfactant protein; ABCA3, ATP-binding cassette transporter A3; ARDS, acute respiratory distress syndrome

reticulogranular "ground glass" appearance (resulting from alveolar atelectasis) with superimposed air bronchograms. Oxygen support and mechanical ventilation are typically required.

Surfactant replacement therapy (SRT) significantly reduces the incidence, severity and mortality associated with RDS, and it has become the standard of care in the management of preterm infants with RDS.[27] SRT reduces the incidence of death, air leak syndromes and intraventricular hemorrhage in premature infants. Surfactant treatments are effective because of complex metabolic interactions between surfactant and the preterm lung. The large treatment dose functions as substrate; it is taken up by the preterm lung and is reprocessed and secreted with improved function. The components of the treatment surfactant remain in the preterm lung for days. If lung injury is avoided, then surfactant inhibition is minimized.[27] Prenatal corticosteroids complement surfactant to further enhance lung function.

Exogenous surfactant preparations, both natural and synthetic, are approved for the treatment and prevention of RDS in infants. Synthetic surfactants differ most notably from natural surfactants in their protein composition. Surfactant preparations containing SPs-B and -C act rapidly, increasing lung volumes and compliance, and thereby decreasing the requirements for positive pressure ventilation and oxygen supplementation. Synthetic surfactant preparations lacking SPs, e.g. colfosceril palmitate, improve lung functions in a delayed manner. However, the overall efficacy of both the type of preparations does not differ much, and are now the standard treatment for RDS. Prophylactic SRT in patients who are at risk for RDS, particularly those infants born at less than 30 weeks gestation, improves neonatal survival and reduces morbidity. For infants in whom RDS develop, SRT early in the course of RDS, before surfactant inactivation plays a prominent role in lung pathophysiology, is superior to later SRT when lung disease is more advanced.[28]

Inherited Defects of Surfactant Metabolism

A variety of inherited defects of surfactant metabolism includes the following:

Hereditary SP-B Deficiency

Homozygous SP-B gene (SFTPB) mutations lead to surfactant dysfunction and lethal respiratory distress. Most infants with SP-B deficiency are present with progressive respiratory failure in the first 24–48 hours of life. Pulmonary function studies and radiographic findings in these infants are consistent with surfactant deficiency. Radiographic findings include alveolar infiltrates and collapse, reticular-granular infiltrates and air bronchograms in term infants. The disorder is usually inherited as an autosomal recessive condition due to mutation in the SFTPB gene located on chromosome 2. SFTPB mutations are detected in approximately 10% of full-term infants with unexplained respiratory failure.[23] The carrier rate for SFTPB mutation is estimated to be approximately 1 in 1,000.[29] SFTPB mutations include nonsense mutations, point mutations, frameshift mutations, splice-site mutations, deletions and insertions in the SFTPB gene. A single mutation, termed "121 ins 2" (a net insertion of two nucleotides in codon 121 that causes a frame shift, unstable SP-B messenger RNA, and a failure to synthesize SP-B precursor protein), accounts for approximately the two-thirds of mutant SFTPB alleles.[23] However, heterozygous relatives of SP-B-deficient infants do not have clinically apparent lung disease.[30]

Surfactant protein-B deficiency disrupts the formation of lamellar bodies and tubular myelin. The normal packaging and routing of SP-C is also disturbed by SP-B deficiency. Misprocessed SP-C precursor protein (proSP-C) accumulates in amniotic fluid and intracellularly in the airway lumen, causing a proteinosis-like syndrome. Detection of this SP-C precursor protein fragment in BAL fluid of affected patients, by immunohistochemistry, is useful in the diagnosis of hereditary SP-B deficiency. The definitive diagnosis is made by the identification of both mutations in alleles of the SFTPB gene by nucleotide sequence analysis. The disorder is refractory to SRT and most infants die within the first month of life, despite maximal medical therapy. The only known treatment is lung transplantation; it has been found that long-term outcomes after lung transplantation for SP-B deficient infants are similar to those of infants transplanted for other indications.[31]

Some other uncommon forms of mutations in SP-B gene that cause partial deficiency of SP-B have been associated with chronic interstitial lung disease (ILD) in childhood. Most of these children often require intermittent oxygen therapy.

Hereditary SP-C Deficiency

Mutations in the human SP-C gene (SFTPC) resulting in the lack of SP-C represent a rare cause of acute and chronic lung disease (CLD) in infants and adults.[23] SP-C deficiency is inherited as an autosomal dominant disorder; and the mutation could be familial or de novo. This is associated with various forms of ILD, including nonspecific interstitial pneumonitis (NSIP), chronic pneumonitis of infancy (CPI), and IPF; and susceptibility to ARDS following lung injury and infection. Both direct toxicity of abnormal proSP-C, and deficiency of mature SP-C are involved in the pathophysiology of the lung disease caused by SFTPC mutations. Since SP-C may have other functions, including reuptake and catabolism of surfactant particles and surfactant function in the alveolus, it is unclear whether all or some of these activities contribute to the pathogenesis of lung disease caused by mutations in SFTPC.[23] Considerable allelic heterogeneity exists, but there is no obvious correlation between genotype and disease severity. Severe cases resulting in death in early infancy and some requiring lung transplantation have been reported.[9]

ATP-binding Cassette Transporter A3 Transporter Gene Mutation

Mutations in the ABCA3 transporter gene have been frequently implicated in severe neonatal lung disease and CLD in older individuals.[32] The genes for ATP-binding cassette (ABC) transporters encode membrane proteins involved in the transport of compounds across biologic membranes, and 14 ABC genes have been associated with distinct genetic diseases in humans till now.[33] Mutations in the gene encoding ABCA3 have been found in children with severe neonatal respiratory disease and older children with some forms of ILD.[34] ABCA3 mutations are not confined to a single group, and infants from several major racial or ethnic groups can be affected. Generally, this disease presents within first few days of life in full-term infants, with clinical and radiographic features suggestive of surfactant deficiency. Newborn infants are present with grunting, chest retractions and cyanosis followed by rapidly progressive respiratory failure. Diffuse air space consolidation, air bronchograms and reticular-granular infiltrates are seen on chest radiographs.

Most of these patients are refractory to conventional therapies like lung-protective ventilation and ECMO, resulting in respiratory failure and death in the first months of life. Respiratory failure does not respond to the SRT, and lung transplantation is the only known treatment for this disease. Some infants can also present with persistent pulmonary hypertension of the newborn.[35] Alveolar proteinosis, interstitial thickening, hyperplasia of alveolar type II cells, loss of normal alveolar structure, and features of desquamating interstitial pneumonia are certain ultrastructural findings associated with ABCA3 mutations.

ABCA3 gene mutation related lung diseases are inherited in an autosomal recessive manner with phenotypic heterogeneity ranging from fatal to milder forms. Certain forms of pediatric ILD particularly desquamative interstitial pneumonia (DIP), CPI, and nonspecific interstitial pneumonia (NSIP) have been related to the ABCA3 mutations.[34] Some of these children may have a family history of neonatal lung disease. The mechanism for decreased severity of lung disease in these children remains unclear, but it is speculated that it may be related to reduced function rather than complete absence of the ABCA3 protein. It has also been suggested that ABCA3 can be a candidate gene for other pulmonary disorders involving surfactant dysfunction, including the neonatal RDS and disorders with a later onset such as asthma and the acute respiratory distress syndrome (ARDS).[32]

Nucleotide sequencing of the gene in infants and children with refractory pulmonary disease may confirm the diagnosis of ABCA3-related lung disease. Nonsense and frameshift mutations, as well as mutations in highly conserved residues and in splice sites of the ABCA3 gene can be identified in the affected group.[32] The E292V mutation in particular is responsible for the genetic etiology of pILD related to abnormal surfactant function.[34] Electron microscopy of lung tissue from affected patients demonstrates the presence of small, atypical lamellar bodies in alveolar type II epithelial cells and the absence of tubular myelin in the airways, indicating an abnormality in intracellular and extracellular lipid homeostasis.

Acute Respiratory Distress Syndrome

Acute respiratory distress syndrome (ARDS) is characterized by sudden onset, impaired gas exchange, decreased static compliance, and by a nonhydrostatic pulmonary edema.[36] Surfactant production decreases due to diffuse lung injury in ARDS, presumably because the alveolar epithelium becomes damaged. Damage to the alveolar Type I cells lead to an influx of protein-rich edema fluid into the alveoli, as well as decreased fluid clearance from the alveolar space. Neutrophils are attracted into the airways by host bacterial and chemotactic factors and express enzymes and cytokines, which further damage the alveolar epithelial cells. Type II epithelial cell injury leads to a decrease in surfactant production, with resultant alveolar collapse. In ARDS, lavage PL, SP-A and SP-B are decreased, and the ratio of small to large aggregates is significantly increased compared with that in non-ARDS patients. Thus, ARDS leads to both deficiency in pulmonary surfactant constituents and inhibition of the activity of the remaining surfactant. This secondary surfactant deficiency may contribute to the disordered mechanical behavior of the lung in ARDS.

Despite the introduction of novel treatments, the mortality from ARDS still remains high. In a single study, the use of surfactant in younger children with acute lung injury (ALI) was effective in reducing ventilator days and increasing survival.[37] However, most other clinical studies of SRT in adults and children have not shown significant improvement in lung functions; perhaps due to the complex nature of the lung injury in ARDS.[38-40] Therefore, routine SRT for adult patients with ARDS cannot be recommended based on the current data.

Meconium Aspiration Syndrome

Meconium aspiration syndrome (MAS) is also a significant cause of respiratory insufficiency in neonates. When aspirated into fetal lungs, meconium particles mechanically obstruct the small airways. Meconium or the chemical pneumonitis causes and inhibits surfactant function, and inflammation of lung tissue contributes further to small-airway obstruction. Acute intrapulmonary meconium contamination induces a concentration-dependent pulmonary hypertensive response, with 15–20% of infants with the MAS demonstrating persistent pulmonary hypertension.

Meconium causes surfactant inactivation by multiple mechanisms. It is now known that the fibrillary structure of surfactant is destroyed by the meconium and its surface adsorption rate also decreases.[41] The presence of elevated cell count and proinflammatory cytokines IL-1β, IL-6 and IL-8 as early as in the first 6 hours suggests that MAS is associated with an inflammatory response. Phospholipase-A_2 (PLA_2) present in meconium has been found to inhibit the activity of surfactant in vitro in a dose-dependent manner through the competitive displacement of surfactant from the alveolar film. PLA_2 is also known to induce hydrolysis of DPPC, releasing free FA and lyso-PC, which damage the alveolar-capillary membrane and induce intrapulmonary sequestration of neutrophils.[42]

Exogenous surfactant replacement either as bolus therapy or with a diluted surfactant lung lavage have been shown to reverse the hypoxemia and reduce pneumothoraces caused by meconium aspiration, decrease requirement for extracorporeal membrane oxygenation (ECMO), decrease duration of oxygen therapy and mechanical ventilation, and reduce the duration of hospital stays.[43] There is no difference in the different surfactant treatment regimens and it may be related to the heterogeneous nature of this form of lung injury.[44]

Pulmonary Hemorrhage

Pulmonary hemorrhage occurs due to the rise in lung capillary pressure, which could be multifactorial, such as due to the effects of hypoxia, volume overload, congestive heart failure, or trauma induced by mechanical suctioning of the airways. There is a build-up of the capillary filtrate in the interstitial space, which can then burst through into the airspaces through the pulmonary epithelium. In addition to the plasma proteins, neutrophils are released, which in turn express proteases, oxygen free radicals and cytokines. The free oxygen radicals damage type II cells, which decreases surfactant production. Serum albumin, globulin and fibrinogen reduce the rate of adsorption, and increase the minimum surface tension of the surfactant film. The probable mechanism for the increase in surface tension is the competition of plasma proteins with the surfactant, for the interface. Elastase, one of the proteases, damages and degrades SP-A, thereby inhibiting SP-A mediated surfactant lipid aggregation and adsorption in vitro.[45] SRT may be partially effective in such cases.

Pulmonary Alveolar Proteinosis

Pulmonary alveolar proteinosis (PAP) is a rare disorder caused by abundant accumulation of surfactant-derived components in the lungs. The characteristic pathological feature is the filling of alveoli and distal bronchioles with surfactant-derived material that is granular, acidophilic, acellular and amorphous. The substrate stains for periodic acid-Schiff and is nearly identical to surfactant. The material consists of approximately 90% lipid (primarily PLs), 10% protein, and 1% carbohydrate and is usually sterile.[26] It has been demonstrated that the interruption of GM-CSF signaling in the lung results in pulmonary alveolar proteinosis.

Granulocyte-macrophage colony-stimulating factor initiated signaling plays unique role in alveolar macrophage function and pulmonary homeostasis, including terminal differentiation and the survival of macrophages, intracellular lipid metabolism, surfactant catabolism and recycling, expression of pathogen receptors, and phagocytosis and killing.[26] Interruption of GM-CSF signaling in the alveolar macrophage either by the absence of the gene encoding GM-CSF or its receptor in mice or, by neutralizing anti-GM-CSF autoantibodies in humans, impairs the catabolism of surfactant by alveolar macrophages. These results in the intracellular build up of membrane-bound concentrically laminated surfactant aggregates. Progressive expansion of the extracellular surfactant pool and accumulation of cellular debris due to the impaired catabolism eventually cause filling of the alveoli, thus reducing the size of the available gas-exchange surface and eventually leading to the clinical syndrome.[7] Current standard of therapy for acquired PAP is whole lung lavage and GM-CSF therapy in selected group of patients.

CONCLUSION

Clinical investigations, research in transgenic mice, and translation of findings from the bench to the bedside have considerably improved our concepts of the pathogenesis and treatment of the diseases linked to the altered surfactant metabolism. Besides, their role in regulating surface activity, the surfactant components may also play in the local immune regulation of the lungs. Except for RDS in the premature infant, where surfactant deficiency has been unequivocally demonstrated and exogenous surfactant substitution is now part of the routine clinical management, the contribution of surfactant therapy is currently under investigation in a variety of disease states.

REFERENCES

1. Frerking I, Günther A, Seeger W, Pison U. Pulmonary surfactant: functions, abnormalities and therapeutic options. Intensive Care Med. 2001;27(11):1699-717.
2. Griese M. Pulmonary surfactant in health and human lung diseases: state of the art. Eur Respir J. 1999;13(6):1455-76.
3. Christmann U, Buechner-Maxwell VA, Witonsky SG, Hite RD. Role of lung surfactant in respiratory disease: current knowledge in large animal medicine. J Vet Intern Med. 2009;23(2):227-42.
4. McCormack F. The structure and function of surfactant protein-A. Chest. 1997;111(6 Suppl):114S-9S.
5. Hamm H, Lührs J, Guzman y Rotaeche J, Costabel U, Fabel H, et al. Elevated surfactant protein A in lavage fluids from sarcoidosis and hypersensitivity pneumonitis patients. Chest. 1994;106(6):1766-70.
6. Kinder BW, Brown KK, McCormack FX, Ix JH, Kervitsky A, Schwarz MI, et al. Serum surfactant protein-A is a strong predictor of early mortality in idiopathic pulmonary fibrosis. Chest. 2009;135(6):1557-63.
7. Trapnell BC, Whitsett JA, Nakata K. Pulmonary alveolar proteinosis. N Engl J Med. 2003;349(26):2527-39.
8. Lesur O, Bernard AM, Bégin RO. Clara cell protein (CC-16) and surfactant-associated protein A (SP-A) in asbestos-exposed workers. Chest. 1996;109(2):467-74.
9. Nkadi PO, Merritt TA, Pillers DA. An overview of pulmonary surfactant in the neonate: genetics, metabolism, and the role of surfactant in health and disease. Mol Genet Metab. 2009;97(2):95-101.
10. Whitsett JA, Wert SE, Trapnell BC. Genetic disorders influencing lung formation and function at birth. Hum Mol Genet. 2004;13(Spec No 2):R207-15.
11. Mazela J, Merritt TA, Gadzinowski J, Sinha S. Evolution of pulmonary surfactants for the treatment of neonatal respiratory distress syndrome and paediatric lung diseases. Acta Paediatr. 2006;95(9):1036-48.
12. Ikegami M, Weaver TE, Conkright JJ, Sly PD, Ross GF, Whitsett JA, et al. Deficiency of SP-B reveals protective role of SP-C during oxygen lung injury. J Appl Physiol. 2002;92(2):519-26.
13. Glasser SW, Detmer EA, Ikegami M, Na CL, Stahlman MT, Whitsett JA. Pneumonitis and emphysema in sp-C gene targeted mice. J Biol Chem. 2003;278(16):14291-8.
14. Holmskov U, Lawson P, Teisner B, Tornoe I, Willis AC, Morgan C, et al. Isolation and characterization of a new member of the scavenger receptor superfamily, glycoprotein-340 (gp-340), as a lung surfactant protein-D binding molecule. J Biol Chem. 1997;272(21):13743-9.
15. Ikegami M, Jacobs H, Jobe A. Surfactant function in respiratory distress syndrome. J Pediatr. 1983;102(3):443-7.
16. Hills BA, Chen Y. Suppression of neural activity of bronchial irritant receptors by surface-active phospholipid in comparison with topical drugs commonly prescribed for asthma. Clin Exp Allergy. 2000;30(9):1266-74.
17. De Sanctis GT, Tomkiewicz RP, Rubin BK, Schürch S, King M. Exogenous surfactant enhances mucociliary clearance in the anaesthetized dog. Eur Respir J. 1994;7(9):1616-21.
18. Koetzler R, Saifeddine M, Yu Z, Schürch FS, Hollenberg MD, Green FH. Surfactant as an airway smooth muscle relaxant. Am J Respir Cell Mol Biol. 2006;34(5):609-15.
19. Wright JR. Immunoregulatory functions of surfactant proteins. Nat Rev Immunol. 2005;5(1):58-68.
20. Wu H, Kuzmenko A, Wan S, Schaffer L, Weiss A, Fisher JH, et al. Surfactant proteins A and D inhibit the growth of Gram-negative bacteria by increasing membrane permeability. J Clin Invest. 2003;111(10):1589-602.
21. Schagat TL, Wofford JA, Wright JR. Surfactant protein A enhances alveolar macrophage phagocytosis of apoptotic neutrophils. J Immunol. 2001;166(4):2727-33.
22. Baritussio A. Lung surfactant, asthma, and allergens: a story in evolution. Am J Respir Crit Care Med. 2004;169(5):550-1.
23. Whitsett JA, Weaver TE. Hydrophobic surfactant proteins in lung function and disease. N Engl J Med. 2002;347(26):2141-8.
24. Ingenito EP, Mora R, Mark L. Pivotal role of anionic phospholipids in determining dynamic behavior of lung surfactant. Am J Respir Crit Care Med. 2000;161(3 Pt 1):831-8.
25. Nishinakamura R, Nakayama N, Hirabayashi Y, Inoue T, Aud D, McNeil T, et al. Mice deficient for the IL-3/GM-CSF/IL-5 beta c receptor exhibit lung pathology and impaired immune response, while beta IL3 receptor-deficient mice are normal. Immunity. 1995;2(3):211-22.
26. Doerschuk CM. Pulmonary alveolar proteinosis--is host defense awry? N Engl J Med. 2007;356(6):547-9.
27. Jobe AH. Mechanisms to explain surfactant responses. Biol Neonate. 2006;89(4):298-302.
28. Stevens TP, Sinkin RA. Surfactant replacement therapy. Chest. 2007;131(5):1577-82.
29. Cole FS, Hamvas A, Rubinstein P, King E, Trusgnich M, Nogee LM, et al. Population-based estimates of surfactant protein B deficiency. Pediatrics. 2000;105(3 Pt 1):538-41.
30. Yusen RD, Cohen AH, Hamvas A. Normal lung function in subjects heterozygous for surfactant protein-B deficiency. Am J Respir Crit Care Med. 1999;159(2):411-4.
31. Palomar LM, Nogee LM, Sweet SC, Huddleston CB, Cole FS, Hamvas A. Long-term outcomes after infant lung transplantation for surfactant protein B deficiency related to other causes of respiratory failure. J Pediatr. 2006;149(4):548-53.
32. Shulenin S, Nogee LM, Annilo T, Wert SE, Whitsett JA, Dean M. ABCA3 gene mutations in newborns with fatal surfactant deficiency. N Engl J Med. 2004;350(13):1296-303.
33. Dean M, Rzhetsky A, Allikmets R. The human ATP-binding cassette (ABC) transporter superfamily. Genome Res. 2001;11(7):1156-66.
34. Bullard JE, Wert SE, Whitsett JA, Dean M, Nogee LM. ABCA3 mutations associated with pediatric interstitial lung disease. Am J Respir Crit Care Med. 2005;172(8):1026-31.
35. Kunig AM, Parker TA, Nogee LM, Abman SH, Kinsella JP. ABCA3 deficiency presenting as persistent pulmonary hypertension of the newborn. J Pediatr. 2007;151(3):322-4.
36. Bernard GR, Artigas A, Brigham KL, Carlet J, Falke K, Hudson L, et al. The American-European Consensus Conference on ARDS. Definitions, mechanisms, relevant outcomes, and clinical trial coordination. Am J Respir Crit Care Med. 1994;149(3 Pt 1): 818-24.
37. Willson DF, Thomas NJ, Markovitz BP, Bauman LA, DiCarlo JV, Pon S, et al. Effect of exogenous surfactant (calfactant) in pediatric acute lung injury: a randomized controlled trial. JAMA. 2005;293(4):470-6.
38. Anzueto A, Baughman RP, Guntupalli KK, Weg JG, Wiedemann HP, Raventós AA, et al. Aerosolized surfactant in adults with

sepsis-induced acute respiratory distress syndrome. Exosurf Acute Respiratory Distress Syndrome Sepsis Study Group. N Engl J Med. 1996;334(22):1417-21.

39. Gregory TJ, Steinberg KP, Spragg R, Gadek JE, Hyers TM, Longmore WJ, et al. Bovine surfactant therapy for patients with acute respiratory distress syndrome. Am J Respir Crit Care Med. 1997;155(4):1309-15.
40. Spragg RG, Lewis JF, Walmrath HD, Johannigman J, Bellingan G, Laterre PF, et al. Effect of recombinant surfactant protein C-based surfactant on the acute respiratory distress syndrome. N Engl J Med. 2004;351(9):884-92.
41. Bae CW, Takahashi A, Chida S, Sasaki M. Morphology and function of pulmonary surfactant inhibited by meconium. Pediatr Res. 1998;44(2):187-91.
42. Kääpä P, Soukka H. Phospholipase A2 in meconium-induced lung injury. J Perinatol. 2008;28(Suppl 3):S120-2.
43. Wiswell TE, Knight GR, Finer NN, Donn SM, Desai H, Walsh WF, et al. A multicenter, randomized, controlled trial comparing Surfaxin (Lucinactant) lavage with standard care for treatment of meconium aspiration syndrome. Pediatrics. 2002;109(6):1081-7.
44. Salvia-Roigés MD, Carbonell-Estrany X, Figueras-Aloy J, Rodríguez-Miguélez JM. Efficacy of three treatment schedules in severe meconium aspiration syndrome. Acta Paediatr. 2004;93(1):60-5.
45. Malloy JL, Veldhuizen RA, Thibodeaux BA, O'Callaghan RJ, Wright JR. Pseudomonas aeruginosa protease IV degrades surfactant proteins and inhibits surfactant host defense and biophysical functions. Am J Physiol Lung Cell Mol Physiol. 2005;288(2):L409-18.

12

Chapter

Respiratory Defenses and Immunology

Padmavathi Ramaswamy, Padma Srikanth, Vijayalakshmi Thanasekaraan

INTRODUCTION

A moderately active person inhales about 20,000 liters (15 kg) of air every 24 hours, while his food and water consumption for the same period are only about 1.5 kg and 2 kg, respectively. Very little selectivity can be exercised over the inhaled materials as compared to the control one has over what is ingested. So, the respiratory tract is constantly exposed to the external ambient environment. The respiratory tract is exposed to environmental toxic substances, such as the smoke, soot, dust and chemicals in the atmosphere, and also to a wide range of organisms such as viruses, bacteria, fungi and parasites. It has been calculated that the average individual inhales about 8 microorganisms per minute or about 10,000 per day. The magnitude of this atmospheric insult on the respiratory tract is much greater in the developing countries. The vulnerability of individuals to these inhaled substances varies widely depending on age, atopic status, nutrition and coexisting conditions. In India, the acute lower respiratory infection (ALRI) is thought to be responsible for about 490,000 deaths annually, responsible for nearly 1.5% of the entire global burden of disease among children under 5 years of age.[1] It is, therefore, vital for respiratory clinicians to have a clear understanding of the normal defenses of the respiratory tract.

The defense against foreign material within the lungs is a critical physiological function. This is accomplished by passive mechanisms, such as the branching nature of the respiratory tract and the regulation of airway lining fluid composition. The first line of respiratory defense consists of mechanisms, such as the physical barrier; reflexes, including sneezing and coughing; production of mucus; mucociliary clearance; transport of immunoglobulin A (IgA) and anti-microbial mediators (defensins, lysozyme, lactoferrin, lectins). The second-line of defense mechanisms include the innate immunity and the acquired immunity **(Table 1)**. These defenses can be overcome by a large number of organisms and inhibitory factors of pathogens, by compromised effectiveness resulting from air pollutants (e.g. cigarette smoke, ozone) or interference with protective mechanisms (e.g. endotracheal intubation or tracheostomy) or genetic defects (e.g. cystic fibrosis). Following exposure to airborne microorganisms (bioaerosols) in air, the defense mechanisms are able to eliminate most of the larger microorganisms; however, smaller particles and spores may be trapped within the lung tissue, which pose health risks. The impact on health depends on the interaction between genetic differences in the host, agent and environments (duration and exposure dose).

Table 1 Defense mechanisms of respiratory tract

Anatomical site	*Defense mechanism*
Conducting zone of respiratory tract (nose, nasopharynx, larynx, tracheobronchial region excluding the respiratory bronchioles)	Mechanical barrier *Lymphoid tissue*: Adenoids, tonsils, Waldeyer's ring NALT, BALT Mucociliary clearance mechanism Secretory IgA Sneeze and cough reflex
Gas exchange region (terminal or respiratory bronchioles and alveoli)	Alveolar macrophages Immunoglobulins (humoral immunity) Cell-mediated immunity Polymorphonuclear granulocytes

Abbreviations: NALT, nasopharynx-associated lymphoid tissue; BALT, bronchus-associated lymphoid tissue

PARTICLE DEPOSITION IN THE RESPIRATORY TRACT

Three regions of respiratory tract have been described based on the deposition of the particles **(Fig. 1)**—the nasopharyngeal region or head airways region (HAR, anterior nares to larynx), the trachea-bronchial region (TBR, trachea, ciliated bronchial airways till terminal bronchioles), and the pulmonary region or gas exchange region (GER, respiratory bronchioles, alveolar sacs and alveoli). The particle deposition in HAR is

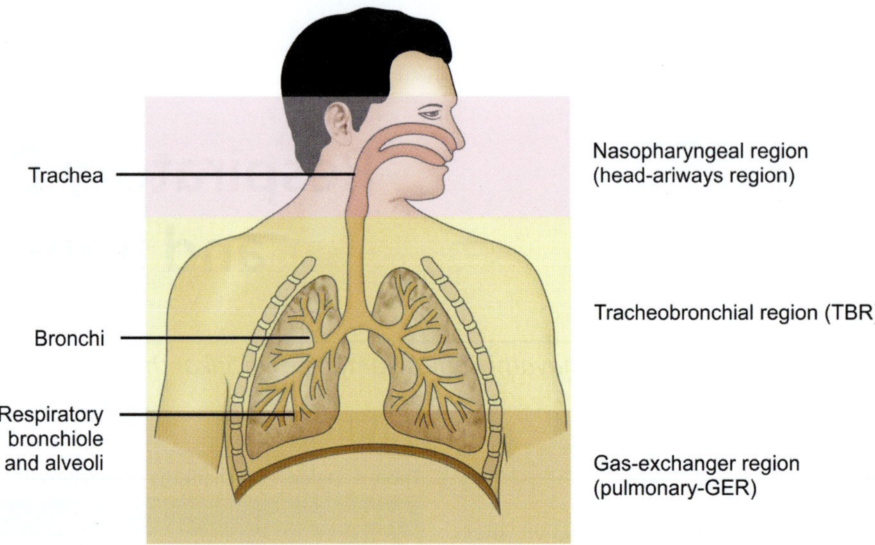

Fig. 1 Regions of respiratory tract

primarily limited to large sized particles that are 10 µm or above. Particles that are 1–10 µm are deposited throughout the respiratory tract, but as the size decreases to 1 µm, these particles can reach the TBR and GER. As the size diminishes below 0.5 µm, the probability of deposition again increases particularly in pulmonary region and to a lesser extent in the TBR.[2,3]

The deposition probability of particles based on the size, in each region can sometimes be used to relate to the anatomical locations of various diseases, e.g. nasal cancer in woodworkers where the airborne particle size is above 10 µm in aerodynamic diameter. The three principal mechanisms for particle deposition are sedimentation, impaction and diffusion. There are several mechanisms of clearance, such as dissolution of relatively soluble material with absorption into the systemic circulation, direct passage of particles into the blood, phagocytosis of particles by macrophages, transfer of particle to lymphatic channels and lymph nodes. A proportion of insoluble particles depositing in GER becomes sequestrated either in immotile macrophages or in fixed tissue over a long period of time contributing to cumulative lung burden.

DEFENSE MECHANISMS OF CONDUCTING ZONE OF THE AIRWAYS

The upper respiratory tract performs several essential physiological functions, such as filtration, olfaction, phonation, microbial defense and conditioning the air that is inhaled, to maintain a suitable temperature and humidity. The mucosal surfaces of the nasal passages are important for conditioning air before it reaches the more delicate alveolar tissue. Many mucosal glands provide moisture for humidification and mucus to adhere the inhaled dust.

Anatomical Defenses

The anatomy of the upper respiratory tract is composed of many features that help to get rid of particles and pathogens. The inside of the nose is lined with hairs, which filters larger particles that are inhaled. The turbinate bones are covered with mucus that collects particles, which are not filtered by nasal hair. Usually, particles 5–10 µm in diameter are either trapped by nasal hair or adhere to the nasal mucosal surfaces. The anatomy of the upper airway is such that it causes many of the larger airborne particles to impinge on the back of the throat.

Most of the surfaces of the upper respiratory tract are colonized by normal flora. These organisms are regular inhabitants of these surfaces and rarely cause disease. The regular inhabitants of the nose, nasopharynx and oropharynx include *Staphylococcus aureus*, *S. epidermidis* and nonencapsulated *Haemophilus influenzae.* The normal flora of these areas play a role in maintaining the healthy state of the host by competing with pathogenic organisms for potential attachment sites and often produce substances (toxins or acids), which are bactericidal. There are no resident bacteria in the lower respiratory tract.

Lymphoid Tissue

The adenoids and tonsils are lymphoid organs in the upper respiratory tract that are important in developing an immune response to pathogens and are located in an area where many of these airborne particles are in contact with the mucosal surface. Tonsils consist of localized lymphoid tissue located in the mucosa of the pharynx. Each tonsil consists of an epithelial crypt surrounded by the dense clusters of lymph nodules. At the center of each lymph nodule is a "germinal center" where the lymphocytes proliferate. Pharyngeal tonsils (also called adenoids) provide sites where immune surveillance cells (lymphocytes) can encounter foreign antigens, which enter the body through inspired air.

The nasal-associated lymphoid tissue (NALT) consists of the lingual, palatine and nasopharyngeal tonsils, the Waldeyer's ring **(Fig. 2)**. Inhaled allergens first encounter the NALT, which is more developed than the bronchus-associated lymphoid tissue (BALT). The NALT drains into the cervical lymph nodes. The respiratory tract contains lymph nodes in the mediastinum, hilar areas of the lung and submucosal aggregates present along the airways at branching points. The lymphoid aggregate with a specialized epithelium in the bronchial lamina propria is called BALT **(Fig. 3)**, similar to the organized lymphoid tissue of the gut [gut-associated lymphoid tissues (GALT)], e.g. Peyer's patches. The BALT at branching points of the airway is likely to contribute to local immunity. BALT formation following pulmonary infections is coordinated by mediators such as macrophages, dendritic cells (DCs), lymphocytes, fibroblasts and endothelial cells.[4] There are DCs present in the airways, which are the antigen-presenting cells that constitutively express a high level of major histocompatibility complex (MHC) (class II) antigen.[5,6] DCs become more numerous in response to inhaled antigens and rapidly decrease in number after treatment with glucocorticoids. DCs after binding with antigens in peripheral airways, migrate via lymphatics to the T cell-dependent areas of regional lymph nodes, such as BALT and lung-associated lymph node (LALN), where they encounter naive lymphocytes and initiate a primary immune response. While BALT performs an essential immunologic function such as sustaining the immunity in airways, hyperplasia of this structure may contribute to bronchial pathology. In the overall immune response, BALT plays a minor role.

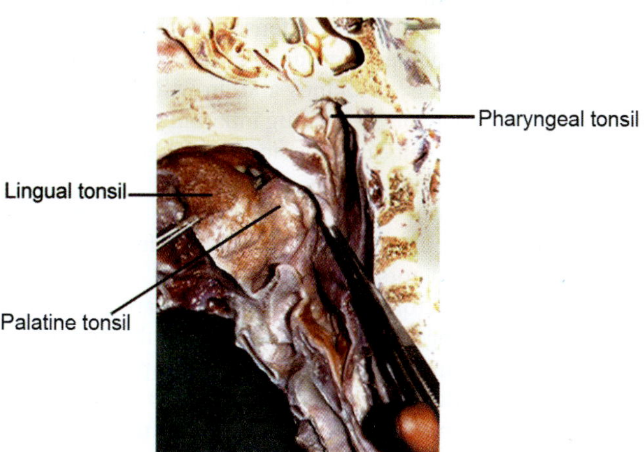

Fig. 2 Lymphoid tissue (Waldeyer's ring)
(*Courtesy:* Dr Melani Rajendran, Department of Anatomy, SRU)

Mucociliary Clearance Mechanism

The respiratory tract, from the nasal cavity through the bronchi, is lined by ciliated, pseudostratified columnar epithelium with goblet cells. Bronchioles are lined by simple cuboidal epithelium and the lung alveoli are lined by very thin simple squamous epithelium. Pseudostratified respiratory epithelium consists primarily of columnar ciliated cells **(Fig. 4)**. Subepithelial cells secrete mucus. The respiratory tract lined with ciliated epithelium is surrounded by thick connective tissue and smooth muscle. Scattered among the ciliated cells are occasional goblet cells. Basal cells are the source of replacement of ciliated and goblet cells.

Respiratory pathogens that reach the respiratory tract are trapped in the mucus layer and are driven upward by ciliary action (the mucociliary elevator or mucociliary escalator) to the back of the throat.[7] The mucus gel acts as a barrier for bacteria wherein these organisms adhere. The mucus may then be swallowed or coughed out. The sneeze and cough reflexes are important mechanisms for clearing material that accumulates in or irritates the respiratory tract.

- *Cilia*: The two human lungs contain approximately 0.5 m^2 of ciliated epithelia, with a total number of cilia in the order of 3×10^{12}. Nasal cavity, paranasal sinuses, pharynx, larynx, trachea are lined by ciliated epithelium. Immediately

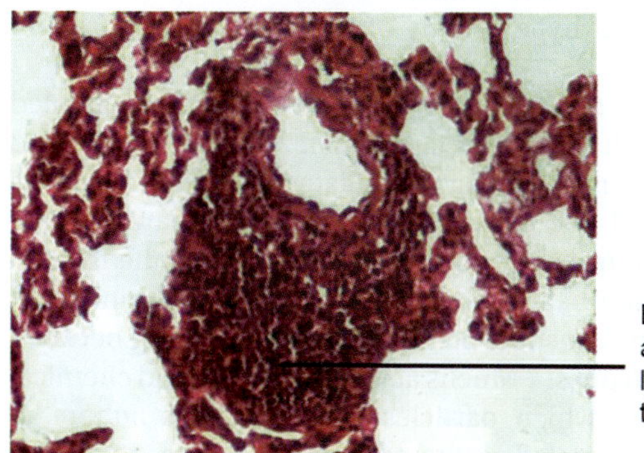

Fig. 3 Lymphoid tissue (BALT)
(*Courtesy:* Dr Melani Rajendran, Department of Anatomy, SRU)

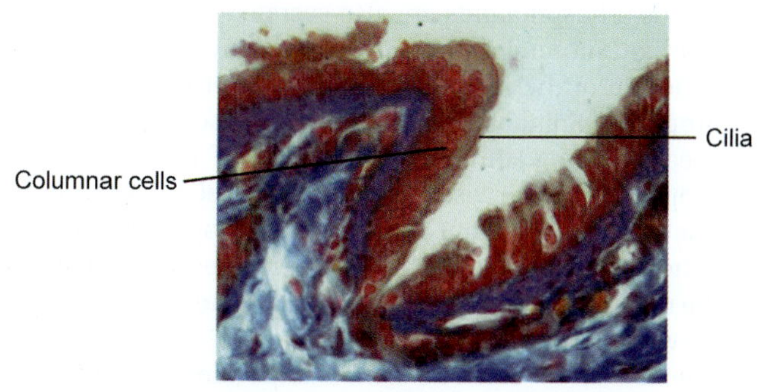

Fig. 4 Pseudostratified ciliated columnar epithelium
(*Courtesy:* Dr Melani Rajendran, Department of Anatomy, SRU)

below the larynx, the tracheobronchial tree is formed by a pseudostratified ciliated columnar epithelium, up to the 16th bronchial division of Weibel.[8] The ciliated cells, characterized by their cytoplasmic projections and numerous microvilli, have about 200 cilia.[1] Each cilium has length of 5–7 μm in the trachea and 2–3 μm in the 7th airway generation and a diameter of 0.25–0.33 μm. Cilia beat 600–1,000 times a minute. Cilia are structurally analogous to flagella, where the motion is dependent on the ATPase dynein. As ATP is metabolized, the structural proteins of the cilium change their configuration so that the cilium moves. Cilia move in a characteristic fashion that makes the overlying mucus to move in one direction only toward the pharynx.[9]

- *Airway mucus:* The airway epithelium is covered by a thin layer of airway surface fluid (ASF). The ASF consists of both a periciliary aqueous layer and an overlying mucus layer. ASF from healthy airways contains approximately 45% Na^+ and Cl^-, and 600% more K^+ than plasma. ASF in normal subjects is hypotonic than plasma.[10] The ionic composition of the ASL is assumed to be important for airway function and may be altered in diseases such as cystic fibrosis and exercise-induced asthma.[11] In patients with sustained airway irritation, infection or cystic fibrosis, the ASF composition becomes more isotonic than that of plasma.[12] The mucus layer is primarily produced by mucus glands in the larger airways and goblet cells in the more peripheral airways. Another type of secretory cell, Clara cell is present in small ciliated bronchioles, which changes to goblet cell in certain disease states.[13,14] Over 125 mL of mucus is secreted each day and forms a continuous sheet like a mucus blanket that covers respiratory tract. The respiratory mucus contains products from several sources, such as the alveolar liquid and secretory products from a variety of cells along the surface of conducting airways. Mucus is composed of greater than 95% of water and approximately 1% of salts and other dialyzable components, 0.5–1% free protein and a similar proportion of carbohydrate-rich glycoproteins or mucins.[15] The physical properties of mucus are provided mainly by mucins, which are mucoglycoproteins and proteoglycans secreted from the surface of epithelial cells and from the glands. Phospholipids are also secreted by the epithelial cells and submucosal glands of the airways weakening the adhesion of the mucus and thereby altering its physical properties. Spinability, non-Newtonian viscosity, elasticity, shear thinning (thixotropy) are some of the rheological properties of the viscoelastic mucus gel of respiratory tract.[16,17] In addition it also possesses properties, such as adhesivity and wettability that determine the capacity of the mucus to protect, hydrate and lubricate the underlying airway epithelium.[18]

Mucus also carries some important bactericidal substances, which contribute to lung defenses such as the secretory immunoglobulin A (IgA), lysozyme, lactoferrin and peroxidases.[19] Lysozyme is a muramidase that degrades a glycosidic linkage of bacterial membrane peptidoglycans. The role of lysozyme as an antibacterial substance is well-known. Besides lysozyme, bronchial secretions contain other antimicrobial substances, such as N-acetylmuramoyl-L-alanine amidase (NAMLAA) and β-defensins such as human beta defensins-1 (hBD-1) and hBD-2, and pulmonary lectins and surfactant collections. At a cellular level, lung epithelial cells express S100a, antileukoprotease and large amounts of major vault protein (MVP). In cells infected with *Pseudomonas aeruginosa*, MVP-1 localizes in lipid raft sections of cell membranes and helps to mediate bacterial clearance. The iron binding proteins, such as lactoferrin may reduce the availability of elemental iron that is a cofactor for bacterial replication. However, in addition, lactoferrin may also be bactericidal by binding to endotoxin. The secretory peroxidases (lactoperoxidases) or those from leukocytes (myeloperoxidases) act on thiocyanate ions or produce oxygen radicals, which are bacteriostatic or bactericidal. Epithelial cells are important sources of compounds, such as glutathione that act as antioxidants. They also produce nitric oxide, which has antimicrobial properties. Epithelial cells also actively participate in host defense against inflammation. These cells are capable of producing and responding to a variety of eicosanoids, cytokines and growth factors, which form a complex network regulating inflammatory responses. They also express cell surface receptors that can interact directly with inflammatory cells.

- *Mast cells:* Mast cells store or generate a number of substances, such as histamine, leukotrienes, specific chemotactic factors and proteases, which have potent inflammatory effects. Mast cells are present in mammalian lung in the bronchial wall, in the epithelium itself, and in airway lumen. Evidence implicating mast cells in the induction of airway muscle constriction and mucosal inflammation includes direct studies of mast cell secretion, measurement of histamine release and inhibition of asthmatic reactions with antihistamines and with the inhibitor of mast cell degranulation, sodium cromoglycate. Definitive evaluation of the role of the mast cell in asthma remains unknown, in part because of the general hyperactivity of airway smooth muscle in asthmatics.
- *Mucociliary transport:* Approximately, 90% of inhaled particles with a diameter larger than 2–3 μm are deposited on the mucus overlying the ciliated epithelium. Mucus is propelled by ciliary movement. The particles are transported from the terminal bronchioles to the trachea by the ciliary beats with the mucus. This motion called mucociliary transport occurs at a speed varying between 100 and 300 $\mu m\ s^{-1}$. Mucus acts as a physical and chemical barrier onto which particles and organisms adhere. It is further propelled to the oropharynx where it is either swallowed or expectorated. Cilia start moving from the resting position by bending sideways and backward.

This is called recovery stroke.[20,21] This is followed by an effective stroke during which the cilia move in a plane perpendicular to the cell surface. During this active phase, the tip of the cilia engages in the overlying mucus and sweeps it in a cephalic direction. The cilium moves in a layer of periciliary fluid whose depth is a little less than the ciliary length. The overlying mucus is only penetrated by the ciliary tips in the effective stroke and not in the recovery stroke, thereby optimizing the propulsive force of the ciliary beating on mucociliary transport. The thickness of the periciliary layer is critical for effective propulsion of mucus. A wide range of ciliary beating frequencies (CBF) is observed in the central airways.[22] Differences in CBF may be attributed to changes in temperature and humidity. The presence or absence of mucus and the load of mucus may also play a role in determining the CBF. CBF decreases with increasing age.

- *Factors affecting mucociliary clearance:* Physiological factors such as age, posture, sleep and exercise affect mucociliary clearance. Number of cilia, their structure, activity and coordinated movement are required for normal functioning of the mucociliary clearance.[23,24] Temperature of 37°C and an absolute humidity of 44 mg/dm^3 corresponding to a relative humidity of 100% is required for optimum functioning of cilia. High humidity enhances the functionality of the mucociliary clearance. Mucociliary clearance is also affected by certain risk factors such as malnutrition, exposure to air pollution and smoking. Malnutrition affects the integrity of mucosal epithelial cells. Air pollutants, such as sulfur dioxide, nitrogen dioxide and ozone are known to affect the functioning of the mucociliary mechanism.[25-27] Hair spray exposure is known to depress the tracheal mucous velocity. Cigarette smoke causes excess mucus production, paralyses the cilia and allows mucus to accumulate so that smokers have to cough to clear the secretions. Chronic smoking induces an increased number of abnormal cilia, which causes impairment of tracheobronchial clearance. The ultrastructural ciliary damage seems to be nonreversible, even after a long period of smoking cessation.[28]

Mucociliary clearance is altered in several airway diseases where structural damage to the epithelium or alteration of the mucus composition increases bacterial adhesiveness. Bacterial products, some of which are ciliotoxic may, furthermore, alter the mucociliary clearance. This is true for the *Pseudomonas aeruginosa* derived elastase.[29] Mucociliary clearance is altered in asthma, chronic bronchitis and cystic fibrosis.[30,31] An abnormal structure of the cilia has been observed in airway diseases, such as chronic bronchitis and in congenital diseases, such as the primary ciliary dyskinesia (PCD) syndrome ciliary immobility and interciliary discoordination with virtually absent mucociliary clearance. In cystic fibrosis, the most common mutation results in a defective transmembrane receptor protein, which is responsible for mediating cyclic AMP-induced increase in chloride secretion. The resulting alterations in the epithelial overlying fluid composition are believed to lead to poor bacterial clearance.[32]

Cough Clearance Mechanism

Cough is an important defense mechanism. Cough is classically described as a very deep breath, followed by a forced expiration against a closed glottis, which opens suddenly to produce the expulsive phase **(Fig. 5)**.

This allows enough turbulence and shearing forces in the major bronchi and trachea to extrude material such as debris, infected mucus or products of epithelial damage. The cough is triggered by a very wide variety of stimuli—mechanical, chemical or inflammatory. It is triggered by irritant receptors in the airways is mediated by the vagus nerve. The cough receptors or rapidly adapting irritant receptors are located mainly on the posterior wall of the trachea, pharynx, at the main carina and at branching points of the large airways. Cough promotes clearance by establishing high shear rates at the epithelial surface. Air forced over the mucosal surface at a sufficiently high velocity, generates lateral force that moves large particles in the direction of airflow. Within certain limits, this process is facilitated by the pliable nature of the walls of peripheral airways. During the forced expiration phase of a cough, the airways are narrowed by the rise in intrathoracic pressure. The medulla regulates the special breathing pattern that characterizes coughing.

Mechanism of cough reflex is also shown in **Flow chart 1**.

Cough serves as a protective mechanism when mucociliary clearance fails especially in patients with PCD, also known as immotile ciliary syndrome or Kartagener syndrome (KS).[13,33] Sneezing is also a protective reflex stimulated when the nasal mucosa is irritated. A series of short inspirations is followed by an explosive expiration, through the mouth, the nose or both. This explosive force carries droplets for long distances, a common means of spreading disease.

DEFENSE MECHANISMS OF RESPIRATORY ZONE OF THE AIRWAYS

Most of the respiratory passageways, from the nasal cavity through the bronchi, are lined by ciliated, pseudostratified columnar epithelium with goblet cells. Bronchioles are lined by simple cuboidal epithelium and the alveoli by very thin simple squamous epithelium **(Fig. 6)**. The squamous epithelial cells of the alveolar walls are sometimes called type I pneumocytes. This epithelium is exceedingly thin to facilitate diffusion of oxygen (O_2) and carbon dioxide (CO_2).

The alveolar walls also contain cuboidal surfactant-secreting cells. The surfactant overcomes the tendency of alveolar walls to adhere to one another (which would obliterate the airspace). As the epithelium of the respiratory or terminal bronchioles and alveoli are not ciliated, immune

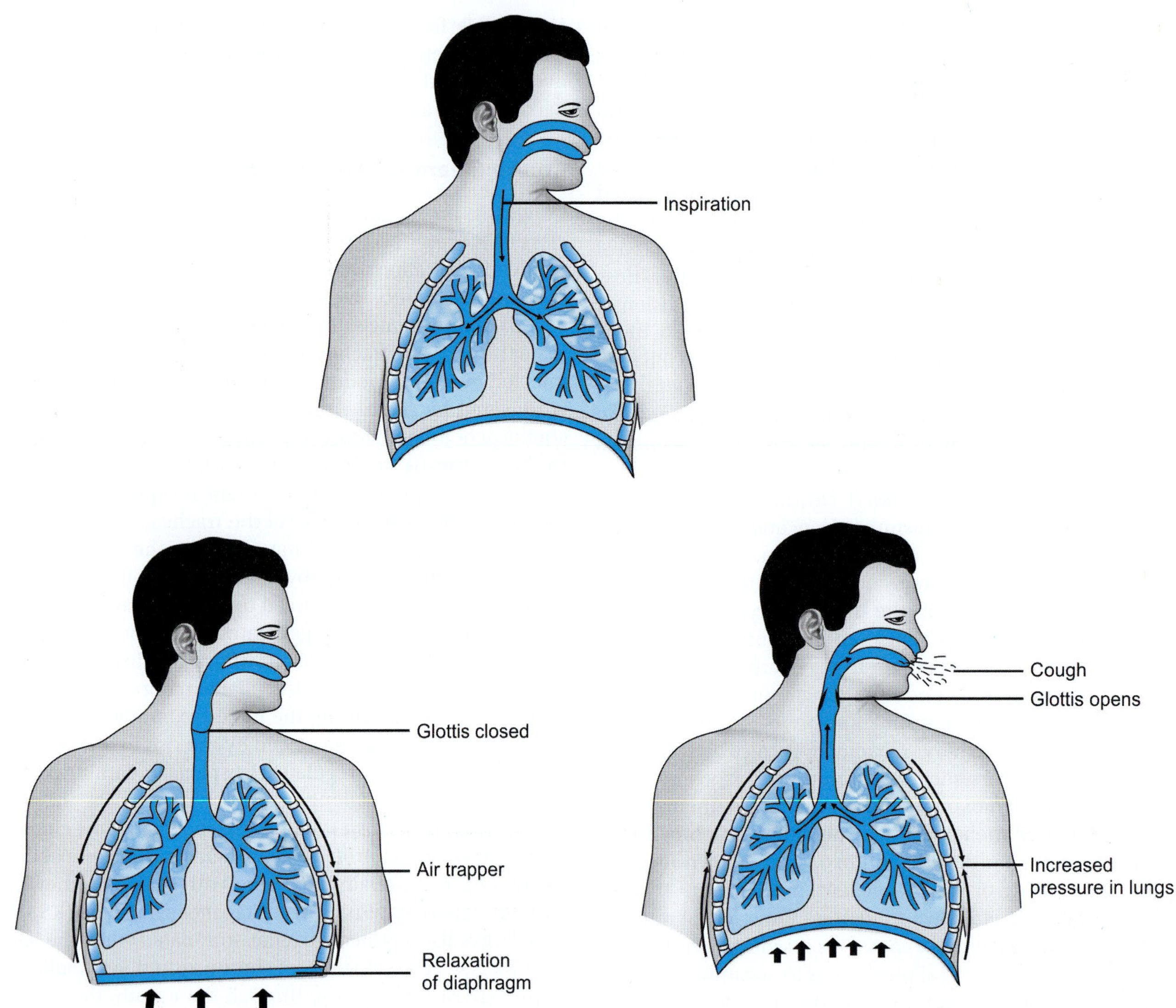

Fig. 5 Mechanism of cough reflex

effector cells, primarily macrophages, are the dominant mechanism for clearance.

Allergens, toxic particles, microorganisms that have escaped the mucociliary transport system are cleared by the alveolar macrophages (AM) by phagocytosis. These AM are sometimes called "dust cells" **(Fig. 7)**. AM provide the defense by phagocytosis, and ingestion of foreign material **(Fig. 8)**. Once they have engulfed the material, they may remain in the alveoli, may be cleared along the mucociliary clearance mechanism or may be cleared by lymphatics.[34,35] AM promote both nonspecific immune responses, such as the production of cytokines (including IL-1, IL-6, tumor necrosis factor, interferon-γ) that mediate an acute-phase response that develops regardless of the inciting microorganism and specific immune response by participating in the production of a variety of antibodies, complex glycoproteins known as immunoglobulins that bind to specific microbial antigenic targets.[36,37] Antibodies can help eradicate the infecting organism by attracting the host's white blood cells (WBCs) and activating the complement system. AM are a phagocyte as well as an effector cell, which initiate immune response. The role of AM in lung immunology is discussed subsequently.

SURFACTANT AND SURFACTANT PROTEIN A (SP-A)

Pulmonary surfactant is a surface-active lipoprotein complex formed by type II pneumocytes. Pulmonary surfactant is critical for maintaining the alveolar stability and gas exchange. SP-A was the first SP identified by its association with surfactant lipid. SPs-B, -C and -D have also been identified. SP-A binds to a variety of microorganisms, including viruses, bacteria,

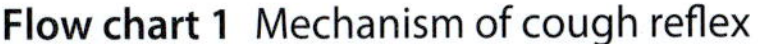

Flow chart 1 Mechanism of cough reflex

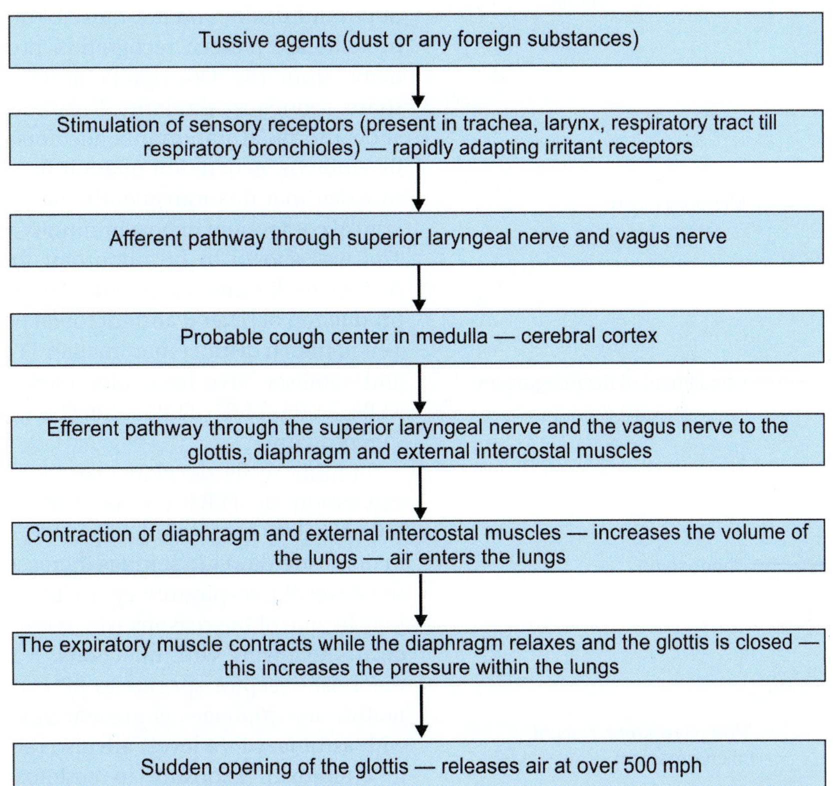
Tussive agents (dust or any foreign substances)
Stimulation of sensory receptors (present in trachea, larynx, respiratory tract till respiratory bronchioles) — rapidly adapting irritant receptors
Afferent pathway through superior laryngeal nerve and vagus nerve
Probable cough center in medulla — cerebral cortex
Efferent pathway through the superior laryngeal nerve and the vagus nerve to the glottis, diaphragm and external intercostal muscles
Contraction of diaphragm and external intercostal muscles — increases the volume of the lungs — air enters the lungs
The expiratory muscle contracts while the diaphragm relaxes and the glottis is closed — this increases the pressure within the lungs
Sudden opening of the glottis — releases air at over 500 mph

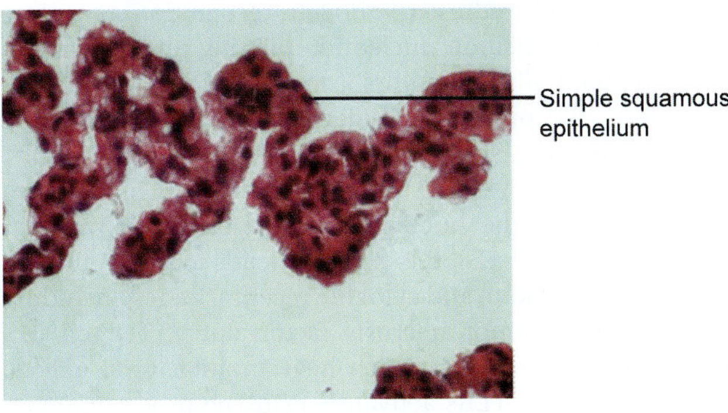
Simple squamous epithelium

Fig. 6 Simple squamous epithelium
(*Courtesy*: Dr Melani Rajendran, Department of Anatomy, SRU)

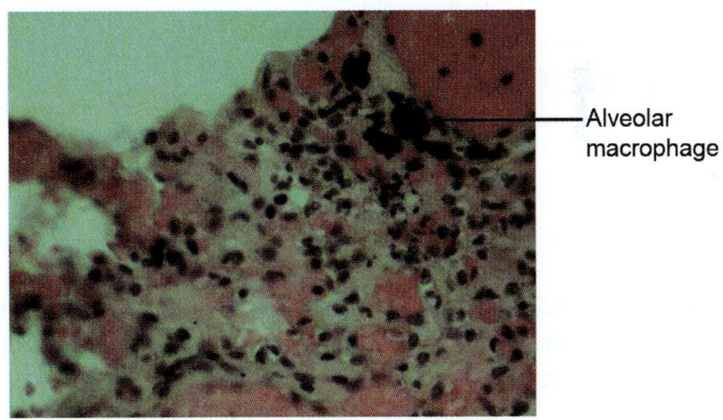
Alveolar macrophage

Fig. 7 Alveolar macrophages
(*Courtesy*: Dr Melani Rajendran, Department of Anatomy, SRU)

mycobacteria, fungi and pneumocystis. Among viruses, SP-A binds influenza, herpes simplex and respiratory syncytial viruses.[38,39] SP-A also binds to and increases phagocytosis of *Streptococcus pneumoniae*, group A *Streptococcus* and *S. aureus*, may bind to peptidoglycan (an important component of the cell wall of gram-positive bacteria). It may not bind to peptidoglycan directly, but inhibits the effect of peptidoglycan by binding to toll like receptor 2 (TLR2).[40] SP-A binds to rough lipopolysaccharide (LPS), aggregates these gram-negative bacteria and increases phagocytosis, however, it poorly binds to the smooth[41] variants of *Escherichia coli.* SP-A enhances the adherence and phagocytosis of mycobacteria and fungi, such as Aspergillus, by binding the conidia, enhancing their phagocytosis and killing, by human neutrophils and AM.[42] SP-A also binds to and inhibits the growth of mycoplasma, but does not clear the infections, even if it binds to Pneumocystis jeroveci.[43]

RESPIRATORY IMMUNE MECHANISMS

The human host is armed with a wide variety of sensors to detect an invading pathogen. The successful clearance

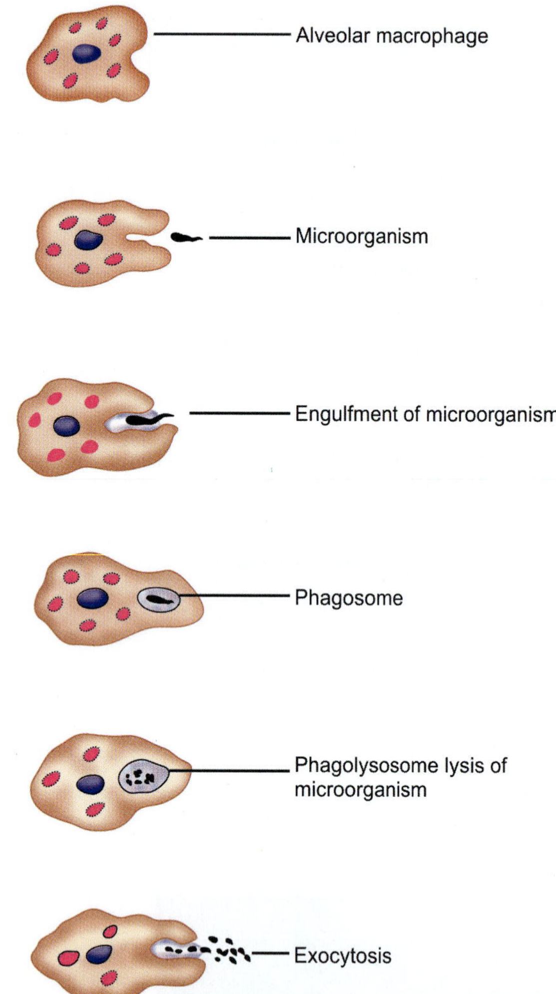

Fig. 8 Stages of phagocytosis

of airborne microorganisms follows pathogen-associated molecular patterns (PAMPs) that bind specific recognition molecules and activate innate immune pathways.

INNATE IMMUNITY AND TOLL-LIKE RECEPTORS

The most frequently detected PAMPs in bioaerosols are endotoxins (present in gram-negative bacteria), peptidoglycan (present in gram-positive bacteria) and glucans,[44] another PAMP recognition molecule, toll like receptors (TLR4), allow for endotoxin signaling to be achieved. Microbes that penetrate an epithelial barrier and enter a tissue site encounter three types of sentinel immune cells in the tissues. These are tissue macrophages, mast cells and immature DCs which act like guards to differentiate between apoptotic particles generated by normal tissue turnover and particles that are infectious.

The molecules mainly responsible for making this important distinction are those of the family of TLRs.[45] TLR proteins are pattern recognition proteins that obtain their name from the Drosophila protein toll with which they share sequence similarity.[46] Although toll was originally shown to be of importance for dorsal-ventral patterning in fly embryos, generation of adult flies expressing mutant toll revealed that this transmembrane receptor also served as a critical component of host immunity against fungal infection. Toll was shown to be important for host defense against pathogens, because engagement of this receptor induced the production of several antimicrobial peptides (e.g. defensins). Ten to fifteen distinct mammalian TLRs have been identified and agonists have been identified for some (TLR2, TLR3, TLR4, TLR5, TLR7, TLR8, and TLR9), but not for all of these TLR proteins.

Immune cells develop tolerance to repeated increased expression of TLR4 on the cell surface which leads to inflammatory response to LPS. RSV present in bioaerosols in domestic-day care settings increases TLR4 expression and sensitizes the respiratory epithelial cells to endotoxin.[47] This may be one of the reasons why secondary bacterial infection occurs following viral infections. A protein called CD14, a mannose receptor specific to LPS and found on surfaces of mature macrophages is present in higher levels in patients with asthma. CD14 levels are also raised in patients exposed to endotoxin. Exposure to endotoxins is associated with increased severity of asthma.

There are a number of cellular receptor families that recognize PAMPs. These pathogen recognition receptors (PRRs) families include nucleotide binding and oligomerization domain like receptors (nod like receptors, NLR), C-type lectin like promoters (CLR) and intracellular receptors to detect double stranded RNA helicase-like receptors. Through various signaling cascades activated TLRs lead to the activation of the nuclear transcription factor, nuclear factor kappa B (NF-κB), this (in turn) leads to the regulation of many host cytokine and cytokine receptor genes, including those for IL-1, tumor necrosis factor-alpha (TNF-α), IL-6, IL-8, IL-10 and IL-12, which have multifactorial effects. Depending on the TLRs activated, cytokine production can result in the full clinical presentation of the acute phase response, including fever. Whether the acute inflammation results from infection or trauma, it is triggered along the same pathway. Adjuvants used for all current vaccines function through the activation of the TLR pathway. The most potent adjuvant, Freund's complete adjuvant is a water-in-oil emulsion containing mycobacterial cell wall components that activate TLR1MTLR2 and TLR4. The simplest adjuvant, alum (aluminum hydroxide) includes molecules involved in antigen presentation in monocytes, MHC class II, CD40, CD54, CD58, CD83 and CD86; drives monocyte differentiation toward a dendritic cell like morphology; and induces secretions of IL-4, a cytokine with potent antibody production enhancing properties.

ALVEOLAR MACROPHAGES

Alveolar macrophages are bone marrow-derived cells that can be differentiated from blood monocytes after they have emigrated into the tissues. AM are located at the air-tissue interface in the lung, and are the first cells, which interact with inhaled organisms and antigens. These cells inhabit the various compartments of the lung, differentiating into mature macrophages, surrounding themselves in phagolysosomes once they engulf ingested material into the alveoli. AM produce lysozyme and defensins, which have bactericidal properties that are capable of destroying gram-positive and gram-negative bacteria and fungi. Reactive oxygen intermediates (superoxide anion, hydrogen peroxide, hydroxyl radicals) or reactive nitrogen intermediates [nitric oxide (NO), nitrites or nitrates] are also involved in destroying microorganisms and tumor cells.

Macrophages also produce macrophage metalloelastases, collagenase, metalloproteases (MMP1, MMP9) fibroblast growth factors, such as transforming growth factor (TGF) or platelet-derived growth factor that help in lung repair and remodeling. Intercellular adhesion molecule-1 (ICAM-1, CD54) and vascular cell adhesion molecule (VCAM-1, CD106) are adhesion molecules of the Ig super-family. Adhesion to the vascular endothelium mediated through ICAM-1/VCAM-1-integrin interactions is a key step in the emigration of white blood cells to the sites of inflammation. It has also been shown that they play an important role in the adherence of effector cells, such as AM to the respiratory epithelium. All these inflammatory mediators together play a crucial role in the orchestration of an inflammatory response, particularly in neutrophil recruitment. Recent studies suggest that cytokines and chemokines originate from AM, and from other cells such as epithelial cells.[48]

The ability of macrophages to interact with microbes is mediated by the surface receptors capable of binding specific ligands, including toxins, polysaccharides, LPSs, complement proteins and globulins. Pulmonary macrophages release the cytokines TNF-α and IL-1β, as well as the chemokines, monocyte chemoattractant protein-1 (MCP-1), macrophage inflammatory protein -1β (MIP-1β), and growth factors.[49] Inflammatory cytokines will favor the activation of the neighboring cells and attract several inflammatory elements from the blood. Stimulation of macrophages or mast cells through their toll-like receptors leads to the synthesis and the secretion of proinflammatory cytokines and lipid mediators, thereby initiating the inflammatory response that recruits both soluble immune components and immune cells from the blood. TLR stimulation of DC induces the initiation of an adaptive immune response.

TLRs are involved in the uptake of pathogens such as bacteria or viruses by alveolar and airway macrophages **(Fig. 9)**. TLRs also play a vital role in the maturation of DC and hence play a key role in the adaptive protection of the lung against bacteria and viruses. TLR2 plays an important role in mediating inflammatory responses to gram-positive microorganisms and mycobacterial products such as peptidoglycan, lipoteichoic acid, lipoproteins and lipoarabinomannan.

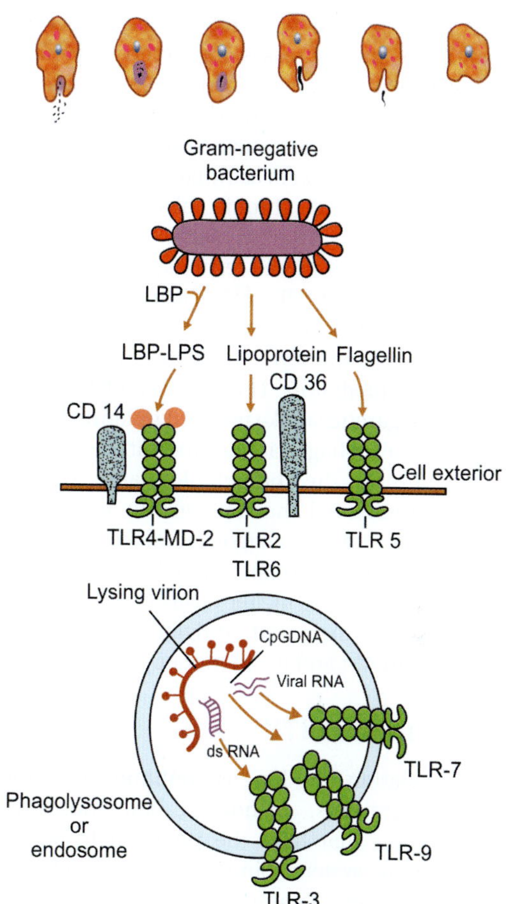

Fig. 9 Toll-like receptors in phagocytosis

Immature DCs express TLR and are activated following infection or inflammation. Allergens may be presented by these DCs to effector T cells which then proliferate and release Th2 cytokines, IL-4,IL-5 and IL -13.[50-53] The pathway for chronic airway inflammation is thus created—Th2 cytokine secretions (especially IL-5 which stimulates the differentiation of eosinophils from bone marrow precursor cells and also prolongs the survival of eosinophils) cause eosinophilic proliferation, infiltration and increases the mucus secretion by the goblet cells.[54-58] TLR4 (tol llike receptor 4) plays a pivotal role in development of allergic asthma. Administration of antagonist to TLR4 by inhalation following parenteral exposure to house dust mite reduced features of asthma such as decreased eosinophilia, decreased levels of Th2 cytokines, decreased goblet cell hyperplasia and also lowered airway hyper responsiveness.[59] LPS can trigger asthma. The role of TLR4 in allergic asthma has been studied extensively using TLR4 agonist LPS. High dose LPS induces a type 1, Th1 response with recruitment of neutrophils into lung tissue and increases interferon gamma (IFN-γ) in bronchoalveolar lavage (BAL) fluid. Low dose LPS and allergen ovalbumin causes increase in eosinophilic and neutrophilic lung inflammation and increases Th2 cytokines and mucus hyper secretion in asthmatic mice.[60]

On the other hand chronic obstructive pulmonary disease (COPD) is characterized by CD8 positive T cells and cytotoxic T-cells and a Th-1 cell response (production of IL-8, IL-12, IL-17, TNF-α and INF-γ.[61,62] Cigarette smoke induced inflammatory response consists of macrophages, neutrophils,monocytes, lymphocyte mediators, and secretion of proinflammatory mediators. TLR2, TLR4 and TLR9 have also been linked to cigarette smoke induced inflammation.[63]

Interstitial macrophages are located within the interstitial tissue surrounding the bronchioles and vessels. The ability of the interstitial macrophages to ingest materials appears variable and the phagocytic activity of interstitial macrophages is reduced compared to that of AM. Interstitial macrophages express the higher levels of MHC class II and CD54 and exhibit increased antigen presenting activity compared to both AM and blood monocytes.

ADAPTIVE IMMUNITY

Following inhalation, the lung is continuously bombarded with inhaled antigens, pathogenic and nonpathogenic particulate matter that have the potential to activate the adaptive immune system. Similar to the development of oral tolerance against commonly encountered antigens and microorganisms in the gut, the lung has developed a mechanism to functionally discriminate between material that can be disposed off through the innate immune system and that necessitates the activation of the adaptive immune system. A state of tolerance to commonly inhaled antigens is induced in the normal lung in which T-cell responses are actively suppressed both at the levels of the T-cell itself and by the down regulation of antigen presenting functions of pulmonary DCs by resident AM.

After the initiation of an inflammatory event or after disruption of the barrier function of the airway or alveolar epithelium, T-cell-mediated responses are rapidly activated to protect the lung. AM suppress T-cell activation in the normal lung and this fine control against commonly encountered nonpathogenic organisms can be down-regulated during lung infections. The mechanisms underlying the induction of macrophage immunosuppressive activity depends on (1) nO, (2) prostaglandin E2 (PGE2), and (3) immunosuppressive cytokines, especially TGF-β and IL-10. However, the relative contribution of each of these molecules is not completely clear.

TH1 OR TH2 RESPONSES (TYPE 1 TYPE 2 RESPONSE)

The helper T-cells produce enormous amount of two types of cytokines—Th1 and Th2 **(Fig. 10)**. Th1 and Th2 responses are polarized responses by the body's T-helper cells when faced by pathogens. T-lymphocytes recognize foreign antigens and produce cytokines that are responsible for the biological effects on the immune system. The Th1 cytokines produced by the helper T-cells produce a proinflammatory response. The Th2 cytokines produce an anti-inflammatory response, but promote allergic responses. The original observation that mouse CD4+ T-cell clones could be divided into two different sets based on their pattern of cytokine expression has become the paradigm for heterogeneity within the T-cell response *in vitro* and *in vivo*.[64] Th1 and Th2 cells are thought to be derived from a nonpolarized, naive Th0 precursor that produced a wide range of cytokines, that can differentiate after activation in the presence of IL-12 and IL-18 (from DCs) into Th1 cells that secrete IL-2.

IFN-γ and lymphotoxin (LT) or in the presence of IL-4 (from B cells or lymphoid DCs) into Th2 cells that secrete IL-4, IL-5 and IL-10. This initial polarization of the response toward Th1 or Th2 is then self-perpetuating as Th1 cytokines enhance further Th1 responses and down regulate Th2 cytokines, and vice versa.

The Th1-type cytokines produce inflammation to kill intracellular organisms (viruses and certain bacteria such as *Listeria* and *Mycobacterium tuberculosis*). These cytokines also perpetuate any form of autoimmune response, and can cause cell-mediated allergies. The Th2 cytokines counteract the effects of the Th1 cytokines—they have an anti-inflammatory action, but they also help to kill extracellular pathogens (which live outside the body's cells and are exposed to antibodies in blood and other body fluids). The Th2 cytokines induce a pronounced allergic response (e.g.) IgE-mediated allergies or asthma **(Fig. 10)**.[65]

ROLE OF IMMUNOGLOBULINS

The respiratory tract immunoglobulins are produced by passive diffusion from the vascular compartment across the lung tissue, and locally in the respiratory tract by the B cells within lung tissue. The bronchial mucosa is the most active site for production. The immunoglobulin reaches the airways lumina either by passive diffusion or by active transport through epithelial cells.

Experiments in animal models indicate that exposure to low doses of antigens usually does not evoke a primary antibody response. The low doses of antigens are cleared by the nonspecific defense mechanisms such as by mucociliary

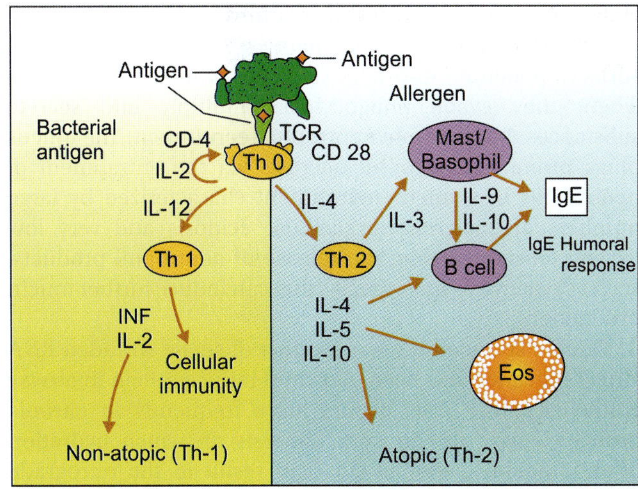

Fig. 10 Production of cytokines by T-cells

blanket and nonspecific phagocytosis. The dose of antigen required to elicit an antibody response has to be large to overcome the nonspecific defense mechanisms and induce pulmonary inflammation leading to the translocation of the antigen from the lung to the draining LALN.[66] DCs play an important role in antigen uptake, transport and presentation to the LALN. The nonspecific pulmonary inflammation allows for the recruitment of antibody forming cells (AFCs), which are generated in the LALN and are released into efferent lymphatics and blood and subsequently reside in the lung parenchyma. It has been demonstrated in a dog model that β-cells recruited to and/or produced in the lung interstitium are able to produce antibody for years after local immunization and challenge because of production of immune memory cells only in the immunized lung lobe.

Immunoglobulin A: Local production and active secretion of total IgA into human respiratory tract can be assessed by BAL specimen analysis. The IgA producing plasma cells are found in large numbers in glands and lamina propria of the major bronchi, small bronchi, bronchioles and alveolar septa. Majority of the BAL IgA is polymeric sIgA. Subclass of IgA, IgA2 constitutes 10–20% of total IgA in blood and about 30% of total IgA in BAL. Free secretory component (SC) **(Fig. 11)** can also be recovered, however, the recovery of SC is markedly reduced in smokers. IgA deficiency, defined as IgA level less than 5 mg/dL, is a relatively common disorder (prevalence estimated as 1/300 to 1/2,000). It may be associated with IgG subclass deficiency, the infections commonly noted include recurrent pneumonia, bronchiectasis, COPD and chronic bronchitis. IgE-mediated allergy is strongly associated with IgA deficiency and allergic asthma frequently occurs in these patients.

- *Immunoglobulin G:* Respiratory tract IgG is mostly serum derived. All IgG subclasses have been identified in human BAL. Increased levels of IgG1 (in both serum and lavage) and of IgG3 has been documented in smokers. IgG subclass deficiency is associated with a variety of infections, the clinical manifestation depends on the subclass or subclasses involved. For example, deficiency of IgG1 is associated with a lifelong increased susceptibility to pyogenic infection and progressive deteriorating lung disease. IgG1 deficiency is most often linked with IgG2 and IgG3 deficiency. IgG2 deficiency results in decreased antibody production to polysaccharide antigen. Such patients frequently have infections with capsulated microorganisms, develop sinusitis, otitis media, and pneumonias leading to chronic lung disease or recurrent meningitis. IgG2 subclass deficiency is associated with IgA deficiency. IgG3 subclass deficiency also results in recurrent respiratory tract infections and chronic lung disease.

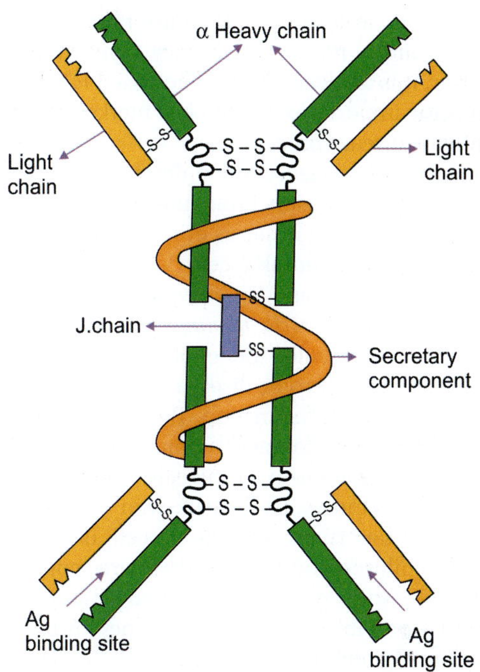

Fig. 11 Structure of immunoglobulin (IgA) with secretory component

It is difficult to demonstrate IgG4 subclass deficiency, since 30% of the general population may have undetectable levels using standard methods. Use of extremely sensitive techniques, that can detect IgG4 levels as low as 0.005 mg/dL, have shown that patients develop recurrent lung infections and/or bronchiectasis. Some individuals with IgG subclass deficiency may be completely normal and healthy in whom a complete evaluation of the patient's ability to make antibody to tetanus toxoid and pneumococcal vaccine must be undertaken.[67]

- *Immunoglobulin E:* IgE appears to be locally produced in the respiratory tract. IgE bound to histamine-containing cells can also be identified in the human lung by BAL. Elevated BAL Ig levels have been noted in hypersensitivity pneumonitis, idiopathic pulmonary fibrosis, sarcoidosis and acquired immunodeficiency syndrome (AIDS). However, it is unclear whether increased IgE levels are of pathogenic importance or simply a marker of some other underlying disease process.

- *Humoral β-cell deficiency:* Sinopulmonary infections (such as otitis media, sinusitis bronchitis and pneumonia and bacteremia resulting in sepsis or meningitis) can occur in individuals with humoral (β-cell) deficiency. Encapsulated organisms, such as *S. pneumoniae, Haemophilus influenzae* and *Neisseria meningitides* or gram-negative organisms are usually the etiologic agents. Recurrent infection leads to chronic diseases such as bronchiectasis and/or respiratory dysfunction. There may be a complete failure of B cell development as characterized by Bruton's agammaglobulinemia to selective IgG subclass deficiency. A number of molecular defects with B cell deficiency have been described. Usually B cell deficiencies are found in children and recently there are reports in older individuals with primary immunodeficiency diseases. Common variable immune deficiency presents as a hypogammaglobulinemia, decreased antigen-specific antibody function and increased recurrent infections.[68]

IMPACT OF BACTERIA AND VIRUSES ON LUNG IMMUNOLOGY

In healthy individuals, the lower airways are sterile and contain very few goblet cells. In patients with mucus hypersecretory diseases, the lower airways are often infected with bacteria or viruses and contain many goblet cells. The importance of bacteria and viruses in the pathogenesis of asthma, chronic bronchitis, cystic fibrosis, and in exacerbations of these diseases has become clear.[69] An important mechanism appears to involve the recruitment of neutrophil chemokines produced by epithelial cells infected with bacteria and viruses. Infection with rhinovirus (RV), the most common respiratory virus, associated with asthma exacerbations induces mucus hypersecretion in airway epithelial cells.[70] RV infection was associated with IL-8 levels and with increased neutrophils in lavage fluid. Virus replication also induces IL8 synthesis by airway epithelial cells.[71,72]

In COPD and cystic fibrosis patients, gram-negative bacteria, such as *P. aeruginosa* and *Chlamydia pneumoniae* colonize the lower airways and cause acute exacerbations of disease. These exacerbations are associated with excessive mucus formation. The elevated sputum levels of IL-8 neutrophils, neutrophil elastase and DNA, suggest the role of bacteria in neutrophil recruitment and destruction in the airway lumen.[73] *P. aeruginosa* and *C. pneumoniae* induce IL-8 production by airway epithelial cells. In addition to its role in neutrophil recruitment, IL-8 inhibits neutrophil apoptosis, (self death) resulting in increased neutrophils within the airways. Infection of mucus plugs in the lower airways where cough is ineffective, further leads to neutrophil-dependent mucin production.[74,75] *P. aeruginosa* deposited on mucus surfaces penetrate into hypoxic zones within mucus plugs, where they evade phagocytosis, multiply and secrete substances that promote neutrophil recruitment. The mucus plugs promote neutrophil necrosis via the entrapment of neutrophils in a microenvironment characterized by large numbers of bacteria, extracellular acidosis and very low oxygen tension causing the release of neutrophil products, such as reactive oxygen species that can induce further mucin production.

Double stranded RNA, a product of single stranded RNA virus replication has been shown to induce mucin in airway epithelial cells.[76] This occurs more frequently in chronic bronchitis and also in cystic fibrosis, in which hydration of submucosal gland mucins can result in the retrograde movement of mucus. Retrograde aspiration of bacteria and mucus into the peripheral airways may lead to bacterial infection, goblet cell formation, goblet cell degranulation and mucus plugging in the periphery.

HUMAN LEUKOCYTE ANTIGENS AND MYCOBACTERIAL DISEASES

There is a possible genetic predisposition to particular bacterial/mycobacterial diseases. Early studies on human leukocyte antigens (HLA) variation established its relevance in susceptibility to tuberculosis (TB) and leprosy, especially in Asian population.[77] Children who are homozygous for mutations in the IFN-α receptor gene have been found to be susceptible to weakly pathogenic mycobacteria, including the Bacillus Calmette-Guérin vaccine, and have a poor prognosis. The role of genetic factors in various lung defenses is a subject of further investigations.

MUCOSAL VACCINES FOR RESPIRATORY INFECTIONS

The approach toward use of mucosal vaccines against respiratory infections caused by viruses (e.g. influenza) has generated considerable interest due to ease of administration, ability to mimic natural infection and because topical application may induce protective immunity. Parenteral route of administration may be effective in causing transudation of serum antibodies. Locally produced sIgA antibodies are important for protection of upper respiratory tract and corresponding IgG for protection of lower respiratory tract and against viremia. Nasal vaccines induce significantly higher local IgA antibodies in nasal washings and local cell mediated immune response but produce less serum antibody titers than injectable vaccines, though the overall efficacy remains about the same.[78] Improving the mode of delivery of mucosal vaccines against respiratory pathogens is under investigation.

REFERENCES

1. Smith KR. Indoor air pollution and acute respiratory infections. Indian Pediatr. 2003;40(9):815-9.
2. Silverman L, Billings CE, First MW. Particle size analysis in industrial hygiene. New York: Academic Press. 1971.
3. Mercer TT. Aerosol Technology in Hazard Evaluation. New York: Academic Press. 1973.
4. Pabst R, Gehrke I. Is the bronchus-associated lymphoid tissue (BALT) an integral structure of the lung in normal mammals, including humans? Am J Respir Cell Mol Biol. 1990;3(2):131-5.
5. McWilliam AS, Nelson D, Thomas JA, Holt PG. Rapid dendritic cell recruitment is a hallmark of the acute inflammatory response at mucosal surfaces. J Exp Med. 1994;179(4):1331-6.
6. Vermaelen K, Pauwels T. Pulmonary dendritic cells. Am J Respir Crit Care Med. 2005;172(5): 530-51.
7. Samet JM, Cheng PW. The role of airway mucus in pulmonary toxicology. Environ Health Perspect. 1994;102(Suppl 2):89-103.
8. West JB. Respiratory physiology, 4th edition. Baltimore, MD: William and Wilkins. 1990.
9. Afzelius BA. Role of cilia in human health. Cell Motil Cytoskeleton and ß in alloreactions induced by human lung dendritic cells and macrophages. Am J Respir Cell Biol. 1995;13:83-90.
10. Widdicombe JH. Regulation of the depth and composition of airway surface liquid. J Anat. 2002;201:313-8.
11. Widdicombe JG. Relationship between the composition of mucus, epithelial lining liquid, and adhesion of microorganisms. Am J Crit Care Med. 1995;151:2088-93.
12. Joris L, Dab I, Quinton PM. Elemental composition of human airway surface fluid in healthy and diseased airways. Am Rev Respir Dis. 1993;148:1633-7.
13. Camner P, Mossberg B, Afzelius BA. Measurements of tracheobronchial clearance in patients with immotile-cilia syndrome and its value in differential diagnosis. Eur J Respir Dis Suppl. 1983;127:57-63.
14. Camner P, Mossberg B. Airway mucus clearance and mucociliary transport. In: Moren F, Dolovich MB, New-house MT, Newman SP (Eds). Aerosols in Medicine. Principles, Diagnosis and Therapy. Amsterdam: Elsevier; 1993. pp. 247-60.
15. Creeth JM. Constituents of mucus and their separation. Br Med Bull. 1978;34(1):17-24.
16. King M, Rubin BK. Mucus physiology and pathophysiology. Therapeutic aspects. In: Derenne JP, Whitelaw WA, Similowski T (Eds). Acute Respiratory Failiure in Chronic Obstructive Pulmonary Disease. Lung Biology in Health and Disease, Vol. 92. New York: Marcel Dekker; 1994. pp. 391-411.
17. King M, Rubin BK. Rheology of airway mucus: relationship with clearance function. In: Takishima T, Shimura S (Eds). Airway secretion: Physiological basis for the control of mucous hypersecretion. Lung Biology in Health and Disease, Vol. 72. New York: Marcel Dekker; 1994. pp. 283-314.
18. Puchelle E, Girod-de Bentzmann S, Jacquot J. Airway defence mechanisms in relation to biochemical and physical properties of mucus. Eur Respir Rev. 1992;2:259-63.
19. Jacquot J, Puchelle E, Zahm JM, Beck G, Plotkowski MC. Effect of human airway lysozyme on the in vitro growth or type 1 Streptococcus pneumoniae. Eur J Respir Dis. 1987;71(4):295-305.
20. Sleigh MA. Ciliary function in transport of mucus. Eur J Respir Dis Supp. 1983;128:287-92.
21. Sanderson MJ, Sleigh MA. Ciliary activity of cultured rabbit tracheal epithelium: beat pattern and metachrony. J Cell Sci. 1981;47:331-47.
22. Svartengren K, Wiman L, Thyberg P, Rigler R. Laser light scattering spectroscopy: a new method to measure tracheobronchial mucociliary activity. Thorax. 1989;44(7):539-47.
23. Mortensen J, Lange P, Nyboe J, Groth S. Lung mucociliary clearance. Eur J Nucl Med. 1994;21(9):953-61.
24. Hasani A, Agnew JE, Pavia D, Vora H, Clarke SW. Effect of oral bronchodilators on lung mucociliary clearance during sleep in patients with asthma. Thorax. 1993;48(3):287-9.
25. Riechelmann H, Maurer J, Kienast K, Hafner B, Mann WJ. Respiratory epithelium exposed to sulfur dioxide—functional and ultrastructural alterations. Laryngoscope. 1995;105(3 Pt1):295-9.
26. Helleday R, Huberman D, Blomberg A, Stjernberg N, Sandström T. Nitrogen dioxide exposure impairs the frequency of the mucociliary activity in healthy subjects. Eur Respir J. 1995;8(10):1664-8.
27. Foster WM, Costa DL, Lagenback EG. Ozone exposure alters tracheobronchial mucociliary function in humans. J Appl Physiol. 1987;63(3):996-1002.
28. Verra F, Escuider E, Lebargy F, Bernaudin JF, De Crémoux H, Bignon J. Ciliary abnormalities in bronchial epithelium of smokers, ex-smokers, and non smokers. Am J Respir Crit Care Med. 1995;151(3):630-4.
29. Wilson R, Pitt T, Taylor G, Watson D, MacDermot J, Sykes D, et al. Pyocyanin and 1-hydroxyphenazine products by *Pseudomonas aeruginosa* inhibit the beating of human respiratory cilia in vitro. J Clin Invest. 1987;79(1):221-9.
30. Moretti M, Lopez-Vidriero MT, Pavia D, Clarke SW. Relationship between bronchial reversibility and trachea-bronchial clearance in patients with chronic bronchitis. Thorax. 1997;52(2):176-80.
31. Bateman JR, Pavia D, Sheahan NF, Agnew JE, Clarke SW. Impaired tracheobronchial clearance in patients with mild stable asthma. Thorax. 1983;38(6):463-7.
32. Boat TF, Boucher RC. Cystic fibrosis. In: Murray JF, Nadel JA (Eds). Textbook of Respiratory Medicine. Philadelphia: Saunders; 1994. pp. 1418-50.
33. Salathe M, O'Riordan TG, Wanner A. Mucociliary clearance. In: Crystal RG, West JB, Weible ER, Barnes PJ (Eds). The Lung: Scientific Foundations. Philadelphia: Lippincott-Raven; 1997. pp. 2295-308.
34. Thepen T, Claassen E, Hoeben K, Brevé J, Kraal G. Migration of alveolar macrophages from alveolar space to paracortical T cell area of the draining lymph node. Adv Exp Med Biol. 1993;329:305-10.
35. Sibille Y, Reynolds HY. Macrophages and polymorphonuclear neutrophils in lung defense and injury. Am Rev Respir Dis. 1990;141(2):471-501.
36. Nicod LP, el Habre F, Dayer JM, Boehringer N. Interleukin-10 decreases tumor necrosis factor alpha and beta in alloreactions induced by human lung dendritic cells and macrophages. Am J Respir Cell Mol Biol. 1995;13(1):83-90.
37. Lacraz S, Nicod L, Galve-de Rochemonteix B, Baumberger C, Dayer JM, Welgus HG. Suppression of metalloproteinase biosynthesis in human alveolar macrophages by interleukin-4. J Clin Invest. 1992;90(2):382-8.
38. LeVine AM, Gwozdz J, Stark J, Bruno M, Whitsett J, Korfhagen T. Surfactant protein-A enhances respiratory syncytial virus clearance in vivo. J Clin Invest. 1999;103(7):1015-21.

39. Li G, Siddiqui J, Hendry M, Akiyama J, Edmondson J, Brown C, et al. Surfactant protein-A—deficient mice display an exaggerated early inflammatory response to a beta-resistant strain of influenza A virus. Am J Respir Cell Mol Biol. 2002;26(3):277-82.
40. Murakami S, Iwaki D, Mitsuzawa H, Sano H, Takahashi H, Voelker DR. Surfactant protein A inhibits peptidoglycan induced tumor necrosis factor alpha secretion in U937 cells and alveolar macrophages by direct interaction with toll-like receptor 2. J Biol Chem. 2002;277(9):6830-7.
41. Van Iwaarden JF, Pikaar JC, Storm J, Brouwer E, Verhoef J, Oosting RS, et al. Binding of surfactant protein A to the lipid A moiety of bacterial lipopolysaccharides. Biochem J. 1994;303 (Pt 2):407-11.
42. Madan T, Eggleton P, Kishore U, Strong P, Aggrawal SS, Sarma PU, et al. Binding of pulmonary surfactant proteins A and D to *Aspergillus fumigatus* conidia enhances phagocytosis and killing by human neutrophils and alveolar macrophages. Infect Immun. 1997;65(8):3171-9.
43. Zimmerman PE, Voelker DR, McCormack FX, Paulsrud JR, Martin WJ. 120-kD surface glycoprotein of Pneumocystis carinii is a ligand for surfactant protein A. J Clin Invest. 1992;89(1):143-9.
44. Hauskrith DW, Sundy JS. Bioaerosols and innate immunity responses in airway diseases. Curr Opin Allergy Clin Immunol. 2004;4(5):361-6.
45. Takeda K, Kaisho T, Akira S. Toll-like receptors. Annu Rev Immunol. 2003;21:335-76.
46. Vasselon T, Detmers PA. Toll receptors: a central element in innate immune responses. Infect Immun. 2002;70(3):1033-41.
47. Monick MM, Yarovinsky TO, Powers LS, Butler NS, Carter AB, Gudmundsson G, et al. Respiratory syncytial virus up-regulates TLR4 and sensitizes airway epithelial cells to endotoxin. J Biol Chem. 2003;278(52):53035-44.
48. Droemann D, Goldmann T, Branscheid D, Clark R, Dalhoff K, Zabel P, et al. Toll-like receptor 2 is expressed by alveolar epithelial cells type II and macrophages in the human lung. Histochem Cell Biol. 2003;119(2):103-8.
49. Bilyk N, Holt PG. Inhibition of the immunosuppressive activity of resident pulmonary alveolar macrophages by granulocyte/macrophage colony-stimulating factor. J Exp Med. 1993;177(6):1773-7.
50. Robinson DS, Hamid Q, Ying S, Tsicopoulos A, Barkans J, Bentley AM, et al. Predominant TH2-like bronchoalveolar T-lymphocyte population in atopic asthma. N Engl J Med. 1992;326:298-304.
51. Krug N, Madden J, Redington AE, Lackie P, Djukanovic R, Schauer U, et al. T-cell cytokine profile evaluated at the single cell level in BAL and blood in allergic asthma. Am J Respir Cell Mol Biol. 1996;14(4):319-26.
52. Wills-Karp M. Interleukin-13 in asthma pathogenesis. Immunol Rev. 2004;202:175-190.
53. Barnes PJ. Cytokine networks in asthma and chronic obstructive pulmonary disease. J Clin Invest. 2008;118(11):3546-56.
54. Chaudhuri N, Dower SK, Whyte MK, Sabroe I. Toll-like receptors and chronic lung disease. Clin Sci. 2005;109:125-33.
55. Schröder NW, Maurer M. The role of innate immunity in asthma: leads and lessons from mouse models. Allergy. 2007;62(6):579-90.
56. Lambrecht BN, De Veerman M, Coyle AJ, Gutierrez-Ramos JC, Thielemans K, Pauwels RA. Myeloid dendritic cells induce Th2 responses to inhaled antigen, leading to eosinophilic airway inflammation. J Clin Invest. 2000;106:551-9.
57. Hammad H, Lambrecht BN, Pochard P, Gosset P, Marquillies P, Tonnel AB, et al. Monocyte-derived dendritic cells induce a house dust mite-specific Th2 allergic inflammation in the lung of humanized SCID mice: involvement of CCR7. J Immunol. 2002;169:1524-34.
58. Lambrecht BN. Dendritic cells and the regulation of the allergic immune response. Allergy. 2005;60:271-82.
59. Hammad H, Chieppa M, Perros F, Willart MA, Germain RN, Lambrecht BN. House dust mite allergen induces asthma via toll-like receptor 4 triggering of airway structural cells. Nat Med. 2009;15:410-16.
60. Dong L, Li H, Wang S, Li Y. Different doses of lipopolysaccharides regulate the lung inflammation of asthmatic mice via TLR4 pathway in alveolar macrophages. J Asthma. 2009;46:229-33.
61. Barnes PJ. Mediators of chronic obstructive pulmonary disease. Pharmacol Rev. 2004;56:515-48.
62. Hodge G, Nairn J, Holmes M, Reynolds PN, Hodge S. Increased intra cellular T helper 1 proinflammatory cytokine production in peripheral blood, bronchoalveolar lavage and intraepithelial T cells of COPD subjects. Clin Exp Immunol. 2007;150:22-9.
63. Karimi K, Sarir H, Mortaz E, Smit JJ, Hosseini H, De Kimpe SJ, et al. Toll-like receptor-4 mediates cigarette smoke-induced cytokine production by human macrophages. Respir Res. 2006;7:66.
64. Szabo SJ, Sullivan BM, Stemmann C, Satoskar AR, Sleckman BP, Glimcher LH. Distinct effects of T-bet in TH1 lineage commitment and IFN-gamma production in CD4 and CD8 T cells. Science. 2002;295(5553):338-42.
65. Kuipers H, Lambrecht BN. The interplay of dendritic cells, Th2 cells and regulatory T cell in asthma. Curr Opin Immunol. 2004;16(6):702-8.
66. Meuwissen HJ, Hussains M. Bronchus-associated lymphoid tissue in human lung: correlations of hyperplasia with chronic pulmonary disease. Clin Immunol Immunopathol. 1982;23(2):548-61.
67. Maguire GA, Kumararatne DS, Joyce HJ. Are there any classical indications for measuring IgG subclasses? Ann Clin Biochem. 2002;39(Pt 4):374-7.
68. Thickett KM, Kumararatne DS, Banerjee AK, Dudley R, Stableforth DE. Common variable immune deficiency: respiratory manifestation of pulmonary infection and high-resolution CT scan findings. QJM. 2002;95(10):655-62.
69. Hill AT, Campbell EJ, Hill SL, Bayley DL, Stockley RA. Association between airway bacterial load and markers of airway inflammation in patients with stable chronic bronchitis. Am J Med. 2000;109(4):288-95.
70. Peebles RS. Viral infections, atopy, and asthma: is there a casual relationship? J Allergy Clin Immunol. 2004;113(1 Suppl): S15-8.
71. Fiedler MA, Wernke-Dollries K, Stark JM. Respiratory syncytial virus increases IL-8 gene expression and protein release in A549 cells. Am J Physiol. 1995;269:L865-72.
72. Yuta A, Doyle WJ, Gaumond E, Ali M, Tamarkin L, Baraniuk JN, et al. Rhinovirus infection induces mucus hypersecretion. Am J Physiol. 1998;274 (6 Pt 1):L1017-23.

73. Massion PP, Inoue H, Richman-Eisenstat J, Grunberger D, Jorens PG, Housset B, et al. Novel Pseudomonas product stimulates interleukin-8 production in airway epithelial in vitro. J Clin Invest. 1994;93(1):26-32.
74. Inoue H, Massion PP, Ueki IF, Grattan KM, Hara M, Dohrman AF, et al. Pseudomonas stimulates interleukin-8 mRNA expression selectively in airway epithelium, in gland ducts, and in recruited neutrophils. Am J Respir Cell Mol Biol. 1994;11(6):651-63.
75. Jahn HU, Krüll M, Wuppermann FN, Klucken AC, Rosseau S, Seybold J, et al. Infection and activation of airway epithelial cells by Chlamydia pneumonia. J Infect Dis. 2000;182(6): 1678-87.
76. Gern JE. Viral respiratory infection and the link to asthma. Pediatr infect Dis J. 2004;23(Suppl 1):S78-86.
77. Singh SP, Mehra NK, Dingley HB, Pande JN, Vaidya MC. Human leucocyte antigen (HLA)-linked control of susceptibility to pulmonary tuberculosis and association with HLA-DR types. J Infect Dis. 1983;148(4):676-81.
78. Jan Holmgren, Cecil Czerkinsky. Mucosal immunity and vaccines. Nature Medicine. 2005;11:545-53.

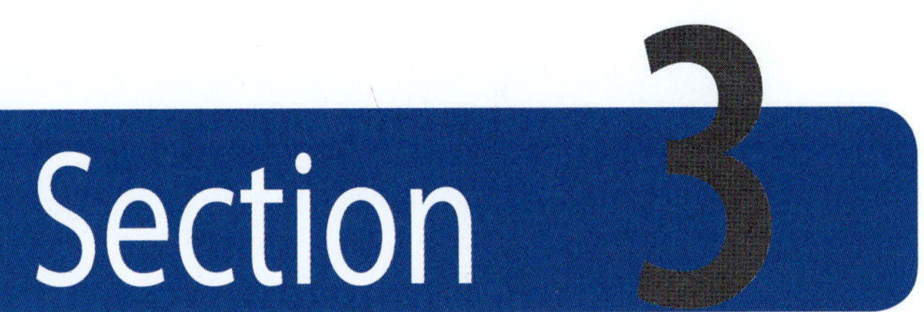

Respiratory Pharmacology

Aditya Jindal, Nusrat Shafiq

13

Chapter

Antimicrobial Agents

Nusrat Shafiq, Samir Malhotra, J Whig, Bharti Mahajan, Rajesh Mahajan

Part I: Antibacterial and Antiviral Drugs

Nusrat Shafiq, Samir Malhotra

Antibacterial Drugs

INTRODUCTION

Antibacterials are commonly, many times inappropriately, used for upper and lower respiratory tract infections. Therapeutic concentrations in respiratory secretions, in excess of the minimum inhibitory concentration (MIC) for that pathogen, are necessary for the successful treatment of pulmonary infections. Concept of blood-lung barrier on the lines of blood-brain barrier has been also proposed. Ability of drugs to penetrate respiratory secretions depends on factors such as molecular size of the antibacterial, lipid solubility and degree of ionization. In order to achieve higher local concentrations, especially those of polymyxins and aminoglycosides, they are often administered as aerosols as well.

Pharmacokinetic properties of the antibiotics, their ability to reach the site of infection, their half-lives (how many times per day) and presence of comorbid conditions (impaired renal or hepatic functions) may also determine the choice of drugs. For instance, the doses of drugs eliminated by kidneys (aminoglycosides, vancomycin, others) or metabolized by liver (chloramphenicol) must be adjusted in the presence of impaired renal or hepatic function, respectively. Moreover, side effect profiles and drug interactions would need further consideration. Some side effects like gastrointestinal (nausea, vomiting and diarrhea) and drug rash can occur with the majority of the antibiotics. Hypersensitivity reactions can occur with most antimicrobials especially, but not exclusively, with parenteral use. Bone marrow suppression has also been reported with most of the antimicrobials. However, some may be typical for a class, e.g. nephrotoxicity for aminoglycosides, and QT prolongation for quinolones like moxifloxacin and sparfloxacin.

Cost factors are important especially in countries with sparse cover of health insurance. Most of the novel antimicrobials must be used sparingly, not only due to cost factors, but also to save the drugs from misuse and development of resistance.

The following chapter focuses on the pharmacological aspects of antibacterials used for the empiric management of respiratory tract infections.

BETA-LACTAMS

Beta-lactam group includes penicillins, cephalosporins, carbapenems and monobactams. The name of this group of agents derives from basic structure of thiazolidine ring connected to a beta-lactam ring to which a side chain is attached. They inhibit the synthesis of peptidoglycan, an important component of cell walls of the bacteria. Specifically, the final step of transpeptidation is inhibited by penicillins. Additionally, penicillins and cephalosporins bind to Penicillin-Binding Proteins (PBPs) bringing about lytic, as well as nonlytic killing. Alteration in PBPs and production of beta-lactamases are the important mechanisms of resistance, which is not inherently present in some bacteria. At least four types of beta-lactamases are known. Class A beta-lactamases, also called extended spectrum beta-lactamases, inhibit penicillins, cephalosporins and carbapenems. Class B beta-lactamases destroy all beta-lactams except aztreonam. Class C beta-lactamases are against cephalosporins while Class D beta-lactamases degrade cloxacillin.

Penicillins

Penicillin G (benzylpenicillin) is the only naturally obtained penicillin used clinically; several semisynthetic penicillins with desired properties are derived from modification of 6-aminopenicillanic acid. Various classes of penicillin are:

- Highly active against sensitive strains of Gram-positive cocci, but ineffective against *Staphylococcus aureus*, which produces penicillinase: Penicillin G, benzathine penicillin, procaine penicillin, penicillin V.
- Penicillinase-resistant penicillins, effective against *S. aureus* and *Staphylococcus epidermidis* that are methicillin susceptible: Methicillin, nafcillin, oxacillin, cloxacillin, dicloxacillin, flucloxacillin.
- Penicillins effective against Gram-negative organisms, such as *Haemophilus influenzae, Escherichia coli* and *P. mirabilis:* Ampicillin, amoxicillin, bacampicillin, metampicillin, pivampicillin.

  The last three are prodrugs and are hydrolyzed to ampicillin *in vivo*.

Penicillins with activity against *Pseudomonas, Enterobacteriaceae* and *Proteus* species (carboxypenicillins): Carbenicillin, ticarcillin. These penicillins are inferior to ampicillin against Gram-positive cocci.

Penicillins with activity against *Pseudomonas, Klebsiella* (ureidopenicillins): Mezlocillin, azlocillin.

Penicillins with activity against *Pseudomonas, Klebsiella* and Gram-positive cocci: Piperacillin.

Individual Penicillins

- *Penicillin G (Crystalline penicillin, benzylpenicillin)*: Susceptible organisms include *Corynebacterium diphtheriae, Peptostreptococcus* spp., nonbeta-lactamase-producing staphylococci and streptococci, including *Streptococcus agalactiae* (group B), *Streptococcus pneumoniae* (pneumococci), *Streptococcus pyogenes* (group A), and some viridans streptococci; of these Group A streptococci are an occasional cause of pneumonia in previously healthy adults. These organisms are responsible for 20–40% cases of exudative pharyngitis in children. Group B streptococci are the most common cause of pneumonia in neonates. Enterococci are relatively insensitive to penicillins. *Pasteurella multocida, Streptobacillus moniliformis* and *Spirillumminus* (or *minor*) are also susceptible to penicillins. *Actinomyces* show good susceptibility to penicillins. Most strains of *S. aureus* are resistant to penicillin. *Bacillus anthracis* and *C. diphtheriae* are other susceptible pathogens, which may cause respiratory tract infections.

  Resistance to *Staphylococcus, S. pneumoniae,* pneumococci and *H. influenzae* are common.

  A survey conducted across 25 countries from 1999 to 2000 reported prevalence of resistance from 7.8% to 71.5%.[1] However, penicillin G remains agent of choice for serious infections like bacteremia, empyema, severe pneumonia, pericarditis, endocarditis, meningitis, and others caused by sensitive strains of the Gram-positive species mentioned above. It may also be considered for sensitive strains of pneumococci. The Drug-Resistant *Streptococcus pneumoniae* Therapeutic Working Group (DRSP) argued that penicillin susceptibility categories should be shifted upward for pneumococcal pneumonia so that the susceptible category includes all isolates with MIC of no greater than 1 μg mL^{-1}, the intermediate category includes isolates with MIC of 2 μg mL^{-1} and the resistant category includes isolates with MIC of no less than 4 μg mL^{-1}. The group suggested the aforementioned classification in order to parallel penicillin resistance categories with clinical outcomes.[2]

  The dose of 20–24 MU of penicillin G should be administered daily by constant intravenous infusion (IV) or 1–2 million units intramuscularly (IM) every 2 hours. Therapy should be continued for three to five days after the patient becomes afebrile. Each million units contains approximately 6.8 mg (0.3 mEq) of sodium and 65.6 mg (1.68 mEq) of potassium. In splenectomized patients with compromised immunity status, phenoxymethylpenicillin (penicillin V) may be offered for lifelong prophylaxis against pneumococcal and *H. influenzae* infections. Penicillin G is the drug of choice for actinomycosis, 12–20 MU of penicillin G are given IV. Combination with aminoglycosides is synergistic and is usually employed for enterococcal infections. However, with bacteriostatic drugs like chloramphenicol and tetracyclines, antagonism may be seen. It is less commonly used due to its limited availability and availability of other drugs.
- *Methicillin*: The antimicrobial spectrum is largely similar to benzylpenicillin. It is active against both penicillinase-producing and nonpenicillinase-producing staphylococci. Since it is no longer in use clinically, it will not be discussed further.
- *Oxacillin*: It is an orally active oxazolyl penicillin. Though it is active against sensitive strains of penicillinase-producing staphylococci, it is not considered for the treatment of serious infections caused by penicillinase-producing staphylococci. It is incompletely absorbed from the gastrointestinal tract (GIT) and the absorption is affected by the presence of food which is why a gap of 1 to 2 hours between food and drug intake is recommended. Peak plasma concentration is achieved in 1 hour after oral administration. Oxacillin is excreted both in the urine and bile. Its indications are similar to flucloxacillin. It is administered orally in a dose of 1 g twice a day. Hepatitis may occasionally occur.
- *Flucloxacillin*: Penicillinase and nonpenicillinase-producing staphylococci and *Strep pneumoniae* are susceptible to flucloxacillin though the activity of benzylpenicillin is more against these organisms as compared to flucloxacillin. In some centers it continues to remain a good choice for the empirical treatment of staphylococcal infections in intensive care units.[3] Absorption through gastrointestinal tract is good and peak plasma concentration is achieved

in 1 hour. It may also be given by intramuscular injection. The oral and parenteral dose is 250 mg four times daily.

Susceptible Gram-positive infections, including the recently important infection due to *Panton-Valentine Leukocidin* (PVL)—producing *S. aureus,* which is emerging as a serious problem worldwide. There has been an increase in the incidence of necrotizing lung infections in otherwise healthy young people with a very high mortality associated with these strains. Flucloxacillin (4 g tid) and rifampicin may be given empirically.[4] The usual dose is 250 mg four times daily orally or intramuscularly. Its IV dose is 0.25-1 g four times daily by slow injection over 3-4 minutes or by IV infusion. The dose may be doubled in severe infections. Hepatitis and cholestatic jaundice may occur occasionally. The side effect may be delayed for more than 2 months after stopping the drug. Flucloxacillin is a pregnane X receptor (PXR) agonist at pharmacologically relevant concentrations, and a functionally significant upstream PXR polymorphism is a risk factor for flucloxacillin-induced liver injury.[5] It should be used with caution in patients with hepatic dysfunction.

- *Cloxacillin*: Its spectrum and other features are similar to those of flucloxacillin. It is incompletely absorbed from the gastrointestinal tract. Peak plasma concentration after oral administration is achieved in 1-2 hours. Food affects its absorption and an interval of half an hour is required between the administration of the drug and food intake. Indications and dosage are similar to flucloxacillin. It is administered in a dose of 250-500 mg 6 hourly. It should be administered slowly over 3-4 minutes. Penicillins are incompatible with aminoglycosides and should not be mixed in the syringe, infusion set or IV fluids.
- *Dicloxacillin*: Absorption from the gastrointestinal tract is better than that of cloxacillin. Rest of the profile is similar to cloxacillin.
- *Ampicillin*: Ampicillin has a broader spectrum of activity than benzyl penicillin. In addition to Gram-positive bacteria, some Gram-negative bacteria such as *H. influenzae* are susceptible to ampicillin. It is well absorbed after oral administration. Food hampers its absorption and hence it should preferably be taken 30 minutes before meals. Peak plasma concentrations are reached in 1-2 hours after oral administration. It undergoes enterohepatic circulation. Dose adjustment is required in renal impairment. It is indicated for the initial treatment of acute tracheobronchitis of I, II and III Class. As a therapy for acute exacerbation of tracheobronchitis, it offers modest benefit at best.[6] Ampicillin in a dose of 1-2 g daily in 3-4 divided doses for 7-10 days orally or IV, either alone or in combination with beta-lactamase inhibitor (sulbactam), is indicated for the empirical therapy of pneumonia in adults—pneumonia with chronic bronchitis and for suspected pneumococcal pneumonia if resistance to ampicillin is not common.

Ampicillin-sulbactam is also indicated for empirical antimicrobial therapy for pneumonia in pediatric patients of less than 1 month of age when Group B *Streptococcus, H. influenzae* and *S. aureus* are the usual pathogens. The combination is also indicated for the empirical therapy of pneumonia in pediatric patients of 3 months to 6 years of age in whom the suspected organisms include *Pneumococcus* or *H. influenzae.* Ampicillin-resistant *H. influenzae* may be susceptible to ampicillin sulbactam combination. Ampicillin for 3 months has been successfully used in patients with actinomycosis or a follow-up therapy to ceftriaxone. Benzyl-penicillin, however, continues to remain the treatment of choice for this condition. Recently, aerosolized ampicillin was reported for the treatment of *S. aureus* lung infection in a 14-year-old patient of cystic fibrosis.[7]

Salient adverse effects: Urticarial and maculopapular rash are known to occur with ampicillin, the former represents hypersensitivity. Maculopapular rash may occur 7 days after the drug administration. Appearance of rash is not necessarily an indication for stopping the use of penicillins. However, sensitivity testing should be undertaken before use. Patients with infectious mononucleosis, lymphatic leukemia and HIV infection are particularly susceptible to ampicillin induced rash. Caution should be exercised with the subsequent use of penicillin. Studies in adults indicate that ampicillin, in a dose-dependent manner, impairs platelet function and moderately prolongs the bleeding time (generally by 60-90 seconds). A similar increase in bleeding time is also noted in pediatric patients.[8] Diarrhea, hepatitis, cholestatic jaundice, erythema multiforme, Stevens-Johnson syndrome and toxic epidermolytic necrosis have all been reported with its use.

- *Amoxicillin*: Amoxicillin is a 4-hydroxy analog of ampicillin. The antimicrobial spectrum of amoxicillin is similar to that of ampicillin. It is not inactivated by gastric acid. Compared to ampicillin, it is absorbed more rapidly and completely. Half-life may increase to nearly 20 hours in severe renal impairment. It crosses the placenta and small amount may be secreted in breast milk. It is largely excreted by tubular secretion and glomerular filtration.

The indications for amoxicillin are similar to those of ampicillin. Addition of beta-lactamase inhibitor, clavulanic acid extends the spectrum of amoxicillin to include *H. influenzae* and *Moraxella catarrhalis.* In a recent Cochrane review done to evaluate effective antibiotics for ambulatory pediatric patients with community acquired pneumonia, amoxicillin had similar failure rates as those of cotrimoxazole.[9] The authors concluded that for severe pneumonia without hypoxia, oral amoxicillin may be an alternative to injectable penicillin in hospitalized children; however, for ambulatory treatment of such patients with oral antibiotics, more studies in community settings are required.[9] Its dose is 250-500 mg three times a day orally. An extended release preparation of amoxicillin is available in some countries. It is generally used for pharyngitis due to *S. pyogenes* and it is given as a single daily dose for 10 days.

The incidence of diarrhea is less than that of ampicillin. Hepatitis and cholestatic jaundice have been reported with the use of amoxicillin. These have largely been seen when it is used in combination with clavulanic acid.

- *Carbenicillin*: The antimicrobial spectrum is similar to that of benzylpenicillin and is penicillinase susceptible. In addition, it is also effective against *P. aeruginosa*. However, it is not effective against most strains of *S. aureus, Enterococcus* and *Klebsiella*. It has largely been superseded by piperacillin and ticarcillin for most of its indications.

It is not absorbed through gastrointestinal tract and needs to be given either intramuscularly or intravenously. However, carbenicillin indanyl is a prodrug, designed for oral administration. The carbenicillin, which is released from this prodrug does not achieve sufficient concentrations in the blood and is used only for the treatment of urinary tract infections. The half-life of carbenicillin is increased in renal impairment.

Indications and dosage are similar as for ticarcillin. Dose-dependent coagulation defect may occur. Congestive heart failure may result due to the sodium ions present in carbenicillin sodium. Carbenicillin sodium contains about 5 mEq Na^+ per gram of drug, and this will result in the administration of more than 100 mEq Na^+ when patients are treated for *P. aeruginosa* infections. Carbenicillin constitutes large amount of nonreabsorbable anion and may cause hypokalemia.

- *Ticarcillin*: It is two to four times more active against *P. aeruginosa* than carbenicillin. It is given by intravenous route. The drug is eliminated renally and caution should be exercised in patients with reduced creatinine clearance. The maintenance dose needs to be modified from 2 g every 12 hours to 2 g every 24 hours for creatinine clearance of 10 mL/min to 30 mL/min, respectively. Half-life of the drug may be shortened in patients with cystic fibrosis.

When given with clavulanic acid, the activity of ticarcillin is extended to beta-lactamase producing organisms such as staphylococci, enterococci and *H. influenzae*. It needs to be noted that addition of clavulanic acid does not increase its activity against *P. aeruginosa*. Ticarcillin-clavulanate is considered for the empirical antimicrobial therapy for pneumonia in adults with a history of alcoholism. The suspected organisms in these cases are *Pneumococcus, Klebsiella pneumoniae, S. aureus, H. influenzae* and possibly mouth anaerobes. More than 70% of *Pseudomonas* isolates obtained from patients of cystic fibrosis may be susceptible to ticarcillin.[10] It is given by injection as the sodium salt in the doses of 200–300 mg/kg daily by intravenous infusion in four or six divided doses. The adverse effects of cholestatic jaundice and hepatitis seen with ticarcillin/clavulanic acid are mainly due to the clavulanic acid component. The defects of platelet aggregation are known to occur.

- *Piperacillin*: Its spectrum includes most strains of *P. aeruginosa,* Enterobacteriaceae (nonbeta-lactamase producing), many *Bacteroides* spp., and *Enterococcus faecalis*. In combination with a beta-lactamase inhibitor (*piperacillin-tazobactam*), it has the broadest antibacterial spectrum out of all penicillins. Peak plasma concentrations are achieved in half to one hour. High biliary concentrations are also achieved. Recently, it has been suggested that the plasma concentrations of piperacillin should be monitored to achieve better outcomes.[11] The combination with tazobactam is indicated for the empiric therapy of pneumonia in adults who have a history of alcoholism and those with nosocomial pneumonia. It is also indicated in patients with community-acquired pneumonia in whom pseudomonas infection is suspected. In life-threatening infections, particularly those caused by *Pseudomonas* or *Klebsiella* spp., it should be given in a dose of not less than 16 g/day up to a maximum dose of 24 g/day. The combination is also indicated for use in *Acinetobacter baumannii* infection, a causative organism of ventilator associated pneumonia.
- *Mezlocillin and azlocillin*: These penicillins do not find recommendations in most guidelines for the treatment of respiratory tract infections. They have good activity against pseudomonas.

Adverse Effects of Penicillins

Hypersensitivity reactions are not only the most common adverse reactions (up to 10%) associated with penicillins, but can also be fatal. The manifestations include the occurrence of maculopapular rash, urticarial rash, fever, bronchospasm, vasculitis, serum sickness, exfoliative dermatitis, Stevens-Johnson syndrome and anaphylaxis. There is a wide variation in their presentation; any history of hypersensitivity reaction to penicillin precludes its use in future.

All types of skin rashes are known to occur with their use. Rarely thrombocytopenic purpura and Henoch-Schönlein purpura may occur. Exfoliative dermatitis (erythema multiforme) may also occur. Serum sickness characterized by fever, leukopenia, splenomegaly, arthralgia, arthritis, purpura, electrocardiographic changes may sometimes occur after 1 week of treatment with penicillin. Skin vasculitis, positive Coomb's reaction and reversible neutropenia may also occur. The latter is more commonly seen with the use of nafcillin. Fever, eosinophilia, reversible interstitial nephritis (mainly with methicillin) are sometimes observed.

Angioedema and anaphylaxis constitute the most serious adverse reactions associated with the use of penicillins. These can occur with any route of administration although more commonly with the parenteral routes. Anaphylactic and anaphylactoid reaction constitute medical emergency and occur with an incidence of 0.004–0.04%. It presents with severe bronchoconstriction, drop in blood pressure, nausea, vomiting, abdominal pain and diarrhea. Prior skin testing with a small amount of penicillin (a few units) is mandatory before the use of penicillins.

Oral penicillins are likely to cause GI adverse effects (diarrhea, nausea) in a significant proportion of patients.

Pseudomembranous colitis can occur with almost all antibiotics, including penicillins (especially ampicillin and amoxicillin). Hematological adverse effects (like hemolytic anemia, neutropenia, abnormal platelet function leading to prolongation of bleeding time), convulsions, encephalopathy (intrathecal administration), and electrolyte imbalance can occur. Hepatitis and cholestatic jaundice are rare (especially with flucloxacillin, oxacillin, and amoxicillin/ticarcillin-clavulanic acid combination). Nephropathy and interstitial nephritis (mainly with methicillin) can occur.

Cephalosporins

The cephalosporins or cephem antibacterials are semi-synthetic antibacterials derived from cephalosporin C, a natural antibacterial produced by the mold *Cephalosporium acremonium*. The hydrolysis product of cephalosporin, 7-aminocephalosporanic acid, has been modified to give various classes of this drug. As a consequence, four generations of cephalosporins are available with differences in their antibacterial and other pharmacological properties.

First-generation Cephalosporins

Included in this group are cefazolin, cephalexin, cephalothin, cephradine and cephadroxil. They are active against Gram-positive cocci like *S. aureus* (including beta-lactamase-producing strains), *S. epidermidis, S. pyogenes, S. agalactiae* and *S. pneumoniae,* but not against enterococci, methicillin-resistant *S. aureus,* and *S. epidermidis*), anaerobes (except *Bacteroides fragilis),* and, to a lesser extent, against Gram-negative microorganisms. Activity against *M. catarrhalis, E. coli, K. pneumoniae* and *P. mirabilis* is quite good.

- *Cefalexin*: It is well absorbed from the GIT, absorption may be delayed by food, but extent of absorption is not affected. Most of it is excreted unchanged in urine. It is useful in respiratory tract infections and otitis media caused by susceptible organisms, especially if penicillin cannot be used. The usual dose is 1–4 g daily in divided doses.
- *Cefazolin*: Its gastrointestinal absorption is poor, thus used parenterally (IM and IV). It is excreted unchanged in the urine. It is used for respiratory tract infections and septicemia caused by *S. pneumoniae, S. aureus* (including beta-lactamase producing strains), *P. mirabilis* and *E. coli.* It is used in doses of 0.5–1 g every 6–12 hours (up to a maximum of 12 g) by deep IM injection or by intravenous infusion.
- *Cefalothin*: It is used only parenterally as it is poorly absorbed from the GIT. About two-thirds is excreted in the urine and the rest is metabolized by the liver.

Second-generation Cephalosporins

The antimicrobial spectrum of second generation cephalosporins (cefamandole, cefoxitin, cefaclor, loracarbef, cefuroxime, cefotetan and cefprozil) extends to include enterobacter, *Proteus* and *Klebsiella* species. *H. influenzae* are also susceptible to this generation.

- *Cefamandole:* It has similar or slightly less activity than cefalothin against Gram-positive bacteria, but greater stability to hydrolysis by beta-lactamases produced by Gram-negative bacteria. Due to its erratic absorption, it is given as an intravenous or intramuscular preparation. It is primarily excreted by the kidneys.

It is effective against infections caused by susceptible organisms and also for surgical prophylaxis. Prophylaxis with cefamandole (3 g/day) for 6 months, followed by amoxicillin/clavulanate for the next 12 months has shown to decrease the incidence of postoperative pneumonia following lung resection.[12]

- *Cefoxitin*: It demonstrates some resistance to beta-lactamases produced by some Gram-negative rods. The hallmark of cefoxitin is its activity against *B. fragilis.* It is used parenterally and almost all of it is excreted unchanged by the kidneys. It does not cross the blood-brain barrier even in the presence of inflammation. Cefoxitin is an alternative for pulmonary disease with rapidly growing opportunistic mycobacteria such as *Mycobacterium abscessus, Mycobacterium chelonae, Mycobacterium fortuitum* and *Mycobacterium gordonae.* It is also a useful antimicrobial for anaerobic and mixed infections.
- *Cefaclor*: It has good activity against Gram-negative bacteria such as *Klebsiella* and *H. influenzae.* It may be active against some beta-lactamase producing strains of *H. influenzae.* It is used in upper and lower respiratory tract infections and otitis media in doses of 250–500 mg three times a day up to a maximum of 4 g/day. It is indicated for empirical therapy of pneumococcal pneumonia in children less than 5 years of age an alternative to amoxicillin. It is considered as an alternative drug for acute exacerbation of bronchitis in otherwise healthy individuals.

Serum sickness-like illness with the repeated use of cefaclor in children has been reported. It may increase the prothrombin time when given concomitantly with warfarin.

- *Loracarbef*: It is actually a carbacephem, which is slightly different structurally from cephalosporin, but has antimicrobial activity similar to that of cefaclor. It is well-absorbed orally. The indications are also same as cefaclor.
- *Cefuroxime:* The antimicrobial spectrum of cefuroxime is similar to that of cefamandole. Cefuroxime is considered for empirical therapy of pneumonia in elderly when the likely pathogens are *Pneumococcus, Klebsiella, H. influenzae* or *M. catarrhalis.* Cefuroxime axetil is a prodrug of cefuroxime, after absorption it is hydrolyzed in the intestinal mucosa to cefuroxime. Cefuroxime is also used parenterally.

The major indications are bronchitis, other lower respiratory tract infections, meningitis, otitis media and sinusitis. It is also commonly used for surgical infection prophylaxis. It may also be used for the empirical antimicrobial therapy for pneumonia in children. It may rarely cause Stevens-Johnson syndrome and toxic epidermal necrolysis.

- *Cefprozil*: The indications for cefprozil are similar to that of cefaclor. It has a good oral bioavailability in a single daily dose. It may also be used for the treatment of pharyngitis caused by *S. pyogenes*.
- *Cefotetan*: It is another second-generation antibiotic, which is seldom used in respiratory tract infections. The antimicrobial spectrum is similar to that of cefoxitin. The N-methylthiotetrazole side chain has the potential to cause hypoprothrombinemia and bleeding.

Third-generation Cephalosporins

These cephalosporins, also called extended spectrum cephalosporins, have good activity against many Gram-positive and Gram-negative bacteria. They are more resistant to hydrolysis by beta-lactamases than the second-generation cephalosporins. Some of these agents have activity against *Pseudomonas.*

- *Ceftriaxone*: Among Gram-negative bacteria, *in vitro* activity is seen against Enterobacteriaceae and *Klebsiella* besides *H. influenzae* and *M. catarrhalis.* There is only moderate susceptibility towards *Pseudomonas.* Among Gram-positive bacteria, it is active against staphylococci and streptococci except methicillin-resistant *S. aureus.* It is not absorbed orally; about two-thirds is excreted by the kidneys and the rest by liver. It crosses the blood-brain barrier even in the absence of inflammation.

It is indicated for the presumptive therapy of pneumonia in elderly patients. It is also indicated in the management of pneumococcal pneumonia in immunocompetent adults for strains with reduced susceptibility to penicillins. In adult patients with community-acquired pneumonia who are admitted in the wards, ceftriaxone or cefotaxime may be combined with a macrolide (or doxycycline). Calcium salt may rarely cause biliary sludge and pseudolithiasis. Administration of calcium salts within 48 hours of ceftriaxone administration should be avoided. Isolated fatal cases have been reported in the neonates due to the deposition of calcium ceftriaxone in the lungs. Hyperbilirubinemia may occur due to the high protein binding associated with its use. Methylthiotriazine side chain may aggravate the action of anticoagulants and disulfiram-like reaction may occur when used concomitantly with alcohol.

- *Cefotaxime*: It is highly resistant to most beta-lactamases, has more activity than first- or second-generation cephalosporins against Gram-negative bacteria. It is active against Gram-negative bacteria like Enterobacteriaceae, *Proteus, Providencia, Salmonella, Serratia, Shigella, H. influenzae, M. catarrhalis,* and *Neisseria meningitidis.* It is also active against Gram-positive bacteria, including *S. aureus (except* methicillin-resistant), *S. epidermidis, Streptococcus agalactiae, S. pneumoniae, S. pyogenes, and* anaerobic bacteria (like some strains of *B. fragilis and Clostridium difficile*).

It is not orally absorbed. The main route of elimination is renal although there is some hepatic metabolism as well that leads to the formation of active metabolite desacetyl-cefotaxime. It is commonly used in intensive care settings to treat serious infections like brain abscess, endocarditis, sepsis, meningitis, peritonitis, pneumonia and typhoid. It is also used for surgical prophylaxis. Cefotaxime/sulbactam combination may be as effective as amoxicillin-clavulanic acid in children with lower respiratory tract infections.

- *Ceftazidime*: Its spectrum is similar to that of cefotaxime, but the activity against *Pseudomonas* is greater. It is given parenterally, the predominant route of elimination is renal.
- *Ceftizoxime*: It is similar to cefotaxime, administered either by intramuscular or slow intravenous injection. It is mainly eliminated by the kidneys.
- *Cefixime*: It is active against Enterobacteriaceae, *H. influenzae, M. catarrhalis* and streptococci. It is slowly and partially absorbed from the gastrointestinal tract and eliminated by the kidneys and liver. It is used for the treatment of otitis media, pharyngitis, and lower respiratory tract infections caused by susceptible organisms.
- *Others*: Cefpodoxime, cefditoren and cefdinir have spectrum similar to that of cefixime, but more active against *S. aureus.*

Fourth-generation Cephalosporins

The fourth-generation cephalosporins have an extended antibacterial spectrum. This group of cephalosporins is largely resistant to beta-lactamases. They are active against many Enterobacteriaceae, which are resistant to type-1 beta-lactamases. These may, however, be hydrolyzed by extended spectrum beta-lactamases. The activity against *H. influenzae* is comparable to that of cefotaxime. These agents are also active against streptococci, including penicillin-resistant streptococci and methicillin-sensitive *S. aureus.* In combination with aminoglycosides, they are indicated for the empiric therapy of nosocomial pneumonia with suspected Gram-negative bacilli (*K. pneumoniae,* enterobacter, *P. aeruginosa*).

- *Cefepime*: It is used in respiratory tract and other serious infections, including in patients with febrile neutropenia caused by susceptible organisms. It has also been used successfully in the treatment of ventilator associated pneumonia.[13] Cases of neurotoxicity manifesting as nonepileptic convulsion have been reported.[14]
- *Cefpirome*: Used in serious infections like pneumonia and sepsis, especially in immunocompromised patients, it is given in the doses of 1–2 g twice a day by IV infusion.

The adverse effects of cephalosporins are similar to those of penicillins. The gastrointestinal (diarrhea, nausea), dermatologic (rash), rash, and electrolyte disturbances (most of them are administered as sodium salts) are seen in ≥1% of patients. Less common are headache, dizziness, antibiotic associated diarrhea, superinfection and fever. Hypersensitivity reactions as seen with penicillins can occur with cephalosporins, but less commonly compared to penicillins. Cross-reactivity with penicillins is seen in about 10% of patients.[15]

Carbapenems

Drugs such as imipenem, meropenem, doripenem and ertapenem of this group structurally resemble penicillins and have similar mechanism of action. Carbapenems are particularly useful for the initial empirical therapy for hospitalized patients with suspected bacterial community-acquired pneumonia, patients with pneumonia in medical wards with or without previous recent history of antibiotic therapy and for patients with pneumonia in intensive care unit with suspected pseudomonas infection. For the latter, ciprofloxacin is usually combined with carbapenems. Further, meropenem may be superior to ceftazidime/aminoglycoside for the empirical treatment of ventilator-associated pneumonia.[16]

- *Imipenem*: It is a broad-spectrum antimicrobial with activity against Gram-positive, Gram-negative (including the beta-lactamase producing), many aerobic and anaerobic bacteria. The sensitive Gram-positive organisms include most streptococci, staphylococci (penicillinase and nonpenicillinase producing), *E. faecalis, Nocardia, Rhodococcus* and *Listeria*. It is not universally active against methicillin-resistant *S. aureus*. The Gram-negative bacteria susceptible to imipenem include Enterobacteriaceae, including the *Citrobacter, Enterobacter, E. coli, Klebsiella, Proteus, Providencia, Salmonella, Serratia, Shigella* and *Yersinia*. It is also active against *P. aeruginosa, Acinetobacter, Campylobacter jejuni, Haemophilus influenzae* and *Neisseria*. It is also active against anaerobes like *Bacteroides* and *Clostridium difficile*. Although it is stable to most beta-lactamases, it is hydrolyzed by metallo-beta-lactamases, which could be an important cause of resistance to carbapenem treatment in ventilator-associated pneumonia.[17] *Acinetobacter baumannii* is also increasingly showing resistance to carbapenems.[18] Carbapenem-resistant *A. baumannii* (CRAB) is often associated with ventilator-associated pneumonia. Cilastatin, commonly coadministered with imipenem (see below), does not have any antimicrobial action.

Imipenem, not absorbed from the GIT, needs to be administered parenterally. It is partly metabolized to toxic metabolites in the kidneys by tubular brush border enzyme (dehydropeptidase-I) and it is given along with cilastatin (inhibitor of dehydropeptidase) to increase imipenem concentrations in urine (but not serum). It is eliminated by the kidneys with a half-life of 1 hour.

The major indications are for infections in febrile neutropenia and other immunocompromised states, for hospital-acquired pneumonia, and sepsis. In anthrax, it is combined with other agents. Combination with cilastatin reduces the nephrotoxicity of imipenem. Seizures may be precipitated with its use in up to 1.5% of patients, especially in those with compromised renal function and prior central nervous system (CNS) disease. Mental disturbances and confusion may also occur. It can cause reddish discoloration of urine, which may be alarming, but not dangerous.

- *Meropenem*: The antimicrobial spectrum of meropenem is similar to that of imipenem, but it may have activity against some imipenem-resistant *P. aeruginosa*, may be more active than imipenem against Enterobacteriaceae and less active against Gram-positive organisms. Meropenem may be particularly useful in aspiration pneumonia.[19] It is similar to imipenem in most aspects, but not metabolized to a significant extent by renal enzymes and not given with cilastatin. It has less potential to cause seizures and is less nephrotoxic than imipenem.
- *Ertapenem*: It is similar to meropenem in most aspects except that it is not active against *P. aeruginosa* and *Acinetobacter*. Its in vitro activity against Enterobacteriaceae carrying plasmid- or chromosomal-mediated beta-lactamases, including AmpC- and extended-spectrum beta-lactamases, is especially clinically significant.
- *Doripenem*: The supposed advantage of doripenem over other carbapenems is its potent activity against pseudomonas. Data from 6 phase 3 multinational doripenem clinical trials on Ciprofloxacin-Resistant Enterobacteriaceae (CIPRE) and Extended-Spectrum Beta-Lactamases (ESBL) were evaluated.[20] Doripenem and meropenem were more potent than other drugs. At the same time it needs to be noted that a warning has been issued for doripenem use in patients with ventilator-associated pneumonia as it increased the risk of death and lower clinical cures.

Monobactams

Aztreonam: Its mechanism is similar to that of penicillins. The important feature of aztreonam is its resistance to most beta-lactamases. It has activity only against aerobic Gram-negative bacteria like *E. coli, Klebsiella, Proteus, Providencia, Salmonella, Serratia, Shigella* and *Yersinia* spp. It has some activity against *P. aeruginosa* and *H. influenzae*.

Its major indications are serious infections caused by Gram-negative organisms, and it is a useful alternative to aminoglycosides and third-generation cephalosporins. It is used in lower respiratory tract infections, including the pseudomonal infections in patients with cystic fibrosis, meningitis and sepsis. Use with an aminoglycoside is of benefit in serious *P. aeruginosa* infections.

It shows little cross-reactivity with penicillins and cephalosporins, with the exception of ceftazidime. Caution should be exercised in patients receiving anticoagulants as prothrombin time may be increased.

Beta-lactamase Inhibitors

Clavulanate, sulbactam and tazobactam are beta-lactamase inhibitors. When given in combination with beta-lactams, they inhibit plasmid-mediated beta-lactamases. Clavulanate is a suicide inhibitor of beta-lactamases produced by both Gram-positive and Gram-negative organisms. Since it is available as both oral and parenteral preparations, it has been combined with amoxicillin and ticarcillin to improve their antimicrobial spectra. Amoxicillin-clavulanic acid combination extends the spectrum of amoxicillin to beta-lactamase-producing strains of staphylococci and *H. influenzae*. Similarly, the antimicrobial spectrum of ticarcillin-clavulanic acid includes Gram-negative bacilli and *S. aureus*.

Sulbactam is another beta-lactamase inhibitor available both as oral and parenteral preparation. Used with ampicillin, it improves the antimicrobial spectrum of ampicillin akin to that of amoxicillin. Tazobactam is available only for parenteral administration. It is not effective against chromosomally mediated beta-lactamases. Though it is coadministered with piperacillin, the effectiveness of the combination against *P. aeruginosa* is doubtful. When given in combination, the dose of piperacillin gets reduced.

Sulbactam has been demonstrated to have bactericidal activity against acinetobacter when given alone also. The mechanism of its action is not known, though.[21]

Macrolides

Erythromycin, the prototype of macrolides is obtained from *Streptomyces erythreus*. Clarithromycin and azithromycin are semisynthetic derivatives of erythromycin. These agents are largely bacteriostatic (may be bactericidal at high concentrations) and inhibit the growth of microorganisms by binding to the 50S ribosomal subunit of sensitive microorganisms. They inhibit the translocation step in the peptide synthesis process wherein the newly formed peptidyl t-RNA moves from donor to acceptor site. Agents in this class also demonstrate postantibiotic effect where the effect persists after the antibiotic is removed from the system.

- *Erythromycin*: The antimicrobial spectrum of erythromycin includes both Gram-positive and certain Gram-negative organisms. It is effective against pneumococci, streptococci, staphylococci and corynebacteria. Certain atypical microorganisms such as mycoplasma, legionella, *Chlamydia trachomatis, Chlamydophila psittaci, Chlamydophila pneumoniae, M. kansasii* and *Mycobacterium scrofulaceum* are also susceptible. Resistance has been seen in penicillin resistant *S. pneumoniae and* mycoplasma. Cross resistance is seen with other groups of these agents.

Erythromycin without an enteric coating is destroyed in the stomach. Erythromycin stearate, ethylsuccinate and estolate provide the requisite enteric coating and the latter is best able to resist destruction in the stomach. Absorption of erythromycin ethylsuccinate and estolate is not affected by the presence of food. Erythromycin gluceptate and lactobionate are available for intravenous administration. Only about 5% of the orally administered drug is excreted in the urine and dose adjustment is not required if the renal functions are compromised.

For pulmonary infections, the indications of erythromycin include acute tracheobronchitis, acute exacerbations of chronic bronchitis with or without complications, and for empirical antimicrobial therapy for pneumonia in previously healthy, ambulatory patients (pneumococcus, *Mycoplasma pneumoniae* being the usual causative organisms). It is also used for the elderly (*Pneumococcus, Klebsiella, S. aureus, H. influenzae* being the most likely causative organisms), empirical therapy of pneumonia in pediatric patients of 1–3 months of age (*Chlamydia, Ureaplasma, Pneumocystis carinii* being potentially causative) and also for empirical therapy of pneumonia in children of more than 6 years of age (in whom pneumococcus and mycoplasma may be causative). Erythromycin is used in *Legionella* infections, and respiratory tract infections such as bronchitis and pneumonia (mycoplasma and other atypical pneumonias as well as streptococcal). It may be used as part of a multidrug regimen for the treatment of inhalational anthrax. It is also used in the prevention of diphtheria in nonimmune patients and of pertussis in non- or partially immune patients. It may be used as an alternative for actinomycosis for patients who are allergic to penicillin. It is also used as an alternative to the tetracyclines in patients with *Chlamydia pneumoniae*.

The adverse effects include gastrointestinal disturbances such as nausea, vomiting and diarrhea. Acute cholestatic hepatitis occurs most commonly with the estolate salt. This is a hypersensitivity reaction, which usually occurs 10–20 days after treatment and is characterized by nausea, vomiting, diarrhea and abdominal cramps. The condition recurs on the readministration of the drug. Reversible sensorineural deafness has been reported with its use. Prolongation of QT interval is known to occur with its administration. Erythromycin may aggravate myasthenia gravis. It inhibits cytochrome P450 enzyme and can lead to the elevated levels of theophylline, oral anticoagulants, cyclosporine and methylprednisolone. It may lead to the elevation of digoxin levels by the inhibition of gastrointestinal and renal P-glycoproteins.

- *Clarithromycin*: Clarithromycin is slightly more potent than erythromycin against the sensitive strains of streptococci and staphylococci, and has modest activity against *H. influenzae* and *Neisseria gonorrhoeae.* Clarithromycin has good activity against *M. catarrhalis, Chlamydia* spp., *Legionella pneumophila, Borrelia burgdorferi, Mycoplasma pneumoniae* and *Helicobacter pylori.* It is more active than erythromycin for *Mycobacterium avium* complex.

The oral absorption of clarithromycin is good. However, it undergoes extensive first pass metabolism. The extended release form is usually given with food to improve its bioavailability. The drug is metabolized in the liver to an active metabolite; 20–40% of the drug is excreted unchanged in the urine. Dosage adjustment is not needed in hepatic or renal impairment. Clarithromycin exhibits nonlinear pharmacokinetics.

The gastrointestinal symptoms are lesser than that of erythromycin. Prolongation of QT interval has been reported rarely with its use. Isolated cases of corneal opacities, progressive cholestatic jaundice have been reported with its use. It inhibits CYP3A4 and has drug interactions similar to that seen with erythromycin. Concomitant use with theophylline, zidovudine, digoxin, statins, colchicine and carbamazepine may lead to the increase of serum levels and toxicity of these drugs. With verapamil, it may lead to hypotension, bradyarrhythmias and lactic acidosis; it may potentiate the effects of the oral anticoagulants. Inducers of the CYP3A4 (efavirenz, nevirapine, rifampicin, rifabutin and rifapentine) may increase clarithromycin metabolism and thus lower its plasma levels. Both clarithromycin and itraconazole (and also saquinavir) are CYP substrates and increase the plasma levels of each other if used together. QT prolongation leading to torsades de pointes has been reported with its concurrent use with other QT prolonging drugs.

- *Azithromycin*: Azithromycin generally is less active than erythromycin against Gram-positive organisms and slightly more active than either erythromycin or clarithromycin against *H. influenzae* and *Campylobacter* spp. Azithromycin is very active against *Moraxella catarrhalis, Chlamydia* spp., *M. pneumoniae and L. pneumophila.* It is also active against some atypical mycobacteria. Its adverse effects and drug interactions are similar to clarithromycin.
- *Roxithromycin*: It is similar to azithromycin in the terms of spectrum and indications. The dose may need to be reduced in patients with hepatic or renal impairment. Gastrointestinal side effects are less as compared to erythromycin.
- *Telithromycin*: It is actually a ketolide, obtained from the structural modification of macrolide structure. Addition of keto group confers its properties, which make it less prone to resistance. It is indicated for mild to moderate community-acquired pneumonia due to *S. pneumoniae*, including multidrug resistant, *H. influenzae, M. catarrhalis, C. pneumoniae* or *M. pneumoniae*. Mild gastrointestinal disturbances occur commonly.

Severe liver injury leading to acute hepatic failure and even death has been reported. Visual disturbances (such as blurred vision, difficulty in focusing and diplopia) and transient loss of consciousness have been reported because of which patients should be advised to be careful while driving or operating machinery. It should not be given to patients with myasthenia gravis as it may lead to disease exacerbation. It may cause clinically significant QT prolongation.

Quinolones and Fluoroquinolones

Quinolones are derivatives of nalidixic acid. A major disadvantage with nalidixic acid and other quinolones (cinoxacin and oxolinic acid—no longer used) was the fact that they did not achieve sufficient concentration in the blood and tissues and were only suitable for very few conditions, like urinary tract infections. Fluorination of nalidixic acid has led to the development of compounds, which can achieve sufficient concentrations in the blood and tissues and have wider antibacterial spectrum.

Mechanism of Action

Fluoroquinolones inhibit two enzymes, Topoisomerase II (DNA gyrase) and Topoisomerase IV. DNA gyrase condenses the large DNA strands into the cell by introducing supercoils into the DNA. During this supercoiling process, both DNA strands are cleaved by DNA gyrase, forming a "quinolone binding pocket".[21,22] Two quinolone molecules enter this pocket and inhibit further supercoiling. This creates gaps in the DNA strands activating exonucleases (DNA repair enzymes) leading to irreversible DNA damage and cell death. The function of Topoisomerase IV is not well understood, but appears to be involved in the separation of the DNA daughter chains.

Quinolones inhibit DNA gyrase in Gram-negative organisms and Topoisomerase IV in Gram-positive bacteria.

Pharmacokinetics

Fluoroquinolones in general are drugs with excellent oral bioavailability and have low-plasma protein binding of about 30% **(Table 1)**. They readily and rapidly penetrate the body tissues, achieving tissue and fluid concentrations that are generally higher than those in plasma. Peak serum concentrations occur within 1–2 hours of oral doses. Longer half-lives (10 hours) of some quinolones (trovafloxacin, grepafloxacin, moxifloxacin) permit once-daily dosing. Although levofloxacin has a short half-life, it is used once daily. Fluoroquinolones are eliminated by both renal and nonrenal mechanisms **(Table 1)**. Dose adjustment is required in the presence of renal or hepatic dysfunction.

Spectrum, Pulmonary Indications and Dosage

Till date four generations of quinolones have been developed **(Tables 2 and 3)**.[23] The first-generation compounds have activity against both Gram-negative and Gram-positive organisms. However, compared to quinolones of subsequent generations, the activity is not very potent. The second-generation agents have good activity against Gram-negative organisms and moderately good activity against Gram-positive organisms. While good activity against *Pseudomonas* (ciprofloxacin in particular) is an advantage, methicillin-

Table 1 Pharmacokinetic features of fluoroquinolones

Drug	*Half-life (hours)*	*Bioavailability (%)*	*With respect to food*	*Route of elimination*
Ciprofloxacin	3–5	60–80	Empty stomach	Renal > hepatic
Ofloxacin	4–5	~ 100	No effect	Renal
Gatifloxacin	7–14	95	No effect	Renal
Gemifloxacin	7	70	No effect	Renal > hepatic
Levofloxacin	7	90	No effect	Renal
Moxifloxacin	13	99	No effect	Hepatic > renal
Lomefloxacin	8	>90	Empty stomach	Renal
Pefloxacin	8–13	>70	Empty stomach	Hepatic
Grepafloxacin	12	70	No effect	Hepatic

Table 2 Classification and spectrum of quinolones[1]

Classification	*Drugs*
First generation	Nalidixic acid, Cinoxacin
Second generation	Norfloxacin, Lomefloxacin, Enoxacin, Ofloxacin, Ciprofloxacin
Third generation	Levofloxacin, Sparfloxacin, Gatifloxacin, Moxifloxacin
Fourth generation	Trovafloxacin

resistant staphylococci and streptococcal infections may not respond to this group, except to levofloxacin, which may have superior efficacy.

Most of the newer fluoroquinolones are effective in sinusitis, acute bacterial exacerbations of chronic bronchitis, and for presumptive therapy for pneumonia in adults with chronic bronchitis or alcoholism. Some of them are also indicated in community- and hospital-acquired pneumonia. Mild-to-moderate respiratory exacerbations owing to *P. aeruginosa* in patients with cystic fibrosis also respond to oral fluoroquinolone therapy. Unlabeled respiratory indications of fluoroquinolones include pulmonary tuberculosis, anthrax, Legionnaires' disease and community-acquired pneumonia in children.

Adverse Drug Reactions and Drug Interactions

Fluoroquinolones are relatively safe drugs; the adverse effects are generally mild and rarely need discontinuation of therapy. The overall incidence of adverse reactions with fluoroquinolones is low (approximately 6% to 7%), the most common are gastrointestinal (mild nausea, vomiting and/or abdominal discomfort) reported in 3–17% of patients. Mild headache and dizziness have been reported in up to 11% of patients. A typical, but rare adverse effect seen with these drugs is the photosensitivity or phototoxicity reaction, which can be moderate to severe. The reaction may present as an exaggerated sunburn reactions (burning, erythema, exudation, vesicles, blistering and edema) on areas exposed to sun or artificial ultraviolet (UV) light. Relative potential of the various fluoroquinolones to cause photosensitivity/phototoxicity is unclear. Patients should be advised to avoid unnecessary or excessive exposure to sunlight and artificial UV light, cover the skin with clothing or use sunscreen. The drug should be discontinued if this adverse reaction occurs.

The effect of quinolones on cartilage has been a matter of debate, precluding their use in immature animals. Ciprofloxacin, norfloxacin and nalidixic acid have been given safely in children with cystic fibrosis with few reports of reversible joint symptoms. Achilles tendon rupture or tendinitis had occurred with their use prompting US Food and Drug Administration to add a black box warning with the use of all fluoroquinolones. Leukopenia, eosinophilia and mild elevations in serum transaminases occur rarely. As with most antimicrobials, *Clostridium difficile*-associated diarrhea and colitis (antibiotic-associated diarrhea or pseudomembranous colitis) have been reported in patients receiving fluoroquinolones.

Rarely, serious and occasionally fatal hypersensitivity and/or anaphylactic reactions have occurred usually after multiple doses. Sometimes there is concomitant cardiovascular collapse, loss of consciousness, tingling, edema (pharyngeal or facial), dyspnea, urticaria or pruritus. Fever, rash or severe dermatologic reactions (toxic epidermal necrolysis, Stevens-Johnson syndrome), vasculitis, arthralgia, myalgia, serum sickness, allergic pneumonitis, interstitial nephritis, acute renal insufficiency or failure, hepatitis, jaundice, acute hepatic necrosis or failure, anemia (including hemolytic and aplastic), thrombocytopenia (including thrombotic thrombocytopenic purpura), leukopenia, agranulocytosis, and pancytopenia have all been reported. They require discontinuation of the quinolones. QTc prolongation has been observed with sparfloxacin (withdrawn in some countries) and to a lesser

Table 3 Approved respiratory indications of fluoroquinolones

Drug	*Indication*	*Dosage*	*Route*
Ciprofloxacin	Ear, nose and throat infections (including otitis externa, otitis media, and sinusitis) Lower respiratory tract infections (including pseudomonal infections in cystic fibrosis, but excluding infections due to *S. pneumoniae)* Respiratory infections in cystic fibrosis patients Anthrax	250–750 mg BD. IV dose is 200–400 mg BD In cystic fibrosis, 40 mg/kg/day PO div q12h In anthrax: 400 mg IV q12h or 500 mg PO q12h	PO, IV
Lomefloxacin	Acute exacerbation of chronic bronchitis caused by *Haemophilus influenzae* or *Moraxella catarrhalis*	400 mg OD for 10 days	PO
Gemifloxacin	Acute exacerbation of chronic bronchitis caused by *S. pneumoniae, H. influenzae, Haemophilus parainfluenzae,* or *M. catarrhalis* Mild-to-moderate community-acquired pneumonia caused by *S. pneumoniae* (including penicillin-resistant strains), *H. influenzae, M. catarrhalis, Mycoplasma pneumoniae, Chlamydia pneumoniae,* or *Klebsiella pneumoniae*	320 mg OD for *5 days* in the treatment of acute exacerbation of chronic bronchitis 320 mg OD for 7 days in the treatment of community-acquired pneumonia	PO
Levofloxacin	Acute mild-to-moderate sinusitis due to *S. pneumoniae, H. influenzae,* or *M. catarrhalis* Mild-to-moderate acute exacerbation of chronic bronchitis due to *S. aureus, S. pneumoniae, H. influenzae, H. parainfluenzae* or *M. catarrhalis* Mild, moderate or severe community-acquired pneumonia caused by *S. aureus, S. pneumoniae* (including penicillin-resistant strains), *H. influenzae, M. catarrhalis, M. pneumoniae, C. pneumoniae, Legionella pneumophila* or *K. pneumoniae*	For sinusitis, 500 or 750 mg OD for 5 days For acute exacerbation of chronic bronchitis, 500 mg OD for 7 days or 750 mg OD for 5 days For community-acquired pneumonia, 500 mg OD for 7–14 days or 750 mg OD for 5 days	PO, IV
	Nosocomial pneumonia due to methicillin-susceptible *S. aureus,* for nosocomial pneumonia, *P. aeruginosa, Serratia marcescens, E. coli, K. pneumoniae,* 750 mg OD for 7–14 days *H. influenzae* or *S. pneumoniae*		
Moxifloxacin	Acute bacterial sinusitis caused by *S. pneumoniae, H. influenzae* or *M. catarrhalis* Acute exacerbations of chronic bronchitis due to *S. pneumoniae, H. influenzae, H. parainfluenzae, K. pneumoniae, S. aureus* (methicillin-susceptible strains), or *M. catarrhalis* Community-acquired pneumonia due to *S. pneumoniae* (including multidrug-resistant strains), *S. aureus* (oxacillin-susceptible strains), *K. pneumoniae, H. influenzae, M. pneumoniae,* or *M. catarrhalis*	For sinusitis 400 mg OD for 10 days Acute exacerbations of chronic bronchitis 400 mg OD for 5 days For community-acquired pneumonia (CAP), 400 OD for 7–14 days	PO, IV
Abbreviations: BD, twice daily; OD, once daily; PO, orally; IV, intravenous			

extent with gatifloxacin and moxifloxacin warranting their use with care in patients on class III (*amiodarone*) and class IA (*quinidine, procainamide*) antiarrhythmics.

In conjunction with theophylline or nonsteroidal anti-inflammatory drugs (NSAIDs), hallucinations, delirium and seizures may rarely occur. Ciprofloxacin and pefloxacin inhibit the metabolism of theophylline, and toxicity from elevated concentrations of methylxanthine may occur. Concomitant use of corticosteroids increases the risk of severe tendon disorders (tendinitis, tendon rupture), especially in geriatric patients of older than 60 years of age. Antacids, sucralfate, metal preparations and multivitamins should be taken at least 2 hours prior or 2 hours after the administration of some of the oral fluoroquinolones (like levofloxacin) and 4–8 hours for moxifloxacin. Quinolones may enhance the effects of warfarin; therefore, it is advisable to closely monitor coagulation parameters.

The antimicrobial spectrum of second-generation quinolones includes Gram-negative organisms (including *Pseudomonas*), some Gram-positive organisms (*S. aureus,* but not *Streptococcus pneumoniae*) and some atypical pathogens. The spectrum of third-generation agents is same as of second-generation agents plus expanded Gram-positive coverage (penicillin-sensitive and penicillin-resistant *S. pneumoniae*) and expanded activity against atypical pathogens. The third-generation agents have the same coverage as of third-generation agents plus broad anaerobic coverage.

Aminoglycosides

Aminoglycosides are bactericidal drugs and their importance lies in their ability to synergize with the action of penicillins especially against enterococci and streptococci. Agents in this class are derived from either *Streptomyces* (framycetin, kanamycin, neomycin, paromomycin, streptomycin and tobramycin) or the genus *Micromonospora* [gentamicin (which is why it is not spelled *gentamycin*) and sisomicin]. They act by several mechanisms, but mainly through the inhibition of 30S and 50S portions of bacterial ribosomes. They are also known to disrupt the integrity of bacterial cell membrane.

Spectrum

The antimicrobial spectrum of aminoglycosides includes aerobic Gram-negative bacilli. As mentioned earlier, their action may be extended to Gram-positive bacteria when given with penicillins. The most clinically important mechanism of resistance is their inactivation by aminoglycoside modifying enzymes acetyltransferases, adenyltransferases or phosphotransferases. The other mechanisms include (i) decreased permeability of the antimicrobial into the cells because of alteration in their transport system, inadequate membrane potential, or modification in the lipopolysaccharides, and (ii) mutations in chromosomal genes encoding ribosomes leading to alteration in their targets. Cross resistance to other aminoglycosides may occur, but is less with amikacin.

Pharmacokinetics

This group of antibiotics is not absorbed orally and needs to be administered either via intramuscular or as intravenous infusion. Aminoglycosides exhibit concentration dependent kinetics and have considerable postantibiotic effect. These two properties make it prudent to administer aminoglycosides as a single large dose rather than multiple small doses. With once a day regimen, the propensity for toxicity is also reduced once daily dosing allows for longer periods for which the drug remains below the threshold concentration. Additionally, once a day administration has the advantage of enabling treatment in an outpatient setting.

The polar nature of these compounds does not allow intracellular penetration, thereby considerably reducing the volume of distribution. Since aminoglycosides are largely eliminated renally, the dose has to be adjusted in accordance with creatinine clearance.

Therapeutic drug monitoring may be required with their use. The doses are adjusted so as to achieve a target concentration of less than 1 µg/mL between 18 hours and 24 hours after the dose administration. Obtaining blood sample 8 hours after drug administration will enable dose adjustment to achieve target concentration at 18 hours. When they are administered in multiple dose regimens, both peak and trough concentrations need to be measured.

They are primarily indicated for infections (including serious infections of the respiratory tract) caused by Gram-negative bacteria, including *Pseudomonas, E. coli, Proteus, Providencia, Klebsiella, Enterobacter, Serratia* and *Acinetobacter*. In spite of a large number of adverse effects associated with their use, they remain important option in many serious infections like septicemia, bacterial endocarditis and other serious infections caused by Gram-negative bacilli.

- *Gentamicin*: It is used in many severe systemic infections caused by susceptible organisms, including pneumonia, septicemia, endocarditis, cystic fibrosis, plague, meningitis, infections in immunocompromised patients and patients admitted in intensive care units. It is seldom used alone and is commonly prescribed with penicillins for streptococcal and enterococcal infections, with antipseudomonal beta-lactams for *Pseudomonas*, and with metronidazole (clindamycin) for mixed aerobic-anaerobic infections.
- *Tobramycin*: It is similar to gentamicin, but has been specifically used in pseudomonal infections.
- *Kanamycin*: It is also similar to gentamicin. Development of resistance is a bigger problem with kanamycin as compared to other aminoglycosides, which has led to a decline in its use.
- *Amikacin*: Its indications are similar to those of gentamicin except that should be reserved for the treatment of gentamicin- and tobramycin-resistant severe infections. It is also useful in nontuberculous mycobacterial infections. It is also used in combination with other antibiotics like gentamicin.
- *Netilmicin*: It is similar to amikacin and can be used as its alternative. It was suggested that it is less nephrotoxic and ototoxic than other aminoglycosides. This has not been substantiated in all studies.
- *Streptomycin*: It is mainly used as an antitubercular drug and is covered elsewhere.

Adverse Effects of Aminoglycosides

Ototoxicity and nephrotoxicity are the major limitations. Ototoxicity manifests as vestibular disturbance and/or auditory dysfunction. The irreversibility of ototoxicity makes it a cause of concern. Mild ototoxicity may be seen in up to 25% patients, but overt ototoxicity occurs in 2–10%. A high pitched tinnitus is the first sign of cochlear toxicity. If the drug is not discontinued, permanent auditory dysfunction may occur. Vestibular toxicity is more difficult to diagnose and headache may precede vestibular toxicity. This progresses onto loss of coordination, mental past pointing and positive Romberg's test. Predisposing factors include extremes of age, higher dose/duration of use, raised peak and trough levels, and concurrent use of other ototoxic drugs. Aminoglycosides constitute the single most common cause of bilateral vestibulopathy, accounting for 15–50% of all cases.[24]

Nephrotoxicity caused due to the accumulation of drugs in proximal convoluted tubule is seen in 8–26% patients, its incidence is similar with different aminoglycosides. Unlike ototoxicity, nephrotoxicity is almost always reversible if treatment is promptly discontinued. Typical picture is that of nonoliguric renal failure; elevation of serum creatinine; albuminuria; presence of red cells, white cells and casts; and development of hypoosmolar urine after several days of therapy. Azotemia and oliguria have also been reported. Predisposing factors include high dose and long duration of drug administration, high peak and trough levels, extremes of age, compromised renal function, dehydration and concurrent use of other nephrotoxic drugs.

The third important adverse effect of aminoglycosides is neuromuscular-blocking action leading to respiratory depression and muscle paralysis. Other adverse reactions (seen rarely) include rash, fever, headache, anaphylaxis, nausea and vomiting, tremor, arthralgia, hypotension, blood dyscrasias, purpura, stomatitis, liver dysfunction, peripheral neuropathy, meningeal irritation encephalopathy, confusion, lethargy, hallucinations and convulsions.

Tetracyclines

Tetracyclines are protein synthesis inhibitors. They are bacteriostatic broad-spectrum antibiotics with susceptibility extending to Gram-positive, Gram-negative, aerobes, anaerobes, rickettsia and mycoplasma. Resistance to the tetracyclines is common, is mediated by plasmids preventing drug accumulation within the cell by decreasing active transport of the drug or by increasing efflux.

Tetracyclines differ amongst each other mainly for pharmacokinetic parameters **(Table 4)**. Antimicrobial spectrum of different tetracyclines is largely the same. However, organisms showing resistance to certain tetracyclines may still be susceptible to doxycycline, minocycline and tigecycline, the new generation tetracycline.

Indications and Dosage

Tetracyclines are broad-spectrum antimicrobials active in rickettsial infections, pharyngitis, sinusitis, or pneumonia due to *C. pneumoniae* and by *M. pneumoniae* **(Table 5)**. They can also be used in community-acquired bacterial pneumonia caused by penicillin-susceptible *S. pneumoniae*, including in patients with associated bacteremia, beta-lactamase negative *H. influenzae* and *L. pneumophila.* They are also used (along with streptomycin) in brucellosis and plague. They are also effective in anthrax and chronic bronchitis.

Doxycycline, minocycline, tetracycline hydrochloride are commonly used for acute respiratory exacerbations of chronic bronchitis.[25] Doxycycline is also used for empirical therapy of pneumonia in previously healthy patients with no history of antibiotic intake. Though not approved for this indication, tigecycline has been shown to be as effective as levofloxacin in hospitalized adult patients with community-acquired pneumonia. Its use for this indication is discouraged. Further, its use for ventilator-associated pneumonia has been shown to be associated with increased mortality and there is a black box warning by the USFDA.

Table 4 Important pharmacokinetic aspects of tetracyclines

Tetracycline	*Oral bioavailability*	*Half-life*	*Duration of action*	*Metabolism and elimination*
Chlortetracycline	30%		Short acting	Mainly eliminated by kidney, though undergoes enterohepatic recirculation
Oxycline	60–80%	6–12 hours	Short acting	Mainly eliminated by kidney, though undergoes enterohepatic recirculation
Demeclocycline	60–80%	16 hours	Intermediate acting	Mainly eliminated by kidney, though undergoes enterohepatic recirculation. Photosensitivity reactions are common. Known to cause nephrogenic diabetes insipidus
Tetracycline	60–80%	6–12 hours	Short acting	Mainly eliminated by kidneys, though undergoes enterohepatic recirculation
Doxycycline	95%	16–18 hours	Long acting	Mainly eliminated by kidneys
Minocycline	100%	16–18 hours	Long acting	Significantly metabolized by the liver. It is also retained in fatty tissues
Tigecycline	Not given orally due to poor oral bioavailability	36 hours	Long acting	59% eliminated by biliary/fecal excretion, and 33% excreted in urine

Table 5 Doses and some features of tetracyclines

Drug	*Dose*	*Remarks*
Tetracycline	250 or 500 mg four times a day (maximum 4 g/day) orally or by slow intravenous (IV) infusion or intramuscularly	1 hour before or 2 hours after meals. Avoid in patients with renal impairment
Demeclocycline	600 mg/day in 2 or 4 divided doses. Preferably for atypical pneumonia, 900 mg/day in 3 divided doses	1 hour before or 2 hours after meals. In patients with liver disease, maximum dose is 1 g/day
Doxycycline	200 mg on day 1, followed by 100 mg/day orally or IV. In severe infections 200 mg/day throughout	May be used in patients with renal impairment
Minocycline	200 mg loading dose followed by 200 mg/day in 2 divided doses orally or by slow IV infusion	More active against *Staphylococcus aureus*, Streptococci, *Acinetobacter*, *Bacteroides*, *Haemophilus*, and some mycobacteria
Tigecycline	100 mg loading dose followed by 50 mg twice daily by IV infusion over 30–60 minutes	Effective against tetracycline-resistant organisms

Adverse Effects

The most common gastrointestinal (nausea, vomiting and diarrhea) adverse effects of tetracycline occur because of mucosal irritation. Esophageal ulceration can occur, therefore, oral preparations should be taken with sufficient water, in sitting or supine position, and a few hours before bedtime.

Glossitis, stomatitis, dysphagia, oral candidiasis, vulvo-vaginitis may occur due to overgrowth with *Candida albicans.* Antibiotic-associated diarrhea can occur as with most antimicrobials. Doxycycline may be less prone to cause GI adverse effects because of better absorption. Other serious complications of tetracycline therapy may include side effects such as, renal dysfunction, especially in patients with pre-existing renal disease; increases in liver enzymes; rarely severe hepatotoxicity; and pancreatitis. They are deposited in both milk teeth and permanent teeth leading to permanent discoloration and enamel hypoplasia. Tetracyclines are also deposited in calcifying areas in bone and nails and may interfere with bone growth.

Abnormal pigmentation of skin, conjunctiva, oral mucosa, tongue, and internal organs such as the thyroid has occurred rarely. Permanent discoloration of cornea has been reported in infants born to mothers given tetracycline in high doses during pregnancy. Intracranial hypertension with headache, dizziness, tinnitus, visual disturbances and papilledema have been reported. Transient myopia, muscle weakness in patients with myasthenia gravis, lupus exacerbation, hypersensitivity reactions, phototoxicity, and rarely agranulocytosis, aplastic anemia, hemolytic anemia, eosinophilia, neutropenia, and thrombocytopenia have been reported. They can also cause hypoprothrombinemia and reduction in serum-vitamin B concentrations. Outdated tetracyclines can cause Fanconi-type syndrome.

Drug Interactions

The absorption of tetracyclines is reduced by antacids, iron, and milk and dairy products. Therefore, it is advisable to have a gap of 1–3 hours in between. Nephrotoxicity and hepatotoxicity of tetracyclines may be increased by other nephrotoxic and hepatotoxic drugs, respectively. Concomitant use with retinoids may lead to an increased incidence of benign intracranial hypertension. Tetracyclines may decrease the efficacy of oral contraceptives. Bactericidal drugs like penicillins should not be used with tetracyclines (bacteriostatic).

Glycopeptides

They include vancomycin, teicoplanin, and others like telavancin, ramoplanin, decaplanin. Their mechanism of action is the inhibition of cell wall synthesis by binding to d-Ala d-Ala terminus of nascent peptidoglycan inhibiting synthesis of peptidoglycan. This group of drugs should be reserved for serious, multidrug-resistant infections since resistance to these drugs is uncommon, and also because of their toxicity profile.

- *Vancomycin*: It is active against *S. aureus, S. epidermidis* (including methicillin-resistant), *S. pneumoniae, S. pyogenes, Viridans streptococci, enterococci, Clostridium, Actinomyces, Bacillus anthracis, Corynebacterium*, lactobacilli and *Listeria.* Like other beta-lactams, it is synergistic with the aminoglycosides. Resistance is plasmid-mediated and may be transferable to other Gram-positive organisms; it has been seen in *Lactobacillus* and enterococci.

Its major indication is serious Gram-positive infections like methicillin-resistant staphylococcal infections which are commonly seen in nosocomial pneumonia, neutropenic and immunocompromised patients when other beta-lactams cannot be used because of microbial resistance, adverse effects or hypersensitivity.

It may cause histamine release leading to erythema, flushing, or rash over the face and upper torso (red man syndrome); rarely hypotension and shock may occur.

Nephrotoxicity and ototoxicity are two other serious adverse effects, which are more likely to occur in patients with renal impairment or with high dose. Ototoxicity (may be irreversible) is more common in patients with pre-existing hearing problems and with concomitant use of other ototoxic drugs. Tinnitus is usually the first sign of impending ototoxicity and warrants stoppage of treatment. Because of its irritant nature, thrombophlebitis can occur, but is rare if it is used diluted and infused slowly. Inhalational use has caused bronchoconstriction, which is treated with inhaled beta agonists.

- *Teicoplanin*: Its spectrum and resistance patterns are similar to vancomycin. Cross-resistance with vancomycin occurs, but may not be complete. It is not orally absorbed and is given parenterally. It is excreted by the kidneys with a half-life of about 60 hours. Incidence of "red man" syndrome is less. It is also less irritant and, therefore, incidence of thrombophlebitis is less.
- Dalbavancin and telavancin are two other glycopeptides under development. The former is characterized by a long half-life permitting once a week administration. Telavancin has activity against Gram-positive bacteria and against strains with intermediate sensitivity to vancomycin. It has dual mechanism of action as it inhibits both cell wall and cell membrane. They are largely being evaluated for skin and soft tissue infections.

Miscellaneous Antimicrobials

Trimethoprim-Sulfamethoxazole

The combination of trimethoprim and sulfamethoxazole is synergistic in action by the virtue of its action on two sequential steps in the synthesis of folic acid. Sulfamethoxazole inhibits the incorporation of para-aminobenzoic acid (PABA) into folic acid while trimethoprim prevents the reduction of dihydrofolate to tetrahydrofolate. Both of these steps are required in the synthesis of folic acid. The antimicrobial spectrum of the combination includes *Chlamydiae diphtheria, S. aureus, S. epidermidis, Streptococcus pyogenes, Klebsiella* spp., pneumocystis and *Yersinia pseudotuberculosis*. Methicillin-resistant strains of *S. aureus* may be susceptible to trimethoprim-sulfamethoxazole. Widespread resistance is common in streptococci. Resistance has been commonly observed in both Gram-positive and Gram-negative organisms.

Indications and dosage: The combination is available as 80 mg trimethoprim and 400 mg sulfamethoxazole and as Double Strength (DS) tablets containing 160 mg trimethoprim and 800 mg sulfamethoxazole. For the treatment of acute exacerbations of chronic bronchitis (it is not first or even second choice) due to susceptible strains of *S. pneumoniae* or *H. influenzae*, it is used as one DS tablet twice daily for 10–14 days. The daily dose for treatment of *P. carinii* pneumonia is 15–20 mg/kg trimethoprim and 75–100 mg/kg sulfamethoxazole in equally divided doses every 6 hours for 14–21 days. For prophylaxis of *P. carinii*, the dose is one DS tablet once daily. Doses will need to be adjusted for creatinine clearance.

Adverse effects: Adverse effects are common, include gastrointestinal disturbances (nausea, vomiting and anorexia) and skin reactions (rash and urticaria). Blood dyscrasias may occur. Caution needs to be exercised in patients with hepatic or renal impairment. It is contraindicated in patients with megaloblastic anemia due to folate deficiency. Folate supplementation is required if the drug is given for a prolonged period or when used in elderly patients with a tendency for folate deficiency. Rarely, fatal reactions like Stevens-Johnson syndrome, toxic epidermal necrolysis, fulminant hepatic necrosis, agranulocytosis, aplastic anemia, other blood dyscrasias, and hypersensitivity of the respiratory tract have occurred. Renal failure, interstitial nephritis, hyperkalemia, hyponatremia, aseptic meningitis, convulsions, peripheral neuritis, ataxia, vertigo, tinnitus, headache, hallucinations, depression, apathy, nervousness, arthralgias, myalgias, cough, shortness of breath, and pulmonary infiltrates have all been reported.

Chloramphenicol

It is a broad-spectrum bacteriostatic antimicrobial effective against Gram-positive and Gram-negative bacteria, as well as several others that acts by binding to the 50S subunit of the bacterial ribosome leading to the inhibition of protein synthesis. Its spectrum includes *H. influenzae, N. meningitidis, S. pneumoniae, S. pyogenes, Viridans streptococci, S. epidermidis, S. aureus* (not all strains), and streptococci such as *S. pneumoniae, S. pyogenes, B. anthracis, C. diphtheriae, Peptococcus, Peptostreptococcus, Bordetella pertussis, Brucella abortus, Campylobacter, Legionella pneumophila* and *B. fragilis*.

Bone marrow depression is the most important and potentially fatal adverse effect. The depression is generally reversible, related to the dose. Rarely, (1 in 50,000) it is dose-independent and irreversible. "Grey baby syndrome" is typically seen in premature infants characterized by ashen color of skin, abdominal distension, vomiting and hypothermia, progressing as to development of cyanosis, disturbed breathing, circulatory collapse and death. Bleeding, hemolytic anemia (especially in G-6-PD deficiency), neuritis (including optic), encephalopathy, headache, and ototoxicity have all been seen with its use.

Linezolid

The oxazolidinone *linezolid* has activity against Gram-positive organisms, including the vancomycin-resistant enterococci and methicillin-resistant *S. aureus*. It is a bacteriostatic drug and acts by the inhibition of ribosomal proteins. It is well absorbed after oral administration. It is an alternative to vancomycin for community-acquired pneumonia due to methicillin-resistant *S. aureus* (MRSA) and for hospital-acquired pneumonia, where the possibility of MRSA infection exists. It is also used for infections of the respiratory tract, including those due to vancomycin-resistant enterococci and methicillin-resistant *S. aureus.* It has been also used in the treatment of nocardiosis.[25]

Lactic acidosis, convulsions, bullous skin eruptions, including Stevens-Johnson syndrome, peripheral neuropathy, optic neuropathy (leading to blindness), and reversible myelosuppression have been rarely reported. It should not be used in Gram-negative infections; increased mortality in patients with Gram-negative or mixed infections was seen in a trial comparing linezolid to vancomycin, oxacillin or dicloxacillin (21.5% vs 16%) leading to an FDA alert in 2007.[26,27] It is a reversible and nonselective inhibitor of enzyme Monoamine Oxidase (MAO) and, therefore, can interact with adrenergic and serotonergic drugs similar to antidepressant MAO inhibitors. Serotonin syndrome may be precipitated when linezolid is used with Selective Serotonin Reuptake Inhibitors (SSRIs). Marked increase in blood may be seen with dopamine or adrenaline, reduction in the doses of these pressor agents may be needed.

Streptogramins

Quinupristin and dalfopristin are semisynthetic derivatives of pristinamycin I and II respectively, used in a ratio of 3:7. They act by inhibiting protein synthesis by binding to the 50S ribosomal subunit. The action of quinupristin and dalfopristin is synergistic. The spectrum includes MRSA, multidrug-resistant *S. aureus,* vancomycin-resistant *Enterococcus faecium* (but not *E. faecalis*), penicillin- and macrolide-resistant *Streptococcus pneumoniae,* and Gram-negative bacteria (*Legionella pneumophila, Moraxella catarrhalis* and *Mycoplasma pneumoniae).* Since it has shown efficacy against *Mycobacterium,* its routine use should be discouraged.

They are not absorbed orally. They are rapidly metabolized, the main route of elimination is fecal (3/4th) and the rest is eliminated in urine with half-lives of about 1 hour. They are approved for use in Europe for the treatment of nosocomial pneumonia and infections caused by MRSA. They are also indicated for the treatment of serious infections caused by Gram-positive organisms, as well as vancomycin-resistant *E. faecium.*

Liver enzyme elevation, myalgias and arthralgias, anemia, neutropenia, eosinophilia and thrombocytopenia may occur. They inhibit CYP3A4 and can increase blood levels of drugs metabolized by these enzymes. They may cause QT interval prolongation when given with other drugs having actions (like astemizole, terfenadine and cisapride).

Lincosamides

Lincomycin and clindamycin are not related structurally to erythromycin and the other macrolide antibacterials, but have similar antimicrobial activity. They act at the same site on bacterial ribosome. The lincosamides have a potential for use as alternatives to penicillin, however, pseudomembranous colitis limits their use for this indication. Currently, they may be considered for the treatment of severe anaerobic infections.

Polymyxins

This group includes polymyxin B and colistin (also known as polymyxin M). In 1962, Edgar and Dickinson wrote, *"Attempts to cure infections caused by Pseudomonas...are often unsuccessful. Many strains of the organism are resistant to almost all chemotherapeutic agents, and strains initially sensitive may become resistant during treatment".* This statement holds true even today and this group of agents have emerged as a "last resort" antimicrobials for Gram-negative infections resistant to all existing drugs. They replace the Ca^{++} and Mg^{++} ions on the LPS layer of Gram-negative cell wall leading to permeability changes and cell death. They also have a unique antiendotoxin activity for which they have been utilized in Gram-negative bacterial sepsis and endotoxin-mediated shock.

They are bactericidal against most Gram-negative bacilli except *Proteus* spp. and are particularly effective against *P. aeruginosa. Acinetobacter, E. coli, Enterobacter* and *Klebsiella, H. influenzae, B. pertussis, Salmonella, Shigella Serratia, Burkholderia, Providencia,* and *B. fragilis* are usually resistant. They are also not active against *Neisseria* spp., obligate anaerobes, and Gram-positive bacteria.

Polymyxins are not absorbed from GIT, through mucous membranes, or intact or denuded skin. They do not cross blood-brain barrier, pleura, synovial fluid, or placenta. The half-life is 6 hours and is prolonged in renal impairment. They can be administered topically for skin, ear and eye infections; orally for selective digestive tract decontamination (SDD); parenterally for systemic infections; intrathecally for meningitis and subconjunctivally for ocular infections.

The dose for polymyxin B is 15,000–25,000 u/kg/day (maximum 2 million u/day). Five lac units should be dissolved in 500 mL of D5 and infused over 24 h or it can be given in two divided doses every day infused over 1 hour. It is also given by aerosolization for Gram-negative nosocomial pneumonia and respiratory failure requiring mechanical ventilation. For this purpose, 25,000 u/kg/day divided into 4 doses as 0.5% solution in NS is administered.

It is important to note that polymyxin B should be stored at controlled room temperature 15–30°C before reconstitution but it should be protected from light for which it may be retained in carton until time of use. After reconstitution it must be stored under refrigeration, between 2° and 8°C and any unused portion should be discarded after 72 hours.

Colistin is administered parenterally as colistimethate, in doses of 6 million u/day in three divided doses. It can be given as direct intermittent injection over 3–5 minute every 12 h or by continuous infusion. For the latter, ½ of total daily dose is given over 3–5 minute and the remaining ½ of total daily dose is dissolved NS or DNS or 5% D or Ringer Lactate and administered by slow IV infusion, starting 1–2 h after the initial dose, over the next 22–23 h. Colistimethate infusion should be freshly prepared and used within 24 h.

The oral dose for colistin is 1.5–3 million units tid; as inhalation it is used in doses of 1–2 million units bid-tid. Colistin can be administered through nebulization along with parenteral administration with some advantage of higher doses reaching the site of action.[28]

The major dose-related toxicity of polymyxins is neurotoxicity and nephrotoxicity for which they were infrequently used until a few years back. They can also cause hypersensitivity reactions including those due to histamine release leading to bronchoconstriction and anaphylactoid symptoms. The neurotoxicity is seen in about 7% of patients with normal renal function and manifests as paresthesias, visual disturbances, dizziness, ataxia, confusion, or drowsiness. Neuromuscular blockade is a serious complication and can lead to respiratory paralysis and apnea for which the only treatment is artificial respiration. Nephrotoxicity is the major adverse effect and older literature quotes the incidence as about 20%. However, it is believed that for the newer more purified polymyxins the incidence may be less.

In conclusion, polymyxins should be reserved only for serious Gram-negative infections by bacteria resistant to all currently available beta-lactams, aminoglycosides and fluoroquinolones. Although both polymyxin B and colistin are similar in most aspects, polymyxin B may be superior to colistin for MDR *P. aeruginosa*. Patients with abnormal renal function test should receive lower doses.

Antiviral Drugs

INTRODUCTION

The development of antiviral drugs has lagged behind that of antibacterial drugs. Although the first antibacterial drugs became available in the 1930s, the discovery of the first antiviral compounds occurred some two decades later. The first antivirals in clinical use were idoxuridine for herpetic keratitis and methisazone for the prophylaxis of smallpox in contacts and the treatment of the infective complications of smallpox in the 1960s.[29]

Advancements in combinatorial chemistry, computer-assisted drug design and elucidation of microorganisms' genomes coupled with the increasing understanding of viral replication mechanisms have provided information on several novel targets for new drug development with the result that we have been able to discover, over the past few years, several new drugs that are effective, selective for viruses and spare the host cells. Many viral infections for which no treatment was available until a few years ago are now amenable to treatment, e.g. HIV, hepatitis C (HCV) and B (HBV) viruses, herpes viruses, papillomavirus and influenza. However, there still exist several viral infections that have no treatment, for instance, poliomyelitis, common cold, rabies, mumps, rubella and others.

There are several reasons for the inability to discover novel, safe and effective antiviral drugs. Viruses are obligate intracellular parasites that, on entry into their host, need metabolic processes of the host cell to replicate. Consequently, the antiviral drug should either be able to block entry of the virus into the host cells or exit or be able to kill the virus within the host cells, but do it without interfering with the functions of the host cells. Therefore, selective inhibitors of these viral processes that do not cause toxicity to the host cells are difficult to develop. Moreover, viruses constantly change their antigens leading to alterations in drug target enzymes that not only makes drug development difficult, but also leads to the emergence of drug resistant strains. Some general features of antiviral chemotherapy are outlined in **Table 6**.

MECHANISM OF ACTION OF ANTIVIRAL DRUGS

The basic processes for viral replication include viral attachment to certain host cell surface receptors followed by viral entry into the cell.[30] The virus then uncoats its nucleic acid and starts to synthesize the regulatory proteins necessary for synthesis of new viral RNA or DNA. With the help of host metabolic machinery, the virus is now capable of synthesizing structural proteins needed for the maturation of new viral

Table 6 General features of antiviral chemotherapy

• None of the antiviral drugs is virucidal; these drugs are only able to inhibit viral replication (virustatic). Therefore, if the immune system of the host is compromised, viruses start replicating once treatment is stopped leading to disease recurrence and drug-resistance
• The antiviral drugs are not effective against latent viruses and need active replication of the viruses to be effective
• Early initiation of antiviral drug treatment is crucial for effectively controlling the infection
• For most viral infections multidrug therapy is needed
• The correlation of culture sensitivity testing with clinical use is weaker as compared to antibacterial drugs mainly for the reason that these tests are not standardized for antiviral agents. Moreover, the antiviral drugs lead to adverse effects because of insufficient selectivity, which may make it difficult to choose a drug even if virus is sensitive to it in the lab
• Antiviral drugs are not substitutes to immunization for prophylaxis of viral infections
• An important property of any antiviral drug is its ability to penetrate the infected cells to be effective
• Because of the relative ineffectiveness of most antiviral drugs, the role of symptomatic, supportive treatment must not be ignored

particles. These newly formed viruses then leave the host cell to infect more cells. Currently available antiviral drugs utilize these steps in the viral replication process.

Anti-influenza Drugs

Influenza is an acute respiratory tract infection caused by Orthomyxoviridae family of RNA viruses. Of the three types of known influenza viruses (A, B and C), type A is the most important as it causes most infections (including the outbreaks) whereas types B and C are less commonly implicated and lead to mild infections. "Bird flu" (first reported in 1997 in Hong Kong) is also a form of influenza (avian or H5N1 influenza), may cause severe illness and has high mortality rates. "Swine flu" (H1N1 and other strains like H1N2, H3N1, etc.), first reported in 1918, had its most recent outbreak in humans in 2009.

There are two main classes of antiviral drugs for influenza: M2 ion channel inhibitors (amantadine, rimantadine) and neuraminidase inhibitors (oseltamivir, zanamivir). None of them is effective against all the types of influenza; and none of them has been proven to be conclusively effective against serious influenza infections when the risk of development of complications is high.

M2 Ion Channel Inhibitors

Amantadine and rimantadine inhibit viral uncoating and may reduce viral assembly probably via hemagglutinin pathway by acting on influenza A virus M2 protein, which is a membrane protein and is basically an ion channel. Although primary drug resistance is seen in less than 2% of viruses, acquired resistance is much more common (1/3rd of cases).[31]

Both these drugs are used for prophylaxis, as well as for the treatment of influenza A virus infections. For prophylaxis, 200 mg/day in one or two divided doses in young adults is about 70–90% protective.[32] For treatment, 200 mg/day for 5 days of either drug is considered useful although it reduces the duration of fever and systemic complaints by just about 1–2 days. They are ineffective against influenza B, or avian influenza H5N1 strain or the H1N1 swine flu.

The most common adverse effects are minor gastrointestinal (GI) disturbances (loss of appetite, nausea) and CNS symptoms (anxiety, light-headedness, difficulty concentrating, insomnia, etc.). The latter are seen in up to 30% of patients on amantadine, but are less common with rimantadine.[33] Rarely, serious adverse effects like cardiac arrhythmias, delirium, hallucinations, seizures and coma may occur.

Neuraminidase Inhibitors

Neuraminidase enzyme is important for the release of virus from infected cells and neuraminidase inhibitors cause a conformational change in the active site of the enzyme leading to its inhibition. Resistance occurs in 5–15% of cases. Oseltamivir is given orally and is rapidly absorbed. Zanamivir is not absorbed after oral administration and is used by inhalation when about 15% is deposited in the lower respiratory tract and about 80% in the oropharynx.[34] The plasma half-life of oseltamivir carboxylate is 6–10 hours and that of zanamivir is 2.5–5 hours after inhalation (1.7 hours after IV). Both the drugs are predominantly eliminated unchanged in the urine.

Both the drugs are effective in prophylaxis and treatment of influenza A and B virus infections. For prophylaxis, oseltamivir is given orally 75 mg or zanamivir intranasally once daily. For treatment, oseltamivir 75 mg twice daily or zanamivir 10 mg twice daily for 5 days are effective in reducing the duration of disease (by 1 day) and may reduce the risk of complications. These drugs also have some efficacy against some strains of avian influenza and swine flu. Interestingly, the benefit of oseltamivir in high risk cases of swine flu also stands controversial. It has been pointed that this conclusion has been drawn from studies which were not free from biases, particularly confounding by indication and survivorship bias.[35]

Oseltamivir causes GI irritation leading to nausea, abdominal discomfort and vomiting, but these symptoms are self-limiting even if treatment is continued. They are also decreased if drug is taken with food. Headache may also occur, but is uncommon. Neuropsychiatric disturbances, which were a concern earlier, have not been found to be occurring with any increased frequency than the controls in the studies. Zanamivir inhalation can cause wheezing and bronchospasm that leads to deterioration in lung function. Occasionally, deaths have been reported especially in patients with underlying lung disease.

Second generation long-acting neuraminidase inhibitors: Single-dose or once weekly treatment may offer several advantages like superior patient compliance and greater protection in a population. The first Long-Acting Neuraminidase Inhibitor (LANI), hence the name *laninamivir*, has recently completed phase 3 of clinical new drug development and may be marketed within a few years of publication in some countries. It is approved for use of prevention and treatment of influenza A or B in Japan. It has been shown to have efficacy similar to that of oseltamivir in patients with influenza A or B. In another study, it reduced the median time to illness alleviation in pediatric patients with oseltamivir-resistant influenza A virus.[36] Besides influenza A and B, it may also have activity against other influenza viruses.

In conclusion, there is some evidence to show that neuraminidase inhibitors may be superior to M2 ion channel inhibitors in the view of their lesser incidence of resistance, fewer adverse effects and greater efficacy against influenza B. Neuraminidase inhibitors may also be effective against strains resistant to M2 ion channel inhibitors. Combination regimens of amantadine, ribavirin and oseltamivir have been shown to be effective for viruses resistant to neuraminidase inhibitors. However, these findings are only experimental and adverse effect profile of such combinations would need consideration.[37]

Antiviral Drugs for Respiratory Syncytial Virus Infection

Respiratory syncytial virus (RSV) is an RNA virus of the Paramyxoviridae family that causes respiratory infections in all age groups, although infants and young children are more susceptible. RSV is an important cause of serious respiratory illness in blood and marrow transplant (BMT) recipients. In some subsets of these immunocompromised patients, RSV upper respiratory illnesses frequently progress to fatal viral pneumonia. The management is primarily supportive. Ribavirin is the only approved specific antiviral drug for RSV and palivizumab is a recently approved humanized monoclonal antibody.

Ribavirin

It is a synthetic nucleoside analog structurally related to guanine and acts by inhibiting viral nucleic acid synthesis. It is rapidly and extensively absorbed after oral administration. Aerosolized ribavirin achieves high concentrations in the respiratory tract, but is also absorbed systemically. It is not metabolized, gets stored in the tissues and is slowly eliminated by the kidneys with a half-life of about 300 hours. It is indicated for severe RSV bronchiolitis and is preferably given by aerosol. It is also active against influenza, parainfluenza, severe acute respiratory syndrome (SARS), measles, mumps, HIV, herpesviruses, adenoviruses and poxviruses. The most common adverse effects of oral ribavirin are flu-like symptoms and neuropsychiatric disturbances (anxiety, depression, insomnia and irritability). Bacterial infections, hemolytic anemia, leukopenia, thrombocytopenia, aplastic anemia and several other complications may also occur. When given by inhalation, it can cause lung function worsening, bacterial pneumonia, pneumothorax and hypotension.

Palivizumab

Produced by recombinant DNA technology, it is an antibody against an epitope in the A antigenic site of F protein of RSV. It was approved for use in infants with high risk for RSV infection. It effectively neutralizes a broad range of clinical isolates of RSV and may be several times more active than RSV-IGIV. Palivizumab is administered in a dose of 15 mg/kg IM once a month during the RSV season, which may occur predominantly between December to February in India. Given with ribavirin, palivizumab has shown improvement in response rate.[38] Side effects include erythema, pain, induration and bruising at the injection site. Vomiting, diarrhea and fever, and mild to moderate elevation of aspartate aminotransferase may also occur.

Antiherpesvirus Drugs

Two types of herpesviruses are common pathogens—herpes simplex virus type 1 (HSV-1) and HSV-2. HSV-1 leads to oral, esophageal, facial, dermatological or brain infections whereas HSV-2 leads to genital, rectal, dermatological or meningeal infections. The major drugs used in these infections are synthetic nucleoside analogs—*acyclovir, valacyclovir, ganciclovir, valganciclovir, famciclovir* and *penciclovir,* and non-nucleoside pyrophosphate *foscarnet.* They inhibit viral DNA synthesis. Resistance is common and occurs by alterations in viral enzymes (thymidine kinase, DNA polymerase) involved in their mechanisms of action.

Nucleoside Analogs

Besides HSV infections, these drugs are also effective against varicella-zoster virus (VZV) and prophylaxis of cytomegalovirus (CMV) in immunocompromised patients, but they are ineffective against established CMV infections. Ganciclovir is also effective against HIV and hepatitis B virus. The dose of oral acyclovir is 200 mg five times daily or 400 mg three times daily for 7–10 days and that of valacyclovir is 1,000 mg twice daily for 7–10 days. Intravenous acyclovir is used in doses of 5–20 mg/kg every eight hours. Ganciclovir is more effective against CMV and is used in doses of 5 mg/kg by IV infusion every 12 hours. Penciclovir is used topically as a 1% cream every 2 hours during waking hours for 4 days in the treatment of herpes labialis.[39] Famciclovir is given orally in doses of 250 mg three times daily, or 500 mg twice daily or 750 mg once daily.

These drugs can lead to nausea, diarrhea, rash, headache, renal insufficiency and neurotoxicity. Confusion and hallucinations can occur with high doses. Thrombocytopenia may also occur especially in immunocompromised patients.[40] Increased liver enzymes, hair loss, rash, Stevens-Johnson syndrome, toxic epidermal necrolysis and anaphylaxis have also been reported. Injection site reactions and even lead to tissue necrosis can occur with IV use. Hematological adverse effects are more common with ganciclovir.

Foscarnet

Besides herpesviruses it is also effective against CMV infections (pneumonia in bone marrow transplant patients and retinitis), including ganciclovir-resistant infections; HSV and VZV (including acyclovir-resistant); Epstein-Barr virus; VZV, HBV and HIV. The usual dose is 40–60 mg/kg infused over 1 hour every 8 hours.

The most common serious dose-limiting toxicity is nephrotoxicity. It can also cause anemia, granulocytopenia and thrombocytopenia. It is a chelator of bivalent metal ions and lead to hypocalcemia with normal plasma levels of calcium. It can also cause injection site reactions, GI symptoms (nausea, vomiting and diarrhea), malaise, fatigue, fever, CNS disturbances (headache, tremors, dizziness, irritability, seizures, hallucinations and mood disorders), paresthesias, rash, increases in liver function tests, blood pressure, ECG abnormalities and pancreatitis.

Idoxuridine

It is a thymidine analog that inhibits replication of various DNA viruses, including (herpesviruses and poxviruses) mainly used for topical treatment of HSV keratitis. *Trifluridine* is a pyrimidine nucleoside that has activity against HSV 1 and 2, CMV, vaccinia, and some adenoviruses. It is used for primary keratoconjunctivitis and recurrent epithelial keratitis owing to HSV types 1 and 2.

Antiviral Drugs for Severe Acute Respiratory Syndrome

Severe acute respiratory syndrome (SARS) is a respiratory illness caused by a newly identified coronavirus.[41] It is a serious disease and the mortality during the 2002–2003 outbreak was about 9.5%. Besides supportive treatment, corticosteroids, ribavirin, interferons, immunoglobulins and ritonavir-lopinavir have been tried, but convincing evidence for their efficacy is lacking.

REFERENCES

1. Felmingham D, Reinert RR, Hirakata Y, Rodloff A. Increasing prevalence of antimicrobial resistance among isolates of Streptococcus pneumoniae from the PROTEKT surveillance study, and comparative in vitro activity of the ketolide, telithromycin. J Antimicrob Chemother. 2002;50 (Suppl) S1: 25-37.
2. Nascimento-Carvalho CM, Cardoso MR, Brandileone MC, Ferrero F, Camargos P, Berezin E, et al. Penicillin/ampicillin efficacy among children with severe pneumonia due to penicillin-resistant pneumococcus (MIC=4 microg ml(-1)). J Med Microbiol. 2009;58(Pt 10):1390-2.
3. Rijnders MI, Deurenberg RH, Boumans ML, Hoogkamp-Korstanje JA, Beisser PS, Stobberingh EE; Antibiotic Resistance Surveillance Group. Flucloxacillin, still the empirical choice for putative *Staphylococcus aureus* infections in intensive care units in the Netherlands. J Antimicrob Chemother. 2009;64(5):1029-34.
4. Jung N, Lehmann C, Hellmann M, Seifert H, Valter MM, Hallek M, et al. Necrotizing pneumonia caused by Panton-Valentine leucocidin-producing *Staphylococcus aureus* originating from a Bartholin's abscess. Infect Dis Obstet Gynecol. 2008;2008:491401.
5. Andrews E, Armstrong M, Tugwood J, Swan D, Glaves P, Pirmohamed M, et al. A role for the pregnane X receptor in flucloxacillin-induced liver injury. Hepatology. 2010;51(5):1656-64.
6. Smucny J, Fahey T, Becker L, Glazier R. Antibiotics for acute bronchitis. Cochrane Database Syst Rev. 2004;(4):CD000245.
7. Máiz L, Lamas A, Fernández-Olmos A, Suárez L, Cantón R. Unorthodox long-term aerosolized ampicillin use for methicillin-susceptible *Staphylococcus aureus* lung infection in a cystic fibrosis patient. Pediatr Pulmonol. 2009;44(5):512-5.
8. Sheffield MJ, Lambert DK, Henry E, Christensen RD. Effect of ampicillin on the bleeding time of neonatal intensive care unit patients. J Perinatol. 2010;30(8):527-30.
9. Kabra SK, Lodha R, Pandey RM. Antibiotics for community-acquired pneumonia in children. Cochrane Database Syst Rev. 2010;3:CD004874.
10. Manno G, Cruciani M, Romano L, Scapolan S, Mentasti M, Lorini R, et al. Antimicrobial use and *Pseudomonas aeruginosa* susceptibility profile in a cystic fibrosis centre. Int J Antimicrob Agents. 2005;25(3):193-7.
11. Blondiaux N, Wallet F, Favory R, Onimus T, Nseir S, Courcol RJ, et al. Daily serum piperacillin monitoring is advisable in critically ill patients. Int J Antimicrob Agents. 2010;35(5):500-3.
12. Schussler O, Dermine H, Alifano M, Casetta A, Coignard S, Roche N, et al. Should we change antibiotic prophylaxis for lung surgery? Postoperative pneumonia is the critical issue. Ann Thorac Surg. 2008;86(6):1727-33.
13. Biernawska J, Zukowski M, Zegan-Barańska M, Zukowska A. [Cefepime in empiric therapy of ventilator-associated pneumonia]. Anestezjol Intens Ter. 2009;41(4):242-5.
14. Thabet F, Al Maghrabi M, Al Barraq A, Tabarki B. Cefepime-induced nonconvulsive status epilepticus: case report and review. Neurocrit Care. 2009;10(3):347-51.
15. Cephalosporins and other beta-lactams. In: British National Formulary, 56th edition. London: BMJ Publishing Group Ltd and Royal Pharmaceutical Society Publishing; 2008. pp. 295.
16. Aarts MA, Hancock JN, Heyland D, McLeod RS, Marshall JC. Empiric antibiotic therapy for suspected ventilator-associated pneumonia: a systematic review and meta-analysis of randomized trials. Crit Care Med. 2008;36(1):108-17.
17. Dwivedi M, Mishra A, Azim A, Singh RK, Baronia AK, Prasad KN, et al. Ventilator-associated pneumonia caused by carbapenem-resistant Enterobacteriaceae carrying multiple metallo-beta-lactamase genes. Indian J Pathol Microbiol. 2009;52(3):339-42.
18. Routsi C, Pratikaki M, Platsouka E, Sotiropoulou C, Nanas S, Markaki V, et al. Carbapenem-resistant versus carbapenem-susceptible *Acinetobacter baumannii* bacteremia in a Greek intensive care unit: risk factors, clinical features and outcomes. Infection. 2010;38(3):173-80.
19. Tokuyasu H, Harada T, Watanabe E, Okazaki R, Touge H, Kawasaki Y, et al. Effectiveness of meropenem for the treatment of aspiration pneumonia in elderly patients. Intern Med. 2009;48(3):129-35.
20. Kaniga K, Flamm R, Tong SY, Lee M, Friedland I, Redman R. Worldwide experience with the use of doripenem against extended-spectrum-beta-lactamase-producing and ciprofloxacin-resistant Enterobacteriaceae: analysis of six phase 3 clinical studies. Antimicrob Agents Chemother. 2010;54(5):2119-24.
21. Lin CH, Su SC, Ho KH, Hsu YW, Lee KR. Bactericidal effect of sulbactam against *Acinetobacter baumannii* ATCC 19606 studied by 2D-DIGE and mass spectrometry. Int J Antimicrob Agents. 2014;44:38-46.
22. Hooper DC, Wolfson JS. Mechanism of quinolone action and bacterial killing. In: Hooper DC, Wolfson JS (Eds). Quinolone Antimicrobial Agents, 2nd edition. Washington DC: American Society for Microbiology; 1993. pp. 53-75.

23. King DE, Malone R, Lilley SH. New classification and update on the quinolones antibiotics. Am Fam Physician. 2000;61(9):2741-8.
24. Halmagyi GM, Fattore CM, Curthoys IS, Wade S. Gentamicin vestibulotoxicity. Otolaryngol Head Neck Surg. 1994;111(5):571-4.
25. Daniels JM, Snijders D, de Graaff CS, Vlaspolder F, Jansen HM, Boersma WG, et al. Antibiotics in addition to systemic corticosteroids for acute exacerbations of chronic obstructive pulmonary disease. Am J Respir Crit Care Med. 2010;181(2):150-7.
26. Moylett EH, Pacheco SE, Brown-Elliott BA, Perry TR, Buescher ES, Birmingham MC, et al. Clinical experience with linezolid for the treatment of nocardia infection. Clin Infect Dis. 2003;36(3):313-8.
27. FDA.Information for health care professionals: Linezolid (marketed as Zyvox) [online] Available from: *http://www.fda.gov/cder/drug/InfoSheets/HCP/linezolidHCP.pdf.* [Accessed 16th March 2007].
28. Linden PK, Paterson DL. Parenteral and inhaled colistin for treatment of ventilator associated pneumonia. Clin Infect Dis. 2006;43:S89-94.
29. Bauer DJ. A history of the discovery and clinical application of antiviral drugs. Br Med Bull. 1985;41(4):309-14.
30. Hayden FG. Antiviral agents (Non retroviral). In: Brunton LL, Lazo JS, Parker KL (Eds). Goodman and Gilman's The Pharmacological Basis of Therapeutics, 11th edition. McGraw Hill Professional; 2005.
31. Hayden FG. Amantadine and rimantadine: Clinical aspects. In: Richman D (Ed). Antiviral Drug Resistance. New York: Wiley; 1996. pp. 59-77.
32. Hayden F, Aoki F. Amantadine, rimantadine, and related agents. In: Yu V, Merigan T, White N, et al. (Eds). Antimicrobial Therapy and Vaccines, illustrated edition. Baltimore: Williams and Wilkins; 1999. pp. 1344-65.
33. Keyser L, Karl M, Nafziger A, Bertino JS Jr. Comparison of central nervous system adverse effects of amantadine and rimantadine used as sequential prophylaxis of influenza A in elderly nursing home patients. Arch Intern Med. 2000;160(10):1485-8.
34. Cass LM, Efthymiopoulos C, Bye A. Pharmacokinetics of zanamivir after intravenous, oral, inhaled or intranasal administration to healthy volunteers. Clin Pharmacokinet. 1999;36 Suppl 1:1-11.
35. Freemantle N, Shallcross LJ, Kyte D, Rader T, Calvert MJ. Oseltamivir: the real world data. BMJ. 2014;348:g2371.
36. Sugaya N, Ohashi Y. Long-acting neuraminidase inhibitor laninamivir octanoate (CS-8958) versus oseltamivir as treatment for children with influenza virus infection. Antimicrob Agents Chemother. 2010;54(6):2575-82.
37. Nguyen JT, Hoopes JD, Le MH, Smee DF, Patick AK, Faix DJ, et al. Triple combination of amantadine, ribavirin, and oseltamivir is highly active and synergistic against drug resistant influenza virus strains in vitro. PLoS One. 2010;5(2):e9332.
38. Tsitsikas DA, Oakervee H, Cavenagh JD, Gribben J, Agrawal SG, Mattes FM. Treatment of respiratory syncytial virus infection in haemopoietic stem cell transplant recipients with aerosolized ribavirin and the humanized monoclonal antibody palivizumab: a single centre experience. Br J Haematol. 2009;146(5):574-6.
39. Spruance SL, Rea TL, Thoming C, Tucker R, Saltzman R, Boon R. Penciclovir cream for the treatment of herpes simplex labialis: a randomized, multicenter, double-blind, placebo-controlled trial. Topical Penciclovir Collaborative Study Group. JAMA. 1997;277(17):1374-9.
40. Feinberg J, Hurwitz S, Cooper D, Sattler FR, MacGregor RR, Powderly W, et al. A randomized, double-blind trial of valaciclovir prophylaxis for cytomegalovirus disease in patients with advanced human immunodeficiency virus infection. AIDS Clinical Trials Group Protocol 204/Glaxo Wellcome 123-014 International CMV Prophylaxis Study Group. J Infect Dis. 1998;177(1):48-56.
41. Peiris JS, Yuen KY, Osterhaus AD, Stöhr K. The severe acute respiratory syndrome. N Engl J Med. 2003;349(25):2431-41.

Part II: Antifungal Drugs

J Whig, Bharti Mahajan, Rajesh Mahajan

INTRODUCTION

Bacterial epidemics were a global and important cause of mortality at the beginning of 20th century. A drastic rise in fungal infections was observed when antibiotic therapies were developed in late 1960s.[1] The use of a large number of antibiotics and the increasing number of immunocompromised patients in hospital-care are the major factors responsible for the rising incidence of fungal infections.[2] Fungi are recognized as the fourth leading pathogen of nosocomial sepsis in USA.[3] Mortality among infected patients may be as high as 75–100%, presenting an enormous challenge for healthcare providers.[4]

There are an estimated several hundred thousand species of fungi, only 150–200 were considered to be pathogenic for humans, which now are increasing at an alarming rate. The endemic fungal infections are acquired from the environmental sources, e.g. coccidioidomycosis, while the opportunistic mycoses are caused by the fungi, which are present in the normal human flora in an immunocompromised host, e.g. *Candida* (yeast) and *Aspergillus* (mold).[5]

All the fungal infections tend to be more aggressive in immunocompromised patients.[6] There is also an increasing incidence of infections with other molds, including *Fusarium* spp., *Scedosporium* spp., (Hyalohyphomycosis), and *Rhizopus* spp. (mucormycosis or zygomycosis).[7] It has intensified the search for newer, safer and more efficacious agents to combat serious fungal infections.[8] The number of agents available to treat fungal infections have increased by 30% since the year 2000.[9]

It is important to know the differences in the antifungal spectrum of activity, bioavailability, drug interactions and adverse effects of the various antifungal agents.[9] They are broadly classified into the following classes. These agents are mainly used for the systemic fungal infections.[10]

- *Polyenes*: Amphotericin B (AMB), nystatin
- *Azoles imidazoles*: Miconazole, ketoconazole, econazole triazoles: fluconazole, itraconazole, voriconazole, posaconazole
- *Antimetabolites/Nucleoside analogs*:
  - Flucytosine
  - *Echinocandins*: Caspofungin, micafungin, anidulafungin
- *Miscellaneous*: Griseofulvin, terbinafine and others.

POLYENES

Amphotericin B and nystatin are the currently available polyenes. They have an important role in antifungal management plans due to their broad spectrum of action against fungi and rarity of resistance.[11]

Amphotericin B: It is an amphoteric polyene macrolide. It is almost insoluble in water, therefore, prepared as a colloidal suspension of AMB and sodium desoxycholate for intravenous (IV) injection.[12] It binds to ergosterol present within the fungal cell wall membrane and leads to the formation of pores resulting in subsequent efflux of potassium and intracellular molecules causing fungal cell death **(Fig. 1)**.[13]

Antifungal spectrum: AMB has useful activity against *Candida* spp., *Cryptococcus neoformans, Blastomyces dermatitidis, Histoplasma capsulatum, Sporothrix schenckii, Coccidioides immitis, Paracoccidioides brasiliensis, Aspergillus* spp., *Penicillium marneffei* and the agents of mucormycosis/zygomycosis.[14] Although conventional AMB (Fungizone in the form of micelles) remains the standard therapy for many invasive or life-threatening mycoses, the use of this drug is often limited by its toxicity, especially drug-induced renal impairment.[15] Consequently, it led to the development of Lipid Formulations of AMB (LFAmBs)—Amphotericin B Lipid Complex (ABLC; in the form of ribbons), Liposomal Amphotericin-B (L-AMB) and Amphotericin-B colloidal dispersion (ABCD; in the form of disks). AMB is complexed to cholesteryl sulfate in all these preparations.[16]

Pharmacokinetics

Amphotericin B is poorly absorbed from the gastrointestinal (GI) tract. Hence, oral AMB cannot be used for systemic fungal infections.[12] The drug is 90% bound to plasma proteins, largely β-lipoproteins. The penetration of AMB is very little into cerebrospinal fluid (CSF), vitreous humor and normal

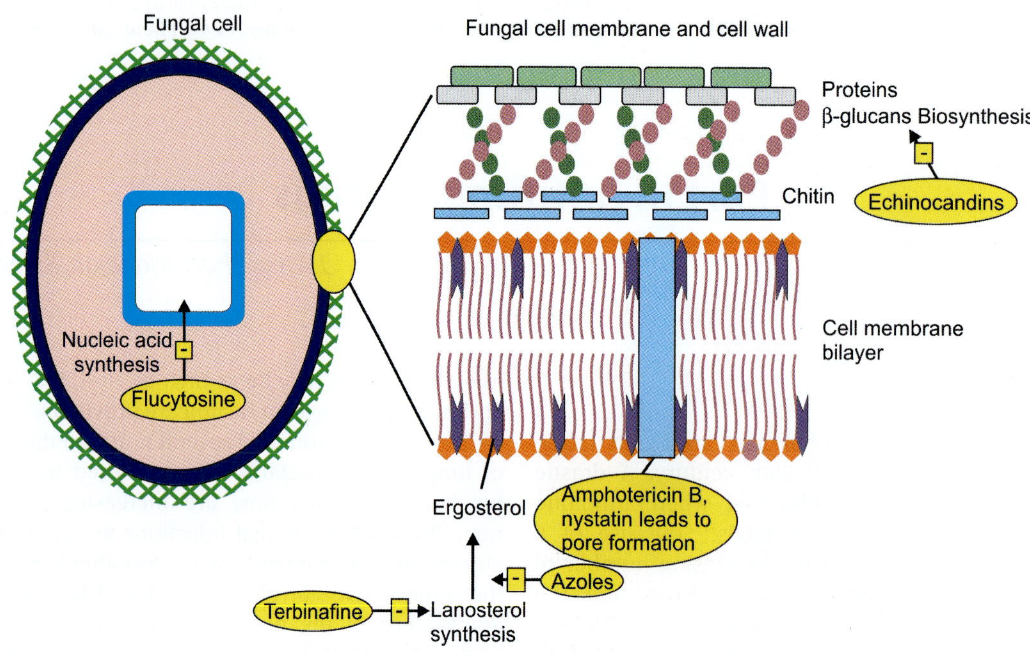

Fig. 1 Antifungal agents: Mechanism of action

amniotic fluid.[14] Most of the drug is excreted unchanged by the kidney or the liver.[17] The half-life is approximately 15 days.[12]

There are striking differences in their plasma pharmacokinetics of lipid formulations. The L-AMB contains rigid, charged phospholipids and cholesterol to retain AMB within the bilayer membranes of the circulating liposomes. This lipid vehicle serves as an amphotericin reservoir, reducing nonspecific binding to human cell membranes. This helps in limiting the adverse effects without sacrificing the efficacy and also allows for the use of a larger dose of the drug.[12] Amongst the various LFAmBs, L-AMB has the greatest renal protection.[18] Different formulations of AMB have been given by the inhalational route also to avoid nephrotoxicity associated with systemic administration.[9]

Adverse Effects

The main adverse effects of conventional AMB include infusion-related events like chills, fever, headache, nausea, vomiting and dose-limiting nephrotoxicity.[19] An increase in intrarenal vascular resistance is the major cause of nephrotoxicity.[14] AMB-associated nephrotoxicity can be reduced by the maintenance of intravascular volume, by avoiding diuretic drugs and saline-loading with 500–1000 mL of normal saline before the infusion of AMB.[20] AMB can also lead to bone marrow depression manifested by anemia.[21] The lipid formulations have several advantages over conventional AMB, such as the increased daily dose of the parent compound (up to 10 fold); high tissue concentration in the lungs, liver and spleen; less infusion related adverse effects (mainly with L-AMB) and marked decrease in nephrotoxicity with L-AMB.[22,23] The three lipid formulations, collectively reduced the risk of the patient's serum creatinine doubling during therapy by 58%.[24] They are now preferred as initial therapy in patients, who are at high risk for nephrotoxicity.[25] They have also proven to be cost-effective as the duration of hospital stay is reduced due to less toxicity.[9]

Indications

The broad antifungal spectrum and experience with the use of AMB accounts for its continued use despite its toxicity problems.[9] It is often used as the initial induction regimen for serious fungal infections and is then replaced by one of the newer azole drugs for chronic therapy or prevention of relapse.[12] AMB is the drug of choice for most forms of invasive candidiasis.[14] LFAmBs are used as second-line or salvage therapy for the treatment of invasive aspergillosis.[26] L-AmB is currently the first-line therapy for disseminated histoplasmosis in HIV-positive or HIV-negative patients, coccidioidomycosis, blastomycosis and sporotrichosis.[9,11] AMB in combination with flucytosine, remains the drug of choice for the treatment of cryptococcal meningitis in patients, whether infected with HIV or not.[11] It is also approved as empiric therapy for the neutropenic patients who have persistent fever despite the use of broad-spectrum antibiotics. High doses of L-AMB represents an effective first-line treatment for zygomycosis or mucormycosis.[11] A delay in therapy in patients infected with one of the zygomycetes has resulted in a twofold greater risk for death.[27]

Dose

The recommended dose of IV conventional AMB ranges between 0.7 mg/kg and 1 mg/kg. Escalating doses of lipid formulations of AMB may be indicated when alternative agents are not available or have been found to be ineffective.[9] The dose range for L-AMB (AmBisome) is 3–5 mg/kg/day; for ABLC (Abelcet) is 5 mg/kg/day and for ABCD (Amphotec) is also 5 mg/kg/day. Intrathecal AMB doses in adults normally range from 0.25 to 0.5 mg diluted in 5 mL of 5% glucose.[28,29]

AZOLES

The azole antifungals include two broad classes, imidazoles and triazoles. Both have same antifungal spectrum and mechanism of action.

Imidazoles

Imidazoles (clotrimazole, miconazole, ketoconazole, econazole, butoconazole, oxiconazole, sertaconazole and sulconazole) are predominantly used.[14] They have been replaced for systemic administration by triazoles,[30] which include terconazole, itraconazole, fluconazole, voriconazole and posaconazole. Triazoles have more favorable pharmacokinetic profile and improved safety profile than imidazoles. They also have enhanced clinical efficacy in the treatment of systemic mycoses.[31-33]

Triazoles

Mechanism of action: They inhibit the Cytochrome P450 enzyme 14 α-sterol demethylase, which prevents the conversion of lanosterol to ergosterol **(Fig. 1)**. Inhibition of this enzyme leads to accumulation of toxic methyl sterols and results in inhibition of fungal cell growth and replication.[9] The spectrum of action of azoles ranges from many *Candida* species, cryptococcus neoformans, and the endemic mycoses (blastomycosis, coccidioidomycosis and histoplasmosis), to the dermatophytes, and even the *Aspergillus* infections.[12]

Fluconazole

It remains one of the most frequently prescribed triazoles because of its excellent bioavailability, tolerability and side effect profile.[9] It is water soluble and well absorbed from the GI tract. Its absorption is not affected by food or gastric pH.[34] It has least protein binding and a long half-life of 27–34 hours (in the presence of normal renal function), which can allow once-a-day administration.[16] It has high penetration into CSF (≥70% of serum levels) and therefore, used for treating cryptococcal and coccidioidal meningitis.[20] It undergoes 90% of elimination by the renal route.[14]

Adverse effects and drug interactions: Nausea and vomiting may occur at high doses above 200 mg daily. More severe toxicity is unusual. Reversible alopecia, hepatic failure or Stevens-Johnson syndrome has been reported.[14] It has fewer drug-drug interactions than other triazoles. It is an inhibitor of CYP3A4 and CYP2C9. It increases the serum levels of phenytoin, glipizide, glyburide, warfarin, amprenavir and cyclosporine.[14]

Indications: Fluconazole is used in the treatment of candidemia in non-neutropenic patients and is shown to be as effective as AMB in two large randomized trials.[35,36] Fluconazole may be inappropriate for the empirical treatment of suspected fungal infection in neutropenic patients, because prior exposure, as treatment or prophylaxis is associated with resistant candidal strains and also because of its lack of activity against molds.[37] It is active against most of the *Candida* spp. except *C. Krusei* and *C. glabrata* isolates. If a *C. glabrata* isolate is found susceptible to fluconazole, higher doses (12 mg/kg/d) should be used.[37,38] There is no appreciable activity against *Aspergillus, Fusarium, Pseudallescheria* or the *Zygomycetes.*[9] It has become the agent of choice for the treatment of coccidioidal meningitis, although relapses have followed therapy with this agent. It is useful for both consolidation and maintenance therapy for cryptococcal meningitis. As, it has greatest penetration into the CSF and vitreous fluid, it is used in the treatment of CNS and intraocular infections.[39,40] Recommended dosage is 50–800 mg once daily, identical for oral and intravenous administration. Children are treated with 3–6 mg/kg once daily.[14]

Itraconazole

It has a wider spectrum than fluconazole.[7] It is active against yeasts and molds, with the exception of *Fusarium* spp., *Scedosporium* spp., and the Zygomycetes.[41,42] There are few data that examine the use of itraconazole in the treatment of invasive candidiasis.[40] It is generally reserved for patients with mucosal candidiasis, especially those who have experienced treatment failure with fluconazole.[43]

Pharmacokinetics

Maximal absorption of itraconazole capsules depend on the acidic pH. The absorption of the drug is erratic and unpredictable on the concomitant administration of H2-receptor antagonists, proton-pump inhibitors or antacids. It is recommended that itraconazole capsules be taken with food or a cola beverage to increase the absorption.[44] The bioavailability is unpredictable, hence, therapeutic drug monitoring (TDM) is recommended. Itraconazole is found in equal amounts in plasma as the native drug and as a metabolite, hydroxyitraconazole, which has equivalent antifungal activity to the parent compound. Both molecules are bound more than 99% to plasma proteins. It does not penetrate the CSF.[30]

Indications

This drug has become the standard treatment for lymphocutaneous sporotrichosis, as well as for mild or moderately severe histoplasmosis, blastomycosis and paracoccidioidomycosis and also in certain types of chromoblastomycosis.[20] The development of newer and more effective antifungal agents like voriconazole has relegated itraconazole to second-line therapy during the treatment of invasive aspergillosis (IA). Itraconazole is licensed in the United States only for salvage therapy of IA.[26] It is also approved for allergic bronchopulmonary aspergillosis.[26] Oral formulations are dosed in adults at 200 mg 3 times daily for 3 days, then 200 mg once or twice daily thereafter.[40]

Adverse Effects and Drug Interactions

The adverse effects include gastrointestinal symptoms (<10%), headache, dizziness, raised hepatic transaminases (5%), menstrual disorders, peripheral neuropathy and allergic reactions (2%).[45,46] The patients on high doses of itraconazole for prolonged periods are reported to have cardiac failure.[7] It is metabolized in liver and is a substrate and strong inhibitor of CYP3A4.[30] An important drug interaction is reduced bioavailability of itraconazole when taken with rifamycins.[12]

Voriconazole

The spectrum of this drug is similar to that of itraconazole, which also extends to several emerging molds, including *Fusarium* spp. and *Scedosporium* spp. with the exception of Zygomycetes.[47,48] It also has in vitro activity against many fluconazole resistant *Candida* spp.[49]

Pharmacokinetics

Genetic variability in metabolism plays an important role in pharmacokinetic variability of voriconazole. Polymorphism in CYP2C-19 encoding gene results in 3 populations of patients who are classified as extensive metabolizers of voriconazole, moderate metabolizers and poor metabolizers. This has led to different rates of nonlinear voriconazole clearance despite the administration of same fixed daily dose. The poor metabolism genotype is more common in patients of Asian or Pan-pacific origin (14–19%) than in patients of African origin or whites (2%).[50] It is formulated as tablets or as a sulfobutyl-ether cyclodextrin (SBECD) solution for IV administration. SBECD and voriconazole dissociate in plasma and follow their own disposition. The cyclodextrin molecule undergoes renal clearance. There are the chances of accumulation of the vehicle in individuals with renal insufficiency.[26]

Significant accumulation of SBECD occurs with a creatinine clearance below 50 mL/minute. As the toxicity of SBECD at high plasma concentration is unclear, oral voriconazole is preferred in azotemic patients.[14] Bioavailability is 96% after oral administration as either tablet or solution. Oral absorption is reduced by 22% when taken with food, while fatty food reduces bioavailability by 80%.[30] The volume of distribution is good (4.6 L/kg), protein binding of the drug is 56%. It is widely distributed in mammalian tissues, with the CSF levels of equivalent to 50% in plasma levels. The elimination half-life is around 6 hours, which warrants twice-daily dosing.[26]

Indications

It is licensed for the primary treatment of invasive aspergillosis and has been compared with AMB in a nonblinded trial.[51] Significantly, more patients experienced adverse effects with AMB than with voriconazole.[7] Voriconazole is as effective as fluconazole, but less well tolerated in the treatment of esophageal candidiasis.[52] It is also approved for use as salvage therapy in patients with *Scedosporium* and *Fusarium* infections.[14] Penicilliosis marneffei also responds well to voriconazole.[53]

Treatment is usually started with IV infusion of 6 mg/kg every 12 hours for 2 doses, followed by 4 mg/kg every 12 hours. It should be administered at 3 mg/kg/hour, not as a bolus. After improvement, the drug is continued as 200 mg every 12 hours. If there is no response, it may be given as 300 mg every 12 hours. It is available as 50 or 200 mg tablets or a suspension of 40 mg/mL when hydrated. Oral drug should be given either 1 hour before or 1 hour after meals, as the bioavailability of the drug is reduced by high fat meals.[14] Pediatric patients are known to hypermetabolize voriconazole and for this reason, an IV dose of 7 mg/kg twice daily and oral dosing of 200 mg twice daily without loading is recommended.

Adverse Effects and Drug Interactions

Voriconazole is usually well tolerated. The most common adverse effects include transient visual disturbances with an incidence of 20–23%, which are mainly characterized by photopsia, blurred vision and color changes 30 minutes to 1 hour after dosing. Other adverse effects include hepatotoxicity, which may be dose limiting and is manifested by elevated serum bilirubin, alkaline phosphatase and hepatic aminotransferase enzyme levels; skin rash (usually in sunlight exposed areas).[54] QTc prolongation and torsades de pointes should be a consideration in patients with predisposing factors.

Coadministration with rifampin, rifabutin or ritonavir is contraindicated because of accelerated voriconazole metabolism. The dose of voriconazole should be doubled when coadministered with phenytoin, cyclosporine, tacrolimus, rifabutin and warfarin. Coadministration with sirolimus is contraindicated, as voriconazole increases its area under curve by 11-fold.[14]

Posaconazole

It is an orally-active, extended spectrum triazole.[55] It is insoluble in water and no IV formulation has yet been developed. It is administered as a cherry-flavored suspension using polysorbate 80 as the emulsifying agent. It has a broad spectrum of antifungal activity against molds like *Aspergillus* spp., zygomycetes like *Rhizopus, Absidia*; dimorphic fungi like blastomyces, coccidioides and *Histoplasma* spp.; *Fusarium* spp. and dermatophytes like *Trichophyton* spp.; and yeasts, e.g. *Candida* spp., *Cryptococcus* spp. This drug is active against *Candida* spp. isolates that exhibited resistance to other triazoles like fluconazole, itraconazole and voriconazole.

It is available only as a suspension for oral use. It has now also been approved as 100 mg delayed-release tablet by FDA.[56]

Absorption is increased when taken with food, especially with fatty meals. Each dose of posaconazole should be administered with a full meal or with a liquid nutritional supplement in patients who cannot eat a full meal. Moreover, oral absorption is better in divided daily doses and optimal when administered four times daily. It exhibits not only linear kinetics, but also saturable absorption; thus, oral loading doses are not possible. It has large volume of distribution indicating extensive tissue penetration and is highly plasma protein bound (>98%), predominantly to albumin. It undergoes hepatic metabolism and minimal glucuronidation. Renal clearance plays a minor role in its clearance. It is predominantly eliminated unchanged by the fecal-oral route.[9]

Indications

It is approved for the prevention of invasive aspergillosis and *Candida* infections in patients aged ≥13 years who are at high risk of developing these infections due to the severely immunocompromised state, such as graft versus host disease (GVHD) in hematopoietic stem cell transplant (HSCT) patients and also in patients with hematological malignancies with prolonged neutropenia from chemotherapy; it can also be used as salvage therapy for refractory invasive aspergillosis.[57,58]

It is administered as an oral suspension for prophylaxis in the dose of 200 mg three times daily. The duration of therapy is based on recovery from neutropenia or immunosuppression. The dosage for salvage treatment is 800 mg administered in two or four divided doses. Improved efficacy is seen with higher posaconazole levels.[57] It is administered in the dose of 100 mg daily or up to 400 mg twice daily for oropharyngeal candidiasis, which is refractory to fluconazole and itraconazole.[59]

Table 7 New triazoles on the frontline

Drug	*Route*	*Spectrum*	*Advantages*	*Disadvantages*
Isavuconazole	Oral and intravenous	*Candida* spp., *Aspergillus* spp., Dermatophytes	Broad spectrum, water soluble (no need for cyclodextrin), long acting (allows OD up to once-weekly dosing), drug tolerability favorable, limited drug interaction	Submitted to FDA by Astellas as a new drug application[62]
Ravuconazole	Oral and intravenous	Similar to isavuconazole and also: *Cryptococcus* spp., *Chaetomium* spp., *Trypanosoma cruzi*	Long-acting drug similar to very isavuconazole	Potential for cross-resistance with other azoles
Albaconazole	Oral	*Candida* spp., *Aspergillus* spp., *Paecilomyces* spp., *Cryptococcus* spp., *Malassezia* spp., *Trypanosoma cruzi*	*Broad spectrum, good pharmacokinetics excellent oral bioavailability azoles*	*Low concentration achieved in the CSF, Potential for cross-resistance with other*

Adverse Effects and Drug Interactions

It is usually a well-tolerated drug and the safety profile seems to be more favorable than that of voriconazole. The most frequent adverse effects are headache, GI complaints like nausea, diarrhea and vomiting (3–12% each in several studies).[57-60] Others include transaminase elevation and hyperbilirubinemia occurring in 3%.[57] QTc prolongation was reported to be as high as 4% in one study.[58] The safety of posaconazole has not been evaluated in children under 13 years old.[30]

Newer Triazoles

Despite the incoming of new effective drugs, there are several therapeutic problems, such as new pathogenic fungal species; slow microbiological diagnosis; variable drug bioavailability; toxicity, lack of oral or IV preparations; significant drug interactions for some agents; the development of resistance; and breakthrough infections. Several newer triazoles are in the advanced stages of development to address some of these problems **(Table 7)**.

ANTIMETABOLITES/NUCLEOSIDE ANALOGS

Flucytosine (5 FC; ANCOBON)

Flucytosine has been used to treat candidiasis and other invasive mycoses since 1968.[61] Although not used as monotherapy, 5 FC can be used as an adjunct to AMB or azoles in the treatment of hematogenous candidiasis because of the rapid emergence of resistance when used alone.[63] It has clinically useful activity against *Cryptococcus neoformans*, *Candida* spp., and the agents of chromoblastomycosis.[14]

It is currently available in only in an oral formulation. More than 90% of the drug is absorbed after an oral dose. The peak plasma concentration is achieved within 1–2 hours. It is poorly protein bound and has a good penetration into all the body fluid compartments, including CSF.[12] The half-life of the drug is 3–6 hours in normal individuals. The half-life may be as long as 200 hours in patients having renal failure.[14] The adverse effects are rare if peak levels are kept below 100 µg/mL.[64] Adverse effects like nausea, diarrhea, hepatotoxicity and bone marrow suppression are reversible on discontinuation of the drug.[64] Cytarabine reduces 5 FC levels, hence, caution must be employed when used with other myelosuppressive drugs.[7]

The combination of AMB with 5 FC has been shown to be effective in randomized controlled trials of patients with cryptococcal meningitis. It is given orally at 100 mg/kg/day, in four divided doses at 6 hour interval. Dosage should be adjusted for decreased renal function.[14] It is also recommended, in combination, in patients having endophthalmitis, meningitis and endocarditis due to *Candida* spp.[37]

Broad spectrum, good low concentration achieved in pharmacokinetics, excellent the CSF, potential for cross-oral bioavailability resistance with other azoles.

Echinocandins

The newest class of antifungal drugs is the echinocandins. They are the only ones that target the fungal cell wall by inhibiting β-1, 3-D glucan polymers which are the key cross-linking structural components of the cell wall **(Fig. 1)**. These drugs are effective against clinically relevant yeasts and molds.[65]

Pharmacokinetics

They are synthetically modified lipopeptides. The molecular weight of all three echinocandins is large, which explains their poor oral absorption. All echinocandins have linear kinetics following single-dose IV administration, and have a terminal half-life of 8–13 hours, so once a day usage is appropriate.[66] They are slowly metabolized in the liver by nonenzymatic peptide hydrolysis and/or N-acetylation to inactive low molecular weight products. A lower dose (35 mg/day) is recommended in patients with hepatic insufficiency. Micafungin is metabolized by nonoxidative metabolism within the liver and anidulafungin undergoes nonenzymatic degradation within the kidney. Both these agents undergo fecal excretion. These agents do not require dose adjustment with hepatic impairment.[67] The concentration of these drugs is almost negligible in CSF, vitreous and urine.[68] The efficacy of echinocandins is predicted by peak to minimum inhibitory concentration (MIC) ratios. Optimal fungicidal activity is obtained when peak concentrations exceed MICs by 5–10 fold.[67] Echinocandin resistance is uncommon, but may develop during therapy.[68]

A number of in vitro studies have shown a "paradoxical effect" of echinocandins. This refers to the growth of echinocandin-susceptible organisms at highly elevated drug concentrations, far in excess of the MIC (>16 µg/mL) showing break through growth. However, a normal susceptibility pattern is seen with a typical low MIC.[69] The exact mechanism has not been fully elucidated and the clinical significance remains uncertain.[70]

Adverse Effects and Drug Interactions

Caspofungin is generally well tolerated. The most frequent adverse effects include phlebitis/thrombophlebitis, fever, chills, headache, nausea, vomiting, abdominal pain, diarrhea and rash.[71] Caspofungin is a poor substrate for the Cytochrome P450 enzyme, so a fewer drug interactions occur with it.[65] Daily caspofungin dose should be increased, when administered along with inducers of hepatic metabolism like phenytoin, rifampicin, carbamazepine and dexamethasone. Tacrolimus blood concentration is reduced by 26% when coadministered with caspofungin. Monitoring of tacrolimus blood concentration is essential and the dosage should be adjusted accordingly.

Indications

These drugs have broad-spectrum antifungal activity against *Candida* and *Aspergillus* spp. without cross-resistance to existing antifungal agents and are effective against azole-resistant yeasts and molds.[65,72] They are highly effective on biofilms.[73] They are less active against zygomycetes, *Cryptococcus neoformans* or *Fusarium* spp.[65]

These drugs have excellent safety and tolerability profiles with few drug-related adverse events, which make them attractive options for various fungal infections over other available antifungals.[9] Caspofungin is licensed for the treatment of invasive candidiasis in non-neutropenic adults. It is as effective as AMB in the treatment of candidemia and is also better tolerated.[74] It has its use in the treatment of patients with esophageal candidiasis and is as effective as AMB and fluconazole.[75,76] Caspofungin can be prescribed in patients of invasive aspergillosis, who are refractory to or intolerant to AMB, lipid formulations of AMB and/or itraconazole.[77] For the empirical treatment of presumed fungal infections in patients with febrile neutropenia, caspofungin (50 mg once daily, followed by a loading dose of 70 mg on the first day) is no less effective than liposomal AMB (3 mg/kg once daily).[78]

Micafungin (100 mg IV daily) has been compared to L-AMB 3 mg/kg IV daily in an international, double-blind trial for candidemia and invasive candidiasis. The patients were assigned to IV treatment of 14 days and successful treatment was equivalent in each group. There were less adverse events with micafungin than there were with L-AMB.[79]

Anidulafungin MIC required to inhibit the growth of 90% of organisms (MIC90) value for *C. albicans* clinical isolates is generally lower than 0.5 µg/mL.[80] Also, the isolates of *C. parapsilosis* are susceptible to anidulafungin, but not to caspofungin or micafungin (MIC90 values 2 mg/L, 8 mg/L and 16 mg/L, respectively).[81] Anidulafungin, also, has in vitro activity against *Candida* spp., growing as biofilms making it a useful addition to the Italian therapeutic armamentarium.[82] Intravenous dosing regimens for invasive candidiasis with the three compounds are as follows: Caspofungin loading dose of 70 mg and 50 mg daily thereafter, anidulafungin loading dose of 200 mg and 100 mg daily thereafter, and micafungin, 100 mg daily.[40]

Candida and *Aspergillus* spp. (Predominantly *C. albicans* and *A. fumigates*) are two of the most common pathogenic fungi and are associated with significant morbidity and mortality in certain patient groups (e.g. neutropenic patients receiving cancer chemotherapy or patients undergoing stem cell transplantation). Mortality rates of up to 95% are being reported in rapidly progressive IA.[83] However, there has been an increased incidence of less common non-*Aspergillus* molds that include zygomycetes, *Fusarium* spp., and *Scedosporium* spp.[84] Reflecting a key need, important advances have been made in the antifungal armamentarium with the availability of lipid formulations of AMB, triazoles and echinocandins. As the number of patients exposed to echinocandin therapy broadens, the chances for the resistance will also increase.

MISCELLANEOUS ANTIFUNGALS[86,87]

Nystatin, a polyene antifungal is too toxic for parenteral administration and is mainly used topically for the suppression of local candidal infection. Imidazoles like clotrimazole, miconazole, econazole and others are used for superficial mycoses. Systemic use of ketoconazole has fallen out of clinical use because of its nonselective inhibition of cytochrome P450. Griseofulvin is used only in the systemic treatment of dermatophytoses and has been largely replaced by other antifungals like itraconazole and terbinafine. Terbinafine is a synthetic allylamine, used for the treatment of dermatophytoses especially onychomycosis.

Table 8 Recommendations for therapeutic drug monitoring of antifungals

Drug	*Indications*	*Toxic level (µg/mL)*	*Goal*
5 FC	Routine during first week of therapy, renal insufficiency, lack of response to therapy	>100	10–50 µg/mL
Itraconazole	Routine during first week of therapy, lack of response to therapy, gastrointestinal dysfunction, comedication	Not established	Therapy: >1 µg/mL Prophylaxis: >0.5 µg/mL
Voriconazole	Lack of response to therapy, gastrointestinal dysfunction, comedication, children; IV to oral switch, nonlinear kinetics	>6.0	>0.5–2 µg/mL
Posaconazole	Lack of response to therapy, gastrointestinal dysfunction, comedication, variable absorption	Not established	>1.5 µg/mL

Table 9 Infectious Diseases Society of America (IDSA) recommendations for the management of fungal infections

Clinical disease	*Therapy*	
Aspergillosis	*Primary*	*Alternative*
Invasive pulmonary aspergillosis (IPA)	Voriconazole (6 mg/kg IV every 12 hours for 1day, followed by 4 mg/kg IV every 12 hours; oral dosage is 200 mg every 12 hours)	L-AMB (3–5 mg/kg/day IV), ABLC (5 mg/kg/day IV), Caspofungin (70 mg/day 1 IV and 50 mg/day IV thereafter), Posaconazole (200 mg QID initially, then 400 mg BID PO after stabilization of disease)
Invasive sinus aspergillosis	Similar to IPA	Similar to IPA
Tracheobronchial aspergillosis	Similar to IPA	Similar to IPA
Chronic necrotizing pulmonary aspergillosis (subacute IPA)	Similar to IPA	Similar to IPA
Aspergillosis of the CNS	Similar to IPA	Similar to IPA
Chronic cavitary pulmonary aspergillosis	Itraconazole or voriconazole	Similar to IPA
Allergic bronchopulmonary aspergillosis (ABPA)	Itraconazole	Oral voriconazole (200 mg PO every 12 hours) or posaconazole (400 mg PO BID)
Candidiasis	*Primary*	*Alternative*
Candidemia: Non-neutropenic adults	Fluconazole 800 mg (12 mg/kg) LD*, then 400 mg (6 mg/kg) daily or an echinocandin#	LFAmB 3–5 mg/kg daily; or AmB-d 0.5–1 mg/kg daily; or voriconazole 400 mg (6 mg/kg) bid for 2 doses, then 200 mg (3 mg/kg) bid
Candidemia: Neutropenic patients	An echinocandin# or LFAmB 3–5 mg/kg daily	Fluconazole 800 mg (12 mg/kg) LD*, then 400 mg (6 mg/kg) daily; or voriconazole 400 mg (6 mg/kg) bid for 2 doses then 200 mg (3 mg/kg) bid
Chronic disseminated candidiasis	Fluconazole 400 mg (6 mg/kg) daily for stable patients; LFAmB 3–5 mg/kg daily or AmB-d 0.5–0.7 mg/kg daily for severely ill patients; after patient is stable, change to fluconazole	An echinocandin# for several weeks followed by fluconazole
CNS candidiasis	LFAmB 3–5 mg/kg with or without 5 FC 25 mg/kg qid for several weeks, followed by fluconazole 400–800 mg (6–12 mg/kg) daily	Fluconazole 400–800 mg (6–12 mg/kg) daily for patients unable to tolerate LFAmB
Blastomycosis	*Preferred therapy*	
Moderately severe to severe pulmonary	LFAmB 3–5 mg/kg per day, or AmB-d 0.7–1 mg/kg /day for 1–2 weeks, followed by itraconazole, 200 mg bid for 6–12 months	

Contd...

Contd...

Mild-to-moderate pulmonary	Itraconazole 200 mg once or twice per day for 6–12 months	
Moderately severe to severe disseminated	LFAmB 3–5 mg/kg/day or AmB-d, 0.7–1 mg/kg/day for 1–2 weeks, followed by itraconazole 200 mg bid for 12 months	
Mild-to-moderate disseminated	Itraconazole 200 mg once or twice per day for 6–12 months	
CNS disease	LFAmB 5 mg/kg/day for 4–6 weeks is preferred, followed by an oral azole for at least 1 year	
Histoplasmosis	*Preferred treatment*	
Acute pulmonary histoplasmosis: Moderately severe or severe	LFAmB (3–5 mg/kg daily) or AmB-d (0.7–1.0 mg/kg daily) weeks, followed by Itraconazole (LD* of 200 mg 3 times daily for the first 3 days, then 200 mg twice daily for a total of 12 weeks) Methylprednisolone (0.5–1.0 mg/kg daily IV for 1–2 weeks)	
Mild-to-moderate	For symptoms of <4 weeks, none; For symptoms of >4 weeks, Itraconazole (200 mg once or twice daily for 6–12 weeks)	
Chronic cavitary pulmonary histoplasmosis	Itraconazole (LD* of 200 mg 3 times daily for the first 3 days, then 200 mg once or twice daily for at least 12 months)	
Progressive disseminated histoplasmosis: Moderately severe to severe	LAmB (3 mg/kg daily), LFAmB (5 mg/kg daily), or AmB-d (0.7–1.0 mg/kg daily) for 1–2 weeks, followed by Itra (200 mg twice daily for at least 12 months)	
Mild to moderate	Itra (200 mg twice daily for at least 12 months)	
CNS histoplasmosis	LAmB (5 mg/kg daily for 4–6 weeks), followed by Itra (LD* of 200 mg 3 times daily for the first 3 days, then 200 mg 2–3 times daily for at least 12 months)	
Sporotrichosis	*Preferred treatment*	*Alternative treatment*
Pulmonary	LFAmB 3–5 mg/kg/day, then Itraconazole 200 mg bid; or Itraconazole 200 mg bid	AmB-d 0.7–1 mg/kg/day, then Itraconazole 200 mg bid; surgical removal
Meningitis	LFAmB 5 mg/kg/day, then Itraconazole 200 mg bid	AmB-d 0.7–1 mg/kg/day, then Itraconazole 200 mg bid
Disseminated	Lipid AmB 3–5 mg/kg/day, then Itraconazole 200 mg bid	AmB-d 0.7–1 mg/kg/day, then Itraconazole 200 mg bid

*LD, Loading Dose; #Echinocandins: Doses given in the text

Agents like undecylenic acid, benzoic acid and salicylic acid (Whitfield's Ointment) are very effective in the treatment of tinea pedis.[12,14]

SPECIFIC ISSUES

Antifungals in Pregnancy

The data on the safety of antifungals for treating patients who are pregnant or lactating are limited. The agents like azoles, griseofulvin and flucytosine should not be used in pregnancy as the risks clearly outweigh the therapeutic benefit. Breastfeeding should be discouraged in women receiving these agents. Successful treatment of systemic mycoses has been documented with AMB in pregnancy with no excess toxicity to either the mother or fetus. Thus, AMB formulations have been the mainstay treatment of antifungal therapy in pregnancy.[85]

Therapeutic Drug Monitoring

There is significant interpatient variability for several available antifungal drugs and exposure-effect relationships have been demonstrated for antifungal compounds. TDM is useful to both reduce drug toxicity and optimize efficacy for the following agents. TDM, very well can be incorporated into the patient management **(Table 8)**.[86-88]

New Frontiers for Antifungal Therapy

Inhaled L-AMB has been found protective against the development of invasive aspergillosis when given twice weekly to neutropenic patients who have malignancy.[89] Lead compounds that appear promising for antimycotic therapy include nikkomycins, sordarins, lytic peptides, hydroxypyridones and cathelicidins. Other less conventional drug discovery approaches include targeting known traditional virulence factors (e.g. adhesions and secreted enzymes). This approach is based on the principle that killing of the microbe need not occur for an anti-infective agent to be efficacious in the reduction of disease.[85]

Clinical decisions about combination therapy should be based on patient-specific in vivo evaluations. Because of the limited clinical data, combination antifungal therapy should be initiated cautiously. Except for the treatment of cryptococcal meningitis and disseminated aspergillosis, combination therapy should be reserved for the cases of treatment failure (disseminated candidiasis) with no other established pharmacologic options for therapy or for mold infections with high mortality rates.[85]

CLINICAL IMPLICATIONS OF THE ANTIFUNGAL DRUGS

Pharmacotherapy of fungal disease has been revolutionized by the introduction of the newer agents. **Table 9** highlights the Infectious Diseases Society of America (IDSA) guidelines for the management of fungal infections.

REFERENCES

1. Vandeputte P, Ferrari S, Coste AR. Antifungal resistance and new strategies to control fungal infections. Int J Microbiol. 2012;2012:713687.
2. Lichtenstern C, Nguyen TH, Schemmer P, Hoppe-Tichy T, Weigand MA. Efficacy of caspofungin in invasive candidiasis and candidemia-de-escalation strategy. Mycoses. 2008;51 (Suppl 1):35-46.
3. Martin GS, Mannino DM, Eaton S, Moss M. The epidemiology of sepsis in the United States from 1979 through 2000. N Engl J Med. 2003;348(16):1546-54.
4. Meyers JD. Fungal infections in bone marrow transplant patients. Semin Oncol. 1990;17(3 Suppl 6):10-3.
5. Edwards JE. Diagnosis and treatment of fungal infections. In: Fauci AS, Braunwald E, Kasper DL, Hauser S, Longo D, Jameson J, Loscalzo J (Eds). Harrison's Principles of Internal Medicine, 17th edition. New York: McGraw Hill Companies, Inc.; 2008. pp. 1242-4.
6. Shelburne SA, Hamill RJ. Mycotic infections. In: McPhee SJ, Papadakis MA, Tierney LM (Eds). Current Medical Diagnosis and Treatment, 47th edition. USA: The McGraw-Hill Companies, Inc.; 2008. pp. 1328-38.
7. Enoch DA, Ludlam HA, Brown NM. Invasive fungal infections: a review of epidemiology and management options. J Med Microbiol. 2006;55(Pt 7):809-18.
8. Ghannoum MA, Rice LB. Antifungal agents: mode of action, mechanisms of resistance, and correlation of these mechanisms with bacterial resistance. Clin Microbiol Rev. 1999;12(4):501-17.
9. Thompson III GR, Cadena J, Patterson TF. Overview of Antifungal Agents. In: Knox KS, Sarosi GA (Guest Eds). Clinics in Chest Medicine: Fungal Diseases; 2009. pp. 203-17.
10. Chapman SW, Sullivan DC, Cleary JD. In search of the holy grail of antifungal therapy. Trans Am Clin Climatol Assoc. 2008;119:197-215.
11. Lanternier F, Lortholary O. Liposomal amphotericin B: what is its role in 2008? Clin Microbiol Infect. 2008;14(Suppl 4):71-83.
12. Sheppard D, Lampiris HW. Antifungal agents. In: Katzung BG (Ed). Basic and Clinical Pharmacology, 10th edition. McGraw-Hill Companies, Inc.; 2007. pp. 781-9.
13. Ben-Ami R, Lewis RE, Kontoyiannis DP. Immunocompromised hosts: immunopharmacology of modern antifungals. Clin Infect Dis. 2008;47(2):226-35.
14. Bennett JE. Antimicrobial agents - antifungal agents. In: Brunton LL, Lazo JS, Parker KL (Eds). Goodman and Gilmans: The pharmacological basis of therapeutics, 11th edition. New York: McGraw-Hill Medical Publishing Division; 2006. pp. 1225-42.
15. Dismukes WE. Introduction to antifungal drugs. Clin Infect Dis. 2000;30(4):653-7.
16. Chander J. Antifungal drugs. In: Chander J (Ed). Textbook of Medical Mycology, 3rd edition. New Delhi: Mehta Publishers; 2009. pp. 71-89.
17. Bekersky I, Fielding RM, Dressler DE, Lee JW, Buell DN, Walsh TJ. Pharmacokinetics, excretion and mass balance of liposomal amphotericin B (AmBisome) and amphotericin B deoxycholate in humans. Antimicrob Agents Chemother. 2002;46(3):828-33.
18. Wingard JR. Lipid formulations of amphotericins: are you a lumper or a splitter? Clin Infect Dis. 2002;35(7):891-5.
19. Gallis HA, Drew RH, Pickard WW. Amphotericin B: 30 years of clinical experience. Ref Infect Dis. 1990;12(2):308-29.
20. Branch RA. Prevention of amphotericin-B induced renal impairment: a review on the use of sodium supplementation. Arch Intern Med. 1988;148(11):2389-94.
21. (2009). Antifungal drugs. [Online]. Available from: *http://www.merck.com/mmpe/sec14/ch180/ ch180b.html.* [Accessed on April 2010].
22. Hiemenz JW, Walsh TJ. Lipid formulation of amphotericin B: recent progress and future directions. Clin Infect Dis. 1996;22 (Suppl 2):S133-44.
23. Wong-Beringer A, Jacobs RA, Guglielmo BJ. Lipid formulation of amphotericin B: clinical efficacy and toxicities. Clin Infect Dis. 1998;27(3):603-18.
24. Barrett JP, Vardulaki KA, Conlon C, Cooke J, Daza-Ramirez P, Evans EG, et al. A systematic review of the antifungal effectiveness and tolerability of amphotericin B formulations. Clin Ther. 2003;25(5):1295-320.
25. Bates DW, Su L, Yu DT, Chertow GM, Seger DL, Gomes DR, et al. Mortality and costs of acute renal failure associated with amphotericin B therapy. Clin Infect Dis. 2001;32(5):686-93.
26. Walsh TJ, Anaissie EJ, Denning DW, Herbrecht R, Kontoyiannis DP, Marr KA, et al. Treatment of aspergillosis: clinical practice guidelines of the Infectious Diseases Society of America. Clin Infect Dis. 2008;46(3):327-60.
27. Chamilos G, Lewis RE, Kontoyiannis DP. Delaying amphotericin B-based frontline therapy significantly increases mortality among patients with hematologic malignancy who have zygomycosis. Clin Infect Dis. 2008;47(4):503-9.
28. Saubolle MA, McKellar PP, Sussland D. Epidemiologic, clinical, and diagnostic aspects of coccidioidomycosis. J Clin Microbiol. 2007;45(1):26-30.
29. Phillips P, Fetchick R, Weisman I, Foshee S, Graybill JR. Tolerance to and efficacy of itraconazole in treatment of systemic mycoses: preliminary results. Rev Infect Dis. 1987;9 (Suppl 1):S87-93.
30. Zonios DI, Bennett JE. Update on azole antifungals. Semin Respir Crit Care Med. 2008;29(2):198-210.
31. Groll AH, Piscitelli SC, Walsh TJ. Clinical pharmacology of systemic antifungal agents: A comprehensive review of agents in clinical use, current investigational compounds, and putative targets for antifungal drug development. Adv Pharmacol. 1998;44:343-500.
32. Kauffman CA, Carver PL. Use of azoles for systemic antifungal therapy. Adv Pharmacol. 1997;39:143-89.
33. Perfect JR, Lindsay MH, Drew RH. Adverse drug reactions to systemic antifungals. Prevention and management. Drug Saf. 1992;7(5):323-63.

34. Brammer KW, Farrow PR, Faulkner JK. Pharmacokinetics and tissue penetration of fluconazole in humans. Rev Infect Dis. 1990;12(Suppl 3):S318-26.
35. Rex JH, Bennett JE, Sugar AM, Pappas PG, van der Horst CM, Edwards JE, et al. A randomized trial comparing fluconazole with amphotericin B for the treatment of candidemia in patients without neutropenia. Candidemia Study Group and the National Institute. N Engl J Med. 1994;331(20):1325-30.
36. Phillips P, Shafran S, Garber G, Rotstein C, Smaill F, Fong I, et al. Multicenter randomized trial of fluconazole versus amphotericin B for treatment of candidemia in non-neutropenic patients. Canadian Candidemia Study Group. Eur J Clin Microbiol Infect Dis. 1997;16(5):337-45.
37. Pappas PG, Rex JH, Sobel JD, Filler SG, Dismukes WE, Walsh TJ, et al. Guidelines for the treatment of candidiasis. Clin Infect Dis. 2004;38(2):161-89.
38. Baddley JW, Patel M, Bhavnani SM, Moser SA, Andes DR. Association of fluconazole pharmacodynamics with mortality in patients with candidemia. Antimicrob Agents Chemother. 2008;52(9):3022-8.
39. Arndt CA, Walsh TJ, McCully CL, Balis FM, Pizzo PA, Poplack DG. Fluconazole penetration into cerebrospinal fluid: implications for treating fungal infections of the central nervous system. J Infect Dis. 1988;157(1):178-80.
40. Pappas PG, Kauffman CA, Andes D, Benjamin DK Jr, Calandra TF, Edwards JE Jr, et al. Clinical practice guidelines for the management of candidiasis: 2009 update by the Infectious Diseases Society of America. Clin Infect Dis. 2009;48(5):503-35.
41. National committee for clinical laboratory standards. Reference method for broth dilution antifungal susceptibility testing of yeasts; approved standard. Document M27-A. Wayne, PA: National committee for clinical laboratory standards; 1997.
42. Johnson EM, Szekely A, Warnock DW. In-vitro activity of voriconazole, itraconazole and amphotericin B against filamentous fungi. J Antimicrob Chemother. 1998;42(6):741-5.
43. Eichel M, Just-Nubling G, Helm EB, Stille W. [Itraconazole suspension in the treatment of HIV-infected patients with fluconazole-resistant oropharyngeal candidiasis and esophagitis]. Mycoses. 1996;39(Suppl 1):102-6.
44. Lange D, Pavao JH, Wu J, Klausner M. Effect of a cola beverage on the bioavailability of itraconazole in the presence of H2 blockers. J Clin Pharmacol. 1997;37(6):535-40.
45. Vardakas KZ, Michalopoulos A, Falagas ME. Fluconazole versus itraconazole for antifungal prophylaxis in neutropenic patients with haematological malignancies: a meta-analysis of randomised-controlled trials. Br J Haematol. 2005;131(1):22-8.
46. Tucker RM, Haq Y, Denning DW, Stevens DA. Adverse events associated with itraconazole in 189 patients on chronic therapy. J Antimicrob Chemother. 1990;26(4):561-6.
47. Diekema DJ, Messer SA, Hollis RJ, Jones RN, Pfaller MA. Activities of caspofungin, itraconazole, posaconazole, ravuconazole, voriconazole and amphotericin B against 448 recent clinical isolates of filamentous fungi. J Clin Microbiol. 2003;41(8):3623-6.
48. Johnson LB, Kauffman CA. Voriconazole: a new triazole antifungal agent. Clin Infect Dis. 2003;36(5):630-7.
49. Pfaller MA, Diekema DJ, Messer SA, Boyken L, Hollis RJ, Jones RN. In vitro activities of voriconazole, posaconazole, and four licensed systemic antifungal agents against *Candida* species infrequently isolated from blood. J Clin Microbiol. 2003;41(1):78-83.
50. Desta Z, Zhao X, Shin JG, Flockhart DA. Clinical significance of the cytochrome P450 2C19 genetic polymorphism. Clin Pharmacokinet. 2002;41(12):913-58.
51. Herbrecht R, Denning DW, Patterson TF, Bennett JE, Greene RE, Oestmann JW, et al. Voriconazole versus amphotericin B for primary therapy of invasive aspergillosis. N Engl J Med. 2002;347(6):408-15.
52. Ally R, Schurmann D, Kreisel W, Carosi G, Aguirrebengoa K, Dupont B, et al. A randomized, double-blind, double-dummy, multicenter trial of voriconazole and fluconazole in the treatment of esophageal candidiasis in immunocompromised patients. Clin Infect Dis. 2001;33(9):1447-54.
53. Perfect JR, Marr KA, Walsh TJ. Voriconazole treatment for less-common, emerging, or refractory fungal infections. Clin Infect Dis. 2003;36(9):1122-31.
54. Boucher HW, Groll AH, Chiou CC, Walsh TJ. Newer systemic antifungal agents: pharmacokinetics, safety and efficacy. Drugs. 2004;64(18):1997-2020.
55. Keating GM. Posaconazole. Drugs. 2005;65(11):1553-67.
56. (2013). FDA approves new formulation of merk antifungal. [online] Drug Discovery & Development website. Available from: *http://www.dddmag.com/news/2013/11/fda-approves-new-formulation-merck-antifungal-drug*. [Accessed on January 2016].
57. Ullmann AJ, Lipton JH, Vesole DH, Chandrasekar P, Langston A, Tarantolo SR, et al. Posaconazole or fluconazole for prophylaxis in severe graftversushost disease. N Engl J Med. 2007;356(4):335-47.
58. Cornely OA, Maertens J, Winston DJ, Perfect J, Ullmann AJ, Walsh TJ, et al. Posaconazole vs. fluconazole or itraconazole prophylaxis in patients with neutropenia. N Engl J Med. 2007;356(4):348-59.
59. Vazquez JA, Skiest DJ, Nieto L. A multicenter randomized trial evaluating posaconazole versus fluconazole for the treatment of oropharyngeal candidiasis in subjects with HIV/AIDS. Clin Infect Dis. 2006;42(8):1179-86.
60. Skiest DJ, Vazquez JA, Anstead GM. Posaconazole for the treatment of azole-refractory oropharyngeal and esophageal candidiasis in subjects with HIV infection. Clin Infect Dis. 2007;44(4):607-14.
61. Tassel D, Madoff MA. Treatment of *Candida* sepsis and Cryptococcus meningitis with 5-fluorocytosine. A new antifungal agent. JAMA. 1968;206(4):830-2.
62. New antifungal as effective as existing drugs with fewer adverse effects. [online] EurekAlert website. Available from: *http://www.eurekalert.org/pub_releases/2014-09/asfm-naa090214.* php. [Accessed on October 2014].
63. Rex JH, Walsh TJ, Sobel JD, Filler SG, Pappas PG, Dismukes WE, et al. Practice guidelines for treatment of candidiasis. Infectious Diseases Society of America. Clin Infect Dis. 2000;30(4):662-78.
64. Vermes A, Guchelaar HJ, Dankert J. Flucytosine: a review of its pharmacology, clinical indications, pharmacokinetics, toxicity and drug interactions. J Antimicrob Chemother. 2000;46(2):171-9.
65. Denning DW. Echinocandin antifungal drugs. Lancet. 2003;362(9390):1142-51.
66. Balani SK, Xu X, Arison BH, Silva MV, Gries A, DeLuna FA, et al. Metabolites of caspofungin acetate, a potent antifungal agent, in human plasma and urine. Drug Metab Dispos. 2000;28(11):1274-8.

67. Dodds Ashley Es LR, Lewis JS, Martin C, Andes D. Pharmacology of systemic antifungal agents. Clin Infect Dis. 2006;43(s1):S28-39.
68. Thompson GR, Wiederhold NP, Vallor AC, Villareal NC, Lewis JS 2nd, Patterson TF. Development of caspofungin resistance following prolonged therapy for invasive candidiasis secondary to *Candida glabrata* infection. Antimicrob Agents Chemother. 2008;52(10):3783-5.
69. Perlin DS. Resistance to echinocandin-class antifungal drugs. Drug Resistance Updat. 2007;10(3):121-30.
70. Wiederhold NP. Attenuation of echinocandin activity at elevated concentrations: a review of the paradoxical effects. Curr Opin Infect Dis. 2007;20(6):574-8.
71. Randhawa GK, Sharma G. Echinocandins: a promising new antifungal group. Indian J Pharmacol. 2004;36(2):65-71.
72. Morrison VA. Echinocandin antifungals: review and update. Expert Rev Anti Infect Ther. 2006;4(2):325-42.
73. Bachmann SP, VandeWalle K, Ramange G, Patterson TF, Wickes BL, Graybill JR, et al. In vitro activity of caspofungin against *Candida albicans* biofilms. Antimicrob Agents Chemother. 2002;46(11):3591-6.
74. Mora-Duarte J, Betts R, Rotstein C, Colombo AL, Thompson-Moya L, Smietana J, et al. Comparison of caspofungin and amphotericin B for invasive candidiasis. N Engl J Med. 2002;347(25):2020-9.
75. Villanueva A, Arathoon EG, Gotuzzo E, Berman RS, DiNubile MJ, Sable CA, et al. A randomized double-blind study of caspofungin versus amphotericin for the treatment of candidal esophagitis. Clin Infect Dis. 2001;33(9):1529-35.
76. Villanueva A, Gotuzzo E, Arathoon EG, Noriega LM, Kartsonis NA, Lupinacci RJ, et al. A randomized double-blind study of caspofungin versus fluconazole for the treatment of esophageal candidiasis. Am J Med. 2002;113(4):294-9.
77. Maertens J, Raad I, Petrikkos G, Boogaerts M, Selleslag D, Petersen FB, et al. Efficacy and safety of caspofungin for treatment of invasive aspergillosis in patients refractory to or intolerant of conventional antifungal therapy. Clin Infect Dis. 2004;39(11):1563-71.
78. Walsh TJ, Teppler H, Donowitz GR, Maertens JA, Baden LR, Dmoszynska A, et al. Caspofungin versus liposomal amphotericin B for empirical antifungal therapy in patients with persistent fever and neutropenia. N Engl J Med. 2004;351(14):1391-402.
79. Kuse ER, Chetchotisakd P, da Cunha CA, Ruhnke M, Barrios C, Raghunadharao D, et al. Micafungin versus liposomal amphotericin B for candidaemia and invasive candidiasis: a phase III randomised double-blind trial. Lancet. 2007;369(9572):1519-27.
80. Pfaller MA, Boyken L, Hollis RJ, Kroeger J, Messer SA, Tendolkar S, et al. In vitro susceptibility of invasive isolates of *Candida* spp. to anidulafungin, caspofungin, and micafungin: six years of global surveillance. J Clin Microbiol. 2008;46(1):150-6.
81. Ghannoum MA, Chen A, Buhari M, Chandra J, Mukherjee PK, Baxa D, et al. Differential in vitro activity of anidulafungin, caspofungin and micafungin against *Candida* parapsilosis isolates recovered from a burn unit. Clin Microbiol Infect. 2009;15(3):274-9.
82. Morace G, Borghi E, Iatta R, Montagna MT. Anidulafungin, a new echinocandin: in vitro activity. Drugs. 2009;69(Suppl 1): 91-4.
83. McCormack PL, Perry CM. Caspofungin: a review of its use in the treatment of fungal infections. Drugs. 2005;65(14):2049-68.
84. Bhatti Z, Shaukat A, Almyroudis NG, Segal BH. Review of epidemiology, diagnosis, and treatment of invasive mould infections in allogeneic hematopoietic stem cell transplant recipients. Mycopathologia. 2006;162(1):1-15.
85. Cleary JD, Stanley W, Pearson CM. Fungal infections. In: Koda-Kimble MA, Young LY, Alldredge BK, et al (Eds). Applied Therapeutics: The Clinical Use of Drugs, 9th edition. Philadelphia: Williams and Wilkins; 2008. pp. 71-128.
86. Smith J, Andes D. Therapeutic drug monitoring of antifungals: pharmacokinetic and pharmacodynamic considerations. Ther Drug Monit. 2008;30(2):167-72.
87. Andes D, Pascual A, Marchetti O. Antifungal therapeutic drug monitoring: established and emerging indications. Antimicrob Agents Chemother. 2009;53(1):24-34.
88. Antifungal Drug Monitoring. Why, When, and How to Measure Serum Concentrations. Available from: *http://www.mayomedicallaboratories.com/articles/communique/2010/11.html*. [Accessed on September 2014].
89. Rijnders BJ, Cornelissen JJ, Slobbe L, Becker MJ, Doorduijn JK, Hop WC, et al. Aerosolized liposomal amphotericin B for the prevention of invasive pulmonary aspergillosis during prolonged neutropenia: a randomized, placebo-controlled trial. Clin Infect Dis. 2008;46(9):1401-8.

14 Chapter

Immunosuppressant Drugs

Nusrat Shafiq, Samir Malhotra

INTRODUCTION

Immunosuppressant drugs are mainly used in the treatment of disorders in which autoimmunity has an important role, some malignancies and for prevention of transplantation rejection. There are four main classes of immunosuppressant drugs: glucocorticoids, calcineurin inhibitors, antiproliferative or antimetabolite drugs, and biologics (antibodies). These are briefly discussed herein, particularly, with reference to their role in pulmonary disorders.

GLUCOCORTICOIDS

Most aspects of glucocorticoids have been discussed in the chapter on antiasthma drugs. Their role as immunosuppressants is known since the 1960s.[1] The exact mechanism(s) behind their immunosuppressant actions is (are) unknown **(Box 1)**. These actions make steroids one of the most effective immunosuppressants and anti-inflammatory drugs. Most of their effects are seen on cell-mediated immunity, they have no or little effect on humoral immunity.

Alone, or in combination with other immunosuppressant drugs, steroids are used in the treatment of interstitial lung diseases, vasculitides, sarcoidosis, asthma, and other allergic disorders (including drug-induced). They are also used in the management of several other autoimmune disorders such as rheumatoid arthritis, other arthritic disorders, systemic lupus erythematosus (SLE), dermatomyositis, psoriasis, other serious dermatological disorders, inflammatory bowel disease, many disorders of the eye, autoimmune disorders of blood, multiple sclerosis, and many other life-threatening disorders. Steroids also constitute the core management of transplant rejection. Prednisone, commonly used as an immunosuppressive agent, is converted to active prednisolone in the body. It is well-absorbed from the gastrointestinal tract (GIT), conveniently given once daily in the usual dose of 1 mg/kg/day and tapered once there is clinical improvement. In many disorders, including in post-transplant cases, it is continued lifelong. It should be taken with food to minimize GI toxicity. In order to mimic the circadian rhythm, administration between 7 a.m. and 8 a.m. is recommended. Methylprednisolone is used in high doses (1 g/day IV) for three days in a month in various immunosuppressive protocols. High doses of methylprednisolone are routinely required for preventing acute graft rejection.

The most important adverse effects of steroids include hypertension, dyslipidemia, hyperglycemia, osteoporosis, avascular necrosis of bone, poor wound healing, increased risk of infections, cataract and growth retardation in children.

BOX 1 Proposed mechanisms for immunosuppressant anti-inflammatory actions of steroids

- Redistribution of lymphocytes leading to decreased lymphocytes in peripheral blood
- Transcription of various genes involved in immune processes
- Decreased activation of nuclear factor kappa-light-chain-enhancer of activated B cells (NF-kappa B) leading to increased apoptosis of activated cells[2]
- Decreased production of interleukin-2 (IL-2) by T lymphocytes
- Downregulation of proinflammatory cytokines (IL-1, IL-6)
- Inhibition of proliferation of T lymphocytes cells
- Inhibition of activation of cytotoxic T lymphocytes
- Decreased neutrophils or monocyte-induced chemotaxis
- Decreased lysosomal enzyme release

CALCINEURIN INHIBITORS

Calcineurin is a protein that activates T lymphocytes. Calcineurin inhibitors (cyclosporine, tacrolimus and pimecrolimus) are among the most efficacious immunosuppressant drugs **(Flow chart 1)**.

Cyclosporine

Cyclosporine is an 11 amino acid cyclic polypeptide obtained from fungus *Beauveria nivea*. It forms a complex with an immunophilin (cyclophilin) and inhibits T cell responses **(Flow chart 1)**. When administered orally, it is slowly and incompletely (20–50%) absorbed. Food has variable effects

Flow chart 1 The calcineurin pathway and site of action of calcineurin inhibitors

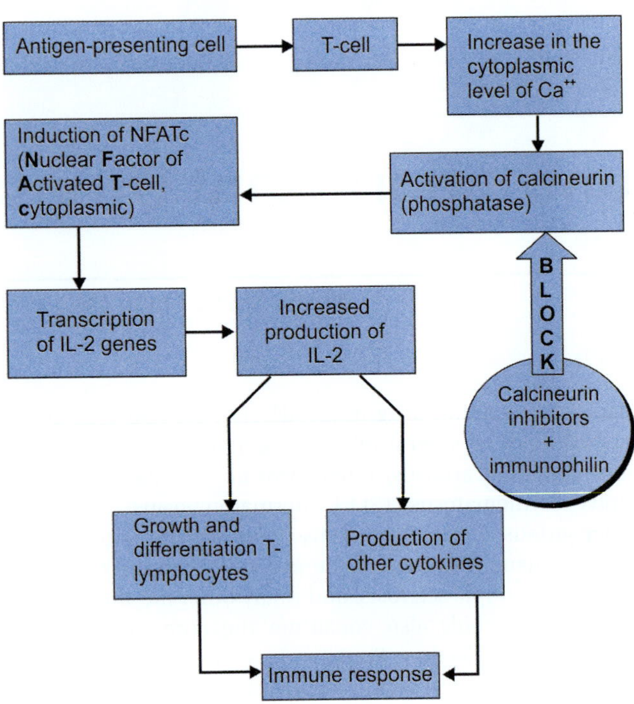

on its absorption. The various oral preparations, which are available in the market, may not be bioequivalent, hence, it is not advisable to switch brands without expert supervision and plasma level monitoring. The absorption also depends on the presence of bile, leading to considerable interpatient and intrapatient variability. The microemulsion formulation of cyclosporine forms a microemulsion spontaneously with aqueous fluids in the GIT, making it less dependent on bile for absorption. The intravenous (IV) formulation in castor oil needs to be diluted in 5% dextrose or normal saline before injection.

It is extensively metabolized by the hepatic CYP3A, the metabolites are eliminated by the kidneys. Its half-life is 5–18 hours with a considerable interindividual variation. Because of this variation, toxicity and specialized use in transplant patients, monitoring of blood levels is recommended. The best time to obtain sample is just before the next dose (trough concentration) or at a designated time point after drug administration, 2-hour postdose sample has been proposed as a better option.[3]

The daily doses of cyclosporine are different for transplant patients from those with autoimmune disorders. In the treatment of most autoimmune disorders, the usual initiating oral dose is 2.5–5 mg/kg/day in two divided doses, which is reduced once remission is achieved to the lowest effective maintenance dose.[4] In most cases, it is not recommended to continue treatment if there is insufficient response within 6–8 weeks. The IV doses are one-third of oral, given by slow infusion over 2–6 hours.

The pulmonary uses include refractory asthma, sarcoidosis and diffuse parenchymal lung disease. In refractory asthma (in doses of 5 mg/kg/day), it has been shown to improve lung function, decreased frequency of exacerbation, and enable reduction in doses of steroids.[5,6] Adverse effects limit its usefulness.[7] The evidence for its use in sarcoidosis and diffuse parenchymal lung disease is limited. It has also been given by inhalation in the management of acute graft rejection in lung transplantation in doses of 300 mg/day via a nebulizer.[8] One case-control study has shown aerosolized cyclosporine to improve survival among lung transplant recipients with bronchiolitis obliterans.[9] A randomized controlled trial showed that prophylactic use of inhaled cyclosporine did not have a beneficial effect on the rate of acute rejection, but improved chronic rejection-free survival and overall survival.[10]

Renal dysfunction, which may be due to arteriolar constriction, is an important complication of cyclosporine. Hypertension, hyperlipidemia, tremors, hyperuricemia, hirsutism, and gum hyperplasia are the other important adverse effects. It can also lead to GI disturbances, fatigue, hepatotoxicity, headache, hyperkalemia, hypomagnesemia, paresthesias, muscle cramps, anemia, weight gain, infections, edema, thrombocytopenia, rash, pancreatitis, neuropathy, anaphylaxis and anaphylactoid reactions, hyperglycemia, and increased incidence of infections and some tumors (particularly lymphoma, skin cancer and Kaposi's sarcoma).[11]

Because of the risk of anaphylaxis, it is recommended that patients should be "under continuous observation for at least the first 30 minutes following the start of the infusion and at frequent intervals thereafter".[12] In case of anaphylaxis, the infusion should be stopped and epinephrine administered.

It has a large number of pharmacokinetic drug-drug interactions. CYP3A inhibitors (verapamil, nicardipine, fluconazole, ketoconazole, erythromycin, glucocorticoids, HIV protease inhibitors and grapefruit juice) can increase its blood concentration whereas CYP3A inducers (nafcillin, rifampin, carbamazepine, phenobarbital, phenytoin, octreotide, ticlopidine, St John's wort) decrease its blood concentrations.

Because of the large number of adverse effects it also has a number of pharmacodynamic drug interactions. Sirolimus and cyclosporine potentiate each other's adverse effects. Nonsteroidal anti-inflammatory drugs (NSAIDs) and other nephrotoxic agents lead to additive nephrotoxicity. It increases the blood levels of methotrexate, digoxin and statins. There also is the increased risk of myopathy and rhabdomyolysis with statins. Hyperkalemia may occur with the concomitant use of potassium-sparing diuretics and potassium supplements. The risk of gingival hyperplasia may be increased, if used along with amlodipine or nifedipine. It may also reduce the efficacy of live vaccines.

Tacrolimus

Tacrolimus is a macrolide antibiotic produced by *Streptomyces tsukubaensis*. It inhibits T-cell activation by inhibiting calcineurin, but acts on a different immunophilin [FK binding proteins-12 (FKBP-12)] than cyclosporine. Gastrointestinal absorption after oral administration is incomplete (20–25%) and variable and food (particularly high fat). It is extensively metabolized by the hepatic CYP3A4 and excreted in feces with a half-life of about 12–16 hours.

Like cyclosporine, it is used for the prophylaxis of solid-organ allograft rejection and for rescue therapy in patients with rejection episodes despite "therapeutic" levels of cyclosporine.[13]

It can be used in autoimmune diseases, but experience with its use is limited. It is currently approved in some countries for the refractory cases of myasthenia gravis, rheumatoid arthritis and lupus nephritis, if steroids are contraindicated. Tacrolimus-releasing stents are commonly used in cardiology to reduce restenosis after coronary artery stent placement.

The adverse effect profile and pharmacokinetic interactions are similar to those of cyclosporine.

ANTIPROLIFERATIVE OR ANTIMETABOLIC DRUGS

Sirolimus

Discovered by an Indian scientist, Dr Suren Sehgal, sirolimus is a macrocyclic lactone produced by *Streptomyces hygroscopicus.* After oral administration, sirolimus is rapidly, but incompletely (15%) absorbed.

Sirolimus is indicated for the prevention of organ transplant rejection in combination with a calcineurin inhibitor and glucocorticoids.[14] In patients experiencing or at high risk for calcineurin inhibitor-associated nephrotoxicity, sirolimus has been used with glucocorticoids and mycophenolate mofetil to avoid permanent renal damage.[1] It is also being evaluated in autoimmune diseases. Sirolimus-releasing stents are used to reduce restenosis after coronary artery stent placement and in peripheral arteries to reduce ischemia in severe claudication. It is well-known that transplant recipients on immunosuppressant drugs are susceptible to the development of malignancies; there is some evidence to show that sirolimus, coupled with the discontinuation of immunosuppressant drugs, may not only lead to reduced incidence of malignancies, but may also cause tumor regression as seen in the case of Kaposi's sarcoma.[15]

Everolimus

Everolimus is a derivative of sirolimus and resembles it in most aspects. Its indications and adverse effects are similar to sirolimus.

Azathioprine

Azathioprine, a 6-mercaptopurine derivative, is an immunosuppressive antimetabolite drug. It is a purine analog, gets converted to a sham nucleotide 6-thioinosine monophosphate (thio-IMP) and inhibits T lymphocytes **(Flow chart 2)**. Azathioprine is well-absorbed from the GIT after oral administration. It is rapidly (half-life 10 minutes) metabolized to active mercaptopurine, which is further broken down to many active metabolites having longer half-lives (5 hours).

Flow chart 2 Mechanism of the action of azathioprine

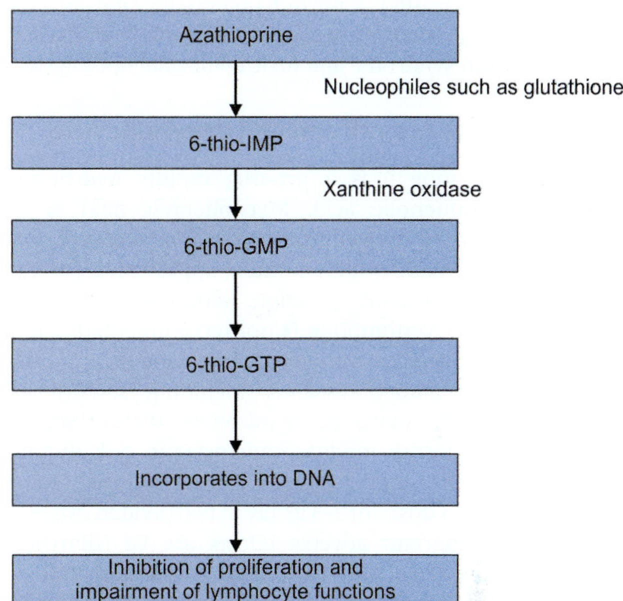

Abbreviations: Thio-IMP, thioinosine monophosphate; thio-GMP, thio-guanosine monophosphate; thio-GTP, thio-guanosine-5'-triphosphate; DNA, deoxyribonucleic acid

Azathioprine is used as an adjunct in autoimmune disorders, such as the interstitial lung disorders and for prevention of organ transplant rejection. Its effects may not be seen for several weeks after administration, but if there is no improvement in 12 weeks, it may be discontinued. The starting dose for the prevention of organ rejection is 3–5 mg/kg/day. For autoimmune disorders the recommended dose is 1 mg/kg/day. It is generally used orally, but may also be given by IV infusion over 30–60 minutes after dilution in normal saline or 5% dextrose. Blood counts and liver function tests should be regularly monitored and it should be withdrawn or the dose reduced if blood counts show a downward trend.

The major side effect of azathioprine is dose-related bone marrow suppression, which is generally reversible. It commonly manifests with leukopenia, thrombocytopenia is less common, anemia is uncommon, and agranulocytosis, pancytopenia or aplastic anemia is rare. Other adverse effects are the GI disturbances, fever, rigors, rash, muscle and joint pains, pneumonitis, pancreatitis, tachycardia, hepatotoxicity (mainly cholestatic), renal dysfunction, hypotension, reversible alopecia, pancreatitis, and increased susceptibility to malignancies and infections (especially varicella and herpes simplex viruses). Rare but potentially fatal adverse effects include the occurrence of veno-occlusive liver disease, Stevens-Johnson syndrome and toxic epidermal necrolysis.

Mycophenolate Mofetil and Mycophenolic Acid

Mycophenolate mofetil is a prodrug rapidly hydrolyzed to active mycophenolic acid. Mycophenolic acid is an immunosuppressant derived from *Penicillium stoloniferum*. It is used along with other immunosuppressants for the prevention of transplant rejection, although its use in combination with azathioprine is not recommended.[16] It is also being investigated in various autoimmune or immune-mediated inflammatory diseases, including sarcoidosis, scleroderma, SLE, vasculitic syndromes (Churg-Strauss syndrome, polyarteritis nodosa, microscopic polyangiitis, Takayasu's arteritis, and Wegener's granulomatosis), some others. It is used in doses of 2–3 g/day in two divided doses.

The most important adverse effects are GI (diarrhea, vomiting; hemorrhage and perforation) and hematologic (leukopenia, thrombocytopenia and anemia). There is an increased incidence of infections [particularly cytomegalovirus (CMV) sepsis] and malignancies (particularly skin cancer). Aplastic anemia and bone marrow depression may also occur and sometimes fatal.

IMMUNOSUPPRESSIVE CYTOTOXIC DRUGS

Drugs discussed in this category are cytotoxic antimetabolites used mainly as antineoplastic agents, but also possess immunosuppressive effects.

Methotrexate

It is an antimetabolite of folic acid. It acts by competitively inhibiting the enzyme dihydrofolate reductase, which is needed for the formation of tetrahydrofolate. It is rapidly absorbed from the GIT after oral, as well after intramuscular administration. Its half-life is 3–10 hours, but increases (8–15 hours) after high-dose administration. It is excreted primarily by the kidneys.

The main indications are the induction and maintenance of remission in acute lymphoblastic leukemia, non-Hodgkin's lymphomas, and solid neoplasms like choriocarcinoma. Among autoimmune disorders it is used in psoriasis, rheumatoid arthritis, asthma,[17] sarcoidosis,[18] SLE, vasculitic syndromes and others. It has steroid-sparing action in some of these diseases. It is also used to prevent graft-versus-host disease after bone marrow transplantation. The most commonly used dose is 15 mg/m^2 once or twice weekly in malignancies and 7.5–20 mg once weekly in other disorders.

Bone marrow depression (leukopenia, thrombocytopenia and anemia) and GI toxicity (oral ulcers, stomatitis, diarrhea, hemorrhagic enteritis and intestinal perforation) are the common dose-related adverse effects. Hepatotoxicity is the next important adverse effect and cirrhosis can also occur. Folinic acid is given to counter some of the adverse effects of methotrexate, particularly on bone marrow (folinic acid rescue).

Salicylates, other NSAIDs, probenecid, and some penicillins decrease its renal excretion leading to increased chances of methotrexate toxicity. Cotrimoxazole or trimethoprim co-administration can cause severe methotrexate toxicity. Concomitant use of other drugs having bone marrow, renal or hepatic toxicity may further increase the risk. Folic acid and its derivatives may decrease its efficacy despite the fact that they are used together to reduce methotrexate toxicity.

Cyclophosphamide

It is an antineoplastic drug belonging to the class of alkylating agents and also has immunosuppressant action. It is used in the treatment of non-Hodgkin's lymphomas, many other cancers and autoimmune diseases.

Chlorambucil

It is an antineoplastic drug that belongs to the class of alkylating agents. Its immunosuppressive properties are sometimes utilized in the treatment of autoimmune disorders like sarcoidosis, amyloidosis and Behçet's syndrome. Its major adverse effects include bone marrow suppression, GI symptoms, azoospermia, amenorrhea, pulmonary fibrosis, seizures, dermatitis and hepatotoxicity.

Because of the risks associated with chronic use of immunosuppressants, patients should be regularly monitored for malignancies and infections **(Table 1)**.

MISCELLANEOUS IMMUNOSUPPRESSANTS

Thalidomide

Introduced many decades ago as a hypnotic, it was found to have immunomodulating actions, but its mechanism of action remains unclear. Thalidomide has been used in several autoimmune diseases like graft-versus-host disease, recurrent aphthous stomatitis in severely and terminally immunocompromised patients (HIV-associated wasting syndrome), AIDS-related Kaposi's sarcoma, treatment of the clinical manifestations of both tuberculous and nontuberculous mycobacterial infection, myelodysplastic syndrome, primary brain malignancies, sarcoidosis, Behçet's syndrome, inflammatory bowel disease, SLE, refractory rheumatoid arthritis and several others. Its major adverse effect is its teratogenic potential for which it was withdrawn in the 1960s. The other adverse effects include peripheral neuropathy, venous thromboembolism, constipation, dizziness, orthostatic hypotension and toxic epidermal necrolysis.

Table 1 Monitoring of patients for malignancies and infections

Drug	*Safety monitoring schedule*
Glucocorticoids	Hematology, glucose, RFT, LFT, lipid profile, eye examination: Every 3–6 months
Calcineurin inhibitors (cyclosporine, tacrolimus)	Hematology, glucose, RFT, LFT, lipid profile: Every 2–3 months Serum calcium, phosphate, magnesium: Every 2–3 months Lipid profile: Every 6 months
Sirolimus or Everolimus	Hematology, glucose, RFT, LFT, lipid profile: Every 2–3 months Body weight: Every 2–3 months Lipid profile: Every 6 months Urine: Every 6 months
Azathioprine	Hematology, glucose, RFT, LFT, lipid profile: Every 2–3 months Lipid profile: Every 6 months
Mycophenolate mofetil	Hematology, glucose, RFT, LFT, lipid profile: Every 2–3 months Lipid profile: Every 6–12 months
Methotrexate	Hematology, glucose, RFT, LFT, lipid profile: Every 2–3 months Lipid profile: Every 6–12 months
Cyclophosphamide or chlorambucil	Hematology, glucose, RFT, LFT, lipid profile: Every month Lipid profile: Every 6 months Urine: Every 6 months

Abbreviations: RFT, renal function tests; LFT, liver function tests

Leflunomide

It is an immunosuppressant antiproliferative mainly used as a disease-modifying drug in the treatment of rheumatoid arthritis. It has been tried in other arthritides like psoriatic arthritis and has been investigated in solid tumors, Crohn's disease and ankylosing spondylitis.

In conclusion, the drugs discussed in this chapter have revolutionized the area or organ transplantation and have made significant contribution to the treatment of diseases that have autoimmune or autoimmune-inflammatory components. Most of the times, several drugs are used together. Importantly, these toxic drugs having a large number of serious adverse effects since they inhibit most of the immune responses nonspecifically leading to increased susceptibility to infections and malignancies. Moreover, many of these drugs are nephrotoxic, diabetogenic and suppress bone marrow. Nevertheless, it is possible to use them sometimes lifelong, relatively safely, provided proper care is taken with respect to adverse drug reactions.

Biological Agents: Interleukin-2 Receptor Antagonists

Two monoclonal antibodies, basiliximab and daclizumab exert their immunosuppressive effect by binding to the alpha chain (CD25) on the surface of activated T-lymphocytes. This binding prevents the proliferation of T-cells. "Muromonab" is a murine monoclonal antibody to the CD3 receptor on mature human T-cells (OKT3). It has been used as an induction therapy in transplant patients. "Alemtuzumab" has been approved for use in B-cell chronic lymphocytic leukemia, its role as an immunosuppressant is increasingly being recognized. Administration of alemtuzumab causes complete lymphocyte depletion. Alemtuzumab, when given as an induction agent along with reduced maintenance doses of immunosuppressants in lung transplant patients led to comparable early survival, rejection and infection rates as compared to conventional high-dose immunosuppression regimens.[19] "Abatacept" has been approved for the treatment of patients with moderate-to-severe rheumatoid arthritis. "Sotrastaurin" is being evaluated primarily in renal transplant patients. Some early studies have also shown efficacy in autoimmune diseases like psoriasis.[20]

REFERENCES

1. Krensky AM, Vincenti F, Bennett WM. Immunosuppressants, tolerogens, and immunostimulants. In: Brunton LL, Lazo JS, Parker KL (Eds). The Pharmacological Basis of Therapeutics, 11th edition. New York: McGraw-Hill; 2006.
2. Auphan N, DiDonato JA, Rosette C, Helmberg A, Karin M. Immunosuppression by glucocorticoids: inhibition of NF-kappa B activity through induction of I kappa B synthesis. Science. 1995;270(5234):286-90.
3. Cole E, Maham N, Cardella C, Cattran D, Fenton S, Hamel J, et al. Clinical benefits of neoral C2 monitoring in the long-term management of renal transplant recipients. Transplantation. 2003,75(12):2086-90.
4. Schreiber SL, Crabtree GR. The mechanism of action of cyclosporin A and FK506. Immunol Today. 1992;13(4):136-42.
5. Alexander AG, Kay AB, Barnes NC. Trial of cyclosporin in corticosteroid-dependent chronic severe asthma. Lancet. 1992;339(8789):324-8.
6. Lock SH, Kay AB, Barnes NC. Double-blind, placebo-controlled study of cyclosporin A as a corticosteroid-sparing agent in corticosteroid-dependent asthma. Am J Respir Crit Care Med. 1996;153(2):509-14.
7. Evans DJ, Cullinan P, Geddes DM, et al. Cyclosporin as an oral corticosteroid sparing agent in stable asthma. Cochrane Database Syst Rev. 2001;2:CD002993.
8. Corcoran TE. Inhaled delivery of aerosolized cyclosporine. Adv Drug Deliv Rev. 2006;58(9-10):1119-27.
9. Iacono AT, Corcoran TE, Griffith BP, Grgurich WF, Smith DA, Zeevi A, et al. Aerosol cyclosporin therapy in lung transplant recipients with bronchiolitis obliterans. Eur Respir J. 2004;23(3):384-90.
10. Iacono AT, Johnson BA, Grgurich WF, Youssef JG, Corcoran TE, Seiler DA, et al. A randomized trial of inhaled cyclosporine in lung-transplant recipients. N Engl J Med. 2006;354(2):141-50.
11. Penn I. Cancers following cyclosporine therapy Transplantation. 1987;43(1):32-5.
12. Novartis Pharmaceuticals Corporation. Products (Sandimmune®). [online] Available from *www.pharma.us.novartis.om/product/pi/pdf/sandimmune.pdf.* [Accessed January, 2016].

13. Mayer AD, Dmitrewski J, Squifflet JP, Besse T, Grabensee B, Klein B, et al. Multicenter randomized trial comparing tacrolimus (FK506) and cyclosporine in the prevention of renal allograft rejection: a report of the European Tacrolimus Multicenter Renal Study Group. Transplantation. 1997;64(3):436-43.
14. Kahan BD, Julian BA, Pescovitz MD, Vanrenterghem Y, Neylan J. Sirolimus reduces the incidence of acute rejection episodes despite lower cyclosporine doses in Caucasian recipients of mismatched primary renal allografts: a phase II trial. Rapamune Study Group. Transplantation. 1999;68(10): 1526-32.
15. Stallone G, Schena A, Infante B, Di Paolo S, Loverre A, Maggio G, et al. Sirolimus for Kaposi's sarcoma in renal-transplant recipients. N Engl J Med. 2005;352(13):1317-23.
16. Kimball JA, Pescovitz MD, Book BK, Norman DJ. Reduced human IgG anti-ATGAM antibody formation in renal transplant recipients receiving mycophenolate mofetil. Transplantation. 1995;60(12):1379-83.
17. Marin MG. Low-dose methotrexate spares steroid usage in steroid-dependent asthmatic patients: a meta-analysis. Chest. 1997;112(1):29-33.
18. Baughman RP, Lower EE. A clinical approach to the use of methotrexate for sarcoidosis. Thorax. 1999;54(8):742-6.
19. Van Loenhout Kc, Groves SC, Galazka M, Sherman B, Britt E, Garcia J, et al. Early outcomes using alemtuzumab induction in lung transplantation. Interact Cardiovasc Thorac Surg. 2010;10(2):190-4.
20. Sommerer C, Zeier M. AEB071—a promising immunosuppressive agent. Clin Transplant. 2009;23(Suppl 21):15-8.

Section 4

Symptom Approach to Respiratory Disease

Richard S Irwin

15 Chapter

Cough in the Adult

Scott E Kopec, Abduljabbar Dheyab, Richard S Irwin

INTRODUCTION

Coughing is an important reflex that helps protect the lungs from the aspiration of upper airway secretions and from inhaled particles and irritants. It is also an important mechanism for clearing airway secretions. When coughing becomes excessive, it can potentially be the primary symptom for a wide variety of pathological conditions. The symptom of cough is common, and it results in significant costs to the healthcare system. Cough is a frequent symptom for many life-threatening diseases, and it can negatively impact a patient's lifestyle and the sense of well-being. Therefore, it is vital for healthcare professionals to understand the etiologies and effective treatments for cough.

The format of this chapter, and its contents, are updates to material that we have previously published on the subject of cough.[1-3]

EPIDEMIOLOGY

Cough is one of the most common symptoms for which patients seek medical attention.[4,5] Questionnaires estimate the prevalence of cough to be between 9% and 33% of the population in the US and Europe.[6,7] A survey in rural India reported a prevalence of cough in patients seeking medical attention to be about 3%.[8]

From March 2012 to March 2013, over $6.8 billion were spent in the US for over-the-counter cough treatments alone.[5] If one adds to this the cost of prescription medications to treat cough, the cost of physician visits, and the lost production in the workplace due to cough, the overall costs are staggering, with estimates approaching $40 billion annually.[9] In addition, there are other costs to the patient. Patients with cough are viewed by the public as being unhealthy, or having a potentially contagious disease. This in turn may result in a patient feeling isolated, embarrassed, or maligned by society. The negative impact that chronic cough has on a patient's quality of life is well documented.[10]

PHYSIOLOGY

There are cough receptors in the hypopharynx, larynx, trachea, bronchi, and probably the esophagus, that when triggered, start the cough reflex. These receptors are either chemical receptors or mechanical receptors.[11-13] Cough can be induced by stimulating the chemical receptors with stimuli such as inflammatory mediators and acid. The mechanical receptors can be stimulated by vibration and temperature. Multiple afferent nerves carry the impulse from the sensory receptors to the brainstem, where the cough response is coordinated. The major afferent nerves are C-fibers, which are located throughout the upper and lower airways and the lungs. In addition to the C-fibers, cough can be triggered by the stimulation of vagal afferent nerves, or a group of receptors called rapidly adapting receptors (RARs). The RARs are mechanoreceptors that respond to physical forces associated with lung inflation and deflation.[14]

The coughing mechanism is divided into three phases. The first phase is the inspiratory phase, which is marked by a deep inspiration. This phase is followed by the compressive phase when the glottis closes, resulting in rising intrathoracic pressure. Finally, the expiratory phase occurs with the sudden opening of the glottis. With an effective cough, expiratory velocities can reach up to 28,000 cm/second (500 mph).[15]

PATHOPHYSIOLOGY

One of the major functions of cough is to clear excessive secretions from the airway when mucociliary function is not adequate. When the cough is not adequate to serve this purpose, complications such as gas exchange abnormalities, atelectasis, pneumonia and bronchiectasis, can occur. Clinical disorders that minimize the effectiveness of cough interfere with either the inspiratory or the expiratory phase, or both. What these clinical disorders have in common is an association with the insufficient strength of the respiratory muscles. Some conditions associated with ineffective cough

BOX 1 Conditions associated with an ineffective cough[1]

Pulmonary disorders
- Asthma, bronchiectasis, chronic obstructive pulmonary disease (COPD), cystic fibrosis, tracheal lesions (extrinsic compression, intraluminal masses, strictures), tracheobronchomegaly

Extrapulmonary disorders
- Paralysis or muscle weakness (cervical or upper thoracic spinal cord injuries, Guillain-Barré syndrome, amyotrophic lateral sclerosis, polymyositis, botulism)
- Pain (rib fractures, postoperative from chest or abdomen surgery)
- Central depression of cough center (drugs, strokes)
- Upper airway obstruction (vocal cord paralysis, laryngeal masses) associated with an ineffective cough.[16] At the bedside, an ineffective cough can be predicted if the patient is unable to, or can barely cough on command.

are listed in **Box 1**.[1] It is estimated that maximal expiratory pressures of less than 40 cm H_2O are associated with an ineffective cough.

BENEFITS OF COUGH

The main benefit of coughing is airway clearance. This benefit is especially important in conditions where the normal mucociliary clearance is overwhelmed such as pneumonia. Not only is coughing beneficial in clearing mucus from the airways, it is also important in protecting the lung from retaining inhaled particles and irritants such as the aspiration of upper airway and gastrointestinal (GI) secretions. Finally, coughing is beneficial in preventing atelectasis that might occur after intubation, general anesthesia, and surgery. Cough has been demonstrated to be highly effective in cardiopulmonary resuscitation, a technique called cough cardiopulmonary resuscitation. In conscious patients with asystole, profound bradycardia and ventricular tachycardia, coughing can convert the patient back to sinus rhythm.[17] Coughing can help support blood pressure and maintain consciousness in patients in ventricular fibrillation, asystole, or high-degree heart block. Forceful coughing at 1-second intervals for 30–90 seconds is commonly employed in the cardiac catheterization laboratory in patients who develop arrhythmias as might occur during contrast injection into the coronary arteries. Studies have demonstrated that vigorous coughing can elevate systolic blood pressures to near 140 mm Hg, compared to systolic pressures of about 75 mm Hg generated with well performed chest compressions.[18]

COMPLICATIONS OF COUGH

During the expiratory phase of vigorous coughing, intrathoracic pressures can reach as high as 300 mm Hg.[19] Therefore, it should come as no surprise that these extreme thoracic pressures can result in numerous complications. **Box 2** lists some of the most common complications of severe coughing.[1,2,20] While coughing can be beneficial in elevating systolic blood pressure, severe coughing can also result in hypotension, most likely due to decreased central venous return that in turn can result in near-syncope or syncope. Patients with cough-induced urinary or fecal incontinence face additional embarrassment that can further worsen their quality of life and self-esteem. In postoperative patients, severe coughing can place the patient at risk for wound dehiscence. Patients undergoing surgeries, such as hernia repair or cataract surgery should have their coughs controlled before surgery in an effort to avoid intraoperative or postoperative complications.

BOX 2 Complications of severe coughing or chronic cough*[1,2,20]

Constitutional
Fatigue or exhaustion, excessive sweating, anorexia

Neurological
Syncope or near syncope, headache, dizziness, seizure, stroke, cerebral air embolism, acute cervical radiculopathy

Cardiovascular
Hypotension, nasal and anal vein rupture, brady- and tachyarrhythmias

Respiratory
Exacerbations of asthma or chronic obstructive pulmonary disease (COPD), lung herniation, pneumothorax, pneumomediastinum, bronchial rupture

Gastrointestinal or Abdominal
Vomiting, gastroesophageal reflux, Mallory-Weiss tears, hernias, splenic rupture, fecal incontinence

Genitourinary
Urinary incontinence, bladder prolapse, vaginal prolapse

Skin or Ophthalmological
Petechiae or purpura, disruption of surgical wounds, subconjunctival or intraocular hemorrhage

Musculoskeletal
Rib fractures, diaphragmatic rupture, costochondritis, pulled or torn chest wall muscles

Psychological
Depression, fear of serious disease, lifestyle changes, decreased self-confidence

**This box includes the most common causes in each category and is not meant to be exhaustive.*

CAUSES OF COUGH

Many diseases and conditions are associated with cough as a symptom. Cough can be the major symptom for disease processes that are of minor consequence, such as the common cold, or the major symptom of life-threatening conditions, such as a pulmonary embolism. A useful way to categorize many causes of cough is to divide them up based on the duration of the cough. For example, acute cough is defined as lasting less than three weeks, subacute cough as lasting between 3 weeks and 8 weeks, and chronic cough as lasting

BOX 3 Common causes of cough, separated into these three groups*

Acute cough (<3 weeks)

Upper respiratory infections (viral, sinusitis) allergic rhinitis, pneumonia, exacerbations of asthma and chronic obstructive pulmonary disease (COPD), congestive heart failure, lung cancer, pulmonary embolism, acute bronchitis, acute environmental exposures (dusts, chemicals)

Subacute cough (3–8 weeks)

Upper respiratory infections, *Bordetella pertussis* infections, exacerbations of asthma, COPD, and bronchiectasis

Chronic cough (> 8 weeks)

Upper airway cough syndrome (UACS), asthma, gastroesophageal reflux disease (GERD), angiotensin-converting-enzyme (ACE) inhibitors, nonasthmatic eosinophilic bronchitis (NAEB), chronic bronchitis, bronchiectasis, lung cancer, sarcoidosis, tuberculosis, somatic cough syndrome, tic cough, unexplained cough.

**This table includes the most common causes in each category and is not meant to be exhaustive.*

more than 8 weeks. **Box 3** lists the most common causes of cough, separated into these three groups.[1,2,20] One should note that several conditions, such as asthma can present as acute, subacute, or chronic cough. Of these groups, acute cough contains the widest spectrum of diseases, including most of the life-threatening conditions.

Acute bronchitis is a condition manifested by cough, with or without phlegm, which lasts for less than 3 weeks.[21] However, it is a diagnosis of exclusion, as conditions that cause identical symptoms, such as pneumonia, asthma and COPD exacerbations, and the common cold, have to be ruled out. Respiratory viruses most commonly cause acute bronchitis, and the routine use of antibiotics is not recommended.[21,22] Antitussive agents may provide some short-term symptomatic relief, and inhaled bronchodilators are sometimes used when patients have wheezing in addition to the cough. If a patient with suspected acute bronchitis does not have resolution of their cough after 3 weeks, an alternative diagnosis should be investigated (see subacute cough below).

The most common cause of a subacute cough is post-infectious cough, especially from infections with *Bordetella pertussis.* Subacute cough from an infection with *B. pertussis* should be considered in patients with cough-induced vomiting, and in patients with the classic whoop (a stridorous sound during inspiration that follows a prolonged episode of coughing). This condition, as well as exacerbations of asthma, bronchiectasis, and chronic bronchitis should be considered when patients present with a biphasic course (cough worsens after appearing to improve).

The most common causes of chronic cough in patients with normal chest radiographs are upper airway cough syndrome (UACS) [previously known as postnasal drip (PND) syndrome], asthma, gastroesophageal reflux disease (GERD), angiotensin-converting-enzyme (ACE) inhibitor-induced cough, nonasthmatic eosinophilic bronchitis (NAEB) (similar to atopic cough that has been described in Japan), and bronchiectasis. These six disorders account for nearly 95% of all the causes of chronic cough. In addition, patients often have more than one cause contributing to their chronic cough.

Work-up and Management of Acute Cough

A complete history and physical examination is most helpful in determining the cause of acute cough. PND and throat clearing with the associated symptoms of nasal congestion, rhinorrhea and sneezing suggest an upper airway cause such as the common cold or allergic rhinitis. Symptoms of chest tightness, wheezing, or dyspnea in a patient with a history of asthma or COPD suggest an exacerbation of these diseases as the cause of the acute cough. Some associated symptoms or signs should raise concern to a potentially life-threatening cause of the acute cough. Patients complaining of fever, chest pain, orthopnea, or hemoptysis with their cough, or who are found to have crackles, focal rhonchi, or an S3 gallop, require further testing, such as a chest radiograph looking for conditions, including pneumonia, congestive heart failure or cancer. We recommend following the diagnostic algorithm published by the American College of Chest Physicians (ACCP) for the work-up of acute cough **(Flow chart 1)**.[3]

Work-up and Management of Subacute Cough

The most common cause of subacute cough is postinfectious. Infections that can leave the patient with a subacute cough include viral upper respiratory infections, such as the common cold, lower respiratory tract infections from respiratory syncytial virus (RSV), and infections with *B. pertussis*. The majority of patients with cough from an uncomplicated common cold will have their cough resolve within 3 weeks. On the other hand, a high index of suspicion is needed to confirm a diagnosis of *B. pertussis*. While the classic "whoop" may be absent in adults, symptoms of vomiting caused by severe cough episodes suggest a *B. pertussis* infection. During the first two weeks of a *B. pertussis* infection, patients will have upper respiratory tract symptoms suggestive of a common cold, associated with an intermittent nonproductive cough, and sometimes fever. This is known as the catarrhal stage. After approximately two weeks, the patient enters the paroxysmal phase, in which the classic coughing is the hallmark. Protracted episodes of cough-induced vomiting can result in dehydration. This phase typically peaks after 2–3 weeks, but the cough may persist for 2–3 months, or longer. The last phase, called the convalescent phase, is marked by less common paroxysmal coughing. During this phase a patient may develop worsening of the paroxysmal coughing if exposed to irritants or another upper respiratory infection.

Flow chart 1 An algorithm for the work-up of acute cough in the adult

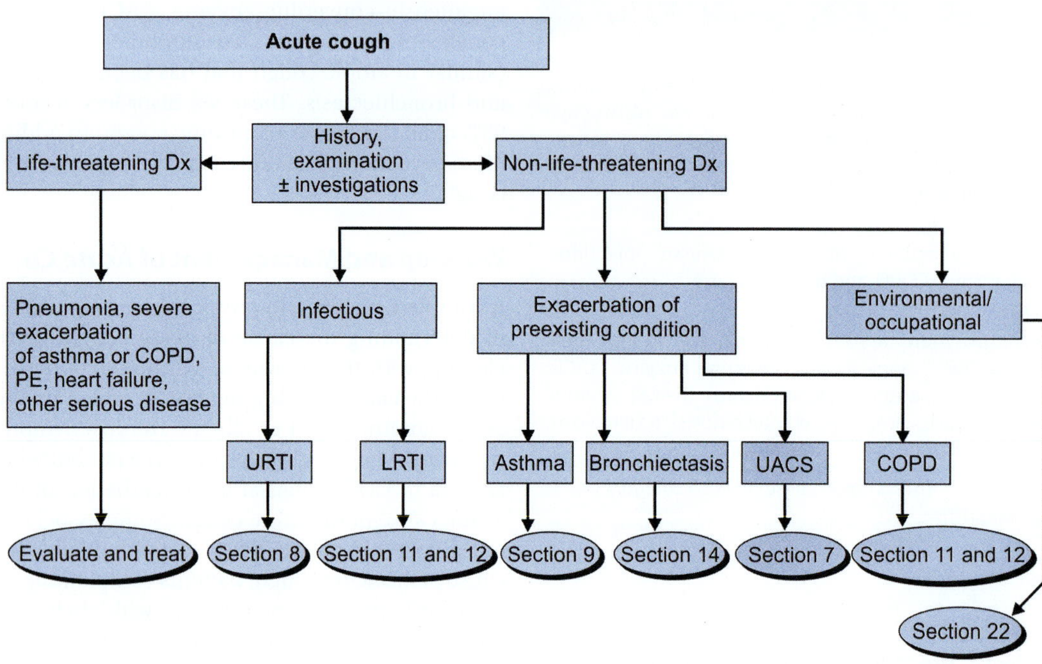

Source: The sections denoted in the algorithm refer the reader to the corresponding sections in the American College of Chest Physician Cough Guidelines, Chest. Reproduced with permission from Irwin RS, Baumann MH, Bolser DC, Boulet LP, Braman SS, Brightling CE, et al. Diagnosis and management of cough executive summary: ACCP evidence-based clinical practice guidelines. Chest. 2006;129(Suppl 1):1-23.
Abbreviations: Dx, diagnosis; COPD, chronic obstructive pulmonary disease; PE, pulmonary embolism; URTI, upper respiratory tract infection; LRTI, lower respiratory tract infection; UACS, upper airway cough syndrome

Common laboratory findings are nonspecific, but may include leukocytosis and an elevated absolute lymphocyte count (>10,000 cells/μL).[23] Diagnosis of pertussis can be confirmed by the isolation of the organism from nasopharyngeal secretions. However, while this has a 100% specificity, the sensitivity of the culture within the first 3 weeks of symptoms can be as low as 15–45%.[24] In addition, culture sensitivity decreases with the duration of the infection.[25] Polymerase chain reaction (PCR) for *B. pertussis* appears to have a higher sensitivity, ranging from 65% to 97%.[25,26] As with the cultures, the sensitivity of the PCR decreases with duration of the infection.[25] Direct fluorescent antibody (DFA) can provide rapid detection of *B. pertussis*, but the sensitivity and specificity are inferior to cultures and PCR. Because no single test has 100% sensitivity, the US Centers for Disease Control (CDC) recommends both cultures and PCR.[27] The CDC has also established guidelines for the method of collecting specimens and the method of testing.[27]

Treatment for *B. pertussis* includes antibiotics, either a microlide or trimethoprim or sulfamethoxazole[28] in the macrolide allergic patient. While quinolones have *in vitro* activity against *B. pertussis*, studies supporting their use are lacking. Some authors also suggest the addition of oral corticosteroids.[29] If patients are treated within eight days of the onset of symptoms, antibiotics are effective at decreasing the severity of the illness and decreasing the risk of exposing other patients. Prophylactic antibiotics are also recommended for people exposed to patients with whooping cough.

Some conditions that cause acute cough can also present as a subacute cough if there is a delay in the patient receiving medical attention. COPD and asthma exacerbations, congestive heart failure, lung cancer, and infections such as tuberculosis (TB) are examples of conditions that can present as either an acute or subacute cough. We recommend following the diagnostic algorithm published by the ACCP for the work-up of subacute cough **(Flow chart 2)**.[3]

Work-up and Management of Chronic Cough

When evaluating a patient with chronic cough, it is best to use a systematic approach such as that published by the ACCP **(Flow chart 3)**.[3] When starting with the history, the character, timing, and quality of the cough are often not helpful in determining the etiology. Factors that are important include: whether the patient is an active smoker; if the patient is taking an ACE inhibitor; if the patient lives in the area where TB or other fungal diseases are endemic; if the patient has a history of cancer, TB, AIDS; and if the patient has systemic symptoms such as fever, night sweats, or weight loss. Other associated symptoms potentially may be helpful. For example, episodic

Flow chart 2 Algorithm for the work-up of subacute cough in the adult

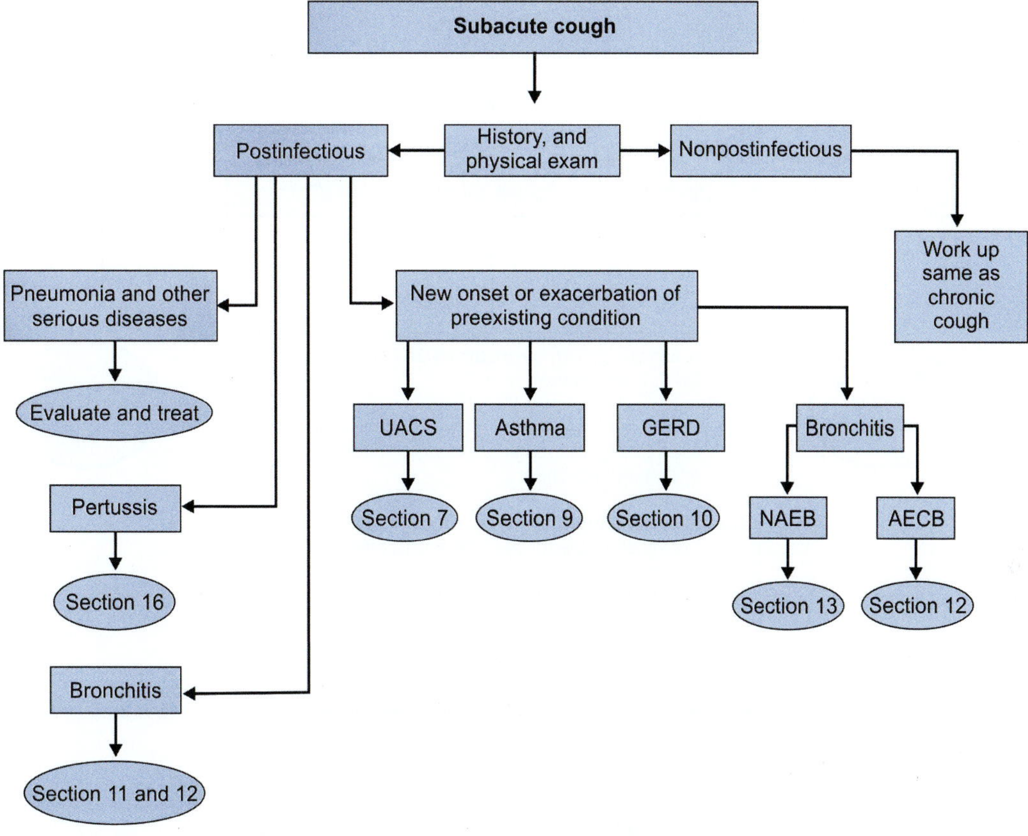

Source: The sections denoted in the algorithm refer the reader to the corresponding sections in the American College of Chest Physician Cough Guidelines, Chest. Reproduced with permission from Reproduced with permission from Irwin RS, Baumann MH, Bolser DC, Boulet LP, Braman SS, Brightling CE, et al. Diagnosis and management of cough executive summary: ACCP evidence-based clinical practice guidelines. Chest. 2006;129 (Suppl 1):1-23.

Abbreviations: UACS, upper airway cough syndrome; GERD, gastroesophageal reflux disease; NAEB, nonasthmatic eosinophilic bronchitis; AECB, acute exacerbation of chronic bronchitis

wheezing, dyspnea, and chest tightness might suggest asthma or COPD, but wheezing alone can also be seen in patients with both asthma and UACS. Other potentially helpful associated symptoms and history will be discussed below with the specific conditions that cause chronic cough. If patients also describe coughing up blood, we suggest following the recommendations in the chapter on hemoptysis.

After a complete history is obtained, a thorough physical examination should be performed. While there are no specific exam findings that are pathognomonic for a specific cause of chronic cough, some findings can help in suggesting a condition contributing to the cough. For example, observing mucopurulent secretions in the oropharynx suggests UACS due to suppurative upper airway disease, while diffuse wheezing might suggest asthma.

One of the most important tests to order when evaluating a patient with chronic cough is a chest radiograph. When the chest radiograph is abnormal and shows more than inconsequential scarring, the abnormality should be felt to be contributing to the patient's cough until proven otherwise. For example, if the chest radiograph demonstrates findings consistent with congestive heart failure, sarcoidosis, or malignancy, further work-up for these conditions followed by the appropriate treatments should be preferentially pursued. One must also keep in mind, however, that an abnormality on chest radiograph may not be associated with the patient's chronic cough (e.g. solitary pulmonary nodule), or the patient may have an additional condition contributing to their cough. In these cases, further investigation, specifically investigating the common causes of chronic cough should be performed, once the conditions suggested by the abnormality have been addressed and the patient continues to complain of cough.

For patients with normal chest radiographs who are not active smokers or taking an ACE inhibitor, the differential diagnosis for chronic cough significantly narrows to one or more of the following: UACS, asthma, GERD, chronic

Flow chart 3 Algorithm for the work-up of chronic cough in the adult

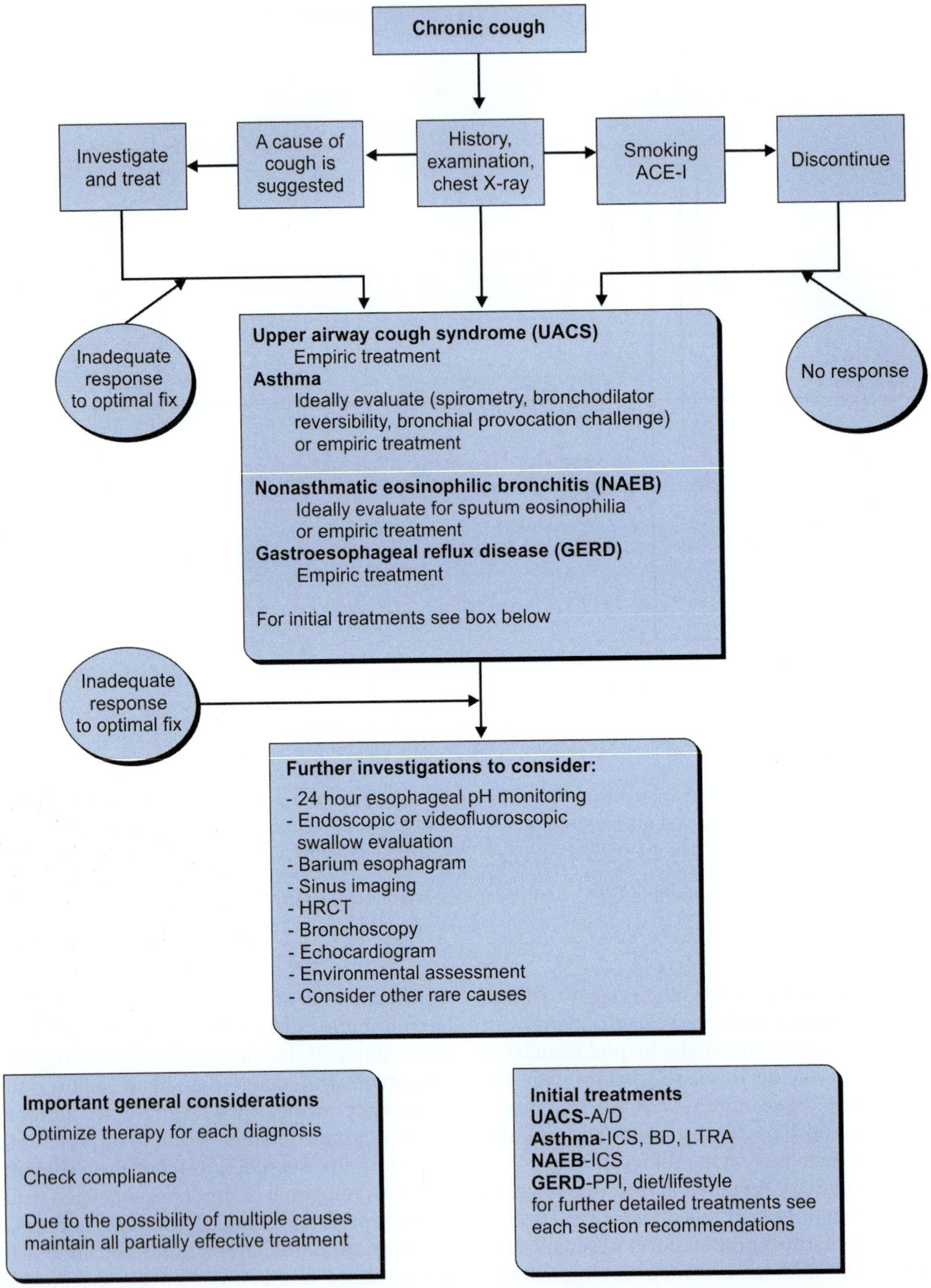

Chronic cough

History, examination, chest X-ray

A cause of cough is suggested → Investigate and treat

Smoking ACE-I → Discontinue

Inadequate response to optimal fix

No response

Upper airway cough syndrome (UACS)
Empiric treatment
Asthma
Ideally evaluate (spirometry, bronchodilator reversibility, bronchial provocation challenge) or empiric treatment

Nonasthmatic eosinophilic bronchitis (NAEB)
Ideally evaluate for sputum eosinophilia or empiric treatment
Gastroesophageal reflux disease (GERD)
Empiric treatment

For initial treatments see box below

Inadequate response to optimal fix

Further investigations to consider:
- 24 hour esophageal pH monitoring
- Endoscopic or videofluoroscopic swallow evaluation
- Barium esophagram
- Sinus imaging
- HRCT
- Bronchoscopy
- Echocardiogram
- Environmental assessment
- Consider other rare causes

Important general considerations
Optimize therapy for each diagnosis

Check compliance

Due to the possibility of multiple causes maintain all partially effective treatment

Initial treatments
UACS-A/D
Asthma-ICS, BD, LTRA
NAEB-ICS
GERD-PPI, diet/lifestyle
for further detailed treatments see each section recommendations

Source: The sections denoted in the algorithm refer the reader to the corresponding sections in the American College of Chest Physician Cough Guidelines, Chest. Reproduced with permission from Irwin RS, Baumann MH, Bolser DC, Boulet LP, Braman SS, Brightling CE, et al. Diagnosis and management of cough executive summary: ACCP evidence-based clinical practice guidelines. Chest. 2006;129(Suppl 1):1-23.
Abbreviations: ACE-I, angiotensin-converting-enzyme inhibitor; HRCT, high-resolution computed tomography; A/D, anti-histamines/decongestants; BD, bronchodilator; LTRA, leukotriene receptor antagonist; ICS, inhaled corticosteroid; PPI, proton-pump inhibitors

bronchitis from environmental irritants such as cigarette smoke or smoke from using biomass fuels, NAEB, and bronchiectasis. In the US and many other parts of the world, such as southeast Asia, UACS, asthma, and GERD are the cause(s) of chronic cough in over 92% of nonsmokers who are not on an ACE inhibitor and who have a normal chest radiographic appearance.[30] Even in areas where TB is endemic, these three conditions tend to be the most common causes of chronic cough.[31] As mentioned earlier, these entities may coexist and the cause of chronic cough may be multifactorial. At least 25% of patients with chronic cough have more than one potential cause.[30] It is also important to realize that each of these conditions may present with cough being the only symptom (silent UACS, cough-variant asthma, silent GERD). If work-up for the common causes of chronic cough is unremarkable, one should consider less common causes that account for less than 6% of cases in patients with normal chest radiographs such as bronchogenic carcinoma, chronic interstitial pneumonia, sarcoidosis, and left ventricular failure, among others.[30]

In the initial evaluation of chronic cough in patients with normal chest radiographs, bronchoscopy has a low diagnostic yield. However, if the patient's initial evaluation is negative for UACS, asthma, NAED, and GERD, or the patient fails to respond to optimal treatment for these conditions, a bronchoscopy can yield a positive result up to 28% of the time.[1]

Here is a more detailed discussion on the most common causes of chronic cough.

Upper Airway Cough Syndrome

In the US, UACS is the most common cause of chronic cough in immunocompetent adults. Patients usually complain of a throat "tickle" or a need to clear the throat, and nasal congestion or discharge. Symptoms may occur after a recent cold and may be accompanied by a wheeze. Approximately, 20% of patients with this condition are unaware of the presence of PND or throat clearing (silent UACS) even though they can be heard to frequently clear their throats in front of loved ones and the physician.[32] The symptoms and physical exam findings reflective of UACS are very sensitive, but not specific, and may include the evidence of nasal discharge, drainage or a cobblestone appearance of the mucosa. The diagnosis of UACS is confirmed if rhinosinus conditions thought to be contributing to PND are treated and cough is subsequently eliminated.

Postnasal drip may be a potential stimulus that irritates the afferent limb of the cough reflex in the hypopharynx and/or larynx. In association with hypersensitivity of the cough reflex in the upper airway, it is presumed that direct physical or chemical irritation stimulates the cough reflex peripherally, leading to increased central reactivity.[32] Why some patients with irritated upper airways cough, but many do not is not known. This situation is analogous to the angiotensin-converting enzyme inhibitor (ACEI) induced cough situation. While all patients taking ACEIs have excessive amounts of substance P and prostaglandins that are thought to cause hypersensitivity of the cough reflex, it is not known why only some patients develop cough while most do not.

Several conditions cause UACS, including allergic rhinitis, rhinitis medicamentosa, environmental irritant rhinitis, perennial nonallergic rhinitis, postinfectious rhinitis (*Mycoplasma, Chlamydia pneumoniae* and *B. pertussis*), vasomotor rhinitis, allergic fungal sinusitis, bacterial sinusitis, anatomic abnormalities, and rhinitis of pregnancy.[30] Of note, chronic bacterial sinusitis may also be silent, so in patients not improving on decongestants in whom UACS is suspected as the etiology of cough, sinus imaging studies may be helpful. UACS is the principal cause of cough associated with the common cold, making it also the most common cause of acute cough.[32]

As far as treatment is concerned, there is evidence to suggest that older generation antihistamine with or without decongestant combination medications are more effective than newer generation relatively nonsedating antihistamines, likely, secondary to their anticholinergic properties. Intranasal steroids and ipratropium nasal spray, cromolyn, and allergen avoidance are also used. For acute sinusitis, antibiotics directed at the most common organisms are recommended (see the chapter on sinusitis). Intranasal decongestants, such as oxymetazoline, may be used in conjunction for symptom relief in the short term. For chronic sinusitis causing cough, a prolonged course of antibiotics (see the chapter on sinusitis) is recommended (at least 2–3 weeks), as well as older generation antihistamine with or without decongestants and intranasal decongestants twice daily for up to 5 days, along with intranasal steroids for 3 months. Allergic fungal sinusitis may require surgical drainage and treatment with oral antifungal agents.

Asthma

In certain patients with asthma, cough may be the primary symptom, or occasionally, the only symptom (i.e. cough-variant asthma).[30] Patients with isolated cough-variant asthma usually have baseline normal spirometry; they have airway hyperresponsiveness and the cough will resolve with asthma treatment.[30] In fact, the diagnosis of asthma as a cause of chronic cough relies upon cough resolution with asthma treatment. A negative methacholine inhalation challenge essentially excludes asthma from the differential of chronic cough. The negative predictive value of a methacholine challenge testing approaches 100% in the symptomatic patient.

Patients with cough-variant asthma respond to the same treatment as patients with other forms of asthma and should be treated with inhaled bronchodilators, both short-acting and long-acting as needed, along with steroids, either inhaled, or oral as needed. Leukotriene receptor agonists may also be effective. Inhaled medications should be either a dry powder or a metered dose inhaler with a spacer. Because inhaled medications may provoke coughing, this possibility should be assessed and oral medications preferentially prescribed if this occurs. Treatment may take 6–8 weeks before maximum symptomatic benefit is achieved. Of note, if a patient's cough is refractory to inhaled corticosteroids, the presence of airway eosinophilia on induced sputum or bronchoalveolar lavage will identify patients who may benefit from more aggressive therapy.[33]

Gastroesophageal Reflux Disease

The prevalence of GERD as a cause of chronic cough has increased dramatically over the years. Studies accounted for reflux as an etiology of chronic cough in 10% of cases in 1981, and up to 36% of cases in 1998.[34] The term reflux disease is actually the preferred nomenclature over acid reflux disease because nonacid reflux can also contribute and will not respond to acid suppression therapy. Interestingly, in up to 75% of cases, there may be no associated GI symptoms.[34]

While reflux disease may cause cough by aspiration or from irritation of the upper respiratory,[34] it most likely causes chronic cough through a vagally mediated distal esophageal-tracheobronchial reflex mechanism.[35] Furthermore, a cough-reflux perpetuating cycle likely exists whereby cough from any cause may precipitate further reflux. Risk factors for GERD are many and include certain medications: bisphosphonates, oral corticosteroids, inhaled bronchodilators, theophylline, progesterone, calcium channel blockers, nitrates, anti-cholinergic agents, and certain narcotics, such as morphine and meperidine; obesity; smoking; vigorous exercise; alcohol; caffeine; fatty foods, chocolate, citrus juices and tomato products; prolonged intubation; after transplant; following pneumonectomy; peritoneal dialysis; and a variety of respiratory diseases such as asthma and obstructive sleep apnea.[34,36-38] At this time, esophageal pH and impedance monitoring appears to be the most sensitive and specific test for linking acid and nonacid reflux disease and coughing in a potential cause and effect manner. An esophageal pH monitoring study by itself is only helpful for evaluating acid reflux, and will not detect episodes of nonacid reflux. A normal esophagoscopy does not rule out reflux disease as a cause of cough, because most patients do not have esophagitis or Barrett's epithelium. For readers interested in reading more about reflux disease in general, we encourage them to read an article on this topic and associated references.[34]

The 2006 ACCP Cough Guideline Committee recommends empiric therapy for GERD for patients with the following clinical profile: cough greater than 8 weeks, the patient is not exposed to environmental irritants and is a nonsmoker, is not on an ACE inhibitor, and chest radiograph is normal or stable,[34] methacholine challenge is negative, cough fails to respond to a first-generation antihistamine with or without decongestant medication, and cough has failed to respond to systemic corticosteroids. This profile means that the following conditions have been ruled out: asthma, UACS, and nonasthmatic eosinophilic bronchitis.[34] The mainstay of treatment for reflux disease is acid suppression, prokinetic therapy, and lifestyle and dietary interventions. It is important to let patients know that they may not see improvement for 2 or 3 months after initiation of this therapy. Occasionally, patients may require antireflux surgery for cases refractory to medical treatment. Failure of medical therapy can be determined by 24-hour esophageal pH or impedance monitoring while the patient continues intensive medical therapy. It is important to keep in mind that GERD may still be the cause if the patient does not respond to treatment because treatment may not be maximal or because medical therapy failed and surgery might be necessary. Up to approximately 85% of patients note improvement in their chronic cough after antireflux surgery.[39]

Nonasthmatic Eosinophilic Bronchitis

Nonasthmatic eosinophilic bronchitis is characterized by a chronic cough, normal airway responsiveness to methacholine challenge, eosinophilic airway inflammation in induced sputum samples, and improvement in cough following corticosteroid therapy.[40] While patients usually present with normal baseline spirometry, airflow obstruction can occur if the inflammation is not suppressed. While the cough usually responds to inhaled corticosteroids, systemic corticosteroids may be necessary. The etiology of NAEB is unclear, although it may be associated with exposure to an inhaled allergen or occupational sensitizer. Whenever possible, avoidance of an offending agent is the best treatment.[40] For unclear reasons, NAEB tends to be diagnosed with greater frequency outside the US. Non-US studies have accounted for NAEB as the cause of chronic cough in up to 33% of cases, whereas some US studies have been able to prospectively report successful treatment of chronic cough without reporting a single case of NAEB.[31] It is unclear whether the prevalence is simply greater outside the US or whether it has been traditionally overlooked as a cause of chronic cough in the US. Regardless, it should be considered in all patients with chronic cough. Histologically, this disease is characterized by mast cells within the airway wall, a sign of epithelial infiltration, as opposed to the smooth muscle and airway inflammation by mast cells that is seen in patients with asthma.[40]

Chronic Bronchitis

Chronic bronchitis is defined as a bronchial disease with cough and sputum expectoration occurring on most days for at least 3 months of the year for at least 2 years when other pulmonary or cardiac causes of a chronic cough-phlegm syndrome are excluded.[41] It is known to be one of the most frequent causes of cough worldwide.[42] It is caused by the inhalation of irritants: tobacco, cigar, pipe smoke, passive smoke exposures, hazardous chemicals, organic dusts, cotton, wood, jute, hemp, flax, sisal, grains, manufactured fibers, oil mist, cement, silica, osmium, vanadium, indium,[43] welding fumes, engine exhausts, fumes of cooking fuels,[41,44] and fumes from burning biomass. In India, the prevalence of chronic bronchitis among *bidi* and cigarette smokers is 8.2% and 5.9%, respectively.[45] Occupational exposure may account for up to 15% of cases. While most smokers have cough, they are not the group of patients who most commonly seek medical attention for this symptom.

Chronic bronchitis is associated with airway inflammation, mucus hypersecretion, and impaired mucociliary clearance. Additionally, the airways of patients with chronic bronchitis are thought to have heightened responsiveness, albeit, not in the range seen in asthmatics. Progressive airflow obstruction can lead to an ineffective cough due to decreased expiratory flow and impaired mucociliary clearance that can cause the retention of secretions, further aggravating the cough reflex, thereby, promoting a cycle of recurrent cough.[41]

There are increased numbers of neutrophils and macrophages seen on bronchoalveolar lavage of patients with chronic bronchitis. The inflammation causes structural changes: mucus gland hyperplasia, bronchiolar edema, smooth muscle hypertrophy, and peribronchiolar fibrosis leading to the narrowing of the small airways.[46]

Treatment should focus on reducing sputum production and the reduction of airway inflammation by removing irritants (e.g. tobacco cessation). In patients without severe airflow limitation, cough has been shown to disappear or markedly decrease in 94–100% of cases with smoking cessation, often within 4 weeks.[18] Mucolytics often do not help. Ipratropium has been shown to decrease sputum production. While anticholinergics and/or inhaled corticosteroids and long-acting bronchodilators have been shown to decrease exacerbations, antibiotics and systemic corticosteroids serve to decrease cough during severe COPD exacerbations. In patients with frequent exacerbations, azithromycin, through anti-inflammatory and immune-modulating effects, has been shown to delay time to and decrease exacerbation rates in patients with COPD.[47]

Bronchiectasis

In prospective studies, bronchiectasis has caused chronic productive cough with sputum production in approximately 4% of cases.[48] Recurrent bacterial colonization and infection or bronchial obstruction causes airway injury, mediated by neutrophils, lymphocytes, and inflammatory mediators that result in the destruction of the elastic and muscular components of bronchial walls. The result is the dilation of involved airways. Some disorders predisposing patients to bronchiectasis include bronchial obstruction, pneumonia, cystic fibrosis, primary ciliary dyskinesia, allergic bronchopulmonary mycoses, rheumatoid arthritis, inflammatory bowel disease, hypogammaglobulinemia, alpha-1 antitrypsin deficiency, HIV infection, and Marfan's syndrome, among others.[48] Diagnosis is based on history, chest radiography, high-resolution chest computed tomography (CT) scans, and the response to targeted therapy. The cough associated with bronchiectatic flares is treated with chest physiotherapy, systemic antibiotics, and drugs to stimulate mucociliary clearance.[48] There has been no proven benefit of oral steroids to treat chronic cough associated with bronchiectasis. A recent small randomized controlled trial (RCT) demonstrated decreased exacerbations of noncystic fibrosis bronchiectasis in patients receiving thrice weekly azithromycin versus placebo.[49] There is some data for chest physiotherapy and high frequency chest wall oscillation in decreasing cough and improving quality of life in patients with noncystic fibrosis bronchiectasis as well.[50] In patients with severe bronchiectasis and frequent exacerbations, there may be a role for regularly scheduled antibiotics in 8-week intervals in reducing frequency and severity of exacerbations, based on one small RCT.[51]

Nonbronchiectatic bacterial suppurative airway disease has also been described as a cause of chronic cough.[52] These patients will have excessive purulent secretions in their central airways and positive bacterial cultures, yet have little to no productive cough, and no radiographic evidence of pneumonia or bronchiectasis. Diagnosis is made by bronchoscopy, and patients often respond to prolonged intravenous antibiotics (3 weeks) after courses of oral antibiotic have been shown to be ineffective.[52]

Bronchogenic Carcinoma

Bronchogenic carcinoma is most commonly due to smoking; cough is present in 65% of patients at the time of lung cancer diagnosis.[53] Chest radiography results have a positive predictive value for bronchogenic carcinoma of 36–38%, and markedly diminish the likelihood of lung cancer when chest radiographs are normal.[30,54] Along with chest radiographs, chest CT scans, sputum cytology, flexible bronchoscopy are all used for diagnosis, particularly, in patients for whom there is a high index of suspicion for cancer (e.g. cigarette smoker). Surgery to remove non-small cell lung cancer (NSCLC) in patients with stage I and II disease is the treatment of choice. For patients with more advanced disease, external beam radiation and/or chemotherapy are the treatments of choice.

Newer chemotherapeutic agents like gemcitabine, can palliate cough.[53] Localized endobronchial treatment options (e.g. brachytherapy) exist for patients with advanced disease and symptoms of dyspnea and hemoptysis. This may palliate concomitant cough; however, this type of treatment would not be an option for patients with cough alone. Some patients require narcotic antitussive agents to control cough associated with lung cancer.

Angiotensin-converting Enzyme Inhibitor-induced Cough

The cough associated with ACE inhibitor use is typically nonproductive and described as an irritating or tickling or scratching sensation in the back of the throat. Cough has been found to be a class effect and not dose related; therefore, in patients who complain of cough who are on ACE inhibitors, switching to a different class of antihypertensives is recommended. Because angiotensin-receptor blockers are not associated with an increased incidence of cough and they have been shown to have many of the same benefits as ACE inhibitors, they are an excellent substitution choice. The incidence of cough due to ACEIs in the series of patients with chronic cough is 0–3% of cases and may appear within a few hours to weeks or months after initiating therapy with an ACE inhibitor.[30] Some symptomatic relief may be obtained by adding sulindac, indomethacin, nifedipine, picotamide, and inhaled sodium cromoglycate when patients are unable to come off of their ACE inhibitors; however, discontinuation of the offending medication is the preferred treatment.[55] Cough secondary to an ACE inhibitor should disappear or markedly improve within the 4 weeks of discontinuing the medication; however, on occasion, cough may take up to 3 months to completely resolve.[56]

Somatic Cough Syndrome and Tic Cough

Somatic cough syndrome and tic cough are diagnoses of exclusion, and should be only considered after exclusion of organic etiologies of cough.[57] Certain qualities of the cough such as a barking or honking cough, or suppression of the cough during sleep, have been suggested to be suggestive for somatic cough syndrome or tic cough, but these features are not specific for the diagnosis of these conditions. While depression and anxiety are conditions that can be associated with somatic cough syndrome, their mere presence is not diagnostic or suggestive of these condition. The core clinical features of a tic cough are suppressibility, distractibility, suggestibility, variability and presence of a premonitory sensation, occurring in repetitive sequence, and sometimes associated with other motor actions. While there are effective treatments for tic disorders in general, we are not aware of any pharmacological treatments that have been adequately studied to target somatic cough syndrome or cough tic. Some nonpharmacological therapies such as hypnosis, suggestion therapy, relaxation technique and psychotherapy were reported to be beneficial in children[57] with cough tic, the evidence of these therapies remain of low quality. Because the terms psychogenic cough and habit cough are not accepted psychological terms, the American College of Chest Physicians Expert Cough Panel has suggested that these terms be abandoned.[57]

Miscellaneous Causes

A variety of unusual causes of cough are listed in **Box 4.**[58] Because the more common causes of cough can be the cause of chronic cough 50% of the time in patients with chronic interstitial lung diseases, chronic interstitial pulmonary disease should not be assumed to be the cause of the cough until the more common causes have been adequately evaluated and treated.

Endobronchial abnormalities (tumors, TB,[59] sarcoidosis, retained sutures) occasionally cause chronic cough. Bronchiolitis (nonbronchiectatic suppurative airway disease) affects the small airways and is caused by infections, toxins, systemic diseases (such as inflammatory bowel disease), drug reactions, and in transplant recipients, and is another less common cause of chronic cough.[60] Because these etiologies are uncommon causes of cough, one needs a strong index of suspicion based on the patient's clinical and laboratory picture to make these diagnoses.

BOX 4 Uncommon causes of chronic cough*[59]

Pulmonary (airway)
Tracheomalacia or bronchomalacia foreign bodies or airway stents, tracheobronchomegaly, tracheobronchopathia osteochondroplastica, broncholithiasis

Pulmonary (interstitial)
Lymphangioleiomyomatosis, langerhans cell histiocytosis, pulmonary alveolar proteinosis, pulmonary alveolar microlithiasis

Connective tissue diseases
Relapsing polychondritis, scleroderma, rheumatoid arthritis, systemic lupus erythematosus, Sjögren's syndrome, giant cell arteritis, granulomatosis with polyangiitis

Gastrointestinal disorders
Tracheoesophageal fistula, inflammatory bowel disease

**This listing is not meant to be exhaustive of cough.*

Unexplained Cough

Unexplained chronic cough is a category of chronic cough that has been described to represent around 5%–10% of patients with chronic cough.[61] This category includes patients who have a refractory chronic cough after all other causes of chronic cough have been excluded. In order to classify a patient as having an unexplained chronic cough (UCC), the following criteria should be met: the cough should be of at least 8 weeks duration; proper investigation of the cough should have been conducted **(Flow chart 3)**; and supervised therapeutic trials of therapy done according to the best practice guidelines.[61]

As an initial approach to UCC, repeating some of the investigations for the cough and ensuring adequate therapy for previously identified causes should be done. Speech therapy is recommended as a nonpharmacological intervention.[62] Trials of medications should be based on data obtained from double-blinded randomized placebo-controlled trials, and include certain opiates and gabapentin.[63, 64] Inhaled steroids in patients with negative bronchial hyper-responsiveness tests are not recommended. The use of opioid medications in treatment of UCC remains a point of contention, as the proposed benefit has to be always weighed against the risk of adverse effects including dependency.[63]

Chronic Cough in the Pediatric Population

Unlike the adult population, a chronic cough in children less than 15-years-old is defined as a cough lasting more than 4 weeks. A comprehensive approach for evaluating a patient less than 15-years-old with a chronic cough is presented in the ACCP Evidence-based Clinical Practice Guideline.[65] For patients 15 years of age and older with a chronic cough, one should follow the above mentioned guidelines for adults **(Flow chart 3)**.

Cough in the Immunocompromised Patient

Cough is a very common symptom in patients with compromised immune systems. The initial evaluation for immunocompromised patients presenting with acute and chronic coughs depends on the degree of their immunosuppression. HIV-positive patients with CD4 counts less than 250 cells/µL who present with acute cough are most likely to have upper respiratory infections, such as acute bronchitis and acute sinusitis, with less than 5% having bacterial pneumonia or *Pneumocystis jiroveci* pneumonia (PJP).[66] For patients with CD4 counts below 250 cells/µL, upper respiratory infections and acute bronchitis still explain almost 45% of cough cases, but the number presenting with *Mycobacterium tuberculosis* and pneumonia increase to over 23%, and includes PJP as well as bacterial pneumonia.[66,67]

When considering the etiology of chronic cough in patients who are immunocompromised, it is also important to assess the nature and severity of their immune defect. A general rule to remember is as follows: If CD4 count is less than 200 cells/µL, evaluate the patient for opportunistic infections. If the CD4 count is greater than 400 cells/µL, evaluate the patient as if they have a normal immune system, as the etiology of chronic cough in these patients is the same as what would be expected for immunocompetent patients. For CD4 counts between 200 and 400 µL, the patient's clinical condition matters. If the patient is cachectic, has evidence of oral thrush, or known prior infections with opportunistic organisms, evaluate the patient for opportunistic infections. If the patient is otherwise healthy appearing, initially evaluate them as if they have a normal immune system.[68]

Although TB has been reported in all countries, it remains a highly prevalent disease in developing countries. In fact, it is estimated that approximately one-third of the world's population is infected with *Mycobacterium tuberculosis*, that approximately 9 million people develop active TB each year, and approximately 1.9 million people die from TB each year.[59] Cough is a cardinal symptom of TB, and contributes to its transmission. Despite the higher prevalence of TB in the developing world, it is still not a common cause of chronic cough.[69] However, because it is highly contagious and causes significant morbidity and mortality for those infected, it should be considered in all patients with chronic cough who are at risk for TB, and patients who are immunocompromised, especially, with HIV. For patients who are at high risk for TB, the World Health Organization recommends that their cough be considered "chronic" after 2–3 weeks and evaluation begun to rule out infections such as TB.[70] Sputum for acid- fast bacilli (AFB) smear and culture, and chest radiograph when possible is recommended for initial evaluation for tuberculosis.

Patients who are immunosuppressed for reasons other than HIV are also at the risk of having infections, such as tuberculosis and *Pneumocystis* pneumonia as the cause of their chronic cough. Such patients include those with neutropenia; chronic disease, such as diabetes, cancer and renal failure; and patients receiving chronic corticosteroids.

Cough due to Parasitic Infections

Special attention is needed when evaluating a patient with chronic cough who resides in an area were certain fungal or parasitic diseases are endemic. While this is especially true when evaluating an immunocompromised patient with chronic cough, immunocompetent patients are also at risk for these infections. For example, paragonimiasis needs to be considered as a potential cause of chronic cough in patients who live or travel in the southeast Asia, especially in Japan, Korea, the Philippines, Taiwan, and parts of China.[71] These patients should be evaluated for the presence of eosinophilia and elevated immunoglobulin E (IgE) levels. The chest radiograph can have various appearances, such as pulmonary nodules, cavitary lesions, lymphadenopathy, pleural effusion or pneumothorax. The diagnosis can be confirmed by identifying *Paragonimus westermani* eggs in stool, sputum, pleural fluid or in bronchoalveolar lavage.

Syngamosis is another rare cause of chronic cough. It is the result of infestation by the nematode *Syngamus laryngeus* in which the parasite lodges itself in the tracheobronchial tree of a human after the ingestion of contaminated food or water. It remains unclear if the parasite migrates from the larynx, or is spread hematogenously after absorption from the GI tract. Symptoms include cough, fever, malaise, leukocytosis and eosinophilia. While uncommon in humans, it tends to occur geographically in the Caribbean islands and Brazil.[72] Diagnosis is established by the visualization of copulating reddish-brown worms in the upper airway on bronchoscopy or in expectorated sputum.[73] Cough and other respiratory symptoms reportedly subside after the removal of parasites from the bronchial tree.

Other parasitic infections associated with a chronic chough include ascariasis,[74] leishmaniasis,[75] malaria,[76] and schistosomiasis.[77]

CONCLUSION

Cough is one of the most common symptoms for which patients seek medical attention. While cough is a normal defense mechanism to clear secretions and foreign material from the airways, it can also result in clinically important complications. Cough is also a common symptom for a wide spectrum of both life-threatening and non-life-threatening illnesses. Dividing cough into acute, subacute and chronic categories, based on its duration, is most helpful in constructing the lists of differential diagnoses. Once the cough is categorized into one of these groups, a systematic approach to evaluating and treating the patient has the best chance of being successful in eliminating cough.

REFERENCES

1. Irwin RS. Cough. In: Irwin RS, Curley FJ, Grossman RF (Eds). Diagnosis and treatment of symptoms of the respiratory tract. Armonk: Futura Publishing Co; 1997. pp. 1-54.
2. Madison JM, Irwin RS. Cough: a worldwide problem. Otolaryngol Clin North Am. 2010;43(1):1-13.
3. Irwin RS, Baumann MH, Bolser DC, Boulet LP, Braman SS, Brightling CE, et al. Diagnosis and management of cough executive summary: ACCP evidence-based clinical practice guidelines. Chest. 2006:129(Suppl 1):1S-23S.
4. Morice AH, Fontana GA, Belvisi MG, Birring SS, Chung KF, Dicpinigaitis PV, et al. ERS guidelines on the assessment of cough. Eur Respir J. 2007;29(6):1256-76.
5. Irwin RS, French CT, Lewis SZ, Diekemper RL, Gold PM. CHEST Expert Cough Panel; CHEST Expert Cough Panel. Overview to the management of cough: CHEST Guideline and Expert Panel Report. Chest. 2014;146(4):885-9.
6. Chung KF, Pavord ID. Prevalence, pathogenesis, and causes of chronic cough. Lancet. 2008;371(9621):1364-74.
7. Morice A. Chronic cough: epidemiology. Chron Respir Dis. 2008;5(1):43-7.
8. Fochsen G, Deshpande K, Diwan V, Mishra A, Diwan VK, Thorson A. Health care seeking among individuals with cough and tuberculosis: a population-based study from rural India. Int J Tuberc Lung Dis. 2006;10(9):995-1000.
9. Fendrick AM, Monto AS, Nightengale B, Sarnes M. The economic burden of non-influenza-related viral respiratory tract infections in the United States. Arch Intern Med. 2003; 163(4):487-94.
10. French CL, Irwin RS, Curley FJ, Krikorian CJ. Impact of chronic cough on quality of life. Arch Intern Med. 1998;158(15):1657-61.
11. Canning BJ, Mori N, Mazzone SB. Vagal afferent nerves regulating the cough reflex. Respir Physiol Neurobiol. 2006; 152(3):223-42.
12. Karlsson JA, Fuller RW. Pharmacological regulation of the cough reflex—from experimental models to antitussive effects in Man. Pulm Pharmacol Ther. 1999;12(4):215-28.
13. Laude EA, Higgins KS, Morice AH. A comparative study of the effects of citric acid, capsaicin, and resiniferatoxin on the cough challenge in guinea-pig and man. Pulm Pharmacol. 1993;6(3):171-5.
14. Canning BJ. Afferent nerves regulating the cough reflex: mechanisms and mediators of cough in disease. Otolaryngol Clin North Am. 2010;43(1):15-25.
15. Comroe JH. Special acts involving breathing. In: Physiology of Respiration: an introductory text, 2nd edition. Chicago, IL: Year Book Medical Publishers Inc; 1974. pp. 230-31.
16. Gracey DR, Divertie MB, Howard FM. Mechanical ventilation for respiratory failure in myasthenia gravis. Two-year experience with 22 patients. Mayo Clin Proc. 1983;58(9):597-602.
17. Conti CR. Coronary arteriography. Circulation. 1977;55:227-37.
18. Schultz DD, Olivas GS. The use of cough cardiopulmonary resuscitation in clinic practice. Heart Lung. 1986;15(3):273-82.
19. Sharpey-Schafer EP. The mechanism of syncope after coughing. Br Med J. 1953;2(4841):860-3.
20. Irwin RS. Complications of cough: ACCP evidence-based clinical practice guidelines. Chest. 2006;129(Suppl 1):54S-58S.
21. Braman SS. Chronic cough due to acute bronchitis: ACCP evidence-based clinical practice guidelines. Chest. 2006:129 (Suppl 1):95S-103S.
22. Llor C, Moragas A, Bayona C, Morros R, Pera H, Plana-Ripoll O, et al. Efficacy of anti-inflammatory or antibiotic treatment in patients with noncomplicated acute bronchitis and discoloured sputum: randomized placebo controlled trial. BMJ. 2013;347:f5762.
23. Hewlett EL. Bordetella species. In: Mandell GL, Bannett JE, Dolin R (Eds). Principles and Practices of Infectious Diseases. Philadelphia: Churchill Livingstone; 2005. pp. 2701-12.
24. Crowcraft NS, Peabody RG. Recent developments in pertussis. Lancet. 2006;367(9526):1926-36.
25. Sotir MJ, Cappozzo DL, Warshauer DM, Schmidt CE, Monson TA, Berg JL, et al. Evaluation of polymerase chain reaction and culture for diagnosis of pertussis in the control of a country-wide outbreak focused among adolescents and adults. Clin Infect Dis. 2007;44(9):1216-9.
26. Dragster DM, Dohn B, Madsen J, Jensen JS. Comparison of culture and PCR for detection of Bordetella pertussis and Bordetella parapertussis under routine laboratory conditions. J Med Microbiol. 2004;53(Pt 8):749-54.
27. Centers for Disease Control and Prevention (2015). Pertussis (Whooping cough). [online] Available from *http://www.cdc.gov/vaccines/pubs/pertussis-guide/ guide.htm*. [Accessed January, 2016].
28. Wood N, McIntyre P. Pertussis: review of epidemiology, diagnosis, management, and prevention. Pediatr Respir Rev. 2008;9(3):201-11.
29. Bettiol S, Thompson MJ, Roberts NW, Perera R, Heneghan CJ, Harnden A. Symptomatic treatment of the cough in whooping cough. Cochrane Database Syst Rev. 2010;1:CD003257.
30. Irwin RS, Curley FJ, French CL. Chronic cough: the spectrum and frequency of causes, key components of the diagnostic evaluation, and outcome of specific therapy. Am Rev Respir Dis. 1990;141(3):640-7.
31. Birring SS, Pavord ID. Idiopathic chronic cough and organ-specific autoimmune disease. Chest. 2006;129(1):213-4.
32. Pratter MR. Chronic upper airway cough syndrome secondary to rhinosinus diseases (previously referred to as postnasal drip syndrome): ACCP evidence-based clinical practice guidelines. Chest. 2006;129(Suppl 1):63S-71S.
33. Dicpinigaitis PV. Chronic cough due to asthma: ACCP evidence-based clinical practice guidelines. Chest. 2006;129(Suppl 1):75S-79S.
34. Irwin RS. Chronic cough due to gastroesophageal reflux disease: ACCP evidence-based clinical practice guidelines. Chest. 2006;129(Suppl 1):80S-94S.

35. Ing AJ, Ngu MC, Breslin AB. Pathogenesis of chronic persistent cough associated with gastroesophageal reflux. Am J Respir Crit Care Med. 1994;149(1):160-7.
36. Richter JE, Castell DO. Drugs, foods, and other substances in the cause and treatment of reflux esophagitis. Med Clin North Am. 1981;65(6):1223-34.
37. Vitale GC, Cheadle WG, Patel B, Sadek SA, Michel ME, Cuschieri A. The effect of alcohol on nocturnal gastroesophageal reflux. JAMA. 1987;258(15):2077-9.
38. Clark CS, Kraus BB, Sinclair J, Castell DO. Gastroesophageal reflux induced by exercise in healthy volunteers. JAMA. 1989;261(24):3599-601.
39. Novitsky YW, Zawacki JK, Irwin RS, French CT, Hussey VM, Callery MP. Chronic cough due to gastroesophageal reflux disease: efficacy of antireflux surgery. Surg Endosc. 2002;16(4):567-71.
40. Brightling CE. Chronic cough due to nonasthmatic eosinophilic bronchitis: ACCP evidence-based clinical practice guidelines. Chest. 2006;129(Suppl 1):116S-121S.
41. Braman SS. Chronic cough due to chronic bronchitis: ACCP evidence-based clinical practice guidelines. Chest. 2006;129 (Suppl 1):104S-115S.
42. Pauwels RA, Buist AS, Calvery PM, Jenkins CR, Hurd SS; GOLD Scientific Committee. Global strategy for the diagnosis, management, and prevention of chronic obstructive pulmonary disease. NHLBI/WHO Global Initiative for Chronic Obstructive Pulmonary Disease (GOLD) Workshop summary. Am J Respir Crit Care Med. 2001;163(5):1256-76.
43. Nakano M, Omae K, Uchida K, Michikawa T, Yoshioka N, Hirata M, et al. Five-year cohort study: emphysematous progression of indium-exposed workers. Chest. 2014;146(5):1166-75.
44. Balmes JR. Occupational airways diseases from chronic low-level exposures to irritants. Clin Chest Med. 2002;23:727-35.
45. Jindal SK, Aggarwal AN, Chaudhry K, Chhabra SK, D'Souza GA, Gupta D, et al. A multicentric study on epidemiology of chronic obstructive pulmonary disease and its relationship with tobacco smoking and environmental tobacco smoke exposure. Indian J Chest Dis Allied Sci. 2006;48(1):23-9.
46. Hogg JC, Chu F, Utokparch S, Woods R, Elliott WM, Buzatu L, et al. The nature of small-airway obstruction in chronic obstructive pulmonary disease. N Engl J Med. 2004;350(26):2645-53.
47. Albert RK, Connett J, Bailey WC, Casaburi R, Cooper JA, Criner GJ, et al. Azithromycin for prevention of exacerbations of COPD. N Engl J Med. 2011;365:689-98.
48. Rosen MJ. Chronic cough due to bronchiectasis: ACCP evidence-based clinical practice guidelines. Chest. 2006;129 (Suppl 1):122S-131S.
49. Wong C, Jayaram L, Karalus N, Eaton T, Tong C, Hockey H, et al. Azithromycin for prevention of exacerbations in non-cystic fibrosis bronchiectasis (EMBRACE): a randomized, double-blind, placebo-controlled trial. Lancet. 2012;380:660-7.
50. Nicolini A, Cardini F, Landucci N, Lanata S, Ferrari-Bravo M, Barlascini C. Effectiveness of treatment with high-frequency chest wall oscillation in patients with bronchiectasis. BMC Pulm Med. 2013;13-21.
51. Mandal P, Sidhu MK, Donaldson LS, Chalmers JD, Smith MP, Turnbull K, et al. Eight-weekly intravenous antibiotics is beneficial in severe bronchiectasis. QJM. 2013;106:27-33.
52. Schaefer OP, Irwin RS. Unsuspected bacterial suppurative disease of the airways presenting as chronic cough. Am J Med. 2003;114(7):602-6.
53. Kvale PA. Chronic cough due to lung tumors: ACCP evidence-based clinical practice guidelines. Chest. 2006;129(Suppl 1):147S-153S.
54. Markowitz DH, Irwin RS. Is bronchoscopy overused in the evaluation of chronic cough? J Bronchol. 1997;4:332-7.
55. Dicpinigaitis PV. Angiotensin-converting enzyme inhibitor-induced cough: ACCP evidence-based clinical practice guidelines. Chest. 2006;129(Suppl 1):169S-73S.
56. Lacourcière Y, Brunner H, Irwin R, Karlberg BE, Ramsay LE, Snavely DB, et al. Effects of modulators of the rennin-angiotensin-aldosterone system on cough. Losartan Cough Study Group. J Hypertens. 1994;12(12):1387-93.
57. Vertigan AE, Murad MH, Pringsheim T, et al. Somatic cough syndrome (Previously referred to as psychogenic cough) and Tic cough (Previously referred to as habit cough) in adults and children: CHEST guideline and Expert Panel Report. Chest. 2015;148(1):24-31.
58. Prakash UB. Uncommon causes of cough: ACCP evidence-based clinical practice guidelines. Chest. 2006;129(Suppl 1): 206S-19S.
59. Rosen MJ. Cough due to tuberculosis and other infections: ACCP evidence-based clinical practice guidelines. Chest. 2006;129(Suppl 1):197S-201S.
60. Brown KK. Chronic cough due to nonbronchiectatic suppurative airway disease (bronchiolitis): ACCP evidence-based clinical practice guidelines. Chest. 2006;129(Suppl 1): 132S-7S.
61. Gibson P, Wang G, McGarvey L, Vertigan AE, et al. Treatment of Unexplained Chronic Cough: CHEST Guideline and Expert Panel Report. Chest. 2016;149:27-44.
62. Vertigan AE, Theodoros DG, Gibson PG, Winkworth AL. Efficacy of speech pathology management for chronic cough: a randomized placebo controlled trial of treatment efficacy. Thorax. 2006;61:1065-9.
63. Morice AH, Menon MS, Mulrennan SA, Everett CF, Wright C, Jackson J, et al. Opiate therapy in chronic cough. Am J Respir Crit Care Med. 2007;175:312-5.
64. Ryan NM, Birring SS, Gibson PG. Gabapentin for refractory chronic cough: a randomized, double-blind, placebo-controlled trial. Lancet. 2012;380:1583-9.
65. Chang AB, Glomb WB. Guidelines for evaluating chronic cough in pediatrics: ACCP evidence-based clinical practice guidelines. Chest. 2006;129(Suppl 1):260S-83S.
66. Wallace JM, Rao AV, Glassroth J, Hansen NI, Rosen MJ, Arakaki C, et al. Respiratory illness in persons with human immunodeficiency virus infection. The Pulmonary Complications of HIV Infection Study Group. Am Rev Respir Dis. 1993;148(6 Pt 1):1523-9.
67. Phair J, Munoz A, Detels R, Kaslow R, Rinaldo C, Saah A. The risk of Pneumocystis carinii pneumonia among men infected with human immunodeficiency virus type 1. Multicenter AIDS Cohort Study Group. N Engl J Med. 1990;332:161-5.
68. Rosen MJ. Cough in the immunocompromised host: ACCP evidence-based clinical practice guidelines. Chest. 2006;129(Suppl 1):204S-5S.
69. Balgos A, Reyes-Pingol R, Siasoco BR, et al. Chronic persistent cough: local experience in the diagnosis using the anatomic and diagnostic protocol, spectrum, and frequency of causes and outcome of specific treatment. Phil J Chest Dis. 1993;1:6-11.
70. Ottomani S, Scherpbier R, Chaulet P, et al. Practical approach to lung health: respiratory care in primary care services: a survey

of 9 countries. Geneva: World Health Organization; 2004. pp. 21.
71. Yokogawa M. Paragonimus and paragonimiasis. Adv Parasitol. 1969;7:375-87.
72. Nosanchuk JS, Wade SE, Landolf M. Case report of and description of parasite in Mammomonogamus laryngeus (human syngamosis) infection. J Clin Microbiol. 1995;33(4): 9981000.
73. Mornex JF, Magdeleine J. Parasitic pulmonary disease: human bronchial syngamosis. Am Rev Respir Dis. 1983;127(4):525-6.
74. Sarinas PS, Chitkara RK. Ascariasis and hookworm. Semin Respir Infect. 1997;12(2):130-7.
75. Magill AJ, Grögl M, Gasser RA Jr, Sun W, Oster CN. Visceral infection caused by Leishmania tropica in veterans of Operation Desert Storm. N Engl J Med. 1993;328(19): 1383-7.
76. Chung HC, Wang JT, Sun HY, Wang JL, Lo YC, Sheng WH, et al. Clinical experience of 17 cases of imported malaria at Taiwan University Hospital, 1999-2005. J Microbiol Immunol Infect. 2007;40(3):209-15.
77. Caldas IR, Campi-Azevedo AC, Oliveira LF, Silveira AM, Oliveira RC, Gazzinelli G. Human schistosomiasis mansoni: immune responses during acute and chronic phases of the infection. Acta Tropica. 2008;108(2-3):109-17.

16 Chapter

Hemoptysis

Andrés F Sosa, J Mark Madison, Paulo J Oliveira

INTRODUCTION

The term hemoptysis refers to the coughing of blood that emanates from the lungs or airways below the larynx.[1] It is an alarming sign for most patients and physicians, the basis of which is the fear that it represents a serious ailment.[2] In 1953, hemoptysis implied tuberculosis for the average medical student[3] and it continues to be so in the developing world;[4] however, bronchiectasis, bronchitis and bronchogenic carcinoma are now the most common causes in the developed world.[5]

Hemoptysis may range from scant streaking of sputum, as often seen in chronic bronchitis, to more severe life-threatening quantities of blood that have the potential to cause significant gas exchange abnormalities.[6] It is useful to categorize the amount of hemoptysis according to the rate of bleeding. Hemoptysis is mild when there are less than 20 mL in 24 hours, moderate or submassive when 20–600 mL and massive when more than 600 mL in a 24 hour period. Gross or frank hemoptysis may be defined as the expectoration of a lesser amount than massive hemoptysis and yet more than mere blood streaking. The faster the bleeding, the greater the risk of mortality, which reaches 37% when bleeding exceeds 600 mL in 48 hours and 52% when more than 600 mL in less than 16 hours.[7-9] The rate of blood loss above 15 mL per hour substantially increase the risk of death due to asphyxiation or exsanguination.[10] These volumetric, quantitative definitions are often quoted in texts, but in practice quantification of the amount of coughed out blood is difficult. What may be more relevant and useful is a qualitative definition based on the magnitude of clinical consequences incurred by the patient with hemoptysis. The vast majority of patients with massive hemoptysis die due to asphyxiation, not exsanguination.[10] The anatomical dead space of the major airways is approximately 100–200 mL. Thus, a brisk bleed of 150 mL, for example, could lead to major airway obstruction and the rapid demise of the patient due to inability to oxygenate and ventilate.

It is important not to confuse hemoptysis with bleeding that originates from sources other than the lower respiratory tract, also referred to as "pseudohemoptysis". Patients may not be able to describe the source of their bleeding and, blood arising from the nares, oral cavity, tongue and pharynx penetrate into the larynx to stimulate the cough reflex.[11-13] Hematemesis, as well, may be aspirated into the respiratory tract to cause pseudohemoptysis.[13] Also, in hospitalized patients who have received broad-spectrum antibiotics and mechanical ventilation, colonization of the oropharynx by *Serratia marcescens* may produce a red pigment, prodigiosin, that can be mistaken for blood.[14] It should be kept in mind, however, that infection with *Serratia marcescens* can lead to necrotizing pneumonia, presenting with true hemoptysis. Overdose with rifamycin antibiotics can imbue tracheobronchial secretions with a reddish hue that can be mistaken for blood-tinged sputum.[15] Finally, there is also the possibility of factitious hemoptysis. In these cases, the episodes of hemoptysis are self-inflicted; this may lead to an unnecessary and extensive diagnostic work-up.[16]

ANATOMY

The lungs have a dual vascular supply. The pulmonary vasculature is a low-pressure system that supplies the lung parenchyma to support gas exchange and the respiratory bronchioles. The bronchial arteries, part of the systemic vasculature, are a high-pressure system that supplies the airways, from the trachea and mainstem bronchi to terminal bronchioles, the peribronchial and perivascular connective tissue, the middle third of the esophagus, the visceral diaphragmatic and mediastinal pleura, intrapulmonary lymphoid tissue, pulmonary vessels and nerves. Bronchial arteries generally originate from the aorta or intercostal arteries. There are usually 2–4 bronchial arteries in total and they tend to be more numerous on the left side.[17,18] Arterial and venous communications between both vascular systems occur at the level of the terminal and respiratory bronchioles and the two systems complement each other by maintaining constant flow. The bronchial circulation is the source of over 90% of cases of hemoptysis.[19]

ETIOLOGY AND PATHOGENESIS

The source of hemoptysis depends on the location of disease. If the disease process is located within the lung parenchyma it will involve the pulmonary circulation, but if it is contained within the airways it will involve the bronchial circulation. Chronic disease processes involving the airways and parenchyma will frequently lead to increased vascularity (neovascularization, engorgement and the enlargement of the local blood supply, increased anastomoses with the pulmonary circulation) and friability/fragility in the compromised areas.[20] There are over 140 causes of hemoptysis, which have been described. For practical purposes the causes can be divided into several major categories **(Table 1)**.[16,21-129]

Nonmassive hemoptysis accounts for the majority of cases (bronchitis being one of the most common causes), but there is a considerable overlap between the massive and nonmassive causes of hemoptysis. The most common causes of massive hemoptysis, accounting for more than 60% of cases, are active tuberculosis, bronchiectasis, mycetoma and bronchogenic carcinoma **(Table 2)**.[130-132] As mentioned previously, categorizing the severity of the hemoptysis has significant implications for prognosis and further management.

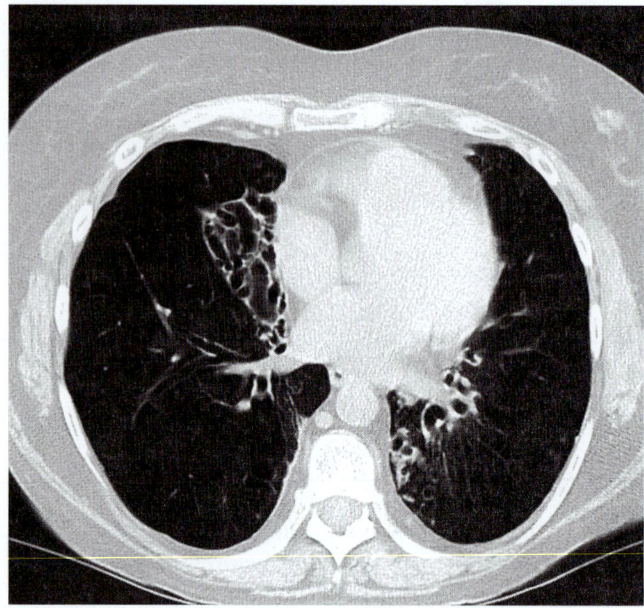

Fig. 1 Computed tomography of the chest showing an axial image of a patient with dysmotile cilia syndrome resulting in severe bronchiectasis

Infection and Inflammation

Patients with chronic bronchitis have increased vascularity beneath the endobronchial surface. The mucosa is friable and prone to bleed, especially in the presence of bacterial or viral infections.[133] Chronic bronchitis is a major cause of hemoptysis in the United States.[134] Bronchiectatic airways are also prone to bleeding episodes due to the proliferation of bronchial vessels and precapillary anastomoses with the pulmonary circulation **(Figs 1 and 2)**. These enlarged vessels are susceptible to injury from the local inflammation and frequent episodes of infection that are the hallmark of bronchiectasis.[135]

Tuberculosis (TB) and its sequelae, such as bronchiectasis, broncholithiasis and recurrent bacterial infections continue to remain the most common causes of hemoptysis in the developing world.[4] Hemoptysis tends to develop in young, female patients with extensive disease, in cases of TB relapse, and in patients with old inactive mycobacterial disease complicated by bacterial superinfection.[136] Early pneumonia from tuberculosis may cause scant hemoptysis resulting from the necrosis of a small vessel; however, later stages of the disease may develop severe parenchymal fibroulcerative lesions that can erode into a bulging arterial aneurysm causing episodes of massive bleeding and respiratory distress **(Figs 3 and 4)**.[137] Also, calcified lymph nodes impinging on the airway can erode into the airway lumen and cause streaky hemoptysis by disrupting vessels in the peribronchial and submucosal plexi; alternatively, they can lead to massive hemoptysis when there is a large bronchial artery in the path of this eroding calcified lymph node or broncholith.[138]

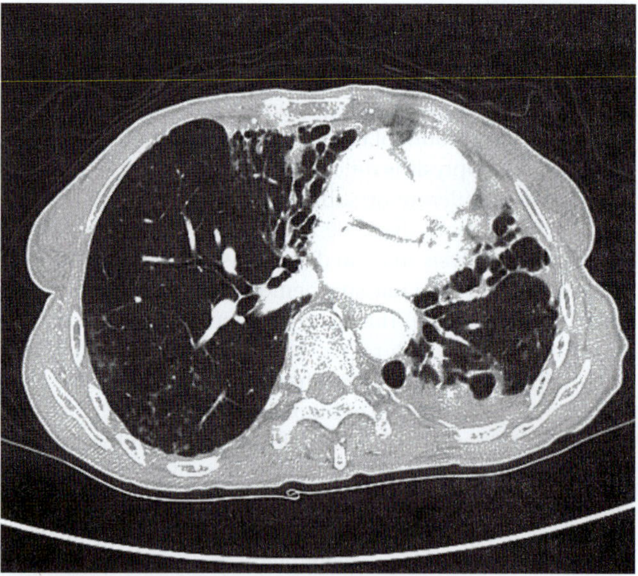

Fig. 2 Computed tomography of the chest showing an axial image of a patient with chronic atypical *Mycobacterium* infection and bronchiectasis

Finally, expanding, thick-walled tuberculous cavities may incorporate pulmonary vessels that are prone to damage and bleeding when exposed to inflammation and mycobacteria. The vessels become ectatic and aneurysmal, as well as may rupture to cause massive hemoptysis.[137,139]

Table 1 Causes of hemoptysis*

- *Infectious and inflammatory*
  - Bronchitis
  - Bronchiectasis
  - Bacterial
    - Lung abscess
    - Necrotizing pneumonia
      - *Staphylococcus*
      - *Pneumococcus*
      - *Klebsiella*
      - *Pseudomonas*
      - *Acinetobacter*
      - *Legionella*
      - *Burkholderia pseudomallei*
  - Fungal
    - Aspergillosis
    - Coccidiomycosis
    - Histoplasmosis
    - Paracoccidiomycosis
    - Candidiasis
    - Cryptococcosis
    - Mucormycosis
    - Sporotrichosis
  - Viral
    - Influenza
  - Mycobacteria
    - *Mycobacterium tuberculosis*
    - Atypical mycobacteria
  - Parasitic
    - Amebiasis
    - Strongyloides
    - Paragonimiasis
    - Ascariasis
    - Echinococcosis
    - Schistosomiasis
- *Neoplastic*
  - Benign
    - Carcinoid
    - Polyps
    - Hamartoma
    - Lymphangioma
  - Malignant
    - Bronchogenic
    - Renal cell carcinoma
    - Breast adenocarcinoma
    - Other metastatic
    - Choriocarcinoma
    - Thyroid carcinoma
    - Melanoma
- *Cardiac*
  - Congestive heart failure
  - Mitral stenosis
  - Congenital heart disease
- *Vascular and embolic*
  - Venous thromboembolism
  - Arteriovenous malformations
  - Fat embolism
  - Pulmonary hypertension
  - Septic emboli
  - Tumor embolization
  - Thoracic endometriosis
  - Aortic aneurysm
  - Bronchial artery rupture
  - Superior vena cava syndrome
  - Dieulafoy's lesion
- *Congenital*
  - Cystic fibrosis
  - Pulmonary sequestration
  - Dysmotile cilia syndrome
  - Duplication cyst
- *Trauma*
  - Pulmonary contusion
  - Pulmonary laceration
  - Thoracic splenosis
  - Pulmonary pneumatocele
  - Tracheobronchial injury
- *Iatrogenic*
  - Central line catheters
  - Pulmonary artery catheterization
  - Tracheotomy
  - Transthoracic needle biopsy of the lung
  - Transbronchial biopsy of the lung
- *Systemic*
  - Amyloidosis
  - Goodpasture's syndrome
  - Idiopathic pulmonary hemosiderosis
  - Vasculitides and collagen vascular disease
- *Drugs and Toxins*
  - Amiodarone
  - Antiplatelet agents
  - Antithrombotic therapy
  - Charcoal lighter fluid
  - Cocaine
  - Isocyanates
  - Penicillamine
  - Trimellitic anhydride
- *Hematologic*
  - Disseminated intravascular coagulation
  - Leukemia
  - Von Willebrand's disease
  - Thrombocytopenia
  - Hemophilia
- *Miscellaneous*
  - Broncholithiasis
  - Cryptogenic
  - Foreign body aspiration
  - Hypersensitivity pneumonitis
  - Lymphangiomyomatosis
  - Gastric acid aspiration
  - Sarcoidosis
  - Factitious

Source: *Modified from Balter MS. Hemoptysis, in Diagnosis and Treatment of Symptoms of the Respiratory Tract. Armonk, New York: Futura Publishing Company, Inc.; 1997. pp. 155-97.

Table 2 Common causes of massive hemoptysis*

- Tuberculosis
- Bronchiectasis
- Mycetoma
- Bronchogenic carcinoma
- Tracheoarterial fistula
- Pulmonary arteriovenous malformation

Source: *Modified from Balter MS. Hemoptysis, in Diagnosis and Treatment of Symptoms of the Respiratory Tract. Armonk, New York: Futura Publishing Company, Inc.; 1997. pp. 155-97.

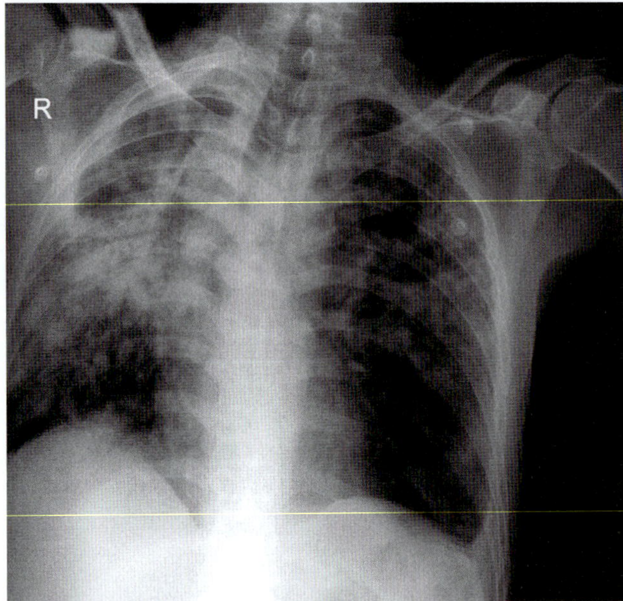

Fig. 3 Chest radiograph of a patient with active tuberculosis

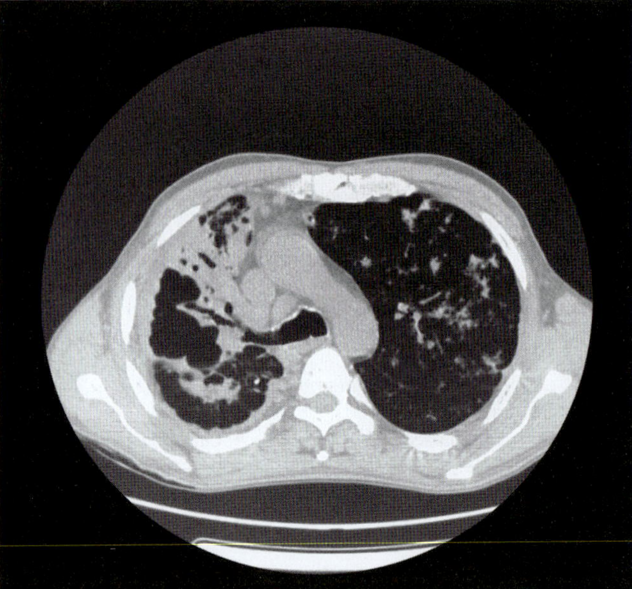

Fig. 4 Computed tomography of the chest showing an axial image of a patient with HIV and active tuberculosis

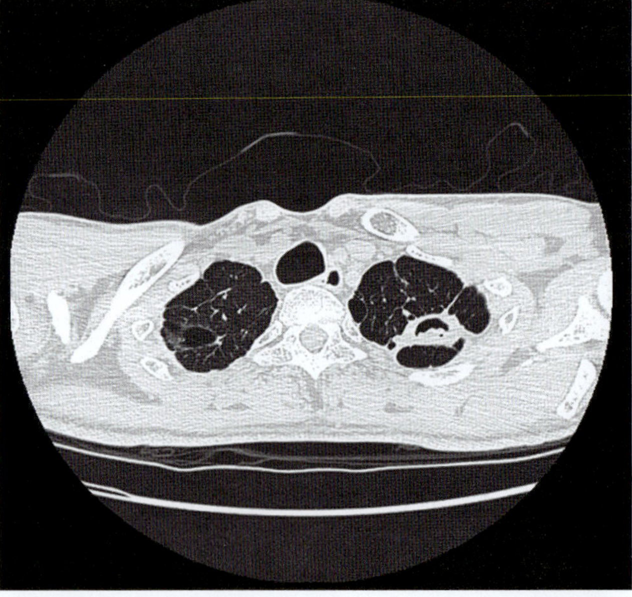

Fig. 5 Computed tomography of the chest showing an axial image of a patient with a mycetoma in a preformed cavity secondary to sarcoidosis

Cavities may develop in pulmonary parenchyma damaged by TB, sarcoidosis, vasculitis, emphysema, neoplasms, pulmonary fibrosis, lung abscess, bronchial cyst, asbestosis, ankylosing spondylitis or pulmonary infarction.[140] These pre-existing cavities may become colonized by Aspergillus to form mycetomas or fungus balls **(Fig. 5)**. These mycetomas are frequently complicated by hemoptysis, up to 85% of the time.[29,141] The fungus ball may cause erosion into a blood vessel by releasing anticoagulant proteolytic enzymes.[142,143]

Melioidosis caused by *Burkholderia pseudomallei* may mimic active tuberculosis. Most cases have been reported in Southeast Asia. Melioidosis, like active tuberculosis, causes protean signs and symptoms that include fever, productive cough, hemoptysis, weight loss, pleuritic chest pain and, typically, necrotizing upper lobe involvement. The disease can also be present acutely with an abrupt onset and rapidly deteriorating course.

Recrudescence has been described up to 26 years after the patient had left the endemic zone.[144]

The ingestion of raw or undercooked shellfish primarily in Southeast Asia may lead to infection with *Paragonimus westermani*. The adult parasite forms cysts near bronchioles and bronchi. Hemoptysis occurs as the cysts erode into the airway.[42,43] Loeffler's syndrome is caused by different types of parasites (e.g. Ascaris, hookworm, Strongyloides) due to the migration of parasite larva through the lungs, most often 1–2 weeks after infection, but the incubation period will vary depending on the species of the parasite.[145] The syndrome is characterized by fever, urticaria, wheeze, dry cough and sometimes, hemoptysis. Typically, the patient has eosinophilia on a complete blood count and the chest radiograph shows migratory pulmonary infiltrates.

Neoplastic Causes

Bronchogenic carcinoma may present with hemoptysis when the tumor invades a blood vessel or becomes necrotic. Hemoptysis can be the presenting symptom in 10% of lung cancer patients,[55] typically mild to moderate.[146] Squamous cell carcinoma seems to be the most likely type of lung cancer to cause massive bleeding because of its typical central location and tendency to cavitate.[55] Squamous cell carcinoma is 10 times more likely to bleed than other types of bronchogenic carcinoma **(Fig. 6)**.[55] Bronchial carcinoids are slow growing endobronchial neuroendocrine tumors that are highly vascularized and may bleed up to 30% of the time.[147,148]

Cardiac Causes

The elevated pressure in the pulmonary circulation that results from congestive heart failure and mitral stenosis may lead to the distension and rupture of pulmonary and bronchial veins. Significant back pressure from mitral stenosis may be transmitted to the bronchial veins, resulting in submucosal varices that are prone to rupture and bleeding.[149,150]

Vascular Causes

Venous thromboembolism can cause hemoptysis when there is the necrosis of pulmonary parenchyma due to infarction, congestive atelectasis or hemorrhagic consolidation. Venous thromboembolism can also cause hemoptysis by increasing bronchial artery blood flow through collaterals that are formed with the pulmonary circulation to bypass the embolized artery.[151,152]

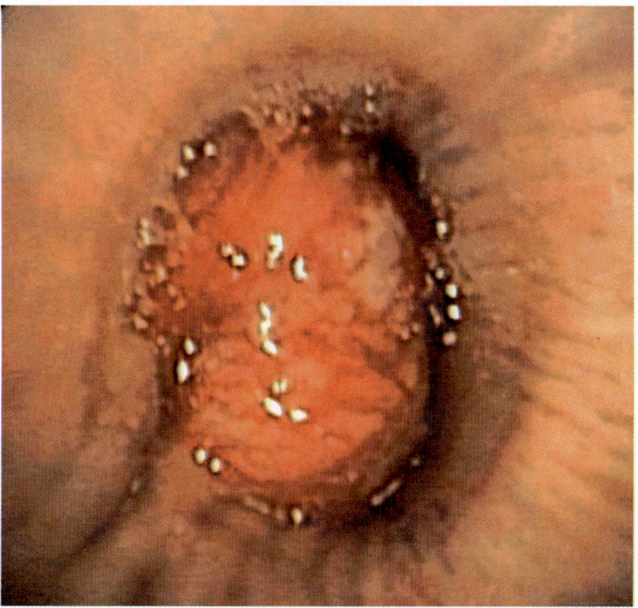

Fig. 6 Bronchoscopy picture showing a highly vascularized squamous cell lung carcinoma

Pulmonary arteriovenous malformation (AVM) is another important cause of hemoptysis that may result in profuse bleeding.[153,154] The majority of hemoptysis caused by AVMs will be seen in the patients with hereditary hemorrhagic telangiectasia or Osler-Weber-Rendu syndrome. The AVMs tend to be numerous and bilateral, bleeding occurs from either rupture of a pulmonary AVM or an endobronchial telangiectasia.[155] The risk of bleeding is higher with feeding vessels of >3 mm.[156]

Dieulafoy's lesion is another type of vascular malformation. In these lesions, there is a bronchial artery draining into a pulmonary artery causing left-to-right shunting of blood. Dieulafoy's disease of the bronchus is associated with the abnormal superficial location of this vascular anomaly contiguous to the epithelium of the bronchial mucosa. Dieulafoy's lesions can appear as sessile tumors covered by endobronchial mucosa or they may have an overlying white cap. If biopsied, these lesions may bleed profusely.[157] Disease of the bronchus is analogous to the Dieulafoy's lesion of the gastric mucosa that can present with severe upper gastrointestinal bleeding due to the superficial location of a dilated, ectopic gastric artery.

Congenital Causes

Cystic fibrosis patients are prone to develop pulmonary abscesses, recurrent pneumonias and bronchiectasis **(Figs 1 and 2)**. Patients may subsequently present with hemoptysis, the risk appears to increase with more advanced age.[158,159] Bronchiectatic airways bleed because they have a higher degree of vascularity in the endobronchial and peribronchial circulation.[78]

Trauma

Both penetrating and blunt chest trauma can cause hemoptysis. Pulmonary lacerations, pneumatoceles and pulmonary hematomas may all be caused by blunt chest trauma. Pulmonary contusions occur when external forces are applied to the pulmonary parenchyma. Pulmonary contusions cause the disruption of the alveolar-capillary membranes, increased permeability and edema, shunting and ventilation-perfusion mismatching. Pulmonary contusions rarely cause hemoptysis since they do not tend to disrupt the pulmonary parenchyma and the bleeding is confined to the alveoli and interstitium.[82] Tracheobronchial injury is another type of traumatic injury that may occur with the sudden compression of the chest and shearing of the mainstem bronchus. Chest compression against a closed glottis can also tear the membranous portion of the cartilaginous rings and cause hemoptysis. Deceleration injuries may cause rupture at fixed points at the cricoid and main carina.[160]

Iatrogenic Causes

Rupture of the pulmonary artery by a balloon flotation catheter may complicate right heart catheterization. This complication tends to occur when there is pulmonary hypertension, a distally located catheter tip, excessive catheter manipulation, a large catheter loop in the right ventricle or advanced age.[23]

Tracheoarterial fistulas usually involving the innominate artery, are complications of tracheotomies and a cause of life-threatening hemoptysis. The fistulas are most likely to form at the stoma in low tracheotomies, at the balloon site, or at the tip of the tracheotomy tube when there is excessive angulation causing pressure necrosis. It usually takes at least 48 hours after tracheotomy to develop a tracheoarterial fistula. A sentinel bleed precedes massive hemoptysis in 35–50% of these cases.[89]

Transbronchial lung biopsies may cause hemoptysis in 2% of cases, the bleeding is usually mild and self-limited. However, some patients are at a higher risk of more profuse bleeding, especially those with thrombocytopenia and uremia, those who are immunocompromised, or those who are on mechanical ventilation.[161] Caution should also be taken when performing transbronchial biopsies in patients with severe pulmonary hypertension [pulmonary artery systolic pressure (PASP) >55–60 mm Hg] as they may be at increased risk for bleeding complications.[162,163]

Systemic and Immune Diseases

Diffuse alveolar hemorrhage (DAH) may occur due to capillary damage by autoimmune diseases, such as Goodpasture's syndrome; Systemic lupus erythematosus (SLE); the ANCA-associated vasculitides [Necrotizing granulomatous vasculitis (NGV), (formerly Wegener's granulomatosis)], microscopic polyangiitis; Churg-Strauss syndrome; and cryoglobulinemia **(Figs 7 and 8)**. All of these diseases may involve the nervous system, gastrointestinal tract, skin, kidneys and joints.[164-168] Thoracic endometriosis is the cause of catamenial hemoptysis, happening within 48–72 hours of menses.[169]

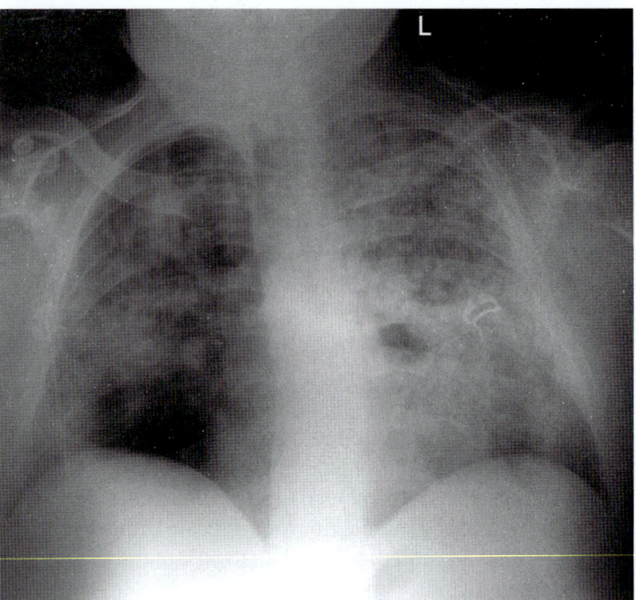

Fig. 7 Chest radiograph of a patient with diffuse alveolar hemorrhage in the setting of necrotizing granulomatous vasculitis

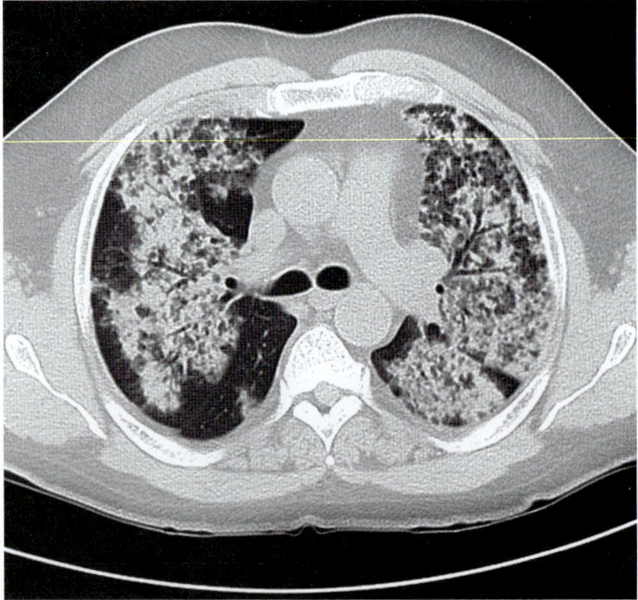

Fig. 8 Computed tomography of the chest showing an axial image of a patient with diffuse alveolar hemorrhage in the setting of necrotizing granulomatous vasculitis

Drugs/Toxins

Anticoagulants and thrombolytics may induce hemoptysis in patients with underlying chronic inflammation (e.g. chronic bronchitis), neoplastic lesions, or structural abnormalities of the lungs and airways (e.g. bronchiectasis).[170] Other, rare causes of toxin-induced DAH and hemoptysis include penicillamine, mitomycin-C, isocyanates, crack cocaine, abciximab, sirolimus, all-trans-retinoic acid and trimellitic anhydride.[118,120,171,172]

Cryptogenic Hemoptysis

Cryptogenic or idiopathic hemoptysis is the term used when no specific cause of hemoptysis can be found after thorough medical, roentgenographic and bronchoscopic evaluations. The incidence at referral centers is about 19%. In general, the prognosis for cryptogenic hemoptysis is favorable with the resolution of any further hemoptysis within 6 months of the initial evaluation.

However, more contemporary data over a 6.6 year period of follow-up, has revealed that the subsequent diagnosis of lung cancer in patients with cryptogenic hemoptysis may be as high as 6%, especially among those patients who smoke and are older than 40 years of age.[122] Interestingly, it was found in a recent report from France, which described 81 patients who were labeled as cryptogenic hemoptysis, that 5 out of the 9 patients in the cohort who presented with massive hemoptysis and required surgical intervention had a Dieulafoy's lesion as the etiology, discovered on surgical specimens. These patients were all smokers and it is postulated that the associated chronic irritation and inflammation from smoking may have participated in the pathological evolution of the ectopically located, superficial bronchial arteries seen in Dieulafoy's disease of the bronchus.[173]

Diagnostic Approach

If one excludes cryptogenic hemoptysis as a distinct diagnosis, the cause of hemoptysis can be determined in 68–98% of cases.[13,174] The diagnostic work-up of hemoptysis involves both standard evaluations that should be performed on most patients **(Table 3)**, and specialized testing to be ordered only if indicated by the specific clinical setting **(Table 4)**. After the initial evaluation, the next steps are determined by each patient's specific clinical picture.

Table 3 The initial evaluation of hemoptysis

History and physical
• Smoking history • Presence of cardiopulmonary disease • History of bleeding from upper airways or gastrointestinal tract • History of aspiration events • Duration of symptoms • Drugs and medications • Travel history
Laboratory evaluation
• Complete blood count, platelets • Blood urea nitrogen (BUN)/Creatinine • Urinalysis • Coagulation studies • Brain natriuretic peptide (BNP)
Sputum
• Acid-fast bacillus (AFB), bacteria and fungus • Cytology
Chest radiograph
+/–Chest CT scan
+/–Bronchoscopy

History

A detailed history and physical examination should always be performed **(Table 3)**. The first step is to confirm the presence of hemoptysis and distinguish it from pseudohemoptysis. The second step is to try to quantify the volume of hemoptysis.

Table 4 List of special tests for the work-up of hemoptysis

Imaging
• High-resolution computed tomography • CT scan with contrast • Bronchial angiogram • Spiral aortogram • Pulmonary angiogram • Magnetic resonance imaging • Ventilation-perfusion scan • Lower extremity venous duplex scan • Echocardiogram
Laboratory values
• Antinuclear antibodies • Rheumatoid factor • Antineutrophilic cytoplasmic antibodies • Complement levels • Cryoglobulins • Anti-glomerular basement membrane antibodies • Urine legionella and urine pneumococcal antigens • Stool exam for ova and parasites
Pathology
Lung or kidney biopsies

The third step involves identifying the most likely broad category of etiology **(Table 1)**. The fourth and final step is to find a specific cause of hemoptysis.

Even though not indicative of severity, the frequency, timing and duration of hemoptysis may be helpful in assessing the cause of hemoptysis. Bronchiectasis may present with recurrent episodes over the course of years.[175] Bronchogenic carcinoma causes the recurrent episodes of mild hemoptysis often developing for a few weeks.[176] The timing can also be misleading in a patient with chronic bronchitis who may subsequently develop a lung cancer. Hemoptysis coinciding with the menstrual period, suggests thoracic endometriosis.[177] Exertion induced and postcoital bloody expectoration is characteristic of pulmonary congestion as seen with cardiogenic pulmonary edema.[66] Acute onset of hemoptysis, fever and chest pain suggests infection or pulmonary infarction from thromboembolism.[1]

The patient's age is another important consideration. Before the third decade of life, the likely causes of hemoptysis include acute tracheobronchitis, congenital cardiac or pulmonary disease, cystic fibrosis and infectious pneumonia. However, persistent hemoptysis after adequately treated pneumonia should raise the suspicion of an endobronchial lesion or a coagulopathy.[178] Bronchogenic carcinoma is very rare in patients younger than 40 years of age; however, germ cell tumors may lead to endobronchial metastases that may bleed. Bronchial adenoma is another consideration in the younger patient population.

Occasionally, the character of the sputum can add some useful information during the diagnostic evaluation.

Pulmonary edema from passive congestion, as seen with left ventricular failure and mitral stenosis, may present with pink frothy sputum in a patient with orthopnea and paroxysmal nocturnal dyspnea. When gritty, white material is seen mixed with blood in the sputum, one should consider the diagnosis of broncholithiasis as seen in tuberculosis and histoplasmosis. Blood and pus in expectorated sputum suggest infection.

A history of hematuria should raise the suspicion of a vasculitis. NGV comes with the characteristic triad of upper and lower airway disease with rapidly progressive glomerulonephritis. SLE may cause DAH anytime during the course of the disease.[104] When the pulmonary and renal manifestations are present in a young male smoker, Goodpasture's syndrome, caused by antibasement membrane antibodies, is a strong possibility;[95] influenza infection,[179] inhalation of hydrocarbons,[177] and penicillamine ingestion should also be considered.[118] DAH may also complicate hematopoietic stem cell transplantation in 5% of allogeneic and autologous recipients, and in this setting, carries a 50–100% mortality rate, with a 38% 6-month mortality rate for those who survive.[180]

Hemoptysis with simultaneous bleeding from the gastrointestinal tract, skin or the nose may point to an inappropriate high dose of anticoagulants or a bleeding disorder such as disseminated intravascular coagulation (DIC). The latter should be suspected in a critically ill patient with bleeding, thrombocytopenia and microangiopathic anemia. Oral contraceptives, prolonged immobilization, long bone fractures and recent surgery should raise the suspicion of deep venous thrombosis and venous thromboembolism.

Tracheoarterial fistulas, though rare, should be considered in a patient with a tracheotomy and hemoptysis. Massive hemoptysis from rupture of these fistulas will have a sentinel or preceding smaller bleed in 34–50% of cases. The peak incidence is between the first and second week after tracheotomy, with 72% occurring within 21 days.[89] During the initial 48 hours of tracheotomy placement, bleeding can result from overly vigorous suctioning.

The travel history should be documented. Bacterial, fungal and parasitic etiologies for hemoptysis can be suspected depending on the geographical area of exposure. Tuberculosis is endemic in the developing world and should always be considered in the differential diagnosis. Melioidosis caused by *Burkholderia pseudomallei* is ubiquitous in the soil and stagnant water of Southeast Asia, as well as it can mimic the clinical presentation and course of tuberculosis.[144] Examples of fungal infections include coccidiomycosis in the Southwest of the United States, Central and South America; histoplasmosis in the Mississippi River valley, as well as in the caves of South America and Africa; and paracoccidiomycosis in the regions of North, Central and South America. Examples of parasitic infections include paragonimiasis in travelers to East Asia, Central and South America, Central and West Africa; and schistosomiasis in all of Africa, the Middle East, Southeast and Central Asia and South America.[145]

Physical Examination

While doing a physical examination, special attention should be paid to the nose, gums, pharynx and skin. The presence of telangiectasia suggests a diagnosis of Osler-Weber-Rendu disease. NGV will frequently involve the nasal passages. Ecchymoses and petechiae raise the concern for a clotting disorder or a vasculitic process. When wheezing is localized, it points to an endobronchial lesion. Stridor is more likely seen with an obstructing lesion of the extrathoracic airway or edema of the larynx. Localized crackles suggest focal airspace disease. Even though the physical examination may be helpful in determining the cause of hemoptysis, it is unreliable in localizing the site of bleeding.

Laboratory Evaluation

Routine laboratory studies may be helpful in specific situations. Iron deficiency anemia may suggest idiopathic pulmonary hemosiderosis; likewise, an elevated white blood cell count in the right clinical setting may support a diagnosis of pneumonia. The urinalysis may show hematuria as seen with the pulmonary-renal syndromes. Coagulation studies and platelet counts may unmask a bleeding disorder. The brain natriuretic peptide (BNP) may aid in the diagnosis of cardiogenic pulmonary edema.

Sputum Gram stain and cultures may aid in the diagnosis of bacterial pneumonia. Acid-fast bacilli smear and cultures can also be obtained from sputum. Serum antiglomerular membrane antibodies help in the diagnosis of Goodpasture's, antineutrophil antibodies and antineutrophil cytoplasmic antibodies (ANCA) will be elevated in SLE and NGV, respectively.

Chest Radiograph

An initial posteroanterior and lateral chest radiograph should always be obtained in patients with hemoptysis. About 30% of patients with hemoptysis will have a normal chest radiograph.[181-184] Aspirated blood may give a false impression of being the source of hemoptysis, and bronchoscopy may reveal other areas causing bleeding that were not evident on the chest radiograph.[102,185,186] The chest radiograph may reveal radiopaque foreign bodies that can cause hemoptysis even years after aspiration. Cavities may be single or several, suggest tuberculosis and other bacterial, fungal or parasitic infections, thromboembolic events, neoplasms or NGV **(Figs 7 and 8)**. The finding of a mass within a preformed cavity is suggestive of a fungus ball, seen with aspergillomas. Squamous cell lung carcinoma is the most likely type of lung cancer to cavitate **(Fig. 6)**. Multiple nodules are seen in septic emboli, miliary TB, lung metastases and NGV. Arteriovenous fistulas may be seen as pulmonary nodules with feeding vessels. Diffuse alveolar filling, sparing the costophrenic angles and apices, is suggestive of pulmonary hemorrhage. Thick, dilated bronchi with an air fluid level may be seen in bronchiectasis. Bilateral pleural effusions, an enlarged cardiac silhouette, Kerley B lines and perihilar edema suggest congestive heart failure.

Bronchoscopy

Bronchoscopy is a very valuable tool for localizing and diagnosing the source of hemoptysis, but not all patients with hemoptysis require a bronchoscopy. Patients who may forgo this procedure include those with strong evidence of a non-neoplastic disease (e.g. congestive heart failure), those with pseudohemoptysis, those whose condition is so debilitating or so far advanced that no change in management will result from the bronchoscopic findings, and lastly those who are younger than 40 years of age with short-lived hemoptysis of less than 1 week in duration.[181]

Bronchoscopy will localize the source of bleeding in 93% of patients if performed within 24 hours.[185,187] However, the rate of success drops to 51% if done within 48 hours.[188] Rigid bronchoscopy is preferred in the cases of massive hemoptysis because an airway is secured and the patient is ventilated during this procedure. The rigid bronchoscope has a large lumen that allows for more vigorous suctioning and more therapeutic options than a flexible bronchoscope. Rigid bronchoscopy must be performed under general anesthesia in the operating room. Flexible bronchoscopy may be performed at the bedside, does not require general anesthesia, and can visualize up to the sixth generation of airways. However, the suctioning capacity of the flexible bronchoscope is limited and it does not secure the airway. To deal with this problem, the patient can be intubated and the bronchoscope advanced through the endotracheal tube. This ensures airway control and makes frequent removal and reinsertion of the bronchoscope possible. Alternatively, the patient could be intubated with a rigid bronchoscope for better suctioning and a flexible bronchoscope can be advanced through it for better overall airway visualization.

Bronchoscopy may also be helpful in the diagnosis of DAH. Bronchoalveolar lavage fluid that becomes progressively bloodier with each aliquot and lavage fluid containing hemosiderin-laden macrophages that number more than 20% of total alveolar macrophages are both suggestive of DAH.[189]

Computed Tomography

Computed tomography (CT) scanning plays an important role in the evaluation of hemoptysis. It has been shown, in some studies, to be as good as bronchoscopy for localizing the bleeding, and superior to bronchoscopy at diagnosing the cause of bleeding.[190] Chest CT is superior to plain films and bronchoscopy in diagnosing bronchiectasis, post-tuberculous lesions, aspergillomas and tumors, together the most common causes of massive hemoptysis. However, CT will fail to identify localized mucosal abnormalities such as bronchitis, telangiectasias, early carcinoma, squamous metaplasia, benign papillomas and Kaposi's sarcoma.[188] Contrast administration appears to be unnecessary for making a diagnosis by CT. In addition, a large number of patients with massive hemoptysis will undergo angiographic embolization. It seems appropriate to consider a CT of the chest without contrast on all cases of massive and moderate hemoptysis.[190]

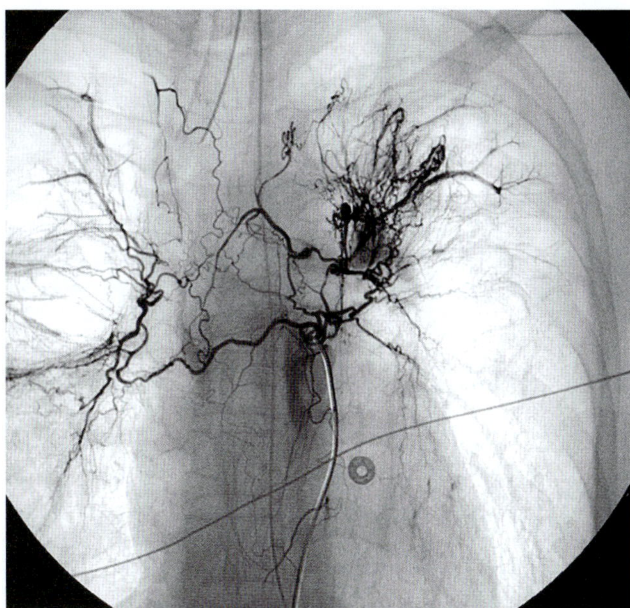

Fig. 9 Selective bronchial angiography showing intense neovascularization and bronchial-pulmonary anastomoses in a patient with a left upper lobe mycetoma

Bronchial Angiography

Bronchial angiography is an excellent method for localizing the site of bleeding in patients with active, submassive and massive hemoptysis. Abnormal bronchial arteries may be hypertrophied, tortuous, increased in size and number, as well as there may be arteriovenous shunts and aneurysms.[191] The site of bleeding can be determined angiographically in up to 90–93% of cases.[192] Angiography may locate a bleeding site in about 4% of cases, when bronchoscopy and other radiographic techniques fail.[187] Once a bleeding vessel is identified, arterial embolization can be performed to stop the bleeding; potential therapeutic intervention represents an additional advantage of arterial angiography **(Figs 9 and 10)**.

TREATMENT

The goals of treatment are to prevent asphyxiation due to the aspiration of large volumes of blood and to stop the bleeding. Both general supportive care and more specific definitive

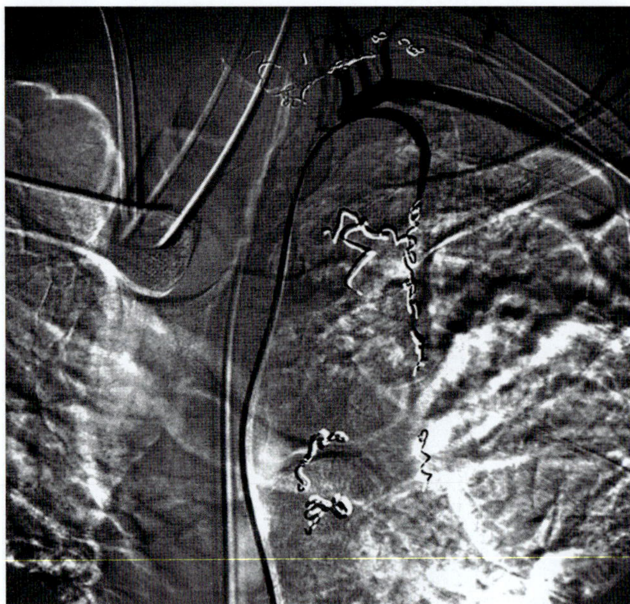

Fig. 10 Angiographic coil embolization of internal mammary artery and thyrocervical artery branches. Notice the acute cutoff of the contrast in the internal mammary artery after the coils

measures are necessary.[193] **Flow chart 1** shows an overview of the therapeutic approach to hemoptysis.

Supportive Care

Patients should be placed on bed rest; if the site of bleeding is known, the affected lung should be placed down in the lateral supine position. Mild sedation can be used to attenuate vigorous coughing that may worsen bleeding by dislodging clots; however, too much depression of cough should be avoided because an effective cough may be necessary to avoid aspiration and asphyxiation. Chest physiotherapy and postural drainage should be avoided.

Patients who experience rapid deterioration with worsening oxygenation may require endotracheal intubation. Whenever intubation is needed, an 8.0 mm or greater endotracheal tube should be used to allow for future bronchoscopy. Another option is to intubate with a double lumen tube and try to isolate the unaffected lung; however, these tubes have a smaller internal diameter that can be more easily obstructed by clots and secretions. They are also difficult tubes to place properly, even by an experienced anesthesiologist, are prone to migrate and lose their isolating effect.[9] Intravenous (IV) fluids and blood products should be administered as needed to reverse any underlying coagulopathy; two large bore peripheral IV lines should be placed for this end. An exception to the avoidance of anticoagulation is patients with venous thromboembolism.[194]

Definitive Care

Nonmassive Hemoptysis

For the definitive care of nonmassive hemoptysis, treatment should be targeted to the specific underlying cause. Suppurative bronchiectasis should be treated with antibiotics and a bronchodilator (e.g. β-adrenergic agonists). Similarly, an exacerbation of chronic bronchitis can be controlled with steroids, antibiotics and a bronchodilator; but most importantly, by smoking cessation. Airway lesions should be resected whenever possible. Congestive heart failure and mitral stenosis can be treated with diuretics and afterload reduction. Venous thromboembolism should be treated with anticoagulation and diuretics.

Massive Hemoptysis

Several bronchoscopic options are available to stop severe bleeding. Placement of an endobronchial balloon can be used for tamponade in all lobes except the right upper lobe where the acute angle of the right upper lobe bronchus prevents placement.[195] Placement is done with a 100 cm long four French Fogarty balloon catheter. The balloon should be positioned in a way that completely occludes the bronchus and causes distal pulmonary collapse. Smaller catheter balloons can also be used and be placed more distally in segmental bronchi. A downside to the use of the Fogarty catheter is its propensity to migrate. Newer catheters have special Y connectors that may be secured to the endotracheal tube to prevent migration.[196] Other interventions include iced saline lavage, laser bronchoscopy,[195] application of topical epinephrine (1:20,000), thrombin, or a fibrinogen-thrombin combination.[197]

Angiographic embolization has a high success rate for the control of massive hemoptysis, being successful in 77–95% of cases **(Fig. 10 and Flow chart 1)**.[19,187] However; there is a 16% incidence of rebleeding within 1–4 days so multiple procedures are frequently necessary.[19,198,199] After proper control of hemoptysis, it may be expected that 20% of patients will rebleed in the next 6 months,[200] and 22% within 3–5 years.[19] The potential complications of angiographic embolization are rare, but spinal artery embolization does occur less than 1% in experienced hands of the time, especially when a spinal artery originates from a bronchial artery.[198]

The combination of endobronchial stenting and angiographic embolization has been done to achieve the equivalent of a "medical pneumonectomy" in a patient with massive hemoptysis due to a pulmonary artery pseudoaneurysm after radiation therapy for nonsmall cell lung cancer.[201]

The role of surgery has decreased significantly due to the high success rate of angiographic embolization procedures. However, surgery remains the preferred treatment of massive hemoptysis due to AVMs, leaky aortic aneurysms, hydatid

Flow chart 1 Proposed algorithm for the management of hemoptysis. The flow chart shows a proposed algorithm for the management of massive versus nonmassive hemoptysis

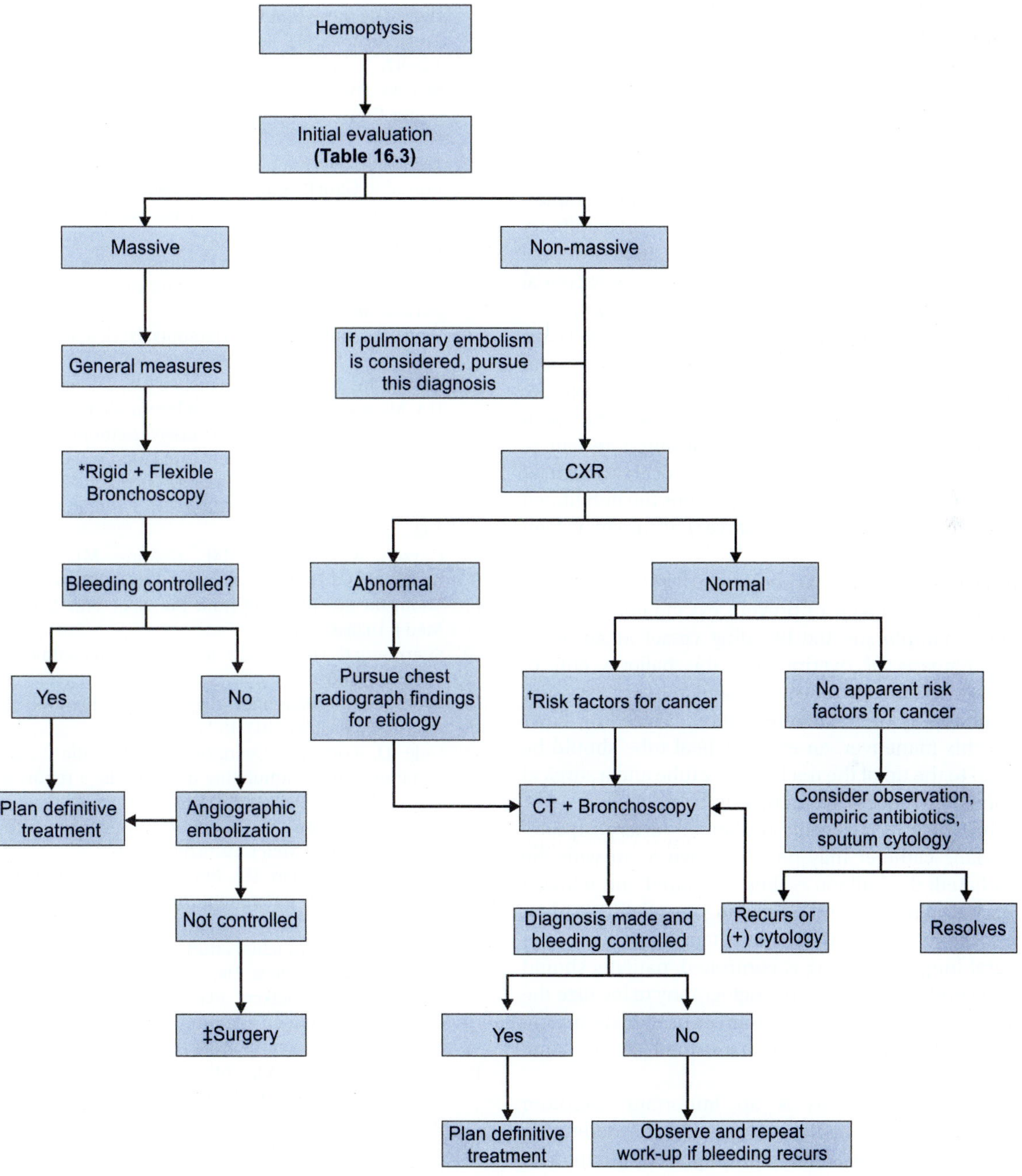

*There may be situations where angiographic embolization is indicated first.
†Age >40-years-old, smoker, previous cancer or other.
‡Surgery may be indicated first when the etiology of bleeding is not amenable to embolization or may have a high likelihood of recurrence, see text.
Abbreviations: CXR, chest radiograph; CT, computed tomography

cysts, pulmonary artery ruptures, chest traumas, bronchial adenomas and fungus balls that have not responded to medical therapy.[198] All these situations involve either a problem not amenable to embolization, or a very likely recurrence after embolization. Because emergency surgery for hemoptysis is associated with higher morbidity and mortality, if possible, bleeding should be controlled by nonsurgical therapies first in order to optimize conditions for surgery and improve outcomes.[202]

Given the complexity and availability of different therapies, in all cases of massive hemoptysis a multidisciplinary approach involving the critical care specialist, interventional pulmonologist, thoracic surgeon and interventional radiologist is likely to achieve the best possible outcomes.[203]

The treatment of DAH generally requires IV corticosteroids, cytotoxic drugs and even plasmapheresis (e.g. NGV and Goodpasture's). Vasculitis-induced DAH will often require combined therapy. Pulmonary aspergillomas have been treated by the intracavitary instillation of amphotericin B, nystatin and sodium iodide solutions.[204,205] Local radiation of fungus balls may be an alternative for patients too debilitated or having such a poor pulmonary reserve that surgery is high risk.[206,207]

When bleeding is due to a tracheoarterial fistula, immediate measures should be taken to prevent exsanguination. One way to try to tamponade the bleeding vessel in an acute emergency consists of overinflating the balloon cuff of the tracheotomy tube as downward and forward pressure is applied on top of the tracheotomy tube. If bleeding slows down with this maneuver, an endotracheal tube should be placed distal to the tip of the tracheotomy tube and a surgical consult should be requested emergently.[89]

In the presence of iatrogenic pulmonary artery rupture, the Swan-Ganz catheter may be withdrawn 5 cm with the balloon deflated; the balloon is then reinflated and allowed to float back to tamponade the bleeding vessel. The patient should also be intubated in the mainstem bronchus of the contralateral lung. If bleeding is controlled, patients should immediately undergo pulmonary angiography to localize the arterial tear and assess for the formation of a pseudoaneurysm. Frequently, embolization can be performed at the same time.[23]

In summary, hemoptysis is an important symptom requiring a thorough medical evaluation to determine the underlying diagnosis. The first step in evaluation is a complete medical history and physical examination. Depending on whether the bleed is massive or nonmassive, subsequent evaluation and treatment may require additional radiographic imaging, flexible bronchoscopy, rigid bronchoscopy, angiographic embolization and surgery. The diagnostic tests and therapeutic interventions required will depend largely on the clinical presentation, rate of bleeding, and the availability of the proper equipment and experienced personnel.

REFERENCES

1. Balter MS. Hemoptysis. In: Irwin RS, Curley FJ, Grossman RF (Eds). Diagnosis and Treatment of Symptoms of the Respiratory Tract. Armonk, NY: Futura Publishing Company, Inc.; 1997. pp. 155-97.
2. Selecky PA. Evaluation of hemoptysis through the bronchoscope. Chest. 1978;73(5 Suppl):741-5.
3. Noehren TH. Ward rounds: hemoptysis. Dis Chest. 1953;24(5):580-1.
4. Prasad R, Garg R, Singhal S, Srivastava P. Lessons from patients with hemoptysis attending a chest clinic in India. Ann Thorac Med. 2009;4(1):10-2.
5. Sakr L, Dutau H. Massive Hemoptysis: An update in the role of bronchoscopy in diagnosis and management. Respiration. 2010;80:38-58.
6. Wolfe JD, Simmons DH. Hemoptysis: diagnosis and management. West J Med. 1977;127(5):383-90.
7. Crocco JA, Roonet JJ, Fankushen DS, DiBenedetto RJ, Lyons HA. Massive hemoptysis. Arch Intern Med. 1968;121(6):495-8.
8. Corey R, Hla KM. Major and massive hemoptysis: reassessment of conservative management. Am J Med Sci. 1987;294(5):301-9.
9. Conlan AA, Hurwitz SS, Krige L, Nicolaou N, Pool R. Massive hemoptysis: a review of 123 cases. J Thorac Cardiovasc Surg. 1983; 85(1):120-4.
10. Garzon AA, Cerruti MM, Golding ME. Exsanguinating hemoptysis. J Thorac Cardiovasc Surg. 1982;84(6):829-33.
11. Thomson SC. Bleeding from the Nose and Throat. Postgrad Med J. 1928;3:73-8.
12. Stiernberg C. Hemoptysis of undetermined etiology. Tex Med. 1964;60:630-5.
13. Lyons HA. Differential diagnosis of hemoptysis and its treatment. Basics of RD. 1976;5:26-30.
14. Gale D, Lord JD. Overgrowth of Serratia marcescens in respiratory tract, simulating hemoptysis; a report of a case. J Am Med Assoc. 1957;164(12):1328-30.
15. Newton RW, Forest AR. Rifampicin overdosage—"the red man syndrome". Scott Med J. 1975;20(2):55-6.
16. Baktari JB, Tashkin DP, Small GW. Factitious hemoptysis. Adding to the differential diagnosis. Chest. 1994;105(3): 943-5.
17. Pump KK. The bronchial arteries and their anastomoses in the human lung. Dis Chest. 1963;43:245-55.
18. Cauldwell EW, Seikert RG, Lininger RE, Anson BJ. The bronchial arteries: an anatomic study of 150 human cadavers. Surg Gynecol Obstet. 1948;86(4):395-412.
19. Rabkin JE, Astafjev VI, Gothman LN, Gothman LN, Grigorjev YG. Transcatheter embolization in the management of pulmonary hemorrhage. Radiology. 1987;163(2):361-5.
20. Wood DA, Miller M. Role of dual pulmonary circulation in various pathologic conditions of lungs. J Thorac Surg. 1938;7:649-70.
21. Coblontz CL, Sallee DS, Chiles C. Aortobronchopulmonary fistula complicating aortic aneurysm: diagnosis in four cases. AJR Am J Roentgenol. 1988;150(3):535-8.
22. Moll HH. A clinical and pathological study of bronchiectasis. Q J Med. 1932;25:457-69.
23. Bartter T, Irwin RS, Phillips DA, Benotti JR, Worthington-Kirsch RL. Pulmonary artery pseudoaneurysm. A potential complication of pulmonary artery catheterization. Arch Intern Med. 1988;148(2):471-3.

24. Hamer DH, Schwab LE, Gray R. Massive hemoptysis from thoracic actinomycosis successfully treated by embolization. Chest. 1992;101(5):1442-3.
25. Hirshberg B, Sklair-Levi M, Nir-Paz R, Ben-Sira L, Krivoruk V, Kramer MR. Factors predicting mortality of patients with lung abscess. Chest. 1999;115(3);746-50.
26. Reyes MP. The aerobic gram-negative bacillary pneumonias. Med Clin North Am. 1980;64(3):363-83.
27. Masher DM, McKenzie SO. Infections due to *Staphylococcus aureus*. Medicine (Baltimore). 1977;56(5):383-409.
28. Camuset J, Nunes H, Dombret MC, Bergeron A, Henno P, Philippe B, et al. Treatment of chronic pulmonary aspergillosis by voriconazole in nonimmunocompromised patients. Chest. 2007;131(5);1435-41.
29. Stevens DA, Kan VL, Judson MA, Morrison VA, Dummer S, Denning DW, et al. Practice guidelines for diseases caused by Aspergillus. Infectious Diseases Society of America. Clin Infect Dis. 2000;30(4):696-709.
30. Masur H, Rosen PP, Armstrong D. Pulmonary disease caused by Candida species. Am J Med. 1977;63(6):914-25.
31. Kerkering TM, Duma RJ, Shadomy S. The evolution of pulmonary cryptococcosis: clinical implications from a study of 41 patients with and without compromising host factors. Ann Intern Med. 1981;94(5):611-6.
32. Barenfanger J, Ramirez F, Tewari RP, Eagleton L. Pulmonary phaeohyphomycosis in a patient with hemoptysis. Chest. 1989;95(5):1158-60.
33. Wheat LJ, Slama TG, Eitzen HE, Kohler RB, French ML, Biesecker JL. A large urban outbreak of histoplasmosis: clinical features. Ann Intern Med. 1981;94(3):331-7.
34. Bigby TD, Serota ML, Tierney LM Jr, Matthay MA. Clinical spectrum of mucormycosis. Chest. 1986;89(3):435-9.
35. Bethlem NM, Lemle A, Bethlem E, WANKE, B. Paracoccidio-mycoses. Semin Respir Med. 1991;12:81-97.
36. Pluss JL, Opal SM. Pulmonary sporotrichosis: review of treatment and outcome. Medicine (Baltimore). 1986;65(3):143-53.
37. Ibarra-Pérez C. Thoracic complications of amebic abscess of the liver: report of 501 cases. Chest. 1981;79(6):672-7.
38. Fraser RG, Pare JAP, Pare PD, et al. Diagnosis of Diseases of the Chest, 3rd edition. Philadelphia: WB Saunders Company; 1989. p. 1097.
39. Gelpi AP, Mustafa A. Ascaris pneumonia. Am J Med. 1968;44(3):377-89.
40. Goodman ML, Gore I. Pulmonary infarct secondary to dirofilaria larvae. Arch Inern Med. 1964;113:702-5.
41. Xanthakis D, Efthimiadis M, Papadakis G, Primikirios N, Chassapakis G, Roussaki A, et al. Hydatid disease of the chest: report of 91 patients surgically treated. Thorax. 1972;27(5):517-28.
42. Barrett-Connor E. Parasitic pulmonary disease. Am Rev Respir Dis. 1982;126(3):558-63.
43. Nana A, Bovornkitti S. Pleuroplumonary paragonimiasis. Semin Respir Med. 1991;12:46-54.
44. Mascarenhas DA, Vasudevan VP, Vaidya KP. Pneumocystis carinii pneumonia. Rare cause of hemoptysis. Chest. 1991;99(1):251-3.
45. Shimazu C, Pien FD, Parnell D. Bronchoscopic diagnosis of Schistosoma japonicum in a patient with hemoptysis. Respir Med. 1991;85(4):331-2.
46. Bruno P, McAllister K, Mathews JI. Pulmonary strongyloides. South Med J. 1982;75(3):363-5.
47. Prince DS, Peterson DD, Steiner RM, Gottlieb JE, Scott R, Israel HL, et al. Infection with Mycobacterium Avium complex in patients without predisposing conditions. N Engl J Med. 1989;321(13):863-8.
48. Plessinger VA, Jolly PN. Rasmussen's aneurysm and fatal hemorrhage in pulmonary tuberculosis. Am Rev Tuberc. 1949;60(5):589-603.
49. Shamsuddin D, Tuazon CU. Massive hemoptysis caused by Mycobacterium xenopi. Tubercle. 1984;65(3):201-4.
50. Louria DB, Blumenfeld HL, Ellis JT, Kilbourne ED, Rogers DE. Studies on influenza in the pandemic of 1957-1958. II. Pulmonary complications of influenza. J Clin Invest. 1959;38(1 Part 2):213-65.
51. Davila DG, Dunn WF, Tazelaar HD, Pairolero PC. Bronchial carcinoid tumors. Mayo Clin Proc. 1993;68(8):795-803.
52. Kleinman J, Zirkin H, Feuchtwanger MM, Hertzanu Y, Walfisch S. Benign hamartoma of the lung presenting as massive hemoptysis. J Surg Oncol. 1986;33(1):38-40.
53. Mittelman M, Fink G, Mor R, Avidor I, Spitzer S. Inflammatory bronchial polyps complicated by massive hemoptysis. Eur J Respir Dis. 1986;69(1):63-6.
54. Holden WE, Morris JF, Antonovic R, Gill TH, Kessler S. Adult intrapulmonary and mediastinal lymphangioma causing haemoptysis. Thorax. 1987;42(8):635-6.
55. Miller RR, McGregor D. Hemorrhage from carcinoma of the lung. Cancer. 1980;46(1):200-5.
56. Benditt JO, Farber HW, Wright J, Karnad AB. Pulmonary hemorrhage with diffuse alveolar infiltrates in men with high-volume choriocarcinoma. Ann Intern Med. 1988;109(8):674-5.
57. Bagwell SP, Flynn SD, Cox PM, Davison JA. Primary malignant melanoma of the lung. Am Rev Respir Dis. 1989;139(6):1543-7.
58. Baumgartner WA, Mark JB. Metastatic malignancies from distant sites to the tracheobronchial tree. J Thorac Cardiovasc Surg. 1980;79(4):499-503.
59. Fitzgerald RH. Endobronchial metastases. South Med J. 1977;70(4):440-1.
60. Weiland JE, de los Santos ET, Mazzaferri EL, Schuller DE, Oertel JE, et al. Hemoptysis as the presenting manifestation of thyroid carcinoma. A case report. Arch Intern Med. 1989;149(7):1693-4.
61. Sakumoto N, Inafuku S, Shimoji H, Nomura K, Honma K, Kawabata T, et al. Endobronchial metastasis from renal cell carcinoma: report of a case. Surg Today. 2000;30(8):744-6.
62. Fournel C, Bertoletti L, Nguyen B, Vergnon JM. Endobronchial metastases from colorectal cancers: natural history and role of interventional bronchoscopy. Respiration. 2009;77(1):63-9.
63. Morehead RS, Dale WJ, Lee EY. A 53-year-old female with haemoptysis following breast cancer resection. Eur Respir J. 2006;28(1):248-50.
64. Wood P. An appreciation of mitral stenosis. I. Clinical features. Br Med J. 1954;1(4870):1051-63.
65. Bansal S, Day JA, Braman SS. Hemoptysis during sexual intercourse. Unusual manifestation of coronary artery disease. Chest. 1988;93(4):891-2.
66. Fuks L, Shitrit D, Amital A, Fox BD, Kramer MR. Postcoital hemoptysis: our experience and review of the literature. Respir Med. 2009;103(12):1828-31.
67. Lee YS, Baek JS, Kwon BD, Kim GB, Bae EJ, Noh CI, et al. Pediatric emergency room presentation of congenital heart disease. Korean Circ J. 2010;40(1):36-41.

68. Sheffield EA, Moore-Gillon J, Murday AR, Addis BJ. Massive hemoptysis caused by spontaneous rupture of a bronchial artery. Thorax. 1988;43(1):71-2.
69. Benatar SR, Ferguson AD, Goldschmidt RB. Fat embolism--some clinical observations and a review of controversial aspects. Q J Med. 1972;41(161):85-98.
70. Villar MT, Wiggins J, Corrin B, Evans TW. Recurrent and fatal haemoptysis caused by an atheromatous abdominal aortic aneurysm. Thorax. 1990;45(7):568-9.
71. Olivari MT. Southwestern primary pulmonary hypertension. Am J Med Sci. 1991;302(3):185-98.
72. Hughes JP, Stovin PG. Segmental pulmonary artery aneurysms with peripheral venous thrombosis. Br J Dis Chest. 1959;53(1):19-27.
73. Morgan JM, Morgan AD, Addis B, Bradley GW, Spiro SG. Fatal haemorrhage from mycotic aneurysms of the pulmonary artery. Thorax. 1986;41(1):70-1.
74. Matsumoto AH, Delany DJ, Parker LA, Ney KA. Massive hemoptysis associated with isolated peripheral pulmonary artery stenosis. Cath Cardiovasc Diagn. 1987;13(5):313-6.
75. Tapson VF. Acute pulmonary embolism. N Engl J Med. 2008;358(10):1037-52.
76. Webb DW, Thadepalli H. Hemoptysis in patients with septic pulmonary infarcts from tricuspid endocarditis. Chest. 1979;76(1):99-100.
77. Parish JM, Marschke RF, Dines DE, Lee RE. Etiologic considerations in superior vena cava syndrome. Mayo Clin Proc. 1981;56(7):407-13.
78. Porter DK, Van Every MJ, Anthracite RF, Mack JW Jr. Massive hemoptysis in cystic fibrosis. Arch Intern Med. 1983;143(2):287-90.
79. Panos RJ, Kumpe DA, Samara N, Petty TL. Recurrent cryptogenic hemoptysis associated with bronchial artery-pulmonary artery anastomoses and cystic lung disease. Am J Med. 1989;87(6):683-6.
80. Faerber EN, Balsara R, Vinocur CD, de Chadarevian JP. Gastric duplication cyst with hemoptysis: CT findings. AJR Am J Roentgenol. 1993;161(6):1245-6.
81. Koyama A, Sasou K, Nakao H, Hirano A, Hachiya H, Iwasaki M, et al. Pulmonary intralobar sequestration accompanied by aneurysm of an anomalous arterial supply. Intern Med. 1992;31(7):946-50.
82. Shackford SR. Blunt chest trauma: the intensivist's perspective. J Intensive Care Med. 1986;1(3):125-36.
83. Cordier JF, Gamondes JP, Marx P, Heinen I, Loire R. Thoracic splenosis presenting with hemoptysis. Chest. 1992;102(2):626-7.
84. Baumgartner R, Sheppard B, de Virgilio C, Esrig B, Harrier D, Nelson RJ, et al. Tracheal and main bronchial disruptions after blunt chest trauma: presentation and management. Ann Thorac Surg. 1990;50(4):569-74.
85. Winkler TR, Hamlin RJ, Hinke TD, et al. Unusual cause of hemoptysis: Hickman-induced cava-bronchial fistula. Chest. 1992;102(4):1285-6.
86. Isaacs RD, Wattie WJ, Wells AU, Rea HH, Bai TR. Massive haemoptysis as a late consequence of pulmonary irradiation. Thorax. 1987;42(1):77-8.
87. Leatherman JW, Davies SF, Haidal JR. Alveolar hemorrhage syndromes: diffuse microvascular lung hemorrhage in immune and idiopathic disorders. Medicine (Baltimore). 1984;63(6):343-61.
88. Feng WC, Singh AK, Drew T, Donat W. Swan-Ganz catheter-induced massive hemoptysis and pulmonary artery false aneurysm. Ann Thorac Surg. 1990;50(4):644-6.
89. Schaefer OP, Irwin RS. Tracheoarterial fistula: an unusual complication of tracheotomy. J Intensive Care Med. 1995;10(2):64-75.
90. Zavala DC. Pulmonary hemorrhage in fiberoptic transbronchial biopsy. Chest. 1976;70(5):584-8.
91. Westcott JL. Percutaneous transthoracic needle biopsy. Radiology. 1988;169(3):593-601.
92. Road JD, Jacques J, Sparling JR. Diffuse alveolar septal amyloidosis presenting with recurrent hemoptysis and medial dissection of pulmonary arteries. Am Rev Respir Dis. 1985;132:1368-70.
93. Kariya ST, Stern RS, Schwatzstein RM, Frank H, Brown RS. Pulmonary hemorrhage associated with bullous pemphigoid of the lung. Am J Med. 1989;86(1):127-8.
94. Bateman ED, Morrison SC. Catamenial hemoptysis from endobronchial endometriosis—a case report and review of previously reported cases. Respir Med. 1990;84(2):157-61.
95. Briggs WA, Johnson JP, Teichman S, Yeager HC, Wilson CB. Antiglomerular basement membrane antibody-mediated glomerulonephritis and Goodpasture's syndrome. Medicine (Baltimore). 1979;58(5):348-61.
96. Soerge KH, Sommers SC. Idiopathic pulmonary hemosiderosis and related syndromes. Am J Med. 1962;32:499-511.
97. Bombardiers S, Paoletti P, Ferri C, Di Munno O, Fornal E, Giuntini C. Lung involvement in essential mixed cryoglobulinemia. Am J Med. 1979;66(5):748-56.
98. Green J, Brenner B, Gery R, Nachoul F, Lichtig C, Better OS, et al. Adult hemolytic uremic syndrome associated with non-immune deposit crescentic glomerulonephritis and alveolar hemorrhage. Am J Med Sci. 1988;296(2):121-5.
99. Kathuria S, Cheifec G. Fatal pulmonary Henöch-Schonlein syndrome. Chest. 1982;82(5):654-6.
100. Border WA, Baehler RW, Bhathena D, Glassock RJ. IgA antibasement membrane nephritis with pulmonary hemorrhage. Ann Intern Med. 1979;91(1):21-5.
101. Zashin S, Fattor R, Fortin D. Microscopic polyarteritis: a forgotten aetiology of haemoptysis and rapidly progressive glomerulonephritis. Ann Rheum Dis. 1990;49(1):53-6.
102. Kim JH, Follett JV, Rice JR, Hampson NB. Endobronchial telangiectasias and hemoptysis in scleroderma. Am J Med. 1988;84(1):173-4.
103. Smith BS. Idiopathic pulmonary hemosiderosis and rheumatoid arthritis. Br Med J. 1966;1(5500):1403-4.
104. Carette S, Macher AM, Nussbaum A, Plotz PH. Severe, acute pulmonary disease in patients with systemic lupus erythematosus: ten years of experience at the National Institutes of Health. Semin Arthritis Rheum. 1984;14(1):52-9.
105. Lopez AJ, Brady Al, Jackson JE. Case report: therapeutic bronchial artery embolization in a case of Takayasu's arteritis. Clin Radiol. 1992;45(6):415-7.
106. Hoffman GS, Kerr GS, Leavitt RY, Hallahan CW, Lebovics RS, Travis WD, et al. Wegener granulomatosis: an analysis of 158 patients. Ann Intern Med. 1992;116(6):488-98.
107. Robboy SJ, Minna JD, Colman RW, Birndorf NI, Lopas H, et al. Pulmonary hemorrhage syndrome as a manifestation of disseminated intravascular coagulation: analysis of ten cases. Chest. 1973;63(5):718-21.

108. Connolly JP. Hemoptysis as a presentation of mild hemophilia A in an adult. Chest. 1993;103(4):1281-2.
109. Smith LJ, Katzenstein AL. Pathogenesis of massive pulmonary hemorrhage in acute leukemia. Arch Intern Med. 1982;142(12):2149-52.
110. Fireman Z, Yust I, Abramov AL. Lethal occult pulmonary hemorrhage in drug-induced thrombocytopenia. Chest. 1981;79(3):358-9.
111. Milman N, Rossel K. Recurrent haemoptysis and pulmonary haemosiderosis associated with granulomatous lung disease and von Willebrand's coagulopathy. Eur J Respir Dis. 1986; 69(3):192-4.
112. Vizioli LD, Cho S. Amiodarone-associated hemoptysis. Chest. 1994;105(1):305-6.
113. Finley TN, Aronow A, Cosentino AM, Golde DW. Occult pulmonary hemorrhage in anticoagulated patients. Am Rev Respir Dis. 1975;112(1):23-9.
114. Vaziri ND, Jeminson-Smith P, Wilson AF. Hemorrhagic pneumonitis after intravenous injection of charcoal lighter fluid. Ann Intern Med. 1979;90(5):794-5.
115. Murray RJ, Albin RJ, Mergner W, Criner GJ. Diffuse alveolar hemorrhage temporarily related to cocaine smoking. Chest. 1988;93(2):427-9.
116. Patterson R, Nugent KM, Harris KE, et al. Immunologic hemorrhagic pneumonia caused by isocyanates. Am Rev Respir Dis. 1990;141(1):226-30.
117. Conetta R, Tamarin FM, Wogalter D, Brandstetter RD. Liquor lung. N Engl J Med. 1987;316(6):348-9.
118. Matloff DS, Kaplan MM. D-penicillamine-induced Goodpasture's-like syndrome in primary biliary cirrhosis--successful treatment with plasmapheresis and immuno-suppressives. Gastroenterology. 1980;78(5 Pt 1):1046-9.
119. Nathan PE, Torres AV, Smith AJ, Gagliardi AJ, Rapeport KB. Spontaneous pulmonary hemorrhage following coronary thrombolysis. Chest. 1992;101(4):1150-2.
120. Ahmad D, Morgan WK, Patterson R, Williams T, Zeiss CR. Pulmonary haemorrhage and haemolytic anemia due to trimellitic anhydride. Lancet. 1979;2(8138):328-30.
121. McLean TR, Beall AC, Jones JW. Massive hemoptysis due to broncholithiasis. Ann Thorac Surg. 1991;52(5):1173-5.
122. Herth F, Ernst A, Becker HD. Long-term outcome and lung cancer incidence in patients with hemoptysis of unknown origin. Chest. 2001;120:1592-4.
123. Adelman M, Haponik EF, Bleecker ER, Britt EJ. Cryptogenic hemoptysis. Clinical features, bronchoscopic findings, and natural history in 67 patients. Ann Intern Med. 1985;102(6):829-34.
124. Pattison CW, Leaming AJ, Townsend ER. Hidden foreign body as a cause of recurrent hemoptysis in a teenage girl. Ann Thorac Surg. 1988;45:330-1.
125. Wynne JW, Modell JH. Respiratory aspiration of stomach contents. Ann Intern Med. 1977;87(4):466-74.
126. Salvaggio JE. Robert A. Cooke memorial lecture. J Allergy Clin Immunol. 1987;79(4):558-71.
127. Ghio AJ, Elliott CG, Crapo RO, Collins MP, Tocino I. A migratory infiltrate in a patient with hemoptysis and chest pain. Chest. 1989;96(1):195-6.
128. Fliegel E, Chitkara RK, Azueta V, Steinberg H. Fatal hemoptysis in lymphangiomyomatosis. NY State J Med. 1991;91(2):66-7.
129. Frymoyer PA, Anderson GH, Blair DC. Hemoptysis as a presenting symptom of pheochromocytoma. J Clin Hypertens. 1986;2(1):65-7.
130. Fartoukh M, Khalil A, Louis L, Carette MF, Bazelly B, Cadranel J, et al. An integrated approach to diagnosis and management of severe haemoptysis in patients admitted to the intensive care unit: a case series from a referral centre. Respir Res. 2007;8:11.
131. Ong TH, Eng P. Massive hemoptysis requiring intensive care. Intensive Care Med. 2003;29(2):317-20.
132. Chan VL, So LK, Lam JY, Lau KY, Chan CS, Lin AW, et al. Major haemoptysis in Hong Kong: aetiologies, angiographic findings and outcomes of bronchial artery embolisation. Int J Tuberc Lung Dis. 2009;13(9):1167-73.
133. Boushy SF, North LB, Trice JA. The bronchial arteries in chronic obstructive pulmonary disease. Am J Med. 1969;46(4):506-15.
134. Johnston H, Reisz G. Changing spectrum of hemoptysis: underlying causes in 148 patients undergoing diagnostic flexile fiberoptic bronchoscopy. Arch Intern Med. 1989;149(7):1666-8.
135. Liebow AA, Hales MR, Lindskog GE. Enlargement of the bronchial arteries and their anastomoses with the pulmonary arteries in bronchiectasis. Am J Pathol. 1949;25(2):211-31.
136. Syabbalo N. Hemoptysis: the Third-World perspective. Chest. 1991;99(5):1316-7.
137. Rasmussen V. On hemoptysis, especially when fatal, in its anatomical and clinical aspects. Edinburgh Med J. 1968;14:385-404.
138. Lin CS, Becker WH. Broncholith as a cause of fatal hemoptysis. JAMA. 1978;239(20):2153.
139. Auerbach O. Pathology and pathogenesis of pulmonary arterial aneurysm in tuberculous cavities. Am Rev Tuberc. 1939;39:99-115.
140. Van Kralingen KW, Hekker TA, Bril H, Strack van Schijndel RJ, Postmus PE. Haemoptysis and an abnormal X-ray after prolonged treatment in the ICU. Eur Respir J. 1994;7(2):419-20.
141. Glimp RA, Bayer AS. Pulmonary aspergilloma: diagnostic and therapeutic considerations. Arch Intern Med. 1983;143(2):303-8.
142. Joynson DH. Pulmonary aspergilloma. Br J Clin Pract. 1977; 31(12):207-21.
143. Zmeili OS, Soubani AO. Pulmonary aspergillosis: a clinical update. QJM. 2007;100(6):317-34.
144. Morrison RE, Lamb AS, Craig DB, Johnson WM. Melioidosis: a reminder. Am J Med. 1988;84(5):965-7.
145. Checkley AM, Chiodini PL, Dockrell DH, Bates I, Thwaites GE, Booth HL, et al. Eosinophilia in returning travelers and migrants from the tropics: UK recommendations of investigation and initial management. J Infect. 2010;60(1):1-20.
146. Hirshberg B, Biran I, Glazer M, Kramer MR. Hemoptysis: etiology, evaluation, and outcome in a tertiary referral hospital. Chest. 1997;112(2):440-4.
147. Hurt R, Bates M. Carcinoid tumors of the bronchus: a 33-year experience. Thorax. 1984;39(8):617-23.
148. McCaughan BC, Martini N, Bains MS. Bronchial carcinoids: Review of 124 cases. J Thorac Cardiovasc Surg. 1985;89(1):8-17.
149. Lunger M, Abelson DS, Elkind AH, Kantrowitz A. Massive hemoptysis in mitral stenosis; control by emergency mitral commisurotomy. N Eng J Med. 1959;261:393-5.
150. Ferguson FC, Kobilack RE, Deitrick JE. Varices of the bronchial veins as a source of hemoptysis in mitral stenosis. Am Heart J. 1944;28:445-6.
151. Dalen JE, Haffajee CI, Alpert JS 3rd, Howe JP, Ockene IS, Paraskos JA. Pulmonary embolism, pulmonary hemorrhage and pulmonary infarction. N Engl J Med. 1977;296(25): 1431-5.

152. Moser KM. Pulmonary embolism. Am Rev Respir Dis. 1977;115(5):829-52.
153. Burke CM, Safai C, Nelson DP, Raffin TA. Pulmonary arteriovenous malformation: a critical update. Am Rev Respir Dis. 1986;134(2):334-9.
154. Bosher LH, Blake DA, Byrd BR. An analysis of the pathologic anatomy of pulmonary arteriovenous aneurysms with particular reference to the applicability of local excision. Surgery. 1959;45(1):91-104.
155. Ference BA, Shannon TM, White RI Jr, Zawin M, Burdge CM. Life-threatening pulmonary hemorrhage with pulmonary arteriovenous malformations and hereditary hemorrhagic telangiectasias. Chest. 1994;106(5):1387-90.
156. Gossage JR, Kanj G. Pulmonary arteriovenous malformations. A state of the art review. Am J Respir Crit Care Med. 1998;158(2):643-61.
157. Löschhorn C, Nierhoff N, Mayer R, Zaunbauer W, Neuweiler J, Knoblauch A, et al. Dieulafoy's disease of the lung: a potential disaster for the bronchoscopist. Respiration. 2006;73(4):562-5.
158. Di Sant'Agnese PA, Davis PB. Cystic fibrosis in adults. Am J Med. 1979;66(1):121-32.
159. Lloyd-Stil JD, Wessel HU. Advances and controversies in cystic fibrosis. Semin Respir Med. 1990;11:197-210.
160. Kshettry VR, Bolman RM. Chest trauma. Assessment, diagnosis, and management. Clin Chest Med. 1994;15(1):137-46.
161. Ahmad M, Livingston DR, Golish JA, Mehta AC, Wiedemann HP. The safety of outpatient transbronchial biopsy. Chest. 1986;9(3):403-5.
162. Wahla AS, Depriest KL, Pascual RM, et al. Bronchoscopic myths and legends: safety of transbronchial biopsy in patients with pulmonary hypertension. Clin Pulm Med. 2009;16:281-3.
163. Diaz-Guzman E, Vadi S, Minai OA, Gildea TR, Mehta AC. Safety of diagnostic bronchoscopy in patients with pulmonary hypertension. Respiration. 2009;77(3):292-7.
164. Germain MJ, Davidman M. Pulmonary hemorrhage and acute renal failure in a patient with mixed connective tissue disease. Am J Kidney Dis. 1984;3(6):420-4.
165. Gómez-Puerta JA, Hernández-Rodríguez J, López-Soto A, Bosch X. Antineutrophil cytoplasmic antibody-associated vasculitides and respiratory disease. Chest. 2009;136(4):1101-11.
166. Ciledağ A, Deniz H, Eledağ S, Özkal C, Düzgün N, Erekul S, et al. An aggressive and lethal course of Churg-Strauss syndrome with alveolar hemorrhage, intestinal perforation, cardiac failure and peripheral neuropathy. Rheumatol Int. 2012;32(2):451-5.
167. Ramos-Casals M, Robles A, Brito-Zerón P, Nardi N, Nicolás JM, Forns X, et al. Life-threatening cryoglobulinemia: clinical and immunological characterization of 29 cases. Semin Arthritis Rheum. 2006;36(3):189-96.
168. Rosen MJ. Dr. Friedrich Wegener, the ACCP, and History. Chest. 2007;132(3):739-41.
169. Alifano M, Trisolini R, Cancellieri A, Regnard JF. Thoracic endometriosis: current knowledge. Ann Thorac Surg. 2006;81(2):761-9.
170. O'Reilly SC, Taylor PM, O'Driscoll BR. Occult bronchiectasis presenting as streptokinase-induced haemoptysis. Respir Med. 1994;88:393-5.
171. Schwarz MI, Fontenot AP. Drug-induced diffuse alveolar hemorrhage syndromes and vasculitis. Clin Chest Med. 2004;25(1):133-40.
172. Panagi S, Palka W, Korelitz BI, Taskin M, Lessnau KD. Diffuse alveolar hemorrhage after infliximab treatment of Crohn's disease. Inflamm Bowel Dis. 2004;10(3):274-7.
173. Savale L, Parrot A, Khalil A, Antoine M, Théodore J, Carette MF, et al. Cryptogenic hemoptysis: from a benign to a life-threatening pathologic vascular condition. Am J Respir Crit Care Med. 2007;175(11):1181-5.
174. Rath GS, Schaff JT, Snider GL. Flexible fiberoptic bronchoscopy. Techniques and review of 100 bronchoscopies. Chest. 1973;63(5):689-93.
175. Souders CR, Smith AT. The clinical significance of hemoptysis. N Eng J Med. 1952;247(21):790-93.
176. Poe RH, Israel RH, Marin MG, Ortiz CR, Dale RC, Wahl GW, et al. Utility of fiberoptic bronchoscopy in patients with hemoptysis and a nonlocalizing chest roentgenogram. Chest. 1988;93(1):70-5.
177. Kleinknecht D, Morel-Maroger L, Callard P, Adhémar JP, Mahieu P. Antiglomerular basement membrane nephritis after solvent exposure. Arch Intern Med. 1980;140(2):230-2.
178. Pratt LW. Hemoptysis. Ann Otol Rhinol Laryngol. 1954;63(2):296-309.
179. Wilson CB, Smith RC. Goodpasture's syndrome associated with influenza A2 virus infection. Ann Intern Med. 1972;76(1):91-4.
180. Lara AR, Schwarz MI. Diffuse alveolar hemorrhage. Chest. 2010;137(5):1164-71.
181. Weaver LJ, Solliday N, Cugell DW. Selection of patients with hemoptysis for fiberoptic bronchoscopy. Chest. 1979;76(1):7-10.
182. Jackson CL, Diamond S. Hemorrhage from the trachea, bronchi and lungs of non-tuberculous origin. Am Rev Tuberc. 1942;46:126-38.
183. Schneider L. Bronchogenic carcinoma heralded by hemoptysis and ignored because of negative chest X-ray results. N Y State J Med. 1959;59(4):637-42.
184. Kallenbach J, Song E, Zwi S. Haemoptysis with no radiological evidence of tumor—the value of early bronchoscopy. S Afr Med J. 1981;59(16):556-8.
185. Smiddy JF, Elliott RC. The evaluation of hemoptysis with fiberoptic bronchoscopy. Chest. 1973;64(2):158-62.
186. Holsclaw DS, Grank RJ, Schwachman H. Massive hemoptysis in cystic fibrosis. J Pediatr. 1970;76(6):829-38.
187. Saumench J, Escarrabill J, Padró L, Montañá J, Clariana A, Cantó A. Value of fiberoptic bronchoscopy and angiography for diagnosis of the bleeding site of hemoptysis. Ann Thorac Surg. 1989;48(2):272-4.
188. McGuinness G, Beacher JR, Harkin TJ, Garay SM, Rom WN, Naidich DP. Hemoptysis: prospective high-resolution CT/bronchoscopic correlation. Chest. 1994;105(4):1155-62.
189. De Lassence A, Fleury-Feith J, Escudier E, Beaune J, Bernaudin JF, Cordonnier C. Alveolar hemorrhage. Diagnostic criteria and results in 194 immunocompromised hosts. Am J Respir Crit Care Med. 1995;151(1):157-63.
190. Revel MP, Fournier LS, Hennebicque AS, Cuenod CA, Meyer G, Reynaud P, et al. Can CT replace bronchoscopy in the detection of the site and cause of bleeding in patients with large or massive hemoptysis? Am J Roentgenol. 2002;179(5):1217-24.
191. Roberts AC. Bronchial artery embolization therapy. J Thorac Imaging. 1990;5(4):60-72.
192. Kalluri S, Petrides S, Wilson CB, Tomaszewski JE, Palevsky HI, Grippi MA, et al. Anti-alpha1(IV) collagen autoantibodies

associated with lung adenocarcinoma presenting as the Goodpasture syndrome. Ann Intern Med. 1996;124(7):651-3.
193. Worrell SG, DeMeester SR. Thoracic emergencies. Surg Clin N Am. 2014;94:183-91.
194. Barritt DW, Jordan SC. Anticoagulant drugs in treatment of pulmonary embolism. A controlled trial. Lancet. 1960;1(7138):1309-12.
195. Dweik RA, Stoller JK. Role of bronchoscopy in massive hemoptysis. Clin Chest Med. 1999;20(1):89-105.
196. Campos J. An update on bronchial blockers during lung separation techniques in adults. Anesth Analg. 2003;97:1266-74.
197. De Gracia J, de la Rosa D, Catalan E, Alvarez A, Bravo C, Morell F. Use of endoscopic fibrinogen-thrombin in the treatment of severe hemoptysis. Respir Med. 2003;97(7):790-5.
198. Jean-Baptiste E. Clinical assessment and management of massive hemoptysis. Crit Care Med. 2000;28(5):1642-7.
199. Yu-Tang GP, Lin M, Teo N, En Shen Wong D. Embolization for hemoptysis: a six-year review. Cardiovasc Intervent Radiol. 2002;25(1):17-25.
200. Stoll JF, Bettmann MA. Bronchial artery embolization to control hemoptysis: a review. Cardiovasc Intervent Radiol. 1988;11(5):263-9.
201. Chawla M, Getzen T, Simoff MJ. Medical pneumonectomy interventional bronchoscopic and endovascular management of massive Hemoptysis due to pulmonary artery pseudoaneurysm a consequence of endobronchial brachytherapy. Chest. 2009;135:1355-8.
202. Andrejak C, Parrot A, Bazelly B, Ancel PY, Djibré M, Khalil A, et al. Surgical lung resection for severe Hemoptysis. Ann Thorac Surg. 2009;88(5):1556-65.
203. Shigemura N, Wan IY, Yu SCH, Wong RH, Hsin MK, Thung HK, et al. Multi-disciplinary approach to life-threatening Hemoptysis: A 10-year experience. Ann Thorac Surg. 2009;87:849-53.
204. Shapiro MJ, Albelda SM, Mayock RL, McLean GK. Severe hemoptysis associated with pulmonary aspergilloma. Percutaneous intracavitary treatment. Chest. 1988;94(6):1225-31.
205. Lee KS, Kim HT, Kim YH, Choe KO. Treatment of hemoptysis in patients with cavitary aspergilloma of the lung: value of percutaneous instillation of amphotericin B. Am J Roentgenol. 1993;161(4):727-31.
206. Glover S, Holt SG, Newman GH, Kingdon EJ. Radiotherapy for a pulmonary aspergilloma complicating p-ANCA positive small vessel vasculitis. J Infect. 2007;54(4):e215-7.
207. Falkson C, Sur R, Pacella J. External beam radiotherapy: a treatment option for massive haemoptysis caused by mycetoma. Clin Oncol (R Coll Radiol). 2002;14(3):233-5.

17 Chapter

Dyspnea

J Mark Madison, Richard S Irwin

INTRODUCTION

Dyspnea is difficult, labored or unpleasant breathing that is distressing to an individual.[1] The symptom of dyspnea, often referred to as shortness of breath, is frequently described vaguely by patients and it is probably not a single sensation given the many qualitative descriptors patients use to describe it. Three distinct sensations of respiratory discomfort have been described to subcategorize dyspnea—air hunger, work and effort related, and chest tightness—and it is possible that different neural pathways underlie each.[2]

PHYSIOLOGY

The neurophysiologic basis of dyspnea is not yet established.[3,4] However, because the cardiorespiratory system is complex and regulated by complex neurophysiology, it is not surprising that functional neuroimaging and other studies suggest that multiple different sensory, efferent, brain stem and cortical neural pathways are involved in mediating the sensation of dyspnea.[1-5] Afferent neural pathways from all thoracic and even upper abdominal organs may potentially modulate or mediate the sensation of dyspnea.[2,6] It is not surprising that many cardiopulmonary disorders can result in dyspnea or that the intensity of the sensation can be modulated by learning, experience, and emotional and behavioral conditions.

Evidence suggests that three different types of neural receptors are involved in the genesis of dyspnea—(1) chemoreceptors, (2) mechanoreceptors and (3) ergoreceptors of skeletal muscle.[7] Afferent signals from these receptors are integrated in the central nervous system, modulated by cortical input, and compared to efferent motor neuron discharge to the respiratory muscles.

Chemoreceptors detect changes in blood carbon dioxide and oxygen levels.[7] Acute increases in arterial carbon dioxide potently stimulate medullary chemoreceptors that lead to dyspnea by increasing ventilation and by mechanisms independent of ventilation as well. The effect of carbon dioxide on these central chemoreceptors is probably indirect and due to changes in pH. Consistent with this, patients with chronic hypercapnia and a compensated respiratory acidosis are less dyspneic at the same partial pressure of carbon dioxide and less sensitive to changes in carbon dioxide as well. Peripheral chemoreceptors in the carotid and aortic bodies are stimulated by decreases in the partial pressure of oxygen in arterial blood and to a lesser extent by increases in carbon dioxide and decreases in pH. Although it would intuitively seem that hypoxemia would be the main stimulus to dyspnea, this has not been supported by clinical observation or experimental evidence. Not all subjects with dyspnea have hypoxemia and not all patients with hypoxemia have dyspnea. Instead, low oxygen is not the main stimulus to dyspnea and is a much less potent stimulus than elevated carbon dioxide. Evidence suggests that, although it is not a potent stimulus, low oxygen does contribute to dyspnea mainly through its effects on increased ventilation.

Mechanoreceptors are neural receptors that detect changes in pressure, stretch and position.[7] The respiratory system has many different types of mechanoreceptors located throughout the airways, lung parenchyma, chest wall and diaphragm. Discordance between the afferent output of these mechanoreceptors and respiratory motor efferent discharge is believed to play a central role in generating the distressing sense that breathing is difficult.[2]

Ergoreceptors (also called metaboreceptors) are believed to underlie the ergoreflex.[7] This is a complex metabolic reflex that originates in skeletal muscles and stimulates ventilation. Ergoreceptors in skeletal muscle are thought to detect metabolic products of active muscle (possibly lactic acid and others) and send afferent signals that stimulate ventilation. There is high research interest in this reflex and its metabolic receptors, particularly the role of the reflex in causing dyspnea in the settings of heart failure and chronic obstructive pulmonary disease (COPD).

DIFFERENTIAL DIAGNOSIS OF DYSPNEA

The causes of dyspnea are numerous. Many diseases and disorders of the cardiorespiratory system and other organ systems can result in dyspnea. However, the causes of dyspnea can be categorized into general areas **(Table 1)**. The frequency with which specific causes of dyspnea are encountered will vary with the clinical setting, the acuity of onset, and the age of the patients. For different clinical settings, it has been estimated that 75–92% of cases of dyspnea in an emergency department or inpatient hospital setting are due to cardiopulmonary diseases and disorders, while in the ambulatory setting that figure is 46–85%.[1,8-11] Pulmonary, cardiac, psychogenic, gastroesophageal reflux disease (GERD) and deconditioning disorders were the most common causes in an ambulatory clinic specializing in pulmonary diseases **(Fig. 1)**.[11] Specifically for chronic dyspnea, the four most common causes were COPD, asthma, interstitial lung disease and cardiomyopathy.[10]

DISEASE-SPECIFIC PATHOPHYSIOLOGY

The pathophysiologic mechanisms underlying dyspnea in asthma, COPD, cardiac disorders, GERD, psychogenic disorders and deconditioning are different and not well-established.[5]

Respiratory mechanical factors, arterial blood gases and psychological factors all contribute to the genesis of dyspnea in asthma. Importantly, the severity of dyspnea in asthma does not always correlate with the degree of airway obstruction. Asthma patients with a prior history of near-fatal exacerbations have a decreased ventilatory response to hypoxia and a decreased sense of dyspnea.[12]

In COPD, respiratory mechanics play an important role similar to that in asthma. However, the role of carbon dioxide and hypoxemia in the genesis of dyspnea appears to be greater in COPD than in asthma. Recently, for COPD, many studies have focused on the important role that dynamic hyperinflation plays in the genesis of dyspnea during exertion. The dynamic hyperinflation causes increased load on inspiratory muscles, places inspiratory muscles at the suboptimal length for effective contraction, restricts the ability of the patient to increase tidal volume (inspiratory capacity is decreased), and causes ventilation perfusion inequalities that impair gas exchange.[2] Afferent signals from mechanoreceptors and chemoreceptors reflect these distortions of muscle mechanics and changes in gas exchange. Because these are discordant with the amount of efferent motor activity emanating from the medulla respiratory center, severe dyspnea results.[2,13]

Interstitial lung diseases probably cause dyspnea by the mechanical effects of the disease on lung compliance, activation of vagal afferents, and abnormal gas exchange.[1,5] Similarly, compressing lung tissue with pneumothorax or pleural effusion and distortions of the thoracic cage by disease processes (e.g. kyphoscoliosis) probably stimulate dyspnea by the way of vagal afferents, changes in thoracic compliance, and alterations of gas exchange.

Nonpulmonary disorders cause dyspnea by mechanisms that also involve the activation of vagal afferents. Congestive

Table 1 General causes of dyspnea with selected examples[5]

Causes
• *Cardiac*
– Congestive heart failure – Cardiac ischemia
• *Deconditioning/obesity*
• *Endocrine*
– Goiter – Hyperthyroidism – Diabetic ketoacidosis
• *Gastrointestinal*
– Gastroesophageal reflux disease
• *Hematologic/oncologic*
– Anemia – Lung cancer
• *Larynx and upper airway*
– Postnasal drip syndrome (now called UACS) due to any rhinosinus disease – Laryngitis – Vocal cord dysfunction – Goiter
• *Neuromuscular disease*
– Amyotrophic lateral sclerosis – Postpolio syndrome – Mitochondrial myopathies – Neuromuscular weakness of any cause
• *Pharmacologic*
– Nonsteroidal anti-inflammatory drugs
• *Pregnancy*
• *Psychiatric*
– Anxiety – Depression – Hyperventilation syndrome
• *Pulmonary*
– Asthma – COPD – Cystic fibrosis – Pneumonia – Interstitial inflammation of any cause and fibrosis – Pneumothorax – Pleural effusion – Compressive lesions of the airways – Tracheobronchial malacia
• *Renal*
– Metabolic acidosis – Renal failure
• *Rheumatologic*
– Amyloidosis – Ankylosing spondylitis – Rheumatoid arthritis scleroderma – Systemic lupus erythematosus – Vasculitis
• *Vascular*
– Pulmonary thromboembolism – Pulmonary hypertension – Right-to-left vascular shunt
Abbreviations: COPD, chronic obstructive pulmonary disease; UACS, upper airway cough syndrome

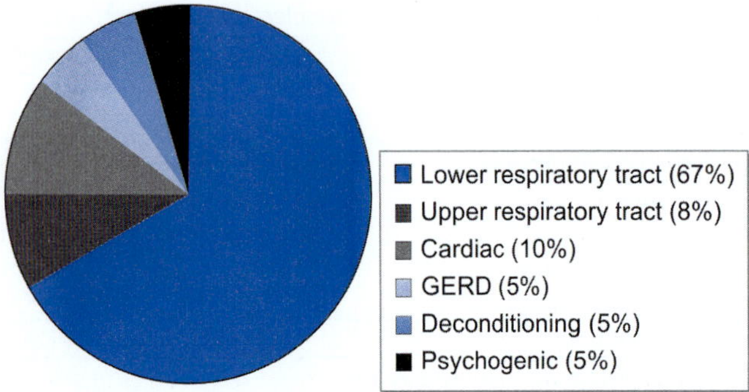

Fig. 1 Spectrum and frequency of the causes of unexplained dyspnea.[11] In this study, 85 patients referred to a pulmonary clinic for difficult to diagnose dyspnea were evaluated. Asthma, chronic obstructive pulmonary disease, interstitial lung disease, and cardiomyopathy accounted for approximately two-thirds of the cases

heart failure probably causes dyspnea by the activation of vagal afferent mechanoreceptors in the lungs and airways and by altering gas exchange. How GERD causes dyspnea is not known, but GERD is commonly associated with respiratory symptoms and has been reported to account for unexplained dyspnea, in up to 5% of cases.[1,11,14,15] Possibly, GERD causes dyspnea by the activation of vagal afferents in the esophagus that secondarily stimulate an increase in minute ventilation to produce the sensation of dyspnea.[16] Of course, in severe GERD, the obstructive effects of laryngospasm or the aspiration of refluxate into the lungs would also be expected to contribute to dyspnea. Deconditioning can stimulate dyspnea by requiring increased minute ventilation for the task performed. Finally, there are psychogenic causes of dyspnea, such as anxiety, panic and hyperventilation. Presumably, dyspnea in these conditions is primarily due to the inappropriate cortical modulation of the neural pathways that integrate and compare the normal afferent and efferent activity driving respiration. However, hyperventilation can lead to the alterations of blood gases and these changes may secondarily contribute as well.

POSITIONAL AND NOCTURNAL DYSPNEA

Trepopnea is dyspnea that increases when one side is dependent. For example, patients with a paralyzed hemidiaphragm may complain that they cannot lie down on one side. However, trepopnea is a nonspecific finding because any asymmetric lung disease can cause trepopnea.[5] It can be seen in common diseases, such as COPD and congestive heart failure.

Orthopnea is dyspnea worse on recumbency. It is not a symptom or sign that is specific for congestive heart failure.[5] It can be seen in congestive heart failure, COPD or neuromuscular weakness. It does not reliably distinguish the cardiac causes of dyspnea from pulmonary causes.

Platypnea is dyspnea that is worsened by an upright position.[5] Classically, it is observed when there is right to left shunting of blood, either intracardiac or pulmonary parenchymal.[17,18] For example, patients with cirrhosis can develop pulmonary arteriovenous malformations at the bases of the lungs. As these shunts become more dependent with the upright position and blood flow through them increases, right to left shunting increases when the patient is upright and this causes orthodeoxia (decrease in arterial oxygen tension when the subject goes from a recumbent position to an upright position) and dyspnea. However, the finding is not specific for right to left shunting of blood and has been reported with ileus and pericarditis as well.[5]

EVALUATING ACUTE DYSPNEA

In evaluating a patient with acute dyspnea, the first priority is to consider potentially life-threatening conditions, such as pulmonary thromboembolism, acute myocardial ischemia or infarction, congestive heart failure, cardiac arrhythmia, an acute exacerbation of asthma or COPD, pneumothorax, upper airway obstruction, pulmonary edema, and pneumonia.[1,5] A history and physical examination should be done, and based on the findings, further testing ordered as appropriate. Commonly useful tests for the evaluation of acute dyspnea include radiographic imaging, electrocardiogram, measurement of serum B-type natriuretic peptide (BNP), complete blood count, arterial blood gases, spirometry or peak flow measures, and computed tomography (CT) angiography or ventilation-perfusion lung scanning, and echocardiography.

EVALUATING CHRONIC DYSPNEA

A systematic approach to diagnosing the underlying cause of dyspnea has been validated in a university hospital, ambulatory or pulmonary clinic.[11] In this setting, respiratory disorders accounted for approximately 75% of cases.

Evaluation begins with medical history and physical examination, concentrating on the anatomy of afferent nerves important in the genesis of dyspnea, especially the vagus nerve that subserves organs of both the thorax and upper abdomen. Also, the focus of the medical history and examination should be on the most common causes of chronic dyspnea, including asthma, COPD, interstitial lung disease and cardiomyopathy. If the initial history and physical examination are not suggestive of these most common diagnoses, additional attention should be directed to the other causes of chronic dyspnea, such as postnasal drip syndrome [now referred to as upper airway cough syndrome (UACS)] and other causes of upper airway obstruction, other respiratory disorders, evidence of deconditioning, psychogenic problems (hyperventilation), and GERD. In practice, the history and physical examination are most helpful in ruling out common diagnoses rather than establishing diagnoses. A history of wheezing or a prior diagnosis of asthma is only 50% predictive of asthma being the cause of the patient's chronic dyspnea. For another example, finding crackles on physical examination has only a modest positive predictive value for interstitial

Table 2 Laboratory tests useful in the evaluation of unexplained dyspnea[5]

- *Pulmonary function tests*
  - Spirometry with flow-volume loops
  - Spirometry before and after bronchodilator
  - Methacholine inhalation challenge
  - Lung volumes
  - Diffusing capacity
  - Arterial blood gas (ABG)
  - Pulse oximetry at rest and during exertion
  - Maximal inspiratory and expiratory mouth pressures
  - Cardiopulmonary exercise testing
  - Hyperventilation provocation testing
- *Radiographic imaging*
  - Chest radiographs
  - Chest and neck computed tomography (CT) scans
- *Noninvasive cardiovascular tests*
  - Blood B-type natriuretic peptide (BNP)
  - D-dimer
  - Electrocardiogram
  - Echocardiography
  - Cardiac stress test
- *Gastrointestinal testing*
  - Modified barium swallow
  - Barium esophagography and/or 24-hour esophageal pH and impedance monitoring
- *Invasive testing*
  - Lung biopsy
  - Cardiac catheterization

For a more complete listing and suggested sequence of testing, see reference.[5]

lung disease or congestive heart failure being the cause of dyspnea, but the absence of crackles essentially rules out both with 98% and 92% confidence, respectively.

The clinical impression based on medical history and physical examination is next supported by objective testing beginning with a chest radiograph. Abnormal findings on chest radiograph should be pursued as potential causes of dyspnea. The absence of findings on chest radiograph has a high negative predictive value (91%) in excluding many thoracic disorders capable of causing dyspnea.[11]

After the chest radiograph, additional objective testing is warranted to establish the cause of the patient's dyspnea. Without objective testing beyond history, examination and chest radiograph, diagnoses may be incorrect approximately 33% of the time.[1] Several tests are important in evaluating the causes of chronic dyspnea and most of them are useful because of their high negative predictive values for ruling out specific diagnoses **(Table 2)**.[11] For example, spirometry is useful for ruling out COPD with 100% confidence and negative bronchial provocation studies (e.g. methacholine inhalation challenge) are useful for ruling out a diagnosis of symptomatic asthma with nearly 100% confidence.

Cardiopulmonary exercise testing (CPET) can be very helpful in identifying the underlying cause of dyspnea.[4,5,19] Observing the ventilatory responses and changes in gas exchange during exercise can help distinguish cardiac from pulmonary causes of dyspnea, provide evidence of deconditioning, and help identify patients with psychogenic causes of dyspnea.

Normal patients will exercise to their predicted maximum heart rate and, at that point, still have substantial breathing reserve (20–40%) compared to their predicted maximum minute ventilation. In cardiac disease, heart rate is maximum at a low workload, there is still substantial pulmonary reserve, the oxygen pulse (oxygen consumption divided by heart rate) is low and the anaerobic threshold is low. Distinguishing a cardiac limitation from deconditioning can be difficult with CPET unless ischemia, arrhythmias, or significant changes in blood pressure are documented by electrocardiography (ECG) and blood pressure monitoring. Typically, deconditioned patients show a low maximum oxygen consumption and low anaerobic threshold. In contrast, patients with a pulmonary limitation to exercise have a low breathing reserve and do not reach maximum predicted heart rate during exercise. They may show oxygen desaturation, show abnormalities of gas exchange, or have evidence of airway obstruction on postexercise spirometry. Patients with psychogenic dyspnea may have a normal CPET study or, with anxiety/hyperventilation syndromes, demonstrate hyperventilation at rest, but an increase in carbon dioxide as exercise first begins.

Determining the underlying cause of dyspnea depends, whenever possible, on observing that specific therapy eliminates or improves the symptom. Because causes of dyspnea may coexist simultaneously, partially successful therapy should not be discontinued as new therapeutic trials are attempted. Instead, add therapies sequentially. To guide management, a measure of dyspnea is useful and recommended by consensus guidelines.[3,4] The Borg scale, the visual analog scale, and the numerical rating scale have utility in assessing the severity of dyspnea in patients with advanced disease.[3]

TREATMENT

Specific

The best treatment of dyspnea is specific treatment directed at the underlying cause of the symptom. In one study, 76% of patients improved with specific therapy.[11] All patients with asthma, UACS, psychogenic causes, deconditioning, or GERD showed improvement with specific therapy. Fewer patients improved with specific therapy for COPD (33%), interstitial lung disease (58%) and cardiomyopathy (78%). It is beyond the scope of this chapter to comprehensively review the treatment of even the most common causes of dyspnea. Readers are referred to the chapters that specifically focus on these diseases.

Specific therapy for obesity/deconditioning, psychogenic causes of dyspnea, and neuromuscular diseases should not be overlooked.[5] For obesity or deconditioning, both respond to diet and exercise. Consultation with a dietician and a regular, daily exercise regimen can decrease dyspnea at maximum treadmill workload, with most patients showing some improvement within 3 months.[5,20] For the psychogenic causes of dyspnea and hyperventilation syndromes, patients often respond to education, reassurance and breathing retraining strategies.[5,21,22] For panic disorder, many patients are helped by counseling, behavioral breathing strategies, and pharmacological intervention if necessary. For neuromuscular diseases, specific interventions designed to increase muscle effectiveness are available. In quadriplegia and potentially other diseases characterized by muscle weakness, patients may benefit from inspiratory muscle trainers aimed to increase muscle hypertrophy and strength in inspiratory muscles still innervated.[23] For patients with cervical injuries resulting in diaphragm paralysis, diaphragmatic pacing can help. Resting weak muscles with nocturnal or intermittent positive pressure mechanical ventilation may help some patients with severe muscle weakness due to diseases, such as amyotrophic lateral sclerosis or muscular dystrophy.[24]

Nonspecific

Nonspecific therapy is aimed at the symptom rather than the underlying cause of dyspnea.[5] Many nonspecific therapies for dyspnea have been proposed and these include nutritional support;[25] conditioning regimens;[26] pursed-lip breathing; stress reduction; teaching coping skills;[27] respiratory muscle training;[28] supplemental oxygen;[29] heliox (helium-oxygen mixture);[30] noninvasive or invasive mechanical ventilation;[30,31] vagotomy; muscle vibration techniques; acupuncture; and pharmacotherapy[32] with narcotics, anxiolytics, phenothiazines; and furosemide. The long-term efficacy of these various treatments for relieving dyspnea has not been well-established with the exception of conditioning regimens (i.e. pulmonary rehabilitation)[4] and nutritional support for patients with COPD.[25]

Supplemental oxygen does have a well-established role for treating resting and exertional hypoxemia in patients with advanced heart and lung disease and also may have a role in relieving the symptom of dyspnea in such patients.[3,4] However, long-term relief of dyspnea with supplemental oxygen has not been established and even studies of dyspnea relief in the short-term have had mixed results.[3] No studies have yet established that supplemental oxygen relieves dyspnea in patients without hypoxemia.

Some evidence suggests that inhaled furosemide may relieve exertional dyspnea in healthy subjects and subjects with COPD,[33-35] although the mechanisms are not clear and probably multifactorial.[36] In 20 subjects with COPD, a single dose of inhaled furosemide decreased dyspnea during exercise and exercise endurance time increased by 1.65 minutes.[36] However, the clinical role of inhaled furosemide is not yet established and awaits larger, multicenter trials.

Although benzodiazepines and opioids[37] have roles in treating dyspnea in terminally ill cancer patients, their roles in the long-term relief of chronic dyspnea are less clear. Benzodiazepines at low doses are prescribed by some physicians to treat intractable, chronic breathlessness, but there is very little clinical evidence to support this practice. Similarly, the use of nebulized opioids to relieve intractable dyspnea has been proposed, but studies show no benefit.[3,23,38] There is more evidence supporting the use of low doses of oral opioids.[32,39,40] In one randomized and controlled 4-day crossover study, 48 patients who mostly had COPD as the cause of intractable dyspnea were given 20 mg of sustained release morphine per 24 hours.[41] There were documented improvements in dyspnea and improved sleep. However, the severity of a patient's baseline dyspnea was not predictive of a response to the opioids. Whether the relief may persist during treatment longer than 4 days is not known. The global initiative for chronic obstructive lung disease (GOLD) states that opioids are effective for relieving dyspnea in patients with very severe COPD, but does caution that there may be serious adverse effects and that responders may be only a limited subgroup.[42] Because of the potential risk for respiratory depression, the use of opioids for intractable dyspnea needs to be done on a case-by-case basis with due respect for potential side effects.

CONCLUSION

In summary, dyspnea is the distressing sensation that breathing is difficult, labored or unpleasant. The symptom is nonspecific because it is caused by many cardiopulmonary disorders. The evaluation of dyspnea in a patient begins by establishing whether the symptom is acute or chronic and this is followed by a detailed medical history and physical examination. Guided by history and physical examination findings, laboratory testing then is used to establish the underlying diagnosis. For this, chest radiographs, pulmonary function tests and CPET are frequently helpful. In general, treatment is aimed at the specific underlying diagnosis. However, nonspecific therapies aimed at the symptom rather than the diagnosis also play a supplementary role in the relief of dyspnea.

REFERENCES

1. Irwin RS. Symptoms of respiratory disease. In: ACCP Pulmonary Medicine Board Review, 25th edition. Northbrook, IL: American College of Chest Physicians; 2009. pp. 415-56.
2. O'Donnell DE, Banzett RB, Carrieri-Kohlman V, Casaburi R, Davenport PW, Gandevia SC, et al. Pathophysiology of dyspnea in chronic obstructive pulmonary disease: a roundtable. Proc Am Thorac Soc. 2007;4(2):145-68.
3. Mahler DA, Selecky PA, Harrod CG, Benditt JO, Carrieri-Kohlman V, Curtis JR, et al. American College of Chest Physicians consensus statement on the management of dyspnea in patients with advanced lung or heart disease. Chest. 2010;137(3): 674-91.
4. Parshall MB, Schwartzstein RM, Adams L, Banzett RB, Manning HL, Bourbeau J, et al. An official American Thoracic Society statement: update on the mechanisms, assessment and management of dyspnea. Am J Respir Crit Care Med. 2012;185(4):435-52.
5. Curley FJ. Dyspnea. In: Irwin RS, Curley FJ, Grossman RF (Eds). Diagnosis and Treatment of Symptoms of the Respiratory Tract. Armonk, NY: Futura Publishing Company; 1997. pp. 55-111.

6. Fisher JT, O'Donnell DE. The clinical physiology and integrative neurobiology of dyspnea: introduction to the Special Issue of Respir Physiol Neurobiol. Respir Physiol Neurobiol. 2009;167(1):1.
7. Gillette MA, Schwartzstein RM. Mechanisms of dyspnoea. In: Ahmedzai SH, Muers MF (Eds). Supportive Care in Respiratory Disease. Oxford: Oxford University Press; 2005. pp. 93-122.
8. Fedullo AJ, Swineburne AJ, McGruire-Dunn C. Complaints of breathlessness in the emergency department: the experience at a community hospital. NY State J Med. 1986;86(1):4-6.
9. Pearson SB, Pearson EM, Mitchell JR. The diagnosis and management of patients admitted to hospital with acute breathlessness. Postgrad Med J. 1981;57(669):419-24.
10. Mustchin CP, Tiwari I. Diagnosing the breathless patient. Lancet. 1982;1(8277):907-8.
11. Pratter MR, Curley FJ, Dubois J, Irwin RS. Cause and evaluation of chronic dyspnea in a pulmonary disease clinic. Arch Intern Med. 1989;149(10):2277-82.
12. Kikuchi Y, Okabe S, Tamura G, Hida W, Homma M, Shirato K, et al. Chemosensitivity and perception of dyspnea in patients with a history of near-fatal asthma. N Engl J Med. 1994;330(19):1329-34.
13. Killian K. Dyspnea. J Appl Physiol. 2006;101(4):1013-4.
14. DePaso WJ, Winterbauer RH, Lusk JA, Dreis DF, Springmeyer SC. Chronic dyspnea unexplained by history, chest roentgenogram, and spirometry: Analysis of a seven-year experience. Chest. 1991;100(5):1293-9.
15. Nordenstedt H, Nilsson M, Johansson S, Wallander MA, Johnsen R, Hveem K, et al. The relation between gastroesophageal reflux and respiratory symptoms in a population-based study: the Nord-Trøndelag Health Survey. Chest. 2006;129(4):1051-6.
16. Field SK, Evans JA, Price LM. The effects of acid perfusion of the esophagus on ventilation and respiratory sensation. Am J Respir Crit Care Med. 1998;157 (4 Pt 1):1058-62.
17. Seward JB, Hayes DL, Smith HC, Williams DE, Rosenow EC, Reeder GS, et al. Platypnea-orthodeoxia: clinical profile, diagnostic workup, management, and report of seven cases. Mayo Clin Proc. 1984;59(4):221-31.
18. Lambrecht GL, Malbrain ML, Coremans P, Verbist L, Verhaegen H. Orthodeoxia and platypnea in liver cirrhosis: effects of propranolol. Acta Clin Belg. 1994;49(1):26-30.
19. Martinez FJ, Stanopoulos I, Acero R, Becker FS, Pickering R, Beamis JF. Graded comprehensive cardiopulmonary exercise testing in the evaluation of dyspnea unexplained by routine evaluation. Chest. 1994;105(1):168-74.
20. Reardon J, Awad E, Normandin E, Vale F, Clark B, ZuWallack RL. The effect of comprehensive outpatient pulmonary rehabilitation on dyspnea. Chest. 1994;105(4):1046-52.
21. Grossman P, de Swart JC, Defares PB. A controlled study of a breathing therapy for treatment of hyperventilation syndrome. J Psychosom Res. 1985;29(1):49-58.
22. Lum LC. The syndrome of chronic habitual hyperventilation. In: Hill OW (Ed). Modern Trends in Psychosomatic Medicine. London, UK: Buttersworth, 1976.
23. Gross D, Ladd HW, Riley EJ, Macklem PT, Grassino A. The effect of training on strength and endurance of the diaphragm in quadriplegia. Am J Med. 1980;68(1):27-35.
24. Meyer TJ, Hill NS. Noninvasive positive pressure ventilation to treat respiratory failure. Ann Intern Med. 1994;120(9):760-70.
25. Rogers RM, Donahoe M, Costantino J. Physiologic effects of oral supplemental feeding in malnourished patients with chronic obstructive pulmonary disease: a randomized control study. Am Rev Respir Dis. 1992;146(6):1511-7.
26. Lindsay J, Goldstein R. Rehabilitation and exercise. In: Ahmedzai SH, Muers MF (Eds). Supportive Care in Respiratory Disease. Oxford: Oxford University Press; 2005. pp. 189-214.
27. MacLeod R. Psychosocial therapies. In: Ahmedzai SH, Muers MF (Eds). Supportive Care in Respiratory Disease. Oxford: Oxford University Press; 2005. pp. 229-38.
28. Folgering H, Heijdra Y. Dyspnoea and respiratory muscle training. In: Ahmedzai SH, Muers MF (Eds). Supportive Care in Respiratory Disease. Oxford: Oxford University Press; 2005. pp. 215-28.
29. Booth S. Oxygen and airflow. In: Ahmedzai SH, Muers MF (Eds). Supportive Care in Respiratory Disease. Oxford: Oxford University Press; 2005. pp. 165-88.
30. Laude EA, Duffy NC, Baveystock C, Douglill B, Campbell MJ, Lawson R, et al. The effect of helium and oxygen on exercise performance in chronic obstructive pulmonary disease: a randomized crossover trial. Am J Respir Crit Care Med. 2006;173: 865-70.
31. Cassanova C, Celli BR, Tost L, Soriano E, Abreu J, Velasco V, et al. Long-term controlled trial of nocturnal nasal positive pressure ventilation in patients with severe COPD. Chest. 2000; 118:1582-90.
32. Davis C. Drug therapies. In: Ahmedzai SH, Muers MF (Eds). Supportive Care in Respiratory Disease. Oxford: Oxford University Press; 2005. pp. 147-64.
33. Moosavi SH, Binks AP, Lansing RW, Topulos GP, Banzett RB, Schwartzstein RM. Effect of inhaled furosemide on air hunger induced in healthy humans. Respir Physiol Neurobiol. 2007;156(1):1-8.
34. Nishino T, Ide T, Sudo T. Inhaled furosemide greatly alleviates the sensation of experimentally induced dyspnea. Am J Resipir Crit Care Med. 2000;161(6):1963-7.
35. Ong KC, Kor AC, Chong WF, Earnest A, Wang YT. Effects of inhaled furosemide on exertional dyspnea in chronic obstructive pulmonary disease. Am J Respir Crit Care Med. 2004;169(9):1028-33.
36. Jensen D, Amjadi K, Harris-McAllister V, Webb KA, O'Donnell DE. Mechanisms of dyspnoea relief and improved exercise endurance after furosemide inhalation in COPD. Thorax. 2008;63(7):606-13.
37. Ben-Aharon I, Gafter-Gvili A, Paul M, Leibovici L, Stemmer SM. Interventions for alleviating cancer-related dyspnea: a systematic review. J Clin Oncol. 2008;26(14):2396-404.
38. Davis CL, Hodder CA, Love S, Shah R, Slevin M, Wedzicha J. Effect of nebulized morphine and morphine 6-glucuronide on exercise endurance in patients with chronic obstructive airways disease. Thorax. 1994;49:393P.
39. Rocker G, Horton R, Currow D, Goodridge D, Young J, Booth S. Palliation of dyspnoea in advanced COPD: revisiting a role for opioids. Thorax. 2009;64(10):910-5.
40. Mahler DA. Opioids for refractory dyspnea. Expert Rev Respir Med. 2013;7:123-35.
41. Abernethy AP, Currow DC, Frith P, Fazekas BS, McHugh A, Bui C. Randomised, double blind, placebo controlled crossover trial of sustained release morphine for the management of refractory dyspnoea. BMJ. 2003;327(7414):523-8.
42. GOLD Executive committee. (2014). Global strategy for diagnosis, management, and prevention of COPD (Revised 2014). [Online] Available from *http://www.goldcopd.com/*. [Accessed Jan 2016].

18

Chapter

Wheeze and Respiratory Disease

J Mark Madison, Richard S Irwin

INTRODUCTION

Wheeze is either a symptom reported by a patient or a sign heard on the auscultation of the chest and neck during physical examination. Wheezes indicate airway obstruction somewhere in the respiratory tract and are defined as continuous musical sounds (approximately 100–1,000 Hz) lasting more than 80–100 msec, but usually not more than 250 msec.[1-4] They can be inspiratory or expiratory, high or low pitched, consist of single or multiple musical tones and originate from any airway, either inside or outside of the thoracic cavity.[1-4] Stridor is a special type of wheeze and refers to inspiratory wheezing heard loudest over the central large airways of the chest and neck.

It is fundamental to understand that wheezing is a nonspecific finding that simply signifies the presence of airway obstruction, not its cause. It is not, by itself, diagnostic of any specific respiratory disease. Evaluation of the cause of wheezing begins with a medical history and physical examination and should be supplemented by diagnostic studies such as pulmonary function tests. In general, treatment of wheezing is specifically directed at the identified, underlying disease causing the airway obstruction, but nonspecific supportive therapy may be needed until definitive therapy is effective.

PHYSIOLOGY OF WHEEZE

Wheezes are caused by obstruction to airflow, but precisely how airway obstruction causes wheeze is not known.[5] Most likely, wheezes are caused by the oscillations or fluttering of airway walls and secretions in the airways.[6,7] In accordance with the Bernoulli's principle describing the relationship between gas flow and pressure, air moving through an airway increases in velocity when it encounters a segment of airway that is narrowed. The higher gas velocity means lower airway pressure in that local region and, therefore, there is a tendency for the airway wall to collapse inward slightly. As the collapse increases, the worsening obstruction decreases airflow and increases pressure in the airway. Higher airway pressure in turn pushes the airway wall outward, partially relieving the obstruction and then the cycle starts again. This inward and outward movement of the airway wall happens cyclically to create an oscillatory vibration that is heard as a musical tone on the auscultation of the chest.

HISTORY AND PHYSICAL EXAMINATION

It is a common error to assume that the site(s) of airway obstruction can be reliably determined by physical examination. Determining the phase of the respiratory cycle (inspiratory versus expiratory) when wheezing is heard and noting the timbre of the wheezing (monophonic versus polyphonic) may be helpful clinically when combined with the other elements of patient evaluation, but these characteristics cannot, by themselves, be used to reliably identify the sites or causes of wheezing.

Inspiratory wheezing is neither a sensitive nor specific indicator of extrathoracic airway obstruction. It is true that extrathoracic obstruction of a large airway tends to produce inspiratory wheezing, because negative airway pressure during inspiration tends to augment the degree of narrowing as airway tissue collapses slightly inward.

However, inspiratory wheezing is an insensitive method of detecting extrathoracic obstruction since the lumen diameter must decrease to approximately 5 mm to produce stridor clinically.[8] Moreover, inspiratory wheezing is a nonspecific finding because inspiratory wheezing is frequently heard with expiratory wheezing due to intrathoracic obstruction in smaller airways such as obstruction due to asthma.[2,9] Moreover, wheezing due to asthma may sometimes be heard only on inspiration.

Expiratory wheezing by history or physical examination is neither sensitive nor specific for diagnosing asthma.[10] Symptomatic asthma can present without wheezing and wheezing caused by other diseases can mimic the wheezing of asthma. In one clinical study, only 35% of patients referred to a pulmonary clinic for a history of difficult to diagnose wheezing ultimately proved to have asthma upon further evaluation.[11] Similarly, only 43% of patients with expiratory wheeze on physical examination proved to have asthma as the underlying cause of the wheeze.

The pitch and timbre of wheeze do not reliably indicate where, in the respiratory tract, the obstruction to airflow is located.[12] Therefore, the pitch and timbre of wheezing may be helpful as additional clinical information, but should not be relied on exclusively for diagnostic decisions.

It should be emphasized that the loudness or amplitude of wheezing is not a reliable indicator of the severity of airway obstruction.[3,9,13,14] Because wheezing depends on airway narrowing and the amount of airflow, the amplitude of wheezing may be low or absent even when there is severe obstruction present because there is very little airflow.[6] For one classic example of this, it is an ominous finding when a patient with a severe exacerbation of asthma has a "silent chest" on physical examination.

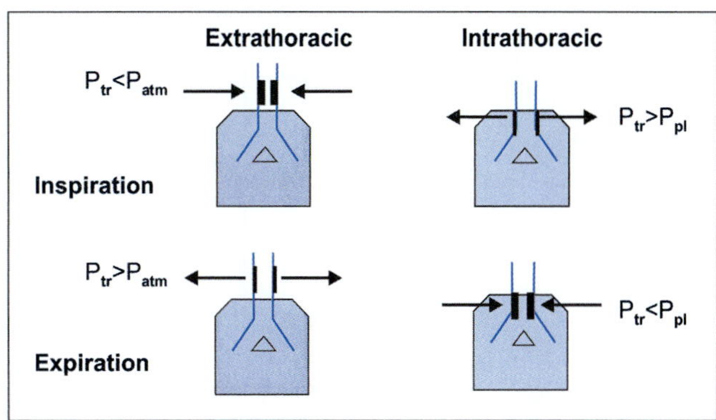

Fig. 1 Physiology of upper airway obstruction. Transmural pressure changes during inspiration and expiration affect the diameter of the airway lumen differently depending on whether the single site of obstruction is inside the chest cavity (intrathoracic) or outside the chest cavity (extrathoracic)

PULMONARY FUNCTION TESTING

Spirometry and flow-volume loops can help a physician determine whether the airway obstruction causing wheeze is located in the extrathoracic upper airways, intrathoracic upper airways, or intrathoracic lower airways.[2,3] These different regions of the airways have distinguishing physiologic characteristics that make pulmonary function testing informative when evaluating the cause of wheeze.[2,3,15,16]

Extrathoracic upper airway lesions can be located in the mouth, pharynx, larynx or extrathoracic trachea.[2,3,5,14] The word "variable" is used to describe an obstructed region of the airway that is pliable or deformable enough that the size of the lumen diameter is variable at the site of the obstruction depending on whether the patient is inspiring or expiring. Outside the thoracic cavity, the lumen diameter of the airway depends on the difference between lumen air pressure and atmospheric pressure. When a patient inspires, the airway lumen pressure becomes negative compared to atmospheric pressure and the pliable tissues of the airway collapse inward slightly **(Fig. 1)**. When the patient expires, extrathoracic lumen air pressure is positive relative to atmospheric pressure and the airway wall is forced outward increasing the lumen diameter **(Fig. 1)**. If there is a partially obstructing lesion narrowing the extrathoracic airway at a single point, this inward collapse during inspiration and outward movement during expiration can produce higher maximal air flows during expiration compared to inspiration. This physiology is best detected by performing flow volume loops during spirometric testing in the pulmonary function laboratory. In the presence of a variable extrathoracic lesion, inspiratory flows are limited and there is, therefore, a flow limitation or "plateau" on the inspiratory limb of the flow-volume loop **(Fig. 2)**. On the expiratory limb of the flow-volume curve, there is no corresponding flow limitation or plateau. When inspiratory and expiratory flow rates at 50% of vital capacity are compared, the ratio of the two is characteristically less than one. The patient having this pattern on the flow volume curve is said to have a variable extrathoracic upper airway obstruction.

A variable intrathoracic upper airway lesion has the opposite pattern on flow-volume loops because lumen diameter in intrathoracic airways is determined by the difference between lumen air pressure and pleural pressure.[2,3,15,16] During inspiration, pleural pressure is negative relative to lumen pressure and the pliable walls of the airways are pulled outward to increase lumen diameter **(Fig. 1)**. During expiration, the opposite is true and the pliable airway walls collapse inward slightly **(Fig. 1)**. If there is a partial narrowing of the airway at a single point, these differences in lumen diameter during inspiration and expiration can produce significant changes in airflow that, again, are best assessed on flow-volume loops. In the presence of a variable intrathoracic lesion, inspiratory flows may be unaffected by the presence of the lesion and so the inspiratory limb of the flow-volume loop appears normal or nearly normal.

However, on expiration, when the airway diameter is smaller due to positive pleural pressure, there is a flow limitation or plateau on the expiratory limb of the flow-volume loop **(Fig. 2)**. The patient having this pattern on the flow-volume loop is said to have a variable intrathoracic upper airway obstruction.

When the single obstructing lesion is "fixed" rather than variable, it means that the tissue at the site of the lesion is not pliable or deformable enough to allow significant changes in airway lumen diameter during inspiration and expiration. Therefore, the pattern on flow-volume loop is characteristically abnormal during both inspiration and expiration and there is a flow limitation or plateau on both limbs of the flow-volume loop **(Fig. 2)**.

Unlike upper airway lesions, obstruction in the smaller caliber central and peripheral intrathoracic airways is almost always at multiple scattered sites impeding airflow in a

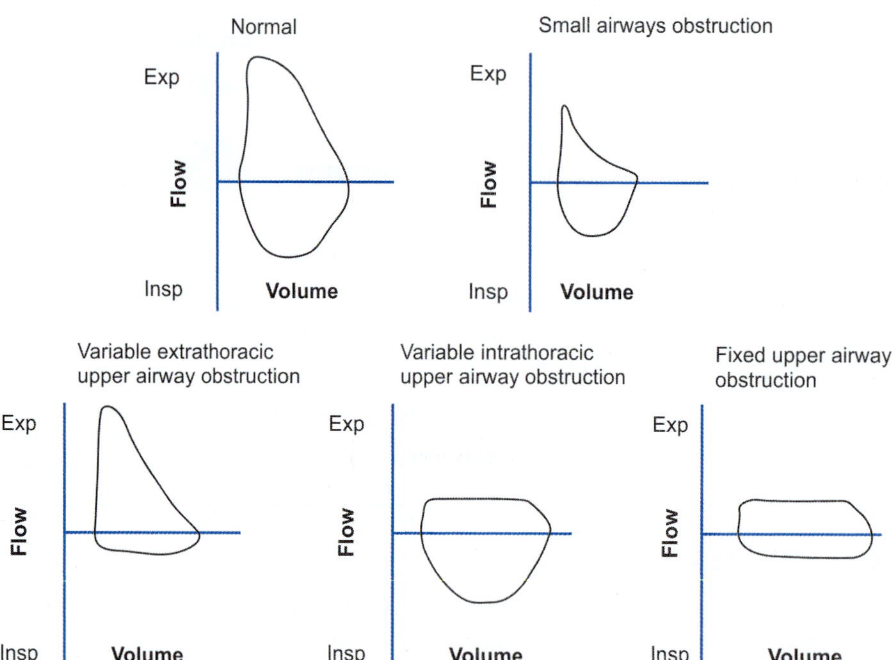

Fig. 2 Flow-volume loop configurations for airway obstruction. Flow-volume loops are useful for identifying the site of airway obstruction causing wheezing. For smaller, lower airways obstruction, there is a characteristic concave upward appearance on the expiratory limb of the flow-volume loop. For obstructions of the large upper airways, distinct patterns are evident for intrathoracic and extrathoracic sites of obstruction

nonuniform manner. Diseases, such as asthma and chronic obstructive pulmonary disease (COPD) are among the most common causes of wheezing due to airway obstruction. Spirometry is the main method of detecting and quantifying this airway obstruction.[17] The forced expired volume in 1 second (FEV_1) and the forced vital capacity (FVC) are both reduced, but the FEV_1 is reduced out of proportion to the FVC such that the FEV_1/FVC ratio is abnormally low (less than the lower limit of predicted normal). For obstruction, an FEV_1 less than 50% of predicted, or less than 1 liter, indicates "severe" airway obstruction. The flow-volume loop of a patient with obstruction of the lower airways characteristically shows a concave upward appearance on the expiratory limb of the flow-volume loop **(Fig. 2)**. Spirometry repeated after the inhalation of drugs or medications or after a treatment course can also be helpful in evaluating the causes of airway obstruction.[2,3] For example, in the presence of airway obstruction, spirometry repeated after the administration of bronchodilator or after a course of corticosteroids may reveal the presence of reversible airway obstruction consistent with a diagnosis of asthma. For another example, in the absence of airway obstruction at baseline, a nonspecific bronchoprovocation challenge test (e.g. methacholine inhalation challenge test) may reveal the presence of bronchial hyperresponsiveness consistent with a diagnosis of asthma.

It is sometimes possible to detect coexisting small and large airway obstructions by taking advantage of the fact that helium is less dense than air. Airflow in small airways, having mainly laminar flow, is unaffected by substituting less dense helium for the nitrogen in air.[2,3,18] However, in large airways, where there is much turbulent gas flow, breathing a helium-rich gas mixture allows higher rates of gas flow compared to breathing air. Therefore, if a comparison of maximal expiratory flows for breathing air versus heliox (20% oxygen/80% helium) shows significantly greater gas flow with the helium mixtures, the patient is likely to have an obstructing lesion in a large airway with turbulent gas flow as part of his/her problem.

DIFFERENTIAL DIAGNOSIS FOR WHEEZING

Because the causes of airway obstruction are multiple, it is not surprising that wheezing appreciated by history or physical examination is a nonspecific finding.[11] Any cause of airway narrowing can result in wheezing and these causes include dynamic collapse of the airways; bronchospasm; airway wall edema, thickening or inflammation; airway secretions; remodeling of the airways; distortions of airway anatomy; and any compressing or partially obstructing mass **(Table 1)**. It is a common error of physicians to mistakenly assume that all wheezing is due to asthma or COPD and this pitfall in evaluation should be avoided.[19,20]

One clinical study examined the spectrum and frequency of the causes of wheezing among patients referred to a pulmonary clinic for evaluation **(Fig. 3)**.[11] Thirty-four

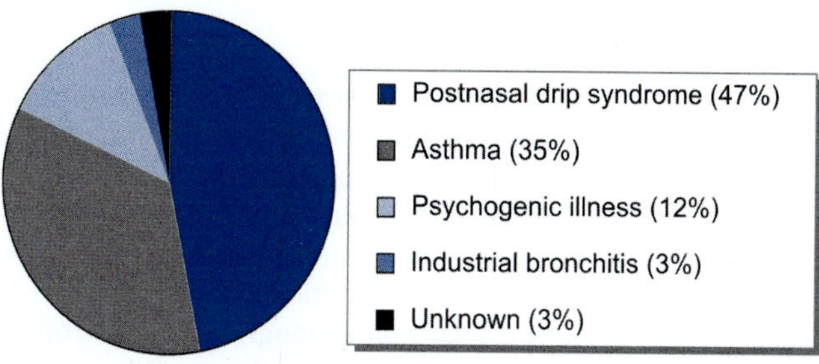

Fig. 3 Spectrum and frequency of the causes of wheezes.[11] In this study, patients referred to a pulmonary clinic for difficult to diagnose wheezing were evaluated. Postnasal drip syndrome [now referred to as upper airway cough syndrome (UACS)] was the most common cause of difficult to diagnose wheezing among these patients. Vocal cord dysfunction syndrome is an example of a potential psychiatric illness presenting as wheeze

Table 1 Causes of wheeze[3]

Extrathoracic upper-airway obstruction
• Anaphylaxis • Cricoarytenoid arthritis • Epiglottitis (supraglottitis) • Hypertrophied tonsils • Laryngeal edema • Laryngocele • Malignancy • Obesity • Postnasal drip due to rhinosinus disease (now referred to as UACS) • Relapsing polychondritis • Retropharyngeal abscess • Vocal cord dysfunction or paralysis
Intrathoracic upper-airway obstruction
• Benign and malignant tracheal and bronchial tumors • Foreign body aspiration • Goiter (intrathoracic) • Herpetic tracheobronchitis • Right-sided aortic arch • Tracheal stenosis postintubation • Tracheobronchomegaly • Tracheomalacia
Intrathoracic lower-airway obstruction
• Anaphylaxis • Aspiration • Asthma • Bronchiectasis • Bronchiolitis • Carcinoid syndrome • Chronic obstructive pulmonary disease • Cystic fibrosis • Lymphangitic carcinomatosis • Parasitic infections • Pulmonary edema • Pulmonary thromboembolism • Tracheobronchitis
Courtesy: See Reference 3 for more details and a referenced list. *Abbreviation*: UACS, upper airway cough syndrome

patients with wheezing of unclear etiology were referred to an ambulatory pulmonary clinic for further evaluation that included methacholine inhalation challenge testing. Interestingly, only 35% of these patients had methacholine challenge tests that were consistent with asthma being the underlying cause of their wheezing. The most common cause of wheeze among these patients was not asthma, but, instead, postnasal drip syndrome (46% of cases).[21] Postnasal drip syndrome (now referred to as upper airway cough syndrome or UACS) is a common condition and known to cause upper airway obstruction so it is not surprising that it can commonly result in wheezing.

Assessing the acuity of wheezing and the patient's overall clinical condition is an important part of the clinical evaluation and this is helpful in narrowing diagnostic possibilities, assessing the urgency of the clinical situation and planning management. For acute onset wheezing, the physician must assess the overall clinical presentation and judge whether there is a life-threatening cause of the wheezing. If so, the physician must rapidly institute specific therapy directed at the underlying disease process and support the patient until that specific therapy has had time to be effective. Obviously, not all acute or recent onset wheezing represents an urgent medical condition and that is why clinical judgment is used to assess the overall clinical presentation. It is beyond the scope of this chapter to comprehensively review the diagnosis and management of the many different diseases that cause wheezing **(Table 1)**. Instead, selected diseases will be emphasized and categorized anatomically as either upper or lower airway conditions.

Upper Airway Conditions

Upper airway cough syndrome is a common cause of upper airway obstruction and therefore a common cause of wheezing.[11] The condition may be either acute or chronic and is caused by many rhinosinus diseases.[21] Acute presentations are most commonly due to the common cold. Chronic presentations can be due to allergic, perennial, nonallergic, postinfectious, environmental irritant, and vasomotor rhinitis and/or sinusitis. For example, among patients with allergic rhinitis, 77.2% report postnasal drip and 19.4% have wheezing as a symptom.[22] Consider the diagnosis of UACS when a patient describes the sensation of secretions or dripping in their throat, the frequent need to clear their throat, or frequent nasal discharge, or if patients are heard to frequently clear their throats even when they are not aware of doing it. Mucoid or mucopurulent secretions in the oropharynx or a cobblestone appearance of the pharyngeal mucosa suggests the diagnosis on physical examination.

Epiglottitis (supraglottitis) is an acute, potentially life-threatening, infection of the supraglottic region of the upper airway.[23] The infection can be caused by bacteria, viruses, or fungi, but *Haemophilus influenzae* is the most common cause. In adults, consider the diagnosis if the complaint of acute or recent onset throat pain is severe and out of proportion to the inflammation seen on physical examination of the posterior oropharynx, especially if there is respiratory distress, fever, drooling, and changed voice. Lateral neck radiographs and computed tomography of the neck can be helpful in further clinical evaluation.

Vocal cord dysfunction syndrome can cause wheeze or stridor because the upper airway is obstructed by the paradoxical adduction of the vocal cords during inspiration.[24-26] The syndrome is thought to be frequently due to emotional distress or trauma and may be difficult to diagnose when the symptoms are intermittent. It can be difficult to distinguish from asthma and, in fact, sometimes coexists with asthma.[24] An arterial blood gas may be helpful in distinguishing wheezing due to vocal cord dysfunction from that due to obstruction of lower airways because the alveolar-arterial oxygen tension difference would be expected to be high in asthma, but not in upper airway obstruction. Early and abrupt decreases in flow rates during inspiration on flow-volume loop can suggest the diagnosis, but usually the diagnosis is confirmed endoscopically by observing the movement of the unanesthetized vocal cords during inspiration. While initially thought to be provoked by psychogenic factors, the syndrome has also been reported in elite athletes during vigorous exercise and associated with UACS and gastroesophageal reflux disease (GERD).

Laryngotracheal injury caused by endotracheal intubation is another potential cause of upper airway obstruction and, therefore, wheezing.[27] The injury can occur during the process of intubation or as a result of an endotracheal tube being in the airway for a prolonged period of time. The tissue injury can lead to obstruction in the supraglottic regions of the upper airway, at the vocal cords, or in the trachea itself. Obstructing tracheal lesions can be due to edema and/or granulation or fibrous tissues that form at the site or near the tip of the endotracheal tube. The condition is often easily missed in patients who were recently intubated for respiratory failure due to asthma or COPD. For example, in follow-up, persistent or poorly resolving respiratory symptoms can be mistakenly ascribed to the patient's underlying asthma or COPD and wheezing due to upper airway obstruction may be missed. The diagnosis should be suspected in any patient who has unexplained or persistent respiratory symptoms, especially wheezing or stridor, following endotracheal intubation. Flow-volume loops and direct endoscopic visualization of the upper airway are frequently helpful in further evaluation; comparing maximal expiratory flows during air and helium/air mixtures may uncover the large airway obstructing component as described above (see section on Pulmonary Function Testing).

Lower Airway Conditions

Asthma obstructs intrathoracic airways due to bronchospasm, secretions, and inflammatory infiltration and edema of the airway walls.[28] Asthma is characterized by partially or fully reversible airway obstruction and bronchial hyper-responsiveness. Wheezing in patients with asthma may be chronic or absent during the periods of remission. It is important to again emphasize that although asthma is strongly associated with wheezing, not all patients with asthma wheeze. Patients suspected of having asthma should be evaluated with pulmonary function testing. If there is airway obstruction evident on baseline testing, then a 12% increase in FEV_1 or FVC upon the inhalation of bronchodilator (e.g. a short and rapidly acting beta-adrenergic agonist) suggests reversible airway obstruction. If there is no airway obstruction present at baseline, then nonspecific bronchoprovocation testing (e.g. methacholine inhalation challenge) is helpful in establishing the presence of bronchial hyperresponsiveness.[21] Because a positive methacholine challenge test, alone, is not diagnostic of asthma, improvement in asthma symptoms must be observed during specific treatment for asthma in order to establish the diagnosis.

Chronic obstructive pulmonary disease is a disease process consisting of varying degrees of emphysema and chronic bronchitis that leads to chronic airway obstruction.[29] Although COPD can be caused by hereditary diseases (e.g. alpha-1-antitrypsin deficiency), air pollutants from the burning of biomass fuels, and exposure to smoke from cook fires, the most common cause of COPD worldwide is tobacco smoking.[29,30] Whether tobacco is consumed by smoking cigarettes, cigars, pipes, *beedi* (bidi), hookahs, kreteks, or even the passive inhalation of tobacco smoke, the toxic products of tobacco combustion are clearly and widely recognized to be linked to the development of COPD (chronic bronchitis and emphysema) worldwide. The history or physical finding of wheezing in a moderate to heavy smoker should raise the possibility of COPD and prompt further evaluation for chronic airflow obstruction by pulmonary function testing. Although exceptions are frequently observed, patients with COPD typically have no, or only very small, responses to inhaled bronchodilators on pulmonary function testing. However, it is important to consider that, because both COPD and asthma are common, these diseases may coexist in an individual patient.

Pulmonary edema due to congestive heart failure is a well-recognized cause of airway obstruction and wheezing—so called cardiac asthma.[20,31] Most likely, the airway obstruction is due to airway wall edema and peribronchial edema that narrows the caliber of the lower airways. However, some evidence suggests that bronchial hyperresponsiveness may also play a role in the airway obstruction.[3] Theoretically, any cause of pulmonary edema, whether cardiac or noncardiac, could lead to airway wall edema, airway obstruction and wheezing. When congestive heart failure is suspected as a cause of wheezing, measurement of serum B-type natriuretic peptide (BNP) levels and/or echocardiography may be helpful in further evaluation.

Aspiration of secretions into the airways is common and can lead to respiratory symptoms, including wheezing, especially when the frequency and/or volume of aspiration is high.[32] The wheezing may be due to laryngeal irritation, tracheobronchitis, obstruction of airways from aspirated material, or peribronchial edema. Aspiration as a cause of wheezing should be suspected when there are predisposing factors associated with aspiration and when wheezing is associated with diffuse or multiple focal infiltrates on chest radiograph, especially in a posterior or inferior location. Predisposing factors the clinician should look for include hiatal hernia, Zenker's diverticulum, esophageal dysmotility, nasogastric feeding tubes, GERD, medications that lower esophageal sphincter pressure (e.g. calcium channel antagonists), pharyngeal dysfunction (e.g. strokes, amyotrophic lateral sclerosis), sedative use, alcohol abuse, and advanced age.[3] Diagnostic tests that can be helpful to further evaluate for aspiration include bedside swallowing evaluation, modified barium swallow, and 24 hour-esophageal pH and impedance monitoring to assess for GERD.

Acute venous thromboembolism (VTE) may result in wheezing and can be confused clinically with the presentation of acute asthma.[33] The wheezing may be due to bronchoconstriction of airways responding to platelet-derived mediators such as thromboxanes, serotonin and histamine. Typically, bronchospasm due to VTE is poorly responsive to bronchodilators.[33] Because the treatment for VTE is immediate systemic anticoagulation, it is important to at least consider the possibility of VTE in any patient presenting with acute wheezing, especially if there are risk factors for deep venous thrombosis.

Anaphylaxis is a systemic allergic reaction that may obstruct the upper (e.g. laryngeal edema) and lower airways (bronchoconstriction, mucosal edema, airway secretions) to produce wheezing.[34] It is typically of abrupt onset and may feature dyspnea, wheezing, urticaria, angioedema, nausea, abdominal pain, diarrhea and hypotension. It may be due to an acute allergic sensitivity to any agent, but is often due to an allergy against drugs or medications and stinging insects or due to a sensitivity to contrast agents.

Parasitic infections may also cause wheezing. Wheezing has been reported with infections due to species of *Strongyloides, Ascaris, Ancylostoma, Necator, Echinococcus, Toxocara, Schistosoma, Brugia, Dirofilaria,* and filarial species.[3] With an incubation period of 1–2 weeks depending on the species of parasite, Löffler's syndrome is seen in parasitic infections that feature the migration of parasite larva through the lungs during an acute infection. It is recognized clinically as fever, urticaria, wheeze, cough and rarely hemoptysis.[35] Laboratory findings include eosinophilia and migratory and transient infiltrates on chest radiograph. Parasites should be suspected as a cause of wheezing when there is wheeze in a patient without a history of asthma or COPD, when there has been travel or residence in an endemic area, fatigue, weight loss, fever, and infiltrates on chest radiograph.

Table 2 Diagnostic tests useful in the evaluation of wheeze

Pulmonary function tests
• Spirometry • Flow-volume loops • Bronchodilator testing • Nonspecific bronchial provocation testing • Spirometry comparing air and oxygen-helium mixtures
Imaging
• Chest radiograph • Sinus radiographs for assessing sinusitis causing UACS • Lateral neck radiograph for assessing upper airway obstruction • Computed tomography (CT) of the chest, neck or sinuses • CT angiography for assessing venous thromboembolism • Echocardiography and other imaging for assessing cardiac function
Endoscopy
• Laryngoscopy • Bronchoscopy
Evaluation for aspiration
• Bedside swallowing observation • Modified barium swallow • 24-hour esophageal pH and impedance monitoring
Blood tests
• Complete blood count and differential to assess for eosinophilia • B-type natriuretic peptide (BNP) • D-dimer
Evaluation for parasites
• Stool for ova and parasites • Microscopic examination of sputum and gastric washings for larva • Serologic testing for parasites (e.g. schistosoma, strongyloides, filaria)

APPROACH TO THE DIAGNOSIS OF WHEEZE

An approach to the diagnosis of wheezing uses a combination of history, physical examination and pulmonary function testing **(Table 2)**. First, identify any associated symptoms or signs that might suggest specific diagnoses. Second, assess whether the wheezing is potentially life-threatening and either acute or chronic, recognize the spectrum and frequency of the causes of wheeze, and then narrow the differential diagnosis by localizing the site of the wheezing to the intrathoracic versus extrathoracic airways.

TREATMENT

Because the causes of wheezes are many, it is beyond the scope of this chapter to review the treatment of all the various diseases and disorders that can cause wheezing. In general, however, treatment of upper or lower airway obstructions should be specific and directed at the underlying disease.

In treating, the severely obstructed patient with impending respiratory failure, supportive measures may be needed until specific therapy has had time to be effective. Supplemental oxygen should be administered and the patient's respiratory status monitored closely by clinical examination and oxygen saturation. Oral endotracheal intubation or tracheostomy may be needed to bypass critical obstruction of an upper airway and/or to support gas exchange and increased work of breathing caused by severe upper or lower airway obstructions.

For severe obstructions of the upper airway, helium and oxygen gas mixtures (40% or 80% helium and 60% or 20% oxygen, respectively) can be helpful in supporting the patient as a bridge to more definitive therapy.[36] The density of helium is low and therefore it lowers the resistance and the work of breathing when airflow is turbulent (as in the upper airways) rather than laminar (as in the lower, smaller airways).[37] In contrast, for asthma and COPD, disease processes that obstruct the smaller intrathoracic airways where airflow is mainly laminar, helium-oxygen mixtures may have a role, but their routine use is controversial and not currently recommended in treatment guidelines.[28,29,38]

In summary, wheezing indicates obstruction to airflow in the lower and/or upper airways. It is important for physicians to recognize that not all wheezing is due to asthma or COPD and not all asthma or COPD produces wheezes. A broad range of cardiopulmonary diseases and a variety of different infections can cause wheezing, whether the onset and timing be acute or chronic. Evaluation for the underlying cause of wheeze in a given patient, starts with a thorough history and physical examination and can be aided by additional laboratory and radiographic studies, especially pulmonary function testing. In general, treatment of wheezing should be specifically aimed at the identified underlying diagnosis. However, in the acute setting, mixtures of helium and oxygen may provide rapid, temporary relief for severe upper airway obstructions.

REFERENCES

1. Pasterkamp H, Kraman SS, Wodicka GR. Respiratory sounds: advances beyond the stethoscope. Am J Respir Crit Care Med. 1997;156(3 Pt 1):974-87.
2. John D Buckley. Symptoms of respiratory disease. In: Irwin RS (Ed). ACCP Pulmonary Medicine Board Review, 25th edition. Northbrook, IL: American College of Chest Physicians; 2009. pp. 415-56.
3. Smyrnios NA, Irwin RS. Wheeze. In: Irwin RS, Curley FJ, Grossman RF (Eds). Diagnosis and Treatment of Symptoms of the Respiratory Tract. Armonk, New York: Futura Publishing Company, Inc; 1997. pp. 117-53.
4. Loudon R, Murphy RL. Lung sounds. Am Rev Respir Dis. 1984;130(4):663-73.
5. Murphy RL, Loudon RG. Lung sounds in health and disease. In: Davis GS (Ed). Medical Management of Pulmonary Diseases. New York: Marcel Dekker, Inc. 1999.
6. Campion EW. Fundamentals of lung auscultation. N Engl J Med. 2014;370:744-51.
7. Nagasaka Y. Lung sounds in bronchial asthma. Allergology Internat. 2012;61:353-63.
8. Geffin B, Grillo HC, Cooper JD, Pontoppidan H. Stenosis following tracheostomy for respiratory care. JAMA. 1971;216(12):1984-8.
9. Shim CS, Williams MH. Relationship of wheezing to the severity of obstruction in asthma. Arch Intern Med. 1983;143(5):890-2.
10. Busse WW. What is the best pulmonary diagnostic approach for wheezing patients with normal spirometry? Resp Care. 2012;57:39-46.
11. Pratter MR, Hingston DM, Irwin RS. Diagnosis of bronchial asthma by clinical evaluation. An unreliable method. Chest. 1983;84(1):42-7.
12. Forgacs P. The functional basis of pulmonary sounds. Chest. 1978;73(3):399-405.
13. Marini JJ, Pierson DJ, Hudson LD, Lakshminarayan S. The significance of wheezing in chronic airflow obstruction. Am Rev Respir Dis. 1979;120(5):1069-72.
14. King KD, Thompson BT, Johnson DC. Wheezing on maximal forced expiration in the diagnosis of atypical asthma. Lack of sensitivity and specificity. Ann Intern Med. 1989;110(6):451-5.
15. Miller RD, Hyatt, RE. Obstructing lesions of the larynx and trachea: clinical and physiologic characteristics. Mayo Clin Proc. 1969;44(3):145-61.
16. Kryger M, Bode F, Antic R. Diagnosis of obstruction of the upper and central airways. Am J Med. 1976;61(1):85-93.
17. Mannino DM, Gagnon RC, Petty TL, Lydick E. Obstructive lung disease and low lung function in adults in the United States: data from the National Health and Nutrition Examination Survey, 1988-1994. Arch Intern Med. 2000;160(11):1683-9.
18. Gelb AF, Klein E. The volume of isoflow and increase in maximal flow at 50 percent of forced vital capacity during helium-oxygen breathing as tests of small airways dysfunction. Chest. 1977;71(3):396-9.
19. Seccombe LM, Polley L, Rogers PG, Ing AJ. All that wheezes is not asthma: the value of curves. Thorax. 2012;67:564-8.
20. Lakticova V, Koenig S. Not all wheezing is from COPD. Chest. 2013;143:e1-e3.
21. Pratter MR. Chronic upper airway cough syndrome secondary to rhinosinus diseases (previously referred to as postnasal drip syndrome): ACCP evidence-based clinical practice guidelines. Chest. 2006;129(1 Suppl):63S-71S.
22. Baran H, Ozcan KM, Selcuk A, Cetin MA, Cayir S, Ozcan M, et al. Allergic rhinitis and its impact on asthma classification correlations. J Laryngol Otol. 2014;128(5):431-7.
23. Glynn F, Fenton JE. Diagnosis and management of supraglottitis (epiglottitis). Curr Infect Dis Rep. 2008;10(3):200-4.
24. Christopher KL, Morris MJ. Vocal cord dysfunction, paradoxic vocal fold motion, or laryngomalacia? Our understanding requires an interdisciplinary approach. Otolaryngol Clin North Am. 2010;43(1):43-66.
25. Newman KB, Mason UG, Schmaling KB. Clinical features of vocal cord dysfunction. Am J Respir Crit Care Med. 1995;152 (4 Pt 1):1382-6.
26. Kenn K, Balkissoon R. Vocal cord dysfunction: what do we know? Eur Respir J. 2011;37:194-200.

27. Jaber S, Chanques G, Matecki S, Ramonatxo M, Vergne C, Souche B, et al. Post-extubation stridor in intensive care unit patients. Risk factors evaluation and importance of the cuff-leak test. Intensive Care Med. 2003;29(1):69-74.
28. National Asthma Education and Prevention Program. Expert Panel Report 3: guidelines for the diagnosis and management of asthma (Publication No. 08-4051). Bethesda, MD: National Institutes of Health; 2007.
29. GOLD Executive committee (2014). Global strategy for diagnosis, management, and prevention of COPD (Revised 2014). [online] Available from *http://www.goldcopd.com/*. [Accessed January, 2016].
30. Bruce N, Perez-Padilla R, Albalak R. Indoor air pollution in developing countries: a major environmental and public health challenge. Bull World Health Organ. 2000;78(9): 1078-92.
31. Jorge S, Becquemin MH, Delerme S, Bennaceur M, Isnard R, Achkar R, et al. Cardiac asthma in elderly patients: incidence, clinical presentation and outcome. BMC Cardiovasc Disord. 2007;7:16.
32. Smith Hammond CA, Goldstein LB. Cough and aspiration of food and liquids due to oral-pharyngeal dysphagia: ACCP evidence-based clinical practice guidelines. Chest. 2006; 129(Suppl 1):154S-68S.
33. Windebank WJ, Boyd G, Moran F. Pulmonary Thrombo-embolism presenting as Asthma. BMJ. 1973;1(5845):90-4.
34. Joint Task Force on Practice Parameters; American Academy of Allergy, Asthma and Immunology; American College of Allergy, Asthma and Immunology; Joint Council of Allergy, Asthma and Immunology. The diagnosis and management of anaphylaxis: an updated practice parameter. J Allergy Clin Immunol. 2005;115(3 Suppl 2):S483-523.
35. Checkley AM, Chiodini PL, Dockrell DH, Bates I, Thwaites GE, Booth HL, et al. Eosinophilia in returning travellers and migrants from the tropics: UK recommendations for investigation and initial management. J Infect. 2010;60(1):1-20.
36. McGarvey JM, Pollack CV. Heliox in airway management. Emerg Med Clin North Am. 2008;26(4):905-20.
37. Madison JM, Irwin RS. Heliox for asthma. A trial balloon. Chest. 1995;107(3):597-8.
38. Valli G, Paoletti P, Savi D, Martolini D, Palange P. Clinical use of Heliox in asthma and COPD. Monaldi Arch Chest Dis. 2007;67(3):159-64.

Section 5

Respiratory Diagnosis

Randeep Guleria, SK Jindal

19 Chapter

History and Physical Examination

Prahlad R Gupta

INTRODUCTION

Rapid advances have been made in the diagnostic tools in the field of medicine. Most such tools are now widely available to help clinicians to resolve complex clinical problems. Yet, clinical history and physical examination will continue to play an important role in the assessment of medical illness in a given patient. Respiratory illnesses are no exception. Optimal time required for history taking, physical examination, formulation of differential diagnosis, decision making and writing the treatment as well as instructions to the patients is about an hour. But in a crowded outpatient department as in India, this has to be accomplished within 5–10 minutes. Quick decisions regarding treatment are often made on the basis of clinical evaluation alone. Hence, it is necessary for every physician to acquire all the necessary skills to obtain complete information, without missing important points, to arrive at a clinical diagnosis in the given time. It is true to a great extent that the clinicians are natural Bayesians and their reasoning about patients is intuitive, probabilistic and reiterative.[1] Such subjective, context dependent reasoning is integral to clinical judgment and is especially useful to diagnose rare diseases.

HISTORY TAKING

The guiding principle to history taking is: "Listen to the patient as if he is revealing the diagnosis." Allow him to speak about his illness in his own words. Avoid unnecessary interruptions except when it becomes essential to seek details on certain issues. In case, a patient is describing his illness aimlessly with irrelevant details, it should be gently curtailed. Selective open ended questions may be asked but leading questions are best avoided. When a patient is too ill to give a coherent account of his illness, history should be taken from a relative or an attendant.

Begin with history of the presenting symptoms. Details of onset, nature and severity of each symptom, are essential. Also, ask for time scale (progressive or static, constant or paroxysmal) of the symptoms as well as aggravating or relieving factors, if any. In respiratory system, common symptoms include cough, chest pain, hemoptysis, shortness of breathing and/or wheezing. (Each of these symptoms has been discussed in greater details in separate chapters.)

Cough

Cough is a reflexive or deliberate explosive expiratory act. It is normally physiological and meant to clear the airways, but may become troublesome at times. It then prompts a patient to visit a physician. Psychogenic stress may cause or aggravate cough due to organic causes.[2] Chronic maxillary sinusitis, asthma, postviral reactive airway disease syndrome (RADS) and inhaled foreign bodies commonly cause persistent cough during childhood. In nonsmoker adults, asthma, postnasal drip, RADS and gastroesophageal reflux predominate, but in the elderly, asthma, cardiac failure and gastroesophageal reflux are the more common causes of cough (all may lead to nocturnal cough). Use of an angiotensin-converting-enzyme (ACE) inhibitor causing dry cough should always be kept in mind.[3] Smokers usually do not complain of cough, but when it is associated with excessive sputum, blood or dyspnea, it may point to an underlying disease, i.e. chronic obstructive pulmonary disease (COPD) or bronchogenic carcinoma.

History should cover the duration and characteristics of cough, whether it is dry or productive of sputum or blood, the provocative factors, i.e. cold, smoke, change of posture or eating and what are the accompanying symptoms to find out its likely cause, i.e. running nose and sore throat (postnasal drip); fever, chills and pleuritic pain chest (pneumonia); heartburn (gastroesophageal reflux); weight loss and night sweats (chronic infection or tumor); choking sensation and difficulty in swallowing while eating or drinking (aspiration).[4]

Sputum

A patient having productive cough should be asked about the time course, amount, character, viscosity, taste and color of the sputum. Early morning sputum in smokers suggests chronic bronchitis but if it occurs while lying down/going to bed, it points to underlying bronchiectasis or lung abscess. Most children and adult females usually do not spit but swallow their sputum; the presence of sputum should be assessed by the sound of their cough. It is usually not possible to measure the exact amount of sputum, but its quantum can be accessed from the number of spits, spoonfuls or cupfuls. Sputum may be very foul smelling in lung abscess or bronchiectasis. It is better to inspect the sample of sputum as the patient may not be able to describe its exact character, viscosity and color.

Sputum may be serous (pulmonary edema, bronchio-alveolar carcinoma), mucoid (chronic bronchitis, COPD, asthma) or mucopurulent/purulent (bronchiectasis, lung abscess, pneumonia). Viscous sputum is often difficult to expectorate (asthma). In anaerobic infections, the sputum is often foul to smell. Sputum is yellow, green or brown in bronchopulmonary infections, green if it contains eosinophils, golden yellow or green in bronchobiliary fistula, rusty in pneumococcal infections, red currant jelly type in *Klebsiella pneumoniae*, anchovy sauce colored in ruptured amoebic liver abscess, and black in coal-workers pneumoconiosis. Sputum may contain brown or black casts in the recovery phase of asthma or allergic bronchopulmonary aspergillosis (ABPA).[5]

Hemoptysis

Hemoptysis is coughing out blood from respiratory tract, mainly the lungs. Mild hemoptysis, often seen as blood streaking, is a common symptom with severe sough. Lungs have been provided with a dual blood supply namely the low pressure pulmonary arteries (95%) and the high-pressure bronchial (systemic) circulation (5%). Hemoptysis mostly originates from the later except in the cases of trauma or erosion of pulmonary arteries or inflammation of pulmonary capillaries. Efforts should be made to differentiate true hemoptysis from hematemesis, epistaxis or bleeding from oral cavity by asking the patient about the temporal pattern of blood spitting.[6] Hematemesis generally follows nausea, vomiting or retching; in epistaxis, the patient feels sensation of postnasal drip or bleeding from nares without coughing but hemoptysis follows coughing. The type of blood in the expectorate can also help to detect the source (bright red often mixed with frothy sputum in hemoptysis versus the dark black, often in clumps and mixed with food, in hematemesis).[6]

History should cover the onset (sudden, recurrent or cyclical), duration, provoking factors (exertion, change of position, exposure to cold, smoke or allergens) and amount (streaking or massive) of hemoptysis. It is seldom a solitary event. Associated symptoms may provide clue to the cause of hemoptysis, i.e. chest pain (pulmonary embolism), dependent edema, orthopnea and paroxysmal nocturnal dyspnea (pulmonary edema), fever and cough (pneumonia), weight loss [tuberculosis (TB) or cancer], bloody nasal discharge [granulomatosis with polyangiitis (GPA)], hematuria (Goodpasture's syndrome, GPA), and bleeding from other sites or easy bruising (coagulopathy). Enquire about a risk factor as it may provide the likely etiology, i.e. human immunodeficiency virus (HIV) infection or use of immune-suppressant drugs (TB and fungal infections), long-standing smoking history (lung cancer) or a recent history of immobilization, travel for long distances, surgery, pregnancy, cancer or use of oral contraceptives (pulmonary thromboembolism).

Chest Pain

Chest pain is a common complaint, but the patient's perception about its gravity may vary. To some, it is a warning of potential life-threatening illness and they may seek repeated consultations even when the symptom is trivial. Others, including those with serious illnesses, may tend to ignore. However, a physician should never discard the symptom without exploring its etiology. Chest pain may have its origin from disorders of chest wall, pleura, lungs, heart/great vessels, esophagus and subdiaphragmatic structures **(Table 1)**.

History of chest pain should include its duration, location, radiation to other areas and character, i.e. heaviness, tearing, burning, stabbing, sharp needle like, urge to eructate or merely a discomfort (dull ache or boring). Precipitating factors, such as physical or psychological stress, respiratory efforts, coughing or swallowing, and relieving factors (such as leaning forward) should be enquired. Associated symptoms like cough, dyspnea, palpitation, syncope, diaphoresis, nausea, vomiting, fever and chills, weakness, malaise and weight loss should be asked for. Leg pain and swelling may point to deep vein thrombosis and pulmonary thromboembolism.

Dyspnea

Dyspnea is an unpleasant or uncomfortable awareness of breathing. In most situations, it occurs due to an imbalance between neurological stimulation and the mechanical changes that occurs in the lungs and the chest wall, the resulting mismatch of ventilation and its demand.[7] A variety of scaling methods have been used to quantify dyspnea, i.e. Borg category scale, visual analog scale and American Thoracic Society Scale, but none can be universally applied to all the patients.[8] For epidemiological purposes, the one suggested by the Medical Research Council, is quite useful.[9]

A host of pulmonary, cardiac or other disorders may lead to dyspnea. History should cover its duration, onset (sudden or insidious), severity and exacerbating or relieving factors, i.e. exertion or rest, supine or sitting position or exposure to cold, dust, smoke and allergens.

Associated symptoms may provide useful clue to the cause of dyspnea, i.e. chest pain (pulmonary embolism, myocardial infarction), dependent edema, orthopnea or paroxysmal nocturnal dyspnea (cardiac failure), wheezing (asthma), fever or cough (pneumonia), black stools or heavy menses (anemia) and weight loss (TB or cancer). A patient with psychogenic dyspnea is symptomatic more often during rest than on exertion.

Table 1 Common causes of chest pain and likely character of pain

Site of lesion	*Cause*	*Likely character of pain*
Pulmonary	Tumors Pneumonia Pulmonary embolism/infarction	Mostly dull aching Often pleural Central, sharp and sinking
Pleural	Pneumothorax/hemothorax/ effusion/empyema/pleuritis Tumors	Sharp, stabbing, worse on coughing Dull ache
Cardiovascular	Myocardial ischemia/infarct Myocarditis Pericarditis Dressler's syndrome Dissecting aortic aneurism Mitral valve prolapsed	Central, sharp and sinking, radiating to left arm Mostly dull ache Sharp and stabbing Sharp, stabbing or dull aching Sharp and tearing Mostly dull ache
Esophageal	Spasm/rupture/esophagitis/ulceration Neoplasm Achalasia/diverticula FB sharp	Central lower chest, sharp Mostly dull ache Burning Stabbing
Gastrointestinal	Liver abscess Pancreatitis Whipple's disease	Sharp and throbbing Sharp, stabbing, radiating to back Mostly dull ache
Chest wall	Herpes zoster Breast lesions Musculoskeletal Infection/tumor/trauma in spine/ribs	Sharp, sometimes throbbing Mostly dull ache Sharp, often with cough, dyspnea and fever Localized and sharp
Mediastinal	Tumors Inflammation	Mostly dull ache Central and sharp
Miscellaneous	Subdiaphragmatic abscess Other diseases of subdiaphragmatic structures Psychoneurosis	Sharp and throbbing Boring Severe, worse in presence of attendants

Abbreviation: FB, foreign bodies

Upper Respiratory Tract Symptoms

A brief history of upper respiratory tract symptoms, more particularly running of nose, itching, sneezing, congestion, discharge of blood or blood mixed secretions or blocked nose, should always be obtained while assessing a patient for respiratory illness. These symptoms may point to specific respiratory (asthma) or systemic illnesses (sarcoidosis, GPA, etc).

General Symptoms

Once the assessment of the respiratory symptoms is over, the patient should be asked for the presence of general symptoms and those pertaining to other systems. Presence of fever, loss of appetite, weight loss or anemia signifies serious illness. History of associated urinary symptoms, dysphasia, joint pain and skin lesions may point to an important systemic illness. Symptoms pertaining to cardiac and neuromuscular diseases may unravel the cause of respiratory illness, particularly of dyspnea.

Past Medical History

Past medical history of the patient may give an important clue to the etiology of the current illness. Ask about childhood illnesses like fever, cough and cold; if recurrent, as these may end up with diagnoses of asthma, COPD or bronchiectasis during adult life. Chest injuries in past (particularly those with hemothorax) may indicate frozen chest. History of loss of consciousness in the past may point to lung abscess. Surgery or pregnancy in recent past suggests pulmonary thromboembolism. Indeed, history of infections, trauma, surgery, malignancies or prolonged bed rest in the past, all may provide important clue to the diagnosis of the current illness. Important lifestyle diseases that may have impact on respiratory system include diabetes mellitus and obesity. History of allergy to food, drugs and/or dust may give an important clue to the diagnosis of rhinitis/asthma. History of wheezy bronchitis in childhood is also helpful in diagnosis of asthma in adults.

HISTORY OF TREATMENT

Most patients visit a pulmonologist only after consulting their family physician. It is therefore, always worthwhile to ask the patient about the details of such consultations, investigations already done, diagnosis made, treatment offered and the outcome thereof. A correct diagnosis may have been missed for want of time and skill and even if a diagnosis was correctly made, the treatment may be wanting in the terms of drugs, dosages and compliance. Past history of incorrect or irregular treatment of TB may point to drug failure (and drug resistance), relapse or sequelae such as bronchiectasis, aspergilloma or chronic necrotizing pulmonary aspergillosis.[10] Drugs taken for other illnesses may be responsible for the current illness, e.g. busulphan causing pulmonary fibrosis, ACE inhibitors causing cough, aspirin and nonsteroidal anti-inflammatory drugs (NSAIDs) causing asthma, and so on.

Personal History

Patient's lifestyle and personal habits like smoking or alcohol consumption, along with the details of the quantity, frequency and its duration, are integral parts of a good history-taking. Exposure to pets and animals may be responsible for a serious or recurrent respiratory illness. Present or past occupational exposure to organic dust like bagasse or hay or inorganic dust like silica, coal or asbestos may at times help to unravel the diagnosis in most difficult clinical situations. Being in a profession that keeps a person away from spouse, i.e. truck drivers, labors in metro cities/brick kilns, invites extramarital or promiscuous sex and predispose to acquired immunodeficiency syndrome (AIDS) and other infectious disease.

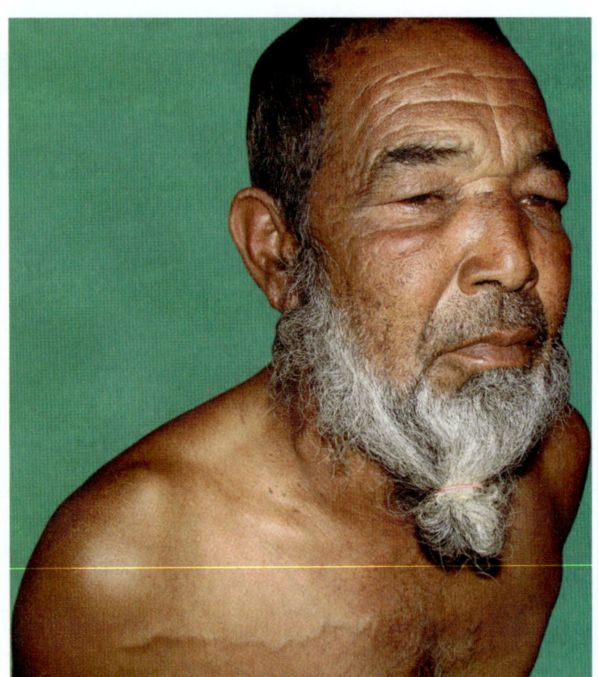

Fig.1 Plethoric appearance of face in a patient with superior vena cava obstruction

PHYSICAL EXAMINATION

After the history-taking, the clinician already has some idea regarding the likely diagnosis and what to expect of the physical examination. Yet a systematic approach to the latter is always rewarding and may obviate the need for unnecessary investigations at a later stage. This chapter briefly highlights the approach to general physical, respiratory system and other systems examination. For details regarding the methodology, the reader is referred to various books on clinical methods in medicine.[11-13]

General Physical Examination

Always begin with assessment of the general appearance, mental faculty and breathing pattern of the patient. Note down the presence of wheeze, stridor or voice abnormality, if any. An anxious look indicates acute illness while the presence of fatigue and cachexia point to a chronic disease or malignancy. A plethoric appearance may be seen in polycythemia, most commonly as a result of chronic lung disease or superior vena cava (SVC) obstruction **(Fig. 1)**. Look at the tongue, soft palate and the nail beds for cyanosis, anemia or polycythemia, at fingers for clubbing, at face, neck, hands and feet for edema (generalized, localized or differential); and neck for any lymphadenopathy or abnormal pulsations/fullness of veins. Record vital signs, i.e. pulse (rate, rhythm and character), respiration (type, rate and regularity), blood pressure and temperature. Also look for nicotine stains on the intertriginous surfaces of the second and third fingers (in cigarette or *bidi* smokers) or the palm (in *chillum* or *hookah* smokers).

Breathing Pattern

Breathing pattern should be observed throughout the clinical examination. Normal breathing is quiet with a frequency of between 12 and 18 per minute. An increased respiratory rate (tachypnea) is seen in the presence of anxiety, anemia, asthma, restrictive lung diseases, pulmonary artery hypertension and hypoxia of any etiology. A slow respiratory rate (bradypnea) may be attributed to decreased respiratory drive as a result of drug overdose or lesions of the central nervous system. Use of the accessory muscles of respiration or pursed lip breathing, which indicate severe illness, should be recorded. Noisy breathing indicates the narrowing of central airways, such as from carcinomatous lesions of vocal cord or trachea, or intrinsic lesions of vocal cords like palsies. When such obstruction is severe, the sound assumes a musical tone during inspiration (occasionally during expiration also). This is then called as croup or strider. Wheezy breath sounds, audible to unaided ears, are produced by the narrowing of intrathoracic airways, e.g. in asthma. Periodic breathing

Table 2 Common causes of cyanosis

Pulmonary	*Cardiac*	*Others*
Pneumonia Atelectasis Asthma/COPD Interstitial lung diseases Pulmonary AV fistulas	Congenital heart disease Pulmonary thromboembolism Decreased cardiac output	High altitude pulmonary edema central apneas
Abbreviations: COPD, chronic obstructive pulmonary disease; AV, arteriovenous		

patterns, including Cheyne-Stokes and Biot's breathing are usually associated with left heart failure and disorders of the central nervous system. In Kussmaul breathing, the depth of respiration is increased more than the rate. This pattern most often occurs in severe metabolic acidosis, but may be seen in an anxious person. The resultant hyperventilation in the latter may lead to respiratory alkalosis, weakness, dizziness and muscle cramps (tetany).

Cyanosis

Cyanosis is the bluish discoloration of the tongue and the soft palate (central, when it mostly reflects arterial hypoxemia) or of nail beds and lips (peripheral, when it may also reflect arterial hypoxemia due to low blood flow). Central cyanosis mostly occurs due to severe chronic hypoxemia of pulmonary or cardiac origin and is often associated with polycythemia **(Table 2)**. Peripheral cyanosis (often with edema) affecting face, neck (and sometimes the upper limbs) may indicate SVC obstruction, and that of lower limbs, the inferior vena cava obstruction. Bluish discoloration of the tongue and the soft palate, the nail beds or the lips may be due to methemoglobinemia or sulfhemoglobinemia. In carbon monoxide poisoning, the organs are discolored as cherry red.

Clubbing

Clubbing is characterized by the diffuse bulbous enlargement of the terminal phalanges **(Fig. 2)**. Early changes consist of thickening of the fibroelastic tissue of the nail bed, which can be detected by the loss of the normal angle between the base of the nail and the adjacent dorsal surface of the finger. This finding is demonstrated best when the finger is viewed from the side. Finger clubbing can occur in various pulmonary, cardiac and abdominal diseases **(Table 3)**. Rarely clubbing may be congenital (familial) in origin. With time, it may progress to hypertrophic pulmonary osteoarthropathy (HPOA). At this stage, the patient may complain of bone or joint pains.

Lymphadenopathy

Lymphadenopathy is abnormal enlargement of lymph glands (mostly less than 0.5 cms in size) at neck, axilla, groin and other external or internal sites. Note down the number, size, consistency and fixity of the lymph nodes to each other, the underlying tissues or to the overlying skin. Large fixed masses indicate metastasis, while firm and matted nodes point to tuberculosis. Lymph nodes in Hodgkin's lymphoma are classically described as large, soft and rubbery in character.

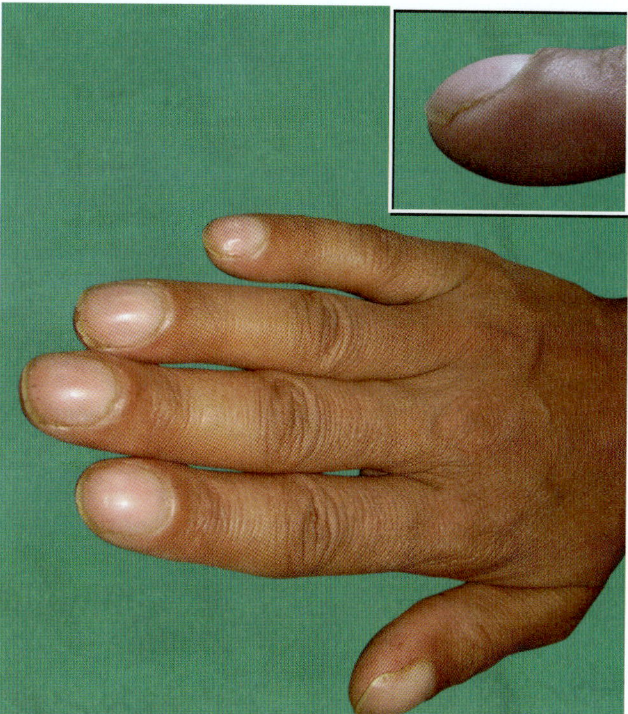

Fig. 2 Clubbed fingers. Insert showing the same in side profile. Note the convexity of nail and the loss of the normal angle between the base of the nail and the adjacent dorsal surface of the finger

Table 3 Common causes of clubbing

Pulmonary	*Cardiac*	*Enteric*
Tumors of lung Mesotheliomas Suppurative lung diseases Idiopathic pulmonary fibrosis	Congenital heart disease Bacterial endocarditis	Cirrhosis liver Ulcerative colitis Coeliac disease Crohn's disease

Miscellaneous Physical Findings

All components of the upper respiratory tract (nasal cavity, nasopharynx, nasal sinuses, oropharynx and the larynx) need to be examined sequentially as this may help clinch the diagnosis, e.g. discharging nasal lesion in GPA (Wegener's granulomatosis). Thyroid gland should also be examined to detect abnormality in its shape, size and consistency. Other lesions that may provide clue to the underlying respiratory pathology include skin lesions such as erythema nodosum in sarcoidosis and TB **(Fig. 3)**; malar rash in systemic lupus

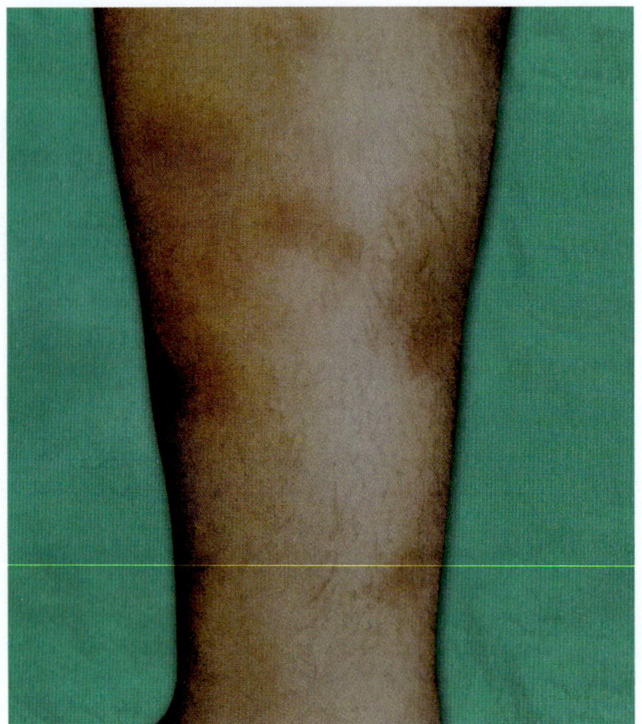

Fig. 3 Erythema nodosum. Note the coppery red and raised skin lesions

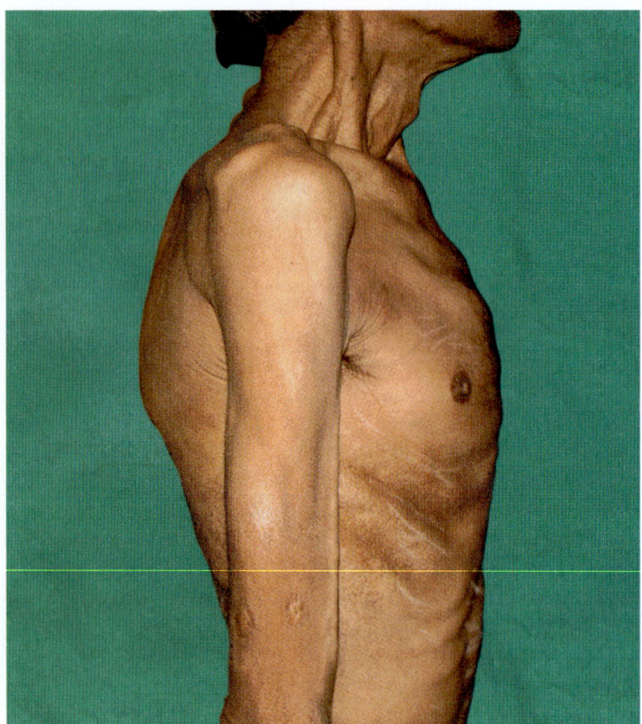

Fig. 5 Pectus carinatum (Pigeon chest)

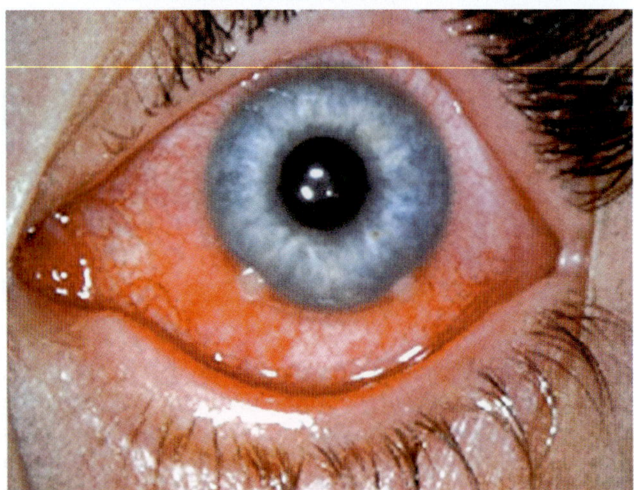

Fig. 4 Phlyctenular conjunctivitis

erythematosus and dermatomyositis; subcutaneous nodules in metastatic carcinoma and eye lesions such as phlyctenular conjunctivitis in TB **(Fig. 4)**; Horner's syndrome in lung cancer; iridocyclitis in TB and sarcoidosis; chemosis in SVC obstruction and flapping tremors in type II respiratory failure (hypercapnea).

Examination of the Chest

Traditionally, the scheme of chest examination includes inspection, palpation, percussion and auscultation in that order, but some physicians combine inspection with palpation. It is best done in good daylight with the patient in the sitting posture and arms at the side.

Inspection

- *Appearance, shape and size of chest*: Normal chest is bilaterally symmetrical and elliptical in cross section but in disease, it may be asymmetrical (generalized or localized flattening or fullness, as is seen in congenital or acquired disorders of lungs, pleura, ribs, vertebra or sternum or chest wall) or abnormal in shape (rickets). The latter includes pectus carinatum or pigeon chest [localized prominence of sternum and adjacent ribs **(Fig. 5)**], pectus excavatum or funnel chest [localized depression of sternum and adjacent ribs **(Fig. 6)**], kyphosis (forward bending), scoliosis (lateral bending), kyphoscoliosis, flattening [decreased anteroposterior (AP) diameter] and hyperinflation or barrel shaped [increased AP diameter **(Figs 7A and B)**]. Also observe for any scar, injection mark, stains or lumps as a consequence of disease or trauma as well as for muscle wasting, if any.
- *Movements of chest wall*: Normally, the two sides of the chest move equally. Decreased or absent movements on one side may indicate disease of chest wall, pleura or of the lung on that side. Symmetrical decrease in the movement of chest wall occurs in emphysema, asthma and end-stage diffuse pulmonary fibrosis. Intercostal recession (indrawing of intercostals spaces) indicates severe upper

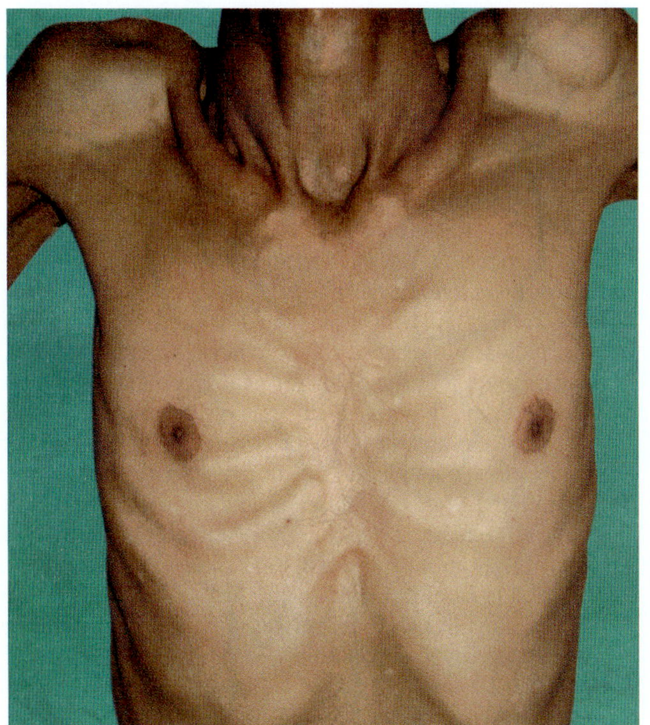

Fig. 6 Pectus excavatum (Funnel chest)

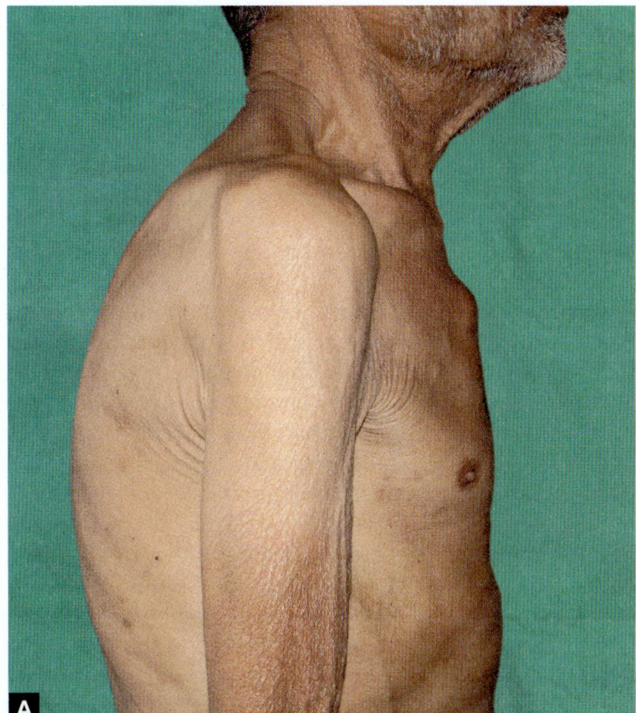

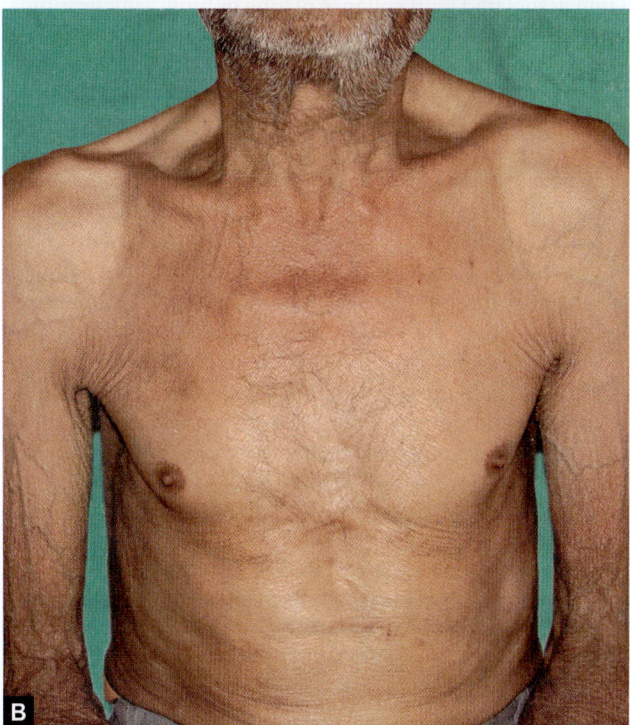

Figs 7A and B Barrel-shaped chest

airway obstruction (laryngeal or tracheal tumor). Inward movement of lower ribs on inspiration (instead of normal outward movement) occurs in emphysema and asthma. Observe for use of alae nasi (pneumonia in childhood) or accessory muscles of respiration (emphysema).

- *Shift of mediastinum*: Observe for prominence of the tendon of sternomastoid muscle at the suprasternal notch. The trachea is shifted to the side of prominence (positive trails sign) and indicate shift of upper mediastinum to the same side (fibrosis or collapse) or the opposite side (pleural effusion, pneumothorax or a mass). Also observe for the cardiac impulse, normally visible as a pulse, synchronous with heartbeat in the 5th intercostal space, half an inch inside the midclavicular line. It may not be visible in emphysema (hyperinflated lung overlying the heart), pericardial effusion or other diffuse cardiac diseases.

Palpation

Palpation is done mostly to confirm the findings of inspection. Gently begin palpating the part of the chest showing obvious swelling on inspection, or at the site where the patient complains of pain to detect—inflammatory edema (fractured ribs, cellulitis, infected cysts or tumors), air (subcutaneous emphysema), pus (abscess, empyema necessitans) or nodules (purpura, sarcoid nodule, metastatic nodule). Assess the position of trachea in suprasternal notch and of apex beat at the lower chest wall. Displacement of these structures indicate shift of the mediastinum, to the same side in collapse or fibrosis but to the contralateral side in effusion or pneumothorax. Assess for symmetry of the movements on the two sides. In general, the side of chest which moves less is pathological (or more pathological than the other side).

Assess for the width of intercostal spaces on the two sides to confirm or deny flattening or fullness, as the case may be. Vocal fremitus is detected by placing the ulnar side of hand over the equivalent areas on the two sides of the patient's chest when he narrates "one, two, three" or "ninety-nine" but it may be done along with vocal resonance at the time of auscultation. At times, a rub or rhonchus may be palpable.

Percussion

Compare the degree of resonance over the equivalent areas on the two sides of chest and then focus on the area of interest to detect a generalized or localized abnormality. Note for an area of tenderness, if any. The character of percussion note may point to the underlying pathology **(Table 4)**. A stony dull percussion note indicates pleural effusion, more so, if the breath sounds and vocal resonance are decreased. A dull note with increased bronchial breath sounds and bronchophony indicates consolidation but with shrunken chest and decreased breath sounds, it indicates atelectasis. Hyper-resonant note indicates pneumothorax, more so when the chest appears fuller and the breath sounds and/or vocal resonance are decreased or absent. Pulmonary tumors cause dullness when peripheral and abut the chest wall or when associated with collapse of lobe or lung. Topographical and tidal percussion has practically lost its value in modern clinical practice.

Auscultation

- *Breath sounds:* Listen to lung sounds for its character and quality over all the parts of the chest wall, on both the sides, using the diaphragm of stethoscope. Breath sounds are vesicular in character (low frequency rustling sound with longer inspiration than expiration and without a pause in between) over the healthy lungs and are best heard at the lung bases. When the breath sound is blowing in character and loud in midexpiration, it is called as bronchovesicular. In a normal person, such a breath sound may be heard over the lung apices. Bronchial breathing is a high-pitched blowing sound, heard during inspiration and expiration and separated by a brief pause and is normal over trachea or larynx. When heard over a part of the chest wall, it is abnormal and indicates consolidation of the underlying lung. It is produced due to the increased transmission of high-pitched breath sounds to the chest wall through the solid lung which now acts as a bridge between the airways and the chest wall. Breath sounds are decreased in intensity when fluid (effusion), air (pneumothorax) or atelectasis interferes with the transmission of sounds from airways to the chest wall.
- *Adventitious sounds:* Normal lung fields are devoid of any extra sounds but wheezes, crackles and/or pleural rub may be heard in disease states. Wheezes are continuous, high-pitched sounds, often musical in character, which arise from air moving in the narrowed airways, e.g. in asthma. They are more marked during expiration and usually associated with prolonged expiratory time. Continuous, but low-pitched sound may be heard at a localized area (rhonchus) such as obstruction of a large airway by a tumor. Crackles are discontinuous, "popping" or bubbling sounds. Coarser, gurgling sounds are caused by secretions in the larger airways and are heard during inspiration as well as expiration. Finer crackles are usually heard during early inspiration. They are commonly heard in the presence of restrictive lung disorders such as the pulmonary edema and pulmonary fibrosis. They may be produced due to sudden opening of the small airways. Rub is a localized cracking or rubbing sound, often associated with chest pain and is heard during inspiration as well as expiration (to and fro character). It may, at times, be felt by the palpating hand. It indicates pleural inflammation. Exclude extraneous or false sounds that may occur due to the movement of stethoscope on skin, hair or clothing, or due to muscle twitching (shivering due to cold).
- *Vocal resonance:* It is the audible perception of the transmitted vibrations from the vocal cords over the chest as the patient narrates "one, two, three" or "ninety-nine." Compare each point on one side with the corresponding point on the opposite side. It is increased in the presence of consolidation but is decreased (or absent) in the presence of atelectasis, pneumothorax or pleural effusion. In consolidation, the spoken words may be perceived as if spoken directly into the listener's ear (bronchophony) or the whispered sounds may be clearly perceived (whispering pectoriloquy); in effusion, the spoken sound may be perceived with nasal or bleating character (egophony).

Table 4 Types of percussion note and likely etiology

Percussion note	*Likely etiology*
Tympanic	Hollow viscus, pneumothorax
Hyper-resonant	Pneumothorax
Resonant	Normal lung
Impaired to dull	Consolidation Collapse Fibrosis Tumors
Stony dull	Effusion Empyema

Systemic Examination

Examination of other systems may provide vital clues in the assessment of a patient with respiratory illness.

Certain skin lesions are an essential part of the pulmonary disease, i.e. erythema nodosum in TB and sarcoidosis; Kaposi's sarcoma in AIDS; larva migrans in Loeffler's syndrome; metastatic nodule in lung carcinoma; and "Mat" telangiectasia in Osler-Weber-Rendu disease. Skin lesions may also manifest as the complication of drugs, i.e. Stevens-Johnson syndrome in a patient of TB on antitubercular treatment or be a part of a systemic disease having pulmonary manifestations, i.e. lupus pernio, flashy papules and erythema nodosum in sarcoidosis, malar rash and discoid lesions (often accompanied by telangiectasia, atrophy and scarring) in systemic lupus erythematosus. Besides, certain primary skin diseases like erythema multiforme may have pulmonary complications.

Examination of the joints may show symmetrical arthritis of small joints (rheumatoid arthritis) or large joints (Behçet's disease). Examination of cardiovascular system may unravel cor pulmonale complicating the hypoxemia of pulmonary diseases or unravel the underlying pericardial, myocardial, endocardial or valvular lesions of the heart or aneurysmal lesions of vessels that complicate the respiratory diseases. Similarly, examination of abdomen may reveal advanced cirrhosis that leads to hepatopulmonary syndrome, while neurological examination may reveal the signs of metastatic brain lesion in an otherwise occult lung cancer.

Systemic examination is important also because a number of systemic diseases may first present with significant pulmonary symptoms and signs.[14] Factually, the respiratory system cannot be seen and assessed in isolation.

Bedside Measurement of Lung Functions

Measurement of forced expiratory time has been used to detect the presence of airway obstruction in a patient at bedside.[15] The length of time taken to walk 6 meter distance (6MWD) is a simple test of lung function.[16] Peak expiratory flow measurements and oxymetry can also be considered as essential components of the initial clinical and physical assessment.

Examination of Chest Skiagrams

Many chest physicians now consider examination of the respiratory system as incomplete without perusal of the recent and past skiagrams of the chest. It provides a visual appreciation of the respiratory illness and helps planning of further investigations. Occasionally, situation may arise where the clinical findings may not correlate with the X-ray findings and the latter will prevail over the former in making clinical judgement.

In summary, the importance of history-taking and physical examination should never be underestimated, in-spite of the ever-expanding diagnostic armamentarium. Patients expect and appreciate some degree of physical examination by the doctor. Besides being a powerful diagnostic tool, it helps as healing-ritual and promotes physician-patient relationship.[17,18] While over-reliance on physical findings and stress on mandatory demonstration of individual physical signs is unnecessary, the importance of history-taking remains critical for diagnosis as well as for comprehensive management.

REFERENCES

1. Gill CJ, Sabin L, Schmid HC. Why clinicians are natural bayesians. BMJ. 2005;330(7499):1080-3.
2. Karlsson JA, Sant'Ambrogio G, Widdicombe J. Afferent neural pathways in cough and reflex bronchoconstriction. J Appl Physiol (1985). 1988;65(3):1007-23.
3. Morice AH, Lowry R, Brown MJ, Higenbottam T. Angiotensin-converting enzyme and the cough reflex. Lancet. 1987; 2(8568):1116-8.
4. Irwin RS, Baumann MH, Bolser DC, Boulet LP, Braman SS, Brightling CE, et al. Diagnosis and management of cough executive summary: ACCP evidence based clinical practice guidelines. Chest. 2006;129(1 Suppl):1S-23S.
5. Campbell MJ, Clayton YM. Bronchopulmonary aspergillosis. A correlation of the clinical and laboratory findings in 272 parients investigated for bronchopulmonary aspergillosis. Am Rev Respir Dis. 1964;89:186-96.
6. Israel RH, Poe RH. Hemoptysis. Clin Chest Med. 1987;8(2):197-205.
7. Cambell EJM, Howell JBL. The sensation of Dyspnoea. BMJ. 1963;2:868.
8. Muza SR, Silverman MT, Gilmore GC, Hellerstein HK, Kelsen SG. Comparison of scales used to quantify the sense of breath in patients with chronic obstructive pulmonary disease. Am Rev Respir Dis. 1990;141(4 Pt 1):909-13.
9. Medical Research Council Committee on etiology of chronic bronchitis. Standardized questionnaire on respiratory symptoms. BMJ. 1960;2:1665.
10. Gupta PR, Vyas Aruna, Meena RC, S Khangarot, Devesh Kanoongo, S Jain. Role of itraconazole in the management of aspergillosis in treated patients of pulmonary tuberculosis. Lung India. 2005;22(3):81-5.
11. Alagappan R. Manual of Practical Medicine, 4th edition, Chennai: Jaypee Brothers Medical Publishers Pvt. Ltd.; 2011. pp. 199-268.
12. Vakil RJ, Golwalla AF. Physical Diagnosis, 14th edition, Mumbai: Media Promoters & Publishers; 2012. pp. 337-92.
13. J Moore-Gillon. The respiratory system. In: Michael Swash (Ed.) Hutchison's Clinical Methods, 21st edition. Philadelphia: Saunders; 2002. pp. 60-78.
14. Jindal SK. Approach to systemic manifestations of pulmonary disease. World Clin Pulm Crit Care Med. 2013;2(2):227-37.
15. Lal S, Ferguson AD, Campbell EJ. Forced expiratory time: a simple test for airways obstruction. Br Med J. 1964;1(5386): 814-7.
16. van Stel HF, Bogaard JM, Rijssenbeek-Nouwens LH, Colland VT. Multivariable assessment of the 6-min walking test in patients with chronic obstructive pulmonary disease. Am J Respir Crit Care Med. 2001;163(7):1567-71.
17. Verghese A, Horwitz RI. In praise of the physical examination. BMJ. 2009;339:b5448.
18. Verghese A, Brady E, Kapur CC, Horwitz RI. The bedside evaluation: ritual and reason. Ann Intern Med. 2011;155: 550-3.

Microbiological Approach to Respiratory Infections

Pallab Ray

UPPER RESPIRATORY TRACT INFECTIONS

Bacterial infections of the upper respiratory tract vary from benign pharyngitis to life-threatening epiglottitis. Infections can be divided into syndromes involving the nasal cavity and its extensions, including the sinuses, the middle ear and the associated tissues.

Normal Flora of the Upper Respiratory Tract

The upper respiratory tract is colonized with a host of organisms. The paranasal sinuses are normally sterile. The anterior nares are colonized by staphylococci, micrococci and *Corynebacterium* species.[1] Continuous evaporation of tear draining into nasal cavities raises the salt concentration locally, favoring colonization by salt-resistant staphylococci, including *Staphylococcus aureus*. The nose is the primary site of carriage of *S. aureus* in nearly a third of the healthy population. The nasopharynx has a more complex flora comprising of resident and transient flora. The resident flora comprises of streptococci (viridans group), *Neisseria* species, members of family *Enterobacteriaceae* and anaerobes, including *Bacteroides* species and *Fusobacterium* species.[2] Additionally, all individuals are transiently colonized by one or more potentially pathogenic bacteria that include group A *Streptococcus* (less frequently groups B, C and G), *Streptococcus pneumoniae*, *Haemophilus influenzae*, *Neisseria meningitidis* and *Moraxella catarrhalis*.

Common Cold

Common cold is an upper respiratory syndrome caused by a variety of viral pathogens. The significance of common cold originates from the sheer frequency of these illnesses in the general population. Although generally mild and self-limited, these illnesses are associated with an enormous economic burden both in lost productivity and in expenditures for treatment.

Etiology

Rhinoviruses cause approximately one-half of all colds. More than 100 serotypes and short-lasting serotype specific immunity results in repeated infections with seasonal predominance in the community. Other important pathogens include the coronaviruses and respiratory syncytial virus (RSV). Influenza, parainfluenza and adenoviruses are often associated with cold-like symptoms though these agents primarily cause lower respiratory or systemic symptoms. Recently identified causes, though uncommon, include metapneumovirus, detected in 2001,[3] and bocavirus, a human parvovirus discovered in respiratory secretions in 2005.[4]

Laboratory Findings

Routine laboratory studies are not helpful for the diagnosis and management of the common cold. A nasal smear for eosinophils may help differentiate allergic rhinitis from a viral etiology. A neutrophilic predominance in nasal secretions is rather characteristic of uncomplicated colds and does not necessarily indicate bacterial superinfection demanding antibiotics. Though it is possible to establish the viral etiological agent of common cold by culture, antigen detection and molecular or serologic methods, the lack of therapeutic relevance generally precludes the necessity of the same. Bacterial cultures or antigen detection is indicated only when group A *Streptococcus* (GAS), *Bordetella pertussis*, or nasal diphtheria is suspected. The isolation of other bacterial pathogens is not an indicator of bacterial nasal infection.

Pharyngitis

Acute pharyngitis classically presents as sore throat, fever and pharyngeal inflammation characterized by redness and edema, frequently with vesicles or ulcerations.[5] It affects all age groups though children are more frequently affected with higher incidence during winter and spring in temperate climates and transitional seasons in tropical climates. Besides pharyngitis as a primary entity, sore throat and pharyngeal erythema may be associated with systemic disorders, such as the acute retroviral syndrome, or part of a more generalized upper respiratory tract infection.

Etiology

Most cases of acute pharyngitis are due to viral infections, and are usually benign, self-limited illnesses. Viruses account for up to one-half of all cases, often associated with other signs or symptoms of upper respiratory tract infection.[6] All viruses implicated in upper respiratory tract infections have been implicated in causation of pharyngitis. Adenovirus is considered as the most common viral cause of pharyngitis, reported in 12–23% of cases.[7] Other respiratory viruses that cause pharyngitis include rhinoviruses, coronaviruses, enteroviruses, influenzavirus A and B, parainfluenza viruses, RSV, coronaviruses, human metapneumovirus (hMPV), and human bocavirus.[8] Human herpesviruses, such as Epstein-Barr virus (EBV), herpes simplex virus (HSV), human immunodeficiency virus type 1 (HIV-1) and human cytomegalovirus have been infrequently reported to cause pharyngitis. A child in the age group of 5–15 years suffers from an average of seven episodes of sore throat in a year, of which six are viral and one is streptococcal.[9] *Streptococcus pyogenes*, also known as lancefield GAS or group A beta-hemolytic *Streptococcus* (GA-BHS), is the most common bacterial etiological agent of highest concern because of its associated nonsuppurative sequelae, acute rheumatic fever and poststreptococcal glomerulonephritis. Group A *Streptococcus* is responsible for approximately 10–15% of cases of pharyngitis in adults[10] and 15–30% of cases in children.[9,11] Developing countries have reported a recent trend of emergence of *Streptococcus* group C and G in pharyngeal carriage and infection.[12] *Arcanobacterium haemolyticum* is a rare cause of bacterial pharyngitis, especially in adolescents and young adults.[13]

Fusobacterium necrophorum, a gram-negative, nonspore-forming anaerobe, is a bacterial cause of sore throat in about 10% of cases of pharyngitis, distinctive by its frequent recurrences.[14] *Corynebacterium diphtheriae* is a cause of pharyngitis and diphtheria in countries without adequate coverage of primary immunization.[15,16] Rare causes of bacterial pharyngitis include *Neisseria gonorrhoeae* in sexually active adolescents and young adults, *Mycoplasma pneumoniae* and *Chlamydophila pneumoniae*.[7]

Diagnosis

Pharyngitis is one of the most common causes for seeking medical attention. Differentiation of bacterial etiology from viral is important for the substantially higher morbidity of the former, serious nonsuppurative sequelae associated with GAS infection and to avoid unnecessary antibiotic therapy in viral cases. In GAS pharyngitis, the risk of development of rheumatic fever or poststreptococcal glomerulonephritis is directly proportional to the delay in the institution of therapy. Symptoms, such as conjunctivitis, coryza, oral ulcers, cough and diarrhea suggest a viral cause. On the other hand, abrupt onset, presence of tonsillar or pharyngeal exudates, tender anterior cervical lymphadenopathy, and fever are more commonly associated with GAS infection. Many clinical prediction rules have been proposed to help differentiate GAS from viral pharyngitis. Scoring systems use clinical and epidemiologic pointers to a quantitative probability that favors GAS over a viral etiology.[17] The clinical predictive efficacy of these scoring protocols are limited by extensive overlap of the signs and symptoms of many viral causes of acute pharyngitis with those of infections caused by GAS. Consequently, the Infectious Disease Society of America, the Committee on Infectious Diseases of the American Academy of Pediatrics, and the American Heart Association recommend guidelines that include confirmation of GAS infection by rapid antigen detection test (RADT), throat culture, or both.[18] In contrast, the guidelines issued by the centers for disease control and prevention and the American College of Physicians—American Society of Internal Medicine suggest empirical treatment based on a pharyngitis score alone with or without microbiologic confirmation.[19] The differences in these guidelines have been debated, and empirical therapy based on these clinical prediction rules has been implicated in the overuse of antibiotics for treatment of pharyngitis.[17] A study of the effectiveness of these strategies concluded that microbiologic confirmation was the most effective and least expensive when all factors were considered.[20] Confirmation of GAS by throat swab culture on sheep blood-agar plate is the most widely accepted practice for diagnosing streptococcal pharyngitis. Selective streptococcal media, less often used, inhibit contaminating normal flora and increase the sensitivity and specificity of culture for GAS,[21] with the attending risk of inhibiting other bacterial etiologic agents. Specimens should be obtained from bilateral tonsillar surfaces and the posterior pharynx while avoiding the mouth and other surfaces of the pharynx. The major disadvantage of culture for the confirmation of GAS pharyngitis is the time period of 24–48 hours required for accurate detection. RADTs have become widely available and the sensitivity and specificity compares well with those of culture. Rapid results help in timely treatment, help reduce the spread of GAS and antibiotic abuse in viral pharyngitis, and, most importantly, minimize suppurative and nonsuppurative sequelae of GAS. Newer assays use molecular biology methods to detect DNA specific to GAS by chemiluminescence or real-time polymerase chain reaction (PCR), but are restricted because of the need to batch specimens and the specialized equipment required. On a properly collected specimen, the sensitivity of RADTs is 70–90% compared with culture, with a specificity of approximately 95%.[22] A negative RADT result, in a child with high index of suspicion for GAS infection, should be confirmed by culture.[23] Culture on either standard blood-agar plate or selective streptococcal media will isolate both group C and G streptococci; however, identification needs further characterization and serogrouping. *Arcanobacterium haemolyticum* also grows on standard blood-agar or selective streptococcal media, but may take as long as 72 hours to grow as small and dry colonies.

Confirmation of pharyngitis, caused by other bacterial agents, requires high degree of clinical suspicion and use of specific media and techniques. If diphtheria is suspected, the laboratory must be informed so that tellurite containing selective and differential media, not routinely used, are used for isolation. Recently, multiplex PCR has been used for the identification of *Corynebacterium diphtheriae* and to differentiate toxin producing from nontoxigenic strains.[24] *Fusobacterium* pharyngitis demands special techniques for the isolation of anaerobic bacteria. The diagnosis of pharyngitis caused by *N. gonorrhoeae* is confirmed by culture on selective gonococcal media like modified Thayer-Martin medium.

Pharyngitis caused by *M. pneumoniae* or *Legionella pneumophila* requires serologic testing demonstrating rising titers in paired, acute and convalescent, serum samples; however, PCR and culture are commonly used in addition to serology for research purposes in advanced laboratories. The diagnosis of EBV infection is also confirmed by serology, by a heterophile antibody test (Monospot® or Monoslide®) or detection of immunoglobulin M antibodies to EBV viral capsid antigen. Common respiratory viruses that cause pharyngitis can be identified by either viral culture of a nasopharyngeal swab or molecular detection techniques such as PCR or reverse transcriptase-PCR (RT-PCR).

Acute Laryngitis

Acute laryngitis is a not-so-uncommon clinical condition, usually mild and self-limiting. The symptoms include recent onset of hoarseness or a husky voice often associated with dry cough.[25] Similar symptoms are frequently associated with an upper respiratory tract infection, rhinorrhea and sore throat. All the major respiratory viruses have been known to cause laryngitis; the most common being parainfluenza virus in one-fifth of the cases. Less frequent agents include the rhinoviruses, influenza virus, the parainfluenza viruses, coronavirus, adenovirus and human metapneumovirus.[26,27] Bacterial respiratory infections have been associated with acute laryngitis. Hoarseness is often associated with acute streptococcal pharyngitis and diphtheria, the latter especially in the developing world. Tubercular laryngitis is a frequent association with tubercular lung infection.[28] The possible etiologic roles of *Moraxella (Branhamella) catarrhalis* and *H. influenzae* in acute laryngitis has been suggested, but remains to be proven. Uncommon causes of acute laryngitis include herpesviruses, parvovirus B19, mucosal candidiasis, *Coccidioides immitis, Cryptococcus neoformans, Sporothrix schenckii,* and group G beta hemolytic streptococci in normal and immunocompromised patients.[29] Hoarseness may also be noted as a component of other laryngeal infections such as croup, acute epiglottitis or supraglottitis.

Acute Laryngotracheobronchitis (Croup)

Croup is a childhood viral infection of the upper and lower respiratory tracts resulting in inflammation in the subglottic area and manifesting as dyspnea with characteristic stridor on inspiration. The term "croup" is derived from an Anglo-Saxon word "kropan" or the old Scottish term "roup," which meant "to cry out in a shrill voice."

Etiology

The predominantly viral etiology of croup has been established with recent molecular diagnostic techniques, including RT-PCR, with the parainfluenza type 1 virus causing one-fourth to one-third of cases followed by parainfluenza type 3 as the second most common agent. Other agents, less frequently incriminated, include the influenza virus, rhinoviruses, enteroviruses, bocavirus, adenoviruses, hMPV, *M. pneumoniae*, human coronavirus and measles virus.[30]

Diagnosis

The diagnosis of croup is primarily clinical and epidemiological. Identification of the specific viral agent is usually unnecessary, and obtaining respiratory tract swabs and secretions is more likely to augment the child's respiratory distress than yield clinically relevant information.

Otitis Externa

Infection of the external auditory canal (otitis externa) resembles those of skin and soft tissue elsewhere and the microbial flora of the external auditory canal resembles flora of skin elsewhere, predominantly composed of *Staphylococcus epidermidis*, *S. aureus*, corynebacteria, and *Propionibacterium acnes*.[31] Otitis externa may be subdivided into acute localized otitis externa, acute diffuse otitis externa, chronic otitis externa and malignant otitis externa, and the causative organisms include those of the normal skin flora and gram-negative bacilli, particularly *Pseudomonas aeruginosa*.

Otitis Media

Acute otitis media (AOM) is an acute illness characterized by inflammation of the mucosa lining the middle ear with exudation. Otitis media with effusion (OME) is characterized by fluid in middle ear without signs of acute inflammation of the middle ear mucosa.

Microbiology

The bacteriology of otitis media documented by the cultures of middle ear effusions obtained by needle aspiration has implicated the importance of *S. pneumoniae* and *H. influenzae* in all age groups, but more recent studies, since the introduction of the pneumococcal conjugate vaccine in developed countries, suggest that *H. influenzae* may replace *Pneumococcus* as the most frequently isolated pathogen of AOM in children.[32] *S. pneumoniae* is the most important bacterial cause of otitis media in most parts of the world. Otitis media caused by *H. influenzae* is associated with nontypeable strains in majority of patients whereas *H. influenzae* type b causes 10% of cases, which are frequently severe and accompanied by bacteremia or meningitis. *M. catarrhalis* has been isolated from approximately 10% of children with AOM[33] and is usually associated with a mild form of disease. Most strains produce beta lactamase and are resistant to penicillin G, ampicillin and amoxicillin. *S. aureus*, including methicillin and multidrug-resistant (MDR) strains, is an uncommon cause of AOM. During the preantibiotic era, GAS was a frequent cause of severe AOM, frequently complicated by mastoiditis and often associated with scarlet fever, but the entity has become rare in the last two decades. Chronic suppurative otitis media cases frequently yield *P. aeruginosa*, *S. aureus* and *aerobic gram-negative bacilli* on culture.[34] Viral infection is frequently the initial event in the development of AOM.[35,36] Respiratory viruses have been isolated from one-fourth of middle ear fluids of children with AOM. RSV, influenza virus, enteroviruses, coronaviruses and rhinoviruses were the most common viruses.[36] Combined viral and bacterial infections are frequent and may be more severe than bacterial infection alone.[35]

Mastoiditis

Most cases of AOM with fluid in the middle ear space are associated with inflammation of the mastoid air cells. Clinically significant mastoiditis has been rare since the introduction of antimicrobial agents. Infection in the mastoid usually follows middle ear infection. The bacteriology of mastoiditis is the same as that of AOM, including *S. pneumoniae* and *H. influenzae* as the major pathogens. Patients with prolonged perforation of the tympanic membrane may have invasion of organisms from the ear canal, including *Pseudomonas spp*. Polymicrobial flora is commonly isolated from the cases of chronic mastoiditis in developing countries.[37] Cultures for bacteria from ear drainage fluid must be interpreted with care to distinguish fresh drainage fluid from material in the external canal. The canal must be cleaned and fresh pus, free of contamination from external canal, obtained. If the tympanic membrane is intact, tympanocentesis should be performed to obtain material from the middle ear.

Sinusitis

Sinusitis may be classified as acute or chronic. Because most cases of acute bacterial sinusitis are secondary to viral infection of the upper respiratory tract or allergic inflammation, nasal inflammation is commonly associated justifying the commonly used term as rhinosinusitis. The preferred term is acute community-acquired bacterial sinusitis.[38,39]

Microbiology

The paranasal sinuses are sterile under normal conditions, unlike the nasal passages, which are heavily colonized with bacteria. Reliability of knowledge of the microbiology of acute community-acquired sinusitis is dependent on proper specimen collection. The nasal cavity is heavily colonized with commensal flora that easily contaminates specimen from the paranasal sinuses. Reliable specimens of sinus secretions have been obtained by puncture of the maxillary antrum, to reduce the risk of nasal contamination. To further discriminate true infection from contamination, quantitative methods have been used to enumerate the microbial load. Attempts have been made to define infection as a bacterial load of at greater than equal to 10^4 colony-forming units per milliliter (CFU/mL) of aspirated material.[39] Cultures obtained from the middle meatus adjacent to the sinus ostia collected by swab or aspiration via an endoscope have been compared to those obtained by sinus aspiration. This is associated with a high risk of contamination of the endoscope while negotiating through the nonsterile anterior nasal cavity. Most studies using endoscopic middle meatal culture in adult patients show a sensitivity of approximately 80%, a specificity of 90%, a positive predictive value of 80–90%, and a negative predictive value of 80–90%, with maxillary sinus aspiration considered the gold standard.[40] In community-acquired bacterial sinusitis, *S. pneumoniae* is the most frequently isolated organism, followed by nontypeable *H. influenzae* and *M. catarrhalis*. Streptococci, *S. aureus*, and anaerobes are isolated less frequently.[41] In children, *M. catarrhalis* is isolated with a greater frequency than in adults. Widespread immunization with pneumococcal conjugate vaccine, in several countries, has diminished the frequency of *S. pneumoniae* with a consequent shifting of the serotypes[42] and a relative increase in the isolation of *H. influenzae*. Viruses have been infrequently isolated from patients with acute sinusitis. This may reflect the delay in the timing of sampling, done after the patient has been symptomatic for a week, when the viral infection may have waned or overshadowed by secondary bacterial pathogens. Respiratory viruses, such as adenovirus, parainfluenza and rhinovirus have been recovered from approximately 10% of sinus aspirates. Fungi have long been recognized as important pathogens in selected patients with acute or chronic sinusitis. Nosocomial sinusitis is a frequent complication; particularly in critical care setting affecting between 7.7% and 32% of patients.[43] Nasal intubation constitutes a risk factor for this infection. Gram-negative organisms, including *P. aeruginosa* and *S. pneumoniae* are frequently isolated in patients with nosocomial sinusitis.

Epiglottitis

Acute epiglottitis is a cellulitis of the epiglottis and adjacent structures leading, in some cases, to sudden airway obstruction. *H. influenzae* type b is the most frequent pathogen isolated from epiglottis in pediatric patients and in up to one-fourth of adult patients.[44] Other agents occasionally implicated include *S. pneumoniae*, staphylococci and streptococci.[45] The role of viruses in epiglottis, other than possibly herpes simplex infections (rarely) has not been established.

LOWER RESPIRATORY TRACT INFECTIONS

Acute Bronchitis

Acute bronchitis refers to a clinical syndrome distinguished by a relatively brief, self-limited inflammatory process of large and mid-sized airways, not associated with pneumonia on chest radiograph.

Microbial Etiology

Acute bronchitis is commonly caused by a wide range of viruses. Approximately 10% of cases are attributed to bacterial pathogens, including *M. pneumoniae, C. pneumoniae,* and *B. pertussis*. The relative prevalence of different pathogens varies according to age, season and the reliability of the diagnostic methods used. Molecular tests, contrary to conventional culture, identify a wider range of viral pathogens, especially in adults, that include RSV, adenovirus, hMPV and parainfluenza viruses.[46] Influenza A and B viruses are commonly associated with winter outbreaks of acute bronchitis.[47] Coronavirus, rhinoviruses, echovirus, coxsackievirus and strains of severe acute respiratory syndrome (SARS) like the SARS-CoV (SARS coronavirus) and middle east respiratory syndrome coronavirus (MARS-CoV) can cause acute bronchitis. Bacteria contribute to a minority of cases and the agents include *M. pneumoniae, C. pneumoniae, B. pertussis* and *Bordetella bronchiseptica*.[47,48]

Diagnosis

Etiologic diagnosis depends on laboratory confirmation. Rapid antigen detection in nasopharyngeal swabs is relatively sensitive for influenza virus and RSV. Identification of other viral pathogens (RSV, hMPV, coronaviruses and parainfluenza viruses) requires tissue culture or RT-PCR assay. Diagnosis of *M. pneumoniae* depends on demonstrating specific immunoglobulin M (IgM) in serum or PCR. *B. pertussis* diagnosis can be made by serology, PCR, or culture. *C. pneumoniae* is difficult to diagnose and requires PCR or serology.

Bronchiolitis

Bronchiolitis, variously named as "acute catarrhal bronchitis", "interstitial bronchopneumonia", "spastic bronchopneumonia", "capillary or obstructive bronchitis" and, more commonly, "wheezy bronchitis" and "asthmatic bronchiolitis", is the most common acute viral lower respiratory tract illness occurring during the first 2 years of life.

Etiology

Respiratory syncytial virus is the cause of about two-thirds of the cases of bronchiolitis.[49,50] Other viruses include hMPV, the parainfluenza viruses, influenza, rhinoviruses, human non-SARS coronaviruses and human bocavirus. Viral agents of upper respiratory tract infections, rhinoviruses and enteroviruses, also are commonly isolated from specimens from children with bronchiolitis. Role of these viruses as primary agents causing bronchiolitis or as coinfecting agents is uncertain.

Diagnosis

Laboratory determination of the specific etiology of bronchiolitis usually is unnecessary and therapeutically irrelevant. Rapid virologic diagnosis may be epidemiologically useful for the implementation of appropriate infection control procedures or, in selected cases with high risk conditions or severe illness with influenza or RSV, for determination of specific antiviral therapy. The specific agent of bronchiolitis can be identified by viral isolation from a nasal wash using shell vial culture techniques. Rapid viral antigen techniques, including immunofluorescent assays, optical immunoassays and enzyme immunoassays are technically nondemanding, cost effective and rapid.[51] These assays are available for RSV, parainfluenza viruses, influenza viruses, and hMPV and many of these commercially available antigen assays allow the simultaneous detection of multiple agents. The use of molecular diagnostic assays, including RT-PCR has enhanced the sensitivity and specificity of the detection of the respiratory viruses associated with bronchiolitis,[51,52] but they are expensive, and are not usually easily available in developing countries.

Acute Pneumonia

Pneumonia, designated by Sir William Osler as the "Captain of the men of death" is among the top ten most common causes of death among all age groups in the United States, the sixth leading cause of death in those 65 years or older, and the single most common cause of infection-related mortality.[53] An understanding of the pathogenesis of the disease, evaluation of relevant data from a careful history and physical examination, recognition of common clinical patterns of infection, and information from the microbiology laboratory all aid in narrowing down the possible etiologic agents of pneumonia, thereby allowing reasonable therapy to be selected empirically.

Acute Community-acquired Pneumonia

A long list of bacterial, fungal, viral and protozoal agents may cause pneumonia. *S. pneumoniae* is undoubtedly the most common cause of acute community acquired pneumonia in developing countries, accounting for one-half of the cases though reliable reports of its actual prevalence are not available. Acute respiratory infections (ARI) are leading causes of high morbidity and mortality in infancy and childhood in developing countries. Such respiratory infections are reported to kill 4 million children every year worldwide, while in India, they account for 14.3% of deaths during infancy and 15.9% during early childhood.[54,55] Of all upper and lower respiratory tract diseases, pneumonia is the most important cause of death accounting for about 3 million deaths in children worldwide. In United States alone, pneumonia rank as the sixth leading cause of death while in India, it is the number one killer disease.[56] Annually 94 out of every 1,000 Indian children develop pneumonia and account for 12–15% of deaths.[57] Pneumonia is a disease caused by a wide variety of microorganisms and has a spectrum of severity that ranges from mild illness to severe disease associated with a high mortality rate. *S. pneumoniae* is the most common pathogen though the relative incidence is rapidly coming down with the implementation of pneumococcal vaccination in developed nations. An estimated 3–38% of cases of acute community acquired pneumonia are caused by *H. influenzae*.[58] In developed countries, the use of the *H. influenzae* conjugate vaccine has decreased the incidence of invasive disease caused by *H. influenzae* type b, with a consequent increased incidence of invasive disease, including pneumonia caused by nontypeable strains.[59] Classically, *S. aureus* has accounted for 2–5% of acute community-acquired pneumonia (CAP) cases[60] commonly in older adults and in those with influenza. Although *Pneumococcus* still represents the most common etiologic agent, staphylococcal disease occurs with a higher frequency than that noted in noninfluenza-related, CAP. In 2002 many cases of CAP caused by *S. aureus* were described in France.[61] Acute respiratory distress syndrome (ARDS) was a frequent complication of infection and mortality rates were higher than in patients with pneumonia caused by *S. aureus* without the Panton-Valentine leukocidin (PVL). Similar disease patterns have been described in the United States with these strains of community-acquired of methicillin-resistant *S. aureus* (CA-MRSA).[62] These CA-MRSA pneumonias are associated with severe pneumonia with mortality rates of 29–60%. CA-MRSA pneumonia has therefore become an important entity to consider in the right clinical setting. Aerobic gram-negative bacteria and mixed aerobic and anaerobic infections cause most of the remaining cases of acute CAP.

Gram-negative rods may cause 7–18% of pneumonia cases. *Klebsiella pneumoniae, P. aeruginosa* and *Enterobacter* species are the most often isolated organisms.[63] Gram-negative bacilli are particularly important pathogens in older adults, especially those with chronic underlying disease and those who are bedridden and recently hospitalized. *Pseudomonas* infection should be suspected in patients with pulmonary comorbidities and recent hospital stays.

Indian investigations have reported *S. pneumoniae* and *H. influenzae* as the most commonly involved organisms in CAP.[64,65] In a study from Shimla,[66] 70 cases of CAP were studied by culture of sputum, blood and pleural fluid and IgM enzyme-linked immunosorbent assay (ELISA) for *M. pneumoniae.* An etiological agent was identified in 53 (76%) cases of which 41 (77%) were monomicrobial and 12 (23%) had a mixed etiology. *S. pneumoniae* was the most common (36%) agent followed by *K. pneumoniae* (22%), *S. aureus* (17%) and *M. pneumoniae* (15%). The role of *M. pneumoniae* in the causation of CAP has been variably reported from various studies in India. One study from Delhi[67] showed evidence of *M. pneumoniae* infection in 36% (10% definitive and 26% probable) of 62 adults studied using IgM ELISA, graduate pharmacy aptitude test (GPAT) and antigen detection by immunofluorescence. Another study from same place has shown *M. pneumoniae* responsible for 27–62 children with CAP.[68] There was evidence of *Chlamydia pneumoniae* in 6% of the children with CAP. From South India, incidence of *M. pneumoniae* have been shown to be 24% amongst children with CAP in Manipal[69] and 30% amongst children with CAP from Vellore.[70] The serological evidence of *L. pneumophila* infection was reported in 60 hospitalized cases of CAP.[71]

Legionella species are the most important water-related pulmonary pathogens in the United States with regard to mortality and morbidity. The importance of *Legionella* species in causing pneumonia has varied greatly in different geographic areas, with incidences ranging from 2% to 30%.[72] *Moraxella catarrhalis* has also been identified as a cause of pneumonia.[73] The overall incidence of disease caused by this bacterium is low, but it is an important pathogen in older adults with chronic obstructive pulmonary disease (COPD) and various forms of immunosuppression. Pneumonia is the second or third most common reason for hospitalization in people who are 65 years old and above; and represents a major cause of morbidity and mortality. In some series, pneumonia represents the leading cause of death in this population. In general, the cause of CAP in the older population follows the general trend of infection in younger populations. *S. pneumoniae* is the predominant organism, accounting for more than half of the cases. *H. influenzae,* mostly nontypeable, is the second most common agent; accounting for up to 10% of episodes.[74] The incidence of other aerobic gram-negative bacilli in causing pneumonia in older adults is variable because the criteria for diagnosis of true pneumonia versus colonization vary. Increased oropharyngeal colonization with aerobic gram-negative bacilli has been documented in the older population. Colonization is an outcome of debility, prior use of antibiotics, decreased activity, diabetes, alcoholism, and incontinence and is thought to be a risk factor of development of pneumonia caused by these organisms.[75] Older adults are at greater risk for infection with group B streptococci, *M. catarrhalis* and *Legionella* species, although the overall incidence of these agents in the older population is relatively low.[73] Polymicrobial infections and pneumonia due to aspiration occur more frequently in older adults.[76] With the development of sensitive nucleic acid amplification tests, the role of viruses as a cause of pneumonia is being more clearly defined.[77] Recent studies have suggested a viral etiology in 15–29% of all patients hospitalized with pneumonia with significantly more viral infections noted in the older age groups (median age of 76).[77,78] Influenza is consistently the most commonly isolated virus usually followed by RSV, human metapneumovirus, parainfluenza virus, enterovirus and coronavirus. SARS-CoV and MERS-CoV are strains of coronavirus that have been associated with outbreaks of pneumonia with considerable mortality. The cause of CAP in patients with acquired immunodeficiency syndrome (AIDS) has changed significantly since the beginning of the epidemic. *Pneumocystis jiroveci (carinii)* remains the most frequent AIDS-defining opportunistic pneumonia in the United States and the rest of the world, although highly active antiretroviral therapy (HAART) and effective prophylactic strategies have more than halved the incidence of *P. jiroveci* pneumonia and its associated mortality. Bacterial pneumonia has a ten times higher incidence in HIV-positive versus HIV negative cohorts.[79] The rate of invasive pneumococcal disease may be three times greater in HIV-infected patients than in non-HIV-infected controls.[80] *H. influenzae* and *S. aureus* are also important pathogens.[80,81] A variety of other bacteria have been implicated, including *Rhodococcus equi, Escherichia coli, Serratia* species and *P. aeruginosa.* Infections with *Pseudomonas* are associated with the late stages of disease with *Mycobacterium tuberculosis,* nontuberculous mycobacteria, *C. neoformans* and cytomegalovirus playing important roles as etiologic agents.[82]

Health Care-associated Pneumonia

An increasing number of patients present to hospital services with pneumonia following contact with various types of the healthcare institutions, resulting in a blurring of the distinction between community-acquired and nosocomial pneumonia. Healthcare associated pneumonia now represents a new syndrome, a hybrid of CAP and hospital-associated pneumonia.[83] Patients with a history of hospitalization within 90 days prior to developing pneumonia; patients attending hemodialysis clinics; patients receiving intravenous therapy, wound care, or chemotherapy at home; and residents of long-term care facilities or nursing homes are the most likely involved. *S. aureus,* including MRSA; aerobic gram-negative bacilli, including *P. aeruginosa*; and mixed aerobic-anaerobic pathogens associated with aspiration have been most commonly reported.

Atypical Pneumonia Syndrome

Atypical pneumonia classically presents with a mild respiratory tract illness followed by pneumonia with dyspnea and cough without sputum, an atypical chest X-ray and a negative routine culture of sputum specimen. Atypical pneumonia in its typical form is rarely encountered today. *M. pneumoniae, C. pneumoniae, L. pneumophila,* and respiratory viruses are the most significant causes of atypical pneumonia. Other agents, such as *Chlamydophila psittaci, Francisella tularensis, M. tuberculosis* and *Coxiella burnetii* may also cause atypical pneumonia. In patients with AIDS, *Pneumocystis* and nontuberculous mycobacteria should also be included. The difficulty in identifying the various etiologic agents associated with atypical pneumonia has made estimates of incidence difficult. *M. pneumoniae* may account for 10–30% of cases of CAP.[84] *C. pneumoniae* has emerged as a cause of atypical pneumonia and may account for approximately 6–20% of CAP cases.[85] Of the viral agents associated with atypical pneumonia in adults, influenza A and B, adenovirus types 3, 4, and 7 (especially in military recruits), human metapneumovirus,[77] RSV (especially in older adult and immunosuppressed patients), and parainfluenza virus are the most common.[78,86]

Aspiration Pneumonia

The bacteriology of aspiration pneumonia reflects the flora of the oropharynx, and presence of periodontal disease. Anaerobic bacteria alone are involved in half of cases[87] and in combination with aerobes in other cases.[88] *Bacteroides* species, *Porphyromonas* species, *Prevotella melaninogenica, Fusobacterium* species and anaerobic gram-positive cocci are the predominant anaerobes isolated. In community-acquired aspiration pneumonia, *Streptococcus* species and *H. influenzae* are the most common aerobic isolates.[87] *M. catarrhalis* and *Eikenella corrodens* may also be involved. In contrast, gram-negative bacilli (including *P. aeruginosa*) and *S. aureus* are the most commonly isolated aerobes from nosocomial aspiration pneumonia, including VAP.[87]

Nosocomial Pneumonia, Hospital-acquired Pneumonia, Ventilator-associated Pneumonia

Nosocomial pneumonia is the second leading type of nosocomial infection and accounts for 13–18% of all such infections. It is the leading cause of infection-related deaths in hospitalized patients with an attributable mortality of 33–50%.[89] Higher mortality rates have been observed when patients are bacteremic or have pneumonia caused by *P. aeruginosa* or *Acinetobacter* species. Ventilator-associated pneumonia (VAP) has been accepted as an important subcategory of nosocomial pneumonia.

Approximately 60–75% of cases of nosocomial pneumonia are caused by aerobic gram-negative bacilli, with members of the family Enterobacteriaceae (*K. pneumoniae, E. coli, Serratia marcescens, Enterobacter* species), *Acinetobacter* species and *Pseudomonas* species accounting for the majority of these. *S. aureus* causes 13–40% of nosocomial pneumonia and appears to be more common in burn units, in patients with wound infections, and in patients recently ventilated after neurosurgery or head trauma.[90] In contrast to the developed western countries, in Indian studies *S. aureus* accounts for less than 10% of VAP. MRSA and MDR organisms now play major etiologic roles. In contrast to its prominent role in CAP,

S. pneumoniae causes only 3–20% of nosocomial pneumonias in most studies and is associated with infection developing early in the hospital course. Anaerobic bacteria have been isolated in up to 35% of the cases of nosocomial pneumonia, although usually less than 5% of infections are thought to be caused by these organisms. They play a role when aspiration is likely to have occurred. Pneumonia caused by *Legionella* species may occur sporadically or as part of outbreaks.

Pleural Effusion and Empyema

Microbiology

In the preantibiotic era, *S. pneumoniae* accounted for 60–70% of cases, *S. pyogenes* for 10–15% of cases, and *S. aureus* for 5–10% of cases. *S. pneumoniae* more recently accounted for less than 10% of cases and many infections are mixed, with anaerobes present in up to 75% of empyemas as sole organisms or in combination with other aerobic or facultative organisms.[91,92] Bartlett and Finegold found that pleural empyema was caused by aerobic bacteria in 24%, anaerobic bacteria in 35%, and both aerobic and anaerobic bacteria in 41% of 83 medical service patients without prior antibiotic therapy or surgical procedures.[93] The most common anaerobes isolated include the *Bacteroides fragilis* group, *Prevotella* species, *Fusobacterium nucleatum,* and *Finegoldia* species. Recently, there has been a shift from conventional pathogens to the *Streptococcus anginosus* group in community-acquired empyema in patients with comorbidities.[93] Hospital-acquired empyemas include more staphylococcal infections and gram-negative organisms.

Predisposing factors and associated comorbidities are important pointers to the most likely pathogens. Pneumonia continues to be the most frequent predisposing factor in the development of empyemas. Otherwise healthy adults with pneumonia, the most common bacteria causing empyema are *S. aureus* and *S. pneumoniae.* The incidence of a parapneumonic effusion in hospitalized patients is estimated to be 40%. Empyema caused by *S. aureus, S. pneumoniae* or *H. influenzae* has been common in children. Most cases of *S. aureus* empyema result from *S. aureus* pneumonia with a tendency to cause cavitation, most often seen in older hospitalized patients with underlying medical problems. In developing countries, tuberculous effusions are common, and they can be secondary to a primary infection or more frequently occur as reactivation tuberculosis. Factors predisposing to aspiration, such as altered mental status, alcoholism and periodontal disease, are common in patients with anaerobic infections of the pleura. Many of these cases tend to be polymicrobial. In addition to anaerobes, viridans group streptococci, aerobic gram-negative bacilli, and occasionally *S. aureus* have been recovered. Pleuropulmonary actinomycosis can result from aspiration leading to a chronic pulmonary infection with chest wall involvement. Nocardia infections occur more frequently in patients with underlying conditions, such as organ transplantation, malignancy, diabetes mellitus, AIDS and long-term use of steroids. Pleural effusions can develop in up to 50% of patients with nocardiosis.

Laboratory Diagnosis

Aspirated pleural fluid should be sent to the microbiology laboratory for Gram stain microscopy and aerobic and anaerobic cultures. Conventional methods can achieve a bacterial diagnosis in approximately 60% of pleural fluid samples.[94] The low detection rate may be due to prior antimicrobial use frequent in developing countries. Antigen detection test by latex agglutination test or immunochromatographic test (ICT) for the detection of *S. pneumoniae* antigen is rapid, highly sensitive and not affected by prior antibiotic therapy.[94] Pleural tuberculosis can be diagnosed by acid-fast stain microscopy of pleural fluid in only 18–23% of patients, but cultures of pleural fluid and histologic examination of pleural biopsy specimens permit the diagnosis in up to 95% of patients. Radiometric culture increases the speed of diagnosis in patients with pleural tuberculosis. Three other diagnostic tests are available to help establish the diagnosis of tuberculous pleural disease—tests for adenosine deaminase (ADA) and interferon-gamma and the PCR assay. In one study, pleural fluid ADA levels above 40 U/L were found in 99.6% of patients with tuberculous pleurisy.[95] Assay of interferon-gamma needs evaluation in developing countries where the disease is more prevalent. Two tests for *M. tuberculosis* nucleic acid are commercially available and nucleic acid amplification tests require rigorous standardization to prevent nonspecific results common with this technique.

Bacterial Lung Abscess

Microbiology

The predominant organisms responsible for lung abscess are bacteria, specifically mouth anaerobes that are normal flora in the gingival crevices.[96] Studies using rigorous sample collection techniques that avoid contamination with oral flora combined with reliable anaerobic culture methods have shown that anaerobes are found in about 90% of lung abscesses and are the only organisms present in about half of cases. The most frequently isolated anaerobes are *Peptostreptococcus* spp. (now identified as *Finegoldia magna*), *Fusobacterium nucleatum* and *Prevotella melaninogenica.*[97] Abscesses usually contain multiple anaerobe species, usually three to four per culture specimen; microaerophilic streptococci and viridans streptococci often are present as well. Lung abscess occasionally may be caused by *S. aureus,* enteric gram-negative rods such as *Klebsiella spp., P. aeruginosa, Burkholderia pseudomallei* (melioidosis), *Pasteurella multocida,* GAS, *H. influenzae* types b and c, *Legionella spp., R. equi, Actinomyces spp.,* and *Nocardia spp.* Oropharyngeal colonization with *P. aeruginosa,* other aerobic gram-negative rods and, less often, *S. aureus* is a common event in hospitalized patients, particularly patients who receive ventilatory support. These bacteria are important pathogens when lung abscess or necrotizing pneumonia develops during hospitalization and may produce infection as the sole pathogen or as one component of a mixed flora infection involving other aspirated oropharyngeal organisms. In patients with impaired cell-mediated immunity (AIDS, transplantation immunosuppression), opportunistic pathogens, such as mycobacteria, *Nocardia*, *Aspergillus*, and *Rhodococcus*, are important causes of cavitary lung lesions. In patients with impaired host defenses caused by granulocytopenia (leukemia, chemotherapy), aerobic bacteria (*P. aeruginosa*, *S. aureus*) and fungi, including *Aspergillus* and Zygomycetes, are important pathogens.

Diagnosis

Sputum Gram stains in these patients show many neutrophils and mixed flora, with many morphologically different bacteria; routine cultures usually grow normal respiratory flora. Because expectorated sputum is contaminated by oral flora containing large numbers of anaerobes, special techniques for obtaining lower tract specimens are necessary to confirm the role of anaerobes. These techniques include transtracheal aspiration, transthoracic aspiration, protected brush fiberoptic bronchoscopy, bronchoalveolar lavage with quantitative cultures,[98] and empyema fluid obtained by thoracentesis. Blood cultures rarely are positive in anaerobic lung abscess. Patients without the classic presentation and patients with secondary lung abscess should have stains and cultures of expectorated sputum for aerobic bacteria, mycobacteria, fungi, and, in some instances, parasites.

REFERENCES

1. Schuster GS. Oral flora and pathogenic organisms. Infect Dis Clin North Am. 1999;13(4):757-74, v.
2. Sutter VL. Anaerobes as normal oral flora. Rev Infect Dis. 1984;6(Suppl 1):S62-6.
3. Walsh EE, Peterson DR, Falsey AR. Human metapneumovirus infections in adults: another piece of the puzzle. Arch Intern Med. 2008;168(22):2489-96.
4. Kesebir D, Vazquez M, Weibel C, Shapiro ED, Ferguson D, Landry ML, et al. Human bocavirus infection in young children in the United States: molecular epidemiological profile and clinical characteristics of a newly emerging respiratory virus. J Infect Dis. 2006;194(9):1276-82.
5. Alcaide ML, Bisno AL. Pharyngitis and epiglottitis. Infect Dis Clin North Am. 2007;21(2):449-69.
6. Huovinen P, Lahtonen R, Ziegler T, Meurman O, Hakkarainen K, Miettinen A, et al. Pharyngitis in adults: the presence and coexistence of viruses and bacterial organisms. Ann Intern Med. 1989;110(8):612-6.
7. Esposito S, Blasi F, Bosis S, Droghetti R, Faelli N, Lastrico A, et al. Aetiology of acute pharyngitis: the role of atypical bacteria. J Med Microbiol. 2004;53(Pt 7):645-51.
8. Choi JH, Chung YS, Kim KS, Lee WJ, Chung IY, Oh HB, et al. Development of real-time PCR assays for detection and quantification of human bocavirus. J Clin Virol. 2008;42(3): 249-53.
9. Nandi S, Kumar R, Ray P, Vohra H, Ganguly NK. Group A streptococcal sore throat in a periurban population of northern India: a one year prospective study. Bull World Health Organ. 2001;79(6):528-33.
10. McIsaac WJ, White D, Tannenbaum D, Low DE. A clinical score to reduce unnecessary antibiotic use in patients with sore throat. CMAJ. 1998;158(1):75-83.
11. Kaplan EL, Top FH, Dudding BA, Wannamaker LW. Diagnosis of streptococcal pharyngitis: differentiation of active infection from the carrier state in the symptomatic child. J Infect Dis. 1971;123(5):490-501.
12. Bramhachari PV, Kaul SY, McMillan DJ, Shaila MS, Karmarkar MG, Sriprakash KS. Disease burden due to *Streptococcus* dysgalactiae subsp. equisimilis (group G and C *Streptococcus*) is higher than that due to Streptococcus pyogenes among Mumbai school children. J Med Microbiol. 2010;59(Pt 2):220-3.
13. Carlson P, Renkonen OV, Kontiainen S. Arcanobacterium haemolyticum and streptococcal pharyngitis. Scand J Infect Dis. 1994;26(3):283-7.
14. Batty A, Wren MW, Gal M. Fusobacterium necrophorum as the cause of recurrent sore throat: comparison of isolates from persistent sore throat syndrome and Lemierre's disease. J Infect. 2005;51(4):299-306.
15. Dittmann S, Wharton M, Vitek C, Ciotti M, Galazka A, Guichard S, et al. Successful control of epidemic diphtheria in the states of the Former Union of Soviet Socialist Republics: lessons learned. J Infect Dis. 2000;181(Suppl 1):S10-22.
16. Saikia L, Nath R, Saikia NJ, Choudhury G, Sarkar M. A diphtheria outbreak in Assam, India. Southeast Asian J Trop Med Public Health. 2010;41(3):647-52.
17. McIsaac WJ, Kellner JD, Aufricht P, Vanjaka A, Low DE. Empirical validation of guidelines for the management of pharyngitis in children and adults. JAMA. 2004;291(13): 1587-95.
18. Committee on infectious diseases: Group A streptococcal infections. In: Pickering LK (Ed.). Red Book, 27th edition. Elk Grove Village, IL: American Academy of Pediatrics; 2006. pp. 610-20.
19. Snow V, Mottur-Pilson C, Cooper RJ, Hoffman JR; American Academy of Family Physicians; American College of Physicians-American Society of Internal Medicine, et al. Principles of appropriate antibiotic use for acute pharyngitis in adults. Ann Intern Med. 2001;134(6):506-8.
20. Neuner JM, Hamel MB, Phillips RS, Bona K, Aronson MD. Diagnosis and management of adults with pharyngitis: a cost-effectiveness analysis. Ann Intern Med. 2003;139(2):113-22.
21. Bellon J, Weise B, Verschraegen G, De Meyere M. Selective streptococcal agar versus blood agar for detection of group A beta-hemolytic streptococci in patients with acute pharyngitis. J Clin Microbiol. 1991;29(9):2084-5.
22. Gerber MA, Shulman ST. Rapid diagnosis of pharyngitis caused by group A streptococci. Clin Microbiol Rev. 2004;17(3):571-80.
23. Dajani A, Taubert K, Ferrieri P, Peter G, Shulman S. Treatment of acute streptococcal pharyngitis and prevention of rheumatic fever: a statement for health professionals. Committee on Rheumatic Fever, Endocarditis, and Kawasaki Disease of the Council on Cardiovascular Disease in the Young, the American Heart Association. Pediatrics. 1995;96(4 Pt 1):758-64.
24. Pimenta FP, Hirata R, Rosa AC, Milagres LG, Mattos-Guaraldi AL. A multiplex PCR assay for simultaneous detection of Corynebacterium diphtheriae and differentiation between

non-toxigenic and toxigenic isolates. J Med Microbiol. 2008; 57(Pt 11):1438-9.

25. Banfield G, Tandon G, Solomons N. Hoarse voice. An early symptom of many conditions. Practitioner. 2000;244(1608):267-71.
26. Thom DH, Grayston JT, Wang SP, Kuo CC, Altman J. *Chlamydia pneumoniae* strain TWAR, *Mycoplasma pneumoniae*, and viral infections in acute respiratory disease in a university student health clinic population. Am J Epidemiol. 1990;132(2):248-56.
27. Freymouth F, Vabret A, Legrand L, Eterradossi N, Lafay-Delaire F, Brouard J, et al. Presence of the new human metapneumovirus in French children with bronchiolitis. Pediatr Infect Dis J. 2003;22(1):92-4.
28. Bhat VK, Latha P, Upadhya D, Hegde J. Clinicopathological review of tubercular laryngitis in 32 cases of pulmonary Kochs. Am J Otolaryngol. 2009;30(5):327-30.
29. Vrabec DP. Fungal infections of the larynx. Otolaryngol Clin North Am. 1993;26(6):1091-114.
30. Hall CB, McBride JT. Acute Laryngotracheobronchitis (Croup). In: Mandell GL, Bennett JE, Dolin R (Eds.). Principles and Practice of Infectious Diseases, 6th edition. Philadelphia, PA: Elsevier Churchill Livingstone; 2005. pp. 760-6.
31. Riding KH, Bluestone CD, Michaels RH, Cantekin EI, Doyle WJ, Poziviak CS. Microbiology of recurrent and chronic otitis media with effusion. J Pediatr. 1978;93(5):739-43.
32. Casey JR, Pichichero ME. Changes in frequency and pathogens causing acute otitis media in 1995-2003. Pediatric Infect Dis J. 2004;23(9):824-8.
33. Van Hare GF, Shurin PA, Marchant CD, Cartelli NA, Johnson CE, Fulton D, et al. Acute otitis media caused by *Branhamella* catarrhalis: biology and therapy. Rev Infect Dis. 1987;9(1): 16-27.
34. Sharma S, Rehan HS, Goyal A, Jha AK, Upadhyaya S, Mishra SC. Bacteriological profile in chronic suppurative otitis media in Eastern Nepal. Trop Doct. 2004;34(2):102-4.
35. Chonmaitree T, Owen MJ, Patel JA, Hedgpeth D, Horlick D, Howie VM. Effect of viral respiratory tract infection on outcome of acute otitis media. J Pediatr. 1992;120(6):856-62.
36. Chonmaitree T, Revai K, Grady JJ, Clos A, Patel JA, Nair S, et al. Viral upper respiratory tract infection and otitis media complication in young children. Clin Infect Dis. 2008;46(6): 815-23.
37. Albert RR, Job A, Kuruvilla G, Joseph R, Brahmadathan KN, John A. Outcome of bacterial culture from mastoid granulations: is it relevant in chronic ear disease? J Laryngol Otol. 2005;119(10):774-8.
38. Clement PA, Bluestone CD, Gordts F, Lusk RP, Otten FW, Goossens H, et al. Management of rhinosinusitis in children. Int J Pediatr Otorhinolaryngol. 1999;49(Suppl 1):S95-S100.
39. Wald ER. Microbiology of acute and chronic sinusitis in children and adults. Am J Med Sci. 1998;316(1):13-20.
40. Benninger MS, Payne SC, Ferguson BJ, Hadley JA, Ahmad N. Endoscopically directed middle meatal cultures versus maxillary sinus taps in acute bacterial maxillary rhinosinusitis: a meta-analysis. Otolaryngol Head Neck Surg. 2006;134(1):3-9.
41. Jain N, Lodha R, Kabra SK. Upper respiratory tract infections. Indian J Pediatr. 2001;68(12):1135-8.
42. Brook I, Foote PA, Hausfeld JN. Frequency of recovery of pathogens causing acute maxillary sinusitis in adults before and after introduction of vaccination of children with the 7-valent pneumococcal vaccine. J Med Microbiol. 2006;55(Pt 7):943-6.
43. George DL, Falk PS, Umberto Meduri G, Leeper KV, Wunderink RG, Steere EL, et al. Nosocomial sinusitis in patients in the medical intensive care unit: a prospective epidemiological study. Clin Infect Dis. 1998;27(3):463-70.
44. John TJ, Cherian T, Raghupathy P. *Haemophilus influenzae* disease in children in India: a hospital perspective. Pediatr Infect Dis J. 1998;17(9 Suppl):S169-71.
45. Frantz TD, Rasgon BM, Quesenberry CP. Acute epiglottitis in adults. Analysis of 129 cases. JAMA. 1994;272(17):1358-60.
46. O'Shea MK, Pipkin C, Cane PA, Gray GC. Respiratory syncytial virus: an important cause of acute respiratory illness among young adults undergoing military training. Influenza Other Respir Viruses. 2007;1(5-6):193-7.
47. MacFarlane J, Holmes W, Gard P, Macfarlane R, Rose D, Weston V, et al. Prospective study of the incidence, aetiology and outcome of adult lower respiratory tract illness in the community. Thorax. 2001;56(2):109-14.
48. Dworkin MS, Sullivan PS, Buskin SE, Harrington RD, Olliffe J, MacArthur RD, et al. Bordetella bronchiseptica infection in human immunodeficiency virus-infected patients. Clin Infect Dis. 1999;28(5):1095-9.
49. Kaur C, Chohan S, Khare S, Puliyel JM. Respiratory viruses in acute bronchiolitis in Delhi. Indian Pediatr. 2010;47(4):342-3.
50. Bush A, Thomson AH. Acute bronchiolitis. BMJ. 2007;335(7628): 1037-41.
51. Henrickson K, Hall C. Diagnostic assays for respiratory syncytial virus disease. Pediatr Infect Dis J. 2007;26(11):S36-40.
52. Weinberg A, Zamora M, Li S, Torres F, Hodges TN. The value of polymerase chain reaction for the diagnosis of viral respiratory tract infections in lung transplant recipients. J Clin Virol. 2002;25(2):171-5.
53. Miniño AM, Heron MP, Murphy SL, Kochanek KD. Centers for Disease Control and Prevention National Center for Health Statistics National Vital Statistics System. Deaths: final data for 2004. Natl Vital Stat Rep. 2007;55(19):1-119.
54. Mohan M, Bhargava SK. Acute respiratory infections. Indian Pediatrics. 1984;21(1):5-7.
55. Gupta BD, Parakh M, Arora A. Management of community acquired respiratory infections. Indian J Pediatr. 2001;68(2): S39-49.
56. Indrayan A, Wysocki MJ, Kumar R, Chawla A, Singh N. Estimates of the years-of-life-lost due to the top nine causes of death in rural areas of major states in India in 1995. Nat Med J India. 2002;15(1):7-13.
57. Srinivas S. Pneumonia in children. IAP J Practical Pediatrics. 1996;4:95-100.
58. Hirschmann JV, Everett ED. *Haemophilus influenzae* infections in adults. Report of nine cases and a review of literature. Medicine (Baltimore). 1979;58(1):80-94.
59. Dworkin MS, Park L, Borchardt SM. The changing epidemiology of invasive *Haemophilus influenzae* disease, especially in persons > or = 65 years old. Clin Infect Dis. 2007;44(6):810-6.
60. Hausmann W, Karlish AJ. Staphylococcal pneumonia in adults. Br Med J. 1956;2(4997):845-7.
61. Dufour P, Gillet Y, Bes M, Lina G, Vandenesch F, Floret D, et al. Community-acquired methicillin-resistant *Staphylococcus aureus* infections in France: emergence of a single clone that produces Panton-Valentine leukocidin. Clin Infect Dis. 2002;35(7):819-24.
62. Hageman JC, Uyeki TM, Francis JS, Jernigan DB, Wheeler JG, Bridges CB, et al. Severe community-acquired pneumonia due to *Staphylococcus aureus*, 2003-04 influenza season. Emerg Infect Dis. 2006;12(6):894-9.

63. Kang CI, Song JH, Oh WS, Ko KS, Chung DR, Peck KR, et al. Clinical outcomes and risk factors for community-acquired pneumonia caused by gramnegative bacilli. Eur J Clin Microbiol Infect Dis. 2008;27(8):657-61.
64. John TJ, Cherian T, Steinhoff MC, Simoes EA, John M. Etiology of acute respiratory infections in children of tropical southern India. Rev Infect Dis. 1991;13(6):S463-9.
65. Patwari AK, Bisht S, Srinivasan A, Deb M, Chattopadhya D. Aetiology of pneumonia in hospitalized children. J Trop Pediatr. 1996;42(1):15-20.
66. Bansal S, Kashyap S, Pal LS, Goel A. Clinical and bacteriological profile of community acquired pneumonia in Shimla, Himachal Pradesh. Indian J Chest Dis Allied Sci. 2004;46(1):17-22.
67. Dey AB, Chaudhry R, Kumar P, Nisar N, Nagarkar KM. Mycoplasma pneumoniae and community-acquired pneumonia. Natl Med J India. 2000;13(2):66-70.
68. Chaudhary R, Nazima N, Dhawan B, Kabra SK. Prevalence of *Mycoplasma pneumoniae* and *Chlamydia pneumoniae* in children with community acquired pneumonia. Indian J Pediatr. 1998;65(5):717-21.
69. Shenoy VD, Upadhyaya SA, Rao SP, Shobha KL. *Mycoplasma pneumoniae* infection in children with acute respiratory infection. J Trop Pediatr. 2005;51(4):232-5.
70. Mathai E, Padmavathy K, Cherian T, Inbamalar U, Varkki S. *Mycoplasma pneumoniae* antibodies in children with acute respiratory infection. Indian Pediatr. 2001;38(2):157-60.
71. Chaudhry R, Dhawan B, Dey AB. The incidence of *Legionella pneumophila*: a prospective study in a tertiary care hospital in India. Trop Doct. 2000;30(4):197-200.
72. Fang GD, Fine M, Orloff J, Arisumi D, Yu VL, Kapoor W, et al. New and emerging etiologies for community-acquired pneumonia with implications for therapy. A prospective multicenter study of 359 cases. Medicine (Baltimore). 1990;69(5):307-16.
73. Nicotra B, Rivera M, Luman JI, Wallace RJ. Branhamella catarrhalis as a lower respiratory tract pathogen in patients with chronic lung disease. Arch Intern Med. 1986;146(5):890-3.
74. Berk SL, Holtsclaw SA, Wiener SL, Smith JK. Nontypeable *Haemophilus influenzae* in the elderly. Arch Intern Med. 1982;142(3):532-9.
75. Valenti WM, Trudell RG, Bentley DW. Factors predisposing to oropharyngeal colonization with gram-negative bacilli in the aged. N Engl J Med. 1978;298(20):1108-11.
76. Kidd D, Lawson J, Nesbitt R, MacMahon J. The natural history and clinical consequences of aspiration in acute stroke. QJM. 1995;88(6):409-13.
77. Johnstone J, Majumdar SR, Fox JD, Marrie TJ. Viral infection in adults hospitalized with community acquired pneumonia: prevalance, pathogens, and presentation. Chest. 2008;134(6):1141-8.
78. Jennings LC, Anderson TP, Beynon KA, Chua A, Laing RT, Werno AM, et al. Incidence and characteristics of viral community-acquired pneumonia in adults. Thorax. 2008;63(1):42-8.
79. Davis LJ, Fei M, Huang L. Respiratory infection complicating HIV infection. Curr Opin Infect Dis. 2008;21(2):184-90.
80. Baril L, Astagneau P, Nguyen J, Similowski T, Mengual X, Beigelman C, et al. Pyogenic bacterial pneumonia in human immunodeficiency virus-infected inpatients. A clinical, radiological, microbiological, and epidemiological study. Clin Infect Dis. 1998;26(4):964-71.
81. Madeddu G, Porqueddu EM, Cambosu F, Saba F, Fois AG, Pirina P, et al. Bacterial community acquired pneumonia in HIV-infected inpatients in the highly active antiretroviral therapy era. Infection. 2008;36(3):231-6.
82. Rosen MJ. Overview of pulmonary complications. Clin Chest Med. 1996;17(4):621-31.
83. Carratalà J, Garcia-Vidal C. What is healthcare-associated pneumonia and how it is managed? Curr Opin Infect Dis. 2008;21(2):168-73.
84. Miyashita N, Ouchi K, Kawasaki K, Oda K, Kawai Y, Shimizu H, et al. *Mycoplasma pneumoniae* pneumonia in the elderly. Med Sci Monit. 2008;14(8):CR387-91.
85. Blasi F, Tarsia P, Aliberti S, Cosentini R, Allegra L. *Chlamydia pneumoniae* and *Mycoplasma pneumoniae*. Semin Respir Crit Care Med. 2005;26(6):617-24.
86. Falsey AR, Cunningham CK, Barker WH, Kouides RW, Yuen JB, Menegus M, et al. Respiratory syncytial virus and influenza A infections in the hospitalized elderly. J Infect Dis. 1995;172(2):389-94.
87. Marik PE, Careau P. The role of anaerobes in patients with ventilator-associated pneumonia and aspiration pneumonia: a prospective study. Chest. 1999;115(1):178-83.
88. Hammond JM, Potgieter PD, Hanslo D, Scott H, Roditi D. The etiology and antimicrobial susceptibility patterns of microorganisms in acute community-acquired lung abscess. Chest. 1995;108(4):937-41.
89. Haley RW, Culver DH, White JW, Morgan WM, Emori TG. The nationwide nosocomial infection rate. A new need for vital statistics. Am J Epidemiol. 1985;121(2):159-67.
90. Rello J, Quintana E, Ausina V, Castella J, Luquin M, Net A, et al. Incidence, etiology, and outcome of nosocomial pneumonia in mechanically ventilated patients. Chest. 1991;100(2):439-44.
91. Maskell NA, Batt S, Hedley EL, Davies CW, Gillespie SH, Davies RJ. The bacteriology of pleural infection by genetic and standard methods and its mortality significance. Am J Respir Crit Care Med. 2006;174(7):817-23.
92. Bartlett JG, Finegold SM. Anaerobic infections of the lung and pleural space. Am Rev Respir Dis. 1974;110(1):56-77.
93. Ahmed RA, Marrie TJ, Huang JQ. Thoracic empyema in patients with community-acquired pneumonia. Am J Med. 2006;119(10):877-83.
94. Porcel JM, Ruiz-González A, Falguera M, Nogués A, Galindo C, Carratalá J, et al. Contribution of a pleural antigen assay (Binax NOW) to the diagnosis of pneumococcal pneumonia. Chest. 2007;131(5):1442-7.
95. Baba K, Hoosen AA, Langeland N, Dyrhol-Riise AM. Adenosine deaminase activity is a sensitive marker for the diagnosis of tuberculous pleuritis in patients with very low CD4 counts. PLoS One. 2008;3(7):e2788.
96. Bartlett JG. Anaerobic bacterial infections of the lung and pleural space. Clin Infect Dis. 1993;16(Suppl 4):S248-55.
97. Davis B, Systrom DM. Lung abscess: pathogenesis, diagnosis and treatment. Curr Clin Top Infect Dis. 1998;18.252-73.
98. Henriquez AH, Mendoza J, Gonzalez PC. Quantitative culture of bronchoalveolar lavage from patients with anaerobic lung abscesses. J Infect Dis. 1991;164(2):414-7.

21 Chapter

Systematic Approach to Interpretation of Plain Chest Radiographs

D Behera

INTRODUCTION

Roentgenographic examination of the chest is an integral part in the diagnostic evaluation of all types of lung diseases. In fact, in the absence of a plain chest skiagram, work-up of any lung disorder is not complete. While chest skiagram itself is not diagnostic of a particular disease, in correlation with clinical history, it provides important clues to the possible etiology and hints at whether any further diagnostic method is necessary or not.[1-11] After clinical examination, it is the first investigation of choice in any lung disease. Anatomical localization of pulmonary lesions is possible most of the time, and always an attempt should be made to collect this information. A lateral view is most often necessary for this purpose for recognizing various segments and lobes although posteroanterior (PA) views are good enough **(Figs 1 to 7)**.

POSTEROANTERIOR VIEW

The standard posteroanterior views are taken, when the X-rays pass through the body in a PA direction with the patient facing the film cassette. The X-ray tube is placed at a distance of 6 feet. Although the standard technique is to use 60–80 kVp, many centers now use the high voltage technique using 120–350 kVp. The advantage with the latter technique is that the roentgenographic density of the bony thorax is reduced with an overall improvement in the quality of other structures, particularly, the pulmonary vasculature and the mediastinum behind the heart. However, the disadvantage

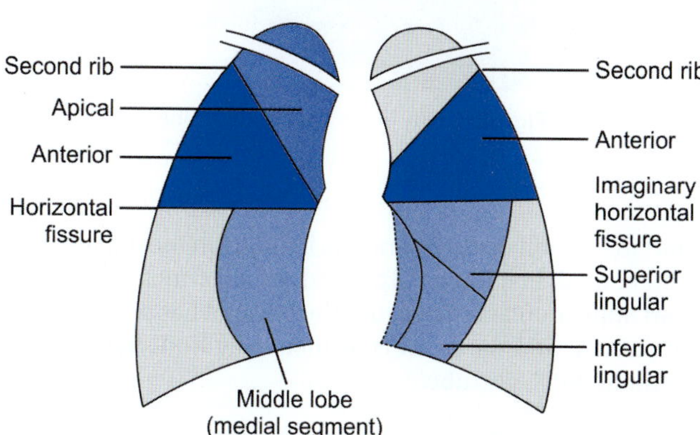

Fig. 1 Posteroanterior (PA) view of the chest skiagram showing different segments of the lungs on both sides. Note that there is no horizontal fissure on the left side. For convenience, however, an imaginary horizontal fissure is drawn. The medial most point is the hilum on the either side

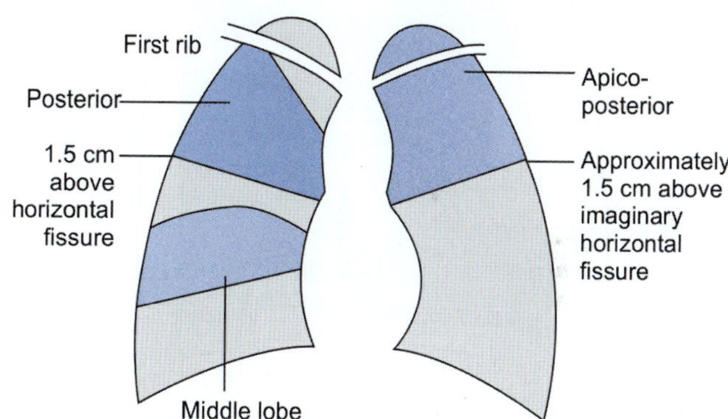

Fig. 2 Posteroanterior (PA) view of the chest skiagram showing the posterior segments on either side. Right middle lobe is also shown

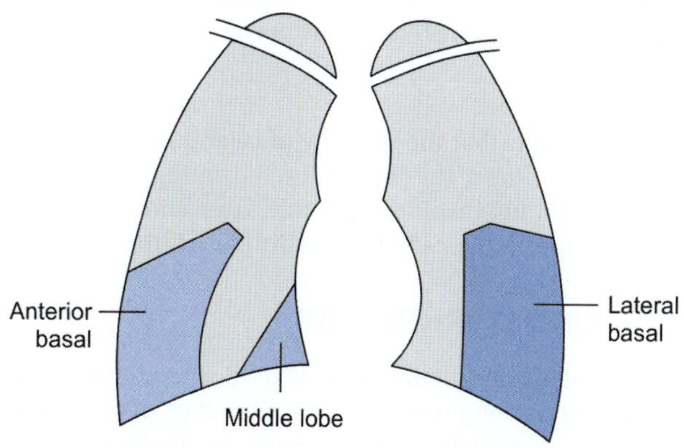

Fig. 3 Basal segments of lower lobes as seen in posteroanterior (PA) view of chest skiagram

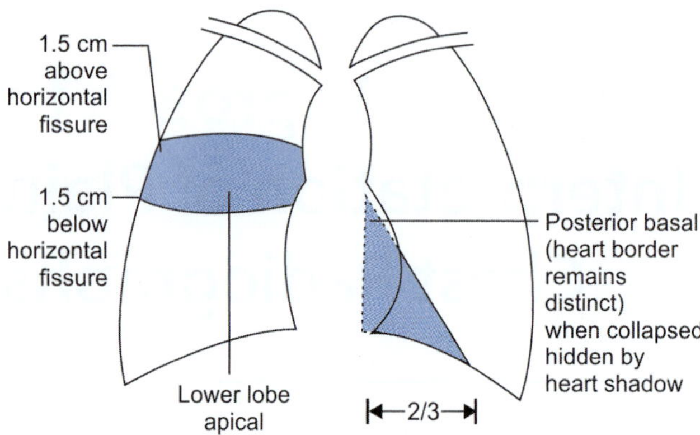

Fig. 4 Apical and posterior basal segments of lower lobes on either side on posteroanterior (PA) view

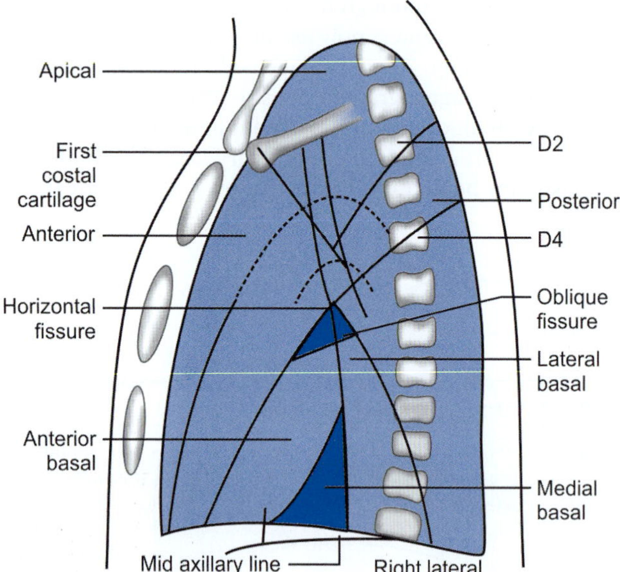

Fig. 5 Right lateral view of the chest skiagram showing different segments of the right upper lobe and lateral and medial basal segments of lower lobe (right). Note the position of oblique fissure. It starts 1.25 cm behind the costophrenic angle and passes through the hilum to touch the body of D4 vertebra. Horizontal fissure is represented by a horizontal line drawn from the hilum

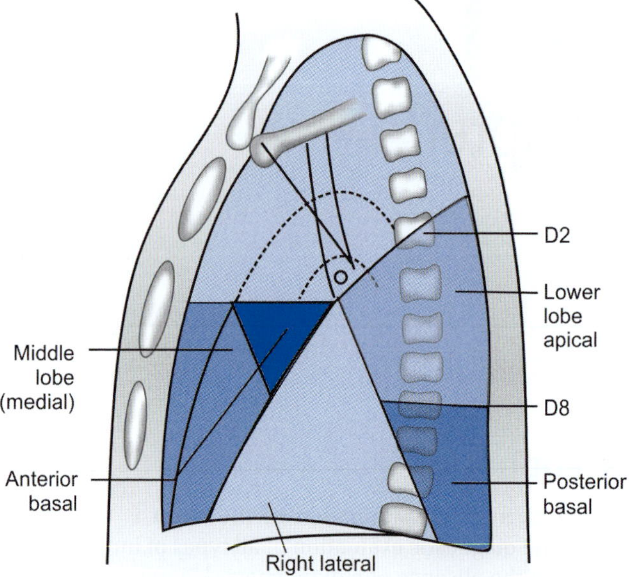

Fig. 6A Right lateral view of the chest radiograph showing segments of middle lobe and apical and posterior basal segments of lower lobe

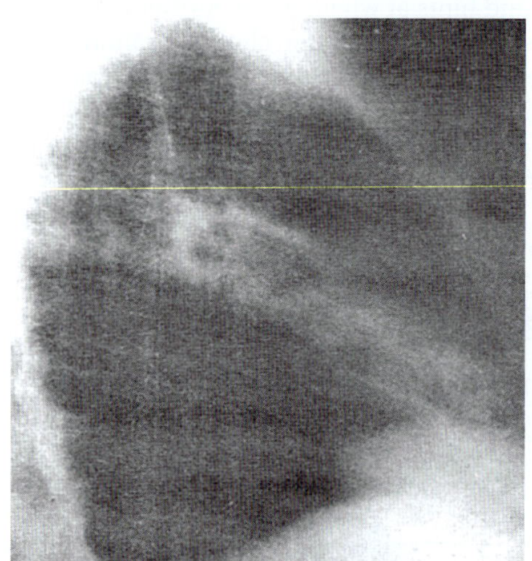

Fig. 6B Cavity in the right middle lobe

of this method is that the visibility of calcium is diminished. Proper positioning of the patient and the timing with phase of respiration [in full inspiration or thin layer chromatography (TLC)] is important for a better quality of PA film.

ANTEROPOSTERIOR VIEW

This view of the chest radiograph is used when the patient is sick and cannot be moved into the radiology department—the so-called "portable X-rays". Such roentgenograms are technically inferior because of the patient's supine position, short focus-film distance and the inability in most patients to achieve a full inspiration. The mediastinal structures and the heart appear enlarged because the cassette lies at the back of the patient, and the heart is further away from the film and nearer to the X-ray tube.

LATERAL VIEW

These chest radiographs are particularly helpful in localizing a mediastinal or pulmonary lesion in its appropriate anatomical compartment. It differentiates a chest wall or

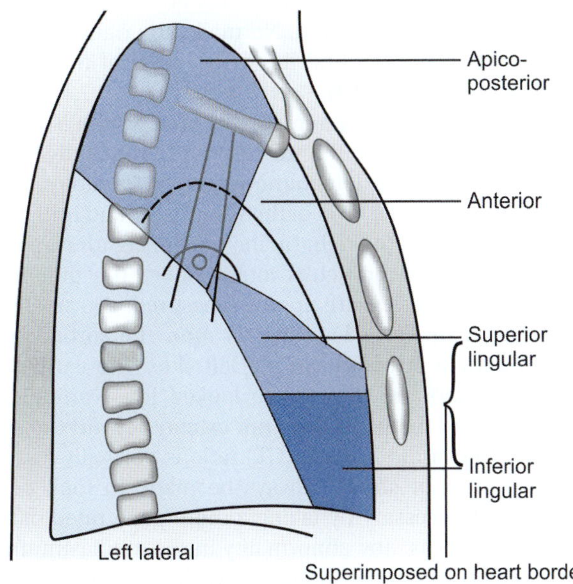

Fig. 7 Left lateral view of the chest skiagram showing segments of the left upper lobe including the lingular segments

cutaneous lesion from that in the lung. Small lesions in the retrocardiac or retrosternal areas or in the curvatures of the diaphragm hidden in the PA films are better seen in a lateral view. However, the lateral film is less easy to interpret than a PA film, as the two lungs and the mediastinum are superimposed one upon the other. The particular side to be X-rayed remains nearer to the film, i.e. in a left lateral view the left side is nearer to the film.[6,7]

APICOGRAM

Apicogram or the apical lordotic view is taken for the better visualization of the lung apices, which tend to be obscured on the standard posteroanterior projections by the upper ribs and the clavicles. The patient assumes a lordotic position arching the back, so that the nape of the neck rests on the top of the cassette, and the X-ray beam remains horizontal. The same view can be taken in an immobile patient in a modified technique. Superior mediastinum and the thoracic inlet can also be better delineated by this method. The minor fissure is better identified in the suspected cases of atelectasis of the right middle lobe in this view.

OBLIQUE VIEW

These skiagrams are infrequently used in respiratory work-up. A standard anterior oblique view is obtained with the anterolateral wall of the chest placed against the cassette at an angle of about 45° and the hands are held in extension above the head. Similarly, the posterior oblique views are taken. These skiagrams are helpful in demonstrating pleural and pulmonary shadows close to the chest wall, pleural plaques in asbestosis and sometimes suspected rib pathology.

LATERAL DECUBITUS FILMS

For this view, the patient lies on one side and the X-ray beam is oriented horizontally. The technique is particularly helpful in detecting small pleural effusions. Fluid collections as little as less than 100 mL can be detected by this method, whereas those taken in erect posture usually do not show pleural effusion of less than 300 mL. A more refined technique can detect fluid as little as 3–5 mL. The lateral decubitus view is also helpful to demonstrate the shifting of air fluid level in a cavity or to demonstrate a freely moving intracavitary loose body as a fungus ball or mycetoma in a tubercular cavity. Another usefulness of this roentgenography is to demonstrate air trapping, characteristic of endobronchial foreign bodies particularly in infants and young children.

EXPIRATORY SKIAGRAMS

These are used (i) to investigate local or generalized air trapping; or (ii) to detect small pneumothoraces. When air trapping is generalized as in bronchial asthma or emphysema, there is little change in the lung density because of symmetrical diminution in the excursion of both diaphragms. However, localized air trapping (bronchial obstruction or lobar emphysema), the expiratory X-ray reveals restricted ipsilateral diaphragmatic elevation, a shift of the mediastinum to the contralateral side and a relative absence of the density change in the involved segment. In small pneumothoraces, when the visceral pleural line is not visible on the standard inspiratory films, an expiratory film may show the line more clearly. This is because of the volume of air in the pleural space being relatively greater in relation to the volume of the lung during expiration, which provides the better separation of the pleural surfaces, and the relationship of pleural line to the overlying ribs change during this maneuver.

Digital radiography: It is a recently introduced technique when the skiagram can be acquired digitally and can be stored like the data in a computer. The picture can be retrieved later. Further areas of particular interest can be studied more thoroughly.[11]

FLUOROSCOPY

Fluoroscopy or screening of the chest is helpful to visualize diaphragmatic excursions in cases of elevated diaphragms, and to distinguish a mass, particularly in the mediastinum whether it is pulsatile or not. In addition, this procedure is used more frequently nowadays for transbronchial biopsy and percutaneous aspiration of lung or mediastinal masses for cytological examination. Loculated or deep-seated lung abscess, empyema or pleural effusions can be easily aspirated under fluoroscopic guidance. This is also used conveniently for other purposes like bronchography, pulmonary angiography and barium swallow examination of the esophagus.

READING A CHEST X-RAY

Normal X-ray

The reading of a standard PA film should proceed in a systematic manner so that no abnormality can be missed. It is always better to read such a film together with a radiologist, a practice most often very helpful. A suggested scheme of reading a chest X-ray is as follows:

First identify the quality and centering of the film. Neither an overpenetrated nor an under penetrated film is good **(Figs 8A and B)**. One may then start looking at the extrapulmonary sites like the soft tissue shadows **(Figs 9 to 11)**, including the breast shadows, skin and subcutaneous tissue thickness, bony cage, supraclavicular areas, scapulae and the areas below the diaphragms. The clavicles and ribs are to be looked for any abnormality **(Figs 12A and B)**.

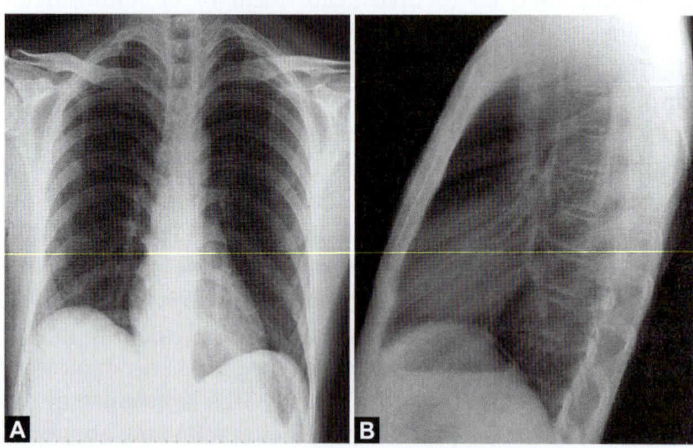

Figs 8A and B Normal chest X-ray

The levels of both the diaphragms and their contour are to be studied and compared. Normally, the right diaphragm is higher than the left and lies at the level of the sixth rib anteriorly **(Figs 8 and 13)**.

The mediastinum is an important area, which is liable to be misread/over-read. The tracheal and bronchial shadows can often be seen. The left pulmonary artery lies above the left main bronchus at the level of the seventh rib and is higher by one rib space than the right (at the level of eighth rib), which overlaps the right bronchus intermedius. The dimensions of both the arteries are to be measured. Normally, the maximum diameter is less than 17 mm. The aortic knuckle is a prominent structure on the left side. The cardiac size and its borders are then to be looked for. Normally, the right border of the heart does not extend beyond the spinal column. The cardiothoracic (CT) ratio is normally less than 50%. An attempt should always be made to look behind the heart, if necessary by taking a more penetrated or a left lateral view. Thus, any abnormality in the mediastinum can be picked up. The spine should always be examined carefully for any evidence of destruction, secondaries or cold abscess. Normally, the spine and the left lower lobe vessels are just visible through the heart shadow.

The lung parenchyma is divided into three radiological zones:

1. Upper zone is the area lying between the apex and the second intercostal space
2. The mid zone between the second and the fourth space
3. The lower zone extends from the fourth space downwards.

Any abnormality in each of these zones on either side should be noted very carefully.

Various deviations from the normal skiagram and few other abnormalities that can be seen are shown in **Figures 14 to 34**.

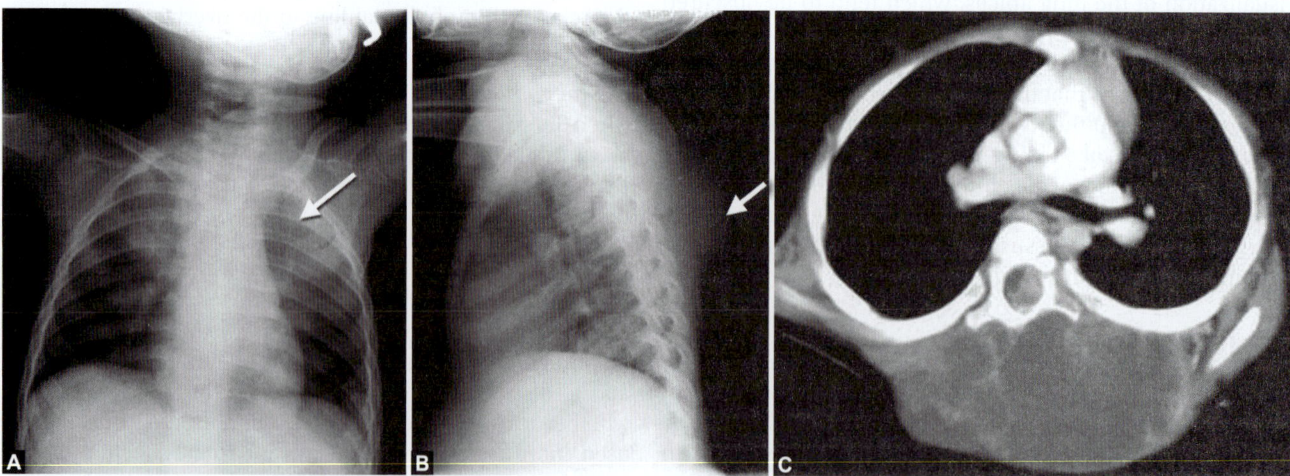

Figs 9A to C Note the external shadow while studying X-ray. Also corresponding computed tomography (CT) scan showing the external shadow

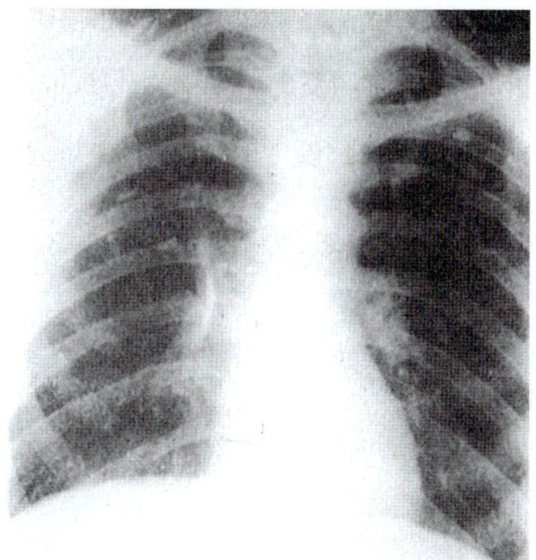

Fig. 10 Cysticerci in the soft tissue of the chest wall

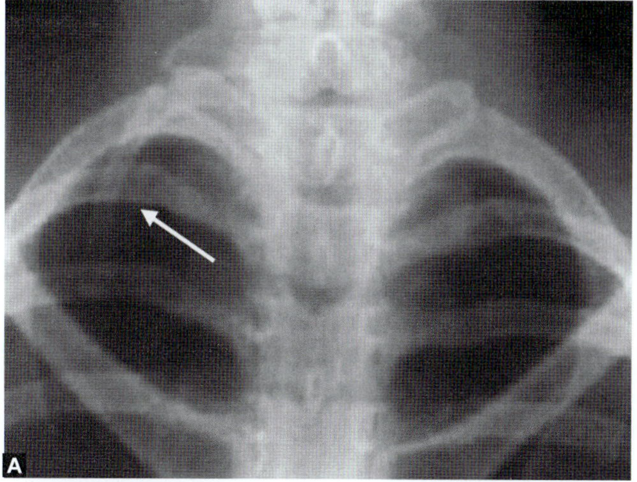

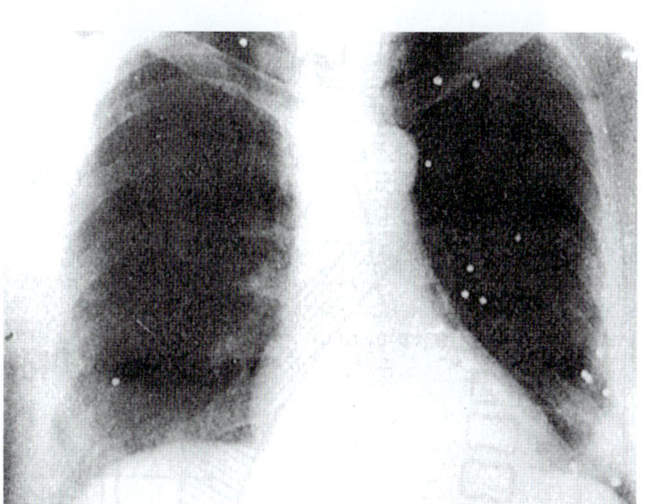

Fig. 11 Multiple bullets in the chest wall

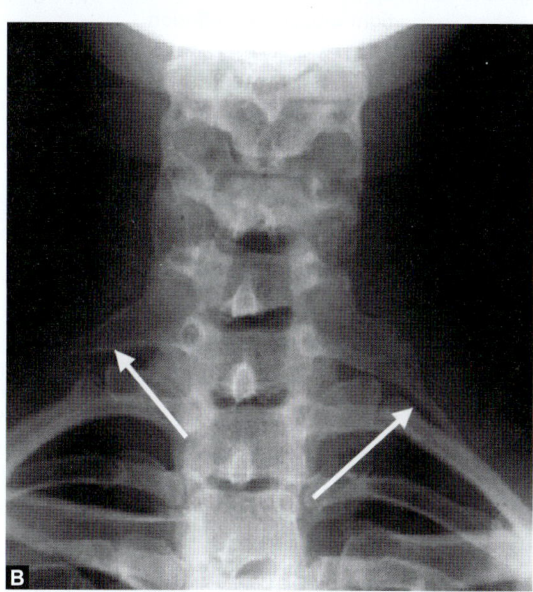

Figs 12A and B Cervical ribs

Limitations of Chest X-rays

About 7–21% of normal chest X-rays reveal abnormalities on computed tomography (CT) scan. Normal chest X-ray does not rule out mediastinal lymphadenopathy. Bronchiectasis, early interstitial lung disease, miliary shadows, nodules less than 5 mm may be missed on chest X-ray.

ABNORMAL RADIOLOGICAL FINDINGS

While it is not possible to describe all the radiological findings of all the pulmonary diseases, a generalized description of possible abnormalities in a chest skiagram will be discussed in brief. The findings may be divided into:

- A solitary nodule
- Parenchymal shadows
- Hilar and mediastinal shadows
- Abnormalities of the pleura.

Solitary Pulmonary Nodule (Figs 35 and 36)

A solitary nodule[12] is defined as a shadow of either 3 cm or less in diameter with distinct borders and is surrounded by relatively normal lung parenchyma. When such a lesion is found in a chest skiagram, it is important to decide whether it is benign or malignant. Three points need special considerations: Age of the patient, doubling time, margins and calcifications, if any. Solitary nodules in subjects below 40 years of age are relatively benign and in patients above the age of 40 years, carcinoma needs to be excluded, particularly,

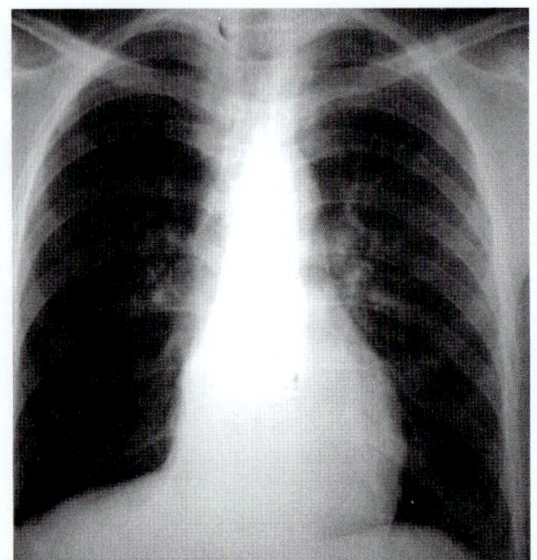

Fig. 13 Chest X-ray: Flattening of right dome of diaphragm—right subpulmonic effusion

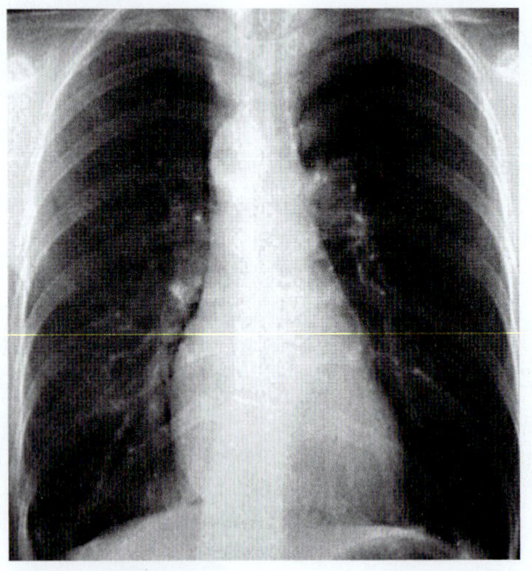

Fig. 14 Right-sided aortic arch

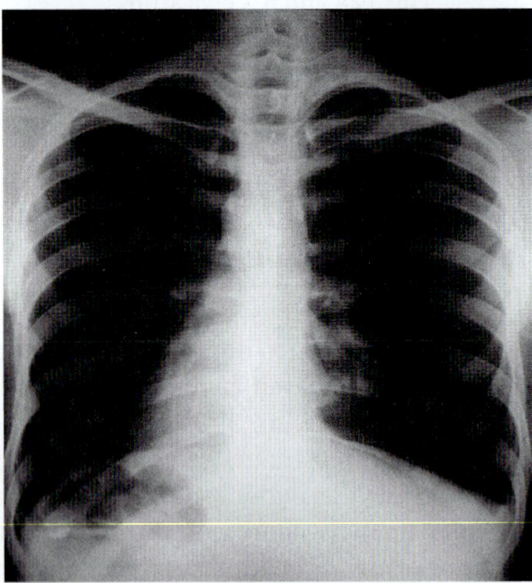

Fig. 15 Dextrocardia

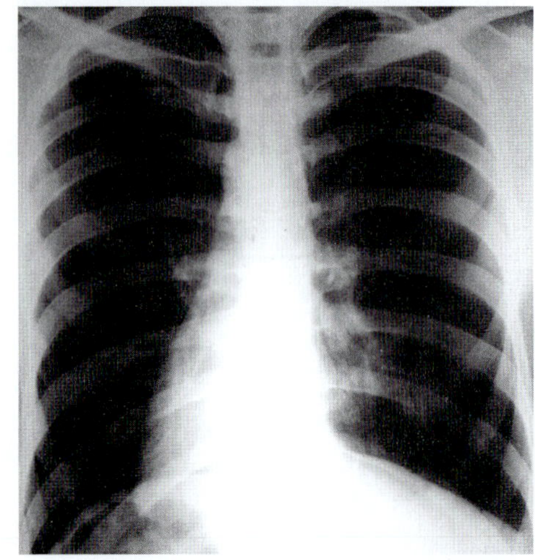

Fig. 16 Chest X-ray—dextrocardia with situs inversus

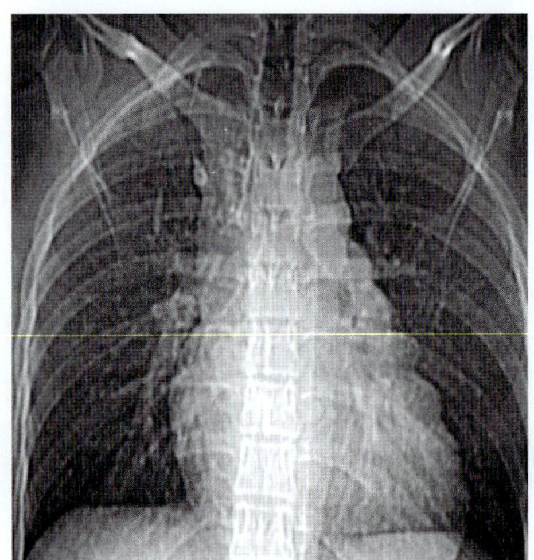

Fig. 17 Azygous fissure

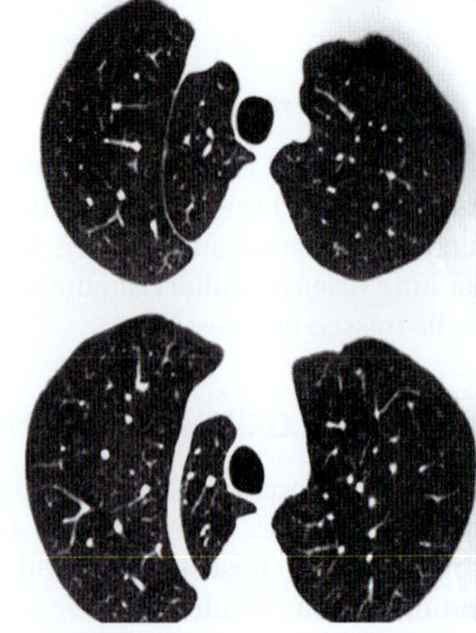

Fig. 18 Azygous fissure [computed tomography (CT)]

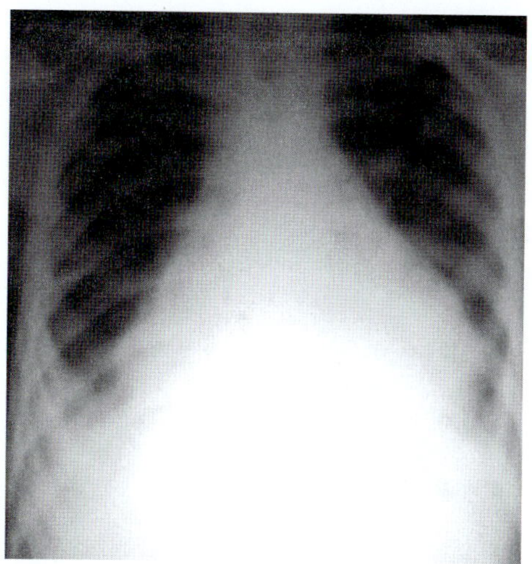

Fig. 19 Chest X-ray—globular-shaped heart shadow (pericardial effusion)

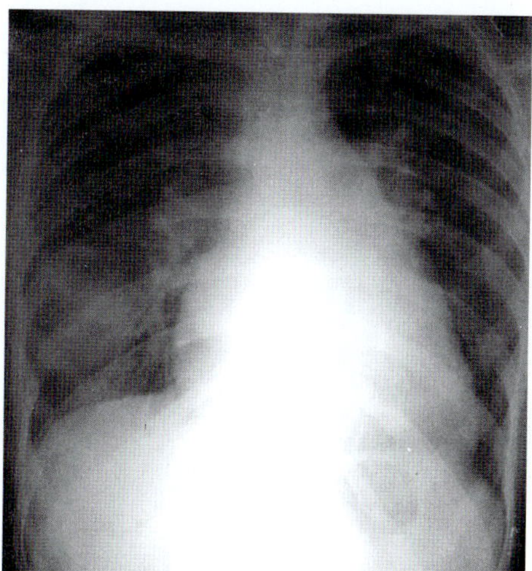

Fig. 22 Fluid in the major fissure in a case of congestive heart failure—pseudotumor

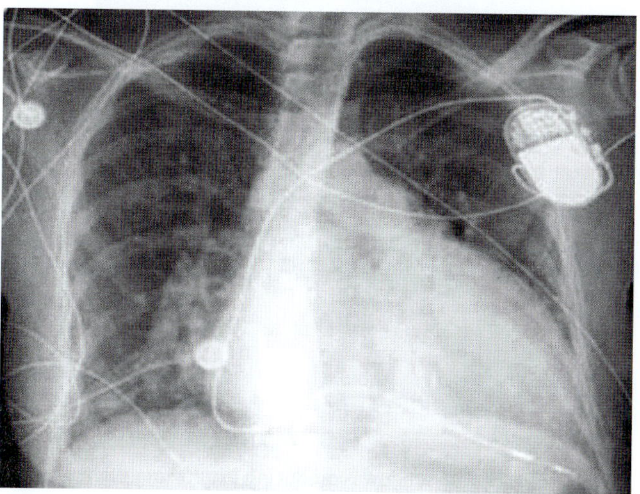

Fig. 20 Left ventriculomegaly

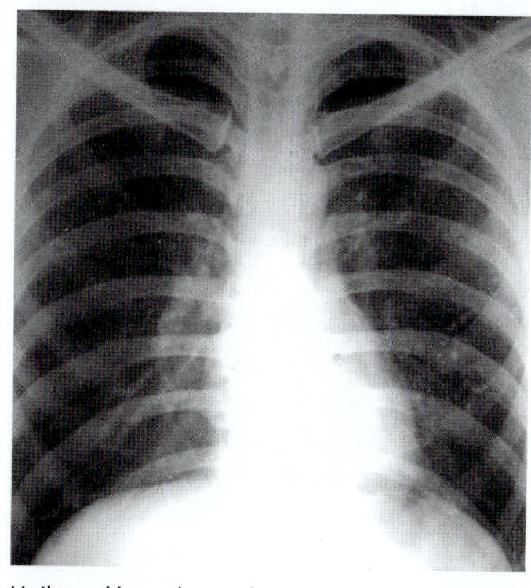

Fig. 23 Unilateral hyperlucent lung on the right side—congenital

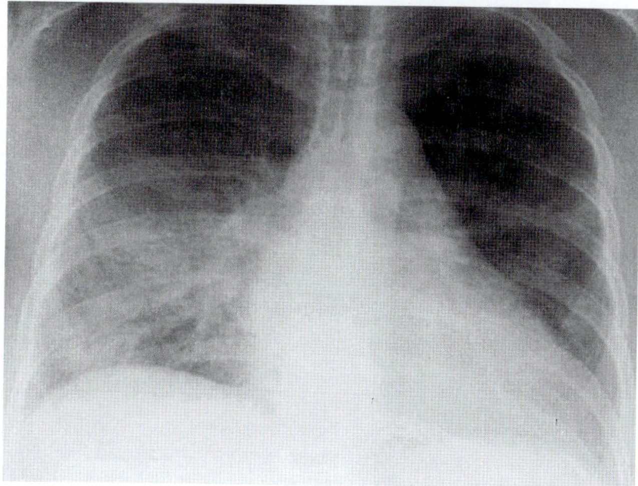

Fig. 21 Pulmonary edema

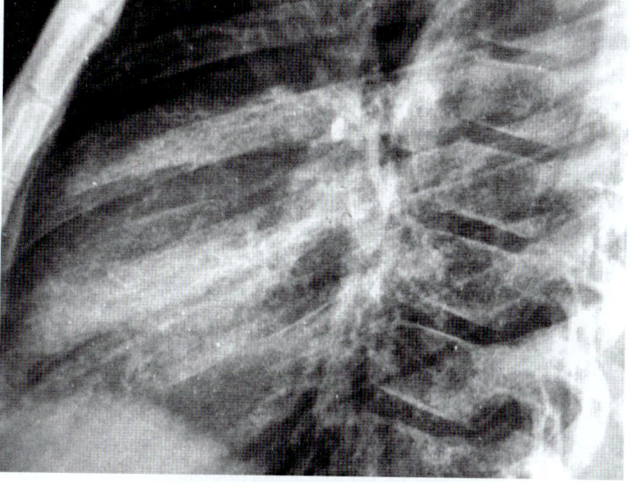

Fig. 24 Tooth in the bronchus—fiberoptic bronchoscopy (FOB) is indicated

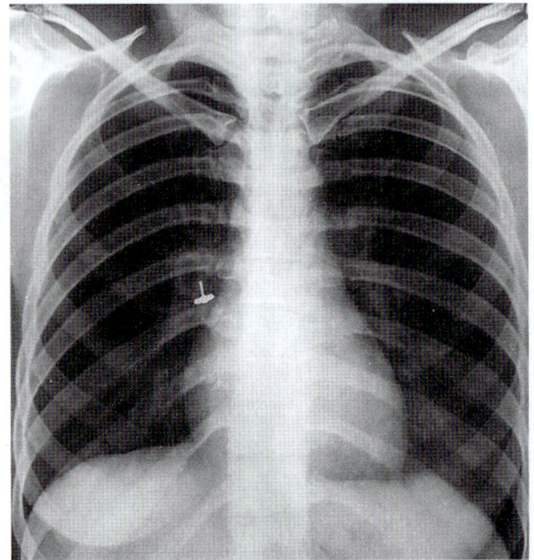

Fig. 25 Ear pendant in the bronchus

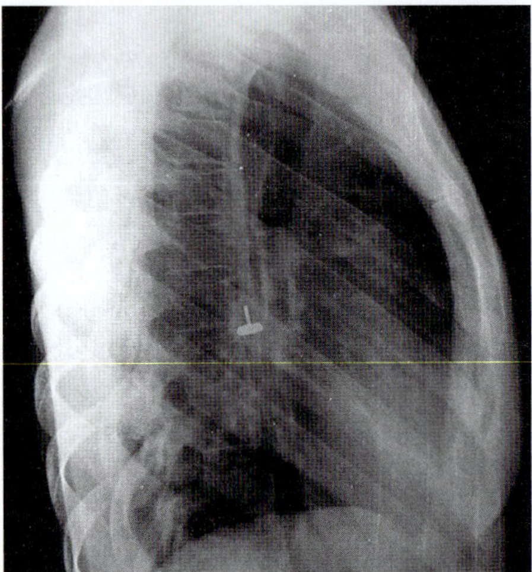

Fig. 26 Lateral view showing ear pendant in the bronchus

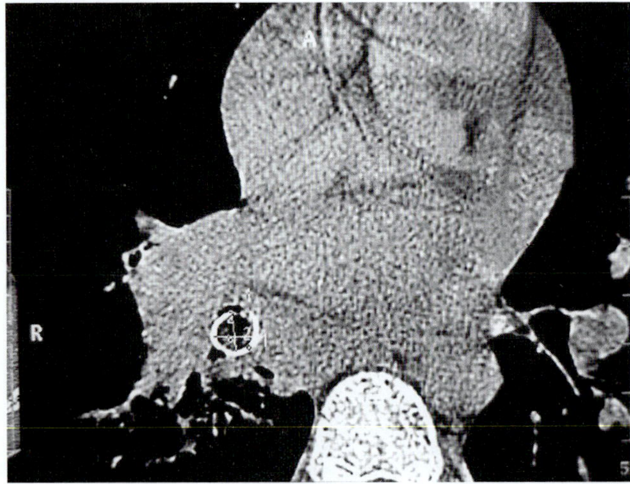

Fig. 27 Ear ring in the bronchus

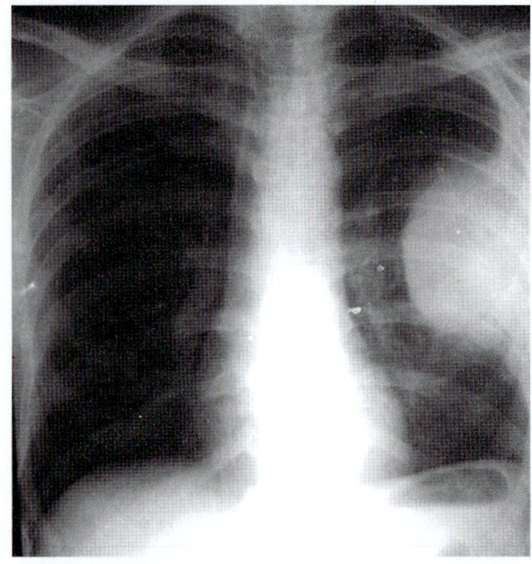

Fig. 28 Extrapulmonary sign—a case of pleural tumor

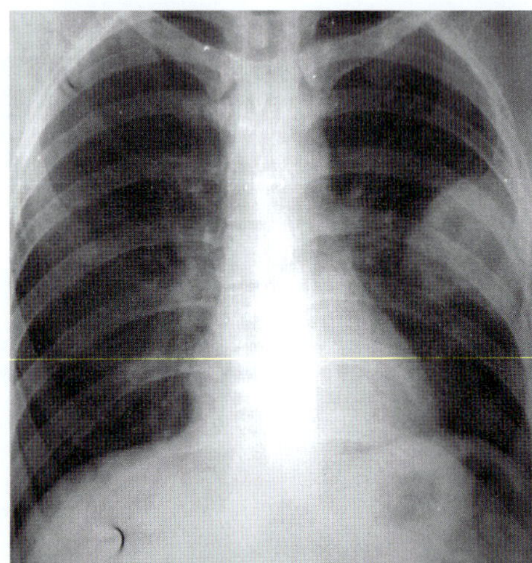

Fig. 29 The shadow is producing extrapleural sign. Note both the angles are obtuse

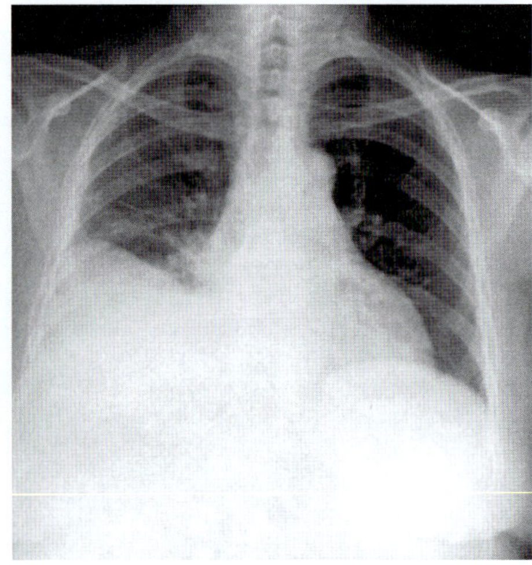

Fig. 30 Right subpulmonic effusion

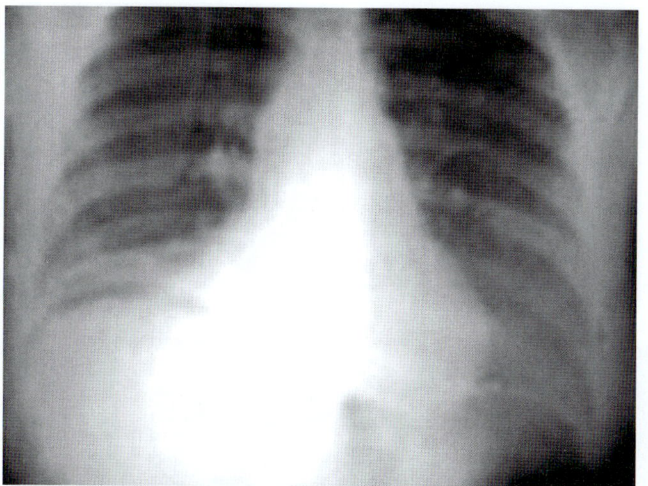

Fig. 31 Free air under right dome of diaphragm

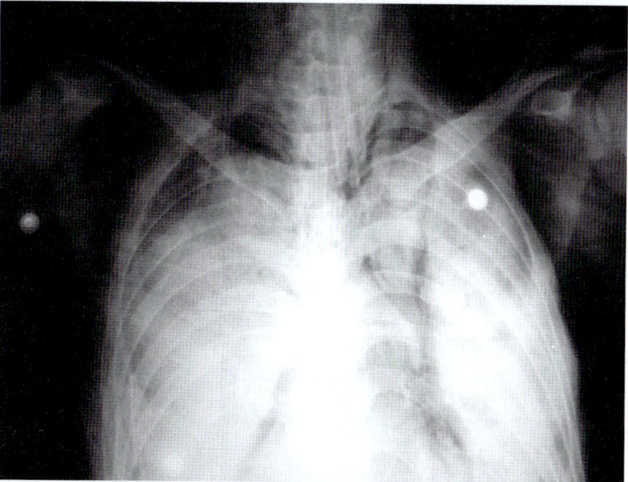

Fig. 34 Alveolar proteinosis

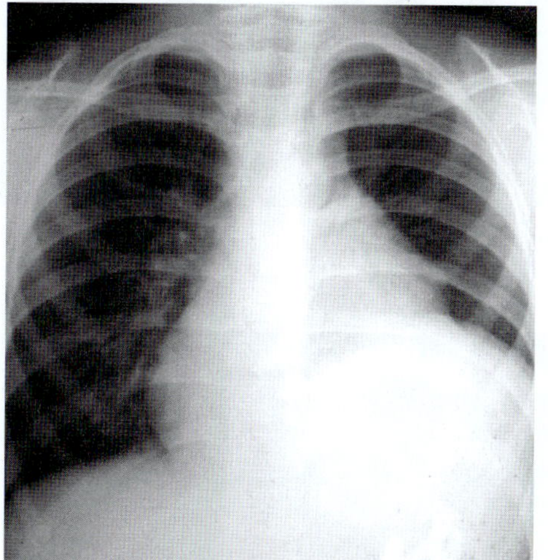

Fig. 32 Chest X-ray. Homogeneous opacity at left cardiophrenic angle (pleural effusion)

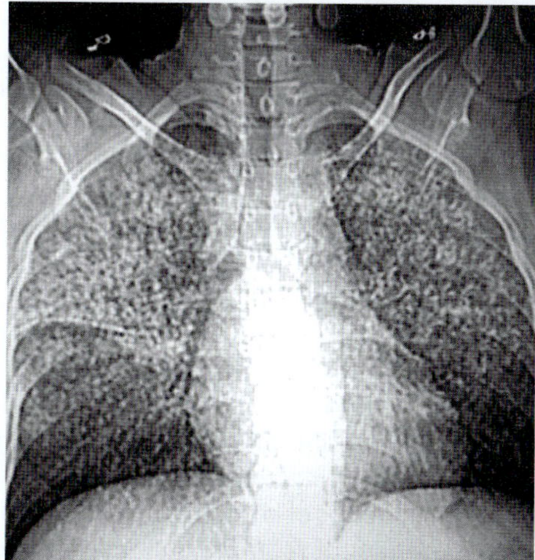

Fig. 33 Chest X-ray—extensive miliary motting

if he is a smoker. All attempts should be made to obtain a previous skiagram, if one was taken, since a lesion lying for few years, is unlikely to be a malignant one. If the lesion in the present skiagram doubles in volume within 7 days, it is more likely to be a benign one. However, secondaries from choriocarcinoma, testicular tumor and osteogenic sarcoma may grow very fast and for these a time limit of 11 days is suggested. On the other hand, lesions having a doubling time greater than 465 days are also benign. Anything outside these limits is more likely to be malignant. If the margins are lobular or nodular in appearance, the chances of malignancy are very high.

A tail is suggestive of a granuloma or arteriovenous malformation. Small satellite lesions accompanying the nodule are common with tubercular lesions. Presence or absence of calcification in the nodule is another indicator of the benign or malignant nature of the lesion. While presence of calcification is taken as a sign of benign lesions, exceptions are there. Calcified nodules may be malignant in the following conditions: (a) A primary carcinoma engulfing a pre-existing calcified granuloma; (b) Solitary metastases from osteogenic sarcoma or chondrosarcoma; (c) Primary peripheral squamous cell carcinoma or papillary adenocarcinoma (primary or metastatic); and (d) Rare cases of carcinoid tumors or metastases from mucinous adenocarcinomas from colon. Benign lesions which usually calcify are: Tuberculoma, histoplasmoma or other fungal diseases **(Fig. 37)**. The pattern of calcification is sometimes characteristic of certain lesions. A small central nidus is seen in granulomas or hamartomas; laminated appearance is almost pathognomonic of granulomas and indicates a benign nature of the disease; popcorn ball calcification is a characteristic feature of hamartomas **(Fig. 38)**; and multiple punctate foci throughout the lesion may be seen either in a granuloma or hamartoma.

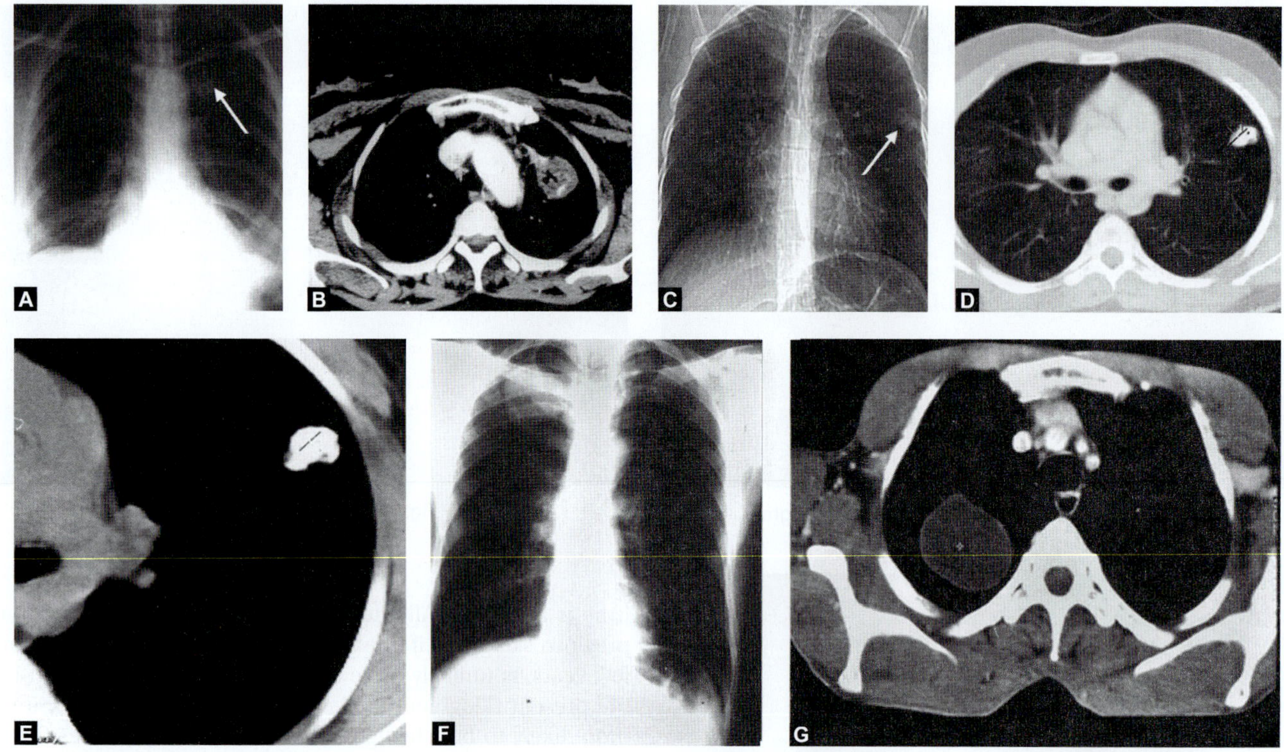

Figs 35A to G Solitary pulmonary nodule

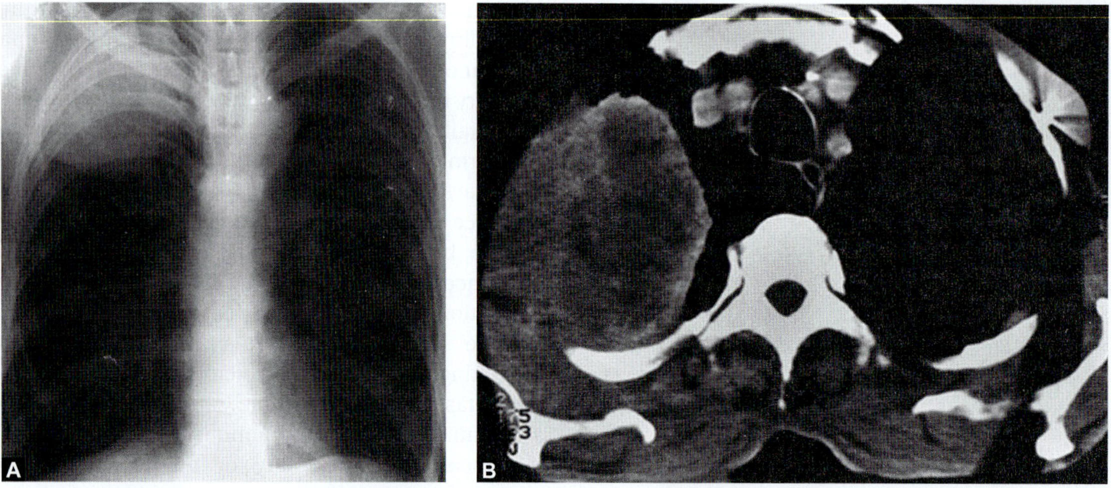

Figs 36A and B Not solitary pulmonary nodule. Not well-defined, invading the surrounding structure

Other spherical lesions seen in a chest skiagram are due to carcinoids, cylindromas, leiomyomas, fibromas, neural tumors, tuberculomas histoplasmomas, cryptococcomas, hydatid cyst, syphilitic gummas, lung abscess, progressive massive fibrosis, Caplan's syndrome, paraffin granulomas, aspiration pneumonias, rheumatoid nodules, Wegener's granulomatosis, bronchocentric granuloma, arteriovenous malformation, sequestration of lung, infarcts and interlobar effusion.

With the availability of different modern diagnostic techniques, assessment of solitary pulmonary nodule (SPN) has become easier. But the problem is of high sensitivity

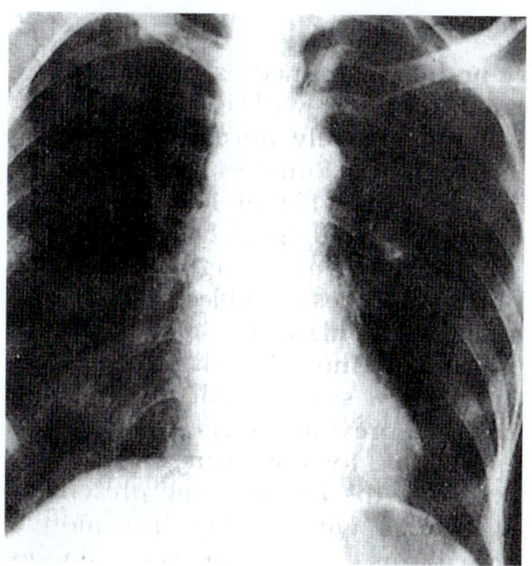

Fig. 37 Calcified solitary nodule on the left mid zone (tuberculoma)

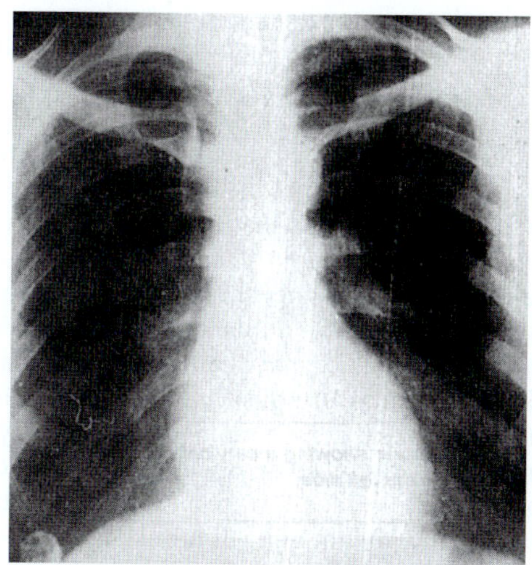

Fig. 38 Note popcorn calcification in a hamartoma in the right lower zone

of these methods. The main concern is the nature of the nodule—whether it is malignant or benign. Too sensitive methods will expose the patients for unnecessary exploration and many benign lesions will be resected unnecessarily.

An SPN diagnostic approach that includes a transbronchial biopsy, then percutaneous needle aspiration (PCNA), clinical observation, repeat CT scans, and repeat biopsies for continued suspicion of malignancy appears to reduce the unnecessary surgical excision of benign nodules from the current rate of 60% to 5% of SPN resections without affecting the survival of patients who have malignant SPNs. Both the ultrasound and radio-guided techniques are accurate to detect SPN, but the radio-guided method yields complications as compared with the ultrasound.[13] Ultra thin section with multislice computed tomography (MSCT) and multiplanar reconstructions (MPR), curved multiplanar reconstructions (CMPR) and surface-shaded display (SSD) reconstruction can improve the demonstration of the patterns of tumor-bronchus relationships, which can reflect the pathological changes of the nodules to some extent and help differentiate malignant from benign tumors. According to one report, CT demonstrated the relationship between the SPN and bronchi in 46 (86.8%) malignant and 18 (75.0%) benign nodules. Five types of tumor-bronchus relationships were identified with MSCT. *Type I*: The bronchus was obstructed abruptly by the SPN; *type II*: The bronchus penetrated into the SPN with tapered narrowing and interruption; *type III*: The bronchial lumen shown within the SPN was patent and intact; *type IV*: The bronchus ran around the periphery of the SPN with intact lumen; *type V*: The bronchus was displaced, compressed and narrowed by the SPN. Malignant nodules were most commonly of type I (58.5%), secondly of type IV (26.4%) and rarely of type V (1.9%). Benign nodules were most often of type V (36.0%), followed by type III (20.0%), type I (16.0%), and there were no type II. Types I, II and IV were more common in malignant nodules, whereas type V was seen more frequently in benign nodules ($p < 0.05$). There was no statistically significant difference between the two groups regarding type III.[14] Dynamic magnetic resonance imaging (MRI) and CT seem to be equally well suited for the differentiation between benign and malignant SPNs.[15] Note popcorn calcification in a hamartoma in the right lower zone computer-aided diagnosis (CAD) has the potential to improve radiologists diagnostic accuracy in distinguishing small benign nodules from malignant ones on high resolution computed tomography (HRCT) **(Fig. 38)**.[16] With a preoperative selection of the patients the rate of secondary thoracotomies due to bronchial carcinoma is low (4%). In patients with a previous history of malignant disease, 22% of the pulmonary lesions are benign. Video-assisted thoracoscopic surgery (VATS) is a safe diagnostic method, with little discomfort for the patient.[17] Thoracoscopic resection of SPN is safely feasible. It results in better patient satisfaction, less nursing care and shorter in-hospital stay and the procedure can be performed without general anesthesia.[18] Ill-defined margins, spiculation, involvement of bronchi or vessels, and tumor enlargement visualized by CT are still important signs of malignancy even for nodules less than 10 mm in size. Tumor size, even for lung cancers measuring less than 10 mm, is not an indication for limited resection.[19] The use of MPR for CT-guided lung biopsy is useful for improving diagnostic accuracy with no significant increase in pneumothorax rate or total procedure time.[20] Recently, Dynamic MRI delineates significant kinetic and morphologic differences in vascularity and perfusion between malignant and benign SPN. Washout seems to be highly specific for malignancy. Malignant nodules show stronger enhancement with a higher maximum peak and a faster slope ($P < 001$). Significant washout (> 0.1% increase in signal intensity per second) is found only in malignant lesions (14 of 27 lesions). Sensitivity, specificity, and accuracy are 96%, 88% and 92%, respectively, for maximum peak; 96%, 75% and 86% for slope; and 52%, 100%, and 75% for washout. When curve profiles and morphologic enhancement patterns are combined, sensitivity increases to 100%.[21]

Established methods (radiography for detection, spiral CT for characterization), after thorough evaluation, will soon be replaced by MRI. Recent experience with MRI points to its potential for the detection and characterization of pulmonary nodules while avoiding ionizing radiation. The development of indications for MRI of the lung (e.g. pediatric radiology) is not yet clear.[22] Pulmonologists are frequently asked to evaluate the CT-detected, small, noncalcified nodule invisible on standard chest radiography. Immediate biopsy is justified, if the likelihood of cancer is high, but if that likelihood is low or intermediate, a period of observation by CT is appropriate. VATS or thoracotomy are rarely necessary for a diagnosis of lung cancer in the CT-detected small pulmonary nodule.[23]

The challenge of diagnosis and management of SPN is among the most common yet most important areas of pulmonary medicine. Ideally, the goal of diagnosis and management is to promptly bring to surgery all patients with operable malignant nodules while avoiding unnecessary thoracotomy in patients with benign disease. Effective management of the SPN depends upon an understanding of decision analysis principles so that diverse technologies can be integrated into a systematic approach. In almost all patients, CT is the best first step. Three key questions can then help to guide the work-up of the SPN. These are what is the pretest probability of cancer, what is the risk of surgical complications, and does the appearance of the nodule on CT scan suggest a benign or malignant etiology. In patients with average surgical risk, positron emission tomography (PET) scan is warranted when there is discordance between the pretest probability of cancer and the appearance of the nodule on CT scan. Thus, when either the patient has a low risk of cancer and the CT suggests a malignant origin, or when there is high risk of cancer and the CT appears benign, PET scan will be cost-effective. In most other situations, PET scanning is only marginally more effective than CT and fine needle aspiration strategies, but costs much more.[24]

Pulmonary hamartoma is the most common type of benign lung tumor. The vast majority of pulmonary hamartomas represent as SPN. Definite diagnosis and the treatment can be achieved by surgical resection with minimal morbidity. Tumor recurrence is very rare.[25]

Airspace Disease

Either liquid, or cells, or both replace the air within the acinus. Typically, many contiguous acini are involved producing a homogeneous opacity **(Fig. 39)**. The size may vary from few centimeters to a whole lobe. Usual causes of such airspace opacities include: Alveolar edema, both cardiac and noncardiogenic, pneumonic consolidations bleeding into the acinus; aspiration of blood or lipid; neoplastic infiltrations

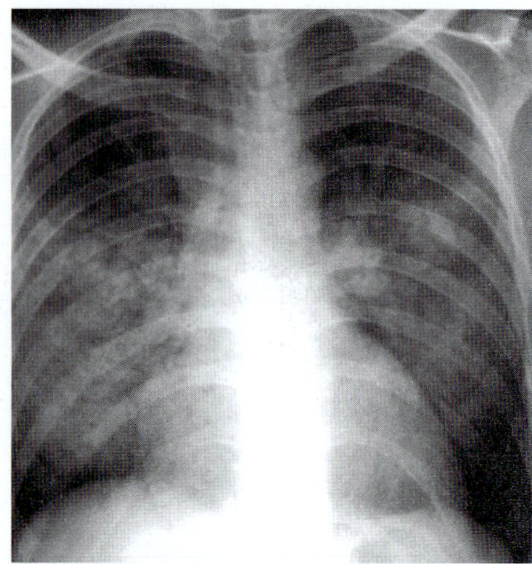

Fig. 39 Alveolar versus interstitial pathology

(bronchoalveolar cell carcinoma and lymphomas); alveolar proteinosis and early stages of fibrosing alveolitis. The classical findings of airspace disease include alveolar nodules or alveolar shadows, coalescence, poor margination, presence of airless bronchograms or bronchiolograms, air alveolograms, no or minimal atelectasis and the evolution is usually rapid. An alveolar shadow or the alveolar pattern of the shadow is nodular in shape measuring 4–10 mm in diameter with well-defined margins, and there will be the presence of small multiple radiolucencies. Another characteristic feature of airspace consolidation is that it does not respect segmental or subsegmental boundaries as is usual with pneumococcal pneumonias or pulmonary edema. However, diseases produced by vascular route or through the tracheobronchial tree usually have a segmental distribution as in an-aspiration pneumonia. Air bronchogram commonly seen in a consolidation, is due to a patent bronchus containing the air column in the bronchi visible in the skiagram. The area of the lung should be completely airless for visualization of air bronchogram, as in collapse or consolidation **(Figs 39 to 46)**.

Parenchymal Atelectasis

The basic difference between a consolidation and an atelectasis (collapse) is that while in the former the lung volume is maintained, in the latter, there is a volume loss **(Figs 47 to 56)**. Common types of atelectasis described are: Resorption atelectasis and compression or passive atelectasis. A resorption atelectasis is mainly due to bronchial obstruction and consequent absorption of air from the alveoli distal to the obstruction rendering the alveoli airless. However, this type of atelectasis can occur without bronchial obstruction as in bronchiectasis. The only definite roentgenographic sign of this type of collapse is a loss of lung volume evidenced radiologically as the displacement of interlobar fissures. Other features are an increase in density locally, elevation of

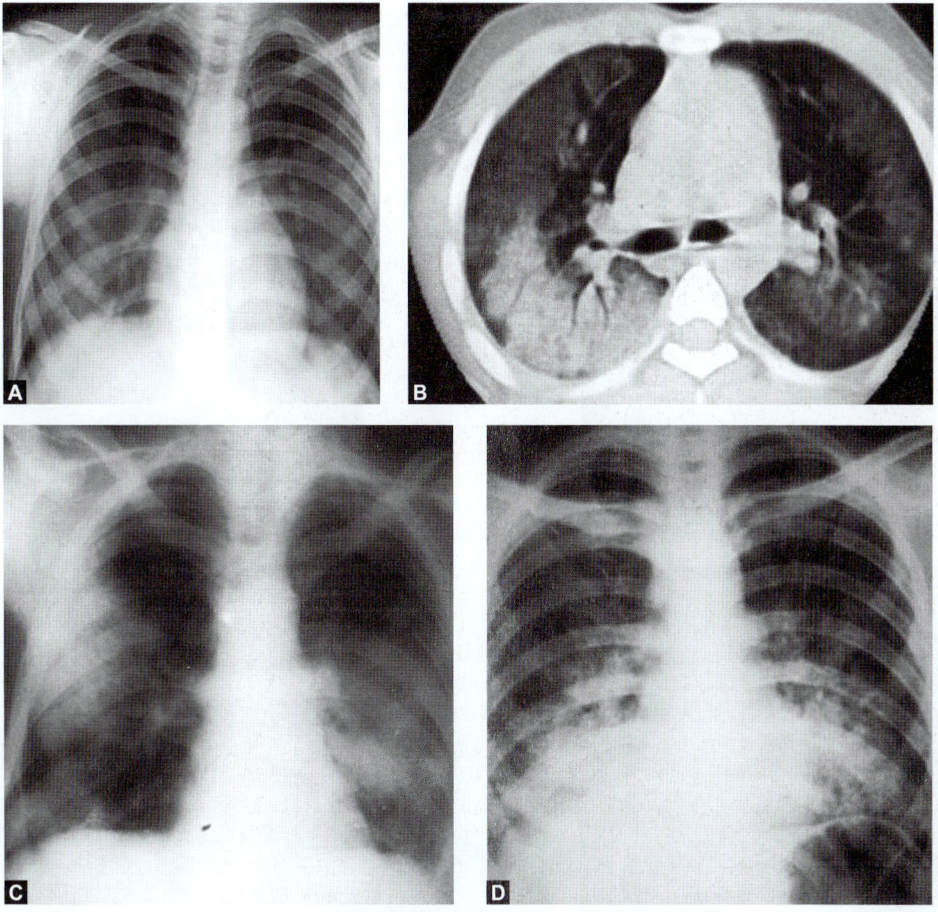

Figs 40A to D Consolidation

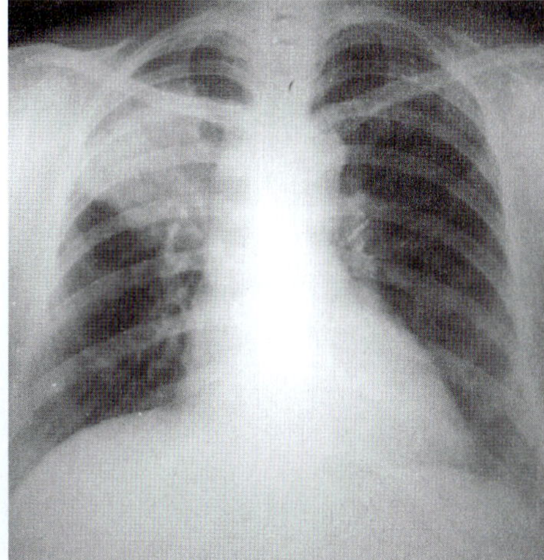

Fig. 41 Consolidation of right upper lobe. Note air bronchogram

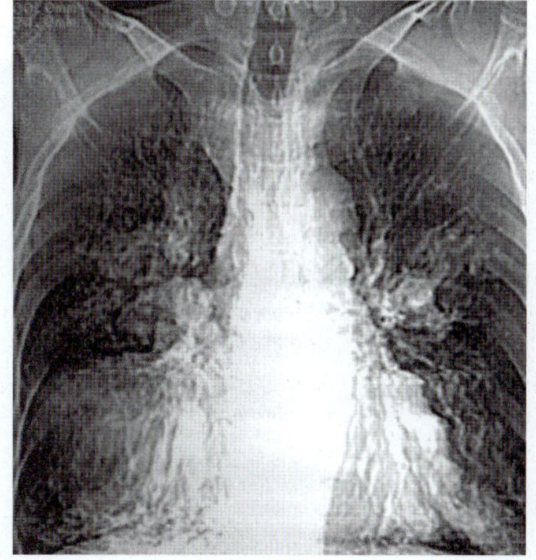

Fig. 42 Chest X-ray-Basal consolidation with air-bronchograms—Bronchiolitis obliterans organizing pneumonia (BOOP)

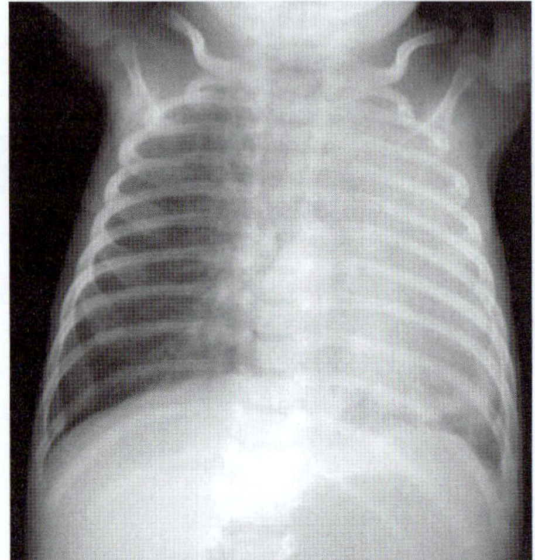

Fig. 43 Left upper lobe consolidation. Anteroposterior (AP) view

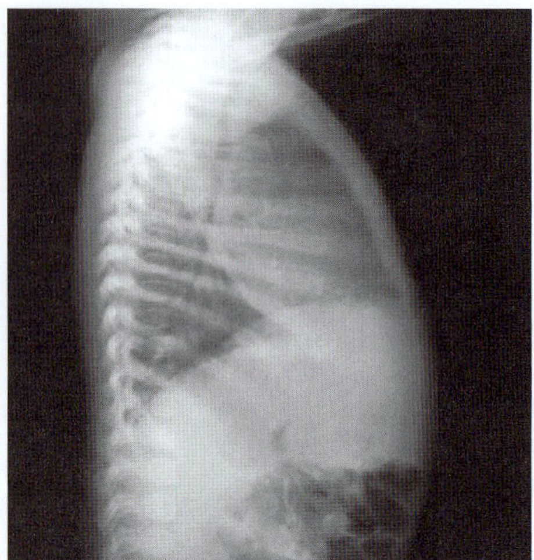

Fig. 44 Left upper lobe consolidation—lateral view

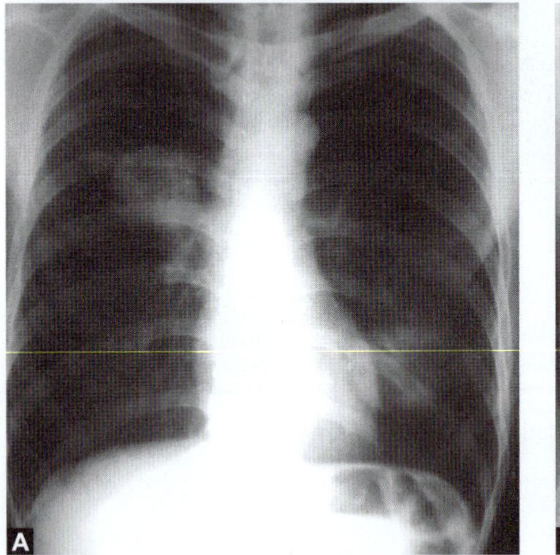

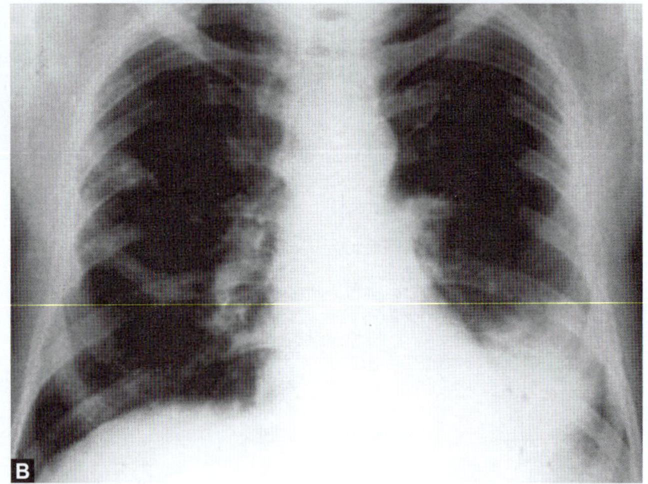

Figs 45A and B (A) Round pneumonia in both the lungs; (B) Consolidation in left lower zone

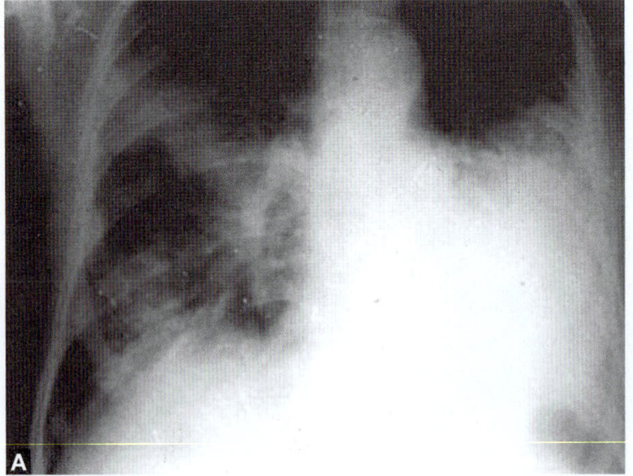

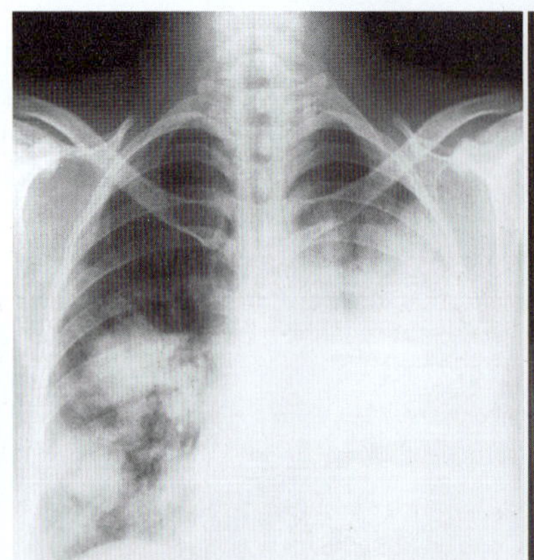

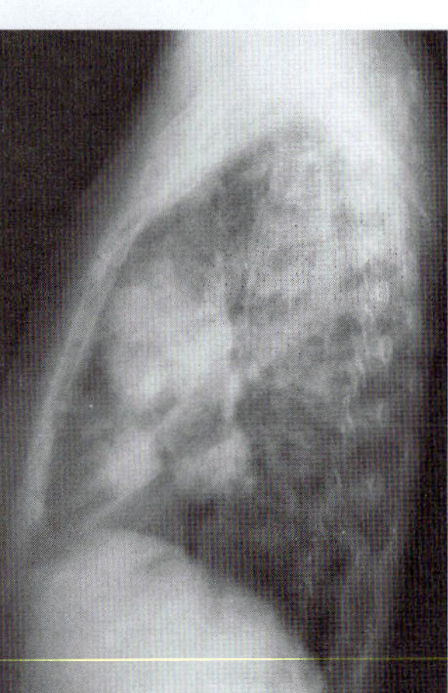

Figs 46A and B Nonresolving consolidation

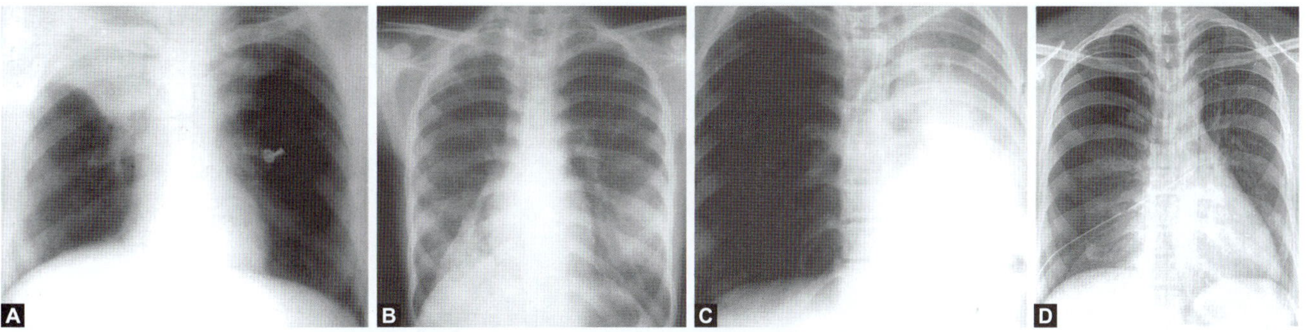

Figs 47A to D Pulmonary collapse

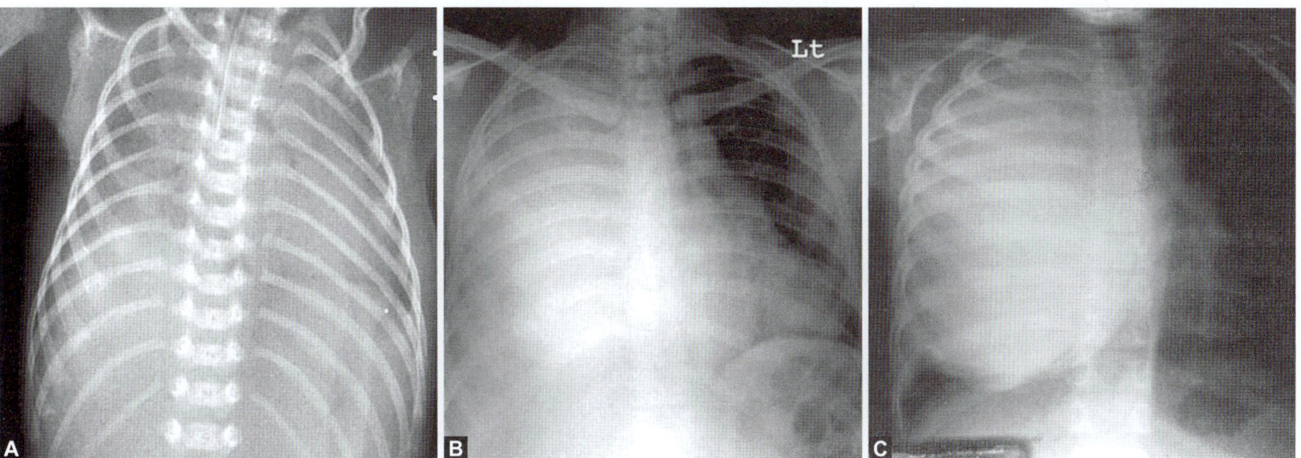

Figs 48A to C Opaque hemithorax

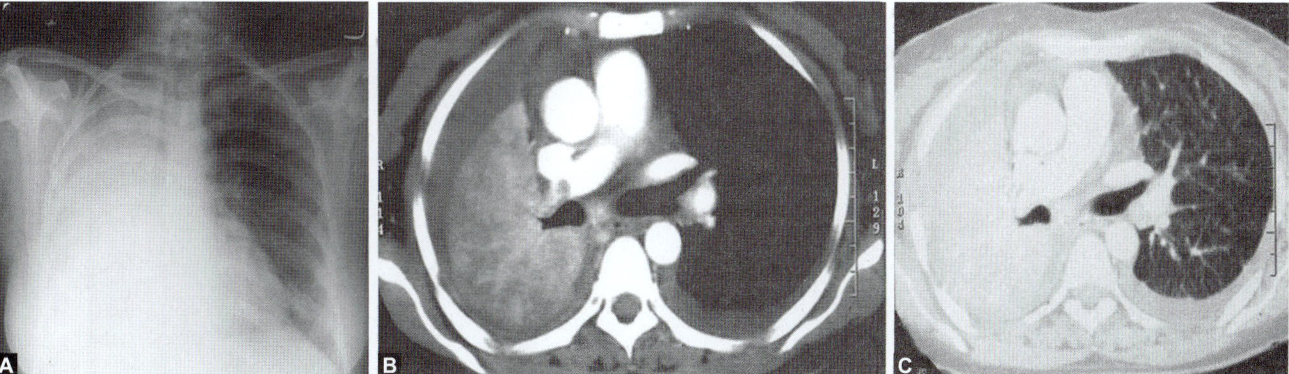

Figs 49A to C Opaque hemithorax. Due to collapse of right lung

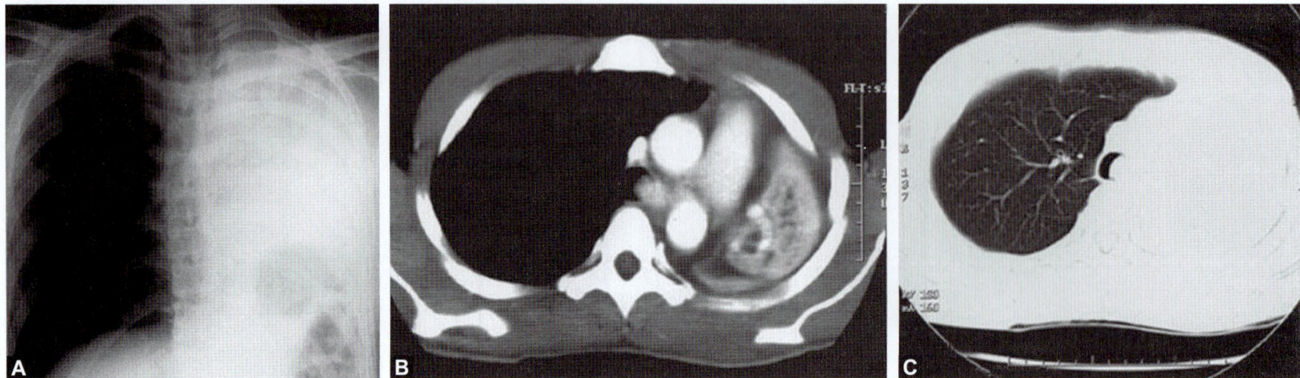

Figs 50A to C Opaque hemithorax. Due to collapse of left lung

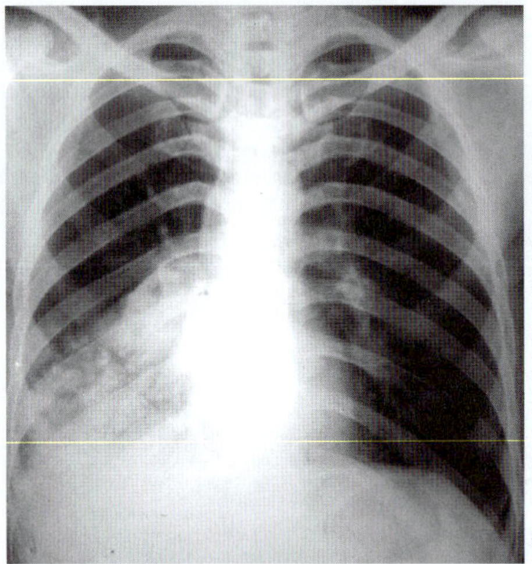

Fig. 51 Postobsturctive collapse consolidation on the right lower lobe

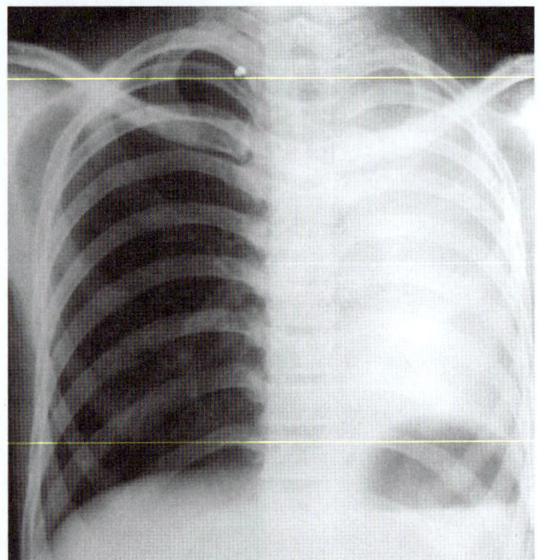

Fig. 52 Entire left lung collapse

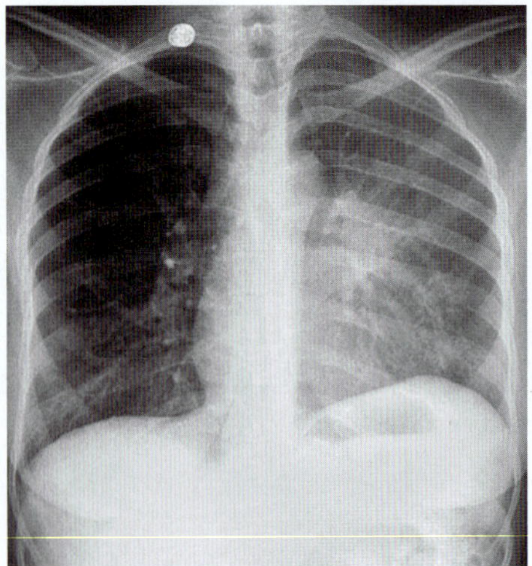

Fig. 53 Left upper lobe collapse—anteroposterior view

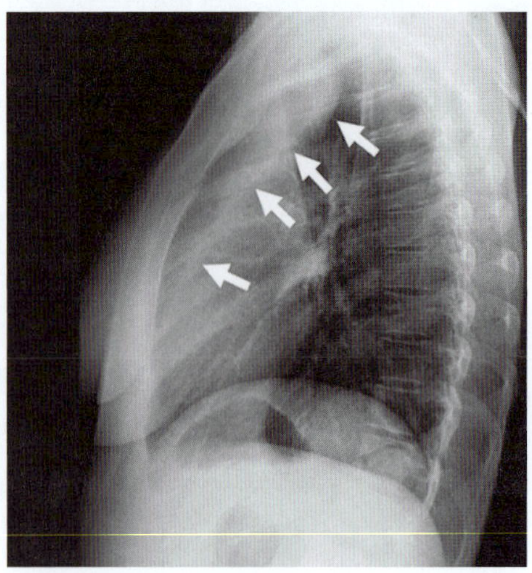

Fig. 54 Left upper lobe collapse—lateral view

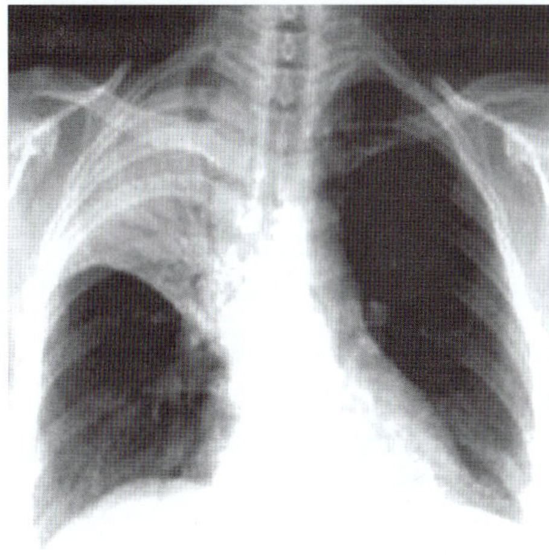

Fig. 55 Right upper lobe collapse

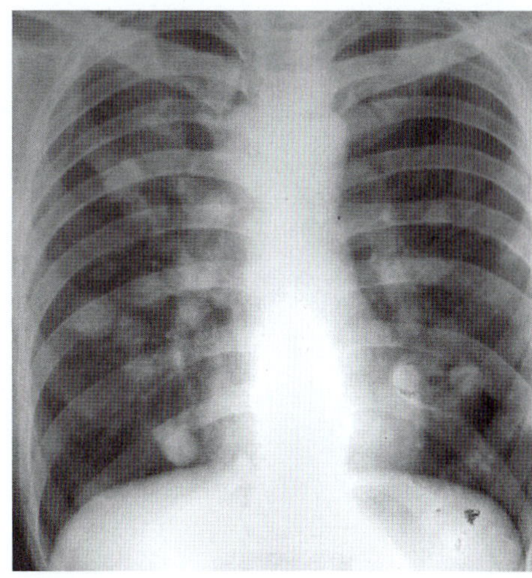

Fig. 57 Cannonball metastasis

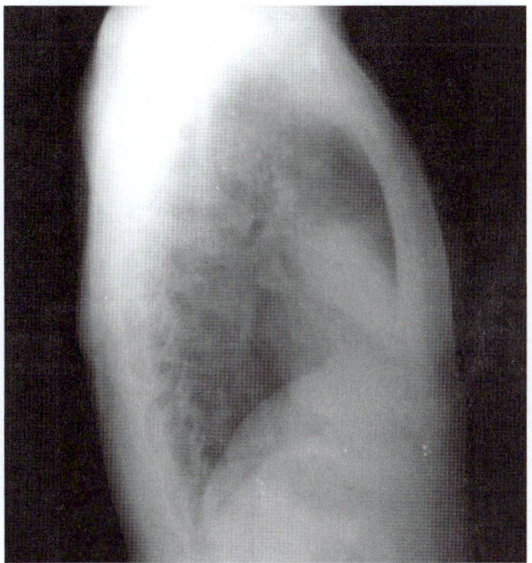

Fig. 56 Right middle lobe collapse. Note the shadow is bound by the two fissures which are also displaced

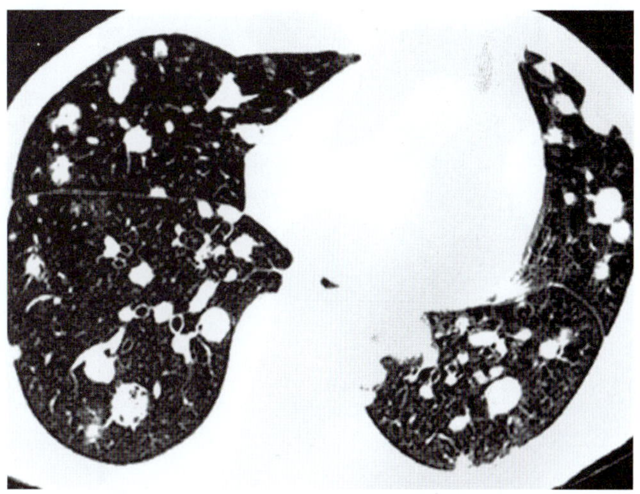

Fig. 58 Computed tomography—metastatic lesions in lungs

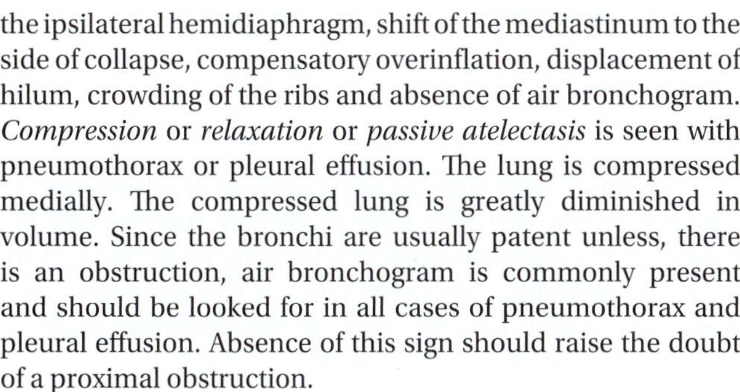

the ipsilateral hemidiaphragm, shift of the mediastinum to the side of collapse, compensatory overinflation, displacement of hilum, crowding of the ribs and absence of air bronchogram. *Compression* or *relaxation* or *passive atelectasis* is seen with pneumothorax or pleural effusion. The lung is compressed medially. The compressed lung is greatly diminished in volume. Since the bronchi are usually patent unless, there is an obstruction, air bronchogram is commonly present and should be looked for in all cases of pneumothorax and pleural effusion. Absence of this sign should raise the doubt of a proximal obstruction.

Rounded or helical atelectasis: It is a recently described unusual radiological shadow. On conventional roentgenograph, the lesion is a fairly homogeneous ill-defined pleural-based opacity, 6–7 cm in diameter, most commonly situated in the posterior portions of the lower lobes. The bronchovascular bundles in the vicinity of the mass are gathered together in a curvilinear fashion as they pass towards the mass simulating the tail of a comet (Comet tail sign). The round opacity is due to a chronic inflammatory process in the parenchyma and most often confused with malignancy. The pathogenesis of this is due to pleural fibrosis, which contracts resulting in the compression of the nearby lung parenchyma.

Metastasis

Metastatic lesions to the lungs are common from many parts of the body because blood from all parts of the body comes to the lungs and because of the rich vascular supply in the lungs. Though typically, the metastatic lesions are rounded, multiple and more abundant in the lower lung fields **(Figs 57 to 59)**, many atypical forms can be seen. This can be in the form of lymphangitic carcinomatosis (linear

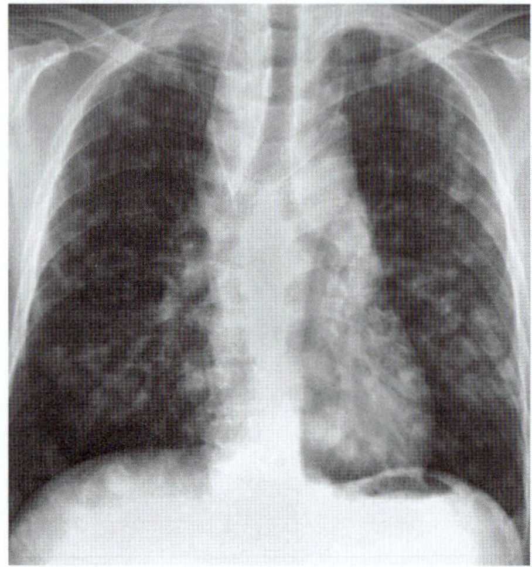

Fig. 59 Metastasis in lungs

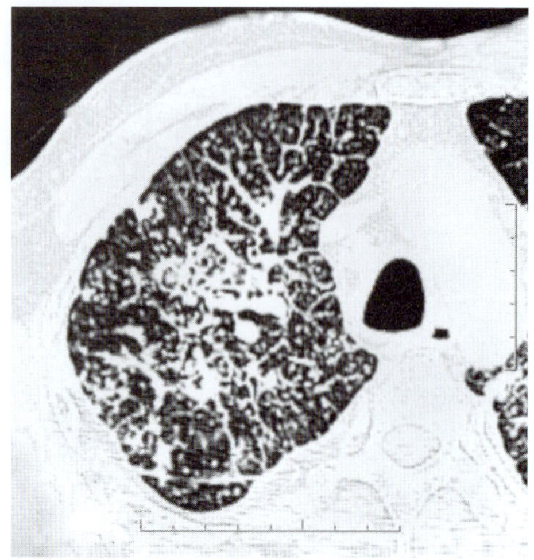

Fig. 61 Computed tomography of lymphangitis carcinomatosis

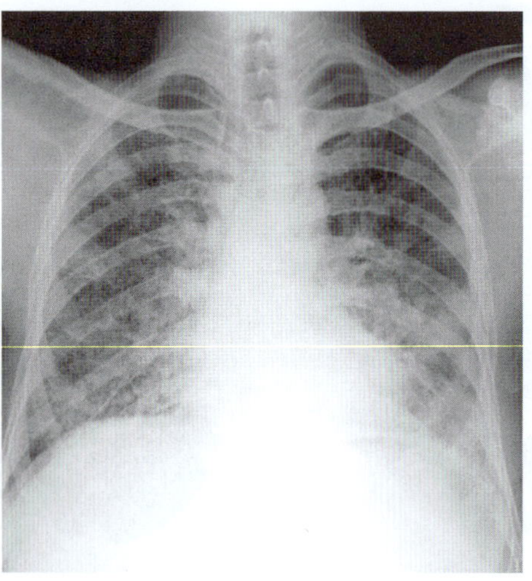

Fig. 60 Lymphangitis carcinomatosis

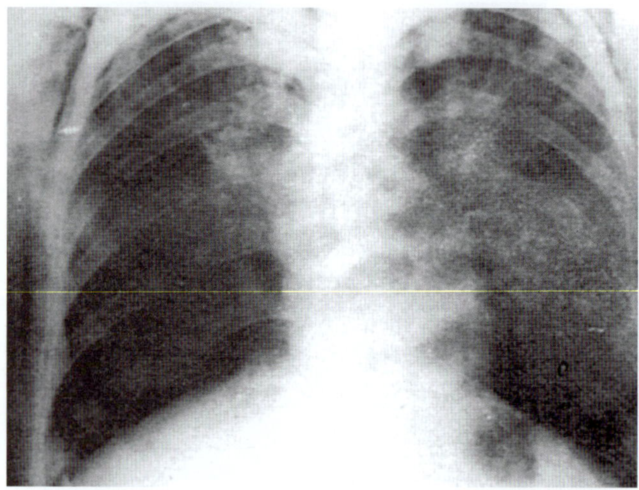

Fig. 62 Fibrosis with cavities in both upper zones because of pulmonary tuberculosis (TB). Note the subcutaneous emphysema. Rounded hyperlucent areas overlying heart and mediastinum are due to air in the tissue plane

streaky shadows) cannonball lesions and cavitating lesions **(Figs 60 and 61)**. Pulmonary metastases typically present as mostly multiple and bilateral, well-defined, noncalcified pulmonary nodules with predominantly basal and peripheral location. Ill-defined, cavitating, calcified and endobronchial metastases are uncommon. In the absence of pathognomonic findings precise differentiation from other even benign pulmonary nodules is almost impossible. Demonstration of contrast enhancement at CT or MRI or evidence of growth at serial examinations supports the diagnosis of pulmonary metastases. In uncertain cases, percutaneous fine-needle aspiration or cutting needle biopsy will allow diagnosis with the acceptable risk of complications and patient discomfort. The only relatively common complication of pneumothorax can and should be controlled by the interventional radiologist by aspiration or drainage.[26]

Fibrosis

Parenchymal fibrosis has the same findings as in a resorption collapse except that it is a more chronic process and the opacity is not uniform. Signs of chronicity in the form of rib crowding and alterations of the thoracic shape may be there. Associated cavity may be seen, as the common cause of fibrosis is tuberculosis (TB) **(Fig. 62)**.

Interstitial Disease

Four radiological patterns have been described:

1. *Reticular pattern* ***(Fig. 63)****:* These are a network of curvilinear opacities surrounding spaces of air density and are due to the thickening of the interstitium due to

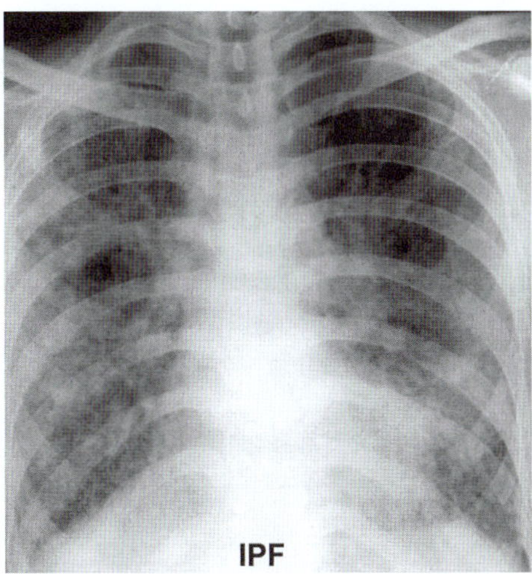

Fig. 63 Interstitial pathology

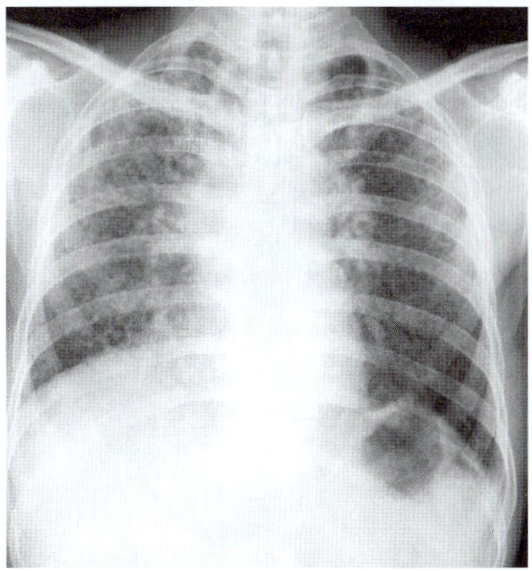

Fig. 64 Reticulonodular shadows

an increase in the total amount of tissue. It may be fine, medium or coarse. Fine reticulation is a prominence of interstitial shadows. Coarse reticulation is characterized by large cystic spaces, 1 cm or more in diameter ringed by soft tissue shadows. Medium reticulation lies between these two extremities and is characterized by 3–10 mm cystic spaces. Honeycombing or honey-comb pattern denotes cystic spaces in the range of medium and coarse reticulation.

2. *Nodular pattern:* A nodular pattern is produced when spherical lesions accumulate within the interstitium. Interstitial nodules differ from airspace nodules in that these are homogeneous, well circumscribed and are of variable size. Such nodular diseases are common in miliary TB, early disseminated hematogenous carcinomatosis, silicosis and sarcoidosis.
3. *Reticulonodular pattern **(Fig. 64)**:* When both the reticular and nodular patterns are seen in the X-ray, it is called as a reticulonodular pattern. This is commonly seen in sarcoidosis and interstitial pneumonitis.
4. *Linear pattern:* This pattern is due to thickening in or around the bronchoarterial bundle, perivenous interstitium or interlobular septa (Kerley A and B lines). Besides early pulmonary edema, lymphangitic carcinomatosis produces these types of shadows **(Figs 65 and 66)**.

Miscellaneous Radiological Features

The smoothness of contour of a shadow in general suggests a benign nature of the lesion, whereas nodularity or lobulation indicates malignancy. "Satellite lesions" are small punctate opacities in close proximity to a larger lesion, usually a SPN, and are thought to suggest an inflammatory nature of the lesion and are most common in TB.

The contour and margin of an opacity are important to decide whether it is a mediastinal, intrapulmonary or extrapulmonary mass. If the medial border is contiguous with the mediastinum and the mediastinal margin cannot be distinguished, it is usually a mediastinal mass **(Fig. 67)**.

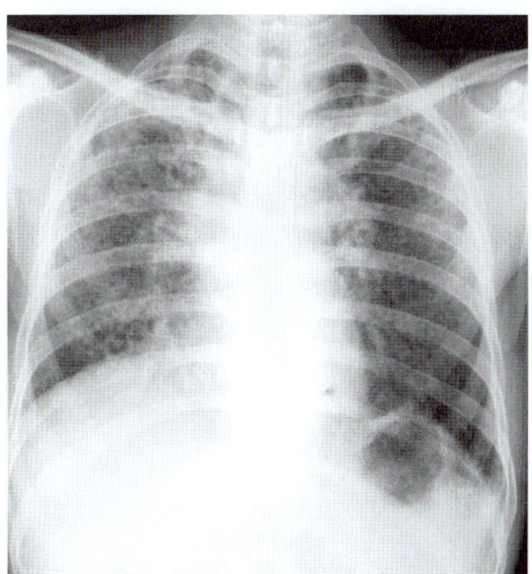

Fig. 65 Lymphangitis carcinomatosis

A mass that originates within the pleural space or extrapleurally displaces the pleura and the underlying lung inwards such that the angle formed by the margins of the mass and the chest wall is obtuse. By contrast, an intrapulmonary mass tends to relate to contiguous pleura with an acute angle. This is called the "extrapleural sign" **(Figs 68A and B)**. Occasionally, there are exceptions to this rule.

Position of the interlobar fissures provides important clues to the underlying pathology **(Figs 69 to 71)**. As mentioned earlier, displacement of the fissure towards a zone of opacity indicates volume loss and usual with atelectasis. Displacement to the opposite direction and bulging of fissure indicates an increase in the volume of the lobe and

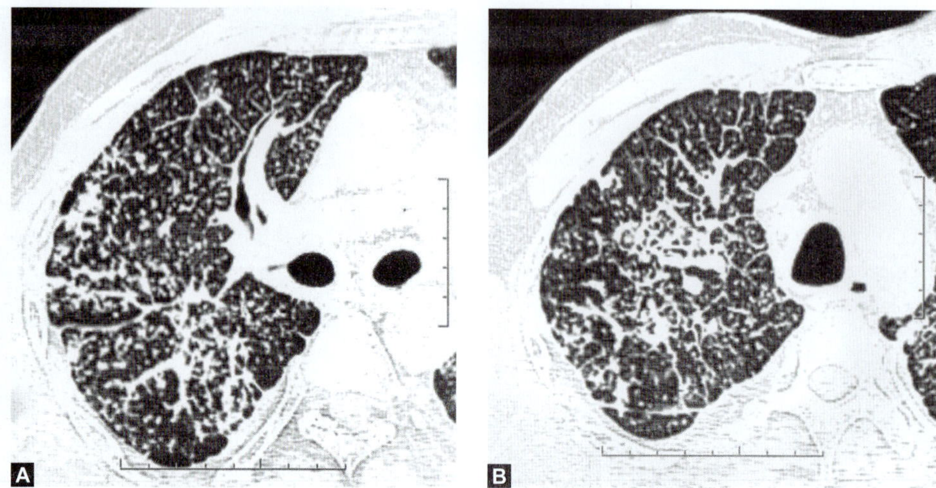

Figs 66A and B Computed tomography of lymphangitis carcinomatosis

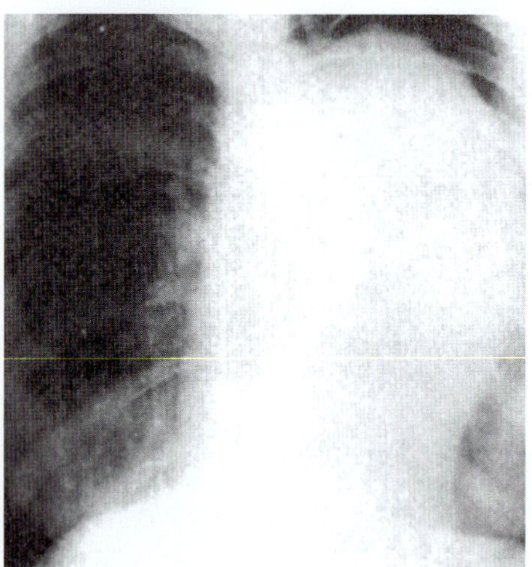

Fig. 67 Mediastinal mass. Note the medial border is merged with mediastinum

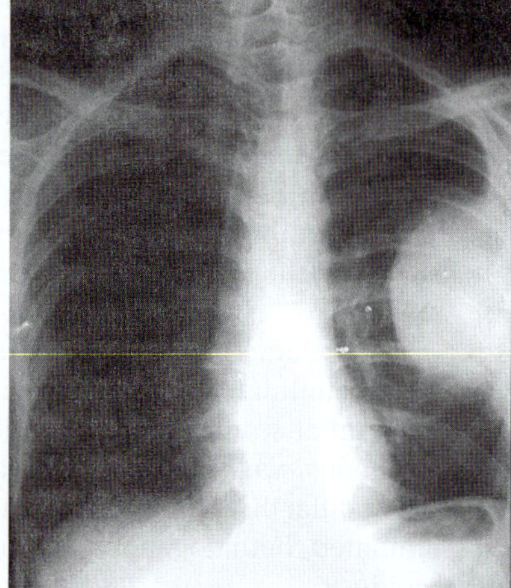

Fig. 68A Extrapulmonary sign—a case of pleural tumor

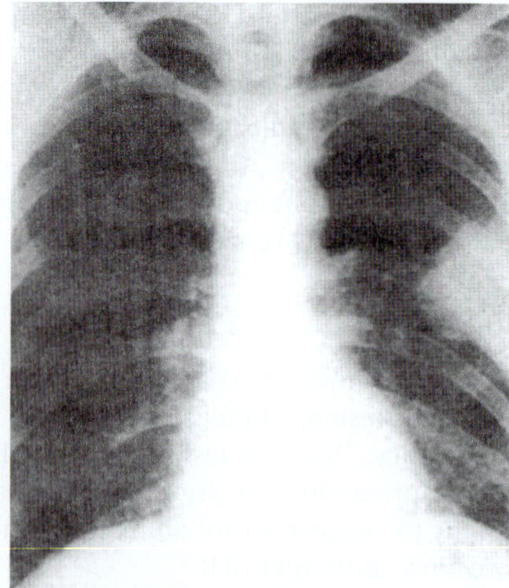

Fig. 68B Extrapleural sign. Note the obtuse angle the shadow produces

is a characteristic feature of *Klebsiella pneumonia*. Rarely, Staphylococcal pneumonia, *Yersinia pneumonia*, acute lung abscess and space-occupying lesions produce this bulging of the fissure. Transgression of the fissure is very uncommon in many lung diseases as the fissure behaves as a barrier; however, such transgression is not uncommon in fungal infections and in actinomycosis.

Cavity

A cavity is a gas-containing space with a wall thickness of greater than 1 mm **(Figs 72 to 75)**. An abscess is a cavity containing fluid. It may even be solid when there is no necrosis or communication with the bronchial tree. In any cavity, the wall, regularity of its inner lining, contents, and the number should be noted. The cavity wall is usually thick in acute lung abscess, primary and secondary carcinomas,

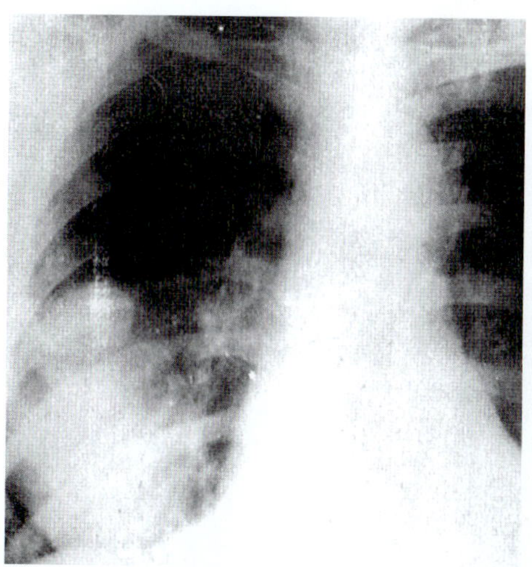

Fig. 69 Two homogeneous opacities in the right mid and lower zones. The shadows are confused with secondaries or cysts. Lateral chest skiagram (*see* Fig. 70) reveals the true diagnosis

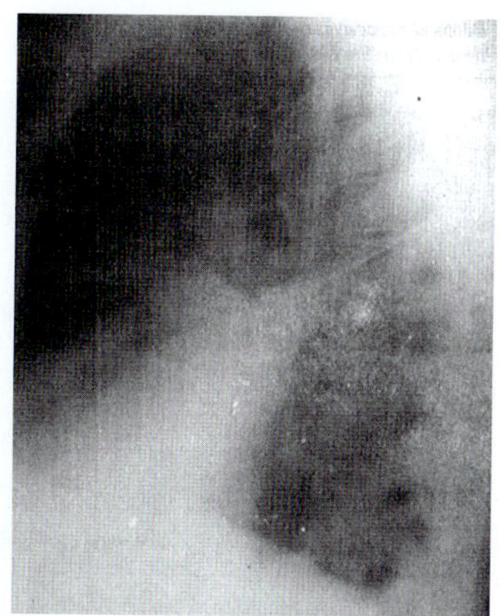

Fig. 70 Pleural effusion (encysted) in the oblique (major) and horizontal (minor) fissures

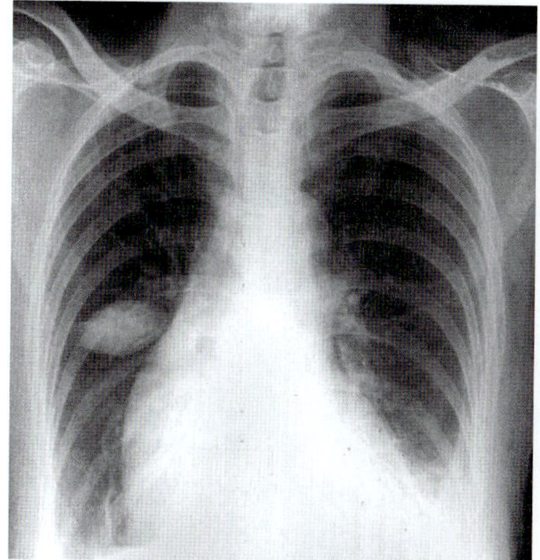

Fig. 71 Pleural effusion—loculation in the fissure

and Wegener's granulomatosis. The wall is thin in infected bullae, post-traumatic cysts and isonicotinyl hydizide (INH) cavities **(Fig. 76)**. It is observed that all lesions in which the thickest part of the cavitary wall is 1 mm, are benign; when 4 mm or less, 92% are benign; between 5 mm and 15 mm the chances of benign and malignant are equal; and when greater than 15 mm, 92% chance is that the lesion is malignant. It is important to measure at the thickest part of the wall. The inner lining is irregular and nodular in malignant cavities **(Fig. 77)**, shaggy in acute lung abscess and smooth in most other cavitary diseases. The content of the cavity is mostly liquid (pus) in infective conditions. A fungus ball or blood clots in a cavity may give rise to a crescent around the mass, and they change their position **(Fig. 78)**. The collapsed membrane of a ruptured hydatid cyst float on top of the fluid within the cyst giving rise to the "waterlily sign" **(Fig. 79)**. Pulmonary gangrene may also be present as a floating mass inside a cavity, seen sometimes in *Klebsiella pneumonia*.

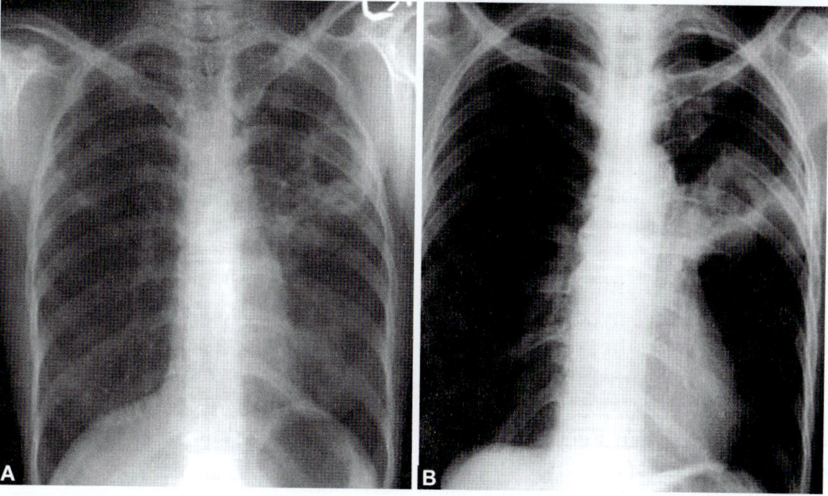

Figs 72A and B Cavities in left upper zone

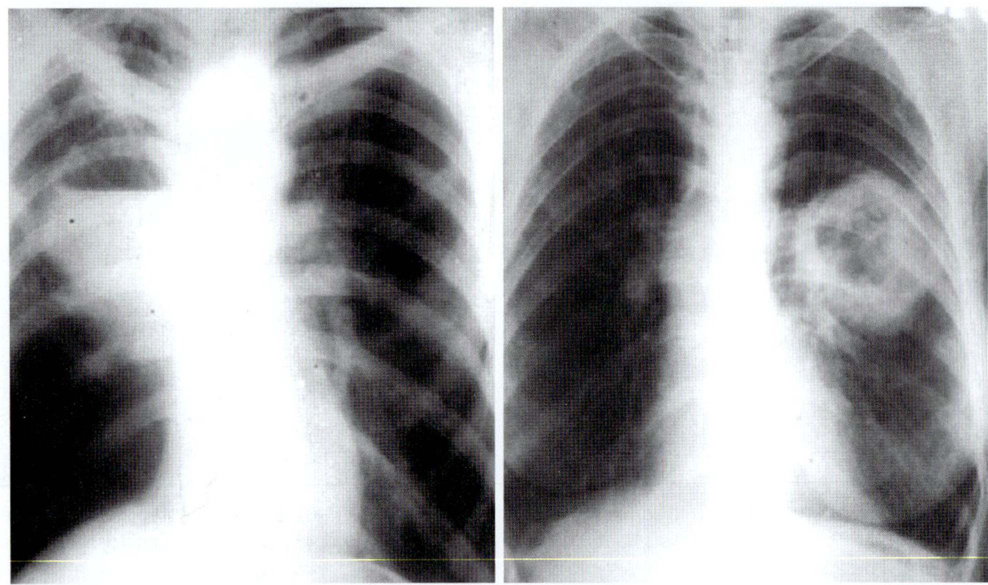

Fig. 73 Note cavities

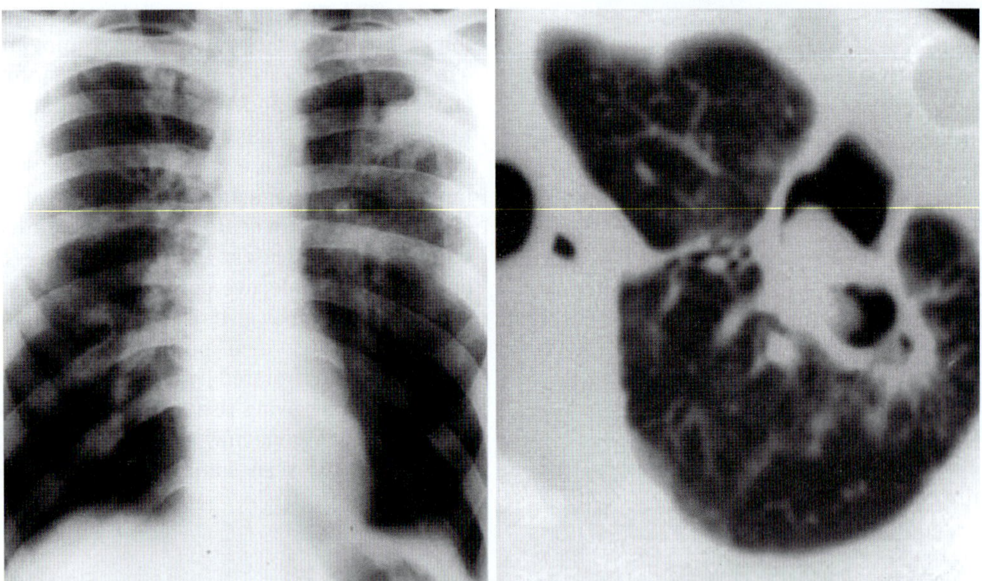

Fig. 74 Pulmonary cavitation

A solitary cavity is usually seen in acute lung abscess **(Fig. 80)**, primary cavitary carcinoma and post-traumatic cavities.

Multiple cavities are, seen in cavitating secondaries, Wegener's granulomatosis and acute pyemic abscesses secondary to bacterial endocarditis and other septicemia.

Bullae or Cyst

These are air-containing spaces more than 1 cm in diameter and less than 1 mm wall thickness **(Fig. 81)**. Bulla is associated with emphysema **(Fig. 82)**. Acute staphylococcal infections in children produce multiple cystic lesions called pneumatoceles due to a check valve type of obstruction of bronchioles and necrosis of the lung parenchyma. Other diseases producing bullae or cysts are: Bullous emphysema, cystic bronchiectasis, bronchopulmonary dysplasia and Wilson-Mikity syndrome, cystic adenoid malformation of the lung, staphylococcal and Gram-negative pneumonia, necrobiotic nodule of rheumatoid arthritis and traumatic lung cysts.

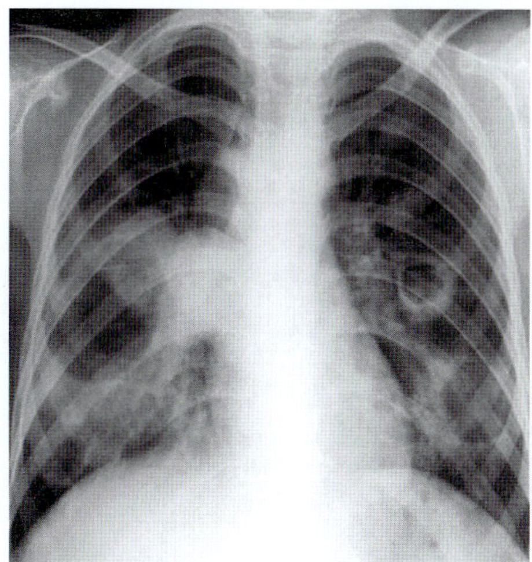

Fig. 75 Multiple cavitation

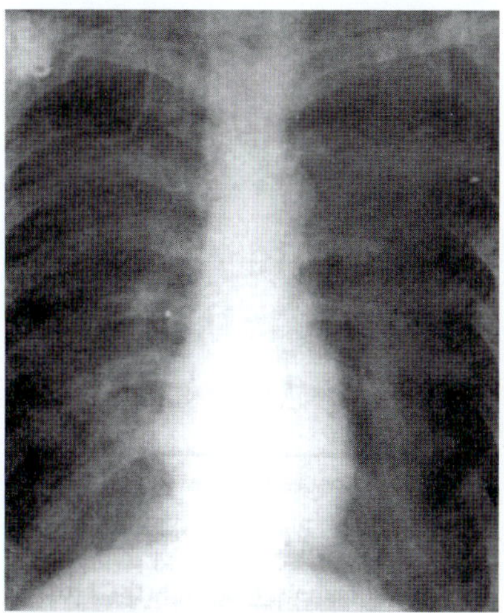

Fig. 76 Thin-walled isonicotinyl hydizide (INH) cavities in the upper zones

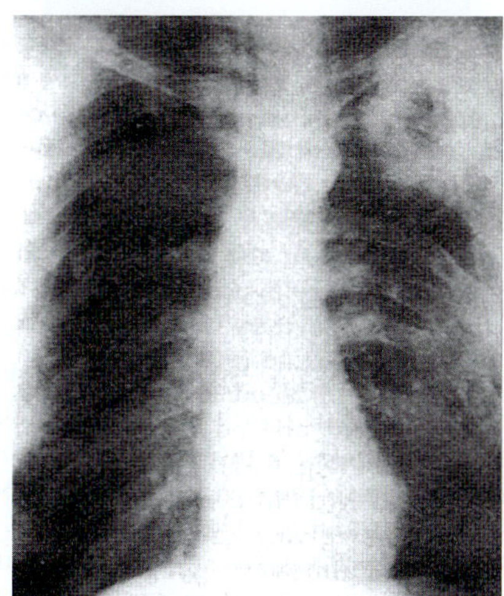

Fig. 77 Cavitating bronchogenic carcinoma (squamous cell type). Note the thick wall of the cavity

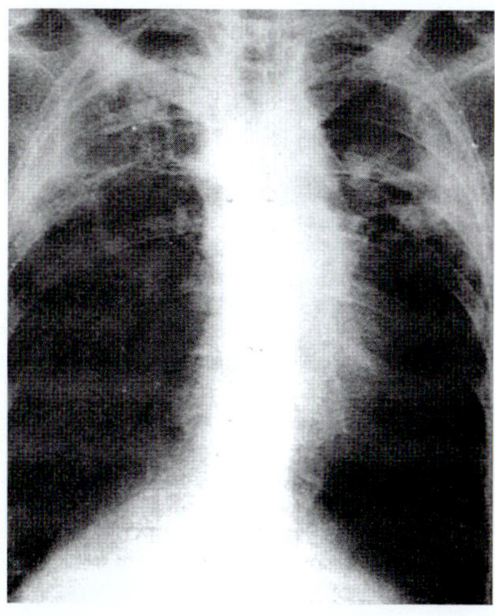

Fig. 78 Bilateral fibrocavitary tuberculosis. A homogeneous opacity is seen in the cavity on the left upper zone (mycetoma)

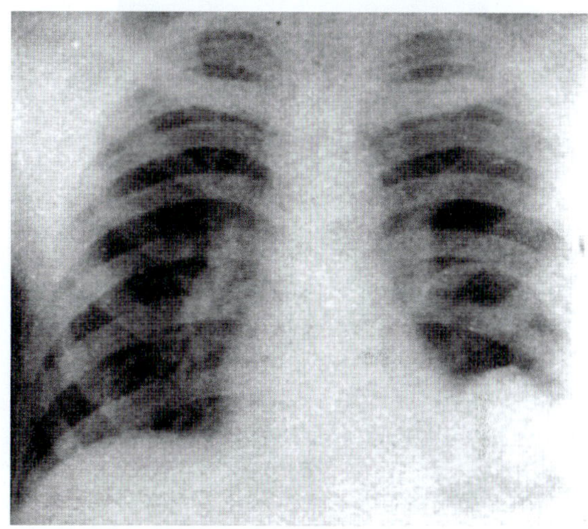

Fig. 79 Hydatid cyst in the left lower lobe. Note the "water-lily" sign

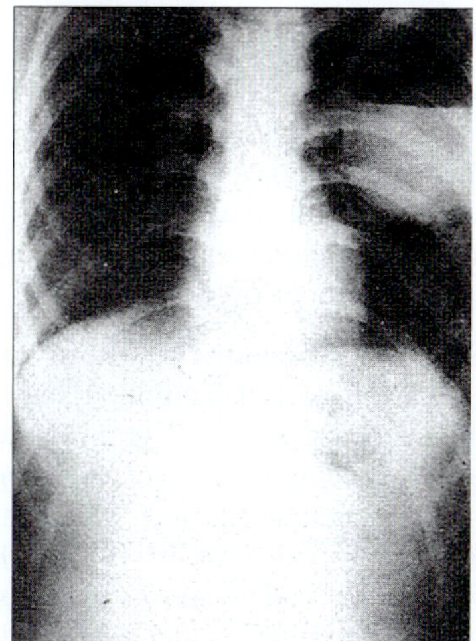

Fig. 80 Lung abscess in the left upper lobe

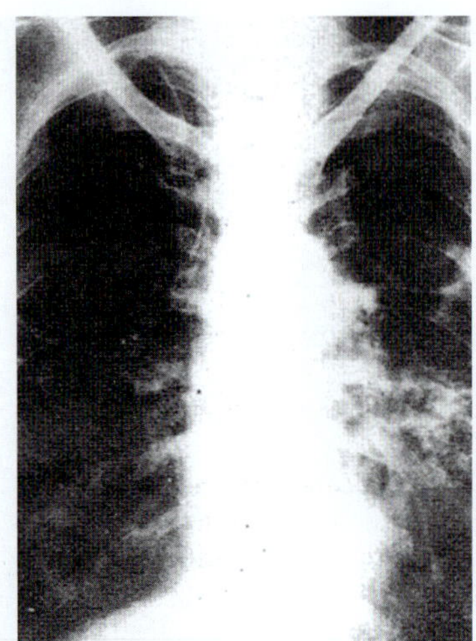

Fig. 81 Thin-walled cysts in both upper zones

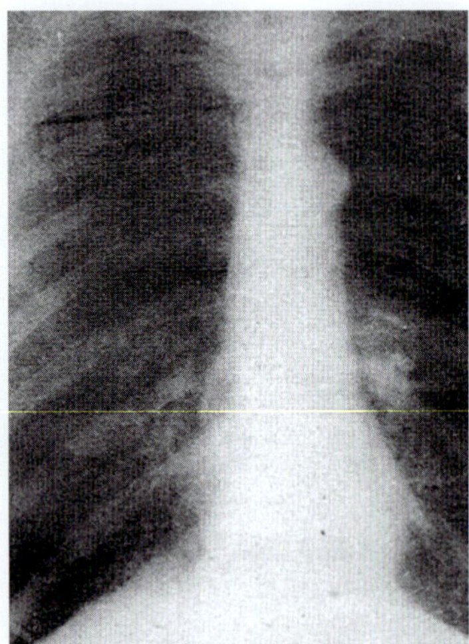

Fig. 82 Bullae seen on both upper lobes in a case of emphysema

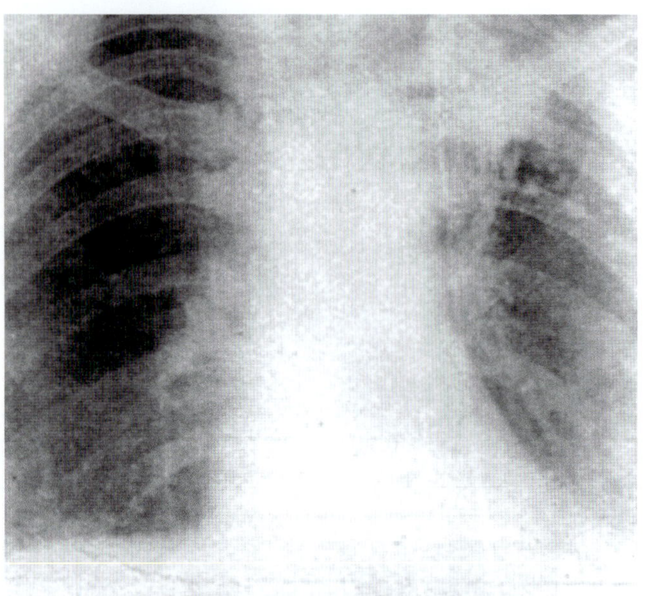

Fig. 83 Dense calcification in left upper zone after healed tuberculosis

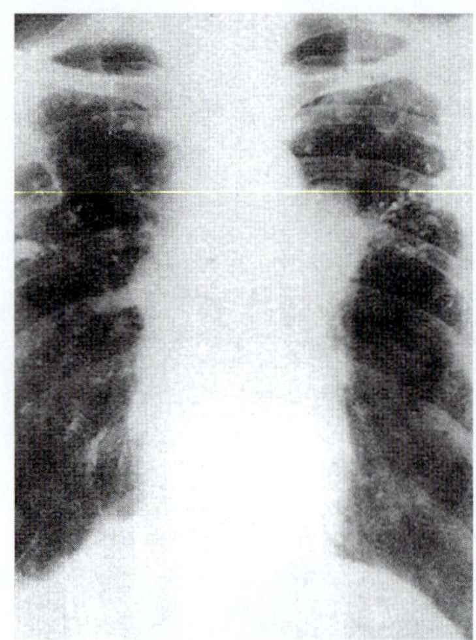

Fig. 84 Discrete parenchymal calcification following pulmonary tuberculosis

Calcification

It is an important radiological sign and should always be looked for. Most commonly, they are of dystrophic type (calcification in dead or damaged tissue) and less commonly, they are metastatic in nature (calcification of living tissue) as in hypercalcemia. Calcification may be either: (a) Pulmonary, (b) Pleural, (c) Lymph nodal, or (d) Mediastinal.

Pulmonary: Single calcifications are more common than multiple diffuse areas of calcification. Usual causes of a densely calcified focus are healed granulomatous lesions **(Fig. 83)** like TB, histoplasmosis, coccidioidomycosis and blastomycosis. Calcification in SPN has been discussed earlier. Diffuse patchy calcification **(Fig. 84)** is seen in healed disseminated TB, alveolar microlithiasis (typically tiny punctate calcospherites), silicosis (multiple nodular calcification or ossification), mitral stenosis (larger sized; greater than 8 mm in size, may even ossify), disseminated histoplasmosis and varicella pneumonia. Intensive ossification of the pulmonary tissue is rare and may occur in fibrosing alveolitis, following busulfan therapy and it may be idiopathic. Metastatic calcification can occur in long-standing hypercalcemia due to secondary hyperparathyroidism as in chronic renal failure, and specifically in those who are maintained on hemodialysis. Other causes can be diffuse myelomatosis and in conditions of elevated serum calcium and phosphorus. Metastatic type of calcification has a predilection for the apical and subapical zones.

Lymph node calcification: The calcification in the lymph nodes is irregularly distributed throughout the node and the usual causes include healed TB, and histoplasmosis **(Fig. 85)**. Egg-shell type of calcification is uncommon, and typically is a ring of calcium at the periphery of the lymph node **(Fig. 86)**. Silicosis and coalworkers pneumoconiosis are the usual causes. Rarely, sarcoidosis, irradiation of the lymph nodes, particularly due to Hodgkin's disease, blastomycosis, histoplasmosis, progressive systemic sclerosis and amyloidosis can produce this type of calcification.

Pleural calcification ***(Figs 87 to 89)****:* The common causes of this type of calcification are: Hemothorax, pyothorax, tubercular empyema and all other causes associated with a thickened pleura and fibrothorax **(Fig. 90)**. They may form a broad, continuous sheet or multiple discrete plaques.

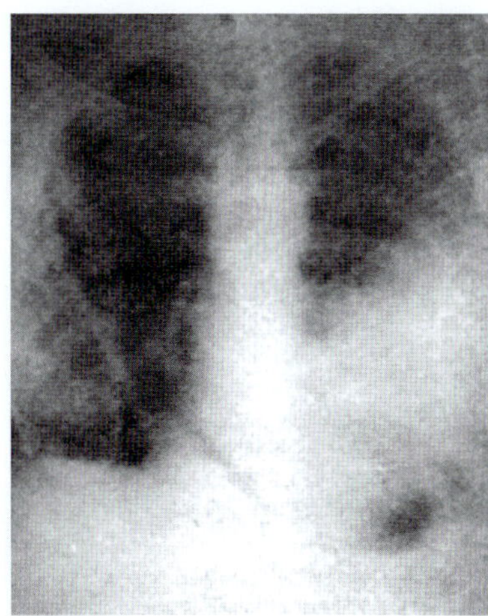

Fig. 87 Sheet-like calcification in the right pleura. An encysted empyema is seen on the left side

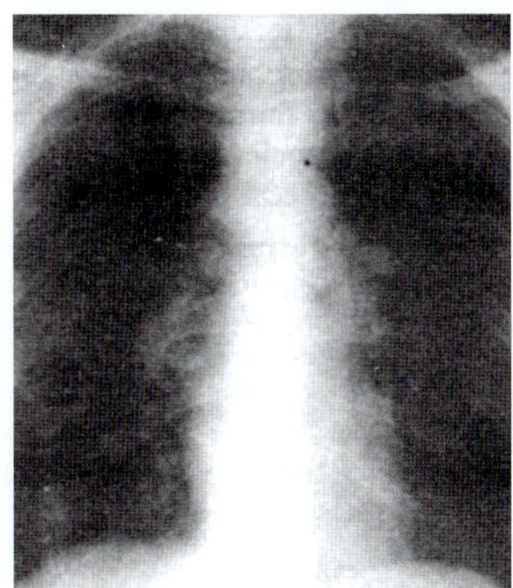

Fig. 85 Lymph node calcification in both hilar areas

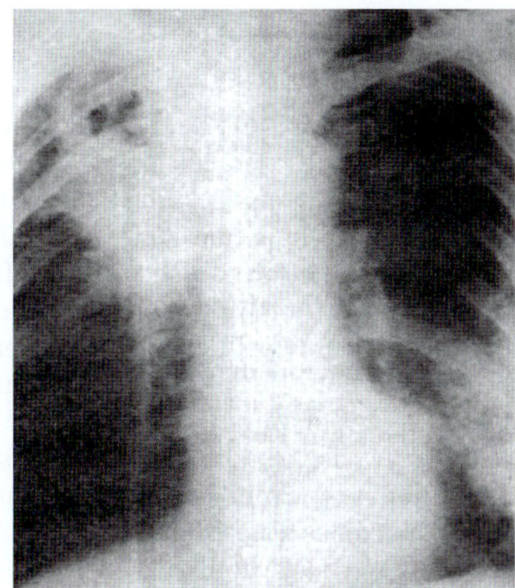

Fig. 88 Pleural calcification (left) with a cavitating carcinoma on the right side

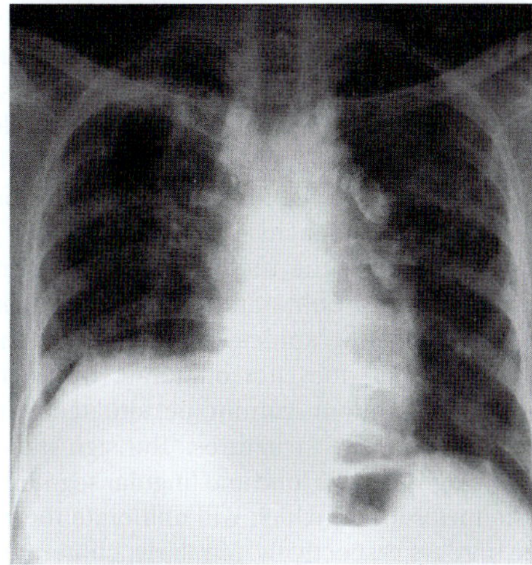

Fig. 86 "Egg-shell" calcification in a case of silicosis

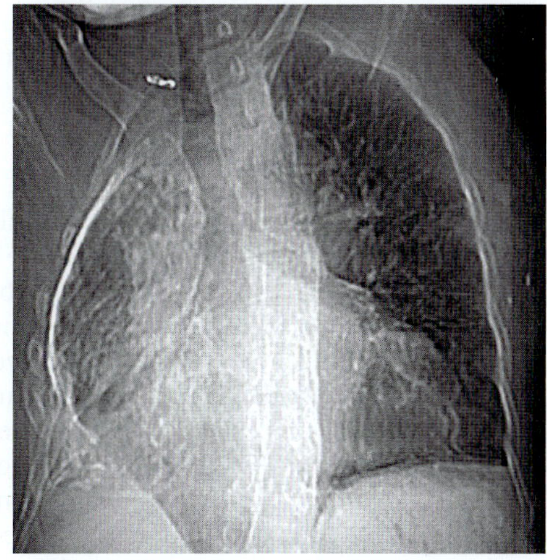

Fig. 89 Chest X-ray—dense right pleural calcification

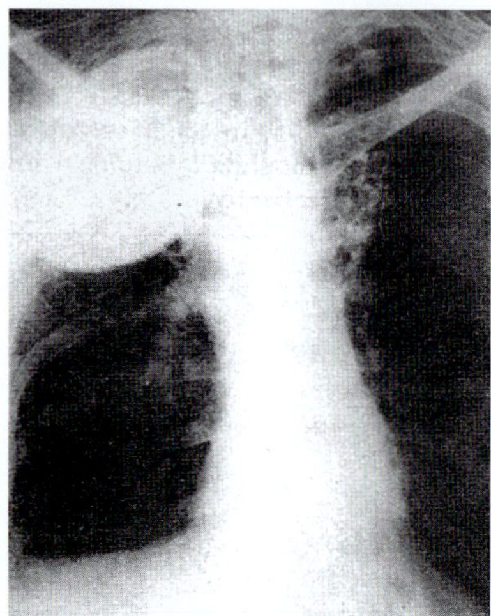

Fig. 90 Calcification in an encysted empyema. Note hilar calcification on left side

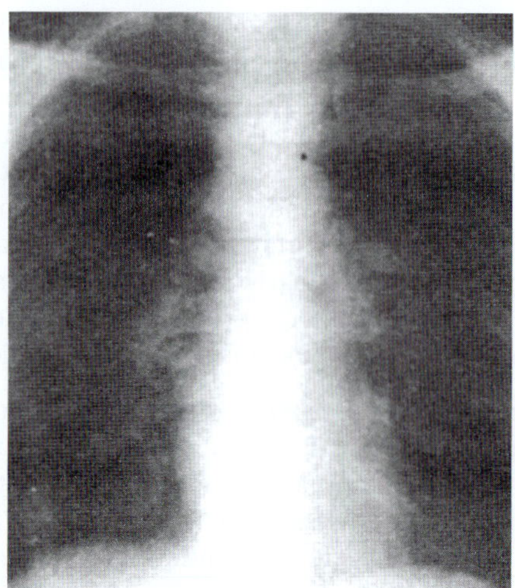

Fig. 91 Cannonball secondaries in the lungs from a testicular seminoma

The calcification usually extends from about the level of the midthorax posteriorly around the lateral lung margin going inferiorly and roughly runs parallel to the major fissures. Calcification may be on the inner surface of the thickened visceral or parietal pleura. Other causes of pleural calcification include silicatoses (asbestosis and talcosis). Calcification in asbestosis is characteristically present as bilateral plaques involving the parietal pleura with extensive thickening. It is rarely associated with pulmonary fibrosis or carcinoma, the two other complications of asbestos exposure. The exposure to asbestos for such calcification may be very short and mechanical irritation is the probable underlying mechanism of pleural calcification of asbestosis.

Other rare sites of calcification may be the cartilages of trachea, bronchi and is common in elderly women. Tracheobronchopathica osteochondroplastica is a rare condition where nodules or spicules of cartilages and bones are formed in the submucosa of trachea and bronchi and is associated with chronic airflow limitation. The pulmonary arteries can rarely be calcified.

Anatomic Distribution

Certain lesions have characteristic anatomic distribution. Aspiration pneumonia is gravity dependent and in the supine position, the posterior segments of the upper lobes are commonly affected than the anterior segments. In the erect posture, lower lobes are the common sites to be involved. The right lung is most often involved than the left one. Pulmonary infarction is more common in the lower lobes than the upper lobes because of the pattern of blood flow being more to the former. Similarly, metastatic lesions are more common in the lower lobes **(Fig. 91)** and a solitary mass in the upper lobes is rarely metastatic. However, in a bed-ridden patient the upper lobe is the common site of metastasis. Primary and cavitary carcinomas are more often seen in upper lobes. Postprimary TB in adults is more common in the apical and posterior segments of the upper lobes and superior segments of the lower lobes possibly because of a high ventilation-perfusion ratio and high PO_2 in the upper lobes. TB is rare in lateral lung zones. However, it must be remembered that this may not be true always. Primary TB commonly involves the anterior segments of the right upper lobe and middle lobe. Radiological changes in interstitial fibrosis are more evident in the lower lobes. Silicosis, sarcoidosis and eosinophilic granuloma involve the upper lobes more frequently.

Silhouette Sign

This is another important radiological sign **(Figs 92 to 94)** helpful to localize the lesion in the lungs. Although anatomical localization of most pulmonary lesions is possible in most cases from a PA and lateral views, it may not be possible when there are multiple segments of both lungs involved and when only an anteroposterior (AP) view is available for study. In these circumstances. Silhouette sign is very helpful. Normally, the mediastinum and the diaphragm are radiologically visible because of the contrast with the contiguous air-containing lungs. However, when opacity is situated in any position of the lung adjacent to the mediastinal or diaphragmatic border, that border is obliterated and can no longer be distinguished roentgenographically. Accordingly, an opacity within the lungs that does not obliterate the mediastinal or diaphragmatic contour cannot be situated within the lung contiguous to these structures. The sign is helpful in distinguishing right middle lobe and lingular segments on the left from the lower lobes, which will obliterate the right and left cardiac borders respectively. Similarly, obliteration of the aortic knuckle indicates involvement of the posterior segment of the left upper lobe; obliteration of the ascending aorta and

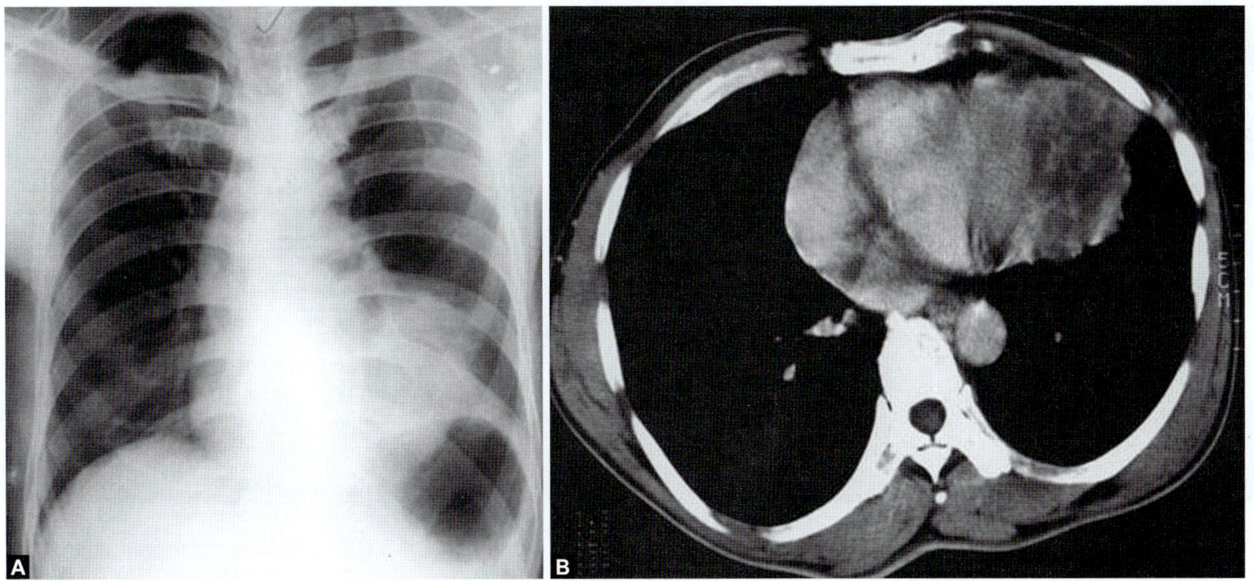

Figs 92A and B Note obliteration of left cardiac border and part of diaphragm

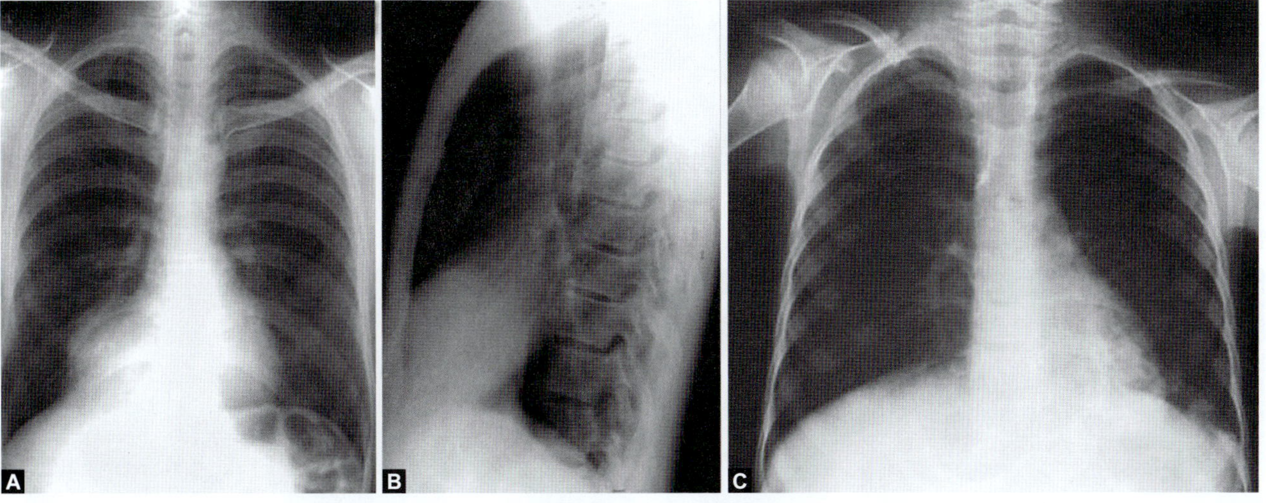

Figs 93A to C Silhouette sign

superior vena cava indicates involvement of the anterior segment of the right upper lobe and the posterior paraspinal gutter is obliterated by opacities in the left posterior gutter.

Mediastinal and Hilar Shadows

All suspected mediastinal and hilar shadows must be confirmed by lateral X-rays. Common causes of hilar enlargements are bronchogenic carcinoma, lymph node enlargement and dilatation of pulmonary arteries. Lymph node enlargement is typically lobulated and may extend up to the paratracheal glands. Bronchogenic carcinoma, tuberculosis, lymphoma and sarcoidosis may cause hilar lymphadenopathy. Whereas, sarcoidosis causes bilateral symmetrical lymph node enlargement, in lymphoma, there will be bilateral and asymmetrical enlargement of the nodes. Tuberculosis and metastatic carcinoma will produce unilateral lymph node enlargement. Rarely, silicosis, glandular fever, fungal infections, generalized drug reactions and berylliosis can produce hilar lymph node enlargement. Enlarged pulmonary arteries are due to *cor pulmonale* secondary to chronic obstructive pulmonary disease, mitral valve disease, and left to right shunts, multiple pulmonary thromboembolism, aneurysms and poststenotic dilatation

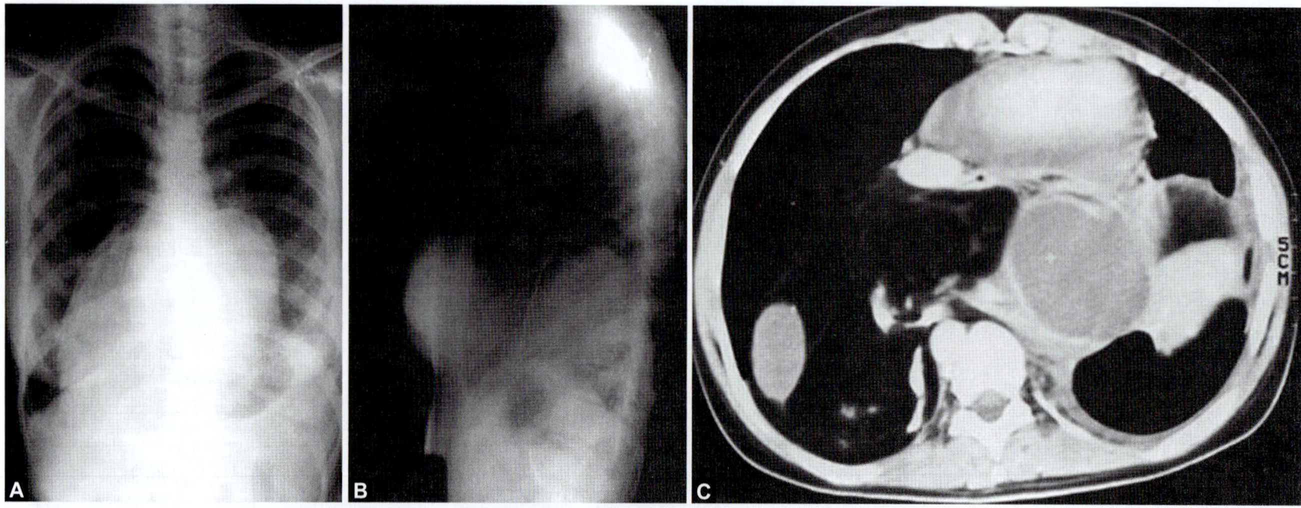

Figs 94A to C No Silhouette sign

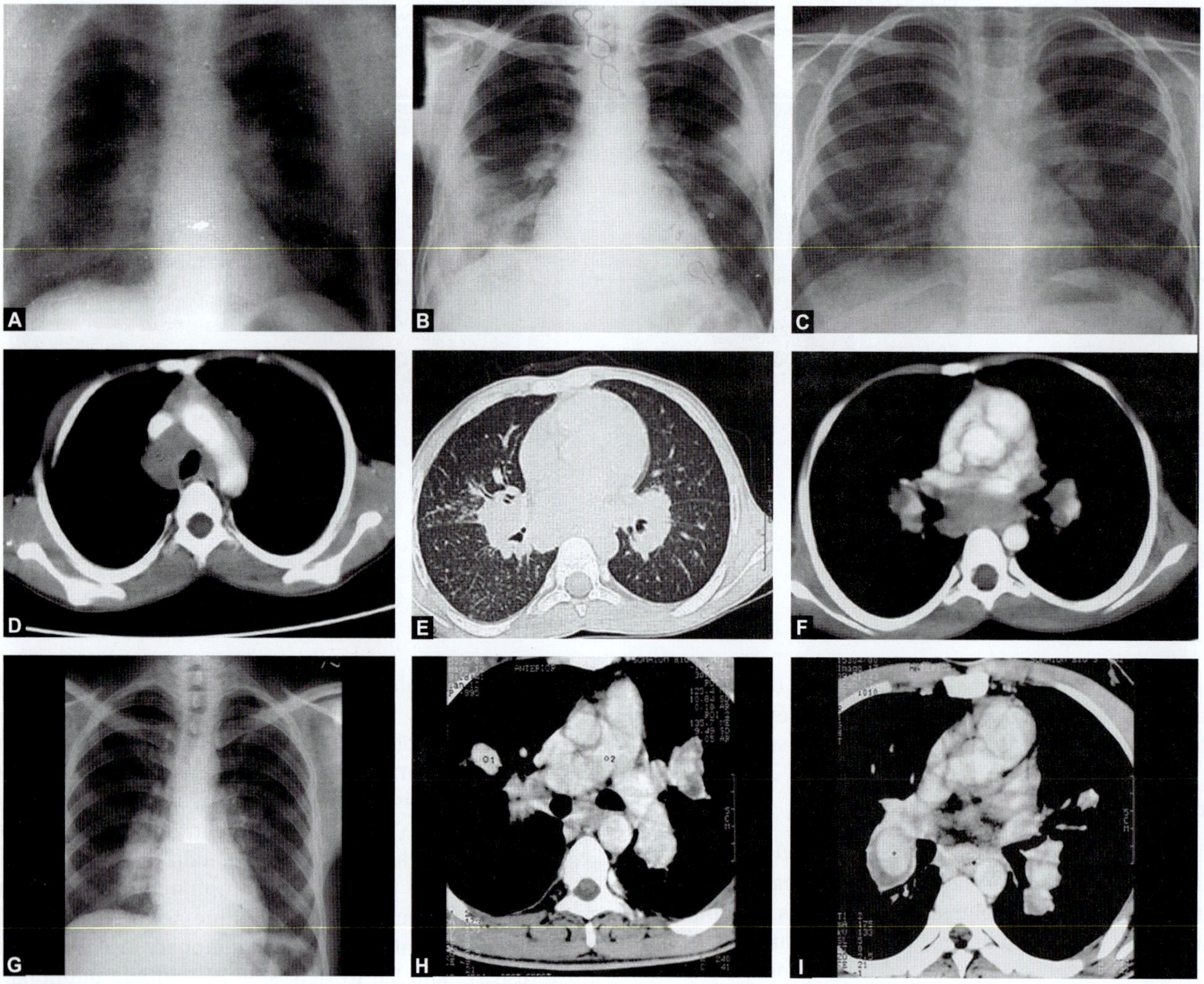

Figs 95A to I Hilar enlargement

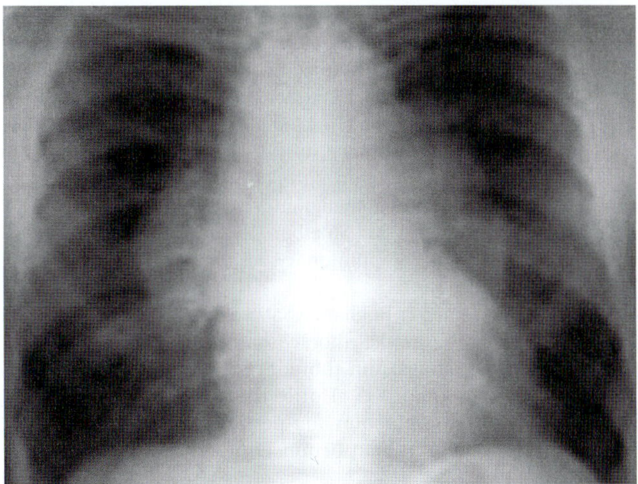

Fig. 96 Bilateral hilar lymphadenopathy

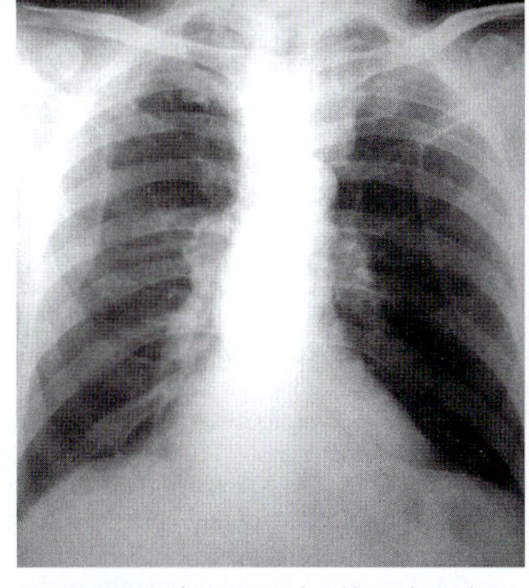

Fig. 98 Right paratracheal lymph node

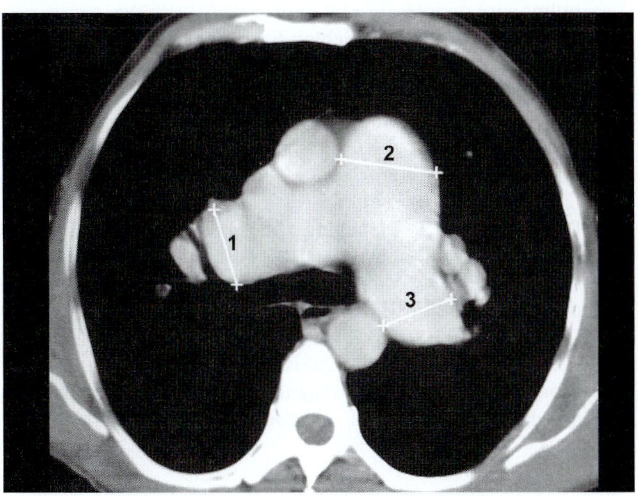

Fig. 97 Pulmonary hypertension dilated pulmonary artery: 1. Right main branch, 2. Main trunk and 3. Left main branch

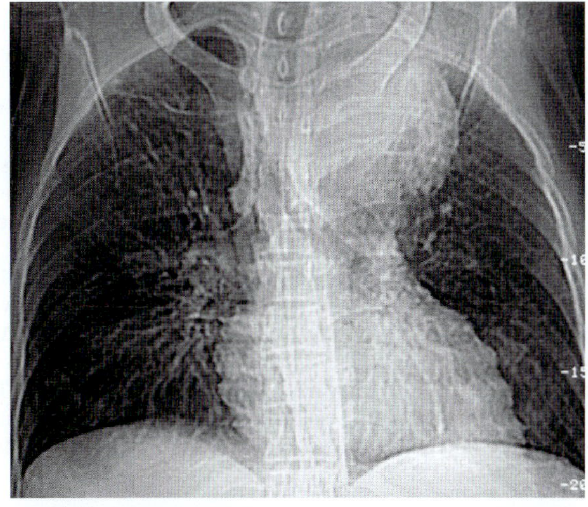

Fig. 99 Chest X-ray—Left paratracheal mass: Castleman disease

in pulmonary stenosis. It may be idiopathic also. Some of the X-ray pictures of hilar enlargement are shown in **Figures 95 to 99**.

Mediastinal enlargement will be dealt with in more detail in the chapter on mediastinum. Briefly, the anterior mediastinal shadows are due to dermoid cyst, thymoma, intrathoracic goiter, hernia through the foramen of Morgagni, bronchogenic carcinoma and lymphoma; middle mediastinal lesions include hilar nodes, bronchogenic cyst, cystic hygroma, pericardial cyst **(Fig. 100)** and lipomas; and lesions in the posterior mediastinum are mostly neurogenic tumors. Other lesions in the posterior mediastinum are hiatus and Bochdalek's hernia, esophageal dilatation due to achalasia and aneurysm of the aorta.

Pleural lesions will be discussed in the chapter on pleural diseases.

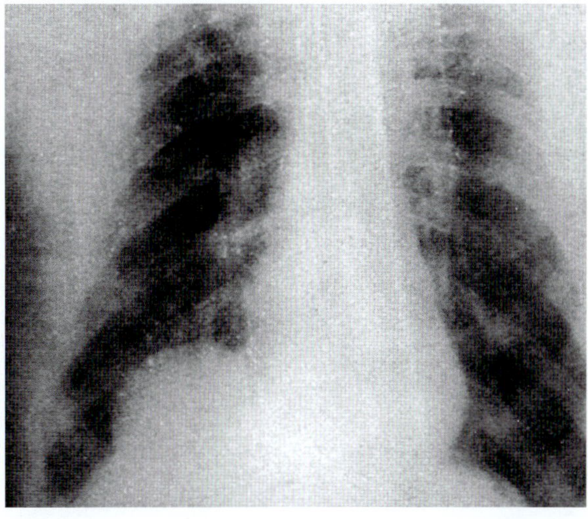

Fig. 100 Pericardial cyst right common site in the cardiophrenic angle

REFERENCES

1. Fraser RG, Pare JA, Pare PD, et al. Diagnosis of diseases of the chest, 3rd edition. Philadelphia: WB Saunders Company; 1988. p. 316.
2. Milne EN. Correlation of physiologic findings with chest roentgenology. Radiol Clin North Am. 1973;11(1):17-47.
3. Felson B. Chest roentgenology. Philadelphia: WB Saunders; 1973. pp. 22-38.
4. Simon G. Principles of chest X-ray diagnosis. London: Butterworth-Heinemann; 1978.
5. Friedman PJ. Practical radiology of the hila and mediastinum. Postgrad Radiol. 1981;1:269.
6. Vix VA, Klatte EC. The lateral chest radiograph in the diagnosis of hilar and mediastinal masses. Radiology. 1970;96(2):307-16.
7. Sagel SS, Evens RG, Forrest JV, Bramson RT. Efficacy of routine screening and lateral chest radiographs in a hospital-based population. N Eng J Med. 1974;291(19):1001-4.
8. Wilkinson GA, Fraser RG. Roentgenography of the chest. Appl Radial. 1975;4:41.
9. Tuddenham WJ. Rationale for high kVp chest radiography. Am J Roentgenol. 1980;134:200.
10. Trout ED, Keily JP, Larson VL. A comparison of an air gap and a grid in roentgenography of the chest. Am J Roentgenol Radium Ther Nucl Med. 1975;124(3):404-11.
11. Goodman LR, Wilson CR, Foley WD. Digital radiography of the chest: promises and problems. AJR. 1988;150(6):1241-52.
12. Welker JA, Alattar M, Gautam S. Repeat needle biopsies combined with clinical observation are safe and accurate in the management of a solitary pulmonary nodule. Cancer. 2005;103(3):599-607.
13. Sortini D, Feo CV, Carcoforo P, Carrella G, Pozza E, Liboni A, et al. Thoracoscopic localization techniques for patients with solitary pulmonary nodule and history of malignancy. Ann Thorac Surg. 2005;79(1):258-62.
14. Qiang JW, Zhou KR, Lu G, Wang Q, Ye XG, Xu ST, et al. The relationship between solitary pulmonary nodules and bronchi: multi-slice CT-pathological correlation. Clin Radiol. 2004;59(12):1121-7.
15. Kim JH, Kim HJ, Lee KH, Kim KH, Lee HL. Solitary pulmonary nodules: a comparative study evaluated with contrast-enhanced dynamic MR imaging and CT. J Comput Assist Tomogr. 2004;28(6):766-75.
16. Li F, Aoyama M, Shiraishi J, Abe H, Li Q, Suzuki K, et al. Radiologists' performance for differentiating benign from malignant lung nodules on high-resolution CT using computer-estimated likelihood of malignancy. AJR. 2004;183(5):1209-15.
17. Ludwig C, Zeitoun M, Stoelben E. Video-assisted thoracoscopic resection of pulmonary lesions. Eur J Surg Oncol. 2004;30(10):1118-22.
18. Pompeo E, Mineo D, Rogliani P, Sabato AF, Mineo TC. Feasibility and results of awake thoracoscopic resection of solitary pulmonary nodules. Ann Thorac Surg. 2004;78(5):1761-8.
19. Ohtsuka T, Nomori H, Horio H, Naruke T, Suemasu K. Radiological examination for peripheral lung cancers and benign nodules less than 10 mm. Lung Cancer. 2003;42(3):291-6.
20. Ohno Y, Hatabu H, Takenaka D, Imai M, Ohbayashi C, Sugimura K. Transthoracic CT-guided biopsy with multiplanar reconstruction image improves diagnostic accuracy of solitary pulmonary nodules. Eur J Radiol. 2004;51(2):160-8.
21. Schaefer JF, Vollmar J, Schick F, Vonthein R, Seemann MD, Aebert H, et al. Solitary pulmonary nodules: dynamic contrast-enhanced MR imaging—perfusion differences in malignant and benign lesions. Radiology. 2004;232(2):544-53.
22. Abolmaali ND, Vogl TJ. Modern diagnosis of lung nodules. Radiology. 2004;44(5):472-83.
23. Libby DM, Smith JP, Altorki NK, Pasmantier MW, Yankelevitz D, Henschke CI. Managing the small pulmonary nodule discovered by CT. Chest. 2004;125(4):1522-9.
24. Ost D, Fein A. Management strategies for the solitary pulmonary nodule. Curr Opin Pulm Med. 2004;10(4):272-8.
25. Lien YC, Hsu HS, Li WY, Wu YC, Hsu WH, Wang LS, et al. Pulmonary hamartoma. J Chin Med Assoc. 2004;67(1):21-6.
26. Diederich S. Radiological diagnosis of pulmonary metastases: imaging findings and diagnostic accuracy. Radiology. 2004;44(7):663-70.

Systematic Approach to Interpretation of CT of the Chest

Rubal Patel, Rakesh Shah, Sabiha Raoof, Suhail Raoof

INTRODUCTION

Computed tomography (CT) was discovered independently by Sir Godfrey Hounsfield and Dr Alan Cormack in the 1970s and has undergone substantial advancement corresponding to the progression of modern computer technology. CT has become a fundamental part of clinical decision making. Technological developments in CT have significantly influenced the diagnostic approach to many clinical diseases. This chapter focuses on a comprehensive review of the diagnostic and interpretative findings seen on CT imaging. It is broken down into three general parts: (1) the technical aspects of CT imaging with a summary of the special features and clinical indications of each technique; (2) normal components of the pulmonary parenchyma, airways and pulmonary vasculature with descriptions of specific radiographic signs pertaining to each component; (3) diseases involving the tracheobronchial tree, pulmonary parenchyma, mediastinum and a few miscellaneous conditions.

TECHNICAL ASPECTS

In general, CT provides comparatively more information than plain radiography. It provides good contrast between tissues allowing for detection of even subtle differences between tissues. Plain radiographs detect differences in contrast of about 5%, whereas CT can detect differences of less than 0.5%. Images on CT are free of superimposition of structures, thereby eliminating the effects of overlapping anatomy. Images can be obtained rapidly with a wide field of view and an ability to provide cross-sectional images of the thorax. CT can localize diseases seen on conventional radiography, assist in guidance of interventional procedures, contribute new information or detect unsuspected abnormalities.

Disadvantages of CT include the exposure to more radiation that plain chest radiography, requirement of patient transport to the CT scanner, which may be difficult in critically ill patient, and the risk of intravenous contrast administration. The wide range of indications for CT and unlimited variation of pathologic presentations make it essential to alter each CT examination to the clinical diagnosis in question. There are several technical parameters such as slice thickness, scan times, pitch, reconstruction intervals and window settings that can be selected. In general, three modes of CT imaging are currently in practice: (1) conventional CT, (2) high-resolution CT and (3) volumetric or spiral/helical CT.

Conventional CT

Conventional CT provides multiple contiguous cross-sectional images (greater than 2 mm thick) through the thorax while the patient is stationary with table position incremented between acquisitions. Narrower collimation of 5 mm may be utilized when scanning through the hilar regions; 1–2 mm to demonstrate small pulmonary nodules and high resolution CT of lung parenchyma. The conventional CT is broadly accepted and available for the work-up of many pulmonary conditions. Disadvantages of the conventional CT are motion artifact and loss of detail from volume averaging.

Multislice CT

Multislice CT has largely replaced single slice scanners and allows for extended anatomic coverage and shorter examination times.[1] Several 100-image slices are generated in less than a minute. Depending on the type of a multislice CT scanner, images can be scanned up to 64 times faster than single slice CT scanners. Consequently, they can cover more patient length per unit time, a predetermined scanning volume, or the same volume in the same time with thinner slices. The entire chest can be scanned in less than 10 seconds. There is improved temporal and spatial resolution with thinner sections and greater contrast enhancement. Diagnosis of vascular abnormalities such as subsegmental pulmonary emboli, characterization of small pulmonary nodules and recognition of airway disease are significantly improved. The distribution and morphology of diffuse lung disease is better illustrated with 1 mm collimation, can be viewed in the coronal and sagittal planes.

Reconstruction images are created by workstations that have a range of computer software programs and processing tools, which determine the quality or characteristics of the image. The reconstruction of CT data sets obtained on multislice scanners may result in several (1,000–5,000) images per examination. This makes it difficult to extract all the information presented by using standard two-dimensional techniques. Postprocessing volume imaging and 3D image display are crucial to volume visualization. Various software and workstation designs are available to improve volume visualization. Techniques such as volume rendering and maximum intensity projection, which are computer-implemented algorithms, are used to transform serially acquired axial CT image data into 3D images.

High-resolution CT

High-resolution CT (HRCT) shows very thin (less than 2 mm) cross-sectional images at 10 mm or 20 mm intervals (noncontiguous) with high spatial resolution, allowing for detailed analysis of lung structure. This provides more details than conventional CT scanning. The basic lung unit that is visible on HRCT is the secondary pulmonary lobule, around which many pathologic processes can also be visualized.[2] HRCT is particularly helpful in the detection of metastatic lesions, solitary pulmonary nodules (SPNs), bronchiectasis and characterization of interstitial lung diseases, where detailed assessment is necessary.[3] It can provide an accurate assessment of the configuration, distribution, and even the degree of disease activity and potential reversibility of diffuse lung disease. HRCT scans provide a good correlation between radiographic and histopathologic appearances. The pattern of scanning may be specified to the suspected diagnosis. For instance, scanning should be performed at 1 cm intervals for diffuse lung disease but should be limited to the involved area in focal lung diseases and SPNs.

Helical (Spiral or Volumetric) CT

Helical (spiral or volumetric) CT scanning is one major technical development in CT scanning. It provides multiplanar images of the entire chest during a single breath-hold (8–10 sec), while the patient is moved continuously through the CT gantry with continuous rotation of the X-ray tube and detector assembly. The main advantages include speed, less radiation exposure, and an ability to retrospectively construct 3D images. Respiratory motion is eliminated and volumetric data can be manipulated to obtain overlapping axial sections without additional radiation to the patient.[4] However, the requirement for breath-holding may not be feasible for patients with symptomatic pulmonary disease. It is useful in the evaluation of mediastinal abnormalities.

CT Angiography

CT angiography is obtained during a 15–30 second helical scan. The influx time of the contrast medium and the degree of vascular and parenchymal enhancement are dependent upon the concentration of contrast material, the rate of injection, and the cardiac output. It is exceedingly effective in diagnosis of pulmonary embolism. Several studies have confirmed comparable results of CT angiography to conventional pulmonary angiography.

Low-dose CT

Low-dose CT limits the radiation exposure to the patient and produces high-resolution three dimensional images. It is indicated for use in screening for lung cancer in high-risk populations.[5] The radiation dose of a low-dose CT scan is equivalent to approximately 15 chest X-rays and five times lower than the dose from a conventional CT scan. The disadvantage of low-dose CT is higher false positive results.

The special features, advantages and disadvantages and clinical indications of these techniques are summarized in **Table 1**.

NORMAL COMPONENTS OF PULMONARY PARENCHYMA

A good knowledge of lung anatomy is necessary to understand the CT features of lung diseases. It allows for better understanding of the pattern of disease as well as the specific distribution in the lung. The lung is composed of anatomical elements of similar architecture at gradually smaller sizes. These include lungs, lobes, segments, subsegments, secondary lobules and acini. Each division is organized around central supporting structures such as airways and arteries and peripheral supporting structures such as pleura and connective tissue septa.[6]

The support system of the lung consists of a network of connective tissues, which forms the interstitium. This structure not only maintains a strong structural support for the airways, blood vessels and alveoli, but also is thin enough to allow for gas exchange. The interstitium can be divided into three components that communicate freely: (1) the peripheral, (2) axial and (3) parenchymal connective tissue[7] **(Fig. 1)**. The peripheral connective tissue extends from the lung pleura to the lung septa. The septa are incomplete partitions within the lung that divide the lung segments, subsegments and secondary pulmonary lobules and acini. The axial connective tissue stems from the hilum and surrounds the bronchovascular structures, extending peripherally. The parenchymal connective tissue is located in between the alveoli and capillaries, where gas exchange takes place. It extends to the axial and peripheral connective tissues.[7]

The normal segmentation of pulmonary lobes includes three (upper, middle and lower) in the right lung and two (upper and lower) in the left lung. They are separated by interlobar fissures. Lobes are identified on CT by visualization of interlobar fissures or an avascular plane on which they lie or by identifying bronchial branches that lead to the

Table 1 Clinical indications, special features, advantages and disadvantages of various techniques of CT chest imaging

CT technique	*Indications*	*Special features*	*Advantages/Disadvantages*
Conventional	Work-up of many pulmonary conditions: • Localization and characterization of mediastinal mass • Staging of lung cancer • Detection of pulmonary metastases • Approach for biopsy	• Provides multiple contiguous cross-sectional images • Allows for scanning throughout the thorax	• Susceptible to motion artifact • Loss of detail from volume averaging
Multislice	Diagnosis of vascular abnormalities: • Subsegmental pulmonary emboli • Characterization of small pulmonary nodules • Evaluation of airway disease	• Improved resolution • Improved contrast enhancement • Ability to create retrospective reconstructions • Thinner sections	• Faster imaging • Less motion artifacts • Greater anatomic coverage
HRCT	Evaluation and detailed characterization of: • Solitary pulmonary nodule • Interstitial lung disease • Bronchiectasis • Metastatic lesions	• Thinner cross-sectional images • Provides more detail than conventional CT scanning	• Accurately assessment of the pattern and distribution of diffuse lung disease • Characterization of disease activity • Guidance for lung biopsy • Does not provide contiguous images–skips areas between the thin sections
Helical	Evaluation of various thoracic injuries: • Aortic dissection • Pneumothorax • Pulmonary contusions and lacerations • Tracheobronchial injury • Skeletal injuries such as rib, sternal, vertebral fractures • Diaphragmatic injuries	• Increased scanning speed • Improved vascular enhancement • Thinner collimation • Acquires volumetric data of the thorax, allowing for manipulation of image data • Able to generate high quality multiplanar 2-D and 3-D reconstructions	• Capable of scanning large volumes of tissue during a single breath hold • Minimizes motion artifact • Generates high quality images with the ability to show branching or oblique airway or vascular anatomy • Assists in surgical planning
CT Angiogram	Detection and evaluation of vascular abnormalities: • Aortic disease • Pulmonary embolism	• Requires rapid intravenous injection of contrast material • Ability to use volume rendering to improve diagnostic accuracy • Technical details may be manipulated to obtain optimal vascular studies	• Proper injection timing is essential to ensure imaging at the time of peak intravascular enhancement • The volume of contrast used should be adequate to maintain maximal vascular opacification throughout the spiral acquisition • With optimal technique, CT angiography can provide accurate images, eliminating the need for conventional angiography
Low-dose CT	Used for lung cancer screening	• Reduced radiation dose	• Faster scanning speed • Loss of detail • Increased false positive results

corresponding lobes.[8] Pulmonary segments and subsegments are not as easily discerned as lobes. Of the three units of lung structure, i.e. the primary pulmonary lobule, acinus and secondary pulmonary lobule, the secondary lobule is the smallest unit of lung structure that is seen on HRCT bordered by interlobular septa[9] **(Figs 2 and 3)**. The secondary lobules are the building blocks around which CT patterns are constructed. These structures are extremely important in the interpretation of lung changes seen on CT.

The interpretation of HRCT is exceptionally useful for the diagnosis of various diffuse and focal lung diseases, which are centered around the secondary pulmonary lobule. Therefore a good knowledge of the anatomy of the secondary lobule is essential to determine the distribution pattern of the disease. Differential diagnosis of lung disease can be limited by evaluation of whether the disease is located in or around the airways, the blood vessels, the lymphatics or the lung interstitium.[10]

Secondary Pulmonary Lobule

The secondary pulmonary lobules are polyhedral in shape and differ in size from 1.0 cm to 2.5 cm and are formed by a collection of acini.[2,7,10] The reported number of acini that

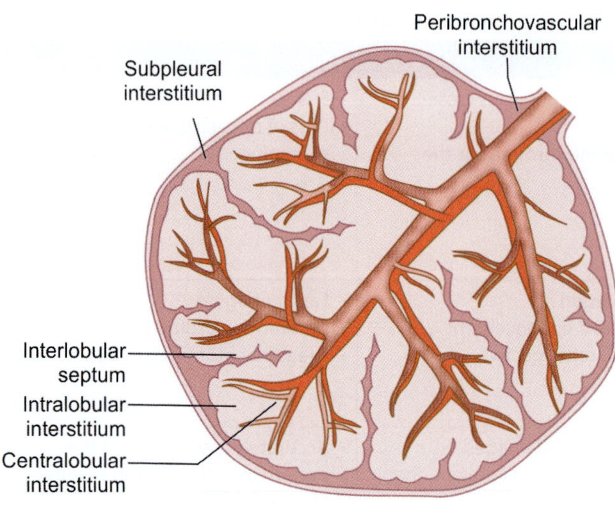

Fig. 1 Divisions of the pulmonary interstitium. The interstitium can be divided into three components that communicate freely: the peripheral, axial and parenchymal connective tissue. The peripheral support system consists of the subpleural and interlobular septa. The axial support system consists of the peribronchial and centrilobular interstitium

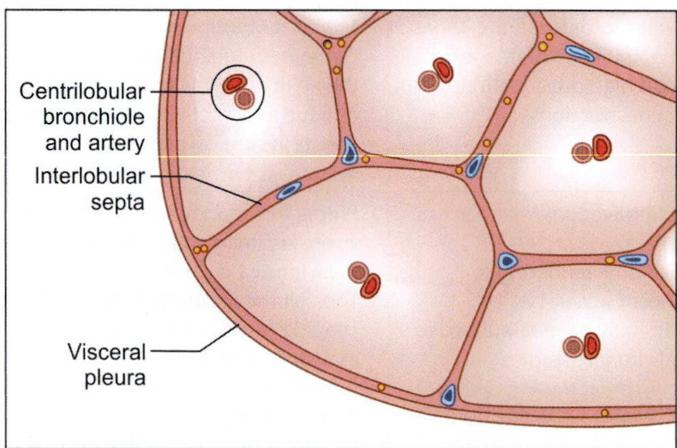

Fig. 2 The secondary pulmonary lobule. The central structures include the intralobular pulmonary artery and terminal bronchiole. The septal structures include the pulmonary venules, lymphatics and fibrous septa

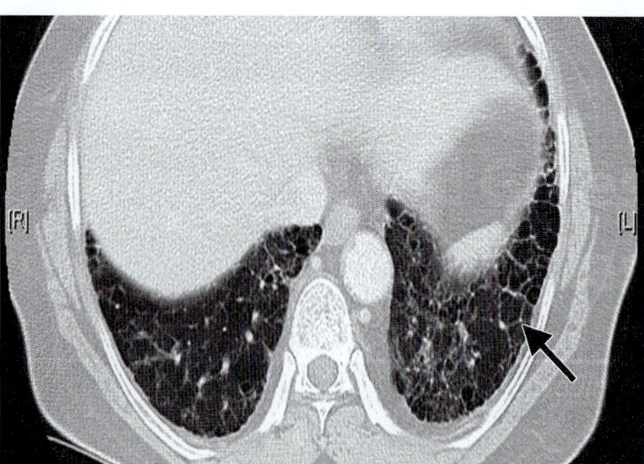

Fig. 3 HRCT chest performed at the lung base, showing interlobular septal thickening (arrow), reticular opacities and some honeycombing changes

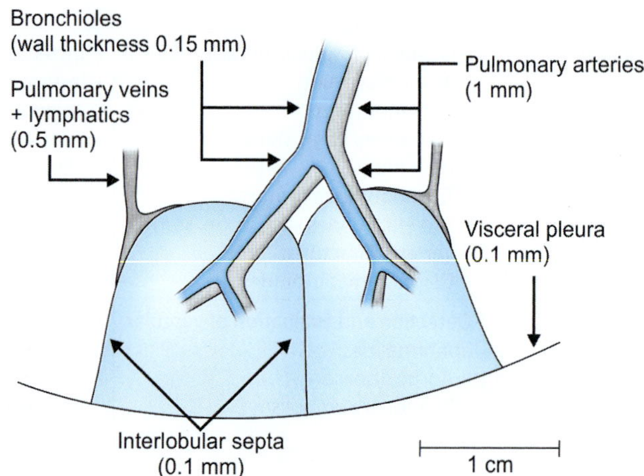

Fig. 4 The secondary pulmonary lobule. Each secondary lobule is made up of a small bronchiole and pulmonary artery and bordered by interlobular septa, where a pulmonary vein and lymphatic branches reside[10]

Source: Raoof S, Amchentsev A, Vlahos I, et al. Pictorial essay: mulitinodular disease: a high-resolution CT scan diagnostic algorithm. Chest. 2006;129(3):805-15.

form a secondary pulmonary lobule vary considerably and a range of 3–12 has been described. An acinus is the largest lung unit where all airways participate in gas exchange. Each secondary lobule is made up of a small bronchiole and pulmonary artery and bordered by interlobular septa, where a pulmonary vein and lymphatic branches reside **(Fig. 4)**.[10,11]

Interlobular Septae

The secondary lobules are surrounded by interlobular septae made by connective tissue. The lymphatic system draining the visceral pleura, courses within the interlobular septae along with the septal veins leading to the lymphatics and nodes within the hila. The interlobular septae measure 0.1 mm in the subpleural location, are much thinner and less defined in the center.[2] The thickness of the peripheral interlobular septa is at the lower limit of HRCT resolution, hence may or may not always be seen, especially in CT scans of normal patients.

Centrilobular Region

The central part of the secondary lobule contains the peribronchovascular interstitium that surrounds the terminal pulmonary artery and the terminal bronchial branches.[10]

It is difficult to discern the bronchial or arterial structures and the HRCT appearance of these structures is dependent on their size. A linear branching or dot-like opacity usually seen within the center of the lobule represents the intralobular artery branch and its distributions.[2] The centrilobular arteries are not seen to extend to the pleural surface. The airway wall thickness determines the visibility on HRCT. The wall thickness of a normal terminal bronchiole measures 0.1 mm, which is below the resolution of HRCT.[12] Therefore on HRCT imaging, intralobular bronchioles are not usually identified, and not normally seen within 1 cm of the pleural surface.

Specific Signs

The diagnostic approach for HRCT relies upon a good understanding of lung anatomy in general, particularly the secondary pulmonary lobule, the pattern and the distribution of disease, and on associated findings such as pleural plaques, calcifications, thickening, effusions, lymph node enlargement, and the clinical history.

The principal parenchymal patterns seen on HRCT include "reticular and nodular structures, increased opacity (ground-glass and air space filling or consolidation), and decreased opacity, including cystic lesions, mosaic attenuation, and air trapping".[6] Accompanying findings include linear opacities, parenchymal bands and architectural distortion **(Fig. 5)**.

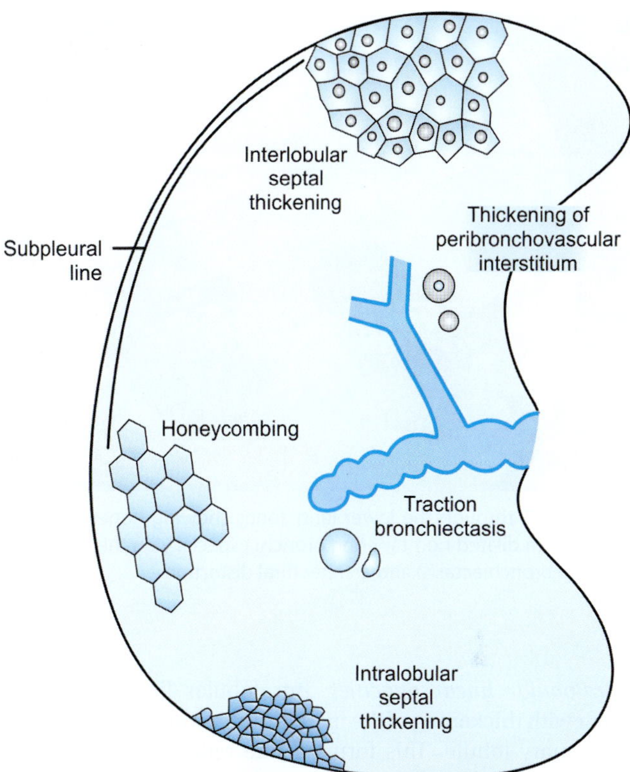

Fig. 5 Pictorial representation of reticular opacities: Thickening of the peribronchovascular interstitium, interlobular septal thickening, honeycombing and traction bronchiectasis

Reticular Patterns

Reticular opacities occur with thickening of the pulmonary interstitium by fluid, fibrosis, or other infiltrative processes **(Fig. 6)**. The reticular pattern can be coarse, intermediate or fine. The coarse reticular pattern (1 cm) occurs due to thickening of interlobular septae, intermediate reticular changes are seen with honeycombing, and fine reticular changes are seen with intralobular septal thickening. The reticular pattern may be smooth, nodular or irregular.

Interface sign: The interface sign is the most common and earliest HRCT abnormality found in interstitial disease with an irregular and thickened appearance of the normally smooth septae bordering the parenchyma with vessels, bronchi and visceral pleura.[6] This is, however, a nonspecific sign of interstitial diseases. Other findings include interlobular septal thickening, peribronchial thickening, intralobular linear opacities and cysts.

Interlobular septal thickening: Interlobular septal thickening is a characteristic finding of interstitial lung disease. They appear as 1–2 cm lines that are perpendicular to the pleura and extend out to the pleural space. Centrally they form polygonal structures outlining the secondary lobules **(Figs 3 and 5)**.

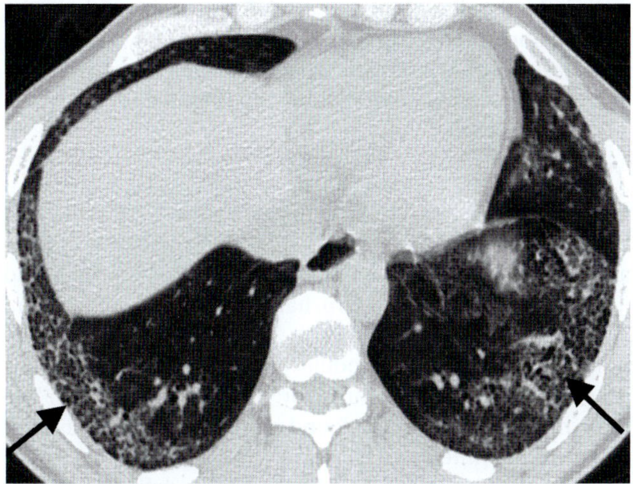

Fig. 6 HRCT through the lung bases showing subpleural reticulation in a patient with idiopathic pulmonary fibrosis. Also visible are small cysts (arrows) from honeycombing

Peribronchial or perivascular interstitial thickening: Peribronchial or perivascular interstitial thickening results from thickening of the connective tissue surrounding the bronchi or pulmonary vessels. The thickening may be smooth or irregular. Dilatation of the bronchi may result in cases where surrounding fibrosis results in traction, known as traction bronchiectasis **(Figs 5 and 7)**.

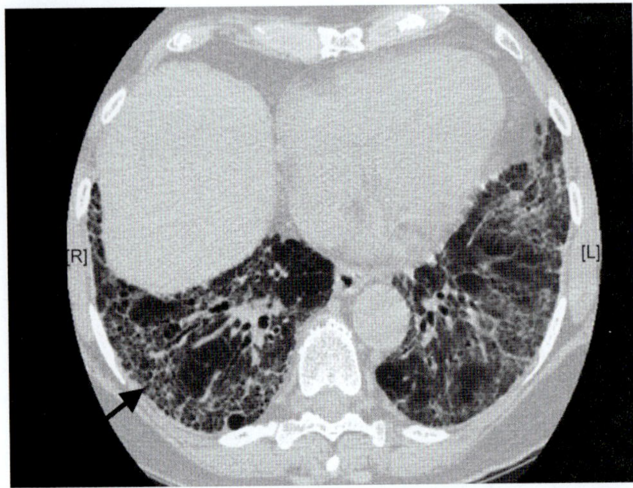

Fig. 7 HRCT through the lower lung zones showing honeycombing (arrow) with dilated non-tapering bronchi especially on the right side (traction bronchiectasis) and architectural distortion

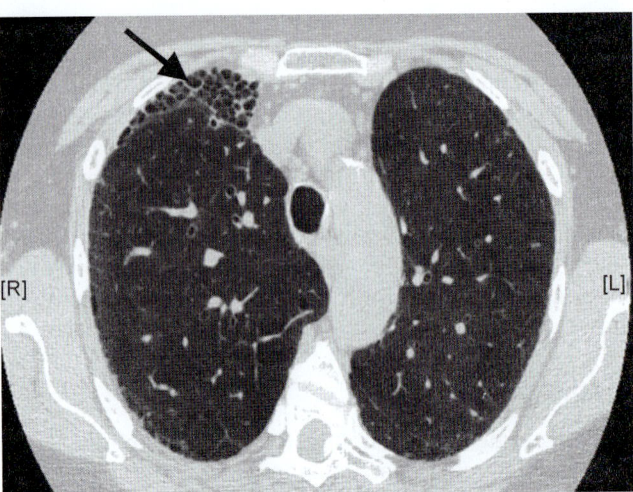

Fig. 8 HRCT through the upper lung zones demonstrating numerous cysts (arrow) involving the subpleural regions resulting in honeycombing. Note dilated bronchi adjacent to branches of the pulmonary artery

Intralobular linear opacities: Intralobular linear opacities occur with thickening of the interstitium within the secondary pulmonary lobule. This forms a fine reticular pattern with small irregular lines separated by only a few millimeters. This pattern is most commonly caused by fibrosis. The distribution (upper vs lower lobes) and associated findings vary with different diseases.

Cysts: Cysts are rounded air-containing spaces surrounded by well-defined walls. When they are 4–5 mm in size and present in the subpleural region, they represent honeycombing in end-stage fibrosis and are associated with traction bronchiectasis and architectural distortion **(Figs 8 and 9)**.

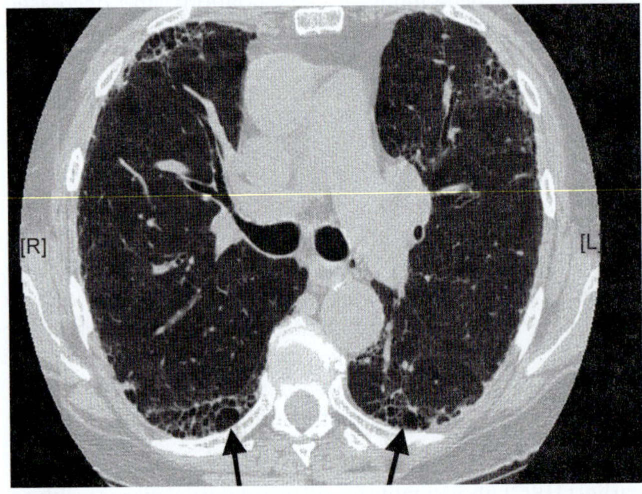

Fig. 9 HRCT demonstrating cystic changes in the subpleural regions (arrows) resulting in a honeycombing pattern in a patient with idiopathic pulmonary fibrosis. Note dilated bronchi (right upper lobe dilated bronchi) and paucity of ground glass opacity

Nodules

Nodules less than 1 cm may be seen in several acute and chronic infiltrative lung diseases. Nodular patterns include airspace lesions with ill-defined or ground-glass borders, and interstitial nodules with sharp, hazy, or stellate margination.[8] The distribution of nodules is useful in narrowing the differential diagnosis.[11] Nodules may predominantly follow a perilymphatic, centrilobular or random distribution. The perilymphatic nodules are found along the bronchovascular interstitium, interlobular septa and subpleural areas. Centrilobular nodules are usually poorly defined and are seen in the center of the secondary lobule. Random nodules occur due to hematogenous spread and thus well-defined and randomly situated in the lung.

Increased Opacities

Ground glass opacification: A ground glass opacity refers to the presence of either a "focal or diffuse and hazy", increased attenuation of the lung, which does not obscure the vascular or bronchial structures, and not associated with air-bronchograms[13,14] **(Figs 10 and 11)**. It is caused by partial filling of the air-space. Although ground glass attenuation is a nonspecific sign, it represents an active process, which may potentially be treated or reversed.[15]

Consolidations or airspace filling defects: Parenchymal consolidation or airspace filling causes opacification with obscuration of vascular structures accompanied by air bronchograms. These two features differentiate it from ground-

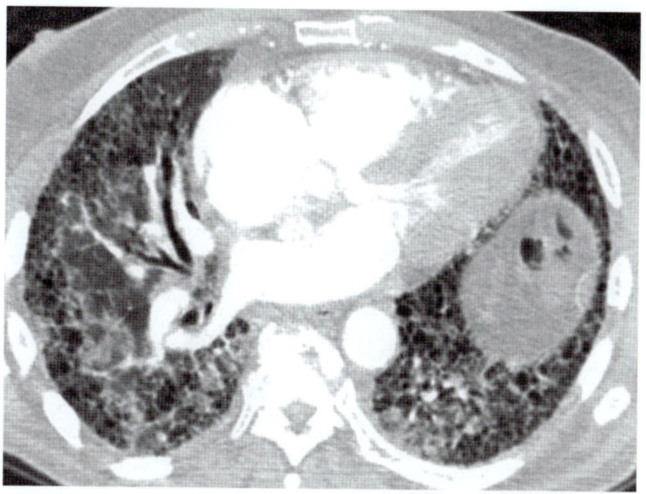

Fig. 10 HRCT through the basilar lung showing areas of extensive ground glass attenuation, honeycombing and peribronchial thickening

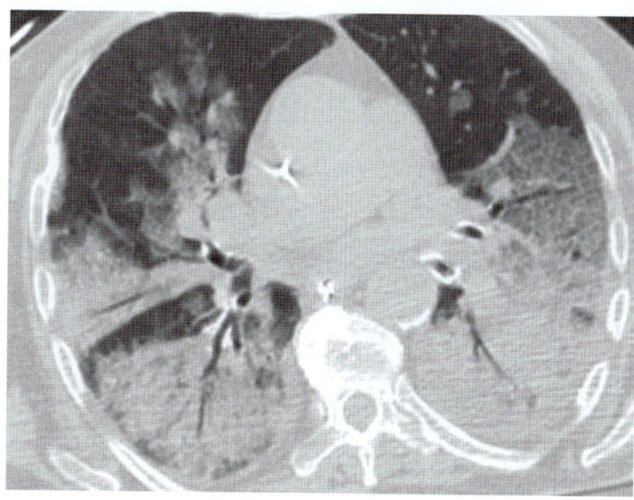

Fig. 12 CT chest through mid-lung showing bilateral dense opacity with air bronchograms. This is typical of air space disease

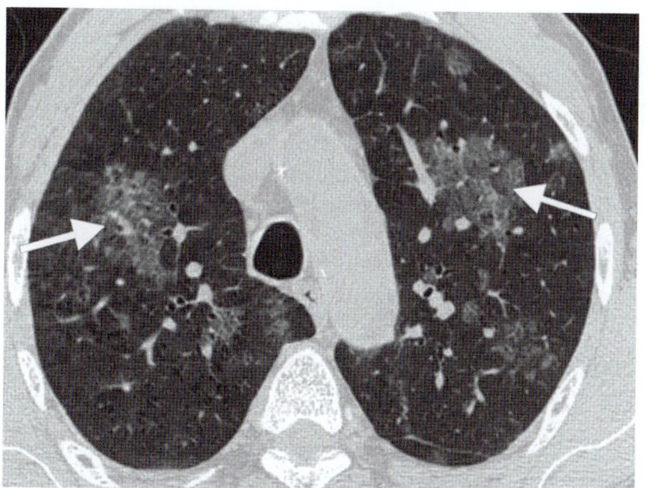

Fig. 11 High resolution CT scan of the upper lung zone demonstrating patchy ground glass attenuation (arrows) in a patient with desquamative interstitial pneumonia

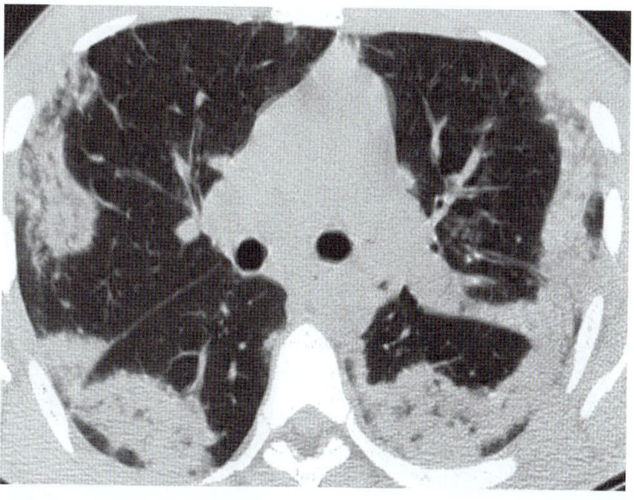

Fig. 13 HRCT chest at the level of the main stem bronchi illustrating dense bilateral opacities in a peripheral distribution. The patient had chronic eosinophilic pneumonia

glass changes **(Figs 12 and 13)**. These changes result from replacement of alveolar gas by pus, edema, blood, or cells.[15]

Decreased attenuation: Decreased lung attenuation can occur from lung damage, e.g. emphysema or diminished blood flow, e.g. pulmonary vasculature or airway abnormalities.

In emphysema, areas of abnormally low attenuation develop that may have no identifiable walls **(Figs 14 and 15)**.[16] There are three main forms of emphysema: (1) centrilobular, (2) panlobular, and (3) distal acinar emphysema.

Low-attenuated areas may also result from decreased perfusion arising from blood flow redistribution in vascular obstruction or airway abnormalities. Redistribution of blood flow away from areas of vascular obstruction or airway obstruction leads to increased attenuation in areas of normal lung parenchyma. This pattern of variable regional areas of decreased and increased attenuation due to regional differences in perfusion is termed mosaic attenuation **(Fig. 16)**.[12] The two processes, i.e. vasculature versus airway abnormalities may be differentiated by performing expiratory CT.[17] Airway disease will show no change in the lucent areas where there is air trapping, whereas in primary vascular disease, the attenuation in both the hyperlucent and hypolucent areas will increase equally on end expiration.

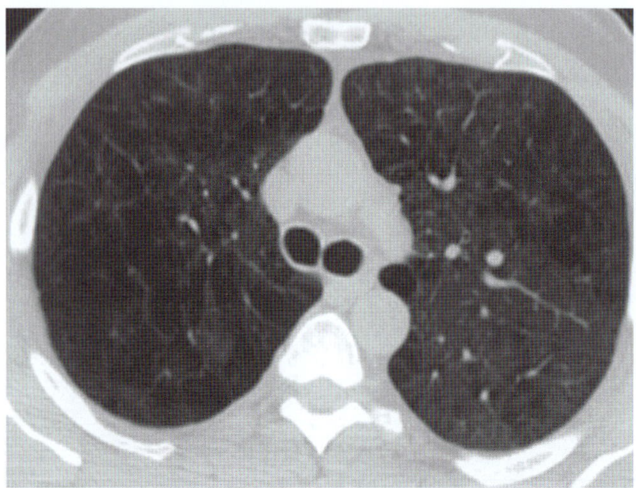

Fig. 14 CT chest through the upper lobes showing focal areas of decreased attenuation. No definable walls are visible in these focal areas of hyperlucency. This patient was a smoker with centrilobular emphysema

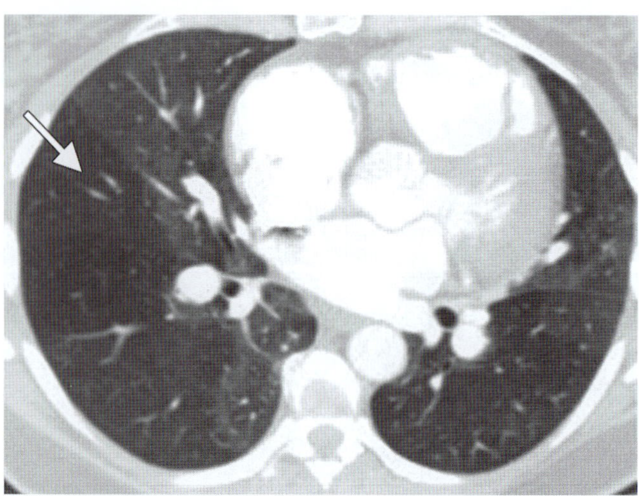

Fig. 16 CT chest through the lower lobes demonstrating a pattern of variable regional areas of decreased and increased attenuation, also known as mosaic attenuation. This patient had chronic thromboembolism. Note the decreased vascularity in the hypolucent areas of the lung (arrow)

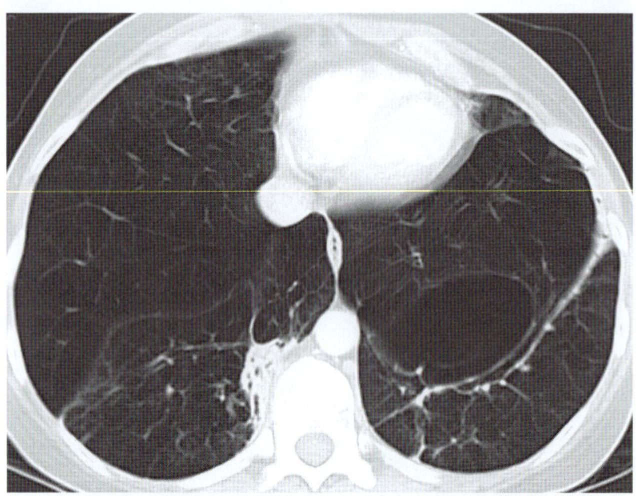

Fig. 15 CT chest through the lower lobes showing extensive panlobular emphysema in a patient with alpha 1 antitrypsin deficiency
Courtesy: Dr A Soleh

Differentiation of mosaic attenuation (due to blood flow redistribution) from true ground-glass attenuation can be accomplished by evaluating the vessel size in the increased and decreased areas. In infiltrative lung disease, the vessel size and number will be equal in areas of increased and decreased attenuation. In airways or vascular disease, vessel size and number will be decreased in regions of hypoattenuation.[17] These findings are summarized in **Table 2**.

NORMAL LUNG COMPONENTS OF THE AIRWAYS

The airways divide by asymmetric dichotomous branching with approximately 23 generations of branches from the trachea to the alveoli that become thin walled as they branch. The accuracy of CT to evaluate the central airways is well established.[18]

Table 2 Differential diagnosis of mosaic attenuation

Abnormality	*Causes*	*Caliber of vessels*	*Effect of exhalation*
Small airways disease	• Asthma • Bronchiolitis obliterans • Cystic fibrosis	Decreased size and number of vessels in hypo-attenuated areas due to regional air trapping and hypoxic vasoconstriction	Unequal attenuation in the hyperlucent and hypolucent areas No change in hypolucent areas (air-trapping)
Small vessel disease	• Chronic pulmonary embolism	Decreased size and number of vessels in hypo-attenuated areas due to obliteration of small vessels	Attenuation in both the hyperlucent and hypolucent areas will increase equally (no air-trapping)
Infiltrative disease	• *Pneumocystis jiroveci* pneumonia • Eosinophilic pneumonia • Hypersensitivity pneumonia	Equal size and number of vessels in areas of increased and decreased attenuation	Attenuation in both the hyperlucent and hypolucent areas will increase equally (no air-trapping)

Trachea

The trachea is a cartilaginous structure extending from the inferior border of the cricoid to the carina. It may be divided into extrathoracic and intrathoracic segments along the manubrium and is approximately 10–12 cm in length.[19] There are 16–22 cartilaginous horseshoe-shaped rings that form the trachea anteriorly. The posterior portion of the trachea consists of a thin fibromuscular membrane, without cartilage. The blood supply to the trachea comes superiorly from the branches of inferior thyroid artery and right intercostal artery and inferiorly from the bronchial arteries and third intercostals artery. The cross-sectional appearance of the trachea may be oval, rounded or horseshoe shaped **(Fig. 17)**. The average tracheal diameter in men is 19.5 mm and in women 17.5 mm.[20] The shape of the trachea may vary with expiration, resulting in a crescentic shape during forceful expiration, due to posterior tracheal bowing.[21]

The trachea splits into main bronchi, which divide into lobar bronchi. The lobar bronchi divide into segmental bronchi, which ultimately branch into subsegmental bronchi. After several more divisions at this level, the terminal bronchi emerge to give rise to the bronchioles.

Bronchi

The bronchi are also composed of cartilaginous and fibromuscular structures but the distribution is less regular than the trachea. They become more difficult to see in the periphery of the lung. Bronchi contain cartilage and glands within their walls, unlike bronchioles. Bronchioles can be divided into membranous bronchioles, which solely conduct air, and respiratory bronchioles, which have alveoli in their wall and are involved in gas exchange. Bronchioles along with corresponding pulmonary artery branches lie within the center of the secondary pulmonary lobule.

Evaluation of the airways should be done using spiral CT technique with thin collimation. The ability of CT to image a particular bronchus depends on its size and orientation relative to the scan plane. The main bronchi and bronchus intermedius are easily detected due to their large size. The origin of the proximal lobar and segmental bronchi can also be identified in most cases. **Table 3** illustrates the nomenclature of the bronchial tree.[22] **Figures 18 to 24** illustrate the division of the bronchial anatomy as seen on spiral CT. The bronchi and large arteries usually run together, with their diameter of approximate equal size. In general, airways less than 2 mm in diameter or close to 1–2 mm to the pleural surface are below the resolution of HRCT images.[2] The presence of visible bronchial structures in the lung periphery signifies pathologic thickening or ectasia.

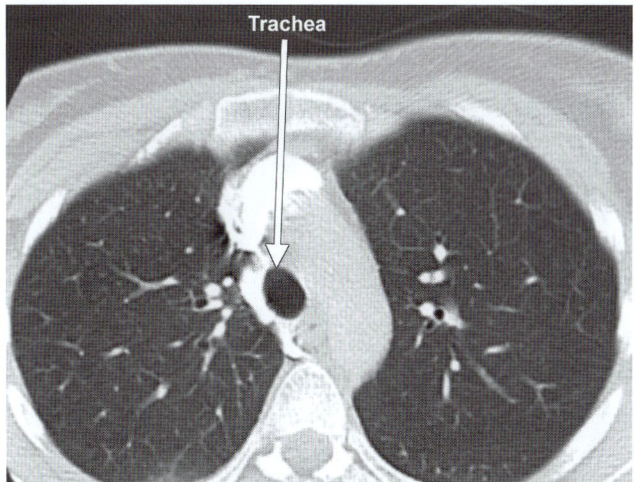

Fig. 17 CT chest through the upper lobes demonstrating normal oval tracheal lumen during inspiration

Specific Signs

Saber-sheath Trachea

A saber-sheath trachea is a condition with marked reduction in the transverse diameter of the intrathoracic trachea greater than half of the sagittal diameter **(Fig. 25)**. It results from conditions such as chronic obstructive pulmonary disease.[23]

Tracheobronchomegaly

Tracheobronchomegaly results when the tracheal diameter increases and can be due to congenital or acquired disease **(Fig. 26)**.[24] It is also known as Mounier-Kuhn syndrome

Table 3 Nomenclature of the bronchial tree

	Right lung			*Left lung*		
Lobes	*Upper*	*Middle*	*Lower*	*Upper*		*Lower*
Segments	Apical	Lateral	Superior	Upper division	Lower (Linguar division)	Superior
	Posterior	Medial	Medial basal	Apical posterior	Superior	Anterior-medial basal
	Anterior		Anterior basal Lateral basal Posterior basal	Anterior	Inferior	Lateral-basal Posterior-basal

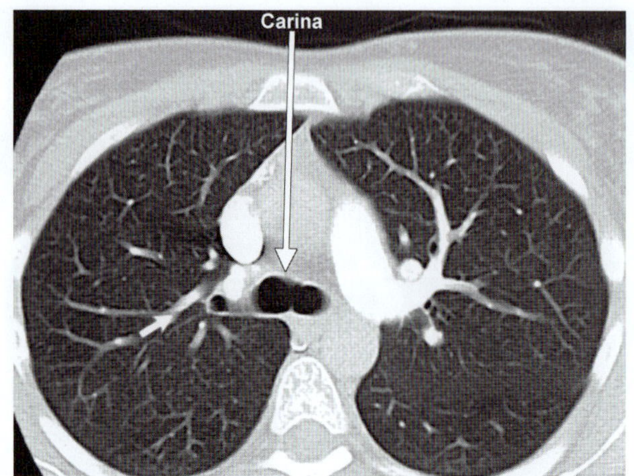

Fig. 18 CT chest showing tracheal division into the right and left main stem bronchi. Note the cross-sectional cut of the right upper lobe (thick arrow). Of note, a patchy area of hazy opacity is seen in the left upper lobe laterally

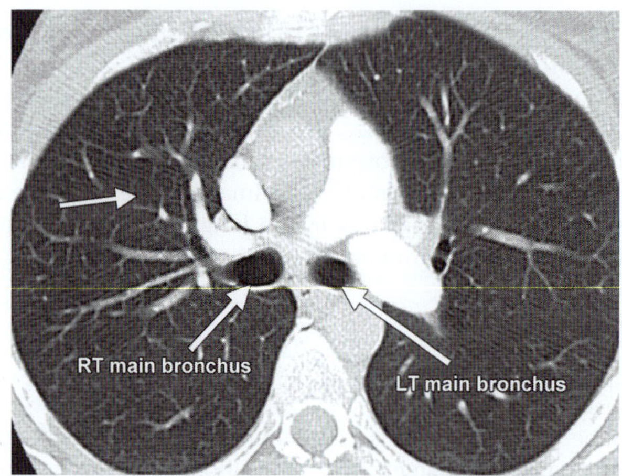

Fig. 19 CT chest showing the right and left main stem bronchi. Note the illustration of the right upper lobe (thick arrow), which almost always lies in the plane of scan

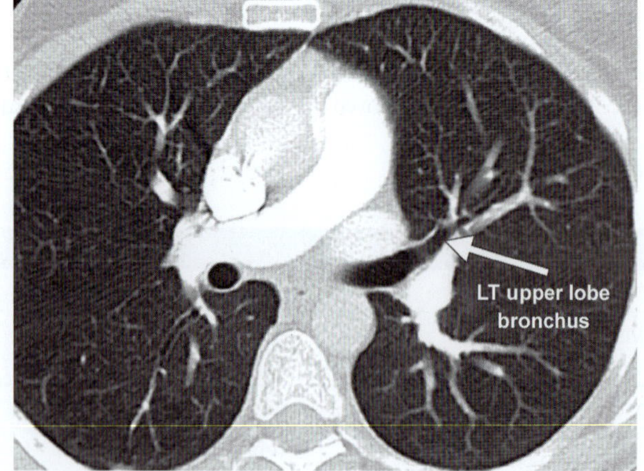

Fig. 20 CT chest at the level of the left main stem bronchus showing the left upper lobe and bronchus

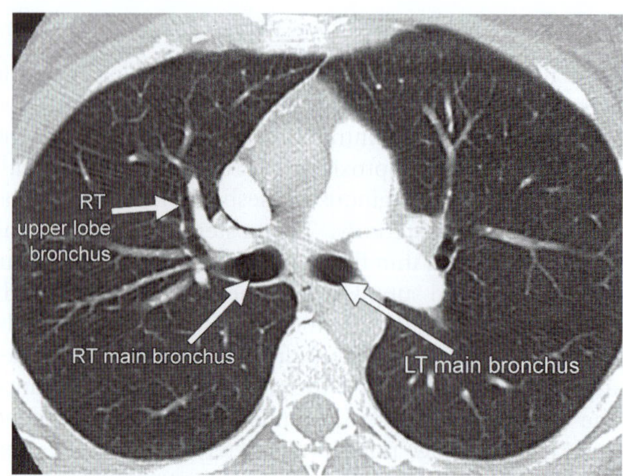

Fig. 21 CT chest showing left and right main stem bronchi with the take off of the right upper lobe bronchus

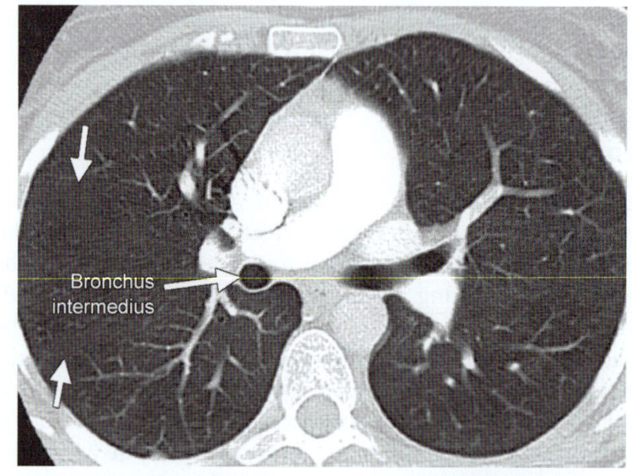

Fig. 22 CT chest illustrating a cross-sectional image of the bronchus intermedius and the left upper lobe bronchus. Note the presence of the minor fissure in the left lung, which is visible as an area with relative paucity of bronchovascular markings (thick arrows)

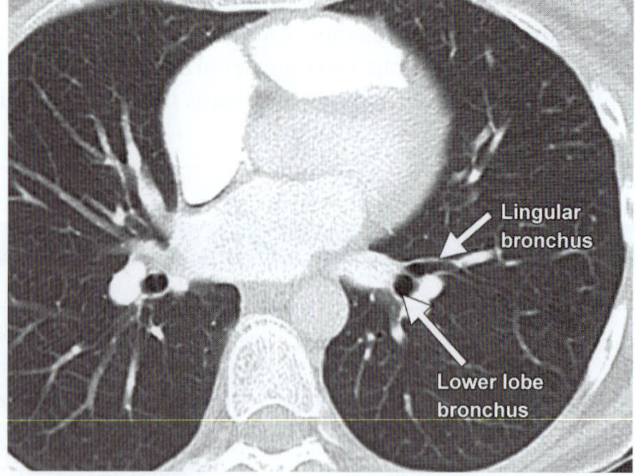

Fig. 23 CT chest showing the origin of the lingular and left lower lobe bronchus

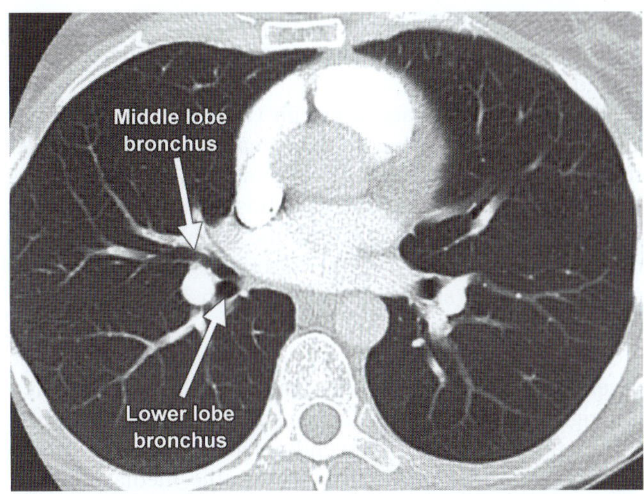

Fig. 24 CT chest illustrating right middle lobe and right lower lobe bronchi

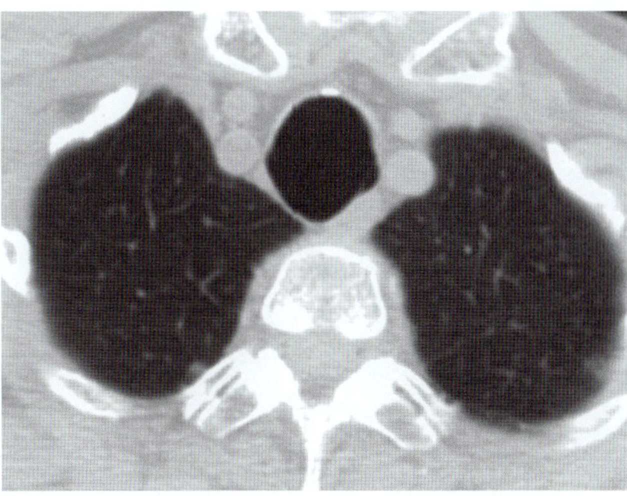

Fig. 26 CT chest showing an increased trachea diameter, resulting in tracheomegaly or Mounier-Kuhn syndrome. The normal tracheal diameter is 19.5 mm in a male and 17.5 mm in a female

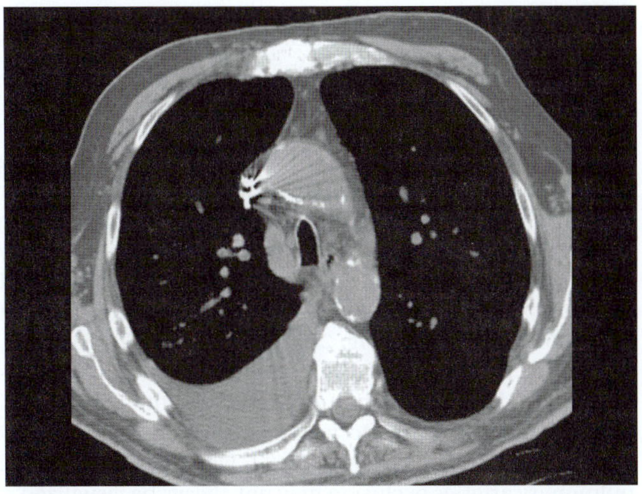

Fig. 25 CT chest showing marked reduction in the coronal diameter of the trachea as compared to the sagittal diameter indicating the characteristic appearance of a saber-sheath trachea. Of note, there is a moderate sized pleural effusion on the right

and is commonly associated with tracheal diverticulosis, bronchiectasis and recurrent infections.

Tracheal Diverticulosis

Tracheal diverticulosis results from outpouching of the posterolateral tracheal wall secondary to weakness in the trachealis muscle. It may be congenital or acquired and is associated with recurrent infections and hemoptysis.[25] On CT imaging, a small focal paratracheal air column is a classic appearance for a tracheal diverticulum.[26]

Tracheobronchopathia Osteochondroplastica

Tracheobronchopathia osteochondroplastica (TBO) is a rare benign condition of unknown etiology characterized by multiple submucosal osteocartilaginous nodules involving the trachea and main stem bronchial walls **(Fig. 27)**. On CT, there is tracheal scalloping and nodularity with irregular narrowing of the trachea. It spares the posterior tracheal membrane.[27]

Tracheobronchomalacia

Tracheobronchomalacia (TBM) is a common, under-recognized cause of dyspnea and cough. It is a condition that results in excessive airway collapse of the tracheal and bronchial walls. By definition, in patients with TBM, the cross-sectional area of the trachea shows a reduction of at least 50% during quiet breathing, forming a crescent-shaped airway **(Fig. 28)**. It can result from several etiologies including but not limited to external trauma, postintubation, chronic obstructive pulmonary diseases and chronic inflammatory diseases such as relapsing polychondritis. It is best diagnosed by paired inspiratory and expiratory dynamic CT imaging.[28]

Tracheal Bronchus

A tracheal bronchus is an uncommon anomaly in which an ectopic bronchus arises from the trachea above the carina. It is more common on the right but can occur on either side.[26]

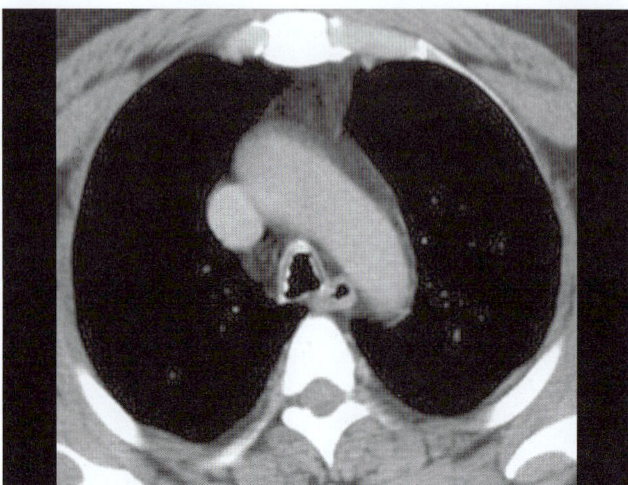

Fig. 27 CT chest section through the mid-trachea showing nodularity of the trachea with calcifications and sparing of the posterior tracheal wall, a characteristic finding in tracheobronchopathia osteochondroplastica

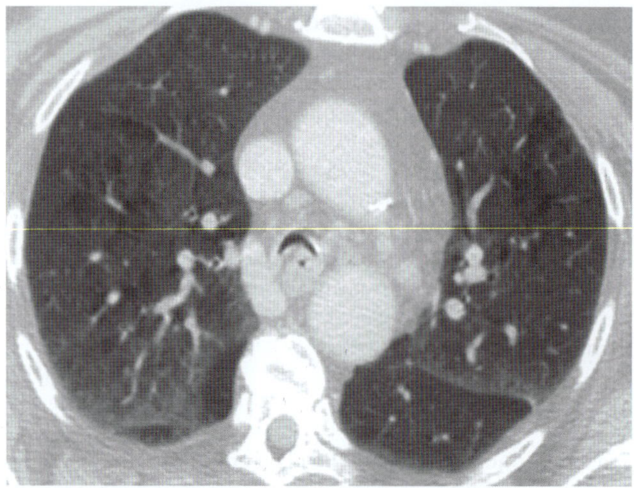

Fig. 28 CT chest in exhalation, showing excessive airway collapse with posterior bowing resulting in tracheomalacia

NORMAL LUNG COMPONENTS OF PULMONARY VASCULATURE

A comprehensive knowledge of the cross-sectional anatomy of pulmonary arteries and veins is imperative in the diagnosis of vascular abnormalities and interpretation of CT images. The arteries accompany the airways and their pattern of division is similar to the branching of airways.

Pulmonary Arterial Anatomy

The main pulmonary artery begins from the base of the right ventricle and extends superiorly dividing into the right and left pulmonary arteries. These central pulmonary arteries are intrapericardial. Pulmonary arteries are elastic and thin-walled vessels.

The main pulmonary artery on CT is the most anterior vascular structure arising from the heart. It is slightly smaller than the ascending aorta in normal subjects, measuring on average 28 mm in diameter.[29] This measurement is best taken at its bifurcation, lateral to the aorta in the short axis of the pulmonary artery. CT measurements of the pulmonary artery have been shown to correlate with pulmonary artery pressure.[29]

The main pulmonary artery divides lateral to the ascending aorta into the right and left pulmonary arteries. The right pulmonary artery arises nearly at a right angle and passes posteriorly to the ascending aorta and anteriorly to the right main bronchus as it crosses the mediastinum. It is seen along its length on CT since it lies in the scan plane. The left pulmonary artery appears in direct communication of the main pulmonary artery. It passes slightly to the left of its origin and arches over the left main bronchus as it enters the hilum. The right and left pulmonary arteries are usually of equal size.

Similar to bronchial division, the pulmonary arteries divide by dichotomous branching. There are approximately 17 divisions from the bifurcation of the main pulmonary artery to arteries of a diameter of 10–15 mm.[30]

The right main pulmonary artery divides into an ascending trunk, truncus anterior, primarily supplying the right upper lobe, and a descending trunk, interlobar branch, supplying mainly the right middle and lower lobes. The left pulmonary artery continues as the descending or interlobar left pulmonary artery, giving rise to segmental branches of the left upper and lower lobes **(Fig. 29)**. The branching of the lobar, segmental and subsegmental pulmonary artery branches show considerable variation and are sometimes identified by associated bronchi. Occlusion of segmental pulmonary arteries can be easily identified on CT, whereas subsegmental pulmonary arteries occlusion may not always be visualized.

Pulmonary Veins

The pulmonary veins arise from alveolar capillaries where pulmonary venules form. Pulmonary veins run through the interlobular septa and then through the more central connective tissue sheaths to the left atrium.[31] The branching patterns of veins are more variable; generally two superior and two inferior pulmonary veins are found on each side.

Bronchial Arteries

The bronchial arteries belong to a different arterial system that originates from the systemic circulation. They accompany the bronchi to the level of the terminal bronchi, where they ramify into pulmonary plexus and are drained by the pulmonary venous system.

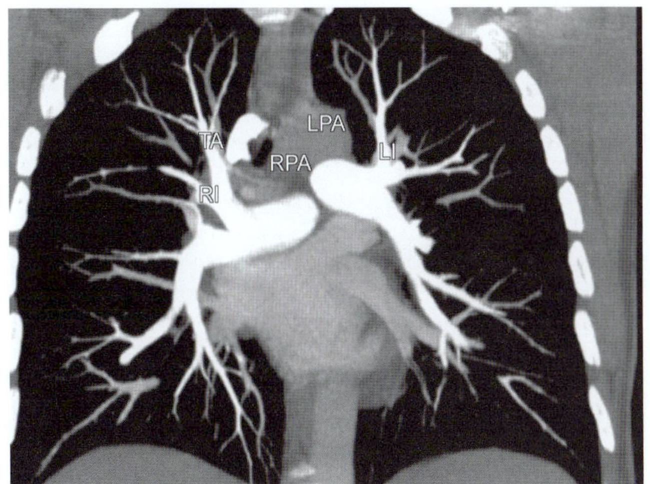

Fig. 29 Coronal image of CT chest showing normal hilar pulmonary artery branching. The right main pulmonary artery (RPA) divides into an ascending trunk, truncus anterior (TA), primarily supplying the right upper lobe, and a descending trunk, interlobar branch (RI), supplying mainly the right middle and lower lobes. The left pulmonary artery (LPA) continues as the descending or interlobar left pulmonary artery (LI), giving rise to segmental branches of the left upper and lower lobes

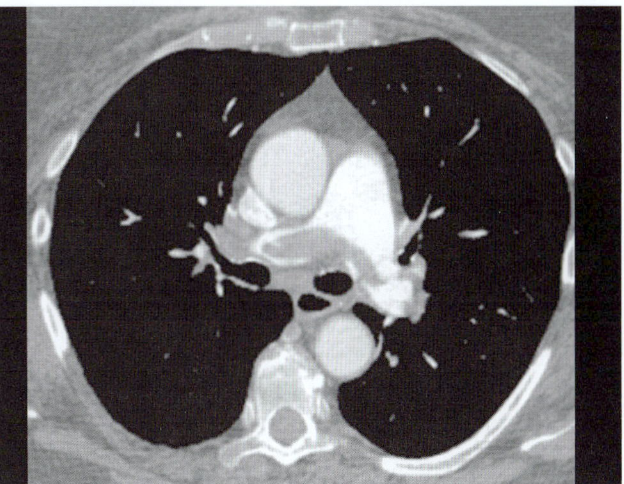

Fig. 30 CT angiogram showing a large filling defect at the division of the right and left main pulmonary arteries. This is also known as a saddle embolism. Note the acute angle formed by the embolus and the contrast-filled lumen

Abnormalities

Pulmonary Artery Agenesis

Congenital abnormalities resulting in embryonic disappearance of proximal segments of the right and the left sixth arch may result in agenesis of either the right or left pulmonary artery respectively. It may occur as an isolated condition or along with cardiac abnormalities. Features seen on CT include a small hemithorax, ipsilateral displacement of the mediastinum and absence of the analogous pulmonary artery.[32]

Anomalous Pulmonary Artery

An anomalous retrotracheal left pulmonary artery is seen on CT to arise from the right pulmonary artery, looping behind the trachea and right main stem bronchus before reaching the left hilum. This can result in symptomatic compression of the right main stem.[33]

Anomalous Pulmonary Vein

Anomalous pulmonary vein abnormalities result in drainage of blood completely or partially into the right atrium.[34] In Scimitar syndrome, there is aberrant drainage of the right pulmonary vein into the inferior vena cava.

Pulmonary Embolism

Knowledge of the hilar vascular anatomy is crucial for the recognition of an acute pulmonary embolism. The identification of pulmonary arteries is done using the bronchial anatomy as reference since the arteries tend to lie adjacent to the airways. The most consistent CT finding of pulmonary embolism is an intraluminal filling defect **(Fig. 30)**. Depending on the plane of the CT and orientation of the artery, these defects may appear as spherical, eccentric or serpiginous filling defects.[35] In large arteries, they may also appear as free-floating masses. An acute pulmonary embolus forms an acute angle with contrast-filled lumen. In chronic pulmonary embolism, the thrombi are smooth or irregular eccentric mural defects, representing organization of the thrombus.[36]

Pulmonary Artery Aneurysm

Pulmonary artery aneurysms have been associated with a spectrum of conditions, such as—in infections, congenital heart conditions, atrial and ventricular septal defects and vasculitis.[37] The primary cause of pulmonary artery aneurysm is cystic medial necrosis. A false aneurysm may be seen as also develop as a result of a pulmonary artery catheter. CT findings are often nonspecific and erroneously identified as masses, nodules or adenopathy.

Pulmonary Varix

Pulmonary varices may be easily identified on CT as an enlarged mass with aneurysmal dilatation of the pulmonary vein[38] **(Fig. 31)**.

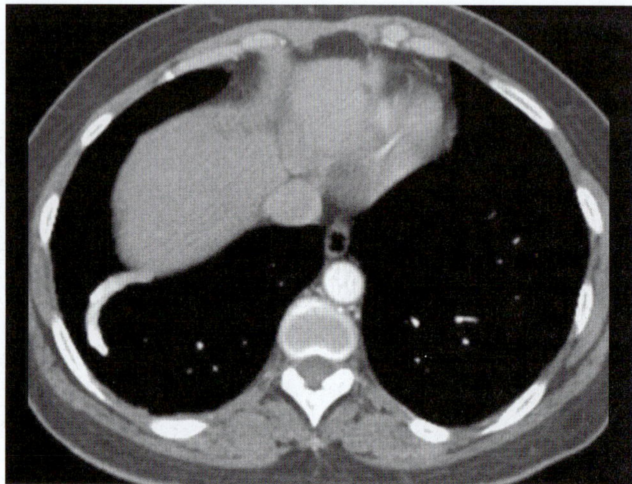

Fig. 31 CT chest with contrast showing a dilatation of the pulmonary vein from a pulmonary varix

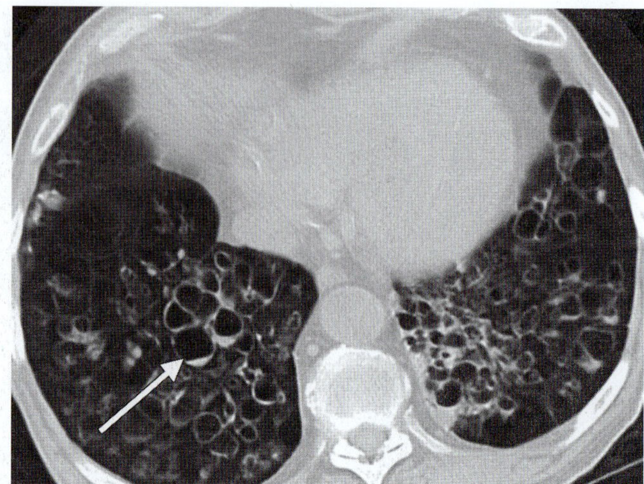

Fig. 32 CT chest through the lower lobes showing saccular bronchiectasis. Some of the bronchi have fluid (arrow) in them. This patient developed bronchiectasis from repeated childhood infections
Source: Dr A Saleh

TRACHEOBRONCHIAL DISEASES

Bronchiectasis

The definition of bronchiectasis is localized, irreversible dilatation of the bronchial tree.[39] Several conditions have been associated with bronchiectasis.[40] These include postinfectious causes following early childhood infections, tubercular sequela, allergic bronchopulmonary aspergillosis, immunodeficiency states and congenital causes. This commonly arises from acute, chronic or recurrent infections. Symptoms usually develop with severe disease and include a history of recurrent pulmonary infections, persistent productive cough or hemoptysis. The radiographic manifestations of bronchiectasis have been well studied. They include loss of clarity of vascular markings in specific lung segments, bronchial wall thickening and in advanced bronchiectasis, distinct cystic masses, frequently demonstrating air-fluid levels.[41]

Bronchiectasis is classically described as "cylindrical, varicose, or cystic" based on appearance and other various terms have also been used **(Fig. 32)**. "Tram-tracks" are dilated airways coursing the scan plane. "Signet rings" describe cross-sectional dilated airways with adjacent pulmonary blood artery branches. "Beading airways" are saccular airways seen along their length. There are direct and indirect methods of diagnosing bronchiectasis on CT. Direct methods include bronchial dilatation, lack of normal bronchial tapering, and presence of airways in the periphery of the lungs. Indirect signs consist of bronchial wall thickening and irregularity and the presence of mucoid impaction within the airways.[41]

Bronchiolar Diseases

The introduction of HRCT on assessing small airway disease has significantly impacted the diagnosis and classification of bronchiolar disease.[42] Normal intralobular structures are beyond the resolution of CT; however, direct and indirect signs of bronchiolar disease may be apparent **(Table 4)**.[43] Direct signs include bronchiolar secretions, distinguished as branching Y-shaped linear densities, peribronchiolar inflammation, characterized by poorly defined centrilobular nodules or bronchiolar wall thickening represented by focal small centrilobular lucencies. Indirect signs manifest as either areas of mosaic attenuation on inspiration or as areas of decreased attenuation on expiration.[44] Bronchiolar disease may be categorized on CT into four groups based on other associated signs.

Tree-in-Bud and Bronchiolar Disease

The characteristic finding in this category of bronchiolar disease is the finding of dilated, mucus-filled bronchioles which result in a pattern of centrilobular nodular, branching or Y-shaped densities which imitate the appearance of a tree-in-bud.[45] This pattern is typically seen in infectious bronchiolitis of several etiologies such as bacterial, viral and fungal causes. Common infections resulting in the tree-in-bud representation include *Mycobacterium tuberculosis* infections, atypical mycobacterial infections, bacterial infections related to immunosuppressive conditions, such as HIV and cystic fibrosis.[44] It was initially described in patients with panbronchiolitis,[46] common in Asia. These patients have clinical symptoms of productive cough and dyspnea, with an obstructive impairment on pulmonary physiologic testing and characteristic ill-defined nodules and tree-in-bud appearance on CT. Other proximal airway infection may also depict the tree-in-bud sign in association with other findings. Examples include cystic fibrosis, tuberculosis, postinfectious bronchiectasis and allergic bronchopulmonary mycoses.[47]

Table 4 Conditions associated with bronchiectasis

Disorders	*Description*
Focal distribution Bronchial obstruction Previous pneumonia	 Foreign body Tumor Broncholithiasis Compression by peribronchial lymph nodes
Diffuse distribution CF Reduced host immunity	 Congenital and acquired hypogammaglobulinemia (especially IgG and/or IgG subclasses) HIV infection
Primary ciliary dyskinesia Allergic bronchopulmonary mycoses Chronic MAC infection Aspiration or toxic inhalation Rheumatoid arthritis Inflammation bowel disease	
Other congenital disorders	α_1-antitrypsin deficiency Tracheobronchomegaly (Mounier-Kuhn syndrome) Cartilage deficiency (Williams-Campbell syndrome) Young syndrome Pulmonary sequestration Marfan syndrome
Yellow nail syndrome	

Source: Rosen M. Chronic cough due to bronchiectasis ACCP evidence-based clinical practice guidelines. Chest. 2006;129:122S-31S.

Flow chart 1 summarizes disorders associated with tree-in-bud opacities with individual characteristic features.[43]

Poorly Defined Centrilobular Nodules and Bronchiolar Disease

As compared to infectious bronchiolitis, the distinguishing finding of this group of bronchiolar disease is the presence of ill-defined centrilobular nodules in the absence of a tree-in-bud picture. A variety of diseases with peribronchiolar inflammation without the tree-in-bud patterns have been described. This includes subacute hypersensitivity pneumonitis, lymphocytic interstitial pneumonitis, follicular bronchiolitis, respiratory bronchiolitis-interstitial lung disease and mineral dust-induced bronchiolitis.[44]

Focal Ground Glass Attenuation or Consolidation and Bronchiolar Disease

This presentation of focal ground glass attenuation is the main characteristic of cryptogenic organizing pneumonia (COP) or bronchiolitis obliterans with organizing pneumonia (BOOP).[48] Patients usually complain of symptoms of nonproductive cough for several months, low-grade fever and increasing dyspnea. The most common radiologic finding on HRCT in COP is patchy bilateral consolidation commonly with peribronchial and subpleural distribution.[49] Small, poorly formed peribronchiolar nodules and irregular linear opacities are seen in a smaller percentage of patients. However, the tree-in-bud pattern is clearly uncommon. Areas of ground glass consolidation may be seen in immunocompromised patients with COP.

Flow chart 1 HRCT signs of bronchiolar disorders[43]

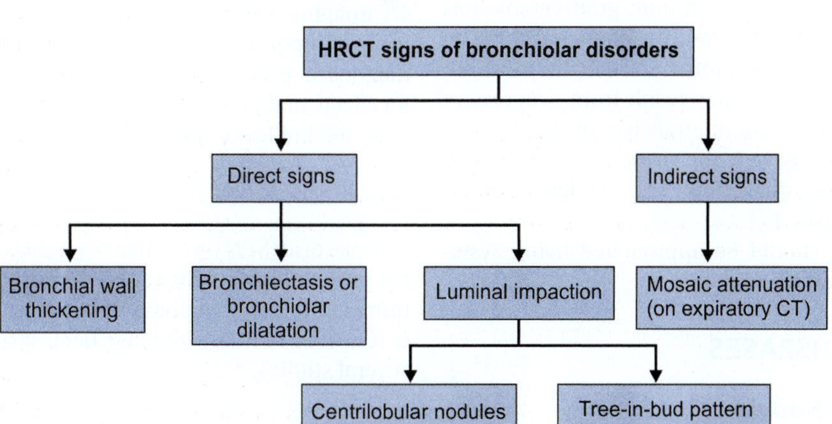

Source: Devakonda A, Raoof S, Sung A, et al. Bronchiolar disorders. A clinical-radiological diagnostic algorithm. Chest. 2010;137:938-51.

Table 5 Characteristic features of bronchiolar diseases with tree-in-bud opacities[43]

	Characteristic clinical features	*Causes and/ or associated conditions*	*HRCT features*	*Histopathologic features*
Infection	Wheezing with concomitant signs of respiratory tract infection	Viral, bacterial, parasitic, mycobacterial, fungal	Tree-in-bud pattern, centrilobular nodules, dense consolidation	Acute and chronic inflammation of small bronchioles with epithelial necrosis and sloughing
Immunologic disorders (allergic bronchopulmonary aspergillosis)	Cough, fever, wheezing; recurrent episodes of bronchial obstruction	Asthma	Tree-in-bud pattern, central bronchiectasis, mucoid impaction, upper lobe predominance	Mucoid impaction of bronchi, eosinophilic infiltration, bronchocentric granulomatosis
Congenital disorders (CF, dyskinetic cilia syndrome)	Recurrent purulent cough, airway hyperactivity	Genetic predisposition, multisystem disease	Tree-in-bud pattern, bronchial wall thickening, bronchiectasis, bronchiolectasis	Cellular infiltration
Neoplasms	Symptoms and signs of upper respirtory tract obstruction (hoarseness, stridor)	Juvenile laryngotracheo-bronchial papillomatosis	Tree-in-bud pattern, multiple solid or cystic nodules	Varies from multiple clusters of squamous cells within alveoli to large cavitary lesions
Diffuse aspiration bronchiolitis	Nonspecific	Elderly, bed bound	Tree-in-bud pattern, centrilobular nodules	Foreign body giant cell reaction
Idiopathic diffuse panbronchiolitis	Mainly in Japanese adults; subacute onset of cough, dyspnea	Associated sinusitis, HLABw54 antigen	Tree-in-bud pattern, thickened ecstatic bronchi, centrilobular nodules	Infiltration of lymphocytes, plasma cells and foamy macrophages at the level of respiratory bronchiole

Abbreviations: CF, cystic fibrosis; HRCT, high-resolution CT
Source: Devakonda A, Raoof S, Sung A, Travis WD, Naidich D. Bronchiolar disorders. A clinical-radiological diagnostic algorithm. Chest. 2010;137:938-51.

Decreased Parenchymal Attenuation and Bronchiolar Disease

This category includes patients with constrictive or obstructive bronchiolitis. Conditions associated with obstructive bronchiolitis include lung transplant, chronic graft-versus-host disease from allogeneic bone marrow transplant and collagen vascular disease.[50] Clinical symptoms are usually mild but severe respiratory compromise may result from progressive airway obstruction. Mosaic attenuation is commonly seen in obstructive bronchiolitis with the presence of bronchial dilatation, peribronchial thickening and evidence of air trapping on expiratory HRCT.[51]

Bronchiolar disease should be approached using systematic method as illustrated in **Table 5.**[43]

PARENCHYMAL DISEASES

Solitary Pulmonary Nodule

The evaluation of focal lung disease in patients poses an imperative challenge in the diagnosis of pulmonary disorders. There is lack of consensus leading to several controversies in the definition, assessment and diagnostic techniques including imaging and mode of pathologic confirmation of focal lung diseases. For the purpose of this chapter, we will define an SPN as a single, rounded lesion in the lung parenchyma, which is not associated with atelectasis or pneumonia. The SPNs are a common, incidental finding on CT imaging. Characterization of the pulmonary nodule is of utmost importance and may aid in narrowing the differential diagnosis, preventing unnecessary procedures or missing localized malignancy. The differential diagnosis of SPNs is depicted in **Flow chart 2.**[52]

Size

The size of an SPN on CT has been shown to directly influence the probability of malignancy.[53] Nodules larger than 3 cm are more apt to being malignant. However, smaller lesions, even of less than 1 cm in size, have been shown to be malignant in several studies.[54]

Location

Primary lung cancers have been shown to be more commonly located in the upper lobes, particularly on the right side.[55] The SPNs have also been reported to be identified in the lung

Flow chart 2 A stepwise approach to bronchiolar disease.[43] History, physical findings, evidence of hyperinflation on chest radiograph or airflow obstruction on pulmonary function testing suggestive of bronchiolar disease, should trigger a request for obtaining an HRCT scan of the chest performed at the end of inspiration and expiration. An HRCT scan of the chest further classifies bronchiolar diseases. The presence of a tree-in-bud pattern largely suggests either an infectious bronchiolitis, if a focal distribution is noted, or diffuse panbronchiolitis or congenital disease related bronchiolitis, if a diffuse pattern is noted. If centrilobular nodules are predominantly seen, then RB-ILD should be suspected in a smoker or HP in a non-smoker. Mosaic attenuation suggests either a constrictive bronchiolitis or obliterative bronchiolitis. Histology is ultimately required for the final confirmation

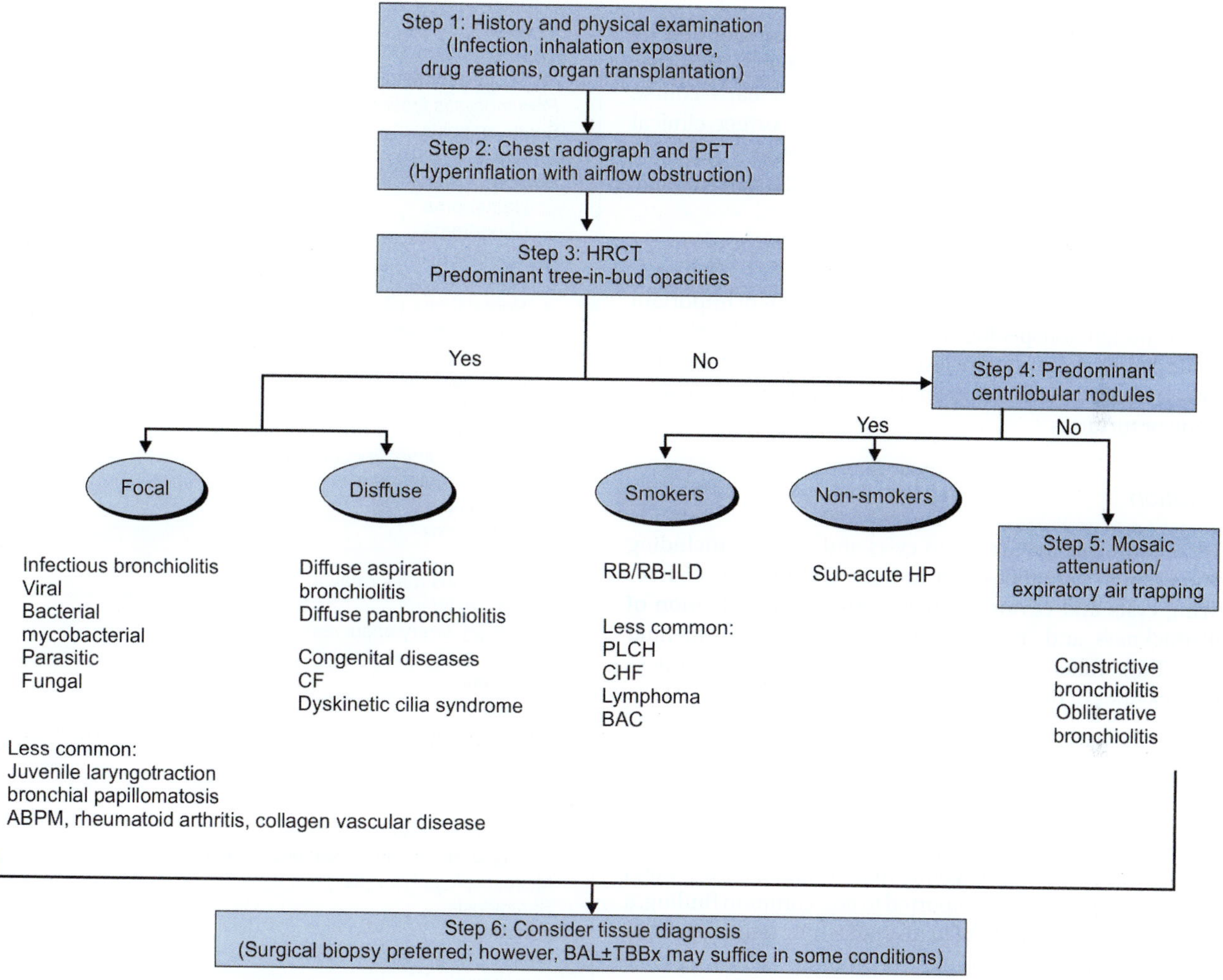

Abbreviations: ABPM, allergic bronchopulmonary mycosis; BAC, bronchoalveolar cell carcinoma; CF, cystic fibrosis; CHF, congestive heart failure; HP, hypersensitivity pneumonitis; PFT, pulmonary function test; PLCH, pulmonary Langerhans cell histiocytosis; RB-ILD, respiratory bronchiolitis-inetrstitial lung disease; TBBx, transbronchial biopsy

Source: Devakonda A, Raoof S, Sung A, Travis WD, Naidich D. Bronchiolar disorders. A clinical-radiological diagnostic algorithm. Chest. 2010;137:938-51.

periphery, rather than the medial third of the lung. Metastatic lesions are predisposed to be subpleural in location, predominantly seen in the lower lobes.[56] Nevertheless, several other lesions, such as lymph nodes, are also seen in the subpleural distribution.[57]

Margin and Contour

Benign nodules tend to demonstrate a round, smooth contour with a sharply defined margin. Malignant lesions are more likely to exhibit an irregular lobulated or ragged shape and a vague, irregular, or spiculated edge.[58] Malignant lesions have been reported to demonstrate a smooth appearance and benign conditions have shown lobulated or spiculated contours.[59] **Table 6** illustrates margin characteristics in benign and malignant processes.[52]

Halo Sign

A halo sign is defined as a distinct nodule surrounded by a circular margin of ground glass attenuation.[60] This sign has been most commonly associated with the early course of invasive pulmonary aspergillosis in the correct clinical context. It has also been reported in Wegener's granulomatosis, Kaposi's sarcoma and bronchoalveolar carcinoma.

Bronchus Sign

The identification of an air bronchogram on CT is of important value. Although nonspecific, the presence of bronchial lumen surrounded by a pulmonary lesion is likely to be malignant. Airways related to lung cancer tend to be abnormal, appearing ecstatic or tortuous.[61]

Cavitation

Several etiologies may result in cysts and cavities, including septic emboli, vasculities and tumors. CT helps in characterizing cysts and cavities, allowing for closer evaluation of wall thickness and intracavitary findings such as air-fluid levels. Thin-walled cavities tend to be benign and thick-walled cavities of uncertain etiology.[62]

Feeding Vessel Sign

A focal lesion with an adjacent vessel is known as a feeding vessel sign or vessel-mass sign, has been described in various conditions such as arteriovenous malformations, metastasis or infarcts.[63] Although, not reported to be a common finding, a feeding vessel sign is helpful in distinguishing hematogenous metastasis from either primary or granulomatous lesions. It is also useful in diagnosing septic emboli and pulmonary vasculitis in the appropriate clinical situation.

Growth Rates

One of the most important radiographic factors allowing for distinction between benign and malignant disease is the growth rate of the SPN. It is, therefore, paramount to review prior chest images in the evaluation of an SPN. The absence of detectable growth over a 2-year period is highly suggestive of a benign etiology.[64] The doubling time for an SPN is the time it takes to double in size which can be determined using the changes in diameter. A 26% increase in diameter will result in a doubling volume of an SPN. A majority of malignant SPNs have a doubling time of 20–400 days.

Table 6 Differential diagnosis of solitary pulmonary nodules[52]

Infections
Tuberculosis (TB)
Round pneumonia, organizing pneumonia
Lung abscess
Fungal: aspergillosis, blastomycosis, cryptococcosis, histoplasmosis, coccidioidomycosis
Parasitic amoebiasis, echinococcosis, Dirofilaria immitis (Dog heartworm)
Measles
Nocardia
Atypical mycobacteria
Pneumocystis jiroveci
Septic embolus
Neoplastic
Benign
Hamartoma
Chondroma
Fibroma
Lipoma
Neural tumor (Schwannomna neurofibroma)
Sclerosing hemangioma
Plasma cell granuloma
Endometriosis
Malignant
Lung cancer
Primary pulmonary carcinoid
Solitary metastasis
Teratoma
Leiomyoma
Vascular
Arteriovenous malformation
Pulmonary infarct
Pulmonary artery aneurysm
Pulmonary venous varix
Hematoma
Congenital
Bronchogenic cyst
Lung sequestration
Bronchial atresia with mucoid impaction
Inflammatory
Rheumatoid arthritis
Granulomatosis with polyangiitis (Wegener)
Microscopic polyangiitis
Sarcoidosis
Lymphatic
Intrapulmonary lymph node
Lymphoma
Outside lung fields
Skin nodule
Nipple shadows
Rib fracture
Pleural thickening, mass or fluid [pseudotumor, (i.e. loculated fluid)]
Miscellaneous
Rounded atelectasis
Lipoid pneumonia
Amyloidosis
Mucoid impaction (mucocele)
Infected bulla
Pulmonary scar

Source: Patel VK, Naik SK, Naidich DP, Travis WD, Weingarten JA, Lazzaro R, et al. A practical algorithm approach to the diagnosis and management of solitary pulmonary nodules: part 1: radiologic characteristics and imaging modalities. Chest. 2013;143(3):825-39.

Table 7 Margin characteristics of solitary pulmonary nodules[52]

Margin	*Etiology*
Smooth	Suggests a benign lesion. However, may be malignant in up to one-third of cases[50,51]
Lobulated	Suggests uneven growth; a PPV of 80% for malignancy.[45,46] Up to 25% of benign lesions, such as hamartomas can have lobulated margins
Spiculated	A spiculated margin (the so-called corona radiata sign) is highly predictive of malignancy, with a PPV of 88% to 94%. A few exceptions of benign SPNs that could have spiculated margins include lipoid pneumonia, focal actelectasis, tuberculoma, and progressive massive fibrosis[45,54]
Ragged	Suggests growth pattern along the alveolar wall; lepidic pattern of adenocarcinoma
Tentacle or polygonal	Seen in fibrosis, alveolar infiltration, and collapsed alveoli
Halo	SPN surrounded by a "halo" of ground glass attenuation, also called the " CT halo sign". Seen in aspergillosis, Kaposi sarcoma, granulomatosis with polyangiitis (Wegener), and metastatic angiosarcoma. Adenosarcoma in situ (previously known as bronchoalveolar carcinoma) can also produce a halo due to its lepidic growth
Notches	SPN with notches or concavity in the margin is seen in some SPNs with tumor growth. These notches are frequently found in adenocarcinomas with overt invasion and are associated with poor prognosis[17]
Source: Patel VK, Naik SK, Naidich DP, Travis WD, Weingarten JA, Lazzaro R, et al. A practical algorithm approach to the diagnosis and management of solitary pulmonary nodules: part 1: radiologic characteristics and imaging modalities. Chest. 2013;143(3):825-39.	

Calcification

The radiographic presence of calcification can suggest that a pulmonary lesion is benign.[65] Four patterns of benign calcification have been studied: (1) laminated and concentric; (2) dense central core; (3) diffuse and solid; and (4) punctuate. There is no specific pattern of calcification associated with malignant nodules. Calcification classically appears speckled or eccentric and usually within large central lesions.[66] Refer to **Table 7** for patterns of calcifications in benign and malignant processes.[52]

Fat

The appearance of fat is suggestive of two key conditions: hamartoma or exogenous lipoid pneumonia. A hamartoma is a benign condition which contains connective tissue, cartilage, smooth muscle, bone and variable amounts of fat and represents the third most common cause of an SPN.[67] They can be diagnosed by CT as lesions containing fat or fat and calcification have an even contour with a sharp circumference.

Contrast Enhancement

Due to the fundamental differences in vascularity of focal benign versus malignant lesions, the phenomenon of pulmonary enhancement has been a valuable tool in differentiating the two processes.[68] Malignant lesions are more prone to enhancement following injection of contrast material. It has been reported that malignant lesion may enhance by greater than 15-20 Hounsfield units.[69]

Diffuse Diseases

Diffuse parenchymal lung diseases include chronic and acute infiltrative lung diseases and emphysema. These conditions, in addition to being diffuse in nature, often have patchy or focal distribution. Suggestive findings that indicate parenchymal irregularity in diffuse lung disease include linear and reticular opacities, nodular opacities, and increased attenuation seen as consolidation or ground glass opacities and decreased attenuation seen in emphysema and cystic diseases.

Several acute and chronic pulmonary conditions result in diffuse infiltration of the lungs. They can be classified based on the predominant radiographic pattern on CT **(Table 8)**.[70] There are seven distinct histologic types of idiopathic interstitial pneumonias: (1) Usual interstitial pneumonia/ idiopathic pulmonary fibrosis (UIP/IPF), (2) nonspecific interstitial pneumonia (NSIP), (3) desquamative interstitial pneumonia (DIP), (4) respiratory bronchiolitis interstitial pneumonia (RBILD), (5) acute interstitial pneumonia (AIP), (6) cryptogenic organizing pneumonia/bronchiolitis obliterans organizing pneumonia (COP/BOOP) and (7) lymphocytic interstitial pneumonia (LIP).[71] HRCT evaluation may avoid the necessity for tissue diagnosis and may limit the differential diagnosis in some cases.

Reticular Pattern

Idiopathic pulmonary fibrosis: Idiopathic pulmonary fibrosis has characteristic HRCT findings that can lead to its diagnosis with a high degree of certainty.[72] In the early phase of IPF, patchy peripheral distribution of ground glass opacities is seen with areas of normal lung intermingled in between.

Table 8 Patterns of calcifications in solitary pulmonary nodules[52]

Patterns of calcification	*Etiology*
Laminated and concentric	Usually benign
Dense central core	Usually benign
Diffuse and solid	Usually benign
Popcorn	Hematoma
Punctate	Malignant lesions: scar carcinoma, typical and atypical carcinoids large-cell neuroendocrine carcinoma and metastasis from colon, ovary, breast, thyroid, and osteogenic tumors
Eccentric	Due to necrosis within the malignant nodule or engulfment of adjacent granuloma

Source: Patel VK, Naik SK, Naidich DP, Travis WD, Weingarten JA, Lazzaro R, et al. A practical algorithm approach to the diagnosis and management of solitary pulmonary nodules: part 1: radiologic characteristics and imaging modalities. Chest. 2013;143(3):825-39.

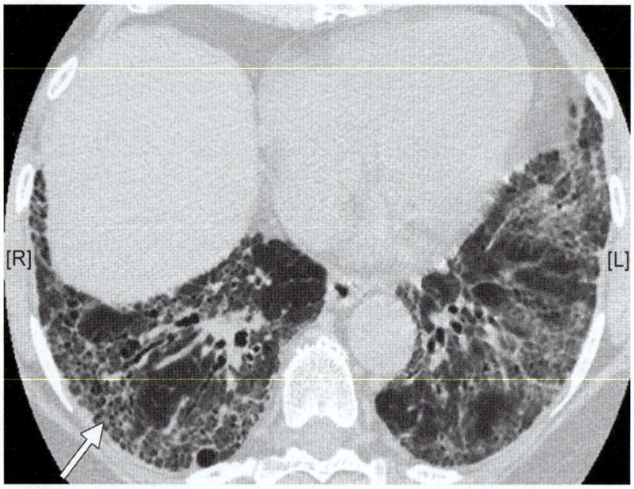

Fig. 33 HRCT showing cuts through the lower lobes showing reticular changes including honeycombing, traction bronchiectasis and architectural distortion

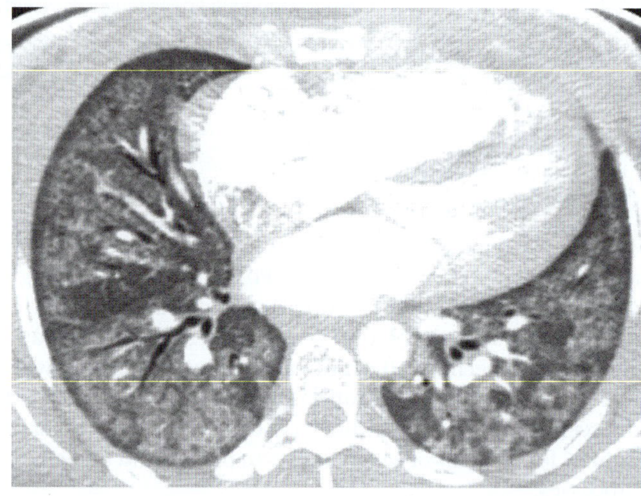

Fig. 34 CT chest features of nonspecific interstitial pneumonia (NSIP) with diffuse, bilateral ground glass attenuation at the lower lung zones. Note the absence of honeycombing

The main pattern of abnormality seen on HRCT in a later stage in patients with IPF include intralobular linear opacities, which correspond to histologic areas of fibrosis, a fine reticular pattern, most pronounced at the lung bases and in the subpleural regions and irregular interfaces between the lung and pulmonary vessels, bronchi and pleural surfaces[73] **(Fig. 33)**. This progression of fibrosis ultimately results in dilatation and tortuosity of bronchi and bronchioles, referred to as traction bronchiectasis. The end stage of IPF is illustrated by honeycombing, noted most severely at the lung bases and in subpleural sites.[74] The IPF is classically represented as a patchy distributed disease, with spatial and temporal heterogeneity. This refers to areas of normal lung, reticular changes or honeycombing seen in the same patient within the same lung section.

Nonspecific interstitial pneumonitis: There are two forms of nonspecific interstitial pneumonia (NSIP) which can occur: "cellular or a fibrotic NSIP". HRCT features of NSIP include ground-glass attenuation in a diffuse or patchy distribution with reticular opacities and traction bronchiectasis.[75] In cellular NSIP, there is prevalence of ground-glass attenuation **(Fig. 34)** and in fibrotic NSIP more reticular changes are noticeable **(Fig. 35)**. Findings of honeycombing are seldom noted. NSIP, unlike UIP, displays temporal and spatial homogeneity, where there is a uniform pattern of HRCT changes within the same lung segment.

Collagen vascular disease: High-resolution CT features similar to IPF may be seen in various collagen vascular diseases such as rheumatoid arthritis, scleroderma, mixed connective tissue disease, polymyositis and systemic lupus erythematosis.[76] Rheumatoid arthritis may result in fibrosis in a small percentage of patients, with a similar lower lung zone distribution as IPF. More commonly seen are pleural manifestations but other findings, such as bronchiectasis or

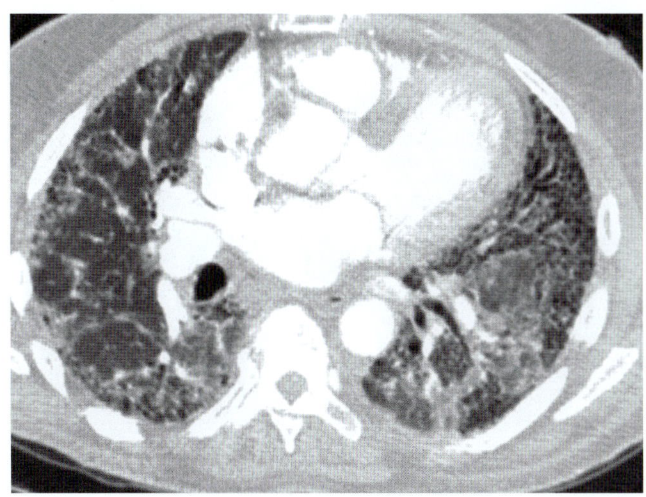

Fig. 35 CT chest through the middle lung zones in a patient with nonspecific interstitial pneumonia (NSIP)

rheumatoid nodules can occur.[77] Scleroderma may result in fibrosis with fine reticulation as well as ground-glass attenuation, honeycombing or pleural thickening.[78]

Asbestosis: Asbestosis leads to predominantly basilar and dorsal lung parenchymal fibrosis. Other characteristic findings include: peribronchiolar fibrosis that forms centrilobular nodules, intralobular and interlobular septal fibrosis that forms subpleural short lines, coarse parenchymal bands, and subpleural curvilinear bands that parallel the pleura and represent fibrotic bridging from one centrilobular region to the next.[79] Coarse honeycombing can be seen in advanced stages. Coexistent pleural plaques are frequently identified, particularly in patients with curvilinear subpleural lines.[80]

Nodular Pattern

The differential diagnosis of nodular disease includes an extensive list of benign and malignant processes. Nodular disease can be further analyzed based on the predominant distribution of nodules: perilymphatic; centrilobular; or random[11] **(Table 9)**.

Perilymphatic Distribution

Sarcoidosis: The characteristic HRCT finding of sarcoidosis includes small nodules and nodular thickening along the bronchovascular bundles, interlobular septa, interlobular fissures, and subpleural lung regions[81] **(Figs 36 and 37)**. The bronchovascular thickening is most pronounced at the hila. The nodules appear irregular and represent coalescence of microscopic granulomas. The "galaxy sign" is a term used to describe an irregularly marginated pulmonary nodule formed by a confluence of multiple smaller nodules. The concentration of smaller nodules becomes less dense towards the periphery resulting in irregular borders and multiple satellite nodules, resembling the appearance of a galaxy.[82] As fibrosis develops, reticular changes, such as intralobular septal thickening occur which ultimately lead to architectural distortion, loss of lung volume and traction bronchiectasis.[83] Honeycombing may also be seen, although it is usually mild

Table 9 Radiographic patterns of diffuse lung disease

Pattern of opacities	*Acute*	*Chronic*
Consolidation	Infection, acute respiratory distress syndrome, hemorrhage, aspiration, acute eosinophilic pneumonia, acute interstitial pneumonia, cryptogenic organizing pneumonia	Chronic infections (tuberculosis, fungal), chronic eosinophilic pneumonia, cryptogenic organizing pneumonia, lymphoproliferative diseases, bronchioloalveolar carcinoma, pulmonary alveolar proteinosis and sarcoidosis
Linear or reticular opacities	Infections (viral, mycoplasma), pulmonary edema	Idiopathic pulmonary fibrosis or usual interstitial pneumonia, connective tissue disease–associated pulmonary fibrosis, asbestosis, sarcoidosis, hypersensitivity pneumonitis, drug-induced lung disease
Small nodules	Infections (disseminated tuberculosis, fungal or viral infections), hypersensitivity pneumonitis	Sarcoidosis, hypersensitivity pneumonitis, silicosis,coal worker's pneumoconiosis, respiratory bronchiolitis, metastases, alveolar microlithiasis
Cystic airspaces	*Pneumocystis carinii* pneumonia, septic embolism	Pulmonary Langerhans cell histiocytosis, pulmonary lymphangioleiomyomatosis, honeycomb lung, metastatic disease
Ground-glass opacities	Infections (*P. carinii*, cytomegalovirus), pulmonary edema, hemorrhage, hypersensitivity pneumonitis, acute inhalational exposures, drug-induced lung diseases, acute interstitial pneumonia	Nonspecific interstitial pneumonia, respiratory bronchiolitis–associated interstitial lung disease, desquamative interstitial pneumonia, drug-induced lung diseases, pulmonary alveolar proteinosis
Thickened interlobular septa	Pulmonary edema	Lymphangitic carcinomatosis, pulmonary alveolar proteinosis, sarcoidosis, pulmonary veno-occlusive disease

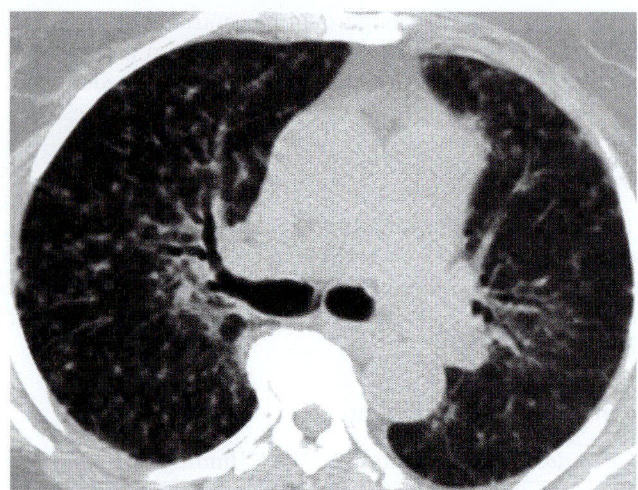

Fig. 36 HRCT at the level of the right upper lobe bronchus showing small nodules and nodular thickening along the bronchovascular bundles, interlobular septa, interlobular fissures, and subpleural lung regions in a patient with sarcoidosis

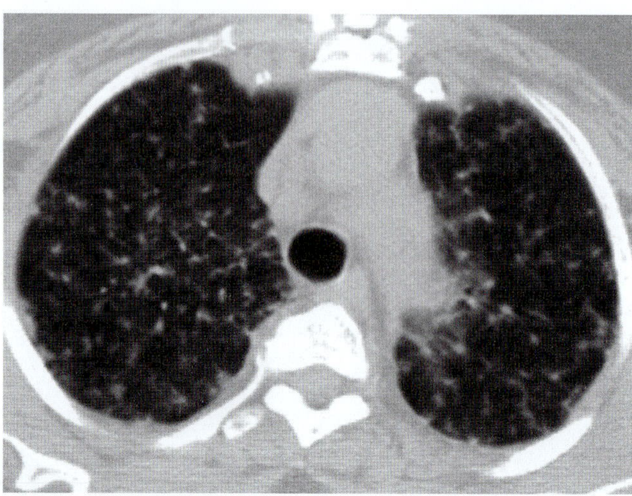

Fig. 37 HRCT through the upper lung zones showing multiple small nodules throughout with nodules seen along the subpleural regions and along the interlobular septa and interlobular fissures

and involves primarily the upper and middle lung zones, with relative sparing of lung bases.[84] Hilar and mediastinal lymphadenopathy is another feature of sarcoidosis seen on CT, with calcification noted in long-standing disease.[85]

Silicosis/Coal Workers Pneumoconiosis: The most characteristic findings in silicosis and coal worker's pneumoconiosis are small nodules predominantly seen in the posterior aspects of the upper lung zones. These nodules vary in size, may be calcified and are distributed largely in the centrilobular pattern.[86] Progressive massive fibrosis is seen as a conglomerate of nodules with an irregular margin, often resulting in architectural distortion.

Lymphangitic carcinomatosis: Pulmonary lymphangitic carcinomatosis refers to lymphangitic or hematogenous spread of tumor to the lungs resulting in infiltration and thickening of the interlobular septa, subpleural interstitium, and bronchovascular bundles and preservation of the normal lung architecture **(Fig. 38)**.[87] The thickening of these structures may be smooth or have a nodular appearance, may be diffuse and bilateral or focal and unilateral in distribution **(Fig. 39)**. The most common primary malignancies resulting in lymphangitic carcinomatosis are adenocarcinoma of the breast, lung, gastrointestinal tract and prostate.

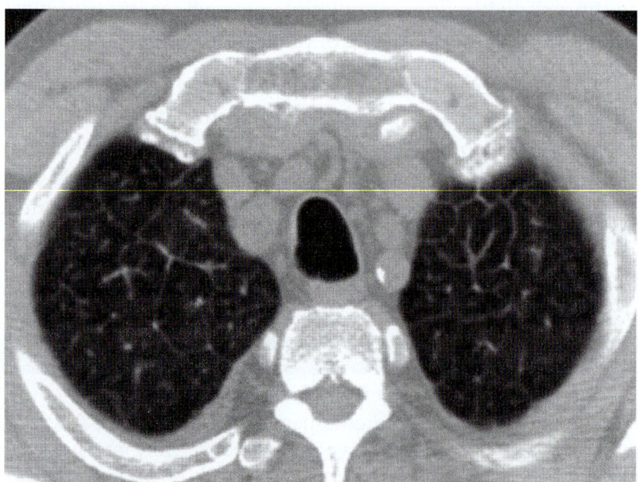

Fig. 38 HRCT through upper lobes demonstrating intralobar septal thickening in a patient with lymphangitis carcinomatosis

Centrilobular Distribution (Ground-Glass Nodules)

Hypersensitivity pneumonitis: Hypersensitivity pneumonitis, also known as extrinsic alveolitis represents a type 3 allergic reaction or immune complex disease. HRCT is most useful in diagnosing subacute hypersensitivity pneumonitis, where it displays diffuse or patchy ground-glass opacification with lobular sparing, lobular air-trapping, and centrilobular poorly defined airspace nodules.[88] The ground-glass attenuation is noted predominantly in the middle and lower lung zones and may be present in combination with mosaic attenuation **(Fig. 40)**. In chronic hypersensitivity pneumonitis, fibrosis, represented by a reticular pattern, architectural distortion and ultimately honeycombing are seen with relative basilar sparing.[89]

Lymphocytic interstitial pneumonitis: Lymphocytic interstitial pneumonitis can be seen in patients with Sjögren's syndrome and is seen commonly in children with acquired immune deficiency syndrome. Dense infiltration of monoclonal or polyclonal T lymphocytes occurs in the interstitium. It can

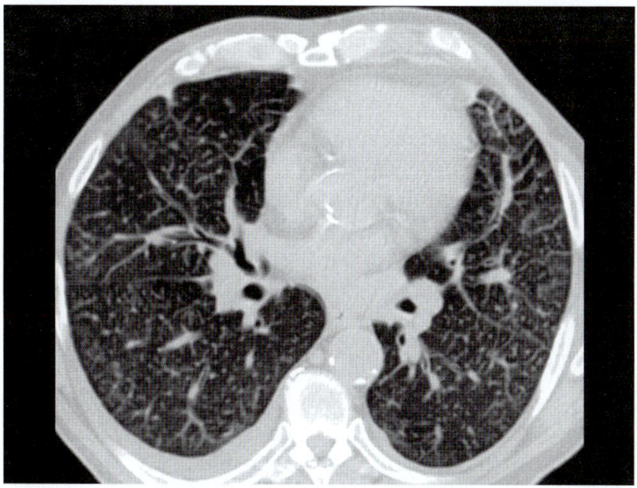

Fig. 39 HRCT at the level of the lower lobe bronchi showing a fine reticular pattern from interlobular septal thickening and multiple tiny nodules in a patient with lymphangitic carcinomatosis. Note the extension of the irregular interlobular septal thickening to the pleural surface

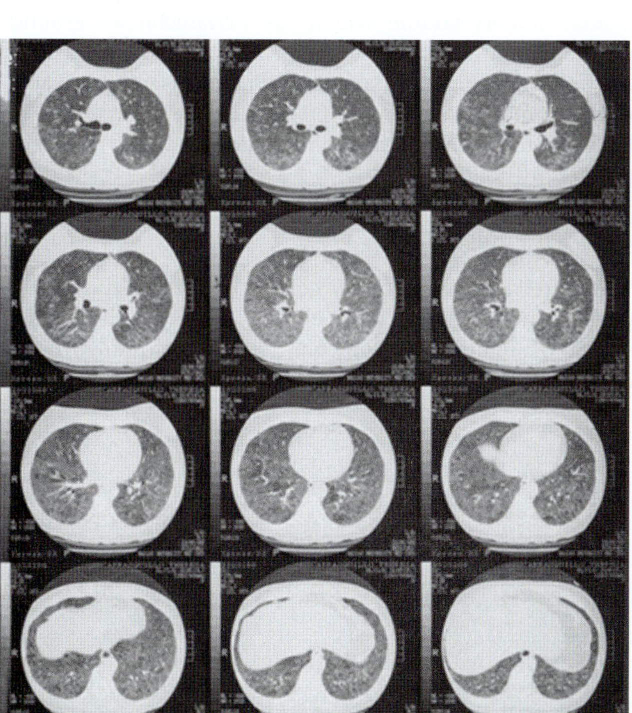

Fig. 40 CT chest representing hypersensitivity pneumonitis. Numerous centrilobular nodules which are poorly defined and shown to extend to the periphery are illustrated

lead to lymphoma of the lung parenchyma. The characteristic features on HRCT include ground-glass opacities, reticular opacities and perivascular cysts **(Figs 41 and 42)**.[90]

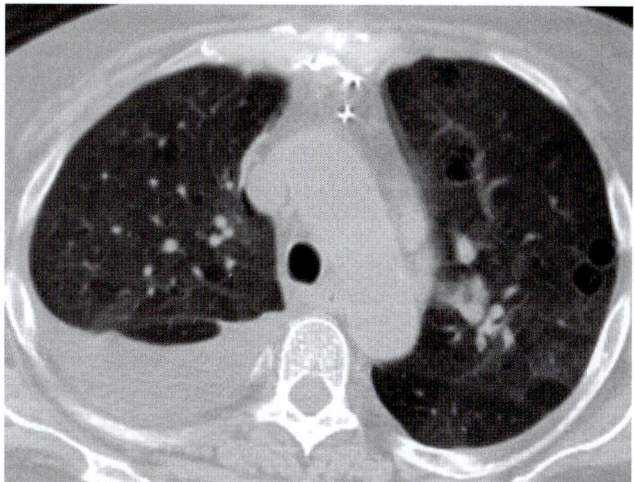

Fig. 41 CT chest through the upper lobes demonstrating cystic changes in a patient with LIP. Also noted is a pleural effusion on the right

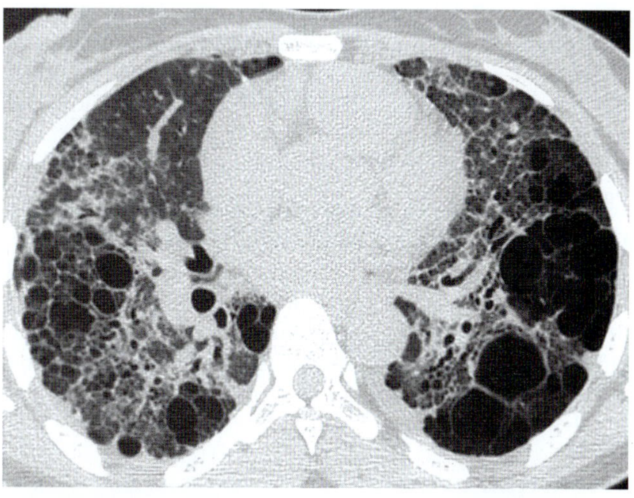

Fig. 42 CT chest through the lower lungs demonstrating cystic changes in a patient with lymphocytic interstitial pneumonitis
Courtesy: Dr A Saleh

Centrilobular Distribution (Tree-in-Bud)

Panbronchiolitis: Panbronchiolitis is a form of diffuse bronchiolitis reported in Asia, especially from Japan and Korea.[91] The characteristic CT features of diffuse tree-in-bud pattern are seen mainly affecting the lower lung zones, with complete resolution after macrolide therapy. Typically seen are centrilobular nodular and linear opacities corresponding to thickened and dilated bronchiolar walls with intraluminal mucous plugs, mosaic attenuation, peripheral air trapping and bronchiectasis, especially in advanced disease.[92]

Infectious etiology: The tree-in-bud pattern is frequently seen in several airway infections of bacterial and viral etiologies;

tuberculosis, *Mycobacterium avium* intracellulare and fungal infections such as allergic bronchopulmonary mycosis (ABPM).[48]

Random Distribution

Hematogenous metastasis: Hematogenous tumor metastasis most commonly results in localized tumor nodules, rather than lymphatic infiltration. Multiple, large, well-defined nodules involving the lower lung zones are seen in a randomly distributed fashion.[93]

Pulmonary Opacities

Ground-Glass Opacities:

Desquamative interstitial pneumonitis/respiratory bronchiolitis interstitial lung disease: Desquamative interstitial pneumonitis (DIP) and respiratory bronchiolitis interstitial lung disease are related disorders exclusively found in smokers. The major HRCT finding in patients with respiratory bronchiolitis is the presence of ill-defined, centrilobular ground-glass nodules, primarily in the upper lobes. DIP may be distinguished from RB-ILD by the presence of ground-glass attenuation, which is predominantly found in the middle and lower lung zones[94] **(Fig. 43)**. Mild fibrosis indicated by irregular linear opacities, architectural distortion and honeycombing may be seen in the subpleural and lower lung regions.

Acute interstitial pneumonitis: Acute interstitial pneumonitis, also known as Hamman-Rich syndrome, is characterized by an acute onset and rapid progression. HRCT findings are of diffuse ground-glass attenuation and consolidation with abnormalities suggestive of fibrosis, such as traction bronchiectasis.[95]

Pulmonary alveolar proteinosis: Pulmonary alveolar proteinosis (PAP) results from ineffective clearance of surfactant from alveoli. The predominant HRCT features of PAP consist of bilateral areas of ground-glass opacification with smoothly thickened interlobular septal lines.[96] There may be lobular or geographic sparing. Other features seen on HRCT include poorly defined nodular opacities and consolidation.[97] The "crazy-paving sign" seen with PAP as well as other interstitial lung conditions is a pattern characterized by reticular markings superimposed on ground glass opacities.[98]

Consolidation

Bronchiolitis obliterans with organizing pneumonia/Cryptogenic organizing pneumonia: HRCT typically shows peribronchial and peripheral areas of consolidation **(Figs 44 and 45)**.[99] Another suggestive finding is the presence of rings or crescents of consolidation surrounding ground-glass opacities, which has been called a "reverse halo" sign.[100]

Bronchoalveolar carcinoma: Bronchoalveolar carcinoma may present with three distinct patterns.[101] It may present as a small solitary nodule, which has a characteristic ground-glass appearance on CT, suggestive of a good prognosis. It may also present as lobar consolidation resembling bacterial pneumonia, where the CT features typically show air bronchograms. Sometimes it presents with multifocal pulmonary nodules.

Cystic Diseases

There are many pulmonary conditions that may result in cystic changes on CT. **Flow chart 3** illustrates the classification of multiple hypolucent lesions according to the distributive pattern.

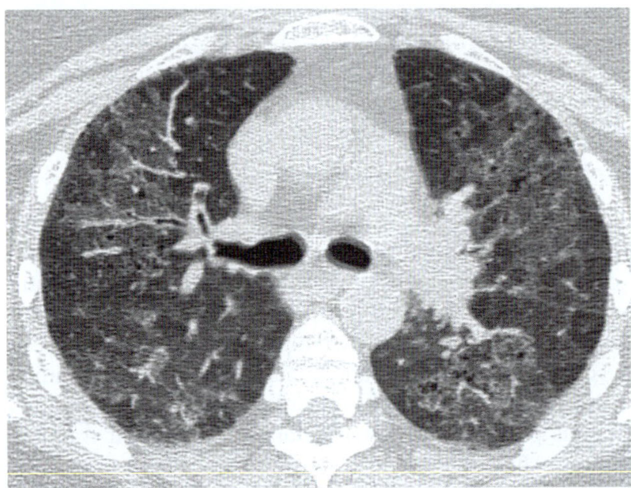

Fig. 43 CT chest through the upper lobes in a patient with desquamative interstitial pneumonitis showing a diffuse ground-glass attenuation

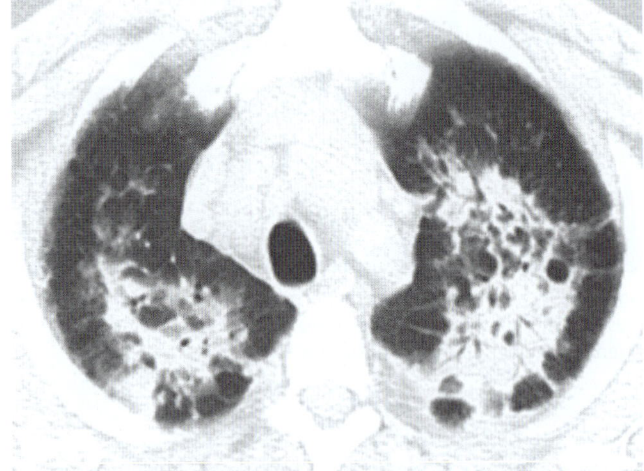

Fig. 44 CT chest showing bilateral dense consolidation in the upper lobes in cryptogenic organizing pneumonia

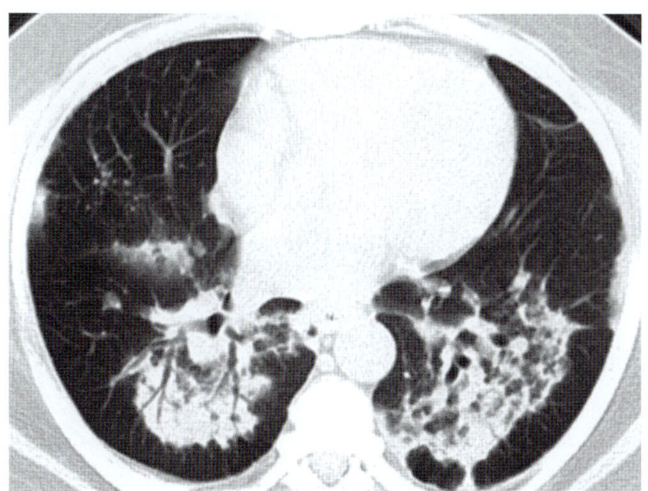

Fig. 45 CT chest through the lung bases showing dense bilateral consolidation with air bronchograms in a patient with cryptogenic organizing pneumonia

Lymphangioleiomyomatosis: Lymphangioleiomyomatosis (LAM) affects women of reproductive age, results from smooth muscle proliferation within the pulmonary interstitium causing thickening of walls of lymphatics, blood vessels and bronchioles. Patients present with spontaneous pneumothorax, chylothorax, hemoptysis and marked hyperexpansion of lungs. Characteristic HRCT features of LAM consist of diffuse thin-walled cysts surrounded by normal lung without regional sparing[102] **(Fig. 46)**. The cysts are rounded, may vary in size but bizarre shaped cysts as those seen in Langerhans cell histiocytosis (LCH) are unlikely[103] **(Fig. 47)**.

Langerhans cell histiocytosis: Langerhans cell histiocytosis also known as eosinophilic granuloma or histiocytosis X is a smoking-related lung disease with 80–100% of cases seen in patients with a history of smoking.[104] It is recognized on CT by the presence of cysts showing an upper lobe predominance, especially in the early stages. The initial changes include

Flow chart 3 Algorithmic approach to multinodular lung disease

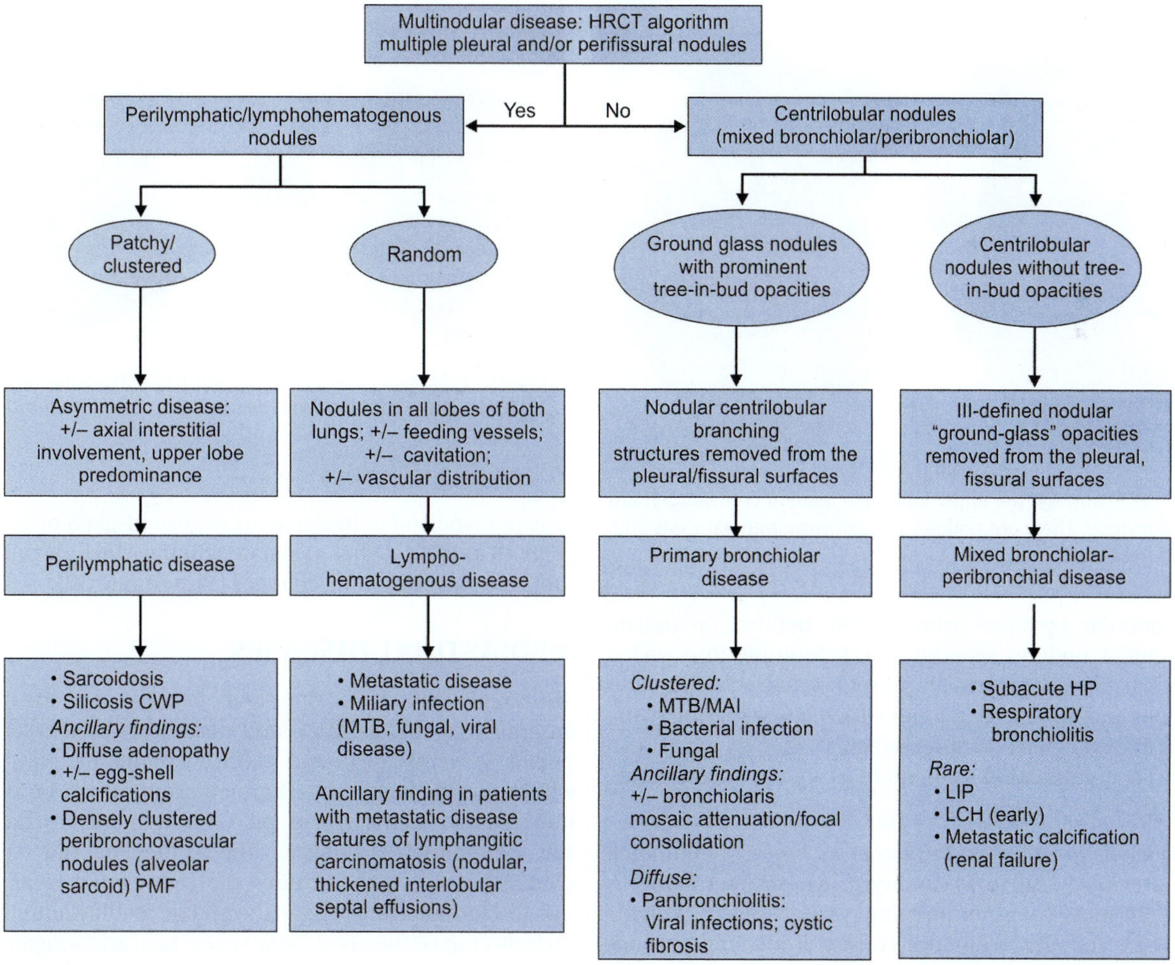

Multinodular disease: HRCT algorithm multiple pleural and/or perifissural nodules

- Yes → Perilymphatic/lymphohematogenous nodules
  - Patchy/ clustered → Asymmetric disease: +/– axial interstitial involvement, upper lobe predominance → Perilymphatic disease →
    - Sarcoidosis
    - Silicosis CWP
    - *Ancillary findings:*
    - Diffuse adenopathy
    - +/– egg-shell calcifications
    - Densely clustered peribronchovascular nodules (alveolar sarcoid) PMF
  - Random → Nodules in all lobes of both lungs; +/– feeding vessels; +/– cavitation; +/– vascular distribution → Lympho-hematogenous disease →
    - Metastatic disease
    - Miliary infection (MTB, fungal, viral disease)
    - Ancillary finding in patients with metastatic disease features of lymphangitic carcinomatosis (nodular, thickened interlobular septal effusions)
- No → Centrilobular nodules (mixed bronchiolar/peribronchiolar)
  - Ground glass nodules with prominent tree-in-bud opacities → Nodular centrilobular branching structures removed from the pleural/fissural surfaces → Primary bronchiolar disease →
    - *Clustered:*
      - MTB/MAI
      - Bacterial infection
      - Fungal
    - *Ancillary findings:* +/– bronchiolaris mosaic attenuation/focal consolidation
    - *Diffuse:*
      - Panbronchiolitis: Viral infections; cystic fibrosis
  - Centrilobular nodules without tree-in-bud opacities → Ill-defined nodular "ground-glass" opacities removed from the pleural, fissural surfaces → Mixed bronchiolar-peribronchial disease →
    - Subacute HP
    - Respiratory bronchiolitis
    - *Rare:*
      - LIP
      - LCH (early)
      - Metastatic calcification (renal failure)

Abbreviations: CWP, coal workers pneumocontosis; MAI, M atrium intracellulare; MTB, M tuberculosis; PMF, progressive massive fibrosis
Source: Raoof S, Amchentsev A, Vlahos I, et al. Pictorial essay: mulitinodular disease: a high-resolution CT scan diagnostic algorithm. Chest. 2006; 129(3):805-15.

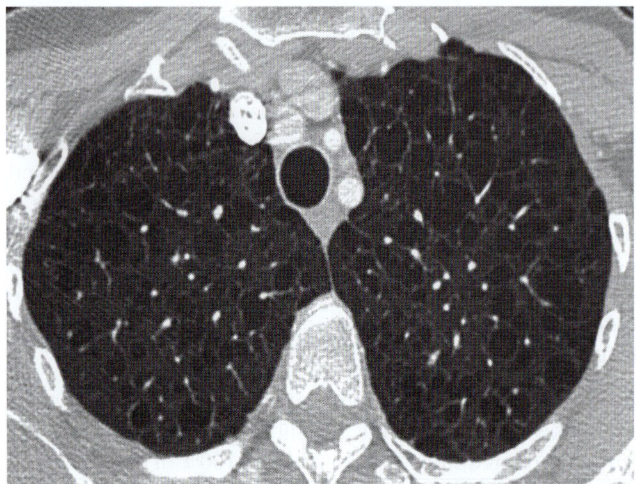

Fig. 46 CT chest through the upper lobes showing diffuse cystic changes in a patient with lymphangioleiomyomatosis. The cysts are evenly distributed and have thin, definable walls. Note the absence of nodules

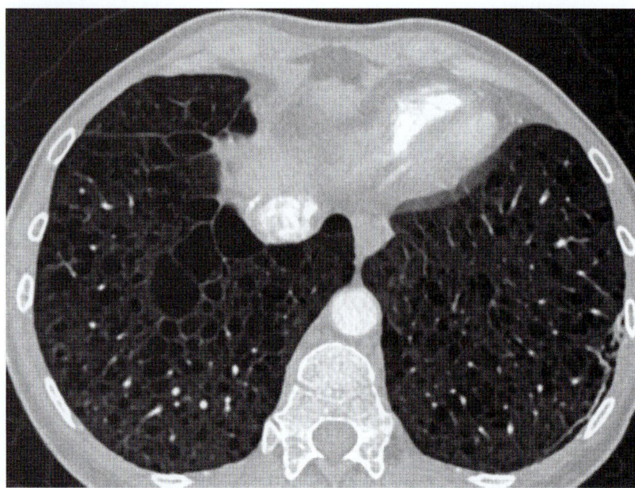

Fig. 47 CT chest in a patient with lymphangioleiomyomatosis showing well-defined, multiple cysts with uniform distribution at the lung bases

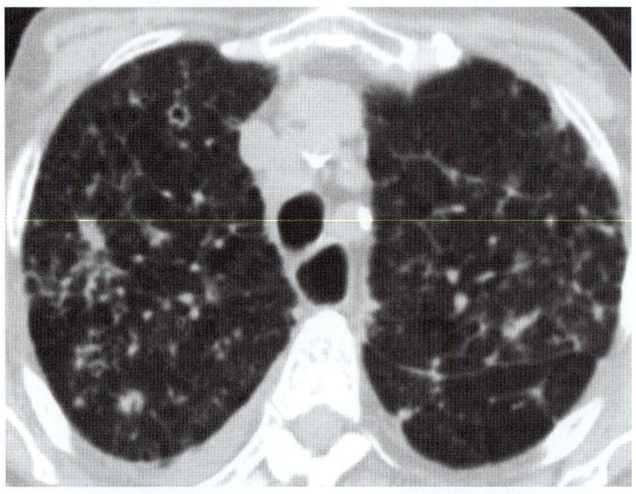

Fig. 48 HRCT through the upper lobes in a patient with Langerhans cell histiocytosis. There are nodules present with irregular cysts with thin and thick walls

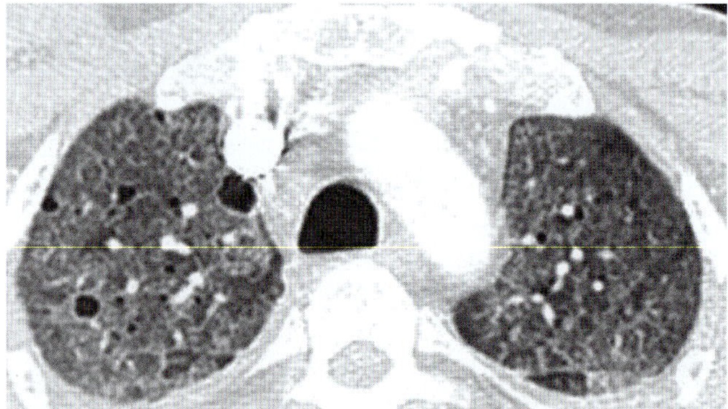

Fig. 49 A classic CT chest representation of diffuse ground glass attenuation in a patient with *Pneumocystic carinii* pneumonia

small nodular opacities with sharply defined or stellate centrilobular nodules seen on HRCT. Multiple thin-walled cysts of varying size are usually present, scattered throughout the upper and middle lung zones with relative sparing of the bases. The cysts have bizarre, irregular shapes, which can appear in combination with nodules in the intermediate stages of the disease **(Fig. 48)**.[105]

Pneumocystis pneumonia: Pneumocystis jiroveci pneumonia (PJP), previously called *Pneumocystis carinii* pneumonia is one of the most common pulmonary infections in patients with AIDS. The HRCT findings consist of bilateral ground-glass attenuation, which appear consolidated with severe disease and a distinct mosaic pattern with areas of normal lung interspersed between areas of ground-glass opacities[106] **(Figs 49 and 50)**. Other associated findings include pneumothoraces and cystic lung changes **(Figs 51 and 52)**.

MEDIASTINAL DISEASES

The mediastinum is bounded laterally by the lungs, anteriorly by the sternum, and posteriorly by the vertebral bodies. Several focal and diffuse conditions may occur within the mediastinum. The mediastinum can be divided into compartments based on CT landmarks to facilitate the differential diagnosis. These include the anterior mediastinum, which includes the retrosternal clear space and the cardiophrenic angle; the middle mediastinum, which includes the retrosternal clear space, subcarinal region, and retrocardiac clear space; and the posterior mediastinum. It should be pointed out that there are no physical boundaries

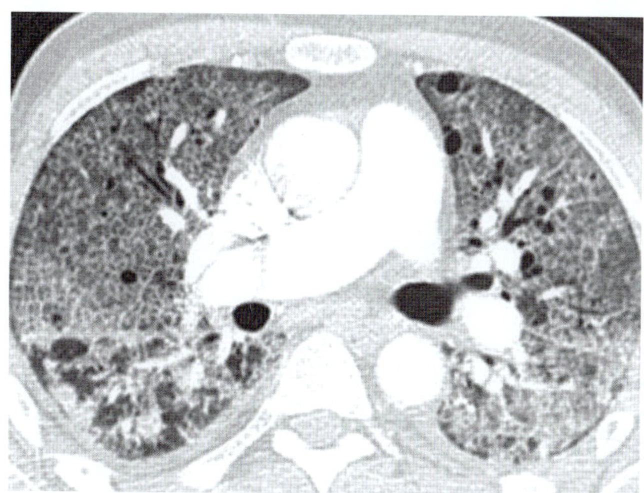

Fig. 50 CT chest showing a diffuse ground glass pattern with a crazy paving appearance in a patient with *Pneumocystic carinii* pneumonia

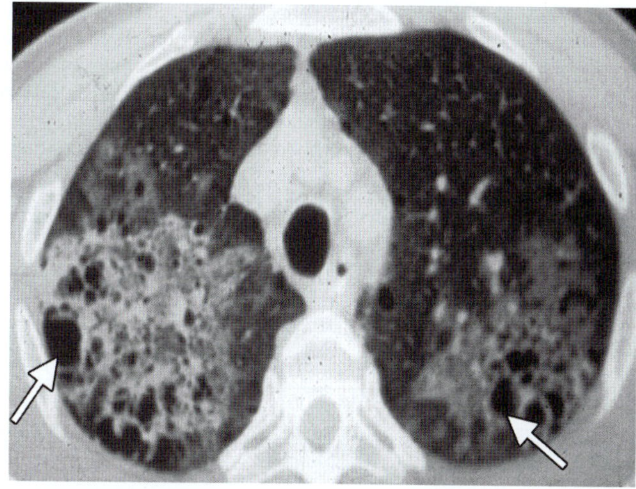

Fig. 52 HRCT through the upper lung zones showing a dense opacity in the right upper lobe, ground glass opacities in the left upper lobe, small and large (arrows) cysts in a patient with *Pneumocystic jiroveci* pneumonia

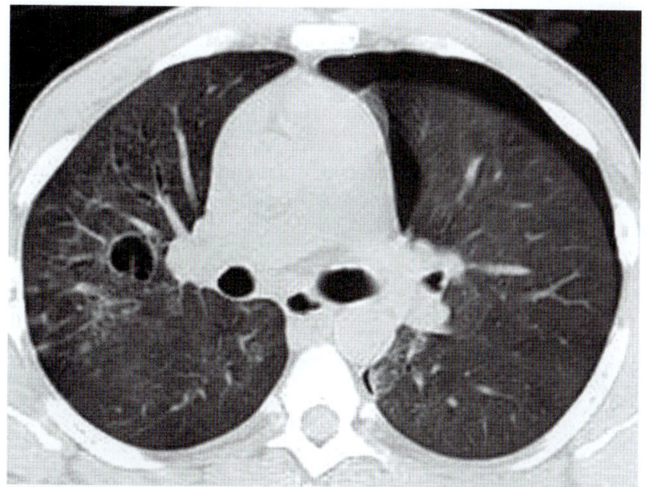

Fig. 51 CT chest in a patient with *Pneumocystic carinii* pneumonia with evidence of pneumothorax and bilateral diffuse haziness

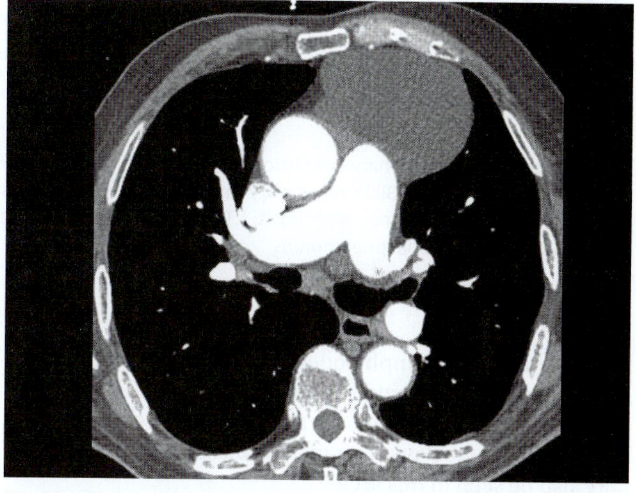

Fig. 53 CT chest (mediastinal window) illustrating a large mediastinal mass in the retrosternal clear space. Note the homogeneous appearance. This is representative of a thymic cyst

between different compartments that may limit any mediastinal disease **(Flow chart 4)**.

Retrosternal Clear Space

This region is bordered anteriorly by the sternum and posteriorly by the aorta and great vessels. The normal structures located in this region include the thymus gland, lymph nodes, and fat. Abnormalities involving the retrosternal clear space include thymoma, thymic cyst, lymphoma, teratoma, aortic aneurysm or lipoma. Thymomas represent a majority of anterior mediastinal lesions in adults. The CT appearance of a thymoma shows a homogeneous soft-tissue rounded or lobulated mass, which is sharply demarcated and does not conform to the normal shape of thymus.[107]

Thymic cysts are thin walled with air fluid levels on CT **(Fig. 53)**. Teratomas are seen with a combination of fluid-filled cysts, fat, soft tissue and calcification.[108]

Cardiophrenic Angle

The cardiophrenic angle is the space anterior to and the right of heart. Usual abnormalities are the benign lesions such as fat, lipoma, pericardial cyst or Morgagni hernia.

Retrotracheal Clear Space

The retrotracheal space includes structures posterior to the trachea, anterior to the thoracic spine and superior to the aortic arch. The normal structures in this area include

Flow chart 4 Multiple lucent lesions are classified according to their distribution pattern as either focal or diffuse. The focal lucencies can further be distinguished into upper lobe, lower lobe or random distribution. Examples of diffuse lucent lesions include panacinar emphysema, LAM, LIP or congenital disease related diffuse bronchiectasis. Examples of focal upper lung lucent lesions include centrilobular or paraseptal emphysema, LCH with presence of small nodules and infectious etiologies. Focal lower lung lucencies are usually seen in interstitial lung diseases such as UIP, DIP and RBILD as cystic changes with ground glass opacities also seen in DIP and RBILD. Randomly distributed focal lucencies may be seen in a braod group of conditions such as rheumatoid arthritis, necrotizing pneumonia and cavitating infarctions after a pulmonary embolism.

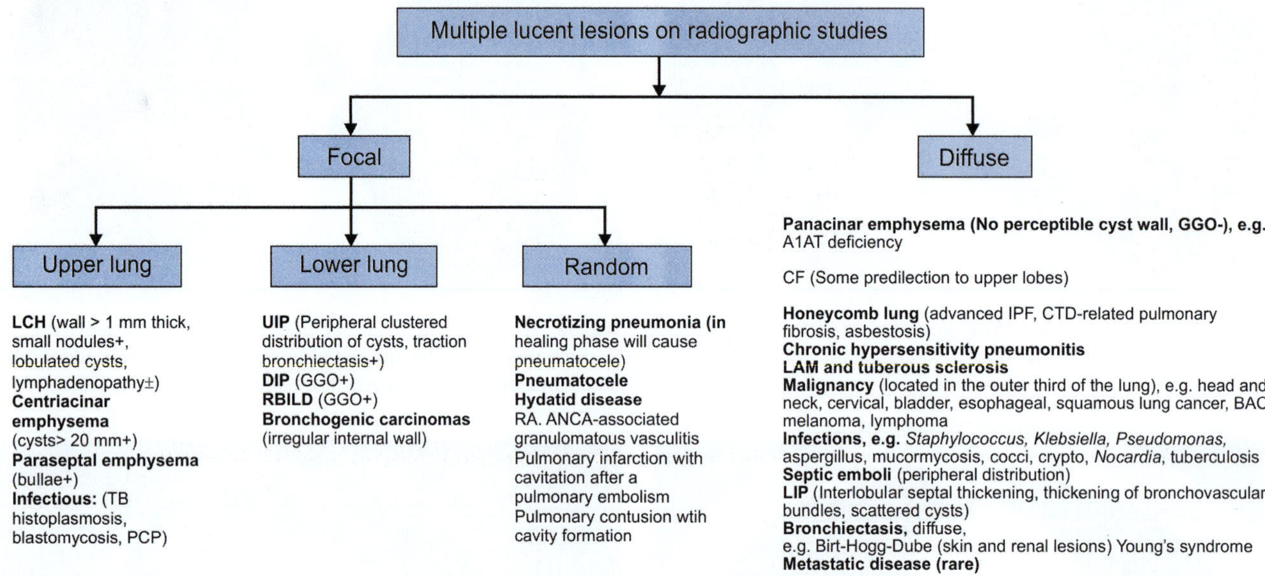

Abbreviations: LCH, Langerhans cell histiocytosis; TB, tuberculosis; PCP, *Pneumocystic jiroveci*; UIP, usual interstitial pneumonitis, DIP, desquamative interstitial pneumonitis; RBILD, respiratory bronchiolitis-interstitial lung disease; RA, rheumatoid arthritis; A1AT, alpha-1-antitrypsin; CF, cystic fibrosis; IFP, idiopathic pulmonary fibrosis; CTD, connective tissue disease; LAM, lymphangioleiomyomatosis; BAC, bronchoalveolar carcinoma; LIP, lymphocytic interstitial pneumonitis

the esophagus and lymph nodes. Abnormalities affecting the esophagus such as tumors, achalasia and Zenkers diverticulum are seen in this region. Vascular structures, such as an aberrant right subclavian, or thyroid masses, such as goiters, may also be seen in this area.[108]

Subcarinal Region

This region is situated below the carina and above the left atrium. Normal structures include fat, lymph nodes and the esophagus. The differential diagnosis of lesions in this location consists of lymphadenopathy, bronchogenic cysts, esophageal diverticulum or tumors **(Fig. 54)**.

Retrocardiac Clear Space

This retrocardiac space exists behind the heart and in front of the thoracic spine. Structures located in this space are the esophagus, aorta, azygous vein, fat, and lymph nodes. Esophageal lesions, such as duplication cyst, varices, hiatal hernia and tumor, aortic aneurysm and lymphadenopathy may arise in this location.

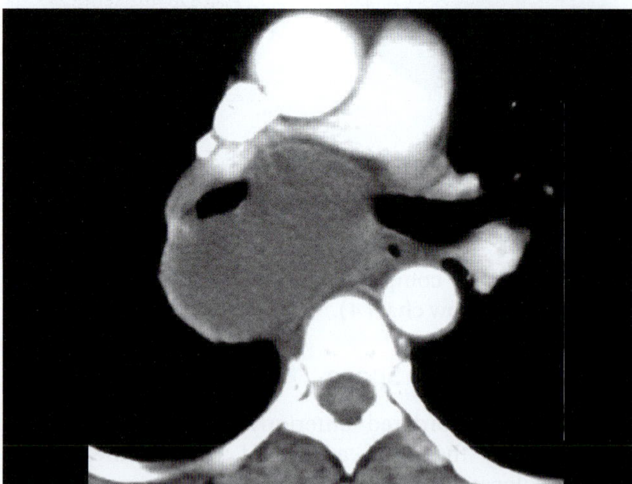

Fig. 54 CT chest (mediastinal window) demonstrating a large bronchogenic duplication cyst in the subcarinal region

Posterior Mediastinum

The posterior mediastinum covers the region posterior to the anterior border of vertebral bodies, where the vertebral

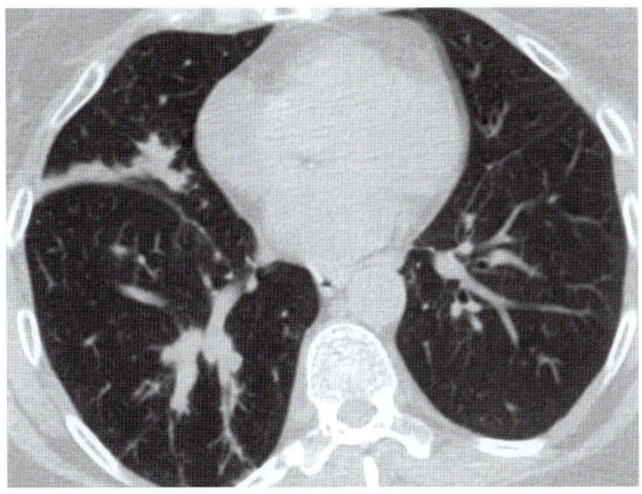

Fig. 55 CT chest showing insipation of bronchi in a patient with allergic bronchopulmonary aspergillosis

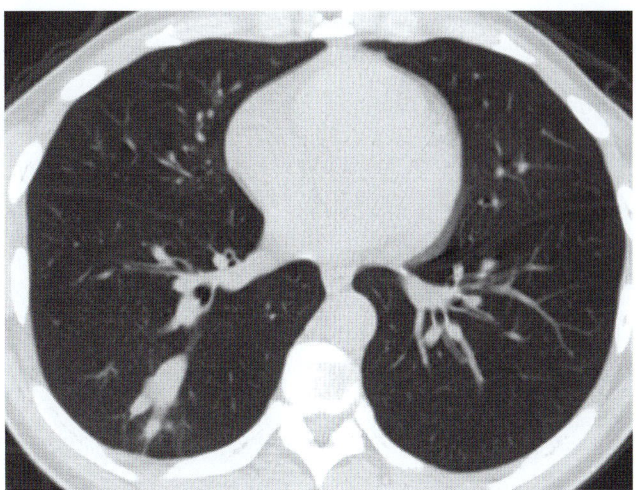

Fig. 56 CT chest in a patient with allergic bronchopulmonary aspergillosis showing insipation of the lower lobe bronchi

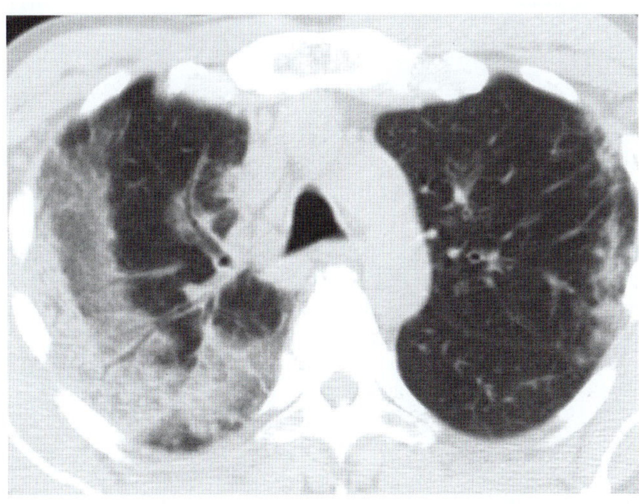

Fig. 57 CT chest with peripherally distributed opacities in a patient with chronic eosinophilic pneumonitis

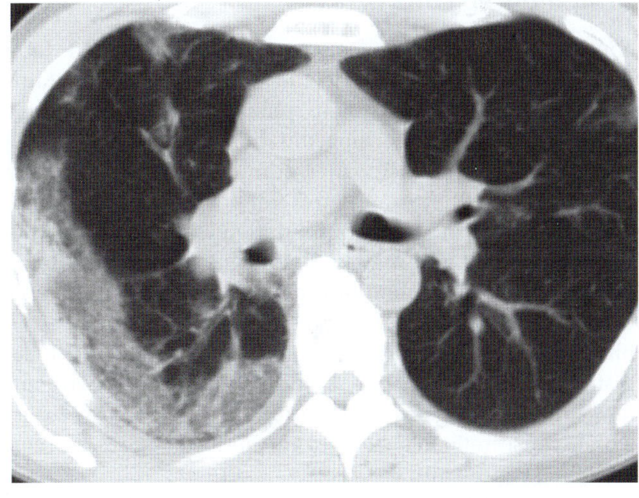

Fig. 58 CT chest in a patient with chronic eosinophillic pneumonitis with peripherally distributed opacities

column, fat and nerves are situated. The most common lesions in the posterior column are neurogenic and best imaged with MRI.

MISCELLANEOUS

Allergic Bronchopulmonary Mycosis

CT findings of ABPM include central airway abnormalities where there is bronchial dilatation with mucus-filled centrilobular bronchioles resulting in a tree-in-bud pattern **(Fig. 55)**.[109] Parenchymal abnormalities, such as consolidation, cavitation, bullae or scarring, and pleural abnormalities including focal pleural thickening may also be evident.[110] Central bronchiectasis and mucoid impaction are specific findings in ABPM **(Fig. 56)**.

Chronic Eosinophilic Pneumonia

The classic HRCT picture of chronic eosinophilic pneumonia is consolidation in a peripheral distribution confined primarily to the outer third of lung, and with an upper lobe distribution **(Figs 57 and 58)**.

Lipoid Pneumonia

CT findings of lipoid pneumonia have been studied in a small number of cases. In the appropriate clinical context, CT may demonstrate a solitary nodule resembling carcinoma, localized area of consolidation or extensive bilateral opacities.[111] HRCT findings of lipoid pneumonia show parenchymal nodules or opacities containing fat **(Fig. 59)**.

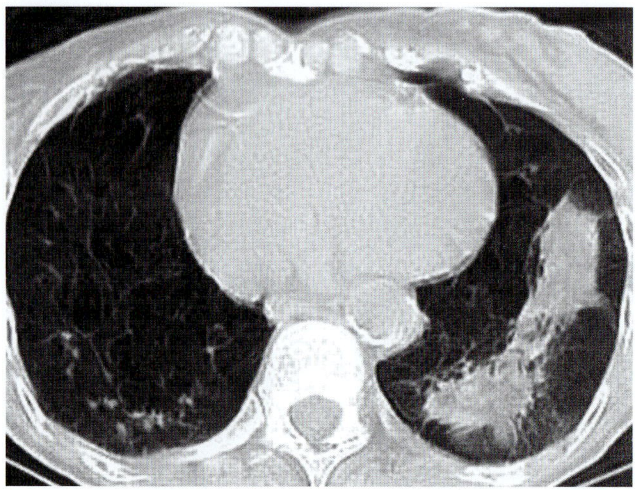

Fig. 59 CT chest representation of lipoid pneumonia

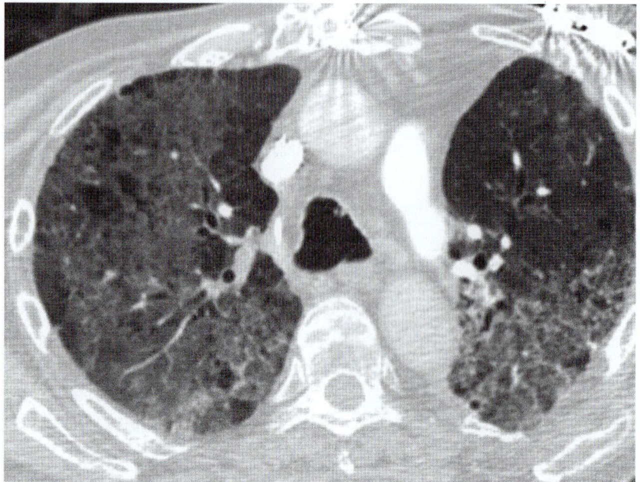

Fig. 60 CT chest showing diffuse fibrosis with ground glass attenuation in a patient with drug-induced lung disease

Drug-induced Lung Disease

There are several manifestations of drug-induced lung disease. The most common include noncardiogenic pulmonary edema, hypersensitivity pneumonitis and chronic pneumonitis.[112] Noncardiogenic pulmonary edema had been described to occur after administration of cytosine arabinoside, methotrexate and cyclophosphamide, resulting in a widespread airspace consolidation with predominance in the dependent lung regions. Hypersensitivity pneumonitis has been seen after methotrexate, cyclophosphamide and bleomycin administration. The HRCT finding consists of bilateral ground-glass attenuation in either patchy or diffuse distribution. Chronic pneumonitis is the most common drug-induced lung disease reported with all cytotoxic drugs which cause reticular changes in the lower lungs as seen with IPF **(Figs 60 and 61)**.

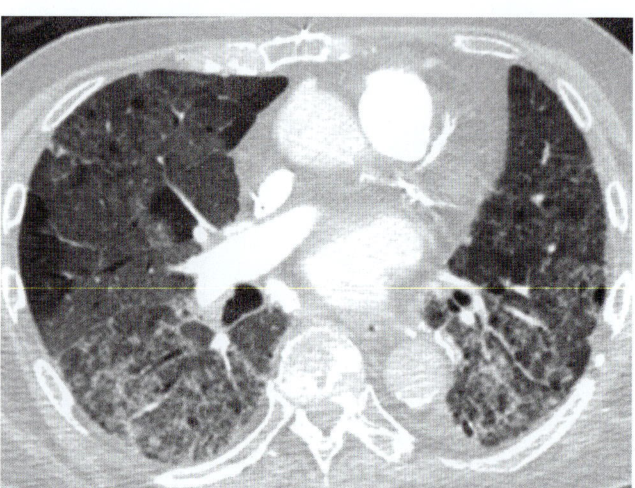

Fig. 61 CT chest showing diffuse fibrosis, increased density in drug-induced lung disease

CONCLUSION

The indications and role of CT imaging in the diagnoses of various thoracic diseases has been influenced immensely by a variety of technologic advancements. CT has become a fundamental part of clinical decision making in a number of conditions involving the lung parenchyma, airways, vasculature and mediastinum. Several characteristic features, such as ground-glass opacification, honeycomb changes and nodular features help to narrow down the differential diagnosis in many situations. These features depict the extent of disease processes and guide the course of management, eliminating the need for invasive diagnostic testing. It is, therefore, of paramount importance to understand and recognize the different CT features in thoracic conditions.

REFERENCES

1. Flohr TG, Schaller S, Stierstorfer K, Bruder H, Ohnesorge BM, Schoepf UJ. Multi-detector row CT systems and image-reconstruction techniques. Radiology. 2005;235(3):756-73.
2. Webb WR. Thin-section CT of the secondary pulmonary lobule: anatomy and the image—the 2004 Fleischner lecture. Radiology. 2006;239:322-38.
3. Müller NL. Clinical value of high-resolution CT in chronic diffuse lung disease. Am J Roentgenol. 1991;157:1163-70.
4. Heiken JP, Brink JA, Vannier MW. Spiral (helical) CT. Radiology. 1993;189(3):647-56.
5. Detterbeck FC, Mazzone PJ, Naidich DP, Bach PB. Screening for lung cancer: Diagnosis and management of lung cancer, 3rd edition. American College of Chest Physicians evidence-based clinical practice guidelines. Chest. 2013;143:e78S-92S.

6. Zerhouni EA, Naidich DP, Stitik FP, Khouri NF, Siegelman SS. Computed tomography of the pulmonary parenchyma: Part 2. Interstitial disease. J Thorac Imaging. 1985;1:54-64.
7. Weibel ER, Gill J. Structure-function relationships at the alveolar level. In: West JB (Ed). Bioengineering aspect of the lung. New York: Marcel Becker, Inc.; 1977. pp. 1-81.
8. Naidich DP, Zerhouni EA, Hutchins GM, Genieser NB, McCauley DI, Siegelman SS. Computed tomography of the pulmonary parenchyma: Part I: Distal air-space disease. J Thorac Imaging. 1985;1:39-53.
9. Miller WS. The Lung. Springfield: Charles C. Thomas; 1947.
10. Heitzman ER, Markarian B, Berger I, Dailey E. The secondary pulmonary lobule: a practical concept to an understanding of roentgen pattern in disease states. Radiology. 1969;93:514-20.
11. Raoof S, Amchentsev A, Vlahos I, Goud A, Naidich DP. Pictorial essay: mulitinodular disease; a high-resolution CT scan diagnostic algorithm. Chest. 2006;129:805-15.
12. Murata K, Itoh H, Todo G, Kanaoka M, Noma S, Itoh T, et al. Centrilobular lesions of the lung: demonstration by high-resolution CT and pathologic correlation. Radiology. 1986;161:641-5.
13. Austin JHM, Müller NL, Friedman PJ, Hansell DM, Naidich DP, Remy-Jardin M, et al. Glossary of terms for CT of the lungs: recommendations of the Nomenclature Committee of the Fleischner Society. Radiology. 1996;200:327-31.
14. Miller WT, Shah RM. Isolated diffuse ground-glass opacity in thoracic CT: causes and clinical presentations. Am J Roentgenol. 2005;184:613-22.
15. Leung AN, Miller RR, Müller NL. Parenchymal opacification in chronic infiltrative lung disease: CT-pathologic correlation. Radiology. 1993;188:209-14.
16. Foster WL, Pratt PC, Roggli VL, Godwin JD, Halvorsen RA, Putman CE. Centrilobular emphysema: CT-pathologic correlation. Radiology. 1986;159:27-32.
17. Stern EJ, Swensen SJ, Hartman TE, Frank MS. Pictorial assay. CT mosaic pattern of lung attenuation: Distinguishing different causes. Am J Roentgenol. 1995;165:813-6.
18. Naidich DP, Harkin TJ. Airways and lung: correlation of CT with fiberoptic bronchoscopy. Radiology. 1995;197:1-12.
19. Gamsu G, Webb WR. Computed Tomography of the trachea: normal and abnormal. Am J Roentgenol. 1983;18:51-60.
20. Breatnach E, Abbott GC, Fraser RC. Dimensions of the normal human trachea. Am J Roentgenol. 1984;141:903-6.
21. Stern EJ, Graham CM, Webb WR, Gamsu G. Normal trachea during forced expiration: dynamic CT measurements. Radiology. 1993;187:27-31.
22. Jackson CL, Huber JF. Correlated applied anatomy of the bronchial tree and lungs with a system of nomenclature. Chest. 1943;9:319-26.
23. Greene R. "Saber sheath" trachea: relation to chronic obstructive pulmonary disease. Am J Roentgenol. 1978;130:441-5.
24. Shin MS, Jackson RM, Ho KJ. Tracheobronchomegaly (Mounier-Kuhn syndrome): CT diagnosis. Am J Roentgenol. 1988;150:777-9.
25. Surprenant EL, O'Loughlin BJ. Tracheal diverticula and tracheobronchomegaly. Dis Chest. 1966;49:345-51.
26. Hartman T. Pearls and Pitfalls in Thoracic Imaging. New York, NY: Cambridge University Press; 2012. p. 234.
27. Restrepo S, Pandit M, Villamil MA, Rojas IC, Perez JM, Gascue A. Tracheobronchopathia osteochondroplastica: helical CT findings in 4 cases. J Thorac Imaging. 2004;19(2):112-6.
28. Baroni RH, Feller-Kopman D, Nishino M, Hatabu H, Loring SH, Ernst A, et al. Tracheobronchomalacia: comparison between end-expiratory and dynamic expiratory CT for evaluation of central airway collapse. Radiology. 2005; 235(2):635-41.
29. Kuriyama K, Gamsu G, Stern RG, Cann CE, Herfkens RJ, Brundage BH. CT-determined pulmonary artery diameters in predicting pulmonary hypertension. Invest Radiol. 1984;19: 16-22.
30. Elliot FM, Reid L. Some new facts about the pulmonary artery and its branching pattern. Clin Radiol. 1965;16:193-8.
31. Webb WR. Radiologic imaging of the pulmonary hila. Postgrad Radiol. 1986;6:145-68.
32. Sondheimer HM, Oliphant M, Schneider B, Kavey RE, Blackman MS, Parker FB Jr. Computerized axial tomography of the chest for visualization of "absent" pulmonary arteries. Circulation. 1982;65:1020-5.
33. Berden WE, baker DH, wung JT. Complete cartilage-ring tracheal stenosis associated with anomalous left pulmonary artery: the ring-sling complex. Radiology. 1984;152:57-64.
34. Dillon EH, Camputaro C. Partial anomalous pulmonary venous drainage of the left upper lobe vs duplication of the superior vena cava: distinction based on CT findings. AJR Am J Roentgenol. 1993;160:375-9.
35. Kuzo RS, Goodman LR. CT evaluation of pulmonary embolism: technique and interpretation. Am J Roentgenol. 1997;169: 959-65.
36. Tiegen CL, Maus TP, Sheedy PF, Johnson CM, Stanson AW, Welch TJ. Pulmonary embolism: diagnosis with electron-beam CT. Radiology. 1993;188:839-45.
37. Bartter T, Irwin RS, Nash G. Review: aneurysms of the pulmonary arteries. Chest. 1988;94:1065-79.
38. Borolowski GP, O'Donovan PB, Troup BR. Pulmonary varix: CT findings. J Comput Assist Tomogr. 1981;5:827-9.
39. Gudjberg CE. Roentgenologic diagnosis of bronchiectasis: an analysis of 112 cases. Acta Radiol. 1955;43:209-26.
40. Rosen M. Chronic Cough Due to Bronchiectasis ACCP Evidence-Based Clinical Practice Guidelines. Chest. 2006;129: 122S-31S.
41. Naidich DP. High resolution computed tomography of cystic lung disease. Semin Roentgenol. 1991;26:151-74.
42. Teel GS, Engeler CE, Tshijian JH, duCret RP. Imaging of small airways disease. Radiographics. 1996;16:27-41.
43. Devakonda A, Raoof S, Sung A, Travis WD, Naidich D. Bronchiolar disorders. A clinical-radiological diagnostic algorithm. Chest. 2010;137:938-51.
44. Hartman TE, Primack SL, Lee KS, Swensen SJ, Mueller NL. CT of bronchial and bronchiolar diseases. Radiographics. 1994;14:991-1003.
45. Im JG, Itoh H, Shim YS, Lee JH, Ahn J, Han MC, et al. Pulmonary tuberculosis: CT findings—early active disease and sequential change with antituberculous therapy. Radiology. 1993;186: 653-60.
46. Akira M, Kitatani F, Lee YS, Kita N, Yamamoto S, Higashihara T, et al. Diffuse panbronchiolitis: evaluation with high-resolution CT. Radiology. 1988;168:433-8.
47. Aquino SL, Gamsu G, Webb WR, Kee ST. Tree-in-bud pattern: frequency and significance on thin section CT. J Comput Assist Tomogr. 1996;20:594-9.
48. Bartter T, Irwin RS, Nash G, Balikian JP, Hollingsworth HH. Idiopathic Bronchiolitis obliterans organizing pneumonia

with peripheral infiltrates on chest roentgenogram. Arch Intern Med. 1989;149:273-9.
49. Epler GR, Colby TV, McLoud TC, Carrington CG, Gaensler EA. Idiopathic Bronchiolitis obliterans with organizing pneumonia. N Engl J Med. 1985;312:152-9.
50. Katzenstein ALA. Major problems in pathology. In: Katzenstein and Askin's surgical pathology of non-neoplastic lung disease, 3rd edition. Philadelphia: WB Saunders; 1997. p. 477.
51. Worthy SA, Flower CDR. Computed tomography of the airways. Eur Radiol. 1996;6:717-29.
52. Patel VK, Naik SK, Naidich DP, Travis WD, Weingarten JA, Lazzaro R, et al. A practical algorithm approach to the diagnosis and management of solitary pulmonary nodules: part 1: radiologic characteristics and imaging modalities. Chest. 2013;143(3):825-39.
53. MacMahon H, Austin JH, Gamsu G, Herold CJ, Jett JR, Naidich DP, et al. Guidelines for management of small pulmonary nodules detected on CT scans: a statement from the Fleischner Society. Radiology. 2005;237(2):395-400.
54. Munden RF, Pugatch RD, Liptay MJ, Sugarbaker DJ, Le LU. Small pulmonary lesions detected at CT: clinical importance. Radiology. 1997;202:105-10.
55. Libby DM, Henschke CI, Yankelevitz DF. The solitary pulmonary nodule: update 1995. Am J Med. 1995;99:491-6.
56. Swensen SJ, Silverstein MD, Ilstrup DM, Schleck CD, Edell ES. The probability of malignancy in solitary pulmonary nodules. Application to small radiologically indeterminate nodules. Arch Intern Med. 1997;157(8):849-55.
57. Bankoff MS, McEniff NJ, Bhadelia RA, Garacia-Moliner M, Daly BDT. Prevelance of pathologically proven intrapulmonary lymph nodes and their appearance on CT. Am J Roentgenol. 1996;167:629-30.
58. Furuya K, Murayama S, Soeda H, Murakami J, Ichinose Y, Yabuuchi H, et al. New classification of small pulmonary nodules by margin characteristics on high-resolution CT. Acta Radiol. 1999;40(5):496-504.
59. Zwirewich CV, Vedal S, Miller RR, Mueller NL. Solitary pulmonary nodule: hight-resoluation CT and radiologic-pathologic correlation. Radiology. 1991;179:469-76.
60. Primack SL, Hartman TE, Lee KS, Mueller NL. Pulmonary nodules and the CT halo sign. Radiology. 1994;190:513-5.
61. Gaeta M, Barone M, Russi EG, Volta S, Casablanca G, Romeo P, et al. Carcinomatous solitary pulmonary nodules: evaluation of the tumor-bronchi relationship with thin-section CT. Radiology. 1993;187:535-9.
62. Woodring JH, Fried AM. Significance of wall thickness in solitary cavities of the lung: a follow up study. Am J Roentgenol. 1983;140:473-4.
63. Mezaine MA, Hruban RH, Zerhouni EA, Wheeler PS, Khouri NF, Fishman EK, et al. High resolution CT of the lung parenchyma with pathologic correlation. Radiographics. 1988;8:27-54.
64. Nathan MH, Collins VP, Adama RA. Differentiation of benign and malignant pulmonary nodules by growth rate. Radiology. 1962;79:221-31.
65. O'Keefe Jr ME, Good CA, Mcdonald JE. Calcification in solitary nodules in the lung. Am J Roentgenol. 1957;77:1023-33.
66. Mahoney MC Sr, Shipley RT, Corcoran HL, Dickson BA. CT demonstration of calcification in carcinoma of the lung. Am J Roentgenol. 1990;154(2):255-8.
67. Siegelman SS, Khouri NF, Scott WW Jr, Leo FP, Hamper UM, Fishman EK, et al. Pulmonary hamartoma: CT findings. Radiology. 1986;160(2):313-7.
68. Littleton JT, Durizch ML, Moeller G, Herbert DE. Pulmonary masses: contrast enhancement. Radiology. 1990;177:861-71.
69. Swensen SJ, Brown LR, Colby TV, Weaver AL, Midthun DE. Lung nodule enhancement at CT: prospective findings. Radiology. 1996;201:447-55.
70. Ryu JH, Olson EJ, Midthun DE, Swensen SJ. Diagnostic approach to the patient with diffuse lung disease. Mayo Clin Proc. 2002;77:1221-7.
71. Katzenstein AL, Myers J. Idiopathic pulmonary fibrosis. Clinical relevance of pathologic classification. Am J Resp Crit Care Med. 1998;157:1301-15.
72. Thomeer M, Demedts M, Behr J, Buhl R, Costabel U, Flower CD, et al. Multidisciplinary interobserver agreement in the diagnosis of idiopathic pulmonary fibrosis. Eur Respir J. 2008;31(3):585-91.
73. Raghu G, Collard HR, Egan JJ, Martinez FJ, Behr J, Brown KK, et al. An official ATS/ERS/JRS/ALAT statement: idiopathic pulmonary fibrosis: evidence-based guidelines for diagnosis and management. Am J Respir Crit Care Med. 2011;183(6): 788-824.
74. Müller NL, Miller RR, Webb WR, Evans KG, Ostrow DN. Fibrosing alveolitis: CT-pathologic correlation. Radiology. 1992;185:91-5.
75. Park JS, Lee KS, Kim JS, Park CS, Suh YL, Choi DL, et al. Nonspecific interstitial pneumonia with fibrosis: radiographic and CT findings in seven patients. Radiology. 1995;195: 645-8.
76. Staples CA, Müller NL, Vedal S, Abboud R, Ostrow D, Miller RR. Usual interstitial pneumonias: correlation of CT with clinical, functional, and radiologic findings. Radiology. 1987;162:377-81.
77. Remy-Jardin M, Remy J, Cortet B, Mauri F, Delcambre B. Lung changes in rheumatoid arthritis: CT findings. Radiology. 1994;193:375-82.
78. Schurawitzki H, Stiglbauer R, Graninger W, Herold C, Pölzleitner D, Burghuber OC, et al. Interstitial lung disease in progressive systemic sclerosis: high-resolution CT versus radiography. Radiology. 1990;176:755-9.
79. Akira M, Yokoyama K, Yamamoto S, Higashihara T, Morinaga K, Kita N, et al. Early asbestosis: evaluation with high-resolution CT. Radiology. 1991;178:409-16.
80. Akira M, Yamatomo S, Yokoyama K, Kita N, Morinaga K, Higashihara T, et al. Asbestosis: high-resolution CT-pathologic correlation. Radiology. 1990;176:389-94.
81. Brauner MW, Grenier P, Mompoint D, Lenoir S, de Cremoux H. Pulmonary sarcoidosis: evaluation with high-resolution CT. Radiology. 1989;172:467-71.
82. Aikins A, Kanne JP, Chung JH. Galaxy sign. J Thorac Imaging. 2012;27:W164.
83. Müller NL, Kullnig P, Miller RR. The CT findings of pulmonary sarcoidosis: analysis of 25 patients. Am J Roentgenol. 1989;152:1179-82.
84. Lynch DA, Webb WR, Gamsu G, Stulbarg M, Golden J. Computed tomography in pulmonary sarcoidosis. J Comput Assist Tomogr. 1989;13:405-10.
85. Sider L, Horton ES. Hilar and mediastinal adenopathy in sarcoidosis as detected by computed tomography. J Thorac Imaging. 1990;5:77-80.
86. Remy-Jardin M, Degreef JM, Beuscart R, Voisin C, Remy J. Coal worker's pneumoconiosis: CT assessment in exposed workers and correlation with radiographic findings. Radiology. 1990;177:363-71.

87. Munk PL, Mueller NL, Miller RR, Ostrow DN. Pulmonary lymphangitic carcinomatosis: CT and pathologic findings. Radiology. 1988;166:705-9.
88. Silver SF, Mueller NL, Miller RR, Lefcoe MS. Hypersensitivity pneumonitis: evaluation with CT. Radiology. 1989;173:441-5.
89. Adler BD, Padley SP, Mueller NL, Remy-Jardin M, Remy J. Chronic hypersensitivity pneumonitis: high-resolution CT and radiographic features in 16 patients. Radiology. 1992;185:91-5.
90. Johkoh T, Muller NL, Pickford HA, Hartman TE, Ichikado K, Akira M, et al. Lymphocytic interstitial pneumonia: thin-section CT findings in 22 patients. Radiology. 1999;212(2):567-72.
91. Sugiyama Y. Diffuse panbronchiolitis. Clin Chest Med. 1993; 14(4):765-72.
92. Akira M, Kitatani F, Lee YS, Kita N, Yamamoto S, Higashihara T, et al. Diffuse panbronchiolitis: evaluation with high-resolution CT. Radiology. 1988;168(2):433-8.
93. Murata K, Takahashi M, Mori M, Kawaguchi N, Furukawa A, Ohnaka Y, et al. Pulmonary metastatic nodules: CT-pathologic correlation. Radiology. 1992;182:331-5.
94. Hartman TE, Primack SL, Swensen SJ, Hansell D, McGuinness G, Müller NL. Desquamative interstitial pneumonia: thin-section CT findings in 22 patients. Radiology. 1993;187:787-90.
95. Primack SL, Hartman TE, Ikezoe J, Akira M, Sakatani M, Müller NL. Acute Interstitial pneumonia: radiographic and CT findings in nine patients. Radiology. 1993;188:817-20.
96. Murch CR, Carr DH. Computed tomography appearance of pulmonary alveolar proteinosis. Clin Radiol. 1989;40:240-3.
97. Godwin JD, Müller NL. Pulmonary alveolar proteinosis: CT findings. Radiology. 1988;169:609-13.
98. Lee CH. The crazy-paving sign. Radiology. 2007;243:905-6.
99. Ujita M, Renzoni EA, Veeraraghavan S, Wells AU, Hansell DM. Organizing pneumonia: perilobular pattern at thin-section CT. Radiology. 2004;232(3):757-61.
100. Kim SJ, Lee KS, Ryu YH, Yoon YC, Choe KO, Kim TS, et al. Reversed halo sign on high-resolution CT of cryptogenic organizing pneumonia: diagnostic implications. Am J Roentgenol. 2003;180(5):1251-4.
101. Trigaux JP. Gevenois PA, Goncette L, Gouat F, Schumaker A, Weynants P. Bronchioloalveolar carcinoma: computed tomography findings. Eur Respir J. 1996;9(1):11-6.
102. Seaman D, Meyer C. Diffuse cystic lung disease at high-resolution CT. Am J Roentgenol. 2011;196:1305-11.
103. Müller NL, Chiles C, Kullnig P. Pulmonary lymphangiomyomatosis: correlation of CT with radiographic and functional findings. Radiology. 1990;175:335-9.
104. Brauner MW, Grenier P, Mouelhi MM, Mompoint D, Lenoir S. Pulmonary histiocytosis X: evaluation with high resolution CT. Radiology. 1989;172:255-8.
105. Bergin CJ, Wirth RL, Berry GJ, Castellino RA. *Pneumocystis carinii* pneumonia: CT and HRCT observations. J Comput Assist Tomogr. 1990;14:756-9.
106. Morgenthaler TI, Brown LR, Colby TV, Harper CM, Coles DT. Thymoma. Mayo Clinic Proc. 1993;68:1110-23.
107. Hoffman OA, Gillespie DJ, Aughenbaugh GL, Brown LR. Primary mediastinal neoplasms (other than thymomas). Mayo Clin Proc. 1993;68:880-91.
108. Franquet T, Erasmus JJ, Giménez A, Rossi S, Prats R. The retrotracheal space: normal anatomic and pathologic appearances. Radiographics. 2002;22:S231-46.
109. Neeld DA, Goodman LR, Gurney JW, Greenberger PA, Fink JN. Computerized tomography in the evaluation of allergic bronchopulmonary aspergillosis. Am Rev Respir Dis. 1990;142: 1200-6.
110. Panchal N, Bhagat R, Pant C, Shah A. Allergic bronchopulmonary aspergillosis: the spectrum of computed tomography appearances. Respir Med. 1997;91:213-9.
111. Wheeler PS, Stitik FP, Hutchins GM, Klinefelter HF, Siegelman SS. Diagnosis of lipoid pneumonia by computed tomography. JAMA. 1981;235:65-6.
112. Padley SPG, Adler B, Hansell DM, Müller NL. High resolution computed tomography of drug induced lung disease. Clin Radiol. 1992;46:232-6.

Pulmonary Function Tests

Ashutosh N Aggarwal

INTRODUCTION

Pulmonary function tests are designed to assess how well the lungs are able to perform their intended role. There is as yet no single test that can provide sufficiently detailed information on all aspects of lung function. Instead, depending on the clinical scenario, one must do one or more procedures to answer a particular question. Further, the available options vary greatly in terms of ease of conducting the test, equipment and technician requirements, test performance characteristics, and procedure cost. As a result, not all investigations may be feasible, or even necessary, in a given setting. Of all pulmonary function tests available, spirometry is by far the most commonly used procedure, in view of its relative simplicity, easy equipment availability, and good standardization of test performance and interpretation algorithms. This chapter provides an overview of the physiologic principles, conduct, and interpretation of commonly used pulmonary function tests. The abbreviations and terminology used herein are outlined in **Table 1**.

Table 1 Glossary of abbreviations and terms describing lung volumes and air flow

Abbreviations		
ERV	Expiratory reserve volume	Difference between the volume of air in lungs at end expiration during quiet breathing [functional residual capacity (FRC)] and after forced exhalation (residual volume)
$FEF_{25-75\%}$	Forced midexpiratory flow	The average airflow in the middle half of a forced expiratory maneuver
FEV_1	Forced expiratory volume in first second	Volume of air exhaled during the first second of a forced vital capacity maneuver
$FEV_1\%$	FEV1/VC	Ratio of forced expiratory volume in first second to the vital capacity (either forced or slow)
FEV_t	Forced expiratory volume in first "t" seconds	Volume of air exhaled during the first 't' seconds of a forced vital capacity maneuver (e.g. FEV_6 is the volume in first 6 seconds)
FRC	Functional residual capacity	Volume of air remaining in lungs at end expiration during quiet breathing
FVC	Forced vital capacity	Volume of air exhaled from a position of full inspiration to full expiration during a forced expiratory maneuver
IRV	Inspiratory reserve volume	Difference between the volume of air in lungs at end inspiration during quiet breathing and after maximal inspiration (TLC)
MVV	Maximal voluntary ventilation	Maximal volume of air that can be breathed in (or out) in 1 minute
PEF	Peak expiratory flow	The maximal air flow generated during a forced expiratory maneuver
RV	Residual volume	Volume of air remaining in lungs even after complete forced expiration
SVC	Slow vital capacity	Volume of air exhaled from a position of full inspiration to full expiration during a slow (or relaxed) expiratory maneuver
TLC	Total lung capacity	Volume of air within lungs at end of full inspiration
VC	Vital capacity	Volume of air exhaled from a position of full inspiration to full expiration
V_E	Minute ventilation	Volume of air exhaled in 1 minute
V_t	Tidal volume	Volume of air breathed in (or out) in each respiratory cycle during quiet respiration

SPIROMETRY

Spirometry is the most common and most widely used lung function test, although its true potential still needs to be realized. In many ways, its utility can be compared to blood pressure measurement, or electrocardiography, in routine cardiac evaluation. However, one needs to pay careful attention to following standard procedures while performing and interpreting the test. Because the residual volume (RV) in lungs cannot be exhaled, spirometric measurements are limited to the vital capacity (VC) and its subdivisions **(Fig. 1)**.

Indications and Contraindications

There are multiple scenarios in which information obtained from spirometry may prove useful. Most, but not all, persons referred for lung function testing suffer from respiratory disorders.[1] The most common indication for doing the test is a functional evaluation of patients with lung disease. The presence of spirometric abnormalities, as well as the degree of impairment, provides useful information about the disease severity and pulmonary reserve of the patient. Often, the test is conducted to narrow the differential diagnosis of a patient being assessed for pulmonary disorder. For instance, documentation of airflow limitation in a smoker being evaluated for breathlessness would increase the probability of the patient having chronic obstructive pulmonary disease (COPD). Because the test can be easily repeated, and the results are quite reproducible for a given patient, serial measurements can provide information about disease progression, as well as response to prescribed treatment. The test also has an important role in clinical trials, as it is the best standardized objective surrogate for true pulmonary function. Spirometry is also used as a screening tool for studies in epidemiologic surveys, as it may provide an objective definition of disease state (such as bronchial asthma). It can also be used to screen at-risk populations for subclinical disease (e.g. preoperative assessment, or detecting COPD among asymptomatic smokers). The test is also utilized in occupational setting, both for detecting work-related respiratory disorders, and for disability assessment in symptomatic people (e.g. as part of compensation procedures). Finally, spirometry is an important research tool for understanding pathophysiology and temporal course of several diseases, as well as for derivation and validation of reference equations.

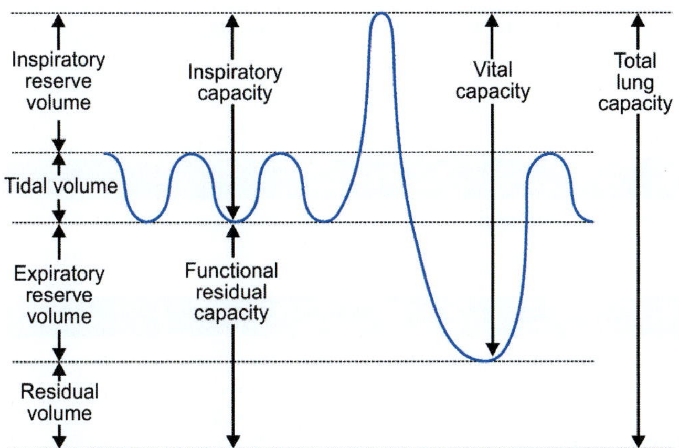

Fig. 1 Various lung volumes and capacities in relation to the spirometry tracing. Note that residual volume (RV) cannot be determined through conventional spirometry

It is also important to understand when not to perform spirometry. Any benefit from the information obtained through this test should be carefully weighed against patient discomfort and risk. The test is better avoided in pregnant and severely dyspneic patients. It should also not be carried out in patients where pressure swings due to a forced expiratory maneuver can worsen existing conditions (such as ruptured tympanic membrane, bronchopleural fistula, ongoing hemoptysis, etc.). Uncooperative patients, and those on life support systems, should also not undergo the test.

Equipment

A wide range of apparatus, ranging from handheld portable devices to large equipment, and from predominantly manual to completely automated systems, is available to perform spirometry. Although many factors such as cost, patient load, clinical requirements, etc. determine the choice of machine, it is important to use one that confirms to some minimum technical specifications necessary to obtain valid results. Such recommendations for equipment performance were laid out by the American Thoracic Society (ATS), and have recently been updated as a joint recommendation from ATS and European Respiratory Society (ERS).[2,3] The important performance criteria relate to accuracy (degree of conformity to the true value), precision (degree of repeatability of the same measurement), and resolution (minimum measurable incremental quantity). It is also advisable to have a system that can be calibrated periodically to ensure optimum performance.

Most commercially available spirometers nowadays are computerized systems that employ a transducer to convert a mechanical signal to an electrical one, and display the output in a fashion understood by the operator. These equipment can be divided into two broad categories: (1) Volume displacement spirometers, and (2) Flow-sensing spirometers. The former work with volume as the primary output, and flow is a derived parameter. Such machines can have a water seal, a dry-rolling seal, or a bellows type design. Flow-sensing devices can either be electronic turbines, or use electronic pneumotachometers (sensors that estimate airflow from the change in pressure occurring across a suitable resistance), which in turn can have a flow-resistive, a heated wire, or an ultrasonic design. As opposed to volume displacement spirometers, these machines measure flow as the primary signal, which is time-integrated to yield volume estimates.

Technique

The basic steps in patient preparation are outlined in **Table 2**. Briefly, the patient is instructed to breathe gently through the mouthpiece from and into the spirometer. This accustoms him to breathing through the machine, and also generates a recording for tidal volume. Thereafter, a maximal inspiratory maneuver starting at tidal end expiration, followed by a forced expiratory maneuver, defines the forced vital capacity (FVC). It is extremely important that the technician supervising the test constantly encourages the patient throughout this procedure, to generate the best possible effort. Failing this, not only will the test remain poor quality, but the end-result may also be a falsely abnormal spirometry report. Several centers routinely perform postbronchodilator assessment as well. Although time-consuming, the additional information from this procedure is quite helpful, especially in characterization of airflow limitation.

Quality assessment involves confirming acceptability and reproducibility of multiple tests in same session. Detailed guidelines are available in this regard, and are summarized in **Table 2**.[3] Acceptability should be tested for each individual maneuver in any spirometry session, whereas reproducibility assesses how well the results of individual "acceptable" maneuvers in any spirometry session match with each other. Each spirometry session should have at least three acceptable maneuvers from which reproducibility can be assessed. If three maneuvers do not meet reproducibility criteria, then testing can be continued till these criteria are met. Normally, no more than eight maneuvers are recommended, as patients

Table 2 A typical spirometry session

Preprocedure preparation
• Ensure equipment integrity (electrical power, tubings, filters, etc.) • Calibrate spirometer • Verify indications/contraindications to the test • Obtain informed consent for procedure • Check personal and clinical details (age, gender, smoking habits, medications, diagnosis, previous tests, results of other investigations, etc.) • Measure weight and standing height • Explain (and preferably demonstrate) test procedure to the subject
Forced expiratory maneuvers
• Apply nose clip • Place appropriately sized mouthpiece in the mouth, and ask subject to tightly close lips around it • Ask subject to breathe gently from and into the mouthpiece for a few breaths • At end-tidal expiration, ask subject to inhale as completely as possible • Ask subject to exhale as rapidly, as completely, as forcefully, and for as long as possible, till no more air can be expelled out from the lungs; provide constant encouragement throughout • Repeat for a minimum of three maneuver
Optimize test quality

• Verify that each maneuvers is technically acceptable
  – Satisfactory start of test (no hesitation)
  – Good duration (expiratory time preferably more than 6 seconds)
  – Free from artefacts (such as cough, submaximal effort, early glottic closure, premature termination of expiration, etc.)
• Check repeatability from among at least three acceptable maneuvers
  – Two largest FVC values within 150 mL of each other
  – Two largest FEV1values within 150 mL of each other
• Perform additional maneuvers if necessary, till repeatability criteria are satisfied

Check for bronchodilator reversibility (BDR) (optional, but recommended)
• Ask patient to inhale 400 µg of salbutamol, preferably through a spacer attached to inhaler • Wait for 15–30 minutes • Repeat forced expiratory maneuvers as above, and verify test quality
Interpretation and reporting
• Compare observed values to predicted norms • Look at shape, size and pattern of flow-volume loop • Review available clinical information • Categorize spirometry data into normal, obstructive or restrictive patterns • Assess severity of pulmonary function impairment (if any) • Generate report, with comments on test quality and interpretation
Abbreviations: FVC, forced vital capacity; FEV1, forced expiratory volume in 1 second

get fatigued beyond that.[4] If reproducibility criteria are not met even after eight attempts, testing should be concluded and interpretation performed from three best tests, making a note of this fact in the final report.

The start of expiration is usually defined by back-extrapolation of the steepest portion of the volume-time curve to zero volume. The end of expiration is reached when the expired volume is less than 25 mL in 1 second or the subject cannot continue exhaling further. Normally, expiratory time should exceed 6 seconds. All measurements should be reported at body temperature and pressure, saturated (BTPS) conditions. This standardizes the readings to barometric pressure at sea level, body temperature, saturated with water vapor. Nomograms are available to derive correction factors based on ambient atmospheric conditions.

Reference Values

The basic purpose of pulmonary function testing is to identify persons with abnormal lung function. To know what is abnormal, we must first define what is normal. Predicted normal values can be obtained from studies carried out in healthy subjects. They are usually in the form of a regression equation describing the predicted value as a function of gender and anthropometric data (e.g. height, weight, etc.), and differ greatly with ethnicity. For instance, the predicted value of forced expiratory volume in 1 second (FEV1) among men is expressed as FEV1 (L) = $-1.90 - 0.025A + 0.00006A^2 + 0.036H$ (*A age in years, H height in cm*) from the regression equation for north Indian adults being used at our laboratory.[5] Any value below the predicted normal is not necessarily reduced, since the normal value is a range rather than a fixed point. This introduces the concept of lower limit of normal (LLN), which can be defined in several ways. The simplest (and most widely used) method is to use a fixed percentage of predicted value. For example, a value less than 80% of predicted FEV1 can be considered abnormal. However, there is very little statistical or physiological basis for such an approach. A more valid approach is to use lower 95% confidence limits of the regression equation, or subtract 1.645 times the standard error of estimate of the regression equation from the predicted value, to define the LLN.[6] Any value below the corresponding LLN is considered abnormal. It is very important to use norms derived from individuals largely similar to the patients being generally tested at any pulmonary function laboratory. Therefore standard Caucasian norms, often incorporated into spirometer softwares, should be avoided, and locally appropriate reference equations preferred wherever available. Reference equations for use in different geographic areas of india are available and should be preferably used.[5,7-14] Due to significant ethnic variability, these equations should not be interchanged with each other.[15] The common practice of using 85% or 90% predicted Caucasian values as the corresponding predicted value for North Indians is also statistically not valid.[16] Recently, the ERS global lung function initiative has developed reference equations that can be applied globally to different ethnic groups. However, data from the Indian subcontinent needs to be added to improve usability of these equations.[17]

Interpretation and Patterns in Common Disorders

Interpreting lung function data is not just about looking at numbers generated by the spirometer. Both the volume-time curve and the flow-volume loop must be also be evaluated with regard to their technical quality, size and shape, and various components, before making a final interpretation. Often such graphical analysis provides additional important information not obtainable from the numerical data. If available, the postbronchodilator graphs should also be similarly evaluated and compared to baseline curves. The clinical data provided in the requisition form is equally important in helping to reach any conclusion, especially in borderline situations.

The most important action is to turn-off computer-based interpretation, even if such software is offered with the machine. The initial step in interpretation is confirming that the test is of reasonably good quality (see earlier). Broadly, the interpretation of spirometric data involves only three numerical variables: FEV1, VC and FEV1/VC.[18] The largest observed values of FEV1 and VC available from among at least three acceptable and reproducible tests should be used as the key parameters for interpretation, even if these individual observations are derived from different test maneuvers. If both forced and relaxed VC maneuvers have been performed, the larger value of VC amongst the FVC and slow vital capacity (SVC) measurements should be used for interpretation. The large number of other variables, often available from computerized spirometer outputs, usually provide no additional information, and are best excluded from a standard interpretative algorithm. It is well recognized that increasing the number of tests for interpretation is likely to increase the probability of falsely abnormal results.[19] These readings may however be used to arrive at a conclusion in borderline or difficult situations. Values clearly above or clearly below their respective LLNs can be interpreted confidently. Borderline values need interpretation with caution, often supplementing clinical information and/or other test results to make decisions.

Any spirometry record with normal FEV1, VC and FEV1/VC (i.e. all values more than their corresponding LLN values) should be interpreted as normal. Any spirometry record with FEV1/VC value below its predicted LLN should be interpreted as having an obstructive abnormality **(Flow chart 1)**. This approach is superior to the use of fixed cutoffs in correctly identifying patients with airflow limitation, especially among the elderly.[20] However, in situations where statistically valid LLN figures are not available (or not practical to use, as in field settings), FEV1/VC ratio less than 70% can be used to define airway obstruction. Such a defect is commonly seen in

Flow chart 1 A basic algorithm for spirometry interpretation

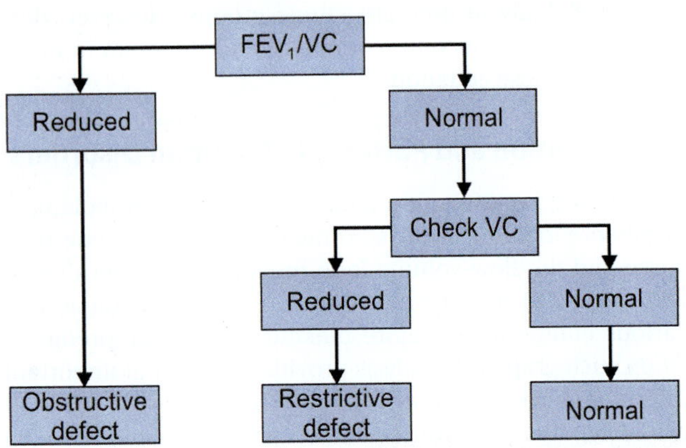

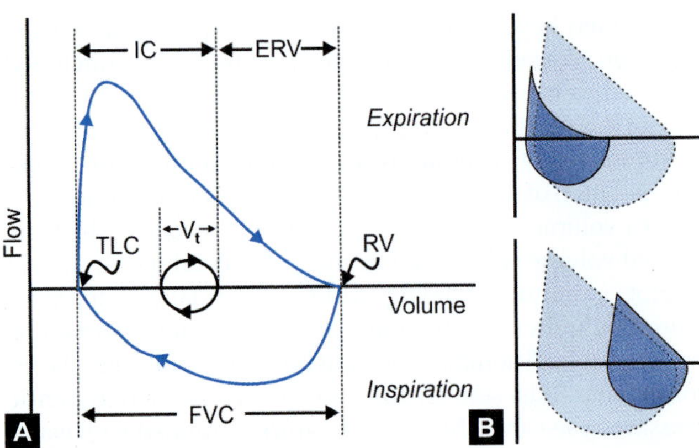

Figs 2A and B Flow-volume loops. (A) A typical flow-volume loop and the various subdivisions of lung volume; (B) Changes in the shape of flow volume loop in obstructive (top) and restrictive (bottom) defects, with the dotted line representing the normal loop

disorders associated with airflow limitation, such as asthma and COPD. It may also be observed in diseases with small airway obstruction (such as bronchiolitis), cystic fibrosis, bronchiectasis, airway tumors, etc. Patients with upper airway obstruction can be further characterized based on appearance of flow volume loops.

Any spirometry record with a normal FEV1/VC (i.e. value above corresponding LLN), coupled with a reduced VC (i.e. value below corresponding LLN), is suggestive of a restrictive abnormality. In situations where statistically valid LLN figures are not available (or not practical to use, as in field settings), observed VC ratio less than 80% of predicted value is often used to define reduction in VC. However, such an approach may result in the substantial misclassification of results.[21] Restrictive defects are common in conditions with loss of functioning lung parenchyma (e.g. diffuse parenchymal lung diseases, lung collapse/atelectasis, pneumonia, after lung resection). Such defects are also observed in neuromuscular diseases (due to reduction in generation of force needed for a FVC maneuver) as well as disorders of chest wall and pleura (e.g. massive pleural effusion, pleural fibrosis, obesity, kyphoscoliosis). It is important to note that spirometry can only suggest, but not confirm, a restrictive defect. True restriction is defined as reduction in total lung capacity. A mixed (obstructive plus restrictive) defect also cannot be diagnosed solely based on spirometry. A disproportionately low VC in face of a reduced FEV1/VC can either represent air trapping (with consequent increase in RV at the expense of VC, as in severe emphysema), or a true reduction in total lung capacity (TLC) (as in COPD with pneumonia). In such situations, it is advisable to estimate TLC (see later) for better characterization. FEV_1, expressed as a percentage of predicted normal value, is used to describe severity of both obstructive and restrictive abnormalities. There is no universally accepted scheme of severity categorization.

More recently, some laboratories are shifting to FEV6 as a substitute for FVC. Forced exhalation up to 6 seconds is a lot easier to perform for many patients. There are much less technical issues with accurate measurement of low flow during prolonged expiratory maneuver, and the end of test can be more easily defined. FEV6 may be more reproducible in several patients, especially those with airflow limitation. Reference equations for FEV6 are also becoming available.[22,23] There is data to suggest that FEV6 may be an acceptable surrogate for FVC in diagnosing both obstructive and restrictive defects on spirometry.[24-26]

The flow-volume loop may also provide a clue to underlying pathology **(Figs 2A and B)**. A small and concave or scooped curve suggests obstructive disorder. A small curve with steep slope suggests restriction. A small and flat curve suggests central airway obstruction. In disorders with variable intrathoracic obstruction, only the expiratory component of the loop is flat, whereas in disorders with variable extrathoracic obstruction, only the inspiratory component is flat. Both components are flat in lesions causing fixed airway obstruction.

Bronchodilator reversibility (BDR) is considered to be present, if the increase in FEV1 and/or VC (15–30 minutes after inhalation of 400 μg salbutamol) in the postbronchodilator study is both more than 12% and more than 200 mL over baseline values.[18] Although an oversimplification, patients with asthma tend to have BDR much more frequently than those with COPD. It must be noted that lack of BDR does not necessarily imply poor clinical response to bronchodilators in either condition.

PEAK EXPIRATORY FLOW

Peak expiratory flow (PEF) is defined as highest flow achieved from a maximum forced expiratory maneuver started without hesitation from a position of maximal lung inflation.[27] It can be measured either as a part of the spirometry procedure on the same instrument (with values derived from the flow volume curve), or separately using peak flowmeters.

The first meter specifically designed to measure this index of lung function was developed more than 50 years ago (Wright meter). Subsequently, a more portable, lower cost version (the "Mini-Wright" peak flow meter) was developed, and other designs and copies have since then become available across the world.

Although PEF is fairly well reproducible for an individual, the normal range of PEF in healthy individuals is rather wide. As a result, predicted values of PEF cannot be used to detect lung disease, since there is substantial overlap between values in patients with lung diseases and normal persons. Further, since PEF recordings are both flow and volume dependant, they tend to get reduced in both obstructive and restrictive disorders. Hence, in general notion that diminished PEF is a marker of airway obstruction is also not correct. While a normal PEF can reliably rule out airway obstruction, a low PEF does not necessarily indicate the same. The degree of reduction in PEF does not correlate well with the severity of obstruction described by the degree of reduction in FEV1. PEF measurements generally underestimate the degree of airway obstruction, as determined from FEV1 measurements.[28] This is partly because PEF predominantly reflects large airway function, while FEV1 reflects both large and peripheral airway function. On the other hand, PEF is an extremely good tool for personal monitoring, especially among patients with bronchial asthma. Once a patient has established his/her personal best value, daily PEF monitoring can provide early clue to worsening airflow limitation due to impending exacerbation or poor control.

To measure PEF using a Mini-Wright meter, the indicator is moved to the bottom of the numbered scale. The subject then inhales deeply, and places the mouthpiece in his/her mouth, tightly closing the lips around it. The mouthpiece should be gripped between the teeth and over the tongue. A nose clip is not necessary. He/she then blows out as hard and fast as possible in a single blow. The procedure is repeated two more times and the highest reading from three successive blows is recorded. The largest two readings should be within 40 L/min of each other. It has been known for some time that the linear scale on the standard mini-Wright PEF meter is an oversimplification, since the scale actually has nonlinear characteristics. As a result, the standard scale can over-record PEF in the midrange by as much as 30%. However, this scale has continued to be used for diagnosing and managing asthma worldwide for nearly half a century. More recently, the requirements for equipment accuracy have been refined in a European Commission standard adopted in 2004.[29] The corresponding new mini-Wright meters have a nonlinear scale that better reflects the true PEF **(Figs 3A and B)**. As predicted values for PEF have been obtained with meters with the old scale, these need to be converted to the new scale for data interpretation using the new meters. Nomograms and online convertors are available for this purpose.

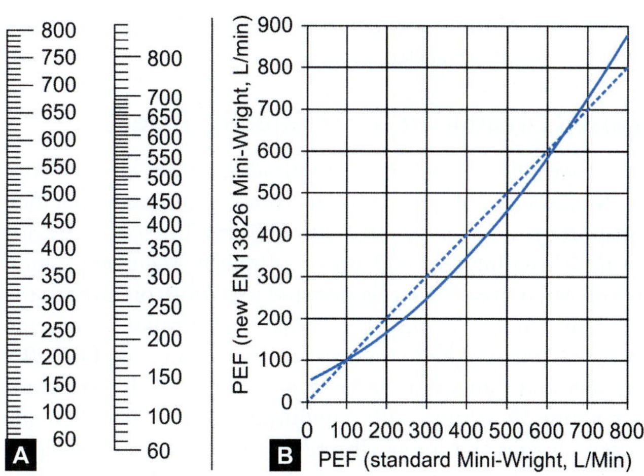

Figs 3A and B Compares the standard and the newer (based on the EN13826 standard) scales used in Mini-Wright peak flowmeters. Note that the standard meter (A) has a linear scale whereas the newer scale (B) is nonlinear. The right panel shows the direction and magnitude of error with the use of the standard scale, in comparison to the newer scale

STATIC LUNG VOLUMES

Since spirometry cannot measure RV, it is not possible to determine functional residual capacity (FRC) and TLC from this test. Other techniques are needed for the purpose. These methods are generally based on principles in which airflow velocity plays no role (in contrast to spirometry), and hence the term "static lung volumes" is often used for these measurements. Three techniques may be used: (1) Open circuit nitrogen washout, (2) Closed circuit inert gas dilution, and (3) Whole body plethysmography. Determination of static lung volumes is helpful in ascertaining true restrictive physiology, and differentiating between obstructive and restrictive disorders. Comparison between TLC estimated through gas dilution and plethysmographic methods can also quantify the extent of air trapping within the lungs.

Open Circuit Nitrogen Washout Technique

In this method, the subject breathes 100% oxygen, starting from end-tidal expiration. This results in washing out of nitrogen from the lungs. The exhaled gas is collected over the next 5–7 minutes, and its volume determined. Nitrogen concentration is measured through an analyzer in the breathing circuit and test stopped once a low plateau (concentration 1–2% for at least three successive breaths) is reached. The initial nitrogen concentration in the lungs is assumed to be similar to that in air. FRC can then be easily computed from the initial and final nitrogen concentrations, and the final collected volume. The technique has the drawback that any lack of precision in measuring nitrogen concentrations or expired volume will result in significant errors.

Closed Circuit Inert Gas Dilution Technique

The method is based on equilibration of air in the lungs with a known volume of gas mixture containing a specified proportion of an inert gas (usually helium). The subject begins by tidal breathing through the mouthpiece. At end expiration of one such breath, he is connected to a reservoir containing a gas mixture with known helium concentration. Thus, the point of starting the maneuver corresponds to the FRC. The subject continues to breathe in and out from this reservoir for about 10 minutes, till equilibration of gas between the reservoir and the lungs. The final concentration of helium is measured, and a simple calculation is used to derive the FRC **(Fig. 4)**. A vital capacity maneuver is performed at the same session to define the other lung volumes, which helps in computing the TLC and RV by addition or subtraction of the spirometrically determined inspiratory capacity (IC) and expiratory reserve volume (ERV) respectively from the FRC. In view of the simple principles and technique, this method is widely used to determine static lung volumes.

Whole Body Plethysmography

In contrast to gas dilution techniques, plethysmography measures the total volume of air in the thoracic cavity, including gas trapped in bullae and other noncommunicating spaces (e.g. air within pleura or esophagus). Plethysmographically determined FRC is therefore often referred to as thoracic gas volume (TGV). Although several different types of body plethysmographs are available, the "volume constant" type is the most widely used. The equipment consists of a large airtight chamber of known (and constant) volume. The subject sits inside this cabin and breathes through a mouthpiece till a stable end-expiratory level is obtained. At end tidal expiration, a solenoid-operated shutter is used to occlude airway at the mouthpiece for 2–3 seconds, and the subject is asked to gently pant against the closed shutter with glottis open. As he breathes, chest expansion and retraction cause small pressure changes within the plethysmograph and at mouthpiece, which are recorded using pressure transducers **(Figs 5A and B)**. Since the plethysmograph volume is constant, these changes can be used to derive changes in

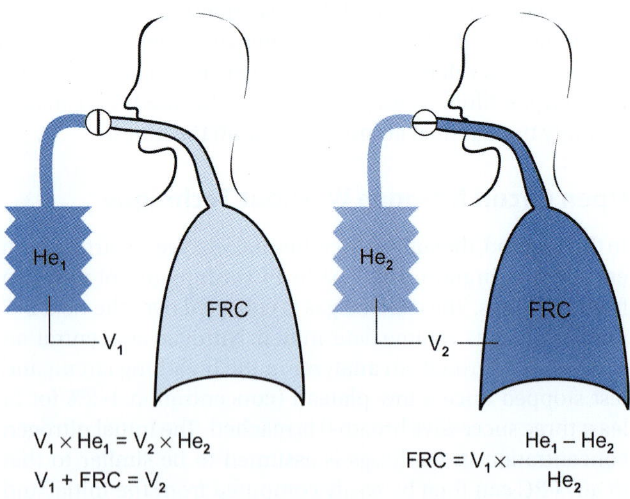

Fig. 4 Helium dilution technique to estimate functional residual capacity (FRC). Gas laws can be used to calculate FRC from initial and final helium concentrations (He_1 and He_2 respectively), and the known volume of helium mixture reservoir (V_1)

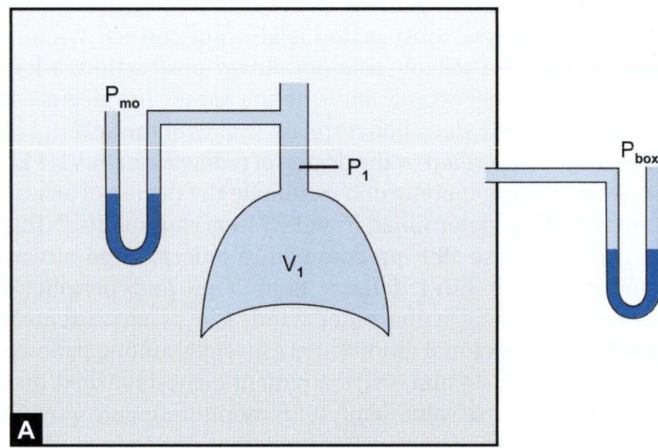

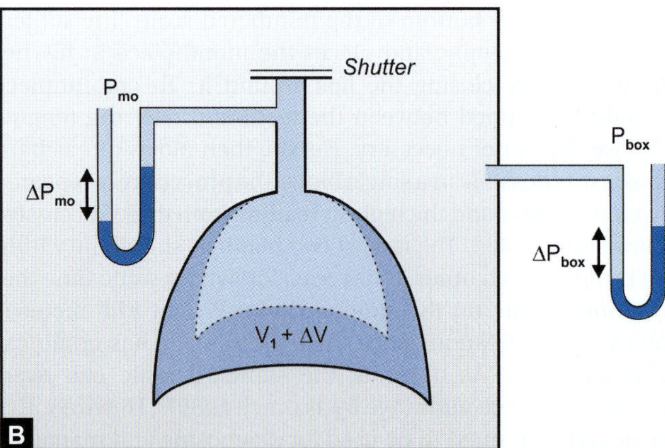

Figs 5A and B Whole body plethysmography to calculate static lung volumes using a constant volume apparatus. Under static conditions, pressure at mouth (P_{mo}) corresponds to the alveolar pressure (P_1), which is atmospheric at baseline. As the subject pants against a closed shutter, small fluctuations in mouth pressure (ΔP_{mo}) reflect alveolar pressure changes, while small fluctuations in lung volume (ΔV) are recorded as corresponding changes in pressure inside the plethysmograph chamber (ΔP_{box}). A standard constant, specific to the plethysmograph being used, can be applied to compute ΔV from ΔP_{box}. If the shutter is closed at tidal end-expiration, then gas laws can be used to compute functional residual capacity (FRC) (V_1) from these data

volume of air within the plethysmograph, and indirectly within the lungs. Pressure changes at the mouthpiece can be considered to directly reflect alveolar pressure changes, as the glottis is open and there is no net gas flow (due to the closed shutter). TGV can be computed from the slope of these pressure-volume curves using Boyle's law. Although the technique is cumbersome, it provides more reproducible measurements than dilution methods.

Interpretation

Reference equations for static lung volumes are used in a fashion similar to spirometry to define population limits of normality. In contrast to spirometry, an increase in TLC beyond the upper limit of normal is also considered pathological. A few regression equations are available in this regard from India as well.[7-11,14]

A decrease in TLC is diagnostic of a restrictive defect. In parenchymal restriction (e.g. lung fibrosis), RV and TLC are reduced proportionately, resulting in a normal RV/TLC ratio. In extrapulmonary restriction (e.g. chest wall or neuromuscular disorders), RV is usually normal (or sometimes even increased), resulting in an increased RV/TLC ratio. On the other hand, TLC might be increased in acromegaly, or in conditions like emphysema, as a result of air trapping. An increase in RV/TLC ratio, with an obstructive defect on spirometry, is a good indicator of air trapping. In conditions characterized by noncommunicating air in the lungs (e.g. emphysema, bullae, etc.), whole body plethysmography provides a better estimate of the lung volume, since gas dilution techniques measure only the volume of air that is freely exchanged during breathing. In fact, the difference in volumes calculated by the two techniques may provide some indication to the volume of noncommunicating air present in the lungs.[30] Estimation of static lung volumes is also necessary to diagnose mixed obstructive-restrictive defects, with a combination of reduced FEV_1/VC ratio and reduced TLC.

DIFFUSING CAPACITY OF LUNGS

Measurement of pulmonary diffusing capacity allows us to assess the ability of lungs to transport gas from inspired air to the red blood cells in pulmonary capillary network. It is however, a misnomer, since gas transfer does not depend solely on diffusion across the alveocapillary membrane, and it is not a "capacity" in that there is no theoretical maximal limit. Many laboratories therefore employ the term "transfer factor" instead.

The diffusing capacity for carbon monoxide (DLCO) is the generally measured index. This is because carbon monoxide uptake is easily measurable, and the gas essentially follows the same pathway as oxygen during transport from alveolar air to red blood cells, and ultimate binding to hemoglobin. DLCO is the uptake of carbon monoxide from lungs per unit time per unit of carbon monoxide driving pressure. The test is usually performed for screening for diffuse lung diseases and pulmonary vascular disorders, precise characterization of airflow limitation, differential diagnosis and severity assessment of restrictive ventilatory defects, disability evaluation, and preoperative assessment. There are no absolute contraindications. However, for technical reasons, most machines cannot measure DLCO in individuals with an extremely low VC (usually <1.5 L) or severely dyspneic patients unable to hold breath for a sufficient time. The test cannot be performed on many patients receiving supplemental oxygen, as this needs to be discontinued before and throughout the test procedure.

Methodology

Diffusing capacity for carbon monoxide can be measured using a single breath method, an intrabreath method, or a rebreathing technique. The first is most commonly used, as it is simpler and better standardized **(Fig. 6)**. The gas mixture used contains 0.3% carbon monoxide, a tracer gas (helium, methane or neon), 21% oxygen, and balance nitrogen. The subject first gently breathes room air through a mouthpiece. Once comfortable, he is instructed to exhale completely (though not forcefully). At RV, he is connected to a reservoir containing the gas mixture, and instructed to inhale fully up to TLC, in less than 2 seconds. At this point, he is asked to hold his breath for approximately 10 seconds, without straining. Thereafter, he exhales fully, smoothly and quickly, and the expired gas is collected. The initial 0.75–1.0 L is discarded as it represents dead space, and the next 0.5–1.0 L is collected for

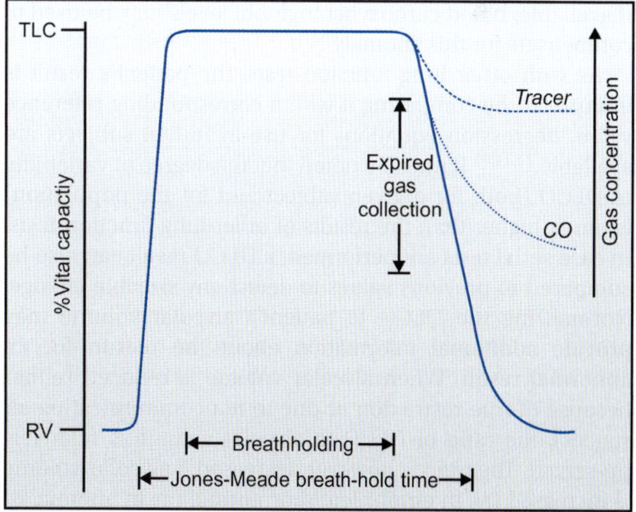

Fig. 6 Schematic representation of the estimation of pulmonary diffusing capacity using the single breath technique. The subject inhales the gas mixture deeply residual volume (RV) to total lung capacity (TLC), and holds breath for 10 seconds. Expired gas is collected after discarding that from dead space. Note that breath-holding time used for calculations[31] is slightly longer than actual breathhold

analysis. Some instruments use rapid analyzers that provide real-time gas concentration curves from the exhaled gas, and allow washout till the tracer gas concentration reaches a plateau, and collection subsequently. The collected mixture is analyzed for final tracer gas concentration and carbon monoxide uptake. For purposes of analysis, the breath hold time is more than the actual breath holding period. The Jones and Meade method measures breath-hold time starting at 30% of inspiratory time and extending to half of the sampling time.[31]

DLCO is calculated from the total lung volume, breath-hold time, and the initial and final alveolar carbon monoxide concentrations. It is a product of the subject's TLC and rate of carbon monoxide uptake during the breath-hold time. An estimate of the total lung capacity and the initial alveolar carbon monoxide concentration is obtained from the tracer gas concentration in exhaled gas.

The test can be repeated after an interval of at least 5 minutes. Generally, a mean value is reported from two acceptable tests whose results agree within 2 mL/min/mm Hg.

Interpretation

In contrast to other pulmonary function tests, observed DLCO values must be normalized to key nonrespiratory variables. Hemoglobin concentration is important as it removes the carbon monoxide from the blood, thus providing a nearly constant gradient for gas transfer. Anemic patients may thus have a lower DLCO, and the measurement should therefore be corrected for this factor in such patients.[32,33] Smokers tend to have a small baseline level of blood carbon monoxide, and thus the transfer gradient may be less than for nonsmokers. If available, blood carboxyhemoglobin levels may be used to compensate for this anomaly.[33,34]

As with other lung function tests, the patient's result is interpreted by comparing it with a corresponding reference value. Regression equations for use in Indian subjects are available.[11,14,35] It must be noted that the degree of variability of DLCO (both for a given subject and for the population) is much higher than the results of other lung function tests. In case serial tests are performed, a DLCO result can also be compared to previous values to detect any sizeable change. Normalizing the DLCO to patient's alveolar volume may provide additional information about the reason for an abnormal result. When alveolar volume is reduced (either because of true restriction or due to noncommunicating air spaces), the ratio of DLCO to alveolar volume is relatively preserved. The ratio is however decreased if alveolar volume is increased (as in emphysema) or normal (as in anemia, or nonperfusion of ventilated alveoli).

EXERCISE TESTING

Exercise testing is generally indicated for: (1) Evaluation of exercise intolerance; (2) Evaluation of unexplained breathlessness; (3) Preoperative assessment; and (4) Formulation of exercise prescriptions. Detailed evaluation can give some clue about whether the underlying disorder is predominantly cardiovascular or respiratory in origin. Exercise testing can range from gross and crude assessments to highly detailed and standardized evaluation using computerized equipment. The two most regularly employed types of exercise testing for evaluating pulmonary diseases are the 6-minute walk test (6MWT) and a formal complete cardiopulmonary exercise testing (CPET).

Basic Modalities

Stair climbing remains the most basic exercise test that asks patients to climb stairs till they get limited by symptoms.[36] There is, however, no consensus on how to standardize the procedure, and several variations (such as climbing at own pace or at brisk pace, climbing with or without holding handrails) are used. Results are generally reported as number of stairs or number of flights of stairs.

Step tests ask the subject to walk up and down on a stool or bench at a specified rate. Several variations exist with regard to height of steps, number of steps, and the frequency of step-ups. The most popular is the Master two-step test.[37] The test is well suited to field use, and subjects can achieve close to their maximal exercise capacity.

The 6MWT is a simple procedure that assesses the maximum distance that a subject can walk on flat surface at his/her own pace in 6 minutes. The test provides a global estimate of functional capacity, but does not provide any specific information on individual systems (cardiac, pulmonary, hematologic, and musculoskeletal) involved in exercise. The test is also sensitive to patient effort. The 6MWT is the most popular among the basic exercise tests as it is simple, practical and well standardized, and involves an activity familiar to almost everyone. A measured corridor, usually about 30 m, is used, and the subject walks to and fro in this space at a self-determined pace. If a long corridor is not available, the test can be performed on a treadmill, although pacing and control are not as optimal and the distance walked is usually less.[38] Guidelines are available regarding the standardization, performance, and interpretation of the 6MWT.[39] The test has good reproducibility and good correlation with other measures of functional status.[40] For this reason, the 6MWT is the preferred investigation when a complete CPET is not available. Norms for healthy Indian men have recently become available.[41]

The shuttle walk test uses an audio signal from a metronome to dictate the walking pace.[42] Walking speed is incrementally increased every minute while the subject walks to and fro on a 10 m straight path. The test is terminated when the subject can no longer maintain the required speed. Hence, the test correlates better with maximal symptom limited tests such as the CPET, rather than the submaximal tests like 6MWT.[43] However, the test is more complicated than 6MWT, and may result in more frequent cardiac complications in the absence of electrocardiographic monitoring.

Exercise testing may sometimes be used to diagnose airway hyper-reactivity due to exercise in patients with unexplained dyspnea. Exercise-induced bronchospasm (EIB) is described as a self-limiting bronchospastic event occurring immediately after strong exercise. Typically, greater than 10–15% reduction in FEV_1 and/or FVC is observed.[44] EIB is caused by loss of heat, water, or both, from the airways during exercise.

Cardiopulmonary Exercise Testing

The cardiopulmonary exercise testing is a more complex investigation that involves exercise at incrementally increasing intensity. The test is terminated when symptoms limit further exercise, or the maximal exercise capacity is achieved. A computerized protocol provides breath-by-breath information on respiratory gas exchange, airflow, oxygen consumption, carbon dioxide production, and cardiac variables (such as heart rate, blood pressure, etc.). The subject exercises on either a treadmill or on a bicycle ergometer; the latter may however be preferable as work rate can be directly measured.

Electrocardiographic and noninvasive blood pressure monitoring accompanies the test. In addition, oxygen saturation is continuously monitored through pulse oximetry. Real-time data on ventilatory and gas exchange parameters is obtained by asking the subject to breathe through a mouthpiece connected to a spirometer and metabolic cart. Flow, volume, and exhaled oxygen and carbon dioxide concentrations are measured. Either incremental or constant work protocol can be used. The test is terminated when the subject (1) gets exhausted, fatigued or distressed, (2) develops signs of cardiovascular instability (ischemia, arrhythmia, substantial blood pressure elevation, etc.), or (3) develops significant hypoxemia.

Although data for a large number of monitored and calculated variables is generated, interpretation and clinical correlation depends on judicious integration of all available information. No single parameter is diagnostic of a cause for exercise limitation. Four basic measurements are critical in describing the response to exercise: oxygen consumption, carbon dioxide production, heart rate, and minute ventilation. Under steady state conditions, measured oxygen uptake (Vo_2) equals metabolic oxygen consumption, and measured carbon dioxide output (Vco_2) is the same as its metabolic production. Both Vo_2 and Vco_2 can be mathematically computed from expired gas concentrations. Vo_2 increases linearly with work intensity until limitations in cardiac output and/or tissue extraction result in a plateau. This level is termed Vo_{2max} and is the best index for aerobic capacity. At lower work levels, Vco_2 increases at a rate similar to Vo_2. However, at higher work levels, bicarbonate buffering of increased lactic acid production (resulting from anaerobic metabolism) causes Vco_2 to rise more steeply. The point where the Vco_2 begins to rise disproportionate to the Vo_2 is termed "anaerobic threshold" **(Fig. 7)**, and is a marker for onset of metabolic acidosis during exercise. It usually occurs at 50–60% of Vo_{2max} with a wide range of normal values. The ratio between Vo_2 and heart rate reflects the amount of oxygen consumed in each cardiac cycle, and is often termed "oxygen pulse".

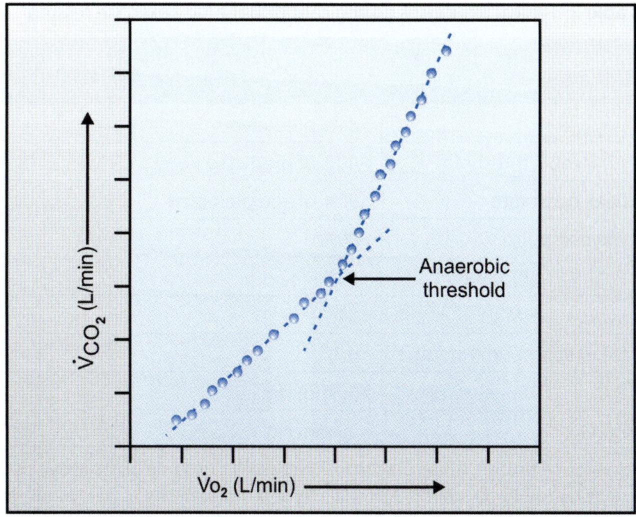

Fig. 7 Anaerobic threshold determined from a plot of oxygen uptake (Vo_2) and carbon-dioxide production (Vco_2) during cardiopulmonary exercise testing

Cardiopulmonary exercise testing is used to find whether or not a subject's maximal exercise capacity is decreased. A reduction in Vo_{2max} is the starting point for evaluating impaired exercise capacity. The quantum of this reduction is a rough indicator to the severity of exercise limitation. If Vo_{2max} is reduced, the other variables are then integrated into decision making to arrive at the most probable cause. In this regard, CPET is not clearly diagnostic of any individual disease process, but can rather only suggest the likely physiologic mechanism of dyspnea or exercise limitation. The cardiovascular response is assessed through anaerobic threshold, oxygen pulse, and relationships of Vo_2 to heart rate and work intensity. The ventilatory response is assessed through respiratory reserve (peak V_E/MVV), maximal respiratory rate, and arterial Pco_2 (if available). Gas exchange is assessed through physiological dead space assessment, oximetry, arterial oxygenation (if available), and calculating alveolo-arterial oxygen gradient ($P_{A\text{-}a}O_2$). Based on these assessments, and taking into account the overall clinical information, the etiology of exercise limitation can be deduced. The three basic causes for exercise limitation are cardiovascular disorders, respiratory disorders, and physical deconditioning **(Table 3)**. However, one must be careful as significant overlap exists between response patterns in different disease conditions.

Table 3 Typical responses during cardiopulmonary exercise testing

Parameter	*Normal value*	*COPD*	*ILD*	*Pulmonary vascular disease*	*Heart failure*	*Obesity*	*Decondition*
Vo_{2max}	>84% predicted	↓	↓	↓	↓	↓	↓
Anaerobic threshold	>40% of predicted Vo_{2max}	↔/↓	↔/↓	↓	↓	↔	↔/↓
Peak heart rate	>90% of age predicted	↓	↓	↔/↓	Variable	↔/↓	↔/↓
Oxygen pulse	>80%	↔/↓	↔/↓	↓	↓	↔	↓
Peak V_E/MVV x 100	<85%	↑	↔/↑	↔	↔/↓	↔/↑	↔
V_E/Vco_2 (at AT)	<34	↑	↑	↑	↑	↔	↔
Dead space/Tidal volume	<0.30	↑	↑	↑	↑	↔	↔
P_aO_2	>80 mm Hg	↔/↓	↓	↓	↔	↔	↔
$P_{A\text{-}a}O_2$	<35 mm Hg	↑	↑	↑	↔	↔/↓	↔

Abbreviations: AT, anaerobic threshold; COPD, chronic obstructive pulmonary disease; ILD, interstitial lung disease; MVV, maximum voluntary ventilation; $P_{A\text{-}a}O_2$, alveoloarterial oxygen gradient; P_aO_2, partial pressure of arterial oxygen; Vco_2, carbon dioxide production; V_E, minute ventilation; Vo_{2max}, maximal oxygen consumption

The test is highly sensitive in identification of subclinical disease than other lung function tests conducted at rest. Therefore, CPET can be performed for preoperative assessment, disability evaluation, and selection of candidates for heart and/or lung transplantation. The test is also useful in determining whether breathlessness results from cardiac or pulmonary component among patients who have disorders of both organ systems.

OTHER TESTS

Airway Hyperresponsiveness

Airway hyperresponsiveness (AHR), a characteristic feature of bronchial asthma, is an increased sensitivity of airways to a variety of inhaled agents. AHR is classically measured using inhalation challenges with airway constrictor agonists, such as histamine or methacholine, which result in direct bronchoconstriction. Recently, inhaled mannitol solution has also become available for this purpose and acts by inducing osmotic changes in the airway.[45] Exercise can also be used to test for AHR (see earlier).

In general, histamine or methacholine solution is freshly prepared in doubling dilutions. After baseline spirometry, the subject inhales progressively increasing concentrations of the provocative agent through a dosimeter or nebulizer. Spirometry is repeated 30–90 seconds after each inhalation, and a rest of up to 5 minutes is provided between two successive inhalations. Several dosing protocols are in vogue, but the two most commonly used are: (1) 2-minute tidal breathing method and (2) five-breath dosimeter method.[44] The results are reported as percentage decrease in FEV_1 from the baseline, and summarized through an index termed PC_{20} (provocative concentration causing 20% reduction in FEV_1). PC_{20} is interpolated from a graph plotting FEV_1 values against logarithm of provocator concentration. For methacholine, values higher than 20 mg/mL are normal, and values less than 4 mg/mL suggest AHR.[44] Resuscitation equipment should be available during testing, as sometimes life-threatening bronchospasm can result from the procedure.

Airway Resistance

Airway resistance can be clinically estimated using several approaches such as interrupter technique, forced oscillation technique, and whole body plethysmography. The interrupter technique is the simplest, and requires monitoring airway pressure and airflow. Flow is abruptly interrupted, and airway resistance is obtained by dividing the pressure change after interruption by the flow obtained immediately before the interruption. Forced oscillation technique measures airway resistance by imposing flow oscillations on the airways during spontaneous breathing. These cyclical waves result in slight shifts in airflow, and consequent changes in airway pressure. Airway resistance is computed from pressure and flow changes, and frequency. The technique can provide added information about contributions from central and peripheral airways to the total airway resistance. When using the plethysmograph, the subject instructed to pant slowly, before and after the shutter at mouth is closed. Airway resistance is computed as the ratio between the slopes of mouth pressure-plethysmograph pressure and air flow-plethysmograph pressure changes.[46] This value can also be standardized to the lung volume by multiplying it by the simultaneously determined TGV. The resultant index is called specific airway resistance, and its reciprocal is termed as specific conductance.

Airway resistance is not normally determined for clinical purposes, but may provide additional information in the evaluation of patients suspected to have obstructive disorders. The range of normal airway resistance is not well defined, and generally values higher than 2.8 cm H_2O/L/sec are considered abnormal.

Pulmonary Mechanics

The elastic properties of the lungs are determined by relating alterations in volume of air in the lungs to the corresponding changes in the lung's recoil. A body plethysmograph is usually used to determine the static pulmonary mechanics. Lung recoil force is measured as the transpulmonary pressure. This is the difference between the alveolar and pleural pressures; the former is measured at mouth under static conditions with shutter at mouth closed and glottis open, and the latter is quantified through pressure measurement from a thin balloon placed in the lower third of esophagus and connected to a pressure transducer. The subject sits in a whole body plethysmograph. After a few tidal breaths, he inspires fully to TLC, then exhales to FRC and again inspires to TLC. During the subsequent exhalation, a shutter at mouth occludes the airway intermittently. Mouth and esophageal pressures are recorded at each occlusion. Since mouth pressure equals alveolar pressure under static conditions, the transpulmonary pressure can be calculated at each shutter closure. This data is integrated with volume measurements to plot the relationship between transpulmonary pressure and lung volume. The slope of this curve over a range corresponding to the tidal volume is the static lung compliance. The whole plot can also be analyzed through a monoexponential analysis to yield a shape constant for the curve.[47] Unlike lung compliance, the shape constant is largely independent of ethnicity, patient effort and lung size. In patients with restrictive ventilatory defects, exponential analysis helps to differentiate restriction due to reduced elastic properties from that due to loss of lung volume.[48]

Respiratory Muscle Function

Estimation of maximal respiratory pressures are a simple technique to assess global respiratory muscle function. A manometer is used to record highest pressures during maximal inhalation and exhalation, which can be sustained for at least 1 second.[49] Maximal expiratory pressure (MEP) is roughly twice as much as maximal inspiratory pressures (MIP). The test is commonly used during evaluation of respiratory muscle weakness in patients with neuromuscular disorders. It is also used as one of the several parameters to assess weaning potential in patients receiving mechanical ventilation. Abnormal muscle strength is identified by comparing observed values to reference data; such data is also available for the Indian population.[50,51] Values are generally higher among men, and decline with age. A reduction in both MIP and MEP indicates generalized skeletal muscle weakness. A low MIP with normal MEP suggests isolated inspiratory muscle weakness (usually diaphragmatic). Isolated expiratory muscle weakness (normal MIP and low MEP) is rare.

The sniff nasal inspiratory pressure (SNIP) is a noninvasive test of inspiratory strength. The test is performed by wedging a catheter into one nostril and asking the subject to sniff through the other nostril. Pressure measured in the obstructed nostril. The SNIP correlates strongly with transdiaphragmatic pressure and the MIP, but provides no information on expiratory muscle function.

Transdiaphragmatic pressure can be measured after insertion of esophageal and gastric balloon catheters. This allows functional assessment during inspiration, expiration, a sniff, a cough, or phrenic nerve stimulation. Although the technique is highly complex and invasive, it is the best measure of respiratory muscle strength. However, a wide normal range limits its clinical utility.[49]

Control of Breathing

The tests available to assess the respiratory control system include: (1) Inhalation of hypoxic or hyperoxic gas mixtures to stimulate chemoreceptors, and (2) Sleep studies to monitor behavior of the control system during sleep.[49] The hypoxic ventilatory response is evaluated by administering a hypoxic gas mixture to the subject over 4–6 minutes through a rebreathing circuit. This results in progressive hypoxemia, stimulation of peripheral chemoreceptors, and an increase in respiratory drive. Blood CO_2 is maintained at the same level by removing CO_2 from the rebreathing bag. The ventilatory response is biphasic, with an initial rapid increase in ventilation followed by a gradual decline to a plateau. Ventilatory response to hypercapnia is determined by asking the subject to rebreathe a hyperoxic gas mixture, thereby causing progressive hypercapnia over 4–6 minutes. This results in stimulation of central chemoreceptors, and an increase in respiratory drive. End-tidal carbon dioxide tension is monitored. The rise in ventilation in response to hypercapnia is linear. In either test, measurements of ventilation or occlusion pressure are used to assess motor output. Occlusion pressure is assessed using $P_{0.1}$, which is the pressure generated in first 100 µsec of inspiration against an occluded airway.

REFERENCES

1. Pretto JJ, Brazzale DJ, Guy PA, Goudge RJ, Hensley MJ. Reasons for referral for pulmonary function testing: an audit of 4 adult lung function laboratories. Respir Care. 2013;58(3):507-10.
2. Standardization of Spirometry, 1994 Update. American Thoracic Society. Am J Respir Crit Care Med. 1995;152(3):1107-36.
3. Miller MR, Hankinson J, Brusasco V, Burgos F, Casaburi R, Coates A, et al. Standardisation of spirometry. Eur Respir J. 2005;26(2):319-38.
4. Ferris BG, Speizer FE, Bishop Y, Prang G, Weener J. Spirometry for an epidemiologic study: Deriving optimum summary

statistics for each subject. Bull Eur Physiopathol Respir. 1978;14(2):145-66.
5. Jindal SK. Pulmonary function laboratory in the tropics: needs, problems and solutions. In: Sharma OP (Eds). Lung disease in the tropics. New York: Marcel Dekker; 1991. pp. 523-42.
6. Lung function testing: selection of reference values and interpretative strategies. American Thoracic Society. Am Rev Respir Dis. 1991;144(5):1202-18.
7. Jain SK, Ramiah TJ. Spirometric studies in healthy women 15-40 years age. Indian J Chest Dis. 1967;9(1):1-12.
8. Jain SK, Ramiah TJ. Influence of age, height and body surface area on lung functions in healthy women 15-40 years old. Indian J Chest Dis. 1967;9(1):13-22.
9. Jain SK, Gupta CK. Age, height and body weight as determinants of ventilatory 'norms' in healthy men above forty years of age. Indian J Med Res. 1967;55(6):606-11.
10. Jain SK, Ramiah TJ. Normal standards of pulmonary function tests for healthy Indian men 15-40 years old: comparison of different regression equations (prediction formulae). Indian J Med Res. 1969;57(8):1453-66.
11. Udwadia FE, Sunavala JD, Shetye VM. Lung function studies in healthy Indian subjects. J Assoc Physicians India. 1987;35(7):491-6.
12. Chatterjee S, Nag SK, Dey SK. Spirometric standards for non-smokers and smokers of India (eastern region). Jpn J Physiol. 1988;38(3):283-98.
13. Chatterjee S, Saha D. Pulmonary function studies in healthy non-smoking women of Calcutta. Ann Hum Biol. 1993;20(1):31-8.
14. Vijayan VK, Kuppurao KV, Venkatesan P, Sankaran K, Prabhakar R. Pulmonary function in healthy young adult Indians in Madras. Thorax. 1990;45(8):611-5.
15. Aggarwal AN, Gupta D, Jindal SK. Comparison of Indian reference equations for spirometry interpretation. Respirology. 2007;12(5):763-8.
16. Aggarwal AN, Gupta D, Behera D, Jindal SK. Applicability of commonly used Caucasian prediction equations for spirometry interpretation in India. Indian J Med Res. 2005;122(2):153-64.
17. Quanjer PH, Stanojevic S, Cole TJ, Baur X, Hall GL, Culver BH, et al. Multiethnic reference values for spirometry for the 3-95-yr age range: the global lung function 2012 equations. Eur Respir J. 2012;40(6):1324-43.
18. Pellegrino R, Viegi G, Brusasco V, Crapo RO, Burgos F, Casaburi R, et al. Interpretative strategies for lung function tests. Eur Respir J. 2005;26(5):948-68.
19. Vedal S, Crapo RO. False positive rates of multiple pulmonary function tests in healthy subjects. Bull Eur Physiopathol Respir. 1983;19(3):263-6.
20. Aggarwal AN, Gupta D, Agarwal R, Jindal SK. Comparison of the lower confidence limit to the fixed-percentage method for assessing airway obstruction in routine clinical practice. Respir Care. 2011;56(11):1778-84.
21. Aggarwal AN, Gupta D, Behera D, Jindal SK. Comparison of fixed percentage method and lower confidence limits for defining limits of normality for interpretation of spirometry. Respir Care. 2006;51(7):737-43.
22. Hankinson JL, Crapo RO, Jensen RL. Spirometric reference values for the 6-s FVC maneuver. Chest. 2003;124(5):1805-11.
23. Hankinson JL, Odencrantz JR, Fedan KB. Spirometric reference values from a sample of the general US population. Am J Respir Crit Care Med. 1999;159(1):179-87.
24. Jing JY, Huang TC, Cui W, Xu F, Shen HH. Should FEV1/FEV6 replace FEV1/FVC ratio to detect airway obstruction? A meta-analysis. Chest. 2009;135(4):991-8.
25. Swanney MP, Jensen RL, Crichton DA, Beckert LE, Cardno LA, Crapo RO. FEV(6) is an acceptable surrogate for FVC in the spirometric diagnosis of airway obstruction and restriction. Am J Respir Crit Care Med. 2000;162(3 Pt 1):917-9.
26. Perez-Padilla R, Wehrmeister FC, Celli BR, Lopez-Varela MV, Montes de Oca M, Muino A, et al. Reliability of FEV1/FEV6 to diagnose airflow obstruction compared with FEV1/FVC: the PLATINO longitudinal study. PLoS One. 2013;8(8):e67960.
27. Quanjer PH, Lebowitz MD, Gregg I, Miller MR, Pedersen OF. Peak expiratory flow: conclusions and recommendations of a Working Party of the European Respiratory Society. Eur Respir J Suppl. 1997;24:2S-8S.
28. Aggarwal AN, Gupta D, Jindal SK. The relationship between FEV1 and peak expiratory flow in patients with airways obstruction is poor. Chest. 2006;130(5):1454-61.
29. European Standard prEN13826 (Peak Flow Meters). London: British Standards Institute; 2000.
30. Agarwal R, Aggarwal AN. Bullous lung disease or bullous emphysema? Respir Care. 2006;51(5):532-4.
31. Jones RS, Meade F. A theoretical and experimental analysis of anomalies in the estimation of pulmonary diffusing capacity by the single breath method. Q J Exp Physiol Cogn Med Sci. 1961;46:131-43.
32. Marrades RM, Diaz O, Roca J, Campistol JM, Torregrosa JV, Barbera JA, et al. Adjustment of DLCO for hemoglobin concentration. Am J Respir Crit Care Med. 1997;155(1):236-41.
33. American Thoracic Society. Single-breath carbon monoxide diffusing capacity (transfer factor). Recommendations for a standard technique: 1995 update. Am J Respir Crit Care Med. 1995;152(6 Pt 1):2185-98.
34. Graham BL, Mink JT, Cotton DJ. Effects of increasing carboxyhemoglobin on the single breath carbon monoxide diffusing capacity. Am J Respir Crit Care Med. 2002;165(11):1504-10.
35. Guleria JS, Sharma MP, Pande JN, Ramchandran K. Pulmonary diffusing capacity in normal Indian subjects. Indian J Physiol Pharmacol. 1970;14(4):245-51.
36. Pollock M, Roa J, Benditt J, Celli B. Estimation of ventilatory reserve by stair climbing. A study in patients with chronic airflow obstruction. Chest. 1993;104(5):1378-83.
37. Master AM, Rosenfeld I. The "two-step" exercise test brought up to date. N Y State J Med. 1961;61:1850-8.
38. Stevens D, Elpern E, Sharma K, Szidon P, Ankin M, Kesten S. Comparison of hallway and treadmill six-minute walk tests. Am J Respir Crit Care Med. 1999;160(5 Pt 1):1540-3.
39. ATS statement: guidelines for the six-minute walk test. Am J Respir Crit Care Med. 2002;166(1):111-7.
40. Cahalin L, Pappagianopoulos P, Prevost S, Wain J, Ginns L. The relationship of the 6-min walk test to maximal oxygen consumption in transplant candidates with end-stage lung disease. Chest. 1995;108(2):452-9.
41. Vaish H, Ahmed F, Singla R, Shukla DK. Reference equation for the 6-minute walk test in healthy North Indian adult males. Int J Tuberc Lung Dis. 2013;17(5):698-703.
42. Singh SJ, Morgan MD, Scott S, Walters D, Hardman AE. Development of a shuttle walking test of disability in patients with chronic airways obstruction. Thorax. 1992;47(12):1019-24.

43. Singh SJ, Morgan MD, Hardman AE, Rowe C, Bardsley PA. Comparison of oxygen uptake during a conventional treadmill test and the shuttle walking test in chronic airflow limitation. Eur Respir J. 1994;7(11):2016-20.
44. Crapo RO, Casaburi R, Coates AL, Enright PL, Hankinson JL, Irvin CG, et al. Guidelines for methacholine and exercise challenge testing, 1999. Am J Respir Crit Care Med. 2000;161(1):309-29.
45. Holzer K, Anderson SD, Chan HK, Douglass J. Mannitol as a challenge test to identify exercise-induced bronchoconstriction in elite athletes. Am J Respir Crit Care Med. 2003;167(4):534-7.
46. Aggarwal AN, Gupta D, Sharma CP, Jindal SK. Effect of household exposure to environmental tobacco smoke on airflow mechanics in asymptomatic healthy women. Indian J Med Res. 2004;119(1):18-23.
47. Colebatch HJ, Greaves IA, Ng CK. Exponential analysis of elastic recoil and aging in healthy males and females. J Appl Physiol. 1979;47(4):683-91.
48. Aggarwal AN, Gupta D, Behera D, Jindal SK. Analysis of static pulmonary mechanics helps to identify functional defects in survivors of acute respiratory distress syndrome. Crit Care Med. 2000;28(10):3480-3.
49. ATS/ERS Statement on respiratory muscle testing. Am J Respir Crit Care Med. 2002;166(4):518-624.
50. Gopalakrishna A, Vaishali K, Prem V, Aaron P. Normative values for maximal respiratory pressures in an Indian Mangalore population: A cross-sectional pilot study. Lung India. 2011;28(4):247-52.
51. Guleria R, Jindal SK. Normal maximal expiratory and inspiratory pressures in healthy teenagers. J Assoc Physicians India. 1992;40(2):108-9.

Respiratory Muscle Function

Randeep Guleria

INTRODUCTION

Breathing, which is essential for life, requires the repetitive contractions of the muscles of respiration. Proper functioning of respiratory muscles is essential and unlike limb muscles, the muscles of breathing have no opportunity to rest and have to work throughout life. Besides breathing, respiratory muscles also play a role in other functions like sneezing, coughing, defecation, urination and parturation. The respiratory muscles are an important component of the "respiratory pump" and this consists of the respiratory center, the conducting nerves, the thoracic cage and the muscles of breathing.[1] Till a few years ago little attention was given to respiratory muscles in the field of pulmonary medicine. A better understanding of respiratory muscles pathophysiology, the realization of the important role of respiratory muscles play in different diseases and the development of newer tests to more accurately assess respiratory muscles function has lead to an increased interest in this area.[2-4] Respiratory muscle training has also emerged as a treatment modality in patient with chronic respiratory diseases. A basic knowledge of the anatomy and physiology of the respiratory muscles is therefore important to properly understand their actions and the tests used to assess their functions.

RESPIRATORY MUSCLES—ANATOMICAL CONSIDERATION

The respiratory muscles can broadly be divided into two categories: those that take part in inspiration and those that are predominantly expiratory in function. In a normal person, during quite inspiration, the respiratory muscles contract in a coordinated manner so that the diaphragm moves down like a piston and the rib cage move upwards and outwards in a bucket handle manner. This increase in the size of the thoracic cage creates a more negative pleural pressure and air is drawn into the lungs. Besides this, during inspiration, as the airway pressure becomes negative other muscles also act and prevent collapse of the conducting structures mainly in the upper airways. These muscles are the pharyngeal constrictor muscles, the genioglossus and the neck strap muscles.[5] These muscles ensure patency of the upper airways during inspiration. Also, the laryngeal abductor muscles contract and open the vocal cords during inspiration. All these muscles must act in synchrony to ensure adequate breathing during inspiration.

Expiration during normal breathing is usually passive. At the end of inspiration, the inspiratory muscles relax and the normal elastic recoil of the lung facilitates expiration. During activities such as exercise and in patients with underlying lung disease expiratory muscles may be recruited for a more active and forceful exhalation.

INSPIRATORY MUSCLES

Diaphragm: The diaphragm is the main muscle of inspiration and during quiet breathing accounts for about 70–80% of the work of breathing.[6] The diaphragm is composed of two distinct muscle components, the costal portion and the crural portion.[7] Both of these are inserted into a central tendon. The costal portion arises anteriorly from the xiphoid process and from the upper margin of the lower six ribs. The thick crural portion consists of muscle fibers that arise from the arcuate ligaments and are inserted into the upper three lumbar bodies on the right side and the upper two lumbar vertebrae on the left side.[7] The costal and crural parts of the diaphragm may be recruited differently especially when an individual is breathing at a high ventilatory rate.

The diaphragmatic curvature is like that of a hemisphere. If the radius of this hemisphere were to be *r*, than as per Laplace's law the pressure inside the sphere (P) would be equal to $2\ T/r$, where T is the tension in the wall. If T is kept constant and r increases, as would happen if the diaphragm flattens and the curvature of the diaphragm decreases, it will lead to a decrease in pressure.[8] This commonly occurs in patients with chronic obstructive pulmonary disease (COPD) were flattening of the diaphragm due to emphysema or air trapping occurs and this decrease the efficiency of the diaphragm to generate pressure. Also, the dome shape of the diaphragm increases diaphragmatic function through the zone of apposition. The zone of apposition is that part of the diaphragm that lies next to the inner aspect to the rib cage. When the diaphragm contracts and descends it increases intra-abdominal pressure. This increased intra-abdominal pressure is transmitted laterally to the rib cage and through the zone of apposition it facilitates the expansion of the lower rib cage.[8,9]

Besides the diaphragm other muscles also contract during normal inspiration. These are mainly the scalene muscles, the intercostals and the triangularis.[10] The scalene muscle originates from the transverse process of the lower five cervical vertebrae. It is inserted on the upper surface of the first and second ribs. These muscles act by lifting and expanding the rib cage during inspiration.

This muscle was initially thought to be an accessory muscle of inspiration, but studies have clearly shown that the scalene are primary and not accessory muscles of inspiration.[10] The intercostals muscles consists of the external and internal intercostals and these muscles run between the ribs. The external intercostals and the parasternal part of the internal intercostals also contract during inspiration. Contraction of these muscles lifts the ribs and thereby increases the anterioposterior diameter of the rib cage.[11]

ACCESSORY INSPIRATORY MUSCLES

As the ventilator demand increases, the accessory muscles of inspiration come into play. The sternocleidomastoid is the most important accessory muscle of inspiration.[11] This muscle runs from the mastoid process and attaches to the medial third of the clavicle, the ribs and the manubrium sterni. Contraction of this muscle leads to the elevation of the first rib and lifting of the sternum. This results in an increase in the anteroposterior diameter of the upper part of the rib cage. The external intercostal muscles may also contract as ventilatory demand increases. Other muscles like the pectoralis major and minor, latissimus dorsi, anterior serratus and trapezius, though not muscles of respiration, actively contract in patients with severe obstructive lung disease.[5]

EXPIRATORY MUSCLES

Expiration in a normal individual is a passive process and is achieved by the elastic recoil of the lung when the muscles of inspiration relax. The abdominal muscles assist expiration. These include rectus abdominis, external and internal oblique and transverse abdominis.[6] Contraction of these muscle decreases the size of the rib cage and the end expiratory lung volume also decreases. Also, as these abdominal muscles contract, the intra-abdominal pressure increase, the abdominal contents get compressed and the diaphragm is pushed upward.[6]

Both the inspiratory and expiratory muscle function in a coordinated manner in a number of activities that an individual performs in day-to-day life. Activities like sneezing, coughing or defecation require the synchronous activity of these muscles to generate a large intrathoracic pressure. In coughing a deep inspiratory effort is required. After this the glottis closes and a very high intrathoracic pressure is generated due to the powerful contraction of the diaphragm and the abdominal muscles. The glottis then opens and this pressure is suddenly released and it leads to an explosive expiratory effort. This causes a very high flow in the airways and a shearing force in the airways is also generated. This helps in removing secretions and other foreign particles which may be present in the airways.

Respiratory Muscles—Basic Physiology

Respiratory muscles generate pressure differences during the cycle of breathing which allow ventilation to occur. It is important to remember that respiratory muscles differ from other skeletal muscles in certain key ways. Firstly, they are the only skeletal muscles on which life depends. Secondly, they are under both voluntary and involuntary control. Also respiratory muscles contract mainly to overcome elastic and resistive loads. This is unlike other skeletal muscles which cope mainly with inertial load. They are also by far the most extensively used skeletal muscles. The force generated by the respiratory muscles, as for any muscle, depends upon its level of excitation, the initial resting length and the mode of contraction.[12]

One important component in the functioning of the respiratory muscles is the length tension relationship. In a muscle, the active force developed is a function of the length of the muscle. As the length of muscle fibers decreases its capacity to generate pressure also decreases. On the other hand, lengthening of a muscle fiber, up to a point, increases its capacity to generate force.[12] This concept is important to understand in relation to the diaphragm. In patients with COPD as the lung hyperinflation, the diaphragm is pushed down and the length of the muscle fibers decrease. This significantly decreases the efficiency of the diaphragm to generate force and there by increases the work of breathing.

Whenever a muscle is stimulated, it contracts and generates a force. As the frequency of the stimulus increases, there occurs an associated increase in the force the muscle can generate. As the stimulus is further increased the force, the muscle can generate continues to increase until it reaches a plateau and above this frequency the force does not increase.[5] This plateau is reached at a frequency above 50 Hz and this association between stimulus and the force a muscle generates is known as force-frequency relationship. Another mechanical properly which is important is the relationship between the force a muscle generates and the velocity of muscle fiber shortening. The greater the force a muscle generates, the slower the velocity of contraction. There is therefore an inverse relationship between the velocity of muscle contraction and the force generating capacity of a muscle.[6]

It has been shown that the respiratory system has been designed in such a way that after some time as the inspiratory demand increases, rather than increasing the force of contraction, newer inspiratory muscles of respiration get recruited. In this way, muscle function is coordinated so that the respiratory muscles are always shortening at a velocity that will lead to optimum function.

Evaluation of Respiratory Muscle Function

Assessment of respiratory muscle function should form a part of routine respiratory system diagnostic work up. Dyspnea occurring when no other pulmonary cause is apparent may occur due to respiratory muscle weakness. Broadly, evaluation of respiratory muscle function would be indicated in two situations: (1) When clinical features suggest respiratory muscle weakness, and (2) If the patient is suffering from a disease where respiratory muscle weakness is known to occur. Respiratory muscle assessment is also being done where muscle weakness may affect other disease processes, as may occur with steroid therapy, prolonged mechanical ventilation and severe malnutrition.[13-16]

HISTORY AND EXAMINATION

Breathlessness is the main symptom of patients with respiratory muscle weakness. In patient with generalized neuromuscular diseases, respiratory muscles are usually involved and these patients may show wasting and fasciculation of the limb muscles. Patients with significant diaphragmatic weakness classically complain of breathlessness when supine, or sitting or standing in water.[2] Breathlessness which occurs immediately on lying supine or on entering a swimming pool is very suggestive of severe diaphragmatic weakness. As the respiratory muscle weakness progresses it lead to nocturnal hypoventilation and disturbed sleep. This leads to day time somnolence and impaired intellect.[17] Ultimately ventilator failure and cor pulmonale develop. Patients with weakness of bulbar and expiratory muscle have poor cough and these patients have a higher chance of developing recurrent aspiration and pneumonia.

Physical examination may at times be helpful. Increase in respiratory rate may occur due to respiratory muscle weakness. Use of accessory muscles and intercostals recession may suggest respiratory distress and muscle weakness. Patients with diaphragmatic weakness or paralyses show a typical paradoxical inward inspiratory abdominal movement. Normally, as the diaphragm contracts during inspiration, the abdominal contents are pushed down and the abdominal wall moves outwards. In patients with diaphragmatic weakness or paralysis, during inspiration the pleural pressure becomes more negative and the weak or paralyzed diaphragm get sucked into the thoracic cage. This leads to the paradoxical inward abdominal movement during inspiration. This movement is better appreciated in the supine position.[3] These physical findings are usually only appreciated when diaphragmatic weakness has progressed to more than 75% and therefore significant respiratory muscle weakness may be missed on clinical examination.[18]

Imaging to Assess Respiratory Muscle Function

A plain chart radiograph may show an elevated hemidiaphragm and this may suggest hemidiaphragmatic paralysis. In patients with bilateral diaphragmatic paralysis both hemidiaphragms are elevated and the X-ray may appear relatively normal.[19] Fluoroscopy is a commonly used test in suspected hemidiaphragmatic palsy and is positive in about 90% of cases.[5] An upward or cephalad movement of the diaphragm is seen. These tests can be falsely positive and do not provide information about the extent of diaphragmatic weakness. A short sharp sub maximal sniff during fluoroscopy is a useful maneuver to assess for diaphragmatic weakness.

Recently ultrasound has emerged as a useful tool to assess movement, thickness and zone of apposition of the diaphragm.[20] Besides this subpulmonary or subdiaphragmatic collections, traumatic rupture and pleural masses can also be detected.[21] It is also a safe method with no radiation exposure and is simple to perform. Ultrasound has also been used for assessing hemidiaphragmatic movements, zone of apposition and the thickness of the diaphragm.[22] Hemidiaphragmatic movement has been evaluated in normal individuals and in with patients with underlying respiratory diseases. By this technique, the normal range of craniocaudal excursion of the posterior hemidiaphragm has been established and an acceptable reliability has been obtained in terms of interobserver and intraobserver reproducibility. It has also been was found to be a reliable quantitative as well as qualitative method for assessing posterior diaphragmatic excursions. Ultrasound has also been used to see the thickness and length of the zone of apposition with good results.[23] The thickness of the zone of apposition at different lung volumes has been measured. This measurement has shown good repeatability in most subjects although it may be difficult to perform in obese individuals.[23] Ultrasound has also been used to evaluate the thickness of the diaphragm in different neuromuscular and respiratory diseases.[22,24] Detailed diaphragmatic function and it movement has been evaluated in patients with COPD, pulmonary fibrosis and emphysema using ultrasound. Ultrasound evaluation of the diaphragm has also been found to be useful in the intensive care unit (ICU) and it has helped in evaluating diaphragm weakness and in predicting success of a weaning trial in patients on a ventilator.[25-28]

Function Testing

At times conventional spirometry provides the first suspicion of respiratory muscle weakness. As spirometry is routinely done and easy to perform it is often used to assess the severity, progression and functional consequence in patients with confirmed respiratory muscle weakness. Patients with inspiratory muscle weakness classically have low vital capacity, decreased total lung capacity (TLC) and near normal residual volume (RV).[23] The functional residual capacity (FRC) is also relatively preserved in patients with respiratory muscle weakness. Usually, the TLC is less markedly reduced than the vital capacity and therefore the RV/TLC ratio and FRC/TLC ratios are often increased.[23] A normal vital capacity makes respiratory muscle weakness highly unlikely. Diffusion capacity to carbon monoxide is reduced but normal or raised when adjusted for volume and this helps to distinguish respiratory muscle weakness from alveolar disorders like pulmonary fibrosis.

In patients with diaphragmatic palsy, the vital capacity falls when the patient is supine and this fall should be more than 25% to be definitely abnormal.[29] Regular monitoring of vital capacity is also useful in patient with progressive muscle weakness or paralysis, i.e. Guillain-Barré syndrome.[30,31] If the vital capacity falls below 50% from baseline, the patient may need ventilator support. It must be remembered that in patient with long standing respiratory muscle weakness, vital capacity will also fall due to reduced chest wall and lung compliance, possibly due to micro atelectasis.[5] Vital capacity maneuver is a patient dependent maneuver and therefore the result depends upon patient's motivation and ability. Moreover, a number of other diseases can lead to a decreased vital capacity. This test is therefore neither specific nor diagnostic.[32]

Flow Rates and Dynamic Spirometry

In patients with pure respiratory muscle weakness, airway resistance is normal. A decrease in both inspiratory and expiratory flow rates occurs in patients with respiratory muscle weakness. These flows are decreased more in the effort dependent part of the flow volume loop. The decrease in expiratory flow rates is less as compared to inspiratory rates and the ratio of maximum mid inspiratory flow rates to maximum mid expiratory flow rates, which is usually greater than one, is less than one is respiratory muscle weakness.[23] However, a similar decrease can occur in extrathoracic upper airway obstruction. Flow volume loop shows a decrease at high lung volumes than at low lung volumes and peak flow is markedly decreased. As residual is approached expiratory muscles cannot overcome the outward elastic recoil of the chest wall flow rapidly decreases and ceases at high RV. Because of this the descending loop of the flow volume curve tends to be convex rather than concave, with an abrupt drop off of flow at the end of expiration.[23]

Maximum voluntary ventilation (MVV) is also reduced.[5] This test is also done and in the past was recommended to assess respiratory muscle weakness. However, it is not a sensitive test and is not useful to diagnose respiratory muscle weakness.[5]

Monitoring overnight pulse oximetry may help in providing evidence to the severity of respiratory muscle weakness.[2] A normal nocturnal oximetry suggests that the muscle weakness is not severe enough to cause ventilatory failure. On the other hand, demonstration of nocturnal hypoventilation suggests severe respiratory muscle weakness which may cause ventilatory failure. Patients with moderate to severe respiratory muscle weakness show fall in oxygen saturation during rapid eye movement sleep.[5] This fall in oxygen saturation is mainly due to hypopneas and these may appear to either central or obstructive or a mixture of both.[33] In patients with pure respiratory muscle weakness, substantial nocturnal desaturation occurs only if respiratory muscle strength is less than one third of normal.[2] As respiratory muscle weakness progresses hypercapnia starts occurring initially during sleep. Many of these patients may have coexisting respiratory disorders which may also contribute to hypoventilation.

Mouth Pressures

These tests give a good estimate of global respiratory muscle strength. The tests most widely used to assess inspiratory and expiratory muscle strength are static maximum inspiratory pressures (MIP) and static maximum expiratory pressure (MEP) at mouth. These tests are simple to perform, fairly accurate, noninvasive and well tolerated by the patients. Also normal values for MIP and MEP have been established in different ethnic groups.[34-37] Portable and inexpensive devices are now available which allows one to measure MIP and MEP at beside, in the outpatient department (OPD) and in the ICU[38] **(Fig. 1)**.

Both MIP and MEP are measured at different lung volumes so that the maximum muscle strength of the muscle can be measured. The length of the respiratory muscles and therefore

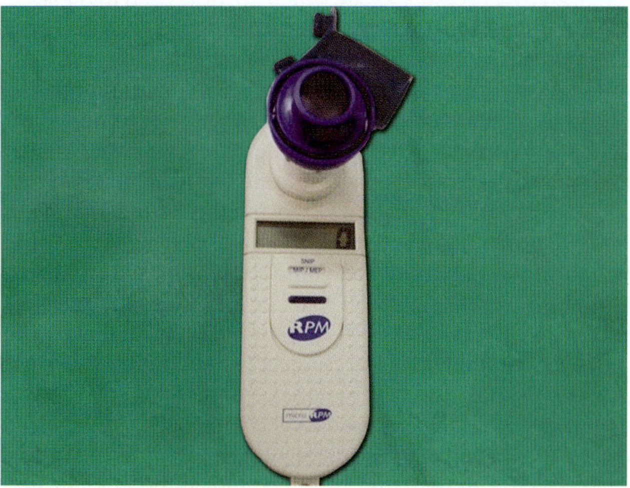

Fig. 1 Simple portable device to measure mouth pressures and sniff nasal inspiratory pressure (SNIP)

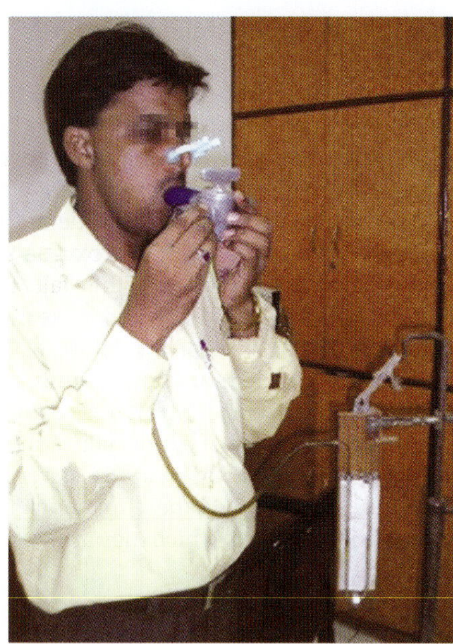

Fig. 2 Traditionally used method to measure mouth pressure using a mercury manometer

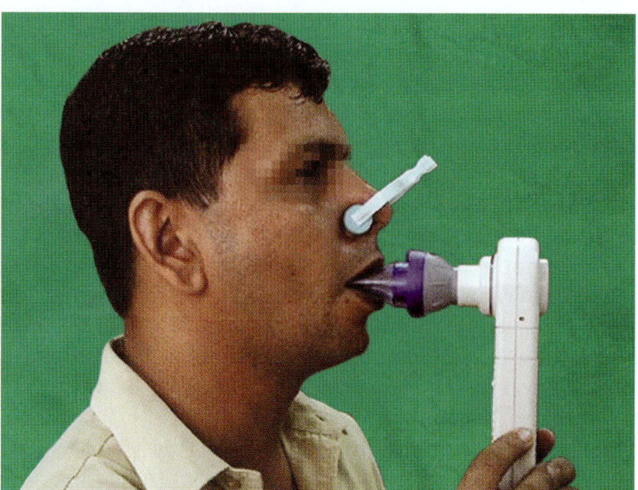

Fig. 3 Pressure meter being used to measure mouth pressure

their contractile force vary with lung volume. The force a skeletal muscle can generate depends on the force-velocity and force-length relationship (see section on respiratory muscle physiology above). The expiratory muscles are longer at high lung volumes and so expiratory muscles contractile force is highest at or near TLC. Conversely, inspiratory muscles are longer at low lung volumes and so inspiratory muscle force is greatest between FRC and RV. Devices used to measure MIP and MEP measure inspiratory and expiratory pressures at mouth when the patient makes a maximum effort against a closed airway. Initially a mercury manometer was used to measure MIP and MEP **(Fig. 2)** but this has been replaced by a pressure gauge which are now used to measure the pressure **(Fig. 3)**. Lips are pursed inside a wide bore mouth piece. This contracts the facial muscles and prevents the cheeks from ballooning during expiration.[34,37] The inspiratory and expiratory pressure must be maintained for at least 1.5 seconds, so that the maximum pressure sustained for at least 1 second can be recorded. For reasons explained above to get the best readings of respiratory muscles strength MEP is measured at or near TLC and MIP between RV and FRC. In females, MIP and MEP are about 65–70% less than that of males. Over the age of 50 years in both sexes the pressure values are about 85–90% of that for younger adults. Also a much greater degree of intrasubject variability in pressure is present as compared to variation in spirometry.

Like the vital capacity, a normal or high MIP (more than 80 cm of H_2O) rules out clinically significant respiratory muscle weakness.[2] Both MIP and MEP are subject dependent and at times it is difficult to ensure that the patient is making a truly maximum effort. Therefore patient's cooperation is very important. A low value may therefore, be due to poor effort and may underestimate the strength of the respiratory muscles. As this test is easy to perform and normal values are available it is widely used to rule out respiratory muscle weakness. Serial measurements over time may give valuable information about progression or improvement in muscle weakness in patient with chronic neuromuscular disease. Also, MIP is useful to assess respiratory muscle strength in the ICU in patients on mechanical ventilator to determine fitness to wean off the ventilator. Patients with an MIP less than in 20 cm H_2O are usually unfit for a weaning trial.[39]

Nasal Pressures

Another method used to assess respiratory muscle strength is by doing the sniff test.[40,41] A sniff is an inspiratory maneuver which is short and sharp in performed through one or both unoccluded nostril. During a sniff, there occurs a sharp contraction of the diaphragm and other inspiratory muscles. Sniff is a natural maneuver, is simple and noninvasive and may patients find it easy to do. It has been shown that in normal subjects the pressure developed in the esophagus during a sniff closely relates to the pressure in the nasopharynx, mouth and nose.[42] Therefore, measurement of the sniff nasal inspiratory pressure (SNIP) provides a good estimate of inspiratory muscle strength. Normal value of SNIP have been established and it has been evaluated in patients with COPD and interstitial lung disease.[43,44]

The tests consist of asking the subject to perform a short sharp maximal sniff through one unobstructed nostril while measuring nasal pressure through a catheter wedged in the contralateral nostril **(Fig. 4)**. Various methods for wedging and occluding the nostril with a small tube are used. These include foam, rubber bung and dental molding material. This test is easy and natural and allows patients to activate

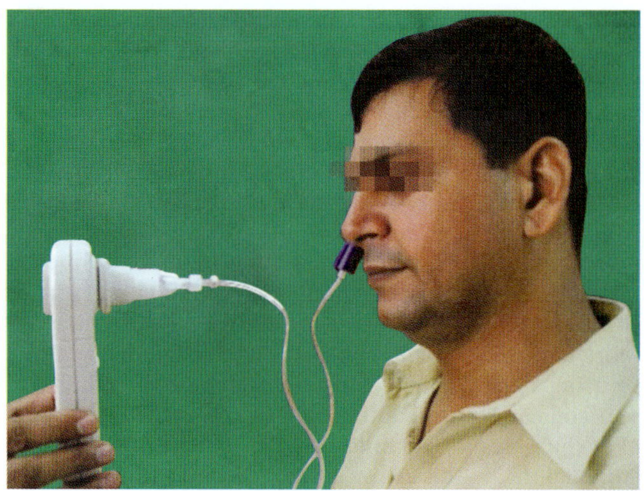

Fig. 4 Sniff nasal inspiratory pressure (SNIP) being measured using a catheter and a nasal bunge to occlude one nostril

inspiratory muscles completely. This test is also relatively reproducible and has a smaller range of normal values than mouth pressures.[41,42] Simple portable devices are available for SNIP recording and this test can now be done at the bedside.[45]

Invasive Tests

Sometime noninvasive tests do not helping in confirming absence of respiratory muscle weakness and at times a more accurate estimation of the degree of muscle weakness is needed for treatment purpose in patients with underlying respiratory muscle weakness. In such situations, tests which are more precise but invasive and where patients own effort is not required are used. These tests require the introduction of two small latex balloons which are sealed over a catheter into the esophagus and stomach. These balloons are thin-walled, usually 5-10 cm long and have a 3.5-5 cm perimeter.[23] The catheter is about 70-100 cm long. The catheter is attached to a transducer which records the pressure. Using local anesthesia these small esophageal and gastric balloons are introduced through the nose and gradually passed through the pharynx into the esophagus. One catheter is positioned at the lower end of the esophagus (esophageal balloons) and the other is positioned in the stomach (gastric balloon). A very small amount of air is introduced into these balloons. One balloon lies just earlier (reflects pleural pressure) and the other just later the diaphragm (reflects abdomen pressure).[23] This allows one to measures the pressure difference across the diaphragm when it contracts and therefore the transdiaphragmatic pressure (Pdi) can be measured.

Maximum Transdiaphragmatic Pressure

Measurement of Pdi maximum (Pdimax) gives an idea of the strength of the diaphragm. Transdiaphragmatic pressure is calculated as the difference in the gastric pressure (pga) and the esophageal pressure (Pes) measured when the subject makes an isotonic contraction during a maximal voluntary effort. The transphragmatic pressure will vary with lung volume and should therefore be recorded at a known lung volume (usually FRC). Normal value for Pdimax and in patients with different lung diseases have been established.[46]

Transdiaphragmatic and Esophageal Pressure during Sniff

Sniff is easy to perform and most subjects are early able to perform a maximal sniff effort. With the gastric and esophaged balloons in place the subject is asked to perform a maximum sniff at FRC without using a nose clip.[2] The sniff transdiaphragmatic pressure (Sniff Pdi) is recorded. Usually the patient is asked to perform a number of these maneuvers till three reproducible tracings are obtained. Sniff Pdi has been studied in normal and in different diseases. It has a narrow normal range and better between day coefficient of variation than MIP.[37]

Studies suggest that clinically useful information about diaphragmatic strength can be obtained by using a single esophageal catheter and measuring sniff esophageal pressure (Sniff Poes).[47] A single esophageal catheter is routinely used in many respiratory laboratories for measuring lung compliance. Esophageal pressure is measured, with a pressure transducer, while the patient makes a short, sharp, maximal sniff. This esophageal pressure during a sniff (Sniff Poes) closely relates to sniff Pdi and is simpler to do **(Fig. 5)**.

All these tests, i.e. Pdimax, Sniff Pdi and Sniff Poes, are useful, accurate and reproducible tests. They provide reliable assessment of and diaphragmatic strength. However, like previous tests they also are dependent on patient's cooperation and low values become difficult to interpret at times.

Tests where Subjects Cooperation not Needed

Phrenic Nerve Stimulation

The diaphragm is innervated by the phrenic nerves only. Thus stimulating the phrenic nerve provides a unique way of assessing diaphragmatic function without the cooperation of the patient. Besides pressure measurement, phrenic nerve stimulation also allows one to record electromyogram of the diaphragm and phrenic nerve conduction time.[48] Phrenic nerve stimulation superimposed on a naturally occurring or voluntary contraction is an important research tool and provides information about the maximal voluntary pressure that the diaphragm can generate.[49]

Electrical Stimulation

Electrical stimulation of the phrenic nerve can be done in the neck and the diaphragmatic contraction can be measured

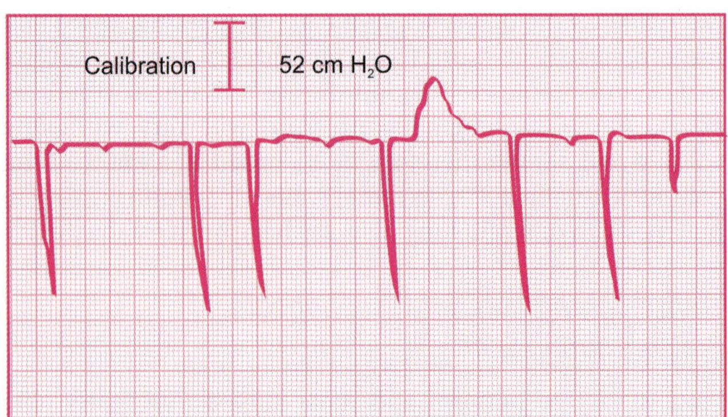

Fig. 5 Tracing of sniff esophageal pressure recorded in a patient using an esophageal balloon catheter. Patient has performed multiple sniff maneuvers. The upward positive wave is due to swallowing

by the esophageal and gastric balloons.[23] The contraction which is the twitch transdiaphragmatic pressure (twitch Pdi) has the advantage that it does not need patient's motivation or cooperation. Both unilateral and bilateral electric stimulation of the phrenic nerve can be done. The phrenic nerve is usually located just beneath the posterior border of the sternocleidomastoid muscle at the level of the cricoid cartilage. Precise location of the nerve is required for electrode placement and to achieve this repeated stimulation near the site are frequently required. Once the nerve is identified the spot is marked and the orientation of the electrode in the neck is observed by the operator.[23] The operator usually stands behind the seated subject and the current intensity is increased to obtained supramaximal stimulation. The procedure is usually done on each side separately and after that bilateral electrical stimulation is applied and twitch Pdi is recorded with the esophageal and gastric balloons. Twitch Pdi has been measured in normal subject and in patients.[50,51] This test can be uncomfortable as the stimulus intensity is increased to achieve supramaximal stimulation. Also sometimes it is difficult to locate the exact site of the nerve and reliable supramaximal stimulus is not obtained. This test is useful when there is severe weakness or the results of the previous tests are not definite as the patient is unwilling or unable to cooperate.

Magnetic Stimulation

It has been known for long that magnetic fields can stimulate the nervous structures.[52] The last decade has seen the extensive use of magnetic stimulation in neurology.[53] Magnetic stimulation by a magnetic coil creates brief and intense magnetic field.[23] This field is only mildly hampered by structures on the surface of the body like skin and bones. It therefore reaches the deeper nervous structures and the rapidly changing magnetic field causes current to flow in the nervous tissue within the field.[54,55] This is turn causes the muscle to contract. Magnetic stimulation overcomes a lot of problems associated with electrical stimulation.[56,57] It is relatively painless and easy to apply in a clinical setting. By placing a circular magnetic over the cervical phrenic nerve routes one can achieve supramaximal bilateral phrenic nerve stimulation once this coil is activated.[58,59] The magnetically measured Pdi is slightly greater than the electrical Pdi possibly due to activation of accessory muscle which may get activated due to the spread of the magnetic field.[2] For the assessment of respiratory muscle function bilateral phrenic nerve stimulation can be achieved by stimulating the phrenic nerve roots in the cervical spine.[58,59] More localized phrenic nerve stimulation can be achieved by using a figure of eight shaped magnetic coil in the neck. This coil can be used unilaterally for unilateral stimulation of the phrenic nerve or bilaterally for bilateral phrenic nerve stimulation.[60,61] This allows easy and accurate assessment of hemidiaphragmatic function. Bilateral anterior stimulation also has the advantage that it can be done in supine position.[60,61] Respiratory muscle assessment using magnetic stimulation is now being done as an OPD procedure, in the ward and even in an ICU setting.[62] This has largely replaced and electric stimulation and has become well established in clinical practice.

Magnetic stimulation of the respiratory muscle is being increasingly used to assess respiratory muscle function and endurance.[60,63,64] The role of abdominal muscle and the pressure changes that occur during abdominal muscle stimulation is being better understood.[60] Also the mechanism of diaphragmatic fatigue, cough, etc. are also being evaluated.[60,65,66]

ELECTROPHYSIOLOGICAL ASSESSMENT OF RESPIRATORY MUSCLES

Electromyography

Electromyography (EMG) has traditionally been used to assess various aspects of skeletal muscle function. Stimulation of the phrenic nerve causes the diaphragm to be activated and the electrical signal generated by this activation is recorded.[67] Recording EMG of the respiratory muscles can help to assess the level and pattern of activation of these muscles. This helps in the diagnosis of neuromuscular diseases and when combined with other tests help to assess the efficacy of the contractile function of the muscle. To record EMG of the diaphragm electrodes can be placed at different sites. Surface electrodes can be placed in the neck, over the chest wall muscles or next to the area of apposition of the diaphragm on the chest wall. Electrodes wound around a small catheter can be swallowed and placed in the lower esophagus to measure a more pure crural diaphragm EMG. Electrodes can also be inserted into the respiratory muscle of interest using needles, wire or hook electrodes. Surface electrodes are commonly used because they are noninvasive, easy to apply and a large number of motor units can be assessed. Surface electrodes have been used to assess activity of the diaphragm, scalene, intercostals, abdominal muscles and accessory muscles. The electrodes are placed over or as close as possible to the muscle to be evaluated. The site is determined by palpation and knowledge of the surface anatomy of the respiratory muscles.

Diaphragmatic EMG can be obtained by needle electrodes introduced with reasonable safety through the 10th intercostals space in the mid axillary line. Placement of surface electrodes in the 7th, 8th and 9th intercostals space can also be used to record diaphragm EMG. Esophageal electrodes are used more for research purpose. They provide a more accurate and pure diaphragm EMG. EMG is useful in distinguishing neuropathic and myopathic diaphragmatic dysfunction. It may also help in detecting diaphragmatic fatigue.

Respiratory Muscle Endurance

Muscle endurance can be defined as the ability to sustain a specific muscular task over time.[23] Although respiratory muscle strength and endurance appear to be closely linked there are many conditions where the endurance of the respiratory muscles cannot be predicted by measuring maximum pressures or maximum ventilator capacity. For example, certain respiratory muscle training protocols used in normal individuals and in patients has a greater effect on endurance than on muscle strength.[68,69] Similarly, some asthmatic patients show an inherent elevation in endurance properties as a faction of strength.[70] Also, patients with COPD or those on acute steroid treatment show significant reduction in endurance properties relative to strength.[71,72] Therefore, measurement of endurance of the respiratory muscles can have important clinical implications. It may also have an important utility in assessing the efficacy of a rehabilitation program. Unfortunately no uniformly accepted and simple method exists for the estimation of endurance.

Endurance may be measured as ventilator endurance or endurance to an applied load.[23] Traditional approach for evaluating ventilator endurance has been to measure the maximum sustainable ventilation (MSV), i.e. the maximum ventilation that can be maintained for 10–15 minutes. MSV is usually expressed as a fraction of MVV. Normal subjects can achieve a MSV which is 60–80% of MVV.[73] Various techniques have been used to calculate MSV. The maximum effort technique requires the subject to breath at a ventilation of approximately 70–90% of their MVV using a visual feedback from either a spirometer or an oscilloscope.[23] Another method that has been used utilizes a 10% incremental increase in target ventilation, every 3 minutes, beginning at 20% of MVV until the subject cannot sustain the target ventilation. MSV is calculated from the last 10 breaths of the last minute of the highest target ventilation. Tests for MSV have been found to be exhaustive and time consuming and are largely impractical.

Various devices have been used to assess endurance against an applied load. Early methods utilized orifice type flow resistance applied to the inspiratory circuit but these have been replaced by threshold resistive loading devices which make it possible to more accurately control the pressure the subject inspires against, independent of flow.[23] Inspiratory threshold devices have also been used to test endurance.[23,74,75] Technique involves inspiring through a device that contains a weighted plunger. To initiate inspiration enough pressure must be generated to lift the plunger out of the socket. Thereafter inspiration remains constant for the entire inspiration. A negative pressure device and a 3 minute incremental protocol has also been described to measure endurance and fatigue.[65,76] The ability to sustain such a breathing effort during an endurance test depends upon the force and the duration of the inspiratory muscle contraction. It has been demonstrated that intense diaphragmatic contractions of brief duration can be sustained for as many breath as could less intense diaphragmatic contractions of brief duration that occupied a larger fraction of breath.[23] Therefore, the tension time index of the diaphragm (TTIdi) is calculated to predict fatigue and is a better marker than either contractile force or duration of contraction. TTIdi is the product of the contractile force and duration and contraction. Force is expressed as Pdi breath/Pdi maximum. The duration of contraction is the inspiration duty cycle (this is TI/TTOT, i.e. the duration of inspiration divided by the duration of a complete breath). It has been shown that the human diaphragm becomes fatigued when the TTIdi exceeds 0.15. Inspiratory threshold devices have also been used to train inspiratory muscles and improve respiratory muscle strength in various conditions including mechanically ventilated patients.[77,78]

CONCLUSION

Respiratory muscles are essential for life. Their assessment and early detection of weakness becomes important. The diaphragm, which is the main muscle of respiration, is unique that it can be assessed by the volume displaced (spirometry), pressure generated (muscle strength) and by the electrical activity of the muscle (EMG). Many different tests have therefore been used to assess diaphragm function. Tests for diaphragmatic endurance and fatigue are also used but these have mainly research implications. Besides respiratory diseases, many systemic illness and disorders cause weakness of the respiratory muscles and their assessment becomes important in these diseases.[14,16,68,79,80] It is therefore important to know when to suspect respiratory muscle weakness in a given patient and how best to test for such weakness.

REFERENCES

1. Epstein S. An overview of respiratory muscles function. Chest Clin North Am. 1994;15:619-39.
2. Polkey MI, Green M, Moxham J. Measurement of respiratory muscles strength. Thorax. 1995;50:1131-5.

3. Laroche CM, Carroll N, Moxham J, Green M. Clinical significance of severe isolated diaphragm weakness. Am Rev Respir Dis. 1988;138:862-6.
4. Goswami R, Guleria R, Gupta AK, Gupta N, Marwaha RK, Pande JN, K, et al. Prevalence of diaphragmatic muscle weakness and dyspnea in Graves disease and their reversibility with carbimazole therapy. Eur J Endocrinol. 2002;147(3):299-303.
5. Flaminiano LE, Celli BR. Respiratory muscle testing. Clinics in Chest Med. 2001;22(4):661-77.
6. Loring SH, DeTroyer A. Action of the respiratory muscles. In: Roussos C, Macklem PT (Eds). Lung biology in health and disease series The Thorax. New York, NY Marcel Dekker Inc.; 1985. pp. 327-49.
7. Leak LV. Gross and ultrastructural morphologic features to of the diaphragm. Am Rev Respir Dis. 1979;19:31-2.
8. Rochester DF. The Diaphragm: contractile properties and fatigue. J Clin Invest. 1985;75:1397-402.
9. Mead J. Functional significance of the area of apposition of diaphragm to rib cage [proceedings]. Am Rev Respir Dis. 1979;119(2 Pt 2):31-2.
10. Campbell EJM. The role of the scalene and sternomastoid muscles in breathing in normal subjects. An study. J Anat. 1955;89:378-86.
11. DeTroyer A, Estenne M. Functional anatomy of the respiratory muscles. In: Belman MJ (Eds). Respiratory Muscles: Function in health and disease. Philadelphia, pa: WB Saunders Co.; 1988. pp. 175-95.
12. Edwaards RHT. Human muscles function and fatigue. In: Porter R, Whelan J (Eds). Human Muscles Fatigue: Physiological Mechanisms. London, Pitman Medical (Ciba Foundation Symposium 82); 1981. pp. 1-18.
13. Ishwar CM, Guleria R, Gupta AK, Pande JN, Sharma SK, Misra A, et al. Does malnutrition affect the strength and thickness of the diaphragm in asymptomatic healthy individuals? Chest. 2006;130:248(S).
14. Panniswami C, Selvaraj DR, Guleria R, Mohan A, Sugunaraj JP, Ramamurthy S, et al. Respiratory muscle strength in rheumatic mitral stenosis improves after balloon valvotomy. J Cardiovasc Med (Hagerstown). 2010;11(6):440-3.
15. Gupta R, Sharma U, Gupta N, Kalaivani M, Singh U, Guleria R, et al. Effect of cholecalciferol and calcium supplementation on muscle strength and energy metabolism in vitamin D deficient Asian Indians: A randomized controlled trial. Clin Endocrinol (Oxf). 2010:73(4):445-51.
16. Guleria S, Agarwal R, Guleria R, Bhomik D, Agarwal SK, Tiwari SC. The effect of renal transplantation on pulmonary function and respiratory muscle strength in patients with end-stage renal disease. Transplantation Proceedings. 2005;37:664-5.
17. Smith PE, Calverley PM, Edwards RH. Hypoxemia during sleep in Duchenne muscular dystrophy. Am Rev Respir Dis. 1988;137:884-8.
18. Meir-Jedzejowicz A, Brophy C, Moxham J, Green M. Assessement of diaphragm weakness. Am Rev Respir Dis. 1988;137:877-83.
19. Alexander C. Diaphragm movements and the diagnosis of diaphragmatic paralysis. Clin Radiol. 1966;17:79-83.
20. Houston JG, Angus RM, Crowan MD, Mcmillan NC, Thomson NC. Ultrasound assessment of normal hemidiphragmatic movement: relation to inspiratory volume. Thorax. 1994;49:500-3.
21. Lipscomb DJ, Flower CDR, Hadfield JO. Ultrasound of the pleura: an assessment of clinical value. Clin Radiology. 1981;32: 289-90.
22. Houston JG, Morris AD, Howie CA, Reid JL, McMillan NC. Technical Report: quantitative assessment of normal hemidiaphragmatic movementa reproducible method using ultrasound. Clin Radiology. 1992;46:405-7.
23. ATS/ERS statement on respiratory muscle testing. Am J Respi Crit Care Med. 2002;166:518-624.
24. Narayanan R, Guleria R, Gupta AK, Pande JN. Ultrasound assessment of diaphragmatic movements and it's correlation with lung function in patients with chronic obstructive airway disease. Chest. 2000;118:201(S).
25. Baria MR, Shahgholi L, Sorenson EJ, Harper CJ, Lim KG, Strommen JA, et al. B-mode ultrasound assessment of diaphragm structure and function in patients with COPD. Chest. 2014;146(3):680-5.
26. He L, Zhang W, Zhang J, Cao L, Gong L, Ma J, et al. Diphragmatic motion studied by M mode ultrasonography in combined pulmonary fibrosis and emphysema. Lung. 2014;192:553-61.
27. DiNino E, Gartman E, Sethi JM, McCool FD. Diaphragm ultrasound as a predictor of successfulextubation from mechanical ventilation. Thorax. 2014;69(5):423-7.
28. Demoule A, Jung B, Prodanovic H, Molinari N, Chanques G, Coirault C, et al. Diaphragm dysfunction on admission to the intensive care unit. Prevalence, risk factors, and prognostic impact-a prospective study. Am J Respir Crit Care Med. 2013;188:213-9.
29. Allen S, Hunt B, Green M. Fall in vital capacity with posture. Br J Dis Chest. 1985;79:267-71.
30. Chevrolet J, Delamont P. Repeated vital capacity measurements as predictive parameters for mechanical ventilation need and weaning success in Guillain Barre syndrome. Am Rev Respir Dis. 1991;144:814-8.
31. Fallat RJ, Jewitt B, Bass M, Kamm B, Norris FH. Spirometry in amyotrophic lateral sclerosis. Arch Neurol. 1979;36:74-80.
32. Black LF, Hyatt RE. Maximual static respiratory pressures in generalized neuromuscular disease. Am Rev Respir Dis. 1971;103(5):641-50.
33. White JES, Drinnan MJ, Smithson AJ, Griffiths CJ, Gibson GJ. Respiratroy muscle activity and oxygenation during sleep in patients with muscle weakness. Eur Respir J. 1995;8:807-14.
34. Guleria R, Jindal SK. Normal Maximal expiratory and inspiratory pressures in healthy teenagers. JAPI. 1992;40:108-9.
35. Pande JN, Verma SK, Singh SP, Guleria R, Khilnani GC. Respiratory pressures in normal Indian subjects. Indian J Chest Dis Allied Sci. 1998;40(4):251-6.
36. Leech J, Ghezzo H, Stevens D, Blecklake M. Respiratory pressures and function in young adults. Am Rev Respir Dis. 1983;128(1):17-23.
37. Black L, Hyatt R. Maximal respiratory pressures: normal values and relationships to age and sex. Am Rev Respir Dis. 1969;99:696-702.
38. Hamnegard CH, Wragg S, Kyoroussis D, Aquilina R, Moxham J, Green M. Portable measurement of maximum mouth pressures. Eur Respir J. 1994;7:398-401.
39. Yang KL, Tobin MJ. A prospective study of indexes predicting the outcome of trials of weaning from mechanical ventilation. NEng J Med. 1991;324:1445-50.
40. Heritier F, Rahm F, Pasche P, Fitting JW. Sniff nasal pressure: a noninvasive assessment of inspiratory muscle strength. Am J Respir Crit Care Med. 1994;150:1678-83.
41. Miller J, Moxham J, Green M. The maximal sniff in the assessment of diaphragm function in man. Clin Sci. 1985;59:91-106.
42. Koulouris N, Mulvey DA, Laroche CM, Sawicka EH, Green M,

Moxham J. The measurement of inspiratory muscle strength by sniff esophageal, nasopharyngeal and mouth pressures, Am Rev Respir Dis. 1989.pp.641-6.
43. Arora N, Guleria R, Pande JN, Sharma SK. Comparison of sniff nasal inspiratory pressure and mouth inspiratory pressure for evaluation of respiratory muscle strength in COPD, ILD and normal subjects. Am J Respir Crit Care Med. 2001;163:A156.
44. Uldry C, Janssens JP, de Meralt B, Fitting JW. Sniff nasal inspiratory pressure in patients with chronic obstructive pulmonary disease. Eur Respir J. 1997;10:1292-6.
45. Hamnegard CH, Wragg S, Kyroussis D, Mills GH, Polkey MI, Moxham J, et al. Sniff nasal pressure measured with a portable meter. Am J Respir Crit Care Med. 1995;415:151.
46. Laporta D, Grassino A. Assessment of transdiaphragmatic pressure in humans. J Appl Physiol. 1985;58:1469-76.
47. Laroche CM, Mier AK, Moxham J, Green M. The value of sniff esophageal pressures in the assessment of global inspiratory muscle strength. Am Rev Respir Dis. 1988;138:598-603.
48. Chen R, Collins S, Remtulla H, Parkes A Bolton C. Phrenic nerve Conductin study in normal subjects. Muscle Nerve. 1995;18:330-5.
49. National Heart Lung and Blood Institute. Respiratory muscle fatigue. NHLBI Workshop. Am Rev Respir Dis. 1990;140:474-80.
50. Bellemare F, Bigland-Ritchie B. Assessment of human diaphragm strength and activation using phrenic nerve stimulation. Respir Physiol. 1984;58:263-77.
51. Mier A, Brophy C, Moxham J, Green M. Phrenic nerve stimulation in normal subjects and in patients with diaphragmatic weakness. Thorax. 1987;42:885-8.
52. d'Arsonaval MA. Production des courants de haute frequence et de grande intensite; leurs effects physiologiques. CR Soc Biol. 1893;45:122-4.
53. Barker AT, Jalinous R, Freeston Il. Non-invasive magnetic stimulation of human cortex. Lancet. 1985;1(8437):1106-7.
54. Machetanz J, Bischoff C, Pilchlmeter R, Meyer BU, Sader A, Conrad B. Magnetically induced muscle contraction caused by motor nerve stimulation and not by direct muscle activation. Muscle Nerve. 1994;17:1170-5.
55. Maccabee PJ, Amassian VE, Cracco RQ, Eberle LP, Rudell, AP. Clin Neurophysiol Suppl. 1991;43:344-61.
56. Schmid UD, Walker G, Schmid Sigron J, Hess CW. Transcutaneous magnetic and electrical stimulation over the cervical spine: excitation of plexus roots rather than spinal roots. Electroencephalogr Clin Neurophysiol Suppl. 1991;43:369-84.
57. Ono S, Oishi M, Du CM, Takasu T. Magnetic stimulation of peripheral nerves: comparison of magnetic stimulaltion with electrical stimulation. Electromyogr Clin Neurophysiol. 1995;35:317-20.
58. Similowski T, Fleury B, Launois S, Cathala HP, Bouche P, Direnne JP. Cervical magnetic stimulation: a new painless method for bilateral phrenic nerve stimulation in conscious humans. J Appl Physiol. 1989;67:1311-8.
59. Wragg S, Aquillina R, Moran J, Ridding M, Hamnegard C, Fearn T, et al. Comparison of cervical magnetic stimulation and bilateral percutaneous electrical stimulation of phrenic nerves in normal subjects. Eur Respir J. 1994;7:1788-92.
60. Man WD, Moxham J, Polkey MI. Magnetic stimulation for the measurement of respiratory and skeletal muscle strength. Eur Respir J. 2004;24:846-60.
61. Mills G, Kyoussis D, Hamnegard C, Polkey M, Green M, Moxham J. Bilateral magnetic stimulation of the phrenic nerves from an anterolateral approach. Am J Respir Crit Care Med. 1996;154:1099-105.
62. Watson AC, Harris ML, Guleria R, Evans T, Moxham J, Green M. Diaphragm and limb muscle strength in the critical care unit. 1997;52(Suppl 6):A19.
63. Kyroussis D, Polkey MI, Mills GH, Hughes PD, Moxham J, Green M. Stimulation of cough in man by magnetic stimulation of the thoracic nerve roots. Am J Respir Crit Care Med. 1997;156: 1696-9.
64. Polkey MI, Lou Y, Guleria R, Hamnegard CH, Green M, Moxham J. Functional magnetic stimulation of the abdominal muscles in humans. Am J Respir Crit Care Med. 1999;160(2):513-22.
65. Guleria R, Lyall R, Hart N, Harris ML, Hamnegard CH, Green M, et al. Central fatigue of the diaphragm and the quadriceps during incremental loading. Lung. 2002;180(1):1-13.
66. Polkey MI, Guleria R, Lou YM, Green M, Moxham J. Cough stimulation by rapid rate magnetic stimulation of the thoracic nerve roots. Thorax. 1997;52(Suppl 6):A80.
67. Sinderby C, Lindstorm L, Grassino AE. Automatic assessment of electromyogram quality. J Appl. Physiol. 1995;79:1803-15.
68. Mancini DM, Henson D, Lamanca J, Levine S. Evidence of reduced respiratory muscle endurance in patients with heart failure. J Am Coll Cardiol. 1994;24:972-81.
69. Leith DE, Bradley M. Ventilatory muscle strength and endurance training. J Appl Physiol. 1976;41:508-16.
70. McKenzie DK, Gandevia SC. Strength and endurance of inspiratory, expiratory and limb muscles in asthma. Am Rev Respir Dis. 1986:134:999-1004.
71. Morrison NJ, Richardson DP, Dunn L, Pardy RL. Respiratory muscle performance in normal elderly subjects and patients with COPD. Chest. 1989;95:90-4.
72. Weiner I, Azgad Y, Weiner M. Inspiratory muscle training during treatment with corticosteroids in humans. Chest. 1995;107:1041-4.
73. Blackie SP, Fairbar MS, McElvancey NG, Wilcox PG, Morrison NJ, Pardy RL. Normal values and ranges for ventilation and breathing pattern at maximal exercise. Chest. 1991;100: 136-42.
74. Nickerson BG, Keens TG. Measuring ventilator muscle endurance in humans as sustainable inspiratory pressure. J Appl Physiol. 1982;52:768-72.
75. Eastwood PR, Hillman DR. A threshold loading device for testing of inspiratory muscle performance. Eur Respir J. 1995;8:463-6.
76. Guleria R, Watson AC, Polkey MI, Moxham J, Green M. Inspiratory muscle performance using negative pressure inspiratory loading. Thorax. 1997;52(Suppl 6):A29.
77. Moodie L, Reeve J, Elkins M. Inspiratory muscle training increases inspiratory muscle strength in patients weaning from mechanical ventilation: a systematic review. J Physiother. 2011;57:213-21.
78. Dixit A, Prakash S. Effects of threshold inspiratory muscle training versus conventional physiotherapy on the weaning period of mechanically ventilated patients. A comparative study. Int J Physiother Res. 2014;2:424-8.
79. Steier J, Kaul S, Seymour J, Jolley C, Rafferty G, Man W, et al. The value of multiple tests of respiratory muscle strength. Thorax. 2007;62:975-80.
80. Rath GP, Bithal PK, Guleria R, Chaturvedi A, Kale SS, Gupta V, et al. A comparative study between preoperative and postoperative pulmonary functions and diaphragmatic movements in congenital craniovertebral junction anomalies. J Neurosurg Anaesthesiol. 2006;18(4)256-61.

Respiratory Disability and Preoperative Evaluation

Gyanendra Agrawal, Dheeraj Gupta

INTRODUCTION

Both disability assessment and preoperative evaluation focus on the accurate assessment of functional state of the respiratory system. The initial part of this chapter is intended to provide a framework for the evaluation of impairment and disability caused by respiratory diseases, including common occupational and environmental respiratory diseases. The later part focuses on a comprehensive clinical assessment and appropriate standardized tests, to objectively assess the risks and the outcomes of patients with lung disease undergoing specific surgeries.

EVALUATION OF RESPIRATORY DISABILITY

The ability of an individual to take part in the gainful employment and activities of daily living are profoundly affected by the respiratory impairment. The common reasons for the evaluation of impairment/disability are to assess fitness for a particular job, to decide compensation on a litigation following a workplace injury, and to assess the eligibility for government entitlement programs in certain countries.

Evaluating physicians generally fit into two categories such as treating (personal) physician and independent medical examiner (IME). Treating physicians know better about health of their patients, but they are often biased. IME, generally appointed by the referring agency, is supposed to provide an unbiased objective evaluation. Evaluation of impairment/disability is a multistep process in which the physician assesses impairment, the award of benefits is decided at an administrative level. Such an assessment is sometimes made by a medical board specifically constituted for this purpose. Although the physician's input is important, the patient must understand that the physician does not have control over the acceptance of claims or level of benefits awarded.

Impairment, Disability and Handicap

Impairment is defined as "a loss, loss of use, or derangement of any body part, organ system or organ function." This is purely a medical condition that objectively measures any loss or abnormality of psychological, physiological, or anatomical structure or function.[1,2]

Disability is a term that indicates the total effect of impairment on a patient's life. It is affected by diverse factors such as age, gender, education, economic and social environment and energy requirements of occupation. Thus, two people with an identical impairment may have different disability.[1,2]

Handicap is the disadvantage for a given individual, resulting from impairment or disability, which limits or prevents fulfilment of a role that is normal (depending upon age, sex, and social and cultural factors) for that individual.

CLINICAL METHODS OF EVALUATING IMPAIRMENT

Accurate assessment of respiratory impairment requires a medical diagnostic evaluation. Decreased lung functions may result totally or in part from nonrespiratory diseases either directly (e.g. neuromuscular diseases, arthritis of the spine) or indirectly, (e.g. congestive cardiac failure). Moreover, the accurate diagnosis and staging of disease is the basis for prognosis and medical prescriptions, which later may bear importantly on determination of disability and impairment. The evaluation of respiratory diseases must include a chest radiograph, in addition to indicated laboratory tests.[2]

History

The most common symptoms that lead to pulmonary disability evaluation are dyspnea, cough and wheezing. Dyspnea or shortness of breath is a distressing sensation of difficult, labored or unpleasant breathing. Dyspnea is entirely subjective and fairly sensitive, but not specific symptom. In all patients, an attempt should be made to rate the severity of patient's dyspnea by means of a scale or classification scheme, such as that suggested by the Medical Research Council (MRC).[3] In the context of disability evaluation only the chronic forms of cough (i.e. lasting for more than 4 weeks) and sputum production are relevant. It is difficult to quantitate the severity of cough and therefore, it is not easy to integrate them into a system of progressive gradation of disability. A history of wheezing may provide important clues during disability evaluation. The temporal correlation of the onset of wheezing, as well as its association with the workplace (or with particular exposures), may help to identify a specific cause of impairment. Wheezing that occurs primarily on workdays and improves during weekends or during vacations is highly suggestive of work-related asthma.

A comprehensive medical history, including the documentation of hospitalizations, allergies and medications, should be obtained, so conditions other than respiratory diseases that contribute to or likely to modify any impairment can be identified. A detailed history of the applicant's employment in chronologic order is required for both attribution and disability evaluation purposes. This history should include even part-time jobs and hobbies. History of exposure to specific respiratory agents at the workplace, like dusts, fumes and vapors should prompt further questioning to clarify the timing, duration and dose of exposure when possible, and the use of respiratory protection. Many work-related abnormalities resemble other diseases and cannot be diagnosed correctly without a validated exposure history. Presence of similar complaints or diseases also in coworkers, is helpful in establishing an occupational etiology.

Inquiries should be made into vocational activities to uncover any potential contributing exposure (e.g. pigeon breeding). An environmental exposure history should include a discussion of potential environmental triggers that include pets in the household, exposures to birds or other organic antigens, such as molds, as well as seasonal or temporal variability of symptoms. Smoking can be the primary cause or a major contributing factor to many respiratory diseases; therefore, a detailed smoking history should be obtained. This includes the age at which the patient started to smoke, estimates of both the average and maximum amount of tobacco smoked per day, whether and when smoking was stopped, as well as second-hand smoke exposure. The cumulative dose of cigarette smoke exposure should be characterized in terms of pack-years (i.e. the number of packages smoked per day multiplied by the number of years of smoking).

Physical Examination

A physical examination that is primarily focused on the cardiopulmonary system should be performed. The patient also should be evaluated for clinical evidence of right heart failure associated with advanced and chronic respiratory disease (cor pulmonale). The physical examination is probably more useful for detecting the signs of nonrespiratory organ system dysfunction that could be contributing to a disability then for characterizing the level of respiratory impairment.

Imaging Studies

The chest radiograph is the most widely used element in the clinical evaluation of patients with respiratory disease. It is more useful in determining the etiologic diagnosis than the level of impairment, because the correlation between radiographic abnormality of the chest and physiologic dysfunction is imperfect, especially among patients with obstructive lung diseases. An asthmatic patient with severe, partially irreversible airflow obstruction may have only minimal abnormality of the chest radiograph. Conversely, patients with a significant amount of bullous emphysema may not have a comparable degree of airflow limitation.[4]

Among patients with pneumoconioses (inorganic dust-related pulmonary interstitial diseases, such as asbestosis, silicosis and coal workers' pneumoconioses), the chest radiographic findings are very important. In fact, the International Labor Organization (ILO) has devised a classification scheme for the standardized interpretation of chest radiographs to objectively characterize and communicate the extent of radiographic abnormalities in the pneumoconioses.[5]

Computed tomography (CT) of the chest is a more sensitive tool than plain radiographs in detecting both parenchymal and pleural abnormalities. They offer considerable insight into the precise anatomic changes that accompany a disease state, but offer little to the evaluation of physiologic impairment. There are no recommendations at present for CT-screening of populations at risk for occupational interstitial lung disease.

Pulmonary Function Testing

Simple pulmonary function tests like spirometry and diffusing capacity measurements are the most commonly used objective measures of respiratory limitation for disability assessment. The equipment used for these tests are widely accessible and adequate standard for repeatability and reproducibility can be easily met. Both these tests should be performed carefully according to the American Thoracic Society (ATS)/the European Respiratory Society (ERS) guidelines.[6,7] Spirometry can distinguish obstructive from restrictive lung physiology and provide the quantification of the degree of pulmonary dysfunction. On the basis of forced vital capacity (FVC), forced expiratory volume in the first second (FEV1), and diffusing capacity, classification of degree of respiratory impairment can be made. The diffusing capacity has particular usefulness in the evaluation of restrictive ventilatory defects and is more sensitive than lung volume measurement as a screening tool for patients at risk for pneumoconiosis.[8]

Arterial Blood Gas Analysis

Arterial blood gas (ABG) studies are rarely used as a criterion of impairment and should be reserved for selected patients. Because of the variability of ABG measurements even in stable patients, arterial hypoxemia should be documented by a minimum of two measurements, at least 4 weeks apart. Resting arterial hypoxemia is considered as a 'modifying condition' in the ATS statement; for example, in a patient whose spirometry and diffusing capacity of the lungs for carbon monoxide (DLCO) results straddle the border between the two categories of impairment, the presence of a low arterial PaO_2 can justify a rating of the higher category of impairment.[2]

Cardiopulmonary Exercise Testing

Majority of the patients being evaluated for respiratory disability do not require exercise testing because there is a good relationship between FEV1 and DLCO and oxygen consumption and work capacity.[9,10] The physician should consider cardiopulmonary exercise testing (CPET) only when there are grounds for believing that the routine tests have underestimated the impairment. The aim of exercise testing in such cases is to determine first, whether or not the person is significantly impaired, and secondly, whether the cause of impairment is due to respiratory disease or some other cause.[2] Because of the later need, the testing must at a minimum include the measurement of ventilation (V_E), maximal oxygen consumption (VO_2 max) and anaerobic threshold. The measurement of oxygen consumption during CPET is considered to be the 'gold standard' assessment of the subject's ability to perform work.[4]

Bronchoprovocation Testing

Bronchoprovocation testing is an important method in the assessment of impairment and disability in the cases of occupational asthma, because routine pulmonary function testing performed between attacks may not reveal the abnormality. The presence of bronchial hyper-reactivity may have significance in judging ability to continue certain types of employment.

DISEASE-SPECIFIC IMPAIRMENT ASSESSMENT

Asthma

Evaluation of impairment in the setting of asthma is a problematic aspect of disability assessment, since asthma is a disorder characterized by variability over time, with airflow obstruction that may revert toward normal, either spontaneously or as a result of medication administration. On the day of evaluation, patient's lung function may not show an accurate reflection of his usual condition, but may be atypically bad or atypically good.[4] Patients with history that is suggestive of asthma and have normal spirometry in the absence of medication for asthma, may be tested for airway hyper-responsiveness with nonspecific bronchodilator challenge.

Workplace exposures frequently exacerbate an underlying asthmatic condition (work-related asthma) or cause sensitization of the respiratory tract to materials found uniquely in the workplace (occupational asthma). Occupational asthma is the most frequently reported occupational lung disease in the industrialized world. It is important to distinguish immunologic occupational asthma from irritant-induced asthma, where continued work may be possible, if irritant exposures are reasonably controlled. Evaluation of impairment in patients with occupational asthma is almost similar to that for patients with atopic asthma. In addition to the pharmacotherapy, nonpharmacological interventions must be addressed such as the control of environment triggers, patient and family education.[11,12]

Pneumoconiosis

A variety of inorganic dust exposure produces pulmonary fibrosis (e.g. asbestosis, silicosis and coal worker's pneumoconiosis) or both granulomatous disease and fibrosis (e.g. beryllium), each with fairly characteristic radiographic appearances. The diagnosis of pneumoconiosis is associated with an increased risk of future impairment, despite normal lung function at the time of testing, because further exposure to the causative agent may increase the risk of progression. Therefore, the recognition of radiologic manifestations of these diseases should prompt removal from mining employment, particularly in relatively young individuals. Such a prohibition is not obviated by showing that current exposure is within legally permissible limits, because such limits are not presumed to provide adequate protection for persons who already manifest the disease.[2]

Hypersensitivity Pneumonitis

With hypersensitivity pneumonitis, continued exposure to the offending agent is likely to lead to either acute attacks or insidious progression of disease, depending on the dose of exposure. Therefore, patients with hypersensitivity pneumonitis should be considered 100% impaired on a permanent basis for any job that involves future exposure to the causative agent.

Obstructive Sleep Apnea

Only some individuals with sleep apnea develop a functional impairment that affects work activity. In severe cases, it can result in the deterioration of daytime cognitive performance, which may interfere with work activities that require constant vigilance like vehicle and machine operators. The development of cor pulmonale indicates 'severe' impairment.[2]

Lung Cancer

Patients with lung cancer are presumed to be severely impaired for at least 1 year following diagnosis, even if surgical resection appears to have been successful in curing the disease. This happens because of the loss of functional lung tissue during resection. It is therefore important to anticipate the postresection lung function.[13]

DISABILITY EVALUATION

Disability evaluation is the determination of the impact of impairment on an individual's ability to meet the demands of his or her own life. Disability evaluation has a broader focus than impairment because factors like the essential requirement of a job, specific tasks, educational level of the individual, individual skills, and potential for retraining must be taken into consideration in determining a specific individual's disability. The American Medical Association (AMA) has developed guidelines for assessing physical impairment that are widely accepted by governments and legal systems as the standard of evaluation for loss of physical function.[14]

Varying percentages of lost function are grouped into four severity classes: Class one constitutes 0% functional loss (for instance, an observable abnormality caused by an anatomic variation); class two indicates that there is objective evidence for a 10–25% impairment of the whole person as result of organ dysfunction; class three indicates a 26–50% impairment of the whole person; and class four is 51–100% impairment of the whole person.

According to the AMA Guides, impairment rating requires that the evaluator first recognize that an abnormality is present, then identify the cause of the abnormality and objectively evaluate the severity of deviation from normal function, and finally, translate the severity of dysfunction into a numerically based classification that estimates how much of an effect the organ dysfunction has on the individual's ability to carry on the activities of daily living. Other steps that may be difficult for the evaluating physician are the work relatedness of the impairment (attribution) and the percentage of the total impairment due to work-related causes (apportionment). Regardless of the evaluating physician's opinions, the final decision concerning the level of disability is made administratively by the responsible agency after the consideration of nonmedical factors.

The evaluation of respiratory disability/impairment is a multistep process. Knowledge of these components of disability evaluation will help physicians to better serve their patients and supply appropriate data to the adjudicating system. Different programs under the social security systems in various countries provide financial and rehabilitative benefits to disabled individuals. However, such programs or specific entitlement systems are lacking in this country. With the introduction of such programs, the community will be better served, ultimately contributing to the growth of nation.

PREOPERATIVE EVALUATION OF RESPIRATORY SYSTEM

Pulmonary physicians are often requested by various surgical departments to do preoperative evaluation of patients. The goals of this consultation are to estimate the risk of postoperative pulmonary complications, to optimize the patient's condition, and to propose strategies to decrease the postoperative pulmonary complications. The second part of this chapter is an attempt to encompass different aspects of preoperative pulmonary evaluation prior to both thoracic and nonthoracic surgeries. It focuses the approach to risk stratification based on patient and procedure-related risk factor analysis, detailed preoperative pulmonary evaluation, and strategies to reduce postoperative pulmonary complications.

Pulmonary Physiology in the Postoperative Period

The knowledge of changes in pulmonary physiology is mandatory to understand the mechanisms of various pulmonary complications that occur in the postoperative period, since many postoperative respiratory complications are related to exaggerations of the expected postoperative changes in pulmonary function that occur as a result of the surgery itself, anesthesia, or various pharmacologic interventions.

The pulmonary functions in the postoperative period are characterized by moderate-to-severe reductions in vital capacity (VC) and smaller reductions in functional residual capacity (FRC). While the FEV1 is decreased, the ratio of FEV1 to the FVC (FEV1/FVC%) remains unchanged, indicating that the overall pattern of pulmonary function abnormalities is restrictive. A significant reduction with up to 70% decrease in VC and up to 50% decrease in and FRC is seen, leading to a high risk of atelectasis and hypoxia, especially in the first 24 hours. This severe reduction in lung function is seen more often with thoracic and upper abdominal procedures than with surgery involving the lower abdomen or extremities; and it gradually recovers within 3 weeks. Reductions in other lung volumes, including total lung capacity (TLC), inspiratory capacity (IC), expiratory reserve volume (ERV), and residual volume (RV) have also been noted.[15] The proposed mechanisms for the reduction in lung volumes consist of the postsurgical pain and associated muscle splinting, which impair lung mechanics; and the diaphragm dysfunction.

The reduction of FRC is of major physiological significance postoperatively, since the decrease of FRC below the closing capacity (CC) leads to the closure of the alveolar units causing atelectasis. FRC is the lung volume at the end of a normal tidal expiration; and CC is the lung volume at which small airways in the lung bases begin to close during expiration because of a reduction in airway radial traction. When CC exceeds FRC, lung volume fails to increase sufficiently during tidal breathing to open all the airways and, consequently, some alveolar units remain closed. This creates an area of low ventilation relative to perfusion, which is the main mechanism of hypoxemia in postoperative patients. Elderly patients, smokers and chronic obstructive pulmonary disease (COPD) patients are at higher risk of getting such complications since the CC is increased in these subset of patients.

Diaphragmatic dysfunction is an important factor, which contributes to the postoperative reduction in lung volumes. Postoperative pain, spasm and paralysis are all known to reduce diaphragm function, although relief of pain does not completely restore function. Rather, diaphragmatic dysfunction has been found to persist even with adequate pain relief.[16] Decreased central nervous system output to the phrenic nerves, possibly as a result of inhibitory reflexes arising from sympathetic, vagal or splanchnic receptors is the proposed mechanism of diaphragmatic dysfunction.

Postoperative hypoxemia is a quite common event and prophylactic oxygen therapy is routinely given to all patients undergoing thoracic and upper abdominal surgeries. The underlying mechanisms are multiple and are largely related to the residual effects of the anesthesia. This includes ventilation-perfusion mismatch, alveolar hypoventilation, anesthetic-induced inhibition of hypoxic pulmonary vasoconstriction, right-to-left shunting, and depressed cardiac output. Microthromboemboli, altered FRC-CC relationships and increased dead space ventilation due to rapid shallow breathing are other mechanisms contributing to postoperative hypoxemia. Respiratory depression either due to the anesthetic agents or narcotic drugs given for postoperative analgesia is a common feature of the postoperative period. These drugs reduce the ventilatory response to hypercapnia and hypoxia, resulting in decreased tidal volume and thereby increasing $PaCO_2$.

Several lung defense mechanisms are compromised after surgery, contributing to an increased risk of pulmonary infection. Ciliary damage from endotracheal intubation and inhalation of dry gases; and reduced tracheal mucus velocity leads to significantly reduced mucociliary clearance. Ineffective cough reflex due to postoperative pain, excessive use of narcotics or altered lung mechanics contributes to the retention of secretions and atelectasis.

Physiologic Changes after Thoracic Surgery

Resection of pulmonary tissue for various indications leads to a number of physiologic changes. VC decreases by about 15% after lobectomy and 35–40% following pneumonectomy.[17] The decrease in lung function is usually less than expected from the number of segments removed, suggesting that the disease had already decreased the function of the resected lung and/or that expansion of the remaining lung had occurred. Serial studies have shown that FEV1 decreases within the first several months following lung cancer resection, but tends to recover to a small extent by 6 months after surgery.[18] The lung becomes stiffer and elastic recoil pressure and transdiaphragmatic pressure at TLC increases after thoracic surgeries. Maximum effort tolerance decreases after pneumonectomy with a normal pulmonary artery pressure at rest and an increase in pulmonary artery pressure and in pulmonary vascular resistance on effort, compared to preoperative values.

Lung volume reduction surgery (LVRS) does not affect the postoperative pulmonary arterial pressure at rest or during exercise.[19] The patients also develop the decrease in arterial oxygen saturation on effort after pneumonectomy, possibly due to the absolute decrease in diffusing capacity. The patients also develop a decrease in oxygen consumption, cardiac output, stroke volume and heart rate at maximum exercise, and they were not able to achieve their preoperative maximal workload.[17] The changes seen after lobectomy are almost similar to the changes seen after pneumonectomy, but the differences are less pronounced.[20]

POSTOPERATIVE PULMONARY COMPLICATIONS

Postoperative pulmonary complications are at least as common as are postoperative cardiac complications and contribute similarly to morbidity, mortality and the length of stay.[21] Pulmonary complications may even be more likely than cardiac complications to predict long-term mortality after surgery.[22] A number of definitions have been proposed for postoperative pulmonary complications. A practical and clinically relevant approach is to include only those complications that contribute directly to morbidity or prolonged length of stay,[23] which will exclude minor complications such as fever and productive cough. Included are the clinically important postoperative pulmonary complications, which are pneumonia, atelectasis, bronchospasm, respiratory failure with prolonged mechanical ventilation, and exacerbation of underlying obstructive lung disease **(Table 1)**. The reported incidence of these

Table 1 Postoperative pulmonary complications

*Nonthoracic surgery**	*Thoracic surgery*
Atelectasis	Bronchopleural fistula
Pneumonia and tracheobronchitis	Empyema
Respiratory failure with prolonged MV	Mediastinitis, osteomyelitis of sternum Phrenic nerve damage
Exacerbation of COPD Thromboembolism	Anastomotic leak during esophagectomy/gastrectomy

*May be associated with thoracic surgeries also.
Abbreviations: MV, mechanical ventilation; COPD, chronic obstructive pulmonary disease

Table 2 Risk factors for postoperative pulmonary complications*

Patient-related risk factors	*Procedure-related risk factors*
Age >60 years	Surgical site
Smoking	Type of anesthesia
General state of health (ASA class >2)	Duration of surgery (>3 hours)
Nutritional status	Type of incision
Obesity	Emergency/elective surgery
COPD/Asthma/OSA	Immobilization
Abnormal chest radiograph	Inadequate pain control
Antecedent respiratory tract infection	

*Modified from reference 20
Abbreviations: COPD, chronic obstructive pulmonary disease; OSA, obstructive sleep apnea

complications ranges from 5% to 90% depending on the variability of the definitions used. In general, pulmonary complications associated with thoracic surgeries are more common and more severe, as compared to nonthoracic surgeries. The mechanisms of postoperative impairment in lung function are multiple, interactive, and at present, incompletely understood.

Risk Factors for Postoperative Pulmonary Complications (Table 2)

A number of risk factors have been associated with the development of postoperative pulmonary complications in various studies. In this chapter, patient and procedure-related risk factors are discussed separately.

Patient-related Risk Factors

The most important patient-related risk factors are the presence of chronic lung diseases, like COPD and asthma, as well as smoking history and the patient's overall state of health. Age and obesity are relatively minor factors; and the precise risks associated with malnutrition and recent viral infections are unknown.

Smoking: Smoking is a risk factor for postoperative pulmonary complications, as has been demonstrated repeatedly since the first report in 1944.[24] Smoking increases risk even among those without chronic lung disease.[25] The available data are mixed, but suggest a modest increase in risk for postoperative pulmonary complications among current smokers, and when the patient is older or has smoked longer. The ill effects of smoking are mainly related to the high level of carboxyhemoglobin in smokers, which usually ranges from 3% to 15%. Carboxyhemoglobin reduces the amount of hemoglobin available to bind with oxygen and shift the oxygen-hemoglobin saturation curve to the left, which facilitates the loading of oxygen onto hemoglobin, but impairs unloading at the tissues. Nicotine can cause systemic vasoconstriction and increase both the heart rate and the systemic blood pressure (BP). A statistically significant reduction in complications occurs only when patients discontinue smoking for at least 8 weeks prior to the surgery.[26]

Chronic lung disease: Among studies reporting multivariable analyses, COPD is the most commonly identified risk factor for postoperative pulmonary complications. While one may consider patients with restrictive lung diseases with severe limitations to have an increased risk for postoperative pulmonary complications, the literature did not support an estimate of the magnitude of this risk in this group.[22] COPD is the single most important patient-related risk factor for the development of postoperative pulmonary complications. The relative risk of pulmonary complications attributable to COPD is three to four folds.[23] Physicians should aggressively treat patients with COPD who, before surgery, do not have optimal reduction of symptoms and airflow obstruction on physical examination and who do not have optimal exercise capacity. Elective surgery should be deferred if acute exacerbation is present. The treatment and preparation of patients who have COPD before elective surgery are the same as those in nonoperative settings.

The increased incidence of postoperative pulmonary complications in patients with COPD is due, in part, to an increase in the CC, favoring the development of the areas of low ventilation-to-perfusion ratios and atelectasis. In addition, in patients who continue to smoke, impaired ciliary function and chronic tracheobronchitis may be contributing factors. Although not precisely quantified in the literature, the risk for postoperative respiratory complications appears to increase significantly (greater than 50%) when the FEV1 is below 65% of predicted. The risk is also increased in patients who are hypercapnic. However, patients with an FEV1 as low as 450 mL have tolerated surgery safely. Therefore, the potential benefits of the operative procedure must be weighed against the operative risk in every individual patient.

Asthma: Patients with acute bronchospasm are probably at increased risk for perioperative complications, since several maneuvers associated with anesthesia may aggravate bronchospasm.[27] However, the same is not true for patients with stable asthma.[22,23] Before surgery, patients should be free of wheezing, with a peak flow greater than 80% of the predicted or personal best value. If necessary, the patient should receive oral corticosteroids to achieve this goal. A short course of perioperative corticosteroids does not increase the incidence of infection.

Obstructive sleep apnea (OSA): It increases the risk for airway management difficulties in the immediate postoperative period. In one case-control study, nonsignificant trends were seen toward the higher rates of reintubation, hypercapnia and hypoxemia for patients with OSA.[28] Pulmonary hypertension is particularly associated with a significant perioperative risk.

As cardiovascular dysfunction in OSA patients can be modified by treatment, it is important to identify patients not known to have OSA and have them treated to improve their perioperative outcomes, as well as to improve their general health.

Restrictive lung diseases: While some experience has been reported with patients undergoing thoracic and corrective orthopedic surgery, very little data exist with regard to abdominal and extremity surgery. Postoperative respiratory complications after corrective surgery in patients with kyphoscoliosis, have been reported in up to 20% of these patients, with pleural space-related processes (e.g. pneumothorax, pleural effusion, bronchopleural fistula and empyema) among the most common. Video-assisted thoracoscopic (VAT) approaches have emerged as good alternatives to open thoracotomy in such patients.

Age: Previous reviews have suggested that age is not a predictor of postoperative pulmonary complications and they are more strongly related to coexisting conditions than to chronologic age.[23] However, a recent review found that the risk of pulmonary complications increases with the advancing age.[22]

These findings appear to hold true when lung tissue is resected. There have been many reports detailing the outcomes of lung resection in the elderly. The general concerns raised by the literature are that the operative mortality is greater in the elderly, operative risks for pneumonectomy are relatively high, and complications may be increased. Despite the study trends, the sum of the evidence suggests that surgery should not be withheld on the basis of age alone.[29]

General health status: Several integrated measures of comorbidity have been evaluated as the potential predictors of postoperative pulmonary complications. The widely used American Society of Anesthesiologists (ASA) classification, which was developed to evaluate the risk of overall perioperative mortality, is strongly predictive of postoperative pulmonary complications.[30] In addition, the Goldman cardiac-risk index, which includes factors from the patient's history, the physical examination, and laboratory data, also predicts pulmonary complications.[31]

Obesity: Despite the changes that occur in pulmonary mechanics and pulmonary functions in obese individuals, studies evaluating clinically meaningful pulmonary complications after surgery have generally found no increased risk attributable to obesity, even for patients with morbid obesity. Obesity is, however, clearly a risk factor for OSA syndrome, which may be unmasked or exacerbated because of the use of postoperative analgesics or narcotics.[22]

Others: The risk of postoperative pulmonary complications in patients with viral upper respiratory infections is unknown. It is reasonable to delay truly elective surgery in patients with upper respiratory infection. Although patients with compromised nutritional status are at higher risk for developing postoperative pulmonary complications, aggressive preoperative nutritional support has not been shown to decrease postsurgical pulmonary morbidity.

Procedure-related Risk Factors

Procedure-related risk factors are as important as patient-related factors in estimating risk for postoperative pulmonary complications. The surgical site is the most important predictor of pulmonary risk. Risk increases as the incision approaches the diaphragm; therefore, upper abdominal and thoracic surgery carries the greatest risk of postoperative pulmonary complications. Studies using multivariable analyses have found that prolonged surgery duration, ranging from 3 to 4 hours, is an independent predictor of postoperative pulmonary complications. The contribution of risk from the type of anesthesia itself has been controversial. Many have reported a lower risk of pulmonary complications among patients receiving spinal or epidural anesthesia than among those receiving general anesthesia, but the results have been inconsistent and the effect small.

Except for the reduced risk of postoperative thromboembolism, there is no clear evidence in the current literature that regional anesthesia results in better intraoperative or postoperative pulmonary function.[32,33] Emergency surgery has been identified as a significant predictor of postoperative pulmonary complications. Abdominal laparoscopic procedures and thoracoscopic lung resection are associated with less postoperative respiratory problems, as compared to open procedures because of reduced patient discomfort, shortened length of hospitalization and faster patient return to full activity. Prolonged bed rest and inactivity following surgery is a major risk factor for deep venous thrombosis and pulmonary embolism.

PREOPERATIVE EVALUATION

This section of the chapter is intended to provide an evidence-based approach to the preoperative physiologic assessment of a patient undergoing either thoracic or nonthoracic surgery. After discussing the initial evaluation, which is to be done in all the patients, the pulmonary specific evaluation is discussed. The task of the preoperative physiologic assessment is to identify patients who are at increased risk for both perioperative complications and long-term disability from surgical resection of lung tissue using the least invasive tests possible.

Initial Evaluation

Initial preoperative pulmonary evaluation is required in almost all elective surgeries. In case of emergency, the surgery should not be delayed for the cause of pulmonary evaluation unless the likelihood of perioperative mortality or

Flow chart 1 Suggested approach for preoperative evaluation

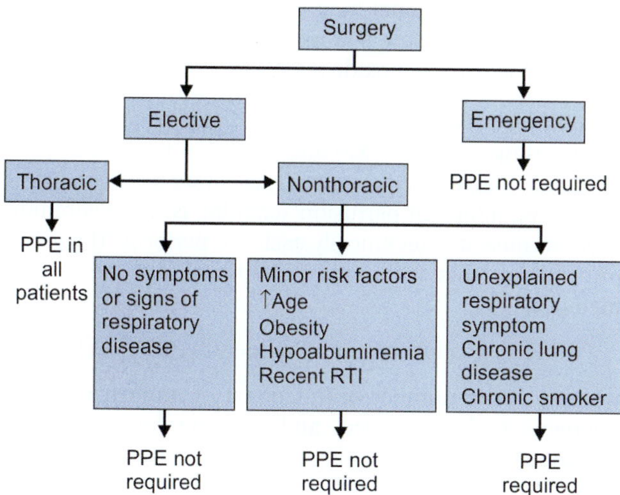

Abbreviations: PPE, preoperative pulmonary evaluation; RTI, respiratory tract infection

postoperative complication is so high that the surgery should not be performed **(Flow chart 1)**. The principal components of preoperative evaluation of the surgical patient are: (a) the history and physical examination, (b) the chest radiograph, (c) spirometry, and (d) arterial blood gas analysis.

History and Physical Examination

A careful history taking and physical examination are the most important parts of preoperative pulmonary risk assessment. One should seek a history of respiratory symptoms (like chronic cough, dyspnea and chest pain) including symptoms of sleep apnea. History should also include the patient's functional capacity and the degree of the limitation of activity. Smoking history should be taken in detail and all patients should be encouraged to quit smoking. If there is history of recent respiratory tract infection, it is advisable to delay the surgery till it gets cured.

The physical examination may identify the findings suggestive of unrecognized pulmonary disease. Among such findings, decreased breath sounds, dullness to percussion, wheezes, rhonchi, and a prolonged expiratory phase predict an increase in the risk of pulmonary complications. It should include an evaluation for signs of metastatic spread, (e.g. lymph node enlargement, hepatomegaly or focal neurologic deficits) and the presence of cardiac failure and pulmonary hypertension.

Chest Radiograph

The current evidence suggests that this test only rarely provides unexpected information that influences preoperative management and clinicians may predict most abnormal preoperative chest radiographs by history and physical examination. Thus, a preoperative chest radiograph is indicated when there are new or unexplained symptoms or signs, when there is a history of underlying lung disease and no recent chest radiograph, or when thoracic surgery is planned.

Spirometry

Spirometry is a simple, inexpensive, standardized, and readily available test, which is used to diagnose the obstructive and restrictive lung diseases. But it does not translate into effective risk prediction for individual patients. There is a consensus that all candidates for lung resection and coronary artery bypass should undergo preoperative spirometry; its value before extrathoracic surgery, however, remains unproven. Moreover, the data do not suggest a prohibitive spirometric threshold below which the risks of surgery are unacceptable. So, preoperative spirometry is reserved for patients undergoing thoracic surgery, or patients having unexplained chest symptoms especially those suggestive of COPD, or history of cigarette smoking.[34,35]

Arterial Blood Gas Analysis

A partial pressure of arterial carbon dioxide ($PaCO_2$) greater than 45 mm Hg is identified as a strong risk factor for pulmonary complications, based on several case series, as it usually indicates chronic respiratory failure.[36,37] Hypercapnia has been a relative contraindication to lung resection.[38] So, it is recommended that the ABG analysis should be done in the patients of chronic lung disease, or who have a significant pulmonary process and patients undergoing lung resection. The routine use of ABG is not recommended in all patients.

Pulmonary-specific Evaluation

Pulmonary-specific evaluation is required in all patients undergoing lung resection surgeries. The two main aims of pulmonary specific evaluation are to assess the perioperative mortality and morbidity to tolerate the surgical procedure; and, to assess the postoperative pulmonary function to allow reasonable quality of life. A number of physiologic tests exist for this purpose, although, there is no single test that is a 'gold standard' in accurately predicting complications.[34,35] This part of preoperative evaluation is divided into the three stages of tests, which are performed in a sequential manner, that help to risk-stratify the patients prior to the planned surgery.

Stage I

The first stage consists of tests to assess the overall functions of both the lungs.

- *Spirometry*: Of all the indices assessed by spirometry, FEV1 is regarded as being the best for predicting the complications of lung resection in the initial assessment, and it is the one most commonly used for decision making. The FEV_1 helps to predict those at risk for postoperative complications, including death. Little evidence exists to utilize one cut-off absolute value of FEV_1 to permit resection of varying extent. Preoperative values of 2 L for pneumonectomy and 1.5 L for lobectomy have been suggested. The risk of postoperative respiratory complications also increases significantly when the FVC or maximal voluntary ventilation (MVV) is less than 50% predicted.

- *Diffusion capacity*: Diffusing capacity of the lung for carbon monoxide (DLCO) reflects alveolar membrane integrity and pulmonary capillary blood flow in the patient's lungs. A retrospective study found DLCO as most important predictor of mortality and was the sole predictor of postoperative pulmonary complications.[39] Absolute cut-offs are not clearly established in the literature. However, individuals with a preoperative DLCO less than 60% predicted were found to have more frequent respiratory complications, hospitalizations for respiratory compromise, and worse median dyspnea scores then individuals with preoperative DLCO more than 60% predicted.[40] Predicted postoperative (PPO) DLCO has been found to be an independent predictor of pulmonary complications, morbidity, and death in other studies.[41,42] A combined value, the predicted postoperative product (PPP), was found to be the best predictor of surgical mortality in one study. The PPP is the product of the PPO FEV_1, and PPO DLCO. A PPP greater than 1650 was found in 75% of those who died and 11% of those who survived surgery.[43]

Stage II

The next stage consists of tests that measure differential lung function and estimate the PPO lung function. There are three techniques to predict the postoperative values—segment method, radionuclide scanning technique and quantitative CT.

Segment method: The simplest methods to predict post-operative pulmonary function involve calculating the portion of all bronchopulmonary segments that will remain after resection. The postoperative lung function should be approximated by the preoperative value multiplied by this portion. The conventional method is to use 19 total segments as the starting value (10 on the right and 9 on the left).

$$\text{PPO FEV}_1 = \text{Preoperative FEV}_1 \times (1 - x/19)$$

where x is the number of lung segments to be removed.

The other method is to use the number of subsegments, corrected for those that were obstructed preoperatively. A regression equation relating the predicted and measured lung function was developed from this method (measured = 0.85 predicted + 0.286 ± 0.296, r = 0.821).[44] A predicted postoperative FEV_1 of 800 mL has been used as a cut-off for withholding resectional lung surgery, based on the clinical impression that below 800 mL many patients are disabled and develop carbon dioxide retention.

Quantitative ventilation-perfusion scan: Ventilation lung scans (using inhaled ^{133}Xe) and perfusion lung scans (using ^{99}Tc macroaggregates) are equally accurate in calculating the PPO FEV_1, although perfusion scanning is more commonly used because it is technically easier to perform. The general principle of this technique is same as for the segment methods.

$$\text{PPO FEV}_1 \text{ postlobectomy} = \text{Preoperative FEV}_1 \times (1 - y/z)$$

where y is the number of functional or unobstructed lung segments to be removed, and z is the total number of functional segments.[18]

$$\text{PPO FEV}_1 \text{ postpneumonectomy} = \text{Preoperative FEV}_1 \times (\text{\% of function of affected lung}).$$

Normally, the right lung contributes 55% of lung function, while the left lung contributes 45% of lung function. The PPO and %PPO DLCO after lung resection can be calculated using the same formula. Using this method, the r-value for correlation between predicted and actual postoperative FEV_1 has been as high as 0.88.[45,46] That for DLCO has been as low as 0.68.[46] The anatomic method can also be applied to segmentectomies because lobectomy does not cause a significantly greater loss of function when compared to segmentectomy.[18]

Quantitative computed tomography: In this technique, the volume of lung with attenuation between 500 and 910. Hounsfield units scale is used to estimate functional lung volume. By calculating the lung volume in the area to be resected as a portion of total lung volume and using the principles stated earlier, the predicted postoperative pulmonary function may be estimated. However, this technique is not widely used despite the evidence of it being better than radionuclide quantitative perfusion imaging.[47]

The PPO FEV_1 can also be calculated without performing a split lung function test. According to Juhl and Frost formula.[48,49]

$$\text{PPO FEV}_1 = \text{Preoperative FEV}_1 \times \{1 - (S \times 5.26)/100\}$$

where S is the number of bronchopulmonary segments involved. Other tests assessing differential lung function include bronchospirometry (the measurement of oxygen uptake in each lung, individually), lateral position testing, and total unilateral pulmonary artery occlusion. These tests are no longer performed in the preoperative evaluation as they are invasive; require specialized equipment, a high level of technical expertise and concerns over the reproducibility of results.[38]

Stage III

The third stage comprises of exercise testing that provide the confirmatory evidence of operability.

Exercise testing: Exercise testing has been used to determine whether individuals with unacceptable lung function by other measures might be able to tolerate resection. Formal testing such as symptom-limited cycle ergometry and simpler tests, including exercise oximetry, stair climbing and shuttle walking, have been studied. Cycle ergometry with incremental workloads, which measures VO_2, VO_2 max, minute ventilation, and carbon dioxide output with concomitant monitoring of electrocardiogram (ECG), BP, oximetry, while the patient exercises to the maximal end point or to the symptom-limited maximum, is probably the best form of exercise testing.

Exercise testing could be fixed exercise challenge, in which a sustained level of work is performed; and incremental exercise testing, in which the work rate is sequentially increased to a desired end point. Exercise capacity, measured as the VO_2 max during CPET, has been shown to be a predictor of postoperative complications, including postoperative and long-term mortality.[50-55] A VO_2 max less than 15–20 mL/kg/min is associated with an increased incidence of postoperative complications.

Other simpler tests can be used in situations where a complete CPET is not possible. In one study, a 4% or greater desaturation during exercise oximetry performed better than FEV_1 and DLCO in predicting postoperative pulmonary complications, including death and respiratory failure.[56] Stair-climbing test and 6-minute walk tests are other technologically simpler tests that have been used to estimate the risk from lung resection. The significant risk of postoperative pulmonary complications has been demonstrated in patients who are unable to climb two flights (where one flight is the equivalent of 12 steps). Patients who are unable to complete a 6-minute walk of more than 500 feet are unacceptable candidates for lung resection. The distance obtained during a shuttle walk test, a type of incremental exercise test, where an individual walks back and forth over a defined distance at an incremental and progressive rate has correlated well with VO_2 max obtained on a treadmill. Walking 25 shuttles (10 m each) approximated a VO_2 max of 10 mL/kg/min.[57]

RECOMMENDED APPROACH

Preoperative pulmonary evaluation for lung resection should be done by a multidisciplinary team. And no patient should be denied surgery on the basis of age alone. Operability for pneumonectomy is determined in the event that this procedure should become necessary, either to remove the tumor completely or because of an intraoperative complication.[58,59] Patients with postbronchodilator FEV_1 (Post BD FEV_1) more than 2 L (or more than 80% predicted normal) and more than 1.5 L are suitable for pneumonectomy and lobectomy respectively without further evaluation, unless there is the evidence of interstitial lung disease or undue dyspnea on exertion. In that case the DLCO should be measured. DLCO should also be measured, if the preoperative FEV_1 is less than these values. The patient is cleared for pneumonectomy and lobectomy, if the DLCO is more than 80% and 60–80% predicted normal respectively.

If an individual is not clearly operable after initial testing (DLCO less than 60% predicted normal), then PPO lung function should be estimated. If the PPO FEV1 and PPO DLCO is less than 30% predicted normal or the product of the PPO FEV1 and PPO DLCO is less than 1650, then there is a very high risk of perioperative death and cardiopulmonary complications. In such cases, surgery should be avoided. The patient can undergo lobectomy and possibly pneumonectomy, if the PPO FEV1 and PPO DLCO is more than 40% predicted. The patient is considered borderline, if this number is between 30% and 40% of the predicted value. In borderline patient, if confirmatory evidence of operability is required, an exercise test should be performed. If the VO_2 max is less than 15 mL/kg/min with both PPO FEV1 and PPO DLCO less than 40% predicted, then the individual is at very high risk for perioperative death and cardiopulmonary complications. The patient is cleared for lobectomy and possibly pneumonectomy if the VO_2 max is more than 20 mL/kg/min. The borderline patients are at high risk for surgery and it is recommended that these patients be counseled about nonoperative treatment options for their disease **(Flow chart 2)**. Individuals with very poor lung function may be considered for combined LVRS and lung cancer resection, if the emphysema is heterogeneous and involves primarily the lobe to be resected, provided both the FEV_1 and the DLCO are more than 20% predicted.[18,29,60]

OPTIMIZING THE CHANCE OF A SUCCESSFUL OUTCOME

Preoperative and intraoperative strategies to reduce the risk of pulmonary complications follow logically from the established risk factors. There has been little rigorous research on how one might increase the chance of a successful outcome in the lung resection candidate. Areas that have been considered include smoking cessation, pulmonary rehabilitation, and the immediate postoperative care regimen includes the use of bronchodilators, corticosteroids and antibiotics **(Table 3)**.

Current and former smoking has been shown to be a risk factor for postoperative pulmonary complications, and an optimal period of abstinence prior to surgery is associated with fewer pulmonary complications, better wound healing, and shorter length of stay in the ICU.[61] Accordingly, the preoperative evaluation of smokers should include enrolling

Flow chart 2 Recommended approach of evaluation for lung resection (See text for details)

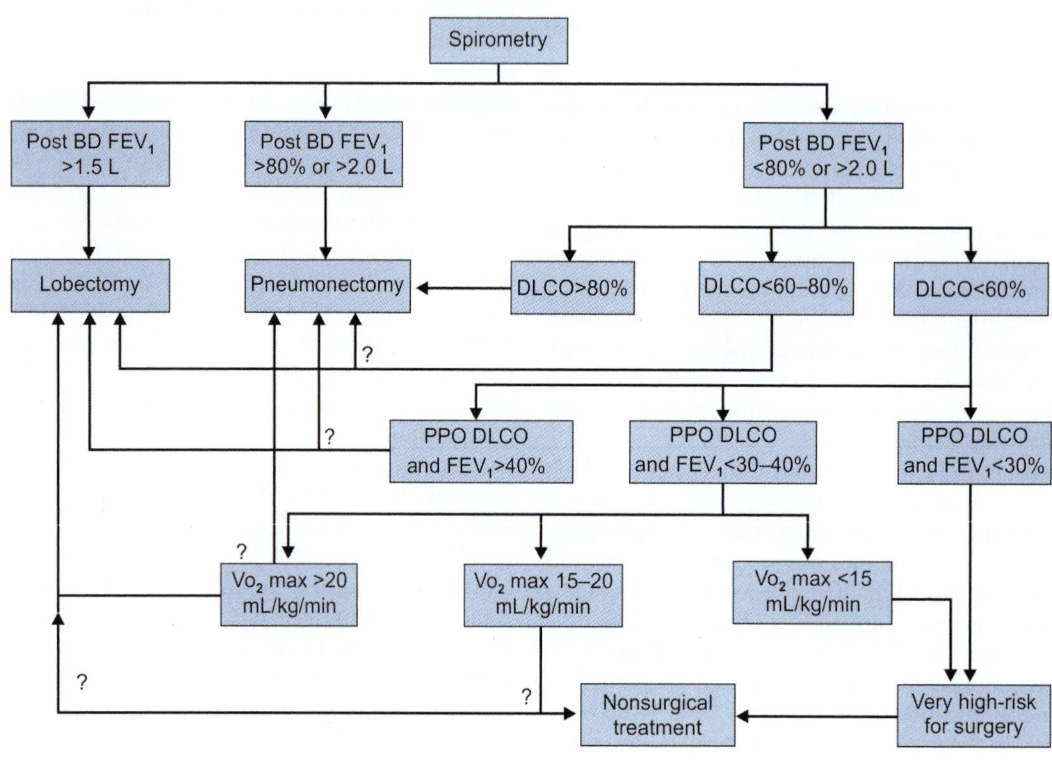

Courtesy: Dr Navneet Singh

Abbreviations: Post BD, postbronchodilator; FEV1, forced expiratory volume in the first second; DLCO, diffusing capacity of the lungs for carbon monoxide; PPO, predicted postoperative; VO_2, oxygen consumption

Table 3 Risk reduction strategies[23]

Preoperative
• Smoking cessation (ideally, a minimum of 8 weeks prior to surgery) • Optimize treatment of COPD/asthma/OSA • Antibiotics for respiratory tract infection • Pulmonary rehabilitation • Weight reduction for severely obese individuals • Lung expansion maneuvers
Intraoperative
• Limit duration of surgery to less than 3 hours • Regional anesthesia • Minimal invasive or laparoscopic surgery
Postoperative
• Early patient mobilization and ambulation • Lung expansion maneuvers (incentive spirometry, deep-breathing exercises) • Adequate analgesia (epidural/intercostal nerve blocks) • Thromboprophylaxis

them in smoking cessation programs or, at a minimum, provide a time when a serious discussion can occur regarding smoking. At least 12–24 hours of preoperative abstinence should be sought to achieve possible cardiovascular benefits and optimally 6–8 weeks of preoperative abstinence to decrease the incidence of postoperative respiratory complications. Pulmonary rehabilitation programs have been shown to improve outcomes and decrease the post-operative pulmonary complications in different studies, whether used before or after the surgery.[62,63] There is no direct evidence to support an additional role for bronchodilators and antibiotics in the lung resection candidate beyond what would be considered the standard use for COPD or asthma.

Intraoperative strategies involve collaboration with anesthesia and surgery colleagues. These strategies include selecting a lower risk or briefer (less than 3 hours) procedure for high-risk patients with few opportunities for risk reduction, recommending laparoscopic rather than open surgeries when possible, using spinal or epidural anesthesia in the lieu of general anesthesia, and avoiding pancuronium.[21]

Lung-expansion maneuvers lower the risk of atelectasis by increasing lung volume. Deep breathing exercises, incentive spirometry and intermittent positive pressure breathing have been studied most extensively. There is no evidence to support a significant difference between any of the three modalities.[64] Preoperative education in lung expansion maneuvers reduces pulmonary complications to a greater degree than instruction that begins after surgery.[65] The advantage of postoperative continuous positive airway pressure (CPAP) and bilevel positive airway pressure (BiPAP) is that, it is not dependent on the patient's effort.[66] It is costly, however, and requires more intensive involvement by hospital personnel than other methods. Because less costly lung-expansion maneuvers are available, physicians should not use CPAP or BiPAP for the primary prevention of complications.

Conventionally, parenteral narcotics have been used for postoperative analgesia. However, concerns over adverse respiratory effects may lead to inadequate dosing and inadequate pain relief. Alternative approaches like patient-controlled analgesia, epidural analgesia and intercostals nerve blocks have been used to overcome this issue. These pain control strategies reduce splinting and promote the ability to take deep breaths after thoracic, aortic and upper abdominal surgeries. While pain control is improved when compared with systemic opioids, studies of their ability to reduce postoperative pulmonary complications have shown conflicting results.

Prophylaxis for thromboembolism constitutes a key management issue in all patients. Finally, careful monitoring for postoperative complications constitutes a key element in all surgical patients. Other perioperative interventions like total parenteral nutrition, pulmonary artery catheterization,[22] chest physiotherapy in the absence of excessive secretions or sputum production, and routine application of positive end-expiratory pressure in mechanically ventilated patients have been shown to be ineffective.

CONCLUSION

The goal of preoperative evaluation of the patient being considered for surgery is to identify everyone who has an acceptable chance of tolerating that procedure, while guiding those found to have the greatest likelihood of major complications about the options that exist. The evaluation of candidates for thoracic surgery differs substantially from the evaluation before general surgery. By using the above described tests and recommendations, the best option for cure to many patients can be provided.

REFERENCES

1. American Thoracic Society. Evaluation of impairment/disability secondary to respiratory disease. J Med Assoc Ga. 1985;74(9):649-54.
2. American Thoracic Society. Evaluation of impairment/disability secondary to respiratory disorders. Am Rev Respir Dis. 1986;133(6):1205-9.
3. Bestall JC, Paul EA, Garrod R, Garnham R, Jones PW, Wedzicha JA. Usefulness of the Medical Research Council (MRC) dyspnoea scale as a measure of disability in patients with chronic obstructive pulmonary disease. Thorax. 1999;54(7):581-6.
4. Taiwo OA, Cain HC. Pulmonary impairment and disability. Clin Chest Med. 2002;23(4):841-51.
5. International Labor Office. Guidelines for the use of the ILO International Classification of Radiographs of Pneumoconioses. Geneva: International Labour Office; 2003.
6. Macintyre N, Crapo RO, Viegi G, Johnson DC, van der Grinten CP, Brusasco V, et al. Standardisation of the single-breath determination of carbon monoxide uptake in the lung. Eur Respir J. 2005;26(4):720-35.
7. Miller MR, Hankinson J, Brusasco V, Burgos F, Casaburi R, Coates A, et al. Standardisation of spirometry. Eur Respir J. 2005;26(2):319-38.
8. Robertson H. Clinical application of pulmonary function and exercise tests in the management of patients with interstitial lung disease. Sem Respir Crit Care Med. 1994;15:1-9.
9. Armstrong BW, Workman JM, Hurt HH, Roemich WR. Clinico-physiologic evaluation of physical working capacity in persons with pulmonary disease. Rationale and application of a method based on estimating maximal oxygen-consuming capacity from MBC and O2ve. II. Am Rev Respir Dis. 1966;93(2):223-33.
10. Wehr KL, Johnson RL. Maximal oxygen consumption in patients with lung disease. J Clin Invest. 1976;58(4):880-90.
11. Guidelines for the evaluation of impairment/disability in patients with asthma. American Thoracic Society. Medical Section of the American Lung Association. Am Rev Respir Dis. 1993;147(4):1056-61.
12. Cowl CT. Occupational asthma: review of assessment, treatment and compensation. Chest. 2011;139:674-81.
13. Von Groote-Bidlingmaier F, Koegelenberg CF, Bolliger CT. Functional evaluation before lung resection. Clin Chest Med. 2011;32:773-82.
14. American Medical Association Guide to the Evaluation of Permanent Impairment, 5th edition. Chicago: American Medical Association; 2001.
15. Fairshter RD, Williams JH. Pulmonary physiology in the postoperative period. Crit Care Clin. 1987;3(2):287-306.
16. Hedenstierna G. Mechanisms of postoperative pulmonary dysfunction. Acta Chir Scand Suppl. 1989;550:152-8.
17. Van Mieghem W, Demedts M. Cardiopulmonary function after lobectomy or pneumonectomy for pulmonary neoplasm. Respir Med. 1989;83(3):199-206.
18. Colice GL, Shafazand S, Griffin JP, Keenan R, Bolliger CT. American College of Chest Physicians. Physiologic evaluation of the patient with lung cancer being considered for resectional surgery: ACCP evidenced-based clinical practice guidelines (2nd edition). Chest. 2007;132(3):161S-77S.
19. Haniuda M, Kubo K, Fujimoto K, Aoki T, Yamanda T, Amano J. Different effects of lung volume reduction surgery and lobectomy on pulmonary circulation. Ann Surg. 2000;231(1):119-25.
20. Larsen KR, Svendsen UG, Milman N, Brenøe J, Petersen BN. Cardiopulmonary function at rest and during exercise after resection for bronchial carcinoma. Ann Thorac Surg. 1997;64(4):960-4.
21. Smetana GW. Preoperative pulmonary assessment of the older adult. Clin Geriatr Med. 2003;19(1):35-55.
22. Qaseem A, Snow V, Fitterman N, Hornbake ER, Lawrence VA, Smetana GW, et al. Risk assessment for and strategies to reduce perioperative pulmonary complications for patients undergoing noncardiothoracic surgery: a guideline from the American College of Physicians. Ann Intern Med. 2006;144(8):575-80.

23. Smetana GW. Preoperative pulmonary evaluation. N Engl J Med. 1999;340(12):937-44.
24. Morton H. Tobacco smoking and pulmonary complications after surgery. Lancet. 1944;1:368-70.
25. Wightman JA. A prospective survey of the incidence of post-operative pulmonary complications. Br J Surg. 1968;55(2):85-91.
26. Warner MA, Divertie MB, Tinker JH. Preoperative cessation of smoking and pulmonary complications in coronary artery bypass patients. Anesthesiology. 1984;60(4):380-3.
27. Bishop MJ, Cheney FW. Anesthesia for patients with asthma. Low risk but not no risk. Anesthesiology. 1996;85(3):455-6.
28. Gupta RM, Parvizi J, Hanssen AD, Gay PC. Postoperative complications in patients with obstructive sleep apnea syndrome undergoing hip or knee replacement: a case-control study. Mayo Clin Proc. 2001;76(9):897-905.
29. Poonyagariyagorn H, Mazzone PJ. Lung cancer: preoperative pulmonary evaluation of the lung resection candidate. Semin Respir Crit Care Med. 2008;29(3):271-84.
30. Gerson MC, Hurst JM, Hertzberg VS, Baughman R, Rouan GW, Ellis K. Prediction of cardiac and pulmonary complications related to elective abdominal and noncardiac thoracic surgery in geriatric patients. Am J Med. 1990;88(2):101-7.
31. Wong DH, Weber EC, Schell MJ, Wong AB, Anderson CT, Barker SJ. Factors associated with postoperative pulmonary complications in patients with severe chronic obstructive pulmonary disease. Anesth Analg. 1995;80(2):276-84.
32. Boutros AR, Weisel M. Comparison of effects of three anaesthetic techniques on patients with severe pulmonary obstructive disease. Can Anaesth Soc J. 1971;18(3):286-92.
33. Ravin MB. Comparison of spinal and general anesthesia for lower abdominal surgery in patients with chronic obstructive pulmonary disease. Anesthesiology. 1971;35(3):319-22.
34. Liang BM, Lam DCL, Feng YL. Clinical applications of lung function tests: a revisit. Respirology. 2012;17:611-9.
35. Bernstein WK. Pulmonary function testing. Curr Opin Anaesthesiol. 2012;25:11-6.
36. Stein M, Koota GM, Simon M, Frank HA. Pulmonary evaluation of surgical patients. J Am Med Assoc. 1962;181:765-70.
37. Milledge JS, Nunn JF. Criteria of fitness for anaesthesia in patients with chronic obstructive lung disease. Br Med J. 1975;3(5985):670-3.
38. Datta D, Lahiri B. Preoperative evaluation of patients undergoing lung resection surgery. Chest. 2003;123(6):2096-103.
39. Ferguson MK, Little L, Rizzo L, Popovich KJ, Glonek GF, Leff A, et al. Diffusing capacity predicts morbidity and mortality after pulmonary resection. J Thorac Cardiovasc Surg. 1988;96(6):894-900.
40. Bousamra M, Presberg KW, Chammas JH, Tweddell JS, Winton BL, Bielefeld MR, et al. Early and late morbidity in patients undergoing pulmonary resection with low diffusion capacity. Ann Thorac Surg. 1996;62(4):968-75.
41. Ferguson MK, Reeder LB, Mick R. Optimizing selection of patients for major lung resection. J Thorac Cardiovasc Surg. 1995;109(2):275-83.
42. Ribas J, Diaz O, Barbera JA, Mateu M, Canalís E, Jover L, et al. Invasive exercise testing in the evaluation of patients at high-risk for lung resection. Eur Respir J. 1998;12(6):1429-35.
43. Pierce RJ, Copland JM, Sharpe K, Barter CE. Preoperative risk evaluation for lung cancer resection: predicted postoperative product as a predictor of surgical mortality. Am J Respir Crit Care Med. 1994;150(4):947-55.
44. Nakahara K, Monden Y, Ohno K, Miyoshi S, Maeda H, Kawashima Y. A method for predicting postoperative lung function and its relation to postoperative complications in patients with lung cancer. Ann Thorac Surg. 1985;39(3):260-5.
45. Bria WF, Kanarek DJ, Kazemi H. Prediction of postoperative pulmonary function following thoracic operations. Value of ventilation-perfusion scanning. J Thorac Cardiovasc Surg. 1983;86(2):186-92.
46. Corris PA, Ellis DA, Hawkins T, Gibson GJ. Use of radionuclide scanning in the preoperative estimation of pulmonary function after pneumonectomy. Thorax. 1987;42(4):285-91.
47. Wu MT, Pan HB, Chiang AA, Hsu HK, Chang HC, Peng NJ, et al. Prediction of postoperative lung function in patients with lung cancer: comparison of quantitative CT with perfusion scintigraphy. Am J Roentgenol. 2002;178(3):667-72.
48. Kearney DJ, Lee TH, Reilly JJ, DeCamp MM, Sugarbaker DJ. Assessment of operative risk in patients undergoing lung resection. Importance of predicted pulmonary function. Chest. 1994;105(3):753-9.
49. Stéphan F, Boucheseiche S, Hollande J, Flahault A, Cheffi A, Bazelly B, et al. Pulmonary complications following lung resection: a comprehensive analysis of incidence and possible risk factors. Chest. 2000;118(5):1263-70.
50. Morice RC, Peters EJ, Ryan MB, Putnam JB, Ali MK, Roth JA. Exercise testing in the evaluation of patients at high risk for complications from lung resection. Chest. 1992;101(2):356-61.
51. Pate P, Tenholder MF, Griffin JP, Eastridge CE, Weiman DS. Preoperative assessment of the high-risk patient for lung resection. Ann Thorac Surg. 1996;61(5):1494-500.
52. Bolliger CT, Jordan P, Soler M, Stulz P, Grädel E, Skarvan K, et al. Exercise capacity as a predictor of postoperative complications in lung resection candidates. Am J Respir Crit Care Med. 1995;151(5):1472-80.
53. Bolliger CT, Wyser C, Roser H, Solèr M, Perruchoud AP. Lung scanning and exercise testing for the prediction of postoperative performance in lung resection candidates at increased risk for complications. Chest. 1995;108(2):341-8.
54. Brutsche MH, Spiliopoulos A, Bolliger CT, Licker M, Frey JG, Tschopp JM. Exercise capacity and extent of resection as predictors of surgical risk in lung cancer. Eur Respir J. 2000;15(5):828-32.
55. Richter Larsen K, Svendsen UG, Milman N, Brenøe J, Petersen BN. Exercise testing in the preoperative evaluation of patients with bronchogenic carcinoma. Eur Respir J. 1997;10(7):1559-65.
56. Rao V, Todd TR, Kuus A, Buth KJ, Pearson FG. Exercise oximetry versus spirometry in the assessment of risk prior to lung resection. Ann Thorac Surg. 1995;60(3):603-9.
57. Singh SJ, Morgan MD, Hardman AE, Rowe C, Bardsley PA. Comparison of oxygen uptake during a conventional treadmill test and the shuttle walking test in chronic airflow limitation. Eur Respir J. 1994;7(11):2016-20.
58. Brunelli A, Kim AW, Berger KI, Addrizzo-Harris DJ. Physiologic evaluation of the patient with lung cancer being considered for resectional surgery: diagnosis and management of lung cancer. American College of Chest Physicians evidence based clinical practice guidelines. Chest. 2013;143(5 Suppl):e166S-90S.
59. Mazzone P. Preoperative evaluation of the lung resection candidate. Cleve Clin J Med. 2012;79(1):e517-22.

60. Beckles MA, Spiro SG, Colice GL, Rudd RM; American College of Chest Physicians. The physiologic evaluation of patients with lung cancer being considered for resectional surgery. Chest. 2003;123(1):105S-14S.
61. Moller AM, Villebro N, Pedersen T, Tønnesen H. Effect of preoperative smoking intervention on postoperative complications: a randomised clinical trial. Lancet. 2002;359(9301): 114-7.
62. Cesario A, Ferri L, Galetta D, Pasqua F, Bonassi S, Clini E, et al. Post-operative respiratory rehabilitation after lung resection for non-small cell lung cancer. Lung Cancer. 2007;57(2):175-80.
63. Spruit MA, Janssen PP, Willemsen SC, Hochstenbag MM, Wouters EF. Exercise capacity before and after an 8-week multidisciplinary inpatient rehabilitation program in lung cancer patients: a pilot study. Lung Cancer. 2006;52(2):257-60.
64. Thomas JA, McIntosh JM. Are incentive spirometry, intermittent positive pressure breathing, and deep breathing exercises effective in the prevention of postoperative pulmonary complications after upper abdominal surgery? A systematic overview and meta-analysis. Phys Ther. 1994;74(1):3-16.
65. Castillo R, Haas A. Chest physical therapy: comparative efficacy of preoperative and postoperative in the elderly. Arch Phys Med Rehabil. 1985;66(6):376-9.
66. Stock MC, Downs JB, Gauer PK, Alster JM, Imrey PB. Prevention of postoperative pulmonary complications with CPAP, incentive spirometry, and conservative therapy. Chest. 1985;87(2):151-7.

26 Chapter

Interpretation of Arterial Blood Gases and Acid-base Abnormalities

Aditya Jindal

INTRODUCTION

Acid-base and oxygenation abnormalities are among the most common clinical problems faced, both in routine medical clinics and in the intensive care units (ICUs). Proper interpretation and analysis of the blood gas report can lead to major changes in the treatment protocols and can be life-saving for the patient. Unfortunately, this is one area where most medical personnel face problems.

This is primarily because of the excessive technical jargon involved in the area. However, one has to make a distinction between clinically relevant analysis and basic pathophysiological processes. The purpose of this chapter is to introduce the relevant pathophysiologic principles and develop a systematic and stepwise approach for the analysis of acid-base disorders.

BASIC CONCEPTS

Definitions

Acids and bases: Acids and bases have been defined variably over the centuries. An acid has been defined based on its sourness quotient, bitter taste and ability to neutralize alkaline solutions. Modern definitions include those of Arrhenius, i.e. ability to produce hydrogen ions when dissolved in water; the Van Slyke definition based on electrolytes; the Bronsted-Lowry definition (an acid is a substance that can donate protons) and finally, the Lewis definition (an acid is a substance that can accept a pair of electrons to form a covalent bond).[1] Conversely, a base is defined as a substance that produces hydroxyl ions when dissolved in water (Arrhenius) or that which can accept protons (Bronsted-Lowry) or that which can donate electrons to form a covalent bond (Lewis).

The familiar Henderson-Hasselbalch equation was based on the Van Slyke definition of acids and bases. This served as the basis of the traditional or physiological approach to acid-base analysis. Further research led to the development of "base excess" and "standard base excess" as a method of description and later on, to the Stewart or physicochemical model.[1-8] In the routine clinical setting, the traditional approach serves well and will be the one that is further explored in this chapter.

Buffer: A buffer is defined as a substance which reacts with acids and bases and minimizes changes in the pH of a solution.

pH: The pH is the negative logarithm of the hydrogen ion concentration in a solution and is used to represent the acid-base status of a solution. The pH of body fluids is maintained in a specific range depending on the anatomical compartment. The accepted normal range for blood is 7.36–7.44.

Henderson-Hasselbalch equation: This equation describes the correlation between the respiratory and metabolic compartments involved in acid-base balance in a mathematical way. Essentially, it relates the hydrogen ion concentration to the balance between carbon dioxide and bicarbonate ions. For the purpose of comprehension it can be expressed simply as:

$$H^+ \propto CO_2 / HCO_3^-$$

This means that the H^+ concentration and the pH is dependent upon these two factors. Any increase in CO_2 would lead to an increase in the H^+/decrease in pH or acidosis, while a decrease would decrease the H^+/increase the pH or alkalosis. Conversely, decrease in HCO_3^- concentration would decrease the pH leading to acidosis, while increase in HCO_3^- would lead to alkalosis. If the pH change is primarily due to change in the CO_2^- it is termed respiratory, while if it is due to change in the HCO_3^- it is termed metabolic.

OVERVIEW OF ACID-BASE PATHOPHYSIOLOGY IN THE BODY

The body is not a static system, but a dynamic one, with continuous changes in the internal and external milieu. From the perspective of acid-base balance the following changes are important:

- *Respiration*: The addition of oxygen and removal of carbon dioxide from the system

- *Nutrition:* The addition of nutrients, like fats, carbohydrates, proteins, etc. to the system which act as acid or alkali loads
- *Excretion:* Both renal and gastrointestinal; removal of acid/base from the body
- *Disease:* Leads to excess or lack of acid/base in the body.

The body has various autoregulatory mechanisms to maintain the acid-base homeostasis. One may ask, what is the need for doing so? Well, most proteins and enzymes in the body function best at their own optimal pH. Change in the pH would lead to disruption in their functioning. Additionally, pH variations would lead to changes in ionization of proteins and other molecules which would further disrupt functioning. The potential impact is huge and widespread almost all body systems would be involved. Thus, despite differing endogenous and exogenous influences the acid-base status (and by default, the pH) needs to be maintained in a stable range which is appropriate for life.

Having understood the need for acid regulation, we will discuss how the body does so. In a normal diet, the majority of calories are provided by fats and carbohydrates with proteins also contributing to some extent. These fats and carbohydrates are metabolized completely to carbon dioxide and water with the help of oxygen. The carbon dioxide so produced may have a significant effect on the acid-base balance because of the following equation:

$$CO_2 + H_2O \leftrightarrow H_2CO_3 \leftrightarrow HCO_3^- + H^+$$

The amount of carbon dioxide in the body is regulated within a normal range by the respiratory system, so as to maintain the pH within a normal range. Any disease process leading to an increase in CO_2 will lead to an increase in H^+ and therefore causes acidosis, while conversely any decrease in CO_2 will lead to alkalosis.

Protein metabolism, in addition to the formation of calories, also leads to the formation of acids, which are not removable by the respiratory system. Examples of these acids include HCl and H_2SO_4, which are also known as "nonvolatile acids". These acids are buffered by the renal system, which uses NH_4^+ to excrete these acid loads and regenerates HCO_3^-, while doing so.

In a typical diet there is an addition of net acid to the body. This includes exogenous and endogenous acid as well as loss of HCO_3^- in feces. This acid is referred to as net endogenous acid production (NEAP). The kidneys maintain the acid-base balance by excreting acid, known as renal net acid excretion (RNAE). This acid is excreted in the form of NH_4^+ or as titratable acid, with the simultaneous generation of HCO_3^- and urinary buffers. The acid-base balance of the body is maintained when the NEAP is equaled by the RNAE.[9] Any disease may impose various acid or base loads; renal and respiratory regulation usually minimize these effects.

TYPES OF ACID-BASE DISORDERS

We have seen that interpretation of the Henderson-Hasselbalch equation lead to categorization of acid-base disorders as either metabolic or respiratory. Metabolic disorders are due to primary changes in HCO_3^-, while respiratory disorders are due to primary changes in CO_2. These may be further categorized as metabolic acidosis and alkalosis, and respiratory acidosis and alkalosis. The normal ranges of the pH, pCO_2 and HCO_3^- are given in **Table 1**.

The pH is normally tightly regulated within the mentioned range. According to the Henderson-Hasselbalch equation this means that the pCO_2/HCO_3^- ratio should not change significantly, i.e. for a primary change in the CO_2 the HCO_3^- would change in the opposite direction and vice versa. This is also known as a secondary or compensatory response. For example, if the HCO_3^- decreases and leads to a primary metabolic acidosis, the CO_2 will also decrease in order to maintain a relatively constant pCO_2/HCO_3^- ratio and thus the pH **(Table 2)**. However, it must be remembered, that in disease conditions the compensatory responses are never strong enough to completely correct the acid-base abnormality, but serve only to limit the change in the pH. The amount of compensation expected in response to any pH change can be calculated and compared with the actual change to have occurred.[10] One must also remember that respiratory compensation for primary metabolic acid-base abnormalities occurs faster (minutes to hours) as compared to metabolic compensation for primary respiratory disorders (hours to days).

It is pertinent to add here that it is entirely possible for two or more separate acid-base disorders to exist simul-

Table 1 Normal ranges of the pH, pCO_2 and HCO_3^-

Parameter	*Normal range*
pH	7.36–7.44
pCO_2	36–44 mm Hg
HCO_3^-	22–26 mEq/L

Table 2 Acid-base abnormalities and compensatory changes based on the Henderson-Hasselbalch equation

Disorder	*Primary change*	*Compensatory response*
Metabolic acidosis	$\downarrow HCO_3^-$	$\downarrow CO_2$
Metabolic alkalosis	$\uparrow HCO_3^-$	$\uparrow CO_2$
Respiratory acidosis	$\uparrow CO_2$	$\uparrow HCO_3^-$
Respiratory alkalosis	$\downarrow CO_2$	$\downarrow HCO_3^-$

Note: HCO_3^-, bicarbonate; CO_2, carbon dioxide; ↓, decrease; ↑, increase

taneously. These can be detected based on calculation of the compensation. As an example, a patient of chronic obstructive pulmonary disease may have both metabolic acidosis due to sepsis and a respiratory acidosis due to the underlying disease.

Respiratory Compensation

Compensation by the respiratory system for metabolic acid-base abnormalities, as mentioned before, is prompt.[10] It is mediated through the peripheral chemoreceptors which are present in the carotid bodies.

Primary Metabolic Acidosis

A primary metabolic acidosis will lead to a fall in the HCO_3^- levels and a fall in the pH. In compensation, the respiratory system will increase ventilation and blow off CO_2 so as to limit this fall, i.e. respiratory compensation. The expected pCO_2 can be calculated by the following equations:[11]

$$\text{Expected } pCO_2 = 1.5 \times [HCO_3^-] + 8 \pm 2 \text{ mm Hg}$$

Or

$$\text{Expected } pCO_2 = [HCO_3^-] + 15 \text{ mm Hg}$$

If the expected pCO_2 is equal to the measured pCO_2, it means that the respiratory compensation is adequate; this is called as compensated metabolic acidosis. If the measured CO_2 is more than the expected it means there is an additional respiratory acidosis; this is called as a primary metabolic acidosis with a superadded respiratory acidosis. If the expected pCO_2 is less than the measured it means there is an additional respiratory alkalosis, and it is known as primary metabolic acidosis with superadded respiratory alkalosis.

Primary Metabolic Alkalosis

A primary metabolic alkalosis will be associated with elevated HCO_3^- levels. In compensation, the CO_2 levels will increase. The compensation can be calculated as below:[11]

$$\text{Expected } pCO_2 = 0.7 \times ([HCO_3^-] - 24) + 40 \pm 2 \text{ mm Hg}$$

Or

$$\text{Expected } pCO_2 = [HCO_3^-] + 15 \text{ mm Hg}$$

Or

$$\text{Expected } pCO_2 = 0.7 \times ([HCO_3^-] + 20 \text{ mm Hg})$$

The calculations for metabolic alkalosis are not as accurate as in metabolic acidosis; however, they do give a general idea of the expected responses. If the expected pCO_2 is equivalent to the measured pCO_2 the response is known as a compensated metabolic alkalosis. If the measures pCO_2 is less than the expected pCO_2 it means that there is additional respiratory alkalosis and this is known as primary metabolic alkalosis with superadded respiratory alkalosis. Similarly, if the measured pCO_2 is more than the expected, there is an additional respiratory acidosis and the condition is known as primary metabolic alkalosis with superadded respiratory acidosis.

Metabolic Compensation

Metabolic compensation to primary respiratory abnormalities is mediated by the kidneys. As mentioned earlier, the time course is somewhat delayed. However, this is also dependent upon the chronicity of the disease. For acute conditions, renal buffering may be started as early as 5–10 minutes, while in chronic conditions buffering may take from 2–3 days and indeed may be continuous as the primary disease continues to worsen.[10]

Clinically, metabolic responses may be divided into acute and chronic; acute before the onset of compensation and chronic after the compensatory response is well established. The kidney generates this compensatory response by varying the reabsorption of HCO_3^-. The kidney respond more effectively over a period of time, therefore the magnitude of the chronic compensatory response is always greater than that of the acute response.

Primary Respiratory Acidosis

The metabolic response to a primary respiratory acidosis will be an increase in the HCO_3^- levels. The expected response can be calculated and compared with the actual to determine the adequacy of compensation and also the coexistence of secondary disorders. The formula for compensation are as follows:[10,11]

For acute conditions:

- $[HCO_3^-]$ is increased by 1 mmol/L for each pCO_2 increase of 10 mm Hg above 40 mm Hg

Or

- Expected $[HCO_3^-] = 24 + [(\text{current } pCO_2 - 40) \times 0.1]$

For chronic conditions:

- $[HCO_3^-]$ is increased by 4–5 mmol/L for each pCO_2 increase of 10 mm Hg above 40 mm Hg

Or

- Expected $[HCO_3^-] = 24 + [(\text{current } pCO_2 - 40) \times 0.35]$

Primary Respiratory Alkalosis

As expected, the metabolic response will be a decrease in the HCO_3^- levels. Also, this can be acute or chronic and can be interpreted as mentioned under the other acid-base disorders.

For acute conditions:

- $[HCO_3^-]$ is decreased by 2 mmol/L for each pCO_2 decrease of 10 mm Hg below 40 mm Hg

Or

- Expected $[HCO_3^-] = 24 - [(40 - \text{current } pCO_2) \times 0.2]$

For chronic conditions:

- $[HCO_3^-]$ is decreased by 4-5 mmol/L for each pCO_2 decrease of 10 mm Hg below 40 mm Hg

Or

- Expected $[HCO_3^-] = 24 - [(40 - \text{current } pCO_2) \times 0.4]$

The expected compensatory responses are summed up in **Table 3**.

ANION GAP

The anion gap is a theoretical concept; it is a value calculated from the concentration of electrolytes in serum. It has been used in the differential diagnosis of acid-base disorders, especially metabolic acidosis.[12] The anion gap reflects the value of the unmeasured anions in serum.

The total negative charge in human plasma must be balanced by the total positive charge to maintain electroneutrality. The total positive charge in the serum is the sum total of the positively charged ions and other particles in the serum. These include cations, such as sodium, potassium, calcium and magnesium and also cationic proteins. As the contribution of the sodium ion to the net positive charge is significantly out of proportion to the other cations, only sodium is considered in the calculation of the anion gap. Similarly, the negatively charged particles include chloride, bicarbonate, anionic proteins, inorganic phosphate, sulfate and organic anions. Only the concentrations of chloride and bicarbonate are considered in the calculation of the net negative charge. Thus,

$$\text{Total positive charge} = \text{Total negative charge}$$
$$Na^+ + UC = Cl^- + HCO_3^- + UA$$

where, UC = unmeasured cations, UA = unmeasured anions

Rearranging the above equation, we get:

$$Na^+ - (Cl^- + HCO_3^-) = UA - UC = \text{anion gap}$$

So, the anion gap, while calculated from the concentrations of sodium, chloride and bicarbonate ions, represents the difference between the unmeasured anions and cations in serum.[13] Traditionally, the normal anion gap value ranges from 8 mEq/L to 16 mEq/L. However, use of ion specific electrodes has led to a decrease in the normal anion gap; it is essential for clinicians to know the normal range from their respective clinical laboratory.[14]

It is obvious from the above equation that the anion gap will change with either decrease or increase in the levels of the unmeasured anions and/or cations. The causes of increased or decreased anion gap are mentioned in **Table 4**.

The anion gap needs to be corrected for hypoalbuminemia before using it to interpret acid-base abnormalities. Albumin is the major unmeasured anion in serum and hypoalbuminemia will therefore lead to the determination of a falsely low anion gap. This is especially important in critically ill patients in the ICU because of the high prevalence of hypoalbuminemia. The equation for the corrected anion gap (cAG) is as follows:[14]

$$cAG = \text{Anion gap} + 2.5\ [\text{normal albumin (g/dL)} - \text{measured albumin (g/dL)}]$$

The most common cause of elevated anion gap is metabolic acidosis. The anion gap can be used for the classification of metabolic acidosis and can also help in the differential diagnosis. Metabolic acidosis involves an increase in the acid load in serum. Addition or underexcretion of organic anions to serum leads to an increase in the unmeasured anion fraction in serum and further on to an elevated anion gap. However,

Table 3 Expected compensatory response to primary acid-base disorders[10,11]

Primary disorder	*Compensatory response*
Primary metabolic acidosis	Expected $pCO_2 = 1.5 \times [HCO_3^-] + 8 \pm 2$ mm Hg Or Expected $pCO_2 = [HCO_3^-] + 15$ mm Hg
Primary metabolic alkalosis	Expected $pCO_2 = 0.7 \times ([HCO_3^-] - 24) + 40 \pm 2$ mm Hg Or Expected $pCO_2 = [HCO_3^-] + 15$ mm Hg Or Expected $pCO_2 = 0.7 \times [HCO_3^-] + 20$ mm Hg
Primary respiratory acidosis	*Acute:* $[HCO_3^-]$ is increased by 1 mmol/L for each pCO_2 increase of 10 mm Hg above 40 mm Hg Or Expected $[HCO_3^-] = 24 + [(\text{current } pCO_2 - 40) \times 0.1]$ *Chronic:* $[HCO_3^-]$ is increased by 4–5 mmol/L for each pCO_2 increase of 10 mm Hg above 40 mm Hg Or Expected $[HCO_3^-] = 24 + [(\text{current } pCO_2 - 40) \times 0.35]$
Primary respiratory alkalosis	*Acute:* $[HCO_3^-]$ is decreased by 2 mmol/L for each pCO_2 decrease of 10 mm Hg below 40 mm Hg Or Expected $[HCO_3^-] = 24 - [(40 - \text{current } pCO_2) \times 0.2]$ *Chronic:* $[HCO_3^-]$ is decreased by 4–5 mmol/L for each pCO_2 decrease of 10 mm Hg below 40 mm Hg Or Expected $[HCO_3^-] = 24 - [(40 - \text{current } pCO_2) \times 0.4]$

Table 4 Abnormalities of the anion gap[12-15]

High anion gap	*Low anion gap*	*Negative anion gap*
Laboratory error	Laboratory error	Laboratory error
Paraproteinemias (usually IgA)	Monoclonal (IgG) or polyclonal gammopathies	Bromide intoxication
Severe volume depletion leading to hyperalbuminemia	Lithium, bromide, iodide intoxication	Multiple myeloma
Metabolic acidosis	Hypoalbuminemia Calcium, magnesium intoxication	Iodide intoxication

Box 1 Causes of and anion gap in metabolic acidosis[12-16]

High anion gap metabolic acidosis

- Ketoacidosis
  - Diabetic
  - Starvation
  - Alcoholic
- Lactic acidosis
- Addition of anions
  - Methyl alcohol
  - Ethyl alcohol
  - Propylene glycol
  - Salicylates
  - Pyroglutamic acid
- Renal failure (both acute and chronic)

Normal anion gap (hyperchloremic) metabolic acidosis

- Gastrointestinal HCO_3^- loss
  - Diarrhea
- Renal HCO_3^- loss
  - Type 2 (proximal) RTA
  - Type 1 (distal) RTA
- Renal dysfunction
  - Some cases of renal failure
  - Hypoaldosteronism (Type 4 RTA)
  - Type 1 (distal) RTA
- Ingestions
  - Ammonium chloride
  - Hyperalimentation fluids
  - Rapid saline administration

Abbreviation: RTA, renal tubular acidosis

some causes of metabolic acidosis are also associated with a normal anion gap. The underlying mechanisms are not entirely clear; however, it is postulated that the retention of chloride by the kidneys to maintain electroneutrality may be responsible **(Box 1)**.

Gap-gap Ratio or Δ Anion Gap

The anion gap can be used further to detect the presence of additional acid-base disorders or triple acid-base abnormalities.[13,14] Patients of high anion gap metabolic acidosis may have superimposed hyperchloremic metabolic acidosis or metabolic alkalosis which can be detected by this ratio. The gap-gap is basically a comparison of the change in the anion gap to the change in the bicarbonate levels which should normally be 1.

The gap-gap ratio or Δ anion gap is calculated as follows:

$$\Delta AG = \text{Measured AG} - \text{normal AG}/\text{normal } HCO_3^- - \text{measured } HCO_3^-$$

where, normal AG = 12 mEq/L and normal HCO_3^- = 24 mEq/L.

In case of a high gap metabolic acidosis, the ratio should be 1, as the amount of fixed acid added to serum should be titrated by HCO_3^-. Therefore, the increase in fixed anion should be equal to the decrease in HCO_3^-. If the ratio is less than 1, it means that the HCO_3^- has decreased to a greater extent than the rise in the anion gap. This indicates a coexisting metabolic acidosis, which is usually a hyperchloremic metabolic acidosis. This condition often occurs in diabetic ketoacidosis or sepsis, where the existing high anion gap metabolic acidosis is often complicated by a hyperchloremic metabolic acidosis due to excessive normal saline (NaCl) administration.

Conversely, if the ratio is more than 1, there is an additional metabolic alkalosis. This is because the anion gap has changed to a greater extent than the bicarbonate. This often occurs in ICU patients who receive multiple drugs including diuretics and corticosteroids and undergo frequent nasogastric suction.

ACID-BASE DISORDERS

The clinical features of acid-base disorders are more dependent on the underlying clinical conditions rather than due the presence of acidosis or alkalosis *per se*. However, severe pH changes will lead to clinical features that are independent and superimposed over that of the underlying disease. Generally, respiratory and metabolic acidosis share common clinical features as do respiratory and metabolic alkalosis.[17,18]

Acidosis

Severe acidosis is considered to exist when the pH falls below 7.20. This can affect multiple systems including the cardiovascular, respiratory and others. The cardiovascular complications include decrease in the blood pressure and cardiac output, reduction in the arrhythmia threshold, decrease in the renal and hepatic blood flow, and shift of blood from the peripheral to the central circulation. These effects, compounded by a decrease in myocardial contractility, predispose to pulmonary edema with even minor fluid shifts. Acidosis also promotes hyperventilation and dyspnea (known as Kussmaul respiration) and also the weakening and early exhaustion of respiratory muscles. The metabolic effects of acidosis include development of insulin resistance, inhibition of anaerobic glycolysis, increase in metabolic demands, depletion of ATP and protein denaturation. Ultimately, severe acidosis may lead to mental obtundation and coma.[17]

Metabolic Acidosis

The causes of metabolic acidosis have been mentioned earlier **(Box 1)**. Metabolic acidosis may be classified into high and normal anion gap metabolic acidosis for purposes of differential diagnosis. The treatment of metabolic acidosis is mainly dependent on the underlying cause. However, in severe acidosis, alkali therapy may be given in order to temporarily increase the pH and prevent the development of the adverse effects of acidosis.

Acidotic conditions where the acidosis is due to the accumulation of metabolizable anions (lactic acidosis and ketoacidosis) need not be given alkali therapy till the acidosis is severe (pH < 7.2). This is because the accumulated anions will be converted to bicarbonate ions in a few hours, if proper treatment is instituted and the kidneys are functioning normally. However, in conditions such as hyperchloremic acidosis, renal failure and acidosis due to accumulation of nonmetabolizable ions (renal failure and toxin ingestion), where the conversion to bicarbonate is not possible and regeneration by the kidneys is either limited or slow in onset, alkali therapy is indicated earlier.[17]

The most common compound used is intravenous sodium bicarbonate. The amount to be given can be calculated by the following formula:

$$(\text{Target } HCO_3^- - \text{Current } HCO_3^-) \times \text{body weight in kg} \times 0.5$$

The amount to be infused is dissolved in saline (because the bicarbonate solution is hypertonic) and infused slowly over a period of hours. The target in case of acidosis due to nonmetabolizable anions is to increase the bicarbonate slowly to the range of 22–24 mEq/L, while it is to increase the bicarbonate to more than 10 mEq/L and the pH to 7.15 in case of acidosis due to metabolizable anions. The use of bicarbonate therapy has been associated with several complications such as fluid overload and pulmonary edema and paradoxical worsening of the acidosis due to conversion of the bicarbonate ion to carbon dioxide. Although, carbon dioxide consuming compounds such as Carbicarb and THAM have been used to prevent the latter complication, they have not shown significant benefit in clinical trials.[17]

Respiratory Acidosis

The causes of respiratory acidosis are mentioned in **Table 5**. The division into acute and chronic is purely for the purposes of diagnostic simplification—it should be remembered that any cause of chronic respiratory acidosis may present acutely due to worsening of the underlying disease and other precipitating factors like infections.

In addition to the general symptoms of acidosis mentioned earlier, respiratory acidosis may have additional symptoms due to the accumulation of carbon dioxide. In the acute settings, these include dyspnea, anxiety, confusion, psychosis and hallucinations with progression to coma and acute respiratory failure as the final event. In the chronic setting symptoms include sleep disturbances with daytime sleepiness, memory loss, personality changes, impairment of coordination, tremors, myoclonic jerks and asterixis (flaps).

Treatment: The treatment is mainly dependent upon the acuteness of presentation and the underlying disease. Patients with rapid onset of respiratory acidosis may require admission in an ICU with intubation and mechanical ventilation. Chronically acidotic patients need to be treated holistically, with realistic treatment end goals and priority given to relief of symptoms. These patients may require long-term noninvasive ventilation, which dramatically increases the quality of life in some cases.

Table 5 Causes of respiratory acidosis

Acute
• Respiratory center depression – Infection – Trauma – *Drugs:* Opioids, general anesthetics, benzodiazepines – Stroke • Airway obstruction – Foreign body – Aspiration – Laryngospasm • Parenchymal disease – Acute exacerbation of COPD – Acute severe Asthma – Barotrauma – ARDS – Pneumonia – Pulmonary edema • Miscellaneous causes – *Electrolyte disturbances:* Hypokalemia, hypophosphatemia • Acute worsening of chronic causes
Chronic
• Neurological/muscular disorders – Stroke – Guillain-Barré syndrome – Myasthenia gravis – Muscular dystrophy – Poliomyelitis – Hypoventilation syndromes • Parenchymal/airway disorders – COPD – Pneumoconiosis • Chest wall restriction – Kyphoscoliosis – Ankylosing spondylitis – Obesity
Abbreviations: ARDS, adult respiratory distress syndrome; COPD, chronic obstructive pulmonary disease

Alkalosis

Both respiratory and metabolic alkalosis may present with similar clinical features. Mild alkalosis is usually asymptomatic; symptoms start to appear as the severity increases (severe alkalosis is defined as a pH > 7.6). At this pH arteriolar constriction occurs, which leads to restriction of cerebral and cardiac circulation. Cardiac effects include reduction in the anginal threshold and predisposition to refractory supraventricular and ventricular arrhythmias. These are more prominent in patients with underlying heart disease.

Alkalosis is associated with electrolyte abnormalities, like hypocalcemia, hypomagnesemia, hypophosphatemia and hypokalemia. Additionally, there may be stimulation of anaerobic glycolysis with anion production, leading to an increase in the anion gap. Alkalosis also leads to hypoventilation, which though a compensatory response, may be life-threatening in patients with inadequate respiratory reserve. Finally, the neurological compilations include tingling, numbness, paresthesia, tetany, lethargy, seizures and mental obtundation progressing on to coma. These may be worsened by the associated electrolyte abnormalities.[18,19]

Metabolic Alkalosis

The causes of metabolic alkalosis are detailed in **Table 6**. The most common causes include vomiting and nasogastric aspiration.

Treatment: The treatment is directed to the underlying cause. Use of antiemetics in vomiting and proton pump inhibitors in cases of pronged gastric aspiration may be sufficient. Likewise, reduction in diuretic dose or addition of potassium sparing diuretics may ameliorate the clinical condition. In severe cases, exogenous acid administration, in the form of 0.1 N hydrochloric acid may be required.

Respiratory Alkalosis

Respiratory alkalosis is the most commonly encountered acid-base abnormality in humans, primary because of its presence in normal pregnancy and at high altitudes, situations in which it is physiological rather than pathological. The causes are listed in **Box 2**.

Treatment: The treatment of respiratory alkalosis is primarily directed toward the cause. However, in cases of anxiety hyperventilation, distressing symptoms can be temporarily ameliorated by rebreathing into a closed bag, in order to increase the carbon dioxide levels.

ARTERIAL VERSUS VENOUS BLOOD FOR BLOOD GAS ANALYSIS

There has been considerable interest in evaluating the use of venous blood for blood gas analysis. The advantages include ease of sampling and less discomfort to the patient. Studies on this subject have shown a good concordance between arterial and venous pH and bicarbonate levels. However, the carbon dioxide levels were highly variable. Moreover, these observations are limited to normal individuals and not in disease states. Further research is needed before venous sampling can be recommended as an alternative to arterial sampling for blood gas analysis.[20]

Stepwise approach to interpretation of arterial blood gases described in Flow chart 1.

Table 6 Casues of metabolic alkalosis[18,19]

Chloride depletion
• Renal loss – Diuretics – Bartter's syndrome – Gitelman's syndrome • Gastrointestinal loss – Vomiting – Nasogastric suction – Villous adenomas – Congenital chloridorrhea
Mineralocorticoid excess
• Primary hyperaldosteronism • Secondary hyperaldosteronism • Apparent mineralocorticoid excess
Miscellaneous causes
• Milk alkali syndrome • Exogenous alkali administration • Severe hypokalemia

Box 2 Causes of respiratory alkalosis

Central hyperventilation

- Pain, anxiety
- Psychotic states
- Fever
- Cerebrovascular accident
- Meningitis, encephalitis
- Tumor
- Trauma

Hypoxia

- High altitude
- Pneumonia
- Pulmonary edema
- Aspiration
- Severe anemia

Drugs or hormones

- Pregnancy
- Progesterone
- Salicylates

Miscellaneous

- Sepsis
- Hepatic failure, cardiac failure
- Mechanical ventilation
- Pulmonary embolism

Flow chart 1 Interpretation of arterial blood gases

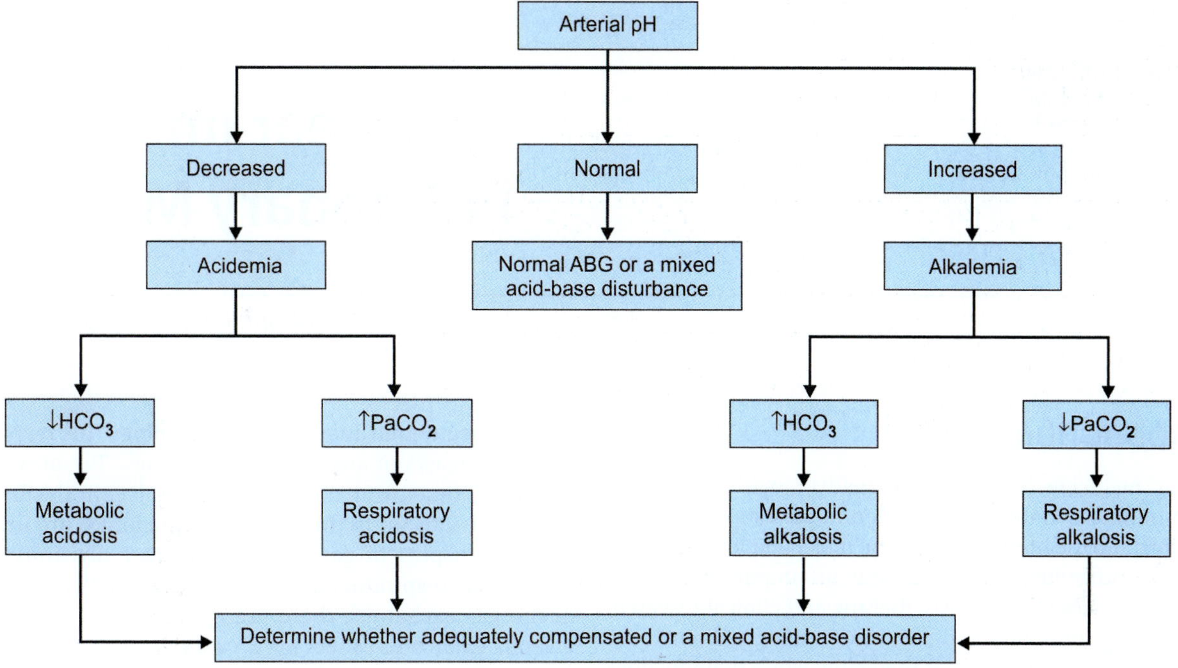

REFERENCES

1. Story DA. Bench-to-bedside review: A brief history of clinical acid-base. Critical care (London, England). 2004;8(4):253-8.
2. Morgan TJ. The Stewart Approach-One Clinician's Perspective. Clin Bioche Rev. 2009;30(2):41-54.
3. Kurtz I, Kraut J, Ornekian V, Nguyen MK. Acid-base analysis: a critique of the Stewart and bicarbonate-centered approaches. Am J Physiol Renal Physiol. 2008;294(5):F1009-31.
4. Seifter JL. Integration of acid-base and electrolyte disorders. New Eng J Med. 2014;371(19):1821-31.
5. Balasubramanyan N, Havens PL, Hoffman GM. Unmeasured anions identified by the Fencl-Stewart method predict mortality better than base excess, anion gap, and lactate in patients in the pediatric intensive care unit. Crit Care Med. 1999;27(8):1577-81.
6. Corey HE. Bench-to-bedside review: Fundamental principles of acid-base physiology. Critical care (London, England). 2005;9(2):184-92.
7. Emmett M. Clinical acid-base disorders: traditional versus "new" analytical models. Kidney Int. 2004;65(3):1112-3.
8. Ghosh AK. Diagnosing acid-base disorders. J Assoc Physicians India. 2006;54:720-4.
9. Koeppen BM. The kidney and acid-base regulation. Adv Physiol Educ. 2009;33(4):275-81.
10. Adrogue HJ, Madias NE. Secondary responses to altered acid-base status: the rules of engagement. J Am Soc Nephrol. 2010;21(6):920-3.
11. Berend K, de Vries AP, Gans RO. Physiological approach to assessment of acid-base disturbances. N Engl J Med. 2014;371(15):1434-45.
12. Forni LG, McKinnon W, Hilton PJ. Unmeasured anions in metabolic acidosis: unravelling the mystery. Critical care. 2006;10(4):220.
13. Kraut JA, Madias NE. Serum anion gap: its uses and limitations in clinical medicine. Clin J Am Soc Nephrol. 2007;2(1):162-74.
14. Kraut JA, Nagami GT. The serum anion gap in the evaluation of acid-base disorders: what are its limitations and can its effectiveness be improved? Clin J Am Soc Nephrol. 2013;8(11):2018-24.
15. Lee S, Kang KP, Kang SK. Clinical usefulness of the serum anion gap. Electrolyte blood pressure. 2006;4(1):44-6.
16. Rastegar A. Use of the DeltaAG/Delta HCO_3- ratio in the diagnosis of mixed acid-base disorders. J Am Soc Nephrol. 2007;18(9):2429-31.
17. Adrogue HJ, Madias NE. Management of life-threatening acid-base disorders. First of two parts. N Engl J Med. 1998;338(1):26-34.
18. Adrogue HJ, Madias NE. Management of life-threatening acid-base disorders. Second of two parts. N Engl J Med. 1998;338(2):107-11.
19. Soifer JT, Kim HT. Approach to metabolic alkalosis. Emerg Med Clin North Am. 2014;32(2):453-63.
20. Kelly AM. Review article: Can venous blood gas analysis replace arterial in emergency medical care. Emerg Med Australas. 2010;22(6):493-8.

Nuclear Imaging in Pulmonary Medicine

BR Mittal, Sunil HV, Kanhaiyalal Agrawal

INTRODUCTION

Nuclear medicine is an exciting field of medical practice where minute quantities of unsealed radioisotopes are used to understand the human body at the molecular level. Nuclear medicine procedures have become an important tool in medical sciences for diagnosis, therapy and clinical research. In general, gamma rays and positron emitting radionuclides are used in diagnostic nuclear medicine, while radionuclides emitting beta and alpha particles are used in therapeutic applications. Radiopharmaceuticals after administration to the patient, emit radiations that are detected externally by sophisticated instruments such as the gamma camera or the positron emission tomography (PET) scanners. This process is unlike a diagnostic X-ray where external radiation is passed through the body to form an image. Planar studies provide a two-dimensional image whereas tomography provides three-dimensional images. The two most widely used emission tomographic studies are single photon emission computed tomography (SPECT) and PET. The anatomical imaging usually gives morphological, whereas nuclear medicine investigations provide functional information. Recently, with wider availability of hybrid imaging like SPECT/CT and PET/CT, both morphological and functional information could be obtained in a single test. Nuclear medicine also plays a pivotal role in the diagnosis and the management of various pulmonary disorders. The various nuclear medicine procedures in pulmonology include ventilation scan, perfusion scan and PET studies. Apart from routinely used 18F-FDG, some of the newer PET tracers include 68Ga DOTATOC for carcinoid tumors to detect somatostatin receptor expression, fluoromisonidazole (18F-MISO) for hypoxia imaging. (This chapter is an outline of the current applications of nuclear medicine in the routine clinical practice. For more details, the reader may refer to specific nuclear medicine books or periodicals).

PULMONARY ANATOMY AND PHYSIOLOGY

Accurate interpretation of ventilation/perfusion (V/Q) lung scans requires proper understanding of the pulmonary vascular segmental anatomy and physiology. The respiratory system consists of airways and two lungs. The airways are divided 23 times from the trachea to the alveoli. The first 16 of these divisions up to the terminal bronchioles are involved in the transport of gas. The remaining 7 divisions which include the respiratory bronchioles and alveoli are involved in the gas exchange. There are approximately 350 million alveoli, each enmeshed by a capillary web, arising from pre-capillary arterioles having a diameter of 10–30 microns. The lower zones of lungs are better ventilated and perfused normally. However, the rate of increase in ventilation from the apex to the base is relatively less compared to increase in the blood flow. In the recumbent position, this hydrostatic gradient decreases and is reoriented to an anteroposterior plane. Effect of posture on regional pulmonary blood flow in rats has also been demonstrated recently using 68Ga-microspheres PET.[1] Increased perfusion to the upper lobes in an upright patient is suggestive of congestive heart failure (CHF), increased left atrial pressure, or α-1-antitrypsin deficiency.

INVESTIGATIONS

Ventilation Imaging

Ventilation in an erect patient is greater at the lung base than at the apex. In supine position, there is relatively a uniform distribution of ventilation. Ventilation scan is primarily used in addition to perfusion scan and the chest X-ray for the diagnosis of pulmonary embolism. Recently, addition of SPECT/CT to ventilation and perfusion study has shown to increase the accuracy of the investigation for detection of pulmonary embolism. Ideally, the ventilation agent should not be cleared too rapidly, because of the need of imaging in multiple views. Broadly, ventilation agents are classified as radioactive gas or radioaerosol. Only ventilation scan is used for studying the transfer of gases across the capillaries. Ventilation studies may be performed using any of the following **(Table 1)**.[2-6]

Table 1 Characteristics of agents used for ventilation

Agent	*Usual dose (MBq)*	*Gamma emission*	*Half-life*	*Advantages*	*Drawbacks*
Radioaerosols					
Tc-99m DTPA	20–30	140 keV	6 hours	Cheaper	Deposition in central airways
Tc-99m Technegas	20–30	140 keV	6 hours	Better images	Expensive, availability
Radioactive gases					
Xe-133	555–740	81 keV	5.24 days	• No central airway deposition • Different energy gamma emission from perfusion agent	Only posterior and single breath hold views are possible
Xe-127	370–740	172, 203, 375 keV	36.4 days	• No central airway deposition • Different energy gamma emission from perfusion agent	Only posterior and single breath hold views are possible
Kr-81m	40–400	190 keV	13 sec	Better image quality	Expensive

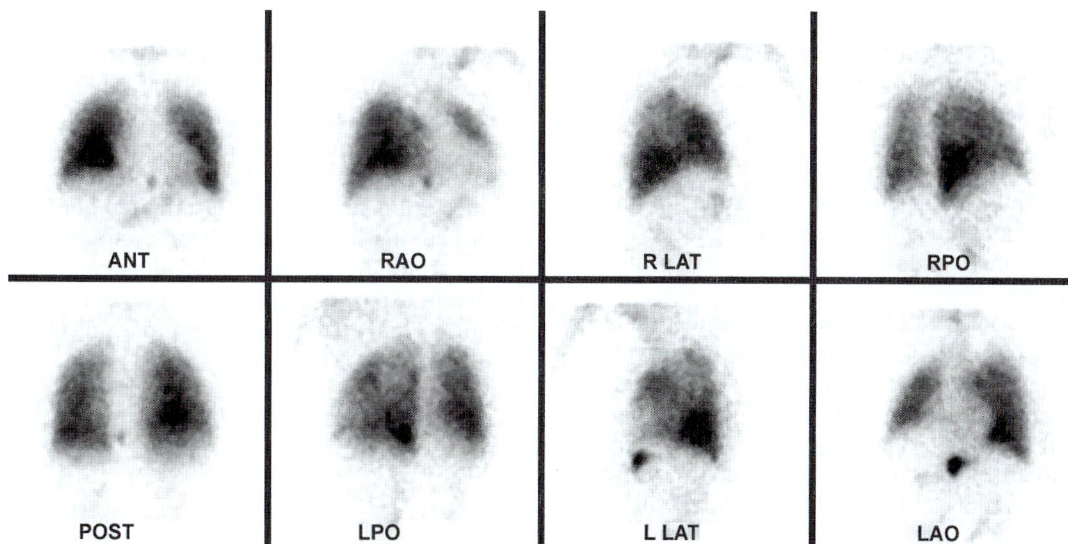

Fig. 1 Normal ventilation study of the lungs performed with Tc-99m DTPA (diethylene triamine penta-acetic acid) aerosols. Uniform distribution of tracer activity is noted throughout both the lungs

Abbreviations: ANT, anterior; RAO, right anterior oblique; RPO, right posterior oblique; POST, posterior; RLAT, right lateral; LPO, left posterior oblique; LAO, left anterior oblique

Tc-99m DTPA Aerosols

The most commonly used ventilation agent in India is Tc-99m diethylene triamine penta-acetic acid (Tc-99m DTPA) aerosol. Technetium produced from a Mo-99–Tc-99m generator system is the main workhorse in nuclear medicine. This decays with gamma energy of 140 keV and half-life of 6 hours. About 25–30 mCi of Tc-99m DTPA is injected into a shielded aerosol system. Aerosols of Tc-99m DTPA are generated by running oxygen through the aerosol system at a rate of 8 L/min. Patient is made to breathe via a face mask for 2–3 minutes with his nose clipped. The expired air is captured in a disposable plastic bag to avoid contamination. Particles produced are generally of 0.5–0.8 microns in diameter, which are delivered to the alveoli like gases during inhalation. Particles larger than 1 micron deposit in the tracheobronchial tree due to inertial impaction and gravitational sedimentation. After sometime, aerosolized Tc-99m DTPA crosses the alveolar capillary membrane and enters the bloodstream where it is filtered by the kidneys and excreted. In normal subjects, the pulmonary clearance of Tc-99m DTPA has a half-time of over 60 minutes (1–1.5 hours).[2] Unlike gases, multiple projections can be obtained due to persistence of activity in the lungs. In patients with obstructive airway disease, excessive tracer in the proximal bronchial tree is often seen due to turbulent airflow, which limits the quality of study. The critical organ is the urinary bladder. The usual radiation exposure to the lungs is about 100 mrad.[2] A normal lung ventilation image performed with Tc-99m DTPA aerosols is shown in **Figure 1**.

Tc-99m Technegas

Technegas and pertechnegas are being used in Australia and some centers in Europe. In this method, Tc-99m gas is passed over heated carbon particles at a high temperature of 2,000–2,500°C in the presence of 100% argon gas. Fine particles of Technegas are generated which provide a uniform distribution over the entire lung field. This property of uniform distribution without central clumping is particularly useful in patients with chronic obstructive pulmonary disease (COPD). However, production of technegas needs onsite generator and is expensive.

Xenon-133

It is a fission product of U-235 having a physical half-life of 5.24 days and a low-energy gamma emission (81 keV).[3,4] The usual dose for inhalation is 15–25 mCi, but it can be administered intravenously in saline. It requires a separate exhaust ventilation system to avoid contamination of the laboratory. Often, only the posterior view is possible. Typical ventilation scan using xenon-133 (Xe-133) consists of three phases:

1. *Single breath (wash in)*: The patient takes a single deep inspiration and holds it for as long as possible. This imparts information about regional ventilation and can detect 50–60% of ventilation defects associated with obstructive airway disease.
2. *Equilibrium*: During this phase, the patient performs normal tidal respirations for 3–5 minutes while rebreathing a mixture of Xe-133 and oxygen. In this view, overall lung volume is demonstrated as tracer equilibrates between all aerated portions of the lungs. It is the least sensitive to detect obstructive airway abnormalities. However, adequate duration of rebreathing ensures diagnostic quality washout phase.
3. *Washout*: Inhalation of Xe-133 is discontinued and the patient breaths room air or oxygen while exhaling the xenon into a charcoal trap. Normally, Xe-133 clears from the lungs in 2–3 minutes. Retention of tracer activity beyond 3 minutes is noticed in obstructive airway disease. The washout phase of the exam can detect about 90% of abnormalities associated with obstructive airway disease. Xenon is overall more sensitive than aerosolized Tc-99m DTPA for detecting obstructive lung disease.

Xenon-127

Xenon-127 has also been used for lung ventilation studies.[5] It is cyclotron produced radionuclide with a physical half-life of 36.4 days. It has three gamma emissions: 172 keV (25%), 203 keV (68%), and 375 keV (18%).

Krypton-81m

It is produced from a Rubidium-81/Krypton-81m generator system. Krypton-81m decays with a gamma emission of 191 keV and a physical half-life of only 13 seconds. This provides an exact comparison of ventilation and perfusion as the ventilation images can be acquired immediately after each perfusion view without moving the patient.[6]

Perfusion Imaging

Lung perfusion scan is typically performed by administration of Tc-99m macroaggregated albumin (Tc-99m MAA) intravenously. The particle size is generally between 10 and 30 microns. These particles are trapped in the pulmonary precapillary arterioles. On an average, typical adult dose contains 500,000 particles which obstruct nearly 0.1–0.3% of the precapillary arterioles.[7] The number of particles need to reduce to about 100,000 in patients with pulmonary arterial hypertension (theoretically acute right heart failure may occur due to limited pulmonary vascular reserve) and in those with known right to left shunts (theoretically may produce symptoms due to lodging of particles in the cerebral/coronary circulations). In neonates, the number of particles should be reduced to 10,000–50,000. The biological half-life of MAA in the lungs is about 4–6 hours. The particles get degraded into smaller particles by enzymatic hydrolysis and are phagocytized by reticuloendothelial (RE) cells.[2] Thus, the occlusion of arterioles is only temporary. The critical organ, i.e. the lung receives a dose of about 1 rad (1 cGy) from a typical 5 mCi dose.[2] The kidneys and bladder receive moderate exposure largely from the excretion of degraded albumin. **Figure 2** represents a normal lung perfusion images performed with Tc-99m MAA.

Ventilation/Perfusion (V/Q) Imaging

Acquisition and Interpretation

Imaging is performed using a large field of view camera coupled with a parallel hole, high-resolution collimator. The scan protocol includes multiple static images in eight standard views (anterior, posterior, right lateral, left lateral, right anterior oblique, left anterior oblique, right posterior oblique and left posterior oblique) with the patient lying in supine position. Each perfusion image is acquired for 500,000–750,000 counts. SPECT imaging is performed wherever deemed necessary. Now-a-days, low dose unenhanced CT may be added to the SPECT at the same time to get combine morphological and functional imaging. The ventilation images are acquired for 100,000 counts or 5 minutes. It may be performed before or after the perfusion study. In a normal scan, all the views show uniform tracer distribution without any defect. Sometimes, one sees a few artifacts on V/Q images.

- *Artifacts on V/Q images*:
  - Trapping of Tc-99m DTPA aerosols in the central airways in patient unable to cooperate with deep breathing or patients with asthma or COPD. This may also produce shine through into the subsequent perfusion study.

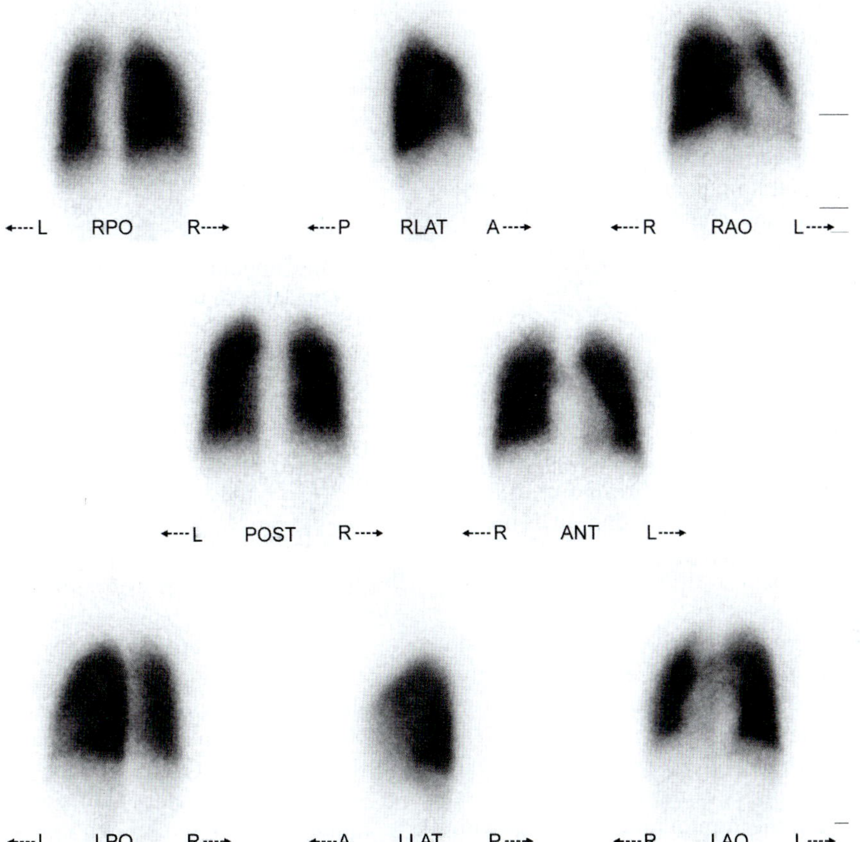

Fig. 2 Normal perfusion study of the lungs performed with Tc-99m MAA (macroaggregated albumin). Uniform distribution of tracer activity is noted throughout both the lungs

Abbreviations: RPO, right posterior oblique; RLAT, right lateral; RAO, right anterior oblique; POST, posterior; ANT, anterior; LPO, left posterior oblique; LLAT, left lateral; LAO; left anterior oblique

- *Liver uptake*: Xenon is fat soluble (somewhat soluble in blood) and may get deposited in the liver, especially in fatty liver.
- *Hot spots*: Which occur due to injection of blood clots inadvertently formed in the syringe. Therefore, the syringe containing Tc-99m MAA should be vigorously shaken before injection. Moreover, at the time of injection, blood should not be withdrawn in the syringe. Further, a 23-gauge or larger needle is recommended to prevent fragmentation of dose.
- *Attenuation defects due to effusions*: When patient scanned supine, effusions may collect posteriorly/superiorly and mimic a defect.

- *Common causes of V/Q mismatch*:
  - *Pulmonary embolism*: Impaired perfusion with normal ventilation. Fat emboli typically produce a mottled appearance due to the presence of many small fat emboli.
  - *Pneumonia/pleural effusion/atelectasis*: Usually more ventilation abnormality with normal or minimally reduced perfusion.
  - *Tumor/hilar lymphadenopathy*: Bronchi are more resistant to extrinsic compression than are the pulmonary arteries because of their rigid cartilaginous rings.
  - *Radiation treatment/vasculitis*: Can reduce regional lung perfusion. Radiation treatment results in the obliteration of the microvasculature. Perfusion defects from radiation are usually geometric and follow the treatment port. They are typically nonsegmental. Ventilation may also be reduced in the irradiated area, but it is usually less affected than perfusion.
  - *Pulmonary artery atresia or hypoplasia.*
  - *Segmental or branch pulmonary artery stenosis.*
  - *Fibrosing mediastinitis*: Can lead to central vascular obstruction.
  - *Aorto-vascular malformation*: Short circuit delivery of the particulate tracer to the regional pulmonary precapillary arterioles.
  - *Congestive heart failure*: Multiple nonsegmental perfusion defects can be seen.

- *Causes of unilateral decreased perfusion:*[8,9] V/Q scans can also show unilateral decreased perfusion in some conditions, viz.
  - *Pulmonary agenesis*: Absent ventilation while X-ray chest may show a small, opaque hemithorax
  - *Hypoplastic lung (pulmonary artery atresia)*: Usually ventilation to a small lung is noted with no evidence of perfusion. On X-ray chest the involved lung is usually small, hyperlucent, and contains few normal pulmonary markings
  - *Swyer-James syndrome*: Characterized by bronchial destruction. It produces a more severe impairment of ventilation than of perfusion in the affected lung. Perfusion typically is decreased and inhomogeneous, but may be severely reduced and nearly inapparent
  - *Tumor/mediastinal mass*: A central mass can compress or occlude the pulmonary artery resulting in absent perfusion. Endobronchial obstruction can produce hypoxic vasoconstriction
  - *Massive pleural effusion*
  - *Pneumothorax*
  - *Pulmonary embolism*: Unilateral decreased perfusion can be secondary to pulmonary embolism. Chronic pulmonary embolism has been shown to be the cause of unilateral hypoperfusion
  - *Aortic dissection*: Unilateral absent perfusion in the right lung due to direct compression of the right pulmonary artery by the intramural hemorrhage within the adjacent ascending aorta.
  - *Fibrosing mediastinitis*: Vessels are occluded by progressive fibrosis prior to occlusion of the bronchi.
  - Shunt procedures for congenital heart disease
  - Lung transplantation with nonperfusion of the native (diseased) lung.

Interpretation Criteria

Prospective investigation of pulmonary embolism diagnosis (PIOPED) criteria: Traditionally, the V/Q scans are interpreted using the PIOPED criteria, though original interpretation was based on Biello's criteria. In PIOPED criteria,[10-12] planar perfusion scan is compared with planar ventilation scan and interpreted along with a recent chest X-ray (<12 hours old). The perfusion defects are classified as small (<25% of a segment), medium (25–75%) and large (>75%) defects.

High-probability Scan

Prospective investigation of pulmonary embolism diagnosis (PIOPED) criteria

- Two or more large mismatched segmental defects (or equivalent in moderate or large defects) with normal radiograph
- Any perfusion defect substantially larger than radiographic abnormality.

Intermediate Probability Scan

Prospective investigation of pulmonary embolism diagnosis (PIOPED) criteria

- Multiple perfusion defects with associated radiographic opacities
- More than 25% of a segment and fewer than two mismatched segmental perfusion defects with normal radiograph:
  - One moderate segmental defect
  - One large or two moderate segmental defects
  - One large and one moderate segmental defects
  - Three moderate segmental defects
- Solitary moderate to large matching segmental defect with matching radiograph (triple match)
- Difficult to characterize as high probability or low probability.

Low Probability Scan

Prospective investigation of pulmonary embolism diagnosis (PIOPED) criteria

- Nonsegmental defects
- Any perfusion defect with substantially larger radiographic abnormality
- Matched ventilation and perfusion defects with normal chest radiograph
- Small subsegmental perfusion defects with normal radiograph.

Normal Scan

Prospective investigation of pulmonary embolism diagnosis (PIOPED) criteria

No perfusion defects

Modifications to PIOPED criteria were suggested on the bases of retrospective PIOPED data review. Gottschalk suggested that a high probability study should be interpreted as pulmonary embolism present and that normal and very low probability exams be interpreted as pulmonary embolism absent for a more conclusive interpretation. All other exams should be interpreted as pulmonary embolism uncertain. The modified PIOPED was based using this type of scheme.

PIOPED II: PIOPED II study compared CT pulmonary angiogram (CTPA) and V/Q scan with pulmonary angiography as the gold standard.[13-16] PIOPED II concluded superiority of CTPA against V/Q scan. The main drawback of V/Q scan as per this study was large number of indeterminate studies. The complicated probabilistic approach and results of PIOPED II study led to the decline in use of V/Q scan. However, it is to be remembered that in PIOPED II, CTPA, an inherently tomographic technique was compared with technically inferior planar V/Q scans.

Prospective investigative study of pulmonary embolism diagnosis (PISAPED) criteria: Alternatively, PISAPED study proposed a simpler way to diagnose or exclude pulmonary embolism by using perfusion scan and recent chest X-ray. It proposed that a wedge-shaped perfusion defect of any size irrespective of the chest X-ray findings should be considered as indicative of PTE.[17] This approach led to the decline in the number of indeterminate scans. The PISAPED criteria did not require ventilation scan. This has sensitivity of 92% and specificity of 87%.

V/Q SPECT: Recently V/Q SPECT has been found to have as accurate as CTPA for diagnosis of pulmonary embolism.[18]

V/Q SPECT/CT: Early reports of perfusion only SPECT/CT for diagnosis of pulmonary embolism on hybrid gamma cameras appears promising. There is the evidence suggesting improved specificity and overall accuracy of ventilation/perfusion scan with addition of SPECT/CT. CT component of the SPECT/CT is usually acquired with lower current avoiding high radiation and is usually noncontrast enhanced.

Applications of Ventilation/Perfusion Scan

Ventilation and perfusion scans are applied in combination with chest X-ray for the diagnosis of pulmonary embolism, to evaluate integrity of the pulmonary alveolar membrane, quantification of lung perfusion prior to a planned pulmonary resection to determine the residual functional lung mass. Various pulmonary disorders in which lung perfusion scan is utilized are discussed below:

Pulmonary embolism: Pulmonary embolism, a potentially fatal condition, is a frequently overlooked diagnosis, which can be associated with significant mortality if untreated. More than 80% of deaths from pulmonary embolism occur in the first 30 minutes and 90% within the first 2–3 hours of the event.[19] It is commonly seen in bedridden hospitalized patients. The common conditions predisposing to this entity are: postoperative states especially following operations on the abdomen and pelvis; trauma including fractures particularly of the lower extremities; neoplasms; prior history of thromboembolic disease; venous stasis; vascular spasm; intimal injury; hypercoagulability states and immobilization. In the PIOPED study, 92% of the patients with pulmonary embolism had at least one of these risk factors.[10]

No single or combination of clinical findings is either specific or sensitive enough to diagnose or exclude pulmonary embolism. Most commonly, the emboli arise from the veins of lower extremity or the pelvis. Patients usually present with acute onset breathlessness, pleuritic chest pain and rarely with haemoptysis. ECG findings may or may not be characteristic of pulmonary embolism.

Diagnosis is straight forward in a patient with predisposing clinical problems and typical manifestations. When the clinical features are atypical, a high index of suspicion is required to diagnose pulmonary embolism. A chest X-ray at presentation is often normal. Classic signs described in a chest X-ray for pulmonary embolism are Hamptom's hump (wedge shaped opacity above the diaphragm) and Westermark's sign (focal oligemia). CTPA (CT pulmonary angiography) is being more frequently used nowadays at the emergency rooms for rapid diagnosis of pulmonary embolism. CTPA has a high negative predictive value. The ready availability of CT has resulted in the modality largely supplanting V/Q scanning, but CTPA is less accurate in detecting subsegmental thrombi. There is additional risk of excessive radiation exposure.[20,21] Breast irradiation from a V/Q scan is approximately 0.28–0.9 mGy-which is less than 5% of the radiation dose to the breast resulting from CTA.[22] It has been determined that approximately 1 of the 300 women in the reproductive age group, who undergo computed tomography pulmonary angiogram (CTPA), has a risk of developing carcinoma breast.[20] CTPA in addition, cannot be used in patients with previously known allergy to iodinated contrast agents and in patients with compromised renal function. Though presently under utilized, V/Q scan offers the advantages of lower radiation exposure.

V/Q scans: V/Q scanning had been the mainstay for screening symptomatic patients for the presence of pulmonar embolism. A normal V/Q scan essentially excludes the possibility of recent significant pulmonary embolus. Ventilation-perfusion mismatch (an area of normal ventilation corresponding to a segmental wedge-shaped area of decreased or absent perfusion) is the hallmark of a pulmonary embolism on V/Q scanning.[11-18,21,22] V/Q lung scan acquired within 4–6 hours of a large (lobar) embolism may show a matched defect due to vascular insult inducing reflex bronchoconstriction. In cases with high clinical concern for pulmonary embolism, SPECT images may help to better define the defect. The false-positive rate of high probability scans is only about 10%. In general, emboli are more frequent in the lower lobes due to the greater blood flow. Emboli are also frequently multiple (in 90%) and bilateral (in 85% of cases). Thus, unilateral decreased/absent perfusion to one lung is uncommonly the result of pulmonary embolism. Injection of Tc-99m MAA into the veins of the feet may help to reveal a DVT. Venous obstruction or collateral flow can be seen. Images recorded several minutes after the injection may also show hot spots where the Tc-99m MAA is adherent to thrombus in the vein.

V/Q scan is also the investigation of choice in women of reproductive age group in patients with renal failure and in patients with allergy to intravenous contrast agents.[23] **Figure 3** is a representative image of pulmonary embolism showing multiple perfusion defects. In patients with prior pulmonary embolism having persistent ventilation-perfusion abnormalities, false-positive interpretation may be made. Pulmonary emboli resolve because of natural thrombolytic processes. A residual perfusion defect can be found in 9–30% of patients and incomplete resolution, more common in patients with an underlying cardiopulmonary disease.

Fat embolism: Classically, a heterogeneous perfusion pattern (multiple small to moderate perfusion defects scattered throughout both the lungs) is observed. Segmental perfusion defects are rarely present. However, in majority

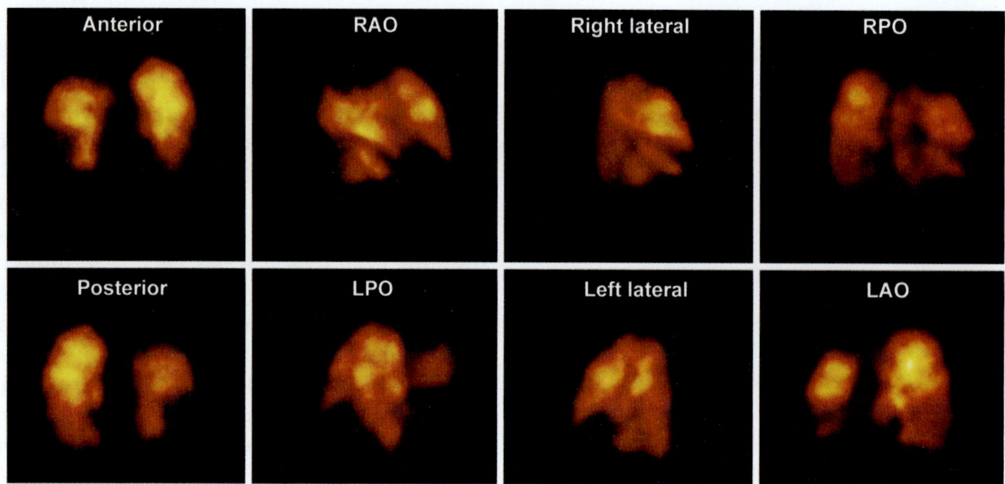

Fig. 3 Lung perfusion study with Tc-99m MAA (macroaggregated albumin) showing multiple large segmental perfusion defects in bilateral lungs, indicating high probability for pulmonary embolism
Abbreviations: RAO, right anterior oblique; RPO, right posterior oblique; LPO, left posterior oblique; LAO, left anterior oblique

of cases due to small size emboli, V/Q scan may be normal. Unfortunately, the lung scan is not very useful in diagnosing fat emboli but can be used to exclude thromboembolic as the cause of the patient's hypoxia in these patients.

Pulmonary infarction: Pulmonary infarction may occur as a complication of pulmonary embolism. The perfusion defect is usually larger than the chest X-ray consolidation.

Pulmonary hypertension: In secondary pulmonary hypertension, perfusion is typically heterogeneous, with small peripheral defects on V/Q scintigraphy. However, the scan may also be normal. In primary pulmonary hypertension, the presence of reverse mismatch (diminished ventilation, normal perfusion) representing failure of hypoxic vasoconstriction has been described.[24] If extensive, this finding is of great physiologic importance as blood shunted through poorly ventilated lung tissue can be a major cause of hypoxia. In patients with primary pulmonary hypertension, high resolution computed tomography (HRCT) demonstrates a characteristic mosaic attenuation pattern. Areas of reverse mismatch on the V/Q scan have been shown to correlate with areas of increased attenuation on HRCT.[25]

Hepatopulmonary syndrome: Tc-99m MAA imaging demonstrates heterogeneous pulmonary perfusion and the presence of right to left shunting **(Fig. 4)** with activity outside the lungs in the brain, liver, and spleen. Scintigraphy can also be used to quantify the shunt, but it cannot distinguish between intracardiac and intrapulmonary shunting (best diagnosed by echocardiography with saline microbubble injection. A geometric mean of counts in brain and lungs is calculated on static images. Steps involved in calculation of lung shunt fraction are shown below:[26]

A lung shut fraction of greater than 6% is considered as significant.

Hemoptysis: Labeled RBCs can also be used in cases of hemoptysis to localize the site of pulmonary hemorrhage. About 50% of patients may show positive scan and bleeding rates as low as 50 mL/day may be detected.

Emphysema: Multiple ventilation defects on the single breath view and abnormal retention on the washout study is visualized on Xe-133 study in patients with emphysema. The late equilibrium images are typically normal as the gas slowly

$$\text{Geometric mean brain counts (GMBC)}$$

$$= \sqrt{\text{right lateral or anterior view brain counts} \times \text{left lateral or posterior view brain counts}}$$

$$\text{Geometric mean lung counts (GMLC)}$$

$$= \sqrt{\text{anterior view lung counts} \times \text{posterior view lung counts}}$$

$$\text{Hepatopulmonary shunt (HPS)} = \frac{\dfrac{\text{GMBC (Brain)}}{0.13}}{\dfrac{\text{GMBC (Brain)}}{0.13} + \text{GMLC (Lung)}}$$

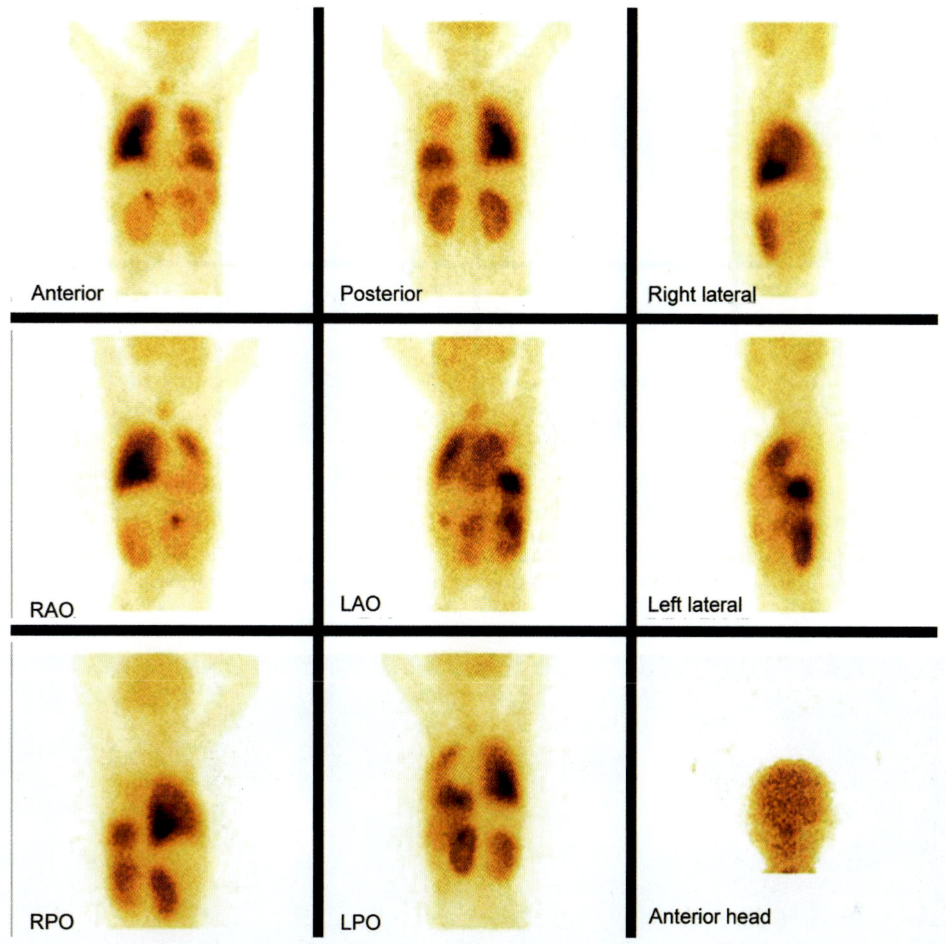

Fig. 4 Lungs, kidneys and brain acquired after intravenous injection of Tc-99m MAA (macroaggregated albumin) showing tracer activity in the lungs and in the systemic circulation suggesting right to left shunting
Abbreviations: RAO, Right anterior oblique; LAO, Left anterior oblique; RPO, Right posterior oblique; LPO, Left posterior oblique

distributes via collateral airways into the abnormal regions. Due to the turbulent air flow, extensive central deposition of the tracer in the large airways may be seen on aerosol ventilation images. Asthmatic patient also demonstrates similar findings on ventilation images **(Fig. 5)**. Xe-133 has also been used to evaluate ventilation before and after lung volume reduction surgery in patients with pulmonary emphysema.[27] Regional ventilation can also be studied using Tc-99m DTPA aerosols.[28] Perfusion scan may be normal or near normal in early or mild COPD. With progression of lung parenchymal destruction, matched nonsegmental ventilation-perfusion defects may be seen. Perfusion defects may also result from bullae themselves or by their compression of adjacent lung tissue. Reduced or absent perfusion in the upper lung zones is seen in the apical bullae.

Preoperative evaluation of regional pulmonary function: It is important to determine the risk of postoperative pulmonary insufficiency in patients with lung cancer. A forced expiratory volume in 1 second (FEV1) > 2L or greater than 60% of the predicted value and FEV1 > 1.5L or over 40% predicted values are essential for pneumonectomy and lobectomy respectively.[29] Lung scintigraphy provides a fairly accurate determination of the patient's ability to undergo surgery. The American college of chest physicians recommends that quantitative perfusion scintigraphy should be used in patients with borderline lung function to predict postoperative lung function.[30] Split function of each lung is determined from the geometric mean of counts obtained from both the anterior and the posterior lung perfusion images **(Fig. 6)**. The post-operative FEV1 can be calculated by multiplying the global preoperative FEV1 by the split function of the remaining lung. Ventilation scintigraphy may be a better predictor of post-operative function, but central airway tracer deposition can potentially limit the results.

Inflammatory lung diseases: Lung epithelial permeability can be evaluated by studying the clearance of inhaled Tc-99m DTPA aerosol from the lungs.[31-33] Clearance of the tracer is mainly dependent on the epithelial permeability and is

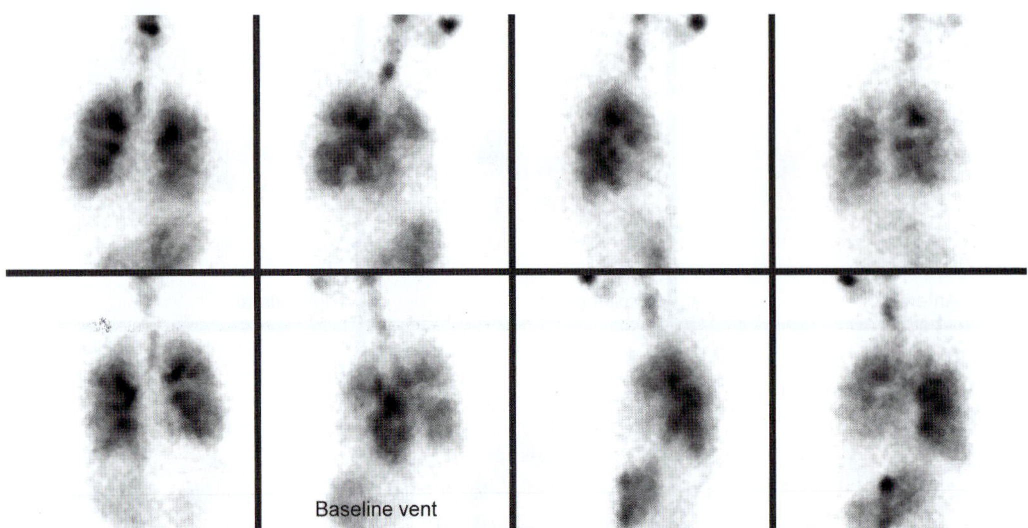

Fig. 5 Lung ventilation study, in a patient with bronchial asthma, performed with Tc-99m DTPA (diethylene triamine penta-acetic acid) aerosol showing central deposition of tracer suggesting obstructive airway disease

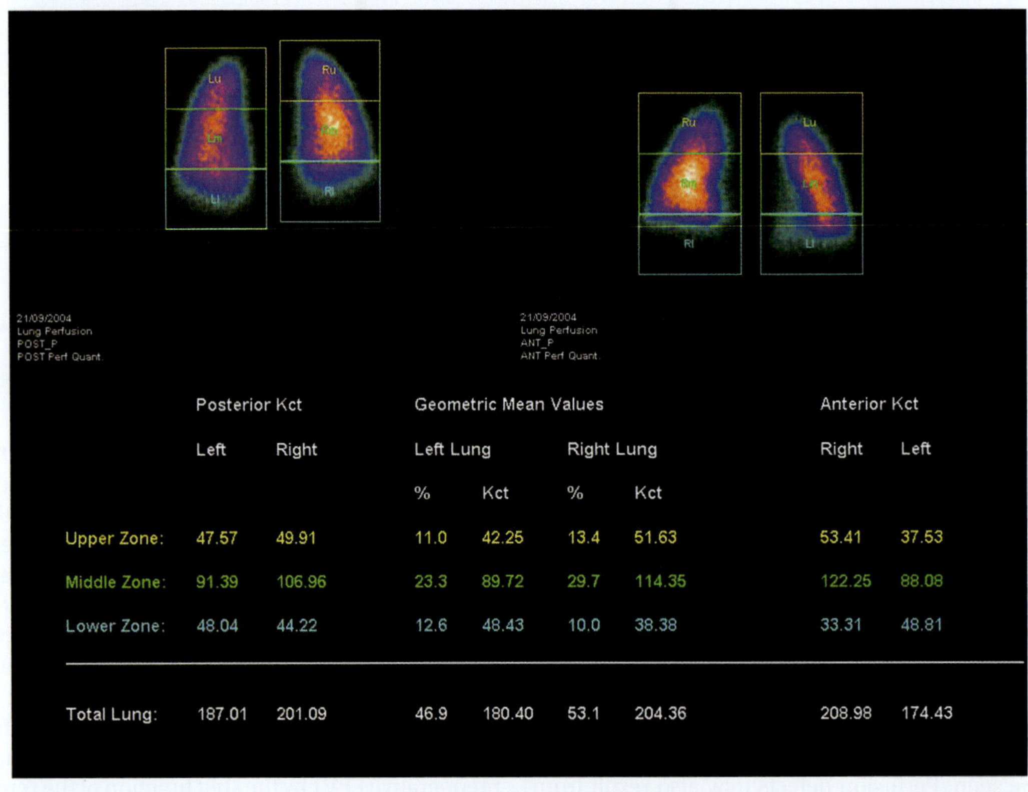

	Posterior Kct		Geometric Mean Values				Anterior Kct	
	Left	Right	Left Lung		Right Lung		Right	Left
			%	Kct	%	Kct		
Upper Zone:	47.57	49.91	11.0	42.25	13.4	51.63	53.41	37.53
Middle Zone:	91.39	106.96	23.3	89.72	29.7	114.35	122.25	88.08
Lower Zone:	48.04	44.22	12.6	48.43	10.0	38.38	33.31	48.81
Total Lung:	187.01	201.09	46.9	180.40	53.1	204.36	208.98	174.43

Fig. 6 Tc99m-MAA (macroaggregated albumin) lung perfusion study with semiquantitative perfusion analysis. Lungs are divided into three zones and their relative function calculated. The example shows normal function of all the three zones of both lungs

only minimally flow dependent. Conditions disrupting the alveolar-capillary membrane such as the acute respiratory distress syndrome (ARDS), hyaline membrane disease, sarcoidosis, idiopathic pulmonary fibrosis, systemic sclerosis, or inhalational lung injury show rapid clearance of Tc-99m DTPA. Biexponential clearance is always abnormal and indicative of greater lung injury than monoexponential clearance. In neonates, biexponential clearance curves are observed shortly after birth and become monoexponential after several days, possibly due to maturation of the surfactant system. Normal Tc-99m DTPA clearance from the lungs is generally between 50 minutes and 80 minutes (T½ approximately 60 minutes).[31] A normal clearance rules out inflammation in the lung from any cause.

Rapid clearance is also observed in active smokers. This is a generalized process throughout the lungs and is proportional to blood carboxyhemoglobin levels. The increased clearance rate is not influenced by the patient's overall smoking history, but rather by their immediate use. Clearance rates can return to normal in 3–7 days after cessation of smoking. Ventilated patients on positive end expiratory pressure (PEEP) or high levels of oxygen (50%) also show more rapid alveolar clearance. Particle deposition in the airways will tend to slow the clearance rates. Patients with primary alveolar proteinosis or congestive heart failure with pulmonary edema also have decreased clearance rates. It is important to exclude extrapulmonary sites of activity (stomach, airways) from the region of interest when determining clearance rates.

Thrombus Imaging

Thrombus imaging may be performed using either of the following tracers:[34-36]

- Tc-99m apcitide (AcuTect)
- In-111 platelets
- Tc-99m antiplatelet antibodies
- Radiolabeled fibrinogen
- Antifibrin antibodies
  - Antifibrin (T2G1s) antibodies F(ab)'2
  - Antifibrin DD-3B6/22 Fab'

Positron Emission Tomography

Positron emission tomography has virtually created a revolution in oncology imaging. F-18 FDG [2-fluoro-2-deoxy-D-glucose] is the most studied PET agent for evaluation of malignant tumors. FDG competes with glucose for facilitated transport into tumor cells and also competes with glucose for phosphorylation by hexokinase. Unlike glucose; however, the phosphorylated form is not further metabolized and it gets trapped within the cell. Tumor cells show increased cellular uptake of FDG due to increased number of surface glucose transport proteins (increased GLUT-1 glucose transporter expression) and a higher rate of glycolysis in comparison to non-neoplastic cells. FDG uptake is related to the degree of cell differentiation and increased FDG uptake is generally associated with greater degrees of de-differentiation. The highly sensitive functional information from PET scan is acquired now in combination with diagnostic quality CT scan for anatomical localization and interpretation.

Lung cancer is the leading cause of cancer death across the world, in part because the disease is usually diagnosed so late. F-18 FDG PET scan finds use in almost all stages of lung cancer. PET/CT is more accurate with fewer equivocal findings and higher specificity than CT alone for characterizing pulmonary nodules. It is useful in the evaluation of a solitary pulmonary nodule measuring more than 8 mm.[37] In a patient with low clinical probability of malignancy, a negative PET scan has a high negative predictive value. The sensitivity of PET/CT for lung cancer is more than 90%, so low to intermediate risk nodules that are metabolically inactive can be followed radiographically to ensure stability or resolution. Because of the FDG uptake in benign disorders as well a positive PET scan in a clinically low probability patient has to be followed with biopsy. In a patient with a high preclinical probability of malignancy, direct biopsy is found to be useful.

Both non-small cell carcinoma (NSCLC - squamous cell carcinoma and adenocarcinoma) and small cell carcinoma (SCLC) are FDG avid. However, well-differentiated adenocarcinoma, carcinoid tumor and bronchoalveolar carcinoma (BAC) show variable FDG uptake and may yield false-negative interpretation. PET is more sensitive than CT for staging of NSCLC, as well as for differentiating lung malignancy from benign lung findings, such as postobstructive atelectasis.[38-40] PET scan has a higher diagnostic accuracy for the detection of metastasis in the mediastinal lymph nodes and the presence of distant metastasis (bone, adrenal, liver). For stage I and II lung cancer, PET does not replace mediastinoscopy and biopsy. The false-negative rate is still higher with PET scan compared with mediastinoscopy. PET is useful in differentiating stage IIIa (resectable disease) from Stage IIIb (unresectable disease). Published data indicate that PET/CT provides additional information in almost 40% of patients, with increased accuracy for T stage as well as the N stage.[41] It is reported that PET/CT detected distant metastases in 92% of patients and was more accurate than CT alone. FDG-PET/CT has become an integral component of NSCLC staging because it improves the detection of nodal and distant metastases and frequently alters patient management **(Figs 7 and 8)**. Magnetic resonance imaging (MRI) is the investigation of choice to detect cerebral metastasis though they may also be seen in an FDG-PET study. Because of the FDG uptake by the background normal brain, it is a less sensitive investigation for detection of cerebral metastasis. Detection of recurrent disease is another indication in which PET/CT is useful. Recurrence if detected at a time when the disease volume is less, offers a chance for curative resection. There are several changes in lung cancer staging in the new American Joint Committee on Cancer (AJCC) staging seventh edition.[42,43] These changes have to be kept in mind while interpreting the FDG-PET/CT images. The mediastinal lymph nodal stations are now named as per the revised International Association for the Study of Lung Cancer (IASLC) classification.[44]

Differentiation of primary tumor (FDG avid) from atelectactic lung (less/non-FDG avid) is an issue of concern

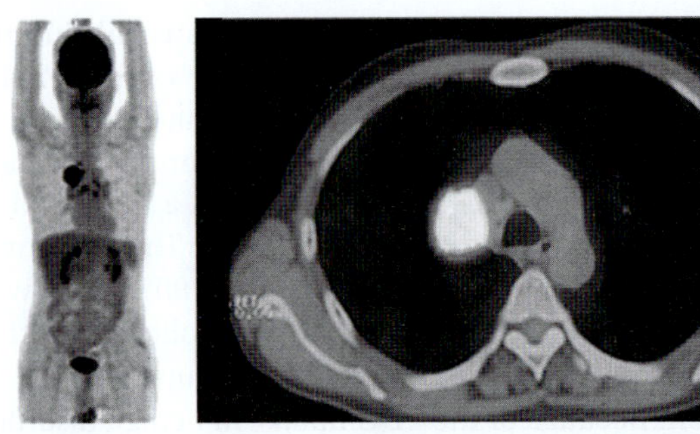

Fig. 7 Whole body F-18 FDG PET/CT image (MIP and transaxial) in a patient with lung cancer showing the hypermetabolic lung tumor with no nodal or distant metastasis thereby enabling curative resection

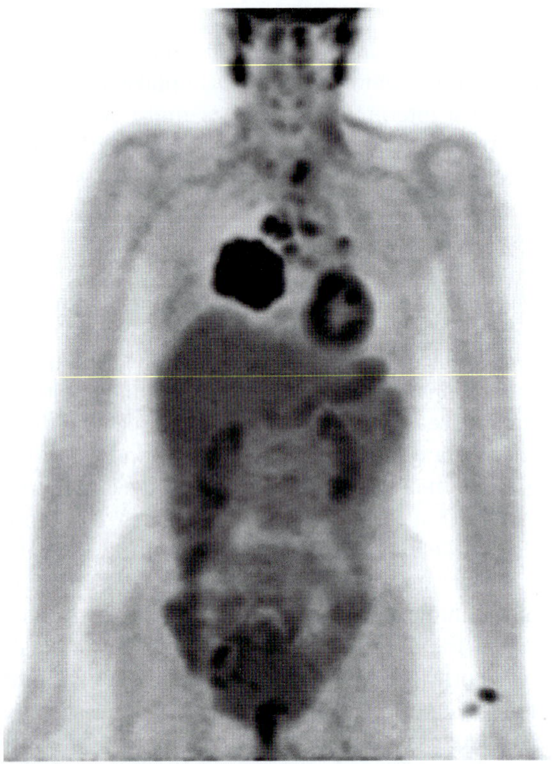

Fig. 8 Maximum intensity projection (MIP) image of F-18-FDG PET/CT showing primary tumor in the right lung with multiple ipsilateral and contralateral mediastinal lymph nodal metastases. The contralateral mediastinal lymph nodes were missed on CT scan because they were sub-centimeter in size. Inclusion of PET prevented a futile thoracotomy

in planning external beam radiotherapy for NSCLC. Often it is difficult to diagnose chest wall invasion in a case of NSCLC on CT scan. Use of radiation therapy for curative treatment of lung cancer is limited by the radiosensitivity of surrounding normal structures. This differentiation is easily possible on PET scan. Incorporation of FDG-PET images into radiation therapy treatment planning resulted in a 15–60% increase or decrease in treated volumes.[45] In 30–60% of patients treated with definitive radiotherapy, PET simulation enhanced precision in coverage of the GTV.[46] PET/CT simulation for radiation therapy treatment planning requires the patient to be aligned using the same set up that will be utilized during radiation therapy. Four-dimensional CT respiratory gating can also be utilized. Four-dimensional radiotherapy using PET scan is the optimum method of delivering precisely targeted dose avoiding normal tissues in the chest.

The assessment of response to therapy with conventional anatomical imaging modalities has inherent limitations. To assess response for example using the response evaluation criteria in solid tumors (RECIST) 1.1 criteria, it requires reduction in tumor volume/diameter. These changes are often difficult to appreciate on a CT scan and take longer time to become perceptible. Metabolic imaging with FDG-PET/CT helps in an early assessment of response to therapy.[47,48] PET scan should be performed after 4–6 weeks of completion of chemotherapy and between 8 weeks and 12 weeks after completion of radiotherapy. As per the proposals of recent PET response criteria in solid tumors (PERCIST criteria), the total disappearance of FDG avid disease is the complete metabolic response; a reduction of >30% in standardized uptake value (SUL Peak) is considered as partial metabolic response; reduction of <30% in SUL is stable disease, and appearance of new FDG avid lesions or increase in >30% is progressive disease.[49]

Most patients with SCLC have advanced metastatic disease at presentation. There are only a few studies on the role of PET scan in SCLC. These have shown some benefit in terms of better staging of the patients and in the assessment of response to therapy.

Carcinoid tumors of the lung are rare and account for 1–2% of lung cancers. Carcinoid tumors typically present as well-defined nodule or mass lesion in relation to the central bronchus often with distal postobstructive subsegmental atelectasis. Well-differentiated carcinoid tumors exhibit somatostatin receptors. This property is made of use in imaging using 68Ga DOTATOC which is a somatostatin receptor analog. 68Ga DOTATOC PET CT is useful in staging carcinoid tumors and assessing their response to therapy.

Malignant mesothelioma is a tumor arising from the parietal pleura. There is an association between exposure to asbestos and development of pleural mesothelioma. These patients usually present with chest pain, breathlessness and recurrent pleural effusions. FDG-PET CT is the most accurate imaging modality for staging pleural malignant mesothelioma. The lesion is seen as a hypermetabolic circumferential nodular thickening in the pleura. FDG-PET CT helps in detection of invasion into the mediastinum and rare distant metastasis. This is helpful for the surgical planning of extrathoracic pneumonectomy **(Fig. 9)**.

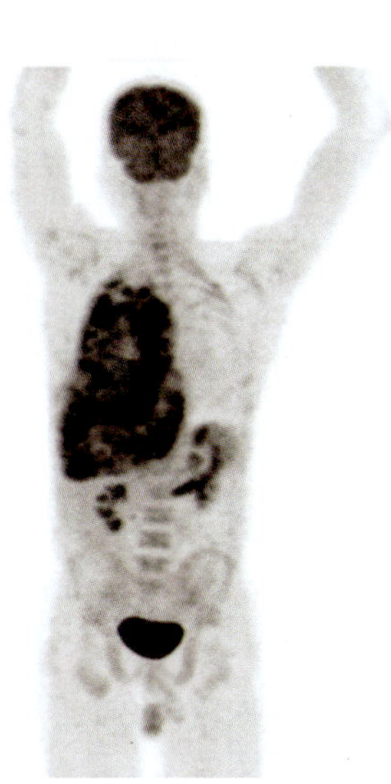

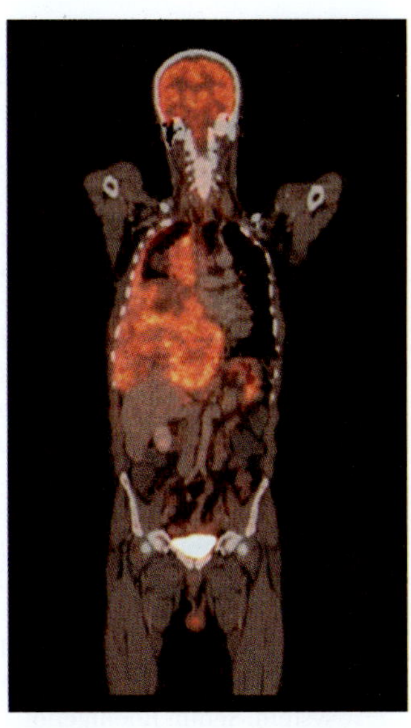

Fig. 9 Maximum intensity projection image and fused coronal image of a patient with mesothelioma showing FDG avid circumferential thickening in the entire pleural lining of the right hemithorax. Distant metastasis was ruled out in this scan thus enabling extrathoracic pneumonectomy

REFERENCES

1. Richter T, Bergmann R, Pietzsch J, Közle I, Hofheinz F, Schiller E, et al. Effects of posture on regional pulmonary blood flow in rats as measured by PET. J Appl Physiol (1985). 2010;108(2):422-9.
2. Stein PD, Gottschalk A. Critical review of ventilation/perfusion lung scans in acute pulmonary embolism. Prog Cardiovasc Dis. 1994;37(1):13-24.
3. Milic-Emili J. Radioactive xenon in the evaluation of regional lung function. Semin Nucl Med. 1971;1(2):246-62.
4. Suga K. Technical and analytical advances in pulmonary ventilation SPECT with xenon-133 gas and Tc-99m-Technegas. Ann Nucl Med. 2002;16(5):303-10.
5. Atkins HL, Susskind H, Klopper JF, Ansari AN, Richards P, Fairchild RG. A clinical comparison of Xe-127 and Xe-133 for ventilation studies. J Nucl Med. 1977;18(7):653-9.
6. Nimmo MJ, Merrick MV, Millar AM. A comparison of the economics of xenon 127, xenon 133 and krypton 81m for routine ventilation imaging of the lungs. Br J Radiol. 1985;58(691): 635-6.
7. Dworkin HJ, Gutkowski RF, Porter W, Potter M. Effect of particle number on lung perfusion images: concise communication. J Nucl Med. 1977;18(3):260-2.
8. Sutter CW, Stadalnik RC. Unilateral absence or near absence of pulmonary perfusion on lung scanning. Semin Nucl Med. 1995;25(1):72-4.
9. Pickhardt PJ, Fischer KC. Unilateral hypoperfusion or absent perfusion on pulmonary scinitgraphy: Differential diagnosis. Am J Roentgenol. 1998;171(1):145-50.
10. Worsley DF, Alavi A. Comprehensive analysis of the results of the PIOPED Study. Prospective Investigation of Pulmonary Embolism Diagnosis Study. J Nucl Med. 1995;36(12):2380-7.
11. Gottschalk A, Juni JE, Sostman HD, Coleman RE, Thrall J, McKusick KA, et al. Ventilation-perfusion scintigraphy in the PIOPED study. Part I. Data collection and tabulation. J Nucl Med. 1993;34(7):1109-18.
12. Gottschalk A, Sostman HD, Coleman RE, Juni JE, Thrall J, McKusick KA, et al. Ventilation-perfusion scintigraphy in the PIOPED study. Part II. Evaluation of the scintigraphic criteria and interpretations. J Nucl Med. 1993;34(7):1119-26.
13. Gottschalk A, Stein PD, Goodman LR, Sostman HD. Overview of Prospective Investigation of Pulmonary Embolism Diagnosis II. Semin Nucl Med. 2002;32(3):173-82.
14. Gottschalk A, Stein PD, Sostman HD, Matta F, Beemath A. Very low probability interpretation of V/Q lung scans in combination with low probability objective clinical assessment reliably excludes pulmonary embolism: data from PIOPED II. J Nucl Med. 2007;48(9):1411-5.
15. Stein PD, Woodard PK, Weg JG, Wakefield TW, Tapson VF, Sostman HD, et al. Diagnostic pathways in acute pulmonary embolism: recommendations of the PIOPED II investigators. Radiology. 2007;242(1):15-21.
16. Wittram C, Waltman AC, Shepard JA, Halpern E, Goodman LR. Discordance between CT and angiography in the PIOPED II study. Radiology. 2007;244(3): 883-9.
17. Miniati M, Sostman HD, Gottschalk A, Monti S, Pistolesi M. Perfusion lung scintigraphy for the diagnosis of pulmonary embolism: a reappraisal and review of the prospective investigative study of acute pulmonary embolism diagnosis methods. Semin Nucl Med. 2008;38(6):450-61.
18. Roach PJ, Bailey DL, Harris BE. Enhancing lung scintigraphy with single-photon emission computed tomography. Semin Nucl Med. 2008;38(6):441-9.
19. Costantino MM, Randall G, Gosselin M, Brandt M, Spinning K, Vegas CD, et al. CT angiography in the evaluation of acute pulmonary embolus. Am J Roentgenol. 2008;191(2):471-4.
20. Einstein AJ, Henzlova MJ, Rajagopalan S. Estimating risk of cancer associated with radiation exposure from 64-slice computed tomography coronary angiography. JAMA. 2007;298(3):317-23.
21. Freeman LM. Don't bury the V/Q scan: it's as good as multidetector CT angiograms with a lot less radiation exposure. J Nucl Med. 2008;49(1):5-8.
22. Sostman HD, Miniati M, Gottschalk A, Matta F, Stein PD, Pistolesi M. Sensitivity and specificity of perfusion scintigraphy combined with chest radiography for acute pulmonary embolism in PIOPED II. J Nucl Med. 2008;49(11):1741-8.
23. Freeman LM, Stein EG, Sprayregen S, Chamarthy M, Haramati LB. The current and continuing important role of ventilation perfusion scintigraphy in evaluating patients with suspected pulmonary embolism. Semin Nucl Med. 2008;38(6):432-40.
24. Fukuchi K, Hayashida K, Nakanishi N, Inubushi M, Kyotani S, Nagaya N, et al. Quantitative analysis of lung perfusion in patients with primary pulmonary hypertension. J Nucl Med. 2002;43(6):757-61.
25. Engeler CE, Kuni CC, Tashjian JH, Engeler CM, du Cret RP. Regional alteration in lung ventilation in end stage primary pulmonary hypertension: correlation between CT and scintigraphy. Am J Roentgenol. 1995;164(4):831-5.
26. Krishnamurthy GT, Krishnamurthy S. Nuclear Hepatology. In: A Textbook of Hepatobiliary Disease, 2nd edition. New York: Springer; 2009.
27. Kurose T, Okumura Y, Sato S, Yamamoto Y, Akaki S, Takeda Y, et al. Functional evaluation of lung by Xe-133 lung ventilation

scintigraphy before and after lung volume reduction surgery (LVRS) in patients with pulmonary emphysema. Acta Med Okayama. 2004;58:7-15.

28. Cabahug CJ, McPeck M, Palmer LB, Cuccia A, Atkins HL, Smaldone GC. Utility of technetium-99m-DTPA in determining regional ventilation. J Nucl Med. 1996;37(2):239-44.
29. Mineo TC, Schillaci O, Pompeo E, Mineo D, Simonetti G. Usefulness of lung perfusion scintigraphy before lung cancer resection in patients with ventilation obstruction. Ann Thorac Surg. 2006;82(5):1828-34.
30. Win T, Tasker AD, Groves AM, White C, Ritchie AJ, Wells FC, et al. Ventilation-perfusion scintigraphy to predict postoperative pulmonary function in lung cancer patients undergoing pneumonectomy. Am J Roentgenol. 2006;187:1260-5.
31. Caner B, Ugur O, Bayraktar M, Ulutuncel N, Mentes T, Telatar F, et al. Impaired lung epithelial permeability in diabetics detected by technetium-99m-DTPA aerosol scintigraphy. J Nucl Med. 1994;35(2):204-6.
32. Rinderknecht J, Shapiro L, Krauthammer M, Taplin G, Wasserman K, Uszler JM, et al. Accelerated clearance of small solutes from the lungs in interstitial lung disease. Am Rev Respir Dis. l980;121(1):105-17.
33. Ugur O, Caner B, Balbay MD, Ozen HA, Remzi D, Ulutuncel N, et al. Bleomycin lung toxicity detected by Tc-99m diethylene triamine penta acetic acid aerosol scintigraphy. Eur J Nucl Med. 1993;20(2):114-8.
34. Stratton JR, Cerqueira MD, Dewhurst TA, Kohler TR. Imaging arterial thrombosis: comparison of technetium-99m-labeled monoclonal antifibrin antibodies and indium-111-platelets. J Nucl Med.1994;35(11):1731-7.
35. Knight LC. Scintigraphic methods for detecting vascular thrombus. J Nucl Med. 1993;34(3 Suppl):554-61.
36. Blum JE, Handmaker H. 1999 plenary session: Friday imaging symposium: Role of small-peptide radiopharmaceuticals in the evaluation of deep venous thrombosis. Radiographics. 2000;20(4):1187-93.
37. Diagnosis of pulmonary nodules, PET professional resources and outreach source, SNM PET centre for excellence. [online] Available from *http://interactive.snm.org/index.cfm?PageID=8761* [Accessed Feb, 2016].
38. NCCN Practice Guidelines in Oncology. Non-Small Cell Lung Cancer v.1.2009. [online] Available from: *http://www.nccn.org/professionals/physician_gls/PDF/nscl.pdf.* [Accessed Feb, 2016].
39. Pauls S, Buck AK, Halter G, Mottaghy FM, Muche R, Bluemel C, et al. Performance of integrated FDG-PET/CT for differentiating benign and malignant lung lesions-results from a large prospective clinical trial. Mol Imaging Biol. 2008;10(2):121-8.
40. Ung YC, Maziak DE, Vanderveen JA, Smith CA, Gulenchyn K, Lacchetti C, et al. 18Fluorodeoxyglucose positron emission tomography in the diagnosis and staging of lung cancer: a systematic review. J Natl Cancer Inst. 2007;99(23):1753-67.
41. De Wever W, Vankan Y, Stroobants S, Verschakelen J. Detection of extrapulmonary lesions with integrated PET/CT in the staging of lung cancer. Eur Respir J. 2007;29 (5):995-1002.
42. Edge S, Byrd DR, Compton CC, Fritz AG, Greene FL, Trotti A. AJCC cancer staging manual, 7th edition. New York: Springer; 2010.
43. Rakheja R, Ko JP, Friedman K. Lung cancer: positron emission tomography/computed tomography and the new staging system. Semin Roentgenol. 2013;48(4):308-22.
44. Terán MD, Brock MV. Staging lymph node metastases from lung cancer in the mediastinum. J Thorac Dis. 2014;6(3):230-6.
45. Macapinlac HA. Clinical applications of positron emission tomography/computed tomography treatment planning. Semin Nucl Med. 2008;38(2):137-40.
46. Bradley J, Thorstad WL, Mutic S, Miller TR, Dehdashti F, Siegel BA, et al. Impact of FDG-PET on radiation therapy volume delineation in non-small-cell lung cancer. Int J Radiat Oncol Biol Phys. 2004;59(1):78-86.
47. Eschmann SM, Friedel G, Paulsen F, Reimold M, Hehr T, Budach W, et al. Repeat 18F-FDG PET for monitoring neoadjuvant chemotherapy in patients with stage III non-small cell lung cancer. Lung Cancer. 2007;55(2):165-71.
48. Nahmias C, Hanna WT, Wahl LM, Long MJ, Hubner KF, Townsend DW. Time course of early response to chemotherapy in non-small cell lung cancer patients with 18F-FDG PET/CT. J Nucl Med. 2007;48(5):744-51.
49. Wahl RL, Jacene H, Kasamon Y, Lodge MA. From RECIST to PERCIST: Evolving considerations for PET response criteria in solid tumors. J Nucl Med. 2009;50(Suppl 1):122s-50s.

Role of Cytology in Lung Lesions

Nalini Gupta, Arvind Rajwanshi

CYTOLOGICAL TECHNIQUES IN RESPIRATORY CYTOLOGY

Over the past two decades, there have been dramatic developments in the understanding of pulmonary disease, in the techniques available to identify, define, quantify and evaluate clinical signs and symptoms, radiographic and pulmonary pathology. Technological developments in recent years have rapidly increased the use of less invasive diagnostic techniques in medicine. This trend has influenced the practice of pathology by increasing the use of cytologic material for definitive diagnosis.

The major types of cytologic preparations that are used for the diagnosis of respiratory pathology in laboratories are:

- Sputum
- Bronchial washings and aspirates
- Bronchial brushing
- Bronchoalveolar lavage (BAL)
- Aspirations:
  - *Fine-needle aspiration cytology (FNAC)*: Transthoracic fine needle aspirations (TTNAs)-Transbronchial needle aspirations (TBNAs)
  - Pulmonary microvascular cytology
  - Pleural aspirations
- Imprint cytology of
  - Bronchial biopsy obtained by forceps on bronchoscopy
  - Lung biopsy obtained by transthoracic needle biopsy
  - Mediastinoscopic biopsy.

Sputum

Although largely replaced by fine-needle aspiration (FNA) and bronchoscopy, cytological examination of sputum for exfoliated malignant cells still is considered a valuable, initial diagnostic test, in patients presenting with a lung mass. Exfoliation of cancer cells in sputum from secondary tumors in the lung is a rare phenomenon in current-day practice, with metastatic colonic adenocarcinoma seen most commonly. Sputum is a specialized product of the respiratory tract, which is the result of an interaction between the mucociliary apparatus and immune system against animate and inanimate invaders from the environment.[1]

- Sputum may be obtained *spontaneously* or may be *induced*:
  - *Spontaneous*: Early morning deep cough sputum is taken.
  - *Induced*: Indicated when patient cannot produce spontaneous deep cough sputum.
  - Inhalation of a solution stimulates mucous production. Usual solution used is 15% NaCl + 20% propylene glycol. Heated to 37°C inhaled for 20 minutes.
  - Postbronchoscopy sputum.
- Sputum can be sent to the laboratory in a *fresh state*, in a *prefixed state*, in *saccomanno fixative* or in CytoLyt® solution.
- *Number of samples*: The optimum number of specimens to diagnose cancer is three, and to exclude cancer is five. By using five specimens, the detection rate (sensitivity) can be as high as 90–95%.[2,3]
- *Satisfactory specimen*: For a sputum sample to be considered satisfactory, the sample should have:
  - Alveolar macrophages (dust cells)
  - Respiratory cells in induced sputum and sputum is raised following bronchoscopy or other invasive procedures.
- *Impact of specimen collection on the morphology of diagnostic cancer cells*: Cancer cells that are expectorated by coughing originate from tumor close to the lumen of bronchi and from necrotic tumor cells which are discohesive. The diagnostic criteria, like nuclear pyknosis in epidermoid carcinoma and nucleolar prominence in adenocarcinoma are actually artifacts due to degenerative changes. These changes can be appreciated in sputum and bronchial wash aspirates rather than bronchial brushing and FNACs.

  These artifacts are specific and constant enough for typing the tumor as squamous cell and adenocarcinoma, respectively.

Bronchoscopy

Gastav Killian[4] in 19th century developed the rigid bronchoscope to directly visualize the mucosal surface of bronchi and obtain samples for cellular evaluation.

Indications

- Evaluate lung lesions of unknown etiology which appear on X-rays as density, infiltrate, atelectasis or localized by unexplained hemoptysis.
- Origin of unexplained positive sputum cytology.
- Stage lung carcinoma and evaluate response to therapy.
- Obtain microbiologic material for suspected pulmonary infections.
- Diffuse and focal lung disease.
- Investigate unexplained paralysis of vocal cord, superior vena cava (SVC) syndrome, chylothorax or unexplained pleural effusion.

Fiberoptic bronchoscope permits the visualization of the lower respiratory tract and a variety of samples can be obtained:

- Bronchial aspirations and washings
- Bronchial brushings of the suspected lesion
- BAL
- Transbronchial fine-needle aspirates
- Imprint cytology of bronchial forceps biopsy.

Bronchial Aspirate and Bronchial Washings

- *Bronchial aspirates* are obtained by introducing the bronchoscope in the lower respiratory tract and aspirating the secretions by suction apparatus.
- *Bronchial washings* from the visualized areas are collected by instilling 3–5 mL of a balanced salt solution through the bronchoscope and reaspirating.

Bronchial Brushings

Cell samples are obtained with small brushes under visual control by fiberoptic bronchoscope or by employing imaging guidance technique.

Brushings should be done prior to biopsy procedure to prevent contamination of the specimen by blood.

Bronchoscopic Findings

It is very important to know the bronchoscopic findings before interpreting the bronchial brush cytology **(Table 1)**.

Forceps biopsy can be done for histopathology. Preceding the biopsy, an imprint cytology or "wash technique" (biopsy is put in normal saline, taken out to be sent for histology, while the saline is sent to the cytology lab) can be used and processed for cytology.

Table 1 Bronchoscopic findings

Bronchoscopy appearance	*Interpretation*
Pale pink	Normal
Granulation tissue	Inflammatory mucosal reaction
Irregularity of mucosa	Early malignancy
Raised lesion	Malignancy
Cauliflower like with pale yellow or white color	Squamous cell carcinoma
Mulberry	Adenocarcinoma
Necrotic appearance of mucosa	Small cell carcinoma
Narrowing of airway	Extrinsic compression by mediastinal nodes

Complications

- Bronchospasm
- Laryngospasm
- Pneumothorax
- Breaking of brushes and forceps
- Fever.

Bronchoalveolar Lavage

Bronchoalveolar lavage (BAL) is based on the concept that cells and noncellular components on the epithelial surface of the alveoli are representative of the inflammatory and immune systems of the entire lower respiratory tract. It is a relatively noninvasive means of sampling the representative cellular component in the alveolar and bronchiolar air spaces. The technique was initially introduced as a therapeutic procedure to remove accumulated secretions in diseases, like alveolar proteinosis, cystic fibrosis and asthma. But over the years, this technique has proved to be of immense value in the diagnosis of the following disorders:[5]

- Detecting opportunistic infections in immunocompromised individuals.[6]
- Diagnosis and staging of interstitial lung diseases.[7]
  - Specific interstitial lung diseases.
    - Idiopathic pulmonary fibrosis (IPF)[8]
    - Pulmonary fibrosis associated with collagen vascular disorders (PF-CV)
    - Hypersensitive pneumonitis (HSP)
    - Extrinsic allergic alveolitis (EAA)
    - Asbestos-related interstitial disease
    - Silicosis
    - Berylliosis
    - Sarcoidosis
    - Lipoid pneumonia[9]
  - Rare interstitial lung disease
    - Histiocytosis-X
    - Chronic eosinophilic pneumonia[10]
    - *Alveolar hemorrhage:* Hemosiderin-laden macrophages

Table 2 Normal constituents of bronchoalveolar lavage in a non-smoker

Constituents	*Percentage*
Alveolar macrophages	≥ 85%
Lymphocytes	10–15%
Neutrophils	≤ 1%
Eosinophils	≤ 1%
Ciliated columnar cells	≤ 2%
T4 : T8 ratio	0.9–2.5

- Obliterative bronchiolitis
- Detection of lung cancer
- Lepidic pattern adenocarcinoma (LAP)
- Lymphangitic carcinomatosis.

Technique and Processing

The middle lobe or lingula is lavaged routinely in the absence of any localized lesion. The tip of the bronchoscope is wedged into a subsegmental bronchus at the level of fourth or fifth branching. 0.9% sterile saline is inserted at room temperature and reaspirated in 20–50 mL aliquots. This is repeated five times at each site.

Lavage procedure is considered invalid if:

- There is a presence of purulent secretions in the airways.
- Bronchoscope is not maintained in wedge position during lavage.
- Volume of fluid recovered is less than 40% of the volume infused.

Normal Constituents of BAL (Table 2)[11,12]

In smokers, the cell yield is four times greater, with slightly increased number of neutrophils.

- *BAL*: Cell counts are useful in the diagnosis and prognosis of certain disorders.
- *Cell count*: The presence of increased nucleated cells is of no diagnostic or prognostic value. The reason for increase in various types of inflammatory cells is shown in **Table 3**.
- *Diagnosis*:
  - Infective agent
  - Malignant cells
- *Diagnosis aided by special stains or additional studies*:
  - Langerhans cell histiocytosis (S100)
  - Alveolar proteinosis [periodic acid-Schiff (PAS)]
  - Pneumoconiosis
  - *Berylliosis*: Positive lymphocyte transformation test
- *Cell count in evaluating prognosis of the disease*:
  - IPF (idiopathic pulmonary fibrosis):
    - *T-lymphocytes*: Good prognosis
    - *Eosinophils in IPF*: Poor prognosis

Table 3 Increase in inflammatory cells

↑ Lymphocytes	*↑ Eosinophils*	*↑ Neutrophils*
Sarcoidosis (active) (T4–T8↑) >1	Eosinophilic pneumonia	Collagen vascular disorders
Berylliosis hypersensitivity pneumonitis (T4 : T8 ↓) <1	Collagen vascular disorders	Idiopathic pulmonary fibrosis
Silicosis	Infection due to helminths, fungi	Bacterial and fungal infections
TB and viral infections	Asthma	Bronchitis
	Allergic bronchopulmonary aspergillosis	Asbestosis and ARDs

Abbreviations: TB, tuberculosis; ARDs, asbestos-related disorders

  - *Collagen vascular diseases:*
    - ↑ *Neutrophils*: Presence of interstitial involvement
    - ↑ *Lymphocytes*: Clinically stable collagen vascular disease
  - *HSP:*
    - ↑ T8 protects against pulmonary fibrosis
  - *Sarcoidosis*: Ratio T4:T8 normal, stable course of diseases:
    - Ratio T4: T8 ↑ deterioration in clinical course
    - BAL lymphocytes >35%; Poor response to therapy
    - BAL lymphocytes <35%; Good response to therapy
  - *Asbestosis*: Presence of asbestos body—indicates exposure
  - Asbestos body with increase lymphocytes, neutrophils and eosinophils indicates subclinical pulmonary involvement.
  - *Berylliosis*: Similar to sarcoidosis.

Aspirations

First report of needle biopsy of the lung was by Leyden in 1883, who used it for the diagnosis of pneumonia. In 1886, Menetrier used it for lung cancer. In 1930, Martin and Ellis used this technique with the thin needle followed by Grover and Bindley in 1939.[13,14] X-ray enhanced television screen was used by Sonderstorm in 1966, followed by Sinner and Nordenstorm in 1975.[15,16] Since most lung masses are carcinomatous in origin, depending on various factors (age, sex, smoking habit and size), the recommendation of FNA as the first-line investigation is warranted because of high yield to risk for complication ratio.[17]

Transbronchial Needle Aspiration

Transbronchial needle aspiration (TBNA) is a special modification of fine-needle aspiration for those cases in which lung neoplasm has not invaded the mucosa, and is therefore, inaccessible by sputum or brushing washings.[18-20]

This aspiration is done under bronchoscopic, fluoroscopic and computed tomography (CT) guidance and the samples processed through conventional techniques.

Indications of TBNA:
- *Mediastinum*: Diagnosis and staging of lung carcinoma
- Hilar lesions
- Intraluminal lesions which are necrotic (so as to sample non-necrotic areas) or submucosal (carcinoids, bronchial gland tumor)
- Parenchymal coin lesions
- Pancoast tumor
- Benign parenchymal lesions, like sarcoidosis or other granulomatous conditions.

Transthoracic Fine-needle Aspiration Cytology

In this technique, a fine needle (with external diameter 0.6 mm, length 10–20 cm) is passed through the chest wall into the pulmonary mass, usually visualized by fluoroscopy or CT. Air dried and wet fixed smears are made from aspirated material and stained by May-Grünwald Giemsa (MGG) and Papanicolaou (PAP) stains.

If the lesion is very deep and small (≤2 cm), then wider bore needle with 0.9–1 mm external diameter should be used. If the lesion is hard and solid (Hamartoma and calcified granulomas), the "screw biopsy" is indicated, where as a stylet with screw tip is introduced through the needle into the lesion and fixed, which facilitates penetration of the hard tumor by the needle.

Indications for TTNA:
- Suspected lung cancer patient with negative results for malignant cells, on five consecutive sputum samples, bronchial brush or wash.
- Other indications are: inoperable lung cancer, solitary pulmonary mass, multiple pulmonary masses, superior sulcus tumor, refusal to undergo exploratory thoracotomy, failure to respond to antituberculosis treatment (ATT) or suspected infectious process.

Contraindications:
- Debilitated uncooperative patients who have uncontrollable cough
- Vascular lesion, pulmonary hypertension, bleeding diathesis or anticoagulant therapy
- Echinococcal cyst.

Complications:
- Pneumothorax[21]
- Air embolism
- Hemothorax
- Hemoptysis.

Pulmonary Microvascular Cytology

Pulmonary microvascular cytology is the examination of a blood sample drawn through a wedged pulmonary artery catheter to diagnose lymphatic carcinomatosis. The blood must be collected in a heparinized tube. In the laboratory, the specimen is placed on a Ficoll-Hypaque gradient to remove the blood and concentrate diagnostic cells.[22]

Pleural Aspirations

A proper cytopreparatory technique for effusions is very important for correct interpretation of the disease process occurring in the pleura. A poorly prepared smear causes diagnostic problems and may result in both false positive and false negative diagnosis.

To ensure an optimal cytopreparation certain prerequisites should be fulfilled.

Immediate submission of unfixed specimen to the cytology lab with immediate processing of the material is mandatory. The fluid is processed by *wet mount technique* where, one drop of centrifuged sediment is added to one drop of toluidine blue solution (0.5 mg of toluidine blue +20 mL 95% alcohol, 80 mL distilled water).

This technique is performed for:
- Rapid diagnosis of malignancy.
- *Judge cellularity*: If the specimens are very cellular, they should be stained separately to prevent cross-contamination, while poorly cellular specimens are processed by cytocentrifugation or filtration techniques.
- Liquid-based cytology (LBC) preparation is of utmost importance in hemorrhagic and paucicellular samples.
- *Ancillary tests*: Additional smears or cell block may be prepared for special stains, immunochemistry, flow cytometry and electron microscopy.

Imprint Cytology

Imprint can be made from bronchoscopic biopsy, obtained by forceps or transthoracic needle biopsy or mediastinoscopic biopsy. The smears are wet-fixed and can be stained by rapid hematoxylin and eosin (H&E) or PAP.

The sensitivity (tumor detection) and specificity (tumor typing) of sputum and BAL/bronchial brushings is approximately 70–80%.

The sensitivity when all three (brush, biopsy, imprint) methods are used together may be as high as 97%; the specificity approaches 100%.[23]

Endoscopic Ultrasonography-guided Fine-needle Aspiration and Endobronchial Ultrasound Fine-needle Aspiration

Endoscopic ultrasonography (EUS) is a novel method for staging of the mediastinum in lung cancer patients. The recent development of linear scanners enabled safe and accurate FNA of mediastinal and upper abdominal structures under real-time ultrasound guidance.[24] EUS-FNA may replace CT-guided biopsies and reduce the number of exploratory thoracotomies.[25] Bronchoscopy can fail to establish a diagnosis in up to 30% of patients with suspected lung cancer. Intrapulmonary tumors located near or adjacent to the esophagus can be visualized and biopsied under real-time ultrasound guidance by EUS-FNA.[26] EUS-FNA is a minimally invasive procedure that can be used as an adjunct or alternative to mediastinoscopy.[27] The technique is safe and it greatly reduces the number of surgical interventions.[28-30]

Endobronchial ultrasound with real-time transbronchial needle aspiration offers improved sensitivity and accuracy for staging of the middle mediastinum, and, combined with endoscopic ultrasound, should allow investigation of the majority of the mediastinum.[31-33]

INFLAMMATORY DISEASES OF THE LUNG

Acute Inflammation

Acute inflammation is characterized by presence of neutrophils, histiocytes, debris and necrosis in pneumonia, abscess, and purulent bronchitis, resulting in tissue destruction.

Chronic Inflammation

Nonspecific: Nonspecific chronic inflammation is common.

Follicular bronchitis: An abundance of immature lymphocytes can point towards follicular bronchitis. This should be distinguished from non-Hodgkin's lymphoma or small cell carcinoma.

Granulomatous Inflammation

Collections of epithelioid histiocytes along with giant cells indicate granulomatous inflammation **(Fig. 1)**. In sputum, epithelioid histiocytes may be shaped, like elongated cones that stain pink to orange when degenerated and look like carrots, hence are termed "carrot cells". These should be differentiated from bronchial epithelial cells, especially in bronchial brushings or aspiration cytology.

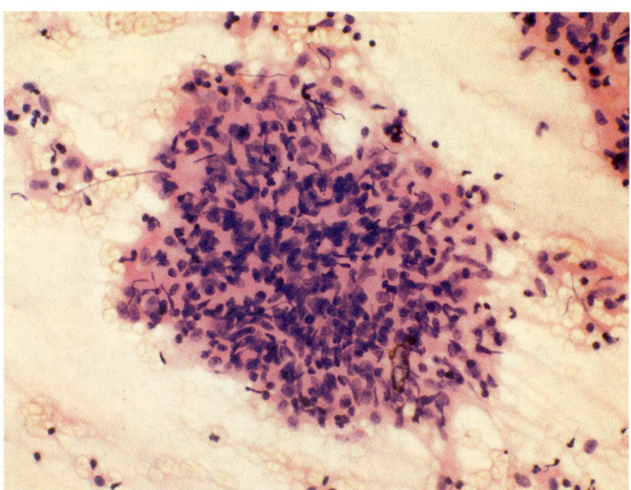

Fig. 1 Collection epithelioid cells and lymphocytes forming a granuloma (H&E, 20x)

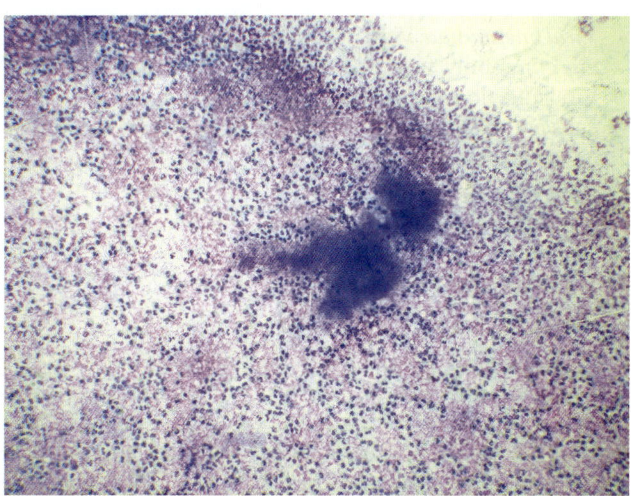

Fig. 2 Sheets of degenerated acute inflammatory cells in a necrotic background (MGG, 10x)

Tuberculosis

Epithelioid histiocytes, giant cells (Langhans' type), lymphocytes, and a necrotic caseous background is diagnostic of tuberculosis **(Fig. 2)**.[34]

Giant cells are seen in sputum in up to half of cases of pulmonary tuberculosis, however, typical Langhans' giant cells are present in only as few as 5% of cases.[35] In tuberculosis, epithelioid histiocytes are found in about 25–50% of sputum specimens.[36] In sputum specimens in which either Langhans' giant cells or epithelioid histiocytes are seen, almost 60% of the patients have tuberculosis, depending upon the patient population.[37,38] Identification of beaded acid-fast bacilli or a positive culture clinches the definitive diagnosis of tuberculosis. The differential diagnosis of necrotizing granulomas includes fungal infections and Wegener's granulomatosis.[39]

Sarcoidosis: It is a chronic granulomatous disease of unknown etiology. Epithelioid histiocytes or giant cells are seen with absence of caseation necrosis **(Fig. 3)**.

Rheumatoid granulomas can also exfoliate epithelioid histiocytes with bizarre shapes. Background may have marked inflammation and necrotic debris.

Specific Infections

Cytologic methods are increasingly being used to diagnose opportunistic infections, especially in immunosuppressed patients.

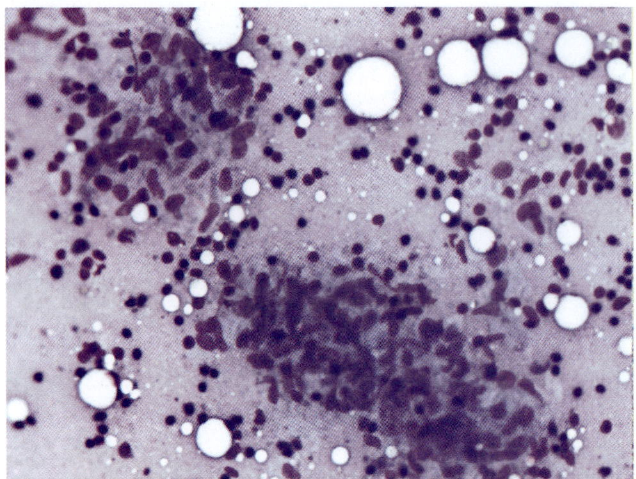

Fig. 3 Epithelioid cell collections along with lymphocytes in a case of sarcoidosis (MGG, 40x)

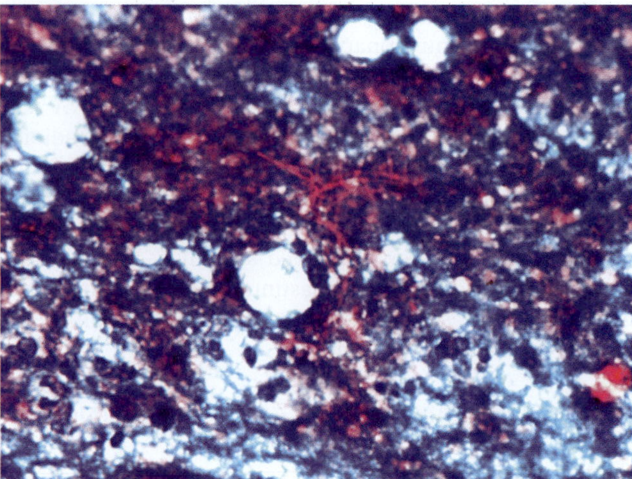

Fig. 4 Multiple thin long filamentous branching filamentous structures (Nocardia) in an inflammatory background (Modified from Ziehl-Neelsen stain, 100x)

- *Viral pneumonia*: Viral infections, such as cytomegalovirus are commonly seen in immunocompromised patients.[40] Viral infection can also cause reactive changes in bronchial cells and it becomes difficult to distinguish the same from adenocarcinoma.
- *Candida, bacterial colonies*: First rule out oral contamination, and overgrowth.

Miscellaneous Infections

Miscellaneous infections are fungi, pneumocystis, toxoplasma, etc. are mostly seen in immunosuppressed patients.[41-43]

Hemophilus, *Staphylococcus* and *Streptococcus* species, *Klebsiella*, anaerobic, or mixed flora are common and can cause lung abscess.[44,45] Fungi, especially *Mucor* or *Aspergillus*, as well as *Actinomyces* or *Nocardia* **(Fig. 4)**[46,47] can also cause pulmonary abscesses.[48]

Reactive atypia and squamous metaplasia associated with epithelioid granulomas, particularly due to tuberculosis or *Aspergillus* can lead to a false-positive diagnosis of cancer.[49,50] Also, granulomas can coexist with cancer.

When an infectious disease is suspected, left over sample should be submitted for cultures and special stains.[51] Culture in FNA specimens is a useful adjunct to diagnosis and impacts care in patients cultured at FNAB. This method can be used to triage patients with suspected infectious diseases and can aid in managing patients who may have recurrent infections.[52]

- *Echinococcus granulosus (hydatid disease)* is considered a contraindication due to possible anaphylaxis,[53] however, the FNA is done accidently for a mass lesion not typical of hydatid radiologically. Hydatid "sand" aspirated from a hydatid cyst shows both scoleces of *Echinococcus* and their hooks **(Fig. 5)**.

  In lung FNA specimens, culture and special stains should be restricted to specimens with acute inflammation or necrosis. Gram's stain and fungal culture are insensitive and not cost-effective, and fungi are often identifiable with routine stains.[54]

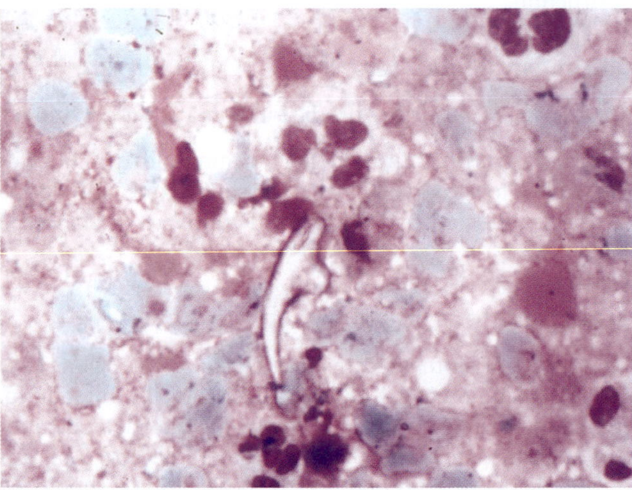

Fig. 5 Hooklet of hydatid in a necrotic background (MGG, 100x)

- *Cytomegalovirus infection* leads to presence of large cells with a nucleus having a large, smooth, amphophilic intranuclear inclusion **(Fig. 6)**. The inclusion has a prominent halo, and thin strands of chromatin connect the inclusion with the inner nuclear membrane.[55]
- *Herpes simplex*: Herpes simplex virus (HSV) pneumonia is a disease of immunocompromised individuals. It is characterized by intranuclear inclusions with nuclear enlargement with basophilic ground-glass alterations in the nucleoplasm. Later, the inclusions may coalesce to form single eosinophilic inclusion body surrounded by a halo.
- *Aspergillus (fumigatus, niger)* is characterized by 45° angle branching of true, septate fungal hyphae of 3–6 µm

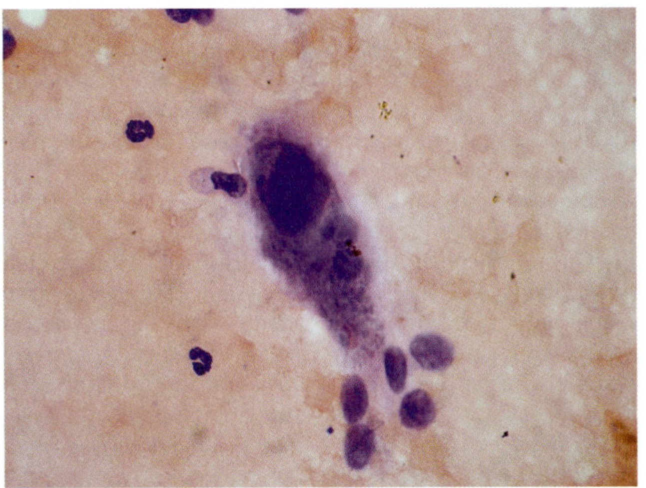

Fig. 6 A single cell showing marked nucleomegaly with a basophilic nuclear inclusion in a case of CMV infection (MGG, 100x)

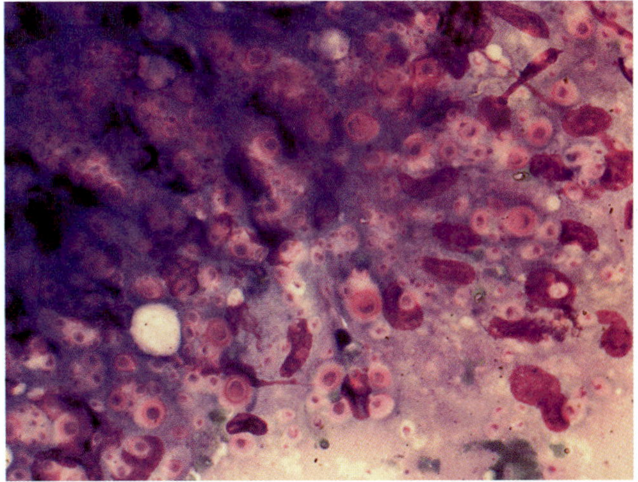

Fig. 8 Many extracellular organisms of varying sizes 5–15 µm in diameter with evidence of budding in a case of cryptococcosis (MGG, 100x)

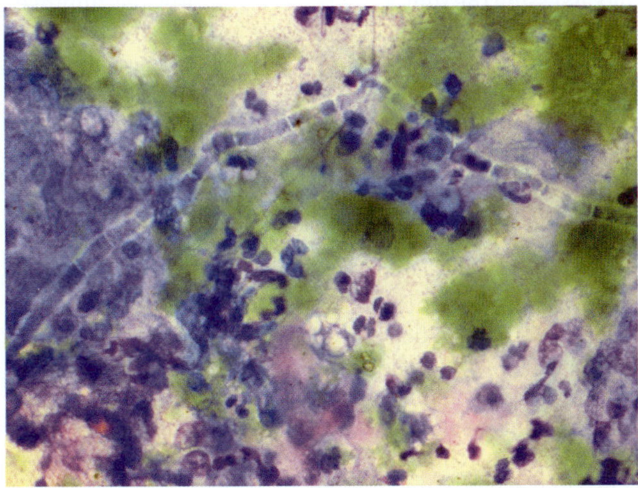

Fig. 7 A long septate hyphae with parallel cell walls of the fungus-aspergillus in a necrotic inflammatory background (MGG, 40x)

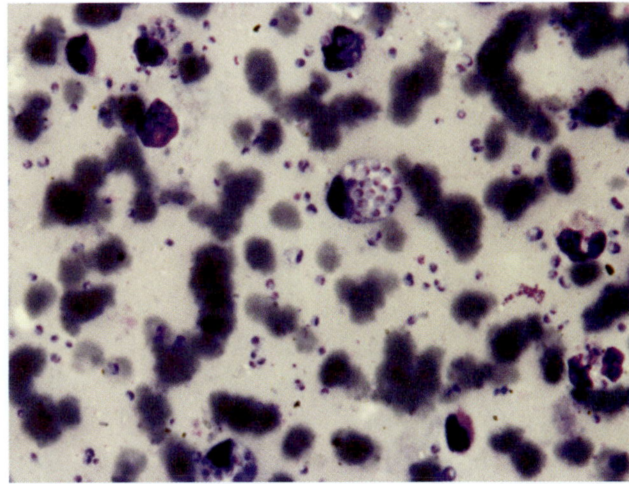

Fig. 9 Numerous round to oval, 2–4 µm in diameter, budding yeasts of histoplasma present both extracellularly as well as intracellularly within histiocytes (MGG, 100x)

uniform width **(Fig. 7)**. Fruiting bodies (conidiophores) are rarely seen.

- *Coccidioides immitis* is marked by nonbudding, thick-walled spherules, measuring 20-60 µm and round, non-budding endospores measuring 1-5 µm.
- *Cryptococcus neoformans* measures 5-20 µm and have a very thick, gelatinous capsule which stains well with special stains, such as mucicarmine, alcian blue, or PAS. Single, teardrop-shaped budding is quite characteristic **(Fig. 8)**.
- *Histoplasma (capsulatum)* is a round to oval, budding yeast, measuring 1-5 µm which should be identified within cytoplasm of a histiocyte or neutrophil to be diagnostic **(Fig. 9)**.
- *Zygomycetes (Mucor, Rhizopus, etc.)* exhibit broad (from 5-20 µm), irregular, thin-walled, folding on themselves, ribbon-like aseptate hyphae that branch at irregular intervals, often at 90° angles **(Fig. 10)**.
- *Pneumocystis jirovecii* is seen more commonly in the acquired immune deficiency syndrome (AIDS) patients.[56] Organisms are seen in foamy/flocculent alveolar casts (rounded masses of organisms). In GMS, the cell wall of the cyst stains black, often with a central dark dot. Cysts are 4-8 µm in diameter and spherical or cup-shaped **(Fig. 11)**. Trophozoites can be up to 8 per cyst, are about 0.5-1.0 µm in diameter. Trophozoites stain in Romanovsky (tiny purple dots).

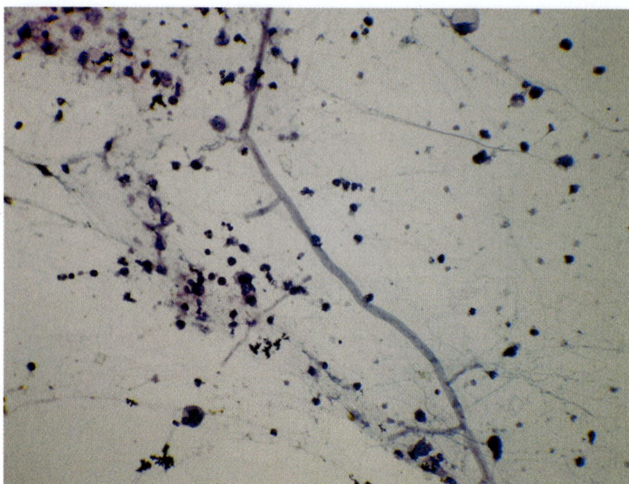

Fig. 10 Mucormycosis-broad (from 5–20 µm), irregular, thin-walled, folding on themselves, ribbon-like aseptate hyphae that branch at irregular intervals, often at 90° angles (PAP, 40x)

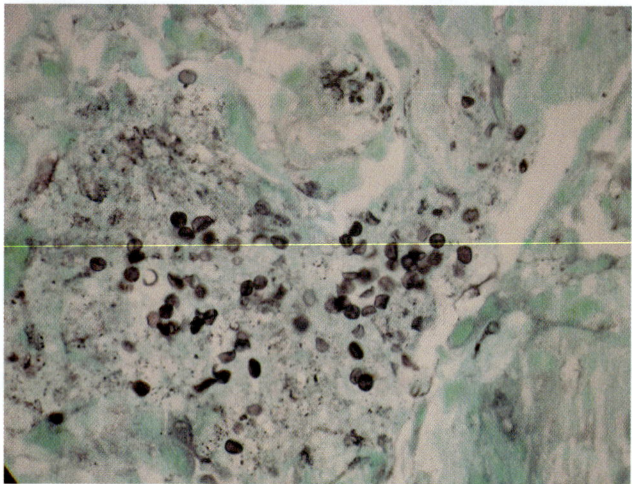

Fig. 11 Many cysts 4–8 µm in diameter and spherical to cup-shaped in a case of *Pneumocystis jirovecii* (Methanamine Silver stain, 100x)

FINE-NEEDLE ASPIRATION CYTOLOGY

Fine-needle aspiration cytology is a simple, relatively safe, rapid reliable technique for the diagnosis of pulmonary lesions, particularly with aid of CT scan. This procedure is almost minimum painful, nonoperative procedure as compared to biopsy for diagnosis of pulmonary lesion and outweighs the single major rare complication of pneumothorax. The published reports revealed that the sensitivity of fine-needle aspiration cytology (FNAC) for the diagnosis for lung cancer ranges from 50% to over 90% whereas specificity is close to 100%. In nearly all these studies the overall positive predictive value is nearly 99%. While the false positive rate is generally less than 1%, a negative test is less reliable with more studies reporting a false negative rate of around 10%.[57,58] The major contribution to the relatively high false negative rate is failure to obtain diagnostic material, most common due to sampling error. Studies have shown that rapid on-site evaluation (ROSE) for cellularity is valuable in minimizing false negative diagnoses due to nondiagnostic material.[59]

Fine-needle aspiration cytology is also a well-established method for providing excellent material for ancillary studies, such as immunochemistry, fluorescence in-situ hybridization (FISH), cytogenetics, cell culture preparations, ultrastructural examination, and molecular studies. The repertoire of molecular tests applied on cytology samples is growing steadily. The current trend is to obtain more information from less material acquired through minimally invasive procedures, such as FNAC. *FNAC also offers several other advantages* over core biopsies for molecular testing, such as (1) FNAC allows multiple passes for wider representation of tumor; (2) FNAC allows acquiring higher proportion of tumor cells with less amount of stroma; (3) rapid on-site evaluation is possible in FNA for further triaging the sample and assessing the tumor tissue; (4) FNAC provides improved archival deoxyribonucleic acid (DNA) quality due to the use of air-dried and/or alcohol-based fixatives, as compared to formaldehyde-based fixatives used in histological sections.

Fine-needle aspiration cytology is effective in routine morphological diagnosis and can differentiate between small cell carcinoma and non-small cell lung cancer (NSCLC) in over 90% cases. In 10–40% of NSCLC cases, it is not possible to ascribe a NSCLC subtype by morphology alone, which applies for both small biopsies as well as cytology samples. The percentage of unclassifiable non-small cell lung cancer-not otherwise specified (NSCLC-NOS) cases is usually falls to about 10% after using immunohistochemistry (IHC) panel. Immunochemistry can be applied in small diagnostic samples, such as effusion samples; transcutaneous FNAC or TBNA either as conventional smears, liquid-based cytology (LBC) or cell block preparations.

Cell block: It is mini formalin fixed paraffin embedded (FFPE) biopsy obtained from fine-needle aspirate or fluid sediment. Preservation of cytological material as cell block for IHC and molecular studies adds to its diagnostic accuracy[60] and enables long-term archiving for future analyses.

Lung Cancer

Lung cancer is the most common cause of cancer-related mortality worldwide. It accounts for one million of five million deaths in world and 2.5 million deaths in developing countries. In India, approximately 63,000 new lung cancer cases are reported each year.[61] More than 70% of lung cancers are unresectable and present in advanced stage. Therefore, many a times only a small biopsy or cytology samples, such as FNAC and fluid specimens are available for diagnostic work-up and molecular characterization. Lung cancer is broadly divided into small cell carcinoma and non-small cell carcinoma.

Non-small Cell Carcinoma

NSCLS accounts for approximately 85% of lung carcinoma. NSCLCs are further classified into lung adenocarcinoma (LADC), squamous cell carcinoma (SCC) and large cell carcinoma, the latter being composed of poorly differentiated LADC and a few uncommon cell types. Historically, all subtypes of NSCLCs were given same chemotherapy, so further categorization of NSCLCs into LADC and SCC was not important on FNAC. But now treatment for lung cancer is personalized and is based on subtype of lung cancer (LADC vs. SCC) and molecular status, i.e. epidermal growth factor receptor (EGFR) mutations and anaplastic lymphoma kinase (ALK) rearrangements. Accurate subtyping of NSCLCs to LADC and SCC, and identification of molecular status is mandatory for administration of appropriate therapy.

International association of the study of lung cancer/ American Thoracic Society/European Respiratory Society (IASLC/ATS/ERS)[62] international multidisciplinary classification of lung cancer proposed classification of lung cancer for small biopsies/cytology samples in 2011 **(Table 4)**.

Adenocarcinoma: Invasive adenocarcinoma is the most common primary peripheral lung cancer and occurs more commonly in nonsmokers. These are classified based on predominant pattern with lepidic, acinar, papillary, micropapillary and solid variants. Other variants include invasive mucinous, colloid, fetal and enteric adenocarcinoma.[62]

Cytologically: The tumors' cells can be singly scattered or loosely clustered. The key diagnostic feature is the formation of acini or papillae, or evidence of mucin production by the malignant cells. The cells are large with classical parameters of malignancy including variable size and shape, coarse chromatin and prominent nucleoli **(Fig. 12)**. The cytoplasm is pale gray thin and sparsely vacuolated. At times it may be abundant.

The main differential diagnosis includes non-keratinizing SCC, large cell carcinoma and metastatic adenocarcinoma. Benign reactions due to pneumonia; infarcts; or physical, chemical, or infectious agents can also lead to false-positive results.

Squamous cell carcinoma: This is a common lung cancer, but its incidence is decreasing.[63] It is strongly associated with cigarette smoking. Most SCC arises in the mucosa of the larger bronchi and therefore, are generally located in the perihilar or central area.[64]

Cytologically, the tumors may be composed of large, pleomorphic to bizarre, poorly cohesive cells to small, uniform, cohesive cells. The nuclei of the cells show hyperchromasia, pyknosis and a coarse chromatin **(Fig. 13)**. A typical background may consist of many degenerated cell with blurred outlines and the malignant cells.

The differential diagnosis of non-keratinizing SCC with poorly differentiated adenocarcinoma may be difficult. Very poorly differentiated SCC should also be distinguished from small cell carcinoma. Benign reactive changes due to infectious agents, particularly tuberculosis or fungi, or infarction, can mimic SCC.

Necessity to Subtype NSCLC into LADC and SCC

Lung cancer therapy has become personalized based on specific subtype of lung cancer. Number of recent clinical studies has shown that:

- *The response rate and survival with the chemotherapeutic agent*: Pemetrexed[65-67] is significantly better in patients with adenocarcinoma (LADC) and other "non-squamous NSCLC".
- Severe life-threatening pulmonary hemorrhage with Bevacizumab [a recombinant humanized monoclonal antibody inhibitor of vascular endothelial growth factor (VEGF)], treatment of advanced lung cancer is associated with SCC.[68]
- NSCLCs with EGFR mutations are more responsive to EGFR tyrosine kinase inhibitors (TKI) than wild-type tumors.[69-73] As almost all EGFR mutant NSCLCs are adenocarcinomas, histological subtyping is important in determining which cases are appropriate to undergo mutation testing.
- NSCLC harboring EML4-ALK (echinoderm microtubule associated protein-like 4-anaplastic lymphoma kinase) translocations are sensitive to ALK kinase inhibitors.[74-76] EML4-ALK is found almost exclusively in LADC.

So, it is very important to subclassify NSCLCs into adenocarcinoma and SCC for the benefit of patients to receive therapy with low adverse effect and high therapeutic response and for further diagnostic workup, i.e. analysis of EGFR mutation and ALK rearrangement.

Immunochemistry: Immunochemistry can be done on alcohol-fixed cytology smears or cell blocks. The IHC done on cell blocks offers better results.

Use of Immunochemical Stains to Distinguish LADC and SCC

In those cases, where a specimen shows NSCLC lacking either definite squamous or adenocarcinoma morphology, immunochemistry may refine the diagnosis. Most of the studies recommend use of panel of antibodies rather than a single antibody to increase sensitivity and specificity. There are several markers for LADC and SCC with different sensitivity and specificity.

TTF-1: Thyroid transcription factor 1 is a 38-kDa homeodomain protein that shows nuclear specific staining. It regulates gene expression in the thyroid, lungs, and

Table 4 Proposed IASLC/ATS/ERS classification of lung cancer for small biopsies/cytology[62]

2004 WHO classification	*Small biopsy/cytology: IASLC/ATS/ERS*
Adenocarcinoma Mixed subtype Acinar Papillary Solid	*Morphologic adenocarcinoma patterns clearly present:* Adenocarcinoma, describe identifiable patterns present (including micropapillary pattern not included in 2004 WHO classification) *Comment*: If pure lepidic growth—mention an invasive component cannot be excluded in this small specimen
Bronchioloalveolar carcinoma (nonmucinous)	Adenocarcinoma with lepidic pattern (if pure, add note: an invasive component cannot be excluded)
Bronchioloalveolar carcinoma (mucinous)	Mucinous adenocarcinoma (describe patterns present)
Fetal	Adenocarcinoma with fetal pattern
Mucinous (colloid)	Adenocarcinoma with colloid pattern
Signet ring	Adenocarcinoma with (describe patterns present) and signet ring features
Clear cell	Adenocarcinoma with (describe patterns present) and clear cell features
No 2004 WHO counterpart—most will be solid adenocarcinomas	*Morphologic adenocarcinoma patterns not present (supported by special stains)*: Non-small cell carcinoma, favor adenocarcinoma
Squamous cell carcinoma Papillary Clear cell Small cell Basaloid	*Morphologic squamous cell patterns clearly present*: Squamous cell carcinoma
No 2004 WHO counterpart	*Morphologic squamous cell patterns not present (supported by stains)*: Non-small cell carcinoma, favor squamous cell carcinoma
Small cell carcinoma	Small cell carcinoma
Large cell carcinoma	Non-small cell carcinoma, not otherwise specified (NOS)
Large cell neuroendocrine carcinoma (LCNEC)	Non-small cell carcinoma with neuroendocrine (NE) morphology (positive NE markers), possible LCNEC
Large cell carcinoma with NE morphology (LCNEM)	Non-small cell carcinoma with NE morphology (negative NE markers)—see comment *Comment*: This is a non-small cell carcinoma where LCNEC is suspected, but stains failed to demonstrate NE differentiation
Adenosquamous carcinoma	*Morphologic squamous cell and adenocarcinoma patterns present*: Non-small cell carcinoma, with squamous cell and adenocarcinoma patterns *Comment*: This could represent adenosquamous carcinoma
No counterpart in 2004 WHO classification	Morphologic squamous cell or adenocarcinoma patterns not present but immunostains favor separate glandular and adenocarcinoma components Non-small cell carcinoma, NOS, (specify the results of the immunohistochemical stains and the interpretation) *Comment*: This could represent adenosquamous carcinoma
Sarcomatoid carcinoma	Poorly differentiated NSCLC with spindle and/or giant cell carcinoma (mention if adenocarcinoma or squamous carcinoma are present)

Abbreviation: IASLC/ATS/ERS, International Association of the Study of Lung Cancer/American Thoracic Society/European Respiratory Society

diencephalon during embryogenesis. It is normally expressed in alveolar pneumocytes, Clara cells, ciliated respiratory epithelial cells, and basal cells of the lung.[77,78] The use of TTF-1 has been well established for differentiation between primary and metastatic LADC of lung.[79] *TTF-1* is a nuclear stain which is reported in 87% of LADC and 2% of SCC.

p63: p63 is a member of the p53 family, located on chromosome 3q27–29. It is involved in the regular growth and development of epithelial tissue. In normal tissues, p63 has been reported to be positive in basal cells of all squamous epithelia, in basal cells of urothelium, and in basal cells of prostate epithelium.[80,81] p63 is detectable in most SCCs of various primary sites, including SCCs of lung, with reported

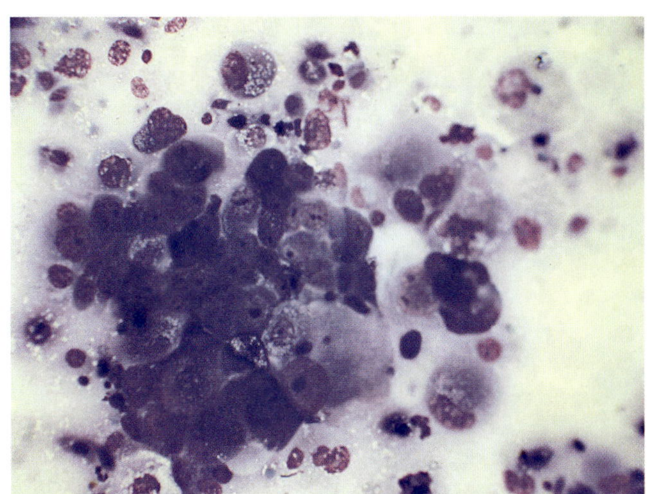

Fig. 12 Loosely cohesive cluster of malignant cells with moderate amount of vacuolated cytoplasm, coarse chromatin and prominent nucleoli (MGG, 100x)

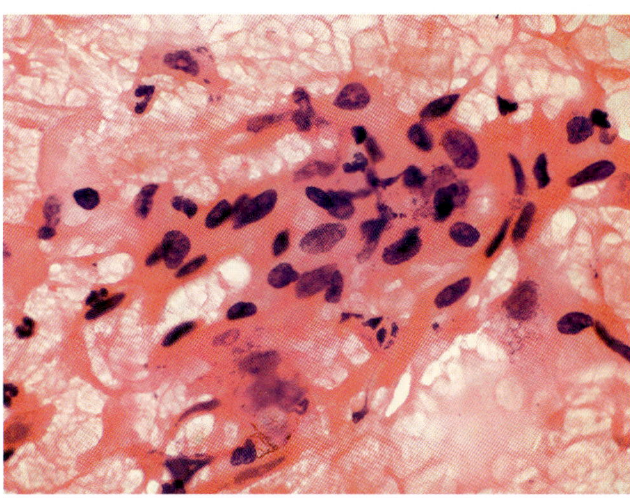

Fig. 13 Keratinized highly pleomorphic squamous cells with irregular shapes and staining reactions with many spindle shaped cells (H&E, 40x)

positivity of 80–97% in most studies. In the lung, however, p63 has been shown to have some overlap in LADCs, with reported positivity in up to 18%.[80-82] To correctly interpret p63, only nuclear staining should be considered as positive.

Cytokeratins: Cytokeratins are intermediate filament cytoskeletal proteins essential to development and differentiation of epithelial cells. Approximately, twenty different cytokeratins have been identified and are classified and numbered according to molecular weight and isoelectric points. In general, most low molecular weight cytokeratins (40-54 kDa) are distributed in non-squamous epithelium, Moll's catalog numbers 7-8 and/or 17-20. High molecular weight cytokeratins (48-67 kDa) are found in the squamous epithelium, Moll's catalog numbers 1-6 and/or 9-16. *Cytokeratin 7* is one of the basic type II cytokeratins and is found in most glandular epithelia and in transitional epithelia. Anti-CK7 is valuable as a histodiagnostic tool for the subtyping of various carcinomas and tumors of epithelial origin.

Cytokeratins 5/6 are related proteins that can be detected in normal cells, including breast myoepithelial cells, prostate basal cells, and the basal layer of the epidermis and salivary glands. Positive IHC staining displays a membranous staining pattern. Marson et al.[83] described positive staining in 100% of primary lung SCCs.

There are number of studies done with panel of IHC markers to differentiate adenocarcinoma and SCC. Use of six-antibody panel consists of (Napsin A, Desmoglein 3, TTF-1, CK5/6, p63 and tripartite motif-containing 29) in one study[84] classified 96% and 87% of moderately and poorly differentiated lung cancer, respectively.

Napsin A is a cytoplasmic stain that is relatively specific for LADC and stains approximately 80% of cases. A dual staining for TTF-1 and Napsin A has been shown in LADC cell blocks in previous reports.[85]

Immunohistochemistry panel: Thrombomodulin (CD141), p63, 34βE12 and CK5/6 have been shown to be sensitive markers for SCC. TTF-1 and Napsin A are considered to be specific markers for LADC **(Figs 14A to D)**. The coexpression of p63 and CK5 has high sensitivity with 100% specificity for SCC **(Figs 15A to D)**. Therefore, a preferred panel of immunostains comprising of TTF-1, p63, CK5/6, CK7 and Napsin A should provide high specificity and sensitivity in differentiating SCC versus LADC.

EPIDERMAL GROWTH FACTOR RECEPTOR MUTATION ANALYSIS

The presence of mutations in exons 18–21, deletions in exon 19 (52%) and a missense mutation L858R in exon 21 (26%) are the most predominant. Mutations in the TK domain of EGFR are common in most NSCLC in Asian population.[86] The most common mutation seen in about 46% cases with EGFR mutations is a short in-frame deletion of 9, 12, 15, 18, or 24 nucleotides in exon 19. The second common mutation, seen in about 43% of cases with EGFR mutations, is a point mutation (CTG to CGG) in exon 21 at nucleotide 2573, that results in substitution of leucine by arginine at codon 858 (L858R). EGFR molecular testing on cytology samples can well be done with availability of cell blocks. Depending on the methods used, authors in previous reports were able to detect these mutations in cytologic material containing as little as 0.1–10% of tumor cells or in specimens containing at least 100 tumor cells. Failure of EGFR molecular testing on cytology samples ranges from 2% to 8% to approximately a quarter of cases in some studies. The latter failure rates are more likely

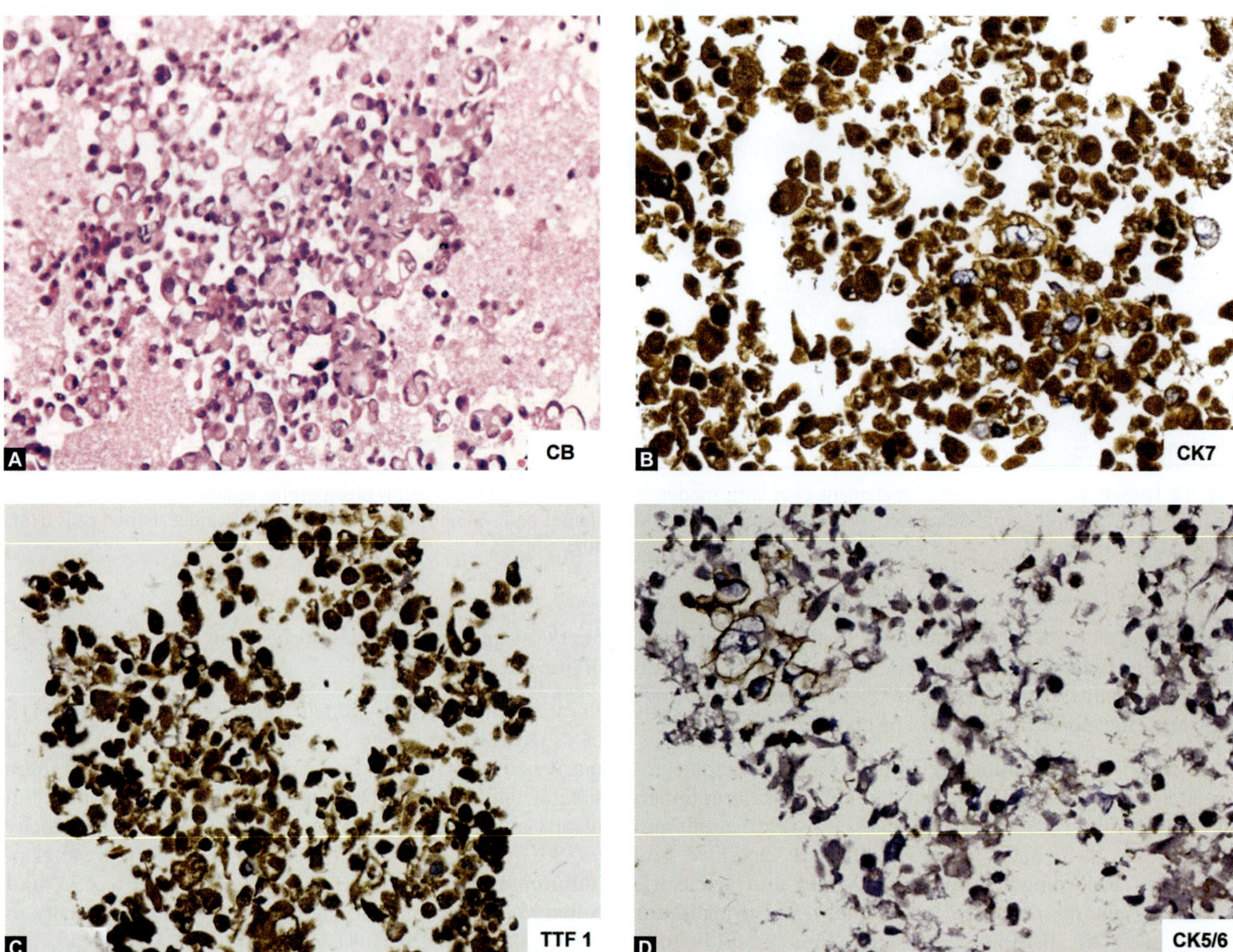

Figs 14A to D A panel of microphotographs of LADC: (A) Dispersed population of atypical cells with eccentrically placed nuclei (MGG, 40x); (B) Strong nuclear positivity for TTF-1 (TTF-1, 100x); (C) Cytoplasmic positivity for CK7 (CK7, 100x); (D) Tumor cells negative for CK5/6 (CK5/6, 40x)

to be technique dependent. The main reasons for test failure in cytology samples are scant cellularity and necrotic tissue.[87]

Epidermal Growth Factor Receptor Mutation by Immunochemistry

Recent reports have shown that immunochemistry using monoclonal antibodies specific to exon 19 E746-A750 (15bp) deletion and exon 21 L858R mutation is available. These antibodies were used on cytology samples (FNA and effusion fluid), small biopsies, cell blocks, LBC samples and resection specimens.[87] IHC with these antibodies can be used as a screening method for EGFR mutations and all negative cases can be sent for molecular analysis to confirm mutation status.

Echinoderm Microtubule-associated Protein-like 4-Anaplastic Lymphoma Kinase Rearrangement Testing

The *EML4-ALK* fusion gene is present in approximately 5% of LADC. Patients with the EML4-ALK fusion gene do not harbor *EGFR* or *KRAS* mutations, hence demonstrating mutual exclusion of these mutations. FISH using break-apart probes is the gold standard for the detection of EML4-ALK. It has been suggested in previous reports that due to relatively high cost, limited availability and technical complexity of FISH, IHC can be done as screening method and FISH may be reserved for cases with equivocal results. Sakairi et al.[88] examined 109 specimens obtained by endobronchial ultrasound-transbronchial needle aspiration (EBUS-TBNA)

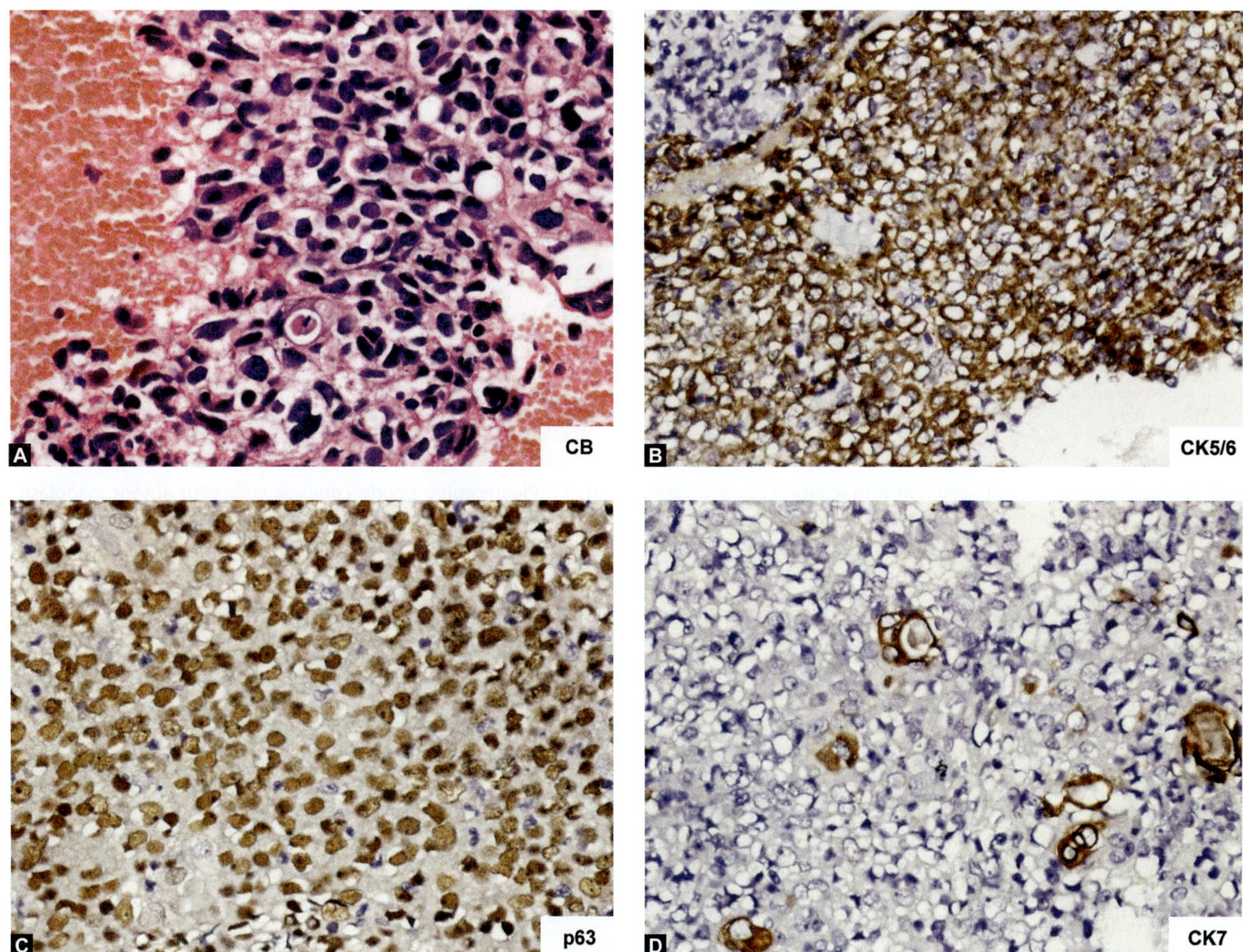

Figs 15A to D A panel of microphotographs of lung SCC: (A) Cell block of SCC (H&E, 40x); (B) Cytoplasmic positivity for CK5/6 (CK5/6, 40x); (C) Strong nuclear positivity for p63 (p63, 40x); (D) Tumor cells negative for CK7 (CK7, 40x)

and found that material obtained was adequate for *ALK* fusion gene assessment by IHC, FISH and reverse transcription polymerase chain reaction (RT-PCR). Cell block can provide persevered cytology material for such studies including IHC, FISH and RT-PCR.

FLUORESCENCE IN-SITU HYBRIDIZATION IN RESPIRATORY CYTOLOGY

Fluorescence in-situ hybridization is the gold standard to identify ALK rearrangements for treatment with the ALK inhibitor Crizotinib. FISH can be applied to almost all types of cytologic specimens such as conventional smears, Cytospins, or LBC preparations and cell blocks.

Large Cell Carcinoma

Most of these tumors occur in men and are associated with smoking. These grow rapidly and have poor prognosis. These types of tumors yield irregular groups and dispersed population of obviously malignant cells. The texture of nucleus is finely granular with gray blue cytoplasm. The cells are generally in groups and consist of cell population with large irregular, single nucleus or multinucleation may be seen. The diagnosis of large cell carcinoma should not be offered on small biopsies/cytology samples and should only be reserved for resection specimens.[62]

Some cases of NSCLC may suggest neuroendocrine morphology; these cases should be subjected to neuroendocrine markers (CD56, Chromogranin, and/Synaptophysin),

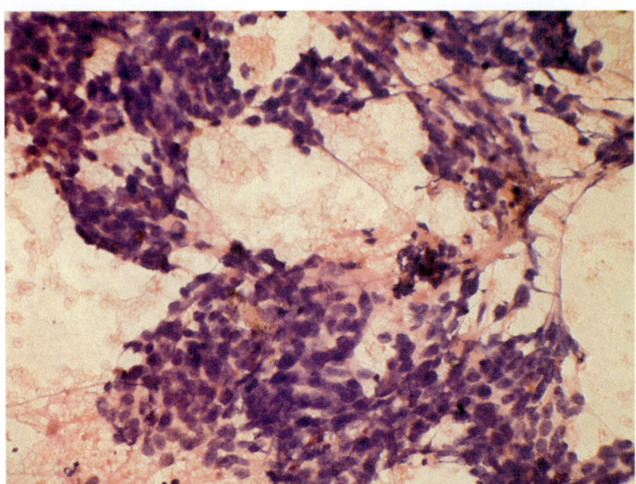

Fig. 16 Poorly cohesive small-sized cells with scanty or no cytoplasm and prominent crushing artifact (H&E, 40x)

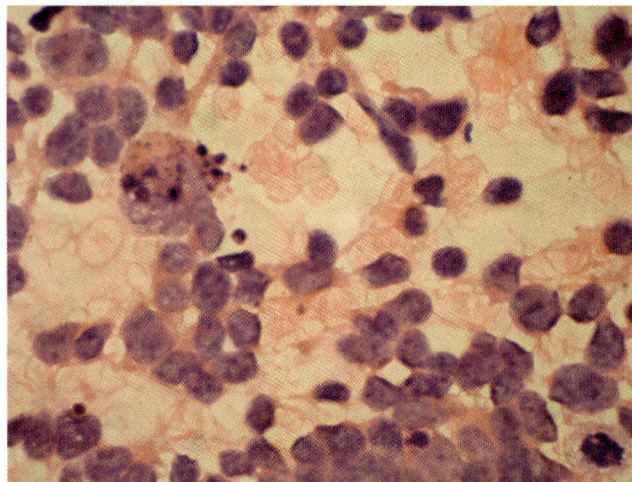

Fig. 17 Pleomorphic poorly cohesive cells with absent cytoplasm, nuclear molding, tear drop cells and inconspicuous nucleoli (H&E, 100x)

so that a diagnosis of large cell neuroendocrine carcinoma (LCNEC) can be suggested.[62]

Small Cell Carcinoma

It is thought to arise from primitive cells that have the capacity for Kulchitsky (neuroendocrine) cell differentiation. Small cell carcinoma has the strongest relationship to cigarette smoking and rarely occurs in nonsmokers.[89,90] Small cell carcinoma is usually centrally located. The tumor characteristically metastasizes extensively to hilar and mediastinal lymph nodes.[91] FNAC is accurate and reliable in the diagnosis of small cell carcinoma.[92,93]

The aspirated material is abundant and semisolid. The smears are thick and the cells are easily traumatized. The cells have superficial resemblance to lymphocytes but are large round to oval or elongated. They form clusters and have classical tendency towards molding. Crushing artifact is quite characteristic of small cell carcinoma in FNA biopsy specimens **(Figs 16 and 17)**. Small cell carcinoma usually demonstrates features of neuroendocrine origin immunocytochemically, including neuron-specific enolase, neurofilament proteins, synaptophysin, Leu-7, and sometimes chromogranin, and may also be positive for keratin.[94]

The differential diagnosis includes a carcinoid, poorly differentiated squamous and adenocarcinoma, non-Hodgkin's lymphoma or malignant small blue round cell tumors.

Carcinoid Tumor

Carcinoid tumor accounts for about 5% of cases of lung cancer.

Central carcinoid tumor usually presents with a slow-growing polypoid mass within a major bronchus, can be non-hormone producing tumor, and some produce carcinoid syndrome. It is common in young adults and children. Infiltration in the surrounding tissues from the bronchus may occur. Cytologically, it shows a loosely cohesive population of monotonous cells **(Fig. 18)**.[95] Rosettes, palisades, or small clusters may also be seen. If there is extensive crush artifact, confusion with small cell carcinoma may occur.

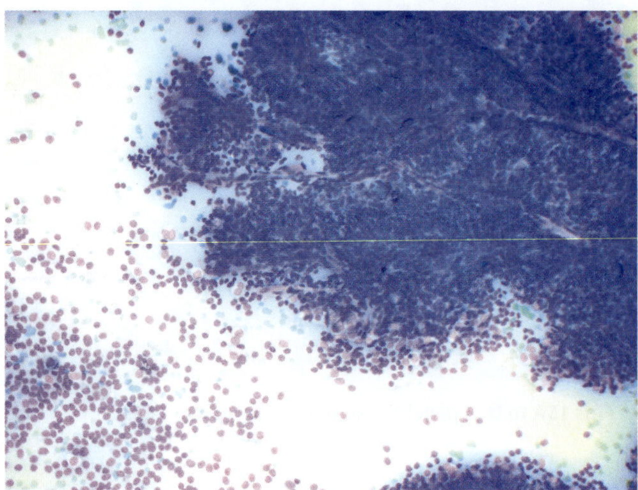

Fig. 18 A highly cellular smear showing tumor cells with prominent pericapillary arrangement and dispersed population of monomorphic tumor cells (MGG, 10x)

Metastases to regional lymph nodes are occasionally reported in about 5% cases. Rarely metastases in bones occur which are of osteoblastic type. Surgery is the treatment of choice and the prognosis is excellent. Oncocytic carcinoid is a variant of central carcinoid in which the tumor cells have abundant, granular acidophilic cytoplasm. Electron

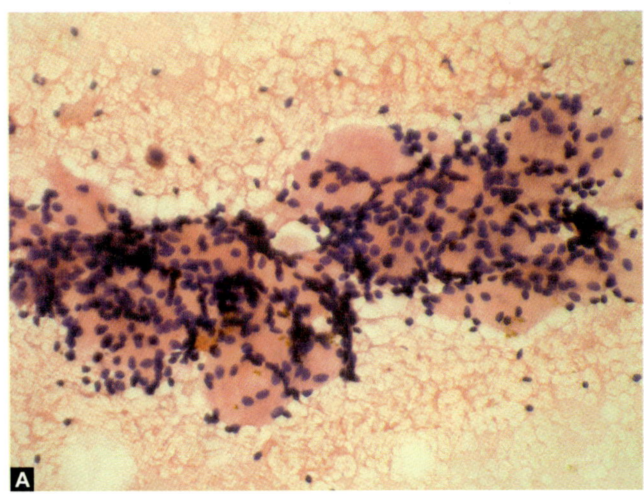
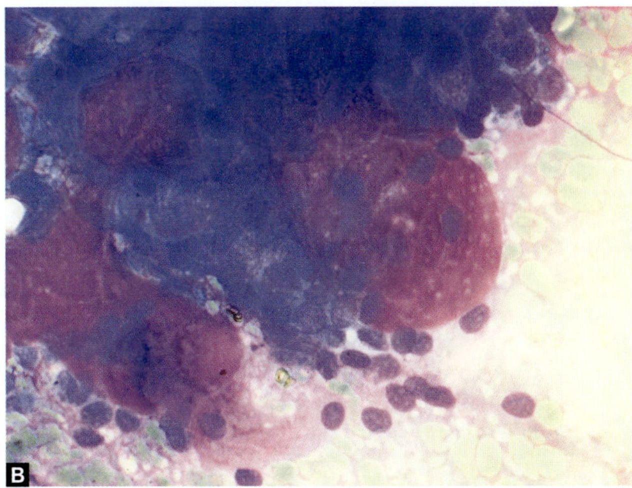

Figs 19A and B (A) Small uniform cells with hyperchromatic nuclei embedded in hyaline stromal globules in a case of adenoid cystic carcinoma (PAP, 40x); (B) Tumor cells embedded in metachromatically staining hyaline stromal globules (MGG, 100x)

microscopy (EM) shows numerous mitochondria with dense core secretory granules.

Peripheral carcinoid tumor usually occurs in peripheral lung beneath pleura and is discovered incidentally. Peripheral carcinoids tend to be more aggressive than central carcinoids, especially when the tumor is composed of spindle cells.[96] Pleomorphism and mitosis are present. The prognosis is excellent after surgical removal.

Atypical carcinoid tumor: This type of tumor possibly represents a link between typical carcinoid tumor and small cell carcinoma. These have been associated with smoking.[97] Cytologically, the tumor cells are larger than those of either typical carcinoid or small cell carcinoma **(Figs 19A and B)**. Single cells are present with atypical features, like increased mitosis, necrosis and nuclear hyperchromasia. Extensive metastasis occurs in lymph nodes. The behavior is aggressive.

Pulmonary Hamartoma

Hamartoma accounts for about 75% of benign lung tumors. It is usually solitary and presents as an asymptomatic clear cut small shadow just beneath the pleura in the lung parenchyma. Radiologically, calcification is seen which may be of popcorn type. Cytologically, the key diagnostic feature is the presence of cartilaginous or fibromyxoid fragments. Immature cartilage, or fibromyxoid matrix, characteristically has wispy, frayed, or irregularly feathered outlines **(Fig. 20)**. It stains variably, but is usually basophilic in Pap and intensely metachromatic (magenta) in Diff-Quik.[98,99]

Grossly, it is sharply delineated and lobulated. Cut surface shows glistening cartilage with cleft. Microscopy shows cartilage, fat, smooth muscle and the clefts are lined by respiratory epithelium. The cartilage may be calcified or ossified. The lesion is acquired and represents primary overgrowth of mesenchymal tissues with secondary entrapment of bronchial epithelium. The treatment is conservative surgery in the form of wedge resection.

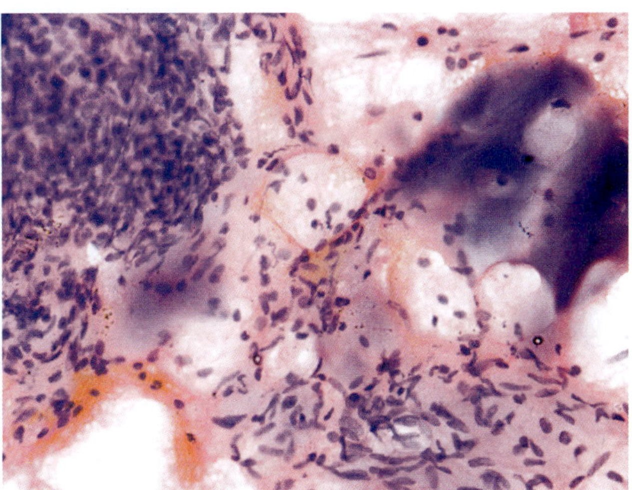

Fig. 20 Chondroid and adipose tissue fragments along with bland spindle shaped cells and scattered benign epithelial cells in pulmonary hamartoma (H&E, 40x)

Inflammatory Pseudotumor

Inflammatory pseudotumors are a quite rare and include fibroxanthoma (xanthogranuloma) and plasma cell granuloma. These are mostly asymptomatic, slow-growing, well-circumscribed, small peripheral lung masses.[100] Cytological features are nonspecific and may show admixture of plasma cells, lymphocytes, eosinophils, neutrophils, mast cells, histiocytes, and myofibroblasts,[101] which can be seen in varying proportions. The stroma can be edematous to myxoid to fibrous to hyalinized. Excision is curative.

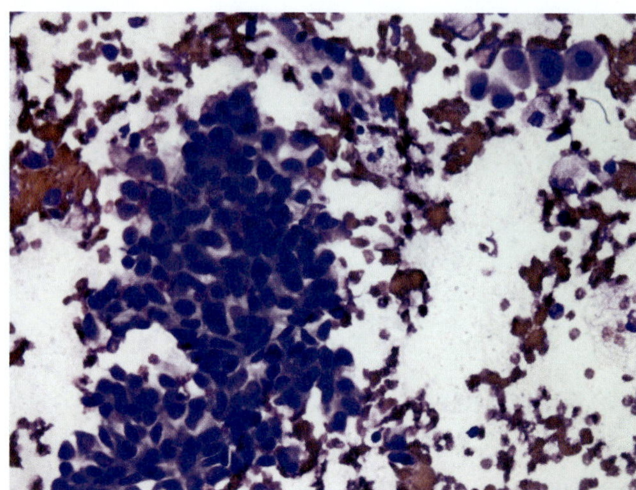

Fig. 21 Sheets and single oval to spindle cells in a bloody background with histiocytes in a case of sclerosing hemangioma (MGG, 40x)

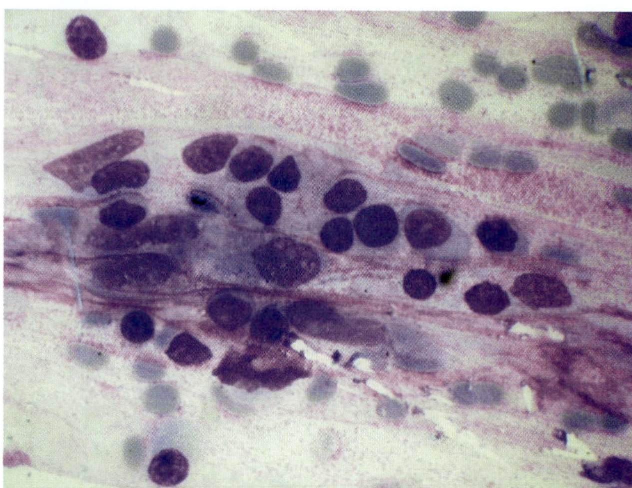

Fig. 22 A biphasic epithelial and spindle cell pattern in a case of pulmonary blastoma (MGG, 100x)

Sclerosing Hemangioma (Type II Pneumocytoma)

It is a rare, benign tumor of the lung. This occurs frequently in women (4:1). This tumor is usually solitary and located near the pleura with a predilection for the lower lobes. Cytosmears show abundant material in the form of sheets or single cells in a bloody background. Finding is aggregates of cells surrounding small blood vessels or sclerotic cores is characteristic **(Fig. 21)**.[102]

Salivary Gland Analog Tumors

These probably arise from submucosal bronchial glands, the pulmonary counterpart of minor salivary glands. Mostly occur in the main bronchi.

Adenoid cystic carcinoma is the most common tumor which usually occurs in a major bronchus. On FNAC, smears show bland, uniform cells, with scant cytoplasm.[103] The cells can be present singly or form tight, globular, honeycomb arrangements. The characteristic feature is the presence of mucoid (basement membrane) material, which is seen as rounded, acellular balls or cylinders, sometimes surrounded by tumor cells **(Figs 19A and B)**.

This material is transparent and lightly cyanophilic in Papanicolaou, but is brightly metachromatic (magenta) in Diff-Quik.

Mucoepidermoid carcinoma (MEC) of the lung can be high or low grade. On FNAC, the smears may show variable numbers of three cell types: (1) mucus-secreting glandular cells, (2) squamous cells and (3) intermediate cells.

Pulmonary Blastoma

Pulmonary blastoma is also known as peripheral carcinosarcoma of embryonal type, or embryoma and can occur at any age. The average age of diagnosis is about 40 years with male to female ratio being 3:1. This is usually located peripherally, but is rarely found intrabronchially. Microscopically, the tumor is reminiscent of fetal lung, the pulmonary counterpart of Wilms' tumor. FNAC shows a biphasic epithelial and spindle cell growth pattern **(Fig. 22)**. The cells of the epithelial component are cuboidal to columnar and may be present in sheets, acini, or three-dimensional glandular structures. The cytoplasm usually contains glycogen vacuoles, which may give the cells a clear appearance. The nuclei are round to variable depending on the degree of differentiation of the tumor. The sarcomatous component is usually cellular or myxoid malignant stroma composed of monotonous, small spindle mesenchymal cells (blastemal cells). The nuclei are slightly irregular with fine chromatin and indistinct nucleoli and scant cytoplasm.[104]

The differential diagnosis includes small cell carcinoma, large cell undifferentiated carcinoma or sarcoma, and the features sometimes overlap with those of carcinosarcoma.

Carcinosarcoma: This tumor usually occurs in adults, on average 10–20 years later than pulmonary blastomas. Most cases of carcinosarcoma are located centrally and have a worse prognosis. FNAC shows a biphasic pattern of epithelial and spindle elements. The cells tend to be more intermixed and in majority of these tumors, the epithelial component is represented by non-keratinizing SCC, but can also be adenocarcinoma or undifferentiated carcinoma.[105] The sarcomatous component is usually resembles a fibrosarcoma or malignant fibrous histiocytoma. Occasionally, foci of chondrosarcoma, osteosarcoma, rhabdomyosarcoma, or angiosarcoma may be seen and osteoclastic giant cells may also be present.[106] The differential diagnosis includes SCC, non-small cell carcinoma, large cell undifferentiated carcinoma, giant cell carcinoma, and pure sarcoma.[107]

Lymphoma: The lymphomas arising in the respiratory tract are rare. The mediastinum is more often involved. The primary lymphoma of this area can be diagnosed by cytological examination or FNAC. The criteria applied are same as described for other organs. The cells in lymphomas are monomorphic, round and sometimes with anaplastic features. Primary Hodgkin's disease is exceedingly rare; however, the metastatic lesions are more often seen.

Vascular Tumors

These tumors in lung are extremely rare and include hemangioma, hemangiopericytoma, angiosarcoma, lymphangioma and epithelioid hemangioendothelioma. Epithelioid hemangioendothelioma presents as multiple nodules. Cytologically, the smears may be hemorrhagic and may show loosely cohesive clusters of plump acidophilic endothelial cells. The tumor grows in slow fashion and remains restricted to thoracic cavity. The subtyping of these tumors is difficult in cytology because of compromised aspirated material in majority of cases and considerable cytomorphological overlap.

Primitive Neuroectodermal Tumor

The term primitive neuroectodermal tumor (PNET) is used to include a variety of tumors which may include malignant small cell tumor of the thoracopulmonary region (Askin's tumor). The immunocytochemistry and immunophenotyping can be applied to these malignant tumors to categorize them.[108]

Fine-needle aspiration cytology smears show small cells in small clusters or discrete cells. The cells are small monotonous primitive cells with scanty cytoplasm. The nuclei are round to oval with inconspicuous nucleoli. Rosette formation is common feature **(Fig. 23)**. These rosettes may be focally present and careful search is required to locate them.

METASTASIS

Lung metastases develop in up to 50% of all patients dying of cancer. The most common sources of lung metastases are breast, colon, pancreas, stomach, melanoma, kidney **(Fig. 24)**, germ cell tumors[109] and sarcomas **(Fig. 25)**; however, almost any malignant tumor can metastasize to the lung.

Usually, the metastases are multiple and described as cannon-ball deposits. Both lung fields are usually involved by well delineated, multiple rapidly growing masses. Sometimes there are military nodules. Rarely, it may present as solitary nodule and may be mistaken for a primary tumor of lung. There are no reliable cytomorphological features that can distinguish primary from metastatic adenocarcinoma.[110] The

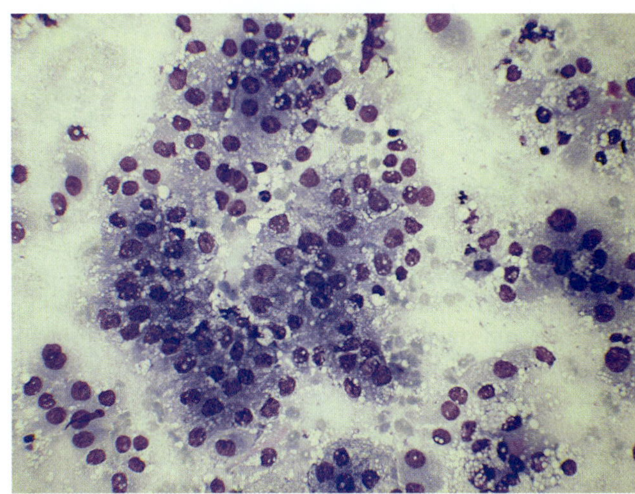

Fig. 24 A loosely cohesive clusters of tumor cells with low N:C ratio, abundant vacuolated to clear cytoplasm and conspicuous nucleoli in a case of metastatic renal cell carcinoma (H&E, 100x)

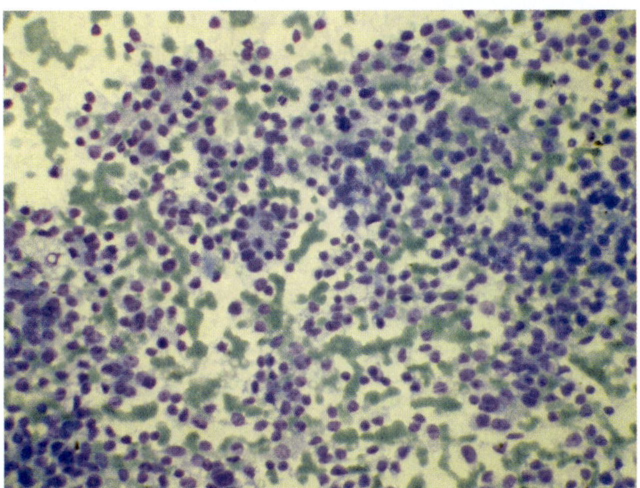

Fig. 23 Cellular smear with dispersed population of small round cells with coarse chromatin and occasional rosette formation in a case of Askin's tumor (MGG, 20x)

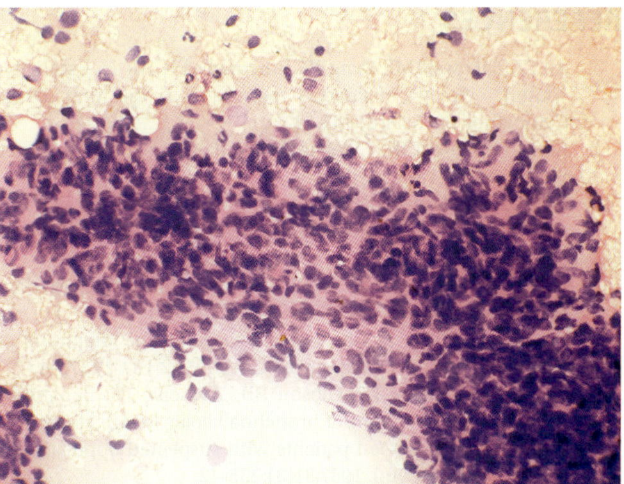

Fig. 25 Highly cellular smear with small fascicles of oval to spindle-shaped cells with blunt ends in a case of metastatic sarcoma (H&E, 20x)

Table 5 Immunocytochemistry of primary and metastatic tumors of lung

	TTFI/Napsin A	*CK7*	*CK20*	*PCEA*	*CD15*	*Others*
Lung adenocarcinoma	+	+	–	+	+	
Colon	–	–	+	+	+	
Breast	–	+	–	+	+	ER/PR+
Kidney	–	–	–	–	+	Vim + EMA +
Mesothelioma	–	+	–	–	–	Calretinin+ Vim+ CK5/CK6 +
Pancreas	–	+	+	+	+	CA 19-9 +
ALCL	–	–	–	–	–	LCA + CD30 + EMA +
Germ cell tumors Seminoma Nonseminoma	–	–	–	–	–	PLAP + CAM 5.2 – CAM 5.2 + EMA

Abbreviation: ALCL, anaplastic large cell lymphoma

cytology of few metastatic lesions is fairly characteristics, e.g. in malignant melanoma and renal cell carcinoma.

Finally, a clear distinction between NSCLC, including subgroups and small cell lung cancer, and between primary lung cancer and metastases has therapeutic impact, but the distinction may be difficult at times on smears. In case additional smears are not available, a cytoscape (CS) technique can be used on virtually any smear to produce material useful for ancillary methods, including IHC. The CS technique improves the diagnostic information from FNA in a clinically relevant way. Immunochemistry of primary and metastatic tumors of lung is shown in **Table 5**.

REFERENCES

1. Ali TZ, Zakowski MF, Yung RC, Burroughs FH, Ali SZ. Exfoliative sputum cytology of cancers metastatic to the lung. Diagn Cytopathol. 2005;33(3):147-51.
2. Erozan YS, Frost JK. Cytopathologic diagnosis of lung cancer. Semin Oncol. 1974;1(3):191-8.
3. Koss LG, Melamed MR, Goodner JT. Pulmonary cytology—a brief survey of diagnostic results from July 1st 1952 until December 31st, 1960. Acta Cytol. 1964;8:104-13.
4. Newman Dorland WA. The American Illustrated Medical Dictionary, 18th edition. USA: South Lyon, MI; 1938.
5. Pirozynski M. Bronchoalveolar lavage in the diagnosis of peripheral, primary lung cancer. Chest. 1992;102(2):372-4.
6. DeFine LA, Saleba KP, Gibson BB, Wesseler TA, Baughman R. Cytologic evaluation of bronchoalveolar lavage specimens in immunosuppressed patients with suspected opportunistic infections. Acta Cytol. 1987;31(3):235-42.
7. Richard A. Helmens, Hunninghake Gary W. Bronchoalveolar lavage. In: Ko Pen Wans (Ed). Biopsy techniques in pulmonary disorders. New York: Raven Press; 1989. pp. 15-28.
8. Behera D, D'Souza G, Rajwanshi A, Jindal SK. Bronchoalveolar lavage—cellular characteristics in patients with idiopathic pulmonary fibrosis and sarcoidosis. Indian J Chest Dis Allied Sci. 1990;32(2):107-10.
9. Khilnani GC, Hadda V. Lipoid pneumonia: an uncommon entity. Indian J Med Sci. 2009;63(10):474-80.
10. Marchand E, Cordier JF. Idiopathic chronic eosinophilic pneumonia. Orphanet J Rare Dis. 2006;1:11.
11. de Gracia J, Bravo C, Miravitlles M, Tallada N, Orriols R, Bellmunt J, et al. Diagnostic value of bronchoalveolar lavage in peripheral lung cancer. Am Rev Respir Dis. 1993;147(3):649-52.
12. Reynold HY. Bronchoalveolar lavage. Am Rev Respir Dis. 1987;135(1):250-63.
13. Diamantis A, Magiorkinis E, Koutselini H. Fine-needle aspiration (FNA) biopsy: historical aspects. Folia Histochem Cytobiol. 2009;47(2):191-7.
14. Rosa M. Fine-needle aspiration biopsy: a historical overview. Diagn Cytopathol. 2008;36(11):773-5.
15. Nordenström B. New instruments of biopsy. Radiology. 1975;117(2):474-5.
16. Söderström N. Cytologic clinical puncture-biopsy. Lakartidningen. 1966;63(26):2497-503.
17. Tscheikuna J, Suttinont P. Is cytology necessary in diagnosis of mediastinal mass? J Med Assoc Thai. 2009;92(Suppl 2):S24-9.
18. Ko Pen Wang. Flexible bronchoscopy with transbronchial needle aspiration biopsy for cytology specimens. In: Ko Pen Wans (Ed). Biopsy Techniques in Pulmonary Disorders. New York: Raven Press; 1989. pp. 73-80.
19. Rajwanshi A, Jayaram N, Behera D, Gupta SK, Malik SK. Fine needle aspiration cytology of intrathoracic lesions—a repraisal. Indian J Pathol Microbiol. 1989;32(4):306-9.
20. Gupta D, Gulati M, Rajwanshi A. Fluoroscopic transbronchial fine needle aspiration for diagnosis of peripheral pulmonary nodules. Indian J Chest Dis Allied Sci. 1996;38(3):163-7.
21. Halloush RA, Khasawneh FA, Saleh HA, Soubani AO, Piskorowski TJ, Al-Abbadi MA. Fine needle aspiration cytology

of lung lesions: a clinicopathological and cytopathological review of 150 cases with emphasis on the relation between the number of passes and the incidence of pneumothorax. Cytopathology. 2007;18(1):44-51.
22. Abati A, Landucci D, Danner RL, Solomon D. Diagnosis of pulmonary microvascular metastases by cytologic evaluation of pulmonary artery catheter-derived blood specimens. Hum Pathol. 1994;25(3):257-62.
23. Popp W, Rauscher H, Ritschka L, Redtenbacher S, Zwick H, Dutz W. Diagnostic sensitivity of different techniques in the diagnosis of lung tumors with the flexible fiberoptic bronchoscope. Comparison of brush biopsy, imprint cytology of forceps biopsy, and histology of forceps biopsy. Cancer. 1991;67(1):72-5.
24. Kramer H, van Putten JW, Douma WR, Smidt AA, van Dullemen HM, Groen HJ. Technical description of endoscopic ultrasonography with fine-needle aspiration for the staging of lung cancer. Respir Med. 2005;99(2):179-85.
25. Annema JT, Veseliç M, Rabe KF. EUS-guided FNA of centrally located lung tumours following a non-diagnostic bronchoscopy. Lung Cancer. 2005;48(3):357-61.
26. Larsen SS, Vilmann P, Krasnik M, Dirksen A, Clementsen P, Skov BG, et al. Endoscopic ultrasound guided biopsy versus mediastinoscopy for analysis of paratracheal and subcarinal lymph nodes in lung cancer staging. Lung Cancer. 2005;48(1):85-92.
27. Caddy G, Conron M, Wright G, Desmond P, Hart D, Chen RY. The accuracy of EUS-FNA in assessing mediastinal lymphadenopathy and staging patients with NSCLC. Eur Respir J. 2005;25(3):410-5.
28. Tournoy KG, Praet MM, Van Maele G, Van Meerbeeck JP. Esophageal endoscopic ultrasound with fine-needle aspiration with an on-site cytopathologist: high accuracy for the diagnosis of mediastinal lymphadenopathy. Chest. 2005;128(4):3004-9.
29. Ang TL, Tee AK, Fock KM, Teo EK, Chua TS. Endoscopic ultrasound-guided fine needle aspiration in the evaluation of suspected lung cancer. Respir Med. 2007;101(6):1299-304.
30. Eckardt J, Petersen HO, Hakami-Kermani A, Olsen KE, Jørgensen OD, Licht PB. Endobronchial ultrasound-guided transbronchial needle aspiration of undiagnosed intrathoracic lesions. Interact Cardiovasc Thorac Surg. 2009;9(2):232-5.
31. Herth FJ, Krasnik M, Kahn N, Eberhardt R, Ernst A. Combined endoscopic-endobronchial ultrasound-guided fine-needle aspiration of mediastinal lymph nodes through a single bronchoscope in 150 patients with suspected lung cancer. Chest. 2010;138(4):790-4.
32. Rintoul RC, Skwarski KM, Murchison JT, Wallace WA, Walker WS, Penman ID. Endobronchial and endoscopic ultrasound-guided real-time fine-needle aspiration for mediastinal staging. Eur Respir J. 2005;25(3):416-21.
33. Peric R, Schuurbiers OC, Veseliç M, Rabe KF, van der Heijden HF, Annema JT. Transesophageal endoscopic ultrasound-guided fine-needle aspiration for the mediastinal staging of extrathoracic tumors: a new perspective. Ann Oncol. 2010;21(7):1468-71.
34. Rajwanshi A, Bhambhani S, Das DK. Fine-needle aspiration cytology diagnosis of tuberculosis. Diagn Cytopathol. 1987;3(1):13-6.
35. Roger V, Nasiell M, Nasiell K, Hjerpe A, Enstad I, Bisther A. Cytologic findings indicating pulmonary tuberculosis. II. The occurrence in sputum of epithelioid cells and multinucleated giant cells in pulmonary tuberculosis, chronic non-tuberculous inflammatory lung disease and bronchogenic carcinoma. Acta Cytol. 1972;16(6):538-42.
36. Tani EM, Schmitt FC, Oliveira ML, Gobetti SM, Decarlis RM. Pulmonary cytology in tuberculosis. Acta Cytol. 1987;31(4): 460-3.
37. Nasiell M, Roger V, Nasiell K, et al. Cytologic Findings Indicating Pulmonary Tuberculosis: I. The Diagnostic Significance of Epithelioid Cells and Langhans' Giant Cells Found in Sputum or Bronchial Secretions. Acta Cytol. 1972;16:146-51.
38. Das DK, Bhambhani S, Pant JN, et al. Superficial and Deep-Seated Tuberculous Lesions: Fine-Needle Aspiration Cytology Diagnosis of 574 Cases. Diagn Cytopathol. 1992;8:211-5.
39. Granados R, Constantine NM, Cibas ES. Nasal Scrape Cytology in the Diagnosis of Wegener's Granulomatosis: A Case Report. Acta Cytol. 1994;38:463-6.
40. Miles PR, Baughman RP, Linnemann CC Jr. Cytomegalovirus in the Bronchoalveolar Lavage Fluid of Patients with AIDS. Chest. 1990;97:1072-6.
41. Gordon SM, Gal AA, Hertzler GL, Bryan JA, Perlino C, Kanter KR. Diagnosis of pulmonary toxoplasmosis by bronchoalveolar lavage in cardiac transplant recipients. Diagn Cytopathol. 1993;9(6):650-4.
42. Hsu CY. Cytologic diagnosis of pulmonary cryptococcosis in immunocompetent hosts. Acta Cytol. 1993;37(5):667-72.
43. Wheeler RR, Bardales RH, North PE, Vesole DH, Tricot G, Stanley MW. Toxoplasma pneumonia: cytologic diagnosis by bronchoalveolar lavage. Diagn Cytopathol. 1994;11(1):52-5.
44. Peña Griñan N, Muñoz Lucena F, Vargas Romero J, Alfageme Michavila I, Umbria Dominguez S, Florez Alia C. Yield of percutaneous needle lung aspiration in lung abscess. Chest. 1990;97(1):69-74.
45. Palmer DL, Davidson M, Lusk R. Needle aspiration of the lung in complex pneumonias. Chest. 1980;78(1):16-21.
46. Busmanis I, Harney M, Hellyar A. Nocardiosis diagnosed by lung FNA: a case report. Diagn Cytopathol. 1995;12(1):56-8.
47. Onuma K, Crespo MM, Dauber JH, Rubin JT, Sudilovsky D. Disseminated nocardiosis diagnosed by fine needle aspiration biopsy: quick and accurate diagnostic approach. Diagn Cytopathol. 2006;34(11):768-71.
48. Stanley MW, Deike M, Knoedler J, Iber C. Pulmonary mycetomas in immunocompetent patients: diagnosis by fine-needle aspiration. Diagn Cytopathol. 1992;8(6):577-9.
49. Dahlgren SE. Aspiration biopsy of intrathoracic tumours. Acta Pathol Microbiol Scand. 1967;70(4):566-76.
50. Sterrett G, Whitaker D, Glancy J. Fine-needle aspiration of lung, mediastinum, and chest wall. A clinicopathologic exercise. Pathol Annu. 1982;17(2):197-228.
51. Wallace JM, Batra P, Gong H Jr, Ovenfors CO. Percutaneous needle lung aspiration for diagnosing pneumonitis in the patient with acquired immunodeficiency syndrome (AIDS). Am Rev Respir Dis. 1985;131(3):389-92.
52. Granville LA, Laucirica R, Verstovsek G. Clinical significance of cultures collected from fine-needle aspiration biopsy. Diagn Cytopathol. 2008;36(2):85-8.
53. Ingram EA, Helikson MA. Echinococcosis (hydatid disease) in Missouri: diagnosis by fine-needle aspiration of a lung cyst. Diagn Cytopathol. 1991;7(5):527-31.
54. Krane JF, Renshaw AA. Relative value and cost-effectiveness of culture and special stains in fine needle aspirates of the lung. Acta Cytol. 1998;42(2):305-11.

55. Buchanan AJ, Gupta RK. Cytomegalovirus infection of the lung: cytomorphologic diagnosis by fine-needle aspiration cytology. Diagn Cytopathol. 1986;2(4):341-2.
56. Chaudhary S, Hughes WT, Feldman S, Sanyal SK, Coburn T, Ossi M, et al. Percutaneous transthoracic needle aspiration of the lung. Diagnosing *Pneumocystis carinii* pneumonitis. Am J Dis Child. 1977;131(8):902-7.
57. Nizzoli R, Tiseo M, Gelsomino F, Bartolotti M, Majori M, Ferrari L, et al. Accuracy of fine needle aspiration cytology in the pathological typing of non-small cell lung cancer. J Thorac Oncol. 2011;6(3):489-93.
58. Stewart CJ, Stewart IS. Immediate assessment of fine needle aspiration cytology of lung. J Clin Pathol. 1996;49(10):839-43.
59. Zakowski MF, Bibbo M. Lung carcinoma in the era of personalized medicine: the role of cytology. Acta Cytol. 2012;56(6):587-9.
60. Sanz-Santos J, Serra P, Andreo F, Llatjós M, Castellà E, Monsó E. Contribution of cell blocks obtained through endobronchial ultrasound-guided transbronchial needle aspiration to the diagnosis of lung cancer. BMC Cancer. 2012;12:34.
61. Noronha V, Dikshit R, Raut N, Joshi A, Pramesh CS, George K, et al. Epidemiology of lung cancer in India: focus on the differences between non-smokers and smokers: a single-centre experience. Indian J Cancer. 2012;49(1):74-81.
62. Travis WD, Brambilla E, Noguchi M, Nicholson AG, Geisinger KR, Yatabe Y, et al. International Association for the Study of Lung Cancer/American Thoracic Society/European Respiratory Society International multidisciplinary classification of lung adenocarcinoma. J Thorac Oncol. 2011;6(2):244-85.
63. Matthews MJ, Mackay B, Lukeman J. The pathology of non-small cell carcinoma of the lung. Semin Oncol. 1983;10(1):34-55.
64. Woolner LB, Fontana RS, Sanderson DR, Miller WE, Muhm JR, Taylor WF, et al. Mayo Lung Project: evaluation of lung cancer screening through December 1979. Mayo Clin Proc. 1981;56(9): 544-55.
65. Ciuleanu T, Brodowicz T, Zielinski C, Kim JH, Krzakowski M, Laack E, et al. Maintenance pemetrexed plus best supportive care versus placebo plus best supportive care for non-small-cell lung cancer: a randomised, double-blind, phase 3 study. Lancet. 2009;374(9699):1432-40.
66. Scagliotti G, Hanna N, Fossella F, Sugarman K, Blatter J, Peterson P, et al. The differential efficacy of pemetrexed according to NSCLC histology: a review of two Phase III studies. Oncologist. 2009;14(3):253-63.
67. Scagliotti GV, Parikh P, von Pawel J, Biesma B, Vansteenkiste J, Manegold C, et al. Phase III study comparing cisplatin plus gemcitabine with cisplatin plus pemetrexed in chemotherapy-naive patients with advanced-stage non-small-cell lung cancer. J Clin Oncol. 2008;26(21):3543-51.
68. Johnson DH, Fehrenbacher L, Novotny WF, Herbst RS, Nemunaitis JJ, Jablons DM, et al. Randomized phase II trial comparing bevacizumab plus carboplatin and paclitaxel with carboplatin and paclitaxel alone in previously untreated locally advanced or metastatic non-small-cell lung cancer. J Clin Oncol. 2004;22(11):2184-91.
69. Maemondo M, Inoue A, Kobayashi K, Sugawara S, Oizumi S, Isobe H, et al. Gefitinib or chemotherapy for non-small-cell lung cancer with mutated EGFR. N Engl J Med. 2010;362(25):2380-8.
70. Mitsudomi T, Morita S, Yatabe Y, Negoro S, Okamoto I, Tsurutani J, et al. Gefitinib versus cisplatin plus docetaxel in patients with non-small-cell lung cancer harbouring mutations of the epidermal growth factor receptor (WJTOG3405): an open label, randomised phase 3 trial. Lancet Oncol. 2010;11(2):121-8.
71. Mok TS, Wu YL, Thongprasert S, Yang CH, Chu DT, Saijo N, et al. Gefitinib or carboplatin-paclitaxel in pulmonary adenocarcinoma. N Engl J Med. 2009;361(10):947-57.
72. Rosell R, Carcereny E, Gervais R, Vergnenegre A, Massuti B, Felip E, et al. Erlotinib versus standard chemotherapy as first-line treatment for European patients with advanced EGFR mutation-positive non-small-cell lung cancer (EURTAC): a multicentre, open-label, randomised phase 3 trial. Lancet Oncol. 2012;13(3):239-46.
73. Zhou C, Wu YL, Chen G, Feng J, Liu XQ, Wang C, et al. Erlotinib versus chemotherapy as first-line treatment for patients with advanced EGFR mutation-positive non-small-cell lung cancer (OPTIMAL, CTONG-0802): a multicentre, open-label, randomised, phase 3 study. Lancet Oncol. 2011;12(8):735-42.
74. Sasaki T, Jänne PA. New strategies for treatment of ALK-rearranged non-small cell lung cancers. Clin Cancer Res. 2011;17(23):7213-8.
75. Shaw AT, Solomon B. Targeting anaplastic lymphoma kinase in lung cancer. Clin Cancer Res. 2011;17(8):2081-6.
76. Kwak EL, Bang YJ, Camidge DR, Shaw AT, Solomon B, Maki RG, et al. Anaplastic lymphoma kinase inhibition in non-small-cell lung cancer. N Engl J Med. 2010;363(18):1693-703.
77. Nakamura N, Miyagi E, Murata S, Kawaoi A, Katoh R. Expression of thyroid transcription factor-1 in normal and neoplastic lung tissues. Mod Pathol. 2002;15(10):1058-67.
78. Lau SK, Luthringer DJ, Eisen RN. Thyroid transcription factor-1: a review. App Immunohistochem Mol Morphol. 2002;10(2):97-102.
79. Ng WK, Chow JC, Ng PK. Thyroid transcription factor-1 is highly sensitive and specific in differentiating metastatic pulmonary from extrapulmonary adenocarcinoma in effusion fluid cytology specimens. Cancer. 2002;96(1):43-8.
80. Massion PP, Taflan PM, Jamshedur Rahman SM, Yildiz P, Shyr Y, Edgerton ME, et al. Significance of p63 amplification and overexpression in lung cancer development and prognosis. Cancer Res. 2003;63(21):7113-21.
81. Pelosi G, Pasini F, Olsen Stenholm C, Pastorino U, Maisonneuve P, Sonzogni A, et al. p63 immunoreactivity in lung cancer: yet another player in the development of squamous cell carcinomas? J Pathol. 2002;198(1):100-9.
82. Sheikh HA, Fuhrer K, Cieply K, Yousem S. p63 expression in assessment of bronchioloalveolar proliferations of the lung. Mod Pathol. 2004;17(9):1134-40.
83. Marson JV, Mazieres J, Groussard O, Garcia O, Berjaud J, Dahan M, et al. Expression of TTF-1 and cytokeratins in primary and secondary epithelial lung tumours: correlation with histological type and grade. Histopathology. 2004;45(2):125-34.
84. Tacha D, Yu C, Bremer R, Qi W, Haas T. A 6-antibody panel for the classification of lung adenocarcinoma versus squamous cell carcinoma. App Immunohistochem Mol Morphol. 2012;20(3):201-7.
85. Fatima N, Cohen C, Lawson D, Siddiqui MT. TTF-1 and Napsin A double stain: a useful marker for diagnosing lung adenocarcinoma on fine-needle aspiration cell blocks. Cancer Cytopathol. 2011;119(2):127-33.
86. Sahooa R, Harini VV, Babu VC, Patil Okaly GV, Rao S, Nargunda A, et al. Screening for EGFR mutations in lung cancer, a report from India. Lung Cancer. 2011;73(3):316-9.

87. Moreira AL, Hasanovic A. Molecular characterization by immunocytochemistry of lung adenocarcinoma on cytology specimens. Acta Cytol. 2012;56(6):603-10.
88. Sakairi Y, Nakajima T, Yasufuku K, Ikebe D, Kageyama H, Soda M, et al. EML4-ALK fusion gene assessment using metastatic lymph node samples obtained by endobronchial ultrasound-guided transbronchial needle aspiration. Clin Cancer Res. 2010;16(20):4938-45.
89. Hoffman PC, Albain KS, Bitran JD, Golomb HM. Current concepts in small cell carcinoma of the lung. CA Cancer J Clin. 1984;34(5):269-81.
90. Stayner LT, Wegman DH. Smoking, occupation, and histopathology of lung cancer: a case-control study with the use of the Third National Cancer Survey. J Natl Cancer Inst. 1983;70(3):421-6.
91. Sinner WN, Sandstedt B. Small-cell carcinoma of the lung. Cytological, roentgenologic, and clinical findings in a consecutive series diagnosed by fine-needle aspiration biopsy. Radiology. 1976;121(2):269-74.
92. Johnston WW. Percutaneous fine needle aspiration biopsy of the lung. A study of 1,015 patients. Acta Cytol. 1984;28(3):218-24.
93. Mitchell ML, King DE, Bonfiglio TA, Pattern SF Jr. Pulmonary fine needle aspiration cytopathology. A five-year correlation study. Acta Cytol. 1984;28(1):72-6.
94. Tabatowski K, Vollmer RT, Tello JW, Iglehart JD, Shelburne JD, Schlom J, et al. The use of a panel of monoclonal antibodies in ultrastructurally characterized small cell carcinomas of the lung. Acta Cytol. 1988;32(5):667-74.
95. Suen KC, Quenville NF. Fine needle aspiration cytology of uncommon thoracic lesions. Am J Clin Pathol. 1981;75(6):803-9.
96. Bonikos DS, Bensch KG, Jamplis RW. Peripheral pulmonary carcinoid tumors. Cancer. 1976;37(4):1977-98.
97. Warren WH, Faber LP, Gould VE. Neuroendocrine neoplasms of the lung. A clinicopathologic update. J Thorac Cardiovasc Surg. 1989;98(3):321-32.
98. Hamper UM, Khouri NF, Stitik FP, Siegelman SS. Pulmonary hamartoma: diagnosis by transthoracic needle-aspiration biopsy. Radiology. 1985;155(1):15-8.
99. Saqi A, Shaham D, Scognamiglio T, Murray MP, Henschke CI, Yankelevitz D, et al. Incidence and cytological features of pulmonary hamartomas indeterminate on CT scan. Cytopathology. 2008;19(3):185-91.
100. Matsubara O, Tan-Liu NS, Kenney RM, Mark EJ. Inflammatory pseudotumors of the lung: progression from organizing pneumonia to fibrous histiocytoma or to plasma cell granuloma in 32 cases. Hum Pathol. 1988;19(7):807-14.
101. Thunnissen FB, Arends JW, Buchholtz RT, ten Velde G. Fine needle aspiration cytology of inflammatory pseudotumor of the lung (plasma cell granuloma). Report of four cases. Acta Cytol. 1989;33(6):917-21.
102. Krishnamurthy SC, Naresh KN, Soni M, Bhasin SD. Sclerosing hemangioma of the lung: a potential source of error in fine needle aspiration cytology. Acta Cytol. 1994;38(1):111-2.
103. Nguyen GK. Cytology of bronchial gland carcinoma. Acta Cytol. 1988;32(2):235-9.
104. Francis D, Jacobsen M. Pulmonary blastoma. Preoperative cytologic and histologic findings. Acta Cytol. 1979;23(6):437-42.
105. Cagle PT, Alpert LC, Carmona PA. Peripheral biphasic adenocarcinoma of the lung: light microscopic and immunohistochemical findings. Hum Pathol. 1992;23(2):197-200.
106. Takeda S, Nanjo S, Nakamoto K, Imachi T, Yamamoto S. Carcinosarcoma of the lung. Report of a case and review of the literature. Respiration. 1994;61(2):113-6.
107. Ro JY, Chen JL, Lee JS, Sahin AA, Ordóñez NG, Ayala AG. Sarcomatoid carcinoma of the lung. Immunohistochemical and ultrastructural studies of 14 cases. Cancer. 1992;69(2):376-86.
108. Akhtar M, Iqbal MA, Mourad W, Ali MA. Fine-needle aspiration biopsy diagnosis of small round cell tumors of childhood: A comprehensive approach. Diagn Cytopathol. 1999;21(2):81-91.
109. Brahmi U, Rajwanshi A, Joshi K, Dey P, Vohra H, Ganguly NK, et al. Flow cytometric immunophenotyping and comparison with immunocytochemistry in small round cell tumors. Analyt Quant Cytol Histol. 2001;23(6):405-12.
110. Arabi H, Shah M, Saleh H. Aspiration biopsy cytomorphology of primary pulmonary germ cell tumor metastatic to the brain. Diagn Cytopathol. 2009;37(10):715-9.

Bronchoscopy

R Narasimhan, AR Gayathri

INTRODUCTION

Endoscopic visualization of the tracheobronchial tree has evolved tremendously from the initial rigid technique originally described by Gustav Killian **(Fig. 1)** in 1867,[1] when an aspirated pork bone was removed from the right main bronchus, to the path breaking invention of the flexible fiberoptic bronchoscope by Professor Ikeda, in the 1960s. Over the subsequent years, newer technologies have been developed and introduced, such as the color video camera by Ikeda and Ono in 1971, bronchoalveolar lavage (BAL) by Reynolds in 1974, video endoscope by Ikeda in 1987, stents by Dumon in 1989 and endobronchial ultrasound (EBUS) by Becker in 1999. The bronchoscopic practice is now widespread in India.[2] More interventional procedures are being done for both diagnostic and therapeutic purposes.

TYPES OF BRONCHOSCOPY

Rigid Bronchoscopy

The procedure is performed under general anesthesia in the supine position with hyperextended neck, using a rigid bronchoscope (usually a ventilating bronchoscope), visualization is made better with the use of various telescopes and circumferential illumination **(Fig. 2)**. Once the preliminary examination is done, the various diagnostic and therapeutic interventions (e.g. stent insertion, laser ablation, dilatation, foreign body removal) can be carried out.[3] The introduction of charge coupled device (CCD) cameras, help in the transmission of images on to the monitors.

Flexible Fiberoptic Bronchoscopy

The flexible fiberoptic bronchoscopy has the advantage over the rigid bronchoscopy technique because it is easy to manipulate, simple to use, does not require general anesthesia and can be done as an outdoor procedure. Various sizes of bronchoscopes are available, which include the ultrathin bronchoscope (for the visualization of neonatal and smaller airways), pediatric bronchoscopes (2.8 mm outer diameter and 1.2 mm working channel), adult bronchoscopes (outer diameters ranging from 4.9 to 6.0 mm and channel sizes of at least 2.0 mm) and therapeutic bronchoscopes (outer diameter 6.0 mm and working channel of 2.8 mm). The video bronchoscope helps in the better visualization of lesions and data storage.

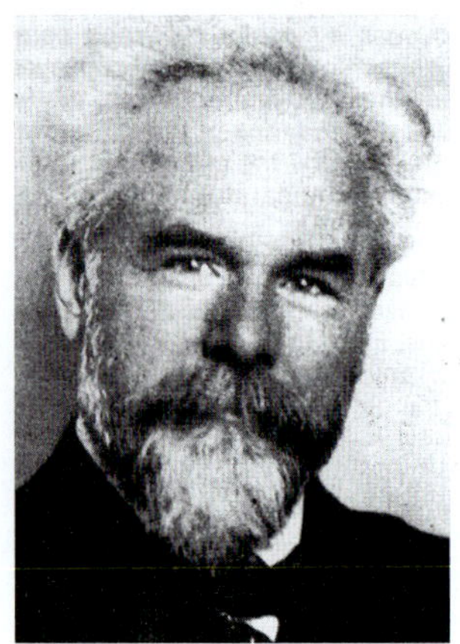

Fig. 1 Gustav Killian

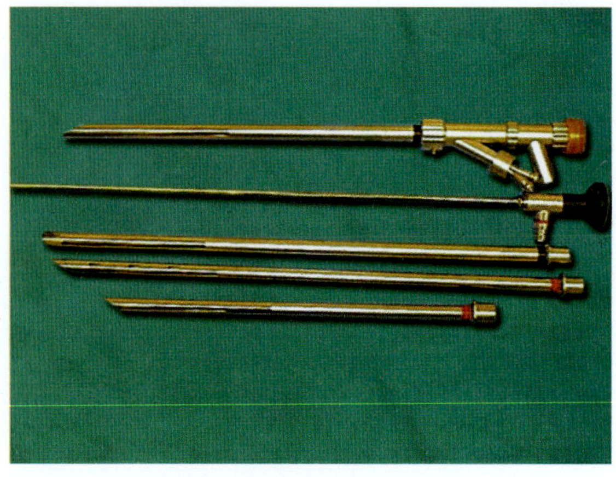

Fig. 2 Rigid bronchoscope

PATIENT PREPARATION AND ANESTHESIA

General and systemic examination of the patient is mandatory. Any medical condition especially cardiac or pulmonary should be identified and appropriate measures should be taken. There are varying opinions with regard to the use of sedation and premedication, prior to the procedure. In our series of patients undergoing transbronchial lung biopsy (TBLB), there was no administration of either premedication or sedation, the patient comfort and cooperation for the procedure were found to be excellent.[4] Several bronchoscopists favor the use of sedation for routine bronchocopies.[5-7] With more interventional procedures being performed the world over, short-acting benzodiazepines (e.g. midazolam) and fentanyl are commonly used. The performance of an effective bronchoscopy requires the use of appropriate local anesthetics. Either 2% or 4% lidocaine is used, mainly for the fast onset of action, wide safety margin and the long duration of action. There is a word of caution with regard to the toxicity due to the amount of local anesthetic used, in view of a high systemic absorption of local anesthetic agent from the nasal passages and tracheobronchial tree because of the high vascularity of those regions. It is therefore, essential to know the amount of lignocaine of the formulation used **(Table 1)**, so as not to exceed the recommended maximum single dose of lidocaine (4.0 mg/kg).

DIAGNOSTIC BRONCHOSCOPY—ACCESSORIES

The working channel of the bronchoscope is designed to allow the use of various diagnostic and therapeutic accessories.

Biopsy Forceps

The alligator and the cupped forceps **(Fig. 3)** are the two principle types of blade design. Alligator forceps have a greater tissue tearing action than its cupped counterpart **(Fig. 4)**. However, it is the cupped forceps, which obtains the larger sample size. Despite these facts, neither type of forceps has been shown to have a greater diagnostic accuracy than the other.[5] A forceps with a needle **(Fig. 5)** helps to prevent slippage and allows for the performance of tangential biopsies.

Table 1 Lignocaine content in various formulations

	Each mL of 2% lidocaine	*Each mL of 4% lidocaine*	*Xylocaine viscous*	*Lidocaine topical aerosol 15% - each actuation*
Lidocaine hydrochloride IP	21.3 mg	42.7 mg	21.3 mg	7.5 mg

Bronchial Brushes

The bronchial brush consists of a central rigid wire surrounded at the tip by brushes, only 0.001 m of specimen is collected during bronchial brushings. The material has to be immediately transferred on to a slide (for cytology sampling) and either sprayed with a fixative or immersed in a slide container of 95% absolute ethyl alcohol.

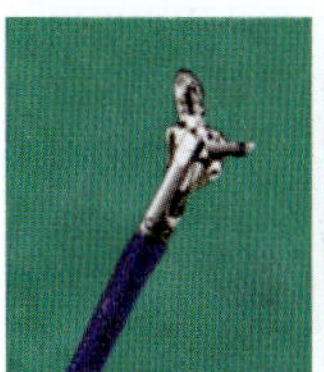
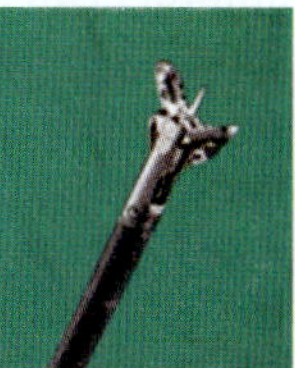
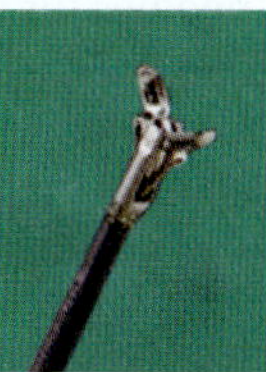
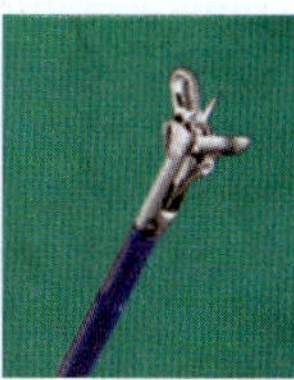

Fig. 3 Types of biopsy forceps

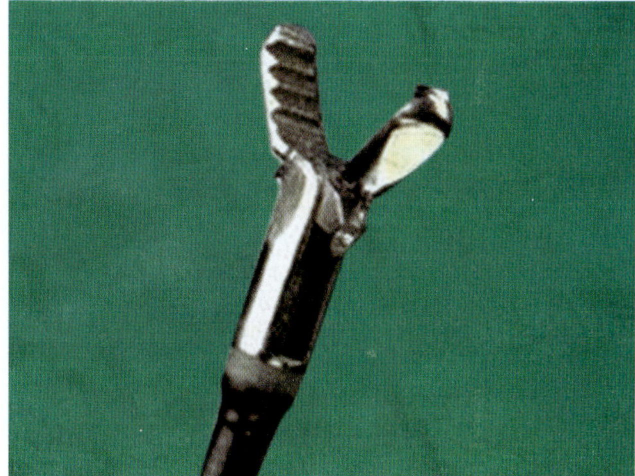

Fig. 4 Alligator forceps

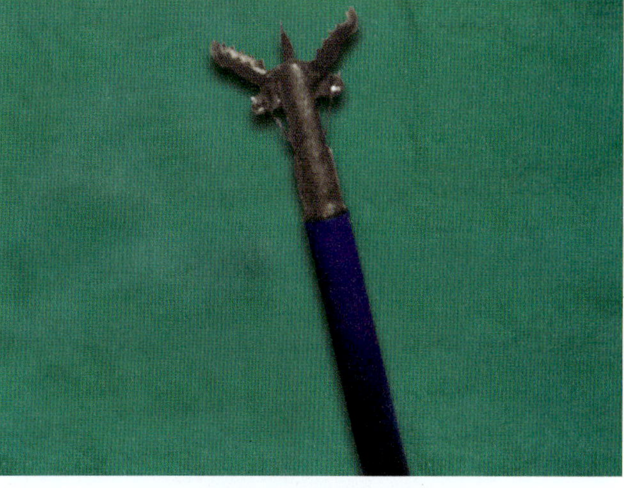

Fig. 5 Needle forceps

For microbiological analysis, the brush has to be agitated in 5–10 mL of sterile saline. The yield of the bronchoscopic brushing procedure increases with the proper method, collection and processing of the samples. It has also been found to be a superior technique in comparison to BAL in the diagnosis and morphological typing of lung cancer.[6]

Transbronchial Needles for Aspiration and Biopsy

Transbronchial needles for aspiration (TBNA) is a minimally invasive, nonsurgical technique by which the diagnosis and staging of bronchogenic carcinoma can be done by sampling the mediastinal lymph nodes. In addition, it is useful for accessing peripheral lesions, submucosal and endobronchial lesions, as well as for the sampling of intrathoracic lymph nodes.[7] There are two types of needles available—the cytology needle and the histology needle. Four insertion techniques have been described as follows:

1. The jabbing technique
2. The piggyback method
3. Hub-against-the-wall method
4. The cough method.[8]

The major complication of TBNA is the perforation of the working channel of the bronchoscope. This can be avoided by careful attention to technique and needle position.

Catheters and Balloons

Selective, protected catheters are available to collect uncontaminated specimens from the bronchial tree. The balloons available are either double lumened or low-pressure balloon catheters.

INDICATIONS FOR DIAGNOSTIC BRONCHOSCOPY

Bronchoscopy is one of the most important investigation for the diagnosis of a large number of clinical conditions and their evaluation **(Table 2)**.

Assessment of Airway Anatomy

The bronchoscopic assessment of the airways begins with the visualization of the upper airways and with special reference to the vocal cords **(Fig. 6)**, their appearance and mobility. The inspection of the lower airways is done with specific regard to their normal anatomy, anatomical variations and pathological involvement. Specific inspection of the airway lumen can be done during inspiratory and expiratory movements. Congenital, post-traumatic, postsurgical and/or pathological disruptions in the integrity of the bronchial lumen can be visualized, e.g. bronchoesophageal fistula **(Fig. 7)**.

Assessment of Tracheobronchial Mucosa

The normal mucosa of the tracheobronchial tree is pale-pink **(Fig. 8)**. The presence of changes like hypervascularity **(Fig. 9)**, ulcerations and granulation tissue point towards the pathological involvement. The use of photosensitizers has been used for cancer detection. The laser imaging fluorescence endoscope (LIFE), which is used in autofluorescence bronchoscopy, generates images which are about 30,000 more times powerful than images taken with usual endoscopic cameras, by which the detection and

Table 2 Indications for diagnostic bronchoscopy

Bronchogenic carcinoma
• Diagnosis
• Staging
• Follow-up after treatment
Other malignancies
• Evaluation of esophageal cancer
• Metastatic carcinoma
• Mediastinal mass
Mediastinal lymph nodes
Interstitial lung disease
Chronic cough
Wheeze–localized
Stridor
Infections
• Nonresolving pneumonias
• Immunocompromised host
• In critical care unit patients
Lung collapse
Vocal cord paralysis
Foreign body aspiration
Chest trauma
Pleural effusion
Superior vena cava syndrome
S/P lung transplantation
Fistula
• Bronchopleural
• Tracheoesophageal
• Bronchoesophageal
Postoperative evaluation following lung surgeries
Tracheal stenosis and strictures
Inhalational injury

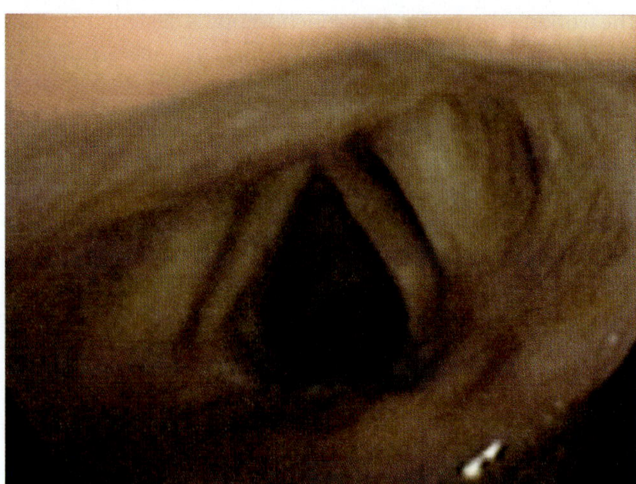

Fig. 6 Vocal cords

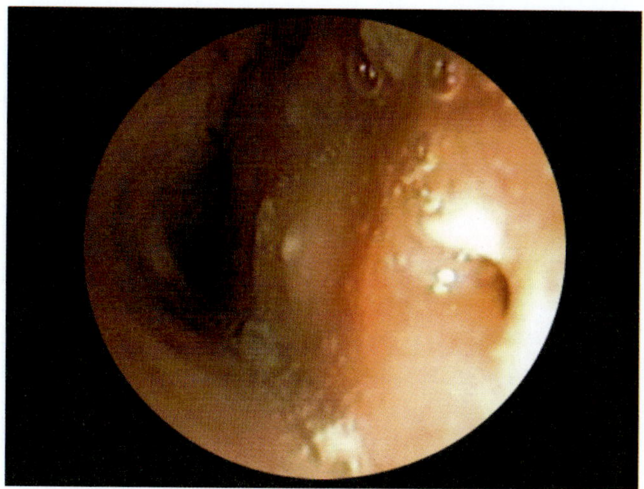

Fig. 7 Fistula between left main bronchus and esophagus

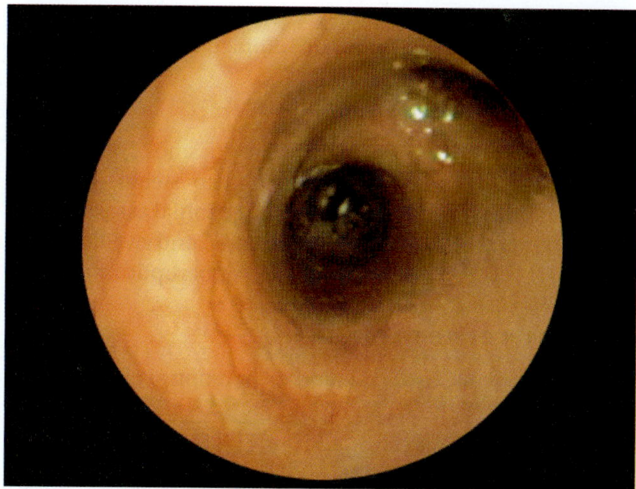

Fig. 9 Hypervascularity of bronchial mucosa

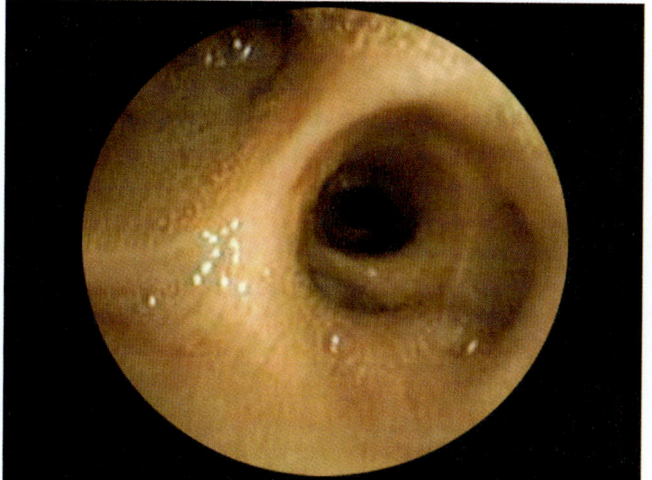

Fig. 8 Normal bronchial mucosa

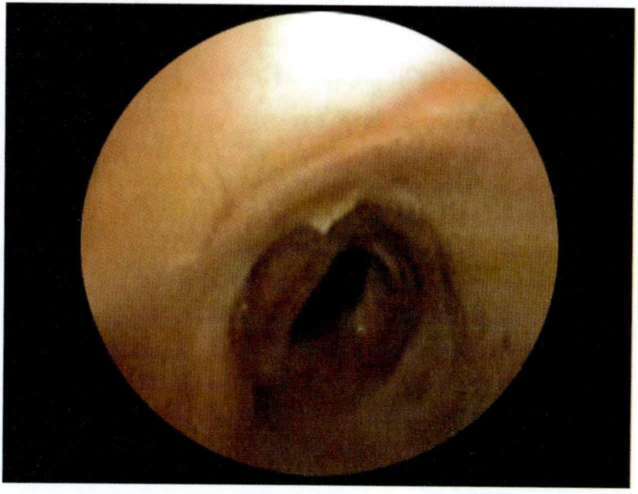

Fig.10 Tracheal stenosis of lower one-third of trachea

subsequent biopsy of lesions leads to the early diagnosis of dysplasia and carcinoma *in situ*. Optical coherence tomography (OCT), is a technique similar to ultrasound imaging, uses infrared rather than acoustic waves.

Evaluation of Cough

Bronchoscopy is one of the recommended investigations in evaluation of patients with chronic cough especially when there is a change in the character of the cough and with an association of smoking.

Evaluation of Wheezing

Lesions like foreign bodies, tracheomalacia, vascular abnormalities, tracheal stenosis **(Fig. 10)**, extrinsic or intrinsic tracheal obstructions due to mass lesions may present clinically with wheeze and may require further evaluation by bronchoscopy.

Evaluation of Stridor

Stridor is a life-threatening sign of upper airway obstruction. Prior to the evaluation of likely causes (in adults), such as infections, Wegener's granulomatosis, bilateral vocal cord paralysis, tracheal tumors, tracheal compression due to mediastinal and esophageal lesions, the bronchoscopist must ensure that adequate facilities are available for emergency intubation and tracheotomy, if required.

Evaluation of the Hoarseness of Voice

It has been found that 36% of vocal cord paralysis were due to neoplastic diseases of which, 55% were from lung cancer.[9]

Left hilar lesions, which may contribute to left recurrent laryngeal nerve paralysis may be sampled by TBNA.

Evaluation of Inhalational Injury

Inhalational injuries may occur due to smoke inhalation, toxin exposure or thermal injury due to steam or superheated air. Bronchoscopy is done for the initial assessment of inflammation, mucosal edema, ulceration and swelling of the laryngeal airway. It can also be used for fiberoptic intubation.

Evaluation of Hemoptysis

Bronchoscopy in the evaluation of hemoptysis helps in the identification of the location and source of bleeding. Early bronchoscopy (within 48 hours) has a greater diagnostic yield than late bronchoscopy, but an overall impact of timing on the patient management has not been found.[10] Though the rigid bronchoscope has better control of the airways and greater suction capacity, the flexible fiberoptic bronchoscope makes visualization of the smaller airways possible.

Evaluation of Superior Vena Cava Syndrome

TBNA of the mediastinal masses or lymph nodes causing superior vena cava syndrome (SVCS) can be done. Diagnosis can be established by bronchoscopic biopsy in about 60–70% of cases.[11]

Evaluation of Peribronchial Structures

The changes, pathological or developmental, of the mediastinal structures and their effects on the tracheobronchial tree can be appreciated through bronchoscopy **(Fig. 11)**. Procedures like TBNA and transbronchial needle biopsy (TBNB) can be done to sample the mediastinal lymph nodes. Diagnosis and staging of lung cancer is an important indication of TBNA. The use of rapid onsite evaluation (ROSE) of TBNA samples, where a cytopathologist is present in or near the bronchoscopy suite, ensures that the material is prepared in the best possible manner, with improvement in yield, and reduction in the number of inadequate specimens. It also avoids the need for further sampling, if the samples are satisfactory. Use of methods like computed tomography (CT) fluoroscopy, EBUS and electromagnetic guidance, increase the yield of TBNA. Newer generation EBUS bronchoscopes allow for concurrent lymph node visualization and performance of TBNA.

Evaluation of Interstitial Lung Disease

Procedures like BAL have been found to be useful in studying the cells causing inflammatory response in idiopathic pulmonary fibrosis (IPF). Use of BAL and bronchoscopic lung biopsy (BLB) have increased the diagnostic yield in diffuse parenchymal conditions such as sarcoidosis, histiocytosis X and lymphangitis carcinomatosa.

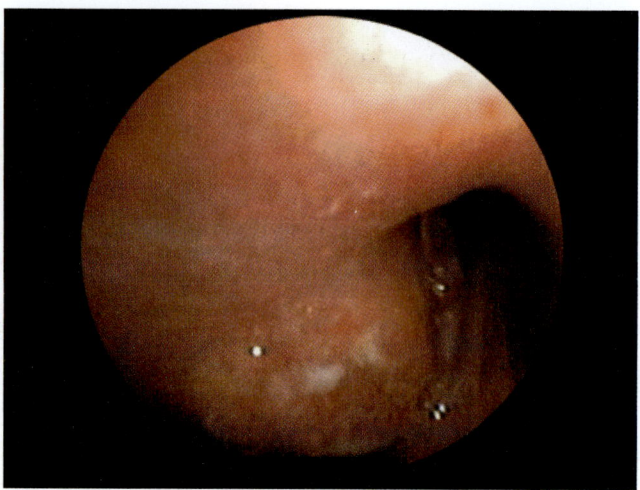

Fig. 11 Right hilar lymph node eroding into bronchial lumen

Evaluation of Infections

Bronchoscopy with BAL is a safe method of sampling the lower respiratory tract secretions. Bronchoscopy is more likely to have a better yield if the radiological infiltrates have been present for more than 30 days, are multilobar or segmental and if the patient is less than 55 years of age.[12]

Evaluation of Lobar Collapse

The yield of diagnostic bronchoscopy is highest, when lobar collapse is being investigated, up to 65% of patients undergoing bronchoscopy for lobar collapse had endobronchial masses.[13]

Evaluation of Pleural Effusions

Presence of hemoptysis, cough, a parenchymal lesion in addition to the pleural effusion, increase the yield of bronchoscopy in pleural effusion.

Evaluation of Chest Trauma

In patients with both blunt and penetrating thoracic trauma, bronchoscopy is an essential tool to assess the airway damage. It is also useful for fiberoptic intubation of patients, as well as to deal with post-trauma complications like mucous plugging and aspiration.

Evaluation of Lung Masses

Lung masses, especially those which present with endobronchial lesions **(Figs 12 to 14)** can be visualized through the bronchoscope and biopsied with forceps. Three to four samples have been found to be sufficient for diagnosis.[14] The use of a combination of sampling techniques, including wash, brush, forceps and TBNA have shown to increase the yield of the diagnosis of bronchogenic carcinoma.[15]

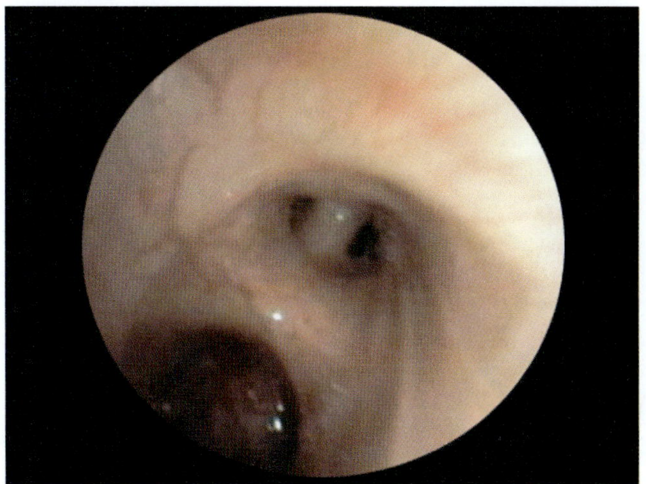

Fig. 12 Endobronchial mass occluding right bronchus intermedius

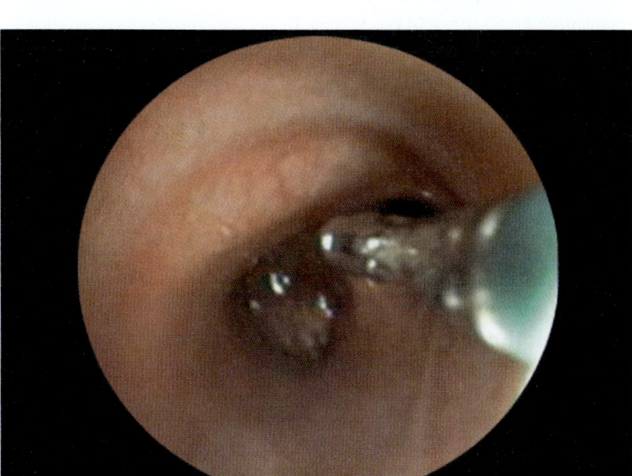

Fig. 13 Endobronchial mass in right bronchus intermedius being biopsied

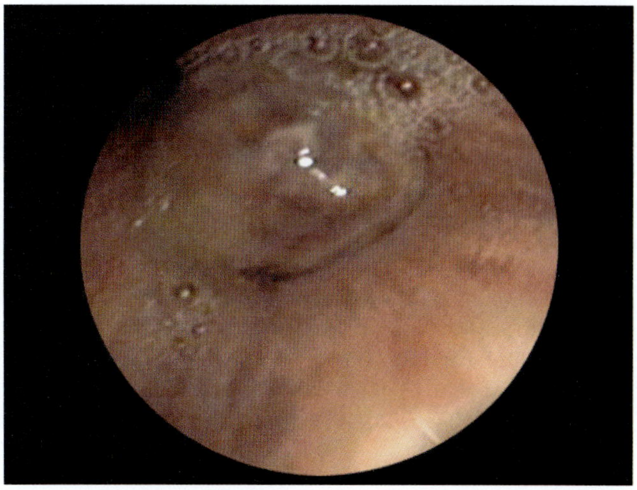

Fig. 14 Endobronchial mass in right lower lobe common basal segment

Table 3 Contraindications to bronchoscopic lung biopsy (BLB)

Absolute contraindications
1. Inability of patient to cooperate with the procedure
2. Inability to undergo general anesthesia (when required) for obtaining BLB
3. Unstable cardiovascular status
4. Acute severe asthma
5. Severe hypoxemia
6. Inadequately trained bronchoscopist or bronchoscopy team
7. Inadequate instruments for procedure performance
Relative contraindications
1. Uncontrollable cough, during procedure
2. Untreated hemorrhagic diathesis
3. Advanced renal failure
4. Significant hypoxemia in a patient with single lung
5. Extensive bullous changes in areas to biopsied
6. Radiological suggestion of vascular malformations adjacent to areas to be biopsied

Evaluation in Lung Transplantation

Bronchoscopy plays a valuable role in patients undergoing lung transplantation. It is useful in evaluating the presence and treatment of various airway complications like infection and stenosis, and also to differentiate between rejection and infection.

DIAGNOSTIC PROCEDURES

Bronchoscopic Lung Biopsy

Bronchoscopic lung biopsy is the technique by which biopsy of the lung parenchyma can be obtained by either the rigid or the flexible fiberoptic bronchoscope. It is also referred to as transbronchial or BLB. Although found to be useful in diffuse parenchymal diseases, its use has generally declined.

The use of CT imaging in the diagnosis of diffuse lung disease has lead to a decrease in the number of bronchoscopic lung biopsies. Moreover, there are several contraindications for BLB **(Table 3)**.[16] EBUS has shown promise in accessing peripheral pulmonary nodules, may even throw light on differences in the nodule architecture of malignant and benign lesions.

Pulmonary hypertension has been considered as a contraindication to BLB, but no significant difference was found in post-BLB complications in the patients of interstitial lung disease with latent pulmonary hypertension in comparison to those patients without pulmonary hypertension.[17]

Sampling of Airway and Alveolar Constituents

The techniques used for sampling the tracheobronchial tree include the bronchial washing, bronchial brushing and BAL. The specimens can be sent for various microbiological and cytological analyses.

Bronchoalveolar Lavage

This is a relatively safe and easy procedure, which involves the instillation of measured aliquots of saline and its recovery through the bronchoscope so as to get a sample of the epithelial lining fluid of the small airways and alveoli. It is useful in the diagnosis of conditions like pulmonary alveolar proteinosis (PAP), eosinophilic granuloma and eosinophilic pneumonia.

Quantitative Microbiological Techniques

In the setting of patients with ventilator associated pneumonias, it is essential to get a sample from the bronchial tree, which is free from the contamination or colonization of organisms. Procedures like protected specimen brush (PSB) and quantitative BAL help in acquiring representative samples.

THERAPEUTIC BRONCHOSCOPY

Bronchoscopy is also employed for several therapeutic indications **(Table 4)**.

Foreign Body Aspiration and Removal

Bronchoscopy finds a major role in the removal of foreign bodies. Traditionally, the rigid bronchoscope had been the instrument of choice for foreign body removal, but now the flexible fiberoptic bronchoscope is being increasingly used. It offers greater access to the periphery and can be used with ease in patients on mechanical ventilator and those who have unstable neck. The various instruments used for foreign body removal include snares, balloon catheters, retrieval baskets and grasping forceps **(Fig. 15)**.

Table 4 Therapeutic bronchoscopy—indications

Removal of foreign bodies
Pulmonary toilet
Stent placement
Bronchoalveolar lavage
Lobar collapse
Intubation
Airway maintenance
Management of malignant and benign endobronchial tissue
• Electrocautery
• Argon plasma coagulation
• Laser photodynamic therapy
• Cryotherapy brachytherapy
Endobronchial valve placement
Bronchial thermoplasty
Thoracic trauma
Pneumothorax

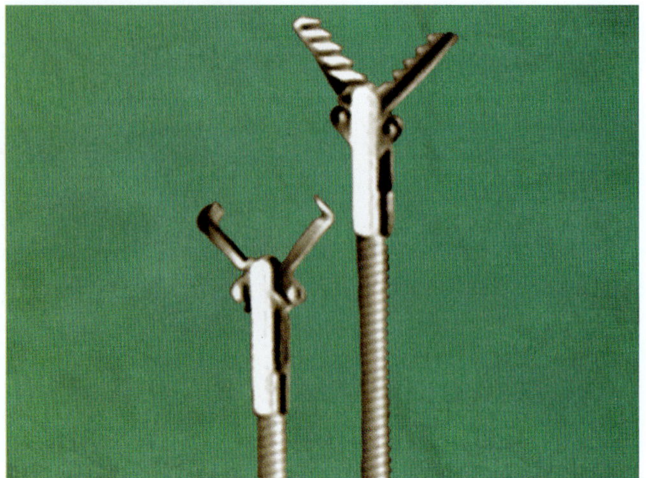

Fig. 15 Foreign body grasping forceps

Control of Hemoptysis

Bronchoscopy is useful for both diagnosis and emergency management of hemoptysis. An instrument with a larger working channel is required, the use of rigid bronchoscopy is recommended. Various measures like instillation of iced saline solution and epinephrine, may be tried. Catheters to offer tamponade on bleeding segments, including Fogarty balloon catheter may be tried. In the event, a visible source of bleeding is seen and laser photocoagulation can be attempted.

Pulmonary Toilet

Clearing of tracheobronchial tree of secretions called toileting, is the most common application of therapeutic bronchoscopy. Bronchoscopes with large suction channel are to be used. This is commonly required in intensive care unit (ICU) practice.

Bronchoalveolar Lavage

Whole lung lavage in patients with PAP has a therapeutic, as well as diagnostic role. About 50% of patients will suffice with a single treatment **(Fig. 16)**, multiple lavages are required in other patients.[18]

Electrocautery and Argon Plasma Coagulation

Electrocautery can be used via the bronchoscope channel in a contact or noncontact mode. It has the advantage over laser because it requires a shorter procedure time and lesser investment for instrument overheads. Indications for

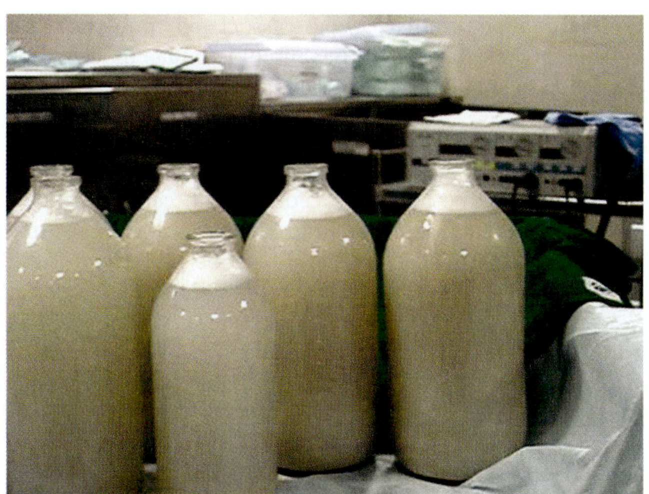

Fig. 16 Lavage fluid from the whole lung lavage of pulmonary alveolar proteinosis (PAP)

electrocautery include the treatment of malignant and benign lesions, debulking of tumors and removal of granulation tissue, hemoptysis management, immediate hemostatic control and coagulation.

Cryotherapy

It is one of the modalities used for the treatment of malignant endobronchial lesions. The principle of treatment is to create the fastest possible cooling of the target tissue in order to provoke intracellular freezing. The cooling agents used are liquid nitrogen, nitrous oxide and carbon dioxide.

Laser Photoresection

The use of laser in obstructive endobronchial lesions allows the establishment of airway patency and the subsequent ventilation of the distal lung and drainage of the postobstructive pneumonia. Other lesions treated by laser photoresection include tracheal granulomas, tracheal stenosis, endobronchial amyloidosis and tracheopathia osteoplastica.

Photodynamic Therapy

Photosensitizers are used to cause tissue necrosis. The likely indications for this therapy include the treatment of early lung cancer or palliation of unresectable bronchogenic carcinoma causing tracheobronchial obstruction.

Balloon Dilatation

It is used to establish airway patency in patients with retention pneumonia, atelectasis, lung abscess or the symptomatic stenosis of tracheobronchial tree.

Tracheobronchomalacia

Tracheobronchomalacia is diagnosed by flexible bronchoscopy. The treatment of choice for diffuse involvement is the insertion of standard or bifurcated silicone tracheobronchial stents. Pneumatic stent with concomitant noninvasive ventilation is another treatment option.

Fistula Closure/Repair

Identification of fistulae beyond the reach of flexible fiberoptic bronchoscope is done by the serial insertion of occluding balloons and checking for air leak. Various sealants like gel foam, autologous blood patches, cryoprecipitate and silver nitrate can be used to close the fistula. Up to 83% of tracheoesophageal fistulas can be detected by bronchoscopy, further treatment can be planned by concomitant esophagoscopy.[19]

Stents

Stents are placed bronchoscopically, to relieve endoluminal obstruction. Both flexible and rigid bronchoscopes are used for stent placements. Patients with primary airway tumors may benefit from endoluminal stenting, if surgery is not indicated. Other tumors that occur adjacent to the airway and produce obstruction by direct invasion or extrinsic compression, may also be successfully palliated with endoluminal treatments combined with stent placement. Patients with postintubation tracheal stenosis are occasionally good candidates for airway dilation and stenting.

Endobronchial Valves

Bronchoscopic lung volume reduction using endobronchial valves (EBV) for selected patients with hyperinflated lung from heterogeneous emphysema has been attempted. The use of EBV to treat persistent pulmonary air leaks has been shown as an effective and minimally invasive procedure.[20]

ELECTRONAVIGATION BRONCHOSCOPY

It is a procedure, which incorporates the patient's CT chest images into a special computer software program, to mark the exact site of lesion by placing electronic markers. It is done for virtual guidance for the bronchoscopist to sample the specific lesion by biopsy, brush or TBNA. The procedure is done under conscious sedation, with the patient lying on a low frequency electromagnetic bed.

SAFETY FACTORS IN BRONCHOSCOPY

Bronchoscopy is a technique, which requires expertise and training. Knowledge of airway anatomy is essential. Adequate equipment, trained personnel and means of handling complications, which may arise are essential. Standard safety

Table 5 Complications of bronchoscopy

Complications related to anesthesia
• Hypersensitivity to local anesthetic agents
• Oxygen desaturation
– Fever
– Infection
– Airway obstruction
– Airway perforation
– Pneumothorax
– Hemorrhage
– Air embolism

precautions when handling the equipment and performance of procedures are essential.

COMPLICATIONS OF BRONCHOSCOPY

Bronchoscopy has a potential of hazards of anesthesia, as well as of the procedure and associated interventions **(Table 5)**. The complications are more likely if the basic prerequisites like patient selection and preparation are not appropriate.

Anesthesia-related Complications

The importance of having a limit on the amount of local anesthetic, which is used, has been mentioned earlier. It is essential to remember that oxygen desaturation may occur during the procedure, especially when done under conscious sedation or general anesthesia. Significant desaturation occurs during BAL. An essential prerequisite therefore, is the administration of supplemental oxygen.

Fever and Infection

The occurrence of transient fever, after bronchoscopy especially after the performance of BAL has been noted. The use of prophylactic antibiotic prior to procedure, as recommended by the American Heart Association, is for patients with a predisposition to endocarditis and those with valvular heart problems. Prophylactic antibiotics are not required prior to flexible bronchoscopy.

Airway Perforation and Obstruction

Various airway complications, including burns, perforation and airway obstruction, may occasionally occur when lasers, stents or valves are used, and when the procedures are inappropriately performed.

Pneumothorax

The incidence of pneumothorax following a transbronchial biopsy is about 4%. The risk increases when the patient is immunocompromised with associated pneumocystis infection, when the patient has multiple bullae in the lungs and when the patient is on a mechanical ventilator.

Hemorrhage

Its occurrence due to the procedure itself, can be avoided by proper selection and evaluation. As per standard recommendations, bronchoscopy should not be performed if the platelet count is less than 50,000/mm^3. Other interventional procedures, including TBLB, laser and stents should be done only if the platelet counts are more than 75,000/mm^3.

Air Embolism

This a serious and fatal complication, which rarely occurs, especially after laser photoresection.

Inspite of the likelihood of several complications, which have been enumerated, the procedure of bronchoscopy is generally safe and risk free. It is however important that it is done by trained personnel with ready availability of backup facilities to handle any complication.

REFERENCES

1. Killian G. Removal of a bone splinter from the right main bronchus with the help of direct laryngoscopy. Munch Med Wschr. 1897;4:44-86.
2. Nanjundiah S. Bronchoscopy in India 2005: a survey. J Bronchol. 2006;13:194-200.
3. Miller JI. Rigid bronchoscopy. Chest Surg Clin N Am. 1996;6(2):161-7.
4. Narasimhan R, Gayathri AR, Illangho RP. Transbronchial Lung Biopsy-A Retrospective Analysis. Pulmon. 2004;6(2):44-9.
5. Shure D. Transbronchial biopsy and needle aspiration. Chest. 1989;95(5):1130-8.
6. Gaur DS, Thapliyal NC, Kishore S, Pathak VP. Efficacy of broncho-alveolar lavage and bronchial brush cytology in diagnosing lung cancers. J Cytol. 2007;24(2):73-7.
7. Gay PC, Brutinel WM. Transbronchial needle aspiration in the practice of bronchoscopy. Mayo Clin Proc. 1989;64(2):158-62.
8. Dasgupta A, Mehta AC. Transbronchial needle aspiration. An underused diagnostic technique. Clin Chest Med. 1999;20(1):39-51.
9. Terris DJ, Arnstein DP, Nguyen HH. Contemporary evaluation of unilateral vocal cord paralysis. Otolaryngol Head Neck Surg. 1992;107(1):84-90.
10. Gong H, Salvatierra C. Clinical efficacy of early and delayed fiberoptic bronchoscope in patients with hemoptysis. Am Rev Respir Dis. 1981;124(3):221-5.
11. Chen JC, Bongard F, Klein SR. A contemporary perspective on superior vena cava syndrome. Am J Surg. 1990;160(2):207-11.
12. Feinsilver SH, Fein AM, Niederman MS, Schultz DE, Faegenburg DH. Utility of fiberoptic bronchoscopy in nonresolving pneumonias. Chest. 1990;96(6):1322-6.
13. Su WJ, Lee PY, Perng RP. Chest roentographic guidelines in the selection of patients for fiberoptic bronchoscopy. Chest. 1993;103(4):1198-201.

14. Shure D, Astarita RW. Bronchoscopc carcinoma presenting as an endobronchial mass. Chest. 1983;83(6):865-7.
15. Shure D, Fedullo PF. Transbronchial needle aspiration in the diagnosis of submucosal and peribronchial bronchogenic carcinoma. Chest. 1985;88(1):49-51.
16. McDougall JC, Cortese DA. Bronchoscopic Lung Biopsy. In: Prakash UB (Eds). Bronchoscopy. New York: Raven Press; 1994. pp. 141-6.
17. Morris MJ, Peacock MD, Mego DM, Johnson JE, Gregg T. The risk of hemorrhage from bronchoscopic lung biopsy due to pulmonary hypertension in interstitial lung disease. J Bronchol. 1998;5:117-21.
18. Murray MJ, DeRuyter ML, Harrison BA. "How I do it": bilateral lung washings for pulmonary alveolar proteinosis. J Bronchology. 1998;5:324-6.
19. Campion JP, Bourdelat D, Launois B. Surgical treatment of malignant esophagotracheal fistulas. Am J Surg. 1983;148(5):641-6.
20. Travaline JM, Mckenna RJ, De Giacomo T, Venuta F, Hazelrigg SR, Boomer M, et al. Treatment of persistent pulmonary air leaks using endobronchial valves. Chest. 2009;136(2):355-60.

Interventional Bronchoscopy

Praveen N Mathur, FD Sheski

DEFINITION OF INTERVENTIONAL PULMONOLOGY

Interventional pulmonology is a relatively new and rapidly growing field within pulmonary medicine which is focused on the use of advanced bronchoscopic and pleuroscopy techniques. This was first defined in 1995 and subsequently by the European Respiratory Society (ERS)/the American Thoracic Society (ATS) guidelines.[1,2] Interventional pulmonology can be defined as "the Art and Science of Medicine as related to the performance of diagnostic and invasive therapeutic procedures that require additional training and expertise beyond that required in a standard pulmonary medicine training program".

Disease processes encompassed within this discipline include complex airway management problems, benign and malignant central airway obstruction, pleural diseases, and pulmonary vascular procedures. Diagnostic and therapeutic procedures pertaining to these areas include, but are not limited to, rigid bronchoscopy, transbronchial needle aspiration (TBNA), autofluorescence (AF) bronchoscopy, endobronchial ultrasound (EBUS), transthoracic needle aspiration and biopsy, laser bronchoscopy, endobronchial electrosurgery, argon-plasma coagulation, cryotherapy, airway stent insertion, balloon bronchoplasty and dilatation techniques, endobronchial radiation (brachytherapy), photodynamic therapy (PDT), percutaneous dilatational tracheotomy, transtracheal oxygen catheter insertion, medical thoracoscopy, and imaging-guided thoracic interventions.[1,2]

Although this definition was established in 1995 there has been a surge of new procedures that now can be performed with a bronchoscope. This area continues to thrive with new innovation and venture capital. Some such techniques include endoscopic lung volume reduction for advanced emphysema, bronchothermoplasty for asthma, and newer spectroscopic imaging techniques.

RIGID BRONCHOSCOPY

Bronchoscopy was first performed with a rigid bronchoscope in 1897 by Gustav Killian to remove a pork bone impacted in the airway of a farmer. Killian used a Mikulicz-Rosenheim rigid esophagoscope.[3] Killian continued to use rigid metal tubes in cadavers. He subsequently described the extraction of foreign bodies from the airways. Chevalier Jackson in Philadelphia was responsible for the development of rigid bronchoscopy in the United States. He improved and developed the modern rigid bronchoscope.[4]

The development of the flexible bronchoscope led to the decrease of the use of rigid bronchoscope. However, rigid bronchoscopy has regained usefulness due to increasing use of interventional bronchoscopy.[5]

The rigid bronchoscope, also known as the open tube bronchoscope, is a rigid, straight, and hollow metallic tube made of stainless steel. The tube comes in various external diameters varying from 2–14 mm. They have the same diameter from proximal to distal ends but most have a beveled tip to facilitate lifting of the epiglottis during intubation and also to core out and endobronchial lesion.

Telescopes were initially made with 0° and multitude of angles, allowing visualization of upper and lower lobe bronchi. Many of the angled telescopes are not used since the fiberoptic bronchoscope is used through the rigid tube. Light sources using xenon or halogen lamps are currently used. Video cameras can be easily connected to the eyepiece of a rigid telescope. Accessory instruments often used during rigid bronchoscopy include biopsy forceps, suction tubing, specific forceps that may become necessary for removal of foreign-body.

Procedure

This procedure is performed under general anesthesia. The teeth must be protected, a rolled blanket is placed between the shoulder blades which enables to move the upper trachea forward. Anesthesia could be intravenous, or if inhaled anesthetic gases are to be used, it is necessary to pack the nose and mouth with gauge to avoid gas leakage. Ventilatory support is provided using assisted spontaneous ventilation or closed-circuit positive pressure ventilation. Several techniques of rigid bronchoscope intubation are used:

- Direct intubation,
- Intubation with the help laryngoscope, or
- Intubation alongside a small endobronchial tube.

Direct intubation is the method of choice for intubation. In this technique, the rigid telescope is placed inside the bronchoscope, and the laryngeal structures are viewed directly through the telescope. The bronchoscope is inserted with its tip facing forward; the bronchoscopist identifies the uvula. The bronchoscope is then gently lifted upwards and the epiglottis comes into the view. Once the arytenoids are identified, the bronchoscope is lifted anteriorly and the vocal cords are seen. The bronchoscope is then rotated 90° as vocal cords traversed. The bronchoscope is advanced and rotated to enter the trachea.

Complications are related to poor insertion technique, such as trauma to gum, teeth, lip and laryngeal swelling.

ADVANCED IMAGING BRONCHOSCOPY

Fluorescence Bronchoscopy

Lung cancer progresses through several stages, including metaplasia, dysplasia, carcinoma *in situ* (CIS), microinvasive carcinoma, and invasive carcinoma.[6] In order to identify the abnormal mucosa, a variety of techniques have been used. When a suitable wavelength is used to excite tissue to fluoresce, infiltrating tumor will alter tissue fluoresce. This difference in fluorescence is used to help detect abnormal mucosa in the airways. Photosensitizing fluorescent compounds were used to increase the intensity of the fluorescence, but this approach has been limited by skin photo toxicity.[7-10] Advances in image processing have improved the detection of subtle differences in fluorescence. CIS and microinvasive carcinoma exhibit a weaker red fluorescence and slightly weaker green fluorescence for normal tissues, when illuminated by light with a wavelength of 380–440 nm **(Figs 1A and B)**. Several reasons have been suggested for this phenomenon. This may be due to increased epithelial thickness, increased blood flow, and/or a reduced concentration of fluorophores in abnormal tissue.[11,12]

The first fluorescence bronchoscopy system that was commercially available was the light-induced fluorescence endoscopy (LIFE) device (Xillix Technologies Corporation, Vancouver, Canada).[13,14] This device used blue light from a helium-cadmium laser and collected fluorescence images via its imaging bundles. The red and green wavelengths reflected by the tissue were filtered and amplified by cameras.

A variety of different color schemes have been used by different manufactures. Fluorescence and white light bronchoscopy (WLB) is performed during the same session. In most of the studies, the investigators have performed conventional WLB, followed by AF bronchoscopy. Biopsies were taken from abnormal and normal areas. AF bronchoscopy is better at detecting airway lesions than WLF.[15] But it is also more likely to give false positive results.[16] In one study, 95 out of 285 (33%) biopsies taken from areas with abnormal fluorescence contained abnormal histology, a positive predictive value of only 33%.[17] There are no accepted indications for AF. It has a role in radiological occult sputum atypia, for surveillance in patient with known CIS or high grade dysplasia. As there are no formal early lung cancer detection programs, the role of AF bronchoscopy is not clearly defined. AF bronchoscopy may be helpful in the evaluation of patients with invasive carcinoma, who are being considered for curative endobronchial or surgical treatment.

Not all high-grade lesions are premalignant and progression is confirmed histological in fewer than 100 patients.[15,18] In addition, one study found that such progression probably occurred in 1 out of 3 patients; the rest regressed to normal.[18] The natural history is not well understood as there are difficulties due to lack of agreement among the pathologist.

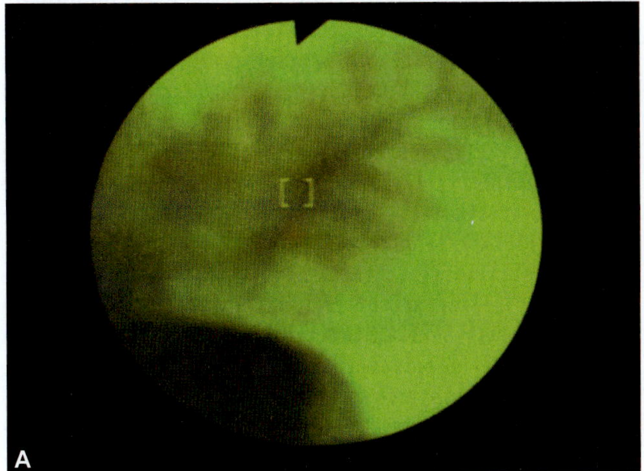

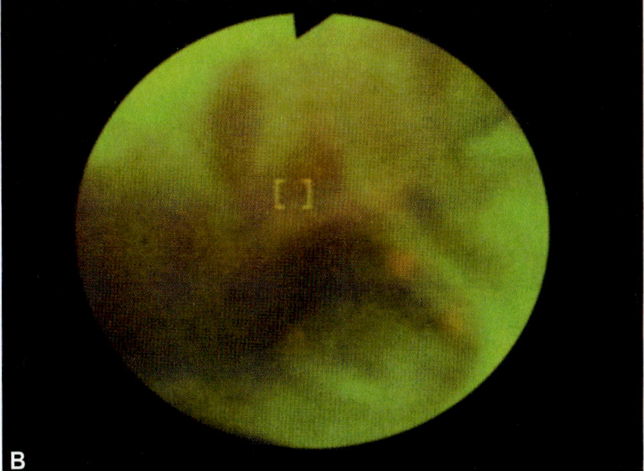

Figs 1A and B (A) Carcinoma *in situ* (CIS) and microinvasive carcinoma exhibit a weaker red fluorescence; (B) Slightly weaker green fluorescence for normal tissues

A variety of other bronchoscopic techniques which include high magnification bronchoscopy (HMB), narrow band imaging (NBI), confocal microscopy and optical coherence tomography (OCT), have been used with variable success rates.

High-magnification Bronchoscopy

Neovascularization or increased mucosal microvascular growth is a hall mark of early lung cancer.[19,20] HMB uses this principal to identify abnormal mucosa. This system can provide information about the bronchial mucosa with a maximum magnification of 110 times. Such increased vascularity in the bronchial mucosa is also seen in asthma and chronic bronchitis. Areas of complex networks of tortuous vessels in the bronchial mucosa that are detected using HMB at sites of abnormal fluorescence may enable discrimination between bronchitis and dysplasia. The sensitivity and specificity of HMB is 70% and 90%, respectively.[19] This promising work has not been duplicated at any other institution.

Narrowband Imaging

This neovascularization or increased mucosal microvascular growth can be observed if a new narrowband filter is used instead of the conventional red/green/blue broadband filter. This narrowband imaging (NBI) technique uses a 415 nm blue light, which is absorbed by hemoglobin contained in the capillary network on the mucosal surface and a 540 nm green light that is absorbed by blood vessels located a bit deeper below the capillary layer.[21] NBI was shown to increase the rate of detection of dysplasia or malignancy by 23% when compared to WLB, however when combined with AF bronchoscopy, there was no increase in yield.[22,23]

Optical Coherence Tomography

This is also a noninvasive technique for endoscopic imaging of *in vivo* tissue structures. OCT resembles ultrasound but uses light rather than acoustic waves. In ultrasound, the resolution of the quality of image is often obscured due to the presence of air. OCT overcomes this problem. Velocity of light is 200,000 times greater than the velocity of sound, thus the resolution is much improved, but the depths is only of up to 2 mm.[24,25] The procedure can be performed with a standard bronchoscopy. OCT can localize preneoplastic changes in the bronchial epithelium once identified by AF bronchoscopy. CIS and invasive carcinoma can be identified from normal bronchial epithelium.[26,27] It may have a role in understanding the airway remodeling in chronic obstructive pulmonary disease (COPD) and asthma as the details of airway can be visualized up to 2 mm depth.[28]

Confocal Endoscopy

This optical technology has the capabilities for submicrometer-level resolution imaging, but has further limitations in depth of penetration (approximately, 0.5 mm compared with approximately 2–3 mm with OCT.[29] It is envisioned that in the sometime soon in the future, the optical technologies will provide a window to intracellular structures *in vivo*, replacing traditional *in vitro* analyzes of cellular components using conventional tissue biopsy specimens.

ADVANCED BIOPSY TECHNIQUES

Transbronchial Needle Aspiration

Needle aspiration of mediastinal lymph nodes was initially described in 1949 and its application via flexible bronchoscopy was later described in 1981.[30,31] The TBNA has been utilized in diagnosis of endobronchial lesions, peripheral nodules, and mediastinal abnormalities.[32-34] The most common application of TBNA is the diagnosis and staging of lung cancer.

Technique

In order to perform optimal TBNA, a computed tomography (CT) of the chest is performed with contrast prior to TBNA. The relationships of the tracheobronchial tree to the lymph nodes and blood vessels are essential to know. The needle must reach the core of the lymph node to get optimal biopsy while avoiding nearby vascular structures. TBNA of lymph nodes in the subcarinal and right paratracheal regions detects metastasis with a higher sensitivity than TBNA of left paratracheal lymph nodes.[35]

When someone is going to perform TBNA, he must first learn and understand the mediastinal anatomy. As the bronchoscope is passed to the right of the distal third of the trachea, the superior vena cava and the azygos vein is found. Directly anterior to the trachea, above the level of the primary carina, is the innominate artery and the aortic arch. They cross the origin of the left main stem bronchus and then lie anterior and to the left of the distal third of the trachea, making an easily recognizable pulsatile imprint.[36] The main pulmonary artery divides into the right and left branches within the concavity of the aortic arch. The left pulmonary artery runs anterosuperiorly in close approximation (within 3–5 mm) to the left main stem bronchus, while the right pulmonary artery lies anterior to the right main stem bronchus and the origin of the upper lobe bronchus. The esophagus lies in close approximation (within 2–3 mm) to the posterior wall of the trachea and the left main stem bronchus.[36]

Retractable needles should be the only one used, as the damage to the working channel is common and costly. The commonly used size is 22 G needle to obtain cytology. There is a larger 19 G needle that is used for histology; however, it is a cumbersome system with poor performance record. During insertion of the catheter, the flexible bronchoscope should be kept as straight as possible, with its distal tip in the neutral position in order to prevent damage to the working channel. The tip of the needle should be kept within the metal hub during its passage through the working channel.[37]

The catheter should be retracted, and the tip of the needle kept in view distal to that of the fiberoptic bronchoscope. The bronchoscope is then advanced as a single unit to the target area, and the tip of the needle is anchored in the intercartilaginous space so as to penetrate the airway wall. The needle should be inserted with the metal hub against the trachebronchial wall. When the needle inserted, suction is applied at the proximal side port using a 60 mL syringe. The catheter is then agitated to and fro to obtain cytology with continuous suction. The needle is withdrawn from the target site after releasing suction.

The specimen for cytology is prepared by using air from a 60 mL empty syringe to spray the specimen onto the slide, smearing it by using another slide, and immediately placing it in a 95% alcohol solution. If rapid on site evaluation (ROSE) service is available, then feedback from the cytologist is extremely helpful and reduces the number of punctures.[38] The cytopathologist reviewing the sample for adequacy has been demonstrated to increase the diagnostic yield.[38] A trained assistant is essential for the success of TBNA and proper tissue handling.

Complications following TBNA are uncommon if appropriate precautions are taken and the proper technique is employed. The most common complication is the damage to the working channel of the bronchoscope. There are no firm recommendations on antibiotic prophylaxis. Oozing of a minimal amount of blood from the puncture site may be encountered; infrequent complications include pneumothorax, pneumomediastinum, and hemomediastinum.

Outcomes

A meta-analysis of 42 studies examining the accuracy of CT in detecting mediastinal nodes infiltrated with malignancy reported a sensitivity and specificity of 79 and 78%, respectively, while another large meta-analysis of 113 studies found that the sensitivity and specificity of TBNA for the diagnosis of non-small cell lung cancer was 39% and 99%, respectively.[39,40] TBNA establishes the diagnosis and provides staging information from a single procedure. Positive N2 or N3 lymph nodes for non-small cell lung cancer avoid surgical intervention. Positron emission tomography (PET) helps in defining which lymph nodes should be sampled.

The utility of TBNA in the diagnosis of lymphoma has been limited, since this usually requires larger samples of nodal tissue, using both cytology needles with flow cytometry. Several reports have confirmed an increase in the diagnostic yield when both transbronchial lung biopsies and TBNA are performed in patients with suspected sarcoidosis.[41,42]

Endobronchial Ultrasound

This bronchoscopic technique uses ultrasound to visualize structures of the mediastinal adjacent to the airway wall to perform TBNA. Therefore, EBUS can be used to guide bronchoscopic sampling of mediastinal lymph nodes, hilar lymph nodes, or peripheral pulmonary nodules.[43] EBUS is different than endoscopic ultrasound (EUS). While both visualize and guide sampling of mediastinal lymph nodes, EBUS is performed during bronchoscopy and EUS is performed during upper endoscopy.

Techniques

Radial probe-endobronchial ultrasound: Radial probe EBUS (RP-EBUS) provides 360° images of the airway wall and surrounding structures, and visualize the layers of the airway wall. RP-EBUS with a surrounding inflatable balloon, can clearly define tracheal and bronchial wall layers, making it an excellent tool to assess tumor invasion. Assessment of tumor depth correlates well with histopathologic findings and this measurement determines appropriate therapy.[44] Tumors that invade through the cartilage layer, require radiotherapy or surgery, whereas those with an intact cartilage layer can be treated endoscopically.

Herth et al. studied 131 consecutive patients with central thoracic malignancies potentially involving the central airways.[45] All patients underwent chest CT followed by WLB and RP-EBUS, with subsequent surgical evaluation and radiology results blinded from the bronchoscopists and surgeons. CT reported 77% of lesions invading airways, but RP-EBUS showed invasion in only 47% of cases. When using surgical assessment as the gold standard, RP-EBUS had a specificity of 100%, sensitivity of 89%, and accuracy of 94%, for assessing tumor invasion.

Miniature radial probe (20 MHz or 30 MHz) are available which provide a depth of penetration of 5 mm. An ultra-miniature radial probe can be extended into subsegmental bronchi allowing peripheral pulmonary nodules to be visualized. The probe and the guide sheath are advanced through the working channel of the bronchoscope until the nodule is visualized, radial probe is removed, leaving the guide sheath in position. Biopsy forceps or a bronchial brush is then inserted through the guide sheath for the nodule to be biopsied. When RP-EBUS is used for TBNA, the radial probe is removed from the working channel before the TBNA can be inserted, thus, it is not performed in real-time.

Convex probe-endobronchial ultrasound: Convex Probe EBUS (CP-EBUS) give a view which is parallel to the shaft of the bronchoscope. This allows real-time TBNA and color flow Doppler will help identify vascular and cystic structures. A 7.5 MHz convex ultrasound probe is a part of the bronchoscope at it tip. The ultrasound image and conventional bronchoscopy image can be displayed on the same monitor bur two separate monitors are preferred. A transbronchial needle system which contains a 22 gauge retractable sharp beveled needle with an internal sheath, is inserted through the working channel, just proximal to the ultrasound probe. Once the catheter emerges from the bronchoscope, the needle is advanced from the catheter and locked into position. It is then pushed through the inter cartilage space and into the target lymph node under ultrasound visualization **(Figs 2A to C)**. Suction is applied

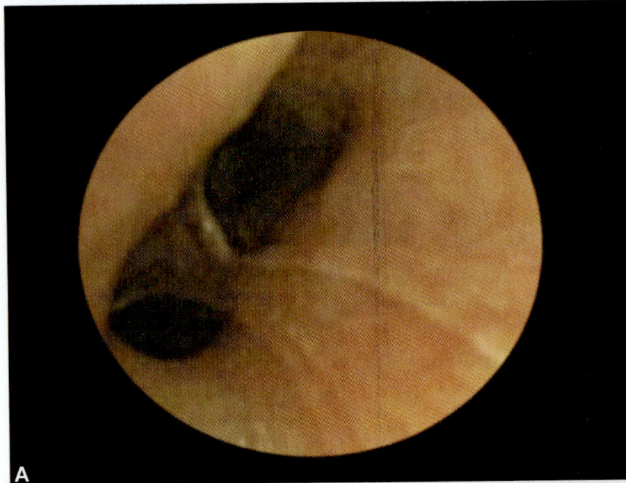

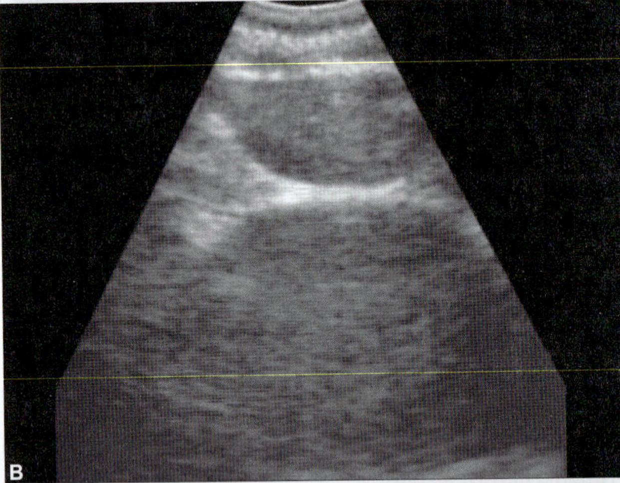

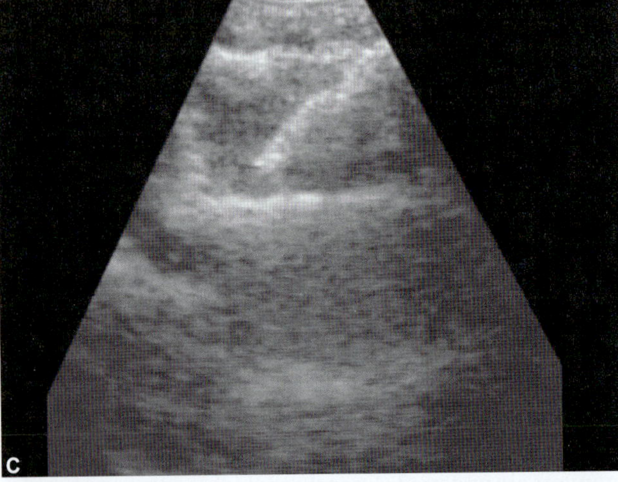

Figs 2A to C (A) Extrinsic compression; (B) Endobronchial ultrasound (EBUS) view of the lymph node; (C) Endobronchial ultrasound (EBUS) needle visible in the lymph node

to the syringe and the catheter is slowly agitated. Suction is released and the needle is pulled into the flexible catheter. The specimen is prepared in a similar manner as TBNA.

Outcomes

Mediastinal lesions

- Enlarged mediastinal lymph nodes are identified by CT scan or are metabolically active on a PET: In an initial clinical trial, RP-EBUS was used in suspected lung cancer.[46,47] Patients with lymphadenopathy were randomized to RP-EBUS and TBNA. Positive result was defined as yielded lymphocytes or a specific abnormality on cytology. In patients with lymph nodes which were other than subcarinal, RP-EBUS-guided TBNA had a better yield (84 versus 58%) when compared to TBNA. RP-EBUS did not add any further value when subcarinal lymph nodes were analyzed.
- In order to demonstrate the proof of principal that CP-EBUS-guided TBNA can successfully sample mediastinal or hilar lymph nodes: Malignancy was detected with a sensitivity 95%, specificity 100%, and diagnostic accuracy of 96%.[48] A large meta-analysis of 11 studies showed similar sensitivity and specificity.[49] When a combination of EBUS-guided TBNA and EUS-guided-fine needle aspiration (EUS-FNA) is used to access mediastinum, there is good possibility of making the entire mediastinum accessible, thus deceasing the need for more invasive procedures. The combination appears to improve the diagnostic yield, when compared to either procedure alone.[50,51]

Mutational analysis is also possible from CP-EBUS TBNA samples; 154 out of 156 cases were successfully analysed (98.7%) for epidermal growth factor receptor (EGFR) mutations using the polymerase chain reaction (PCR) clamp technique on cell-pellets derived from needle-washed solution.[52] Garcia-Olive et al. showed EGFR analysis was possible in 72.2% of patients undergoing CP-EBUS TBNA with metastatic nodal specimens.[53] In a different study, analysis for EGFR and k-ras sequences using co-amplification of lower desaturation temperature (COLD) PCR was achieved in 95.5% and 98.4% of samples respectively.[54] A UK group found that 88% of their CP-EBUS TBNA samples were adequate for mutational analysis using the Scorpion amplification refractory mutation system (ARMS) kit.[55]

CP-EBUS-TBNA has been used to diagnose sarcoidosis. This has been demonstrated by a randomized study where EBUS has been shown to be advantageous than conventional TBNA.[56] EBUS had a sensitivity of 83% and specificity of 83%; conventional TBNA had a sensitivity 61% and specificity 100%. Similarly, EBUS is an effective method for diagnosis of mediastinal lymphoma.[57]

Economic analyses validate the viability of CP-EBUS TBNA.[58] Improved cost efficacy mainly by reducing mediastinoscopies and unnecessary thoracotomies, was also found in a health technology assessment involving hospitals from the United Kingdom, Belgium, and the Netherlands.[59]

The EBUS does have certain disadvantage since the bronchoscope is larger than conventional bronchoscope with a poorer image quality. As the vision is 30° above, it is technically difficult to maneuver and requires some practice. Due to it poorer quality images it should not be used for initial inspection. There is no histology needle available for use, the needle size used is the same size as for TBNA of 22 gauge. The addition of EBUS to perform TBNA does not add to complications which are similar to those of conventional TBNA.

Pulmonary Nodules

In a prospective study of 150 patients with peripheral pulmonary nodules, RP-EBUS-guided forceps biopsy, using a guide sheath, was diagnostic in 77% of cases.[60] The yield was not impacted by lesion size. In comparison, prior studies when a guide sheath was not used, reported a diagnostic yield of up to only 28%. Other studies have similarly reported a diagnostic yield of approximately 79% when a guide sheath is used.[61] In a large randomized trial, assigning patients to RP-EBUS-guided or conventional transbronchial biopsy, nodules that were smaller than 3 cm, RP-EBUS-guided transbronchial biopsy identified malignant disease with a sensitivity of 75% and accuracy 83%.[62] In contrast, conventional transbronchial biopsy identified malignant disease with a sensitivity of 31% and accuracy of 50%. However, the yield was lower than CT-guided percutaneous transthoracic needle aspiration. The RP-EBUS only gives an advantage if the lesion is smaller than 3 cm.

Navigational Bronchoscopy

Navigational bronchoscopy provides a virtual three-dimensional map to enable a physician to perform biopsy or place markers for radiation therapy or facilitate the surgeon to remove a small peripheral lesion. Bronchoscopic lung biopsy has been one of the methods to obtain tissue from a peripheral lesion. The yield for lesion of less than 2 cm is very poor. Transthoracic needle aspiration with CT-guidance is commonly used where variable reports of diagnosis are reported. Similarly, the complication rates are also variable.

Navigational systems use either an electromagnetic navigation assistance or computer assistance to identify the air columns to reach the final destination. Several manufactures are using either of the methods. This procedure requires several steps prior to the bronchoscopy. A CT is performed to the specification of the manufacturer. These images are transferred to laptop containing specific proprietary software and the planning is performed. Depending on the software, the virtual plan is generated. This virtual plan is placed in the navigational computer; finally bronchoscopy is performed with fluoroscopic assistance. A variety of steerable catheters can be placed in the working channel. Using an extended working channel and the navigational catheter the target is approached with help of the navigation system. Once the target is reached, forceps or brushes are used to obtain tissue or fiducial markers are placed.

Several studies have reported a diagnostic yield of 64–69%; if the lesion was more than 2 cm, the yield was 74% and if the lesion was less in size, the yield was 66%. In another study, the yield obtained was 67%.[63,64] In a multicenter, randomized, controlled trial where EBUS, navigation system or EBUS combined with navigation system were used, the diagnostic yield was only 72%. There were poorer results with EBUS alone, i.e. 69% and with navigation, only 59%. The combined yield of EBUS with electromagnetic navigation bronchoscopy (ENB) was 88%. This has not been reproduced anywhere else.[65]

The capital equipment cost is above 200,000 US $ and disposable equipment for every case is above 1000 US $ which make this system currently prohibitive. The majority of navigational bronchoscopy publications do not describe selection/inclusion criteria, and do not randomize patients to competing modalities. There is a high cost and requirement of considerable preprocedure planning [both to obtain the digital imaging and communications in medicine (DICOM) images of recommended parameters, as well as pathway planning]. Therefore, navigational bronchoscopy is only likely to become the mainstream procedure if consumable prices fall and high level evidence demonstrates the diagnostic equivalence to that of transthoracic needle biopsy or RP-EBUS. Navigational bronchoscopy and RP-EBUS may have complimentary roles, however, this combined approach is likely to increase cost and procedure time.

Nonmagnetic Navigation Bronchoscopy

Virtual bronchscopy (VB) is aimed to guide the bronchoscopist to the target lesion. VB allows CT reconstruction of the bronchial tree allowing "virtual" bronchoscopic animation, enabling more accurate procedure planning. Newer scopes have external diameters of only 2.8 mm, and allow direct visualization of up to the 9th generation bronchus.[66]

Asahina et al. assessed the utility of combining VB with RP-EBUS in 29 patients with l peripheral pulmonary lesions (PPLs) less than or equal to 30 mm, 80% of lesions were visualized ultrasonographically and diagnostic sensitivities were 44.4% for lesions of less than 20 mm, and 91.7% for lesions of more than or equal to 20 mm.[67] In a randomized trial of 199 patients with PPLs less than or equal to 30 mm undergoing RP-EBUS with and without VB, the VB group demonstrated higher diagnostic yield (80.4% vs. 67%, P=0.032).[68]

Recently though, a randomized controlled multicenter trial of ultrathin bronchoscopy with and without VB found no difference in diagnostic yield.[69]

The disadvantages are in the ability to obtain sufficient tissue for molecular analysis due to small biopsy forceps size. Virtual bronchoscopy quality is dependent on CT source data and rely on a skilled second operator to manipulate the VB image to the same orientation as the real-time bronchoscopic image; without this, the risk of disorientation is high.[70]

ENDOSCOPIC PALLIATIVE CARE

Introduction

Begin or malignant tracheobronchial obstruction can lead to acute respiratory distress or even asphyxia and death. Endobronchial obstruction may present as an endobronchial lesion, or an extraluminal obstruction or sometimes a combined lesion.

If curative resection is not possible, various endoscopic methods for palliation are available, such as neodymium yttrium aluminium garnet (Nd:YAG) laser, cryotherapy, electrocautery, and argon plasma coagulation (APC) PDT. In case of extraluminal lesions, palliation is performed by balloon dilatation, stent placement, and/or external beam radiation.

These patients present with dyspnea, cough, chest discomfort, hemoptysis, stridor, or a localized wheeze. The history may include known cancer, aspiration of a foreign body, prior airway surgery or intubation, recurrent pneumonia, or other underlying illnesses that may involve the airways, such as sarcoidosis or tuberculosis (TB).

Nd:YAG Laser

Using theories proposed on radiant energy in 1917, Schawlow and Townes formulated the hypothesis of laser light and the subsequent development of a ruby laser reported by Maimon in 1960.[71-73]

Laser technology makes use of the power of radiant energy and properties of light amplification, laser being an acronym for "light amplified by the stimulated emission of radiation". For the stimulated emission of light to occur, there must be an adequate population of excited electrons with subsequent release of photons to produce the lasers light. This phenomenon is termed population inversion and requires an outside energy source. Almost any solid, liquid, or gas may act as a medium; placing the substance to be excited in a chamber with mirrors at either end further facilitates population inversion. The effectiveness of laser light as opposed to naturally occurring light has to do with three important properties: wavelength, spatial coherence and temporal coherence.[74]

The amount of energy that is delivered to a lesion depends on the power setting of the laser expressed in Watts, the distance from the laser tip to the target, and the duration of impact.[75] Light directed at a surface may also be reflected, scattered, transmitted, or absorbed.[75] The depth of penetration, therefore, depends not only on the properties of light but also the inherent properties of the tissue; the characteristics of the light produced, also on the medium used.

In the CO_2, laser light is produced in the infrared spectrum at a wavelength of 10,600 nanometers. The CO_2 laser can be used as a precise cutting tool, with only minimal blood loss owing to a relatively shallow depth of penetration. The most widely used laser light for tracheobronchial lesions is the Nd: YAG laser, which is produced by the stimulation of an YAG glass, coated with ND. The Nd:YAG laser has a wavelength of 1064 nm and is easily transmitted through pale tissues, with sizeable scatter and a potential penetration of up to 5–10 mm from the focal point.

The CO_2 laser therapy is most commonly used in the management of laryngeal lesions involving the area around the glottic opening. The CO_2 laser serves as an excellent scalpel since scattering is minimal; tissue vaporization is rapid and minimal damage to tissue. The Nd:YAG lasers unlike the CO_2 laser, can cause deep tissue vasoconstriction, with a penetration depth of up to 10 mm but has very good coagulation properties.

Indications and Contraindications

The indications and contraindication are listed in **Tables 1 and 2**. Clinical contraindications are relevant in patients who may not tolerate the conscious or general anesthesia because of comorbid diseases. In addition, patients in whom atelectasis distal to the obstruction has been present for more than 4–6 weeks, will probably not benefit from endoscopic laser resection because re-expansion of the involved lung is unlikely.

Complications

Complications of laser therapy are related to the laser equipment or instruments, the anesthesia used, and perioperative causes. Despite the possibility of severe, complications, the overall risk is low. In one series, there were only 60 complication and 12 deaths associated with Nd:YAG laser therapy in 2,610 resection.[76]

A potential catastrophic intraoperative complication of laser therapy is endotracheal fire. The use of combustible anesthetic gases must be avoided, the use of supplemental

Table 1 Contraindications for laser/cryotherapy/electrocautery/argon plasma coagulation (APC)

Anatomic contraindications
• Extrinsic obstruction without endobronchial lesion
• Lesion incursion into bordering major vascular structure (e.g. pulmonary artery) with potential for fistula formation
• Lesion incursion into bordering esophagus with potential for fistula formation
• Lesion incursion into bordering mediastinum with potential for fistula formation
Clinical contraindications
• Candidate for surgical resection
• Unfavorable short-term prognosis without hope for palliation of symptoms
• Inability to undergo conscious sedation or general anesthesia
• Coagulation disorder
• Total obstruction more than 4–6 weeks

Table 2 Indications for laser/cryotherapy/electrocautery/argon plasma coagulation (APC)

Benign or malignant airway lesion associated with:
• Dyspnea
• Uncontrolled cough
• Impending asphyxiation
• Stridor
• Inability to wean from ventilator owing to obstruction
• Postobstructive pneumonia
• Symptomatic or unresolving atelectasis
• Nearly complete (>50%) obstruction of one major bronchus
• Recurrent hemoptysis
• Closure of bronchopleural fistula not responsive to conventional therapy

oxygen should be less than 40%. Although, the metal rigid bronchoscope cannot catch fire, the use of the Nd:YAG laser through an endotracheal tube deserves special consideration. An immediate danger to the patient and operating room personnel is that of intratracheal explosion, with the anesthetic gases or oxygen producing a "torch effect" with ignition of the endotracheal tube; longer-term complication may result from the subsequent lower airway inhalation injury, with mucosal sloughing and airway obstruction caused by granulation tissue. Similarly, a silicone stent should be removed prior to use of laser therapy.

Fatal hemorrhage is associated with perforation into an involved or contiguous vascular structure. Perforation may also occur into adjacent structures with development of pneumothorax, pneumomediastinum, and trachea-esophageal fistula. Systemic air embolism has been reported and is associated with the development of vascular communication with the tracheobronchial tree.

Technique

Physicians prefer to use rigid bronchoscopy with general anesthesia, although procedures can be performed through the flexible fiberoptic bronchoscope using topical anesthesia alone.[77,78] Laser resection is performed first with photocoagulation of the tumor. Coagulated tissue is then removed by the use of the beveled edge of the rigid bronchoscope, forceps, and suction. Complete laser vaporization of tissue may also be performed, but has high-risk of endobronchial fire. The laser beam should always be aligned parallel to the bronchial wall and never be discharged perpendicular to the airway wall. Laser pulses of 1 second or less are usually employed. When using a flexible bronchoscope the removal of devitalized tissue can be slow and difficult due to a small forceps. In addition, the flexible bronchoscope is combustible.

Precautions

The patient's eyes should be protected with saline-soaked pads and aluminum foil to avoid injury from accidental laser scatter, and all personnel should wear protective goggles. Fraction of inspired oxygen should be kept below 40%, Flammable materials should be removed such as endotracheal tubes, silicon stents should be removed prior to the use of laser. If a flexible bronchoscope is employed, the laser must be kept a sufficient distance beyond the tip of the bronchoscope. Power settings greater than 40 watts should not be used.

Outcomes

The indications depend on the anatomic characteristics of the obstructing lesion and the clinical conditions outlined in **Table 2.**[78,79]

Benign and malignant airway endobronchial lesions causing symptomatic or obstructive complications do benefit from endoscopic laser photo resection.[80-84] Laser therapy has also been performed for stenosis related to prolonged intubation, stricture produced by mycobacteral infection, anastomosis granulation tissue following lung transplantation, suture granulomas, and in systemic inflammatory conditions such as Wegner's granulomatosis, Bechet's syndrome, and relapsing polychondritis.[85-89] Laser therapy has also been used in symptomatic obstruction secondary to broncholithiasis.[90]

Benign or low-grade tumors such as hamartomas, spindle cell carcinomas, endobronchial Kaposi's sarcomas, and even diffuse papillomatosis have also benefited from Nd:YAG laser photoablation. Shah reported a large series of benign tumor resections of the tracheobronchial tree in the 185 patients with benign tumors, 317 procedures were performed with the results of laser resection thought to be very good in 62% and good in 38%, with minimal complications.[91]

Hetzel in their experience reported 100 patients referred for palliative treatment of tracheabronchial malignancy.[92] There was objective improvement in the peak flow and alleviation of hemoptysis in 63% of patients with airway obstruction and 29% of those patients with collapsed lung.

Eichenhorn performed Nd:YAG laser therapy in 19 patients with inoperable nonsmall cell carcinoma and symptomatic bronchial obstruction, with the goal of debulking the airways before conventional external-beam radiation therapy.[79] Patients with satisfactory debulking and subsequent radiation therapy had a significantly better outcome (mean survival 340 days compared with less than 100 days; $P < 0.006$) than those with unsatisfactory laser therapy.

Desai showed a significant increase in survival among the subset of 15 patients who underwent emergency palliative photo-resection as the initial therapeutic intervention, compared with the subset of 11 patients who received palliative radiation alone.[93]

Mehta outlined the use of lasers with the flexible bronchoscope, in the group of patients who underwent a combination of Nd:YAG photo-resection with subsequent external-beam radiation therapy or external-beam radiation therapy plus brachytherapy.[94] Although the number of such patient was small (17 of 300 patients), their survival rate was significantly greater than that of historical controls treated with radiation therapy only (P = 0.022).

Cavaliere supplemented their earlier extensive case series experience outlining the treatment of 2008 patients with malignant airway obstructions using combined therapy with Nd:YAG laser, stents, and brachytherapy.[76] In patients treated with laser resection, 93% achieved immediate airway patency and consequent improvement in the quality of life.

Electrocautery

Electrocautery uses an electric current, to produce heat and to destroy tissue. Strauss used electrocautery for treating gastrointestinal (GIT) tumors in 1913 and in 1935 reported their experience on over 40 cases.[95]

Electrocautery uses alternating current at a high frequency (105–107 Hz) to generate heat that coagulates, vaporizes, or cuts tissue depending on the power. The power applied to the electrocautery device (measured in Watts) corresponds to the heat generated in the tissue, as related by the equation, power = $(\text{current})^2 \times$ resistance. Coagulation involves high amperage and low voltage, whereas vaporization uses high voltage and low amperage. Cutting tissue with the ability to coagulate blends these 2 settings. At the temperature of approximately 70°C tissue coagulates and over 200°C tissue carbonizes. The degree of destruction depends on the applied power, the electrical properties of the tissue, the device-tissue contact time, and the device-tissue contact surface area.

When a tissue is heated sufficiently, cellular water evaporates, thereby destroying the cell and then the tissue. Heating to higher temperatures leads to chemical breakdown of the cell and tissue constituents and eventual vaporization/carbonization. Electrocautery devices are monopolar; that is, they require the bronchoscope, the generator, and the patient to be grounded to complete the circuit, or otherwise shocks and burns may occur. The bronchoscope should be insulated. The generator should at least have an isolated power output to minimize current leakage and possible injury, if it is not grounded.

Indications

The indications and contraindications for electrocautery are similar to those of Nd:YAG laser **(Tables 1 and 2)**. Similarly, laser therapy electrocautery produces rapid debulking of a tumor but at a lower cost.[96,97]

Equipment and Technique

Insulated flexible bronchoscopes with working channels of 2.0 or 2.6 mm are used. Electrocautery blunt-tip probe, snare is compatible with the flexible bronchoscopes most commonly used. The generator should regulate the high-frequency current, so that operator can adjust the setting depending on whether the procedure is intended to coagulate, cut, cut and coagulate, or vaporize. The monopolar unit must be grounded with an electrode pad.

The operator can use either a closed forceps or the blunt electrocautery probe to manipulate the lesion and thus to assess its size, mobility, friability/bleeding potential, and to locate any attachment to the airway. Polypoid lesions may be amenable to the snare. The snare is used to cut and remove tissue and a blended current is used to cut and coagulate but not vaporize.

Outcomes

Homasson showed that hemoptysis was controlled in 75% of the cases, dyspnea alleviated in 67%, and cough or stridor relieved in 55%.[98] Petrou reported that 28 of 29 patients had symptomatic improvement after removal of a lesion, with a snare.[99] Sutedja showed that 15 of 17 treated patients had immediate restoration of a patent airway; eight had relief of dyspnea, and four had control of hemoptysis.[100] Most series involve predominantly malignancies, and success is defined as removal of greater than 50% of the tumor; success rates of 70–95% have been reported.[101-103]

Complications

Two endobronchial fires have been reported during the electrocautery procedure; both were associated with high-inspired oxygen concentrations, and in one, a silicon stent also ignited.[102] Several investigators have reported minor hemorrhage in most cases, one death occurred secondary to hemorrhage. Operator and patient burns and electrical shocks are mentioned frequently as possible complications; however, published data are scant. Another concern is using electrocautery in a patient with a pacemaker or an automatic implantable defibrillator because the devices may malfunction. Airway stenosis, and cartilage damage can occur with electrocautery, when used in animal models.

Argon Plasma Coagulation

Argon plasma coagulation (APC) is an electrosurgical technique similar to laser or electrocautery used to remove an obstructing lesion and/or to achieve homeostasis. The indications and contraindication are similar as in **Tables 1 and 2**. APC was developed more than 20 years ago to improve surgical hemostasis. In the early 1990s, a flexible probe was introduced that facilitated its use during endoscopic procedures. APC was initially used during GIT endoscopy to achieve hemostasis during polypectomy.[104] APC has been used during bronchoscopic procedures to debulk malignant airway tumors, control hemoptysis, remove granulation tissue from stents or anastomoses, and treat a variety of other benign disorders.[105-109] This is a form of electrocautery of a

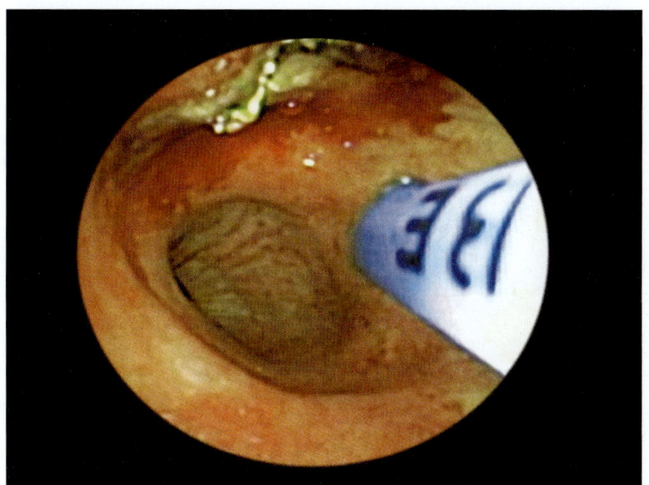

Fig. 3 Argon plasma coagulation (APC) use with an Escher formation

noncontact form. The indications and contraindications are similar to laser and electrocautery.

Procedure

As for electrocautery, a grounding pad should be placed on the patient back. The settings should consist of power of 30 Watts and an argon flow rate of 0.8–1 L/minute. Argon flow rate will determine the length of the flame. As the argon will seek biological tissue or any combustible object, the flame length is important in its airway application. This piece of equipment is generally shared by multiple operators, therefore prior to the use the setting should be fixed for your own needs. The probe tip should be several centimeters beyond the bronchoscope's tip. This ensures that the bronchoscope will not be burned. The probe tip should be within 1 cm of the target lesion. The electric current will not be conducted if the probe is farther from the target lesion. The probe tip should not contact the target lesion.

Argon gas is expelled from the probe and then a high voltage electric current is passed along the probe. When the electric current contacts the argon gas, the gas becomes ionized and conducts a monopolar current to the target lesion.[106,107] This argon plasma is applied to the surface in 1–3 second bursts. The net tissue effect is similar to electrocautery.

In the process of debulking a endobronchial lesion, the eschar is first formed **(Fig. 3)** with the application of APC and then removed with forceps or a cryotherapy probe. APC is then applied to the underlying fresh tissue. This process is repeated until the tumor is removed. If brisk bleeding is encountered, the argon gas can used without the ignition of the gas to blow blood away thus improving visualization.

Outcomes

In a prospective cohort study of 364 patients who underwent APC (482 procedures), a success rate of 67%, defined as hemostasis and/or full or partial airway recanalization was reported.[108] Rigid bronchoscopy was used in 90% of the interventions. In a retrospective cohort study of 60 patients who underwent APC (70 procedures), treatment was immediately successful in 59 patients.[108] All of the patients had either hemoptysis or airway obstruction, with treatment success defined as resolution of hemoptysis and/or decreased airway obstruction. Hemoptysis did not recur over a mean follow-up of 97 days and improved dyspnea persisted over a mean follow-up of 53 days. A similar study of 47 patients reported a success rate of 92%, which was maintained over a mean follow-up of 6.7 months.[106] However, an average of more than three sessions per patient were required to achieve this result. APC has successfully treated benign disorders such as granulation tissue due to stents or airway anastomosis.[107,108]

Complications

Complications of APC are infrequent (less than 1% of procedures). They include airway burn and airway perforation, which can cause pneumomediastinum, subcutaneous emphysema, and pneumothorax.[110] Gas embolism has also been described in a case series, leading to three cases of cardiovascular collapse and one case of death.[111] Such a complication is a reflection of the lack of experience by the operator. A burned bronchoscope has also been reported. Similar to laser and electrocautery limiting the inspired oxygen concentration, the 'd' power (less than 40 Watts), and the application time (less than 5 seconds) probably minimizes the risk of airway fire. Keeping the probe tip several centimeters away from any combustible material likely prevents airway fire.

Cryotherapy

Cryotherapy deals with the destruction of biological materials through the cytotoxic effects of freezing. The damage induced by freezing occurs at several levels, including the molecular level, the cellular level, structural level and the whole tissue. Documents from 3500 BC described the use of cold as treatment for swelling and war wounds.[112] Hippocrates described the use of cold to treat orthopedic injuries.[112] Arnott described the use of salt solutions containing crushed ice at a temperature of about –8°C to –12°C to freeze advanced cancers in accessible sites, producing reduction in tumor size and improvement of pain.[113,114] The Joule-Thomson effect, which is the sudden expansion of a gas from a high to a low-pressure region, is the basis for how the current cryoprobes function, especially in pulmonary medicine.

The destructive effect of cold had been confirmed also by the healing of the tracheobronchial tree, with the restoration of a normal ciliated epithelium without stenosis in mongrel dogs.[115-122] The first study from the Mayo Clinic, consisting of 28 patients with endobronchial

Table 3 Cryosensitive and cryoresistant tissues

Cryosensitive	*Cryoresistant*
Skin	Fat
Mucous membrane	Cartilage
Nerve	Nerve sheath
Endothelium	Connective tissue
Granulation tissue	Fibrosis

tumors concluded that cryotherapy did serve as a good alternative for palliation.[122]

The effect of freeze injury is influenced by many factors and the survival of cells is dependent on the cooling rate, the thawing rate, the lowest temperature achieve and repeated freezing-thawing cycles.[123-129] Certain tissues are cryosensitive (skin, mucous membrane, granulation tissue), and others cryoresistant, such as fat, cartilage, fibrous or connective tissue **(Table 3)**. The cryosensitivity depends on the water content of the cells. Tumor cells may be more sensitive than normal cell.[130]

Cooling Agents

Several cooling agents can be used as cryogens. These are generally used in the liquid phase so that on vaporization, they remove heat at a constant temperature (heat of vaporization). Several studies have shown that the core temperature needed for a lesion to be destroyed is between -20°C and -40°C. Freezing to -40°C or below at the rapid rate of -100°C per minute will cause more than 90% cell death.

Nitrous oxides (N_2O) are most common cooling agents used. The vapor haze of N_2O occurs at the metal tip of the cryoprobes where it expands from a high pressure to atmospheric pressure (Joule-Thomson effect). This expansion lowers the temperature of the fluid and produces droplets of liquid and reaches equilibrium of -89°C at atmospheric pressure.

Cryotherapy Equipment

The cryoprobes are rigid, semirigid or flexible; rigid and semirigid cryoprobes can only be used through a rigid bronchoscope, but flexible cryoprobes can be used through the channel of the fiberoptic bronchoscope. The diameter of the flexible probes requires larger working channel fiberoptic bronchoscope (2.6-3.2 mm).

The monitoring of the freezing remains a problem and there is no ideal solution.[131] The empirical method relies on the experience of the operator, and the operator relies on the change in color/consistency of the frozen tissue, and the length of freezing. In clinical studies, using rigid, semirigid or flexible, each freeze-thaw cycle is about 30 second.[132-135] The thaw phase is almost immediate with rigid probes that have a system of reheating; but with the flexible probes thawing is by body temperature, thus increasing the freeze-thaw cycle timing.

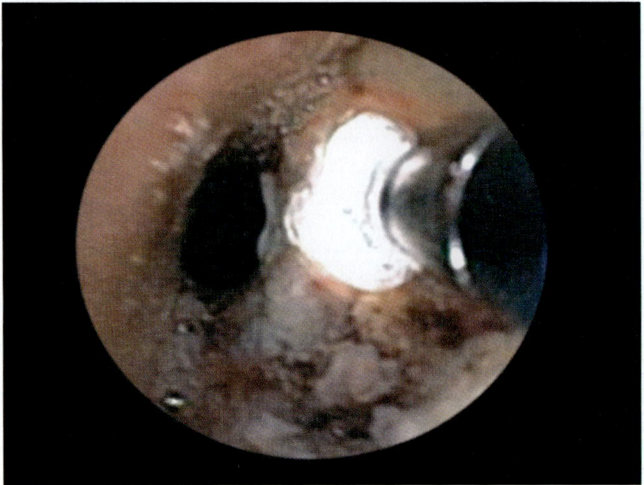

Fig. 4 Use of the cryotherapy

Indications

Cryotherapy is indicated for tracheobronchial obstruction **(Fig. 4)**. The selection criteria are similar to those of laser, APC or electrocautery **(Tables 1 and 2)**, except when there is an urgency to treat. In addition, cryotherapy can be used for extraction of foreign bodies, blood clots, mucous plugs.

Technique

The flexible cryoprobe is passed through the working channel which is visualized and directly applied to the tumor area. The cryoprobe is activated with a foot pedal. An ice ball appears within 30 seconds on the tip of the probe; 2–3 freeze thaw cycles, each lasting for 1 minute are applied to the same or near-by area. The tip of the probe can be applied perpendicularly, tangentially or driven into the tumor mass. The tissues are frozen at -30 to -40°C. The cryoprobe is deactivated by removal of the foot from the foot pedal.

The metallic tip of the cryoprobe that produces circumferential freezing of maximal volume is placed on or pushed into the tumor. 2–3 freeze-thaw cycles are carried out at each site. The probe is then moved 5-6 mm and another 3 cycles carried out in the adjoining area. The hemostatic effect of freezing is often sufficient to stop hemoptysis.

Outcomes

Walsh reported the effects of cryotherapy on dyspnea, hemoptysis, cough, and stridor.[136] In his study, symptoms, lung function, chest radiography, and bronchoscopic findings were recorded serially before and after 81 cryotherapy sessions in 33 consecutive patients. Most patients improved in the overall symptoms, stridor, dyspnea and hemoptysis.

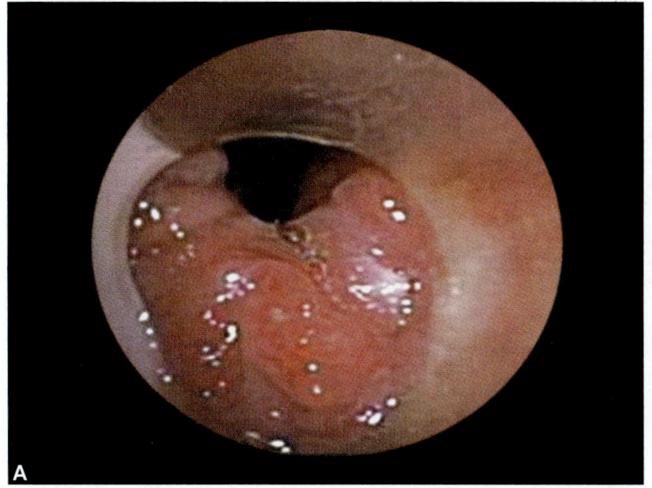

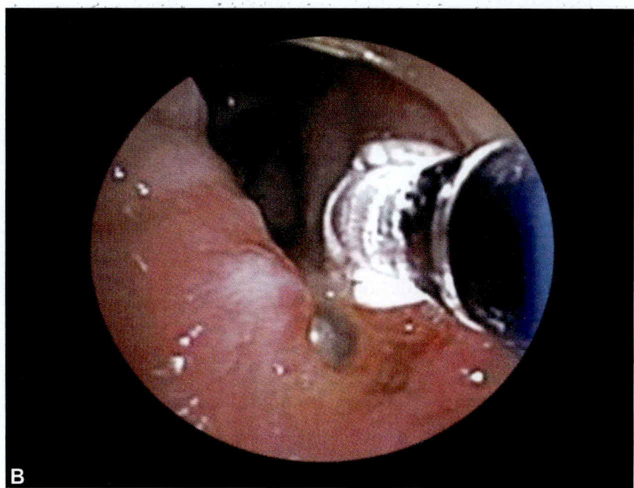

Figs 5A and B Use of cryotherapy in granulation tissue formed after a stent placement

Maiwand reported 600 patients with cryotherapy; following cryotherapy, 78% of the patients noticed a subjective improvement in their condition.[137] These patients had less coughs (64%), dyspnea (66%) hemoptysis (65%) and stridor (70%) following cryotherapy. Homasson described that hemoptysis stopped in 80% of cases and dyspnea was less in 50% of case.[138] Mathur reported similar findings in a smaller number of patients when cryotherapy was used with a fiberoptic bronchoscope.[135,139]

Hetzel demonstrated cryorecannalization of 60 patients with endobronchial tumors.[140] Tumor tissue was frozen on the tip of the probe and subsequently removed from the surrounding respiratory tract tissue through retraction of the probe; 83% patients were completely or partially treated with success. Bleeding occurred in 6 patients but required treatment with argon plasma coagulator. The same group extended their experience in a larger group of patients (225 patients) with symptomatic airway stenosis.[141] Successful cryo-recanalization was achieved in 91.1%. APC was used in 16.4% for bleeding. A bronchus blocker was required in 8.0% patients.

The flexible cryoprobe for treatment of symptomatic endobronchial tumor stenosis is successful for immediate treatment but the safety has to questioned. This can be potentially dangerous in inexperienced hands. This method has been helpful in getting a bigger biopsy sample.[141]

Forty-one patients with diffuse lung disease were selected for transbronchial biopsy.[142] Conventional transbronchial biopsies using forceps were done first. Then a flexible cryoprobe was introduced into the selected bronchus under fluoroscopic guidance. Once brought into position, the probe was cooled and then retracted with the frozen lung tissue being attached on the probe's tip. Bigger samples could be obtained. Two patients had a pneumothorax which resolved with tube thoracostomy.

There has been a renewed interest in treatment of early stages of lung cancers. The French experience reported by the GECC (study group on cryosurgery) is based on 36 patients with 44 lesions ("*in situ*" or microinvasive tumors); 42% of these patients had been treated for an invasive ENT or bronchial cancer.[143] At 1 year, there was complete clinical and histological control of the tumor in 88.8 % with a mean follow-up of 32 months. The mean survival of this population was 30 months.

Benign Tracheobronchial Lesions

Benign lesions have been treated with cryotherapy with very good results, particularly for granulomatous tissues; 100% had favorable results with no recurrence months or even years after treatment (**Figs 5A and B**). Granulation tissue is very sensitive to the effects of cold. Nevertheless, when surgery is not possible, treatment with cryotherapy can yield good results, and several cases of carcinoid, cylindromas, and laryngotracheal papillomas have been successfully treated.

Removal of Foreign Bodies

Foreign bodies have been extracted with success using cryotherapy, most useful to remove friable matter, biological matter, such as pills, peanuts, tooth, chicken bones, etc. This is extremely helpful in the removal blood clots mucus plugs, and slough.

In the treatment of lung cancers, local cryotherapy has been used for palliative care.[144] Forest has demonstrated differential biological effects of these therapies and the benefit to combine them.[145-149] As vascular changes occur after cryotherapy, intratumoral angiogenesis was also studied. Tumors were treated by cryotherapy and chemotherapy by injection of vinorelbine or both. Tumor growth was studied in each group and the treatment/control (T/C) ratios were compared. Tumors treated by cryochemotherapy presented a significantly reduced volume and the lower T/C ratio, confirming the benefit of a combined treatment.

Photodynamic Therapy

Photodynamic therapy is used for endobronchial destruction of tumor and also in treatment of early superficial lung cancer. The only available agent Porfimer (Photofrin®), in a dose of 2 mg/kg is injected intravenously, slowly over 5–10 minutes. There is preferential retention in tumor cells and in vascular endothelium, the cytotoxic reaction of Porfimer is selective for neoplastic cells.[150] After 48 hours, the tumor is exposed to light energy, which triggers the cytotoxic reaction. The absorption peak occurs at a wavelength of 405 nm. For adequate penetration and destruction, a wavelength of 630 nm is used to a depth of 5–10 mm.[151]

The most commonly used design is a cylindrical diffuser which emitts light in a 360° arc near its tip. It is recommended initially to apply 200 Joules/cm treated; additional energy may be applied during a follow-up bronchoscopy, 2 days later and 200 J generally applied with a dye laser. Tumor is visualized, the light fiber is introduced through the working channel and the light is delivered to produce the cytotoxic reaction. A repeat bronchoscopy is performed in 48 hours. First the debris and secretion are removed, then a second treatment is applied.

The most common adverse event of PDT is photosensitivity of the skin. The patient is at risk 4–6 weeks after injection and protective gear must be worn till then.

Outcomes

Photodynamic therapy has shown to have an excellent cure rate in early stage endobronchial cancer, i.e. CIS. In a large study with 175 patients who underwent PDT of stage 0, the 5 years disease-related survival rate was 93%. Other studies have shown similar data.[152-156] PDT has been used for palliation with similar results with other endoscopic techniques but with significant skin photo toxicity. In a randomized control trial, when PDT was compared to Nd:YAG laser, the relief of the symptom were similar.[157] Our preference has been to limit the use of PDT only in superficial early lung cancer.

Brachytherapy

Endobronchial radiation therapy by the use of an implanted source of ionizing radiation (brachytherapy) was first used in the 1920s. Yankauer reported on the implantation of radium into an endobronchial tumor using a bronchoscope and leaving the radium in capsules attached to a string that exited through the mouth.[158] In the mid-1980s publications appeared which distinguished low-dose-rate (LDR) from high-dose-rate (HDR) brachytherapy. LDR brachytherapy is usually defined as less than 2 gray (Gy)/hour and a total dose between 1,500 and 5,000 Gy, given over 3 days. HDR involves more than 10 Gy/hour, in which the total dose and the dose per session (fraction) varies. Fractions have varied anywhere from approximately 300–1,000 Gy, and total dose from approximately 500–4,000 Gy.

Henschke developed the remote after-loading device, thereby reducing radiation exposure to the healthcare staff.[159] Almost 20 years later, the use of the flexible bronchoscope and the polyethylene catheter that holds the radioactive material for brachytherapy was described.[160,161] Iridium-192, the current radiation source was also first described at this time.[160]

Techniques and Dosage

Currently intraluminal brachytherapy uses fiberoptic bronchoscopy for the placement of polyethylene catheter adjacent to the tumor. The placement is verified by bronchoscopy and by radiograph. The catheter can be loaded with the radiation source manually or with a remote after loader. The dose rate of brachytherapy depends on the radioactivity of the radionuclide used. The apparatus designed to deliver HDR brachytherapy uses iridium-192 which is the radionuclide of choice. HDR brachytherapy is usually delivered as fractionated doses to maximize its safety and effectiveness. Treatment schedules vary in clinical practice because the procedure requires bronchoscopy and placement of endobronchial catheters during each session. Most patients are treated once a week or once every 2 weeks rather than once a day to minimize patient discomfort.

Indications and Contraindications

The indications are similar to those of any endobronchial therapy discussed earlier. The goal of brachytherapy is for palliation of symptoms caused by airway obstruction by the tumor. Brachytherapy however, can also be used as an adjunct to external beam radiotherapy for treatment of otherwise unresectable lung cancer. Some investigators have used it in patients who have histologically positive surgical margins after resection.[162]

Absolute contraindications for endobronchial brachytherapy include the presence of known fistulas to nonbronchial tissue areas and lesions that are not proven malignancies. Patients with endotracheal carcinoma causing high-grade obstruction should be treated with Nd:YAG laser and possible placement of stent before brachytherapy because of the potential for postradiation edema and total airway obstruction.

Outcomes

Most studies of brachytherapy have reported on its use in combination with external beam radiation therapy. Subjective improvement after brachytherapy has ranged from 20 to 100% depending on the symptoms. Hemoptysis is relieved in more than 90% of the treated patient. Cough and dyspnea had moderate to minimal relief, probably owing to the underlying chronic bronchitis or radiation fibrosis. In most of studies, there was a greater than 50% improvement in the patency of the airway. The positive response of most studies persisted for 6 months or more.[163-170]

Conventional external-beam radiation therapy relieves symptoms of hemoptysis, dyspnea, or chest pain in 50–80% of patients for 3–4 months.[168] There are no studies directly comparing the external-beam radiation therapy with endobronchial brachytherapy. Based on existing data, however, endobronchial brachytherapy is the second-line treatment option to offer effective palliation.

Complications

Brachytherapy has both early and late complications. The two most serious complications of endobronchial brachytherapy are massive hemoptysis and fistula formation to the mediastinum. Serious complications range from 0 to 42% in several large series. Risk of massive pulmonary hemorrhage is likely related to the proximity of pulmonary arteries to the left upper lobe bronchus. Bedwinek found a 32% rate of massive hemoptysis with recurrent tumors in the right upper lobe, right main stem, and left upper lobe bronchus.[169,170]

Flexible Fiberoptic Balloon Dilation

The successful use of a balloon to dilate a benign airway stricture was first reported in an 18 weeks infant with a postsurgical stricture.[171] These initial reports utilized fluoroscopy or rigid bronchoscopy to guide the dilation procedure. Flexible fiberoptic bronchoscopy with balloon dilation was not described until 1991, since that time relatively few reports with small numbers of patients have been published.[171-178] This technique is useful in the treatment of benign strictures due sequela of long-term endotracheal intubation, bronchial reimplantation, anastomosis of transplanted lungs, granulomatous disease (e.g. TB, Wegener's granulomatosis) or smoke inhalation. A suitable lesion for balloon dilation is a web-like stenosis. The success is poor if there is loss of supporting structures. Medical treatment for the cause of the stricture should be performed prior to attempts at dilation. As an example, the local treatment of patients with strictures secondary to TB should not be attempted until adequate antimicrobial treatment has been given.

Technique

Bronchoscopic balloon dilation is a simple method to dilate a stenosis. A flexible fiberoptic bronchoscope is used in a standard manner with topical anesthesia and conscious sedation. After identification of the stenosis, a 0.89 mm diameter guidewire is passed through the working channel, advanced beyond the stenosis and monitored fluoroscopically. Once the guidewire is in place, the bronchoscope is removed and the guidewire is left in place. Next, a balloon catheter which has been selected based upon diameter of the stenosis, is passed. The balloon has variable diameters, the dilation can be started with small size and then increased in size. The marking on the balloon, which is radiologically opaque, should protrude beyond each end of the stenosed segment for the dilatation of the entire lesion. If the balloon does not extend distally, it tends to slip out of the stenosis upon inflation. If the balloon is ineffective it should be replaced by a larger one. Repeated inflations can be performed with the same balloon if the result is inadequate. Immediate success or failure will be visible to the bronchoscopist **(Figs 6A to C)**.

Complications

Excessive balloon inflation or a larger length may lacerate or rupture the airway, but these complications have not been reported.

Outcomes

Several case series of fiberoptic bronchoscopic balloon dilation in adults have been reported. The largest series involved 19 stenosis in 16 patients. Initial success was achieved in 13 of 19 bronchial stenosis; six dilations were unsuccessful because the stenosis were caused by localized bronchomalacia.[176-178] On an average, about 50% success rate has been reported without reinterventions. Surgical treatment of the stenotic segment is technically feasible in most patients. Endobronchial cryotherapy in conjunction with balloon dilation has been used in two cases of benign airway stenosis with success.[178] An airway stent is usually needed if there is damage to the cartilage in the trachea or bronchi, resulting in bronchomalacia.[178]

Airway Stents

The term "stent" honors a late nineteenth century British dentist, Charles R Stent, who developed a dental impression material that was later used as a template to support healing skin grafts.[179] Today, the term stent connotes an artificial support that maintains patency of a hollow tubular structure. Airway stents can play an important role when the large airway is compressed by an extraluminal lesion **(Figs 5A and B)**. There is no ideal stent but some characteristics make it more valuable, such as ease of insertion and removal, infrequent migration, resistance to external forces, minimal tissue reaction, improved mobilization of secretions, etc.

Indications

Stent may be used alone or with other techniques for palliation of dyspnea, cough, or respiratory insufficiency due to central airway obstruction. An airway stent supports the airway wall against collapse or external compression and can impede

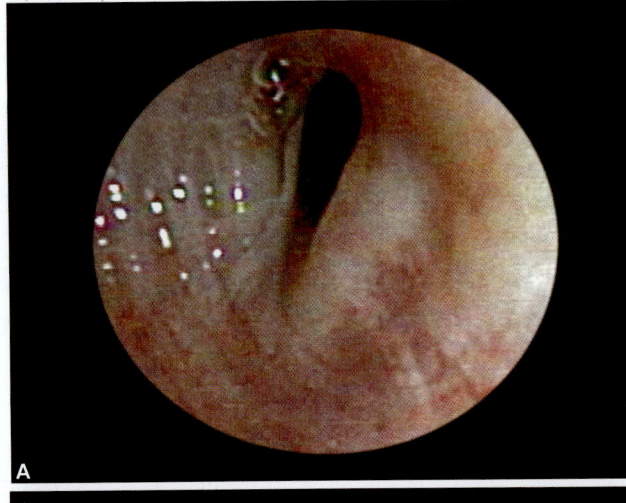

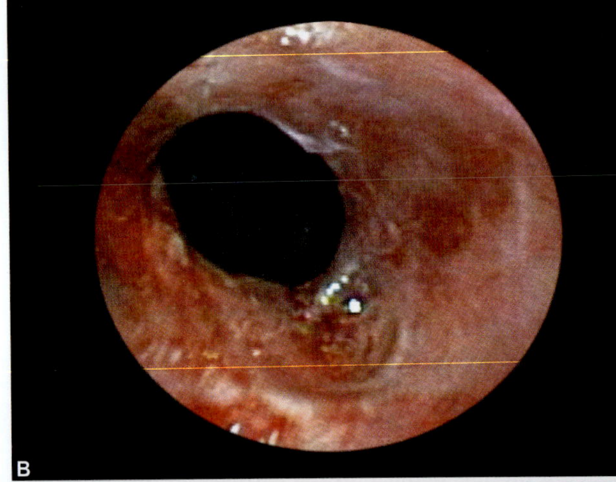

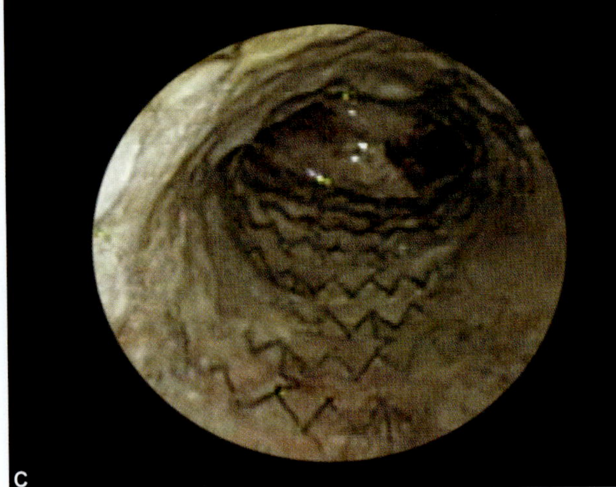

Figs 6A to C (A and B) Web-like stenosis which has been improved by a balloon dilation; (C) A metal stent

extension of tumor into the airway lumen. Stents can be safely used in patients undergoing external-beam radiation therapy or brachytherapy.[76]

Table 4 Airways stents

Silicone stents	*Metal stents*
Rigid bronchoscopy	Flexible bronchoscopy
Removable	Extremely difficult to remove
High migration rate	Low migration rate
Thick caliber	Thin caliber
Infections	Infections
Mucostasis	Mucostasis
Granulation tissue formation	Granulation tissue formation

There is no survival difference between those patients without malignant airway obstruction who received palliative chemotherapy (median survival, 8.4 months) and others with airway obstruction, who received treatment with laser, stent, or both followed by chemotherapy.[180] Surgical repair is the first choice to treat a benign strictures due prolonged intubation, infectious or inflammatory diseases. Stenting is required if there are comorbid conditions that do not allow surgery. There is US Food and Drug Administration (FDA) black box warning against placing metal stent in a patient with be benign strictures.

Types of Stents

Tracheobronchial stents can be grouped as silicone, metal or hybrid stents. Silicone stents include montgomery T-tube, Dumon, Polyflex, Noppen, and Hood **(Table 4)**. The metal stents are available as covered or uncovered which include Palmaz, Wall Stent Wallgraft and Ultraflex. The hybrid stents are a combination of both such as Orlowski and Dynamic stents.

Silicone stents: The most widely used type of stent for central airway obstruction is the silicone stent **(Figs 7A and B)**. Silicone rubber is a synthetic substance made of silicone elastomers; it is firm, stable at high temperatures, and repels water. Silicone stents are relatively inexpensive and well tolerated. They can be repositioned and removed without difficulty. Disadvantages include: Stent migration, granuloma formation, mucous plugging, insufficient flexibility to conform to irregular airways, interference with mucociliary clearance, and a need for rigid bronchoscopy for their placement.

Types and Outcomes

Montgomery t-tube: Montgomery T-tube, introduced in 1965, is the original stent used for the treatment of subglottic and tracheal stenosis.[181] A tracheotomy is needed to place this stent during operation or via rigid bronchoscopy. The limb protruding out of the tracheostoma for cricoid or glottic stenosis is left open, unplugged transiently for bronchial toilet, or closed to allow speech. Radial force is not required to hold this stent in position. Montgomery T-tube a safe stent and is used for sub glottis stenosis.

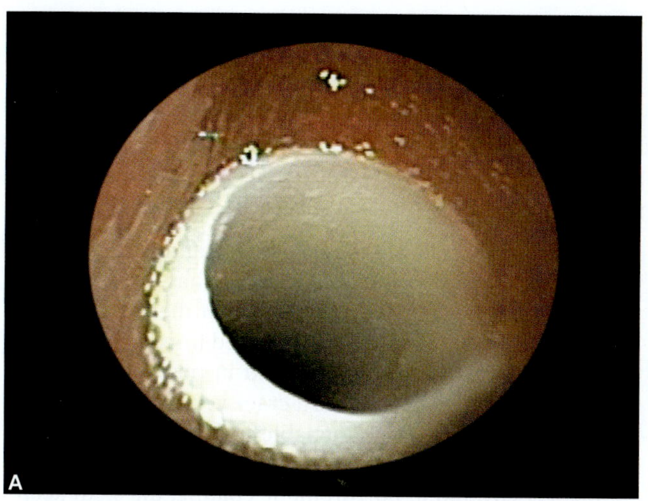
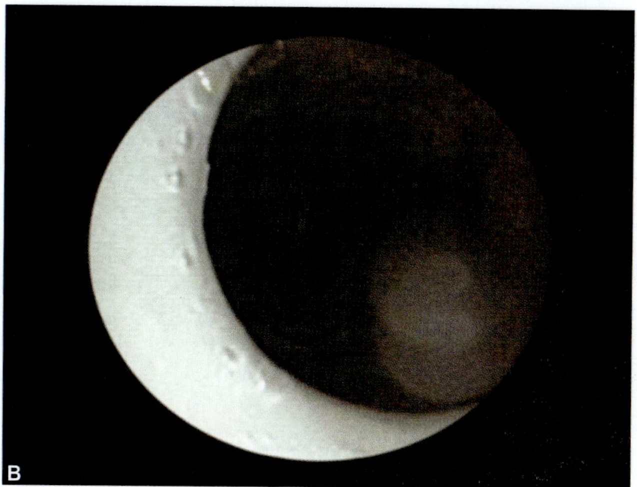

Figs 7A and B Silicone stent on the proximal end as well passing through the silicone stent

Smooth-walled hood stent: The smooth-walled hood stent is one of the first silicone stents designed for use in the airway. It is a straight, smooth-walled silicone tube that can he ordered in varying lengths and diameters, or in the shape of a Y. This stent does easily migrate, the design has been now modified to include a small flange on its proximal and distal aspects. Nevertheless, stent migration still occurs.

Studded Dumon stent: Dumon initially described his experience with a new dedicated tracheobronchial prosthesis made of silicone with studs to decrease the migration.[182] The studded Dumon stent has become the most widely used airway stent in the world since its introduction and now is considered by many as the gold standard. The stent is manufactured in various diameters, lengths, and shapes, including a straight, L-shaped, and Y-shaped.

A multicenter trial followed 1,058 patients in whom 1,574 stents were placed, of which 698 were for malignant airway obstruction.[183] Stent migration occurred in 9.5% of the patients and granuloma formation in 8%. In a similar study by Diaz-Jimenez silicone stents were placed in 60 patients with malignant disease and 30 patients with benign tracheobronchial disease.[137,184] Migration was observed in 13% and granuloma in 6%. The stent stays in place due to radial force and the studs, but still has a significant migration rate.

Reynders-Noppen Tygon stent: The Reynders-Noppen Tygon stent is not commercially available in the United States. It is a cylindrical tygon plastic tube molded into a screw-thread form. This stent is far more rigid than the silicone stents. It must be pushed into place along the outside of a specific introducer; it cannot be folded into an applicator for bronchoscopic introduction. One study compared the outcome of 50 patients treated with either studded Dumon silicone stents or screw-thread stents. Stent migration occurred in more patients who received Dumon stent (24% vs. 5%), although the difference was not statistically significant.[185]

Polyflex stent: Polyflex stent is a self-expanding stent made of cross-woven polyester threads embedded in silicone. Stents of different lengths and diameters and tapered models are available for sealing stump fistula. In one study of 12 patients, who received 16 stents, the migration rate was at 75%. These investigators have abandoned the use of Polyflex stents.[186]

Metal stents: Various metals such as stainless steel, tantalum or alloys incorporating cobalt, chromium, and molybdenum (Vittalium, Nobelium) are inherently inert and can be safely placed into living tissues **(Fig. 6C)**. All metal stents are radiopaque, exhibit varying degrees of radial force, are easy to insert, and maintain ventilation when placed across lobar orifices. These stents can be further divided into fixed-diameter stents which require balloon dilatation, and self-expandable stents which spring to a predetermined diameter once released. These stents could be either made of bare metal or have a thin coating with silicon, nylon, or polyurethane. They can be placed in an outpatient setting via flexible bronchoscopy and under local anesthesia.[187,188]

Due to the ease of use, it has led to significant abuse and harm to patients. Advantage of metallic stents include that their walls are thinner than a silicone stent and are able to conform to tortuous airway. Similar to the silicone stent granulation tissue formation does take place. The disadvantage is the difficulty in removing and repositioning the stent. Fractures of the wires may occur due the constant movement and metal fatigue **(Fig. 8)**. Metal stents rarely migrate (<1%).

Palmaz and strecker stents: The Palmaz and Strecker stents are fixed-diameter balloon-expandable stents. These stents do not exhibit any intrinsic radial force; there by compressive forces such as breathing and coughing leads to collapse of the stent which in turn obstructs the airway. The plastic behavior of the Palmaz stents makes it unsuitable for use.

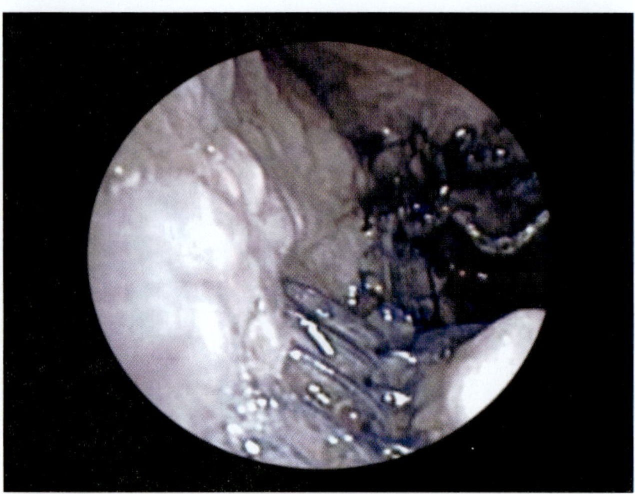

Fig. 8 Broken wire of a metal stent and granulation tissue

Gianturco stent: The Gianturco stent is made of a continuous loop of stainless steel wire and can be compressed into a narrow cylinder before bronchoscopic placement. Once expanded, the stent maintains an expansive force, and small hooks embed in the airway mucosa to retard migration. Complications lead to trachea-pharyngeal fistula and fatal erosion of pulmonary artery. The combination of high radial force exerted over the airway mucosa at selected contact points where there are hooks can lead to mucosal ischemia and perforation.[189] Due to the severity of reported complications, this stent should not be used.

Wall stent: Wall stent is a self-expanding device made of cobalt alloy braided filaments in the form of a tubular mesh. It has a special feature of outward radial force provided by its integral design. It is inserted in a constrained form, and once deployed, it expands to a preset diameter. The stent can be loaded into a delivery catheter, it expands and shortens upon placement. Stents of various lengths and diameters are available. The covered form of the wall stent prevents tumor and granulation growing through the spaces between the thin wire mesh. Dasgupta used 52 uncovered Wall stents in 37 patients, 20 with malignant airway obstruction and 17 with benign disease. Stent-related obstructive granuloma occurred in 11% of patients and stent migration not found.[190]

Ultraflex: The ultraflex is a self-expanding stent made of nitinol which is an alloy with shape memory, which deforms at low temperatures and regains its original shape at higher temperatures. Miyazawa deployed 54 ultraflex stents through flexible or rigid bronchoscopy. Immediate relief of dyspnea was achieved in 82% of the patients and migration was not observed.[191] Herth further demonstrated that the ultraflex stents could be placed satisfactorily without fluoroscopy.[192] Long-term outcome of patients with malignant and benign airway strictures treated with either wall stents and ultraflex stents was analyzed. Median follow-up was 42 days for patients with lung cancer, 329 days for lung transplant recipients. The complication rate was 0.06 complication per patient-month. The most common complication were infectious tracheoabronchitis, obstructing granulomas requiring interventions to restore airway patency. Tumor growth and stent fracture were also seen.[192]

Alveolus stent: Alveolus stent is also self-expanding, completely polyurethane-covered metallic stent. It has been claimed that the stent can be easily removed, but there are no data on this. The Alveolus stent is constructed from a single piece of nitinol, with concentric rings held in position by nitinol strands, this feature also makes it crack vertically, very easily. Due to its structure, it is amenable to length modification. Because it does not foreshorten with deployment and is completely covered in polyurethane coating, the stent keeps to its trimmed length and structural integrity.[193]

Hybrid stents: Several stents incorporating both silicone and metal have been designed in an attempt to remedy some of the drawbacks of purely silicone or metal devices. Hybrid stents consist of expandable metal struts that resist compression but are covered by a silicone membrane, which limits infiltration by tumor or granulation tissue.

The Rusch Y-stent: The Rusch Y-stent it is a Y-shaped stent made of silicone with a firm anterior wall that consists of horseshoe-shaped metal struts which simulate the anterior trachea wall; the posterior wall is made of soft silicone, simulating the pars membranosa of the trachea. The stent can be difficult to insert. It is placed during rigid laryngoscopy by means of a specially designed forceps, and the two distal limbs are inserted into the left and right main bronchi.[194] However, its length makes it difficult for patients to effectively clear airway secretions, and removal can be difficult if it becomes obstructed. It is used for strictures of the trachea, main carina and/or main bronchi; trachea-bronchomalacia; trachea bronchomegaly, and esophageal fistula.

Choice of Stent

The first issue to be addressed is the proper selection of stent size. The length and diameter in relation to the dimensions of the trachea or bronchus are also important to avoid stent-related complications, such as migration, granulation formation, retention of secretions or airway perforation due to excessive radial force **(Figs 5A and B, 9)**. Metal stents are more expensive than silicone. They are difficult, if not impossible, to remove. Silicone stents require specialized equipment, along with rigid bronchoscope, whereas metal stents can be inserted via flexible bronchoscopy. The ease of placement should not lead to the erroneous choice of the easiest stent over the best one to treat a given condition. The immediate and long-term complications should be thought of before a stent is placed.

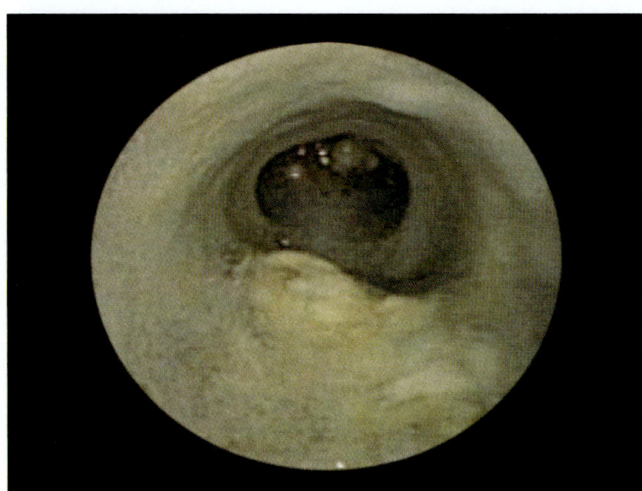

Fig. 9 Retained secretion in a metal stent

A checklist suggested by Lee is as follows:[195]

- "Is a stent required?
- Will the patient benefit from stent placement in terms of quality of life or prognosis?
- Does the stent interfere or prohibit a curative surgical procedure later?
- Do I have the expertise, equipment, and team to place the stent?
- What is the underlying airway pathology and which stent is ideal?
- Is it safe to place a stent in this anatomic site?
- What are the required stent dimensions (length and diameter)? and
- Do I have the optimal stent or should I order a more appropriate one?"

This checklist will avoid errors and also do less harm to the patient. In benign strictures, only silicone stent should be used as they are easy to remove and replace.

Technique

Bronchoscopy should be first performed in a patient with tracheobronchial stenosis. When a stenosis is evaluated, the distance from the vocal cords and the length and diameter of the lesion should be documented. A spiral CT scan with 3-dimensional reconstruction is extremely helpful in the sizing of the stent that will be needed. The largest possible prosthesis should be selected.

If a lesion is not amenable to endoscopic removal, bronchial dilatation should be done so that the stent of greatest diameter can be inserted.

The self-expanding stent that is mounted on an introduction catheter with crochet knots or is pushed out from the delivery system. The distal release model is easier to deploy than the proximal release design. The Polyflex stent with its pusher system is deployed with the help of a rigid bronchoscope. Insertion of the Dumon stent is facilitated by the use of the dedicated Dumon-Efer rigid bronchoscope and stent applicator set. Placement of dynamic and other bifurcated stents is facilitated with dedicated forceps.

Airway stenting is a valuable adjunct to other therapeutic bronchoscopic techniques used for relieving central airway obstruction. Each stent has it unique feature and complications. The technology is still in evolution, and design modifications strive to find the perfect stent. The Dumon stent remains the gold standard against which the all other stents.

REFERENCES

1. Mathur PN, Beamis J. Interventional Pulmonology. Chest Clinics of North America: WB Saunders; 1995.
2. Bolliger CT, Mathur PN, Beamis JF, Becker HD, Cavaliere S, Colt H, et al. ERS/ATS statement on interventional pulmonology. European Respiratory Society/American Thoracic Society. Eur Respir J. 2002;19:356-73.
3. Tyson EB. The development of the bronchoscope. J Med Soc N J. 1957;54:26-30.
4. Jackson C. Bronchoscopy: past, present and future. N Engl J Med. 1928;199:759-63.
5. Dumon JF, Shapshay S, Bourcerau J, Cavaliere S, Meric B, Garbi N, et al. Principles for safety in application of neodymium-YAG laser in bronchology. Chest. 1984;86:163-8.
6. Hirsch FR, Franklin WA, Gazdar AF, Bunn PA. Early detection of lung cancer: clinical perspectives of recent advances in biology and radiology. Clin Cancer Res. 2001;7:5-22.
7. Sutro CJ, Burman MS. Examination of pathologic tissue by filtered ultraviolet radiation. Arch Pathol. 1933;16:346-9.
8. Herly L. Studies in selective differentiation of tissues by means of filtered ultraviolet light. Cancer Res. 1943;1:227-31.
9. Lipson RL, Baldes EJ. The photodynamic properties of a particular hematoporphyrin derivative. Arch Dermatol. 1960;82:508-16.
10. Kato H, Cortese DA. Early detection of lung cancer by means of hematoporphyrin derivative fluorescence and laser photoradiation. Clin Chest Med. 1985;6:237-53.
11. Qu J, MacAulay C, Lam S, Palcic B. Laser induced fluorescence spectroscopy at endoscopy: tissue optics; Monte Carlo modeling and *in vivo* measurements. Opt Eng. 1995;34:3334-43.
12. Qu J, MacAulay C, Lam S, Palcic B. Mechanisms of ratio fluorescence imaging of diseased tissue. Society of Photo-optical Instrumentation Engineers. 1995;2387:71.
13. Lam SC, MacAulay C, Hung JY. Riche JL, Profio AE, Palcic B. Detection of dysplasia and carcinoma *in situ* by a lung imaging fluorescence endoscope (LIFE) device. J Thorac Cardiovasc Surg. 1993;105:1035-40.
14. Lam S, Macaulay C, Leriche JC, Ikeda N, Palcic B. Early localization of bronchogenic carcinoma. Diagn Ther Endosc. 1994;1:75-8.
15. Kennedy TC, McWilliams A, Edell E, Sutedja T, Downie G, Yung R, et al. Bronchial intraepithelial neoplasia/early central airways lung cancer: ACCP evidence-based clinical practice guidelines (2nd edition). Chest. 2007;132:221S-33S.
16. Edell E, Lam S, Pass H, Miller YE, Sutedja T, Kennedy T, et al. Detection and localization of intraepithelial neoplasia and invasive carcinoma using fluorescence-reflectance

bronchoscopy: an international, multicenter clinical trial. J Thorac Oncol. 2009;4:49-54.
17. Lam S, Kennedy T, Unger M, Miller YE, Gelmont D, Rusch V, et al. Localization of bronchial intraepithelial neoplastic lesions by fluorescence bronchoscopy. Chest. 1998;113:696-702.
18. Banerjee AK. Preinvasive lesions of the bronchus. J Thorac Oncol. 2009;4:545-51.
19. Shibuya K, Hoshino H, Chiyo M, Yasufuku K, Iizasa T, Saitoh Y, et al. Subepithelial vascular patterns in bronchial dysplasias using a high magnification bronchovideoscope. Thorax. 2002;57:902-7.
20. Yamada GI, Takahashi H, Shijubo N, Itoh T, Abe S. Subepithelial microvasculature in large airways observed by high-magnification bronchovideoscope. Chest. 2005;128:876-80.
21. Shibuya K, Hoshino H, Chiyo M, Iyoda A, Yoshida S, Sekine Y, et al. High magnification bronchovideoscopy combined with NBI could detect capillary loops of angiogenic squamous dysplasia in heavy smokers at high risk for lung cancer. Thorax. 2003;58:989-95.
22. Vincent BD, Fraig M, Silvestri GA. A pilot study of narrow-band imaging compared to white light bronchoscopy for evaluation of normal airways and premalignant and malignant airways disease. Chest. 2007;131:1794-9.
23. Herth FJ, Eberhardt R, Anantham D, Gompelmann D, Zakaria MW, Ernst A. Narrow-band imaging bronchoscopy increases the specificity of bronchoscopic early lung cancer detection. J Thorac Oncol. 2009;4:1060-5.
24. Drexler W, Morgner U, Kärtner FX, Pitris C, Boppart SA, Li XD, et al. *In vivo* ultrahighresolution optical coherence tomography. Opt Lett. 1999;24:1221-3.
25. Fujimoto JG1, Brezinski ME, Tearney GJ, Boppart SA, Bouma B, Hee MR, et al. Optical biopsy and imaging using optical coherence tomography. Nat Med. 1995;1:970-2.
26. Tsuboi M, Hayashi A, Ikeda N, Honda H, Kato Y, Ichinose S, et al. Optical coherence tomography in the diagnosis of bronchial lesions. Lung Cancer. 2005;49:387-94.
27. Lam S, Standish B, Baldwin C, McWilliams A, leRiche J, Gazdar A, et al. *In vivo* optical coherence tomography imaging of preinvasive bronchial lesions. Clin Cancer Res. 2008;14:2006-11.
28. Coxson HO, Quiney B, Sin DD, Xing L, McWilliams AM, Mayo JR, et al. Airway wall thickness assessed using computed tomography and optical coherence tomography. Am J Respir Crit Care Med. 2008;177:1201-6.
29. Thiberville L, Moreno-Swirc S, Vercauteren T, Peltier E, Cavé C, Bourg Heckly G. *In vivo* imaging of the bronchial wall microstructure using fibered confocal fluorescence microscopy. Am J Respir Crit Care Med. 2007;175:22-31.
30. Schieppati E. La puncion mediastinal a traves del espolon traqueal. Rev As Med Argent. 1949;663:497-9.
31. Wang KP, Marsh BR, Summer WR, Terry PB, Erozan YS, Baker RR. Transbronchial needle aspiration for diagnosis of lung cancer. Chest. 1981;80:48-50.
32. Shure D, Fedullo PF. Transbronchial needle aspiration of peripheral masses. Am Rev Respir Dis. 1983;128:1090-2.
33. Shure D, Fedullo PF. Transbronchial needle aspiration in the diagnosis of submucosal and peribronchial bronchogenic carcinoma. Chest. 1985;88:49-51.
34. Dasgupta A, Jain P, Minai OA, Sandur S, Meli Y, Arroliga AC, et al. Utility of transbronchial needle aspiration in the diagnosis of endobronchial lesions. Chest. 1999;115:1237-41.
35. Patelli M, Agli LL, Poletti V, Trisolini R, Cancellieri A, Lacava N, et al. Role of fiberscopic transbronchial needle aspiration in the staging of N2 disease due to non-small cell lung cancer. Ann Thorac Surg. 2002;73:407-11.
36. Kavuru MS, Mehta AC. Applied anatomy of the airways. In: Wang KP, Mehta AC (Eds). Flexible Bronchoscopy. UK Blackwell Science, Cambridge MA; 1995. p. 6.
37. Minai OA, Dasgupta A, Mehta AC. Transbronchial needle aspiration of central and peripheral lesions. In: Bolliger CT, Mathur PN (Eds). Progress in Respiratory Research-Interventional Bronchoscopy. Berlin: Karger; 1999.
38. Baram D, Garcia RB, Richman PS. Impact of rapid on-site cytologic evaluation during transbronchial needle aspiration. Chest. 2005;128:869-75.
39. Dales RE, Stark RM, Raman S. Computed tomography to stage lung cancer. Approaching a controversy using meta-analysis. Am Rev Respir Dis. 1990;141:1096-101.
40. Holty JE, Kuschner WG, Gould MK. Accuracy of transbronchial needle aspiration for mediastinal staging of non-small cell lung cancer: a meta-analysis. Thorax. 2005;60:949-55.
41. Ketai L, Chauncey J, Duque R. Combination of flow cytometry and transbronchial needle aspiration in the diagnosis of mediastinal lymphoma. Chest. 1985;88:936.
42. Bilaceroglu S, Perim K, Gunel O, Cağirici U, Büyükşirin M. Combining transbronchial aspiration with endobronchial and transbronchial biopsy in sarcoidosis. Monaldi Arch Chest Dis. 1999;54:217-23.
43. Hurter T, Hanrath P. Endobronchial sonography: feasibility and preliminary results. Thorax. 1992;47:565-7.
44. Kurimoto N, Murayama M, Yoshioka S, Nishisaka T, Inai K, Dohi K, et al. Assessment of usefulness of endobronchial ultrasonography in determination of depth of tracheobronchial tumor invasion. Chest. 1999;115:1500-6.
45. Herth F, Ernst A, Schulz M, Becker H. Endobronchial ultrasound reliably differentiates between airway infiltration and compression by tumor. Chest. 2003;123:458-62.
46. Hwangbo B, Kim SK, Lee HS, Kim MS, Lee JM. Application of endobronchial ultrasound-guided transbronchial needle aspiration following Integrated PET/CT in mediastinal staging of potentially operable non-small cell lung cancer. Chest. 2009;135:1280-7.
47. Herth FJ, Becker HD, Ernst A. Conventional vs endobronchial ultrasound-guided transbronchial needle aspiration: a randomized trial. Chest. 2004;125:322-5.
48. Yasufuku K, Chiyo M, Koh E, Moriya Y, Iyoda A, Sekine Y, et al. Endobronchial ultrasound guided transbronchial needle aspiration for staging of lung cancer. Lung cancer. 2005;50: 347-54.
49. Gu P, Zhao YZ, Jiang LY, Zhang W, Xin Y, Han BH. Endobronchial ultrasound-guided transbronchial needle aspiration for staging of lung cancer: a systematic review and meta-analysis. Eur J Cancer. 2009;45:1389-96.
50. Rintoul RC, Skwarski KM, Murchison JT, Wallace WA, Walker WS, Penman ID. Endobronchial and endoscopic ultrasound-guided real-time fine-needle aspiration for mediastinal staging. Eur Respir J. 2005;25:416-21.
51. Wallace MB, Pascual JM, Raimondo M, Woodward TA, McComb BL, Crook JE, et al. Minimally invasive endoscopic staging of suspected lung cancer. J Am Med Assoc. 2008;299:540-54.
52. Nakajima T, Yasufuku K, Nakagawara A, Kimura H, Yoshino I. Multigene mutation analysis of metastatic lymph nodes in non-small cell lung cancer diagnosed by endobronchial ultrasound-guided transbronchial needle aspiration. Chest. 2011;140:1319-24.

53. Garcia-Olivé I, Monsó E, Andreo F, Sanz-Santos J, Taron M, Molina-Vila MA, et al. Endobronchial ultrasound-guided transbronchial needle aspiration for identifying EGFR mutations. Eur Respir J. 2010;35:391-5.
54. Santis G, Angell R, Nickless G, Quinn A, Herbert A, Cane P, et al. Screening for EGFR and KRAS mutations in endobronchial ultrasound-derived transbronchial needle aspirates in non-small cell lung cancer using COLD-PCR. PLoS One. 2011;6:e25191.
55. Esterbrook G, Anathhanam S, Plant PK. Adequacy of endobronchial ultrasound transbronchial needle aspiration samples in the subtyping of non-small cell lung cancer. Lung Cancer. 2013;80:30-4.
56. Tremblay A, Stather DR, Maceachern P, Khalil M, Field SK. A randomized controlled trial of standard vs endobronchial ultrasonography-guided transbronchial needle aspiration in patients with suspected sarcoidosis. Chest. 2009;136:340-6.
57. Kennedy MP, Jimenez CA, Bruzzi JF, Mhatre AD, Lei X, Giles FJ, et al. Endobronchial ultrasound-guided transbronchial needle aspiration in the diagnosis of lymphoma. Thorax. 2008;63: 360-5.
58. Grove DA, Bechara RI, Josephs JS, Berkowitz DM. Comparative cost analysis of endobronchial ultrasound-guided and blind TBNA in the evaluation of hilar and mediastinal lymphadenopathy. J Bronchology Interv Pulmonol. 2012;19:182-7.
59. Sharples LD, Jackson C, Wheaton E, Griffith G, Annema JT, Dooms C, et al. Clinical effectiveness and cost-effectiveness of endobronchial and endoscopic ultrasound relative to surgical staging in potentially resectable lung cancer: results from the ASTER randomised controlled trial. Health Technol Assess. 2012;16:1-75.
60. Kurimoto N, Miyazawa T, Okimasa S, Maeda A, Oiwa H, Miyazu Y, et al. Endobronchial ultrasonography using a guide sheath increases the ability to diagnose peripheral pulmonary lesions endoscopically. Chest. 2004;126:959-65.
61. Kikuchi E, Yamazaki K, Sukoh N, Kikuchi J, Asahina H, Imura M, et al. Endobronchial ultrasonography with guide-sheath for peripheral pulmonary lesions. Eur Respir J. 2004;24:533-7.
62. Chao TY, Chien MT, Lie CH, Chung YH, Wang JL, Lin MC. Endobronchial ultrasonography-guided transbronchial needle aspiration increases the diagnostic yield of peripheral pulmonary lesions: a randomized trial. Chest. 2009;136:229-36.
63. Gildea TR, Mazzone PJ, Karnak D, Meziane M, Mehta AC Electromagnetic navigation diagnostic bronchoscopy: a prospective study. Am J Respir Crit Care Med. 2006;174(9):982-9.
64. Eberhardt R, Anantham D, Herth F, Feller-Kopman D, Ernst A. Electromagnetic navigation diagnostic bronchoscopy in peripheral lung lesions. Chest. 2007;131(6):1800-5.
65. Eberhardt R, Anantham D, Ernst A, Feller-Kopman D, Herth F. Multimodality bronchoscopic diagnosis of peripheral lung lesions: a randomized controlled trial. Am J Respir Crit Care Med. 2007;176(1):36-41.
66. Dolina MY, Cornish DC, Merritt SA, Rai L, Mahraj R, Higgins WE, et al. Interbronchoscopist variability in endobronchial path selection: a simulation study. Chest. 2008;133:897-905.
67. Asahina H, Yamazaki K, Onodera Y, Kikuchi E, Shinagawa N, Asano F, et al. Transbronchial biopsy using endobronchial ultrasonography with a guide sheath and virtual bronchoscopic navigation. Chest. 2005;128:1761-5.
68. Ishida T, Asano F, Yamazaki K, Shinagawa N, Oizumi S, Moriya H, et al. Virtual bronchoscopic navigation combined with endobronchial ultrasound to diagnose small peripheral pulmonary lesions: a randomised trial. Thorax. 2011;66:1072-7.
69. Asano F, Aoe M, Ohsaki Y, Okada Y, Sasada S, Sato S, et al. Complications associated with endobronchial ultrasound-guided transbronchial needle aspiration: a nationwide survey by the Japan Society for Respiratory Endoscopy. Respir Res. 2013;14:50.
70. Asano F, Matsuno Y, Tsuzuku A, Anzai M, Shinagawa N, Yamazaki K, et al. Diagnosis of peripheral pulmonary lesions using a bronchoscope insertion guidance system combined with endobronchial ultrasonography with a guide sheath. Lung Cancer. 2008;60:366-73.
71. Einstein A. The quantum theory of radiation. Phy Jour. 1917; 18:121-8.
72. Schawtow AL, Townes CH. Infrared and optical masers. Phy Rev. 1958;112:1940-9.
73. Maimon TI. Stimulated optical radiation in ruby. Nature. 1960;187:493-4.
74. Herd RM, Dover JS, Amdt KA. Lasers in dermatology. Dermatol Clin. 1997;15:355-73.
75. Dumon MC, Dumon JF. Laser bronchoscopy in Feinsilver SH, Fein AM (Eds): textbook of Bronchoscopy. Baltimore: Williams & Wilkins. 1995. pp. 393-9.
76. Prakash UBS, Offord KP, Stubbs SE. Bronchoscopy in North America: the ACCP survey. Chest. 1991;100:1668-75.
77. Ramser ER, Beamis JF. Laser bronchoscopy. Clin Chest Med. 1995;16:415-26.
78. Cavaliere S, Venuta F, Foccoli P, Toninelli C, La Face B. Endoscopic treatment of malignant airway obstructions in 2,008 patients. Chest. 1996;110(6):1536-42.
79. Eichenhorn MS, Kvale PA, Miks VM, Seydel HG, Horowitz B, Radke JR. Initial combination therapy with YAG laser photoresection and irradiation for inoperable non-small cell carcinoma of the lung. Chest. 1986;89:782-5.
80. Gelb AF, Epstein JD. Neodymium-yttrium-aluminum-garnet laser in lung cancer. Ann Thorac Surg. 1987;43:164-7.
81. Macha HN, Becker KO, Kemmer HP. Pattern of failure and survival in endobronchial laser resection. Chest. 1994;105:1668-72.
82. Kvale PA, Eichenhom MS, Radke JR, Miks V. YAG laser photoresection of lesions obstructing the central airways. Chest. 1985;87:283-8.
83. Ross DJ, Mohsenifar Z, Koemer SK. Survival characteristics after neodymium: YAG laser photoresection in advanced stage lung cancer. Chest. 1990;98:581-5.
84. Stanopoulos IT, Beamis JF, Martinez FJ, Vergos K, Shapshay SM. Laser bronchoscopy in respiratory failure from malignant airway obstruction. Crit Care Med. 1993;21:386-91.
85. Toty L, Personne C, Colchen A, Vourc'h G. Bronchoscopic management of tracheal lesions using the neodymium yttrium aluminum garnet laser. Thorax. 1981;36:175-8.
86. Madden BP, Kumar P, Sayer R, Murday A. Successful resection of obstructing airway granulation tissue following lung transplantation using endobronchial (Nd:YAG) therapy. Eur J Cardiothorac Surg. 1997;12:480-5.
87. Brutinel WM, Cortese DA, Edell ES, McDougall JC, Prakash UBS. Complications of Nd:YAG laser therapy. Chest. 1988;94(5): 903-4.
88. Sacco O, Fregonese B, Oddone M, Verna A, Tassara E, Mereu C, et al. Severe endobronchial obstruction in a girl with relapsing polychondritis: treatment with Nd: YAG laser and endobronchial silicon stent. Eur Respir J. 1997;10:494-6.

89. Witt C, John M, Martin H, Hiepe F, Ewert R, Emslander HP, et al. Bechet's syndrome with pulmonary involvement-combined therapy for endobronchial stenosis using neodymium-YAG laser, balloon dilation and immunosuppression. Respiration. 1996;63:195-8.
90. Cahill BC, Harmon KR, Sumway SJ, Mickman JK, Hertz MI. Tracheobronchial obstruction due to silicosis. Am Rev Respir Dis. 1992;145:719-21.
91. Shah H, Garbe L, Nussbaum E, Dumon JF, Chiodera PL, Cavaliere S. Benign tumors of the tracheobronchial tree. Endoscopic characteristics and role of laser resection. Chest. 1995;107:1744-51.
92. Hetzel MR, Nixon C, Edmondstone WM, Mitchell DM, Millard FJ, Nanson EM, et al. Laser therapy in 100 tracheobronchial tumors. Thorax. 1985;40:341-5.
93. Desai SJ, Mehta AC, VanderBrug Medendorp S, Golish JA, Ahmad M. Survival experience following Nd:YAG laser photoresection for primary bronchogenic carcinoma. Chest. 1988;94(5):939-44.
94. Mehta AC, Lee FYW, DeBoer GE. FlexIble bronchoscopy and the use of lasers. In: Wang KP, Mehta AC (Eds): flexible bronchoscopy Cambridge. UK Blackwell Science; 1995. pp.247-74.
95. Strauss AA, Strauss SF, Crawford RA. Surgical diathermy of carcinoma of the rectum, Its clinical end results. J Am Med Assoc. 1935;104:1480-4.
96. Hooper RG, Jackson FN. Endobronchial electrocautery. Chest. 1985;87:712-4.
97. Hooper RG, Jackson FN. Endobronchial electrocautery. Chest. 1988;94:595-8.
98. Homasson JP. Endobronchial electrocautery. Semin Respir Crit Care Med. 1997;18:535-43.
99. Petrou M, Kaptan D, Goldstraw P. Bronchoscopic diathermy resection and stent insertion: a cost effective treatment for tracheobronchial obstruction. Thorax. 1993;48:1156-9.
100. Sutedja C, Van Kralingen K, Schramet FM, Postmus PE. Fiberoptic bronchoscopic electrosurgery under local anesthesia for rapid palliation in patients with central airway malignancies: a preliminary report. Thorax. 1994;49:1243-6.
101. Carpenter RJ, Neel T, Sanderson DR. Comparison of endoscopic cryosurgery and electrocoagulation of bronchi. Trans Am Acad Ophthalmol Otolaryngol. 1977;84:313-23.
102. Sutedja G, Schramel FM, Smit HJ, Postmus PE. Bronchoscopic electrocautery as an alternative for Nd:YAG laser in patients with intraluminal tumor. Eur Resp. 1996;9(Supp 23):258-9s.
103. Lavandier M, Carre T, Rivoire B. High frequency electrocautery in the management of tracheobronchial disorders. Respir Crit Care Med. 1998;75:A477.
104. Grund KE, Storek D, Farin G. Endoscopic argon plasma coagulation (APC) first clinical experiences in flexible endoscopy. Endosc Surg Allied Technol. 1994;2:42-6.
105. Crosta C, Spaggiari L, De Stefano A, Fiori G, Ravizza D, Pastorino U. Endoscopic argon plasma coagulation for palliative treatment of malignant airway obstructions: early results in 47 cases. Lung Cancer. 2001;33:75-80.
106. Morice RC, Ece T, Ece F, Keus L. Endobronchial Argon Plasma Coagulation for Treatment of Hemoptysis and Neoplastic Airway Obstruction. Chest. 2001;119:781-7.
107 Vonk-Noordegraa A, Postmus PE, Sutedja TG. Bronchoscopic treatment of patients with intraluminal microinvasive radiographically occult lung cancer not eligible for surgical resection: a follow-up study. Lung Cancer. 2003;39:49-53.
108. Reichle G, Freitag L, Kullmann HJ, Prenzel R, Macha HN, Farin G. [Argon plasma coagulation in bronchology: a new method-alternative or complementary?]. Pneumologie. 2000;54: 508-16.
109. Platt RC. Argon Plasma Electrosurgical Coagulation. Biomed Sci Instrum. 1997;34:332-7.
110. Colt HG. Bronchoscopic resection of Wallstent-associated granulation tissue using argon plasma coagulation. J Bronchol. 1998;5:209.
111. Reddy C, Majid A, Michaud G, Feller-Kopman D, Eberhardt R, Herth F, et al. Gas embolism following bronchoscopic argon plasma coagulation: a case series. Chest. 2008;134:1066-9.
112. Breasted JH. The Edwin Smith surgical papyrus. Chicago: University of Chicago Oriental Institute. 1930;3:217.
113. Arnott J. On the treatment of cancer by regulated application of an anaesthetic temperature. London: J Churchill; 1851.
114. Arnott J. On the treatment of cancer by congelation and an improved mode of pressure. London: J Churchill; 1855.
115. Grana L, Kidd J, Swenson O. Cryogenic techniques within tracheobronchial tree. J Cryosurg. 1969;2:62.
116. Thomford NR, Wilson WH, Blackburn ED, Pace WG. Morphological changes in canine trachea after freezing. Cryobiology. 1970;7:19.
117. Skivolocki WP, Pace WG, Thomford NR. Effect of cryotherapy on tracheal tumors in rats. Arch Surg. 1971;103:341.
118. Neel HB, Farrell KH, Payne WS, De Santo LW, Sanderson DR. Cryosurgery of respiratory structures 1. Cryonecrosis of trachea and bronchus. Laryngoscope. 1073;8s3:1062.
119. Gorenstein A, Neel HB, Sanderson DR. Transbronchoscopic cryosurgery of respiratory strictures. Experimental and clinical studies. Ann Otol Rhinol Laryngol. 1976;85:670-8.
120. Carpenter RJ, Neel HB, Sanderson DR. Cryosurgery of broncho-pulmonary structures. An approach to lesions inaccessible to the rigid bronchoscope. Chest. 1977;72:279-84.
121. Gage AA. Cryotherapy for cancer. In: Rand R, Rinfret R, Rinfret A, Von Leden H (Eds). Cryosurgery. Springfield: Thomas Charles C; 1968. pp. 376-87.
122. Sanderson DR, Neel HB, Payne WS, Woolner LB. Cryotherapy of bronchogenic carcinoma. Report of a case. Mayo Clin Proc. 1975;50(8):435-7.
123. Fahy GM, Saur J, Williams RJ. Physical problems with the vitrification of large biological systems. Cryobiology. 1990;27: 492-510.
124. Gage AA, Guest K, Montes M, Garuna JA, Whalen DA. Effect of varying freezing and thawing rates in experimental cryosurgery. Cryobiology. 1985;22:175-82.
125. Smith JJ, Fraser J. An estimation of tissue damage and thermal history in cryolesion. Cryobiology. 1974;11(2):139-47.
126. Miller RH, Mazur P. Survival of frozen-thawed human red cells as a function of cooling and warming velocities. Cryobiology. 1976;13:404-14.
127. Gage AA. Critical temperature for skin necrosis in experimental cryosurgery. Cryobiology. 1982;19:273-82.
128. Rand RW, Rand RP, Eggerding FA, Field M, Denbesten L, King W, et al. Cryolumpestomy for breast cancer: an experimental study. Cryobiology. 1985;22:307-49.
129. Rubinsky B, Ikeda M. A cryomicroscope using directional solidification for the controlled freezing of biological tissue. Cryobiology. 1985;22:55.
130. Homasson JP, Thiery JP, Angebault M, Ovtracht L, Maiwand MO. The operation and efficacy of cryosurgical, nitrous oxide-

driven cryoprobe. Cryoprobe physical characteristics: their effects on cell cryodestruction. Cryobiology. 1994;31:290.

131. Le Pivert P, Binder P, Ougier T. Measurement of intratissue bioelectrical low frequency impedance: a new method to predict per-operatively the destructive effect of cryosurgery. Cryobiology. 1977;14:245.
132. Homasson JP, Renault P, Angebault M, Bonniot JP, Bell NJ. Bronchoscopic cryotherapy for airway strictures caused by tumors. Chest. 1986;90:159-64.
133. Maiwand MO. Cryotherapy for advanced carcinoma of the trachea and bronchi. Br Med J. 1986;293:181-2.
134. Astesiano A, Aversa S, Ciotta D, Galietti F, Gandolfi G, Giorgis GE, et al. Cryotherapeutic destruction of invasive trachea-bronchial tumors. Personal case histories. Casistica personale Min Med. 1986;77(45-46):2159-62.
135. Mathur PN, Wolf KM, Busk MF, Briete WM, Datzman M. Fiberoptic bronchoscopic cryotherapy in the management of tracheobronchial obstruction. Chest. 1996;110:718-23.
136. Walsh DA, Maiwand MO, Nath AR, Lockwood P, Lloyd MH, Saab M. Bronchoscopic cryotherapy for advanced bronchial carcinoma. Thorax. 1990;45:509-13.
137. Maiwand MO, Homasson JP. Cryotherapy for tracheobronchial disorders. In: Mathur PN, Beamis JF (Eds). Clinics in chest medicine. Philadelphia: WB Saunders Company; 1995. pp. 427-43.
138. Homasson JP. Cryotherapy in pulmonology today and tomorrow. Eur Resp J. 1989;2:799-801.
139. Sheski FD, Mathur PN. Endobronchial cryotherapy for benign tracheobronchial lesions. Chest. 1998;114:261-2s.
140. Hetzel M, Hetzel J, Schumann C, Marx N, Babiak A. Cryorecanalization: a new approach for the immediate management of acute airway obstruction. A J Thorac Cardiovasc Surg. 2004;127(5):1427-31.
141. Schumann C, Hetzel M, Babiak AJ, Hetzel J, Merk T, Wibmer T, et al. Endobronchial tumor debulking with a flexible cryoprobe for immediate treatment of malignant stenosis. J Thorac Cardiovasc Surg. 2010;139(4):997-1000.
142. Franke KJ, Szyrach M, Nilius G, Hetzel J, Hetzel M, Ruehle KH, et al. Xperimental study on biopsy sampling using new flexible cryoprobes: influence of activation time, probe size, tissue consistency, and contact pressure of the probe on the size of the biopsy specimen. Lung. 2009;187(4):253-9.
143. Deygas N, Froudarakis ME, Ozenne G, Jouve S, Fournel P, Vergnon JM. Cryotherapy in Early superficial bronchogenic carcinoma. Eur Respir J. 1998;12(28):266S.
144. Vergnon JM, Schmitt T, Alamartine E, Barthelemy JC, Fournel P, Emonot A. Initial combined cryotherapy and irradiation for unresectable non-small cell lung cancer. Chest. 1992;102: 1436-40.
145. Forest V, Peoc'h M, Campos L, Guyotat D, Vergnon JM. Effects of cryotherapy or chemotherapy on apoptosis in a non-small-cell lung cancer xenografted into SCID mice. Cryobiology. 2005;50(1):29-37.
146. Forest V, Campos L, Péoc'h M, Guyotat D, Vergnon JM. [Development of an experimental model for the study of the effects of cryotherapy on lung tumours]. Pathol Biol (Paris). 2005;53(4):199-203.
147. Forest V, Peoc'h M, Ardiet C, Campos L, Guyotat D, Vergnon JM. *In vivo* cryochemotherapy of a human lung cancer model. Cryobiology. 2005;51(1):92-101.
148. Forest V, Peoc'h M, Campos L, Guyotat D, Vergnon JM. Benefit of a combined treatment of cryotherapy and chemotherapy on tumour growth and late cryo-induced angiogenesis in a non-small-cell lung cancer model. Lung Cancer. 2006;54(1): 79-86.
149. Forest V, Hadjeres R, Bertrand R, Jean-François R. Optimisation and molecular signalling of apoptosis in sequential cryotherapy and chemotherapy combination in human A549 lung cancer xenografts in SCID mice. Br J Cancer. 2009;100(12): 1896-902.
150. Gomer CJ, Dougherty TJ. Determination of [3H] and [14C] hematoporphyrin derivative distribution in malignant and normal tissue. Cancer Res. 1979;39:146-51.
151. Dougherty TJ, Marcus SL. Photodynamic therapy. Eur J Cancer. 1992;28A:1734-42.
152. McCaughan JS. Photodynamic therapy of endobronchial and esophageal tumors: an overview. J Clin Laser Med Surg. 1996;14:223-33.
153. Kato H, Okunaka T, Shimatani H. Photodynamic therapy for early stage bronchogenic carcinoma. J Clin Laser Med Surg. 1996;14:235-8.
154. Cortese DA, Edell ES, Kinsey JH. Photodynamic therapy for early stage squamous cell carcinoma of the lung. Mayo Clin Proc. 1997;72:595-602.
155. Moghissi K, Dixon K, Stringer M, Freeman T, Thorpe A, Brown S. The place of bronchoscopic photodynamic therapy in advanced unresectable lung cancer: experience of 100 cases. Eur J Cardiothorac Surg. 1999;15:1-6.
156. McCaughan JS, Williams TE. Photodynamic therapy for endobronchial malignant disease: a prospective fourteen-year study. J Thorac Cardiovasc Surg. 1997;114:940-6.
157. Diaz-Jimenez JP, Martinez-Ballarin JE, Llunell A, Farrero E, Rodríguez A, Castro MJ. Efficacy and safety of photodynamic therapy versus Nd-YAG laser resection in NSCLC with airway obstruction. Eur Respir J. 1999;14:800-5.
158. Yankauer S. Two cases of lung tumor treated bronchoscopically. N Y Med J. 1922;21:741-2.
159. Henschke UK, Hilaris BS, Mahan G. Remote afterloading with intracavitary applicators. Radiology. 1964;83:344-5.
160. Mendiondo DA, Dillon M, Beach U. Endobronchial brachytherapy in the treatment of recurrent bronchogenic carcinoma. Int J Radiat Oncol Biol Phys. 1983;9:579-82.
161. Moylan D, Strubler K, Unal A, Mohiuddin M, Giampetro A, Boon R. Work in progress. Transbronchial brachytherapy of recurrent bronchogenic carcinoma: a new approach using the flexible fiberoptic bronchoscope. Radiology. 1983;147:253-4.
162. Sutedja G, Bans G, Van Zandwijk N, Postmus PE. High-dose rate brachytherapy has a curative potential in patients with intraluminal squamous cell lung cancer. Respiration. 1993;61:167-8.
163. Burt PA, O'Driscoll BR, Notely HM, Barber PV, Stout R. Intraluminal irradiation for the palliation of lung cancer with the high dose rate microselectron. Thorax. 1990;45:765-8.
164. Chang LL, Harvath J, Peyton W, Ling SS. High dose rate after loading intraluminal brachytherapy in malignant airway obstructions of lung cancer. Int J Radiat Oncol Biol Phys. 1994;28:589-96.
165. Golling SW, Burt PA, Barber PV, Stout R. High dose rate intraluminal radiotherapy for carcinoma of the bronchus: outcome of treatment of 406 patients. Radiother Oncol. 1994;33:310-49.
166. Speiser B, Spratling L. Remote afterloading brachytherapy for the local control of endobronchial carcinoma. Int J Radiat Oncot Biol Phys. 1993;25:579-87.

167. Nori D, Allison R, Kaplan B, Samala E, Osian A, Karbowitz S. High dose-rate intraluminal irradiation in bronchogenic carcinoma. Chest. 1993;104:1006-11.
168. Murren JR, Buzaid AC. Chemotherapy and radiation for the treatment of non-small cell lung cancer. A critical review. Clin Chest Med. 1993;14:161-71.
169. Bedwinek J, Petty A, Bruton C, Sofield J, Lee L. The use of high dose rate endobronchial brachytherapy to palliate symptomatic endobronchial recurrence of previously irradiated bronchogenic carcinoma. Intl Radiat Oncol Biol Phys. 1991;22:23-30.
170. Khanavka B, Stern P. Alberti W, Nakhosteen JA. Complication associated with brachytherapy alone or with laser in lung cancer. Chest. 1991;99:1062-5.
171. Cohen MD, Weber TR, Rao CC. Balloon dilation of tracheal and bronchial stenosis. AJR Am J Roentgenol. 1984;142:477-8.
172. Nakamura K, Terada N, Matsushita T, Matsushita T, Kato N, Nakagawa T. Tuberculous bronchial stenosis: treatment with balloon bronchoplasty. AJR Am J Roentgenol. 1991;157:1187-8.
173. Hautman H, Gamarra F, Pfeifer KJ, Huber RM. Fiberoptic bronchoscopic balloon dilatation in malignant tracheobronchial disease: indications and results. Chest. 2001;120: 43-9.
174. Noppen M, Schlesser M, Meysman M, D'Haese J, Peche R, Vincken W. Bronchoscopic balloon dilatation in the combined management of postintubation stenosis of the trachea in adults. Chest. 1997;112:1136-40.
175. Keller C, Frost A. Fiberoptic bronchoplasty. Description of a simple adjunct technique for the management of bronchial stenosis following lung transplantation. Chest. 1992;102: 995-8.
176. Ferretti G, Jouran FB, Thony F, Pison C, Coulomb M. Benign noninflammatory bronchial stenosis: Treatment with balloon dilation. Radiology. 1995;196:831-4.
177. Mayse ML, Greenheck J, Friedman M, Kovitz KL. Successful bronchoscopic balloon dilation of nonmalignant tracheobronchial obstruction without fluoroscopy. Chest. 2004;126:634-7.
178. Sheski FD, Mathur PN. Long-term results of fiberoptic bronchoscopic balloon dilation in the management of benign tracheobronchial stenosis. Chest. 1998;114:796-800.
179. Bond CJ. Note on the treatment of tracheal stenosis by a new T-shaped tracheotomy tube. Lancet. 1891;137:539.
180. Chhajed PN, Baty F, Pless M, Somandin S, Tamm M, Brutsche MH. Outcome of treated advanced non-small cell lung cancer with and without airway obstruction. Chest. 2006;130:1803-7.
181. Montgomery WW. T-tube tracheal stent. Arch Otolaryngol. 1965;82:320-1.
182. Dumon JF. A dedicated tracheobronchial stent. Chest. 1990;92:328-32.
183. Dumon JF, Cavaliere S, Diaz-Jimenez JP, Vergnon JM, Venuta F, Dumon MC, et al. Seven-year experience with the Dumon prosthesis. J Bronchol. 1996;31:6-10.
184. Diaz-Jimenez JP, Munoz EF, Martinez Ballarín JI, Kovitz KL, Manresa Presas F. Silicone stents in the management of obstructive tracheobronchial lesions. J Bronchol. 1994;1(1):15-8.
185. Noppen M, Meysman M, Claes I, D'Haese J, Vincken W. Screw-thread vs Dumon endoprosthesis in the management of tracheal stenosis. Chest. 1999;115:532-5.
186. Gildea TR, Murthy SC, Sahoo D, Mason DP, Mehta AC. Performance of a self-expanding silicone stent in palliation of benign airway conditions. Chest. 2006;130:1419-23.
187. Mehta AC, Dasgupta A. Airway stents. Clin Chest Med. 1999;20:139-51.
188. Rafanan AL, Mehta AC. Stenting of the tracheobronchial tree. Radiol Clin North Am. 2000;38:395-408.
189. Nashef SAM, Droiner C, Velty FJ, Labrousse L, Couraud L. Expanding wire stents in benign tracheobronchial disease: Indications and complications. Ann Thorac Surg. 1992;54: 937-40.
190. Dasgupta A1, Dolmatch BL, Abi-Saleh WJ, Mathur PN, Mehta AC. Self-expandable metallic airway stent insertion employing flexible bronchoscopy: preliminary results. Chest. 1998;114:106-9.
191. Miyazawa T, Yamakido M, Ikeda S, Furukawa K, Takiguchi Y Tada H, et al. Implantation of ultraflex nitinol stents in malignant tracheobronchial stenosis. Chest. 2000;118:959-65.
192. Herth F, Becker HD, LoCicero J, Thurer R, Ernst A. Successful bronchoscopic placement of tracheobronchial stents without fluoroscopy. Chest. 2001;119:1910-12.
193. Saad CP, Murthy S, Krizmanich G, Mehta AC. Self-expandable metallic airway stents and flexible bronchoscopy. Chest. 2003;124:1993-9.
194. Hoag JB, Juhas W, Morrow K, Lund ME. Predeployment length modification of a self-expanding metallic stent. J Bronchol. 2008;15:185-90.
195. Lee P, Kupeli E, Mehta AC. Airway stents Clin Chest Med. 2010;31(1):141-50.

31 Chapter

Thoracoscopy

C Ravindran, Jyothy E

INTRODUCTION

Medical thoracoscopy or pleuroscopy is a minimally invasive procedure to explore the pleural space through an incision in the chest wall. Thoracoscopy together with laparoscopy was introduced in 1910 by Hans-Christian Jacobaeus, who at that time worked as an internist in Stockholm, Sweden. He published his first experiences in a paper entitled "On the possibility to use cystoscopy in the examination of serous cavities."[1] Jacobaeus himself initiated the therapeutic application of thoracoscopy for the lysis of pleural adhesions by means of thoracocautery to facilitate pneumothorax treatment of tuberculosis (Jacobaeus operation).[2]

Between 1950 and 1960, a generation of chest physicians already familiar with the therapeutic application of thoracoscopy began to use the technique on a much broader basis for pleuropulmonary biopsy even for localized and diffuse pulmonary diseases. The excellent results of laparoscopic surgery and the tremendous advances in endoscopic technology stimulated many thoracic surgeons to develop minimally invasive techniques, which were termed therapeutic or surgical thoracoscopy, as well as video-assisted thoracoscopic surgery (VATS).[3-5]

Thoracoscopy is now classified as:

- *Medical thoracoscopy:* This is a minimally invasive procedure, carried out mainly for diagnostic purposes by physicians, generally under local anesthesia and conscious sedation[6]
- *Surgical thoracoscopy:* Popularly known as VATS, is done by surgeons under general anesthesia for both diagnostic and therapeutic applications.[2]

MEDICAL THORACOSCOPY

Medical thoracoscopy is a minimally invasive technique that should be used only when other, simpler procedures are not helpful. The technique is similar to chest-tube insertion by means of a trocar. In addition, the pleural cavity can be visualized and biopsy specimens taken from all the areas of the pleural cavity, including the chest wall, diaphragm, mediastinum and lung. An absolute prerequisite for thoracoscopy is the presence of an adequate pleural space, which should be at least 6–10 cm in width. If not present, a pneumothorax is induced under fluoroscopic or sonographic control, immediately or the day before thoracoscopy.

Medical thoracoscopic examination can be performed under local anesthesia or conscious sedation after premedication, without the support of an anesthesiologist. Furthermore, medical thoracoscopy is less expensive, can be safely performed with nondisposable instruments in an endoscopy suite.

Different techniques used by the pulmonologists are:[7,8]

- *Single-puncture technique*: This technique consists of a single entry with a 9 mm thoracoscope with a working channel for accessory instruments, optical biopsy forceps and local anesthesia.
- *Double-puncture technique*: This technique involves two entries, one with a 7 mm trocar for the examination telescope and the other with a 5 mm trocar for accessory instruments, including the biopsy forceps. Recently, mini thoracoscopy was introduced mainly for the diagnostic purposes. The mini thoracoscopy requires a rigid thoracoscope of 3 mm size, done under local anesthesia. For taking biopsy, a second port of entry is required unlike with the standard equipment.[9,10] Ultrasound can safely and reliably identify entry sites for the trocar placement during medical thoracoscopy, even in patients with pleural adhesions. The use of ultrasound may replace the practice of pneumothorax induction before medical thoracoscopy.[11]

Apart from the conventional white light, other imaging procedures that are said to yield more information especially for the presence of a pleural tumor, have been investigated, but the evidence has remained limited.[12-14] Narrow band imaging (NBI) is a new alternative light wavelength capture system that takes advantage of the altered blood vessel morphology.

Wavelengths of light in the visible spectrum are filtered from the illumination source with the exemption of narrow bands in the blue and green spectrum centered at 415 nm and 540 nm, coinciding with the peak absorption spectrum of oxyhemoglobin making blood vessels more pronounced when viewed in NBI mode.[15] Imaging of vascular structures in deeper layers of thickened pleura can give some indication of where from the biopsy should best be taken. Moreover, NBI facilitates detection of any previously unobserved pleural dissemination.

Electrocoagulation is useful for the cauterization of adhesions and blebs or in the cases of bleeding after biopsy. For pleurodesis of effusions, 8–10 g of sterile, dry, asbestos-free talc is insufflated through a rigid or flexible suction catheter with a pneumatic atomizer. Alternatively, 3 g of talc may be used as slurry for nonmalignant effusion. Use of talc slurry is convenient and associated with excellent outcome and minimal complications.[16] For pneumothorax, 2–3 g of talc is generally sufficient. Immediate suction through the chest tube is always applied following the procedure.

Equipment

Rigid instruments as they were from the beginning are still in use **(Fig. 1)**. They are preferred over the flexible instruments, which have several disadvantages compared to the rigid thoracoscope. The flexible instruments provide less adequate orientation within the pleural cavity and the biopsy specimens are small and frequently inadequate. A recently developed modification with a semiflexible tip can become an acceptable alternative.[17]

Medical thoracoscopy can be performed either under direct vision through the endoscopic optics or indirectly by video transmission.[18] Single entry-site technique is usually done with a 9 mm diameter trocar and a cannula with a valve. Optical devices exist with various fields of view (0°, 30°and 90°). Trocars are also available with diameters of 5 and 3.75 mm for performing thoracoscopy in children. Biopsy forceps with straight optical devices, as well as accessory instruments, such as the puncture needle, cautery electrode, probe, combined suction and cautery cannula with valves and various biopsy forceps and scissors, are available.

A talc atomizer **(Fig. 2)** is used for talc pleurodesis.[19,20] In the case of semirigid pleuroscope, the design including the handle is similar to a standard flexible bronchoscope, the proximal part being stiff (22 cm) with a bendable distal end (5 cm with angulation of 100 and 130 degrees). The outer diameter of the shaft is 7 mm. A working channel with a diameter of 2.8 mm allows the use of standard instruments that are available for flexible bronchoscope.

The semirigid pleuroscope has the advantage that the skills involved in operating the instrument are generally familiar to the practicing bronchoscopist. Moreover, it is compatible with the existing video processors and light sources, so that little additional equipment is required to be added to the endoscopy suite.

A thorough digital examination should be done through the intercostal space before introducing semirigid pleuroscope in to the pleural cavity to look for any adhesions as this can result in acute angulation and damage to the equipment. Its main disadvantage compared to the rigid thoracoscope is the smaller biopsy specimen. However, the flexible tip allows very homogeneous distribution of talc on all pleural surfaces where pleurodesis is required. In a study comparing rigid versus semirigid thoracoscopy, the diagnostic accuracy was 100% for rigid thoracoscopy compared with 97.6% for semirigid thoracoscopy.[21] In another comparative study, the diagnostic yield of rigid thoracoscopy was superior to semirigid thoracoscopy (97.8% versus 73.3%),but was similar (100% versus 94.3%) in those with a successful biopsy.[22] According to the operator rated visual analog scale score, the ease of taking biopsy specimen was higher with rigid

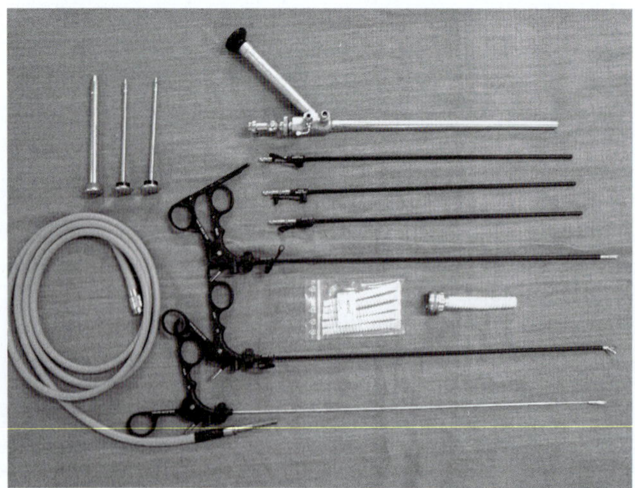

Fig. 1 Rigid thoracoscope and accessories

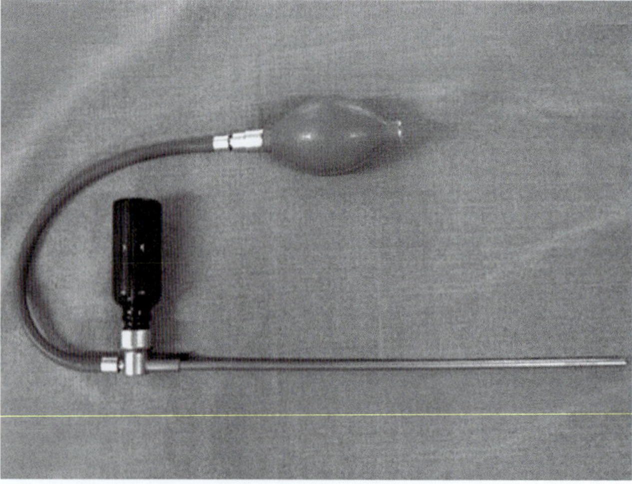

Fig. 2 Talc atomizer for pleurodesis

thoracoscope. In this study, the advantage of semirigid thoracoscope was superior image quality, lesser use of sedative/analgesic agents and scar size.[22]

Procedure

Basic monitoring for medical thoracoscopy involves electrocardiography (ECG) and pulse oximetry. Patient should lie in lateral decubitus position with the healthy lung on the dependent side. Ipsilateral arm should be placed above the head, so that the intercostal spaces become wider. Medical thoracoscopy is done by combining conscious sedation and local anesthesia.

The recommended site for introduction of thoracoscope is the fourth or fifth intercostal space in the midaxillary line. It is also advisable to do a thoracic ultrasound before the procedure, to identify the safest site for trocar insertion. Ultrasound helps to avoid areas of lung adhesion to chest wall. Adequate local anesthesia should be given. The trocar is introduced with a rotating motion perpendicular to the chest wall. Once the trocar is introduced, suction is applied in the case of pleural effusion to remove the fluid. Air should be allowed to enter the thoracic cavity to create pneumothorax and prevent lung re-expansion.

In case of large pleural effusion, 1.5-3 L of pleural fluid may be aspirated 1-2 days prior to thoracoscopy. Air should be allowed to enter the pleural space at the end of pleural aspiration to create hydropneumothorax. A partially collapsed lung is ideal for introduction of thoracoscope. If there is no significant pleural effusion, a pneumothorax should be induced prior to thoracoscopy, and this may be done with Boutin needle, a blunt pleural puncture needle. Once the thoracoscope is introduced, adhesions can be lysed with a biopsy forceps or cautery. Exploration of the pleural space should be done by a slow circular motion of the scope. Biopsy can be taken from any abnormal lesion. At the end of the procedure, a chest drain is introduced in all patients.

Indications

The mostly accepted indications of medical thoracoscopy are:

- Diagnosis of idiopathic pleural effusions
- Staging of lung cancer and mesothelioma
- Pleurodesis
- Biopsy of parietal pleura.

Medical thoracoscopy unlike surgical thoracoscopy, is primarily used as a diagnostic procedure, but can be applied for certain therapeutic indications also **(Table 1)**. The most common indications include the evaluation of the unknown exudative pleural effusion, staging of diffuse malignant mesothelioma or lung cancer, and treatment by talc pleurodesis of malignant or other recurrent effusions and empyema.[23] Medical thoracoscopy is also used for pleurodesis in recurrent pneumothorax. Other diagnostic indication is to obtain biopsies of the diaphragm, lung, mediastinum and pericardium. These procedures are safe in experienced hands, at the same time physicians should be aware of their limitations when indulging in procedures requiring more time and dissection.

Table 1 Indications of medical thoracoscopy

A. *Diagnostic* • Evaluation of undiagnosed exudative pleural effusion • Staging of malignant mesothelioma and lung cancer • Biopsy from lung, diaphragm, mediastinum and pericardium
B. *Therapeutic* • Pleurodesis for malignant/recurrent pleural effusion/ pneumothorax • Lysis of adhesion in pneumothorax/empyema • Sympathectomy

Pleural Effusions

Even after extensive diagnostic evaluation of a patient with pleural effusion, the etiology often remains unclear.[24] Thoracoscopy is the standard diagnostic procedure for investigating exudative pleural effusion, it leads to a conclusive diagnosis for 95% of patients.[23] This should be performed in patients with undiagnosed effusions because of its high diagnostic sensitivity for malignant and tuberculosis etiologies. The tissue obtained will usually provide a higher yield of the positive tubercular cultures, and greater histological proof of lung and pleural malignancies.

Medical thoracoscopy has a diagnostic yield of 86.2% with a complication rate of 10.3% as compared to a diagnostic yield of 62.1% and a complication rate of 17.2% respectively in closed pleural biopsy group.[25] The application of medical thoracoscopy allows the simultaneous insufflation of talc powder which currently offers the best results in pleurodesis. Talc was used in 65% of 110 reported cases of nonmalignant pleural effusion that were treated with chemical pleurodesis, with a success rate of nearly 100%.[16] Further, therapeutic advantages include complete fluid removal and adhesiolysis in tuberculous effusion and empyema.

Malignant effusion: Malignant pleural effusion is the leading diagnostic and therapeutic indication for medical thoracoscopy.[26] Medical thoracoscopy shows a significantly higher sensitivity than needle biopsy plus cytology. All methods taken together are diagnostic in 97% of cases of malignant pleural effusions.[26-28]

The reasons for false negative thoracoscopy results include insufficient and nonrepresentative biopsies, experience of the thoracoscopist, and the presence of adhesions (which denied access to neoplastic tissue).

Medical thoracoscopy is helpful in the staging of lung cancer, diffuse malignant mesothelioma and metastatic cancer.[29] In the case of concomitant pleural effusion in lung cancer that otherwise appears resectable, medical thoracoscopy is indicated as a staging procedure to distinguish malignant from paramalignant effusion.[30] The latter condition would allow for the resection of the tumor; however, in 80–95% of the patients, the effusion is due to the tumor spread and surgical cure is not possible. Thus, medical thoracoscopy can avoid unnecessary thoracotomy.

In diffuse malignant mesothelioma, medical thoracoscopy provides an earlier diagnosis, more precise histologic classification due to a larger, more representative biopsy, and more accurate staging.[29,30] This may have important therapeutic implications, as better responses to local immunotherapy or chemotherapy in stages I and II have been observed.

Thoracoscopy is also helpful in the diagnosis of benign asbestos-related pleural effusion, which is a diagnosis of exclusion. Fibrohyaline or calcified, thick, pearly white pleural plaques indicate probable asbestos exposure. Thoracoscopic biopsies from lung and from certain lesions on the parietal pleura may demonstrate high concentrations of asbestos fibers, providing further support to the diagnosis of asbestos disease.[31]

In metastatic pleural effusions, biopsies of the visceral and diaphragmatic pleura are possible only under direct vision. Because the chest wall pleura are often not involved (in approximately 30% of cases) in early stages, it is not possible in these cases to provide a diagnosis by blind needle biopsy. With the large size of biopsy specimens obtained by thoracoscopy, it may be easier for the pathologist to suggest the origin of the tumor. In metastatic breast cancer, tissue can be obtained for the determination of hormone receptors. Even with lymphomas, the diagnostic yield, as well as the morphologic classification, is improved.[32]

Local treatment of pleural malignancies: The main therapeutic option offered by medical thoracoscopy is the prevention of recurrent effusion with pleurodesis. Under direct visual control, 8–10 g of asbestos-free, sterilized talc (French talc) is insufflated into the pleural space so that the powder is equally distributed on the parietal and visceral pleura. Talc poudrage is probably the most effective, conservative option for pleurodesis.[19,20]

Tuberculous pleural effusion: Tuberculosis remains an important cause of pleuropulmonary involvement in developing countries. In extrapulmonary tuberculosis, pleural involvement is second only to lymph nodes. Although the yield of blind needle biopsy is higher than in pleural malignancies, the diagnostic accuracy of thoracoscopy is greater, because the pathologist is provided with multiple, selected biopsy specimens, and because the bacteriological culture proof of tubercle bacilli is more frequently positive.

In a prospective intrapatient comparison, the histologic diagnosis of 100 patients with tuberculosis (TB) was established by thoracoscopy in 94%, compared with only 38% with needle biopsy, allowing an early start of antituberculous chemotherapy. The combined yield of pleural histology and mycobacterial culture was 99% for medical thoracoscopy, 51% for needle biopsy, and 61% when combined with fluid culture. The percentage of positive TB cultures was twice as high from thoracoscopic biopsy specimens, including cultures from fibrinous membranes (78%), compared with the percentage in pleural effusions and needle biopsy specimens combined (39%). This had the advantages of an early bacteriologic confirmation and drug susceptibility testing. Resistance against one or multiple antituberculous drugs, which influenced therapy and prognosis, was found in 5 of the 78 positive cases (6.4%).[7]

In a prospective study of 40 patients from South Africa, thoracoscopy had a diagnostic yield of 98%, in comparison with an 80% diagnostic yield with Abram's needle biopsies (three biopsy specimens were obtained, each examined histologically and microbiologically).[33] This led to the conclusion that in areas with a high prevalence of TB, Abrams' needle biopsy could contribute significantly to the diagnosis. In a further study on the effect of corticosteroids in the treatment of tuberculous pleurisy, the same authors found that the initial complete drainage of the effusion, performed during thoracoscopy, was associated with greater symptomatic improvement than with any subsequent therapy.[33]

Other pleural effusions: Thoracoscopy may provide clues to the etiology when effusions are neither malignant nor tuberculous as in the cases of rheumatoid arthritis, effusions following pancreatitis, hepatic hydrothorax, extension of disease from the abdominal cavity, or in effusion related to trauma. Although the history, pleural fluid analysis, physical and other examinations are usually diagnostic in these conditions, thoracoscopy is indicated in problematic cases.

When pleural effusions are secondary to an underlying lung disease (such as pulmonary infarction or pneumonia), the diagnosis can frequently be made based on macroscopic examination, confirmed microscopically on lung biopsy. Thoracoscopy is also useful for the diagnosis of benign asbestos-related pleural effusions, which by definition is a diagnosis of exclusion.[34]

By virtue of thoracoscopy, the proportion of so called idiopathic pleural effusions usually decreases to less than 10%, whereas studies in which thoracoscopy was not applied, diagnosis is not established in more than 20% of cases. These figures will also depend on the selection of patients and the definition of an "idiopathic effusion".[35] In the selected cases of the recurrent pleural effusions of nonmalignant etiology, including chylothorax, pleurodesis may be induced by applying talc poudrage during medical thoracoscopy.[32]

The diagnostic accuracy of thoracoscopy in the setting of undiagnosed pleural effusions, varies widely with a range of about 60–90%.[31] Because of its high diagnostic accuracy, thoracoscopy is an excellent option in exudative effusion in which the etiology remains undetermined after pleural fluid analysis **(Fig. 3)**. In a case series of 42 patients who underwent thoracoscopy at our center, 29 were done for diagnostic purposes, of whom 15 were diagnosed as malignant, 3 tuberculous and 10 of nonspecific inflammatory origin.[36]

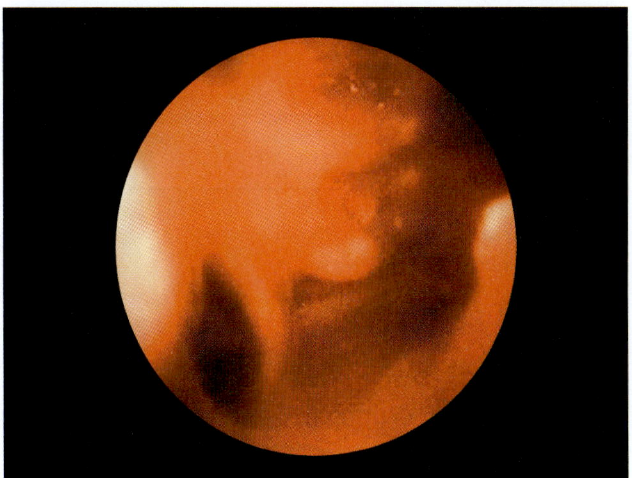

Fig. 3 Multiple nodules on visceral pleural surface in a case of hemorrhagic pleural effusion

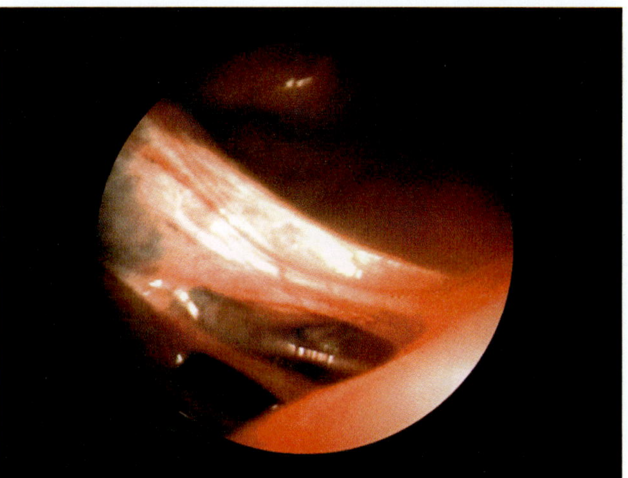

Fig. 5 Thick adhesion in tuberculous pleural effusion

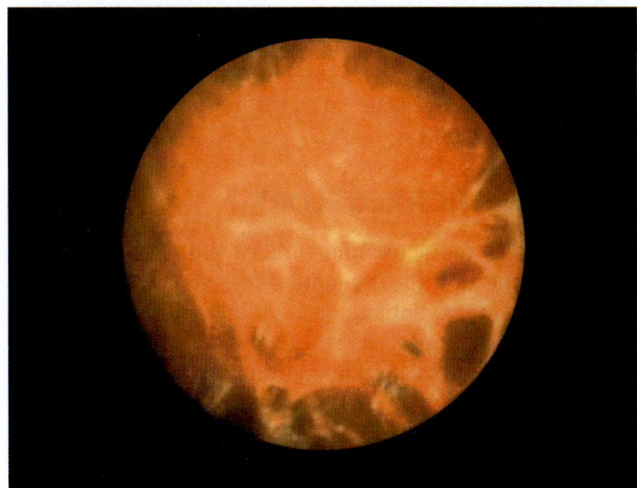

Fig. 4 Thoracoscopic view showing multiple thin adhesions

Empyema

Medical thoracoscopy can be effectively used in the management of empyema.[27] This can help in breaking thin fibrinopurulent adhesions to remove multiple loculations and create a single cavity that can be drained and irrigated more successfully **(Fig. 4)**.[37] This treatment should be instituted early in the course of empyema, before adhesions become too fibrous and adherent **(Fig. 5)**. If chest tube drainage is indicated and if the facilities are available, medical thoracoscopy should be performed at the time of chest-tube insertion itself. Medical thoracoscopy is a procedure similar to that of chest-tube insertion, at the same time it helps in visualizing the pleural cavity and allows better local treatment. In carefully selected cases, medical thoracoscopy can be useful, especially when performed early after the failure of chest tube drainage.[38] In more complex cases, VATS would be the preferred choice.[39,40]

Spontaneous Pneumothorax

In spontaneous pneumothorax, medical thoracoscopy can be used for both diagnostic and therapeutic purposes.[41] In particular, if a chest tube is introduced by a trocar technique, it is easy to visually inspect the lung and the pleural cavity before inserting the chest tube through the cannula. On inspection during medical thoracoscopy, the underlying lesions can be directly assessed according to the classification of Vanderschueren: Stage I with an endoscopically normal lung; Stage II with pleuropulmonary adhesions; Stage III with small bullae and blebs (<2 cm in diameter); and Stage IV with numerous large bullae (>2 cm in diameter).[42] Although the detection rates of blebs and bullae are higher in the series with VATS or thoracotomy, larger bullae, blebs or fistulae are likely to be detected during medical thoracoscopy.[41,42]

Medical thoracoscopy offers the possibility of combining pleural cavity drainage with the coagulation of blebs and bullae, as well as of pleurodesis by talc poudrage. Talc poudrage achieves the best conservative treatment results with the recurrence rates of less than 10%. In stage IV with numerous large bullae, VATS or thoracotomy should usually be performed. Talc poudrage and/or coagulation of bullae are performed only in patients in whom surgery is contraindicated because of the respiratory insufficiency secondary to advanced pulmonary disease.[16]

Medical thoracoscopy is justified in all patients with spontaneous pneumothorax when tube drainage is indicated, as it provides a chance to assess the underlying lesions under direct vision; direct treatment by coagulation of blebs and bullae; severance of adhesions; administration of talc

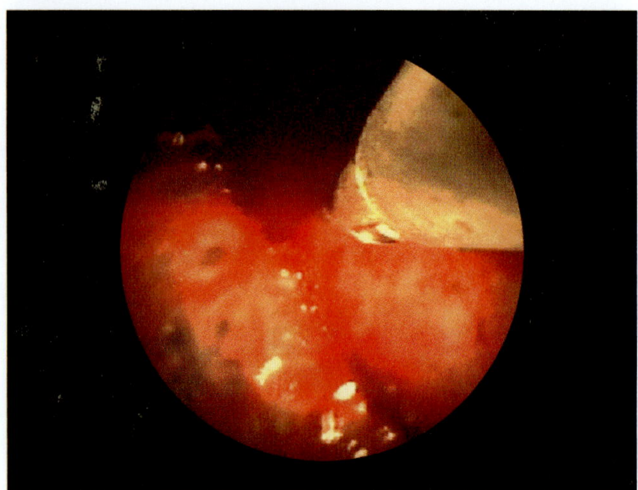

Fig. 6 Thoracoscopic pleural biopsy

poudrage; and selection of the best location for chest-tube placement.

Advanced Indications

Lung biopsy: Forceps lung biopsy with or without electrocautery can be performed by pulmonologists using medical thoracoscopy **(Fig. 6)**.[43] The results are comparable with surgical VATS biopsies in the diagnosis of diffuse lung diseases. Larger VATS biopsies are superior for conditions where lung vascular examination is necessary (e.g. vasculitis).

Other thoracoscopic procedures: Such as sympathectomy for the control of severe hyperhidrosis can be easily performed by a well-trained thoracoscopist. Short- and long-term results are similar to those obtained by typical VATS interventions with a lesser degree of mortality.[4]

Contraindications

An obliterated pleural space is an absolute contraindication.[44] Relative contraindications include the presence of bleeding disorders, hypoxemia, unstable cardiovascular status, and persistent, uncontrolled cough.

Complications

The reported mortality rates are very low (<0.01%) **(Table 2)**. Several liters of fluid can be removed during thoracoscopy with a little risk of pulmonary edema, since immediate equilibration of pressures is provided by the direct entrance of air through the cannula into the pleural space. If lung re-expansion appears to diminish, only low-pressure suction should be applied through the pleural drainage tube, which is always placed at the conclusion of the thoracoscopic procedure.

Table 2 Complications of thoracoscopy

1. *During the procedure* • Significant bleeding • Hypoxemia, cardiac arrhythmias, hypotension, occasionally death • Subcutaneous emphysema
2. *Later complications* • Local site infection • Empyema • Bronchopleural fistula • Respiratory failure • Neoplastic invasion of thoracoscopic tract

Complications with a rigid scope include prolonged air leak, hemorrhage, subcutaneous emphysema, postoperative fever, empyema, and seeding of chest wall from mesothelioma. Most dreaded complications are bleeding after a parietal pleural biopsy, lung perforation, and infections. These are seldom observed. Complication rate reported in one of the randomized controlled study is 10.3% for medical thoracoscopy and 17.2% for closed pleural biopsy.[25] After talc poudrage, fever may occur. Local site infection is uncommon and empyema is rare.

SURGICAL THORACOSCOPY

Video-assisted thoracoscopic surgery, often referred to as VATS, is done in a theater-suite under general anesthesia, with single lung ventilation. It is a minimally invasive thoracic surgery employed in the management of pulmonary, pleural diaphragmatic and mediastinal disease. It avoids the thoracotomy incision and hence shorter operative time and lesser postoperative morbidity. Surgeons often use multiple ports to introduce the thoracoscope, biopsy forceps and suction cannulae. VATS is used to examine the chest cavity from within and to perform diagnostic procedures such as the lung, diaphragmatic and pleural biopsies.[45]

Increasingly complex procedures are now being performed such as the lung resections including lobectomy and pneumonectomy, evaluation of mediastinal tumors and adenopathy, lung biopsy in diffuse parenchymal lung disease, bullectomy, evacuation of pleural based problems, decortication, antireflux procedures, diaphragmatic plication and repair of bronchopleural fistula.[45,46]

Thoracoscopic approach for the microsurgical removal of herniated thoracic disks is also described.[47] In non-small cell lung cancer (NSCLC), thoracoscopy helps in evaluating the extent of invasion by the primary tumor, chest wall invasion, pleural and mediastinal involvement.[48] In a study by Tiziano et al. 64 patients with suspected stage IIIB NSCLC, thoracoscopy improved the preoperative staging. Among 30 patients with mediastinal infiltration based on CT scan, 11 were down staged to stage IIIA or II. VATS can also be used to sample azygos, subaortic, para-aortic, paraesophageal and pulmonary ligament lymph nodes. This invasive lymph node sampling helps in appropriate preoperative staging in selected patients with NSCLC.[49] Compared to medical thoracoscopy, VATS is used for more complex, and time consuming procedures, and replaces thoracotomy in many instances.

Post-thoracoscopic Management

Following thoracoscopy, a chest tube should be introduced into the pleural space. The tube is fixed in place by a skin suture. The tube is removed when there is no further air leakage or when the fluid production is less than 100 mL/day.[10] In uncomplicated cases, intercostal drain is removed after 48–72 hours.

REFERENCES

1. Hatzinger M1, Kwon ST, Langbein S, Kamp S, Häcker A, Alken P. Hans Christian Jacobaeus: Inventor of human laparoscopy and thoracoscopy. J Endourol. 2006;20:848-50
2. Jacobaeus HC. The cauterization of adhesions in artificial pneumothorax therapy of tuberculosis. Am Rev Tuberc. 1922;6: 871-97.
3. Miller JI. Therapeutic thoracoscopy: New horizons for an established procedure. Ann Thorac Surg. 1991;52(5):1036-7.
4. Tape TG, Blank LL, Wigton RS. Procedural skills of practicing pulmonologists: a national survey of 1,000 members of the American College of Chest Physicians. Am J Respir Crit Care Med. 1995;151:282-7.
5. Landreneau RJ, Mack MJ, Hazelrigg SR, Dowling RD, Acuff TE, Magee MJ, et al. Video-assisted thoracic surgery: basic technical concepts and intercostals approach strategies. Ann Thorac Surg. 1992;54(4):800-7.
6. Bhatnagar R, Maskell NA. Medical pleuroscopy. Clin Chest Med. 2013;34:487-500.
7. Loddenkemper R. Thoracoscopy—state of art. Eur Respir J. 1998;11(1):213-21.
8. Seijo LM, Sterman DH. Interventional pulmonology. N Engl J Med. 2001;344(10):740-9.
9. Mathur PN, Boutin C, Loddenkemper R. Medical thoracoscopy: Technique and indications in pulmonary medicine. J Bronchol. 1994;1:228-39.
10. Rodríguez-Panadero F. Medical Thoracoscopy. Respiration. 2008;76(4):363-72.
11. Hersh CP, Feller-Kopman D, Wahidi M, Garland R, Herth F, Ernst A. Ultrasound guidance for medical thoracoscopy: a novel approach. Respiration. 2003;70(3):299-301.
12. Prosst RL, Winkler S, Boehm E, Gahlen J. Thoracoscopic fluorescence diagnosis (TFD) of pleural malignancies: experimental studies. Thorax. 2002;57:1005-9.
13. Chrysanthidis MG, Janssen JP. Autofluorescence videothoracoscopy in exudative pleural effusions:preliminary results. Eur Respir J. 2005;26(6):989-92.
14. Baas P1, Triesscheijn M, Burgers S, van Pel R, Stewart F, Aalders M. Fluorescence detection of pleural malignancies using 5-aminolevulinic acid. Chest. 2006;129(3):718-24.
15. Vincent BD, Fraig M, Silvestri GA. A pilot study of narrow band imaging compared to white light bronchoscopy for evaluation of normal airways premalignant and malignant airways disease. Chest. 2007;131(6):1794-9.
16. Rodriguez-Panadero F, Antony VB. Pleurodesis: state of the art. Eur Respir J. 1997;10(7):1648-54.
17. Ravindran C, Durga B, Mohammed MA. Medical Thoracoscopy-An interventional procedure for the Pulmonologists. Pulmon. 2006;8:6-9 (Online edition *www.pulmoneonline.org*).
18. Davidson AC, George RJ, Sheldon CD, Sinha G, Corrin B, Geddes DM. Thoracoscopy: assessment of a physician service and comparison of a flexible bronchoscope used as a thoracoscope with a rigid thoracoscope. Thorax. 1988;43(4):327-32.
19. Viallat JR, Rey F, Astoul P, Boutin C. Thoracoscopic talc pouldrage pleurodesis for malignant effusions: A review of 360 cases. Chest. 1996;110(6):1387-93.
20. Diacon AH, Wyser C, Bolliger CT, Tamm M, Pless M, Perruchoud AP, et al. Prospective randomized comparison of thoracoscopic talc poudrage under local anaesthesia versus bleomycin instillation for pleurodesis in malignant pleural effusions. Am J Respir Crit Care Med. 2000;162(4 Pt 1):1445-9.
21. Rozman A, Camlek L, Marc-Malovrh M, Triller N, Kern I. Rigid versus semi-rigid thoracoscopy for the diagnosis of pleural disease: a randomized pilot study. Respirology. 2013;18(4): 704-10.
22. Dhooria S, Singh N, Aggarwal AN, Gupta D, Agarwal R. A randomized trial comparing the diagnostic yield of rigid and semirigid thoracoscopy in undiagnosed pleural effusions. Respir Care. 2014;59(5):756-64.
23. Menzies R, Charbonneau M. Thoracoscopy for the diagnosis of pleural disease. Ann Intern Med. 1991;114(4):271-6.
24. Light RW. Diagnostic principles in pleural disease. Eur Respir J. 1997;10(2):476-81.
25. Haridas N, Suraj KP, Rajagopal TP, James PT, Chetambath R. Medical thoracoscopy vs closed pleural biopsy in pleural effusions: A randomized controlled study. J Clin Diagn Res. 2014;8(5):1-4.
26. Thomas JM, Musani AI. Malignant pleural effusions: a review. Clin Chest Med. 2013;34:459-71.
27. American Thoracic Society. Management of malignant pleural effusions. (ATS/ERS statement). Am J Respir Crit Care Med. 2000;162(5):1987-2001.
28. Boutin C, Viallat JR, Cargnino P, Farisse P. Thoracoscopy in malignant pleural effusions. Am Rev Respir Dis. 1981;124(5): 588-92.
29. Boutin C, Rey F. Thoracoscopy in pleural malignant mesothelioma: a prospective study of 188 consecutive patients. Part 1: Diagnosis. Cancer. 1993;72(2):389-93.
30. Boutin C, Rey F, Gouvernet J, Viallat JR, Astoul P, Ledoray V. Thoracoscopy in pleural malignant mesothelioma. Part 2: Prognosis and staging. Cancer. 1993;72(2):394-404.
31. Jamssen JP, Ramlal S, Mravuma M. The long term follow up of exudative pleural effusion after non diagnostic thoracoscopy. J Bronchol. 2004;11:169-74.
32. Ryan CJ, Rodgers RF, Uni UK, et al. The outcome of patients with pleural effusion of indeterminate cause at thoracotomy. Mayo Clin Proc. 1981;56(3):145-9.
33. Colt HG. Thoracoscopy: A prospective study of safety and outcome. Chest. 1995;108(2):324-9.
34. Hillerdal G, Ozermi M. Benign asbestos pleural effusions: 73 exudates in 60 patients. Eur J Respir Dis. 1987;71(2):113-21.
35. Loddenkemper R, Boutin C. Thoracoscopy: Present diagnostic and therapeutic indications. Eur Respir J. 1993;6(10):1544-55.

36. Dhanya TS, Ravindran C. Medical thoracoscopy-minimally invasive diagnostic tool for a trained Pulmonologist. Calicut Medical J. 2009;7:e4 (Open access Journal:*www.calicut-medicaljournal.org*).
37. Janssen JP, Boutin C. Extended thoracoscopy: A biopsy method to be used in case of pleural adhesions. Eur Respir J. 1992;5(6):763-6.
38. Harris RJ, Kavuru MS, Rice TW, Kirby TJ. The diagnostic and therapeutic utility of thoracoscopy. A review. Chest. 1995;108(3):828-41.
39. Lewis RJ, Caccavale RJ, Sisler GE, Mackenzie JW. One hundred consecutive patients undergoing video-assisted thoracic operations. Ann Thorac Surg. 1992;54(3):421-6.
40. Lo Cicero J. Minimally invasive thoracic surgery and thoracoscopy. Chest. 1992;102(2):330-1.
41. Boutin C, Astoul P, Rey F, Mathur PN. Thoracoscopy in the diagnosis and treatment of spontaneous pneumothorax. Clin Chest Med. 1995;16(3):497-503.
42. Schramel FM, Postmus PE, Vanderschueren RG. Current aspects of spontaneous pneumothorax. Eur Respir J. 1997;10(6):1372-9.
43. Bensard DD, McIntyre RC Jr, Waring BJ, Simon JS. Comparison of video-thoracoscopic lung biopsy to open lung biopsy in the diagnosis of interstitial lung disease. Chest. 1993;103(3):765-70.
44. Ernst A, Hersch CP, Herth F, Thurer R, LoCicero J 3rd, Beamis J, et al. A novel instrument for the evaluation of the pleural space: an experience in 34 patients. Chest. 2002;122(5):1530-4.
45. McKenna RJ Jr. Lobectomy by video-assisted thoracic surgery with mediastinal node sampling for lung cancer. J Thorac Cardiovasc Surg. 1994;107(3):879-81.
46. Miller DL, Allen MS, Deschamps C, Trastek VF, Pairolero PC, et al. Video-assisted thoracic surgical procedure: management of a solitary pulmonary nodule. Mayo Clin Proc. 1992;67(5):462-4.
47. Oskouian RJ, Johnson JP, Regan JJ. Thoracoscopic microdiscectomy. Neurosurgery. 2002;50(1):103-9.
48. Roberts JR, Blum MG, Arildsen R, Drinkwater DC Jr, Christian KR, Powers TA, et al. Prospective comparison of radiologic, thoracoscopic and pathologic staging in patients with early non-small cell lung cancer. Ann Thorac Surg. 1999;68(4):1154-8.
49. Tiziano De Giacomo, Erino A Rendina, Federico Venuta, et al. Thoracoscopic staging of IIIB non-small cell lung cancer before neoadjuvant therapy. Ann Thorac Surg. 1997;64:1409-11.

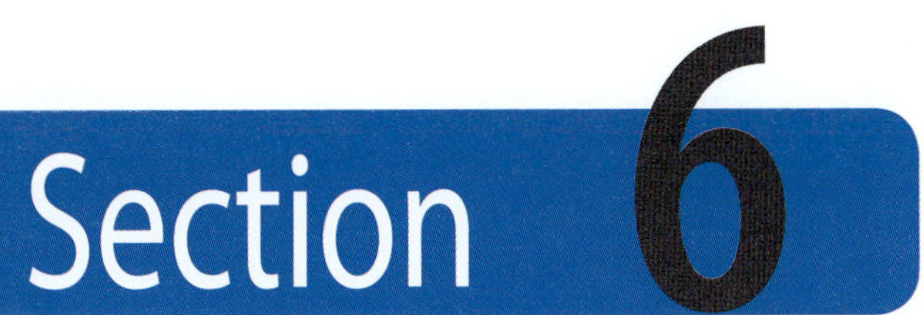

Tuberculosis

D Behera, SK Jindal

Epidemiology of Pulmonary Tuberculosis and Trends in Disease Burden

VK Chadha

INTRODUCTION

Tuberculosis (TB) has been known to afflict the mankind since times immemorial. Information on the magnitude of disease occurrence is available only from the beginning of 18th century when very high rates of morbidity and mortality were recorded in most western countries.[1,2] In these countries, the TB epidemic peaked during the 19th century and due to improvements in living conditions thereafter, the morbidity and mortality rates declined considerably by the first half of the 20th century.[2-4] The declining trend hastened when anti-TB drugs became available from the middle of 20th century.[5] Though control programs were also introduced in developing countries from 1960s, TB continued to be major public health menace in these countries due to ineffective implementation of planned strategies and insufficient resources.[5]

From 1980s, the declining trend in industrialized countries also witnessed a reversal primarily due to the advent of human immunodeficiency virus (HIV) epidemic and immigration from high endemic countries and there was further worsening of the TB problem in developing countries.[4-13] This prompted the World Health Organization (WHO) to declare TB a global emergency in 1993. To give impetus to TB control activities, directly observed treatment, short-course (DOTS) strategy was introduced worldwide during 1990s and further energized by implementation of Stop TB Strategy from 1996. To evaluate the progress in TB control, the Millennium Development Goals (MDGs) of the United Nations provided a framework and specific targets for TB control which were set during a meeting of the group of eight (G-8) industrialized countries in the year 2000. The principal target of MDGs for TB control was to ensure that the incidence rate of TB which was increasing at that time started to decline by 2015 and the supplementary targets were to halve its prevalence and mortality rates by 2015 when compared to 1990.[14] Post 2015 global TB strategy framework envisages further reduction in TB deaths and incidence to the extent of 75% and 50%, respectively by the year 2025 compared to 2015 with the ultimate goal of ending the global TB epidemic by 2035.[15]

The study of epidemiology of any infectious disease is crucial to formulate appropriate control strategies as it generates knowledge about natural dynamics of disease occurrence in communities, modes of transmission, magnitude of the disease burden, its distribution and the impact of control interventions. Therefore, this chapter dwells on the agent, host and environmental factors responsible for disease causation, describes the methods to estimate TB burden and its trends, and reviews the present magnitude and progress towards MDGs for 2015 globally and in India.

AGENT, HOST AND ENVIRONMENTAL FACTORS

The transmission of *Mycobacterium tuberculosis* (MTB) occurs through air when a person suffering from sputum smear positive pulmonary or laryngeal TB coughs or sneezes producing airborne droplet nuclei containing tubercle bacilli; smear negative patients are only one-fifth as infectious.[16] Most of the transmission occurs indoor. In outdoor, the airborne droplets are dispersed rapidly reducing the numbers of droplets per unit volume of air but transmission can take place if the infectious patient coughs or talks in close proximity of the susceptible person.

Once exposed, the risk of becoming infected depends on the size of infectious droplet nuclei and their density in the air. Droplets larger than 10 microns (μ) in diameter settle to the ground faster but smaller droplets remain suspended in the air for a long time. Once inhaled, droplets larger than 5 μ get trapped in the upper respiratory tract and only those less than 5 μ reach the lower tract to establish infection.[17]

The extent of transmission of infection in a given community depends upon the incidence rate of TB, average duration of infectiousness and number of susceptible individuals who come in contact with an infectious patient. Though people in high endemic countries are anyway at high risk of acquiring infection, those living in the same household as an infectious patient are at added risk.[18] An untreated patient remains infectious for a longer period of time than the one diagnosed early and rendered noninfectious through effective treatment. It has been observed that on an average, each point prevalent case of smear positive pulmonary TB (PTB) infects 7–10 persons in a year.[19,20] Infection gets established in about 30–40% of household contacts before the infectious index patient is diagnosed, given the average delay between onset of disease and diagnosis.[21,22]

Overcrowding increases the risk of infection.[23] Recently, restriction fragment length polymorphism (RFLP) based molecular epidemiological studies have demonstrated that even casual contact may be sufficient for some individuals to get infected.[24,25] Therefore, contact tracing which generally focuses on house hold members fails to identify nonhouse hold individuals who might have acquired infection/disease from an infectious patient. It has been demonstrated that TB cases who smoke are more infectious due to increased frequency of coughing, longer delay in seeking diagnosis and poorer rates of success with anti-TB treatment.[26,27]

The transmission of *Mycobacterium bovis* (*M. bovis*) generally occurs through consumption of raw (without boiling or pasteurization) milk from cattle suffering from TB disease.

The nontuberculous mycobacteria (NTM) being present in air, water and soil can enter the body through lungs, gut or skin while breathing, eating, drinking or through cuts and wounds in the skin but are not transmitted from person to person or animal to man.

The bacilli after establishing the infection in the human body remain dormant for variable period of time. Most (about 90%) of the infected immunocompetent individuals remain disease free during the course of their life. The risk of developing disease is higher during the period immediately following infection;[28-30] the other half develop the disease after variable and sometimes very long period of latency. While the average lifetime risk of a young child newly infected with MTB to develop TB is about 10%, half of this risk occurs within the first 5 years of infection.[28] Even though, the individual risk of developing TB is highest among the recently infected,[29,30] majority of the disease incidence is contributed by the remotely infected people because of their numbers being many times more than the recently infected.

In developed countries, most of the disease incidence was hitherto believed to be attributable to reactivation of the dormant bacilli but recent molecular epidemiological studies that characterize the MTB strains within a cluster (a cluster is defined as two or more cases attributable to same strain) in a given community (village/locality/closed institution) indicate that a substantial proportion of cases may be due to recent infection.[31,32] Such studies have also shown that a significant proportion of recurrent cases may be due to reinfection with a different strain rather than relapse of disease caused by the strain responsible for a previous episode.[32] Overall, the proportion of cases attributable to recent infection is more in high transmission set ups of high incidence developing countries.

Of all incidence cases of TB, more than 80% suffer from PTB.[33] In HIV nonreactive adult patients, about 70% of PTB patients are smear positive; this proportion is significantly lower among those who are HIV-reactive and in children.[34]

Community based surveys generally reveal increasing trends in incidence of PTB with age, attributable to increase in the prevalence of infection with age.[35,36] Higher incidence rates in males compared to females by about 2–4 times are also attributed to differences in risk of exposure.[35,36] However, when the level of exposure to infectious cases is similar, the risk of developing TB following infection has been observed to be higher among females especially in early adulthood period.[28,37] The risk of developing TB each year in individuals co-infected with HIV is about 30 times higher than the HIV uninfected.[38] The synergism between TB and HIV pathogens also facilitates faster HIV replication and progression to AIDS.[39]

Though the individual risk of TB is increased 2–3 times among smokers and diabetics, especially those with poor glycogenic control, the total fraction of TB disease occurring in the population due to these risk factors individually is about the same as due to HIV.[40-46] Higher risks of relapse have also been observed in people living with HIV (PLHIV) and diabetics.[47] Silicosis, under-nutrition, malignancy and alcohol consumption are other major risk factors for developing TB.[48-50] Poor socio-economic and living conditions, indoor air pollution and homelessness are also associated with higher incidence of TB.[42,51-54] Ecological studies indicate a close relationship between TB incidence and gross development product (GDP).[54] This is also reflected by the notification rates which are in general several times higher in low income countries compared to the high income countries, despite the poorer efficiency of routine surveillance in the former.[38]

A proportion of TB patients get naturally cured even without treatment. In a longitudinal study carried by the National TB Institute, Bangalore (NTI), about 31% of smear positive cases of PTB having chest X-ray film suggestive of TB had become culture negative after 1.5 years.[55] In this study, the 5-year case fatality among the untreated bacteriologically positive PTB patients was 47%. According to a recent systematic review encompassing studies from the pre-chemotherapy era, fatality was found to be the highest in the initial years of disease and declined with time;[56] about 55% of untreated smear positive PTB patients died over 5 years and almost all of TB associated deaths occurred within 10 years of disease occurrence.[56] The risk of case fatality over 10 years among the untreated, by smear and HIV status was estimated as under **Table 1**.

Besides HIV infection, the time interval between disease onset and diagnosis, poor treatment adherence, drug susceptibility pattern, recurrent TB, smear negativity in HIV reactive TB patients, poor diabetic control, malnutrition and noninfective comorbidities have been found to be independent risk factors for death during anti-TB treatment.[47,57] Significantly, higher mortality rates have also

Table 1 Estimation of fatality from TB over 10-year-period according to HIV status

Smear positive HIV negative TB	72%
Smear negative HIV negative TB	20%
Smear positive HIV positive TB	83%
Smear negative HIV positive TB	74%
Abbreviations: HIV, human immunodeficiency virus; TB, tuberculosis	

been observed in TB patients in the post-treatment period compared to in the general population.[58-61] HIV positivity, advanced immune-suppression, malnutrition, poor socio-economic status and drug and alcohol abuse have been found to be independent risk factors for such post-treatment mortality.[57]

ESTIMATING TUBERCULOSIS BURDEN

Prevalence of Tuberculosis Disease

Prevalence is defined as the proportion of people suffering from TB disease at a given point of time and is commonly expressed as a proportion per 100,000 populations. There are two methods to estimate prevalence.

Direct Estimation from Community Based Surveys

Surveys are useful to estimate prevalence of bacteriologically positive (positive on smear and/or culture) PTB.

The following steps are involved in conducting a TB prevalence survey:

- Selection of a representative sample of the population. Cluster sampling is employed for selection of villages and urban areas. Surveys usually involve a large sample size. For example, about 100,000 individuals would be required to be included in the survey to estimate prevalence within 20% of the true value if the expected prevalence is 200 per 100,000 population.
- Screening the study population for presence of symptoms suggestive of PTB and by radiography of the chest. A significant proportion of TB patients would be missed if only one screening tool is employed.
- Collecting sputum specimens (one spot, one early morning) in wide mouth presterilized bottles from those having symptoms and/or any abnormal pulmonary shadow.
- The sputum specimens are properly packed in sputum boxes and transported to quality assured certified laboratory within 72 hours and examined by smear microscopy and culture for acid fast bacilli (AFB).
- Analysis to estimate prevalence and its confidence intervals, after adjusting for sampling design and coverage of the study population for screening and sputum examination.

Surveys are not suitable for finding out the prevalence of bacteriologically negative radiologically active PTB because of low specificity of X-ray based diagnosis. It has been revealed in earlier studies that about two-thirds of such patients diagnosed on the basis of X-ray picture alone are not true TB cases. Surveys are also not useful for estimating prevalence of extra-pulmonary TB (EPTB) and childhood TB due to non-specific nature of presenting illness and impracticability of performing required investigations in field conditions.

Indirect Estimation

Prevalence can be estimated by using the following equation:

$$\text{Prevalence} = \text{Incidence (I)} \times \text{Mean duration of disease (D)}$$

This equation may be employed if a reliable estimate of incidence is available. Theoretically, "D" can be estimated from prevalence surveys but its precise estimation is limited due to following factors:

- Exact time of onset of disease is unknown
- Many TB patients are asymptomatic or mildly symptomatic when detected during the surveys
- Detection of cases during surveys interferes with the usual course of the disease leading to under estimating the duration
- Patients need to be followed up for relapse.

The duration if measured in notified TB patients would ignore the duration in non-notified and untreated patients. Therefore, "D" is often assumed. Values of "D", used by WHO for estimating prevalence using the above equation are as under **Table 2**.[38]

In a recent systematic review, the mean duration of untreated HIV negative PTB patients (including bacteriologically positive/negative PTB) was estimated at 3 years.[56]

Incidence of Tuberculosis Disease

Incidence of TB is defined as the number of new and recurrent cases arising in a given period of time (usually one year) in a given community and is expressed as a rate per unit population, usually 100,000.

Theoretically, incidence can be measured through prospective cohort studies wherein a representative population is

Table 2 Mean duration of disease, used by WHO for estimating prevalence

Non-notified HIV negative TB	4 years
Non-notified HIV positive TB	0.2 years
Notified HIV negative TB	2 years
Notified HIV positive TB	1 year
Abbreviations: HIV, human immunodeficiency virus; TB, tuberculosis	

Table 3 Reasons and methods employed to estimate the proportion of missed cases

Patients do not have access to health care	There might be already available information about the proportion of the population that lack access to health care facilities. Otherwise, such information may be obtained by piggy backing on other surveys, such as Census, National Family Health survey and socio-economic surveys conducted by the national sample survey organization in India
Patients do not seek care in spite of having access	Proportion of such patients may be determined during TB prevalence surveys and finding out health seeking pattern among person found during the surveys to be having symptoms suggestive of TB
Patients remain undiagnosed in spite of seeking care	The proportion may be estimated through carefully designed research among persons who present to different types of health providers
Patients diagnosed by non-RNTCP providers but not reported	This proportion may be determined by conducting "Inventory study" in which TB cases diagnosed by all providers are counted. If such data do not exist, then special efforts are made to collect the information prospectively
A proportion of patients are diagnosed by RNTCP and collaborating providers but not reported	Determined by inventory study

Abbreviations: TB, tuberculosis; RNTCP, Revised National Tuberculosis Control Program

repeatedly surveyed over short intervals (3–12 months) of time to find out the new cases among persons found to be free of TB disease at the baseline survey. Information should also be obtained about any additional cases in the study population that might be diagnosed at health centers during the period between two consecutive surveys. However, a significant proportion of cases occurring in the intervening period might be missed due to migration, natural cure or death. No country till date has estimated TB incidence using this method since it is too cumbersome, requires a large sample size and is cost prohibitive.

Hitherto, incidence was estimated in many countries by applying Styblo's equation according to which every 1% of annual risk of infection (ARTI) among children corresponded to 50 smear positive incidence cases of PTB per 100,000 populations per year.[62] This equation was derived from data obtained mostly during the prechemotherapy era and is no longer valid in DOTS era when the mean duration of infectiousness is reduced and thus a larger number of incidence cases are needed to infect 1% of the population.[63] Similarly, in communities where significant proportions of TB cases are HIV co-infected, a shorter survival reduces the average duration of infectiousness.[64,65]

Presently, the methods used to estimate incidence are as under.

Direct Estimation of Incidence from Tuberculosis Notification Data

In countries where entire populations have access to TB diagnostic services and almost all incidence cases are reported to National Tuberculosis Programmes (NTPs), the annual case notification rates may be equated with incidence rates after examining the surveillance data for completeness, duplications and misclassifications. Case based electronic recording and reporting systems recently introduced in many countries are expected to address these aspects in the coming years. Nonetheless, full potential of reliable diagnosis in public as well as private health facilities has to be realized before routine surveillance data can be used for estimating incidence. Presently, majority of TB patients diagnosed/treated by health providers outside the ambit of NTPs are not notified to public health authorities in majority of high burden countries (HBCs). In India, compulsory notification has been introduced through a Gazette notification by Ministry of Health in the year 2012. However, intensive efforts are required to improve efficiency of notification by the private sector.

Indirect Estimation

Incidence can be estimated by using the following equation:

$$\text{Incidence} = \frac{\text{Number of notified new TB cases}}{\text{1- Fraction of cases missed by the notification data}}$$

The reasons for which cases are missed from notification and the methods that can be employed to estimate the proportion of missing cases are as under **Table 3**.

The fractions of cases missed at various stages as above are added to find out the total proportion of cases missed by the notification data. In the absence of reliable information on the proportion of missing cases at one or more stages, the opinion of experts may be relied upon till such time reliable information is obtained through special investigations as listed above. The final estimate of incidence should also be corrected for over-diagnosis and over-reporting of cases if any.

Tuberculosis Mortality

Tuberculosis mortality rate is defined as the proportion of HIV-negative individuals in the community who die of TB during a course of one year. Deaths among HIV positive, TB cases are not counted as TB deaths, since these are recorded as HIV deaths as per the International Classification of Diseases (ICD-10).[66]

Direct estimation of TB mortality rate through prospective cohort studies is operationally difficult. Further, routine TB surveillance systems in most HBCs do not provide accurate information on TB mortality rates due to less than 100% case detection rate and nonascertainment of the cause of death (COD) among cases who died during treatment. Moreover, the fate of TB cases that default from treatment or are transferred out is usually not known and some cases may die due to TB even after having completed treatment.[58-61] Thus, the routine surveillance data at best throw light on case fatality rates (CFRs) during the period of treatment. In such situations, the commonly used practical approaches to measure TB mortality are as under.

Direct Estimation Using Vital Registration Data

The most cost effective approach would be to have an efficient system of vital registration in place wherein the underlying cause for every death occurring in the community is identified and coded as per ICD-10 and reported. The advantage of this system over routine TB surveillance system is that it would include deaths occurring before TB diagnosis as well as in defaulters and after completion of treatment. However, these systems are constrained in most high burden TB countries by lack of universal population coverage and inaccuracy in assigning COD.[67] Many countries have introduced vital registration systems in representative samples of their populations as interim solutions till the full time coverage of vital registration system is achieved.

Direct Estimation from Verbal Autopsy Studies

Verbal autopsy (VA) method is being increasingly used to find out the COD.[68-70] In this method, the information on events of deaths taking place in a community during a given period is obtained from various sources, such as hospital data, religious places, crematoria and community-based volunteers. The workers trained in VA visit the houses of the diseased and conduct interviews with their close relatives using a standardized questionnaire. Information is obtained from family members on symptoms, duration of disease, anatomical site and COD as known to them and from available hospital and other records. The interviewer also writes a narrative of events starting from the onset of illness till death. Subsequently, each filled-in questionnaire is reviewed independently by two medical officers trained in ICD to assign and code the COD; disagreement if any is resolved by referring to an umpire. Sensitivity and specificity of the survey tool in assigning causes of death should be validated before undertaking these studies in a specific area.

Table 4 Case fatality rates used by World Health Organization[38]

Non-notified TB patients in high-income countries	12%
Non-notified TB patients in other countries	32%
Notified TB patients in high income countries	3.9%
Notified TB patients in other countries	7.4%
Abbreviation: TB, tuberculosis	

Indirect Estimation

Mortality rate may be estimated by using the following equation: Mortality rate = incidence rate × CFR

The CFRs used by WHO are as under **Table 4**.[38]

This method may be made more accurate by applying specific CFRs observed for cases stratified by source of treatment (DOTS/non-DOTS/untreated), disease classification (pulmonary/extrapulmonary), type of TB patient (new/previously treated), drug sensitivity status, HIV status, and subsequently pooled to estimate the average mortality rate.

Prevalence of Infection

Prevalence of infection in the community is directly measured through tuberculin surveys carried out in a representative sample of the population.[71] Such surveys are generally carried out among children below 10 years of age because the high prevalence of infection with NTM in older age groups interferes with interpretation of data. The magnitude of prevalence of infection among children depends on the prevalence of infectious cases in the community.

A tuberculin survey to estimate prevalence of infection involves the following steps:

- Selection of a representative sample of children.
- Subjecting study population to tuberculin testing by intra-dermal administration of 0.1 mL of tuberculin dilution containing 2 TU of purified protein derivative (PPD) RT23 with Tween 80 on the volar aspect of forearm. Children suffering from high fever, history of measles in the recent past and those with known immune compromised condition, such as HIV and corticosteroid therapy are excluded. PPD vials should be stored at 2–8 C, transported in vaccine carriers and protected from heat and sunlight.
- Measuring maximum transverse diameter of induration at the test site after 48–96 hours and recording the same in millimeters.
- The data on tuberculin reaction sizes obtained during the survey is plotted as a frequency distribution graph with reaction size on X-axis and percentage of reactors on Y-axis. A classical graph of tuberculin survey data is bi-modal with two distinct modes and an easily identifiable antimode **(Fig. 1)**. Reactions to the left of antimode represent cross-reactions to infection with NTM or Bacillus

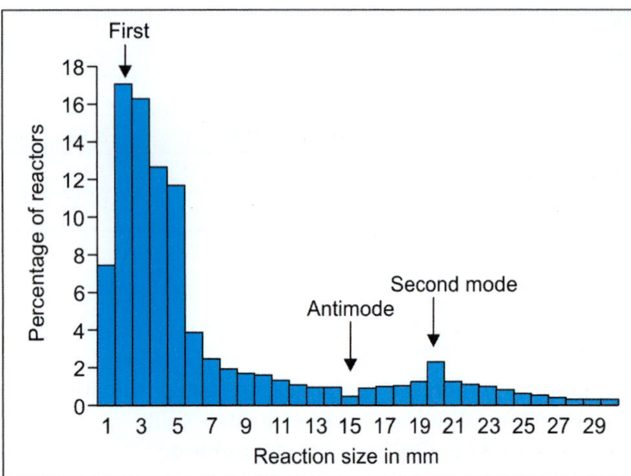

Fig. 1 An example of frequency distribution of tuberculin reaction sizes obtained in a survey

Calmette-Guérin (BCG) vaccination and reactions to its right represent the subgroup of children infected with tubercle bacilli. In case the antimode is clearly discernible, prevalence of infection is estimated as the proportion of children having reactions equal to or larger than the antimode. However, the antimode is usually not clearly identifiable in areas where NTM infections are common and when BCG vaccinated children are included in the survey. In such a scenario, prevalence of infection is estimated by mirror-image technique in which proportion of reactions larger than the second mode is doubled and added to the proportion at this mode. This technique is based on the assumption that reactions due to infection with tubercle bacilli are distributed normally around the mode. With this technique, influence of BCG-induced tuberculin sensitivity on estimate of prevalence of infection is minimal since BCG induced reactions are generally smaller than the second mode.

Sometimes, it is possible that neither the antimode nor the mode can be made out on the graph. In such a scenario, the mode of tuberculin reactions in smear-positive TB patients is applied to the frequency distribution of surveyed children to estimate prevalence of infection among them. This approach is based on the observations that in any given community, the mode of tuberculin reactions among TB patients is generally found to be at the same reaction size as the second mode among apparently healthy children. Thus, it is desirable that about 100–150 newly diagnosed sputum positive cases are also tested at the time of the survey.

Incidence of Tuberculous Infection

Direct Estimation

Theoretically, incidence of infection can be measured through repeat tuberculin surveys to identify the individuals that were uninfected at the previous survey and to find out their proportion that get infected during the interval between the two surveys. This approach is limited by the fact that the first test per se may boost the reaction to the second test.[72]

Indirect Estimation

To overcome the problem of direct estimation, the incidence of infection is computed indirectly from the estimate of prevalence of infection using the following equation:[71]

$$\text{ARTI} = 1 - (1 - \text{P})^{1/a}$$

where ARTI is the *annual risk of tuberculous infection* (termed so, to distinguish it from direct estimation of incidence of infection), "P" is the prevalence of infection and "a" denotes mean age of children tested. This equation is based on the assumption that a person once infected remains infected for the rest of life. Though tuberculin sensitivity may wane with time in a proportion of individuals,[71] the proportion that experience waning may not be significant to influence the prevalence of infection estimates among the child population.

The estimated ARTI represents the overall effect of incidence of infectious TB cases, their average duration of infectiousness and the average number of susceptible individuals that come in contact with an infectious case.

ESTIMATING TRENDS OF TUBERCULOSIS BURDEN

The study of trends of TB burden is more important than precise estimation of disease prevalence, incidence and mortality.

When efficient case finding and treatment programs are in place, the prevalence, mortality and risk of infection start declining earlier and it takes much longer for incidence of disease to decline. This is because of the fact that about one third of the population is already infected with *M. tuberculosis*[73] and thus TB patients will continue to emerge from the infected pool of people for a prolonged period of time. Incidence of disease would start declining only when the pool of infected people is significantly reduced as a result of sustained and effective implementation of control measures. However, the smaller component of incidence due to reinfection as a risk factor may decline earlier.

Trends of prevalence of disease can be measured directly by repeat surveys carried out at intervals of not less than 7–8 years or indirectly through mathematical modeling. The surveys must be comparable in terms of age group, survey tools, quality of data collection and analytical methods. WHO has estimated trends of prevalence of disease for the period 1990–2012 using the indirect method for most countries,[38] except where national level data were available from repeat surveys.

The most practical way to estimate trends in incidence rates of TB is to have an efficient notification system in place so that the trends in annual case notification rates directly reflect the trends in incidence. Any changes in case finding efforts and introduction of new diagnostic tools resulting in variation in case definitions may be kept in mind while analyzing case notification data for this purpose. It is desirable to analyze the data by age groups since in presence of an efficient control program it is the younger age groups in which the incidence would decline first. WHO estimated the trends for 1990–2012 indirectly by first estimating the level of under-reporting for reference years 1990, 1997 and 2011 followed by applying this trajectory of change to subsequent years.[38]

Changes in mean age of notified TB patients also point to the direction of the epidemic. Mean age would decline in a situation of declining notification rates in younger age groups and increase if the epidemic worsens. However, such data should be interpreted carefully, since an expanding program increases the access of services especially to the elderly and the very young. Increasing life expectancy per se may also lead to increase in mean age of TB patients.

Trends in mortality have been measured by WHO using the indirect method.

Trends of ARTI in children have generally been observed to run parallel to the trends in prevalence of TB disease among adults.[35,74-76] However, study of trends in ARTI is losing its importance due to increased difficulty in interpretation of tuberculin survey data. In the presence of DOTS-based programs, with decrease in levels of transmission of infection, it becomes challenging to segregate the infected sub-group from cross-reactors, on the frequency distribution curve.

ESTIMATED TUBERCULOSIS BURDEN

Global

There were an estimated 12 million [confidence interval (CI): 11–13 million] prevalent TB patients during 2012, at 169 (CI: 149–190) per 1,00,000 population.[38] While India followed by China and Indonesia harbor the highest absolute numbers of prevalent cases, the rates per unit population were highest in South Africa, Cambodia and Mozambique followed by Myanmar and Bangladesh.

The absolute incidence of all types of TB cases globally during the year 2012 was estimated at 8.6 million (range: 8.3–8.9 million), at the rate of 122 (CI: 117–127) per 1,00,000 population.[38] Twenty-two countries collectively comprise 80% of the global incident cases and are called high burden countries. India and China together account for 38% of the global incidence. South Africa, Indonesia and Pakistan are the other leading nations in terms of absolute number of TB cases. However, the highest incidence rates in excess of 400 per 1,00,000 populations were estimated for countries of the African region, being exceptionally high in South Africa and Swaziland at 1,000 per 1,00,000 population and in Timor-Leste.

Tuberculosis is the second leading COD among adults from a single infectious agent after HIV.[77] In 2012, about 1 million people (excluding deaths due to TB among HIV reactive patients) are estimated to have died due to TB at the rate of 13 (range: 11–16) per 100,000.[38] About 83% of these deaths occurred in HBCs. India and South Africa accounted for about one third of global TB deaths. An additional 0.3 million deaths among HIV-TB co-infected individuals were counted as HIV deaths.[38] The TB mortality rates were highest in the countries of Africa and South East Asia.

Of all the incidence cases, about 1.1 million (13%) were HIV positive.[38] About 75% of them were concentrated in Africa alone where 43% of all TB cases were HIV positive. Highest rates of HIV prevalence among TB cases were observed in Swaziland, South Africa, Mozambique, Zimbabwe, Uganda and Kenya.

About 2.9 million of all the incident cases occurred in females and 0.41 million women including 0.16 million HIV positive died with TB making it the single largest infectious COD in women.[38]

The precise estimate of TB burden in children is lacking.

Tuberculosis Burden in India

Results of prevalence surveys carried out in the country since 1990 are summarized at **Table 5**.[78-89] Surveys carried out during 2007–09 to estimate prevalence of bacteriologically positive PTB in 8 districts have been used to derive the present estimate of prevalence. While both the screening tools: (1) interview and (2) chest X-ray were used in three sites, only symptom screening by interview was employed in the other five sites. Thus, a correction factor of 1.3 obtained from the sites that employed both screening tools was applied to estimate adjusted prevalence at other sites which did not have measles, mumps, and rubella (MMR) screening. The district level estimates were pooled, after excluding data from one district with implausibly low prevalence rate, to find out the prevalence of bacteriologically positive PTB at national level and further corrected for EPTB and TB in children. The point prevalence of all TB was thus estimated 283 (CI: 207–395) per 1,00,000 population for the year 2008. For projecting the trends, the nationally representative survey conducted during 1956 was considered.[90] A flat trend was assumed from 1956 to 2001 [prior to good level of Revised National Tuberculosis Control Program (RNTCP) implementation]. The data adjusted for ageing population and the trend calculated from 2001 to 2008 has been applied to subsequent years. Thus estimated prevalence in 2012 was 230 (CI: 155–319) per 1,00,000 population.[38]

The national level estimate for ARTI among children for the year 2007 estimated through zonal level surveys was 1%.[91] It varied between 0.6% and 1.2% in the four zones of the country. The results of all tuberculin surveys carried out in the countries since 1990 to estimate ARTI are summarized at **Table 6**.[80, 91-98]

The incidence for India for the year 2012 has been estimated by adding to the cases notified by RNTCP the proportion of cases treated in the private sector as observed during a population based study in 30 districts and the proportions of undiagnosed and/or unreported cases as ascertained

Table 5 Prevalence of PTB per 100 000 population-surveys, carried out during 1990–2009

State and District	*Study period*	*Age (years)*	*Sample size*	*Screening method*	*Prevalence of PTB cases 100000 population*		
					Culture positive	*Smear positive*	*Culture and/or smear positive*
Delhi[79]	1991	>4	27,838	MMR	–	–	330
Jawadhu hill tribes, North Arcot (TN)[80]	1992–93	≥15	5755	Symptoms		209	
Car Nicobar (A and N)[81]	2000–2001	>14	10,570	Symptoms	–	729	–
Thiruvallur (TN)[82]	1999–2001 2001–2003 2004–2006 2007–2008	>14	83,425 85,474 89,413 92,255	MMR + symptoms	609 451 311 391	326 257 169 182	–
Karhal Block, Morena district (MP)[83]	1991–1992	>14	11,097	Symptoms	–	–	1270 (1060–1480)
Karhal Block (Saharia Tribes), Sheopur district, MP[84]	2007–08	≥15	11116	Symptoms	–	–	1518 (1208–1829)
Tribal areas, 11 selected districts (MP)[85]	2006–07	≥15	22 270	Symptoms	–	–	387 (273–502)
Nelamangala, Rural Bengaluru -Sub-district level[86]	2007–09	≥15	71874[@]	MMR + symptoms	152 (108–197)	83 (57–109)	196 (145–246)
Jabalpur (MP) -District level[87]	2008–09	≥15	95,071	Symptoms	–	172 (124–220)	255 (195–315)
Mohali (Punjab) -District level[88]	2008–09	≥15	91,030	Symptoms	–	6.2	24.1
Wardha (Maharashtra) -District level[89]	2007–09	≥15	55,096	MMR + symptoms	–	132	199.1
Faridabad (Haryana) -District level[89]	2008–09	≥15	98,599	Symptoms	–	105	129
Kanpur (UP)-District level[89]	2007–2009	≥15	49,766	Symptoms	–	322.7	361.2
Banda (UP)-District level[89]	2007–2009	≥15	46,709	Symptoms	–	245.4	398.6
Gujarat (State level)[90]	2011–2012	≥15	96,125	MMR + symptoms	–	267 (212–323)	382 (314–451)

through expert opinion. The incidence thus estimated was 2.2 (CI: 2.0–2.4) million at a rate of 176 (CI: 159–193) per 100,000 population, amounting to 26% of the incidence cases worldwide.[38] The country is ranked number 1 among 22 HBCs in terms of the absolute numbers of incidence cases that occur each year.[38]

The present mortality rate has been estimated by pooling the data of limited number of recently carried out VA studies during the period 2002–08 in the selected areas: urban slums in Kolkata city, rural areas of Thiruvallur district in Tamil Nadu and state level mortality surveys in Orissa and Andhra Pradesh (AP). The observed TB mortality rates in these studies varied between 28 and 76 per 1,00,000 populations per year.[99-101] Proportions of all deaths attributable to TB varied between 3.7% and 11.9%. The national level estimate was derived by pooling the data from these surveys after excluding the unexpected high mortality rate of 76 per 1,00,000 population in AP. Applying the expected trajectory from the mid-year of these surveys, the mortality rate for 2012 has been estimated at 22 (14–32) per 1,00,000 population which translates into about 2,70,000 (CI: 1,70,000–3,90,000) TB deaths (excluding TB deaths in HIV reactive patients).[38]

The data obtained in VA studies had some notable limitations: there were high proportion of deaths with

Table 6 ARTI surveys carried out in India, since 1990

Area	*Year of survey*	*Sample size*	*Age group*	*ARTI (%)*
Bengaluru city[93]	1998 2006	4936 3354	5–8 5–8	2.2 1.5
Rural areas, Thiruvallur district, Tamil Nadu[94]	1999–01 2004–05 2001–03	12854 8668 8329	0–9 0–9 0–9	1.6 1.4 1.2
Car Nicobar[81]	2001–02	2708	0–9	2.1
Orissa- state level survey[95]	2002	10626	1–9	1.7
Andhra Pradesh-state level survey[96]	2005–06	3636	5–9	1.4
Khammam, Andhra Pradesh[97]	2001–02		5–7	1.5
Zonal level surveys (4 zones)[92]	2000–03	N. Zone-51380 W. Zone-51733 E. Zone-42836 S. Zone-52300	0–9	N. Zone-1.9 (1.7–2.1) W. Zone-1.7 (1.5–1.9) E. Zone-1.2 (1.0–1.3) S. Zone-1.1 (1.0–1.2) National average 1.5 (1.4–1.6)
Zonal level surveys (4 zones)[92]	2009–10	N. Zone-13309 W. Zone-16065 E. Zone-19563 S. Zone-23343	0–9	N. Zone-1.1 (0.8–1.3) W. Zone-0.6 (0.4–0.7) E. Zone-1.2 (0.9–1.5) S. Zone-1.0 (0.8–1.1) National average 1.0 (0.8–1.1)
Kerala-state level survey[98]	2006	4821	5-9	Not available*
Chennai city[99]	2006	7008	1-9	2.0
Tribal areas, Madhya Pradesh[100]	2006	4802	1-9	1.3

*Due to absence of a cut-off point on frequency distribution of tuberculin reactions.

unspecified cause and crude death rates found out in all of these surveys were significantly lower than the Sample Registration System data for the corresponding periods.[102] Therefore, further standardization of the VA tool is necessary in order to obtain more precise estimates. The one million death study carried out under the aegis of the Registrar General of India during 2003–14 is expected to provide more information on TB specific mortality rates in the country.[70]

About 5% of the incident cases in the country are estimated to be HIV positive.[103]

PROGRESS TOWARDS MILLENNIUM DEVELOPMENT GOALS FOR 2015

Global Trends

According to estimates by WHO, prevalence rate at the global level has declined by 37% from 1990 to 2012; however, the target of 50% reduction at the global level is unlikely by 2015.[38] Region wise, American and Western Pacific regions have already achieved halving of prevalence and South-east Asia and European regions are projected to attain 50% reduction by 2015. But Africa and Eastern Mediterranean region are unlikely to attain the target. The trends in prevalence of PTB from repeat national level surveys available from few countries revealed declines of 41% in Cambodia between 2002 and 2011, 30% in Philippines between 1997 and 2007, 67% in Indonesia between 1980 and 2004 and 35% in Myanmar from 1994 to 2009.[104-107] In China, three rounds of national surveys revealed about three-fold decline in prevalence from 1990 to 2010.[108] While the decline was restricted during the period 1990–2000 only to provinces implementing DOTS, it declined in all provinces of China after 2000.[108] Drastic decline has also been observed in Bangladesh between two rounds of surveys carried out 10 years apart in 1987–88 and 2007–09 respectively.[109]

Tuberculosis mortality rate is estimated to have declined globally by 45% during the period 1990–2012 and is on target for 50% reduction by 2015.[38] By region, the target has been achieved in American, Western Pacific and Eastern Mediterranean regions, seems likely by 2015 in South East Asia region but unlikely in Africa and European region. Mortality rates are estimated to be declining in most countries including HBCs.

Globally, the target for reversing the previously increasing trend in incidence of TB has already been achieved; the incidence rate was estimated to be stable during 1990–2000 and started falling from 2001.[38] Region wise, declining trends were observed first in the America, Eastern Mediterranean and Western Pacific regions during 1990s followed by Europe and South East Asia around the year 2000 and in Africa in 2003. Incidence is also estimated to be declining in most of the 22 HBCs.

Trends in India

There has been a significant decline in the trends in prevalence of TB from 470 in 1990 to 230 per 1,00,000 populations in 2012.[38] This is supported by observations from repeat surveys which revealed decline of 35% in Thiruvallur from 1999 to 2008 and 56% in rural Bangalore from 1975 to 2008.[81,85] In Wardha also, there was a decline of 35% in 2008 when compared to a previous survey in 1985.[88,110] In Thiruvallur, a simultaneous decline in ARTI @ 6% per year was also observed among children.[74] An average decline in ARTI rates @ 4.5% per year was observed at the national level from 1998 to 2007, through two rounds of tuberculin surveys.[91] These trends may be related to a combination of improvements in living conditions and implementation of RNTCP.

Based on a modeling approach, TB mortality rates are estimated to have declined by 39% from 1990 to 2012;[38] the target of 50% reduction might just be achieved by 2015.

Although WHO estimates that TB incidence has started declining, there is no direct evidence as the notification rates of new smear positive cases have continued to increase due to increase in efforts at case finding. WHO projections are based on the reduction in total TB case notification which may primarily be due to reduction in notification rate of smear negative PTB which is more likely to be due to change from a direct X-based diagnosis to an algorithm-based diagnosis; thus, reducing the component of over diagnosis. Trends towards under-diagnosis of smear negative cases were observed during a recently carried out study in the State of Karnataka.[111]

PROSPECTS FOR TUBERCULOSIS CONTROL

Despite increased commitment to control efforts, TB continues to be a major public health problem. Though considerable progress has been made towards reducing the prevalence and mortality rates, TB cases will continue to emerge in large numbers in the years to come since about a third of the world's population is presently infected with tubercle bacillus.

The ultimate aim of the control activities is to reduce the number of people who get afflicted with the disease. Thus, reducing the incidence is the prime target of control programs and it will decline significantly only when the current generation with high levels of prevalence of infection is replaced by the generation of people with low level of infection prevalence. Thus continuous efforts are required for faster reduction in transmission rates by further improving early case finding and treatment efficiency and dedicated airborne infection control activities in health care and congregate settings. Molecular epidemiological studies to identify hotspots of transmission would be further useful to device appropriate strategies focused on such set ups.

Enhanced efforts are also required to engage all health providers including those in the private sector and facilitate them in timely diagnosis and checking poor treatment practices that fuel the multidrug resistant tuberculosis (MDRTB) epidemic, besides strengthening the MDRTB diagnostic cum treatment facilities, collaboration with HIV control programs and community participation in TB control activities. Intra and inter-sector collaboration is needed not only to reduce the prevalence of risk factors of TB, like smoking, HIV, diabetes mellitus but also effective treatment of concomitant diseases besides improving the living conditions especially for the poor people.

CONCLUSION

In conclusion, efficient control programs would need to be further strengthened and sustained for a prolonged period of time in order to significantly reduce the TB burden. More efficient newer diagnostic tools that facilitate early detection and shortened more efficacious therapeutic regimens are needed in order to eliminate TB in a reasonable time frame.

REFERENCES

1. Grigg ER. The arcana of tuberculosis with a brief epidemiologic history of the disease in the USA. Am Rev Tuberc. 1958;78(2): 151-72.
2. Benatar SR, Upshur R. Tuberculosis and poverty: what could (and should) be done? Int J Tuberc Lung Dis. 2010;14(10): 1215-21.
3. Stýblo K, Meijer J, Sutherland I. Tuberculosis Surveillance Research Unit Report No. 1: the transmission of tubercle bacilli; its trend in a human population. Bull Int Union Tuberc. 1969;42:1-104.
4. Raviglione MC, Sudre P, Reider HL, Spinaci S, Kochi A. Secular trends of tuberculosis in western Europe. Bull World Health Organ. 1993;71(3-4):297-306.
5. Styblo K. Selected Papers: Epidemiology of Tuberculosis: Epidemiology of Tuberculosis in HIV Prevalent Countries (Vol. 24). Holland: Royal Netherlands Tuberculosis Association; 1991.
6. Rom WN, Garay SM (Eds). Tuberculosis. Boston: Little Brown & Company; 1996.

7. Narain JP, Raviglione MC, Kochi A. HIV-associated tuberculosis in developing countries: epidemiology and strategies for prevention. Tuber Lung Dis. 1992;73(6):311-21.
8. Dye C. Global epidemiology of tuberculosis. Lancet. 2006; 367(9514):938-40.
9. Date AA, Vitoria M, Granich R, Banda M, Fox MY, Gilks C. Implementation of co-trimoxazole prophylaxis and isoniazid preventive therapy for people living with HIV. Bull World Health Organ. 2010;88(4):253-9.
10. Oxlade O, Schwartzman K, Behr MA, Benedetti A, Pai M, Heymann J, et al. Global tuberculosis trends: a reflection of changes in tuberculosis control or in population health? Int J Tuberc Lung Dis. 2009;13(10):1238-46.
11. Dye C, Lönnroth K, Jaramillo E, Williams BG, Raviglione M. Trends in tuberculosis incidence and their determinants in 134 countries. Bull World Health Organ. 2009;87(9):683-91.
12. Hans L Rieder, International Union against Tuberculosis and Lung Disease. Epidemiologic Basis of Tuberculosis Control. Paris, France: International Union against Tuberculosis and Lung Disease. 1999;1:50-2.
13. Siriarayapon P, Yanai H, Glynn JR, Yanpaisarn S, Uthaivoravit W. The evolving epidemiology of HIV infection and tuberculosis in northern Thailand. J Acquir Immune Defic Syndr. 2002;31(1):80-9.
14. Dye C, Maher D, Weil D, Espinal M, Raviglione M. Targets for global tuberculosis control. Int J Tuberc Lung Dis. 2006;10(4):460-2.
15. World Health Organization. (2013). Landmark meeting on post-2015 TB targets held in Geneva. [online] Available from *http://www.who.int/tb/features_archive/post_2015_targets_meeting/en/* [Accessed March 2016].
16. Behr MA, Warren SA, Salamon H, Hopewell PC, Ponce de Leon A, Daley CL, et al. Transmission of Mycobacterium tuberculosis from patients smear-negative for acid-fast bacilli. Lancet. 1999;353(9151):444-9.
17. Sonkin LS. The role of particle size in experimental air-borne infection. Am J Hyg. 1951;53(3):337-54.
18. Hoa NB, Cobelens FG, Sy DN, Nhung NV, Borgdorff MW, Tiemersma EW. First national tuberculin survey in Viet Nam: characteristics and association with tuberculosis prevalence. Int J Tuberc Lung Dis. 2013;17(6):738-44.
19. Styblo K, Flenely DC, Petty TL. Tuberculosis control and surveillance. In: Trevor Bannister Stretton. Recent Advances in Respiratory Medicine. London: Churchill Livingstone. 1986;4:77-108.
20. Chadha VK, Anjinappa SM. Gowda U, Srivastava R, Ahmed J, Kumar P. Annual risk of tuberculous infection in a rural population of South India and its relationship with prevalence of smear positive pulmonary tuberculosis. Indian J Tuberc. 2013;60:227-32.
21. Rouillon A, Perdrizet S, Parrot R. Transmission of tubercle bacilli: The effects of chemotherapy. Tubercle. 1976;57(4):275-99.
22. Grzybowski S, Barnett GD, Styblo K. Contacts of cases of active pulmonary tuberculosis. Bull Int Union Tuberc. 1975;50(1):90-106.
23. Singh M, Mayank ML, Kumar L, Mathew JL, Jindal SK. Prevalence and risk factors for transmission of infection among children in household contact with adults having pulmonary tuberculosis. Arch Dis Child. 2005;90(6):624-8.
24. Small PM, Hopewell PC, Sing SP, Paz A, Parsonnet J, Ruston DC, et al. The epidemiology of tuberculosis in San Francisco. A population-based study using conventional and molecular methods. N Engl J Med. 1994;330(24):1703-9.
25. Bishai WR, Graham NM, Harrington S, Pope DS, Hooper N, Astemborski J, et al. Molecular and geographic patterns of tuberculosis transmission after 15 years of directly observed therapy. JAMA. 1998;280(19):1679-84.
26. Slama K, Chiang CY, Enarson DA, Hassmiller K, Fanning A, Gupta P, et al. Tobacco and tuberculosis: a qualitative systematic review and meta-analysis. Int J Tuberc Lung Dis. 2007;11(10):1049-61.
27. Godey P, Caylà JA, Casmona G, Camps N, Álvarez J, Alsedà M, et al. Smoking in tuberculosis patients increases the risk of infection in their contacts. Int J Tuberc Lung Dis. 2013;17(6):771-6.
28. Horsburgh CR Jr. Priorities for the treatment of latent tuberculosis infection in the United States. N Engl J Med. 2004;350(20):2060-7.
29. Ferebee SH. Controlled chemoprophylaxis trials in tuberculosis. A general review. Bibl Tuberc. 1970;26:28-106.
30. Hart PD, Sutherland I. BCG and vole bacillus vaccines in the prevention of tuberculosis in adolescence and early adult life. Br Med J. 1977;2(6082):293-5.
31. Alland D, Kalkut GE, Moss AR, McAdam RA, Hahn JA, Bosworth W, et al. Transmission of tuberculosis in New York City. An analysis by DNA fingerprinting and conventional epidemiologic methods. N Engl J Med. 1994;330(24):1710-6.
32. Vynnycky E, Fine PE. The natural history of tuberculosis: the implications of age-dependent risks of disease and the role of re-infection. Epidemiol Infect. 1997;119(2):183-201.
33. Lawn SD, Zumla AI. Tuberculosis. Lancet. 2011;378(9785):57-72.
34. Boehme CC, Nicol M, Nabeta P, Michael JS, Gotuzzo E, et al. Feasibility, diagnostic accuracy, and effectiveness of decentralised use of the Xpert MTB/RIF test for diagnosis of tuberculosis and multidrug resistance: a multicentre implementation study. Lancet. 2011;377(9776):1495-505.
35. Radhakrishna S, Frieden TR, Subramani R, Kumaran PP. Trends in the prevalence and incidence of tuberculosis in south India. Int J Tuberc Lung Dis. 2001;5(2):142-57.
36. Tuberculosis in a rural population of South India: a five-year epidemiological study. Bull World Health Organ. 1974;51(5):473-88.
37. Groth-Petersen E, Knudsen J, Wilbek E. Epidemiological basis of tuberculosis eradication in an advanced country. Bull World Health Organ. 1959;21:5-49.
38. World Health Organization. (2013). Global tuberculosis report 2013. WHO press Geneva. WHO/HTM/TB /2013.15. [online] Available from *http://apps.who.int/iris/handle/10665/91355* [Accessed March 2016].
39. Whalen C, Horsburgh CR, Hom D, Lahart C, Simberkoff M, Ellner J, et al. Accelerated course of human immunodeficiency virus infection after tuberculosis. Am J Respir Crit Care Med. 1995;151(1):129-35.
40. Gajalakshmi V, Peto R. Smoking, drinking and incident tuberculosis in rural India: population-based case-control study. Int J Epidemiol. 2009;38(4):1018-25.
41. Rao VG, Bhat J, Yadav R, Muniyandi M, Bhondeley MK, Sharada MA, et al. Tobacco smoking: a major risk factor for pulmonary tuberculosis—evidence from a cross-sectional study in central India. Trans R Soc Trop Med Hyg. 2014;108(8):474-81.
42. Lin HH, Ezzati M, Murray M. Tobacco smoke, indoor air pollution and tuberculosis: a systematic review and meta-analysis. PLoS Med. 2007;4(1):e20.

43. Jeon CY, Murray MB. Diabetes mellitus increases the risk of active tuberculosis: a systematic review of 13 observational studies. PLoS Med. 2008;5(7):e152.
44. Leung CC, Lam TH, Chan WM, Yew WW, Ho KS, Leung GM, et al. Diabetic control and risk of tuberculosis: a cohort study. Am J Epidemiol. 2008;167(12):1486-94.
45. Dooley KE, Chaisson RE. Tuberculosis and diabetes mellitus: convergence of two epidemics. Lancet Infect Dis. 2009;9(12):737-46.
46. Lönnroth K, Castro KG, Chakaya JM, Chauhan LS, Floyd K, Glaziou P, et al. Tuberculosis control and elimination 2010-50: cure, care and social development. Lancet. 2010;375(9728): 1814-29.
47. Harries AD, Lin Y, Satyanarayana S, Lönnroth K, Li L, Wilson N, et al. The looming epidemic of diabetes-associated tuberculosis: learning lessons from HIV-associated tuberculosis. Int J Tuberc Lung Dis. 2011;15(11):1436-44.
48. Corbett EL, Charalambons S, Moloi VM, Fielding K, Grant AD, Dye C, et al. Human immunodeficiency virus and prevalence of undiagnosed tuberculosis in African gold miners. Am J Respir Crit Care Med. 2004;170(6):673-9.
49. Cegielski JP, McMurray DN. The relationship between malnutrition and tuberculosis: evidence from studies in humans and experimental animals. Int J Tuberc Lung Dis. 2004;8(3):286-98.
50. Feld R, Bodey GP, Gröschel D. Mycobacteriosis in patients with malignant disease. Arch Intern Med. 1976;136(1):67-70.
51. Muniyandi M, Ramachandran R, Gopi PG, Chandrasekaran V, Subramani R, Sadacharam K, et al. The prevalence of tuberculosis in different economic strata: a community survey from South India. Int J Tuberc Lung Dis. 2007;11(9):1042-5.
52. Lopez De Fede A, Stewart JE, Harris MJ, Mayfield-Smith K. Tuberculosis in socio-economically deprived neighborhoods: missed opportunities for prevention. Int J Tuberc Lung Dis. 2008;12(12):1425-30.
53. Bamrah S, Yelk Woodruff RS, Powell K, Ghosh S, Kammerer JS, Haddad MB. Tuberculosis among the homeless, United States, 1994-2010. Int J Tuberc Lung Dis. 2013;17(11):1414-9.
54. Millet JP, Moreno A, Fina L, del Baño L, Orcau A, de Olalla PG, et al. Factors that influence current tuberculosis epidemiology. Eur Spine J. 2013;22(Suppl 4):539-48.
55. Narain R, Rao GR, Chandrasekhar P, Lal P. Fate of cases diagnosed in a survey. Proceedings of Tuberculosis and Chest Diseases Workers Conference, Calcutta 1966. Summaries of NTI Studies. 1997;7.
56. Tiemersma EW, van der Werf MJ, Borgdorff MW, Williams BG, Nagelkerke NJ. Natural history of tuberculosis: duration and fatality of untreated pulmonary tuberculosis in HIV negative patients: a systematic review. PLoS One. 2011;6(4):e17601.
57. Waitt CJ, Squire SB. A systematic review of risk factors for death in adults during and after tuberculosis treatment. Int J Tuberc Lung Dis. 2011;15(7):871-85.
58. Vijay S, Balasangameswara VH, Jagannatha PS, Saroja VN, Kumar P. Treatment outcome and two and half years follow-up status of new smear positive patients treated under RNTCP. Indian J Tuberc. 2004;51:199-208.
59. Kolappan C, Subramani R, Karunakaran K, Narayanan PR. Mortality of tuberculosis patients in Chennai, India. Bull World Health Organ. 2006;84(7):555-60.
60. Kolappan C, Subramani R, Kumaraswami V, Santha T, Narayanan PR. Excess mortality and risk factors for mortality among a cohort of TB patients from rural south India. Int J Tuberc Lung Dis. 2008;12(1):81-6.
61. Sadacharam K, Gopi PG, Chandrasekaran V, Eusuff SI, Subramani R, Santha J, et al. Status of smear-positive TB patients at 2-3 years after initiation of treatment under a DOTS programme. Indian J Tuberc. 2007;54(4):199-203.
62. Styblo K. The relationship between the risk of tuberculous infection and the risk of developing infectious tuberculosis. Bull Int Union Tuber Lung Dis. 1985;60:117-9.
63. Van Leth F, van der Werf MJ, Borgdorff MW. Prevalence of tuberculous infection and incidence of tuberculosis: a re-assessment of the Styblo rule. Bull World Health Organ. 2008;86(1):20-6.
64. Crampin AC, Floyd S, Glynn JR, Sibande F, Mulawa D, Nyondo A, et al. Long-term follow-up of HIV-positive and HIV-negative individuals in rural Malawi. AIDS. 2002;16(11):1545-50.
65. Lohse N, Hansen AB, Pedersen G, Kronborg G, Gerstoft J, Sørensen HT, et al. Survival of persons with and without HIV infection in Denmark, 1995-2005. Ann Intern Med. 2007; 146(2):87-95.
66. World Health Organization. International classification of diseases, 10th revision. Geneva, Switzerland: World Health Organization; 1990.
67. Mathers CD, Fat DM, Inoue M, Rao C, Lopez AD. Counting the dead and what they died from: an assessment of the global status of cause of death data. Bull World Health Organ. 2005;83(3):171-7.
68. Setel PW, Sankoh O, Rao C, Velkoff VA, Mathers C, Gonghuan Y, et al. Sample registration of vital events with verbal autopsy: a renewed commitment to measuring and monitoring vital statistics. Bull World Health Organ. 2005;83(8):611-7.
69. Gajalakshmi V, Peto R. Verbal autopsy of 80,000 adult deaths in Tamilnadu, South India. BMC Public Health. 2004;4:47.
70. Jha P, Gajalakshmi V, Gupta PC, Kumar R, Mony P, Dhingra N, et al. Prospective study of one million deaths in India: rationale, design, and validation results. PLoS Med. 2006;3(2):e18.
71. Rieder HL, Chadha VK, Nagelkerke NJ, van Leth F, van der Werf MJ, KNCV Tuberculosis Foundation. Guidelines for conducting tuberculin skin test surveys in high-prevalence countries. Int J Tuberc Lung Dis. 2011;15(Suppl 1):S1-256.
72. Menzies D. Interpretation of repeated tuberculin tests. Boosting, conversion, and reversion. Am J Respir Crit Care Med. 1999;159(1):15-21.
73. World Health Organization. (2005). Ait-Khaled N, Enarson DA. Tuberculosis: a manual for medical students. WHO/CDS/TB/99.272.
74. Gopi PG, Subramani R, Narayanan PR. Trend in the prevalence of TB infection and ARTI after implementation of a DOTS programme in south India. Int J Tuberc Lung Dis. 2006;10(3):346-8.
75. Tupasi TE, Radhakrishna S, Rivera AB, Pascual ML, Quelapio MI, Co VM, et al. The 1997 Nationwide Tuberculosis Prevalence Survey in the Philippines. Int J Tuberc Lung Dis. 1999;3(6):471-7.
76. Tupasi TE, Radhakrishna S, Pascual ML, Quelapio MI, Villa ML, Co VM, et. al. BCG coverage and the annual risk of tuberculosis infection over a 14-year period in the Philippines assessed from the Nationwide Prevalence Surveys. Int J Tuberc Lung Dis. 2000;4(3):216-22.
77. Lozano R, Naghavi M, Foreman K, Lim S, Shibuya K, Aboyans V, et al. Global and regional mortality from 235 causes of death for 20 age groups in 1990 and 2010: a systematic analysis for the Global Burden of Disease Study 2010. Lancet. 2012;380(9859):2095-128.
78. New Delhi TB Centre. Study of epidemiology of tuberculosis in an urban population of Delhi-report on 30 year follow up. Indian J Tuberc. 1999;46:133-4.

79. Balasubramanian R, Sadacharam K, Selvaraj R, Xavier T, Gopalan BN, Shanmugam M, et al. Feasibility of involving literate tribal youths in tuberculosis case-finding in a tribal area in Tamil Nadu. Tuber Lung Dis. 1995;76(4):355-9.
80. Murhekar MV, Kolappan C, Gopi PG, Chakraborty AK, Sehgal SC. Tuberculosis situation among tribal population of Car Nicobar, India, 15 years after intensive tuberculosis control project and implementation of a national tuberculosis programme. Bull World Health Organ. 2004;82(11):836-43.
81. Kolappan C, Subramani R, Radhakrishna S, Santha T, Wares F, Baskaran D, et al. Trends in the prevalence of pulmonary tuberculosis over a period of seven and half years in a rural community in south India with DOTS. Indian J Tuberc. 2013;60(3):168-76.
82. Chakma T, Vinay Rao P, Pall S, Kaushal LS, Datta M, Tiwary PS. Survey of pulmonary TB in a primitive tribe of Madhya Pradesh. Indian J Tuberc. 1996;43:85-9.
83. Rao VG, Gopi PG, Bhat J, Selvakumar N, Yadav R, Tiwari B, et al. Pulmonary tuberculosis: a public health problem amongst the Saharia, a primitive tribe of Madhya Pradesh, Central India. Int J Infect Dis. 2010;14(8):e713-6.
84. Bhat J, Rao VG, Gopi PG, Yadav R, Selvakumar N, Tiwari B, et al. Prevalence of pulmonary tuberculosis amongst the tribal population of Madhya Pradesh, central India. Int J Epidemiol. 2009;38(4):1026-32.
85. Chadha VK, Kumar P, Anjinappa SM, Singh S, Narasimhaiah S, Joshi MV, et al. Prevalence of pulmonary tuberculosis among adults in a rural sub-district of South India. PLoS One. 2012;7(8):e42625.
86. Rao VG, Bhat J, Yadav R, Gopi PG, Nagamiah S, Bhondeley MK, et al. Prevalence of pulmonary tuberculosis--a baseline survey in central India. PLoS One. 2012;7(8):e43225.
87. Aggarwal AN, Gupta D, Agarwal R, Sethi S, Thakur JS, Anjinappa SM, et al. Prevalence of pulmonary tuberculosis among adults in a north Indian district. PLoS One. 2015;10(2);e0117363.
88. World Health Organization. Regional Office for South-East Asia. (2012). Tuberculosis Control in the South-East Asia Region: The Regional Report 2012, New Delhi; SEA/TB/338. [online] Available from *http://www.searo.who.int/tb/documents/sea_tb_338/en/*[Accessed March 2016].
89. Government of India, Central Tuberculosis Division, Directorate General of Health Services, Ministry of Health and Family Welfare. TB India 2013. Revised National TB Control Programme Annual Status Report 2013. pp. 83-5. [online] Available from *http://www.tbcindia.nic.in/index1.php?page=1&ipp=10&lang=1&level=1&sublinkid=4160&lid=2807* [Accessed March 2016].
90. Indian Council of Medical Research. Tuberculosis in India: a National Sample Survey. ICMR special report series No.34, 1955-1958.
91. Chadha VK, Sarin R, Narang P, John KR, Chopra KK, Jitendra R, et al. Trends in the annual risk of tuberculous infection in India. Int J Tuberc Lung Dis. 2013;17(3):312-9.
92. Chadha VK, Jithendra R, Kumar P, Kirankumar R, Shashidharan AN, Suganthi P, et al. Change in the risk of tuberculous infection over an 8-year period among schoolchildren in Bangalore City. Int J Tuberc Lung Dis. 2008;12(10):1116-21.
93. Shashidhara AN, Chadha VK, Jagannatha PS, Ray TK, Mania RN. The annual risk of tuberculous infection in Orissa State, India. Int J Tuberc Lung Dis. 2004;8(5):545-51.
94. Chadha VK, Kumar P, Satyanarayana AV, Chauhan LS, Gupta J, Singh S, et al. Annual risk of tuberculous infection in the Andhra Pradesh, India. Indian J Tuberc. 2007;54(4):177-83.
95. Chadha VK, Banerjee A, Ibrahim M, Jaganatha PS, Kumar P. Annual risk of tuberculous infection in Khammam a tribal district of Andhra Pradesh. J Commun Dis. 2003;35(3):198-205.
96. Kumar S, Chadha VK, Radhakrishnanan, Jitendra R, Kumar P, Chauhan LS, et al. Annual risk of tuberculosis infection in Kerala. Indian J Tuberc. 2009;56:10-6.
97. Gopi PG, Prasad VV, Vasantha M, Subramani R, Tholkappian AS, Sargunan D, et al. Annual risk of tuberculosis infection in Chennai city. Indian J Tuberc. 2008;55(3):157-61.
98. Rao VG, Gopi PG, Yadav R, Subramani R, Bhat J, Anvikar AR, et al. Annual risk of tuberculosis infection among tribal population of central India. Trop Med Int Health. 2008;13(11):1372-7.
99. Joshi R, Cardona M, Iyengar S, Sukumar A, Raju CR, Raju KR, et al. Chronic diseases now a leading cause of death in rural India—mortality data from the Andhra Pradesh Rural Health Initiative. Int J Epidemiol. 2006;35(6):1522-9.
100. Kanungo S, Tsuzuki A, Deen JL, Lopez AL, Rajendran K, Manna B, et al. Use of verbal autopsy to determine mortality patterns in an urban slum in Kolkata, India. Bull World Health Organ. 2010;88(9):667-74.
101. Personal communication. Soumya Swaminathan, Director, National Institute of Research in tuberculosis. General and Tuberculosis Mortality in two states of India: a population based survey.
102. Registrar General, India. (2006). SRS Bulletin, Sample Registration System. [online] Available from *http://censusindia.gov.in/vital_statistics/SRS_Bulletins/SRS_Bulletins_links/SRS_Bulletin-October-2006.pdf* [Accesses March 2016].
103. Dewan PK, Gupta D, Williams BG, Thakur R, Bachani D, Khera A, et al. National estimate of HIV seroprevalence among tuberculosis patients in India. Int J Tuberc Lung Dis. 2010;14(2):247-9.
104. World Health Organization. (2012). Global tuberculosis report 2012. WHO/HTM/TB/2012;6:1-272.
105. Tupasi TE, Radhakrishna S, Chua JA, Mangubat NV, Guilatco R, Galipot M, et al. Significant decline in the tuberculosis burden in the Philippines ten years after initiating DOTS. Int J Tuberc Lung Dis. 2009;13(10):1224-30.
106. Soemantri S, Senewe FP, Tjandrarini DH, Day R, Basri C, Manissero D, et al. Three-fold reduction in the prevalence of tuberculosis over 25 years in Indonesia. Int J Tuberc Lung Dis. 2007;11(4):398-404.
107. Ministry of Health, Department of Health, Government of Myanmar. Report on national TB prevalence survey 2009-10, Myanmar. [online] Available from *http://www.searo.who.int/myanmar/documents/TB_Prevelence_Survey_report.pdf* [Accessed March 2016].
108. Wang L, Zhang H, Ruan Y, Chin DP, Xia Y, Cheng S, et al. Tuberculosis prevalence in China, 1990-2010; a longitudinal analysis of national survey data. Lancet. 2014;383(9934):2057-64.
109. Zaman K, Hossain S, Banu S, Quaiyum MA, Barua PC, Salim MA, et al. Prevalence of smear-positive tuberculosis in persons aged ≥ 15 years in Bangladesh: results from a national survey, 2007-2009. Epidemiol Infect. 2012;140(6):1018-27.
110. Narang P, Nayar S, Mendiratta DK, Tyagi NK, Jajoo U. Smear and culture positive cases of pulmonary tuberculosis found among symptomatics surveyed in Wardha District. Indian J Tuberc. 1992;39:159-64.
111. Chadha VK, Praseeja P, Hemanthkumar NK, Shivshankara BA, Sharada MA, Nagendra N, et al. Implementation efficiency of a diagnostic algorithm in sputum smear-negative presumptive tuberculosis patients. Int J Tuberc Lung Dis. 2014;18(10): 1237-42.

Risk Factors for Tuberculosis

Parvaiz A Koul, Nargis K Bali

INTRODUCTION

Tuberculosis (TB) develops as a result of the progression of primary infection, exogenous reinfection or endogenous reactivation. Risk of active disease is highest immediately (within 24 hours) after infection is acquired, the accepted principle being that the risk of disease is greatest within first 2 years following infection, which starts to level off after about 7 years, remaining low and unchanged over the following decade and usually during lifetime. Also, if the infection is acquired during childhood, the lifetime risk of progression from infection to disease is around 10%.[1] The development of tuberculosis in man is essentially a two-stage process in which a susceptible person exposed to an infectious *tuberculosis* case becomes infected and may later develop the disease. In individuals infected with *Mycobacterium tuberculosis,* any condition modifying the balance established in the body between the host's immune defenses and the tubercle bacilli can have an impact on the risk of developing the disease. Different factors both "intrinsic" and "extrinsic" to the host can variously affect an individual's susceptibility to develop tuberculosis **(Box 1)**.[2,3]

RISK FACTORS OF DEVELOPING TUBERCULOSIS

Some of the known important risk factors are discussed below:

Underlying Medical Illnesses

Human Immunodeficiency Virus Infection

Worldwide, tuberculosis is the most common human immunodeficiency virus (HIV)-associated disease of public health importance and HIV infection is the strongest risk factor for the reactivation of tuberculosis infection and progression to active disease. The effect of the HIV epidemic on tuberculosis has been well-documented, with incident rates of tuberculosis, particularly in Africa, rising rapidly as a result of HIV.[4,5] Of the 8.6 million people who fell ill with tuberculosis in 2012, an estimated 1.1 million cases (12.7%) occurred among people living with HIV; of the 1.3 million deaths from tuberculosis, 3,20,000 deaths were seen in HIV-positive cases; of the overall tuberculosis deaths among HIV-positive people, 50% were among women. Of the 4,10,000 women who died from tuberculosis in 2012, 1,60,000 women were HIV-positive. Tuberculosis, thus, is one of the top killers of women of reproductive age. Among the children, an estimated 5,30,000 children became ill with tuberculosis

BOX 1 Risk factors for tuberculosis

Underlying medical illness:
- HIV infection
- Diabetes
- Transplantation
- Silicosis
- Malignancy
- Gastrectomy
- Jejunoileal bypass surgery
- Chronic renal failure
- Malnutrition
- Immunosuppressant/corticosteroid treatment.

Sociodemographic factors:
- Age
- Overcrowding
- Homelessness
- Correctional facilities and prisons
- Intravenous drug abuse
- Alcohol abuse
- Immigration from endemic areas
- Smoking
- Poverty
- Malnutrition.

Host-genetic factors:
- Polymorphism in *NRAMP1* gene
- Vitamin D receptor gene
- Gamma interferon signaling
- TNF receptor gene.

Abbreviations: NRAMP, natural-resistance-associated macrophage protein 1; TNF, tumor necrosis factor

of whom 74,000 children HIV-negative died of tuberculosis in 2012. The tuberculosis mortality rate has decreased 45% since 1990, and the 2015 global target of a 50% reduction in mortality is now within reach.

In 2007, as in previous years, the African region accounted for most (79%) HIV-positive tuberculosis cases, followed by the South-East Asian Region (mainly India) with 11% of total cases. South Africa accounted for 31% of cases in the African Region.[4] Around 0.45 million patients coinfected with HIV died of tuberculosis in 2007; tuberculosis is also the leading cause of death in patients living with HIV, even in those receiving antiretroviral therapy.[4,6]

Direct estimates of the prevalence of HIV in tuberculosis provide strong evidence that the risk of developing tuberculosis in HIV-positive compared with HIV-negative (the incidence rate ratio or IRR) is higher than previously estimated. The IRR was estimated as 20.6 in 2007 in countries with a generalized HIV epidemic (i.e. countries where the prevalence of HIV was above 1% in the general population), and 26.7 in countries where the prevalence of HIV in the general population was between 0.1% and 1%; and 36.7 in countries where the prevalence of HIV in the general population was less than 0.1%. These IRR estimates compare with previous estimates of 6, 6 and 30, respectively.[4]

The impact of HIV infection on tuberculosis pandemic is multifold. The risk of active tuberculosis doubles in the first year of HIV coinfection while the risk of developing active disease in those who have latent tuberculosis infection (LTBI) is 10% per year.[7,8] However, the impact of HIV infection on tuberculosis is not limited to the reactivation of LTBI. It has been shown in several studies that HIV-infected patients, who at any point of time, become infected or reinfected with *M. tuberculosis,* progress faster to full-blown disease than HIV-negative individuals who develop tuberculosis.[9-12] Thankfully, however, HIV-infected tuberculosis patients do not appear to be potent transmitters of *M. tuberculosis*, the fact being substantiated by numerous household contact studies which have consistently shown that HIV-infected patients with tuberculosis are less likely to transmit tubercle bacilli to their close contacts than HIV uninfected individuals with tuberculosis.[13-16] HIV-TB coinfected individuals have reduced survival[17] and are at higher risk for subsequent opportunistic infections.[18] In overcrowded and poor living conditions, the combined effect of the two epidemics is magnified as evidenced by more than 2,000 per 1,00,000 population prevalence rates in certain South African communities.[19,20]

In 2012, 46% of notified tuberculosis patients had a documented HIV test result with the African region having the highest tuberculosis or HIV burden. Added complications in coinfected individuals include drug-resistant tuberculosis and immune reconstitution inflammatory syndrome.[21] The emergence of drug-resistant tuberculosis in countries with a high HIV prevalence poses an additional public health threat, not only to people with HIV, but also to the broader community.[8]

Tuberculosis is the prototype of infections that require a cellular immune response for their control.[22] All persons have a native population of lymphocytes, mostly $CD4^+$ cells bearing $\alpha\beta$ T-cell receptors, capable of recognizing mycobacterial antigens, processed and presented by macrophages. In tuberculin-positive patients (those who have been infected with *M. tuberculosis*), endogenous foci may reactivate repeatedly and active CD4 surveillance is mandatory to maintain quiescence. As the CD4 levels fall in HIV-infected patients, both in early (CD4 > 300 cells/mm^3) and late (<200 cells/mm^3) stage of the disease, the chances of both endogenous reactivation and exogenous reinfection increase substantially. The earliest description of tuberculosis in acquired immunodeficiency syndrome (AIDS) patients emphasized the increased risk of reactivation of remote infection due to progressively compromised immunity. Studies carried out in Haitians, all of whom were likely to be infected with *M. tuberculosis* in childhood, showed that AIDS was associated with development of active tuberculosis in 60%.[23] Subsequent studies in methadone clinic patients in the New York city who were HIV-positive and tuberculin-positive revealed, that tuberculosis developed in 8% of the clinic patients per year.[8] These studies thus suggest that nearly all tuberculin-positive patients with HIV infection eventually develop active tuberculosis unless either HIV or tuberculous infection or both are effectively treated or some other fatal complication of AIDS occur.

The clinical picture of tuberculosis in HIV infection is defined by the degree of immunocompromise.[24] The clinical spectrum ranges from a negative-tuberculin sensitivity test result, greater incidence of extrapulmonary disease (>50%), middle and lower lung zone involvement and absence of cavitation to positive-tuberculin test result, cavitatory disease (< 10–15%), predominant extrapulmonary involvement and a diffuse rapidly progressive disease, which is often fatal. Management of these patients may be further complicated by concomitant intravenous drug use and homelessness. Failure to isolate and treat these patients under supervision is a major contributor to the outbreak of multidrug-resistant tuberculosis (MDR-TB) in this population. Directly observed treatment short-course (DOTS) is especially important in coinfected individuals to ensure drug compliance, which is otherwise poor.

Diabetes

Physicians have noted the relationship between diabetes and tuberculosis since ancient times; perhaps the earliest was by Susruta, the Indian physician in 600 AD. Avicenna too had noticed phthisis complicated diabetes and that the presence of diabetes resulted in an increased risk of developing tuberculosis.[25] However, it has gone unnoticed and in the most recent national guidelines, has only been mentioned as something needing more research.[26] If not acknowledged appropriately, the association is believed to pose a threat, both to the successful tuberculosis control and to the treatment of diabetes.[27] Several large studies have demonstrated the increased risk of tuberculosis in patients with diabetes. In Korea, a 3-year longitudinal study involving 8,00,000 civil servants showed that the risk-ratio of tuberculosis in diabetic patients versus nondiabetic controls was 3.47 (95% CI 2.98–4.03).[28] From the UK General Practice Research Database, which included records from over 2 million patients, Jick and colleagues[29] identified all cases of tuberculosis reported between 1990 and 2001 and found that the adjusted odds ratio (adjusted for age, sex and practice) for tuberculosis was 3.8 (95% CI 2.3–6.1) for diabetic patients compared with those without diabetes. In Hong Kong,[30] in a 5-year study of 42,000 elderly individuals, the adjusted hazard of active tuberculosis was higher in diabetic patients than in individuals without diabetes (1.77; 95% CI 1.41–2.24), but this increased risk was only present in those with hemoglobin A1c (HbA1c) concentrations greater than 7%. Indeed, a recent large meta-analysis[31] showed that diabetic patients were 3.1 times (95% CI 2.27–4.26) more likely to have tuberculosis than controls with higher effect sizes in non-North American population. The presence of diabetes was found to increase the risk of contracting tuberculosis by 1.5-fold to 7.8-fold in various studies, being highest in the younger age group without any influence of gender.[32,33] Stevenson et al.[34] estimated that the population attributable risk for tuberculosis from diabetes was 14.8% of incident tuberculosis cases and about 20% of sputum-positive cases in India. Insulin dependence suggestive of a severe diabetes and a higher HbA1c as a marker of poor glycemic control have been found to be associated with a higher risk of tuberculosis.[32,35] In the setting of the increasing overlap of population at risk for both diseases, the combination of tuberculosis and diabetes mellitus represents a worldwide health threat.[36]

Several mechanisms have been put forward to explain the phenomenon of increased risk of tuberculosis in diabetes **(Box 2)**. Alterations in pulmonary immune cell function reduced activity of monocytes or macrophages; impaired activation, chemotaxis and antigen presentation leading to ineffective phagocytosis of intracellular organisms, reduced lymphocyte function and impaired T-cell growth, proliferation and function may all be responsible. The varied effects of diabetic microangiopathy on the capillaries of alveolar septa and arterioles may also affect the local response to infection.[37-39]

Evolution of the symptoms and signs of tuberculosis in diabetic patients are same as that in nondiabetic patients. The coexistence is expectedly known to result in greater complications. The mortality of tuberculosis has been reported to be higher when complicated by diabetes and the disease tends to have increased severity characterized by cavitations, lower lobe involvement and smear positivity.[40,41] A higher risk of MDR-tuberculosis has also been reported in diabetics even as some other studies have shown no significant risk of drug resistance.[42-48]

BOX 2 Possible mechanisms underlying increased risk to tuberculosis in diabetics

- Impaired phagocytic activity of monocytes/macrophages
  - Impaired chemotaxis
  - Impaired phagocytosis
  - Impaired activation
  - Impaired antigen presentation by phagocytes in response to *M. tuberculosis*
- Altered polymorphonuclear cell function
- Impairment in T-cell production of gamma interferon
- Impaired T-cell growth, proliferation and function
- Diabetic microangiopathy induced alteration of local response.

It is unclear, whether the aggressive management of diabetes mellitus (DM) would improve treatment response. Since the causes of death are not reported in most studies, we do not know whether excess mortality is explained by increased severity of tuberculosis in diabetic or by the existence of comorbidities attributable to diabetes mellitus compounded by more advanced age.[36] People with diabetes mellitus may also be important targets for interventions such as active case finding and the treatment of latent tuberculosis.[27]

Organ Transplantation

Procedures employed to minimize the risk of rejection in transplant recipients produce an alteration of immune status in them, predisposing such patients to infections caused by both common and rare organisms. Tuberculosis associated with organ transplantation, occurs in an estimated 0.35–6.5% of organ recipients post-transplantation in the United States and Europe, the risk of tuberculosis in transplant recipients is estimated to be 20–50 times higher than in general population and mortality rates vary from 20–40%.[49] Nearly, 49% of the US transplant recipients with tuberculosis have disseminated disease and 38% of them die.[49]

Risk factors for the development of tuberculosis in transplant recipients include previous tuberculosis infection, immunosuppressive treatment with OKT3 or anti-T-cell antibodies, diabetes mellitus, chronic liver disease and coexisting infections.[49-52] Tuberculosis is rare after hematopoietic stem cell transplantation (HSCT) and ten times less frequent than in solid organ transplantation (SOT), as HSCT recipients do not receive lifelong immunosuppression. Undergoing transplant in a country with a high endemic rate of tuberculosis is also an important risk factor.[53] Unrelated or mismatched related transplants, graft-versus-host disease (GVHD) and total body irradiation increase the risk of tuberculosis reactivation after HSCT.[54] The majority of tuberculosis cases among organ transplant recipients are caused by the activation of LTBI in the recipient. Once immunosuppressive medications are started to prevent organ rejection; a minority are attributed to donor transmission. In one international study, 4% of tuberculosis infections in recipients were considered donor derived.[49]

Clinical aspects of the disease includes a high incidence of extrapulmonary or disseminated tuberculosis (49%).[49] Among extrapulmonary cases presentations include gastrointestinal, hepatic, skin, muscle, osteoarticular, genitourinary, ganglia, central nervous system and other more uncommon sites of disease such as the larynx, tonsils or eyes.[49,55] In transplant patients, tuberculosis should be considered in the differential diagnosis of persistent fever, pneumonia, meningitis, septic arthritis, pyelonephritis, septicemia, graft rejection or bone marrow suppression. Clinicians should recognize that the presence of an unusual constellation of symptoms, particularly during the first few weeks after transplantation, raises the possibility of donor-transmitted infection or activation of LTBI. Even with a high index of suspicion, tuberculosis in an organ recipient can be challenging to diagnose 75–80% of organ recipients who developed tuberculosis, had a false-negative pretransplantation tuberculin skin test (TST).[56] It is important to recognize that in this immunosuppressed population, symptoms of tuberculosis might be attributed to other potential complications, including organ rejection or other infectious diseases. Diagnosis of tuberculosis in an organ recipient, in the absence of clear risk factors or other evidence from pretransplantation screening, should prompt the investigation of possible transmission from the donor. Other recipients from a common donor might be at risk and should be evaluated for tuberculosis.

Investigation of epidemiological risk for LTBI is mandatory in transplant recipients. LTBI can be evaluated through TST. The sensitivity of TST is lower in immunocompromised hosts, induration of ≥ 5 mm, is considered positive.[57] In SOT, around 20% of the recipients test positive, the positivity being greater in liver transplant recipients (around 70%).[49] Positivity of 23% was observed among HSCT recipients.[58] It is important to highlight that the specificity of TST may be impaired in transplant patients from developing countries since a positive test may indicate infection with nontuberculous mycobacteria or previous vaccination with the Bacille Calmette-Guérin (BCG).[59] The role of TST, as well as of the new interferon-gamma release assays (IGRAs), such as the QuantiFERON test, in the evaluation of LTBI in transplant recipients has not been fully investigated. A recent meta-analysis suggests that IGRAs may be more sensitive than TST in immunocompromised patients suspected of having tuberculosis.[60]

Pretransplant evaluation of epidemiological risk of tuberculosis should be made for donors and recipients. Previous tuberculosis infection or contact with infected persons should be particularly investigated, as well as careful radiological evaluation should be done to check for images suggestive of previous healed tuberculosis.[61] TST with 5 tuberculin units of purified protein derivative is recommended for transplant candidates, a negative test should not exclude the possibility of LTBI. If LTBI is suspected, treatment with isoniazid (INH) should be started. A full 9-month course is recommended. Alternative schedules may be considered on individual basis. In HSCT recipients, the combination of pyrazinamide and rifampicin has shown significant liver toxicity and its use is not recommended.[62]

Silicosis

Silicosis, a fibrosing lung disease caused by the inhalation and deposition of crystalline silica particles, is the most prevalent pneumoconiosis.[63] The risk of developing pulmonary tuberculosis is reported to be 2.8–3.9 times higher for patients with silicosis than for healthy controls.[64-66] Patients with silicosis are also at a higher risk for extrapulmonary tuberculosis, the estimated risk being about 3.7 times higher.[65,67]

Local alterations in the lungs together with unfavorable conditions in the mines, inability to diagnose the disease rapidly and the high prevalence of tuberculosis in the population, are some of the factors responsible for the high incidence of this disease in this group of people. Important local alterations include the impairment of macrophage function (which plays a major role in the pathogenesis of the disease). Sublethal doses of silica dust also affect the ability of macrophages to inhibit the growth of *M. tuberculosis.*[68] Silica is reported to modify the immune response of the lungs, impair the metabolism or function of pulmonary macrophages and with frequent exposure, cause macrophage apoptosis.[67,68] These findings are consistent with observations that the incidence of tuberculosis is higher in dust-exposed workers, even in those without established silicosis, than in workers not so exposed. Surfactant protein A is also found to be high in bronchoalveolar lavage (BAL) fluid of patients with silicosis. An excess of this protein seems to be associated with higher susceptibility to tuberculosis, possibly because it allows mycobacteria to enter the alveolar macrophages without triggering cytotoxicity and inhibits the formation of reactive nitrogen species by the activated macrophages.[69,70] The tubercle bacilli are also believed to remain encapsulated within the silicotic nodules, which would be responsible for the reactivation of tuberculosis in such patients.

Diagnosis of tuberculosis in silicotic patients is difficult since the symptoms are nonspecific. Moreover acid-fast stains of sputa of these patients are usually negative, probably because the tubercle bacilli do not reach the bronchial tree due to fibrotic changes. Chest roentgenogram can be of great value in the diagnosis. Radiographic criteria strongly suggestive of tuberculosis include the appearance of new infiltrates, cavities, pleural effusion, coalescence of nodules and development of bronchial stenosis.[68] Patterns suggestive of silicotuberculosis have also been recognized on chest computed tomography (CT) scans. The principal findings consistent with active tuberculosis superimposed on silicosis are thick-walled cavities, consolidations, images presenting a tree-in-bud pattern, nodular image asymmetry and rapid disease progression.[71-73]

Longer therapeutic regimens with conventional antitubercular drugs are employed for the treatment of tuberculosis in these patients; the longer duration is necessitated because of the low penetration of the drugs into silicotic nodules. A study conducted in Hong Kong showed that 22% of the patients in the 6-month therapy group had bacteriological relapse in comparison to 7% relapses seen in patients in the 8-month therapy group, thus suggesting that the standard 6-month short-course therapy is inadequate for these patients.[74] As a general recommendation, the sterilizing phase in these patients should be prolonged and they should be treated for at least 9 months. Moreover, therapy with rifampicin and INH must be given for a minimum of 12 months, if pyrazinamide is not incorporated in the regimen.[68] Preventive chemoprophylaxis with INH has also been considered of great value in reducing the rates of active disease. One such study compared the treatment of 825 silicotic patients with 2,408 untreated silicotic patients. It was shown that preventive therapy with INH decreased the risk of developing active tuberculosis from 2.66–0.32%.[68]

The American Thoracic Society (ATS) recommends that TSTs should be performed in patients with silicosis. In cases of positive results (induration ≥ 10 mm) and after excluding active tuberculosis, the society recommends that chemoprophylaxis should be instituted, using one of the four possible regimens: INH for 9 months; INH for 6 months; rifampicin and pyrazinamide for 2–3 months; or rifampicin for 4 months. The determination of bilirubin and hepatic enzyme levels in the initial evaluation is indicated only for individuals considered to be at high-risk for liver disease such as alcoholics, pregnant women and HIV-infected individuals.[57]

Malignant Disease

The synchronous occurrence of tuberculosis and carcinoma is unusual and the association of the two has baffled surgeons and physicians for over two centuries. Bayle first described the association of tuberculosis and carcinoma in 1810. He described "cavitation cancer use" as one of the six types of tuberculosis, which appears to be the first published description of coexistence of the two.[75] The association of tuberculosis and cancer has been recorded in most of the organs. Kaplan et al. (1974)[76] reviewed 58,245 patients with cancer and identified 201 cases of coexisting tuberculosis. The highest prevalence was seen in patients with Hodgkin's disease (96/10,000 cases) followed by lung cancer (92/10,000), lymphosarcoma (88/10,000) and reticulum cell sarcoma (78/10,000). Hematological malignancies have a higher incidence of tuberculosis than solid organ cancers.[77,78] Patients with hematological malignancies have impaired immunity, partly due to the disease process itself and partly due to cancer treatment, including chemotherapy, radiotherapy, long-term corticosteroid regimes, etc. Patients with leukemia are more prone to develop disseminated or extrapulmonary disease as compared to those with other hematological tumors.[77,79] Patients suffering from hairy cell leukemia have increased chances of developing tuberculosis, with incidences as high as 50%.[80] Lymphomas, notably Hodgkin lymphoma also placed an individual at greater risk of having these manifestations, although extrapulmonary tuberculosis in these patients is usually a focal disease.[81]

Tuberculosis in solid organ malignancies is mainly pulmonary, extrapulmonary or disseminated disease being less common.[77] Highest incidence has been seen in head and neck cancers, lung cancers and gastrointestinal malignancies.[77,81] In a recent case control study from Korea, the incidence of active tuberculosis was 3.07 per 1,000 persons per year against 0.7 amongst controls, showing an increased risk of developing tuberculosis (incidence ratio of 4.46).[82] The authors concluded that immune suppression by cancer or by anticancer chemotherapy increased vulnerability to reactivation of tuberculosis, especially in cancer patients with old healed tuberculosis. Lung cancer and pulmonary tuberculosis have been known to coexist. In some series, the relationship between these two entities was found to be more frequent than other associations.[77] The location of tuberculosis and lung cancer can either be same or different. Interestingly, if HIV infection is associated with lung cancer and tuberculosis, a normal radiographic pattern can be seen. Except for the increased incidence of the disease, tuberculosis in cancer patients does not seem to have different characteristics as compared to the general population.[77] A more severe pattern of disease is noted, if cancer and tuberculosis appear in a sequential pattern, the reason being a greater debilitation of the patient during cancer.[77]

Gastrectomy and Jejunoileal Bypass Surgery

Subtotal gastrectomy and other gastric surgical procedures have been reported to be associated with an increased risk for tuberculosis since 1920s. The association was initially recognized at a time when gastric resection was widely performed for the treatment of refractory peptic ulcer disease. In recent decades, following the introduction of histamine type 2 blockers and proton pump inhibitors, gastric surgery has come to play a minor role in treating peptic ulcer disease. However, evidence that gastrectomy predisposes to the increased incidence of tuberculosis is highly suggestive, but not conclusive. Recent data suggest that gastrectomy patients are more predisposed to develop tuberculosis with an estimated two-fold to five-fold relative risk.[83-86]

Jejunoileal bypass surgery has been used increasingly in the recent decades to cause weight loss in patients of morbid obesity who do not respond to less drastic weight reduction measures. The average annual incidence of tuberculosis among bypass patients has been reported to be 27-fold and 63-fold higher than the incidence in comparison population.[87,88] Presumably, patients who are at greatest risk of developing tuberculosis are those who are already infected with tuberculosis at the time of the operation. However, none of the published reports provides data on the incidence or prevalence of disease among those infected or those uninfected, preoperatively. Nonpulmonary tuberculosis accounts for only 15% of the total cases in the general population, but 82% of cases in bypass patients have involved nonpulmonary sites. The reason for the increased risk of tuberculosis after bypass operation is unknown. Many patients become protein and zinc deficient postoperatively; both conditions are reported to adversely affect the cell-mediated immune responses.[89] The pathogenesis of the increased risk for tuberculosis after gastrectomy and bariatric surgery remains speculative. Confounding, attributed to factors, such as age, poverty, crowded living conditions, heavy ethanol consumption, nosocomial infection after surgery, severe weight loss caused by malabsorption and alkaline reflux gastritis, has been proposed.[83,84] The most widely cited hypothesis is that the increased risk of tuberculosis is attributed to rapid weight loss, malnutrition, and in some individuals, malabsorption. Tuberculosis occurs frequently in persons with protein-calorie malnutrition and resultant impaired cell-mediated immunity.[90]

As per the ATS or Centers for Disease Control and Prevention (CDC) guidelines,[57] individuals with weight loss of more than 10% of ideal body weight and those with gastrectomy or jejunoileal bypass surgery are considered at increased risk and should be offered treatment for LTBI, if they have a purified protein derivative (PPD) skin test reaction of 10 mm or more induration. Nine months of INH is now the preferred regimen for treatment of LTBI for most persons. Clinicians caring for patients, who have had gastric bypass surgery, need to be aware of the increased risk of tuberculosis in this patient population. Prompt diagnostic evaluation with chest roentgenogram, sputum examination, tissue biopsy and other appropriate studies should be initiated in patients with unexplained malaise, fever, cough and lymphadenopathy. In particular, a high level of clinical suspicion is needed for the diagnosis of extrapulmonary tuberculosis. Finally, because of potential problems with the malabsorption of oral drugs in patients after weight-reduction surgery, treatment should be coordinated with experienced tuberculosis control staff and monitoring of serum drug concentrations should be considered.

Sociodemographic Factors

Overcrowding

The most important determinant of infection is the closeness and the infectiousness of the source. *M. tuberculosis* infection is usually airborne; almost all infections are due to the inhalation of droplet nuclei that are infectious particles aerosolized by coughing, sneezing or talking. These particles are dry while airborne, remain suspended for long periods, get inhaled and reach terminal air passages. A sneeze can generate up to 40,000 droplets, which can evaporate to produce droplets of 0.5–12 mm in diameter. A cough can generate about 3,000 droplet nuclei, the same number as talking for 5 minutes (from Elsevier journal). A single cough, talking for 5 minutes and sneezing can generate equal number of droplet nuclei, which may be equal to 3,000 infectious droplet nuclei, or more.[91] The air in a room, occupied by a person with pulmonary tuberculosis, may remain infectious even after his or her absence.

Pulmonary tuberculosis fortunately is a disease with low infectiousness. Generally, prolonged contact and multiple aerosol inocula are required to establish infection. However, *M. tuberculosis* strains may vary widely in their transmissibility. In an outbreak in Kentucky, it was seen that people were infected in spite of the brief casual contact with the index case.[92] Closed spaces with little or no air circulation at all, favors the spread of tuberculosis. In USA, around 27% of household contacts of smear positive cases became infected, whereas rates as high as 80% were seen to occur in closed environments.[93]

Homelessness

With estimated prevalence of 1.6–6.8%, homelessness is regarded as one of the important risk factors for the development of tuberculosis.[94] The factors that contribute to an increased risk for tuberculosis among homeless persons include insufficient access to preventive services and health care as a result of financial, geographical and cultural barriers. Point prevalence of active tuberculosis as high as 968/1,00,000 homeless adults has been reported, nearly 100–300 times the nation wide prevalence.[95] Among homeless persons, the increased prevalence of conditions, which can suppress the immune system (like HIV infection, poor nutrition, untreated diabetes, chronic obstructive pulmonary disease (COPD), alcoholism, illicit drug use and psychological stress) may increase the risk for active tuberculosis if infected.[96-99] Homeless persons also lack access to good health care and are highly mobile, they do not complete tuberculosis therapy and the likelihood of relapse, drug resistance and further transmission of tuberculosis among shelter residents thus increased. [97,99-101]

Clinical characteristics of tuberculosis in this group are similar to those in the general population and variations, if any, are due to the presence of concomitant factors such as HIV infection. Treatment of tuberculosis in this group of people should be using common therapeutic regimes.[94] Measures to curtail the spread of infection in these settings should be directed at rapid diagnosis and treatment of infectious cases, since establishing an effective prevention program is difficult in shelters.[102,103] Structural measures in shelters have also been considered as useful to prevent transmission of the disease; use of ultraviolet lamps to disinfect air and enhanced ventilation systems to reduce airborne transmission of the disease in some of them.[94] As seen with drug abusers, outcome of these homeless is dependent on compliance of therapy, which as expected is very low. Directly observed treatment, short course (DOTS) is indicated for these difficult cases. Several incentives have been recommended, aimed at increasing the adherence to therapy, such as travel tickets, food, clothes or even money and have proven to be effective in increasing the compliance to drug therapy amongst these patients.[94]

Correctional Facilities and Prisons

Tuberculosis is a problem in correctional facilities and prisons; 3.7% of all the cases of tuberculosis in the United States in 1996 occurred amongst the residents of correctional facilities, with incidence rates of new cases in prison systems as high as 200 per 1,00,000 against the general population incidence of 8.0 per 1,00,000.[104-109]

Transmission of tuberculosis from prisons into surrounding communities has also been documented and therefore, correctional facilities may be important reservoirs of infection.[106] A prison was potentially linked to 9% of a state's tuberculosis cases during a 5-year period.[106] Incarcerated inmates have high rates of substance abuse, HIV infection, latent tuberculous infection, low socioeconomic status and other risk factors associated with active tuberculosis and hence have multiple factors operating for a higher risk of developing tuberculosis.

Drug Abuse

In recent years, drug abuse has emerged as a significant risk factor for the development of tuberculosis Close association between HIV infection and intravenous drug abuse makes it difficult to differentiate between the independent roles of the two risk factors in the progression of tuberculosis. Apart from HIV infection, other factors that put drug abusers at increased risk include malnutrition, bad hygienic practices, antisocial behavior (e.g. criminality, auto-medication, and trading of pills to obtain money or drugs). Relation between tuberculosis and intravenous drug abuse has been well-known for many years.[104-113] A positive TST has been reported in up to 44% of HIV negative IV drug users and tuberculous disease has been reported in 6.8%.[104,105] On the other hand, several studies have shown drug abuse to be a statistically significant risk factor for tuberculosis in the general population.[106,107]

In HIV-infected drug abusers, the effects of HIV infection on the immune system often over-shadow other possible defects, which are contributory to increased risk of tuberculous disease. Nonetheless, immune defects can be found in HIV noninfected patients too. Due to the presence of concomitant HIV infection and several other infections, a high index of suspicion is required to diagnose tuberculosis in intravenous drug abusers. It should be a dictum to rule out tuberculosis in any such patient who presents with fever.[114] Screening of these patients for tuberculosis is also difficult owing to their energy status because of HIV infection. A single skin test has previously been reported to be an unreliable predictor of development of tuberculosis and as such is not advocated in this patient population.[115] Instituting chemoprophylaxis in infected patients has been proved to prevent the development of active disease.[116-118] However, the same does not hold true for HIV anergic patients, in whom chemoprophylaxis does not reduce the incidence of disease; hence it is not indicated in these cases.[110,118]

Treatment of active disease has also been shown to be effective with some modifications in HIV patients keeping in view the possible drug interactions among the antiretroviral drugs and the antitubercular drugs.[16,44] Another major issue in treatment is that of noncompliance, which leads to increased chances of therapeutic failure among them with prolonged infectivity, increased rates of transmission and development of drug-resistant strains.[119] Measures for ensuring compliance in this group of patients have included forced confinement during treatment, but by far is the most effective and promising strategy.[119]

Alcohol Abuse

Alcoholism and alcohol intake are closely associated with tuberculosis.[120,121] In one hospital-based study, 49% prevalence of alcoholism was seen in patients with newly diagnosed tuberculosis.[122] The rate of active tuberculosis among alcoholics and drug abusers was 28 times higher than in general New York City population.[120] Alcohol intake was found to be associated with increased risk as well as poor compliance to treatment. These facts call for alcohol intervention campaigns along with tuberculosis control programs.[123]

Age

Among persons with tuberculous infection, rates of occurrence of diseases vary markedly with age. The case-rates are considerably increased amongst infants, young adults and elderly subjects. The reasons for the variations in age are as yet undetermined, but may relate to influences on the effectiveness of the immune response. Infection acquired early in life can progress to typical disease as the age advances. In the past, almost all patients were adolescents and young adults, but the recent years have witnessed a marked change in the clinical pattern of disease.

Infection in infants often results in disease; the younger the patient, the greater is the risk of progressive disease, until the age of 5 years. From this age onwards until puberty, there is relative resistance to the development of progressive disease, but not to infection. Disease confined to lungs in this age group usually heals spontaneously. Nonetheless, lymph nodes and bones may be involved. Short-term prognosis in these patients is good, although the frequency of relapse with chronic cavitary tuberculosis is high, especially during the more disease prone periods of adolescence and young adulthood.[118] Clinical disease that develops in adolescence and young adulthood may resemble childhood infection, but with less parenchymal and hilar calcification, this being particularly the case in dark-skinned races and immunocompromised patients, including those with AIDS.[24] Disease in this age group appears as chronic upper lobe tuberculosis with no clinical features of childhood disease. Tendency towards apical cavitation immediately after childhood infection appears after puberty and is marked in young adults.[57] Mostly, pulmonary tuberculosis in this age group is due to recent new infection rather than due to the progression of childhood infection, which is being substantiated by the fact that most young people in industrialized countries are tuberculin negative.

Infection acquired during the middle years of life has a much better prognosis, both long and short-term, than infection acquired in teens and in early 20s, presumably because of a reduced tendency to tissue necrosis.[118] The incidence among women peaks at 25–34 years of age, rates being usually higher in women in this age group, while in older age groups, the opposite is true.

Immigration

Prevalence of tuberculosis is higher in the African and the Asian countries. Migratory movements of people between countries have become more frequent, favoring the transmission of infectious diseases from one place to another. These unrestricted movements from high prevalence areas can affect the control programs of other countries. As a matter of fact, immigration has been considered as a major cause of resurgence of tuberculosis in the Western countries.

Illegal immigration poses more threats to the control of potentially infected population. A study conducted in Spain showed that 78% were amongst illegal immigrants with active disease. Other factors that complicate the management of tuberculosis in this population include the language barriers, overcrowding, poverty, fear to seek professional advice and frequent imprisonment. All these factors affected compliance since adherence to therapy was even lower in infected patients without active disease.[124] However, strict follow-up and other complementary measures (e.g. use of patient's language for examination) increased the compliance of tuberculous patients to 78%.[124,125]

The potential transmission of tuberculosis from immigrants to local population is a theoretical risk. A molecular epidemiology analysis, making use of restriction fragment length polymorphism (RFLP) and spoligotyping, found only nine minor clusters in both Danish and immigrant patients, thus depicting only minor transmission between these population.[126] However, many other clusters were found suggesting the existence of predominant strains between immigrants and transmission between them.[125,126] A possible explanation is the low social contact between these two communities. Several other reports suggest that tuberculosis in immigrants is the result of reactivation and not of primary disease due to recent infection.[113,126-128] Drug resistance is an additional problem in infected immigrants on account of the multidrug resistance in their native countries. Antimicrobial testing may hence be indicated in such patients for appropriate therapy.

OTHER RISK FACTORS

There are numerous other factors that favor the progression of infection to active disease, notable among them being smoking, poverty and malnutrition, renal failure, immunosuppression and host-genetic factors. Each of these factors places an individual at an increased risk of developing tuberculosis; nonetheless even in the same person, interplay of all or some of the above mentioned factors are seen on occasion.

Tobacco Smoking

An association between tobacco smoking and tuberculosis has been debated for over a hundred years and there is considerable evidence confirming the presence, strength and consistency of this association and the different levels at which it operates. Recent research demonstrates a direct connection between smoking and tuberculosis. Smoking increases the risk of latent tuberculosis infection by nearly two times, as well as increasing the risk of active tuberculosis by around two and a half times.[129] The basis of these findings was a large-scale meta-analysis, in which studies from 14 different countries were assessed.[129] Other research has produced similar results, with smokers having a relative risk of around twice that of nonsmokers for acquiring tuberculosis.[129-131] Smoking has also been found to lead to increased severity of the disease, longer hospital stays and decreased survival rates.[132,133]

Many physical and social factors associated with cigarette smoking are also known to contribute in the development of tuberculosis;[130] immunosuppression, old-healed fibrotic lesions, unemployment, and lower socioeconomic and education status being some of them. It has been shown that tobacco smoking causes pulmonary impairment and smoking would be expected to increase the risk of pulmonary impairment due to tuberculosis.[134] Indoor air pollution from passive smoking is another strong factor in causing tuberculosis. Chronic exposures to smoke from biomass fuels is another contributory risk for tuberculosis, as well as other lung diseases particularly in immigrants.[135-139] A history of such biomass smoke exposure may be an important risk factor for pulmonary tuberculosis and abnormal pulmonary function following its microbiological cure. However, these possibilities need to be substantiated with further research.

Poverty

Growing poverty is an important variable that globally prevents the decline in the number of cases due to tuberculosis. Poverty has always been associated with tuberculosis.[140] A decline in the incidence of tuberculosis seen in the European countries in 19th century was parallel to the reduction of poverty. Economic downfall in Russia in the last decades has been linked to the increased incidence of tuberculosis in that country.[141] Along with HIV or AIDS and malaria, tuberculosis is implicated as one of the three major diseases associated with poverty.

Malnutrition and Immunosuppression

Immunosuppression and malnutrition form the basis for many, if not all, the factors to produce the varied effects of this disease. The population of patients whose host defences are compromised by the underlying diseases or by the medical treatments continue to increase; posing new and complex threats to the ongoing control measures. Both these factors play a pivotal role, not only in the reactivation of latent infection, but also in acquiring primary infection. Contributions of these variables in the development and progression of tuberculosis have already been described under the relevant headings.

Chronic Renal Failure

Chronic renal failure impairs immune function and is associated with an increased incidence of tuberculosis. Rates of tuberculosis are 10-fold to 25-fold amongst patients of renal failure on renal replacement therapy (hemodialysis or continuous ambulatory peritoneal dialysis), equating to incidence rates of approximately 250 per 1,00,000 per year.[142-145]

ETHNIC AND GENETIC FACTORS

It has long been recognized that certain population appears to have a high degree of vulnerability to tuberculosis. Extreme susceptibility to the disease has been observed in Eskimo population in North America, Yanomami Indians in the Brazilian Amazon and black population in the United States.[146-148] Host-genetic factors also influence disease expression, with reports from India suggesting a clear association between HLA-DR2 and increased risk of progression to advanced disease.[149] It has also been shown that DRB1*1501 allele correlates with advanced disease and treatment failure and that DRB1*1502 correlates with decreased risk.[150] A clue to the genetic basis of resistance was provided by the studies of Gros and colleagues who identified a strain of mice with exquisite vulnerability to overwhelming infection with certain bacteria and some strains of mycobacteria, particularly *M. bovis*.[151,152] Eventually, the genetic basis of this susceptibility was mapped to a locus encoding a gene on murine chromosome 1, initially called *Bcg*, then renamed natural resistance-associated macrophage protein 1 (*Nramp1*), responsible for the production of a so-called natural resistance-associated macrophage protein.[152]

Several polymorphisms of the human *Nramp1* gene have been identified and population-based studies in several regions have been conducted, which have identified increased relative risk for moving from latent infection to active disease associated with certain polymorphisms.[153] However, the risk attributable to these polymorphisms is relatively small, and it is clear that *Nramp* alone explains only a portion of genetic susceptibility to tuberculosis. Several other genes and gene families, including those for vitamin D receptors and the components of IFN-γ-signaling pathways, have also been studied for their role in susceptibility to tuberculosis.[154-155] A recent study has concluded that a variation in the 3' untranslated region of the tumor necrosis factor receptor superfamily member 1B gene, which has been shown to be implicated in messenger ribonucleic acid destabilization, contributes to tuberculosis susceptibility.[156]

A recent Russian study involving whole genome sequencing of 1,000 isolates of *M. tuberculosis* showed that common rpoB mutation was associated with fitness-compensatory mutations in rpoA or rpoC, and a new intragenic compensatory substitution.[157] The combination of drug resistance and compensatory mutations displayed by the major clades, thus confers clinical resistance without a compromise of fitness and transmissibility.[157]

These investigations clearly suggest that resistance or susceptibility to tuberculosis is a complex genetic trait and it is highly unlikely that there is a single dominant genetic factor involved.

In conclusion, the fact that more than a quarter of the world's population is infected with *M. tuberculosis* and the active disease remains a worldwide pandemic in spite of the availability of effective antitubercular drugs, bears testimony to the fact that risk factors of tuberculosis continue to pose a big challenge. The presence of a large number of these variables is an important determinant of the occurrence of tuberculosis, as well as of its clinical spectrum and course.

REFERENCES

1. Comstock GW, Livesay VT, Woolpert SF. The prognosis of a positive tuberculin reaction in childhood and adolescence. Am J Epidemiol. 1974;99(2):131-8.
2. Comstock GW. Epidemiology of tuberculosis. Am Rev Respir Dis. 1982;125(3 Pt 2):8-15.
3. Lienhardt C, Fielding K, Sillah JS, Bah B, Gustafson P, Warndorff D, et al. Investigation of the risk factors for tuberculosis: a case-control study in three countries in West Africa. Int J Epidemiol. 2005;34(4):914-23.
4. World Health Organization. Global tuberculosis control: Epidemiology, Strategy, Financing. WHO report 2009. WHO/HTM/TB/2009.411. Geneva, World Health Organization, 2009.

5. World Health Organization. Global Tuberculosis Report 2013. [Online] Available from *http://www.who.int/tb/publications/global_report/en/*, [Accessed September 2014] .
6. Van Zyl Smit RN, Pai M, Yew WW, Leung CC, Zumla A, Bateman ED, et al. Global lung health: The colliding epidemics of tuberculosis, tobacco smoking, HIV and COPD. Eur Respir J. 2010;35(1):27-35.
7. Sonnenberg P, Glynn JR, Fielding K, Murray J, Godfrey-Faussett P, et al. How soon after infection with HIV does the risk of tuberculosis start to increase? A retrospective cohort study in South African gold miners. J Infect Dis. 2005;191(2):150-8.
8. Selwyn PA, Hartel D, Lewis VA, Schoenbaum EE, Vermund SH, Klein RS, et al. A prospective study of the risk of tuberculosis among intravenous drug users with human immunodeficiency virus infection. N Engl J Med. 1989;320(9):545-50.
9. Di Perri G, Cruciani M, Danzi MC, Luzzati R, De Checchi G, Malena M, et al. Nosocomial epidemic of active tuberculosis among HIV-infected patients. The Lancet. 1989;2(8678-79):1502-4.
10. Daley C, Small PM, Schecter GF, Schoolnik GK, McAdam RA, Jacobs WR, et al. An outbreak of tuberculosis with accelerated progression among persons with the human immunodeficiency virus. An analysis using restriction-fragment-length polymorphism. N Engl J Med. 1992;326(4):231-5.
11. Girardi E, Raviglione MC, Antonucci G, Godfrey-Faussett P, Ippolito G. Impact of the HIV epidemic on the spread of other diseases: the case of tuberculosis. AIDS. 2000;14:S47-56.
12. Sonnenberg P, Murray J, Glynn JR, Shearer S, Kambashi B, Godfrey-Faussett P. HIV-1 and recurrence, relapse, and reinfection of tuberculosis after cure: a cohort study in South African mineworkers. Lancet. 2001;358(9294):1687-93.
13. Klausner JD, Ryder RW, Baende E, Lelo U, Williame JC, Ngamboli K, et al. *Mycobacterium tuberculosis* in household contacts of human immunodeficiency virus type-1 seropositive patients with active pulmonary tuberculosis in Kinshasa, Zaire. J Infect Dis. 1993;168(1):106-11.
14. Elliot AM, Hayes RJ, Halwiindi B, Luo N, Tembo G, Pobee JO, et al. The impact of HIV-1 on infectiousness of pulmonary tuberculosis: a community study in Zambia. AIDS. 1993;7(7):981-7.
15. Cauthen GM, Dooley SW, Onorato IM, Ihle WW, Burr JM, Bigler WJ, et al. Transmission of mycobacterium tuberculosis from tuberculosis patients with human immunodeficiency virus infection or AIDS. Am J Epidemiol. 1996;144(1):69-77.
16. Espinal MA, Peréz EN, Baéz J, , Hénriquez L, Fernåndez K, Lopez M, et al. Infectiousness of *Mycobacterium tuberculosis* in HIV-1 infected patients with tuberculosis: a prospective study. Lancet. 2000;355(9200):275-80.
17. Whalen C, Horsburgh CR, Hom D, Lahart C, Simberkoff M, Ellner J. Accelerated course of human immunodeficiency virus infection after tuberculosis. Am J Respir Crit Care Med. 1995;151(1):129-35.
18. Dheda K, Lampe FC, Johnson MA, Lipman MC. Outcome of HIV-associated tuberculosis in the era of highly active antiretroviral therapy. J Infect Dis. 2004;190(9):1670-6.
19. Munsiff SS, Alpert PL, Gourevitch MN, Chang CJ, Klein RS. A prospective study of tuberculosis and HIV disease progression. J Acquir Immune Defic Syndr Hum Retrovirol. 1998;19(4):361-6.
20. Wood R, Middelkoop K, Myer L, Grant AD, Whitelaw A, Lawn SD, et al. Undiagnosed tuberculosis in a community with high HIV prevalence: implications for tuberculosis control. Am J Respir Crit Care Med. 2007;175(1):87-93.
21. Dhasmana DJ, Dheda K, Ravn P, Wilkinson RJ, Meintjes G. Immune reconstitution inflammatory syndrome in HIV-infected patients receiving antiretroviral therapy: pathogenesis, clinical manifestations and management. Drugs. 2008;68:191-208.
22. Orme IM, Anderson P, Boom WH. T cell response to *Mycobacterium tuberculosis*. J Infect Dis. 1993;167(6):1481-97.
23. Pitchemk AE, Cole C, Russell BW, Fischl MA, Spira TJ, Snider DE. Tuberculosis, atypical mycobacteriosis and acquired immunodeficiency syndrome among Haitian and non-Haitian patients in South Florida. Ann Intern Med. 1984;101(5):641-5.
24. Murray JF. Cursed duet: HIV infection and tuberculosis. Respiration. 1990;57(3):210-20.
25. Barach JH. Historical facts in diabetes. Ann Med Hist. 1928;10:387.
26. Ramadoss A. TB INDIA 2009 RNTCP Status Report 'I am Stopping TB'. (Central TB Division), New Delhi: Ministry of Health and Family Welfare; 2009.
27. Young F, Critchley J, Unwin N. Diabetes and Tuberculosis: a dangerous liaison and no white tiger. Indian J Med Res. 2009;130(1):1-4.
28. Kim SJ, Hong YP, Lew WJ, Yang SC, Lee EG. Incidence of pulmonary tuberculosis among diabetics. Tuber Lung Dis. 1995;76(6):529-33.
29. Jick SS, Lieberman ES, Rahman MU, Choi HK. Glucocorticoid use, other associated factors, and the risk of tuberculosis. Arthritis Rheum. 2006;55(1):19-26.
30. Leung CC, Lam TH, Chan WM, Yew WW, Ho KS, Leung GM, et al. Diabetic control and risk of tuberculosis: a cohort study. Am J Epidemiol. 2008;167(12):1486-94.
31. Jeon CY, Murray MB. Diabetes mellitus increases the risk of active tuberculosis: a systematic review of 13 observational studies. PLoS Med. 2008;5(7):e152.
32. Patel JC. Complications in 8793 cases of diabetes mellitus 14-year study in Bombay Hospital. Ind J Med Sci. 1989;43:177-83.
33. Stevenson CR, Critchley JA, Forouhi NG, Roglic G, Williams BG, Dye C, et al. Diabetes and the risk of tuberculosis: a neglected threat to public health? Chronic Illn. 2007;3(3):228-45.
34. Stevenson CR, Forouhi NG, Roglic G, Williams BG, Lauer JA, Dye C, et al. Diabetes and tuberculosis: the impact of the diabetes epidemic on tuberculosis incidence. BMC Public Health. 2007;7:234.
35. Swai AB, McLarty DG, Mugusi F. Tuberculosis in diabetic patients in Tanzania. Trop Doct. 1990;20(4):147-50.
36. Dooley KE, Chaison RE. Tuberculosis and diabetes mellitus: the convergence of two epidemics. Lancet Infect Dis. 2009;9(12):737-46.
37. Koziel H, Kozeil MJ. Pulmonary complications of diabetes mellitus. Pneumonia. Infect Dis Clin North Am. 1995;9(1):65-96.
38. Geerlings SE, Hoepelman AI. Immune dysfunction in patients with diabetes mellitus. FEMS Immunol Med Microbiol. 1999;26(3-4):259-65.
39. Tsukaguchi K, Yoneda T, Yoshikawa M, Tokuyama T, Fu A, Tomoda K, et al. Case study of nterleukin-1 beta, tumor necrosis factor alpha and interleukin-6 production by peripheral blood monocytes in patients with diabetes mellitus complicated by pulmonary tuberculosis. Kekkaku. 1992;67(12):755-60.
40. Fielder JF, Chaulk CP, Dalvi M, Gachuhi R, Comstock GW, Sterling TR, et al. A high tuberculosis case-fatality rate in

a setting of effective tuberculosis control: implications for acceptable treatment success rates. Int J Tuberc Lung Dis. 2002;6(12):1114-7.

41. Singla R, Osman MM, Khan N, Al-Sharif N, Al-Sayegh MO, Shaikh MA. Factors predicting persistent sputum smear positivity among pulmonary tuberculosis patients 2 months after treatment. Int J Tuberc Lung Dis. 2003;7:58-64.
42. Bashar M, Alcabes P, Rom WN, Condos R. Increased incidence of multidrug-resistant tuberculosis in diabetic patients on the Bellevue Chest Service, 1987 to 1997. Chest. 2001;120(5): 1514-9.
43. Alisjahbana B, Sahiratmadja E, Nelwan EJ, Purwa AM, Ahmad Y, Ottenhoff TH, et al. The effect of type 2 diabetes mellitus on the presentation and treatment response of pulmonary tuberculosis. Clin Infect Dis. 2007;45(4):428-35.
44. Fisher-Hoch SP, Whitney E, McCormick JB, Crespo G, Smith B, Rahbar MH, et al. Type 2 diabetes and multidrug-resistant tuberculosis. Scand J Infect Dis. 2008;40(11-12):888-93.
45. Suárez-García I, Rodríguez-Blanco A, Vidal-Pérez JL, García-Viejo MA, Jaras-Hernández MJ, López O, et al. Risk factors for multidrug-resistant tuberculosis in a tuberculosis unit in Madrid, Spain. Eur J Clin Mircobiol Infect Dis. 2009;28(4): 325-30.
46. Tanrikulu AC, Hosoglu S, Ozekinci T, Abakay A, Gurkan F. Risk factors for drug resistant tuberculosis in southeast Turkey. Trop Doct. 2008;38(2):91-3.
47. Singla R, Khan N. Does diabetes predispose to the development of multidrug-resistant tuberculosis? Chest. 2003;123(1):308-9.
48. Subhash HS, Ashwin I, Mukundan U, Danda D, John G, Cherian AM, et al. Drug resistant tuberculosis in diabetes mellitus: a retrospective study from south India. Trop Doct. 2003;33(3):154-6.
49. Singh N, Patterson DL. *Mycobacterium tuberculosis* infection in solid-organ transplant recipients: impact and implications for management. Clin Infect Dis. 1998;27(5):1266-77.
50. Aguado JM, Herrero JA, Gavaldá J, Torre-Cisneros J, Blanes M, Rufí G, Moreno A, et al. Clinical presentation and outcome of tuberculosis in kidney, liver, and heart transplant recipients in Spain. Spanish Transplantation Infection Study Group, GESITRA. Transplantation. 1997;63(9):1278-86.
51. John GT, Shankar V, Abraham AM, Mukundan U, Thomas PP, Jacob CK. Risk factors for post-transplant tuberculosis. Kidney Int. 2001;60(3):1148-53.
52. Muñoz P, Rodríguez C, Bouza E. *Mycobacterium tuberculosis* infection in recipients of solid organ transplants. Clin Infect Dis. 2005;40(4):581-7.
53. Budak-Alpdogan T, Tangün Y, Kalyoglu-Besisisk S, Ratip S, Akan H, Baslar Z, et al. The frequency of tuberculosis in adult allogeneic stem cell transplant recipients in Turkey. Biol Blood Marrow Transplant. 2000;6(4):370-4.
54. Cordonnier C, Martino R, Trabasso P, Held TK, Akan H, Ward MS, et al. Mycobacterial infection: a difficult and late diagnosis in stem cell transplant recipients. Clin Infect Dis. 2004;38(9):1229-36.
55. Patel R, Paya CV. Infections in solid organ transplant recipients. Clin Microbiol Rev. 1997;10(1):86-124.
56. American Society of Transplantation. *Mycobacterium tuberculosis*. Am J Transplant. 2004;4(Suppl 10):S37-S41.
57. Targeted tuberculin testing and treatment of latent tuberculosis infection. American Thoracic Society. MMWR Recomm Rep. 2000;49(RR-6):1-51.
58. Tavil B, Gulhan B, Ozcelik U, Cetin M, Tezcan I, Tuncer M, et al. Tuberculin skin test positivity in pediatric allogenic BMT recipients and donors in Turkey. Pediatr Transplant. 2007;11(4):414-8.
59. Pai M, Zwerling A, Menzies D. Systematic review: T-cell-based assays for the diagnosis of latent tuberculosis infection: an update. Ann Intern Med. 2008;149(3):177-84.
60. Menzies D, Pai M, Comstock G. Meta-analysis: new tests for the diagnosis of latent tuberculosis infection: areas of uncertainty and recommendations for research. Ann Intern Med. 2007;146(5):340-54.
61. Macahdo CM, Martins TC, Colturato I, Leite MS, Simione AJ, Souza MP, et al. Epidemiology of neglected tropical diseases in transplant recipients. Review of the literature and experience of a Brazilian HSCT center. Rev Inst Me Trop S Paulo. 2009;51(6):309-24.
62. Tomblyn M, Chiller T, Einsele H, Gress R, Sepkowitz K, Storek J, et al. Guidelines for preventing infectious complications among hematopoietic cell transplantation recipients: a global perspective. Biol Blood Marrow Transplant. 2009;44(8):453-5.
63. Barboza CE, Winter DH, Seiscento M, Santos Ude P, Terra Filho M. Tuberculosis and silicosis: epidemiology, diagnosis and chemoprophylaxis. J Bras Pneumol. 2008;34(11):959-66.
64. Corbett EL, Churchyard GJ, Clayton T, Herselman P, Williams B, Hayes R, et al. Risk factors for pulmonary mycobacterial disease in South African gold miners. A case-control study. Am J Respir Crit Care Med. 1999;159(1):94-9.
65. Cowie RL. The epidemiology of tuberculosis in gold miners with silicosis. Am J Respir Crit Care Med. 1994;150(5 Pt 1): 1460-2.
66. Tewaternaude JM, Ehrlich RI, Churchyard GJ, Pemba L, Dekker K, Vermeis M, et al. Tuberculosis and silica exposure in South African gold miners. Occup Environ Med. 2006;63:187-92.
67. A double-blind placebo-controlled clinical trial of three anti-tuberculosis chemoprophylaxis regimens in patients with silicosis in Hong Kong. Hong Kong Chest Service/Tuberculosis Research Centre, Madras/British Medical Research Council. Am Rev Respir Dis. 1992;145(1):36-41.
68. Snider DE. The relationship between tuberculosis and silicosis. Am Rev Respir Dis. 1978;118(3):455-60.
69. Pasula R, Wright JR, Kachel DL, Martin WJ 2nd. Surfactant protein A suppresses reactive nitrogen intermediates by alveolar macrophages in response to *Mycobacterium tuberculosis*. J Clin Invest. 1999;103(4):483-90.
70. Gold JA, Hoshino Y, Tanaka N, Rom WN, Raju B, Condos R, et al. Surfactant protein A modulates the inflammatory response in macrophages during tuberculosis. Infect Immun. 2004;72(2):645-50.
71. Bombarda S, Figueiredo CM, Funari MB, Soares Jr J, Seiscento M, Filho MT. Imagem em tuberculose pulmonar. J Pneumol. 2001;27(6):329-40.
72. Lee KS, Hwang JW, Chung MP, Kim H, Kwon OJ. Utility of CT in the evaluation of pulmonary tuberculosis in patients without AIDS. Chest. 1996;110(4):977-84.
73. Chong S, Lee KS, Chung MJ, Han J, Kwon OJ, Kim TS. Pneumoconiosis: comparison of imaging and pathologic findings. Radiographics. 2006;26(1):59-77.
74. A controlled clinical comparison of 6 and 8 months of antituberculosis chemotherapy in the treatment of patients with silicotuberculosis in Hong Kong. Hong Kong Chest

Service/Tuberculosis Research Centre, Madras/British Medical Research Council. Am Rev Respir Dis. 1991;143(2):262-7.

75. Bayle GI. Recherches sur la phthisie pulmonaire. Gabon, Paris. 1810.
76. Kaplan MH, Armstrong D, Rosen P. Tuberculosis complicating neoplastic disease: a review of 201 cases. Cancer. 1974;33(3): 850-8.
77. Libshitz HI, Pannu HK, Elting LS, Cooksley CD. Tuberculosis in cancer patients: an update. J Thorac Imaging. 1997;12(1): 41-6.
78. Melero M, Gennaro O, Dominguez C, Sánchez Avalos JC. Tuberculosis in patients with lymphomas. Medicina (Beunos Aires). 1992;52(4):291-5.
79. Morri T, Narita N. Mycobacterial infections in patients with haematologic disorders. Nippon Rinsho. 1998;56(12):3209-11.
80. Advani SH, Banavali SD. Pattern of infection in hematologic malignancies: an Indian experience. Rev Infect Dis. 1989;11(Suppl 7):S1621-8.
81. Kumar RR, Shafiulla M, Sridhar H. Association of tuberculosis with malignancy at KIMIO-an oncology centre. Indian J Pathol Microbiol. 1999;42(3):339-43.
82. Kim HR, Hwang SS, Ro YK, Jeon CH, Ha DY, Park S, et al. Solid-organ malignancy as a risk factor for tuberculosis. Respirology. 2008;13(3):413-9.
83. Snider DE. Tuberculosis and gastrectomy. Chest. 1985;87(4): 414-5.
84. Yagi T, Yamagishi F, Sasaki Y, Itakura M, Fujikawa A, Kuga M, et al. A study on cases developed pulmonary tuberculosis after receiving gastrectomy. Kekkaku. 2004;79(5):355-9.
85. Thorn PA, Brookes VS, Waterhouse JAH. Peptic ulcer, partial gastrectomy, and pulmonary tuberculosis. Brit Med J. 1956;1(4967):603-8.
86. Steiger Z, Nickel WO, Shannon GJ, et al. Pulmonary tuberculosis after gastric resection. Am J Surg. 1976;131(6):668-71.
87. Pickleman JR, Evans LS, Kane JM, Freeark RJ. Tuberculosis after jejunoileal bypass for obesity. JAMA. 1975;234(7):744.
88. Bruce RM, Wise L. Tuberculosis after jejunoileal bypass for obesity. Ann Intern Med. 1977;87:3514-76.
89. Snider DE. Jejunoileal bypass for obesity: a risk factor for tuberculosis. Chest. 1982;81(5):531.
90. Law DK, Dudrick SJ, Abdou NI. The effects of protein calorie malnutrition on immune competence of the surgical patient. Surg Gynecol Obstet. 1974;139(2):257-66.
91. Bates JH, Stead WW. The history of tuberculosis as a global epidemic. Med Clin North Am. 1993;77(6):1205-17.
92. Valway SE, Sanchez MP, Shinnick TK, Orme I, Agerton T, Hoy D, et al. An outbreak involving extensive transmission of a virulent strain of *Mycobacterium tuberculosis*. N Engl J Med. 1998;338(10):633-9.
93. Stead WW. Tuberculosis among elderly persons: An outbreak in a nursing home. Ann Intern Med. 1981;94(5):606-10.
94. Center for Disease Control (1992a) Prevention and control of tuberculosis among homeless persons. Recommendations of the advisory council for the elimination of tuberculosis. [Online] MMWR 41. Available from http://*www.cdc.gov/mmwr/preview/mmwrhtml/00019922. htm.* [Accessed September 2010]
95. Wright JD. Poor people, poor health: The health status of the homeless. J Soc Issues. 1990;46(4):49-56.
96. Torres RA, Mani S, Atholz J, Brickner PW. Human immunodeficiency virus infection among homeless men in a New York shelter: association with *Mycobacterium tuberculosis* infection. Arch Intern Med. 1990;150(10):2030-6.
97. Brudney K, Dobkin J. Resurgent tuberculosis in New York city: Human immunodieficiency virus, homelessness and the decline of tuberculosis control programs. Am Rev Respir Dis. 1991;144(4):745-9.
98. Reichman LB, Felton CP, Edsall JR. Drug dependence, a possible new risk factor for tuberculosis disease. Arch Intern Med. 1979;139(3):337-9.
99. Brown SM, Stimmel B, Taub RN, Kochwa S, Rosenfield RE. Immunologic dysfunction in heroin addicts. Arch Intern Med. 1974;134(6):1001-6.
100. Slutkin G. Mangement of tuberculosis in urban homeless indigents. Public Health Rep. 1986;101(5):481-5.
101. Barry MA, Wall C, Shirley I, Bernardo J, Schwingl P, Brigandi E, et al. Tuberculosis screening in Boston's homeless shelters. Public Health Rep. 1986;101(5):487-94.
102. Stead WW, Kerby GR, Schlueter DP, et al. The clinical spectrum of primary tuberculosis in adults. Confusion with reinfection in the pathogenesis of chronic tuberculosis. Ann Intern Med. 1968;68(4):731-45.
103. Moss AR, Hahn JA, Tulsky JP, Daley CL, Small PM, Hopewell PC, et al. Tuberculosis in the Homeless. A prospective study. Am J Resp Crit Care Med. 2000;162(2 Pt 1):460-4.
104. Hammett TM, Harmon MP, Rhodes W. The burden of infectious disease among inmates of and releasees from US correctional facilities, 1997. Am J Public Health. 2002;92:1789-94.
105. Hutton MD, Cauthen GM, Bloch AB. Results of a 29-state survey of tuberculosis in nursing homes and correctional facilities. Public Health Rep. 1993;108(3):305-14.
106. Valway SE, Greifinger RB, Papania M, Kilburn JO, Woodley C, DiFerdinando GT, et al. Multidrug-resistant tuberculosis in the New York State prison system, 1990-1991. J Infect Dis. 1994;170(1):151-6.
107. Braun MM, Truman BI, Maguire B, DiFerdinando GT, Wormser G, Broaddus R, et al. Increasing incidence of tuberculosis in a prison inmate population. Association with HIV infection. JAMA. 1989;261(3):393-7.
108. Stead WW. Undetected tuberculosis in prison. Source of infection for community at large. JAMA. 1978;240(23): 2544-7.
109. Bergmire-Sweat D, Barnett BJ, Harris SL, Taylor JP, Mazurek GH, Reddy V. Tuberculosis out-break in a Texas prison, 1994. Epidemiol Infect. 1996;117:485-92.
110. Koo DT, Baron RC, Rutherford GW. Transmission of *Mycobacterium tuberculosis* in a California state prison. Am J Public Health. 1991;87(2):279-82.
111. Daley CL, Hahn JA, Moss AR, et al. Incidence of tuberculosis in injection drug users in San Francisco: impact of energy. Am J Respir Crit Care Med. 1998;157(1):19-22.
112. Friedman LN, Williams MT, Singh TP, Frieden TR. Tuberculosis, AIDS, and death among substance abusers on welfare in New York City. N Engl J Med. 1996;334(13):828-33.
113. Iñigo Martínez J, Chaves Sánchez F, Arce Arnáez A, Alonso Sanz M, Palenque Mataix E, Jaén Herreros F, et al. Recent transmission of tuberculosis in Madrid (Spain): usefulness of molecular techniques. Med Clin (Barc). 2000;115(7):241-5.
114. Gourevitch MN, Alcabes P, Wasserman WC, Arno PS. Cost-effectiveness of directly observed chemoprophylaxis of tuberculosis among drug users at high risk for tuberculosis. Int J Tuberc Lung Dis. 1998;2(7):531-40.

115. Selwyn PA, Sckell BM, Alcabes P, Friedland GH, Klein RS, Schoenbaum EE, et al. High risk of active tuberculosis in HIV-infected drug users with cutaneous energy. JAMA. 1992;268(4):504-9.
116. Snyder DC, Paz EA, Mohle-Boetani JC, Fallstad R, Black RL, Chin DP, et al. Tuberculosis prevention in methadone maintenance clinics. Effectiveness and cost-effectiveness. Am J Respir Crit Care Med. 1999;160(1):178-85.
117. Moro ML, Salamina G, Gori A, Penati V, Sacchetti R, Mezzetti F, et al. Two-year population based molecular epidemiological study of tuberculosis transmission in the Metropolitan Area of Milan, Italy. Eur J Clin Microbiol Infect Dis. 2002;21(2):114-22.
118. Hamburg MA, Frieden TR. Tuberculosis transmission in the 1990s. N Engl J Med. 1994;330(24):1750-1.
119. Halvir DV, Barnes PF. Tuberculosis in patients with Human Immunodeficiency Virus infection. N Engl J Med. 1999;340(5):367-73.
120. Perlman DC, Salomon N, Perkins MP, Yancovitz S, Paone D, Des Jarlais DC. Tuberculosis in drug users. Clin Infect Dis. 1995;21:1253-64.
121. Friedman LN, Sullivan GM, Bevilaqua RP, Loscos R. Tuberculosis screening in alcoholics and drug addicts. Am Rev Respir Dis. 1987;136(5):1188-92.
122. Brown KE, Campbell AH. Tobacco, alcohol and tuberculosis. Br J Dis Chest. 1961;55:150-8.
123. Feingold AO. Association of tuberculosis with alcoholism. South Med J. 1976;69(10):1336-7.
124. Huerga H, López-Vélez R, Navas E, Gomez-Mampaso E. Clinico-epidemiological features of immigrants with tuberculosis living in Madrid, Spain. Eur J Clin Microbiol Infect Dis. 2000;19(3):236-7.
125. Durán E, Cabezos J, Ros M, Terre M, Zarzuela F, Bada JL. Tuberculosis in recent immigrants in Barcelona. Med Clin (Barc). 1996;106(14):525-8.
126. Lillebaek T, Andersen AB, Bauer J, Dirksen A, Glismann S, de Haas P, et al. Risk of *Mycobacterium tuberculosis* transmission in a low-incidence country due to immigration from high incidence areas. J Clin Microbiol. 2001;39(3):855-61.
127. Chin DP, DeRiemer K, Small PM, de Leon AP, Steinhart R, Schecter GF, et al. Differences in contributing factors to tuberculosis incidence in US-born and foreign-born persons. Am J Respir Crit Care Med. 1998;158(6):1797-803.
128. Samper S, Iglesias MJ, Rabanaque MJ, et al. The molecular epidemiology of tuberculosis in Zaragoza, Spain: a retrospective epidemiological study in 1993. Int J Tuberc Lung Dis. 1998;2(4):281-7.
129. Bates MN, Khalakdina A, Pai M, Chang L, Lessa F, Smith KR. Risk of tuberculosis from exposure to tobacco smoke: a systematic review and meta-analysis. Archives of Internal Medicine. 2007;167(4):335-42.
130. Arcavi L, Benowitz N. Cigarette smoking and infection. Arch Intern Med. 2004;164(20):2206-16.
131. Bothamley G. Smoking and tuberculosis: a chance or causal association? Thorax. 2005;60(7):527-8.
132. Hussain H, Akhtar S, Nanan D. Prevalence of and risk factors associated with *Mycobacterium tuberculosis* infection in prisoners, North West Frontier Province, Pakistan. Int J Epidemiol. 2003;32(5):794-9.
133. Altet-Gômez M, Alcaide J, Godoy P, Romero MA, Hernández del Rey I. Clinical and epidemiological aspects of smoking and tuberculosis: a study of 13,038 cases. Int J Tuberculosis Lung Dis. 2005;9(4):430-6.
134. Wang J, Hsueh PR, Jan IS, Lee LN, Liaw YS, Yang PC, et al. The effect of smoking on tuberculosis: different patterns and poorer outcomes. Int J Tuberc Lung Dis. 2007;11(2):143-9.
135. Pelkonena M, Tukiainenb H, Tervahautaa M, Notkola IL, Kivelä SL, Salorinne Y, et al. Pulmonary function, smoking cessation and 30-year mortality in middle aged Finnish men. Thorax. 2000;55(9):746-50.
136. Smith KR, Mehta S, Maeusezahl-Feuz M. Indoor smoke from solid fuels. In: Ezzati M, Rodgers AD, Lopez AD, et al (Eds). Comparative quantification of health risk: global burden of disease due to selected major risk factors. Geneva, Switzerland: World Health Organization; 2004. pp. 1437-95.
137. Zuber PL, McKenna MT, Binkin NJ, Onorato IM, Castro KG. Long-term risk of tuberculosis among foreign-born persons in the United States. JAMA. 1997;278(4):304-7.
138. Talbot EA, Moore M, McCray E, Binkin NJ. Tuberculosis among foreign born persons in the United States, 1993-1998. JAMA. 2000;284(22):2894-900.
139. Mishra VK, Retherford RD, Smith KR. Biomass cooking fuels and prevalence of tuberculosis in India. Int J Infect Dis. 1999;3(3):119-29.
140. Moore-Gillon JC. Tuberculosis and poverty in the developed world. In: Davies PDO (Ed). Clinical Tuberculosis, 2nd edition. Cambridge: Cambridge University Press; 1998. pp. 383-93.
141. Dye C. Tuberculosis, 2000-2010: control, but not elimination. Int J Tuberc Lung Dis. 2000;4:S146-52.
142. Andrew OT, Schoenfeld PY, Hopewell PC, Humphreys MH. Tuberculosis in patients with end-stage renal disease. Am J Med. 1980;68(1):59-65.
143. Chia S, Karim M, Elwood RK, FitzGerald JM. Risk of tuberculosis in dialysis patients: a population-based study. Int J Tuberc Lung Dis. 1998;2(12):989-91.
144. García-Leoni ME, Martín-Scapa C, Rodeño P, Valderrábano F, Moreno S, Bouza E. High incidence of tuberculosis in renal patients. Eur J Clin Microbiol Infect Dis. 1990;9(4):283-5.
145. Malhotra KK, Parashar MK, Sharma RK, Bhuyan UN, Dash SC, Kumar R, et al. Tuberculosis in maintenance haemodialysis patients. Study from an endemic area. Postgrad Med J. 1981;57(670):492-8.
146. Hoeppner VH, Marciniuk DD. Tuberculosis in aboriginal Canadians. Can Respir J. 2000; 7(2):141-6.
147. Stead WW, Senner JW, Reddick WT, Lofgren JP. Racial differences in susceptibility to infection by *Mycobacterium tuberculosis*. N Engl J Med. 1990;322(7):422-7.
148. Sousa AO, Salem JI, Lee FK, Verçosa MC, Cruaud P, Bloom BR, et al. An epidemic of tuberculosis with a high rate of tuberculin anergy among a population previously unexposed to tuberculosis, the Yanomami Indians of the Brazilian Amazon. Proc Natl Acad Sci, USA. 1997;94(24):13227-32.
149. Brahmajothi V, Pitchappan RM, Kakkanaiah VM, Sashidhar M, Rajaram K, Ramu S, et al. Association of pulmonary tuberculosis and HLA in south India. Tubercle. 1991;72(2): 123-32.
150. Mehra NK, Rajalingam R, Mitra DK, Taneja V, Giphart MJ. Variants of HLA-DR2/DR51 group haplotypes and susceptibility to tuberculoid leprosy and pulmonary tuberculosis in Asians Indians. Int J Lepr Other Mycobact Dis. 1995;63(2):241-8.

151. Vidal SM, Malo D, Vogan K, Skamene E, Gros P. Natural resistance to infection with intracellular parasites: isolation of a candidate for Bcg. Cell. 1993;73(3):469-85.
152. Vidal S, Tremblay ML, Govoni G, Gauthier S, Sebastiani G, Malo D, et al. The Ity/Lsh/Bcg locus: natural resistance to infection with intracellular parasites is abrogated by disruption of the Nramp1 gene. J Exp Med. 1995;182:655-66.
153. Bellamy R, Ruwende C, Corrah T, McAdam KP, Whittle HC, Hill AV, et al. Variations in the NRAMP1 gene and susceptibility to tuberculosis in West Africans. N Engl J Med. 1998;338(10):640-4.
154. Dorman SE, Picard C, Lammas D, Heyne K, van Dissel JT, Baretto R, et al. Clinical features of dominant and recessive interferon gamma receptor 1 deficiencies. Lancet. 2004;364(9451):2113-21.
155. Dorman SE, Holland SM. Mutation in the signal-transducing chain of the interferon-gamma receptor and susceptibility to mycobacterial infection. J Clin Invest. 1998;101(11):2364–9.
156. Möller M, Flachsbart F, Till A, Thye T, Horstmann RD, Meyer CG, et al. A functional haplotype in the in the 3'untranslated region of TNFRSF1B is associated with tuberculosis in two African populations. Am J Resp Crit Care Med. 2010;181(4):388-93.
157. Casali N, Nikolayevskyy V, Balabanova Y, Harris SR, Ignatyeva O, Kontsevaya I, et al. Evolution and transmission of drug-resistant tuberculosis in a Russian population. Nat Genet. 2014;46(3):279-86.

Mycobacteria: An Overview

Stuti Agarwal, Romica Latawa, Indu Verma

INTRODUCTION

Mycobacterium tuberculosis (*M. tuberculosis*) is a Gram-positive, nonmotile acid-fast bacillus (retention of carbol fuchsin dye even after treatment with acidic alcohol due to the presence of waxy mycolipids in its cell wall), which grows in the form of pleomorphic nonsporulated rods.[1] It belongs to the actinomycetes group with a length of approximately 1–4 μm and diameter of 0.3–0.6 μm. In smears stained with carbol fuchsin and examined under light microscope, the *tubercle bacilli* typically appear as pink colored straight or slightly curved rods.[2] *M. tuberculosis*, like any other bacteria, has a life cycle consisting of a lag, log, stationary and death phase. It is an obligate intracellular, slow growing aerobe that divides every 16–20 hours and has DNA with a high guanine-cytosine (GC) content (60–70%).

ROUTE AND SPREAD OF INFECTION

Mycobacterium tuberculosis commonly transmits through aerosols, enters the host via mucosal surface of the respiratory tract and harbors the lung rich in oxygen supply, which provides a suitable environment for this slow replicating pathogen. The complex immune responses mounted against *M. tuberculosis* are well defined at cellular level involving both innate and adaptive immune responses. The phagocytic cells engulf the bacteria, rapid inflammatory response is induced followed by adaptive immune response leading to accumulation of a variety of immune cells followed by the formation of granulomas, characterized by a relatively small number of infected phagocytes surrounded by activated monocytes/macrophages and activated lymphocytes.[3] One of the most remarkable features of non-sporulating *M. tuberculosis* is its ability to remain dormant within an individual for decades before reactivating into active tuberculosis (TB).[4]

Latent TB is a clinical syndrome caused by exposure to *M. tuberculosis* followed by the establishment of infection and host's immune response to control bacillary growth, forcing it into a quiescent state in the infected tissue. It is a state of mycobacteria surviving in closed necrotic lesions, characterized by reduction of bacterial metabolism, as a consequence of the action of cellular immune response. *M. tuberculosis* can surpass the immune response and breach the protective barrier and can disseminate into various organs of the body through blood and lymph. Mycobacterium can also establish itself within tissues other than lung such as lymph nodes, eye, bone, meninges, etc. causing extra-pulmonary TB. Newer sites of mycobacterial infection have also been elucidated showing presence of viable mycobacterium in kidney, liver and spleen.[5] Further, viable mycobacteria have been recovered from bone marrow mesenchymal stem cells suggesting that stem cells in bone marrow can act as favorable and protective niche for survival and persistence of mycobacteria.[6]

MYCOBACTERIAL GROUPS

The most important of mycobacterial group is *M. tuberculosis* complex (MTC), which includes *M. tuberculosis, M. leprae, M. bovis* and *M. africanum. M. tuberculosis* and *M. leprae* cause TB and leprosy respectively, in humans. *M. bovis* causes TB in cattle and humans. Some mycobacteria are saprophytes (living on decaying organic matter), while others are obligate parasites. Most are found as free-living forms in soil, water or diseased tissues of animals. The other group atypical mycobacteria that is different from typical MTC, depending upon *in vitro* characteristics is the nontuberculous mycobacteria (NTM). In 1950s, it was divided into four categories on the basis of Runyon classification: Photochromogens (pigment producing on light exposure), e.g. *M. kansasii, M. marinum*; Scotochromogens (pigment producing), e.g. *M. scrofulaceum, M. xenopi*; Nonchromogens (no pigment production), e.g. *M. avium* complex (MAC), *M. terrae* complex; and rapidly growing mycobacteria, e.g. *M. chelonae, M. fortuitum.*

Mycobacterium avium and *M. intracellulare* are closely related species commonly grouped to form MAC that is implicated as a potential pathogen for both animals and humans. Atypical mycobacteria like MAC, *M. kansasii,*

M. fortuitum and *M. chelonae* cause opportunistic infections in patients with human immunodeficiency virus (HIV)/acquired immunodeficiency syndrome (AIDS) or systemic immunosuppression of which MAC is the most common; *M. avium* being highly significant clinically. In patients with HIV infection and/or AIDS, opportunistic infections, caused by atypical mycobacteria, include the MAC, *M. kansasii, M. fortuitum* and *M. chelonae,* although these species are essentially saprophytic. *M. avium* is the most clinically significant of the environmental mycobacteria that opportunistically infects susceptible humans having systemic immunosuppression.[7] *Mycobacterium abscessus, M. massiliense* and *M. bolletii* together comprise *M. abscessus* complex, has been implicated as most common NTM in developed countries after MAC.[8]

CELL WALL STRUCTURE

Mycobacterium has an extremely uncommon cell wall structure; up to 60% of mycobacterial cell wall is composed of lipids that consist of uncommonly long-chain fatty acids with 60–90 carbons, denominated as mycolic acids. These fatty acids are covalently linked to polysaccharide, the arabinogalactan that composes the cell wall, which in turn is attached to peptidoglycan by a phosphodiester link.[9] Mycolic acids act as lipid barrier for majority of stressful conditions like osmotic shock or desiccation[2] as well as resistance to drugs.[1] Various cell envelope glycoconjugates and lipids such as phthiocerol dimycocerosate, cord factor/dimycolyltrehalose, the sulfolipids, the phosphatidylinositol mannosides, etc. intercalate with mycolic acids.[10] The unique structure and translocation of these components within the mycobacterial cell wall contribute to the antigenicity and pathogenesis of *M. tuberculosis.*[11] The mycolic acid biosynthesis and cell wall structure differ in *M. tuberculosis* lineages thus conferring variation in their pathogenic potential.[12] Majority of anti-TB drugs target mycolic acids and arabinogalactan and many compounds are synthesized that can inhibit other aspects of cell envelope metabolism such as peptidoglycan synthesis and synthesis of various glycolipids.[13] The cell wall of NTMs exhibit glycopeptidolipids that are highly specific and their absence from the cell surface confers altered colony morphology, hydrophobicity and inability to grow as biofilms.[14]

MYCOBACTERIAL GENOME

Sequencing of *M. tuberculosis* H37Rv (a virulent laboratory strain) in 1998 revealed it to possess 4,411,532 bp, the second largest microbial genome sequenced at that time.[15] Mycobacterial genome is comprised of approximately 4,000 genes and around 4% of the genome is composed of Insertion Sequences (IS) and phages. Specificity of these IS elements act as a fundamental tool for identification of different mycobacterial species. For example, IS 6,110 is the IS that is most abundantly present in *M. tuberculosis* whereas IS 1,110 and IS 1,245 are specific to *M. avium.* Approximately 8% of the total genome is involved in encoding the enzymes of lipid metabolism. On the contrary, the genome also encodes a number of lipolytic proteins that may be important in host pathogen interactions. Large novel gene families such as PE and PPE were identified which have a conserved N-terminal region with the characteristic motifs ProGlu and ProProGlu respectively. Another such class of novel mycobacterial proteins is PE proteins that belong to polymorphic guanosine-cytosine rich sequence (PGRS) family that has glycine as half of its amino acid content. These genes are considered to be important as a source of genetic diversity in *M. tuberculosis.*

Mycobacterium pathogenicity is attributed to various genes and cellular components they encode, which are known as virulence factors. The most important of these are the transcription regulators that constitute approximately 0.6% of the total mycobacterial genome and other are genes that encode for various cell surface components particularly unique to pathogenic mycobacteria. Another important functional genomic region of *M. tuberculosis* is dormancy regulon that encodes for dormancy and stress-related genes. This region is regulated by transcription factor termed as dormancy survival regulator (DosR) along with two component sensor system DosS/DosT and is responsible for persistence of bacteria in dormant state under the stress conditions such as hypoxia.[16] Another class of proteins termed as resuscitation promoting factors (Rpfs) comprises of five Rpfs (Rpf A-E) that are secretory in nature and play a role in reactivation of latent/dormant bacteria into active bacilli that can cause the disease.[17] The *in vitro* attenuation of BCG was accompanied by the loss of several major deleted regions that include 129 open reading frames (ORFs), termed as region of deletion (RD) comprising RD1-RD16.[18,19] These proteins are either secreted proteins or enzymes that have an important role in synthesis of various cell surface components and play an important role in virulence. The secreted proteins are also called as culture filtrate proteins (CFPs) due to their release in the culture media in which *M. tuberculosis* is grown.

MYCOBACTERIAL IDENTIFICATION

The most common laboratory identification of *M. tuberculosis* complex species includes smear microscopy based on Ziehl-Neelsen (ZN) staining and culture on solid egg-based LJ medium coupled with phenotypic characterization such as the growth rate, colony morphology, pigmentation and antibiotic susceptibility testing (AST). Several highly sensitive broth-based fully automated culture system (BACTEC 460 and MGIT 960) are now routinely being used in many mycobacteriology laboratories to complement microscopy as well as to increase the speed and accuracy of TB diagnosis. It is also possible to distinguish *M. tuberculosis* and *M. avium* using culture and a battery of biochemical tests, but these are complicated and time consuming. The biochemical tests, which are specific for *M. tuberculosis* are niacin reduction test, nitrate test and urease test. On the other hand, tellurite reduction and catalase tests are positive specifically for MAC species. Recently, there has been a marked increase in the development, validation and implementation of novel assays not only for the identification of *M. tuberculosis* complex but also for detection of drug resistance. A more sensitive alternative to ZN stain is auramine-rhodamine fluorochrome stain that has been introduced in many TB diagnostic laboratories throughout the world.[20]

For the identification of isoniazid (INH) and rifampin (RIF) drug resistant isolates, microscopic observation drug susceptibility (MODS) assay is an inexpensive and simple broth-microtiter method. However, the assay requires training and technical expertise along with infrastructure (BSL3 laboratory) and equipment. In addition to various nonmolecular methods, number of molecular assays had been developed to detect the presence of *M. tuberculosis* as well as resistance to INH/RIF. Line Probe Assay (LPA) involves the extraction of DNA from mycobacterial isolates followed by polymerase chain reaction (PCR) and hybridization of labelled PCR products with oligonucleotide probes immobilized on strip that are visualized colorimetrically. The assay has been recommended by World Health Organisation (WHO) in 2008 for detection of drug resistance in mycobacteria. Loop-mediated isothermal amplification assay (Eiken Chemical Company) is another molecular method for detection of *M. tuberculosis* in clinical samples. The GeneXpert *MTB*/RIF (Cepheid), which is considered as most efficient mycobacterial identification technique and being endorsed by WHO is a self-enclosed rapid PCR device that can detect *M. tuberculosis* complex and rifampin resistant mycobacterial species but is unable to detect isoniazid resistance. Lack of technical expertise and infrastructure required for these advanced molecular methods for mycobacterial identification impedes their successful implementation in developing countries.

MYCOBACTERIAL DRUG RESISTANCE

Comparative genomic analysis has revealed that *M. tuberculosis* complex has evolved by extensive horizontal gene transfer and recombination events creating several genomic and molecular changes in the *M. tuberculosis* complex. This has lead to the emergence of more host-adapted pathogenic and virulent *M. tuberculosis.* Many gene gain/loss events, mutation and conversion have arisen leading to *M. tuberculosis*-specific genetic elements that contribute to its virulence.[21,22] The gene content evolution in *M. tuberculosis* is mostly driven by uneven gene gain/loss in gene families, e.g. transposable elements and fatty acid metabolism related gene families,[23] large number of insertions and deletions (Indels) in drug-resistance associated loci and PE-PGRS related genes (contribute to antigenic variabili),[24] lineage specific changes within the amino-acid sequences of transcription regulators and nucleotide sequences of promoter sites,[25] over expression of genes related to drug efflux pumps[26] as well as chromosomal mutations like single nucleotide polymorphism.[24]

The adaptation of mycobacteria within the host leads to selection of mutations within species making it more pathogenic and virulent.[27] Whole-genome based approaches have elucidated that multi/extremely drug resistant (MDR/XDR) strains and more virulent strains of *M. tuberculosis* with enhanced resistance and fitness like Beijing are consequence of gene expansion.[28] This suggests that the development of drug resistance within clinical isolates is a highly diversified and complex process involving variations in the selection intensity of mutations. It also depends on distribution of SNPs and Indels within the genome contributing to nucleotide diversity.[24,27] As a result of these mutations, there is altered expression of various genes as well as encoding of novel functional proteins which further leads to phenotypic diversity within clinical isolates and different levels of drug resistance.[25]

To sum up, considerable information is now available regarding the chemical structure of *M. tuberculosis* unique cell envelope and *M. tuberculosis* genome which has provided a wealth of information that can be important for the understanding of the molecular basis of *M. tuberculosis* pathogenicity. This in turn can be translated into the development of new drugs, diagnostic tests and vaccines to combat TB.

REFERENCES

1. Hett EC, Rubin EJ. Bacterial growth and cell Division: a mycobacterial perspective. Microbiol Mol Biol Rev. 2008; 72(1):126-56.
2. Brennan MJ, Fruth U. Global Forum on TB Vaccine Research and Development. World Health Organization, June 7-8 2001, Geneva. Tuberculosis (Edinb). 2001;81(5-6):365-8.
3. Gonzalez-Juarrero M, Orme IM. Characterization of murine lung dendritic cells infected with *Mycobacterium tuberculosis.* Infect Immun. 2001;69(20):1127-33.
4. Cardona PJ. New insights on the nature of latent tuberculosis infection and its treatment. Inflamm Allergy Drug Targets. 2007;6(1):27-39.
5. Barrios-Payán J, Saqui-Salces M, Jeyanathan M, Alcántara-Vazquez A, Castañon-Arreola M, Rook G, et al. Extrapulmonary locations of *Mycobacterium tuberculosis* DNA during latent infection. J Infect Dis. 2012;206:1194-205.
6. Das B, Kashino SS, Pulu I, Kalita D, Swami V, Yeger H, et al. CD271(+) bone marrow mesenchymal stem cells may provide a niche for dormant *Mycobacterium tuberculosis.* Sci Transl Med. 2013;5(170):170ra13.
7. Todd JL, Lakey J, Howell D, et al. Portal hypertension and granulomatous liver disease in a lung transplant recipient due to disseminated atypical mycobacterial infection. Am J Transplant. 2007;7:1300-3.
8. Sassi M, Drancourt M. Genome analysis reveals three genomospecies in Mycobacterium abscessus. BMC Genomics. 2014;15:359.
9. Bloom WH. Gamma delta T cells and *Mycobacterium tuberculosis.* Microbes Infect. 1999;1:187-95.

10. Brennan PJ. Structure, function, and biogenesis of the cell wall of *Mycobacterium tuberculosis*. Tuberculosis. 2003;83(1-3): 91-7.
11. Angala SK, Belardinelli JM, Huc-Claustre E, Wheat WH, Jackson M. The cell envelope glycoconjugates of *Mycobacterium tuberculosis*. Crit Rev Biochem Mol Biol. 2014; 49(5):361-99.
12. Portevin D, Sukumar S, Coscolla M, Shui G, Li B, Guan XL, et al. Lipidomics and genomics of *Mycobacterium tuberculosis* reveal lineage-specific trends in mycolic acid biosynthesis. Microbiology open. 2014;3(6):823-35.
13. Jackson M, McNeil MR, Brennan PJ. Progress in targeting cell envelope biogenesis in *Mycobacterium tuberculosis*. Future Microbiol. 2013;8(7):855-75.
14. Mukherjee R, Chatterji D. Glycopeptidolipids: immunomodulators in greasy mycobacterial cell envelope. IUBMB Life. 2012;64(3):215-25.
15. Cole ST, Brosch R, Parkhill J, Garnier T, Churcher C, Harris D, et al. Deciphering the biology of *Mycobacterium tuberculosis* from the complete genome sequence. Nature. 1998;393(6685): 537-44.
16. Kumar A, Toledo JC, Patel RP, Lancaster JR Jr, Steyn AJ. *Mycobacterium tuberculosis* DosS is a redox sensor and DosT is a hypoxia sensor. Proc Natl Acad Sci USA. 2007;104(28): 11568-73.
17. Biketov S, Potapov V, Ganina E, Downing K, Kana BD, Kaprelyants A. The role of resuscitation promoting factors in pathogenesis and reactivation of *Mycobacterium tuberculosis* during intra-peritoneal infection in mice. BMC Infect Dis. 2007;7:146.
18. Behr MA, Wilson MA, Gill WP, Salamon H, Schoolnik GK, Rane S, et al. Comparative genomics of BCG vaccines by whole-genome DNA microarray. Science. 1999;284(5419):1520-3.
19. Gordon SV, Brosch R, Billault A, Garnier T, Eiglmeier K, Cole ST. Identification of variable regions in the genomes of tubercle bacilli using bacterial artificial chromosome arrays. Mol Microbiol. 1999;32:643-55.
20. Wilson ML. Recent advances in the laboratory detection of *Mycobacterium tuberculosis* complex and drug resistance. Clin Infect Dis. 2011;52(11):1350-5.
21. Wang J, Behr MA. Building a better bacillus: the emergence of *Mycobacterium tuberculosis*. Front Microbiol. 2014;5:139.
22. Boritsch EC, Supply P, Honoré N, Seemann T, Stinear TP, Brosch R. A glimpse into the past and predictions for the future: the molecular evolution of the tuberculosis agent. Mol Microbiol. 2014;93(5):835-52.
23. Librado P, Vieira FG, Sánchez-Gracia A, Kolokotronis SO, Rozas J. Mycobacterial phylogenomics: an enhanced method for gene turnover analysis reveals uneven levels of gene gain and loss among species and gene families. Genome Biol Evol. 2014;6(6):1454-65.
24. Liu F, Hu Y, Wang Q, Li HM, Gao GF, Liu CH. Comparative genomic analysis of *Mycobacterium tuberculosis* clinical isolates. BMC Genomics. 2014;15:469.
25. Graham Rose, Teresa Cortes, Iñaki Comas, Mireia Coscolla, Sebastien Gagneux, Douglas B. Young. Mapping of genotype-phenotype diversity amongst clinical isolates of *Mycobacterium tuberculosis* by sequence-based transcriptional profiling. Genome Biol Evol. 2013;5(10):1849-62.
26. Anirvan Chatterjee, Dhananjaya Saranath, Purva Bhatter, Nerges Mistry. Global transcriptional profiling of longitudinal clinical isolates of *Mycobacterium tuberculosis* exhibiting rapid accumulation of drug resistance. Plos one. 2013;8(1):e54717.
27. McGrath M, Gey van Pittius NC, van Helden PD, Warren RM, Warner DF. Mutation rate and the emergence of drug resistance in *Mycobacterium tuberculosis*. J Antimicrob Chemother. 2014;69(2):292-302.
28. Niemann S, Supply P. Diversity and evolution of *Mycobacterium tuberculosis*: moving to whole-genome-based approaches. Cold Spring Harb Perspect Med. 2014;4(12): a021188.

Immunology and Pathogenesis

Madhur Kalyan, Krishna K Singh, Indu Verma

INTRODUCTION

Mycobacterium tuberculosis, the causative agent of tuberculosis (TB) is one of the most successful human pathogens, which continues to kill worldwide more people than ever before. In approximately 5–10% of individuals who get infected with *M. tuberculosis*, the bacteria continue to replicate, resulting into clinical TB. In the remaining 90–95% of infected individuals, effective immune responses are elicited, which contain the bacteria in granulomas where they persist latently for several years. Thus, it is clear that immune responses elicited in majority of *M. tuberculosis* infected individuals are sufficient to inhibit the development of TB. This chapter is focused on providing the current understanding of the role of immune responses in pathogenesis of TB.

MYCOBACTERIUM TUBERCULOSIS INFECTION AND OVERVIEW OF IMMUNOPATHOGENESIS

Despite several recent advancements, the pathogenesis of TB is still not clearly defined. The current view of TB pathogenesis in humans can still be pictured as a multiple-stage process, which was described over a decade ago using the rabbit model of TB.[1] Overall, it is a kind of tug of war between host immune system and tubercle bacillus **(Flow chart 1)**.

The first stage starts with the inhalation of small airborne droplet (1-5 μm) containing *M. tuberculosis* expectorated by an individual with pulmonary or laryngeal TB while coughing, sneezing or talking.[2] These droplets can remain in the environment for several hours. The infectious droplets pass through the upper parts of the airways where the majority of bacilli are trapped in mucus and removed by cilia. The remaining droplets containing bacteria settle in the alveoli of distal airways where they are engulfed nonspecifically by activated alveolar macrophages, dendritic cells (DCs) and probably by alveolar epithelial cells also.[3,4]

Flow chart 1 Various stages in the pathogenesis of tuberculosis

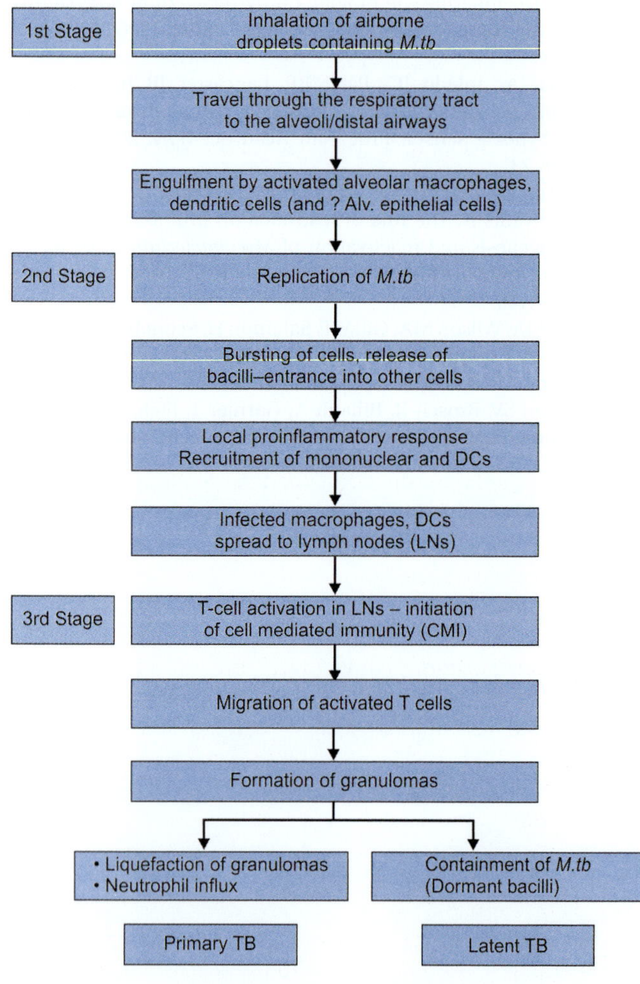

Abbreviation: DCs, dondritic cells

Being a successful human pathogen, *M. tuberculosis* has developed various strategies to avoid the intracellular killing mechanisms of host cells. Thus, the second stage begins with the replication of *bacilli* in alveolar macrophages, to some extent in DCs and possibly in alveolar epithelial cells. The bacilli multiply in these cells until they burst, the released bacilli are ingested by other alveolar macrophages. It is followed by a localized proinflammatory response leading to recruitment of mononuclear and DCs from neighboring blood vessels thus providing new host cells for the expansion of bacterial population and also inducing the alveolar macrophages to invade the lung epithelium.[5-8] The accumulation of these cells at the site of infection initiates the early lesion formation in the lung.[1,6,7] Simultaneously, the bacilli ingested macrophages and DCs disseminate to lymph nodes via the lymphatic system[2,6] or probably by the direct breaching of alveolar wall.[9]

The arrival of bacilli containing macrophages and DCs to the lymph nodes initiate the cell-mediated immunity (CMI), which is the beginning of the third stage of pathogenesis. Studies have shown that T cell activation starts in lymph nodes draining the lung and the development of CMI occurs between 2 weeks and 8 weeks post-infection in the majority of individuals.[2,10] The activation of T cells lead to their expansion followed by migration to the infection site in the lung where they activate macrophages and induce the formation of granulomas. In humans, the granuloma is a hallmark of pulmonary TB, characterized by a central acellular eosinophilic region of caseous necrosis surrounded by concentric layers of macrophages, large epithelioid cells, multinucleated giant Langhan's cells and lymphocytes.[11,12] The central necrotic core of the granuloma with sparse mycobacteria is surrounded by two layers of cells.[12] The inner layer consists of mycobacteria containing $CD68^+$ antigen presenting cells (APCs), epithelioid cells and giant Langhan's cells. This layer is also rich in $CD4^+$ T cells and $CD45RO^+$ memory cells, but $CD8^+$ T cells are rarely present.[12] The outer layer is found to contain mycobacteria infected APCs, numerous $CD4^+$ and $CD8^+$ T cells and different types of B cells ($CD23^+$ naive, $CD27^+$ memory and plasma B cells).[12] Foamy macrophages (macrophages filled with lipid containing bodies) infected with mycobacteria have been demonstrated in the interface region flanking the necrotic core in the granulomas of TB patients.[13]

During the early phase of granuloma formation, the structure is highly vascularized, however at the late stages, the caseous portion of the granuloma becomes hypoxic, bacilli stop replicating and enter into a dormant phase.[14] The infected individuals at this stage show no overt sign of disease and categorized as individuals with latent TB. Recently, a study with non-human primate model of latent TB with no clinical signs or symptoms of disease revealed the presence of metabolically active *M. tuberculosis* in the host tissues that had replicative potential.[15] Although it seems that formation of granuloma leads to containment of the pathogen, some recent studies have demonstrated that granuloma is a population of immunologically altered APCs and T lymphocytes. These populations have distinguished reduction in ability to produce type 1 cytokines such as interferon-gamma (IFN-γ) and bactericidal products such as nitric oxide (NO) while remaining proficient to produce increased levels of interleukin-10, an immunosuppressive cytokine. Hence, human granuloma seems to be not only aiding in the persistence of *M. tuberculosis* but also in bacterial transmission whenever situation is favorable.[15,16]

Although it is well known that *M. tuberculosis* may remain in a non-replicating dormant states for years together, exact niche for its survival and maintaining such a state is still not precisely known. A recent study suggested that *M. tuberculosis* may persist in a mesenchymal subpopulation of human bone marrow stem cells from patients previously treated for pulmonary TB and of mouse bone marrow stem cells from a mouse model of non-replicating *M. tuberculosis* infection.[17]

In the majority of latently infected individuals, the bacilli remain dormant for their entire life and never cause TB. Unfortunately, in some of these individuals, at the time when their immune system becomes weak, the tubercle bacilli outsmart the host immune response and start undergoing intracellular replication. This results into extensive macrophage death and necrosis and the granuloma starts liquefying to form cavity, which permits the spill of numerous viable bacilli into airways.[11,18] In late stage disease, neutrophil influx has also been implicated in the tissue damage and the dissemination of infectious bacteria into the airways in TB patients. This final stage of TB pathogenesis completes with development of productive cough, which promotes the spread of viable bacilli in the aerosol droplets to other individuals.

It is also noteworthy that although most cases of reactivation of dormant *M. tuberculosis* involves the pulmonary site, there might also be a possibility that it persists in and reactivates from other sites distinct from lungs which can subsequently cause extrapulmonary TB. Evidence of extrapulmonary reservoirs of *M. tuberculosis* came from a recent study on autopsy samples of different tissues of patients who died from causes other than TB. The presence of mycobacteria was confirmed on the basis of presence of mycobacterial deoxyribonucleic acid (DNA) in kidney, spleen and liver tissues. In addition to this, presence of ribosomal 16S ribonucleic acid (RNA) confirmed the viability of *M. tuberculosis* in these tissues.[19]

IMMUNE RESPONSES TO TUBERCULOSIS

As described above, during the entire life cycle of *M. tuberculosis* from inhalation of a few bacteria in the lung to the generation of large number of bacilli in the airway by liquefaction of granuloma, there is a constant battle between *M. tuberculosis* and immune system. Although, immune system is able to control infection in a majority of infected individuals, a small proportion of them looses this battle and develops TB. Currently, the mechanism of immune defense against mycobacteria is not clearly known; however, our understanding has considerably increased due to elegant studies performed in the past decade. These studies have demonstrated that both innate and adaptive immune systems are involved in providing immunity against *M. tuberculosis* **(Table 1)**. The following sections are aimed to describe current knowledge about innate and adaptive immunity to TB.

Table 1 Different components of immune responses in tuberculosis

- Innate immunity
  - Role of receptors
  - Role of phagocytic and other cells
- Cytokines and chemokines bridging the innate and adaptive immunity
- Adaptive immunity
  - Cell-mediated immunity
    - i. Role of $CD4^+/CD8^+$ T-cells
    - ii. Role of regulatory T (T_{reg}) cells
    - iii. Role of γδ T-cells
    - iv. Role of memory T (T_M) cells
    - v. Role of unconventional T-cells
  - Humoral immunity – Role of B-cell

Innate Immunity

In general, innate immune system recognizes microbe immediately after infection by using receptors and induces secretion of a range of chemokines and cytokines, which direct the recruitment of various immune cells, including the phagocytic cells to the site of infection to kill the microbes. Although, the mechanism of innate immunity during *M. tuberculosis* infection is poorly understood, the contribution of different components of innate immune system is discussed.

Role of Receptors

M. tuberculosis interacts with many host receptors once it enters into the lungs, the most important being pattern recognition receptors (PRRs). These PRRs include toll-like receptors (TLRs), nucleotide-binding and oligomerization domain (NOD)-like Receptors (NLRs) and dectin-1.[6,20] Other receptors involved in this interaction include complement receptor 3 (CR3), mannose receptor (MR), scavenger receptor, DC-specific intercellular adhesion-molecule-3-grabbing non-integrin (DC-SIGN) on the surface of macrophages and DCs. TLRs are transmembrane receptors present on macrophages, DCs, B cells, specific types of T cells, as well as on fibroblasts and epithelial cells.[21] The role of various TLRs in *M. tuberculosis* infection is not clearly understood, but it is likely that TLR2, TLR4 and TLR9 are involved in signaling innate immune responses against *M. tuberculosis* infection and mycobacterial proteome and lipids.[6] TLR9 is found to recognize mycobacterial DNA and signals synthesis of proinflammatory cytokines.[6] Activation of TLRs also leads to upregulated expression of the vitamin D receptor (VDR) and the vitamin D-1-hydroxylase genes resulting in the induction of the antimicrobial peptides cathelicidin and β-defensin to kill intracellular mycobacteria.[22,23] It has been demonstrated by in vivo infections and human genetic studies that TLRs are not critical for restricting *M. tuberculosis* growth, since they have partially redundant nature in controlling the TB infection. In addition, it has also been demonstrated that MYD88, which is involved in TLRs signaling, and not TLR 2, 4 or 9, plays an essential role in protection against TB.[14,24]

Another transmembrane PRR, dectin-1 is found on macrophages and DCs and binds to β-glucan.[21] Although, dectin-1 plays an important role in antimicrobial response in fungal infections, involvement of dectin-1 in mycobacterial infection is not well studied.[21] It has also been demonstrated that NOD2, which belongs to NLRs family of cytosolic receptor proteins recognizes muramyl dipeptide and induces the production of proinflammatory cytokines following interaction with *M. tuberculosis*.[20] NOD2 and dectin-1 cooperate with TLR-2 during interaction with *M. tuberculosis* to activate NF-κB and induce proinflammatory cytokines. Amongst complement receptors, the phagocytosis of *M. tuberculosis* via CR3 has been found to prevent respiratory burst leading to phagosomal arrest of early endosomes and no inflammatory response.[6] Mannose receptor mediates phagocytosis by binding to mannosylated lipoarabinomannan (ManLAM) of *M. tuberculosis*, which results in the inhibition of phagosome-lysosome fusion leading to increased survival of *M. tuberculosis* in macrophages.[6] Number of host components, such as surfactant protein-A (SP-A) and D (SP-D) also affect the uptake and survival of *M. tuberculosis* in macrophages.[6]

Role of Phagocytic and Other Cells

Macrophages and DCs comprise the major phagocytic cells in immunity against TB. The uptake of *M. tuberculosis* by alveolar macrophages represents the first step in the innate host defense against TB. Following mycobacterial infection, macrophages can differentiate either into type 1 or type 2 macrophages producing IL-23 or IL-10 respectively. Thus, leading to either protection or suppression of immunity to TB.[25] The type 2 macrophages that produce IL-10 can also promote adoption of T-regulatory (T_{reg}) phenotype by $CD4^+$ T cells.[26] Antimycobacterial potential of macrophages is triggered by an important stimulating mediator IFN-γ.[27,28] A key effector mechanism responsible for the anti-mycobacterial action of IFN-γ is by the induction of NO and related reactive nitrogen intermediates via the activity of inducible form of nitric oxide synthase (NOS).[29,30] Along with IFN-γ, TNF-α and IL-1α also stimulate the production of NO in macrophages. The precise mechanism by which NO and other reactive nitrogen species antagonize *M. tuberculosis* is not known. Recently, it has been demonstrated that NO controls the tissue damaging effects of IL-1β via inhibition of inflammasome, a component of innate immune system, since it is involved in production of IL-1β from macrophages and DCs following activation of caspase-1 which leads to maturation and activation of this cytokine.[31-33]

In spite of the potent bactericidal activity of macrophages, *M. tuberculosis* is able to survive and replicate in these cells by avoiding the killing mechanisms. It has been shown that *M. tuberculosis* survive inside macrophage by avoiding the fusion of phagosomes with lysosomes.[6,34] Retention of early endosomal markers by *M. tuberculosis* vacuole longer than normal maturing phagosomes suggested a defect in maturation of *M. tuberculosis* phagosome.[35] *M. tuberculosis* phagosomes are shown to be deficient in lysosomal hydrolases and vesicular proton-adenosine triphosphatase (v-ATPase) required for the acidification of phagosomes.[6,35] Furthermore, *M. tuberculosis* is observed to prevent the accumulation of phosphatidylinositol-3-phosphate (PI3P) on phagosome, which is a host membrane protein and essential for the biosynthesis of phagolysosome.[35-39]

It has been proposed that as a consequence of binding of a mycobacterial lipoprotein, known as LprG, to lipoarabinomannan (LAM) facilitates its movement into the cell envelop from plasma membrane thus increasing LAM exposed on the surface and hence integrity of the cell envelop. This subsequently inhibits the phagosome-lysosome fusion and hence enhanced survival of *M. tuberculosis* inside the macrophages.[40] Another escape mechanism involves enhanced intracellular survival (EIS) protein, secreted by *M. tuberculosis,* which prevents natural killer (NK) cell-dependent reactive oxygen species (ROS) generation via its aminoglycosyl aminotransferase activity.[41]

It has also been shown that plasma membrane cholesterol is essential for the phagocytosis of *M. tuberculosis* by macrophages and it aids in preventing phagosome-lysosome fusion by mediating the phagosomal association with tryptophan aspartate-containing coat protein (TACO), which avoid lysosomal degradation of *M. tuberculosis.*[42] Although, these studies provide a glimpse of the *M. tuberculosis* components involved in the blocking of phagosome-lysosome fusion, more research is needed to completely understand the role of *M. tuberculosis* molecules in its survival inside the macrophages.

M. tuberculosis enters DCs via binding with DC-SIGN receptors.[4] Mycobacterial ManLAM has been found to be ligand for DC-SIGN and binding of ManLAM with DC-SIGN inhibits the maturation of DCs.[43] In vivo, it seems that similar to *M. tuberculosis* receptor, DC-SIGN is also utilized by human immunodeficiency virus (HIV) for its entry in these cells and might account for several pathological and immunological aspects of *M. tuberculosis* infection in subjects coinfected with HIV.[44] Both macrophages and DCs can inhibit mycobacterial growth in NO dependent manner; however, in vitro studies have demonstrated that macrophages are more efficient in killing *M. tuberculosis* than DCs.[45]

Amongst the other cells that are involved in immunity against TB are the NK cells and neutrophils. NK cells are one of the major components of innate immune system and provide the first line of defense against infection.[46] Role of human NK cells in protection against *M. tuberculosis* infection is demonstrated by in vitro studies, which showed that NK cells can directly lead to lysis or apoptosis of *M. tuberculosis* infected monocytes and macrophages.[20]A recent study showed that NK cells restrict the growth of *M. tuberculosis* in macrophages via production of IL-22, which increases the phagosome-lysosome fusion.[47] NK cells can also regulate the expansion and cytotoxicity of $CD8^+$ T cells for lysis of *M. tuberculosis* infected monocytes. These cells have also been found to be a potent early source of cytokines particularly IFN-γ, IL-5, IL-13 and IL-10[46] that play important roles such as in increasing phagosome-lysosome fusion and in regulating expansion of cytotoxicity of $CD8^+$ T cells for lysis of *M. tuberculosis* infected monocytes.[20,46] Another study has demonstrated the direct killing effects of NK cells through the release of perforins and granulysins.[48]

Just like NK cells, neutrophils also have been shown to have a protective role in against *M. tuberculosis,* at least in the early stages of TB infection, as these are attracted to the site of infection thereby restricting the growth of *M. tuberculosis* and secreting various chemokines and cytokines on interaction with *M. tuberculosis.*[20] It is also observed that the ingestion of apoptotic neutrophils by macrophages enhances *M. tuberculosis* killing.[20,49]

Antimicrobial peptides, known as naturally occurring antibiotics, are not only one of the important constituents of innate immunity but also serve as signaling molecules in regulation of both innate and adaptive immune system. Cathelicidin, defensin, and hepcidin are the AMPs that have anti-mycobacterial actions. In addition to direct killing cathelicidin has also been shown to act as an immunomodulator.[50] The defensins are the most profuse type of peptides present in mammals. Majority of peptides produced by neutrophils are human neutrophil defensins or human neutrophil peptides. These peptides have been shown to co-localize with *M. tuberculosis* in the early endosomes, following engulfment of infected neutrophils by macrophages, as a result of which bacterial burden is reduced. In addition to the direct killing effects, defensins also trigger the T Helper Cells (Th1) response resulting in enhanced production of proinflammatory cytokines (TNF-α, IL-12, IFN-γ) and hence protection against TB.[51]

Cytokines and Chemokines Bridging the Innate and Adaptive Immunity

An efficient control of mycobacterial infection requires an effective balance between innate and adaptive immune responses mediated by cytokines and chemokines that develop proper inflammatory response. The control of *M. tuberculosis* infection depends on the appropriate development of inflammatory responses because improper responses can cause chronic infection and associated pathology. IL-12 secreted from infected macrophages and DCs induces IFN-γ which ultimately leads to down modulation of IL-10 and IL-4 and hence results in differentiation of T cells to Th1 cells. Infected macrophages and DCs produce IL-12, a crucial cytokine in controlling early *M. tuberculosis* infection.[52,53] IL-12 induces the secretion of IFN-γ and down modulation of IL-10 and IL-4 that results in the differentiation of naive T cells to Th1 cells. IL-12 therefore provides an important link between innate and adaptive immune system.[53] Secretion of IFN-γ from activated T cells as well as NK cells can promote bacterial killing through reactive nitrogen intermediates (RNI) and ROS production from macrophages as well as by induction of autophagy in macrophages.[54-57]

Role of IFN-γ in human TB has been demonstrated by studies which show that those individuals are more susceptible to infections with mycobacteria having defect in either IFN-γ or IFN-γ receptor genes.[58] Besides IFN-γ, TNF-α, a proinflammatory cytokine secreted by macrophages, DCs and T cells also enhance the killing of mycobacteria intracellularly as well as formation of granuloma by induction of RNI and IFN-γ.[52,59] The role of TNF-α in protective immunity against *M. tuberculosis* in human is suggested by studies showing increased susceptibility to develop TB in Crohn's disease and rheumatoid arthritis patients using anti-TNF-α antibodies.[54] IL-10 is shown to be upregulated in TB and inhibition of IL-10 has been shown to partially restore the suppression of T cell proliferation.[54] In anergic TB patients, increased production of IL-10 also suggests its role in effective suppression of host immune response.[6]

IL-4 is another anti-inflammatory cytokine that has been implicated in various intracellular infections including *M. tuberculosis* for its harmful effects by suppressing IFN-γ production and macrophage activation.[60]Another anti-inflammatory cytokine that is implicated in suppressing protective immunity to *M. tuberculosis* is transforming growth factor (TGF)-β.[61] Production of TGF-β by monocytes and DCs is induced by mycobacterial components specifically by ManLAM.[60,61] An increased production of TGF-β is observed in blood mononuclear cells and lung lesion of TB patients.[61] TGF-β is also found to promote production and deposition of macrophage collagenases and collagen matrix suggesting its role in tissue damage and fibrosis during TB.[60] Inhibition of IFN-γ induced NOS2 production is shown to be responsible for deactivation of macrophages by TGF-β.[52] Also, TGF-β induces secretion of another anti-inflammatory cytokine IL-10 and both the cytokines have been observed to act in synergy for suppression of IFN-γ production.[60]

In addition to the above mentioned cytokines, several investigators have shown that *M. tuberculosis* or its components induce chemokines from monocytes, macrophages, multinucleated giant cells, DCs, granulocytes, etc.[6,62,63] Evidence for in vivo production of chemokines in humans during *M. tuberculosis* infection is provided by studies showing increased levels of CCL2, CCL5, CCL7, CCL12, CXCL8 and CXCL10 in bronchoalveolar lavage (BAL) fluid from TB patients.[63] Various in vitro and in vivo studies suggest that cytokine TNF-α regulates the expression of chemokines during *M. tuberculosis* infection.[62,63] Since, TNF-α is shown to play a crucial role in granuloma formation, whether chemokines are also involved in granuloma formation is not known.

Adaptive Immunity

Although, *M. tuberculosis* infection elicits both humoral and cell mediated immune responses, due to intracellular residence of *M. tuberculosis*, it is well accepted that only cell-mediated immunity provides protection against TB.[52,64] In recent years, it has been shown that humoral immune responses also play important role in protection to TB.[65,66]

Cell-mediated Immunity

The T cells which comprise of $CD4^+$ T Helper Cells (Th), $CD8^+$ Cytotoxic T cells (CTLs), γδT cells, regulatory T cells (T reg cells), memory T cells and unconventional CD1 restricted T cells play main role in providing CMI.

Role of $CD4^+$/$CD8^+$ T cells: In human, the protective role of $CD4^+$ T cells during *M. tuberculosis* infection has been suggested by enhanced occurrence of both primary and reactivated TB in HIV infected individuals showing loss of these cells.[52,64]Although, the mechanism of protection by $CD4^+$ T cells is not clear, so far studies suggest that during *M. tuberculosis* infection, $CD4^+$ T cells of Th1 type activate macrophages primarily through IFN-γ production, which results in the induction of enzymes inducible nitric oxide synthase or nitric oxide synthase 2 (iNOS or NOS2) and phagocyte oxidase (NOX2/ gp91phox) to produce mycobactericidal RNI and ROI respectively.[55,67] Although, these studies suggested that $CD4^+$ T cells controls *M. tuberculosis* infection via IFN-γ production, other antimycobacterial mechanisms suggested for these cells include apoptosis of infected macrophages, release of ATP and Lymphotoxin α3 (LTα3) or TNF-β for control of *M. tuberculosis* infection.[55,68]

Th17 is a newly identified subset of Th cells which secrete proinflammatory cytokine IL-17. Recruitment of neutrophils for pulmonary inflammatory responses, IFN-γ production by T cells and efficient granuloma formation in lungs are attributed to IL-17 in response to infection with *Bacillus Calmette-Guérin* (BCG). Subsequent exposure of the vaccinated mice to *M. tuberculosis* increases Th1 responses mediated by IL-17.[69] Evidences also suggest that IL-17 produced by γδT cells is important during the early stages of infection, is associated with accelerated recruitment of neutrophils that is dependent on the presence of IL-23, a cytokine produced mainly by DCs.[70] In a recent study, it was found that when mice were infected with hypervirulent *M. tuberculosis* HN878, IL-17 was found to be protective as a result of stout production of IL-1β which leads to strong IL-17 responses.[71]

Despite potent abilities of $CD4^+$ T cells to control *M. tuberculosis* infection, existence of persistent infection in the majority of *M. tuberculosis* infected individuals suggests that these cells are ineffective in eliminating the *M. tuberculosis* infection. Although, reasons are not clearly known, it has been shown that *M. tuberculosis* infection leads to the reduction in expression of MHC class II molecules on the macrophage surface and hence the process of antigen presentation to $CD4^+$ T cells.[52] *M. tuberculosis* infection of mice with either β2-microglobulin or transporter associated with antigen processing (TAP) gene disruption, which results in the lack of both major histocompatibility complex (MHC) class I (class Ia and class Ib) molecules and $CD8^+$ T cells has demonstrated that control of *M. tuberculosis* infection also requires $CD8^+$ T cells.[52,72,73] Since *M. tuberculosis* resides in phagosomes, it is still unclear how *M. tuberculosis* antigens gain access to the MHC class I processing system. It has been suggested that *M. tuberculosis* perforates the membrane of phagosome by which its antigens translocate to MHC class I pathway.[52,55]

Other studies have provided evidence against the translocation of molecules from phagosomes to cytoplasm.[55] Although, the main function of the $CD8^+$ T cells is the lysis of infected cells, it is also most likely that IFN-γ from $CD8^+$ T cells activates macrophages and participates in the killing of *M. tuberculosis* as described above for $CD4^+$ T cells. However, unlike $CD4^+$ T cells, very low spontaneous IFN-γ production by $CD8^+$ T cells is observed.[52] The $CD8^+$ T cells can lyse the infected cells by using perforin and granulysin or Fas/FasL pathway.[52] Perforin forms pore and granulysin is required to kill the intracellular organism.[55] It has also been suggested that the infected cell lysis by $CD8^+$ T cells promotes the control of *M. tuberculosis* infection by the release of *M. tuberculosis* from incapacitated cells and their subsequent phagocytosis by activated macrophages.[55]

Role of regulatory T (T_{reg}) cells: T_{reg} cells express CD4, CD25 and foxp3 and are found to suppress the proliferation and function of $CD4^+CD25$ cells and inhibit the production of IFN-γ by secreting IL-10 and TGF-β.[74] Besides $CD4^+CD25^+foxp3^+$ T_{reg} cell subsets, $CD8^+$ T_{reg} cells that inhibit the T cell proliferation and production of cytokines are also described.[75] During *M. tuberculosis* infection in mice, T_{reg} cells proliferate and accumulate at the site of infection and prevent efficient clearance of infection.[76] It has also been described by a study that TB patients have more T_{reg} cells than healthy tuberculin responders and these cells inhibit BCG induced IFN-γ production by $CD4^+$ T cells.[76,77] Furthermore, expansion of T_{reg} cells in response to *M. tuberculosis* infection is shown to be dependent on ManLAM and production of prostaglandin E2 by monocytes.[76] *M. tuberculosis* infection promotes the expansion of T_{reg} cells that are able to suppress the protective immune responses developed against its own infection. Simultaneous inhibition of Th2 and T_{reg} cells by using the pharmacological inhibitors suplatast tosylate and D4476 respectively, not only enhanced *M. tuberculosis* clearance and induced superior Th1 responses but also increased the vaccine efficacy of BCG in studies with mouse.[78]

Role of γδT cells: During mycobacterial infection, γδT cells are rapidly recruited to lung, secrete IFN-γ and kill *M. tuberculosis* infected cells.[79,80] In humans, γδT cells recognize mycobacterial non-peptidic phosphoantigens without any requirement for MHC molecules leading to the secretion of Th1 cytokines primarily IFN- and killing of *M. tuberculosis* infected cells.[79] The occurrence of increased size of granuloma and enhanced numbers of neutrophils in granuloma of *M. tuberculosis* infected γδT cell receptor-knockout mice suggested that γδT cells are involved in the regulation of granuloma formation.[80] The involvement of γδT cells in providing protection against *M. tuberculosis* infection in humans has been demonstrated by studies, which showed decreased number of Vγ9Vδ2 T cells in the blood and lung of pulmonary TB patients, as well as diminished ability of Vγ9Vδ2 T cells from TB patients to expand in response to *M. tuberculosis* or its antigens.[80] Together these studies suggest that γδT cells contribute to protective immunity against *M. tuberculosis* infection.

Role of memory T (T_M) cells: Although, role of T_M cells in providing protection against *M. tuberculosis* infection is poorly defined, persistence of latent *M. tuberculosis* infection in most of the infected individuals suggest the involvement of these cells in controlling *M. tuberculosis* infection during latency. In humans, there are two types of T_M cells; Effector memory T cells (T_{EM}) with CCR7, CD62L, CD69 and central memory T cells (T_{CM}) with CCR7, CD62L, CD69.[81] *M. tuberculosis* infection in mice induces antigen specific T_M cells; however, these memory responses provide only short term protection.[64,72] Similarly, occurrence of *M. tuberculosis* reinfection in cured TB patients suggests that either no T_M cells are induced or these cells are unable to provide protection. It has been proposed that efficient activation of effector T cells for long time by persistent antigens can exhaust memory and cause no memory in extreme cases like in TB patients.[81] Vaccination with BCG and MVA85A has been shown to induce long lasting polyfunctional *M. tuberculosis* specific $CD4^+$ T_M cells.[82]

Role of unconventional T cells: In addition to MHC class I restricted $CD8^+$ T cells, presence of non-classically restricted $CD8^+$ T cells have also been observed during *M. tuberculosis* infection in humans.[52,55] Group I CD1 molecules, which are structurally similar to MHC class I molecules have been found to present several lipids and glycolipid antigens of mycobacterial cell wall to non-classically restricted $CD8^+$ T cells resulting into release of IFN-γ and expression of cytolytic activity.[52,55] Group I CD1a and CD1c can easily have access to mycobacterial antigens in phagosomes whereas group I CD1b molecules can primarily interact with those mycobacterial antigens that are shed inside the phagosomes and enter into late endosomes/lysosomes.[52,55] As group I CD1 molecules are primarily found on DCs and almost absent on macrophages, the CD1 presentation therefore requires transfer of mycobacterial antigens from infected macrophages to bystander DCs.[55] The natural killer T cells (NKT) are also unconventional T cells that are group II CD1d restricted and stimulated by glycolipid antigens of mycobacterial cell wall. In vitro studies showed that human activated NKT cells express granulysin and can kill *M. tuberculosis.*[83]

Another non-classical antigen presenting molecules H2-M3, a type of murine MHC class Ib molecules have been reported in mouse TB model and shown to present N-formylated peptides to $CD8^+$ T cells.[52,55] It is also shown that lysis of *M. tuberculosis* infected macrophages is brought about by IFN-γ produced by $CD4^+$ and $CD8^+$ cells that are specific for mycobacterial N-formylated peptides. The $CD8^+$ and $CD4^+$ T cells specific for mycobacterial N-formylated peptides are shown to produce IFN-γ and lyse *M. tuberculosis* infected macrophages.[52] Since homologues of H2-M3 molecules in humans are not identified, their role in human TB is not known.[55] $CD8^+$ T cells restricted by non-classical molecules, but not CD1 restricted have been found in *M. tuberculosis* infected humans.[52] Another class of unconventional T cells are the mucosal associated invariant T cells (MAIT). It has been shown in an aerosol low dose *M. bovis* BCG model of infection that MAIT cell deficient mice had higher bacterial loads at early times after infection. The inhibition of intracellular growth of *M. bovis* BCG, inside the macrophages, by MAIT cells is thought to be brought about through the production of IFN-γ.[84]

Humoral Immunity

Historically, it is accepted that B cells play no significant role in providing protection against *M. tuberculosis* infection.[65,66,85,86] Although, studies of *M. tuberculosis* infection in B cell deficient mice have yielded variable results, data from *M. tuberculosis* infected B cell deficient mice and polymeric immunoglobulin (Ig) receptor knockout mice deficient in secretory IgA have convincingly demonstrated a role of B cells and antibodies in protection against *M. tuberculosis* infection.[65,66] Protection observed by the administration of intravenous immunoglobulin (IVIg) against *M. tuberculosis* infection in mice and by passive serum therapy with anti-*M. tuberculosis* polyclonal antibodies to reactivation of TB in severe combined immunodeficiency (SCID) mice further, support the role of humoral components in host defense to TB.[65,66] Monoclonal antibodies against several mycobacterial antigens, such as arabinomannan (AM), LAM, 16-kDaα-crystallin, heparin-binding hemagglutinin (HBHA) and MPB83 have been demonstrated to provide protection against TB in mice.[65,86] Following *M. tuberculosis* infection, B cells have also been found to influence the T cell activation by regulating antigen presentation, as well as the modulation of cytokine profile thereby influencing the disease outcome.[66,87]

Interestingly, an *M. tuberculosis* AM-Ag85B conjugated vaccine that induce both humoral and cellular immune responses has been observed to provide protection against *M. tuberculosis* infection in mice, rabbits and guinea pigs similar to BCG.[65,66] Although, in humans, evidence for the role of B cells in immunity against *M. tuberculosis* infection is not available, presence of follicle like B cell aggregates in the periphery of granuloma in the lung of TB patients suggest their role for maintaining the granuloma during *M. tuberculosis* infection.[12,66] A study conducted on non-human primate demonstrated that B cells, plasma cells and antibodies are enriched within the granuloma. These antibodies might have the ability to amend local control of infection in tissues. Still the role of these antibodies in protection, disease pathology or immune modulation in TB is not understood and hence further studies are required.[88] The demonstration of significantly enhanced internalization and growth inhibition of BCG by neutrophil and monocyte/macrophages in the presence of serum from BCG vaccinated individuals and reversal of these effects by the depletion of IgG from serum suggest the involvement of antimycobacterial antibodies in protection against *M. tuberculosis* infection in humans.[65] Together studies conducted in recent years, support the role of humoral immune responses in defense against *M. tuberculosis* infection.

In conclusion, a complex interaction of multiple cell types of host immune system is important for optimal immunity against mycobacteria. The cross talk between *M. tuberculosis* and the host immune system determines the infection outcome. Once *M. tuberculosis* is taken up by alveolar macrophages, possibly by other cells too, and if infection is established, activation of macrophages, DCs, NK cells and T cells lead to production of various chemokines and cytokines that regulate a central non-specific inflammatory immune response. Fate of infection is determined by this initial response which either leads to progressive growth of *M. tuberculosis* or the containment of infection. An efficient means of developing better anti-TB vaccines and treatment strategies is dependent on the understanding of complex network of immune response elicited by the host against this pathogen. Additionally, better animal model and human oriented studies as well as genetic manipulation of mycobacteria could be important for the understanding of such a successful pathogen.

REFERENCES

1. Dannenberg AM, Rook G. Pathogenesis of pulmonary tuberculosis: an interplay of tissue-damaging and macrophage activating immune responses-dual mechanisms that control bacillary multiplication. In: Bloom B. (Ed). Tuberculosis: Pathogenesis, Protection and Control. Washington, DC: American Society for Microbiology; 1994. pp. 459-83.
2. Frieden TR, Sterling TR, Munsiff SS, Watt CJ, Dye C. Tuberculosis. Lancet. 2003;362(9387):887-99.

3. Hernández-Pando R, Jeyanathan M, Mengistu G, Aguilar D, Orozco H, Harboe M, et al. Persistence of DNA from *Mycobaterium tuberculosis* in superficially normal lung tissue during latent infection. Lancet. 2000;356(9248):2133-8.
4. Herrmann JL, Lagrange PH. Dendritic cells and *Mycobacterium tuberculosis*: which is the Trojan horse? Pathol Biol (Paris). 2005;53(1):35-40.
5. Russell DG, Barry CE 3rd, Flynn JL. Tuberculosis: what we don't know can, and does, hurt us. Science. 2010;328(5980):852-6.
6. Tsolaki AG. Innate immune recognition in tuberculosis infection. In: Kishore U (Ed). Target pattern recognition in innate immunity. New York: Landes Bioscience and Springer Science Business Media; 2009. pp. 185-97.
7. Russell DG. *Mycobacterium tuberculosis*: here today, and here tomorrow. Nat Rev Mol Cell Biol. 2001;2(8):569-77.
8. Russell DG, Cardona PJ, Kim MJ, Allain S, Altare F. Foamy macrophages and the progression of the human tuberculosis granuloma. Nat Immunol. 2009;10(9):943-8.
9. Pethe K, Alonso S, Biet F, Delogu G, Brennan MJ, Locht C, et al. The heparin-binding haemagglutinin of *M. tuberculosis* is required for extrapulmonary dissemination. Nature. 2001;412(6843):190-4.
10. Cooper AM, Khader SA. The role of cytokines in the initiation, expansion, and control of cellular immunity to tuberculosis. Immunol Rev. 2008;226:191-204.
11. Saunders BM, Britton WJ. Life and death in the granuloma: immunopathology of tuberculosis. Immunol Cell Biol. 2007;85(2):103-11.
12. Ulrichs T, Kosmiadi GA, Trusov V, Jörg S, Pradl L, Titukhina M, et al. Human tuberculous granulomas induce peripheral lymphoid follicle-like structures to orchestrate local host defence in the lung. J Pathol. 2004;204(2):217-28.
13. Peyron P, Vaubourgeix J, Poquet Y, Levillain F, Botanch C, Bardou F, et al. Foamy macrophages from tuberculous patients' granulomas constitute a nutrient-rich reservoir for *M. tuberculosis* persistence. PLoS Pathog. 2008;4(11):e1000204.
14. Via LE, Lin PL, Ray SM, Carrillo J, Allen SS, Eum SY, et al. Tuberculous granulomas are hypoxic in guinea pigs, rabbits, and nonhuman primates. Infect Immun. 2008;76(6):2333-40.
15. Yuk JM, Jo EK. Host immune responses to mycobacterial antigens and their implications for the development of a vaccine to control tuberculosis. Clin Exp Vaccine Res. 2014;3(2):155-67.
16. Shaler CR, Horvath CN, Jeyanathan M, Xing Z. Within the enemy's camp: contribution of the granuloma to the dissemination, persistence and transmission of Myco*bacterium tuberculosis*. Front Immunol. 2013;4:30.
17. Das B, Kashino SS, Pulu I, Kalita D, Swami V, Yeger H, et al. CD271 (+) bone marrow mesenchymal stem cells may provide a niche for dormant *Mycobacterium tuberculosis*. Sci Transl Med. 2013;5(170):170ra13.
18. Russell DG. Who puts the tubercle in tuberculosis? Nat Rev Microbiol. 2007;5(1):39-47.
19. Barrios-Payán J, Saqui-Salces M, Jeyanathan M, Alcántara-Vazquez A, Castañon-Arreola M, Rook G, et al. Extrapulmonary locations of *Mycobacterium tuberculosis* DNA during latent infection. J Infect Dis. 2012;206(8):1194-205.
20. Korbel DS, Schneider BE, Schaible UE. Innate immunity in tuberculosis: myths and truth. Microbes Infect. 2008;10(9):995-1004.
21. Medzhitov R. Recognition of microorganisms and activation of the immune response. Nature. 2007;449(7164):819-26.
22. Liu PT, Stenger S, Li H, Wenzel L, Tan BH, Krutzik SR, et al. Toll-like receptor triggering of a vitamin D-mediated human antimicrobial response. Science. 2006;311(5768):1770-3.
23. Liu PT, Stenger S, Tang DH, Modlin RL. Cutting edge: vitamin D mediated human antimicrobial activity against *Mycobacterium tuberculosis* is dependent on the induction of cathelicidin. J Immunol. 2007;179(4):2060-3.
24. Hölscher C, Reiling N, Schaible UE, Hölscher A, Bathmann C, Korbel D, et al. Containment of aerogenic *Mycobacterium tuberculosis* infection in mice does not require MyD88 adaptor function for TLR2, -4 and -9. Eur J Immunol. 2008;38(3): 680-94.
25. Verreck FA, de Boer T, Langenberg DM, Hoeve MA, Kramer M, Vaisberg E, et al. Human IL-23- producing type 1 macrophages promote but IL-10-producing type 2 macrophages subvert immunity to (myco)bacteria. Proc Natl Acad Sci USA. 2004;101(13):4560-5.
26. Savage ND, de Boer T, Walburg KV, Joosten SA, van Meijgaarden K, Geluk A, et al. Human anti-inflammatory macrophages induce Foxp3+ GITR+ CD25+ regulatory T cells, which suppress via membrane-bound TGFbeta-1. J Immunol. 2008;181(3):2220-6.
27. Rook GA, Steele J, Ainsworth M, Champion BR. Activation of macrophages to inhibit proliferation of *Mycobacterium tuberculosis*: comparison of the effects of recombinant gamma interferon on human monocytes and murine peritoneal macrophages. Immunology. 1986;59(3):333-8.
28. Flesch I, Kaufmann SH. Mycobacterial growth inhibition by interferon-gamma-activated bone marrow macrophages and differential susceptibility among strains of *Mycobacterium tuberculosis*. J Immunol. 1987;138(12):4408-13.
29. Chan J, Xing Y, Magliozzo RS, Bloom BR. Killing of virulent *Mycobacterium tuberculosis* by reactive nitrogen intermediates produced by activated murine macrophages. J Exp Med. 1992;175(4):1111-22.
30. Denis M. Interferon-gamma-treated murine macrophages inhibit growth of tubercle bacilli via the generation of reactive nitrogen intermediates. Cell Immunol. 1991;132(1):150-7.
31. Mishra BB, Rathinam VA, Martens GW, Martinot AJ, Kornfeld H, Fitzgerald KA, et al. Nitric oxide controls the immunopathology of tuberculosis by inhibiting NLRP3 inflammasome-dependent processing of IL-1β. Nat Immunol. 2013;14(1):52-60.
32. Rayamajhi M, Miao EA. Just say NO to NLRP3. Nat Immunol. 2013;14(1):12-4.
33. Briken V, Ahlbrand SE, Shah S. *Mycobacterium tuberculosis* and the host cell inflammasome: a complex relationship. Front Cell Infect Microbiol. 2013;3:62.
34. Armstrong JA, Hart PD. Response of cultured macrophages to *Mycobacterium tuberculosis*, with observations on fusion of lysosomes with phagosomes. J Exp Med. 1971;134(3 Pt 1): 713-40.
35. Philips JA. Mycobacterial manipulation of vacuolar sorting. Cell Microbiol. 2008;10(12):2408-15.
36. Via LE, Deretic D, Ulmer RJ, Hibler NS, Huber LA, Deretic V. Arrest of mycobacterial phagosome maturation is caused by a block in vesicle fusion between stages controlled by rab5 and rab7. J Biol Chem. 1997;272(20):13326-31.
37. Vergne I, Chua J, Deretic V. Tuberculosis toxin blocking phagosome maturation inhibits a novel Ca2+/calmodulin-PI3K hVPS34 cascade. J Exp Med. 2003;198(4):653-9.
38. Vergne I, Chua J, Lee HH, Lucas M, Belisle J, Deretic V. Mechanism of phagolysosome biogenesis block by viable

Mycobacterium tuberculosis. Proc Natl Acad Sci USA. 2005;102(11):4033-8.
39. Pieters J. *Mycobacterium tuberculosis* and the macrophage: maintaining a balance. Cell Host Microbe. 2008;3(6):399-407.
40. Shukla S, Richardson ET, Athman JJ, Shi L, Wearsch PA, McDonald D, et al. *Mycobacterium tuberculosis* lipoprotein LprG binds lipoarabinomannan and determines its cell envelope localization to control phagolysosomal fusion. PLoS Pathog. 2014;10(10):e1004471.
41. BoseDasgupta S, Pieters J. Striking the right balance determines TB or not TB. Front Immunol. 2014;5:455.
42. Gatfield J, Pieters J. Essential role for cholesterol in entry of mycobacteria into macrophages. Science. 2000;288(5471):1647- 50.
43. Geijtenbeek TB, Van Vliet SJ, Koppel EA, Sanchez-Hernandez M, Vandenbroucke-Grauls CM, Appelmelk B, et al. Mycobacteria target DC-SIGN to suppress dendritic cell function. J Exp Med. 2003;197(1):7-17.
44. Nicod LP. Immunology of tuberculosis. Swiss Med Wkly. 2007;137(25-26):357-62.
45. Bodnar KA, Serbina NV, Flynn JL. Fate of *Mycobacterium tuberculosis* within murine dendritic cells. Infect Immun. 2001;69(2):800-9.
46. Culley FJ. Natural killer cells in infection and inflammation of the lung. Immunology. 2009;128(2):151-63.
47. Dhiman R, Indramohan M, Barnes PF, Nayak RC, Paidipally P, Rao LV, et al. IL-22 produced by human NK cells inhibits growth of *Mycobacterium tuberculosis* by enhancing phagolysosomal fusion. J Immunol. 2009;183(10):6639-45.
48. Lu CC, Wu TS, Hsu YJ, Chang CJ, Lin CS, Chia JH, et al. NK cells kill mycobacteria directly by releasing perforin and granulysin. J Leukoc Biol. 2014;96(6):1119-29.
49. Tan BH, Meinken C, Bastian M, Bruns H, Legaspi A, Ochoa MT, et al. Macrophages acquire neutrophil granules for antimicrobial activity against intracellular pathogens. J Immunol. 2006;177(3):1864-71.
50. Shin DM, Jo EK. Antimicrobial peptides in innate immunity against mycobacteria. Immune Netw. 2011;11(5):245-52.
51. Padhi A, Sengupta M, Sengupta S, Roehm KH, Sonawane A. Antimicrobial peptides and proteins in mycobacterial therapy: current status and future prospects. Tuberculosis (Edinb). 2014;94(4):363-73.
52. Flynn JL, Chan J. Immunology of tuberculosis. Annu Rev Immunol. 2001;19:93-129.
53. Trinchieri G. Interleukin-12 and the regulation of innate resistance and adaptive immunity. Nat Rev Immunol. 2003;3(2):133-46.
54. Kaufmann SH. How can immunology contribute to the control of tuberculosis? Nat Rev Immunol. 2001;1(1):20-30.
55. MacMicking JD, North RJ, LaCourse R, Mudgett JS, Shah SK, Nathan CF. Identification of nitric oxide synthase as a protective locus against tuberculosis. Proc Natl Acad Sci USA. 1997;94(10):5243-8.
56. Gutierrez MG, Master SS, Singh SB, Taylor GA, Colombo MI, Deretic V. Autophagy is a defense mechanism inhibiting BCG and *Mycobacterium tuberculosis* survival in infected macrophages. Cell. 2004;119:753-66.
57. Alonso S, Pethe K, Russell DG, Purdy GE. Lysosomal killing of *Mycobacterium* mediated by ubiquitin-derived peptides is enhanced by autophagy. Proc Natl Acad Sci USA. 2007;104(14):6031-6.
58. Berrington WR, Hawn TR. *Mycobacterium tuberculosis*, macrophages, and the innate immune response: does common variation matter? Immunol Rev. 2007;219:167-86.
59. Flynn JL, Chan J. Tuberculosis: latency and reactivation. Infect Immun. 2001;69(7):4195-201.
60. Van Crevel R, Ottenhoff TH, van der Meer JW. Innate immunity to *Mycobacterium tuberculosis.* Adv Exp Med Biol. 2003;531:241-7.
61. Hernandez-Pando R, Orozco H, Aguilar D. Factors that deregulate the protective immune response in tuberculosis. Arch Immunol Ther Exp (Warsz). 2009;57(5):355-67.
62. Méndez-Samperio P. Expression and regulation of chemokines in mycobacterial infection. J Infect. 2008;57(5):374-84.
63. Algood HM, Chan J, Flynn JL. Chemokines and tuberculosis. Cytokine Growth Factor Rev. 2003;14(6):467-77.
64. Cooper AM. Cell-mediated immune responses in tuberculosis. Annu Rev Immunol. 2009;27:393-422.
65. Abebe F, Bjune G. The protective role of antibody responses during *Mycobacterium tuberculosis* infection. Clin Exp Immunol. 2009;157(2):235-43.
66. Maglione PJ, Chan J. How B cells shape the immune response against *Mycobacterium tuberculosis.* Eur J Immunol. 2009;39(3):676-86.
67. Ehrt S, Schnappinger D. Mycobacterial survival strategies in the phagosome: defence against host stresses. Cell Microbiol. 2009;11(8):1170-8.
68. Roach DR, Briscoe H, Saunders B, France MP, Riminton S, Britton WJ. Secreted lymphotoxin-alpha is essential for the control of an intracellular bacterial infection. J Exp Med. 2001;193(2):239-46.
69. Cowan J, Pandey S, Filion LG, Angel JB, Kumar A, Cameron DW. Comparison of interferon-γ-, interleukin (IL)-17- and IL-22-expressing CD4 T cells, IL-22-expressing granulocytes and proinflammatory cytokines during latent and active tuberculosis infection. Clin Exp Immunol. 2012;167(2):317-29.
70. Pedroza-Roldán C, Barba J, Flores-Valdez MA. Th17: A new player to be considered in tuberculosis studies. J Bacteriol Parasitol. 2012;3:9.
71. Gopal R, Monin L, Slight S, Uche U, Blanchard E, Fallert Junecko BA, et al. Unexpected role for IL-17 in protective immunity against hypervirulent *Mycobacterium tuberculosis* HN878 infection. PLoS Pathog. 2014;10(5):e1004099.
72. Winslow GM, Cooper A, Reiley W, Chatterjee M, Woodland DL. Early T-cell responses in tuberculosis immunity. Immunol Rev. 2008;225:284-99.
73. North RJ, Jung YJ. Immunity to tuberculosis. Annu Rev Immunol. 2004;22:599-623.
74. Vignali DA, Collison LW, Workman CJ. How regulatory T cells work. Nat Rev Immunol. 2008;8(7):523-32.
75. Joosten SA, Ottenhoff TH. Human CD4 and CD8 regulatory T cells in infectious diseases and vaccination. Hum Immunol. 2008;69(11):760-70.
76. Vankayalapati R, Barnes PF. Innate and adaptive immune responses to human *Mycobacterium tuberculosis* infection. Tuberculosis (Edinb). 2009;89(Suppl 1):S77-80.
77. Cooper AM. T cells in mycobacterial infection and disease. Curr Opin Immunol. 2009;21(4):378-84.
78. Bhattacharya D, Dwivedi VP, Kumar S, Reddy MC, Van Kaer L, Moodley P, et al. Simultaneous inhibition of T helper 2 and T regulatory cell differentiation by small molecules enhances bacillus calmette-guerin vaccine efficacy against tuberculosis. J Biol Chem. 2014;289(48):33404-11.
79. Martino A. Mycobacteria and innate cells: critical encounter for immunogenicity. J Biosci. 2008;33(1):137-44.

80. Boom WH. Gammadelta T cells and *Mycobacterium tuberculosis*. Microbes Infect. 1999;1(3):187-95.
81. Kaufmann SH. Recent findings in immunology give tuberculosis vaccines a new boost. Trends Immunol. 2005;26(12):660-7.
82. Beveridge NE, Price DA, Casazza JP, Pathan AA, Sander CR, Asher TE, et al. Immunisation with BCG and recombinant MVA85A induces long-lasting, polyfunctional *Mycobacterium tuberculosis*-specific CD4+ memory T lymphocyte populations. Eur J Immunol. 2007;37(11): 3089-100.
83. Cohen NR, Garg S, Brenner MB. Antigen presentation by CD1 Lipids, T cells, and NKT cells in microbial Immunity. In: Alt FW (Ed.). Advances in Immunology. Boston: Elsevier Inc; 2009. pp. 1-59.
84. Jiang J,Wang X, An H, Yang B, Cao Z, Liu Y, et al. Mucosal-associated invariant T-cell function is modulated by programmed death-1 signaling in patients with active tuberculosis. Am J Respir Crit Care Med. 2014;190(3):329-39.
85. Glatman-Freedman A, Casadevall A. Serum therapy for tuberculosis revisited: Reappraisal of the role of antibody-mediated immunity against *Mycobacterium tuberculosis*. Clin Microbiol Rev. 1998;11(3):514-32.
86. Glatman-Freedman A. The role of antibody-mediated immunity in defense against *Mycobacterium tuberculosis*: advances toward a novel vaccine strategy. Tuberculosis (Edinb). 2006;86(3-4):191-7.
87. Maglione PJ, Xu J, Casadevall A, Chan J, et al. Fc gamma receptors regulate immune activation and susceptibility during *Mycobacterium tuberculosis* infection. J Immunol. 2008;180(5):3329-38.
88. Phuah JY, Mattila JT, Lin PL, Flynn JL. Activated B cells in the granulomas of nonhuman primates infected with *Mycobacterium tuberculosis*. Am J Pathol. 2012;181(2):508-14.

Pulmonary Tuberculosis: Clinical Features and Diagnosis

Surender Kashyap, Malay Sarkar

INTRODUCTION

The clinical features of tuberculosis (TB) depend upon the site and the type of involvement. They are rarely diagnostic. Nonetheless, diagnosis in most of the patients is first suspected on the basis of clinical symptoms and signs. The primary site of implantation of bacilli in the lung parenchyma is called Ghon focus, which together with the draining lymphatics and enlarged draining lymph nodes, constitute the primary complex, also known as the Ranke or Ghon complex. In an immunocompetent host, development of specific immunity is usually able to arrest the bacillary proliferation within the primary lesion with little or no signs of illness, the initial lesion eventually resolves or calcifies. These healed lesions may contain dormant and viable *bacilli*, maintaining continuous hypersensitivity to tuberculous antigen, producing a state of latent TB infection. In a minority of infected individuals (10%), the disease progresses during the initial weeks or months after infection, and the patient develops the typical symptoms of progressive primary TB. In patients with little or no host response and overwhelming infection, disseminated/miliary TB may develop.

POST-PRIMARY PULMONARY TUBERCULOSIS

Most common cause of post-primary TB is the endogenous reactivation of dormant *bacilli* lying in residual foci. Coinfection with human immunodeficiency virus (HIV) is the strongest known risk factor for progression from latent infection to active TB.[1] Other known risk factors are malnutrition, drug and alcohol abuse, coexistent medical conditions, corticosteroid or other immunosuppressive and biological therapies.[1]

Another emerging risk factor in developing countries for TB is biomass fuel exposure. More than 80% population in developing countries use solid fuels for cooking purpose.[2] Several case control studies conducted in India and Brazil has shown firewood or biomass smoke as an independent risk factor for TB disease.[3-5] Various mechanisms proposed are smoke-induced impaired macrophage phagocytic function, surface adherence, and bacterial clearance. Biomass combustion also releases large particulate matter (PM) which can deposit deep into the alveoli and can cause considerable damage.[6] Exogenous reinfection can also be responsible for post-primary TB, although less frequently. In endemic countries, using molecular genotyping methods, it has been demonstrated that reinfection with novel *Mycobacterium tuberculosis* strains may occur in 40% of relapsing cases of TB.[7] Animal study has demonstrated that many T cells harvested from the lungs of mouse showed evidence of exhaustion. Therefore, memory T cell response to reinfection may not be as stable and long lived as was previously thought.[8]

Reactivation can occur at any site; however, lung is the most common site of reactivation.[9] Post-primary disease differs from primary TB in its preferential apical localization, a strong immune response, marked presence of caseation necrosis and cavities.[10] Traditionally, primary and post-primary TB are described in children and adults respectively. Due to the presence of a large number of immunocompromised patients and aging populations, atypical and mixed radio-clinical patterns are frequently observed in adults, with the consequent fading of the age-related distinction between primary and post-primary TB.

SYMPTOMS AND SIGNS

Pulmonary Tuberculosis (PTB) is a disease with protean manifestations, often associated with nonspecific constitutional and specific respiratory signs and symptoms. Constitutional symptoms include tiredness, malaise, weight loss, fever, night sweats, anorexia and headache. They are generally attributed to the release of various cytokines in the systemic circulation. Symptoms are minimal or absent until the disease is in an advanced stage. Complete absence of symptoms has been reported in 4.9% of active adult PTB cases, majority of patients are from countries with endemic TB.[11,12] Most patients develop symptoms insidiously; although, acute manifestations have been also reported.

Fever

Fever is an inconsistent symptom in PTB. Cowie et al.[13] reported fever in only 40% of 300 admitted patients. Similarly, Wang et al.[14] in a recent study reported fever in 33.3% and 15.4% of sputum positive and sputum negative PTB cases, respectively. Absence of fever does not exclude the diagnosis of tuberculosis. Fever in PTB historically has been described by the typical evening rise of temperature. The evening spike of fever may be due to increase in the bacillary multiplication related to the diurnal pattern of adrenal gland steroid release.

In miliary tuberculosis, fever can have morning spikes.[15] The other two conditions associated with morning temperature elevations are typhoid fever and periarteritis nodosa.[16] Initially, fever in PTB is of low grade, but it becomes high grade with the progression of disease. TB is also an important cause of fever of unknown origin (FUO) in several studies.[17,18] In a combined (prospective and retrospective) study of 150 cases of FUO infections, particularly TB, were the most common (50%) cause.[18] Extrapulmonary TB is more common in such a situation.

Cough

Cough is the most predominant symptom in TB.[19] In the initial stages, cough is dry, but subsequently there occurs the production of mucoid or mucopurulent sputum, generally in small amounts. Sometimes, sputum may also be streaked with blood. At the onset, it is more in the early morning; with progressions of disease, it becomes persistent throughout day and night. Cough is less frequent in tubercular pleural effusion. A typical harsh, barking cough is often present in endobronchial TB, which responds to steroids and anti-TB treatment, has poor response to antitussive medication.[20] As per ACCP guidelines, in the high prevalence areas of TB, chronic cough should be defined as cough of two to three weeks duration similar to that recommended by the World Health Organization (WHO).[21]

Hemoptysis

Hemoptysis is usually mild in TB, but occasionally it can be massive. When massive, it is mostly of bronchial artery or nonpulmonary systemic artery origin. Rarely, hemoptysis can also be the presenting symptom. Both active and inactive TB can produce hemoptysis. TB is the most common cause of hemoptysis in endemic countries.[22] It was reported in 79.2% of 476 admitted patients of a chest department.[23] Similarly, in another report, approximately one-third of the patients of TB had hemoptysis of various grade at different stages of their disease.[24] However, the incidence of significant hemoptysis was 8% and fatal hemoptysis was reported in 1 to 5% cases.[24]

There are several mechanisms, which can cause hemoptysis in PTB **(Table 1)**.

Table 1 Mechanisms of hemoptysis in tuberculosis

- Necrosis of pulmonary venules and capillaries in early stages
- Rupture of *Rasmussen's aneurysm*
- Post-tubercular bronchiectasis
- Mycetoma in tubercular cavity
- Broncholiths
- Scar carcinoma very rarely

Usually, massive bleeding is seen in inactive TB with cavitary and bronchiectatic sequelae. Bleeding occurs less commonly in patients of active cavitary disease with associated granulomatous vasculitis, since vascular thrombosis within necrotic areas causes the obliteration of pulmonary vessels.[25] However, it can be seen in active TB if adequate chemotherapy is not given and radiograph shows thick walled cavities.[26] After achieving cure, if the patient complains of recurrent hemoptysis, evaluation for bronchiectasis and/or mycetoma should be done. Pulmonary mycetoma is the fungal colonization, mainly by *aspergillus* species, in a pre-existing pulmonary cavity and without the evidence of invasion into the surrounding structures. Mycetomas have also been reported in other pulmonary conditions such as sarcoidosis, bronchiectasis, lung abscess, neoplasms, pulmonary infarcts, nontuberculous mycobacteria and various mycoses.[27-30] Severe hemoptysis may occur in up to one-third of the cases of mycetoma.[29] In HIV-infected patient with pulmonary mycetoma, significant hemoptysis is less likely observed as compared to immunocompetent patient, but these patients have a high risk of disease progression to more invasive disease.[30]

Rasmussen's aneurysm is a rare complication of cavitary PTB caused by granulomatous weakening of a pulmonary arterial wall. It can present as the repeated episodes of minor hemoptysis or occasionally as major hemoptysis. Incidence of Rasmussen's aneurysm is 4% in patients with advanced cavitary disease.

Breathlessness

Breathlessness, which is a late symptom in PTB may result from extensive pulmonary involvement, bronchial obstruction, pneumothorax and pleural effusion. Rarely, patients with miliary TB or TB bronchopneumonia may present with the symptoms of respiratory failure. The incidence of respiratory failure secondary to PTB is 1.5–1.9%.[31-33] Diagnosis of TB is more likely delayed or missed in patients presenting with acute respiratory failure.[34] Destroyed lung due to TB is also a common cause of respiratory failure in endemic area.[35] The prognosis of TB presenting with respiratory failure is dismal with hospital mortality of 60%.[36]

Chest Pain

Involvement of pleural surface can cause pleuritic chest pain. Pain is referred to ipsilateral shoulder in diaphragmatic pleurisy and to upper abdomen in costal pleural involvement. Pneumothorax due to TB can also cause acute pleuritic chest pain. Sometimes, chest pain can be dull and poorly localized. Chest pain is an early and relatively frequent symptom and it disappears within two or three weeks after effective treatment is started.

Hoarseness

The most common cause of hoarseness of voice in PTB is due to the associated laryngeal TB. Rarely, inflamed TB nodes or the retraction of left upper lobe bronchus by cicatrization atelectasis can cause recurrent laryngeal nerve palsy and hoarseness of voice.[37]

In TB endemic countries, *M. tuberculosis* can have community-acquired pneumonia (CAP) like presentation. Empirical therapy with fluoroquinolones in this condition, misdiagnosed as acute bacterial pneumonia, can suppress the early symptoms of TB and often delay the diagnosis of TB. Therefore, in endemic area for TB, fluoroquinolones should be judiciously used. In a multivariate analysis involving patients presenting with CAP like manifestations, features, such as the longer duration of symptoms (more than two weeks before hospital admission), history of night sweats, upper lobe involvement, cavitary infiltrates, lower total white blood cell (WBC) count and lymphopenia, have been reported as more predictive of PTB.[38]

Primary TB in children is mostly asymptomatic and recognized solely through contact investigation. Some children may experience a symptomatic pneumonia like presentation. Progressive primary TB patients may present with cough, hemoptysis and weight loss. Because of smaller diameter airways, younger children are more prone to airway compression.[39]

In an analysis of data from an international, multicenter phase three trial,[40] fever was the most common symptom to undergo resolution. After the first two months of treatment, 94% of subjects showed resolution of fever, 59% for cough, 77% for chest pain, 94% for sweats, and 81% for dyspnea. Fever, sweats, and dyspnea decreased most rapidly, while chest pain and cough resolved more slowly. 13% of subjects reported cough even at the end of therapy and persistent of cough after completion of successful treatment may be due to post-tubercular bronchiectasis.

TUBERCULOSIS IN THE ELDERLY

The elderly population is particularly susceptible to TB because of the age-induced decline in cell-mediated immunity.[41] More specifically, impairment of helper T-lymphocyte functions and subsequently defects in secretion and response to different cytokines are particularly important in increasing the susceptibility of TB in elderly subjects.[42] Elderly individual is also more likely to suffer from various immunosuppressive conditions. There are several characteristic features of TB in the elderly.[43] After exposure, elderly subjects are more likely to become infected with *M. tuberculosis* than younger subjects, they also develop tuberculous diseases more easily after contracting infection. Mortality from TB is also high in this population.

Delayed diagnosis is not uncommon as the clinico-radiological presentations of TB are often atypical in the elderly.[44] Some patients may present with only nonpulmonary symptoms such as unexplained weight loss, weakness or change in cognitive status.[45] Classical symptoms, such as night sweats, fever and hemoptysis, are less frequently observed in the elderly.[11] Fever is infrequent because of age associated decrease in pyrogenic response. There is decreased responsiveness of the hypothalamic thermoregulatory center to prostaglandin E2 (released by interleukin-1) and an increased sensitivity to natural occurring antipyretics such as α-melanocyte stimulating hormone.[46] Cavitation is less common in elderly age group, which can explain the lower frequency of hemoptysis. Lower lobe involvement is also common.[47] Potential of adverse drug reactions is also high in elderly subjects.

MILIARY TUBERCULOSIS

Miliary tuberculosis contributes 1 to 2% of all cases of TB and about 8% of all the forms of extrapulmonary tuberculosis (EPTB) in the immunocompetent individuals.[48] It is estimated that miliary TB accounts for about less than 2% of all cases of TB in immunocompetent persons and up to 20% of all EPTB cases. It is more common in immunosuppressed individuals. Clinical manifestations are nonspecific and the typical chest radiographic finding of miliary nodules may not be apparent till late in the course of the disease. Classical miliary pattern is detected in 50% cases.[49]Atypical presentations are more common and often delay the diagnosis. Associated TB meningitis has been described in 10 to 30% of adult patients with miliary TB.[41] Choroidal tubercles and cutaneous findings (TB cutis acuta generalisata) are highly specific, but insensitive for miliary TB.[50] Choroidal tubercles are bilateral, pale, gray-white, or yellowish lesions usually less than one-quarter of the size of the optic disk and are located within 2 cm of the optic nerve. Therefore, all patients with suspected miliary TB should be subjected to a systematic ophthalmoscopic examination.[49]

Cutaneous manifestations are more commonly seen in HIV-infected patients with advanced immunosuppression ($CD4^+$ cell counts <100 cells/cmm).[51] TB through hematogenous dissemination can occasionally lead to sepsis and septic shock, it was known as Landouzy septicemia or sepsis tuberculosa acutissima in the past.[52] It is most commonly noted in immunocompromised patients, especially in patients with HIV, but may also occur in immunocompetent patients.[53]

HUMAN IMMUNODEFICIENCY VIRUS AND TUBERCULOSIS

Tuberculosis can involve HIV-infected patients at all the levels of CD4 T lymphocyte counts, but clinical and radiological manifestations depend on the severity of immunosuppression.[54] Majority of patients with CD4 counts >200 cells/cmm have disease limited to the lungs with common chest radiographic findings, such as upper lobe infiltrates with or without cavitation, not substantially different from HIV-negative patients. On the other hand, patients with advanced HIV disease (CD4 T lymphocyte count <200 cells/cmm) are more likely to have atypical presentation such as the lower lobe predominance, adenopathy and absence of cavities. Extrapulmonary and disseminated disease is common in advanced HIV infection, occurring in 63% of patients.[55] Severely immunocompromised patients can have sepsis like syndrome with high fever.[56]

PLEURAL EFFUSION

In primary TB, effusions typically develop three to six-months after infection, are due to hypersensitivity response to a small amount of tuberculoprotein released into the pleural space.[57] Pleural effusion is less commonly seen in post-primary TB, it is due to the rupture of a cavity or adjacent parenchymal focus into pleural space, releasing large number of bacteria in contrast to primary TB. In patients of PTB, pleural involvement appears to be more common in HIV-coinfected individuals. Tuberculous pleuritis often presents acutely, shows significantly higher frequency of chest pain, dyspnea and abdominal pain, whereas hemoptysis and weight are less commonly noticed (See Chapter 156 for details).[58]

PARADOXICAL RESPONSE

Paradoxical response in TB includes the unusual expansion of old lesions or formation of new tuberculous lesion during anti-TB therapy.[59] Paradoxical response is known to occur in tuberculous pleural effusion, PTB, tuberculous lymphadenopathy and intracranial tuberculoma. Paradoxical worsening occurs with rapid mycobacterial killing and release of products that stimulate the T helper subtype 1 (Th1) lymphocyte subpopulation, which in turn, liberates various proinflammatory cytokines, including TNF-α, interleukin IL-2, IL-6 and IL-8, responsible for worsening of tuberculous lesions.[60] Paradoxical reaction is particularly common in up to 30% patients with cervical lymphadenopathy whereas it is rare in those with intrathoracic lymphadenopathy.[61]

PHYSICAL EXAMINATIONS

There are several reactive immunologic phenomena, such as erythema nodosum, erythema induratum, reactive arthritis and amyloidosis, associated with *M. tuberculosis* infections.[62] These are more common in primary TB. Erythema nodosum usually occurs acutely and is clinically characterized by the sudden eruption of erythematous tender nodules and plaques located predominantly over the extensor aspects of the lower extremities. It may occur in a disseminated form in severe reaction and heal without scarring. Erythema induratum, on the other hand, presents with a more indolent course, often precipitated by cold weather, tends to form blue plaques and heal with atrophic scars. Histologically, it is associated with vasculitis and granuloma formation.[63]

Poncet's disease is a reactive arthritis characterized by aseptic inflammatory polyarthritis in the patients of active PTB, which tends to affect knees, ankles and elbows.[64] Amyloidosis (AA type) may complicate chronic infections and TB is a common cause of secondary amyloidosis in the developing countries, can occur as early as two to four weeks after the diagnosis of active TB.[65] The pathogenesis of secondary amyloidosis involves the release of proinflammatory cytokines (such as interleukin IL-1, IL-6, and TNF-α) which stimulate the synthesis of serum amyloid in the liver and its subsequent deposition in various organs. This stimulation occurs even during the inactive stage of the disease.[66]

Wasting is a classic feature of TB, caused by a combination of factors, e.g. lack of appetite, increased losses and altered metabolism as part of the inflammatory and immune responses.[67]

Wasting also carries poor prognosis by causing increased mortality in patients with TB.[68] It is usually seen in advanced disease and indicates the loss of both fat and lean tissues.[67] A major constraint of physical examination of respiratory system is its failure to detect mild or even moderate illness despite apparent radiographic abnormalities. Post-tussive rales constitute an important sign, demonstrated on deep inhalation followed by full exhalation and coughing at the end of exhalation. Fine rales are heard over the areas of TB infiltrations, particularly at the apices. In endobronchial TB, localized wheezing may be heard. In tubercular consolidation, high pitched bronchial breathing, whereas in superficial large cavities, cavernous breathing may be audible. In tubercular pleurisy, pleural rub is often detected. Signs of volume contraction are often present in advanced disease with extensive fibrosis.

DIAGNOSIS OF TUBERCULOSIS

Routine Laboratory Testing

Mild anemia and leukocytosis are the most common hematologic abnormalities in TB. Anemia is caused by the inflammatory cytokines mediated suppression of erythropoiesis, most often described as normochromic, normocytic anemia, while some patients may show leukemoid reactions. Pancytopenia with hypocellular bone marrow has also been reported with *M. tuberculosis* infection.[69] Hematological manifestations are more common in disseminated/military TB patients. Patients of disseminated/miliary TB with granuloma in bone marrow showed significantly higher incidence of severe anemia, peripheral monocytopenia and bone marrow histiomonocytosis as compared to patients without granuloma.[70] In countries where TB is endemic, including in India, TB should be carefully excluded in patients presenting with various hematological manifestations.

Hyponatremia and hypercalcemia have been observed in TB. Hyponatremia is more commonly noticed in tubercular meningitis than in PTB, is due to syndrome of inappropriate antidiuretic hormone secretion (SIADH). It has been reported in 7–10% of active TB cases.[71,72] In addition, hyponatremia in TB can be due to Addison's disease. Adrenal TB was reported in 6% of patients with active TB and bilateral adrenal involvement in 70% cases.[73]

Hypercalcemia is the other electrolyte abnormality in active TB, but symptoms of hypercalcemia are uncommon. Prevalence rate of hypercalcemia in different studies varies from 15 to 51%.[74] The most plausible theory is extrarenal production of 1, 25-dihydroxycholecalciferol. Unfortunately, all these findings are nonspecific. Erythrocyte sedimentation rate (ESR) estimation is also an unreliable indicator of disease activity. Early diagnosis of TB and initiation of optimal therapy is important not only for the patient, but is also equally so for the community to decrease the possibility of transmission of infection to others. *Any diagnostic modality for TB should have certain desirable features:*

- It should have acceptable sensitivity, specificity and predictive value.
- It should be quantitative and reproducible.
- Its turn-around time should be rapid.

Further, the test should be cost-effective, safe, easy-to-use, and should perform equally well in resource-poor settings and HIV prevalent areas. Laboratory testing for TB includes tests for latent TB infection as well as for TB disease. In latent TB infection, individuals are harboring live *M. tuberculosis,* but do not show any clinical evidence or signs and symptoms of active disease. TB, on the other hand, is the clinically manifested illness caused by *M. tuberculosis* complex. Tests for latent tuberculosis infection (LTBI) include tuberculin skin test (TST) and interferon-gamma release assays (IGRA).

Latent Tuberculosis

Tuberculin Skin Test

Tuberculin skin test is the oldest diagnostic test still in use in the modern medical practice. The material used for this purpose is purified protein derivative (PPD). It is injected intradermally, indicates delayed type hypersensitivity response in exposed individuals. In tuberculin test, the area of induration (not erythema is measured after 48–72 hours of administration of PPD). In India, induration of >15 mm is taken as positive TST in immunocompetent person with no known risk factors for TB. PPD despite being in use for a century possesses many shortcomings, including low sensitivity particularly in immunocompromised individuals (elderly, malnourished, HIV-infection and other immunosuppressive conditions). In HIV-infected patients, a cut-off of ≥5 mm of induration is considered as positive response. Overall, 75–90% of patients with active TB react to TST.[75]

Tuberculin testing also lacks specificity since PPD is a mixture of more than 200 proteins derived from *M. tuberculosis,* many of which are shared by other mycobacteria, including the nontuberculous mycobacteria (NTM) and *bacillus calmette guérin* (BCG) strain.[76] A systematic meta-analysis, showed minimal effect of BCG vaccination received in infancy on TST, the effect was virtually nil beyond 10 years of vaccination.[77] NTM usually produce induration smaller than 10 mm in diameter and are a cause of false-positive TST only in areas with the high prevalence of NTM infections.

Despite the diminished specificity of the TST in BCG vaccinated individuals, the American Thoracic Society recommends to ignore vaccination history when interpreting TST.[78] Other shortcomings are the inter-reader and intra-reader variability in reporting and the need for a return visit. Tuberculin skin test does not distinguish between the latent infection and the active disease. To increase the specificity of TST, we need to purify antigens that are specific to *M. tuberculosis* complex. Recently, a recombinant antigen (DPPD, not present in NTM) encoded by a gene unique to the *M. tuberculosis* complex organisms, has shown some promise in increasing the specificity of skin testing in the diagnosis of TB.[79] Another potential antigen that has shown promise in skin testing is the *M. tuberculosis* early secreted antigenic target-6 (ESAT-6).[80]

Interferon Gamma Release Assays

Interferon gamma release assays (IGRA) are the new T cell-based assays that measure the interferon gamma release, by sensitized lymphocytes in response to specific *M. tuberculosis* antigens such as the ESAT-6 and culture filtrate protein 10 (CFP10).[78] These antigens, encoded by genes in the region of difference-1(RD1), are present in *M. tuberculosis,* but are absent in BCG vaccine strain and most nontuberculous mycobacteria except *M. marinum, M. szulgai* and *M. kansasii.*[81]

Two commercially available tests are approved by the US Food and Drug Administration, QuantiFERON-TB Gold In-Tube (QFT-GIT) (Cellestis/Qiagen, Venlo, Limburg) and T-SPOT.TB (Oxford Immunotec, Abingdon, UK).[82,83] Both QFT-GIT and T-SPOT.TB assays use ESAT-6 and CFP-10 whereas QFT-GIT also uses a third antigen, TB 7.7. IGRAs testing methods also include internal control, termed the nil. It determines the amount of interferon gamma detected after incubation without antigens. Interferon gamma level from the nil control is subtracted from the interferon gamma level detected after stimulation with the TB antigens to determine the interferon gamma that is attributable to TB. In addition to nil control, mitogen control is also used to confirm that an individual's cells are capable of responding to antigen stimulation. Phytohemagglutinin (PHA) is used as a nonspecific antigen stimulant and failure to respond appropriately suggests an inadequate number of functional effector T cells or an error in processing the blood or performing the test.[84] QFT-GIT measures interferon gamma produced in heparinized whole blood after stimulation with antigen, while T-SPOT. TB determines the quantity of effector T cells responding to antigen stimulation.

In general, these tests are more specific and potentially more sensitive than the traditional TST.[85] Result of IGRA is not affected by prior BCG vaccination. The IGRA does not require a return visit, has no variability of skin test readings and there is no induction of boosting phenomenon on repeat testing. High diagnostic sensitivity has also been observed in young children for T-SPOT. TB test and in immunosuppressed populations for both T-SPOT. TB test and to a lesser extent to QFT-GIT.[86] Use of IGRA tests cannot differentiate latent infection from active disease. This is particularly problematic in high TB burden countries where the prevalence of latent infection is very high.

Reactivation of latent TB infection reflects an impaired immune response, at least temporarily; so IGRAs may be falsely negative at the time of the development of the disease.[87] Sensitivity in active TB ranges from 64% to 92%. Thus, IGRAs can potentially miss 10–30% of active TB cases and are hence unsuitable for use as rule-in tests.[88] Sensitivity of IGRAs also varies between high and low burden countries clearly emphasizing the need to perform large studies in different settings.[88] The higher cost and need for sophisticated instruments prohibit their widespread use in the developing countries. Chemokine inducible protein 10 (IP-10) is another potential biomarker, which can be used in the immunodiagnosis of *M. tuberculosis* infection. Combination of IP-10 and IFN-γ also increases the detection rate for LTBI.[89] However, these expensive tests do not differentiate latent infection from active disease, these tests are not recommended for use in the diagnostic algorithm for TB in India.

Diagnosis of Pulmonary Tuberculosis

Chest Radiology

Chest radiography is an important tool in suspecting the diagnosis of PTB. Chest X-rays are mostly abnormal in immunocompetent patients, but may be normal in about 10–15% of HIV-infected patients. No radiological features are typical of TB various other lung diseases can radiologically mimic TB. Radiological manifestations have been traditionally described in children and adults on the basis of primary and post-primary TB.[90] Recently, these age-wise distinctions of radiological manifestations have been blurred due to several reasons. Primary infection can occur at any age in an endemic area, further, primary TB accounts for 23–34% of all adult cases of TB.[91] Cavitation generally considered as a sign of reactivation, can occur even after primary infection.

HIV infection is also responsible for atypical radiographic manifestations. Two recent studies based on genotyping *M. tuberculosis* isolates with restriction fragment length polymorphism (RFLP) also show that the radiographic features are often similar in both primary and reactivation TB.[92,93] In primary TB, classical radiological features include the presence of parenchymal disease, lymphadenopathy, pleural effusion, miliary disease and atelectasis. Parenchymal disease affects the areas of greatest ventilation in the lung and the most common sites are the middle lobe, lower lobe and anterior segment of upper lobe; however, it can affect any segment.[94] Dense and homogeneous consolidations are generally observed, but nodular and linear pattern are also occasionally seen.[95,96]

A right-sided predominance of parenchymal lesion is often seen, reflecting greater statistical probability of an airborne infection involving the right lung. Lymphadenopathy usually unilateral is the most common radiological feature in primary TB.[97] Hilar and paratracheal regions are most commonly affected. In adults, lymphadenopathy without a parenchymal infiltrate is unusual except in patients with acquired immune deficiency syndrome (AIDS). The combination of paren-chymal focus and lymphadenopathy is called Ghon complex.[98] On contrast-enhanced computed tomography (CT) scan, TB lymphadenopathy, particularly when more than 2 cm in diameter, shows the characteristic Rim sign consisting of the central areas of low attenuation associated with peripheral rim enhancement and obliteration of surrounding perinodal fat.[99] This corresponds to central caseation necrosis with inflammatory, hypervascular capsular and perinodal reaction and is highly suggestive of active disease.[100] However, rim sign may also be present in other conditions, such as atypical mycobacterial infection, lymphoma, metastases, particularly from testicular carcinoma, Whipple's disease and Crohn's disease.[96]

The radiological features of post-primary TB can be broadly classified as the parenchymal miliary disease, cavitation **(Figs 1 and 2)**, tracheobronchial TB, and pleural extension of parenchymal disease and complications. The most common sites for parenchymal opacities are apical and posterior segments of the upper lobe and the superior segment of the lower lobe. Multiple segments are affected in about 88% of cases, bilateral upper lobe disease observed in 32–64% cases.[101] Poorly defined nodules and linear opacities are seen adjacent to parenchymal opacities in approximately 25% of patients.[102] Cavities are most commonly seen within the areas of consolidation and are reported in 40–50% cases of post-primary TB.[98] Cavitation usually indicates active disease. The number of *bacilli* are in the order of 10^7–10^9; therefore, a high

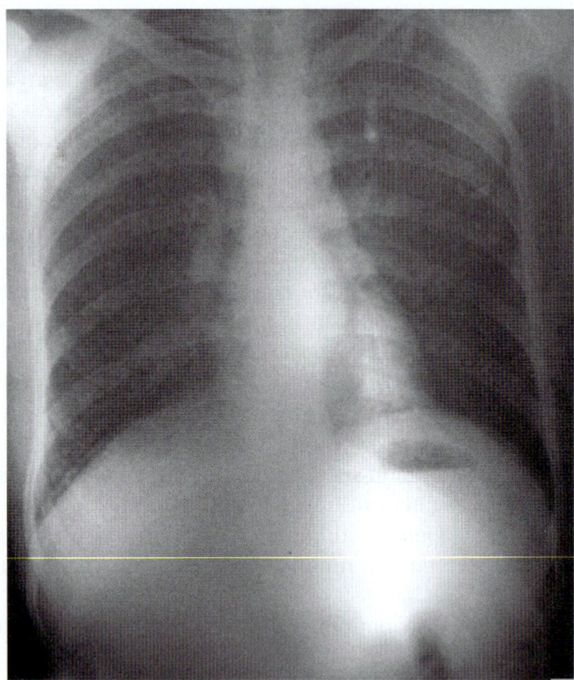

Fig. 1 Chest X-ray showing miliary shadow through both the lung fields

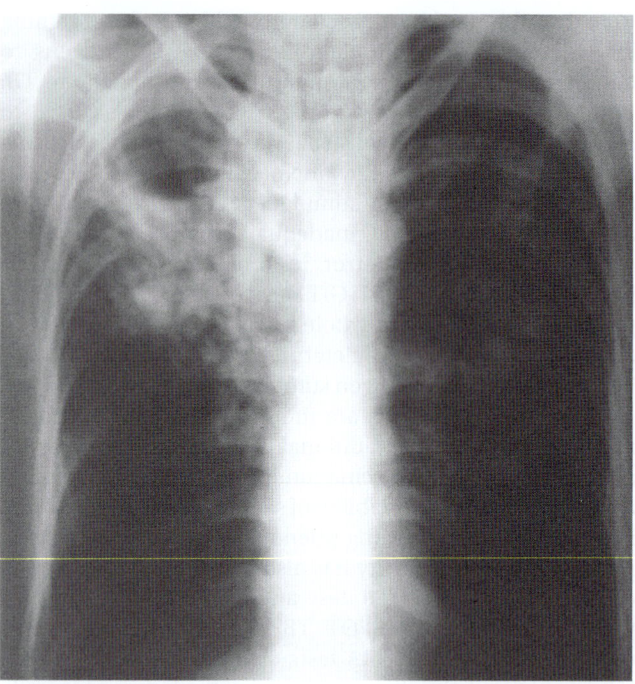

Fig. 2 Chest X-ray showing right upper lobe cavity with infiltration

likelihood of sputum positivity is there in cavitary lesions.[103] One important feature, which differentiates TB from other cavitary diseases is the presence of clearly defined, nodular opacities around the cavity.[94]

Most common complication of cavitation is the bronchogenic spread due to the liquefaction of caseous necrotic material and subsequent communication with the bronchial tree. On chest radiography, bronchogenic spread is detected in approximately 20% of cases, but on CT scans, it can be identified in 95% of cases with post-primary TB.[96]

Characteristics high resolution computed tomography (HRCT) finding of bronchogenic spread is a tree-in-bud appearance, i.e. centrilobular nodules of 2–4 mm in size and sharply marginated linear branching opacities corresponding to the tuberculous involvement of the small airways. Air fluid level within tuberculous cavities may be seen in 9–21% of cases and usually indicates superimposed bacterial or fungal infection.[104-106] Hilar and mediastinal lymphadenopathy are not a common manifestation of post-primary TB, occurs in only 5% of cases.[107] PTB with normal chest radiograph is increasingly being reported in the literature.[108] This is much more so in HIV positive persons (7–14%).[109-111]

The radiographic appearance of PTB is often atypical in HIV-infected patients. It most commonly resembles with that of primary disease. Miliary disease and pleural effusion have been reported in up to 19% and 10% patients respectively.[111,112] Normal chest radiographs have been reported in 12–14% of HIV-infected patients with smear or culture positive pulmonary tuberculosis.[111,112]

Radiological manifestations may also depend on the degree of immunosuppression at the time of overt disease.

Chest CT is required in patients with high clinical suspicion of TB, but normal or nonspecific chest radiography. CT is more sensitive than chest radiography in detecting cavities, intrathoracic lymphadenopathy, miliary disease, bronchiectasis, bronchial stenosis and pleural disease. High resolution computed tomography (HRCT) is superior to standard CT in the evaluation of pulmonary parenchymal disease.[113] In HRCT thorax, most commonly detected abnormalities in PTB are micronodules (100%) followed by tree-in-bud appearance (87%) and cavitation (73%).[114] The micronodules are typically centrilobular in location having indistinct margins. They are usually 5–6 mm in diameter, located in the peripheral parts of consolidations or cavities. Detection of micronodule is indeed highly suggestive of active TB.[113] Their presence indicates inflammatory lesions in the bronchioles and the peribronchiolar alveoli. Micronodules and tree-in-bud appearance are not detected by standard chest radiography. There is a significant correlation between consolidation and cavitation on conventional CT with increase in a number of *bacilli* in the sputum.[115] Consolidation pattern is also suggestive of active PTB, detected in 82% of patients.[114]

Tuberculoma is a sharply marginated round or oval lesion of 0.5–4.0 cm in diameter, detected in approximately 5% of patients with post-primary TB. The location of tuberculoma has been variably reported in upper and lower lobes.[116] About 20–30% of tuberculomas in adults may ultimately calcify. In up to 80% of cases, smaller satellite lesions were seen in the immediate vicinity of the main lesion.[117] Tuberculomas are generally multiple, of similar size in 20% of cases.[118]

Miliary disease is less common in post-primary than in primary TB.[91] Plain chest radiography can be normal in 25–40% of patients at initial presentation since typical miliary lesions need 3–6 weeks after hematogenous dissemination to manifest radiographically.[119] The typical radiological appearance is myriad, 1–3 mm, noncalcified nodules distributed throughout both the lungs, with mild basal predominance **(Fig. 3)**. Other associated radiological features include consolidation, cavitation, calcified lymph nodes and lymphadenopathy observed in up to 30% of patients.[119] HRCT can detect miliary disease before it becomes apparent on standard chest radiography. Intralobular and interlobular septal thickening and areas of ground glass opacity may also be present. A diffuse alveolar pattern has been described in the patients of adult respiratory distress syndrome due to miliary TB.[120]

The differential diagnosis of miliary pattern on chest radiography includes miliary TB, histoplasmosis, sarcoidosis, pneumoconiosis, pulmonary alveolar microlithiasis, tropical pulmonary eosinophilia, bronchoalveolar carcinoma, pulmonary siderosis, and hematogenous metastases from primary cancers of thyroid, kidney, trophoblast, and some of the sarcomas. Another important radiological characteristics of PTB is sequelae of TB. It includes open-healed cavity, mycetoma within cavity and tubercular destroyed lung (TDL). TDL has been a recognized entity and is usually unilateral. It may occur after primary disease or reinfection.[121] TDL is seen more commonly on left side. Various reasons include longer and narrower left main bronchus and the tight mediastinum through which it travels. Drainage of secretions is also poor from left main bronchus due to its more horizontal course.[122] Another important impact of TDL is persistence of mycobacteria leading to relapse of TB and treatment failure with development of MDR-TB *bacilli*. It occurs in TDL due to cessation of pulmonary arterial blood flow to the destroyed lung resulting in reduced levels of chemotherapeutic agents reaching affected sites and thus, ineffective killing of *tubercle bacilli*.[123,124]

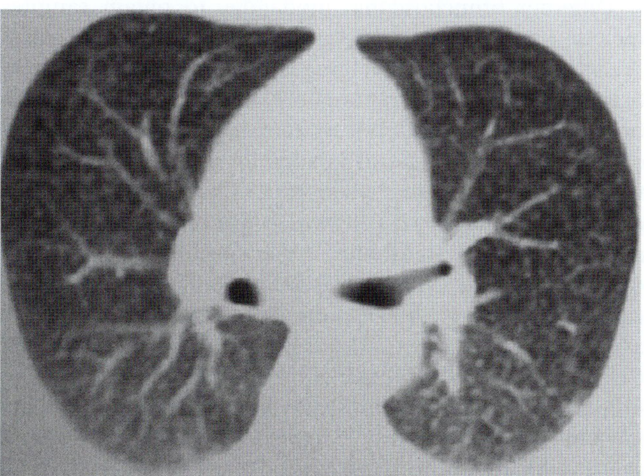

Fig. 3 HRCT thorax showing miliary shadow through both the lung fields

Sputum Microscopy

Sputum microscopy, the most widely available test for active TB, is the diagnostic centerpiece of the directly observed treatment short course (DOTS) strategy. It is cheap, rapid, easy-to-perform and widely available diagnostic procedure to detect mycobacteria in clinical specimens. However, there are certain limitations of sputum microscopy. Sputum microscopy is not a highly sensitive tool, it requires a minimal of 5,000–10,000 *bacilli* per mL of sputum to reliably identify the *bacilli*.[125] It cannot differentiate *M. tuberculosis* from other mycobacteria. Sputum microscopy may also fail to diagnose paucibacillary and EPTB, the incidence of which is disproportionately higher in high HIV prevalent areas. The sensitivity of sputum microscopy ranges from 34–80%.[126] The smear is more likely to be positive in patients who have cavitary disease and multilobar infiltrates. The result of smear microscopy is influenced by several variables like type of the specimen, thickness of the smear, technical preparation of the slide and experience of the laboratory personnel examining the smear.

Sensitivity of sputum microscopy is increased if sputum is liquefied and concentrated by centrifugation or sedimentation prior to acid-fast staining.[127] In a systematic review of 83 studies, it has been demonstrated that sputum processed by centrifugation and use of various chemicals increased the sensitivity of microscopy by 18% compared to direct smear microscopy.[128] The most widely studied sputum processing method is liquefaction of sputum with sodium hypochlorite (NaOCl) usually known as household bleach, followed by centrifugation or sedimentation. There are several advantages of using NaOCl, it is widely available and kills both the mycobacteria and HIV; therefore, tends to increase the safety and acceptability in the laboratory. However, this technique is not suitable for sample intended to be used for culture. Studies done in Ethiopia have reported that a single digested smear can equal the sensitivity of three direct smears.[129] Furthermore, there are certain limitations of these procedures, particularly in the context of resource limited, high prevalence countries. Irregular power supply, potential biohazard of centrifugation, and limited human and financial resources may impede its widespread applicability in the developing countries. Moreover, there is insufficient data to determine the value of sputum processing methods in HIV-infected patients.

There are several staining methods such as the Ziehl-Neelsen, Kinyoun's (cold staining) and fluorescent staining methods.[130] The core principle of these methods is based on the avidity of the lipid rich cell wall to different dyes. In

Ziehl-Neelsen method, heat is applied to encourage the cell wall to take up the stain followed by decolorization with acid or acid alcohol and finally counterstaining with methylene blue or malachite green. In cold Kinyoun's method, higher concentrations of phenol and basic fuchsin are used.[130] The mycobacteria in these staining methods appear red against blue or green background. Performance of Kinyoun's stain has been reported to be inferior to that of Ziehl-Neelsen stain in several studies.[131,132]

Other microorganisms that may take up acid-fast stains, albeit weakly, are *Rhodococcus, Nocardia, Legionella micdadei,* and cysts of *Cryptosporidium, Isospora,* and *Cyclospora.* Fluorescence microscopy requires staining with the dye auramine rhodamine. The mycobacteria appear bright yellow rods against inky black background. *There are several advantages of fluorescent microscopy over conventional staining methods:*[133]

- Rapid turnaround time with fluorescence microscopy as it uses a lower power objective lens (typically 25X) than conventional microscopy (typically 100X), allowing much faster reading of specimens than smears stained with the Ziehl-Neelsen method. It takes one to two minutes per slide in contrast to 15 minutes required for Ziehl-Neelsen staining method.
- It is more sensitive than conventional microscopy. In comparison with Ziehl-Neelsen microscopy, fluorescence microscopy has shown a 10% increase in sensitivity. The major problem of its implementation in the developing countries is the cost of fluorescent bulb, which is costly and is of a short lifespan (typically 200–300 hours). The use of light emitting diodes as a light source is an attractive, inexpensive alternative to mercury vapor lamps.[134]

In recently revised policies on smear microscopy, the WHO now recommends two sputum specimens examination instead of three for screening of TB cases in places, where a well-functioning external quality assurance system exists and where the workload is very high and human resources are limited. Smear microscopy is likely to retain its pivotal role in the diagnosis of TB in major parts of the world.

Optimization of smear microscopy should be an important goal of any TB control program. Smear negative patient who is unable to produce sputum, should undergo further diagnostic testing such as sputum induction (SI), fiberoptic bronchoscopy (FOB) and sometimes gastric washings (GW).

Induced Sputum Examination

There are several advantages of sputum induction:

- Diagnostic yield of single induced sputum is at least equivalent to that of one bronchoscopy with broncho-alveolar lavage (BAL) in the terms of positivity on both smear and culture for mycobacteria.[135,136]
- The diagnostic yield of induced sputum can be increased with significantly higher detection rates than with bronchoscopy alone when multiple (three or more) specimens are used.
- Smear microscopy and culture positivity rates of 91–98% and 99–100% respectively, have been reported with multiple specimens.[137]
- Induced sputum is a very safe procedure with extremely few adverse events, unlike invasive procedure such as bronchoscopy. Most common adverse events are headache, bronchospasm/cough and the risk of transmission of TB to attending staff, if appropriate protection measures are not applied, cost analysis studies also favor sputum induction over bronchoscopy.[138]
- Sputum induction performs equally well in both resource-poor and resource-rich countries and is also useful in HIV positive and negative patients.[130]

Therefore, sputum induction should be used as the primary modality in patients who are either unable to provide spontaneous sputum samples or who are acid-fast *bacilli* (AFB) smear negative.[139] Sputum induction has been shown to improve sputum microscopy result by 29% in patients with suspected TB who previously had negative smear.[140] It is also superior to gastric aspirate specimens in terms of sensitivity and speed to culture positivity.[141]

Fiberoptic Bronchoscopy

The main role of fiberoptic bronchoscopy (FOB) in diagnosing PTB includes patients who are sputum smear negative for AFB or who do not produce adequate sputum, particularly if an immediate diagnosis is required or if alternative diagnoses are being entertained. It is also useful for follow-up studies in endobronchial TB to detect bronchostenosis. Sputum smear negative TB should be declared when sputum microscopy is done in a quality assured and periodically accredited laboratory. This is particularly relevant to developing countries like India, where, commercial laboratories with varying standards still provide sputum examination results in spite of the widespread availability and accessibility to quality microscopy center under the revised national TB control programme (RNTCP).

Different bronchoscopic modalities to obtain samples include the bronchial aspirate, bronchoalveolar lavage, brushings, transbronchial lung biopsy (TBLB) and trans-bronchial needle aspiration (TBNA). Among the various bronchoscopic procedures to retrieve samples, the yield of BAL for *M. tuberculosis* is superior to that of bronchial washings.[141] The higher yield in BAL is due to the large quantity of saline used in BAL, which lowers the concentration of aspirated local anesthetic, which can inhibit the growth of *M. tuberculosis.* A small amount of 2 mL of 2% lignocaine can produce a bronchial aspirate concentration of up to 1% at which most strains of *M. tuberculosis* are inhibited.[142,143] Culture of TBLB and bronchial brushing specimens provide little additional yield. Various studies using FOB as a modality have demonstrated early diagnosis in 4–79% cases and exclusive diagnosis in 2–52% cases.[126]

FOB use in high prevalent areas of TB has successfully led to early diagnosis in a larger percentage of patients (72–73%).[144,145] Use of FOB in miliary TB seems particularly attractive because of inherent problems with conventional diagnostic procedures. Presence of miliary mottling on chest radiography varies from 50% to 93% of cases.[146,147] Smear microscopy and sputum cultures are positive in one-third and less than two-third of patients, respectively.[131] Delay in diagnosis can be associated with significant mortality in miliary TB. Using FOB, immediate (or early) diagnosis (positive AFB smear, transbronchial biopsy specimens revealing caseating granulomas with or without AFB) can be achieved.

Fiberoptic bronchoscopy is also useful in the diagnosis of tuberculous intrathoracic lymphadenopathy by using TBNA technique. Incidence of isolated intrathoracic tuberculous lymphadenitis varies from 0.25% to 5.8%, poses a diagnostic challenge. FOB in tuberculous intrathoracic lymphadenopathy also helps because of the presence of endobronchial involvement in a large percentage of patients (75%), which also explains frequent erosion of bronchial tree by intrathoracic tuberculous lymphadenopathy.[148] Endobronchial ultrasound is another tool, which can further ease the procedure of TBNA.

Post-bronchoscopy sputum is also helpful in increasing the diagnostic yield in TB. It can increase culture yield by 7%.[149]

Use of FOB should consider the scenario in which patient is being evaluated as it is a costly test, an invasive procedure, and is not widely available in the developing countries and resource-poor settings. In developed countries with no resources constraint, best course of action in a patient with suspected sputum negative PTB is early use of FOB, whereas, in resource-poor settings, sputum induction with hypertonic saline should be considered first. If the patient still remains sputum smear negative and pretest probability of the patient having PTB is high, anti-TB treatment should be started and patient should be closely monitored. Consider FOB if patients do not seem to improve/deteriorate on anti-TB treatment or if the pretest probability of PTB is low.[150]

Mycobacterial Cultures

Mycobacterial culture is the gold standard for the diagnosis of TB. It is more sensitive than sputum microscopy, requires 10–100 organisms/mL to detect *M. tuberculosis.*[126] About 25–60% of patients with culture positive PTB may show negative smears. Sensitivity and specificity of culture is 80–93% and 98%, respectively.[126,151] Culture not only increases the sensitivity of *M. tuberculosis* diagnosis, but also helps in species identification, drug susceptibility testing and genotyping. Culture media are of various types: solid media, which can be egg-based (Lowenstein-Jensen) or agar-based (Middlebrook 7H10 and 7H11) media and liquid media (Middlebrook 7H12 and other broths). Most laboratories in the developing countries use solid media for mycobacterial culture. The greatest isolation rates are obtained from a combination of solid and liquid media.

The main constraint of solid media in long time is required for growth (mean time of at least four weeks). Other problems in the developing countries are the nonavailability and the inaccessibility of reliable laboratories for good quality cultures. Liquid culture media based on Middlebrook 7H12 broth give faster results than the solid media. They are also more sensitive than solid media for the detection of mycobacteria and may increase the diagnostic yield by 10%.[152,153] Disadvantages of liquid culture media include a high risk of contamination and cross-contamination and also the lack of colony morphology examination, which may help in detecting unexpected growth of non-TB mycobacteria. *Following are the rapid culture methods which are available:*

- *BACTEC (Becton Dickinson) culture medium:* A BACTEC 460 radiometric system (Becton Dickinson Instrument Systems, Sparks, MD, USA) is an automated method. It is based on the measurement of $^{14}CO_2$ liberated from ^{14}C palmitic acid by metabolizing mycobacteria. There is a rapid turnaround time with 87% of positive cultures recorded at 7 days and 96% by 14 days.[154] Major constraints with this method are the high cost and the problem of disposal of radioactive materials.
- *Mycobacterial Growth Indicator Tube (MGIT):* MGIT is a nonradiometric system. It contains Middlebrook 7H9 broth and a fluorescent compound embedded in a silicone sensor, which is sensitive to oxygen consumption in the medium emitting luminescence. Growth is detected visually using the ultraviolet light. Both manual and automatic (BACTEC MGIT 960) systems are available. Results are comparable to that of BACTEC 460 radiometric system.[155] The mean time for the detection of growth of mycobacteria in MGIT ranges from 8 days to 16 days.
- *Microcolony detection on solid media:* Growth of mycobacteria is detected by microscopic examination of plates covered with the thin layer of Middlebrook 7H11 agar medium. Though this technique is less expensive and requires lesser time than conventional culture, recovery of mycobacteria is less efficient and labor intensive.
- *Septi-chek AFB method:* It is biphasic culture system made up of a modified Middlebrook 7H9 broth with a three-sided paddle containing chocolate, egg-based, and modified-7H11 solid agar. The growth is observed by the three-sided paddle. The main characteristic of this system is the simultaneous detection of *M. tuberculosis*, nontubercular mycobacteria and even, contaminants.
- *MB/BacT system:* This is a nonradiometric system based on the colorimetric detection of CO_2. The disadvantages are the increased contamination and slightly longer time required for the detection of growth as compared to BACTEC 460 system.[156]
- *ESP II culture system:* This is a fully automated continuously monitoring system based on the detection of pressure changes in the culture medium of a sealed vial during mycobacterial growth. It should be used in combination with solid medium only.
- *Microscopic Observation of in-broth Culture (MODS):* It is suitable for high TB burden country, but it requires high laboratory biosafety, relatively costly media, antimicrobial

supplements and high technical skills. Drawback of the MGIT 960 system is that it does not support direct blood or bone marrow aspirate inoculation unlike Bactec 460 system and BacT system.

EXTRAPULMONARY TUBERCULOSIS

In immunocompetent adults, EPTB constitutes about 15–20% of all cases of TB, whereas in HIV positive patients, it accounts for more than 50%.[157] The commonly reported extrapulmonary sites of tuberculous involvement are the lymph nodes, pleura, bones or joints, and central nervous system (CNS). However, it can involve any organ. Lymph node TB is the most common form of EPTB in India and other developing countries.[146] Diagnosis of EPTB can pose a challenge to the clinicians due to various reasons.

- Signs and symptoms are most often nonspecific
- Paucibacillary nature of samples decreases the sensitivity of diagnostic tests
- EPTB involves relatively inaccessible sites so the retrieval of samples for diagnosis is a difficult job.

In a retrospective study done in Tanzania involving patients with EPTB, bacteriological or histological confirmation of diagnosis was possible in only 18% cases.[158] So misdiagnosis is common in almost all countries, which may lead to unnecessary presumptive treatment in patients without TB, or greater morbidity and mortality if the diagnosis of TB is delayed, especially in persons with concomitant HIV infection. Microscopic examination of sputum and culture lacks sensitivity in extrapulmonary disease. In a prospective study in Malawi, sputum positivity rate in EPTB patients was dismal (1.7%).[159]

In some form of EPTB, e.g. pleural TB, sputum samples may be beneficial. Conde et al.[160] reported a remarkably high yield of mycobacterial culture (52%) in a single specimen of induced sputum with sputum smear positivity in 12% of cases. Therefore, resource limited countries where invasive diagnostic procedures are less accessible, sputum induction should be advised.[161] Chest radiology may sometimes provide useful clue of the presence of associated PTB and may obviate the need for further invasive diagnostic modality in the developing countries. Abnormal chest radiography has been reported in 5–44% of lymph node TB, 30–50% of pleural effusion, 20–28% of abdominal TB and 32% of pericardial TB patients respectively.[161] Adenosine deaminase (ADA) enzyme estimation especially in pleural fluid has shown great promise in the diagnosis of tubercular pleural effusion. In pleural effusion, sensitivity and specificity of ADA have varied from 85% to 100% and 80% to 97%, respectively.[162]

Some patients in the early phase of tuberculous pleurisy may have low pleural fluid ADA levels; however, repeat testing may show elevated level.[163] A retrospective study revealed that older age and current smoking are predictive of TB pleural effusion with a low ADA level. Physicians should be careful in elderly patients and/or current smokers with TB pleural effusion when interpreting pleural fluid ADA levels.[164] False positive ADA level has been reported in patients with parapneumonic effusion (PPE) and empyema, rheumatoid pleurisy and malignant pleural effusion. ADA isoenzyme estimation may improve the specificity of the test. ADA2 is the predominant form in TB pleural effusion and is produced by monocytes and macrophages, while ADA1 is mainly elevated in pleural empyemas. The second approach to increase specificity is to ADA level and the pleural fluid lymphocyte/neutrophil ratio. The combination of elevated ADA and pleural fluid lympocyte/neutrophil ratio greater than 0.75 is a more specific diagnostic test than a high ADA level alone.[165] ADA levels are also elevated in a number of extrapulmonary sites in patients with TB, including cerebrospinal fluid (CSF) and BAL. However, the utility of measuring ADA levels in these fluids has not been rigorously studied.

REFERENCES

1. Wallis RS, Johnson JL. Adult tuberculosis in the 21st century: pathogenesis, clinical features, and management. Curr Opin Pulm Med. 2001;7(3):124-32.
2. Smith KR. Indoor air pollution in developing countries: recommendations for research. Indoor Air. 2002;12(3):198-207.
3. Mishra VK, Retherford RD, Smith KR. Biomass cooking fuels and prevalence of tuberculosis in India. Int J Infect Dis. 1999;3(3):119-29.
4. Pérez-Padilla R, Pérez-Guzmán C, Báez-Saldaña R, Torres-Cruz A. Cooking with biomass stoves and tuberculosis: a case control study. Int J Tuberc Lung Dis. 2001;5(5):441-7.
5. Kolappan C, Subramani R. Association between biomass fuel and pulmonary tuberculosis: a nested case-control study. Thorax. 2009;64(8):705-8.
6. Narasimhan P, Wood J, Macintyre CR, Mathai D. Risk factors for tuberculosis. Pulm Med. 2013;2013:828939.
7. Verver S, Warren RM, Beyers N, Richardson M, van der Spuy GD, Borgdorff MW, et al. Rate of reinfection tuberculosis after successful treatment is higher than rate of new tuberculosis. Am J Respir Crit Care Med. 2005;171(12):1430-5.
8. Henao-Tamayo M, Obregón-Henao A, Ordway DJ, Shang S, Duncan CG, Orme IM. A mouse model of tuberculosis reinfection. Tuberculosis (Edinb). 2012;92(3):211-7.
9. American Thoracic Society. Diagnostic standards and classification of tuberculosis. Am Rev Respir Dis. 1990;142(3):725-35.
10. Yoder MA, Lamichhane G, Bishai WR. Cavitary pulmonary tuberculosis: The holy grail of disease transmission. Curr Sci. 2004;86:74-81.
11. Korzeniewska-Kosela M, Krysl J, Müller N, Black W, Allen E, FitzGerald JM. Tuberculosis in young adults and the elderly. A prospective comparison study. Chest. 1994;106(1):28-32.
12. Breen RA, Leonard O, Perrin FM, Smith CJ, Bhagani S, Cropley I, et al. How good are systemic symptoms and blood inflammatory markers at detecting individuals with tuberculosis? Int J Tuberc Lung Dis. 2008;12(1):44-9.
13. Cowie RL, Escreet BC. Patterns of pyrexia in pulmonary tuberculosis. S Afr Med J. 1981;59(1):17-8.
14. Wang CS, Chen HC, Chong IW, Hwang JJ, Huang MS. Predictors for identifying the most infectious pulmonary tuberculosis patient. J Formos Med Assoc. 2008;107(1):13-20.

15. Cunha BA, Krakakis J, McDermott BP. Fever of unknown origin (FUO) caused by miliary tuberculosis: Diagnostic significance of morning temperature spikes. Heart Lung. 2009;38(1):77-82.
16. Cunha BA. Fever of unknown origin: focused diagnostic approach based on clinical clues from the history, physical examination, and laboratory tests. Infect Dis Clin North Am. 2007;21(4):1137-87.
17. Kent A Sepkowitz. Tuberculosis as the Cause of Fever of Unknown Origin: A Review. Int J Infect Dis. 1997;2:47-51.
18. Sharma BK, Kumari S, Varma SC, Sagar S, Singh S. Prolonged undiagnosed fever in Northern India. Trop Geogr Med. 1992;44(1-2):32-6.
19. Gopi PG, Subramani R, Narayanan PR. Evaluation of different types of chest symptoms for diagnosing pulmonary tuberculosis cases in community surveys. Indian J Tuberc. 2008;55(3):116-21.
20. Kashyap S, Mohapatra PR, Saini V. Endobronchial tuberculosis. Indian J Chest Dis Allied Sci. 2003;45(4):247-56.
21. Rosen MJ. Chronic cough due to tuberculosis and other infections: ACCP evidence-based clinical practice guidelines. Chest. 2006;129(1Suppl):197S-201S.
22. Mahouachi R, Kehder AB. Arterial bilateral embolisation in an evolutive tuberculosis. Respiratory Medicine Extra. 2006;2:42-4.
23. Prasad R, Garg R, Singhal S, Srivastava P. Lessons from patients with hemoptysis attending a chest clinic in India. Ann Thorac Med. 2009;4(1):10-2.
24. Telku B, Felleke G. Massive hemoptysis in tuberculosis. Tubercle. 1982;63(3):213-6.
25. Winer-Muram HT, Rubin SA. Thoracic complications of tuberculosis. J Thorac Imaging. 1990;5(2):46-63.
26. Crocco JA, Rooney JJ, Fankushen DS, DiBenedetto RJ, Lyons HA. Massive hemoptysis. Arch Intern Med. 1968;121(6):495-8.
27. Solit RW, McKeown JJ Jr, Smullens S, Fraimow W. The surgical implications of intracavitary mycetomas (fungus balls). J Thorac Cardiovasc Surg. 1971;62(3):411-22.
28. Aslam PA, Eastridge CE, Hughes FA Jr. Aspergillosis of the lung-an eighteen-year experience. Chest. 1971;59(1):28-32.
29. Battaglini JW, Murray GF, Keagy BA, Starek PJ, Wilcox BR. Surgical management of symptomatic pulmonary aspergilloma. Ann Thorac Surg. 1985;39(6):512-6.
30. Greenberg AK, Knapp J, Rom WN, Addrizzo-Harris DJ. Clinical presentation of pulmonary mycetoma in HIV-infected patients. Chest. 2002;122(3):886-92.
31. Levy H, Kallenbach JM, Feldman C, Thorburn JR, Abramowitz JA. Acute respiratory failure in active tuberculosis. Crit Care Med. 1987;15(3):221-5.
32. Choi D, Lee KS, Suh GY, Kim TS, Kwon OJ, Rhee CH, et al. Pulmonary tuberculosis presenting as acute respiratory failure: radiologic findings. J Comput Assist Tomogr. 1999;23(1): 107-13.
33. Agarwal MK, Muthuswamy PP, Banner AS, Shah RS, Addington WW. Respiratory failure in pulmonary tuberculosis. Chest. 1977;72(5):605-9.
34. Heffner JE, Strange C, Sahn SA. The impact of respiratory failure on the diagnosis of tuberculosis. Arch Intern Med. 1988;148(5):1103-8.
35. Park JH, Na JO, Kim EK, Lim CM, Shim TS, Lee SD, et al. The prognosis of respiratory failure in patients with tuberculous destroyed lung. Int J Tuberc Lung Dis. 2001;5(10):963-7.
36. Erbes R, Oettel K, Raffenberg M, Mauch H, Schmidt-Ioanas M, Lode H. Characteristics and outcome of patients with active pulmonary tuberculosis requiring intensive care. Eur Respir J. 2006;27(6):1223-8.
37. Radner DB, Snider GL. Recurrent laryngeal nerve paralysis as a complication of pulmonary tuberculosis. Am Rev Tuberc. 1952;65(1:1):93-9.
38. Liam CK, Pang YK, Poosparajah S. Pulmonary tuberculosis presenting as community-acquired pneumonia. Respirology. 2006;11(6):786-92.
39. Goussard P, Gie R. Airway involvement in pulmonary tuberculosis. Paediatr Respir Rev. 2007;8(2):118-23.
40. Bark CM, Dietze R, Okwera A, Quelapio MI, Thiel BA, Johnson JL. Clinical symptoms and microbiological outcomes in tuberculosis treatment trials. Tuberculosis (Edinb). 2011;91(6):601-4.
41. Ben-Yehuda A, Weksler ME. Host resistance and the immune system. Clin Geriatr Med. 1992;8(4):701-11.
42. Castle S, Uyemura K, Wong W, Modlin R, Effros R. Evidence of enhanced type 2 immune response and impaired upregulation of a type 1 response in frail elderly nursing home residents. Mech Ageing Dev. 1997;94(1-3):7-16.
43. Van den Brande P. Revised guidelines for the diagnosis and control of tuberculosis: impact on management in the elderly. Drugs Aging. 2005;22(8):663-86.
44. Lee JH, Han DH, Song JW, Chung HS. Diagnostic and therapeutic problems of pulmonary tuberculosis in elderly patients. J Korean Med Sci. 2005;20(5):784-9.
45. Rajagopalan S. Tuberculosis and aging: a global health problem. Clin Infect Dis. 2001;33(7):1034-9.
46. Wakefield KM, Henderson ST, Streit JG. Fever of unknown origin in the elderly. Prim Care. 1989;16(2):501-13.
47. Morris CD. Pulmonary tuberculosis in the elderly: a different disease? Thorax. 1990;45(12):912-3.
48. Sharma SK, Mohan A, Sharma A, Mitra DK. Miliary tuberculosis: new insights into an old disease. Lancet Infect Dis. 2005;5(7):415-30.
49. Ray S, Talukdar A, Kundu S, Khanra D, Sonthalia N. Diagnosis and management of miliary tuberculosis: current state and future perspectives. Ther Clin Risk Manag. 2013;9:9-26.
50. Chapman C, Whorton C. Acute generalized miliary tuberculosis in adults: a clinico-pathologic study based on sixty-three cases diagnosed at autopsy. N Engl J Med. 1946;235:239-48.
51. Daikos GL, Uttamchandani RB, Tuda C, Fischl MA, Miller N, Cleary T, et al. Disseminated miliary tuberculosis of the skin in patients with AIDS: report of four cases. Clin Infect Dis. 1998;27(1):205-8.
52. Landouzy L. A note on la typho-bacillose. Lancet. 1908;172: 1440-1.
53. Barber TW, Craven DE, McCabe WR. Bacteremia due to *Mycobacterium tuberculosis* in patients with human immunodeficiency virus infection. A report of 9 cases and a review of the literature. Medicine (Baltimore). 1990;69(6):375-83.
54. Johnson MD, Decker CF. Tuberculosis and HIV infection. Dis Mon. 2006;52(11-12):420-7.
55. Lee MP, Chan JW, Ng KK, Li PC. Clinical manifestations of tuberculosis in HIV-infected patients. Respirology. 2000; 5(4):423-6.
56. Barnes PF, Bloch AB, Davidson PT, Snider DE Jr. Tuberculosis in patients with human immunodeficiency virus infection. N Engl J Med. 1992;324(23):1644-50.
57. Wallgren A. The time-table of tuberculosis. Tubercle. 1948; 29(11):245-51.

58. Qiu L, Teeter LD, Liu Z, Ma X, Musser JM, Graviss EA. Diagnostic associations between pleural and pulmonary tuberculosis. J Infect. 2006;53(6):377-86.
59. Smith H. Paradoxical responses during the chemotherapy of tuberculosis. J Infect. 1987;15(1):1-3.
60. Gupta RC, Dixit R, Purohit SD, Saxena A. Development of pleural effusion in patients during anti-tuberculous chemotherapy: analysis of twenty-nine cases with review of literature. Indian J Chest Dis Allied Sci. 2000;42(3):161-6.
61. Al-Majed SA. Study of paradoxical response to chemotherapy in tuberculous pleural effusion. Respir Med. 1996;90(4):211-4.
62. Franco-Paredes C, Díaz-Borjon A, Senger MA, Barragan L, Leonard M. The ever-expanding association between rheumatologic diseases and tuberculosis. Am J Med. 2006; 119(6):470-7.
63. Cho KH, Lee D, Chun HS, Eun HC, Han SK. Erythema induratum with pulmonary tuberculosis: report of three cases. J Dermatol. 1995;22(2):143-8.
64. Dall L, Long L, Standford J. Poncet's disease: tuberculous rheumatism. Rev Infect Dis. 1989;11(1):105-7.
65. Malhotra P, Agarwal R, Awasthi A, Jindal SK, Srinivasan R. How long does it take for tuberculosis to cause secondary amyloidosis? Eur J Intern Med. 2005;16(6):437-9.
66. Triger DR, Joekes AM. Renal amyloidosis—a fourteen-year follow-up. Q J Med. 1973;42(165):15-40.
67. Paton NI, Chua YK, Earnest A, Chee CB. Randomized controlled trial of nutritional supplementation in patients with newly diagnosed tuberculosis and wasting. Am J Clin Nutr. 2004;80(2):460-5.
68. Zachariah R, Spiehnann MP, Harries AD, Salaniponi FM. Moderate to severe malnutrition in patients with tuberculosis is a risk factor associated with early death. Trans R Soc Trop Med Hyg. 2002;96(3):291-4.
69. Kashyap S, Puri DS, Bansal SK, Dhawan A, Prasher N, Grover PS. *Mycobacterium tuberculosis* infection presenting as pancytopenia with hypocellular bone marrow. J Assoc Physicians India. 1991;39(6):497-8.
70. Singh KJ, Ahluwalia G, Sharma SK, Saxena R, Chaudhary VP, Anant M. Significance of haematological manifestations in patients with tuberculosis. J Assoc Physicians India. 2001;49: 788,790-4.
71. Chung DK, Hubbard WW. Hyponatremia in untreated active pulmonary tuberculosis. Am Rev Respir Dis. 1969;99(4): 595-7.
72. Hill AR, Uribarri J, Mann J, Berl T. Altered water metabolism in tuberculosis: role of vasopressin. Ann J Med. 1990;88(4):357-64.
73. Lam KY, Lo CY. A critical examination of adrenal tuberculosis and a 28-year autopsy experience of active tuberculosis. Clin Endocrinol (Oxf). 2001;54(5):633-9.
74. Dosumu EA, Momoh JA. Hypercalcemia in patients with newly diagnosed tuberculosis in Abuja, Nigeria. Can Respir J. 2006;13(2):83-7.
75. Huebner RE, Schein MF, Bass JB Jr. The tuberculin skin test. Clin Infect Dis. 1993;17(6):968-75.
76. Albini TA, Karakousis PC, Rao NA. Interferon-gamma release assays in the diagnosis of tuberculous uveitis. Am J Ophthalmol. 2008;146(4):486-8.
77. Farhat M, Greenaway C, Pai M, Menzies D. False-positive tuberculin skin tests: what is the absolute effect of BCG and non-tuberculous mycobacteria? Int J Tuberc Lung Dis. 2006;10(11):1192-204.
78. Targeted tuberculin testing and treatment of latent tuberculosis infection. This official statement of the American Thoracic Society was adopted by the ATS Board of Directors, July 1999. This is a Joint Statement of the American Thoracic Society (ATS) and the Centers for Disease Control and Prevention (CDC). This statement was endorsed by the Council of the Infectious Diseases Society of America. (IDSA), September 1999, and the sections of this statement. Am J Respir Crit Care Med. 2000; 161(4 Pt 2):S221-47.
79. Campos-Neto A, Rodrigues-Júnior V, Pedral-Sampaio DB, Netto EM, Ovendale PJ, Coler RN, et al. Evaluation of DPPD, a single recombinant *Mycobacterium tuberculosis* protein as an alternative antigen for the Mantoux test. Tuberculosis (Edinb). 2001;81(5-6):353-8.
80. Arend SM, Franken WP, Aggerbeck H, Prins C, van Dissel JT, Thierry-Carstensen B, et al. Double-blind randomized Phase I study comparing rdESAT-6 to tuberculin as skin test reagent in the diagnosis of tuberculosis infection. Tuberculosis (Edinb). 2008;88(3):249-61.
81. Shingadia D, Novelli V. The tuberculin skin test: a hundred, not out? Arch Dis Child. 2008;93(3):189-90.
82. Cellestis. (2011). QuantiFERON-TB Gold Package Insert. [online]. Available from *www.cellestis.com/IRM/Content/pdf/QuantiFeron%20US%20VerJ_JULY2011_ttf.pdf*. [Accessed may 2014].
83. Oxford Immunotec. T-SPOT.TB Package Insert. 2013. Available at: *http://www.tspot.com/wp-content/uploads/2012/01/PI-TB-US-v4.pdf*. Accessed may 28, 2014.
84. Belknap R, Daley CL. Interferon-gamma release assays. Clin Lab Med. 2014;34(2):337-49.
85. Marais BJ, Pai M. New approaches and emerging technologies in the diagnosis of childhood tuberculosis. Paediatr Respir Rev. 2007;8(2):124-33.
86. Lalvani A. Diagnosing tuberculosis infection in the 21st century: new tools to tackle an old enemy. Chest. 2007;131(6):1898-906.
87. Andersen P, Munk ME, Pollock JM, Doherty TM. Specific immune-based diagnosis of tuberculosis. Lancet. 2000; 356(9235):1099-104.
88. Dheda K, van Zyl Smit R, Badri M, Pai M. T-cell interferon-gamma release assays for the rapid immunodiagnosis of tuberculosis: clinical utility in high-burden vs. low-burden settings. Curr Opin Pulm Med. 2009;15(3):188-200.
89. Ruhwald M, Ravn P. Biomarkers of latent TB infection. Expert Rev Respir Med. 2009;3(4):387-401.
90. McAdams HP, Erasmus J, Winter JA. Radiologic manifestations of pulmonary tuberculosis. Radiol Clin North Am. 1995; 33(4):655-78.
91. Miller WT, Miller WT Jr. Tuberculosis in the normal host: radiological findings. Semin Roentgenol. 1993;28(2):109-18.
92. Jones BE, Ryu R, Yang Z, Cave MD, Pogoda JM, Otaya M, et al. Chest radiographic findings in patients with tuberculosis with recent or remote infection. Am J Respir Crit Care Med. 1997;156(4 Pt 1):1270-3.
93. Geng E, Kreiswirth B, Burzynski J, Schluger NW. Clinical and radiographic correlates of primary and reactivation tuberculosis: a molecular epidemiology study. JAMA. 2005; 293(22):2740-5.
94. Fujita J, Higa F, Tateyama M. Radiological findings of mycobacterial diseases. J Infect Chemother. 2007;13(1):8-17.
95. Havlir DV, Barnes PF. Tuberculosis in patients with human immunodeficiency virus infection. N Engl J Med. 1999; 340(5):367-73.

96. Leung AN. Pulmonary tuberculosis: the essentials. Radiology. 1999;210(2):307-22.
97. Andreu J, Cáceres J, Pallisa E, Martinez-Rodriguez M. Radiological manifestations of pulmonary tuberculosis. Eur J Radiol. 2004;51(2):139-49.
98. Andronikou S, Vanhoenacker FM, De Backer AI. Advances in imaging chest tuberculosis: blurring of differences between children and adults. Clin Chest Med. 2009;30(4):717-44.
99. Curvo-Semedo L, Teixeira L, Caseiro-Alves F. Tuberculosis of the chest. Eur J Radiol. 2005;55(2):158-72.
100. Moon WK, Im JG, Yeon KM, Han MC. Mediastinal tuberculosis lymphadenitis: CT findings of active and inactive disease. AJR Am J Roentgenol. 1998;170(3):715-8.
101. Woodring JH, Vandiviere HM, Fried AM, Dillon ML, Williams TD, Melvin IG. Update: the radiographic features of pulmonary tuberculosis. AJR Am J Roentgenol. 1986;146(3):497-506.
102. Krysl J, Korzeniewska-Kosela M, Müller NL, FitzGerald JM. Radiologic features of pulmonary tuberculosis: an assessment of 188 cases. Can Assoc Radiol J. 1994;45(2):101-7.
103. Canetti G. Present aspects of bacterial resistance in tuberculosis. Am Rev Respir Dis. 1965;92(5):687-703.
104. Hadlock FP, Park SK, Awe RJ, Rivera M. Unusual radiographic findings in adult pulmonary tuberculosis. AJR Am J Roentgenol. 1980;134(5):1015-8.
105. Kuhlman JE, Deutsch JH, Fishman EK, Siegelman SS. CT features of thoracic mycobacterial disease. Radiographics. 1990;10(3):413-31.
106. Palmer PE. Pulmonary tuberculosis–usual and unusual radiographic presentations. Semin Roentgenol. 1979;14(3):204-43.
107. Woodring JH, Vandiviere HM, Lee C. Intrathoracic lymphadenopathy in postprimary tuberculosis. South Med J. 1988;81(8):992-7.
108. Marciniuk DD, McNab BD, Martin WT, Hoeppner VH. Detection of pulmonary tuberculosis in patients with a normal chest radiograph. Chest. 1999;115(2):445-52.
109. FitzGerald JM, Grzybowski S, Allen EA. The impact of human immunodeficiency virus infection on tuberculosis and its control. Chest. 1991;100(1):191-200.
110. Long R, Maycher B, Scalcini M, Manfreda J. The chest radiograph in pulmonary tuberculosis patients seropositive for human immunodeficiency virus type 1. Chest. 1991;99(1):123-7.
111. Greenberg SD, Frager D, Suster B, Walker S, Stavropoulos C, Rothpearl A. Active pulmonary tuberculosis in patients with AIDS: spectrum of radiographic findings (including a normal appearance). Radiology. 1994;193(1):115-9.
112. Pitchenik AE, Rubinson HA. The radiographic appearance of tuberculosis in patients with the acquired immune deficiency syndrome (AIDS) and pre-AIDS. Am Rev Respir Dis. 1985;131(3):393-6.
113. Hatipoðlu ON, Osma E, Manisali M, Uçan ES, Balci P, Akkoçlu A, et al. High resolution computed tomographic findings in pulmonary tuberculosis. Thorax. 1996;51(4):397-402.
114. Lee JJ, Chong PY, Lin CB, Hsu AH, Lee CC. High resolution chest CT in patients with pulmonary tuberculosis: characteristic findings before and after antituberculous therapy. Eur J Radiol. 2008;67(1):100-4.
115. Matsuoka S, Uchiyama K, Shima H, Suzuki K, Shimura A, Sasaki Y, et al. Relationship between CT findings of pulmonary tuberculosis and the number of acid-fast bacilli on sputum smears. Clin Imaging. 2004;28(2):119-23.
116. Cherian MJ, Dahniya MH, al-Marzouk NF, Abel A, Bader S, Buerki K, et al. Pulmonary tuberculosis presenting as mass lesions and simulating neoplasms in adults. Australas Radiol. 1998;42(4):303-8.
117. Sochocky S. Tuberculoma of the lung. Am Rev Tuberc. 1958; 78(3):403-10.
118. Bleyer JM, Marks JH. Tuberculomas and hamartomas of the lung; comparative study of 66 proved cases. Am J Roentgenol Radium Ther Nucl Med. 1957;77(6):1013-22.
119. Kwong JS, Carignan S, Kang EY, Müller NL, FitzGerald JM. Miliary tuberculosis. Diagnostic accuracy of chest radiography. Chest. 1996;110(2):339-42.
120. Piqueras AR, Marruecos L, Artigas A, Rodriguez C. Miliary tuberculosis and adult respiratory distress syndrome. Intensive Care Med. 1987;13(3):175-82.
121. Palmer PE. Pulmonary Tuberculosis–usual and unusual radiographic presentations. Semin Roentgenol. 1979;14(3):204-43.
122. Rajasekaran S, Vallinayagl V, Jeyaganesh D. Unilateral lung destruction: a computed tomographic evaluation. Ind J Tub. 1999;46:183-87.
123. Thomason CB, Rao BR. Lung Imaging–Unilateral absence or near absence of pulmonary perfusion on lung scanning. Semin Nucl Med. 1983;13(4):388-90.
124. Pomerantz M, Brown JM. Surgery in the treatment of multidrug-resistant tuberculosis. Clin Chest Med. 1997;18(1):123-30.
125. Diagnostic Standards and Classification of Tuberculosis in Adults and Children. This official statement of the American Thoracic Society and the Centers for Disease Control and Prevention was adopted by the ATS Board of Directors, July 1999. This statement was endorsed by the Council of the Infectious Disease Society of America, September 1999. Am J Respir Crit Care Med. 2000;161(4 Pt 1):1376-95.
126. Brodie D, Schluger NW. The diagnosis of tuberculosis. Clin Chest Med. 2005;26(2):247-71.
127. Getahun H, Harrington M, O'Brien R, Nunn P. Diagnosis of smear-negative pulmonary tuberculosis in people with HIV infection or AIDS in resource-constrained settings: informing urgent policy changes. Lancet. 2007;369(9578):2042-9.
128. Steingart KR, Ng V, Henry M, Hopewell PC, Ramsay A, Cunningham J, et al. Sputum processing methods to improve the sensitivity of smear microscopy for tuberculosis: a systematic review. Lancet Infect Dis. 2006;6(10):664-74.
129. Yassin MA, Cuevas LE, Gebrexabher H, Squire SB. Efficacy and safety of short-term bleach digestion of sputum in case-finding for pulmonary tuberculosis in Ethiopia. Int J Tuberc Lung Dis. 2003;7(7):678-83.
130. Katoch VM. Smear microscopy to diagnose tuberculosis. Indian J Med Res. 2006;123(6):735-8.
131. Somoskövi A, Hotaling JE, Fitzgerald M, O'Donnell D, Parsons LM, Salfinger M. Lessons from a proficiency testing event for acid-fast microscopy. Chest. 2001;120(1):250-7.
132. Van Deun A, Hamid Salim A, Aung KJ, Hossain MA, Chambugonj N, Hye MA, et al. Performance of variations of carbolfuchsin staining of sputum smears for AFB under field conditions. Int J Tuber Lung Dis. 2005;9(10):1127-33.
133. Bennedsen J, Larsen SO. Examination for tubercle bacilli by fluorescence microscopy. Scand J Respir Dis. 1966;47(2):114-20.
134. Marais B, Brittle W, Painczyk K, Hesseling AC, Beyers N, Wasserman E, et al. Use of light-emitting diode fluorescence microscopy to detect acid-fast bacilli in sputum. Clin Infect Dis. 2008;47(2):203-7.
135. Anderson C, Inhaber N, Menzies D. Comparison of sputum induction with fiber-optic bronchoscopy in the diagnosis of tuberculosis. Am J Respir Crit Care Med. 1995;152(5 Pt 1):1570-4.

136. Conde MB, Soares SL, Mello FC, Rezende VM, Almeida LL, Reingold AL, et al. Comparison of sputum induction with fiberoptic bronchoscopy in the diagnosis of tuberculosis: experience at an acquired immune deficiency syndrome reference center in Rio de Janeiro, Brazil. Am J Respir Crit Care Med. 2000;162(6):2238-40.
137. Al Zahrani K, Al Jahdali H, Poirier L, René P, Menzies D. Yield of smear, culture and amplification tests from repeated sputum induction for the diagnosis of pulmonary tuberculosis. Int J Tuberc Lung Dis. 2001;5(9):855-60.
138. McWilliams T, Wells AU, Harrison AC, Lindstrom S, Cameron RJ, Foskin E. Induced sputum and bronchoscopy in the diagnosis of pulmonary tuberculosis. Thorax. 2002;57(12):1010-4.
139. McCallister JW, Chin R, Conforti J. Bronchoscopic Myths and Legends: Bronchoscopy in the Diagnosis of Pulmonary Tuberculosis. Clin Pulm Med. 2006;13:271-3.
140. Hartung TK, Maulu A, Nash J, Fredlund VG. Suspected pulmonary tuberculosis in rural South Africa–sputum induction as a simple diagnostic tool? S Afr Med J. 2002;92(6):455-8.
141. Venkateshiah SB, Mehta AC. Role of flexible bronchoscopy in the diagnosis of pulmonary tuberculosis in immunocompetent individuals. J Bronchol. 2003;10:300-8.
142. Bartlett JG, Alexander J, Mayhew J, Sullivan-Sigler N, Gorbach SL. Should fiberoptic bronchoscopy aspirates be cultured? Am Rev Respir Dis.1976;114(1):73-8.
143. Schmidt RM, Rosenkranz HS. Antimicrobial activity of local anesthetics: lidocaine and procaine. J Infect Dis. 1970;121(6):597-607.
144. Sarkar SK, Sharma GS, Gupta PR, Sharma RK. Fiberoptic bronchoscopy in the diagnosis of pulmonary tuberculosis. Tubercle. 1980;61(2):97-9.
145. Chawla R, Pant K, Jaggi OP, Chandrashekhar S, Thukral SS. Fibreoptic bronchoscopy in smear-negative pulmonary tuberculosis. Eur Respir J. 1988;1(9):804-6.
146. Proudfoot AT, Akhtar AJ, Douglas AC, Horne NW. Miliary tuberculosis in adults. Br Med J. 1969;2(5652):273-6.
147. Munt PW. Miliary tuberculosis in the chemotherapy era: with a clinical review in 69 American adults. Medicine (Baltimore). 1972;51(2):139-55.
148. Chang SC, Lee PY, Perng RP. Clinical role of bronchoscopy in adults with intrathoracic tuberculous lymphadenopathy. Chest. 1988;93(2):314-7.
149. George PM, Mehta M, Dhariwal J, Singanayagam A, Raphael CE, Salmasi M, et al. Post-bronchoscopy sputum: improving the diagnostic yield in smear negative pulmonary TB. Respir Med. 2011;105(11):1726-31.
150. Mohan A, Sharma SK. Fibreoptic bronchoscopy in the diagnosis of sputum smear-negative pulmonary tuberculosis: current status. Indian J Chest Dis Allied Sci. 2008;50(1):67-78.
151. Dalovisio JR, Montenegro-James S, Kemmerly SA, Genre CF, Chambers R, Greer D, et al. Comparison of the amplified *Mycobacterium Tuberculosis* (MTB) direct test, Amplicor MTB PCR, and IS6110-PCR for detection of MTB in respiratory specimens. Clin Infect Dis. 1996;23(5):1099-106.
152. Dinnes J, Deeks J, Kunst H, Gibson A, Cummins E, Waugh N, et al. A systematic review of rapid diagnostic tests for the detection of tuberculosis infection. Health Technol Assess. 2007;11(3):1-196.
153. Cruciani M, Scarparo C, Malena M, Bosco O, Serpelloni G, Mengoli C. Meta-analysis of BACTEC MGIT 960 and BACTEC 460 TB, with or without solid media, for detection of mycobacteria. J Clin Microbiol. 2004;42(5):2321-5.
154. Venkataraman P, Herbert D, Paramasivan CN. Evaluation of the BACTEC radiometric method in the early diagnosis of tuberculosis. Indian J Med Res. 1998;108:120-7
155. Palomino JC. Nonconventional and new methods in the diagnosis of tuberculosis: feasibility and applicability in the field. Eur Respir J. 2005;26(2):339-50.
156. Rohner P, Ninet B, Metral C, Emler S, Auckenthaler R. Evaluation of the MB/BacT system and comparison to the BACTEC 460 system and solid media for isolation of mycobacteria from clinical specimens. J Clin Microbiol. 1997;35(12):3127-31.
157. Sharma SK, Mohan A. Extrapulmonary tuberculosis. Indian J Med Res. 2004;120(4):316-53.
158. Richter C, Ndosi B, Mwammy AS, Mbwambo RK. Extrapulmonary tuberculosis–a simple diagnosis? A retrospective study at Dar es Salaam, Tanzania. Trop Geogr Med. 1991;43(4):375-8.
159. Kwanjana IH, Harries AD, Hargreaves NJ, Van Gorkom J, Ringdal T, Salaniponi FM. Sputum-smear examination in patients with extrapulmonary tuberculosis in Malawi. Trans R Soc Trop Med Hyg. 2000;94(4):395-8.
160. Conde MB, Loivos AC, Rezenda VM, Soares SL, Mello FC, Reingold AL, et al. Yield of sputum induction in diagnosis of pleural tuberculosis. Am J Respir Crit Care Med. 2003;167(5):723-5.
161. Gopi A, Madhavan SM, Sharma SK, Sahn SA. Diagnosis and treatment of tuberculous pleural effusion in 2006. Chest. 2007;131(3):880-9.
162. Gorguner M, Cerci M, Gorguner I. Determination of adenosine deaminase activity and its isoenzymes for diagnosis of pleural effusions. Respirology. 2000;5(4):321-4.
163. Krenke R, Korczyński P. Use of pleural fluid levels of adenosine deaminase and interferon gamma in the diagnosis of tuberculous pleuritis. Curr Opin Pulm Med. 2010;16(4):367-75.
164. Lee SJ, Kim HS, Lee SH, Lee TW, Lee HR, Cho YJ, et al. Factors influencing pleural adenosine deaminase level in patients with tuberculous pleurisy. Am J Med Sci. 2014;348(5):362-5.
165. Burgess LJ, Maritz FJ, Le Roux I, Taljaard JJ. Combined use of pleural adenosine deaminase with lymphocyte/neutrophil ratio. Increased specificity for the diagnosis of tuberculous pleuritis. Chest. 1996;109(2):414-9.

37

Chapter

Molecular Diagnosis of Tuberculosis

Ramamurthy Sakamuri, Mamta Kalra, Indu Verma, Suman Laal

INTRODUCTION

Only 5–10% of the individuals who get infected with *Mycobacterium tuberculosis* progress to clinical tuberculosis (TB),[1,2] the remaining individuals develop immune responses that arrest the progression of infection to clinical tuberculosis, although they continue to harbor latent tuberculosis infection (LTBI). Approximately, 10% of latently infected subjects reactivate their LTBI and progress to clinical tuberculosis sometime later during the years or decades postinfection. Despite this relatively limited progression of *M. tuberculosis* infection to clinical disease, more than 8 million new cases of tuberculosis occur every year and approximately two million individuals die because of tuberculosis.[3,4] The spread of human immunodeficiency virus (HIV)-infection in the tuberculosis endemic countries and the synergistic relationship between HIV and tuberculosis is further accelerating the morbidity and mortality caused by tuberculosis.[4] The WHO has implemented directly-observed therapy short-term (DOTS) programs for tuberculosis diagnosis and treatment in most parts of the world. However, the success of the DOTS programs is hampered by the lack of rapid and accurate diagnostic tools.

DIAGNOSIS OF TUBERCULOSIS IN LOW-INCOME COUNTRIES

Tuberculosis is a chronic, slow-progressing infection (except in immunocompromised individuals), which can manifest as pulmonary or extrapulmonary disease. Even pulmonary tuberculosis is not a single-stage acute disease and patients present with a spectrum of clinical, radiological and bacterial indications.

There is no single diagnostic test that can detect tuberculosis at all the different stages or the different forms of tuberculosis, a combination of clinical suspicion, microscopic examination of smears made directly from sputum for presence of acid-fast bacilli (AFB) and radiological findings are used for diagnosis. Clinically, tuberculosis can present with symptoms that vary from mild cough or chest pains in an otherwise asymptomatic patient to fever, night sweats, wasting, hemoptysis, (etc.) and therefore, often does not provide unambiguous diagnosis. AFB microscopy is highly specific and low-cost,[5,6] but visualizing bacteria in smears made without processing and concentration of sputum specimens requires the presence of 5–10 thousand AFB per mL of sputum; this occurs only when the patient has progressed to advanced disease.

Microscopy requires careful examination of multiple specimens from each patient, which is tedious and requires good microscopes; factors that decrease sensitivity in settings that have high patient burden and meager resources. As a result, the sensitivity of the AFB smear test varies from 30% to 80% in culture confirmed tuberculosis in different laboratories. Microscopy fails to identify about 50% of patients who have less advanced disease (smear-negative), performs poorly in pediatric cases, patients with extrapulmonary tuberculosis and HIV-infected tuberculosis patients. Thus, AFB smear-based diagnosis results in significant underdiagnosis of tuberculosis, resulting in increased morbidity and mortality and continued transmission into the communities.[6] Chest X-rays can aid diagnosis when the disease is advanced, but their utility is limited by patient variability in that there may be no pulmonary involvement, or patients may have a typical infiltration or progressed to different levels of cavitation and pulmonary damage. Culture of AFB although can enhance the sensitivity of diagnosis, permits identification and drug sensitivity testing of isolated mycobacterial species. However, because *M. tuberculosis* is a slow-growing pathogen, cultures require several weeks (6–8 weeks) and are significantly more expensive than microscopy. In developing countries, culture is not a feasible option because of the high patient burden, the requirement for expensive laboratory infrastructure and the associated expenses. Rapid and simple tests that can replace AFB microscopy, and can improve diagnosis of paucibacillary tuberculosis are urgently required.

DIAGNOSIS OF TUBERCULOSIS IN HIGH-INCOME COUNTRIES

The speed and accuracy of tuberculosis diagnosis is significantly better in the resource-rich countries (e.g. US, Western Europe) that have a low incidence of tuberculosis. Microscopy has significantly improved sensitivity because the smears are prepared from sputum samples that are digested, decontaminated and concentrated; fluorescence microscopy, which is more sensitive, is routinely used. Culture of bacteria on solid (Middlebrook, Lowenstein-Jensen) and/or liquid media complements microscopy and several sensitive broth-based culture systems are routinely used (Becton, Dickinson and Company, Sparks; MB/BacT, Organon Teknika Corporation, NC; ESP, TREK Diagnostic systems Inc, Cleveland, OH; Wampole laboratories, Princeton, NJ, etc.). Fully automated systems where the vials inoculated with the patient specimen are monitored continuously for bacterial growth, are available in most mycobacteriology laboratories. Coupled with the highly sensitive and specific nucleic acid amplification tests (NAAT) that are available for confirmation of *M. tuberculosis*, the sensitivity of tuberculosis diagnosis of multibacillary tuberculosis cases in these countries is very high (95–98%) and a large proportion of paucibacillary cases (48–53%) are also detected.[7,8]

Despite the use of multiple diagnostic methods, diagnosis of smear-negative tuberculosis cases can take several weeks since chest X-rays or computed tomography (CT) scans and microscopy take several days and another 7–14 days are required for culture confirmation even in smear-positive patients. Additional sensitive methods for identification of *M. tuberculosis* from liquid cultures are available [High-performance liquid chromatography (HPLC), gas-liquid chromatography (GLC)] and may be useful for the difficult-to-diagnose cases, but the costs and complexity limit their use in routine diagnosis. Despite the use of multiple tests, no bacteriological confirmation can be obtained for approximately 10–20% of tuberculosis patients, who are determined to have tuberculosis based on clinical and/or radiological improvement while on anti-TB medications.[9] Clearly, there is a definite need for improved diagnostic tests even for the resource-rich countries and tests that can rapidly identify paucibacillary tuberculosis would be an asset to tuberculosis control.[1,10]

Detection and treatment of LTBI is an integral component of tuberculosis control in the high-income settings. The detection of LTBI is based on the tuberculin skin test [TST; also called the purified protein derivative (PPD) skin test], which measures delayed hypersensitivity responses elicited by the mycobacterial antigens.[2] Because PPD is actually a crude mixture of more than 200 different secreted and somatic proteins of *M. tuberculosis*, many of which are shared among nontuberculosis mycobacteria (NTM) and *M. bovis* Bacillus Calmette-Guérin (BCG), the specificity of the PPD test is low, especially in individuals vaccinated with BCG or cross-sensitized with nonpathogenic environmental mycobacteria. The sensitivity of the PPD test is also suboptimal and fails to identify approximately 20–30% of confirmed tuberculosis cases. Although PPD testing is relatively inexpensive, it fails to differentiate between a latent infection that may never progress to active, subclinical or clinical tuberculosis[11-13] and can neither predict if and when the infection will progress to clinical tuberculosis. As a result, even though approximately 5–10% of *M. tuberculosis* infected individuals actually progress to clinical tuberculosis, all PPD-positive individuals require clinical, bacteriological and radiological evaluation, while individuals believed to be infected and at risk for tuberculosis are required to take preventive therapy with isoniazid (INH) for 6–9 months.[2] Thus, PPD test-based decisions are erroneous since they result in treatment of latent infection in individuals who may never progress to clinical tuberculosis, monotherapy in individuals who may have an active but subclinical infection or are infected with INH-resistant *M. tuberculosis* and no treatment in infected individuals with false-negative responses.[2]

According to the CDC estimates, there are approximately 15 million latently infected individuals in the US, and better diagnostic tests that can accurately identify *M. tuberculosis* infection and discriminate between latent and incipient subclinical tuberculosis in high-risk populations are required to eliminate tuberculosis from the US.[10,14] More accurate diagnostic tests for *M. tuberculosis* infection, the interferon gamma release assays (IGRAs; described below) have become available in recent years and are increasingly being used in these countries instead of TST.

TUBERCULOSIS DIAGNOSIS IN HUMAN IMMUNODEFICIENCY VIRUS-POSITIVE INDIVIDUALS

The immune dysfunction caused by HIV infection leads to increased reactivation of latent tuberculosis, increased incidence of primary tuberculosis and accelerated course of disease progression in HIV+ individuals.[15-19] The risk of developing tuberculosis doubles as early as the first year after HIV infection and continues to increase in subsequent years.[20] As a result, in the sub-Saharan Africa and Southeast Asia where tuberculosis is endemic, approximately 50–70% of the HIV+ individuals develop tuberculosis.[4,21-24] Concomitant tuberculosis accelerates the progression of HIV infection. The dysfunctional cellular immune responses in HIV+ patients result in reduced pulmonary pathology and progression to cavitary lesions, which in turn results in reduced smear positivity. For these reasons, the limitations of the current diagnostic tests for tuberculosis are amplified in HIV coinfected individuals.[25] Tuberculosis is thus the single most important cause of morbidity and mortality in HIV+ patients in TB-endemic countries. As in non-HIV *M. tuberculosis* infected individuals, preventive therapy with INH in HIV coinfected individuals with latent *M. tuberculosis* infection has also been shown to reduce the risk for developing tuberculosis.[1]

In TB-endemic countries, the rates of latent infection are high, preventive treatment with anti-TB drugs, and the accompanying clinical, bacteriological and adherence monitoring is impossible, and treatment of unrecognized active tuberculosis with one or two drugs enhances the risk of fostering drug resistance.[26-28] For these reasons, preventive treatment for HIV-infected persons is not recommended in these settings unless active tuberculosis can be ruled out on the basis of clinical evaluation.[29,30] No diagnostic tests that can discriminate between latent tuberculosis and incipient, subclinical tuberculosis in HIV-infected individuals are currently available. This is problematic because undiagnosed active tuberculosis in asymptomatic HIV+ patients with no clinical, radiological or bacteriological indications of tuberculosis has been reported from several settings.[18,19] Thus, tests that can rapidly discriminate between LTBI and incipient subclinical tuberculosis and identify patients with subclinical tuberculosis prior to progression to bacteriologically detectable, clinical tuberculosis, are urgently required. Such a test would prevent progression of *M. tuberculosis* infection to clinical tuberculosis, contribute to interruption of transmission into communities, and retard the progression of HIV-infection in patients who are unable to obtain antiretroviral therapy.[27]

DIAGNOSIS OF TUBERCULOSIS: BEYOND MICROSCOPY

Direct sputum microscopy has been used for tuberculosis diagnosis since the 1880s, it remains the primary tool for tuberculosis diagnosis, 120 years later. More sensitive and specific diagnostic tests have emerged in the last few decades, but are too expensive and technically challenging for implementation in the high burden, low-resource settings. While an unprecedented interest has arisen in devising new diagnostic tools for tuberculosis in the last decade or so, and some new tests have been devised, there is still a significant lack of tools that will be required to control and eliminate tuberculosis. An overview of the diagnostic tests that are used in the developed world or are currently under development is provided **(Table 1)**.

Table 1 Molecular methods used for diagnosis of tuberculosis

- Nucleic acid amplification (NAA) detection-based tests
  - In-house NAA tests
  - Amplified MTB direct test (MTD)
  - Amplicor MTB test (Amplicor)
  - COBAS amplicor MTB test
  - COBAS TaqMan test MTB
  - BD ProbeTec MTB test
  - Loop-mediated isothermal amplification: Loopamp® TB detection, EasyNAT TB assay, Alere q TB diagnostic system, TRCRapid *M. tuberculosis* assay
  - New real-time PCR-based TB products under development: TrueNAT MTB assay, m2000 RealTime MTB assay, and Lap chip G2-3
- Molecular tests for species identification
  - MicroSeq 500 system
  - AccuProbe assay
  - INNO-LiPA Mycobacteria
  - Geno type MTBC and Geno type Mycobacterium
  - New real time PCR-based TB products under development: Anyplex plus MTB/NTM/MDR TB and fluoroType MTB assays
  - Microarray products under development
- Tests for drug-resistance
  - INNO-LiPA RifTB Assay
  - Geno type MTBDR-Plus
  - Cepheid GeneXpert system
  - Bacteriophage-based tests and in-house phage amplification tests
  - New real-time PCR-based TB products under development
  - Microarray products under development.

Abbreviations: MTB, *Mycobacterium tuberculosis*; TB, tuberculosis; PCR, polymerase chain reaction; NTM, non-tuberculous mycobacteria; MTBC, *Mycobacterium tuberculosis* complex.

Nucleic Acid Amplification Detection-based Diagnostic Tests for Tuberculosis

The use of nucleic acid amplification (NAA)-based diagnosis has led to significant improvement in rapid diagnosis of tuberculosis in the resource-rich countries. Initially, hybridization assays such as in-situ hybridization and restriction fragment length polymorphism were devised for *M. tuberculosis* diagnosis. Subsequently, several laboratories worked on devising NAA-based diagnostic tests. In-house assays were developed to amplify *M. tuberculosis* gene targets like 16S rRNA,[31] 23S rRNA,[32] *rpoB*,[33, 34] *gyrB*,[35] *dnaJ*,[36] *devR*,[37] MPT-64,[38] *SodA*,[39] *RecA*,[40] *hupB*,[41] MTP-40,[42] *pncA*[43] and *PPE8*[44]; genes encoding 65KDa heat shock protein,[45] 38 KDa protein,[46] and antigen 85B,[46] insertion sequence elements (*IS6110*,[47] *IS986*[48]); and repetitive elements chromosomal direct repeats (TRC4,[49] PGRS[50]) using different NAA methods such as a simple polymerase chain reaction (PCR), PCR-single strand confirmation polymorphism,[43] dideoxy fingerprinting,[51] heminested PCR,[52] PCR heteroduplex analysis,[53] PCR combined with restriction enzyme assay,[34,54] isothermal amplification methods,[55] multiplex PCR[56] and real time PCR.[57] These in-house tests used agarose or acrylamide gel electrophoresis or hybridization as the read out.[58-61]

According to the latest report by UNITAID, WHO on tuberculosis diagnostics technologies, NAA-based diagnostic tests are currently the largest group of tests for tuberculosis; 123 out of 191 products or tests for tuberculosis diagnosis that are currently available or in development.[62] These tests use different methods to extract nucleic acids from the specimens, amplify specific regions in *M. tuberculosis* genome and to detect the amplified product. Most of the currently commercially available or in development tuberculosis NAA diagnostics products are based on PCR-hybridization, real-time PCR or isothermal amplification.

The first NAAT approved by the United States Food and Drug Administration (USFDA) in 1995 for *M. tuberculosis* detection in AFB smear-positive respiratory specimens was Amplified *M. tuberculosis* direct test (MTD, Gen-Probe Inc, USA). The MTD test is based on isothermal amplification of 16S rRNA transcripts [transcription mediated amplification, (TMA)] that is detected using acridinium ester labeled *M. tuberculosis* complex-specific DNA probes in a hybridization protection assay.[55] These isothermal amplification methods use a single reaction temperature so the entire process can be carried out at 42°C, unlike PCR which requires different temperatures for DNA denaturation, primer annealing and extension and needs a thermocycler. Although entirely manual, the test is rapid with a turn around time of about 2.5 hours. The results require a luminometer for interpretation. Several studies have confirmed the sensitivity and specificity of MTD test; the sensitivity ranges between 90% and 100% in smear-positive and 63–100% in smear-negative specimens. [63] Later, in 1999, a second-generation MTD (enhanced MTD or E-MTD) test was approved for use in respiratory specimens from all patients suspected to have tuberculosis regardless of their smear status.[64,65] Both MTD and E-MTD are highly specific (> 95%) moreover, the sensitivity of E-MTD has been shown to be higher than the original MTD test.[66,67]

The amplicor *M. tuberculosis* test was approved by the FDA in 1996 for testing in AFB smear-positive tuberculosis patients using respiratory specimens only.[64] The amplicor is a DNA-based test which amplifies 16S rRNA gene using genus-specific primers followed by hybridization to specific probes. The binding of probes is detected by a colorimetric reaction in a microwell plate format.[68] Turn around time for the amplicor test is 6–7 hours. The amplicor MTB *(Mycobacterium tuberculosis)* test provides 90–100% sensitivity in smear-positive sputum samples and 50–95.9% in smear-negative samples. Overall specificity has been reported in the range of 90–100%.[32,63] An automated version of the test, the COBAS amplicor is also available that uses the COBAS amplicor analyzer and allows rapid amplification and detection in one system.[69]

Real-time PCR is a quantitative method that combines the two steps, i.e. amplification and detection into one step and is based on hybridization of the amplified segments (DNA) with different fluorescent probes, such as TaqMan probes fluorescence resonance energy transfer (FRET) probes, molecular beacons and bioprobes.[60,70,71] The intensity of fluorescence is detected in a thermal cycler and is directly proportional to the amount of amplified product in the reaction tube. The main advantage of real-time PCR is its ability to yield the results in 1.5–2 hours after DNA extraction and its high sensitivity. In addition, problems with cross-contamination are reduced because the detection occurs in a closed system. A qualitative COBAS TaqMan MTB test based on integration of real-time PCR technology with standard hybridization is now available, replacing both the amplicor *M. tuberculosis* and COBAS amplicor *M. tuberculosis* assays. The turn around time for analyzing 48 samples simultaneously using COBAS TaqMan is 2.5 hours.[32] Recent studies suggest that accuracy of COBAS TaqMan is superior to amplicor for detecting *M. tuberculosis*, the test is CE-in vitro diagnostics (CE-IVD) marked but not yet approved by FDA.[57,72] This COBAS TaqMan can be integrated with COBAS AmpliPrep instrument for sample preparation to automate.

BD ProbeTec MTB test (Becton Dickinson, USA) is another FDA approved (2001) *M. tuberculosis* diagnostic test. It utilizes strand displacement isothermal amplification method for amplification of target sequences located in IS 6110 and 16s rRNA genes.[73] The products of amplification are detected using a luminometer. The test has shown high sensitivity in both smear-positive (100%), as well as smear-negative (92–100%) patients using respiratory samples.[73-75] However, the sample preparation is time consuming. An improved version of BD ProbeTec ET that includes an internal amplification control to detect the presence of inhibitors showed higher sensitivity in smear-positive than smear-negative samples.[75]

A loop-mediated isothermal amplification (LAMP) (Loopamp® tuberculosis, Eiken Chemical Co., Japan) test has recently been developed for simple and sensitive detection for tuberculosis.[76] The Loopamp® tuberculosis detection assay is based on insertion sequence IS *6110* as the gene target.[77] The technique involves autocycling strand displacement DNA synthesis using the large fragment of *Bacillus stearothermophilus* DNA polymerase; pyrophosphate produced as a byproduct during DNA synthesis in LAMP assay is visible as a white precipitate of magnesium pyrophosphate in the reaction vial. DNA detection is based on presence or absence of the precipitate.[77,78] Moreover, the turbidity of the reaction mixture is directly proportionate to the amount of DNA synthesized. The entire procedure is carried out in a single tube by incubating very small volume of DNA at 63°C for 1 hour. A prototype assay (Loopamp® tuberculosis detection) with simplified manual DNA extraction method to detect *M. tuberculosis* in respiratory samples has been used for clinical evaluation in peripheral microscopy centers in Peru, Bangladesh and Tanzania.[79] In these studies the Loopamp® tuberculosis detection test was found to have higher sensitivity (81.4–92.7%) compared to microscopy with slightly lower specificity (80.4–98.3%). Importantly, these studies demonstrated the feasibility of performing the assay without the use of sophisticated equipment and specialized training.[76,79] The sensitivity of the Loopamp® tuberculosis is lower (48–56%) in smear-negative samples. The WHO expert panel recently reviewed this assay, but did not recommend due to insufficient data. If future studies are promising, the assay may soon be released for the diagnosis of tuberculosis worldwide.[76] Currently, several other tuberculosis LAMP assays are being developed with other gene targets like 16S*rDNA*,[80] *gyrB*[77] and rimM.[81]

Since isothermal amplification assays can be performed in a simple inexpensive water bath, and are thus more suitable for low resource settings, several tuberculosis NAA diagnostic tests under development are based on this methods (Ustar EasyNAT TB), (Ustar Biotechnologies, China), Alere q TB diagnostic system (Alere, USA) and TRCRapid *M. tuberculosis* assay (Tosoh Bioscience, Japan). The Ustar EasyNAT tuberculosis assay utilizes cross-priming isothermal amplification, where multiple cross-linked primers are used for strand displacement. The DNA target is amplified at constant temperature, and the amplified products are detected in an inbuilt lateral flow assay. NATeasy TB assay aims to integrate DNA extraction with nucleic acid detection which is currently in development.[71] The sensitivities for the smear-positive and smear-negative sputum samples were found to be 96.9% and 87.5% in the initial evaluation.[82] This test is FDA approved and CE-IVD marked. The Alere q TB diagnostic system is a fully integrated system, from sample processing to reporting of final result. DNA targets are amplified in 5 minutes using isothermal nicking amplification reaction; hence, it only takes 20 minutes from sample collection to result. Currently, the manufacturers are integrating drug-resistance genotyping into this current assay.[62] The gene target for the TRCRapid *M. tuberculosis* assay is 16S rRNA and the assay is based on transcription reverse transcription concerted isothermal amplification method. The assay can also measure the cell viability, since it is dependent on RNA. In initial evaluations, the sensitivities of the TRCRapid *M. tuberculosis* assay for the smear-positive and smear-negative sputum samples is reported as 90.7% and 44.8%, respectively.[83] However, larger multicentric studies reported an overall sensitivity of 86% which is higher than the 80% culture sensitivity when clinical indicators are included.[84]

The use of real time PCR method in the TB-NAA diagnosis is now increasing rapidly. The TrueNAT MTB assay (Molbio, UK), m2000 RealTime MTB assay (Abbott, USA), and Lap chip G2-3 (NanoBioSys Inc. South Korea) are some of the semi-automated platforms which are in development and/or infield evaluation process for *M. tuberculosis* complex detection based on real time PCR.[62] The sensitivity of TrueNAT MTB assay using 226 patients with suspected tuberculosis was found as 99.1% and 75.8% in smear-positive and smear-negative cases, while the specificity of the test was 100%.[85] The m2000 RealTime MTB assay and TrueNAT MTB assays are CE-IVD marked. Initial evaluation of Lap chip G2-3 assay using 247 clinical specimens indicates the 94% sensitivity and 83% specificity in smear-positive; 63% and 95% in smear-negative sputum samples.[86]

The Centers for Disease Control and Prevention (CDC) guidelines recommend that "NAA testing be performed on at least one respiratory specimen from each patient with signs and symptoms of pulmonary tuberculosis for whom a diagnosis of tuberculosis is considered but not established and for whom the test result would alter case management and tuberculosis control activities".[64] Since all the current tests require trained personnel, specialized equipment and are expensive, they are rarely used in the TB-endemic countries and cannot be integrated into routine patient care.

Tests for Species Identification of Mycobacteria

Prompt identification of *Mycobacterium* species has become increasingly important with the increase in NTM infections, especially in HIV-infected individuals.[87] NTMs require a different treatment regimen and a lack of response to standard antituberculous drugs can be confused with drug-resistance.[88] Thus, adequate disease management requires precise classification of mycobacteria. Conventional methods of *Mycobacterium* species identification include biochemical tests and phenotypic characteristics by culturing that are simple and do not require any sophisticated equipment; these tests are laborious and cumbersome, take several days for results, thus delaying prompt and accurate identification of bacteria. Culturing is expensive need a laboratory and not available in most of the developing countries. Newly developed molecular methods are attractive alternatives for rapid identification of mycobacteria, especially *M. tuberculosis* complex. Several molecular commercial tests are currently available for rapid identification of mycobacterial species from culture isolates.[89]

The MicroSeq 500 system (Applied Biosystems, Foster City, CA) is a microbial identification system based on sequencing of a 16S ribosomal DNA. The test has shown high sensitivity with clinical isolates, but is time consuming and requires sophisticated instrumentation for data analysis.[90,91] The AccuProbe GenProbe assay (Gen-Probe Inc, USA), one of the first introduced and the most widely used molecular technique for species identification, utilizes species specific DNA probes. Hybridization of these probes with species-specific target rRNA sequences can differentiate and identify *M. tuberculosis* complex, *M. avium*, *M. intracellulare*, *M. avium* complex, *M. kansasii* and *M. gordonae*.[92-95] The sensitivity and specificity of these probes are reported to be 93.1% and 93.5%, respectively.[96] The turn around time using AccuProbe on culture is 2 hours, but the test can identify only a limited number of species and is unable to differentiate *M. tuberculosis* from the other species in the complex.[97]

The INNO-LiPA Mycobacteria v2 (Fuji-Rebio Europe, Belgium) system for mycobacterial species identification simultaneously detects and identifies the genus *Mycobacterium* along with 16 different species. This line probe assay (LPA) involves PCR amplification followed by hybridization of the amplified products to specific oligonucleotide probes immobilized on the membrane strips. The interpretation is based on the appearance of bands in specific combinations. The assay is based on nucleotide differences in the *16s-23S* rRNA gene spacers. The LPA can be performed on bacteria from liquid or solid cultures and shows high specificity (94%) and sensitivity (100%)[98-100] in a variety of mycobacterial species.

Two other commercially available molecular systems, GenoType *Mycobacterium tuberculosis* complex (MTBC) and GenoType *Mycobacterium* (Hain Lifescience, Germany) use reverse line probe hybridization assays to identify mycobacterial species and differentiate members of the *M. tuberculosis* complex. The GenoType Mycobacterium, based on regions of 23S rRNA, can identify 35 different species of mycobacteria, including *M. tuberculosis*.[101] The GenoType MTBC uses 23S rRNA fragment and gyrB sequence polymorphism to differentiate members of *M. tuberculosis* complex. Further, it targets RD1 deletion for identification of *M. bovis* BCG.[102] The GenoType MTBC test has been widely used for the speciation of mycobacteria in different studies and shows consistently approximately 90% sensitivity and specificity.[103-106] These assays are labor intensive, require extensive training and being culture-dependent, are restricted to use in reference laboratories.

The Anyplex plus MTB or NTM or MDR-TB (Seegene, South Korea) and FluoroType MTB assays (Hain Lifescience, Germany) use real-time PCR for species identification of mycobacteria.[62] The Anyplex plus MTB or NTM TB assay is CE-IVD marked, and in the initial evaluation the assay was found to have the sensitivity and specificity of 100% and 96% for detection of MTBC and 100% and 97% for detection of NTM.[107]

Microarray-based tuberculosis diagnostic tests are in development stages. These tests are being developed to identify or quantify multiple targets in the same assay; the high throughput capability makes these tests important for high-burden settings. Some of the tests being developed include MYCO assay (iCubate, USA), TrueArray MDRTB assay (Akonni Biosystems, USA) and VereMTB detection kit (Veredus Laboratories Pte Ltd, Singapore).[62] In all these products initially gene targets are amplified using PCR, the amplicons are fluorescently labeled, denatured, then hybridized to the complimentary DNA oligonucleotides printed on the arrays and signal intensity is measured using a fluorescence reader. These products not only help to aid in the identification of Mycobacterium species but will also aid in drug-resistance screening.

Diagnostic Tests for Drug-resistance of *Mycobacterium Tuberculosis*

Even as efforts to devise improved diagnostic tests for tuberculosis are ongoing, there has been an alarming increase in the incidence of multidrug-resistant TB (MDR-TB) and extensively drug-resistant tuberculosis (XDR-TB) in several parts of the world.[108-110] MDR-TB is defined as resistance to both INH and rifampicin (RIF) and XDR-TB is defined as MDR-TB with additional resistance to any fluoroquinolone and at least one of the three injectable second-line drugs (SLDs)—capreomycin, kanamycin (KM) and amikacin. As per the WHO estimates, almost 25% of the 5 million cases of MDR-TB that emerged globally in 2012,[111] were from India. Recent studies have reported both MDR-TB and XDR-TB in India.[112-115]

Conventional diagnosis of DR-TB by the proportion method, absolute concentration method or the resistance ratio method takes several weeks even with the rapid-culture (BACTEC 460, MB/BacT, MGIT)-based methods since the primary isolation and culture of *M. tuberculosis* from the clinical specimens is followed by susceptibility testing in cultures. During this time, transmission of resistant bacteria continues and patients are treated with inappropriate regimens, potentially amplifying resistance.

Rifampicin is the key drug in the first-line chemotherapy of tuberculosis, it is estimated that over 90% of the RIF-resistant strains are also INH-resistant. The LPAs were the first *M. tuberculosis* molecular assays that were endorsed by WHO. Initially, two commercial assays for rapid detection of drug resistance in *M. tuberculosis* were developed, the INNO-LiPA RifTB Assay (Innogenetics NV, Belgium) for the detection of resistance to rifampicin and the GenoType MTBDRPlus (Hain Lifescience, Germany) for simultaneous detection of rifampicin and INH resistance. The basis of both assays is reverse solid phase hybridization. As indicated before, the LPAs involve extraction of DNA from *M. tuberculosis* isolates, either from cultures or directly from clinical specimens, followed by PCR-amplification of the resistance-determining region of the gene in question using biotinylated primers.

The PCR products are hybridized with specific oligonucleotide probes that are immobilized on a strip. The captured hybrids are detected by colorimetric development. The mutations are identified by lack of hybridization of the amplified PCR products to wild type probes as well as hybridization to specific probes for most commonly occurring mutations. Results from systematic reviews and meta-analysis commissioned by WHO in 2008[116] showed that the GenoType MTBDRplus is highly sensitive (>97%) and specific (>99%) for the detection of rifampicin resistance, either alone or in combination with INH. The pooled sensitivity and specificity on cultured bacteria for rifampicin resistance were 98% and 99% respectively, and for INH 84% and 99%, respectively.[117,118] The cost of the assay, when performed directly from the sputum is lower than the tuberculosis drug susceptibility testing (DST) culturing. The INNO-LiPA Rif TB assay is no longer commercially available and GenoType MTBDRplus is the only LPA currently available for diagnosing drug-resistant tuberculosis (DR-TB) globally.

The sensitivity of GenoType MTBDRplus assay is lower in smear-negative and HIV-positive individuals, and the test is not approved for use in specimens from these patients.[76] Also, the test requires processing of sputum specimens, use of biosafety level 3 (BSL3) facilities is recommended. Moreover, reagents require refrigeration and/or freezing, which translates into need for regular power supply, molecular grade water and enzyme (Taq polymerase) and several different equipment (thermal cycler, shaker platform, water bath, heating block, sonicator, hybridization chambers, etc.). Clearly, these tests require significant infrastructure and training and will be difficult to implement except in the few sophisticated labs in developing countries. However, currently there are several LPA based products in development or field evaluation for rapid detection of both first-line and second-line drug resistance.[62]

The second tuberculosis NAA test approved by WHO is GeneXpert® MTB/RIF assay (Cepheid, Sunnyvale, CA) which simultaneous detects *M. tuberculosis* and rifampicin resistance.[76] The Cepheid GeneXpert system is an integrated diagnostic system that performs sample processing and real-time PCR analysis test in a single hands-free two-hour step. The assay is designed to perform a heminested molecular beacon assay, which uses six molecular beacons to amplify a sequence of rpoB gene specific to the *M. tuberculosis* complex organisms and probe for mutations in the rifampicin resistance determining region (RRDR) of the rpoB gene. This is an 81bp long region in the rpoB gene, mutations in which occur in 95–98% of the rifampicin-resistant *M. tuberculosis.* Fluorescent dyes and quenchers that allow multiplexing of the different molecular beacons within the same reaction make this system extremely sensitive for the detection of *M. tuberculosis.* The limit of detection of GeneXpert is reported to be 131 CFU/mL using *M. tuberculosis* spiked sputum,[119] which is lower than smear microscopy (5–10 X 10^3 CFU/mL) but higher than liquid culture (<100 CFU/mL)[2].

The GeneXpert MTB or RIF assay is closed system format (cartridge based) and fully automated with nucleic acid extraction, amplification and detection process, hence reduces hands-on time and detection of undesirable nucleic acids.[71] This fully automated approach is first of its kind in tuberculosis diagnosis. Since the sample processing is automated, this assay has fewer biosafety hazards compared to direct smear microscopy. Several studies have demonstrated the diagnostic accuracy of GeneXpert MTB or RIF assay in both the high income and resource limited settings. A recent meta-analysis, reported that the GeneXpert MTB or RIF test has 89% and 99% pooled sensitivity and specificity respectively for tuberculosis diagnosis; the pooled sensitivity and specificity for rifampicin resistance is 95% and 98%, respectively.[120] The sensitivity for tuberculosis diagnosis is lower in smear-negative (67%), extrapulmonary tuberculosis (EPTB) (80%), children (65.1–75.9%) and HIV+ individuals (79%).[120] Despite these promising results, GeneXpert MTB or RIF assay has several limitations including the inability to differentiate live from dead bacteria, the difficulty in detection of mixed infections and operational limitations such as the high cost of the equipment and the cartridges, air-conditioned environment for the machines, requirement for uninterrupted power supply, maintenance and annual calibration of the machine, etc.[121]

Cepheid GeneXpert is a currently developing new test, the Xtend-XDR test for simultaneous screening for drug resistance to INH, fluoroquinolones (FLQ), aminoglycosides (amikacin and kanamycin). Several other manufacturers are also developing new tuberculosis NAA products which not only can identify *M. tuberculosis* but also drug resistance to first-line and second-line drugs using real time PCR. These include Genedrive Mycobacterium identification (iD) test-kit (Epistem, UK), MeltPro DR-TB (Zeesan Biotech, China), MDR-TB test for Enigma mini laboratory system (Enigma Diagnostics, UK), and MTB assay for DiagCORE platform (Stat-Diagnositica, Spain). GenePOC Inc (Canada) and Quidel Inc (USA).[62] Furthermore the Anyplex plus MTB or NTM or MDR-TB (Seegene, South Korea) and FluoroType MTB real-time PCR assays (Hain Lifescience, Germany) that was developed for detection of mycobacteria species can also detect drug resistance.

Microarray technology is also being evaluated for detection of drug resistance in *M. tuberculosis.*[122-124] The microarrays or DNA biochips allow simultaneous detection of multiple mutations. A low-density oligonucleotide chip has been reported to detect mutations associated with INH, RIF, streptomycin (SM), kanamycin and ethambutol (EMB) with sensitivities of 69%, 93%, 86%, 80% and 85%, respectively.[125] Gel-based biochips have been used for epidemiological studies of drug resistance on a large scale in Kyrgyz Republic.[126] The generation of tuberculosis biochips for analysis of second-line fluoroquinolone antibiotics resistance along with rifampicin or INH susceptibility biochip is the first in the world to be certified by a national regulatory agency, Ministry of Public Health of Russian Federation for clinical application.[126] MYCO assay (iCubate, USA) VereMTB detection kit (Veredus Laboratories Pte Ltd, Singapore), TrueArray MDR TB (Akonni Biosystems, USA), INFINITI MTBC-OCTA (AutoGenomics, USA), and HYDRA 1K (Stansford & Insilixa Inc. USA) are some of the microarray-based products that are in development stage for drug-resistance screening.[62]

The usefulness of all molecular tests is limited by the fact that not all drug-resistant isolates have mutations in the hot spots of genes associated with drug resistance. These strains still require phenotype based assays for detection. Secondly, the molecular tests are unable to detect minor populations of drug-resistant organisms in primary culture from clinical samples.[125]

Sample Collection, Processing and Extraction of Nucleic Acids for Nucleic Acid Amplification Tests

The purity and integrity of nucleic acids extracted from clinical sample greatly influence the results of NAA Tests. The sample collection, type of specimen used, nucleic acid extraction method and inhibitors in the nucleic acid after nucleic acid extraction influences the NAA Test results.[127] Although most of the molecular assays are based on sputum sample from pulmonary tuberculosis patients, the clinical samples from EPTB patients are from other body fluids such as cerebrospinal fluid, bronchiolar alveolar lavage, pleural fluid, abscess, lymph, biopsy, fine-needle aspiration for tuberculosis diagnosis.[128]

Acquisition of adequate and quality clinical sample is important for accurate diagnosis. Sputum collection is a challenge in paucibacillary, HIV+, pediatric, and EPTB patients. Sputum induction and concentration methods are used to get improved sample collection. Recently, Medical Acoustics USA developed a small plastic device named "lung flute" which uses sound vibrations for easy production of sputum sample. This device is approved by FDA and CE-IVD marked.[62] Decontamination of the clinical sample is another critical component to remove the contaminants and inactivate *M. tuberculosis* in the clinical sample. N-acetyl cysteine and NaOH decontamination method is commonly used for *M. tuberculosis* culture from sputum sample. Several commercial vendors are offering different products like Decomics (Salubris Inc., USA), OMNIgene SPUTUM (DNA Genotek Inc., Canada) and PrimeStore MTM (Longhorn Diagnostics, USA) to liquefy, decontaminate, neutralize the clinical sample and also stabilize the nucleic acids. To capture and enrich *M. tuberculosis* from sputum samples, Microsens Diagnostics Ltd (UK) developed TB-Beads and Genetein Co Ltd (Japan) developed TRICORE bacterial concentration kit.[62] These products do not require any centrifuge and can be used in microscopy, culture and NAA tests.

The nucleic acids from the clinical samples were extracted by phenol or chloroform method earlier, however NAA Tests reproducibility was greatly affected due to corrosive nature of phenol,[129-131] hence the extraction is now mostly based on column purification, where the nucleic acids are bound to silica matrix membrane after the bacterial lyses, then washed extensively to remove macromolecules, inhibitors and other contaminants and then finally eluted. The *M. tuberculosis* bacteria are lysed in buffer, DNA is captured, and eluted in a pipette tip in the TruTip DNA extraction system developed by Akonni Biosystems (USA). DNA Genotek Inc., (Canada) company's prepIT MAX technology rely on ethanol precipitation, centrifugation for the extraction of DNA from *M. tuberculosis* cells and do not need a mechanical approach to break the cells.[62] Several semi and fully automated NAA test platforms are being designed for nucleic acid extraction from the clinical specimens.[71]

Clinical Impact of the Sensitive Molecular Tests on Tuberculosis Patients

When the Cepheid GeneXpert MTB or RIF assay was commissioned by WHO, it was anticipated as a game changer, since it improved new case detection due to its high sensitivity, and also detected drug resistance. Epidemiological modeling indicated that TB-related mortality could be reduced by 20–35% due to accurate and same day diagnosis.[132] In a recent randomized control study in Africa to examine the clinical effect of GeneXpert MTB or RIF deployed at point of care at the clinics compared to smear microscopy[133] reported that even though GeneXpert detects more tuberculosis cases than smear microscopy and treatment initiation is faster, the overall number of patients on treatment is unaffected. This was primarily due to high rates of empirical tuberculosis treatment, since bacteriological confirmation failed to identify approximately 30% of the pulmonary tuberculosis and approximately 50% of the extrapulmonary tuberculosis patients. There was also no difference in the morbidity and mortality between the patients diagnosed by GeneXpert and smear microscopy.[133,134]

The high burden tuberculosis endemic countries urgently require simple, accurate point-of-care diagnostic tests that can replace and improve upon microscopy without requiring laboratory infrastructure and highly trained personnel. Although multiple new molecular tests for tuberculosis diagnosis are rapidly being developed; several match the sensitivity and specificity of GeneXpert but will be less expensive, their contribution to rapid diagnosis of tuberculosis and slow the tuberculosis epidemic remains to be assessed. Most new molecular tests continue to be too expensive for routine use as point-of-care tests in peripheral facilities. No molecular test as yet matches the sensitivity of liquid culture, and even liquid cultures do not provide bacteriological confirmation in approximately 25–30% of the pulmonary tuberculosis (PTB) patients, and approximately 50% of the patients with extrapulmonary tuberculosis. Furthermore, NAATs and cultures cannot be used for routine screening of high-risk populations. Rapid and simple point-of-care tests that are not based on detection of bacteria or bacterial antigen or nucleic acids are required for screening active tuberculosis, identify different forms of tuberculosis, paucibacillary pulmonary and extrapulmonary tuberculosis.

Optimal Tuberculosis Test

It is important to appreciate the differences between the developed and developing countries in regards to tuberculosis. Unfortunately, the diagnostic tests that are used in the industrialized world as well as the resources required for monitoring treatment are too expensive and technically difficult for routine use in resource-limited countries. The patient burden is enormous; accuracy of microscopy is limited and facilities for culture-confirmation are rarely available.

The ideal diagnostic marker for tuberculosis would be a universal marker that can:

- Replace and improve upon sputum microscopy
- Identify patients with extrapulmonary tuberculosis (tuberculosis meningitis, skeletal tuberculosis, genitourinary tuberculosis, gastrointestinal tuberculosis, tuberculosis lymphadenitis), many of which are not accessible to microscopy[8,128,135,136]
- Identify HIV-infected tuberculosis patients, in whom tuberculosis progresses rapidly and fatally, but the low bacterial burden in the sputum makes detection of bacteria or bacterial molecules difficult, and the immune dysfunction preclude use of cellular immune-based diagnostic assays[4,25]

- Diagnose pediatric tuberculosis patients who rarely produce sputum and are currently diagnosed based on epidemiologic, clinical and radiological suspicion rather than microbiological confirmation[137,138]
- Identify a potential tuberculosis patient during the window period from infection to clinical disease.
- Simultaneously detect drug resistance.

In the absence of a single universal marker, a set of new diagnostic tests may be able to fulfill these criteria. Not only must the new diagnostic tests detect the myriad forms and stages of tuberculosis with high sensitivity, they must be highly specific. Thus, although almost 84% of the *M. tuberculosis* genome encodes proteins that are cross-reactive with other mycobacteria or other prokaryotes,[139] the diagnostic markers must be able to distinguish between infection with *M. tuberculosis* and infection or exposure to other bacteria and mycobacteria. In addition to having high sensitivity and specificity, for any new diagnostic markers to have any impact on the tuberculosis epidemic and to be integrated into the already overburdened tuberculosis control programs in the developing countries, they must be rapid, low-cost, operationally simple requiring minimal laboratory infrastructure and personnel training, robust and stable to withstand the poor storage conditions in these countries and be amenable to large-scale production.

REFERENCES

1. Binkin NJ, Vernon AA, Simone PM, McCray E, Miller BI, Schieffelbein CW, et al. Tuberculosis prevention and control activities in the United States: an overview of the organization of tuberculosis services. Int J Tuberc Lung Dis. 1999;3(8):663-74.
2. Targeted tuberculin testing and treatment of latent tuberculosis infection. This official statement of the American Thoracic Society was adopted by the ATS Board of Directors, July 1999. This is a Joint Statement of the American Thoracic Society (ATS) and the Centers for Disease Control and Prevention (CDC). This statement was endorsed by the Council of the Infectious Diseases Society of America. (IDSA), September 1999, and the sections of this statement. Am J Respir Crit Care Med. 2000;161(4 Pt 2):S221-47.
3. Dye C, Scheele S, Dolin P, Pathania V, Raviglione MC. Consensus statement. Global burden of tuberculosis: estimated incidence, prevalence, and mortality by country. WHO Global Surveillance and Monitoring Project. Jama. 1999;282(7):677-86.
4. Corbett EL, Watt CJ, Walker N, Maher D, Williams BG, Raviglione MC, et al. The growing burden of tuberculosis: global trends and interactions with the HIV epidemic. Arch Intern Med. 2003;163(9):1009-21.
5. Foulds J, O'Brien R. New Tools for the diagnosis of tuberculosis: the perspective of developing countries. Int J Tuber Lung Dis. 1998;2(10):778-83.
6. Perkins MD. New diagnostic tools for tuberculosis. Int J Tuberc Lung Dis. 2000;4(12 Suppl 2):S182-8.
7. Hanna BA. Laboratory Diagnosis, in Tuberculosis. In: Rom WN, Garay SM, (Eds). 2nd edition. Lippincott Williams & Wilkins: Philadelphia; 2004. pp. 163-76.
8. Frieden TR, Sterling TR, Munsiff SS, Watt CJ, Dye C. Tuberculosis. Lancet. 2003;362(9387):887-99.
9. New York City Department of Health NYDH, Tuberculosis in New York City, 2000: Information Summary, Tuberculosis Control Program: New York. 2001. pp. 1-44.
10. CDC. CDC's Response to Ending Neglect: The Elimination of Tuberculosis in the United States Greenspan AL, LA H (Eds). US Department of Health and Human Services, Centers for Disease Control and Prevention. Atlanta, Georgia. 2002. pp.1-62.
11. Huebner RE, Schein MF, Bass JB. The tuberculin skin test. Clin Infect Dis. 1993;17(6):968-75.
12. Fine PE, Bruce J, Ponnighaus JM, Nkhosa P, Harawa A, Vynnycky E, et al. Tuberculin sensitivity: conversions and reversions in a rural African population. Int J Tuberc Lung Dis. 1999;3(11):962-75.
13. American Thoracic Society ATS. The Tuberculin Skin Test, MSotAL Association, (Ed). 1981. pp. 356-63.
14. El-Sadr W. Double scourge: tuberculosis and HIV coinfection. The PRN Notebook. 2001;6(4):4-15.
15. Whalen C, Horsburg CR, Hom D, Lahart C, Simberkoff M, Ellner J. Accelerated course of human immunodeficiency virus infection after tuberculosis. Amer J Respir Crit Care Med. 1995;151(1):129-35.
16. Daley CL, Small PM, Schecter GF, Schoolnik GK, McAdam RA, Jacobs WR, et al. An outbreak of tuberculosis with accelerated progression among persons infected with the human immunodeficiency virus. N Eng J Med. 1992;326(1):231-5.
17. Corbett EL, Charalambous S, Moloi VM, Fielding K, Grant AD, Dye C, et al. Human immunodeficiency virus and the prevalence of undiagnosed tuberculosis in African gold miners. Am J Respir Crit Care Med. 2004;170(6):673-9.
18. Cohn DL. Subclinical tuberculosis in HIV-infected patients: another challenge for the diagnosis of tuberculosis in high-burden countries? Clin Infect Dis. 2005;40(10):1508-10.
19. Mtei L, Matee M, Herfort O, Bakari M, Horsburgh CR, Waddell R, et al. High rates of clinical and subclinical tuberculosis among HIV-infected ambulatory subjects in Tanzania. Clin Infect Dis. 2005;40(10):1500-7.
20. Sonnenberg P, Glynn JR, Fielding K, Murray J, Godfrey-Faussett P, Shearer S, et al. How soon after infection with HIV does the risk of tuberculosis start to increase? A retrospective cohort study in South African gold miners. J Infect Dis. 2005;191(2):150-8.
21. Zumla A, Malon P, Henderson J, Grange JM. Impact of HIV infection on tuberculosis. Postgrad Med J. 2000;76(895): 259-68.
22. Ansari NA, Kombe AH, Kenyon TA, Hone NM, Tappero JW, Nyirenda ST, et al. Pathology and causes of death in a group of 128 predominantly HIV-positive patients in Botswana, 1997-1998. Int J Tuberc Lung Dis. 2002;6(1):55-63.
23. Holmes CB, Losina E, Walensky RP, Yazdanpanah Y, Freedberg KA, et al. Review of human immunodeficiency virus type 1-related opportunistic infections in sub-Saharan Africa. Clin Infect Dis. 2003;36(5):652-62.
24. Cohen J. HIV/AIDS in India. HIV/AIDS: India's many epidemics. Science. 2004;304(5670):504-9.
25. Raviglione MC, Narain JP, Kochi A. HIV-associated tuberculosis in developing countries: clinical features, diagnosis, and treatment. Bull World Health Organization. 1992;70:515-26.
26. Lalvani A, Nagvenkar P, Udwadia Z, Pathan AA, Wilkinson KA, Shastri JS, et al. Enumeration of T cells specific for RD1-encoded antigens suggests a high prevalence of latent *Mycobacterium*

tuberculosis infection in healthy urban Indians. J Infect Dis. 2001;183(3):469-77.
27. Grant AD, Kaplan JE, De Cock KM. Preventing opportunistic infections among human immunodeficiency virus-infected adults in African countries. Am J Trop Med Hyg. 2001;65(6):810-21.
28. Johnson JL, Okwera A, Hom DL, Mayanja H, Mutuluuza Kityo C, Nsubuga P, et al. Duration of efficacy of treatment of latent tuberculosis infection in HIV-infected adults. AIDS. 2001;15(16):2137-47.
29. Mosimaneotsile B, Talbot EA, Moeti TL, Hone NM, Moalosi G, Moffat HJ, et al. Value of chest radiography in a tuberculosis prevention programme for HIV-infected people, Botswana. Lancet. 2003;362(9395):1551-2.
30. National Framework for Joint HIV TB Collaborative Activities. *www.naco.gov.in/policies and guidelines* (Accessed June 2016).
31. Boddinghaus B, Rogall T, Flohr T, Blöcker H, Böttger EC. Detection and identification of Mycobacteria by amplification of rRNA. J Clin Microbiol. 1990;28:1751-9.
32. Palomino JC. Molecular detection, identification and drug resistance detection in *Mycobacterium tuberculosis*. FEMS Immunol Med Microbiol. 2009;56(2):103-11.
33. Somoskovi A, Song Q, Mester J, Tanner C, Hale YM, Parsons LM, et al. Use of molecular methods to identify the *Mycobacterium tuberculosis* complex (MTBC) and other mycobacterial species and to detect rifampin resistance in MTBC isolates following growth detection with the BACTEC MGIT 960 system. J Clin Microbiol. 2003;41(7):2822-6.
34. Lee H, Park HJ, Cho SN, GH, Kim SJ. Species identification of mycobacteria by PCR-restriction fragment length polymorphism of the rpoB gene. J Clin Microbiol. 2000;38(8):2966-71.
35. Goh KS, Fabre M, Huard RC, Schmid S, Sola C, Rastogi N. Study of the gyrB gene polymorphism as a tool to differentiate among *Mycobacterium tuberculosis* complex subspecies further underlines the older evolutionary age of '*Mycobacterium canettii*. Mol Cell Probes. 2006;20(3-4):182-90.
36. Singh A, Kashyap VK. Specific and rapid detection of *Mycobacterium tuberculosis* complex in clinical samples by polymerase chain reaction. Interdiscip Perspect Infect Dis. 2012;2012:654694.
37. Singh KK, Muralidhar M, Kumar A, Chattopadhyaya TK, Kapila K, Singh MK, et al. Comparison of in house polymerase chain reaction with conventional techniques for the detection of *Mycobacterium tuberculosis* DNA in granulomatous lymphadenopathy. J Clin Pathol. 2000;53(5):355-61.
38. Sethi S, Yadav R, Mewara A, Dhatwalia SK, Sharma M, Gupta D, et al. Evaluation of in-house mpt64 real-time PCR for rapid detection of *Mycobacterium tuberculosis* in pulmonary and extra-pulmonary specimens. Braz J Infect Dis. 2012;16(5):493-4.
39. Bull TJ, Shanson DC, Archard LC. Rapid identification of mycobacteria from AIDS patients by capillary electrophoretic profiling of amplified SOD gene. Clin Mol Pathol. 1995;48(3):M124-32.
40. Blackwood KS, He C, Gunton J, Turenne CY, Wolfe J, Kabani AM, et al. Evaluation of recA sequences for identification of Mycobacterium species. J Clin Microbiol. 2000;38(8):2846-52.
41. Verma P, Jain A, Patra SK, Gandhi S, Sherwal BL, Chaudhary M, et al. Evaluation of polymerase chain reaction (PCR) using hupB gene in diagnosis of tuberculous lymphadenitis in fine needle aspirates. Indian J Tuberc. 2010;57(3):128-33.
42. Kathirvel M, Kommoju V, Brammacharry U, Ravibalan T, Ravishankar N, Radhakrishnan B, et al. Clinical evaluation of mtp40 polymerase chain reaction for the diagnosis of extra pulmonary tuberculosis. World J Microbiol Biotechnol. 2014;30(5):1485-90.
43. Scorpio A, Collins D, Whipple D, Cave D, Bates J, Zhang Y, et al. Rapid differentiation of bovine and human tubercle bacilli based on a characteristic mutation in the bovine pyrazinamidase gene. J Clin Microbiol. 1997;35(1):106-10.
44. Srivastava R, Kumar D, Waskar MN, Sharma M, Katoch VM, Srivastava BS, et al. Identification of a repetitive sequence belonging to a PPE gene of *Mycobacterium tuberculosis* and its use in diagnosis of tuberculosis. J Med Microbiol. 2006;55(Pt8):1071-7.
45. Hance AJ, Grandchamp B, Levy-Frebault V, Lecossier D, Rauzier J, Bocart D, et al. Detection and identification of mycobacteria by amplification of mycobacterial DNA. Mol Microbiol. 1989;3(7):843-9.
46. Negi SS, Anand R, Pasha ST, Gupta S, Basir SF, Khare S, et al. Diagnostic potential of IS6110, 38kDa, 65kDa and 85B sequence-based polymerase chain reaction in the diagnosis of *Mycobacterium tuberculosis* in clinical samples. Indian J Med Microbiol. 2007;25(1):43-9.
47. Thierry D, Brisson-Noel A, Vincent-Levy-Frebault V, Nguyen S, Guesdon JL, Gicquel B, et al. Characterization of a *Mycobacterium tuberculosis* insertion sequence, IS6110, and its application in diagnosis. J Clin Microbiol. 1990;28(12):2668-73.
48. Kolk AH, Schuitema AR, Kuijper S, van Leeuwen J, Hermans PW, van Embden JD, et al. Detection of *Mycobacterium tuberculosis* in clinical samples by using polymerase chain reaction and a nonradioactive detection system. J Clin Microbiol. 1992;30(10):2567-75.
49. Barani R, Sarangan G, Antony T, Periyasamy S, Kindo AJ, Srikanth P. Improved detection of *Mycobacterium tuberculosis* using two independent PCR targets in a tertiary care centre in South India. J Infect Dev Ctries. 2012;6(1):46-52.
50. Rahmo A, Hamze M. Characterization of *Mycobacterium tuberculosis* in Syrian patients by double-repetitive-element polymerase chain reaction. East Mediterr Health J. 2010;16(8):820-30.
51. Liu YC, Huang TS, Huang WK, Chen CS, Tu HZ, et al. Dideoxy fingerprinting for rapid screening of rpoB gene mutations in clinical isolates of *Mycobacterium tuberculosis*. J Formos Med Assoc. 1998;97(6):400-4.
52. Whelen AC, Felmlee TA, Hunt JM, Williams DL, Roberts GD, Stockman L, et al. Direct genotypic detection of *Mycobacterium tuberculosis* rifampin resistance in clinical specimens by using single-tube heminested PCR. J Clin Microbiol. 1995;3(3):556-61.
53. Kiepiela P, Bishop K, Kormuth E, Roux L, York DF. Comparison of PCR-heteroduplex characterization by automated DNA sequencing and line probe assay for the detection of rifampicin resistance in *Mycobacterium tuberculosis* isolates from KwaZulu-Natal, South Africa. Microb Drug Resist. 1998;4(4):263-9.
54. Kim HJ, Mun HS, Kim H, Oh EJ, Ha Y, Bai G, et al. Differentiation of Mycobacterial species by hsp65 duplex PCR followed by duplex-PCR-based restriction analysis and direct sequencing. J Clin Microbiol. 2006;44(11):3855-62.
55. Abe C, Hirano K, Wada M, Kazumi Y, Takahashi M, Fukasawa Y, et al. Detection of *Mycobacterium tuberculosis* in clinical

specimens by polymerase chain reaction and gen-probe amplified *Mycobacterium tuberculosis* direct test. J Clin Microbiol. 1993;31(12):3270-4.
56. Sharma K, Ashkin D, Fiorella P, Willis D, Dean S, Sharma A, et al. Evaluation of multiplex polymerase chain reaction utilising multiple targets in *Mycobacterium tuberculosis* direct test negative but culture positive cases: a potential method for enhancing the diagnosis of tuberculosis. Indian J Med Microbiol. 2013;31(4):370-3.
57. Higurashi Y, Satoh T, Hirai T, Moriya K, Koike K, et al. The fundamental evaluation of COBAS TaqMan48 using clinical specimens. Kekkaku. 2009;84(3):117-24.
58. Negi SS, Basir SF, Gupta S, Pasha ST, Khare S, Lal S, et al. Comparative study of PCR, smear examination and culture for diagnosis of cutaneous tuberculosis. J Commun Dis. 2005;37(2):83-92.
59. Cordova J, Shiloh R, Gilman RH, Sheen P, Martin L, Arenas F, et al. Evaluation of molecular tools for detection and drug susceptibility testing of *Mycobacterium tuberculosis* in stool specimens from patients with pulmonary tuberculosis. J Clin Microbiol. 2010;48(5):1820-6.
60. Flores LL, Pai M, Colford JM, Riley LW. In-house nucleic acid amplification tests for the detection of *Mycobacterium tuberculosis* in sputum specimens: meta-analysis and meta-regression. BMC Microbiol. 2005;5:55.
61. Kivihya-Ndugga L, van Cleeff M, Juma E, Kimwomi J, Githui W, Oskam L, et al. Comparison of PCR with the routine procedure for diagnosis of tuberculosis in a population with high prevalences of tuberculosis and human immunodeficiency virus. J Clin Microbiol. 2004;42(3):1012-5.
62. Tuberculosis diagnostic technology and market landscape, 2014. 3rd edition, Geneva. *www.unitaid.org* (Accessed June 2016).
63. Piersimoni C, Scarparo C. Relevance of commercial amplification methods for direct detection of *Mycobacterium tuberculosis* complex in clinical samples. J Clin Microbiol. 2003;41(12):5355-65.
64. Centers for Disease Control and Prevention (CDC). Updated guidelines for the use of nucleic acid amplification tests in the diagnosis of tuberculosis. MMWR Morb Mortal Wkly Rep. 2009;58:7-10.
65. Sloutsky A, Han LL, Werner BG. Practical strategies for performance optimization of the enhanced gen-probe amplified *Mycobacterium tuberculosis* direct test. J Clin Microbiol. 2004;42(4):1547-51.
66. Smith MB, Bergmann JS, Onoroto M, Mathews G, Woods GL. Evaluation of the enhanced amplified *Mycobacterium tuberculosis* direct test for direct detection of *Mycobacterium tuberculosis* complex in respiratory specimens. Arch Pathol Lab Med. 1999;123(11):1101-3.
67. Bergmann JS, Woods GL. Enhanced amplified *Mycobacterium tuberculosis* direct test for detection of *Mycobacterium tuberculosis* complex in positive BACTEC 12B broth cultures of respiratory specimens. J Clin Microbiol. 1999;37(6): 2099-101.
68. Dalovisio JR, Montenegro-James S, Kemmerly SA, Genre CF, Chambers R, Greer D, et al. Comparison of the amplified *Mycobacterium tuberculosis* (MTB) direct test, amplicor MTB PCR and IS6110-PCR for detection of MTB in respiratory specimens. Clin Infect Dis. 1996;23(5):1099-106.
69. DiDomenico N, Link H, Knobel R, Caratsch T, Weschler W, Loewy ZG, et al. COBAS AMPLICOR: fully automated RNA and DNA amplification and detection system for routine diagnostic PCR. Clin Chem. 1996;42(12):1915-23.
70. Garcia de Viedma D. Rapid detection of resistance in *Mycobacterium tuberculosis*: a review discussing molecular approaches. Clin Microbiol Infect. 2003;9(5):349-59.
71. Niemz A, Boyle DS. Nucleic acid testing for tuberculosis at the point-of-care in high-burden countries. Expert Rev Mol Diagn. 2012;12(7):687-701.
72. Yonemaru M, Horiba M, Tada A, Nagai T. Evaluation of COBAS TaqMan: a real-time PCR-based diagnostic kit for mycobacteria. Nihon Kokyuki Gakkai Zasshi. 2009;47(12):1070-6.
73. Bergmann JS, Woods GL. Clinical evaluation of the BDProbeTec strand displacement amplification assay for rapid diagnosis of tuberculosis. J Clin Microbiol. 1998;36(9):2766-8.
74. Pfyffer GE, Funke-Kissling P, Rundler E, Weber R. Performance characteristics of the BDProbeTec system for direct detection of *Mycobacterium tuberculosis* complex in respiratory specimens. J Clin Microbiol. 1999;37(1):137-40.
75. Rusch-Gerdes S, Richter E. Clinical evaluation of the semiautomated BDProbeTec ET system for the detection of *Mycobacterium tuberculosis* in respiratory and nonrespiratory specimens. Diagn Microbiol Infect Dis. 2004;48(4):265-70.
76. Boehme CC, Saacks S, O'Brien RJ. The changing landscape of diagnostic services for tuberculosis. Semin Respir Crit Care Med. 2013;34(1):17-31.
77. Aryan E, Makvandi M, Farajzadeh A, Huygen K, Bifani P, Mousavi SL, et al. A novel and more sensitive loop-mediated isothermal amplification assay targeting IS6110 for detection of *Mycobacterium tuberculosis* complex. Microbiol Res. 2009;165(3):211-20.
78. Mori Y, Nagamine K, Tomita N, Notomi T. Detection of loop-mediated isothermal amplification reaction by turbidity derived from magnesium pyrophosphate formation. Biochem Biophys Res Commun. 2001;289(1):150-4.
79. Boehme CC, Nabeta P, Henostroza G, Raqib R, Rahim Z, Gerhardt M, et al. Operational feasibility of using loop-mediated isothermal amplification for diagnosis of pulmonary tuberculosis in microscopy centers of developing countries. J Clin Microbiol. 2007;45(6):1936-40.
80. Sethi S, Singh S, Dhatwalia SK, Yadav R, Mewara A, Singh M, et al. Evaluation of in-house loop-mediated isothermal amplification (LAMP) assay for rapid diagnosis of *M. tuberculosis* in pulmonary specimens. J Clin Lab Anal. 2013;27 (4):272-6.
81. Zhu RY, Zhang KX, Zhao MQ, Liu YH, Xu YY, Ju CM, et al. Use of visual loop-mediated isotheral amplification of rimM sequence for rapid detection of *Mycobacterium tuberculosis* and *Mycobacterium bovis*. J Microbiol Methods. 2009;78(3):339-43.
82. Fang R, Li X, Hu L, You Q, Li J, Wu J, et al. Cross-priming amplification for rapid detection of *Mycobacterium tuberculosis* in sputum specimens. J Clin Microbiol. 2009;47(3):845-7.
83. Drouillon V, Delogu G, Dettori G, Lagrange PH, Benecchi M, Houriez F, et al. Multicenter evaluation of a transcription-reverse transcription concerted assay for rapid detection of *Mycobacterium tuberculosis* complex in clinical specimens. J Clin Microbiol. 2009;47(11):3461-5.
84. Tanaka H, Hirose H, Kato Y, Kida S, Miyajima E. Clinical evaluation of TRCRapid *M. TB* for detection of *Mycobacterium tuberculosis* complex in respiratory and nonrespiratory specimens. J Clin Microbiol. 2010;48(5):1536-41.
85. Nikam C, Jagannath M, Narayanan MM, Ramanabhiraman V, Kazi M, Shetty A, et al. Rapid diagnosis of *Mycobacterium*

tuberculosis with Truenat MTB: a near-care approach. PLoS One. 2013;8(1):e51121.

86. Lee SH, Kim SW, Lee S, Kim E, Kim DJ, Park S, et al. Rapid detection of *Mycobacterium tuberculosis* using a novel ultra-fast chip-type real-time PCR system. Chest. 2014.
87. Cho SN. Current issues on molecular and immunological diagnosis of tuberculosis. Yonsei Med J. 2007;48(3):347-59.
88. Piersimoni C, Scarparo C. Pulmonary infections associated with non-tuberculous mycobacteria in immunocompetent patients. Lancet Infect Dis. 2008;8(5):323-34.
89. Jagielski T, van Ingen J, Rastogi N, Dziadek J, Mazur PK, Bielecki J, et al. Current methods in the molecular typing of *Mycobacterium tuberculosis* and other mycobacteria. Biomed Res Int. 2014;2014:645802.
90. Hall L, Doerr KA, Wohlfiel SL, Roberts GD. Evaluation of the MicroSeq system for identification of mycobacteria by 16S ribosomal DNA sequencing and its integration into a routine clinical mycobacteriology laboratory. J Clin Microbiol. 2003;41(4):1447-53.
91. Patel JB, Leonard DG, Pan X, Musser JM, Berman RE, Nachamkin I, et al. Sequence-based identification of *Mycobacterium* species using the MicroSeq 500 16S rDNA bacterial identification system. J Clin Microbiol. 2000;38(1):246-51.
92. Lumb R, Lanser JA, Lim IS. Rapid identification of mycobacteria by the gen-probe accuprobe system. Pathology. 1993; 25(3):313-5.
93. Richter E, Niemann S, Rusch-Gerdes S, Hoffner S. Identification of *Mycobacterium kansasii* by using a DNA probe (accuprobe) and molecular techniques. J Clin Microbiol. 1999;37(4):964-70.
94. Louro AP, Waites KB, Georgescu E, Benjamin WH. Direct identification of *Mycobacterium avium* complex and *Mycobacterium gordonae* from MB/BacT bottles using accuprobe. J Clin Microbiol. 2001;39(2):570-3.
95. Ichiyama S, Iinuma Y, Yamori S, Hasegawa Y, Shimokata K, Nakashima N. Mycobacterium growth indicator tube testing in conjunction with the accuprobe or the AMPLICOR-PCR assay for detecting and identifying mycobacteria from sputum samples. J Clin Microbiol. 1997;35(8):2022-5.
96. Guerra RL, Hooper NM, Baker JF, Alborz R, Armstrong DT, Maltas G, et al. Use of the amplified *Mycobacterium tuberculosis* direct test in a public health laboratory: test performance and impact on clinical care. Chest. 2007;132(3):946-51.
97. Scarparo C, Piccoli P, Rigon A, Ruggiero G, Nista D, Piersimoni C. Direct identification of mycobacteria from MB/BacT alert 3D bottles: comparative evaluation of two commercial probe assays. J Clin Microbiol. 2001;39(9):3222-7.
98. Lebrun L, Gonullu N, Boutros N, Davoust A, Guibert M, Ingrand D, et al. Use of INNO-LIPA assay for rapid identification of mycobacteria. Diagn Microbiol Infect Dis. 2003;46(2):151-3.
99. Padilla E, Gonzalez V, Manterola JM, Pérez A, Quesada MD, Gordillo S, et al. Comparative evaluation of the new version of the INNO-LiPA Mycobacteria and genotype Mycobacterium assays for identification of Mycobacterium species from MB/BacT liquid cultures artificially inoculated with Mycobacterial strains. J Clin Microbiol. 2004;42(7):3083-8.
100. Tortoli E, Mariottini A, Mazzarelli G. Evaluation of INNO-LiPA MYCOBACTERIA v2: improved reverse hybridization multiple DNA probe assay for mycobacterial identification. J Clin Microbiol. 2003;41(9):4418-20.
101. Tortoli E, Kirschner P, Bartoloni A, Burrini C, Manfrin V, Mantella A, et al. Isolation of an unusual Mycobacterium from an AIDS patient. J Clin Microbiol. 1996;34(9):2316-9.
102. Richter E, Weizenegger M, Fahr AM, Rüsch-Gerdes S. Usefulness of the GenoType MTBC assay for differentiating species of the *Mycobacterium tuberculosis* complex in cultures obtained from clinical specimens. J Clin Microbiol. 2004;42(9):4303-6.
103. Syre H, Myneedu VP, Arora VK, Grewal HM. Direct detection of mycobacterial species in pulmonary specimens by two rapid amplification tests, the gen-probe amplified *Mycobacterium tuberculosis* direct test and the genotype mycobacteria direct test. J Clin Microbiol. 2009;47(11):3635-9.
104. Somoskovi A, Dormandy J, Rivenburg J, Pedrosa M, McBride M, Salfinger M. Direct comparison of the genotype MTBC and genomic deletion assays in terms of ability to distinguish between members of the *Mycobacterium tuberculosis* complex in clinical isolates and in clinical specimens. J Clin Microbiol. 2008;46(5):1854-7.
105. Gomez MP, Herrera-Leon L, Jimenez MS, Rodríguez JG. Comparison of GenoType MTBC with RFLP-PCR and multiplex PCR to identify *Mycobacterium tuberculosis* complex species. Eur J Clin Microbiol Infect Dis. 2007;26(1):63-6.
106. Singh AK, Maurya AK, Umrao J, Kant S, Kushwaha RA, Nag VL, et al. Role of GenoType (R)) Mycobacterium common Mycobacteria/Additional species assay for rapid differentiation between *Mycobacterium tuberculosis* complex and different species of non-tuberculous Mycobacteria. J Lab Physicians. 2013;5(2):83-9.
107. Lim J, Kim J, Kim JW, Ihm C, Sohn YH, Cho HJ, et al. Multicenter evaluation of Seegene Anyplex TB PCR for the detection of *Mycobacterium tuberculosis* in respiratory specimens. J Microbiol Biotechnol. 2014;24(7):1004-7.
108. Dye C, Williams BG, Espinal MA, Raviglione MC. Erasing the world's slow stain: strategies to beat multidrug-resistant tuberculosis. Science. 2002;295(5562):2042-6.
109. Gandhi NR, Nunn P, Dheda K, Schaaf HS, Zignol M, van Soolingen D, et al. Multidrug-resistant and extensively drug-resistant tuberculosis: a threat to global control of tuberculosis. Lancet. 2010;375(9728):1830-43.
110. Grandjean L, Moore DA. Tuberculosis in the developing world: recent advances in diagnosis with special consideration of extensively drug-resistant tuberculosis. Curr Opin Infect Dis. 2008;21(5):454-61.
111. WHO, Global Tuberculosis Report, 2013. *www.who.int/tb/publications.*
112. Isaakidis P, Das M, Kumar AM, Peskett C, Khetarpal M, Bamne A, et al. Alarming levels of drug-resistant tuberculosis in HIV-infected patients in Metropolitan Mumbai, India. PLoS One. 2014;9(10):e110461.
113. Paramasivan CN, Rehman F, Wares F, Sundar Mohan N, Sundar S, et al. First- and second-line drug resistance patterns among previously treated tuberculosis patients in India. Int J Tuberc Lung Dis. 2010;14(2):243-6.
114. Chakraborty N, De C, Bhattacharyya S, Mukherjee A, Santra S, Banerjee D, et al. Drug susceptibility profile of *Mycobacterium tuberculosis* isolated from HIV infected and uninfected pulmonary tuberculosis patients in eastern India. Trans R Soc Trop Med Hyg. 2010;104(3):195-201.
115. Balaji V, Daley P, Anand AA, Sudarsanam T, Michael JS, Sahni RD, et al. Risk factors for MDR and XDR-TB in a tertiary referral hospital in India. PLoS ONE. 2010;5(3):e9527.
116. WHO, molecular line probe assays for rapid screening of patients at risk of multidrug-resistant tuberculosis (MDR-TB). Policy Statement. 2008.pp.1-9. *www.who.int/tb* Accessed June 2016).

117. Bwanga F, Hoffner S, Haile M, Joloba ML. Direct susceptibility testing for multi-drug resistant tuberculosis: a meta-analysis. BMC Infect Dis. 2009;9:67.
118. Ling DI, Zwerling AA, Pai M. GenoType MTBDR assays for the diagnosis of multidrug-resistant tuberculosis: a meta-analysis. Eur Respir J. 2008;32(5):1165-74.
119. Helb D, Jones M, Story E, Boehme C, Wallace E, Ho K, et al. Rapid detection of *Mycobacterium tuberculosis* and rifampin resistance by use of on-demand, near-patient technology. J Clin Microbiol. 2009;48(1):229-37.
120. Steingart KR, Sohn H, Schiller I, Kloda LA, Boehme CC, Pai M, et al. Xpert(R) MTB/RIF assay for pulmonary tuberculosis and rifampicin resistance in adults. Cochrane Database Syst Rev. 2013;1:CD009593.
121. Boehme CC, Nicol MP, Nabeta P, Michael JS, Gotuzzo E, Tahirli R, et al. Feasibility, diagnostic accuracy, and effectiveness of decentralised use of the Xpert MTB/RIF test for diagnosis of tuberculosis and multidrug resistance: a multicentre implementation study. Lancet. 2011;377(9776):1495-505.
122. Tang X, Morris SL, Langone JJ, Bockstahler LE. Microarray and allele specific PCR detection of point mutations in *Mycobacterium tuberculosis* genes associated with drug resistance. J Microbiol Methods. 2005;63(3):318-30.
123. Gryadunov D, Mikhailovich V, Lapa S, Roudinskii N, Donnikov M, Pan'kov S, et al. Evaluation of hybridisation on oligonucleotide microarrays for analysis of drug-resistant *Mycobacterium tuberculosis*. Clin Microbiol Infect. 2005;11(7):531-9.
124. Park H, Song EJ, Song ES, Lee EY, Kim CM, Jeong SH, et al. Comparison of a conventional antimicrobial susceptibility assay to an oligonucleotide chip system for detection of drug resistance in *Mycobacterium tuberculosis* isolates. J Clin Microbiol. 2006;44(5):1619-24.
125. Cho SN, Brennan PJ. Tuberculosis: diagnostics. Tuberculosis (Edinb). 2007;87(Suppl 1):S14-7.
126. Mikhailovich V, Gryadunov D, Kolchinsky A, Makarov AA, Zasedatelev A. DNA microarrays in the clinic: infectious diseases. Bioessays. 2008;30(7):673-82.
127. Dineva MA, MahiLum-Tapay L, Lee H. Sample preparation: a challenge in the development of point-of-care nucleic acid-based assays for resource-limited settings. Analyst. 2007;132(12):1193-9.
128. Mehta PK, Raj A, Singh N, Khuller GK. Diagnosis of extrapulmonary tuberculosis by PCR. FEMS Immunol Med Microbiol. 2012;66(1):20-36.
129. Santos A, Cremades R, Rodriguez JC, García-Pach0́n E, Ruiz M, Royo G. Comparison of methods of DNA extraction for real-time PCR in a model of pleural tuberculosis. APMIS. 2010;118(1):60-5.
130. Honore-Bouakline S, Vincensini JP, Giacuzzo V, Lagrange PH, Herrmann JL. Rapid diagnosis of extrapulmonary tuberculosis by PCR: impact of sample preparation and DNA extraction. J Clin Microbiol. 2003;41(6):2323-9.
131. Aldous WK, Pounder JI, Cloud JL, Woods GL. Comparison of six methods of extracting *Mycobacterium tuberculosis* DNA from processed sputum for testing by quantitative real-time PCR. J Clin Microbiol. 2005;43(5):2471-3.
132. Keeler E, Perkins MD, Small P, Hanson C, Reed S, Cunningham J, et al. Reducing the global burden of tuberculosis: the contribution of improved diagnostics. Nature. 2006;444 (Suppl 1):49-57.
133. Peter JG, Theron G, Pooran A, Thomas J, Pascoe M, Dheda K. Comparison of two methods for acquisition of sputum samples for diagnosis of suspected tuberculosis in smear-negative or sputum-scarce people: a randomised controlled trial. Lancet Respir Med. 2013;1(6):471-8.
134. Theron G, Pooran A, Peter J, van Zyl-Smit R, Kumar Mishra H, Meldau R, et al. Do adjunct tuberculosis tests, when combined with Xpert MTB/RIF, improve accuracy and the cost of diagnosis in a resource-poor setting? Eur Respir J. 2012;40(1):161-8.
135. Shafer RW, Kim DS, Weiss JP, Quale JM. Extrapulmonary tuberculosis in patients with human immunodeficiency virus infection. Medicine (Baltimore). 1991;70(6):384-97.
136. Shafer RW, Edlin BR. Tuberculosis in patients infected with Human Immunodeficiency Virus: perspective on the past decade. Clin Infect Dis. 1996;22:683-704.
137. de Charnace G, Delacourt C. Diagnostic techniques in paediatric tuberculosis. Paediatr Respir Rev. 2001;2(2):120-6.
138. Eamranond P, Jaramillo E. Tuberculosis in children: reassessing the need for improved diagnosis in global control strategies. Int J Tuberc Lung Dis. 2001;5(7):594-603.
139. Cole ST, Brosch R, Parkhill J, Garnier T, Churcher C, Harris D, et al. Deciphering the biology of *Mycobacterium tuberculosis* from the complete genome sequence. Nature. 1998;393:37-544.

Management of Tuberculosis

D Behera

CHEMOTHERAPY OF TUBERCULOSIS

The modern era of tuberculosis treatment, short-course chemotherapy (SCC) began with the first East-African/British Medical Research Council (BMRC) study in the early 70s and subsequent studies in different parts of the world, which demonstrated that the addition of rifampin (R) to isoniazid (H) and streptomycin (S) allowed a dramatic curtailment from 18 months to 6 months in the duration of drug therapy required to elicit cures in 95% or more of patients, which is considered as the gold standard of the efficacy of any chemotherapy program.[1] Subsequently, a number of clinical trials all over the world done in a wide variety of populations and health service conditions, have confirmed that the duration of treatment can be reduced to 6–9 months from the earlier 12–18 months with the use of suitable combinations of antitubercular drugs.[2-12] Since then, short course chemotherapy is now widely accepted as the treatment of choice for pulmonary tuberculosis. From the results of clinical trials and of complimentary laboratory studies, the mechanisms of action of the main antitubercular drugs and their contributions to regimens are becoming increasingly well understood.

The antituberculosis drugs vary in (1) their bactericidal action, defined as their ability to kill large numbers of actively metabolizing bacilli rapidly; (2) their sterilizing action, defined as their capacity to kill special populations of slowly or intermittently metabolizing semidormant bacilli, the so called "persisters"; (3) their ability to prevent the emergence of acquired resistance by suppressing drug-resistant mutants present in all large bacterial populations and (4) their suitability for intermittent use.[13]

PREVENTION OF DRUG-RESISTANCE

Drugs can be graded according to their activity in preventing the emergence of resistance to a second drug, usually isoniazid. Even populations of tubercle bacilli, which are not exposed to antitubercular drugs, contain small proportions of drug-resistant mutants. The proportion of such mutants in wild strains is 1 in 10^5–10^6 for streptomycin, isoniazid and ethambutol and 1 in 10^7 for rifampicin. If inadequate drug combinations are used, these mutants are likely to replace the killed susceptible bacilli and give rise to drug-resistant disease. The effectiveness of drugs in preventing the emergence of acquired resistance depends upon the extent to which they can inhibit bacilli continuously, whatever their rate of metabolism, even if there is some irregularity in taking drugs. Isoniazid and rifampicin are the most effective at preventing the emergence of resistance to other drugs and streptomycin and ethambutol are only slightly less. Pyrazinamide (Z) is less effective; para aminosalicylic acid (PAS) and thiacetazone are the least effective. Activity of a drug is assessed from the results of clinical studies of the treatment of smear positive pulmonary tuberculosis in which the drug concerned is given in a 2-drug combination with isoniazid. Drug gradings are based on the proportion of patients who fail during treatment with the emergence of isoniazid-resistance. This proportion is about 0.5% for rifampicin (high activity) and 13–15% for thiacetazone (low activity).

EARLY BACTERICIDAL ACTIVITY

Most of the antitubercular drugs (INH, rifampin, streptomycin, pyrazinamide) have bactericidal activity.[14] Of them, isoniazid kills the largest number of bacilli early during the first 2 days of chemotherapy in a rate of 0.72 $\log_{10}$ cfu/mL/day when given alone and the kill of other drugs is increased considerably by 0.36 $\log_{10}$ cfu/mL/day when isoniazid is added to them in treatment. Next in order of bactericidal activity are ethambutol and rifampin with rates of kill of 0.25 $\log_{10}$ cfu/mL/day and 0.19 $\log_{10}$ cfu/mL/day, respectively. They add little or nothing to the activity of second drugs. Streptomycin, thiacetazone and pyrazinamide are just bactericidal with rates of kill of 0.09–0.04 $\log_{10}$ cfu/mL/day.

STERILIZING ACTION

Sterilizing activity is the ability to kill all or virtually all of the bacilli in the lesions as rapidly as possible. As the speed of killing gets progressively slower during chemotherapy, sterilizing activity measures the speed with which the last few viable bacilli are killed. This activity is assessed in man by (1) proportion of sputum cultures that are negative at 2 months, or round about that time, after the start of treatment and (2) the proportion of relapses that occur after chemotherapy has been stopped. The sterilizing activity of a drug indicates its suitability for incorporation in short course regimens. The two drugs with the greatest sterilizing activity are rifampicin and pyrazinamide. Isoniazid is less active, taking longer time to sterilize lesions. Though less active than isoniazid, addition of streptomycin or thiacetazone to a regimen probably increases its sterilizing activity to a very small extent.[15] Ethambutol virtually has no sterilizing activity.

Mitchison in 1979[16] had suggested a special population hypothesis and subsequently an extension of this hypothesis explaining the bactericidal and sterilizing activities of various drugs **(Fig. 1)**. The majority of tubercle bacilli in the lesions at the start of treatment are growing more or less rapidly (population A). Isoniazid kills them during the first few days of chemotherapy. Other drugs contribute to the bactericidal activity, only if INH is not included or the bacilli are resistant. Other bacilli are almost dormant, therefore antitubercular drugs, including INH kill them slowly. Some of these semidormant bacilli are in an acid environment, perhaps inhibited by acidity or by poor oxygen supply because of low pO_2 (inside macrophages or in areas of inflammation) and are best killed by pyrazinamide, because it is active only at a pH of about 5.5 or less (population B). Other semidormant bacilli have occasional spurts of active metabolism, lasting perhaps for few hours (population C). These are killed most efficiently by rifampicin because its bactericidal action starts very quickly during the spurts of metabolism, before isoniazid has a chance to start killing. The organisms may be in neutral or an acid environment, so that there is some overlap between populations B and C. Finally, there is a completely dormant population of bacilli (population D), which is unaffected by any drug. Thus, early bactericidal activity kills population A, while populations B and C are killed by drugs with high sterilizing activity throughout the entire period of chemotherapy.

Subsequent observations proved that the assumptions as above were not entirely correct and therefore, an "extended special population theory" was proposed **(Fig. 2)**. According to this hypothesis, most of the bacilli in the lesions at the start of treatment exist in extracellular sites, including the areas of caseation where they are not closely surrounded by inflammatory cells. These bacilli (corresponding to population A in **Figure 1**) are in a mildly acid environment (6.5–7.0) and most are growing fairly rapidly. These population of bacilli are killed rapidly by INH actively, streptomycin is weakly bactericidal because of overall acidic pH and pyrazinamide is not bactericidal because the pH is not sufficiently acidic.

As further inflammatory reaction proceeds, the pH falls and the organisms are partially inhibited (population B and C of **Figure 1**). Pyrazinamide and rifampicin are now more bactericidal than INH and streptomycin is completely inactive. There is a steady transfer of bacilli from population A to population B in open cavities that contains majority of the bacilli. After several weeks of treatment, the inflammation starts dying down and the pH reverts towards the 6.5–7.0 ranges. The bacilli, corresponding to population C, are persisters and are relatively refractory to chemotherapy. Rifampicin has the greatest activity against them and INH and streptomycin are slow killers. Because of higher pH, pyrazinamide is inactive and therefore, the drug has no sterilizing activity after the first 2 months of short course chemotherapy.[17] If the bacilli again start to multiply, because of any reason (i.e. isoniazid resistance) local inflammation begins again, the pH falls and the situation is repeated

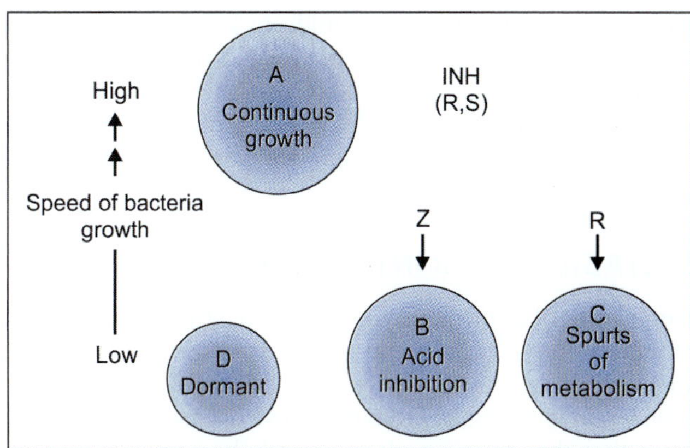

Fig. 1 Special bacterial population hypothesis by Mitchison
Abbreviations: R, rifampin; S, streptomycin; Z, pyrazinamide

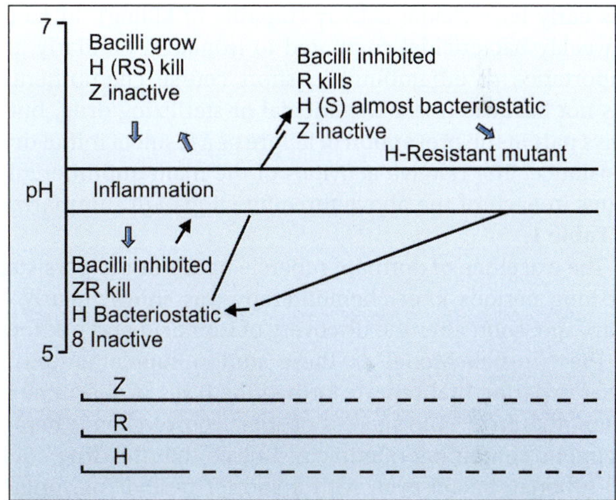

Fig. 2 Role of pH and inflammation in modifying the growth of *M. tuberculosis*. The circulation of periods of rapid killing by ZR and H is indicated in the lower part

with the necessity of pyrazinamide to kill the bacilli. Thus in multidrug short course regimens, the main killing activity of pyrazinamide occurs during the first few weeks of chemotherapy, while killing by rifampicin continues throughout treatment and isoniazid has its main activity during the first few days.

SUITABILITY FOR INTERMITTENT USE

Isoniazid, rifampicin, pyrazinamide, streptomycin and ethambutol are all effective when given twice or thrice a week. Thiacetazone is less effective when given intermittently than when given daily. From the above discussion, it is quite clear that the three functions of early bactericidal activity, sterilizing activity and ability to prevent drug resistance are unrelated. In the combinations, in which they are given, are effective because one or the other drug is having different grade of above activities. For example, while rifampicin has early bactericidal activity (rapidity of killing), in fact it is weakly bactericidal compared to isoniazid. Similarly, the importance of ethambutol in short course chemotherapy lies not because it is a bactericidal or sterilizing drug, but it plays part in the prevention of failure as a result of initial drug resistance. The relative activities of the main antitubercular drugs in each of the above three functions are summarized in **Table 1**.

The existence of dormant tubercle bacilli or the persisters for long periods after chemotherapy was shown nearly 40 years ago, soon after the discovery of isoniazid and is known as the "Cornell Model".[18] These studies supplemented by other experimental reports formed the basis of short course chemotherapy.[19] The success of short course chemotherapy regimens containing rifampicin showed that the drug could kill tubercle bacilli even with a shorter periods of contact, whereas other powerful drugs like isoniazid require about one generation time (24 hours). Based on these explanations and other clinical trials, the established short-course chemotherapy became widely acceptable. Unfortunately, the emergence of new molecular biology techniques like polymerase chain reaction (PCR), single-strand conformation polymorphism (SSCP) analysis, and restriction fragment length polymorphism (RFPL) have shown persistence of mycobacterial DNA in the animal tissues as well as in human material after discontinuation of therapy.[20,21] The relevance of these reports in the context of clinical practice is not clear; whether these may be indicators of re-emergence of tuberculosis, are yet to be answered. With the available information, many countries have developed guidelines for the treatment of tuberculosis.[22-33] The basic principle is the same, i.e. short course chemotherapy of 6 months duration.

Table 1 Grading of activities of antituberculosis drugs

Extent of activity	*Prevention of resistance*	*Early bactericidal*	*Sterilizing*
High	Isoniazid	Isoniazid	Rifampicin
	Rifampicin		Pyrazinamide
		Ethambutol	
	Ethambutol	Rifampicin	Isoniazid
	Streptomycin		
		Streptomycin	Streptomycin
	Pyrazinamide	Pyrazinamide	Thiacetazone
Low	Thiacetazone	Thiacetazone	Ethambutol

A number of National and International guidelines for the treatment of pulmonary tuberculosis are available:

- World Health Organization (2010). Treatment of Tuberculosis: Guidelines - 4th edition.
- WHO/HTM/TB/2009.420; International Standards for Tuberculosis Care
- *www.who.int/tb/ISTC_Report_2ndEd_Nov2009.pdf;*
- *www.cdc.gov/tb/publications/guidelines/treatment.htm* Oct 24, 2013
- *www.cdc.gov/mmwr/PDF/rr/rr5211.pdf.*

The Revised National Tuberculosis Control Program (RNTCP) for drug susceptible as well as MDR/XDR TB developed by the Central TB Division, Directorate General of Health Services, Govt. of India. *www.tbcindia.org.*

The World Health Organization has published guidelines for the treatment of tuberculosis for national programs.[34] In order to standardize short course chemotherapy in national tuberculosis programs, case definitions are required. The main purposes of these case definitions are for the proper patient registration and case notification, to evaluate the trend in the proportions of new smear-positive cases and smear-positive relapse and other treatment cases, to allocate cases to standardized treatment categories and for cohort analysis.

There are four determinants of case definition—the site of tuberculosis, severity of the disease, bacteriology and the history of previous treatment. WHO recommends the following definitions:

An active case of tuberculosis refers to symptomatic disease due to infection with *Mycobacterium tuberculosis* complex.

SITE OF TUBERCULAR DISEASE (PULMONARY OR EXTRAPULMONARY)

In general, recommended treatment regimens are similar for both pulmonary and extrapulmonary tuberculosis and are the same irrespective of the site of disease, although some authorities recommend a prolonged continuation phase for tubercular meningitis. Pulmonary tuberculosis refers to disease involving the pulmonary parenchyma and intrathoracic tuberculous lymphadenitis.

New Patients (Tables 2 and 3)

New patients are defined as those who have no history of prior TB treatment or who received less than 1 month of anti-TB drugs (regardless of whether their smear or culture results are positive or not).

New patients are presumed to have drug-susceptible TB with two exceptions:

1. Where there is a high prevalence of isoniazid resistance in new patients
   or
2. If they have developed active TB after known contact with a patient documented to have drug-resistant TB; they are likely to have a similar drug resistance pattern to the source case and DST should be carried out at the start of treatment. While DST results of the patient are awaited, a regimen based on the DST of the presumed source case should be started.

The 2-month rifampicin regimen (2HRZE/6HE) is associated with more relapses and deaths than the 6-month rifampicin regimen (2HRZE/4HR).

World Health Organization recommends the following treatment regimen for new patients presumed or known to have drug-susceptible TB.

New patients with pulmonary TB should receive a regimen containing 6 months of rifampicin: 2HRZE/4HR (Strong/High-grade of evidence)

This recommendation also applies to extrapulmonary TB except TB of the central nervous system, bones or joints for which some expert groups suggest longer therapy. WHO further recommends that national TB control programs

Table 2 Standard regimens for new TB patients (presumed, or known, to have drug-susceptible TB)

Intensive phase treatment				*Continuation phase*		
2 months of HRZE				4 months of HR		
Dosages of antitubercular drugs						
Daily dosage				*Intermittent dosage*		
	Adults and children	*Adults*		*Adults and children*	*Adults*	
Drug	*mg/kg*	*Weight*	*Dose*	*mg/kg*	*Weight*	*Dose*
H	5	—	300 mg	15	—	—
R	10	<50 kg	450 mg	15	—	600–900 mg
		>50 kg	600 mg			
S	15–20	<50 kg	750 mg	15–20	<50 kg	750 mg
		>50 kg	1 g		>50 kg	1 g
Z	35	<50 kg	1.5 g	50	<50 kg	2.0 g
		>50 kg	2.0 g	3 times/week	>50 kg	2.5 g
				75	<50 kg	3.0 g
				2 times/week	>50 kg	3.5 g
E	25 × 2 mo.	—	—	30	—	—
	then, 15			3 times/week		
				45		
				2 times/week		
T	4 (children)	—	150 mg	—	—	—
P	300	—	10–15 g	—	—	—
ET/PT	15–20	<50 kg	750 mg	—	—	—
		>50 kg	1 g	—	—	—
K	10–15	—	0.5–1 g	—	—	—
C	15	—	1 g	—	—	—
Cy	15	<50 kg	750 mg	—	—	—
		>50 kg	1 g	—	—	—

Abbreviations: H, INH; R, rifampicin; Z, pyrazinamide; S, streptomycin; E, ethambutol; T, thiacetazone; P-PAS; ET, ethionamide; PT, prothionamide; K, kanamycin; C, capreomycin; Cy, cycloserine. Ethambutol and capreomycin are not to be used in children

Table 3 Recommended doses of first-line antituberculosis drugs for adults

Drug	*Recommended dose*			
	Daily		*3 times per week*	
	Dose and range (mg/kg body weight)	*Maximum (mg)*	*Dose and range (mg/kg body weight)*	*Daily maximum (mg)*
Isoniazid	5 (4–6)	300	10 (8–12)	900
Rifampicin	10 (8–12)	600	10 (8–12)	600
Pyrazinamide	25 (20–30)	–	35 (30–40)	–
Ethambutol	15 (15–20)	–	30 (25–35)	–
Streptomycin*		15 (12–18)	15 (12–18)	1000

* Patients aged over 60 years may not be able to tolerate more than 500–750 mg daily, so some guidelines recommend reduction of the dose to 10 mg/kg per day in patients in this age group. Patients weighing less than 50 kg may not tolerate doses above 500–750 mg daily (WHO Model Formulary 2008, *www.who.int/selection_medicines/list/en/*).

provide supervision and support for all TB patients in order to ensure completion of the full course of therapy. Drug resistance surveys (or surveillance) should be carried out for monitoring the impact of the treatment program, as well as for designing standard regimens.

The other important recommendation of WHO is that the 2HRZE/6HE treatment regimen should be phased out. In terms of dosing frequency for human immunodeficiency virus (HIV)-negative patients, the systematic review found little evidence of differences in failure or relapse rates with daily or three times weekly regimens. However, patients receiving three times weekly dosing throughout therapy had higher rates of acquired drug resistance than patients who received drugs daily throughout treatment. In patients with pretreatment isoniazid resistance, three times weekly dosing during the intensive phase was associated with significantly higher risks of failure and acquired drug resistance than daily dosing during the intensive phase.

Other Important Recommendation

Wherever feasible, the optimal dosing frequency for new patients with pulmonary TB is daily throughout the course of therapy (Strong/High-grade of evidence).

There are two alternatives to the above:

New patients with pulmonary TB may receive a daily intensive phase followed by three times weekly continuation phase [2HRZE/4(HR)3] provided that each dose is directly observed (Conditional/High or moderate grade of evidence). Three time weekly dosing throughout therapy [2(HRZE)3/4(HR)3] is another alternative, provided that every dose is directly observed and the patient is NOT living with HIV or in an HIV-prevalent setting (Conditional/High or moderate grade of evidence).

In terms of dosing frequency for HIV-negative patients, the systematic review found little evidence of differences in failure or relapse rates with daily or three times weekly regimens. However, rates of acquired drug resistance were higher among patients receiving three times weekly dosing throughout therapy than among patients who received daily drug administration throughout treatment. Moreover, in patients with pretreatment isoniazid resistance, three times weekly dosing during the intensive phase was associated with significantly higher risks of failure and acquired drug resistance, particularly to rifampicin, than daily dosing during the intensive phase.

There is insufficient evidence to support the efficacy of twice weekly dosing throughout therapy.

Mediastinal lymphadenitis and pleural effusions without radiographic parenchymal involvement are taken as extrapulmonary tuberculosis. A patient with both pulmonary and extrapulmonary tuberculosis constitutes a case of pulmonary tuberculosis. The case definition of an extrapulmonary case with several sites affected depends upon the site representing the most severe form of the disease.

SEVERITY OF DISEASE

Bacillary load, extent of disease and anatomical site of involvement are taken into account in defining the severity of the disease. Involvement of an anatomical site results in classification as severe disease if there is either a significant acute threat to life as in pericardial tuberculosis, or a risk of subsequent severe sequel with handicap as in spinal tuberculosis, or both as in tuberculous meningitis. Thus, the following forms of extrapulmonary tuberculosis are classified as severe: Meningitis, miliary, pericarditis, peritonitis and bilateral or extensive pleural effusion, spinal, intestinal and genitourinary. Other forms of extrapulmonary tuberculosis like lymphadenitis, unilateral pleural effusion and bone (excluding spine), peripheral joint and skin are classified as less severe.

Bacteriology (Result of Sputum Smear)

It is very important to define the smear result in pulmonary cases because smear-positive cases are the most infectious and they have an increased mortality. The positive cases are the only ones for which bacteriological monitoring of cure is possible. A smear-positive pulmonary tuberculosis is one if (i) at least two sputum specimens are positive for acid fast bacilli by microscopy; or (ii) if at least there is one sputum specimen positive for acid fast bacilli by microscopy and radiographic abnormalities consistent with pulmonary tuberculosis and a decision by a physician to treat with a full curative course of antituberculous chemotherapy; or (iii) a patient with at least one specimen positive for acid fast bacilli by microscopy and which is culture positive for *M. tuberculosis*. Under program conditions with available microscopy services, pulmonary tuberculosis smear-positive cases represent about 65% of the total pulmonary tuberculosis cases in adults and 50% or more of all tuberculosis cases when diagnostic criteria are properly applied. This proportion may be high in populations with a high incidence of HIV infection.

A smear-negative pulmonary tuberculosis is one (i) two sets of at least two sputum specimens negative for acid fast bacilli on microscopy, examined at least 2 weeks apart; (ii) radiographic abnormalities consistent with pulmonary tuberculosis and a lack of clinical response despite 1 week of a broad spectrum antibiotic; and (iii) a decision by a physician to treat with a full curative course of antitubercular drugs. The category also includes patients who are severely ill; and at least two sputum specimens negative for acid-fast bacilli by microscopy; and radiographic abnormalities consistent with extensive pulmonary tuberculosis like interstitial or miliary forms of disease; and a decision by a physician to treat with a full curative course of antitubercular chemotherapy. The other group of patients that come under this category are those whose initial sputum were negative, who had sputum sent for culture initially and whose subsequent sputum culture results are positive. Thus, in the absence of culture, standard chest radiography is necessary to document cases of smear-negative pulmonary tuberculosis. Fluoroscopy examination results are not acceptable as documented evidence of pulmonary tuberculosis.

PREVIOUSLY TREATED CASES (TABLES 4 AND 5)

History of Previous Treatment

By this information, a case is defined whether a patient had previous antitubercular treatment or not. By this case-definition, patients who are at increased risk of acquired drug resistance are identified for the prescription of appropriate treatment; and for epidemiological monitoring. *Accordingly, the following five different categories of cases can be identified:*

Table 4 Standard regimens for previously treated patients depending on the availability of routine DST to guide the therapy of individual retreatment patients

DST	*Likelihood of MDR (Patient registration group[a])*	
Routinely available for previously treated patients	High (failure[b])	Medium or low (relapse, default)
Rapid molecular-based method	DST results available in 1–2 days confirm or exclude MDR to guide the choice of regimen	
Conventional method	While awaiting DST	
	Empirical MDR regimen. *Regimen should be modified once DST results are available.*	2HRZES/1HRZE/5HRE *Regimen should be modified once DST results are available.*
None (Interim)	Empirical MDR regimen *Regimen should be modified once DST results or DRS data are available.*	2HRZES/1 HRZE/5HRE for full course of treatment. *Regimen should be modified once DST results or DRS data are available.*

[a]The assumption that failure patients have a high likelihood of MDR (and relapse or defaulting patients a medium likelihood) may need to be modified according to the level of MDR such as in patients who develop active TB after known contact with a patient with documented MDR-TB. Patients who are relapsing or returning after defaulting from their second or subsequent course of treatment probably also have a high likelihood of MDR.

[b]Regimen may be modified once DST results are available (up to 2–3 months after the start of treatment).

Notes:

1. A country's standard MDR regimen is based on country-specific DST data from similar groups of patients
2. In the country's standard regimens, the 8-month retreatment regimen should not be "augmented" by a fluoroquinolone or an injectable second-line drug; this practice jeopardizes second-line drugs that are critical treatment options for MDR patients. Second-line drugs should be used only for MDR regimens and only if quality-assured drugs can be provided by directly observed treatment (DOT) for the whole course of therapy. In addition, there must be laboratory capacity for cultures to monitor treatment response, as well as a system for detecting and treating adverse reactions (on the Green Light Committee Initiative) before embarking on MDR-TB treatment.

Table 5 RNTCP regimen for MDR TB: 6 (9) Km Ofx (Lvx) Eto Cs Z E/18 Ofx (Lvx)Eto Cs E

S. No.	*Drugs*	*16–25 kg*	*26–45 kg*	*>45 kg*
1	Kanamycin	500 mg	500 mg	750 mg
2	Ofloxacin	400 mg	600 mg	800 mg
3	Levofloxacin	200 mg	500 mg	750 mg
4	Ethionamide	375 mg	500 mg	750 mg
5	Ethambutol	400 mg	800 mg	1000 mg
6	Pyrazinamide	500 mg	1250 mg	1500 mg
7	Cycloserine	250 mg	500 mg	750 mg
8	PAS (80% bioavailability)	5 g	10 g	12 g
	Pyridoxine	50 mg	100 mg	100 mg

Abbreviation: PAS, para-aminosalicylic acid

1. *New case*: A patient who has never had treatment for tuberculosis or who has taken antitubercular drugs for less than 4 weeks.
2. *Relapse*: A patient who has been declared cured of any form of tuberculosis in the past by a physician, after one full course of chemotherapy, and has become sputum smear-positive.
3. *Treatment failure*: A patient who, while on treatment, remained or became again smear-positive 5 months or later after commencing treatment. It is also a patient who was initially smear-negative before starting treatment and became smear-positive after the 2nd month of treatment.
4. *Treatment after interruption (TAI) or return after default*: A patient who interrupt treatment for 2 months or more, and returns to the health service with smear-positive sputum or sometimes smear-negative, but still with active disease clinically and radiologically.
5. *Chronic case*: A patient who remained or became again smear-positive after completing a fully supervised retreatment regimen.

Although smear-negative and extrapulmonary cases may also be treatment failures, relapses, or chronic cases, this is rare. The importance of case definitions as above is important for registration, notification and to define treatment categories.

In populations with known or suspected high levels of isoniazid resistance, new TB patients may receive human radiation experiments (HRE) as therapy in the continuation phase as an acceptable alternative to HR. While there is a pressing need to prevent multidrug resistance (MDR), the most effective regimen for the treatment of isoniazid-resistant TB is not known. There is inadequate evidence to quantify the ability of ethambutol to "protect rifampicin" in patients with pretreatment isoniazid resistance. There is no sufficient evidence for ocular toxicity from ethambutol but the risk of permanent blindness exists. Thus, further research is urgently needed to define the level of isoniazid resistance that would warrant the addition of ethambutol (or other drugs) to the continuation phase of the standard new patient regimen in TB Programs where isoniazid drug susceptibility testing is not done (or results are unavailable) before the continuation phase begins. Daily (rather than three times weekly) intensive-phase dosing may also help prevent acquired drug resistance in TB patients starting treatment with isoniazid resistance. Patients with isoniazid resistance treated with a three times weekly intensive phase had significantly higher risks of failure and acquired drug resistance than those treated with daily dosing during the intensive phase.

The RNTCP India is considering to tackle the issue of INH/Ethambutol/Streptomycin/Pyrazinamide resistance, either mono or poly-resistance based on suitable regimens.

TUBERCULOSIS TREATMENT IN PERSONS LIVING WITH HUMAN IMMUNODEFICIENCY VIRUS

Current WHO recommendations support that the antiretroviral therapy in TB patients living with HIV should be put rapidly into practice; the TB control program has already accepted this recommendation. TB patients with known positive HIV status and all TB patients living in HIV-prevalent settings should receive daily TB treatment at least during the intensive phase (Strong/High-grade of evidence). (HIV-prevalent settings are defined as countries, subnational administrative units, or selected facilities where the HIV prevalence among adult pregnant women is ≥1% or among TB patients is ≥5%).

For the continuation phase, the optimal dosing frequency is also daily for these patients (Strong/High-grade of evidence). If a daily continuation phase is not possible for these patients, three times weekly dosing during the continuation phase is an acceptable alternative (Conditional/High and moderate grade of evidence). The WHO recommends that TB patients who are living with HIV should receive at least the same duration of TB treatment as HIV-negative TB patients (Strong/High-grade of evidence). Some experts recommend prolonging TB treatment in persons living with HIV. Previously treated TB patients who are living with HIV should receive the same retreatment regimens as HIV-negative TB patients.

If a patient gains 5 kg or more in weight during treatment and crosses the weight-band range, the DOTS—Plus site committee may consider moving the patient to the higher weight-band drug dosages. Similarly if a patient loses 5 kg or more in weight during treatment and crosses the weight band the DOTS Plus site committee may consider moving the patient to the lower weight band. The new higher/lower dosages are provided whenever the patient is due for the next supply of drugs in the normal course of treatment and not as soon as change of weight is noted.

RATIONALE FOR RECOMMENDED TREATMENT REGIMENS

For new cases, treatment regimens have an initial or intensive phase for 2 months and a continuation phase lasting for 4–6 months. During the initial intensive phase of therapy, four drugs are administered wherein a rapid killing of bacilli takes place. Infectious patients become noninfectious within about 2 weeks and symptoms improve. The vast majority of cases with sputum smear-positive tuberculosis become sputum negative within 2 months. In the continuation phase fewer drugs, usually two, are required, but for a longer period of 4–6 months. The sterilizing effect of the drugs eliminates remaining bacilli and prevent relapse. In smear-positive cases, there is a risk of selecting resistant bacilli as these patients harbor and excrete a large number of bacilli. However, short-course chemotherapy consisting of four drugs initially and two drugs subsequently, reduce this risk of selecting resistant bacilli. These drugs are practically as effective in patients with initial resistant organisms as in those with sensitive organisms. In patients with smear-negative pulmonary tuberculosis and extrapulmonary tuberculosis, there is little risk of selection as these patients carry only a small bacillary load.

SUPERVISION OF CHEMOTHERAPY

Poor compliance by the patient is by far the most important cause of poor results even from the most potent regimens under program conditions. The poor compliance is due to a number of factors, including the unpleasantness of taking tablets and capsules daily, forgetfulness (a common human nature), cost, inconvenience for the patient to collect drugs regularly, side effects of the drugs, etc. The importance of complying with the treatment throughout the whole duration of therapy must repeatedly be emphasized to the patient and to his family. Whenever possible every dose of the regimen should be administered under full supervision. In some countries, this can be achieved by medical service staff on an entirely outpatient basis. In others, service staff can provide full outpatient supervision in the urban, but not in the rural areas, while in others treatment is rarely, if ever, fully supervised by service staff. Paramedical or laypersons, including a member of the patient's family, can be taught to do so.

It is well established that domiciliary therapy is preferable because of many socioeconomic reasons and is fully effective. It is not necessary to admit patients of tuberculosis for better supervision in hospitals except in certain special circumstances like a complication (hemoptysis, respiratory failure, cor pulmonale, etc.); for surgery, severe disease with hypotension, toxemia, complication due to drug therapy (hepatitis), surgery, and in cases of treatment failures for evaluation. It is better to accustom the patient to receive chemotherapy regularly and correctly on an outpatient basis from the start, organizing supervision as efficiently as circumstances allow. Whatever may be the level of supervision; compliance should be monitored by measures like periodic pill counting and surprising urine tests for isoniazid or inspection of the urine for red coloration of rifampicin or can be detected in urine by chloroform extraction. Under program conditions, DOT is now the practice world over including in India.

REFERENCES

1. Controlled clinical trial of four 6-month regimens of chemotherapy for pulmonary tuberculosis. Second report. Second East African/British Medical Research Council Study. Am Rev Respir Dis. 1976;114(3):471-5.
2. Results at 5 years of a controlled comparison of a 6-month and a standard 18-month regimen of chemotherapy for pulmonary tuberculosis. Am Rev Respir Dis. 1977;116(1):3-8.
3. Controlled trial of 6-month and 9-month regimens of daily and intermittent streptomycin plus isoniazid plus pyrazinamide for pulmonary tuberculosis in Hong Kong. The results up to 30 months. Am Rev Respir Dis. 1977;115(5):727-35.
4. Controlled trial of 6-month and 8-month regimens in the treatment of pulmonary tuberculosis. First report. Am Rev Respir Dis. 1978;118(2):219-28.
5. Controlled clinical trial of four short-course regimens of chemotherapy for two durations in the treatment of pulmonary tuberculosis: first report: Third East African/British Medical Research Councils study. Am Rev Respir Dis. 1978;118(1): 39-48.
6. Clinical trial of six-month and four-month regimens of chemotherapy in the treatment of pulmonary tuberculosis. Am Rev Respir Dis. 1979;119(4):579-85.
7. Controlled clinical trial of five short-course (4-month) chemotherapy regimens in pulmonary tuberculosis. Second report of the 4th study. East African/British Medical Research Councils Study. Am Rev Respir Dis. 1981;123(2):165-70.
8. Controlled trial of four thrice-weekly regimens and a daily regimen all given for 6 months for pulmonary tuberculosis. Lancet. 1981;1(8213):171-4.
9. Five-year follow-up of a controlled trial of five 6-month regimens of chemotherapy for pulmonary tuberculosis. Hong Kong Chest Service/British Medical Research Council. Am Rev Respir Dis. 1987;136(6):1339-42.
10. Santha T, Nazareth O, Krishnamurthy MS, Balasubramanian R, Vijayan VK, Janardhanam B, et al. Treatment of pulmonary tuberculosis with short course chemotherapy in South India-- 5-year follow-up. Tubercle. 1989;70(4):229-34.
11. Controlled trial of 2, 4, and 6 months of pyrazinamide in 6 month, three-times-weekly regimens for smear-positive pulmonary tuberculosis, including an assessment of a combined preparation of isoniazid, rifampin, and pyrazinamide. Results at 30 months. Hong Kong Chest Service/British Medical Research Council. Am Rev Respir Dis. 1991;143(4 Pt 1):700-6.
12. Assessment of a daily combined preparation of isoniazid, rifampin, and pyrazinamide in a controlled trial of three 6-month regimens for smear-positive pulmonary tuberculosis. Singapore Tuberculosis Service/British Medical Research Council. Am Rev Respir Dis. 1991;143(4 Pt 1):707-12.
13. Mitchison DA. The action of antituberculosis drugs in short-course chemotherapy. Tubercle. 1985;66(3):219-25.

14. Jindani A, Aber VR, Edwards EA, Mitchison DA. The early bactericidal activity of drugs in patients with tuberculosis. Am Rev Respir Dis. 1980;121(6):939-49.
15. Fox W. Short course chemotherapy for tuberculosis. In: Flenley DC (Ed.). Recent advances in respiratory medicine, 2nd edition. London: Churchill Livingstone; 1980. p. 189.
16. Mitchison DA. Basic mechanisms of chemotherapy. Chest. 1979;76(6 Suppl):771-81.
17. Fox W. The chemotherapy of pulmonary tuberculosis: a review. Chest. 1979;76(6 Suppl):785-96.
18. McCune RM, Feldman FM, Lambert HP, McDermott W. Microbial persistence. I. The capacity of tubercle bacilli to survive sterilization in mouse tissues. J Exp Med. 1966;123(3): 445-68.
19. Gangadharam PR. Mycobacterial dormancy. Tubercle Lung Dis. 1995;76(6):477-9.
20. Dewit D, Wootton M, Dhillon J, Mitchison DA. The bacterial DNA content of mouse organs in the Cornell model of dormant tuberculosis. Tuber Lung Dis. 1995;76(6):555-62.
21. Hellyer TJ, Fletcher TW, Spears PA, et al. Strand displacement amplification (SDA) and the polymerase chain reaction (PCR) for monitoring the response to chemotherapy in patients with tuberculosis. ASM General meeting, Washington DC, May 2125; 1995. Abstract # U97.
22. American Thoracic Society. Treatment of mycobacterial diseases. Am Rev Respir Dis. 1977;115:85.
23. Antituberculosis regimens of chemotherapy. Recommendations from the Committee on Treatment of the International Union against Tuberculosis and Lung Disease. Bull Int Union Tuberc Lung Dis. 1988;63(2):60-4.
24. Iseman MD, Sbarbaro JA. Short-course chemotherapy of tuberculosis. Hail Britannia (and friends)! Am Rev Respir Dis. 1991;143(4 Pt 1):697-8.
25. American Thoracic Society. Medical Section of the American Lung Association: Treatment of tuberculosis and tuberculosis infection in adults and children. Am Rev Respir Dis. 1986; 134(2):355-63.
26. O'Brien RJ. Present chemotherapy of tuberculosis. Semin Respir Infect. 1989;4(3):216-24.
27. Fox W. Whither short course chemotherapy? Br J Dis Chest. 1981;75(4):331-57.
28. Chemotherapy and management of tuberculosis in the United Kingdom: recommendations 1998. Joint Tuberculosis Committee of the British Thoracic Society. Thorax. 1998;53(7): 536-48.
29. Collazos J, Mayo J, Martinez E. The chemotherapy of tuberculosis—from the past to the future. Respir Med. 1995;89(7):463-9.
30. Davidson PT, Le HQ. Drug treatment of tuberculosis--1992. Drugs. 1992;43(5):651-73.
31. Kapoor SC. Chemotherapy-new strategic? Ind J Tuberc. 1995;42:193-4.
32. Tuberculosis Research Centre, Madras. Interim findings on the evaluation of split drug regimens for pulmonary tuberculosis: a randomized controlled clinical trial. Ind J Tub. 1995;42(4):201-6.
33. Tuberculosis Research Centre (Indian Council of Medical Research), Madras. Seven year findings of short-course chemotherapy in 18 districts in India under district tuberculosis program. Ind J Tub. 1996;43(3):131-42.
34. Treatment of tuberculosis: Guidelines for National programs. In: 2nd edition. Geneva: World Health Organization; 1997.

Antitubercular Drugs

SK Katiyar, S Katiyar

INTRODUCTION

Mycobacterium tuberculosis (MTB) is a slow growing organism that has the ability to enter a state of dormancy, which allows it to persist in the host despite adequate treatment. The low oxygen tensions prevailing in solid caseous tissue do not favor rapid multiplication of bacilli. Following liquefaction, caseation and cavity formation, the prevailing oxygen tension becomes higher, favoring extracellular bacillary multiplication. In a patient with tuberculosis (TB), there are 3 kinds of populations of *M. tuberculosis* organisms:[1] (1) the first population is the actively growing extracellular organisms—huge numbers of organisms can grow extracellular in pulmonary cavities within liquefied caseous debris, it is this population, which develops drug-resistance most rapidly; (2) the second population consists of slow growing or intermittently growing organisms (spurts of metabolism), which are inside macrophages and (3) the third population is made up of slow growing organisms, which grow in solid caseous material. This environment is neutral in pH, but the penetration of drugs into this area may be compromised by a poor blood supply.

From studies of the fall in sputum bacterial counts in the early days of treatment with single drugs, it has been established that isoniazid (INH) is the most potent bactericidal agent, rifampicin (RIF) is less bactericidal, while streptomycin (SM), and pyrazinamide (PZA) have only low bactericidal activity.[2] Rifampicin is the only drug that is bactericidal against all three populations. Isoniazid and streptomycin are bactericidal against extracellular organisms (especially in cavity walls) and isoniazid also has bactericidal activity against intracellular bacilli. Pyrazinamide is bactericidal against intracellular organisms and works well in an acidic pH. Ethambutol is a bacteriostatic drug. Finally, a fourth population of totally dormant bacilli, not killed by any drug, is believed to exist. The sterilizing activity of drugs has been particularly studied in the experimentally infected mouse, where rifampicin and pyrazinamide were found to be very potent sterilizing drugs.[3] Among the alternative drugs, the quinolones have the highest bactericidal activity against *M. tuberculosis*.[4]

It has been estimated that the population of slowly growing organisms in macrophages and caseous lesions/tissues is less than 10^5, whereas in cavities, the rapidly growing population numbers 10^7-10^9 organisms.[1] Since mutants resistant to streptomycin, isoniazid and ethambutol in wild strains of tubercle bacilli number 1 per 10^5-10^6 organisms and those resistant to rifampicin 1 per 10^7, such strains could easily be selected by therapy with one drug. Such selection is avoided by multiple drug therapy. Also, the other important factor leading to drug—resistance is adding a single drug to a failing regimen. In such case, the majority of the organisms, which are susceptible to that single drug will be killed, but the small number of organisms, which have spontaneously mutated will survive and multiply. Overtime, selection of drug—resistant organisms will occur. When formulating a therapeutic regimen for TB, it is important to remember that viable organisms from slow growing or intermittently growing population may persist if drugs are not continued for an adequate period of time.

It has now been established that the shortest course of chemotherapy required for adequate sterilization with currently available drugs is 6 months.[5] Modern drug treatment regimens consist of an initial or introductory phase of therapy followed by a maintenance or continuation phase of therapy. In order to prevent relapse and drug—resistance, clinicians must prescribe an adequate regimen and ensure that patients adhere to therapy. To ensure adherence, directly observed therapy (DOT) should be considered for all cases. There are many factors that may influence patients' compliance, which include patients' social characteristics, personality, understanding of the illness and treatment and patient-doctor relationship.[6]

The antitubercular drugs can be grouped into five categories depending upon their pharmacotherapeutic characteristics. Group 1 consists of first line oral agents—isoniazid (INH); rifampicin (R); ethambutol (E); pyrazinamide (Z) and rifabutin (RFB). Group 2 consists of injectable agents streptomycin (S); kanamycin (KM); amikacin (AM) and capreomycin (CM). Group 3 includes—fluoroquinolones levofloxacin (LFX); ofloxacin (OFX); moxifloxacin (MFX). Group 4 features oral bacteriostatic second-line agents ethionamide (ETO); prothionamide (PTO); cycloserine (CS); terizidone (TRD) and para-aminosalicylic acid (PAS). Group 5 consists of agents with unclear efficacy clofazimine (CFZ); linezolid (LZD); amoxicillin/clavulanate (AMX/CLV); thiacetazone (THZ); imipenem/cilastatin (IPM/CLN); high-dose isoniazid (high-dose H) and clarithromycin (CLR). These drugs are not recommended by the World Health Organization (WHO) for routine use in multidrug-resistant tuberculosis (MDR-TB) patients.

First-line drugs are those used in initial and maintenance chemotherapy unless drug resistance is known. Rifabutin is not on the WHO list of essential medicines. It has been added here as it is used routinely in patients on protease inhibitors in several settings. High-dose H is defined as 16–20 mg/kg/day.

ISONIAZID

Domagk, the discoverer of the first sulfonamide, with fox and others synthesized several thiosemicarbazone derivatives in which the benzene ring was replaced with a pyridine ring and found that such derivatives retained antituberculous effects.[7,8] These studies eventually led to the discovery that an intermediate product, isoniazid ($C_6H_7N_3O$) had the most potent antituberculous action. Isoniazid (H or INH), a hydrazide of isonicotinic acid was first synthesized from ethyl isonicotinate and hydrazine hydrate in 1912 by Meyer and Malley in Prague.[9] Its use was not considered until 1945 when the observation of the antituberculous effect of nicotinamide by chlorine[10] stimulated others to test pyridine derivatives for their antimycobacterial effects. The first clinical trial of INH was initiated at sea view hospital, Staten island, New York in 1951, reported in April 1952.[11] INH was the one of the most active compounds used to treat and prevent tuberculosis worldwide. Its low cost, good bioavailability, relatively low-toxicity, excellent intracellular penetration and narrow spectrum of action make it an almost ideal antimicrobial agent.

Isoniazid is readily absorbed after oral or parenteral administration, gets distributed into all body fluids and intracellular compartments.[12] After oral administration, peak plasma concentration is achieved in 1–2 hours. Heavy meals, including both carbohydrate and fatty foodstuffs result in delayed absorption, with maximal concentrations ranging from 9% to 50%.[13,14] Individuals with extensive gastric surgery or those with resected or dysfunctional terminal ileum may fail to have normal absorption. In cerebrospinal fluid (CSF), the concentration reaches about 20% of that in plasma. INH is minimally bound to serum proteins. The dosage of INH for adults is 5 mg/kg if given daily (max 300 mg) and 15 mg/kg if given twice-thrice weekly (max 900 mg). Similarly, for children the dosage is 10–20 mg/kg, 20–40 mg/kg and 15 mg/kg if given daily (max 300 mg), twice-weekly and thrice-weekly (max 900 mg) respectively. In fetus, the serum concentration reaches 50% of that in the mother. INH achieves a concentration of 16.6 mg/mL with 300 mg dose after 3 hours and 12–25% of the usual infant dose of 10–20 mg/day is available to the infant from milk.[15,16] This may be a problem for the infant who is given INH for either treatment or for chemoprophylaxis especially in higher dosage, since about one-fifth of the daily therapeutic dose of INH is also ingested form milk by the infant. Such infants may be predisposed to convulsions due to pyridoxine deficiency.[17]

Minimal inhibitory concentration (MIC) of INH for majority (80%) of susceptible *M. tuberculosis* strains is less than 1 mg/mL (0.025–0.05 mg/mL).[18] The peak serum concentration is 3–5 mg/mL, far in excess of MIC required. The MIC of other pathogenic mycobacterial species (*M. kansasii, M. avium, M. haemophilum*) is higher in the range of more than 1–10 mg/mL, and hence, these may fail to respond to INH.

Most of INH (75–95%) is excreted in metabolized form in urine within 24 hours.[12] The major metabolites are acetylisoniazid formed by acetylation of INH by hepatic acetyltransferase and isonicotinic acid formed by hydrolysis. None of the other biotransformation products have biological activity. The half-life of INH ranges from 0.5 hour to 1.5 hours in rapid acetylators and 2–4.5 hours in slow acetylators. The acetylation rate is related to genetic differences in host acetyltransferase activity. There are 3 groups of acetylation status: (1) fast, (2) intermediate and (3) slow. The *NATZ IZA* allele codes for fast acetylation. Rapid acetylators are homozygous, intermediate acetylators are heterozygous and slow acetylators do not possess this allele.[19] Acetyltransferase is predominantly found in liver and small intestine. Liver disease can reduce acetylation rates. Neither age nor gender influences INH acetylation. Distribution of acetylation genotypes varies by race with approximately 50% of whites, blacks and South Indians being rapid acetylators whereas 80–90% of Chinese, Japanese and Eskimos have this trait.[20-22]

Earlier studies suggested that rapid acetylators who were more likely to have poor therapeutic response developed chronic tuberculosis.[23] However, careful monitoring of drug intake in such patients revealed that acetylation status does not influence treatment outcome.[24,25] This stands true for patients on daily, twice or thrice weekly regimens. By contrast, rapid acetylators have consistently less favorable outcomes in once-weekly regimens. Small amounts of INH are also excreted in saliva, sputum and feces. Isoniazid is removed by hemodialysis and peritoneal dialysis. The half-life of INH can be increased by drugs, such as para-aminosalicylic acid (PAS), procainamide, chlorpromazine, and decreased by ethanol and other drugs that induce cytochrome P-450. Isoniazid may increase phenytoin, warfarin and carbamazepine serum levels.

The mechanism of action of INH consists of the inhibition of mycolic acid synthesis, depletion of nicotinamide adenine dinucleotide (NAD), incorporation of INH derivatives into NAD to form NAD analogs (which lead to nonfunctional coenzymes) and catalase peroxidase.[26-30] Isoniazid is a prodrug, must be activated by a bacterial catalase-peroxidase enzyme called *KatG*.[31] *KatG* couples the isonicotinic acyl with NADH to form isonicotinic acyl-NADH complex. This complex binds tightly to ketoenoylreductase known as *InhA*, thereby blocking the natural *enoyl-AcpM* substrate and the action of fatty acid synthase. This process inhibits the synthesis of mycolic acid, required for the mycobacterial cell wall.

Kruger-Theimer[30] proposed that after uptake, INH is oxidized by the organism's catalase-peroxidase system to isonicotinic acid (INA) and other products incorporated to NAD analog. These NAD analogs are no longer functional as coenzymes, hence the tubercle bacilli become unable to oxidize hydrogen by the usual dehydrogenase-cytochrome oxidase system to form water. Also, a compensatory oxidation of hydrogen by flavin enzymes sets in, which leads to intracellular accumulation of hydrogen peroxide and inhibits bacterial multiplication.

Adverse Effects

The hepatotoxicity associated with INH was reported to result from the toxic effect of the intermediate products monoacetylhydrazine and dimethylhydrazine produced by liver cytochrome P-450 mixed function oxidase. After a standard 300 mg dose of oral INH, rapid acetylators excrete 23% of the drug as monoacetylhydrazine and slow acetylators excrete 5%.[29] Hence, the former phenotype was believed to be associated with increased hepatotoxicity. Larger studies have shown no significant differences in the incidence of hepatotoxicity by host acetylation rate status.[32,33]

The incidence of hepatotoxicity increases with advancing age.[34] It is 0% for persons younger than 20 years, 0.3% for persons 20–34 years of age, 1.2% for persons of age 35–49 years and 2.3% for persons 50 years or older.[35] Other factors that predispose INH associated liver damage include excessive alcohol consumption, intravenous (IV) drug abuse and pre-existing liver disease. Asymptomatic elevation of serum transaminase levels occur in as many as 20% of cases.[36] The incidence of hepatitis was higher in those who were taking both INH and rifampicin than those who took either INH plus other drugs without RIF or RIF plus other drugs without INH.[37] RIF induces an INH degradation pathway whereby more of the INH is hydrolyzed to form increased amounts of hydrazine, a potentially toxic compound.[38] Although, the rate of acetylation does not change in the presence of liver disease, clearance of drug is diminished in severe liver impairment, hence the dose of INH must be reduced to 150–200 mg daily and serum levels monitored.[39,40]

Since only a small proportion of INH is excreted renally, the dose needs to be reduced only in patients with severe renal insufficiency (creatinine clearance <10 mg/dL). However, normal daily doses of INH (300 mg or 5–6 mg/kg) can be given to patients with severe renal impairment as the administration of these doses in such cases will be equivalent to 8–9 mg/kg, which is well tolerated.[41] It has been demonstrated that reducing INH doses to 200 mg/day results in significant reduced therapeutic potency.[42] Keeping this background information in mind, most clinicians do not alter normal doses of isoniazid in the patients of chronic renal failure (CRF). In patients undergoing periodic hemodialysis, INH must be given in usual dose just following hemodialysis for rapid acetylators, a reduced dose may be appropriate for slow acetylators.[43]

Isoniazid has been shown to interfere with the biological functions of the pyridoxine compounds resulting in various toxicities like peripheral neuropathy and anemia.[44] The likelihood of toxicity is related to the nutritional status of the patient, is dosage related, rarely occurring with standard 300 mg daily dose. Conditions that predispose to neuropathy increase the risk of this manifestation in INH therapy. Hence, pyridoxine supplementation must be given for chronically under-nourished persons, chronic alcoholics, pregnant women, adolescent girls, diabetic patients, patients with uremia, seizure disorders, advanced age and cancer patients. Because of the potential for interference by high doses of pyridoxine with the antituberculous activity of INH, no more than 10 mg/ day should be used.[44]

The peripheral neuropathy is characteristically a "stocking-glove" type that commences with numbness and tingling, usually worse in the feet. Untreated, it may progress to disabling paresthesias, pain and weakness. The therapeutic dose of pyridoxine is 100 mg daily in such patients. Other less frequent neurological adverse effects that have been reported with INH are toxic encephalopathy, optic neuritis, cerebellar ataxia and psychiatric disturbances.[45,46] The mechanism by which these side effects occur has not been elucidated. Hypersensitivity reactions to INH are occasionally encountered, manifesting by the way of fever, pruritus, cutaneous eruptions (morbilliform, maculopapular and eruptive rash). The other rare side effects of INH are lupus like reactions, arthralgias and hematological disorders (anemia, agranulocytosis).[47,48]

The ingestion of toxic amounts of isoniazid causes recurrent seizures, profound metabolic acidosis, coma and even death. In adults, toxicity can occur with the acute ingestion of as little as 1.5 g of isoniazid. Doses larger than 30 mg/ kg often produce seizures. When ingested in amounts of 80–150 mg/kg or more, isoniazid can be rapidly fatal. The first signs and symptoms of isoniazid toxicity usually appear 30 minutes to 2 hours after ingestion and include nausea, vomiting, slurred speech, dizziness, tachycardia and urinary retention, followed by stupor, coma and recurrent grandmal seizures. The seizures produced by isoniazid toxicity are often refractory to anticonvulsant therapy. Given in gram-per-gram amounts of the isoniazid ingested, pyridoxine (vitamin B_6) usually eliminates seizure activity and helps to correct the patient's metabolic acidosis. Isoniazid toxicity should be suspected in any patient who presents with refractory seizures and metabolic acidosis.

Mechanisms of Resistance to Isoniazid

- Mutation in *KatG* gene reduces catalase-peroxidase (*KatG*) ability to activate prodrug INH to a range of highly reactive bactericidal species. This mutation is responsible for 22–64% of INH resistant cases.
- *InhA* gene produces NADH-dependent enoyl-ACP reductase, which is necessary for the production of mycolic acid in tubercle bacilli. Mutation of this gene leads to the upregulation of INH A and hence increased the production of mycolic acid. This mutation occurs in 20–34% of INH resistance (low level resistance, MIC ≤1 mg/mL) and this can be overcome by increasing the dosage of INH.
- *KasA* gene produces β-Ketoacyl ACP synthase and mutation of this gene reduces INH ability to interfere with mycolic acid synthesis (low level resistance). Occurs in 14% of INH-resistant cases.
- *AhpC* gene produces alkyl hydroperoxide reductase and mutation of this gene reduces INH activation (in 10% cases).
- Mutation of the gene *ndh* (NADH dehydrogenase) results in the increased competition of NADH with INH-NAD to bind with inhA site.

RIFAMPICIN

Rifampicin is a semisynthetic broad-spectrum bactericidal antibiotic derived from *Amycolatopsis mediterranei (*formerly classified as *Streptomyces mediterranei).*[49] Out of many biologically active compounds identified from the crude extract, rifamycin B was the most stable, least toxic, but with moderate level of therapeutic activity. Further, refinement of rifamycin B led to the synthesis of rifampin (rifamycin B to rifamycin O to rifamycin SV to rifampicin).[50,51] Rifampicin was synthesized initially in Italy in 1957, but introduced in to clinical use only in 1966, employed initially for the retreatment of drug-resistant treatment failure cases.[52] Several large clinical trials have demonstrated that RIF containing regimens effectively reduce the duration of the chemotherapy to less than 9 months.[53-57] Also, RIF has contributed to the success of intermittent therapy.[57,58] Both the shortened duration and increased interval of dosages have improved patient compliance, hence RIF became a standard element of therapy by late 1970s.[59] In addition to its antituberculosis activity, it has a wide range of activity against other bacteria, including *Staphylococcus, Streptococcus, Clostridium,* coliforms, *Pseudomonas, Proteus, Salmonella, Shigella, Bacteroides* and *Legionella.*

Rifampicin's target is β subunit of mycobacterial ribonucleic acid (RNA) polymerase, which read the deoxyribonucleic acid (DNA) target sequence and catalyzing the polymerization of the complementary RNA chain with ribonucleic triphosphate monomers.[60] Binding of RIF with β subunit of RNA polymerase either inhibits the nascent RNA chain form translocating into the polymer site allosterically or decreases the affinity of the active site for short chain RNA transcripts.[61,62] This results in short oligoribonucleotides that rapidly diffuse out of the active center.

Although, RIF has lesser early bactericidal activity (EBA) than INH, it has superior sterilizing activity.[2,63] This sterilization activity has been attributed to RIF's ability to affect semidormant bacilli, which are sporadically active for the short periods of time (population-C).[64] These brief periods of time are insufficient for other equally effective bactericidal agents to work, but sufficient for RIF to exert its effects.[64] Rifampicin is better absorbed in acidic environment, hence both food and antacids must be avoided in relation to the time of its administration. When taken on an empty stomach, peak plasma levels of 6–7 μg/mL are reached at 3 hours and the drug has a half-life of about 5 hours.[65] The MICs of susceptible strains range from 0.06 μg/mL to 0.25 μg/mL.[66]

It is partly deacetylated in the liver, excreted almost entirely in the bile; but there is enterohepatic circulation, some drug does appear in urine.[67] During the first few weeks of therapy, RIF induces accelerated rates at which it is deacetylated in the liver.[68] Since, desacetyl-rifampicin is excreted in the bile more rapidly than plain RIF, the peak concentration and serum half-life reduces during initial few weeks. Thus, the peak levels initially may reach 20 μg/mL or higher, the usual range seen later is between 8 μg/mL and 12 μg/mL. No adjustment in dosage is necessary in patients with renal failure. The dosage of RIF is 10 mg/kg body weight (max 600 mg/day). Dosages of RIF exceeding this limit result in more drug bye-passing the liver and increased serum levels. Divided daily doses of RIF result in lower serum concentration, hence it must be given in a single daily dose. Although, about 75% of the drug is protein bound, it penetrates well into tissues and cells. Therapeutic concentrations are reached in CSF when the meninges are inflamed.

Rifampicin accelerates the hepatic cytochrome P450 pathway and reduces the serum levels of many drugs, including the antifungal agents, corticosteroids, warfarin and oral hypoglycemic agents **(Table 1)**. Rifampicin also reduces the levels of protease inhibitors and non-nucleoside reverse transcriptase inhibitors used to treat human immunodeficiency virus (HIV) infection.[69] This interaction may lead to the rapid development of resistance in HIV strains to the protease inhibitors. Rifampicin reduces the effectiveness of oral contraceptives[70] and patients should be advised to use nonhormonal contraception during and for 1 month after, treatment with rifampicin-containing regimens.

Rifampicin is the most potent inducer of CYP P450 enzyme, rifapentine is about 50% as active and rifabutin about 10%. Maximum induction of the cytochrome P450 pathway may require 7–10 days; conversely these effects do not resolve for 7–14 days following the discontinuation of rifampin. If major drug—drug interactions are feared one may either substitute rifabutin or adjust upward the doses of the other drugs.

Rifampicin may be detected in urine following the extraction of 10 mL urine by analytical-grade chloroform in

Table 1 Drug interactions of rifamycins with other compounds[71-73]

Cytochrome P450 pathway induction, resulting in more rapid elimination of • Corticosteroids • Oral contraceptives • Warfarin • Protease inhibitors • Azole antifungal agents • Anticonvulsants (phenytoin) • Oral hypoglycemic agents • Opiates (methadone) • Benzodiazepines • Antiarrhythmic agents • Chloramphenicol • Theophylline • Cyclosporine
Drugs that inhibit CYP P450, hence retard elimination of rifamycins • Ciprofloxacin • Macrolides • Azole antifungals • Protease inhibitors.

a screw-capped tube by gentle tilting.[74] The test is negative if no color develops, a yellow to orange color in the chloroform layer indicating the presence of rifampicin. The test is valid for up to at least 6 hours and in some patients, up to 12 hours after the ingestion of rifampicin. Tetracyclines, nitrofurantoin and phenothiazine derivatives also give a yellow color.

Adverse Effects

Rifampicin is well-tolerated by most patients at the currently recommended dosages. Unlike other drugs, RIF produces some adverse reactions more frequently with intermittent than with daily regimens. Moreover, the risk of adverse effects increases with the interval between doses, thus toxicity is high, if treatment is taken only once a week.

The drug is excreted in body fluids, all patients should be warned that their urine, sweat and tears may be colored orange-pink. It may also discolorize soft contact lens. Of the gastrointestinal (GI) reactions, nausea, anorexia and mild abdominal pain are most common, vomiting and diarrhea occurring less frequently. The incidence of these effects varies from 0% to 17%, more common in the elderly.[75,76] They may be resolved by giving the drug at night or, if this fails, during a meal. Transient elevations in aspartate aminotransferase levels are common (14–40% of patients), are of no clinical significance.[77] Major elevations of aspartate aminotransferase (>150 IU/L) occur in 4% and hepatitis with jaundice in about 1% patients. Rifampicin can also competitively interfere with the excretion of bilirubin and transiently elevate serum bilirubin.[78] Risk groups for jaundice include elderly women, alcoholics and those with a previous history of liver or biliary disease.[79] Rifampicin should be administered with care to these groups.

Cutaneous reactions are usually mild, consist of flushing with or without itching or a rash, commonly occur 2–3 hours after taking the drug. Patients usually desensitize themselves to these reactions, but occasionally an antihistamine may be required. Severe conjunctivitis and chronic papular acneiform reactions of the head, neck and shoulders have also been described. Cases of osteomalacia, pseudomembranous colitis, pseudoadrenal crisis, light-chain proteinuria with renal failure and cutaneous vasculitis have also been described.[80-82] Several other syndromes may occur with the intermittent regimens of rifampicin.

The "flu syndrome", with flu-like symptoms, lasting for up to 8 hours after administration of the drug, may occur a few months after treatment has been started, attributed to the development of circulating rifampicin-dependent antibodies.[83] It may resolve spontaneously or necessitate a switch to a daily regimen. Thrombocytopenic purpura constitutes an absolute indication for stopping therapy with rifampicin permanently. Asthmatic and hypotensive syndromes, may occur separately or together, require corticosteroid therapy before conversion to a daily regimen. Acute hemolytic anemia and acute tubular necrosis have also been reported. Cutaneous syndromes usually start during the 1st month and GI symptoms are spread over the first 6 months. The "flu" syndrome, observed only with intermittent regimens, generally begins in the 3rd–5th month of the treatment.[84] The incidence of side effects in recent reports of intermittent therapy have been gratifyingly low.[85,86] Anyone, who develops serious allergic drug reactions, such as renal failure, thrombocytopenia or respiratory insufficiency should not receive rifampin again.

Mechanism of Resistance to Rifampicin

Single base pair changes in the central region of the RNA polymerase beta subunit gene (*rpoB*) result in rifampin resistance. These mutations lead to decreased enzyme affinity for RIF.[87,88]

STREPTOMYCIN

Streptomycin (SM) was originally isolated from two strains of an actinomycetes species *(Streptomyces griseus)* by Selman Waksman and coworkers in 1943. Streptomycin was the first clinically effective drug available for the treatment of tuberculosis. Utility of this drug has been limited by the need for large doses that cannot be administered orally; frequent side effects and rapid emergence of resistance. Sole therapy with streptomycin in the late 1940s and early 1950s demonstrated the difficulty of treating TB with a single agent. As many as 80% of patients with cavitary disease harboring the large number of bacilli developed resistance to SM after the 3 months of therapy. It soon became evident that combination chemotherapy with newer agents prevented the emergence of drug resistance, hence, SM was used along with PAS until isoniazid was developed.

Streptomycin does not cross most membranes due to its large size and cationic charge, hence oral absorption is very poor. It must be given by either intramuscular or IV route. It diffuses readily into most body tissues, but penetration into CSF is less, with maximum levels obtained in inflamed meninges, of about 25% of serum levels.[89] For this reason, SM is not usually recommended for TB meningitis. When no other agents are available, intrathecal or intraventricular administration is advisable in life-threatening cases.[90] The peak plasma levels in the range of 40 µg/mL are achieved 1 hour after injection and MICs are maintained for at least 8 hours.[91] Most strains of *M. tuberculosis* are inhibited in vitro at a concentration of 8 µg/mL. The drug is excreted almost entirely by glomerular filtration, dosage must be modified in renal failure to avoid toxicity. A safe rule is to multiply the daily dose by the ratio of the patient's creatinine clearance to normal creatinine clearance.

Streptomycin binds with 30S subunit of ribosomes, reduces protein synthesis and induces misreading of mRNA. Some experts do not feel this sufficiently explains the bactericidal action of SM as agents that affect protein synthesis are generally bacteriostatic, not lethal to cells.[92] The other proposed mechanisms of action include increased permeability of membranes and enhanced uptake of drug.

It crosses the placenta, fetal serum levels are about half those in maternal blood. Use of streptomycin showed increase in the incidence of malformations in infants, 16.9% versus 1.4–6.0% in controls.[93] Aminoglycosides should not be used in pregnancy. The level of the drug in breast milk ranges from 12% to 47% after 6 hours of a dose. Thus, the potential for side effects exist and SM should not be used if alternatives are available. Streptomycin sulfate for intramuscular injection is supplied as a powder in vials and should be reconstituted immediately before use. The dose of SM in adults is 15 mg/kg body weight daily or thrice weekly. The dose should be reduced to 0.5 g/day for patients of age more than 50 years.

Adverse Effects

Streptomycin is toxic to the eighth cranial nerve, with vestibular damage more common than auditory damage. The patient usually complains of the progressive giddiness and unsteadiness of gait. Nystagmus may be present. The damage to the nerve is permanent, but most patients eventually compensate via ocular and proprioceptive compensatory mechanisms. The risk increases with the dose of drug and age.[94,95] The sensorineural deafness is most marked at higher frequencies. The first sign of ototoxicity is usually tinnitus or headache, which should prompt testing for hearing acuity with particular attention to deficits in the higher frequencies.

Streptomycin is ototoxic to the fetus. Other adverse effects include rashes, anaphylaxis, renal tubular damage, precipitation of heart failure, visual scotomas, peripheral neuritis, perioral paresthesia and blood dyscrasias, including hemolytic and aplastic anemia, agranulocytosis and thrombocytopenia. Streptomycin potentiates the neuromuscular block produced by curare, is contraindicated in individuals suffering from myasthenia gravis.

Mechanism of Drug Resistance

Mutation of *rpsL* gene (which encodes for S12 ribosomal protein) reduces the binding of streptomycin to S12 ribosomal protein and leads to the resistance.

PYRAZINAMIDE

Pyrazinamide (PZA), an amide derivative of pyrazine-2-carboxylic acid, was synthesized by Kushner and coworkers and found to be the most active nicotinamide analog against *M. tuberculosis.*[96] The first clinical trial of PZA given as single agent, at an average dose of 2.8 g/day demonstrated bacteriological and clinical improvement in most patients.[97] However, this effect was not sustained and resistance to PZA developed rapidly. In all earlier clinical trials, the dosage of PZA was very high (ranges from 40 mg/kg to 70 mg/kg), which resulted in lethal hepatotoxicity.[98,99] Thus, PZA was used as second line agent until 1970. Trials of short-course chemotherapy for tuberculosis in the 1970s revived interest in PZA and suggested that PZA was essential to reduce the duration of therapy for smear positive pulmonary tuberculosis to 6 months. The relapse rates were very low (1.4–2.4% at 5 years) without increased toxicity. It was also noted in subsequent studies, that there was no additional utility of PZA if used beyond initial 2 months.[100] A modest, but significant reduction in serum RIF level was observed when PZA was given simultaneously.[101] Also, PZA caused a slight reduction in the bactericidal activity of RIF.[102] These studies clearly indicated that PZA need not be used beyond the first 2 months, unless drug resistance was detected.

Currently, PZA is considered a first line agent, is the third most important drug used in the treatment of tuberculosis. The exact mechanism of the antimycobacterial action of PZA is not completely known. It is bactericidal in an acid environment ($pH < 5.0$), hence its activity can be demonstrated *in vitro* only in low pH environment. Initially, it was thought that such acidic milieu was present in the phagolysosomes of macrophages. The tubercle bacilli produces an enzyme called "pyrazinamidase", which converts PZA to pyrazinoic acid (POA),[103] reduces the pH and is inhibitory to tubercle bacilli. At the same time, the bacilli produces ammonia, neutralize pH, hence the effect of PZA on macrophage diminishes 4–7 days after infection.[104] Extreme regional acidity within the localized regions of the diseased host has been offered as another theory to explain PZA's activity. It had been suggested that the local milieu in necrotic, caseating lesions is acidic that results in the inhibition or semidormancy of the tubercle bacilli, therefore PZA may contribute uniquely to chemotherapy by killing bacilli in this state, wherein they are not vulnerable to other agents, which only act on proliferating bacilli.[105,106] However, this activity of PZA was termed as "sterilizing" rather than a classic "bactericidal" effect. *M. bovis* is resistant to this drug.

It is well absorbed from the gastrointestinal tract (GIT), with the peak concentrations of about 50 μg/mL occurring 1.5–2 hours after ingestion. At a pH of 5.5, the minimal inhibitory concentration of pyrazinamide for *M. tuberculosis* is 20 μg/mL. It penetrates well into tissues, including the CSF. The drug is excreted in urine, 40% as pyrazinoic acid and 3% as unchanged PZA. The dose of pyrazinamide is 25–35 mg/kg body weight, daily. Lyophilized form of morphazinamide may be used for IV therapy if required, administered by drip infusion in a dose of 1 g following reconstitution with solvent.

Adverse Effects

Hepatitis was more common when the higher doses of the drug were used than are now recommended. It occurs in about 1% of patients, but milder subclinical derangement of liver function tests is common. The drug should be administered with caution to those with a history of liver or biliary tract disease. There is no significant increase in hepatotoxicity when pyrazinamide in standard dosage is added to a regimen of isoniazid and rifampicin during the initial 2 months of therapy.[107] Unlike RIF or INH-induced hepatitis, wherein values typically normalize in 10–14 days, PZA induced hepatitis may persist for 4–6 weeks after the drug has been discontinued.

Cutaneous reactions in the form of faintly erythematous rash and mild pruritus are rarely reported. Arthralgia is a common adverse effect (occurs in 40% of patients) that appears in the first 2 months of treatment, more frequently in Chinese patients. It is due to the inhibition of renal tubular secretion of uric acid by pyrazinoic acid, the main metabolite of pyrazinamide, can be treated with nonsteroidal anti-inflammatory agents.[108] High serum concentration of uric acid may uncommonly precipitate gout. Rarer adverse effects include anorexia, nausea, vomiting and sideroblastic anemia.

Mechanism of Drug Resistance

Mutation of *pncA* gene (which encodes for pyrazinamidase) results in the blocking of conversion form PZA to pyrazinoic acid (active intermediate).

ETHAMBUTOL

Ethambutol (d-ethylenediimino-di-1-butanol) is a singular compound, not related to any other family of antimicrobial agents. The effectiveness of this drug in tuberculosis was first described in 1961.[109] Ethambutol (EMB) is generally considered as a bacteriostatic drug, although, it is bactericidal *in vitro*.[110] It interferes with synthesis of arabinogalactan and with the transfer of mycolic acids into mycobacterial wall.[111] It has high EBA, reducing the number of bacilli in sputum over 14 days at a rate second only to INH.[2] Studies of EMB activity have indicated that high concentrations of EMB (10 μg/mL) have considerable bactericidal activity against *M. tuberculosis*.[112] Since, these high concentrations were achievable with dosages given in intermittent therapy, there appeared a role for EMB in twice-thrice weekly treatment. However, the available data indicate that EMB has only modest activity in drug susceptible tuberculosis, if given in the regimens containing INH, RIF and PZA. The major utility of EMB was demonstrated in the British Medical Research Council (BMRC) trials for cases with initial drug resistance to INH and/or SM.[113] In such cases, the primary effect of EMB is to prevent the treatment failure and further acquisition of drug resistance. However, SM appears slightly more potent than EMB as a fourth drug to accompany INH, RIF and PZA.

It is well absorbed after ingestion, with the peak plasma levels of 4 μg/mL occurring 2–4 hours after a dose of 15 mg/kg; food does not interfere with EMB absorption. The dose of EMB is 15–20 mg/kg body weight daily, 30 mg/kg thrice weekly and 40 mg/kg if given twice weekly. Peak levels correlate with the dosage. CSF concentrations of EMB are low (1–2 μg/mL with a dose of 25 mg/kg) even in the presence of meningitis. The drug is excreted in the urine, dosage adjustment is required for patients with renal insufficiency.[114] In patients on hemodialysis, a daily dose of 5 mg/kg body weight or a dose of 1.5 mg/kg every 8 hours has been suggested, with the testing of serum EMB levels and visual acuity, the serum levels should not exceed 5 μg/mL.[115] Levels of 1.5 mg/L and 4.6 mg/L have been observed in the milk of lactating mother. Hence, an infant of 3.5 kg body weight would ingest 0.5–0.9 mg/kg/day from breast milk (2.8–6.9% of pediatric therapeutic dose), this is not likely to be toxic for the infant.[116]

Adverse Effects

The principal adverse effect of EMB is retrobulbar neuritis, presenting with blurred vision, central scotomas and disturbance of red-green vision.[117,118] Recovery is the rule if the drug is stopped at the first sign of visual problems, but if these are ignored, optic atrophy may result. This complication is uncommon at a dose of 15 mg/kg, but increases with a daily dose of 25 mg/kg. Preexisting ophthalmic diseases may predispose to EMB toxicity. Patients should be warned to report visual symptoms immediately and to stop treatment if symptoms develop; pretreatment testing and recording of visual acuity is advised for patients taking this drug. The renal clearance of urates is decreased by EMB in a significant number of normal patients and acute attacks of gout have been precipitated in patients at risk.[119] Other adverse reactions of EMB occasionally described are: anaphylaxis, skin rashes, hepatic dysfunction, blood dyscrasias, interstitial nephritis and peripheral neuropathies.

Mechanism of Drug Resistance

Mutation of *embB* gene (which encodes for a membrane protein) reduces the binding of ethambutol with the membrane protein and leads to resistance to EMB. This mutation is responsible for 48–62% of cases resistant to EMB.

QUINOLONES

The quinolones are derivatives of pyridinecarboxylic acid, initially derived from an intermediate in chloroquine synthesis.[120] The 6-fluoroquinolones are potent antibacterial agents that interfere with a wide variety of DNA related processes, primarily through their action on a subunit of DNA gyrase (topoisomerase), the enzyme responsible for introducing supercoils into bacterial DNA. The fluoroquinolones have both bactericidal and sterilizing activities. These are well absorbed in GIT and the bioavailability approaches 100%. It is distributed widely in the body, 30–50% of serum concentration is attained in CSF with inflamed meninges. It has minimal hepatic metabolism; 87% of dose is excreted unchanged in the urine within 48 hours via glomerular filtration and tubular secretion. Dose reduction is necessary in patients with renal failure. Animal data demonstrated arthropathy in immature animals, with erosions in joint cartilage. Quinolones should be used during pregnancy only if the potential benefit justifies the potential risk to the fetus.

Ciprofloxacin is no longer recommended to treat drug-susceptible or drug-resistant tuberculosis.[121] Currently, the most potent available fluoroquinolones in descending order based on *in vitro* activity and animal studies are—moxifloxacin equal to gatifloxacin greater than levofloxacin greater than ofloxacin.[122,123] While ofloxacin is commonly used because of relatively lower cost, the later—generation fluoroquinolones, moxifloxacin and levofloxacin, are more effective and have similar adverse effect profiles. Furthermore, the later—generation fluoroquinolones may have some efficacy against ofloxacin-resistant strains.[124] Although, similar to moxifloxacin in its efficacy against TB, gatifloxacin is associated with serious cases of hypoglycemia, hyperglycemia and new-onset diabetes. If gatifloxacin is used, it should undergo close monitoring; the drug has been removed from the markets of many countries. Levofloxacin is, for the time being, the fluoroquinolone of choice until more data confirm the long-term safety of moxifloxacin. A later-generation fluoroquinolone is recommended for the treatment of extensively drug-resistant tuberculosis (XDR-TB), although there is inadequate evidence on whether this is an effective strategy.

Adverse Effects

The quinolones are generally well-tolerated. GI intolerance, headache, malaise, insomnia, restlessness, dizziness, allergic reactions, diarrhea, photosensitivity, tendon rupture and peripheral neuropathy have been rarely reported. Quinolones have the potential to cause tachycardia and QTc prolongation, can cause serious arrhythmia. This potential has been most marked for gatifloxacin and sparfloxacin, less seen with other quinolones. These drugs should be avoided in the presence of hypokalemia and in those patients taking drugs that can prolong QT such as cisapride, tricyclic antidepressants, phenothiazines, class IA and class III antiarrhythmics and macrolides.

Mechanism of Drug Resistance

Mutation of *gyrA* gene (which encodes for bacterial DNA *gyraseA* subunit) results in the inability of fluoroquinolones to inhibit DNA gyrase.

PARA-AMINOSALICYLIC ACID

Lehman studied 50 related compounds of salicylates and found PAS the most active agent against tubercle bacilli.[125] In a BMRC trial,[126] it was observed that there was no significant difference in the efficacy of streptomycin plus PAS versus streptomycin alone; however, a marked decrease in the development of streptomycin-resistant strains was noticed with addition of PAS. It was considered a first-line agent in combination with INH and SM until 1963 when ethambutol was approved for clinical use and replaced PAS as the first-line agent.

Para-aminosalicylic acid is a structural analog of para-aminobenzoic acid (PABA). It exerts a bacteriostatic effect on *M. tuberculosis* by competitively blocking the conversion of PABA into folic acid (which is essential for DNA synthesis), hence inhibits bacterial growth.[127] The MIC of sensitive strains ranges from 0.5 mg/mL to 2.0 mg/mL.[128] The drug is readily absorbed from the GIT. The peak serum level of 7–8 mg/mL is reached within 1–2 hours after an oral dose of 4 g. About 60–70% of the drug is bound to plasma proteins. PAS is metabolized in the liver by acetylation and excreted in urine as metabolites.[129] It does not cross noninflamed meninges, rapidly diffuses into caseous lesions within 30 minutes, but rapidly disappears from the lesion as soon as drug administration is discontinued.[130] The drug is excreted rapidly, thus larger doses must be given. The dose of PAS is 150 mg/kg daily in divided doses or 10–12 g/day.

Adverse Reactions

Nearly all patients suffer GI upset in the form of nausea, vomiting, anorexia or diarrhea. Many patients stop taking PAS prematurely. Hypersensitivity reactions manifested by fever, rashes, pruritus and hepatic dysfunction occur in about 5–10% of patients. In some patients, lymphadenopathy, joint pains and pulmonary infiltrates with eosinophilia have been reported. Most of these symptoms disappear with the discontinuation of therapy. It can cause fluid retention from excessive sodium load in patients with congestive cardiac failure. Hemolytic anemia has been reported in patients with

G6PD deficiency. PAS partially inhibits the uptake of iodine by thyroid, thus can cause hypothyroidism.[131]

Mechanism of drug resistance to PAS is not known.

ETHIONAMIDE/PROTHIONAMIDE

Ethionamide (alpha-ethyl-thioisonicotinamide) is a thioamide of isonicotinic acid that was synthesized by Lieberman in 1952.[128] The exact mechanism of action is unknown, but it appears to be similar to that of INH. Ethionamide is believed to exert its action on the outer envelope of tubercle bacilli, which includes the inhibition of mycolic acid synthesis.[128] The MIC of susceptible strains of *M. tuberculosis* is 0.3 µg/mL. The drug is well-absorbed from the GIT, the peak serum level is about 1.4 µg/mL after 3 hours of administration. After absorption, the drug gets widely distributed in the body, inactivated by liver and to a lesser extent by the kidney.[132] It is excreted in the kidney mainly as metabolites, about 5% as active drug. The drug readily crosses both the inflamed and the noninflamed meninges, the concentration in CSF equals to the serum concentration.

Prothionamide is the N-propyl derivative of ethionamide, similar to ethionamide in its action, clinical effectiveness and toxicity. However, prothionamide is considered to be unpleasant of the two.

The maximum optimum daily dose of ethionamide and prothionamide is 15–20 mg/kg (max 1 g/day), usually 500–750 mg. The dose must be reduced to 250–500 mg/day in patients with creatinine clearance of less than 30 mL/minute. Resistance develops rapidly if used alone, there is complete cross-resistance between ethionamide and prothionamide (partial cross-resistance with isoniazid and thiacetazone). Thiacetazone resistant organisms are often sensitive to prothionamide, but the reverse does not apply.

Adverse Reactions

The most common side effect of ethionamide/prothionamide is GI upset, which includes nausea, vomiting, unpleasant metallic taste and epigastric burning pain. GI effects may be minimized by decreasing dosage, by changing the time of drug administration, or by the concurrent administration of an antiemetic agent. Most of the symptoms disappear in a week, but in some the symptoms are severe requiring the discontinuation of therapy. Hepatitis with jaundice has been reported to occur in 4.3% of patients. Other side effects include mental depression, psychological disturbances, peripheral neuritis, convulsion, hypoglycemia, photosensitivity, gynecomastia, hypothyroidism, alopecia and acne. The drug is teratogenic in animals, should be avoided in pregnancy (at least during the first trimester) and care should be taken in the presence of diabetes, liver disease, alcoholism or mental illness. Ethionamide is considered to be unsafe in patients with porphyria because it has been shown to be porphyrinogenic in animals and *in vitro* systems.

Mechanism of Drug Resistance

Mutation of *inhA* gene (similar to that in isoniazid) leads to resistance to ethionamide in 40% of resistant cases.

CYCLOSERINE/TERIZIDONE

Cycloserine introduced in 1955, is an antibiotic isolated by Harned and Kropp from the culture of *Streptomyces orchidaceous.* Cycloserine is a structural analog of D-alanine. It competitively blocks the enzymes alanine racemase and D-alanyl-D-alanine synthetase, which are necessary for the synthesis of D-alanine dipeptide. This dipeptide is essential for mycobacterial cell wall synthesis, inhibition of which leads to the inhibition of cell growth.[127] Cycloserine is bacteriostatic, the MIC is 10 µg/mL for susceptible strains. The drug is rapidly absorbed orally, a mean peak serum level of 50 µg/mL is achieved in 4 hours of drug intake. The drug is widely distributed in the body, crosses the meninges promptly regardless of inflammation. There is no cross-resistance with other antituberculosis drugs, 60–70% of the drug is excreted unchanged in the urine via glomerular filtration; small amount are excreted in feces and a small amount is metabolized.

Terizidone contains two molecules of cycloserine. It is used in some countries instead of cycloserine, assumed to be as efficacious; however, there are no direct studies comparing the two drugs. Terizidone is not yet recommended by the WHO. The dosage of cycloserine is 10–15 mg/kg daily (max 1,000 mg), usually 500–750 mg/ day given in two divided doses.

Adverse Reactions

The frequently encountered adverse effects of cycloserine are neurological and psychiatric problems, including headaches, irritability, sleep disturbances, aggression, tremors, gum inflammation, pale skin, depression, confusion, dizziness, restlessness, anxiety, nightmares, severe headache and drowsiness. Occasionally, visual changes, skin rash, numbness, tingling or burning in hands and feet, jaundice, eye pain, rarely seizures and suicidal thoughts may also occur. Neurotoxicity is dose related, monitoring of the blood level is recommended to avoid levels in excess of 30 µg/mL.

CAPREOMYCIN

Capreomycin has a different chemical structure from the aminoglycosides, but the mechanism of antibacterial activity is similar. Polypeptides appear to inhibit the translocation of the peptidyl-tRNA and the initiation of protein synthesis. Capreomycin is bactericidal in action. It has got no cross-resistance with aminoglycosides. It penetrates meninges, only if inflamed. Excretion of 50–60% of the drug is through kidneys and a small amount through biliary excretion. There is no significant oral absorption. Intramuscular absorption may be delayed if the same site is used consistently. Capreomycin is given in a daily dose of 15–20 mg/kg with a usual dose of 1 g in a single daily dose. When necessary, it is possible to give the drug at the same dose 2–3 times weekly during the continuation phase, under close monitoring for adverse effects. Levels should be monitored for patients with impaired renal function. Interval adjustment (12–15 mg/kg 2–3 times per week) is recommended for patients with creatinine clearance of less than 30 mL/min or on hemodialysis.

Adverse Reactions

Animal studies show teratogenic effect, hence it is contraindicated in pregnancy. The frequent side effects are nephrotoxicity (20–25%), tubular dysfunction, azotemia, proteinuria, urticaria or maculopapular rash. The other side effects that have been reported include ototoxicity (vestibular > auditory), electrolyte abnormalities (decreased blood levels of calcium, magnesium and potassium), pain, induration and sterile abscesses at injection sites.

THIACETAZONE

Thiacetazone is a low-potency, cheap drug given orally and frequently used as a companion drug for isoniazid in developing countries. It is bacteriostatic in its action. The mechanism of action is unknown. It is well absorbed in the GIT and excreted in urine. It crosses placental barrier and excreted in milk in a concentration equal to that in the mother's blood. It is given in an oral dose of 150 mg daily.

Adverse Reactions

The most frequent side effect is the GI upset, which includes nausea, abdominal discomfort, vomiting and diarrhea. Other adverse effects include anemia, agranulocytosis, thrombocytopenia, cerebral edema, conjunctivitis, blurred vision and jaundice. Thiacetazone may enhance the ototoxicity of streptomycin. Generalized, reactions are common. Cutaneous hypersensitivity reactions progressing to toxic epidermal necrolysis have been reported in a significant percentage of patients with HIV-associated tuberculosis treated with thiacetazone-containing regimens. HIV-positive patients or those with clinical markers for acquired immunodeficiency syndrome (AIDS) should have ethambutol substituted for thiacetazone in their treatment regimen.

GROUP FIVE DRUGS

Group five drugs are not recommended for routine use in the treatment of drug-resistant tuberculosis because their contribution to the efficacy of multidrug regimens is unclear. Although, they have demonstrated some activity *in vitro* or in animal models, there is little or no evidence of their efficacy in humans for the treatment of drug-resistant tuberculosis. Most of these drugs are expensive, in some cases require IV administration. However, they can be used in cases where adequate regimens are not possible to design with the medicines from group 1 to group 4. They should be used in consultation with an expert in the treatment of drug resistance. If a situation requires the use of group 5 drugs, it is recommended to use at least two drugs from the group, given the limited knowledge of their efficacy.

CLOFAZIMINE

Clofazimine (CFZ) is orally active (40–70% absorbed) and accumulates in many tissues, especially in fat. Usual adult dose is 100–300 mg daily. Some clinicians begin at 300 mg daily and decrease to 100 mg after 4–6 weeks.

The major side effect is reddish-black discoloration of skin, especially on exposed parts. Discoloration of hair, conjunctiva and body secretions can also occur. Dryness of skin and itching is often troublesome. Acneiform eruptions and phototoxicity have been reported. Enteritis with intermittent loose stools, nausea, abdominal pain, anorexia and weight loss can occur at higher dosage. The early syndrome is a reflection of irritant effect of the drug, subsides with dose adjustment and administration along with meals. A late syndrome occurring after the few months of therapy is due to the deposition of clofazimine crystals in the intestinal mucosa. Clofazimine is to be avoided in early pregnancy and in patients with severe liver or renal impairment.

LINEZOLID

Linezolid is a new class antimicrobial agent termed "oxazolidinones", active against resistant gram-positive aerobes and anaerobes. Recently, it has been found to be useful in drug-resistant tuberculosis.[133] It inhibits bacterial protein synthesis by binding to the 23S fraction of 50S ribosome and interferes with the formation of tRNA, stops protein synthesis at an early step. As such, there is no cross resistance with any other class of antimicrobial agents. It is rapidly and completely absorbed orally, partly metabolized nonenzymatically and excreted in urine. The dose at which it is to be used is still under argument. Recent data suggest it should be started at 1,200 mg/day for 4–6 weeks followed by 300–600 mg/day for the remaining period.[133,134] It has been found to have an early sputum culture conversion (78.8% vs 37.6% at 24 months) and early cavity closure rate in a recent study.[133]

Side effects are mostly limited to abdominal pain and bowel upset. It can cause anemia, thrombocytopenia, leukopenia and bone marrow depression. It can also lead to optic and peripheral neuropathy which is reversible on removal of drug. Occasionally, rashes, pruritus, headache and oral/vaginal candidiasis have been reported.

AMOXICILLIN/CLAVULANATE

Amoxicillin/Clavulanate (AMX/CLV) is generally well tolerated, but GI tolerance is poorer especially in children. Dosages for the drug-resistant cases of tuberculosis are not well-defined. Normal, adult dose is 675/125 mg twice a day or 500/125 mg three times a day. Dosages of 1,000/250 have been used, but adverse side effects may limit this dosing. Candida stomatitis/vaginitis, rashes and hepatic injury have been reported.

IMIPENEM/CILASTATIN

Imipenem/Cilastatin (IM/CN) belongs to the subgroup of carbapenem. Imipenem has a broad-spectrum of activity against both sensitive and resistant aerobic and anaerobic gram-positive, as well as gram-negative bacteria. It acts by inhibiting cell wall synthesis. It remains very stable in the presence of beta-lactamase. Usual adult dose is 500–1,000 mg IV every 6 hours. Common adverse drug reactions are nausea and vomiting. Those who are allergic to penicillin and other beta-lactam antibiotics should not take imipenem. It can also cause seizures.

CLARITHROMYCIN

Clarithromycin belongs to the group "macrolide" having a macrocyclic lactone ring with attached sugars. It is rapidly absorbed and has greater tissue distribution. No dose modification is needed in liver disease and in mild-to-moderate renal failure. It inhibits hepatic oxidation of many drugs and leads to rise in the plasma levels of theophylline, carbamazepine, valproate, warfarin, terfenadine, astemizole and cisapride. Usual adult dose of clarithromycin is 500 mg twice daily.

Side effects can occur in the form of GI upset, but it is better tolerated than erythromycin. A few cases of pseudomembranous enterocolitis, hepatic dysfunction or rhabdomyolysis have been reported. Several cases of QT prolongation and serious ventricular arrhythmia are reported due to the inhibition of CYP3A4 resulting in the high blood levels of concurrently administered terfenadine/astemizole/cisapride.

HIGH-DOSE ISONIAZID

Many experts feel that high-dose isoniazid (16–20 mg/kg daily) can still be used in the presence of resistance to low concentrations of isoniazid (>1% of bacilli resistant to 0.2 μg/mL, but susceptible to 1 μg/mL of isoniazid), whereas isoniazid is not recommended for high-dose resistance (>1% of bacilli resistant to 1 μg/mL of isoniazid).[134] One study from a low-resource setting where a standardized regimen was used, suggested that routine inclusion of high-dose isoniazid (16–20 mg/kg/day) could improve outcomes.[135]

BEDAQUILINE

Bedaquiline is the latest addition to the antitubercular drugs class after a hiatus of nearly four decades. It was discovered by Koen Andries team and works by blocking the mycobacterial adenosine triphosphate (ATP) (adenosine 5'-triphosphate) synthase leading to loss of energy generation by the bacteria.[136] The drug is better absorbed with food with a plasma protein binding of greater than 99.9%. It is metabolized by CYP3A4 to form N-monodesmethyl metabolite which has a half-life of 137 hours. Therefore, the drug is discontinued earlier than other second line drugs so as to prevent resistance to it.[137,138] The MIC is 0.002–0.06 μg/mL.[138-140] The dose approved is 400 mg daily for 2 weeks followed by 200 mg thrice weekly for 22 weeks.[19] This drug has been approved specifically for pulmonary MDR tuberculosis and should only be used in adults (>18 years) with documented resistance to rifampicin and isoniazid. It may be used when the regimen suggested by the WHO (consisting of at least pyrazinamide and 4 seconds line drugs) is not possible either due to documented in vitro resistance to any of the drugs or adverse drug reactions. Further, it may also be used in XDR-TB cases in which the WHO category five drugs are required as well as in resistant extrapulmonary tuberculosis.[141] However, it should not be used in pregnancy or in children as no data is available.

The drug was approved by the food and drug administration's (FDA) on the basis of two phase 2b trials (C208 and 209) on 28th December 2012 and currently phase three trials are underway.

Adverse Effects

An increased risk of death is associated with the drug usage. However, the cause of which could not be determined in the trials. Apart from this, other side effects include nausea, arthralgia, headaches and elevation of transaminases as well as blood amylase. Coadministration with rifampicin should not be done due to significant drug interaction. Bedaquiline carries a black box warning for arrhythmia, as it leads to QT prolongation by blocking hERG channel, therefore, it should be used with caution in patients receiving moxifloxacin or clofazimine.[142]

DELAMANID

Delamanid is a new drug which has been synthesized from nitro-dihydro-imidazooxazole class of compounds. It is a bactericidal drug which acts by inhibiting the mycolic acid synthesis.[143,144] Absorption of the drug is better when taken with food. It has a half-life of 36 hours while it is 99.5% protein bound.[145] The dose which is being used is 100–200 mg for 6 months[146,147] but the ideal dose has still not been defined. The recommendation for use remain the same as that of bedaquiline.

Adverse Effects

The risk of adverse events were more at higher dose but were not dose limiting which included nausea, vomiting and palpitations due to QT prolongation.[145]

COTRIMOXAZOLE

Cotrimoxazole is an antibiotic which is used in a variety of infections. It consists of, trimethoprim and sulfamethoxazole (SMX) in a ratio of 1:5. Both the components are individually bacteriostatic while together they become bactericidal.[148] It acts by inhibiting the folic acid synthesis in the bacteria.[149] The MIC is 1/19 µg/mL.[150] The recent hypothesis is that only SMX is active against tubercle bacilli and not trimethoprim.[150,151] SMX has been found to have a synergistic effect with rifampicin and an additive one with ethambutol.[152] It is well distributed in all body fluids as well as the CSF and is 58-66% protein bound.[153,154] It has a half-life of 9 hours and it undergoes partial acetylation and glucuronide conjugation in the liver.[153]

Adverse Effects

Co-trimoxazole is a safe drug with minimal side effects which are mostly related to GI upset like nausea, vomiting, anorexia and diarrhea although it may also cause hyperkalemia, hypernatremia, leukopenia, thrombocytopenia and aplastic anaemia.[155-158]

REFERENCES

1. Grosset J. Bacteriologic basis of short-course chemotherapy for tuberculosis. Clin Chest Med. 1980;1(2):231-41.
2. Jindani A, Aber VR, Edwards EA, Mitchison DA. The early bactericidal activity of drugs in patients with pulmonary tuberculosis. Am Rev Respir Dis. 1980;121(6):939-49.
3. Grosset J. The sterilizing value of rifampicin and pyrazinamide in experimental short course chemotherapy. Bull Int Union Tuberc. 1978;53(1):5-12.
4. Tsukamura M. In vitro antituberculosis activity of a new antibacterial substance ofloxacin (DL8280). Am Rev Respir Dis. 1985;131(3):348-51.
5. Larbaoui D. Present state of chemotherapy of tuberculosis in high prevalence countries. The present state of short course chemotherapy. Bull IUAT. 1985;60:17.
6. Komaroff AL. Editorial: The practitioner and the compliant patient. Am J Public Health. 1976;66(9):833-5.
7. Domagk G, Offe HA, Siefken W. [Additional investigations in experimental chemotherapy of tuberculosis (neoteban)]. Dtsch Med Wochenschr. 1952;77(18):573-8.
8. Fox HH. The chemical attack on tuberculosis. Trans N Y Acad Sci. 1953;15(7):234-42.
9. Meyer H, Mally J. Hydrazine derivatives of pyridine-carboxylic acids. Monatsh. 1912;33:393-414.
10. Chorine V. Action de l'amide nicotinique sur les bacilles du genre mycobacterium. CR Acad Sci (Paris). 1942;220:150-1.
11. Robitzek EH, Selikoff IJ. Hydrazine derivatives of isonicotinic acid (rimifon marsilid) in the treatment of active progressive caseous-pneumonic tuberculosis; a preliminary report. Am Rev Tuberc. 1952;65(4):402-28.
12. Holdiness MR. Clinical pharmacokinetics of the antituberculosis drugs. Clin Pharmacokinet. 1984;9(6):511-44.
13. Männisto P, Mäntylä R, Klinge E, Nykänen S, Koponen A, Lamminsivu U. Influence of various diets on the bioavailability of isoniazid. J Antimicrob Chemother. 1982;10(5):427-34.
14. Zent C, Smith P. Study of the effect of concomitant food on the bioavailability of isoniazid, rifampicin and pyrazinamide. Tuberc Lung Dis. 1995;76(2):109-13.
15. Berlin CM, Lee C. Isoniazid and acetylisoniazid disposition in human milk, saliva and plasma. Fed Proc. 1979;38:426.
16. Tran JH, Montakantikul P. The safety of antituberculosis medications during breastfeeding. J Hum Lac. 1998;14(4):337-40.
17. McKenzie SA, Macnab AJ, Katz G. Neonatal pyridoxine responsive convulsions due to isoniazid therapy. Arch Dis Child. 1976;51(7):567-8.
18. Trinka L, Mison P, Otten H. Experimental evaluation of efficacy. In: Bartmann K (Ed). Handbook of Experimental Pharmacology Antituberculosis drugs. 84 Volume. Berlin: Springer-Verlag; 1988.
19. Parkin DP, Vandenplas S, Botha FJ, Vandenplas ML, Seifart HI, van Helden PD, et al. Trimodality of isoniazid elimination: phenotype and genotype in patients with tuberculosis. Am J Respir Crit Care Med. 1997;155(5):1717-22.
20. Armstrong AR, Peart HE. A comparison between behavior of Eskimos and non-Eskimos to the administration of isoniazid. Am Rev Respir Dis. 1960;81:588-94.
21. Tiitinen H, Mattila MJ, Eriksson AW. Comparison of the isoniazid inactivation in Finns and Lapps. Ann Med Int Fenn. 1968;57(4):161-6.
22. Short EI. Studies on the inactivation of isonicotinyl acid hydrazide in normal subjects and tuberculosis patients. Tubercle. 1962;43:33-42.
23. Teichmann W, Koehler R. Contribution to a quick differentiation of the individual isoniazid metabolism. Prax Pneumol. 1964;18:535-41.
24. Bang HO, Jacobsen LK, Strandgaard E, YDE H. Metabolism of isoniazid and para amino salycilic acid (PAS) in the organism and its therapeutic significance. Acta Tuberc Pnemol Scand. 1962;41:237-51.
25. Gow JG, Evans DA. A study of the influence of the isoniazid inactivator phenotype on reversion in genitourinary tuberculosis. Tubercle. 1964;45:136-43.
26. Middlebrook G. Sterilization of tubercle bacilli by isonicotinic acid hydrazide and the incidence of variants resistant to the drug in vitro. Am Rev Tuberc. 1952;65(6):765-7.
27. Russe HP, Barclay WR. The effect of isoniazid on lipids of the tubercle bacillus. Am Rev Tuberc. 1955;72(6):713-7.
28. Bekierkunst A. Nicotinamide-adenine dinucleotide in tubercle bacilli exposed to isoniazid. Science. 1966;152(3721):525-6.
29. Sriprakash KS, Ramakrishnan T. Comparative study of nicotinamide adenine dinucleotide nucleosidase from Mycobacterium tuberculosis H37Rv and pig brain: effect of isonicotinic acid hydrazide on the enzyme-inhibitor complex. Indian J Biochem. 1966;3(4):211-4.
30. Thiemer-Kruger E. Isonicotinic acid hypothesis of the antituberculous action of isoniazid. Am Rev Tuberc. 1958;77(2):364-7.
31. Suarez J, Ranguelova K, Jarzecki AA, Manzerova J, Krymov V, Zhao X, et al. An oxyferrous heme/protein-based radical

intermediate is catalytically competent in the catalase reaction of Mycobacterium tuberculosis catalase-peroxidase (KatG). J Biol Chem. 2009;284(11):7017-29.
32. Weber WW, Hein DW, Litwin A, Lower GM. Relationship of acetylator status to isoniazid toxicity, lupus erythematosis, and bladder cancer. Fed Proc. 1983;42(14):3080-97.
33. Gurumurthy P, Krishnamurthy MS, Nazareth O, Parthasarathy R, Sarma GR, Somasundaram PR, et al. Lack of relationship between hepatic toxicity and acetylator phenotype in three thousand South Indian patients during treatment with isoniazid with tuberculosis. Am Rev Respir Dis. 1984;129(1):58-61.
34. Kopanoff DE, Snider DE, Caras GJ. Isoniazid-related hepatitis: a U.S. Public Health Service cooperative surveillance study. Am Rev Respir Dis. 1978;117(6):991-1001.
35. Isoniazid associated hepatitis: Summary of the Tuberculosis Advisory Committee and special consultants to the Director. Centers for Disease Control. MMWR. 1974;23:97-8.
36. American Thoracic Society. Medical Section of the American Lung Association: Treatment of tuberculosis and tuberculosis infection in adults and children. Am Rev Respir Dis. 1986;134(2):355-63.
37. Steele M, Burk RF, DesPrez RM. Toxic hepatitis with isoniazid and rifampicin. A meta-analysis. Chest. 1991;99(2):465-71.
38. Sarma GR, Immanuel C, Kailasam S, Narayana AS, Venkatesan P. Rifampicin-induced release of hydrazine from isoniazid. A possible cause of hepatitis during treatment of tuberculosis with regimens containing isoniazid and rifampicin. Am Rev Respir Dis. 1986;133(6):1072-5.
39. Acocella G, Bonollo L, Garimoldi M, Mainardi M, Tenconi LT, Nicolis FB, et al. Kinetics of rifampicin and isoniazid administered alone and in combination to normal subjects and patients with liver disease. Gut. 1972;13(1):47-53.
40. Peloquin CA. Antituberculosis drugs: pharmacokinetics. In: Heifits LB (Ed). Drug Susceptibility in the Chemotherapy of Mycobacterial Infections. Boca Raton, FL: CRC press; 1991. pp. 59-88.
41. First line chemotherapy in the treatment of bacteriological relapses of pulmonary tuberculosis following a shortcourse regimen. Lancet. 1976;1(7952):162-3.
42. East African/British Medical Research Council. Isoniazid with thiacetazone in the treatment of pulmonary tuberculosis in East Africa: second investigation. Tubercle. 1963;ii:283-4.
43. Bowersox DW, Wintebauer RH, Stewart GL, Orme B, Barron E. Isoniazid dosages in patients with renal failure. N Engl J Med. 1973;289(2):84-7.
44. Snider DE. Pyridoxine supplementation during isoniazid therapy. Tubercle. 1980;61(4):191-6.
45. Cheung WC, Lo CY, Lo WK, Ip M, Cheng IK. Isoniazid induced encephalopathy in dialysis patients. Tuber Lung Dis. 1993;74(2):136-9.
46. Pallone KA, Goldman MP, Fuller MA. Isoniazid-associated psychosis: case report and review of the literature. Am pharmacother. 1993;27(2):167-70.
47. Cush JJ, Goldings EA. Drug induced lupus: clinical spectrum and pathogenesis. Am J Med Sci. 1985;290(1):36-45.
48. Claiborne RA, Dutt AK. Isoniazid-induced pure red cell aplasia. Am Rev Respir Dis. 1985;131(6):947-9.
49. Margalith P, Beretta G, Rifomycin XI. Taxonomic study on streptomyces mediterranei nov. sp. Mycopathol Mycol Appl. 1961;13:321-30.
50. Sensi P. History of the development of rifampin. Rev Infect Dis. 1983;5 Suppl 3:S402-6.
51. Furesz S, Timbale MT. Antibacterial activity of rifomycins. Chemotherapy. 1963;257:200-8.
52. Vall-Spinosa A, Lester TW. Rifampin: characteristics and role in the chemotherapy of tuberculosis. Ann Intern Med. 1971;74(5):758-60.
53. A controlled trial of six months chemotherapy in pulmonary tuberculosis. Second report: results during the 24 months after the end of chemotherapy. British Thoracic Association. Am Rev Respir Dis. 1982;126(3):460-2.
54. Five-year follow-up of a controlled trial of five 6-month regimens of chemotherapy for pulmonary tuberculosis. Hong Kong Chest Service/British Medical Research Council. Am Rev Respir Dis. 1987;136(6):1339-42.
55. Long-term follow-up of a clinical trial of six month and four month regimens of chemotherapy in the treatment of pulmonary tuberculosis. Singapore Tuberculosis Service/ British Medical Research Council. Am Rev Respir Dis. 1986;133(5):779-83.
56. Snider DE, Graczyk J, Bek E, Rogowski J. Supervised six-months treatment of newly diagnosed pulmonary tuberculosis using isoniazid, rifampin, and pyrazinamide with and without streptomycin. Am Rev Respir Dis. 1984;130(6):1091-4.
57. Eule H, Beck H, Evers H, Fischer P, Kwiatkowski H, Merkel S, et al. Daily ultrashort chemotherapy and intermittent short-term chemotherapy with 4 drugs of communicable pulmonary tuberculosis treated for the first time. Results of a cooperative multicenter study. Z Erkr Atmungsorgane. 1986;167(1-2):29-41.
58. Clinical trial of three 6-month regimens of chemotherapy given intermittently in the continuation phase in the treatment or pulmonary tuberculosis. Singapore Tuberculosis Service/ British Medical Research Council. Am Rev Respir Dis. 1985;132(2):374-8.
59. Fox W. The current status of short course chemotherapy with particular reference to regimens and mechanisms (author's transl). Kekkaku. 1978;53(10):503-9.
60. Hartmann G, Honikel KO, Knüsel F, Nüesch J. The specific inhibition of the DNA-directed RNA syntheis by rifamycin. Biochim Biophys Acta. 1967;145(3):843-4.
61. McClure WR, Cech CL. On the mechanism of rifampicin inhibition of RNA synthesis. J Biol Chem. 1978;253(24):8949-56.
62. Schutz W, Zillig W. Rifampicin inhibition of RNA synthesis by destabilization of DNA-RNA polymerase-oligonucleotide-complexes. Nucleic Acid Res. 1981;9(24):6889-906.
63. Mitchison D. Mechanisms of the actions of drugs in the short-course chemotherapy. Bull Int Union Tuberc. 1985;60(1-2):36-40.
64. Dickinson JM, Mitchison DA. Experimental models to explain the high sterilizing activity of rifampin in the chemotherapy of tuberculosis. Am Rev Respir Dis. 1981;123(4 Pt 1):367-71.
65. Brouet G, Roussel G. Trial 6.9.12: overall methods and results. Rev Franc Mal Resp. 1977;5(Suppl 1):5.
66. Heifets LB, Lindholm-Levy PJ, Flory MA. Bactericidal activity in vitro of various rifamycins against Mycobacterium avium and Mycobacterium tuberculosis. Am Rev Respir Dis. 1990;141(3):626-30.
67. Acocella G, Conti R, Luisetti M, Pozzi E, Grassi C. Pharmacokinetic studies on antituberculosis regimens in

humans. I. Absorption and metabolism of the compounds used in the initial intensive phase of the short-course regimens: single administration study. Am Rev Respir Dis. 1985;132(3):510-5.
68. Acocella G. Clinical pharmacokinetics of rifampicin. Clin Pharmacokinet. 1978;3(2):108-27.
69. Centers for Disease Control and Prevention (CDC). Updated guidelines for the use of rifabutin or rifampin for the treatment and prevention of tuberculosis in HIV-infected persons taking protease inhibitors or non-nucleoside reverse transcriptase inhibitors. MMWR Morb Mortal Wkly Rep. 2000;49(9):185-9.
70. Skolnick JL, Stoler BS, Katz DB, Anderson WH. Rifampin, oral contraceptives, and pregnancy. JAMA. 1976;236(12):1382.
71. Baciewicz AM, Self TH. Rifampin drug interactions. Arch Intern Med. 1984;144(8):1667-71.
72. Baciewicz AM, Self TH, Bekemeyer WB. Update of rifampin drug interactions. Arch Intern Med. 1987;147(3):565-8.
73. Borcherding SM, Baciewicz AM, Self TH. Update of rifampin drug interactions. II. Arch Intern Med. 1987;152(4):711-6.
74. Eidus L, Ling GM, Harnanansingh AM. Laboratory investigation of rifampicin. Int Z Klin Pharmakol Ther Toxikol. 1969;2(4):296-9.
75. Gomi J, Aoyagi T. Therapeutic effects and side effects of rifampin administered daily or twice-weekly. Scand J Respir Dis Suppl. 1973;84:145-52.
76. Proust AJ. The Australian rifampicin trial. Med J Aust. 1971;2(2):85-94.
77. Cohn HD. Clinical studies with a new rifamycin derivative. J Clin Pharmacol J New Drugs. 1969;9(2):118-25.
78. Capelle P, Dhumeaux D, Mora M, Feldmann G, Berthelot P. Effect of rifampicin on liver function in man. Gut. 1972;13(5):366-71.
79. Grönhagen-Riska C, Hellstrom PE, Fröseth B. Predisposing factors in hepatitis induced by isoniazid-rifampicin treatment of tuberculosis. Am Rev Respir Dis. 1978;118(3):461-6.
80. Long MW, Snider DE, Farer LS. U.S. Public Health Service Cooperative trial of three rifampicin–isoniazid regimens in treatment of pulmonary tuberculosis. Am Rev Respir Dis. 1979;119(6): 879-94.
81. Winter RJ, Banks RA, Collins CM, Hoffbrand BI. Rifampicin induced light chain proteinuria and renal failure. Thorax. 1984;39(12):952-3.
82. Iredale JP, Sankaran R, Wathen CG. Cutaneous vasculitis associated with rifampin therapy. Chest. 1989;96(1):215-6.
83. Poole G, Stradling P, Worlledge S. Potentially serious side-effects of high-dose twice-weekly rifampicin. Br Med J. 1971;3(5770):343-7.
84. Controlled trial of intermittent regimens of rifampin plus isoniazid for pulmonary tuberculosis in Singapore. The results up to 30 months. Am Rev Respir Dis. 1977;116(5):807-20.
85. Dutt AK, Moers D, Stead WW. Undesirable side-effects of isoniazid and rifampicin in largely twice weekly short course chemotherapy for tuberculosis. Am Rev Respir Dis. 1983;128(3):419-24.
86. The management of pulmonary tuberculosis in adults notified in England and Wales in 1988. The British Thoracic Society Research Committee and the Medical Research Council Cardiothoracic Epidemiology Group. Respir Med. 1991;85(4):319-23.
87. Jin DJ, Gross CA. Mapping and sequencing of mutations in the Escherichia coli rpoB gene that leads to rifampicin resistance. J Mol Biol. 1988;202(1):45-58.
88. Telenti A, Imboden P, Marchesi F, Lowrie D, Cole S, Colston MJ, et al. Detection of rifampicin-resistant mutations in *Mycobacterium tuberculosis*. Lancet. 1993;341(8846):647-50.
89. Strausbaugh LJ, Mandaleris CD, Snade MA. Comparison of four aminoglycoside antibiotics in the therapy of experimental E. coli meningitis. J Lab Clin Med. 1977;89(4):692-701.
90. Kaiser AB, McGee ZA. Aminoglycoside therapy of gram-negative bacillary meningitis. N Engl J Med. 1975;293(24):1215-20.
91. Welling PG, Baumueller A, Lau CC, Madsen PO. Netilmicin pharmacokinetics after single intravenous doses to elderly male patients. Antimicrob Agents Chemother. 1977;12(3):328-34.
92. Davis BB. The lethal action of aminoglycosides. J Antimicrob Chemother. 1988;22(1):1-3.
93. Snider DE, Layde PM, Johnson MW, Lyle MA. Treatment of tuberculosis during pregnancy. Am Rev Respir Dis. 1980;122(1):65-79.
94. Bignall JR, Crofton JW, Thomas JA. Effect of streptomycin on vestibular function. Br Med J. 1951;1(4706):554-9.
95. Smith JM, Zirk MH. Toxic and allergic drug reactions during the treatment of tuberculosis. Tubercle. 1961;42:287.
96. Kushner S, Dalalian H, Sanjuro SL. Experimental chemotherapy of tuberculosis. The synthesis of pyrazinamides and related compounds. J Am Chem Soc. 1952;74:3617.
97. Yeager RL, Monroe WE, Dessau FI. Pyrazinamide (aldinamide*) in the treatment of pulmonary tuberculosis. Trans Annu Meet Natl Tuberc Assoc. 1952;48:178-201.
98. McDermott W, Ormond L, Muschenheim C, Deuschle K, McCune RM, Tompsett R. Pyrazinamide-isoniazid in tuberculosis. Am Rev Tuberc. 1954;69(3):319-33.
99. Campagna M, Calix A, Hauser G. Observations on the combined use of pyrazinamide (Aldinamide) and isoniazid in the treatment of pulmonary tuberculosis; a clinical study. Am Rev Tuberc. 1954;69(3):334-50.
100. Controlled trial of 2, 4, and 6 months of pyrazinamide in 6-month, three-times-weekly regimens for smear-positive pulmonary tuberculosis, including an assessment of a combined preparation of isoniazid, rifampin, and pyrazinamide. Results at 30 months. Hong Kong Chest Service/British Medical Research Council. Am Rev Respir Dis. 1991;143(4 Pt 1):700-6.
101. Jain A, Mehta VL, Kulshrestha S. Effect of pyrazinamide on rifampin kinetics in patients with tuberculosis. Tuberc Lung Dis. 1993;74(2):87-90.
102. Sbarbaro JA, Iseman MD, Crowle AJ. The combined effect of rifampin and pyrazinamide within the human macrophage. Am Rev Respir Dis. 1992;146(6):1448-51.
103. Konno K, Feldman FM, McDermott W. Pyrazinamide susceptibility and amidase activity of tubercle bacilli. Am Rev Respir Dis. 1967;95(3):461-9.
104. Crowle AJ, Sbarbaro JA, May MH. Inhibition by pyrazinamide of tubercle bacilli within cultured human macrophages. Am Rev Respir Dis. 1986;134(5):1052-5.
105. Mitchison DA. [Mechanisms of the action of drugs in the short-course chemotherapy]. Bull Int Union Tuberc. 1985;60(1-2):36-40.
106. Hobby GL, Lenert TF. The in vitro action of antituberculosis agents against multiplying and non-multiplying microbial cells. Am Rev Tuberc. 1957;76(6):1031-48.
107. Steele MA, Des Prez RM. The role of pyrazinamide in tuberculosis chemotherapy. Chest. 1988;94(4):845-50.
108. Horsfall PA, Plummer J, Allan WG, Girling DJ, Nunn AJ, Fox W, et al. Double blind controlled comparison of aspirin,

allopurinol and placebo in the management of arthralgia during pyrazinamide administration. Tubercle. 1979;60(1):13-24.

109. Thomas JP, Baughn CO, Wilkinson RG, Shepherd RG. A new synthetic compound with antituberculous activity in mice: ethambutol (dextro-2,2'- (ethylenediimino)-di-1-butanol). Am Rev Respir Dis. 1961;83:891-3.
110. Crowle AJ, Sbarbaro JA, Judson FN, May MH. The effect of ethambutol on tubercle bacilli within cultured human macrophages. Am Rev Respir Dis. 1985;132(4):742-5.
111. Takayama K, Kilburn JO. Inhibition of synthesis of arabinogalactan by ethambutol in Mycobacterium smegmatis. Antimicrob Agents Chemother. 1989;33(9):1493-9.
112. Gangadharam PR, Prat PF, Perumal VK, Iseman MD. The effects of exposure time, drug concentration, and temperature on the activity of ethambutol versus Mycobacterium tuberculosis. Am Rev Respir Dis. 1990;141(6):1478-82.
113. Mitchison DA, Nunn AJ. Influence of initial drug resistance on the response to short course chemotherapy of pulmonary tuberculosis. Am Rev Respir Dis. 1986;133(3):423-30.
114. Varughese A, Brater DC, Benet LZ, Lee CS. Ethambutol kinetics in patients with impaired renal function. Am Rev Respir Dis. 1986;134(1):34-8.
115. Christopher TG, Blair A, Forrey A, Cutler RE. Kinetics of ethambutol elimination in renal disease. Proc Clin Dial Transplant Forum. 1973;3:96-101.
116. Snider DE, Powell KE. Should women take antituberculous drugs during breast-feed? Arch Intern Med. 1984;144(3):589-90.
117. Leibold JE. The ocular toxicity of ethambutol and its relation to dose. Ann NY Acad Sci. 1966;135(2):904-9.
118. Citron KM. Ethambutol: a review with special reference to ocular toxicity. Tubercle. 1969;50(Suppl):32-6.
119. Self TH, Fountain FF, Taylor WJ, Sutliff WD. Acute gouty arthritis associated with the use of ethambutol. Chest. 1977;71(4):561-2.
120. Lesher GY, Froelich EJ, Gruett MD, BAILEY JH, Brundage RP. 1,8-Naphthyridine derivatives. A new class of chemotherapeutic agents. J Med Pharm Chem. 1962;91:1063-5.
121. Moadebi S, Harder CK, Fitzgerald MJ, Elwood KR, Marra F. Fluoroquinolones for the treatment of pulmonary tuberculosis. Drugs. 2007;67(14):2077-99.
122. Alvirez-Freites EJ, Carter JL, Cynamon MH. In vitro and in vivo activities of gatifloxacin against Mycobacterium tuberculosis. Antimicrob Agents Chemother. 2002;46(4):1022-5.
123. Ji B, Lounis N, Maslo C, Truffot-Pernot C, Bonnafous P, Grosset J. In vitro and in vivo activities of moxifloxacin and clinafloxacin against Mycobacterium tuberculosis. Antimicrob Agents Chemother. 1998;42(8):2066-9.
124. Yew WW, Chan CK, Leung CC, Chau CH, Tam CM, Wong PC, et al. Comparative roles of levofloxacin and ofloxacin in the treatment of multidrug-resistant tuberculosis: preliminary results of a retrospective study from Hong Kong. Chest. 2003;124(4):1476-81.
125. Lehman J. Para-aminosalicylic acid in the treatment of tuberculosis. Lancet. 1946;250:15-6.
126. Treatment of pulmonary tuberculosis with streptomycin and para-aminosalicylic acid; a Medical Research Council Investigation. Br Med J. 1950;2(4688):1073-85.
127. Lorian V (Ed). Antibiotics in Laboratory Medicine, 2nd edition. Baltimore:Williams and Wilkins; 1986. pp. 93-150.
128. Youmans GP. Biologic activities of mycobacterial cells and cell components. In: Youmans G (Ed). Tuberculosis. Philadelphia: WB Saunders; 1979. pp. 46-62. pp. 63-193.
129. Kucers A, Bennett N (Eds). The use of antibiotics: a comprehensive review with clinical emphasis, 3rd edition. London, United Kingdom: William Heinemann Medical Books Ltd; 1979. pp. 646-53.
130. Heller A, Ebert RH, Koch-Weser D, Roth LJ. Studies with C14 labelled para-aminosalicylic acid and isoniazid. Am Rev Tuberc. 1957;75(1):71-82.
131. Sutherland D. Antithyroid effect of para-aminosalicylic acid. Transactions of the twelfth conference on the chemotherapy of tuberculosis. Washington, DC: Veterans administration-army-navy; 1953. pp. 314-5.
132. Hamilton EJ, Eidus L, Little E. A comparative study in vivo of isoniazid and alpha-ethylthioisonicotinamide. Am Rev Respir Dis. 1962;85:407-12.
133. Tang S, Yao L, Hao X, Zhang X, Liu G, Liu X, et al. Efficacy, safety and tolerability of linezolid for the treatment of XDR-TB: a study in China. Eur Respir J. 2015;45(1):161-70.
134. Koh WJ, Kwon OJ, Gwak H, Chung JW, Cho SN, Kim WS, et al. Daily 300 mg dose of linezolid for the treatment of intractable multidrug-resistant and extensively drug-resistant tuberculosis. J Antimicrob Chemother. 2009;64(2):388-91.
135. Sikora AG, Rothstein SG, Garay KF, Spiegel R. Tuberculosis of the head and neck. In: Rom WN, Garay SM (Eds). Tuberculosis, 2nd edition. Philadelphia: Lippincott Williams and Wilkins; 2004. p. 751.
136. Katiyar SK, Bihari S, Prakash S, Mamtani M, Kulkarni H. A randomized controlled trial of high-dose isoniazid adjuvant therapy for multidrug-resistant tuberculosis. Int J Tuberc and Lung Dis. 2008;12(2):139-45.
137. Koul A, Dendouga N, Vergauwen K, Molenberghs B, Vranckx L, Willebrords R, et al. Diarylquinolines target subunit c of mycobacterial ATP synthase. Nat Chem Biol. 2007;3(6):323-4.
138. Matteelli A, Carvalho AC, Dooley KE, Kritski A. TMC207: the first compound of a new class of potent anti-tuberculosis drugs. Future Microbiol. 2010;5(6):849-58.
139. Andries K, Verhasselt P, Guillemont J, Göhlmann HW, Neefs JM, Winkler H, et al. A diarylquinoline drug active on the ATP synthase of Mycobacterium tuberculosis. Science. 2005;307(5707):223-7.
140. Van Heeswijk R, Lachaert R, Leopold L, DeBeule K, McNeeley D. The effect of CYP3A4 inhibition on the clinical pharmacokinetics of TMC207. Presented at: the 38th Union World Conference on Lung Health; Cape Town, South Africa. 8-12 November 2007; Poster PS-71358-71311.
141. Huitric E, Verhasselt P, Andries K, Hoffner SE. In vitro antimycobacterial spectrum of a diarylquinoline ATP-synthase inhibitor. Antimicrob Agents Chemother. 2007;51(11):4202-4.
142. The World Health Organization (WHO). 2013. The use of bedaquiline in the treatment of multidrug-resistant tuberculosis, Interim Policy Guidance. [online] Available from *http://apps.who.int/iris/bitstream/10665/84879/1/9789241505482_eng.pdf* [Accessed 07 February, 2016].
143. Matsumoto M, Hashizume H, Tomishige T, Kawasaki M, Tsubouchi H, Sasaki H, et al. OPC-67683, a nitro-dihydro-imidazooxazole derivative with promising action against tuberculosis in vitro and in mice. PLoS Med. 2006;3(11):e466.
144. Barry PJ, O'Connor TM. Novel agents in the management of Mycobacterium tuberculosis disease. Curr Med chem. 2007;14(18):2000-8.

145. Gler MT, Skripconoka V, Sanchez-Garavito E, Xiao H, Cabrera-Rivero JL, Vargas-Vasquez DE, et al. Delamanid for multidrug-resistant pulmonary tuberculosis. N Engl J Med. 2012;366(23):2151-60.
146. Diacon AH, Dawson R, Hanekom M, Narunsky K, Venter A, Hittel N, et al. Early bactericidal activity of delamanid (OPC-67683) in smear-positive pulmonary tuberculosis patients. Int J Tuberc Lung Dis. 2011;15(7):949-54.
147. Jindani A, Aber VR, Edwards EA, Mitchison DA. The early bactericidal activity of drugs in patients with pulmonary tuberculosis. Am Rev Respir Dis. 1980;121(6):939-49.
148. Martindale: The Complete Drug Reference. Co-trimoxazole. London, UK: Pharmaceutical Press; 2011.
149. Medscape. Bactrim, Bactrim DS (trimethoprim/sulfamethoxazole) dosing, indications, interactions, adverse effects, and more. [online] Available from *http://reference.medscape.com/drug/bactrim-trimethoprim-sulfamethoxazole-342543*. [Accessed April, 2016].
150. Forgacs P, Wengenack NL, Hall L, Zimmerman SK, Silverman ML, Roberts GD. Tuberculosis and trimethoprim-sulfamethoxazole. Antimicrob Agents Chemother. 2009;53(11):4789-93.
151. Chick J. Safety issues concerning the use of disulfiram in treating alcohol dependence. Drug Saf. 1999;20(5):427-35.
152. Macingwana L, Baker B, Ngwane AH, Harper C, Cotton MF, Hesseling A, et al. Sulfamethoxazole enhances the antimycobacterial activity of rifampicin. J Antimicrob Chemother. 2012;67(12): 2908-11.
153. Reeves DS, Wilkinson PJ. The pharmacokinetics of trimethoprim and trimethoprim/sulphonamide combinations, including penetration into body tissues. Infection. 1979;7(Suppl 4): S330-S41.
154. Patel RB, Welling PG. Clinical pharmacokinetics of co-trimoxazole (trimethoprim-sulphamethoxazole). Clin Pharmacokinet. 1980;5(5):405-23.
155. Smilack JD. Trimethoprim-sulfamethoxazole. Mayo Clin Proc. 1999;74(7):730-4.
156. Masters PA, O'Bryan TA, Zurlo J, Miller DQ, Joshi N. Trimethoprim-sulfamethoxazole revisited. Arch Intern Med. 2003;163(4):402-10.
157. Mori H, Kuroda Y, Imamura S, Toyoda A, Yoshida I, Kawakami M, et al. Hyponatremia and/or hyperkalemia in patients treated with the standard dose of trimethoprim-sulfamethoxazole. Intern Med. 2003;42(8):665-9.
158. Heimpel H, Raghavachar A. Hematological side effects of co-trimoxazole. Infection. 1987;15(Suppl 5):S248-S53.

40

Chapter

Historical and Nonpharmacological Management of Pulmonary Tuberculosis

KB Gupta

INTRODUCTION

Since ancient time, tuberculosis (TB) has taken a heavy toll of lives. The disease is known for centuries and there have been continuous attempts to find a cure that involves many types of measures such as physical, chemical and others. *The therapy for TB is directed to achieve five major purposes:*

1. To kill the bacilli by adopting specific chemotherapy.
2. To eliminate the diseased tissue by resectional surgery.
3. To assist the healing of lesions by collapse measures.
4. To improve general resistance of the body.
5. To improve quality of life by rehabilitation program.

HISTORY

Tuberculosis is known by different terms, including consumption, phthisis, scrofula, Pott's disease, white plague, Koch's disease, yakshma, consumption, "chaky oncay", each of which makes reference to the "drying" or "wasting" effect of the illness.[1-3]

Signs of the disease have also been found in the Egyptian mummies dated between 3000 BC and 2400 BC.[4] The first reference to TB in Asian civilization is perhaps found in the Hindu "Vedas", the oldest of them (Rigveda, 2000 BC) calls the disease "yakshma." The "Atharvaveda" calls it by another name: "Balasa". It is in the Atharvaveda that the first description of scrofula is given. The "Sushruta Samhita", written around 600 BC, recommends that the disease be treated with breast milk, various meats, alcohol and rest. The "Yajurveda" advises sufferers to move to higher altitudes. The "Manusmriti", written around 1500 BC states that sufferers of yakshma are impure and prohibit "Brahmans" from marrying any women that have a family history of the disease.

The first mention of TB in Chinese literature appears in a medical text written by emperor Shennong of China (2700 BC).·Yellow emperor, wrote "Huangdi Neijing", in which he describes "Xiao Bing" (weak consumptive disease), which is believed to be TB. Hippocrates (460–377 BC) described the characteristics, while Aristotle and Celsus also mentioned about the disease. Galen proposed a series of therapeutic treatments, including opium as a sleeping agent and painkiller, blood-letting and a diet of barley water, fish and fruit.[3] In the famous library of Leipzig there is a folio, which contains information that Jesus had suffered from this illness.

During the dark ages (400–1400 BC), all the knowledge of the disease was lost. With the spread of Christianity, monarchs were seen as religious figures with magical or curative powers. It was believed that "royal touch", the touch of the sovereign of England or France, could cure diseases due to the divine right of sovereigns,[5] King Henry IV of France usually performed the rite once a week. Scrofula became known as the "King's evil". Touching the king's feet for the cure of king's evil (as tuberculous was then known) was prevalent during the 11th centuries and 12th centuries in England and elsewhere. The infectious nature of the disease was described by Girolamo Fracastoro of Verona (1483–1553). Franciscus Sylvius of Leyden (1614–1672) first employed the term "tubercle" and stated that tubercles were seen in patients of consumptives.[5]

Seventeenth and Eighteenth Century

Franciscus Sylvius began differentiating between various forms of TB. He recognized that the skin ulcers caused by scrofula resembled tubercles seen in phthisis, thus, noted that "phthisis is the scrofula of the lung".[4] Thomas Willis concluded that all diseases of the chest must ultimately lead to consumption. Willis did not know the exact cause of the disease, but he blamed it on sugar or an acidity of the blood.[4] Benjamin Marten proposed in a new theory of consumption of the lungs that the cause of TB was some type of animacula: microscopic living beings that were able to survive in a new body. Robert Whytt gave the first clinical description of TB meningitis.[6]

Nineteenth Century

The disease began to represent spiritual purity and temporal wealth, leading many young, upper class women to purposefully pale their skin to achieve the consumptive appearance. Jean-Antoine Villemin demonstrated that the disease was indeed contagious, after conducting an experiment in which tuberculous matter from human cadavers was injected into laboratory rabbits, who then became infected.[3]

Robert Koch revealed for the first time on 24th March 1882, the causal agent of the disease-*Mycobacterium tuberculosis* or Koch's bacillus.[2,3,7] Rudolf Virchow (1821–1902), the founder of cellular pathology described the development of caseation in tuberculous tissue and believed that susceptibility to the disease was inherited and not the disease itself. In 1890, Koch developed tuberculin, a purified protein derivative of the bacteria.[8,9] It proved to be an ineffective means of immunization, but in 1908, Charles Mantoux found it was an effective intradermal test for diagnosing TB.[10]

Vaccine: The first genuine immunization against TB was developed from attenuated bovine-strain TB by Albert Calmette and Camille Guérin in 1906. It was called Bacillus Calmette-Guérin (BCG).[11] The BCG vaccine was first used on humans in 1921 in France, but it was not until after the World War II that BCG received widespread acceptance in the United States, Great Britain and Germany.

Treatment: As the century progressed, some surgical interventions, including the pneumothorax or plombage technique—collapsing an infected lung to "rest" and allow the lesions to heal—were used to treat TB. Giorgio Baglivi reported a general improvement in TB sufferers after they received sword wounds to the chest. F Ramage induced the first successful therapeutic pneumothorax.[6]

In 1944, Albert Schatz, Elizabeth Bugie and Selman Waksman isolated *Streptomyces griseus* or streptomycin (SM), the first antibiotic and the first bacterial agent effective against *M. tuberculosis.* This discovery is generally considered the beginning of the modern era of TB, although the true revolution began some years later in 1952, with the development of isoniazid, the first oral mycobactericidal drug. The advent of rifampin in the 1970s hastened recovery times and significantly reduced the number of TB cases until the 1980s.[6]

ANCIENT DRUGS IN THE TREATMENT OF TUBERCULOSIS

Before the discovery of conventional antituberculosis drugs, treatment of TB was mainly passive in nature. Many drugs, chemical or herbal, had been tried and used for the treatment of TB. Some of them are still in use while others have been abandoned due to their unacceptable benefit to risk ratios.

Drugs Used in the Past

Since ages, drugs like gold, arsenic, calcium, sulfur, plant extracts and animal products have been used in the hope of curing TB.

Gold compounds: Treatment of pulmonary TB with these compounds was introduced first by Robert Koch and later popularized by Danish physicians, in the mid-1920s, despite consistently negative experimental results, based on Paul Ehrlich's theories of antimicrobial drug effects. Although, found as an effective antituberculosis drug, its toxicity resulted in its discard.[12]

Arsenic: Initially introduced by Koch, Burrow found that potassium arsenite prevented the growth of tubercle bacilli in vitro. The results of Burrow were contradicted by Nürnberger who observed no specific action in TB, or on the tubercle bacilli, in vitro.[13]

Calcium: Peterson and Levinson have reported more deaths among tuberculous patients with low blood calcium. Those patients with a higher blood calcium evidenced a healed or healing lesion and, therefore, a good prognosis.[14]

Cod liver oil: Introduced as a treatment for pulmonary TB between the 1770s and the 1930s, cod liver oil was introduced into the British Pharmacopoeia in 1771. By the end of the 18th century, it was a prominent treatment in the Manchester infirmary. Cod liver oil entered medical practice in the United States in the 1840s, quickly gaining widespread use. After the discovery of the tubercle bacillus, some claimed that cod liver oil had specific action against the bacillus.[15]

Copper: Initially started by the Swiss physician Koechlin, based on a Chinese original, it was widely used in central Europe to treat a range of skin, neurological and infectious diseases, including TB. Copper treatment for TB continued until the 1940s and various physicians reported on their success in using copper preparations in intravenous injections.[16]

Antimony: Percy Moxey used intramuscular injections of colloidal antimony for the treatment of TB.[17]

Mercury: It acts as tonic and renders the blood bactericidal, producing an antitoxin, which has direct effect on the bacilli.[18]

Herbal Drugs

In the great Vedas, there has been mention of certain herbs having medicinal properties against *M. tuberculosis.* Herbal drugs are used in ayurvedic medicine, may have some role in the treatment of TB. Several herbal drugs as below, have been used in the past, but none has been shown to have a proven clinical value.

- *Ashwagandha*: Its extract contains at least 13 heterogeneous alkaloids, which are chemically identified as, pyridine, pepindinine, sonine and free amino acids.[19] These alkaloids show:
  - Anti-inflammatory and antipyretic effects
  - Inhibit growth of Gram-positive aerobic and mycobacterial organisms
  - Suppress granuloma formation

- Antitumor activity and immunomodulation
- Increase in T lymphocytes level in TB patients.

Licorice (glycyrrhiza glabra liquorice; family—papilionaceae/fabaceae): The activity guided fractionation of ethanolic extract from the roots of *glycyrrhiza* glabra and subsequent phytochemical analysis resulted in identifying glabridin as the active constituent and hispaglabridin B as inactive constituent against *M. tuberculosis*. The antimycobacterial activity of root ethanolic extract was observed at 500 g/mL against *M. tuberculosis* H37Ra and H37Rv strains through BACTEC assay. The maximal insufflation capacity (MIC) of test compounds was noted on the basis of growth index (GI) value. Further, the ethyl acetate fraction showed better activity at a concentration range of 100–250 g/mL.[20]

- *Allium sativum*: The inhibitory effect of garlic on *M. tuberculosis* has been mentioned in clinical reports for nearly 100 years. Delaha and Vincent studied the inhibitory effect of garlic extract on mycobacteria.[21] In an another study in patients of tubercular lymphadenitis, garlic extracts or compounds have shown a good potential as antitubercular(s) drug, if given as a supplement to antitubercular therapy (ATT).[22]
- *Asparagus racemosus*: Roots of *asparagus racemosus* (Shatavari) are widely used in Ayurveda as "Rasayana" for immunostimulation.[23]

Other Plant Extracts

In South Africa, antimicrobial properties of certain plant extracts, which were used by traditional healers for the treatment of TB like *Artemisia afra* Jacq. ex Willd, *Carpobrotus edulis L, Tulbaghia violacea Harv* were studied for activity against *B. cereus, E. coli, Klebseilla pneumoniae, S. aureus* and *Mycobacterium aurum* A+ strain using two-fold microdilution bioassay.[24]

Astragalus membranaceus is a herb used in traditional Chinese medicine to boost immunity.[25]

Plant extracts obtained from *Euphorbia cerebrosides* and *cetraria* usnic acid have inhibitory activities comparable to standard antituberculosis drugs. *Rhododendron, Melaleuca* and *Leptospermum* essential oils had minimal inhibitory concentration in a range of 0.25–0.025%. Most plant extracts had no toxic effect against human cells in vitro.[26]

Certain plant extracts like emblica officinalis and *Tinospora cordifolia* showed hepatoprotective properties against antituberculosis drug-induced liver injury.[27]

Homeopathic medicines used for the treatment of scrofula TB.[28] For example, calcarea carbonica, sulfur, baryta carbonica, silicea, graphite and mercurius.

Drugs used in Unani system[29] for the symptomatic treatment of

- *Fever*: Tukhm anisoon (*pimpinella anisum*) seeds, rRb-u-soos, persiawashan, barley husk cooked with crab, massage of sandal, camphor and rose water on chest.
- *Cough*: White opium seeds, gum, starch, Kateera and *Bambusa arundinacea.*
- *Hemoptysis*: Curd milk from which cream is removed and hot iron pieces are added to it and cooked.

SANATORIUM TREATMENT

Sanatorium is an institute in good climate. The sanatoria started in 18th century and continued in the 19th century till the development of the concept that domiciliary treatment is as effective as sanatorium treatment **(Table 1)**. *The essential features of sanatorium treatment are the following:*

- Close and skilled supervision in good surroundings
- Proper training of the individual in hygienic living, particularly in respect to breathing fresh air, taking adequate rest, feeding rationally and preventing infection.[30,31]

Role of Sunlight

Throughout history, the sun has been respected for its healing power. In ancient Greece, physicians employed symptom-specific techniques of solar therapy by placing patients in specially constructed healing temples in the sun city of Heliopolis. Early in the 20th century, prior to discovery of antibiotics, European physicians sent their TB patients to hospital in Swiss and Austrian Alps. Sunlight promotes good immune function and helps to fight infection, stimulates

Table 1 Evolution of sanatoria for treatment of tuberculosis

A-Global	
Year	*Name of sanatorium*
19th Century	
1863	Brehmerschen Heilanstalt für Lungenkranke in Gabersdorf (Sokolowski), Silesia
1882	Adirondack cottage sanatorium in Saranac lake, New York
20th Century	
1911	Burkeville, Virginia's Piedmont Sanatorium, United States of America; Waverly Hills Sanatorium, United States of America
1930	Paimio Sanatorium, Finland Heliantia Sanatorium in Valadares, Portugal
B-India	
Year	*Name of sanatorium*
1906	Missionary tuberculosis (TB) sanatorium, Tilonia, Ajmer
1908	Missionary TB sanatorium, Almora
1909	TB sanatorium, Dharampur, Shimla
1912	United mission tuberculosis sanatorium, Madanapalle
1917	TB dispensary, Bombay and Madras[32,33]

metabolism and relieves insomnia and depression. Sunlight is much like a nutrient on which the body depends for smooth functioning of its glandular and metabolic systems. It also acts as an important cofactor in the proper activity of vitamins in the body.[34]

Role of Rest and Exercise

Rest and properly graded exercise are important factors in the treatment of TB. When a patient recovers to full weight with no fever, he should have graded exercise to gradually adjust to considerable endurance. Deep breathing exercise should never be taken while the disease is active and considerably advanced. There is also a reported danger of tearing loose adhesions by such exercise.[35,36]

Nutrition

It is clear that TB affects nutritional status. Many patients with active TB experience severe weight loss and show signs of vitamin and mineral deficiencies. Patients with TB/human immunodeficiency virus (HIV) coinfection are even worse, nutritionally. However, the evidence for best practices for nutritional management is very limited.[37]

Collapse Therapy

The main role of collapse therapy is to provide rest to the diseased part of lung and to facilitate healing.[38]

Surgery

The earlier attempts in the 1880, of removing the affected portion of the lung had been unsuccessful and resection was given up being too dangerous a procedure.[39]

Tuberculin Therapy

It was advised by Robert Koch after his discovery in 1882.

Modern Chemotherapy

It had its beginning with the discovery of streptomycin by Waksman in 1944. Soon other drugs were discovered—para-amino salicylic acid (PAS) (1948) and isoniazid (INH) (1952) followed by rifampicin, pyrazinamide and other drugs. Standard chemotherapy with streptomycin (SM), INH and PAS became the right choice for the treatment of TB after the 1950. Studies conducted at TB research center (TRC), Madras (India) and other countries in 1956 had shown that domiciliary treatment with chemotherapy was as good as sanatorium treatment with chemotherapy.[40,41] Consequently, patients with pulmonary TB who were slightly active were allowed to exercise themselves in the open air.

Sanatorium versus Home Treatment for Pulmonary Tuberculosis

Pulmonary TB is recognized at the present time as the most curable of chronic diseases. The first essential component in the treatment is to control the mental and the emotional state of the patient, without which the physical reactions cannot be controlled. To carry out these essentials, one must first be able and have an opportunity to thoroughly study the patient and his disease processes, and be able to place the patient in an environment that will assist him to the fullest extent in adjusting his psychic reactions to the circumstances.[42]

The patient in a sanatorium profits by the examples and mistakes of other patients. Education and information acquired in such an atmosphere constitute the keystone to the discipline, which is so essential in the proper treatment of pulmonary TB. In the sanatorium, the patient has a much greater opportunity to be protected from the nervous and over-anxious members of his family and the disturbances, which occur in the ordinary routines of the home.

Finally, in the sanatorium the patient learns that flare ups in the course of pulmonary TB are more or less the rule, when these occur, his reaction is entirely different from that of the patient having a similar experience in a home environment.[43-45]

SURGERY

Historically, surgery has played a major role in the treatment of pulmonary TB, while the introduction of multidrug therapy in 1970s significantly reduced its role. However, the increased prevalence of multidrug-resistant (MDR) TB has again renewed the interest in surgery.

Historical Procedures

Cavernostomy Era

During the 18th century, large TB cavities in the lungs were opened through the thoracic wall (cavernostomy)/ Monaldi operation.[45] Others performed "open cavernostomy" in a staged manner, which invariably caused bronchopleurocutaneous fistula which would drain.

Collapse Therapy Era

The period between 19th centuries and 20th centuries, marked the era of bedrest and collapse therapy. Bedrest was introduced by Dettweitter in Germany and Turban in Switzerland around 1880.[46] Collapse therapy was used in 70% of sanatorium patients. The purpose of collapse therapy was relaxation of the diseased lung and a better chance for the scar tissue to contract.

Phrenic Nerve Paralysis

In the 1930s, this was the most common procedure of lung collapse. *It was supposed to help in different ways:*

- Rise of ipsilateral diaphragm reduces the distance between apex and base of lung thus relaxing the diseased portion
- Decreased excursion of diaphragm provides rest to lung
- Cavities at the base of lung responded favorably to this procedure.

Artificial Pneumothorax

The use began in the late 19th century and came into wide use between 1920 and 1940. A specially designed pneumothorax apparatus was used; if there were no intrapleural adhesions, the pneumothorax relaxed the lung effectively. For cases with intrapleural adhesions and intrapleural pneumonolysis was done.

In addition, artificial pneumothorax was found to be useful in achieving culture negativity in new cases with cavitary pulmonary TB and in retreatment cases.[47]

Pneumoperitoneum

For some time, pneumoperitoneum was used as collapse therapy by causing the elevation of diaphragm. The results of pneumoperitoneum alone were unpredictable. Combined procedure of pneumoperitoneum and phrenic nerve paralysis were often effective in the closure of a basal cavity.[48]

Extrapleural Pneumonolysis

In this procedure, a space was created between the apex of lung and the chest wall. This space was filled up with paraffin, which eventually became encapsulated with the fibrous tissue and remained in place permanently.[49]

Thoracoplasty

Alexander is considered to be the father of thoracoplasty in United States of America.[50] He perfected the technique of staged posterior lateral thoracoplasty with an operative mortality of less than 2% and cavity closure and sputum conversion in over 80% of cases.[50] In plombage thoracoplasty, material substances are used to maintain collapse (plombe), including paraffin, polythene sphere and sheets. Recently, a new modality of collapse therapy, which uses percutaneous tissue expanders (the perthese tissue expander) has been described.[51-59]

IMMUNOTHERAPY

Anti-TB drugs are not able to fully eradicate *M. tuberculosis* from all sites because of their relative inactivity against semidormant or persisting organisms, particularly those in lung granulomas. Several immunotherapies are being evaluated in human clinical trials as adjunctive immunotherapy together with chemotherapy having potential to:

- Improve success rates in treatment of MDR-TB and extensively drug-resistant-tuberculosis (XDR-TB)
- Shorter duration of treatment of drug susceptible TB
- Improve immunity
- Reduce the pathology in individuals cured by chemotherapy thereby preventing recurrence.

Immune Protection and Immunopathology

Protective immunity is comprised of bacteriostatic and bactericidal components. Although, a bacteriostatic response may transiently protect the host from an invasive pathogen, it does so at cost of creating dormancy, a source of recurrent infection, which is difficult to eradicate. Thus, the challenge for immunotherapy is to convert a predominantly bacteriostatic response into bactericidal response.

Immune protection results from phagocytosis and killing of mycobacteria by activated macrophages, this cellular response is regulated by antigen-specific T cells that produce IFN-γ, which together with TNF-α and interleukin-15 (IL-15) (referred as type I cellular response) are essential for macrophage activation and immune protection. Other immune mechanisms that lead to bactericidal activity are autophagy, apoptosis and killing by cytotoxic T lymphocytes.

These immunoprotective mechanisms are susceptible to downregulation by combination of Th2 cytokines and TGF-β. Thus, downregulation is dependent on IL-4 expression; IL-4 and TGF-β together downregulate cytotoxic T lymphocyte response. The aim of immunotherapy is to improve the immune response and to optimize the balance between Th1/Th2 immune response by downregulating Th2 response.

Immunotherapy Agents

Various immunotherapeutic agents **(Table 2)** have been used for adjunctive treatment.[60-72]

The role of some immunosuppressive agents, as well as of supplementary effect or cytokines has been also reported, but largely limited to experimental designs for the present.[73-83]

Several other agents that have been tried in the past include the following:

- *Pentoxifylline*:[84] It acts by competitive nonselective phosphodiesterase inhibition, which raises intracellular CAMP, inhibits TNF-α and leukotriene synthesis and reduces inflammation and innate immunity. Combination of pentoxifylline and dexamethasone, when used to treat *M. avium* infected macrophage from normal and HIV-infected person in vitro showed decrease in TNF-α by 48%.[84]
- *Imiquimod*: It is an oral inducer of IFN and other cytokines. It is a low molecular weight compound originally described as potent-inducer of IFN and other cytokines like TNF and IL-12 when given orally to mice and humans.

Table 2 Immunoregulatory approaches for the treatment of tuberculosis (TB)

Agent	*Mechanism of action*	*Supportive studies*	*Results*
For which GMP manufacturing capacity exists			
• High dose IVIg[60,61]	Anti-inflammatory action	Animal experiments	Marked therapeutic effect and excellent safety
• HE 2000 (16 α Bromoepi-and roster one)[62]	Modified form of DHEA that cannot go into sex steroid pathway	Animal experiments	Well-tolerated and safe and reduced the incidence of TB and significant decrease in viral load in HIV patient
• Multidose heat killed (*M. vaccae*)[63-65]	Induce regulatory "T" cells that inhibit Th2 response, a Th1 response that activates CTL that kill *M. tuberculosis* infected macrophages	Chinese Dardar study	Effective as adjective therapy in MDR TB enhanced clearance of sputum and normalization of serum IL-4 and TNF-α Decrease in TB
• Neutralizing antibodies to IL-4 (Pascolizumab)[66]	It reduces IL-4 that causes a secondary decrease in TGF-β	Animal experiments	Have a therapeutic effect and safe
For which GMP manufacturing capacity can be established			
• DNA vaccine (HSP65)[67,68]	Enhance cytotoxic "T" cell while inhibiting IL-4 response, synergy with antibacterials with moxifloxacin	Animal experiment. Development of DNA vaccine, including three other antigens Ag 85B MPT-64 MPT-63, used together with antibacterial	Downregulation of Th2 response. Significant reduction in CFU
Others			
• Dzherelo[69]	Plant extract widely used in Ukraine	Need for definite GCP studies	
• SCV-07 SciClone (r-glutamyltryptophan)[70]	Immunostimulatory peptide with unknown mechanism of action	Small human TB study	Safe and use as an adjunct in MDR-TB, XDR-TB and in HIV-TB
• RUTI—a vaccine made of detoxified fragmented *M. tuberculosis* delivered in liposome[71,72]	Trigger a strong Th1 and Th2 immunity against 13 known *M. tuberculosis* antigens. It enhances the CD8 and IFN-γ	Animal experiment	In latent TB infection. It accelerates bacillary clearance.

Abbreviations: IVIG, intravenous immunoglobulin; DHEA, dehydroepiandrostenedione; TB, tuberculosis; HIV, human immunodeficiency virus; MDR-TB, multidrug-resistant tuberculosis; XDR-TB, extensively drug-resistant

- *Transfer factor*:[85] Transfer factor was first reported in 1949 by Lawrence and named it so because it was the factor that transferred TB immunity from a person who had an active immunity to TB to a naïve individual.[85] Later, it was discovered that this process is naturally accomplished between mammalian mothers and their newborns through mother's colostrums.

Transfer factor products can be both dietary supplements and drugs depending on how they are prepared and marketed. Transfer factor preparations consist of three identifiable fractions.

- *Inducer fraction*: It triggers a general state of readiness in the immune system.
- *Antigen-specific fraction*: Is an array of critical tags used by immune system to identify the host of enemy microbes.
- *Suppressor fraction*: It keeps the immune system from focusing all its strength on a defeated infection while ignoring new microbial threat. It also controls allergic reaction and blocks autoimmune disorder.

Originally, transfer factors were given through infection, later studies showed that transfer factor was equally effective orally.

- *Levamisole*: Mechanism of action for its immuno-stimulating effects is not well understood. It is believed that it restores cell-mediated immune function in peripheral T lymphocytes and stimulates phagocytosis by monocytes. The drug appears to restore depressed immune function rather than to stimulate response to above normal levels. Further, studies are required for its effectiveness as immunomodulator in TB treatment.

Thus, immunotherapies have the potential to improve the outcome in all TB patients, including those with MDR-TB and XDR-TB. Immunotherapy for TB may shorten TB treatment and improve the immunity of individuals cured by chemotherapy, potentially preventing recurrence. Currently, none of the available agents have proof of efficacy for use. Further, development and evaluation of existing immunotherapy agents is required to find the effective agent.

TUBERCULOSIS AND NUTRITION

INTRODUCTION

Nutrition plays an important role in etiology, complications and therapy of TB. Although, many are infected with tubercle bacilli, yet all do not develop the disease, TB recruits many of its candidates from amongst the undernourished, the under-fed or residents of the centers of congestion of urban communities. "The death rates from TB in England rises and falls with the price of bread" was wisely said by Stewart. Young people who are both underweight and undernourished are choice of "candidates" for active TB.[86-89]

Tuberculosis causes malnutrition, which further weakens immunity, thereby increasing the likelihood of active disease in latent TB. Wasting is associated with increased mortality in TB patients.[90] Reduced micronutrient intake, especially of vitamin B and minerals, such as vitamins A, E and C, zinc and selenium, has been associated with impaired immune responses.[91-93]

MALNUTRITION AND IMMUNITY

It is well established that nutritional deficiency is associated with impaired immune functions.[94] Malnutrition limits cell-mediated immunity and increases susceptibility to infection, while infection can lead to nutritional stress and weight loss, thereby weakening the immune function and nutritional status.[95]

Malnutrition and Tuberculosis

Malnutrition enhances the development of active TB, which makes malnutrition worse.[96] It has been suggested that generalized malnutrition by reducing the expression of gamma interferon, tumor necrosis factor alpha and other mycobactericidal substances may selectively compromise portions of the cell-mediated response that are important for containing and restricting TB.[97] During the wasting process, there is usually a loss of both fat and lean muscle tissue with the loss persisting for several months after the initiation of anti-TB therapy.[98,99]

During active TB, catabolic processes that cause wasting usually begin before the patient is diagnosed.[100] Utilization of amino acids and protein synthesis may be inhibited due to the presence of proinflammatory cytokines.[101,102] Cell-mediated immunity is the most important defense against TB. Malnourished individual is more likely to become infected with TB and latent infection is more likely to become active TB when the cell-mediated immune response is impaired in malnutrition.[103] In a larger study conducted in Norway, the incidence of smear-positive and smear-negative TB declined significantly with increasing body mass index (BMI) in all age groups.[104]

Nutritional Status Changes during Tuberculosis Treatment

During drug treatment of active TB, nutritional status usually improves without supplementary nutrition. This happens due to a variety of reasons, including the improved appetite and food intake, reduced energy nutrient demands and improved metabolic efficiency. Most improvements, however, are limited to increase in fat mass.[101,105,106] There are studies to show that the nutritional status may have an effect on relapse of active TB. So, the maintenance of good nutritional status in TB patients all though the life, is important.

Low concentration of serum albumin less than 35 g/L is an indicator of protein status at the time of TB diagnosis.[107] The concentration of micronutrients may have a role in host defense against TB.[92,93,95,104,108,109] In the era before drug management of active TB, administering cod liver oil rich in vitamins A and D was a common therapy to improve the host defense.[110]

Antioxidants

Antioxidants neutralize the free radicals. TB may induce oxidative substances, which in turn, can promote tissue injury and inflammation. Reactive oxygen species (ROS) are highly toxic to lipids, fat cells causing peroxidation, resulting in damage to cell membranes and are also associated with the pathogenesis of lung fibrosis and dysfunction in pulmonary TB.[95,104,109,110]

Vitamin E: It protects cell membranes against lipid peroxidation and oxidative stress. Zinc is essential for deoxyribonucleic (DNA) synthesis and cell differentiation. Zinc deficiency is associated with recurrent infection, decreased phagocytosis, decreased β and T lymphocytes production and depressed macrophage activity. Selenium is an essential part of antioxidative enzymes, such as glutathione peroxidase, which protects cells from oxidative damage.[108-111]

Studies of Micronutrient Status and Tuberculosis

Vitamin A

Because of the acute phase response, serum retinal levels are generally lower in patients with active TB, particularly those who are TB/HIV coinfected and tend to improve with anti-TB therapy.[112]

Ascorbic Acid (Vitamin C)

Vitamin C, together with vitamin E and glutathione, is important for pulmonary antioxidant defense.[92,113] The levels of serum ascorbic acid in TB patients with history of smoking were significantly lower than in the controls.[92]

Pyridoxine (Vitamin B_6)

Isoniazid inhibits the phosphorylation of pyridoxine, which results in an increased excretion of vitamin B_6.[114,115]

Vitamin D

Susceptibility to TB and the severity of active TB may be increased by vitamin D deficiency.[96,97,116] It was hypothesized that immigrants from tropical countries, where latent TB is common, had a marked decrease in their serum vitamin D levels when they lived in cold and cloudy England, with considerably less opportunity for exposure to sunshine. Poverty was not considered the factor since these immigrants communities were generally prosperous.[117]

Effect of Micronutrient Supplementation on Tuberculosis Outcomes

Vitamin A and zinc: The supplementation of vitamin A and zinc improves the effectiveness of the anti-TB treatment in the first 2 months of the therapy, with less improvement seen between 2 months and 6 months of treatment. The major benefit is at the community level because the patient becomes less infectious sooner, with lesser opportunity to infect others.[118]

Anemia is common in patients with pulmonary TB, more so among TB/HIV coinfected patients.[119] However, iron loading may enhance the growth of *M. tuberculosis* by impairing macrophage suppression of invading microorganisms. Elevated dietary iron may increase the risk of activating TB disease. In mild to moderately anemic TB patients, iron supplementation accelerated the normal hematopoiesis.[120]

Malnutrition and Tuberculosis/Human Immunodeficiency Virus Coinfection in Adults

Coinfection may lead to poor appetite with decreased nutrient intake, which may interact with the altered metabolism associated with both infections as part of the immune and inflammatory responses.[94,119] The combination of TB/HIV coinfection and malnutrition has been termed "triple trouble".[120]

Nutritional Support within Tuberculosis Programs

Food assistance is a potentially influential targeted means for increasing adherence to TB treatment, reducing the costs to patients of staying in treatment and improving the nutritional status. Food assistance may influence early case detection and promote full course of the treatment. Both of these are important to decrease TB transmission.[121,122]

World Food Program

The goal of the World Food Program (WFP) is to improve nutrition, quality of life and self-help of individual and communities.[94]

C-SAFE: The Consortium for the Southern Africa Food Security Emergency (C-SAFE) provides food assistance to patients with HIV/acquired immunodeficiency syndrome (AIDS), including those coinfected with TB.[114]

Dietary Management in Tuberculosis Patients

A TB patient requires more food for two reasons: (1) first, he has fever, which causes him to burn up his energy faster than in health. (2) second, he has a destructive process going on in his body, which he must seek to overcome by supplying ample repair material in the form of food.[86] A highly publicized diet is the Hermannsdörfer-Sauerbruch diet for TB given at the ratio of 1.15 g protein, 2.7 g fat, 4 g carbohydrates.[86] Most TB patients have poor appetite, therefore, a meal should be made simple, easily digestible and tempting to encourage the patient to eat. All meals should have cereal-pulse combination with some amount of animal proteins. Some typical examples are: "Khichri" with curd; sweet dalia with milk; "paushtik chapatis" with curd and cheap sources of vitamin C, such as guava, amla and sprouted pulses should be given.[88]

A day's simple diet plan for TB patients **(Tables 3 and 4)** should be able to provide energy equal to 2,787 kcal; protein equal to 75–90 g; vitamin A equal to 600 mg retinal and calcium equal to 400 mg.

REHABILITATION IN TUBERCULOSIS

For many persons with TB, microbiological cure is just the beginning, not the end of their illness. Post-tuberculosis pulmonary impairment has emerged as a distinct clinical entity, which is almost indistinguishable from the other forms.[122,123] Cavitation, extensive fibrosis, bulla formation and bronchiectasis have been implicated in the genesis of chronic obstructive pulmonary disease (COPD) caused by the destroyed lung.[124-126] A definite association between the type of healed lesions present and degree of impairment exists.[127] Pathological changes, such as "emphysematous change" on the radiograph could be considered as an important cause of obstructive ventilatory impairment. Effective chemotherapy decreases the likelihood of development of obstructive lung diseases.[128]

Lung function, such as forced vital capacity (FVC) and postbronchodilator FEV1 of post-tuberculosis patients, was lower compared to those of COPD.[129] Thus, pulmonary impairment associated with obstructive airway disease is

Table 3 Food plan for tuberculosis patients in India

Meal	Menu	Amount
Early morning	Tea	1 cup
Breakfast	"Paushtik chapatis" (besan, spinach, cabbage, onion, wheat, flour and oil) Curd Tea	2 95 g 1 cup
Mid-morning	Sprouted "moong chat" Tea	1 bowl 1 cup
Lunch	Scrambled egg Spinach and potato, vegetable "Chapatis" Peanut "chikki" Amla	1 1 bowl 2–3 1
Evening tea	Tea	1 cup
Dinner	"Upma" (with vegetable) "Sambar" (with brinjal and bottle gourd) Carrot "raita" Rice/"chapatis" cooked/ Guava	1 bowl 1 bowl 1.5 bowl 2–3 1 1.

recognized as a common complication of advanced TB. There is a need of rehabilitation in patient of TB for the restoration of the disabled to maximum physical, mental, social, economic and vocational capacity of which they are capable.

Situation Needing Rehabilitation of Tuberculosis Patients

- Chronically ill and drug failure patients, who continue to excrete TB bacilli in spite of treatment
- Those patients, who have no source of steady income
- Development of complication such as emphysema, bronchiectasis or whose lung functions following surgical intervention is reduced to very low.

Tuberculosis continues to afflict the low-income groups. By the time they seek diagnosis and treatment, the disease is already in the advanced stage. Very often, they become untreatable and secrete drug-resistant bacilli. Some of them have little possibility of returning to work. Joint family system is fast disintegrating in India, but longevity is increasing. People have to rely on their own resources. Other members of the family are reluctant to bear the burden of the incapacitated person. There is thus, need for organized

Table 4 Food choices for inclusion in a meal

Foods high in vitamin B_6 (pyridoxine)	*Foods high in iron*
• Liver, chicken, meats and fish	• Liver and kidney
• Dried fruit (raisins, dates and figs)	• Cream of wheat, whole grain cereals
• Hazelnuts, walnuts and peanuts	• Meats, veal and ham
• Brussels sprouts, cauliflower, peas and broccoli	• Dried peas, beans and lentils
• Chick peas and soybeans	• Prune juice, prunes, dates and dark green leafy vegetables
• Wheat germ, whole grain cereals and oatmeal	
• Bananas, cantaloupe and grapes body best when eaten with foods	*Tip*: Iron is taken up by the high in vitamin C
Foods high in vitamin A	*High protein foods*
• Broccoli, carrots, squash and sweet potatoes	• Meats, lamb, veal and ham
• Spinach and other dark green leafy vegetables	• Milk, yogurt and cheese
• Liver, dairy products and eggs	• Poultry and fish
• Cantaloupe and apricots	• Dried peas, beans and lentils
	• Eggs
Tip: Add skim milk powder to soups, milk and casseroles	
Foods high in vitamin C	*Foods high in calcium*
• Citrus fruit and juice	• Milk, yogurt and cheese
• Tomato and baked potatoes	• Soybeans and tofu
• Broccoli, sweet peppers and kale	• Broccoli and kale
• Cantaloupe, strawberries, cabbage and cauliflower	• Sardines and salmon with bones
	• Baked beans (canned).
Tip: Steam or cook vegetables in a small amount of water just until tender-crisp, will help to get the most amount of vitamin C from the vegetables	

rehabilitation in these situations. Settlements and colonies for such handicapped people were established in the past. Papworth and Preston Hall in the United Kingdom, a township in Saranac lake round the famous trudeau sanatorium in the United States of America and Sheltered work centers like altro shops in New York are some examples.

Rehabilitation is a field in which the TB association of India, other voluntary organizations and social service agencies can play an important role with the help of state governments and the Government of India.

REFERENCES

1. Flick LF. Development of our knowledge of tuberculosis. Philadelphia: Wickersham; 1925.
2. Webb GB. Tuberculosis. New York: Hoeber; 1936.
3. Rubin SA. Tuberculosis. Captain of all these men of death. Radiol Clin North Am. 1995;33(4):619-39.
4. Keers RY. Pulmonary tuberculosis. A journey down the centuries. London: Bailliere Tindall; 1978.
5. Evans CC. Historical background. In: Davies PDO (Ed). Clinical Tuberculosis. London: Chapman and Hall Medical; 1994.
6. University of Medicine and Dentistry of New Jersey. Brief history of tuberculosis. [online] Available from *http://www.umdnj.edu/ntbcweb/history.htm*. [Accessed February, 2016].
7. Rao KN. Textbook of tuberculosis, 2nd edition. 1981. pp. 4-5.
8. Waksman SA. The conquest of tuberculosis. Berkley and Los Angeles: University of California Press; 1964. p. 217.
9. Daniel TM. Robert Koch and the pathogenesis of tuberculosis. Int J Tuberc Lung Dis. 2005;9(11):1181-2.
10. Mantoux C. L'intradermo-reaction a la Tuberculin et son interpretation Clinique. Presse Med. 1910;18:10-3.
11. Calmette A. Tubercle bacillus infection and tuberculosis in man and animal (translated by Soper WB, Smith GB) Baltimore: Williams and Wilkins; 1923.
12. Benedek TG. The history of gold therapy for tuberculosis. J Hist Med Allied Sci. 2004;59(1):50-89.
13. Aaron Arki, HJ Corper. The tuberculocidal action of arsenic compounds and their distribution in the tuberculous organism. The Journal of Infectious Diseases. 1916;18(4):335-48.
14. Goldberg B. The calcium therapy in tuberculosis. Chest. 1936;2:18-20.
15. Grad R. Cod and the consumptive: a brief history of cod-liver oil in the treatment of pulmonary tuberculosis. Pharm Hist. 2004;46(3):106-20.
16. Scientia Press. Medicinal effects of copper bracelets. [online] Available from *(http://www.scientiapress.com/findings/bracelets.htm)*. [Accessed August, 2010].
17. Moxey P. Treatment of tuberculosis: a note on the effect of colloidal antimony. Br Med J. 1927;1(3451):374-5.
18. GG Moseley. Mercury in the treatment of treatment of tuberculosis. Cal State J Med. 1909;7(9):338-40.
19. Chatterjee AM. Role of Ashwagandha in the treatment of difficult tuberculosis. Ind J Tub. 2000;47:171.
20. Gupta VK, Fatima A, Faridi U, Negi AS, Shanker K, Kumar JK, et al. Antimicrobial potential of glycyrrhiza glabra roots. J Ethnopharmacol. 2008;116(2):377-80.
21. Delaha EC, Garagusi VF. Inhibition of mycobacteria by garlic extract (Allium sativum). Antimicrob Agents Chemother. 1985;27(4):485-6.
22. Gupta RL, Jain S, Talwar V, Gupta HC, Murthy PS. Antitubercular activity of garlic (allium sativum) extract on combination with conventional antitubercular drugs in tubercular lymphadenitis. Indian J Clin Biochem. 1999;14(1):12-8.
23. Gautam M, Saha S, Bani S, Kaul A, Mishra S, Patil D, et al. Immunomodulatory activity of Asparagus racemosus on systemic Th1/Th2 immunity: implications for immunoadjuvant potential. J Ethnopharmacol. 2009;121(2):241-7.
24. Buwa LV, Afolayan AJ. Antimicrobial activity of some medicinal plants used for the treatment of tuberculosis in Eastern Cape province, South Africa. African Journal of Biotechnology. 2009;8(23):6683-7.
25. Xu HD, You CG, Zhang RL, Gao P, Wang ZR. Effects of astragalus polysaccharides and astragalosides on the phagocytosis of *Mycobacterium tuberculosis* by macrophages. J Int Med Res. 2007;35(1):84-90.
26. Banfi E, Scialino G, Cateni F. Plants extracts as new antituberculous agents, evaluated by MRA. 16th European congress of clinical microbiology and infectious diseases. France: NICE; 2006. pp. 1-4.
27. Tasduq SA, Kaisar P, Gupta DK, Kapahi BK, Maheshwari HS, Jyotsna S, et al. Protective effect of 50% hydroalcoholic fruit extract of Emblica officinalis against anti-tuberculosis drugs induced liver toxicity. Phytother Res. 2005;19(3):193-7.
28. *http://health.hpathy.com/scofula-swollen-glands.asp.*
29. Jamil S, Jabeen A, Ahmad S. Pulmonary tuberculosis and its management in classical unani literature. Indian J Tradl Knowl 2005;4(2):143-9.
30. Pearson SV. The role of the sanatorium in the treatment of pulmonary tuberculosis. Postgrad Med J. 1928;3:193-7.
31. Rao KN. Textbook of Tuberculosis, 2nd edition. New York: Asia Book Corporation; 1981.
32. Davis AL. History of the sanatorium movement. In: Rom WN, Garay SM (Eds). Tuberculosis. Boston: Little Brown; 1996. pp. 35-54.
33. Ayrazian LF. History of tuberculosis. In: Reichman LB, Hershfield ES (Eds). Tuberculosis: a comprehensive international approach. New York: Marcel Dekker; 1993. p. 1.
34. Warren P. The evolution of the Sanatorium: the first half century, 1854-1904. Can Bull Med Hist. 2006;23(2):457-76.
35. Schaaf HS, Zumla A. Tuberculosis: a comprehensive clinical reference. London, UK: Saunders Elsevier; 2009.
36. Rom WN, Garay SM. Tuberculosis, 2nd edition. Philadelphia, PA: Lippincott Williams & Wilkins; 2003.
37. Styblo K. Selected Papers. 24th Volume. Epidemiology of tuberculosis association; 1991.
38. Carson J. Essays. Physiological and Practical. Liverpool: BF Wright; 1822.
39. Schlossberg D. Tuberculosis and Nontuberculous mycobacterial infections, 4th edition. 1987. pp. 131-6.
40. Satya Sri. Text book of pulmonary and extrapulmonary tuberculosis. 6th edition. 2009.
41. Tuberculosis Chemotherapy Centre Madras. A concurrent comparison of home and sanatorium treatment of pulmonary tuberculosis in South India. Bull World Health Organ. 1959;21:51-144.
42. Hayes EW. Sanatorium versus home treatment for pulmonary tuberculosis. Chest. 1935;1:18-9.
43. Bobrowitz ID. Sanatorium treatment of tuberculosis. Chest. 1940;6:278-80.
44. Monaldi V. Tentatini di aspirazione endocavit area nelle canverne tubercolari del polmone. Lotta Tuberc. 1938;9:910.

45. Pratt JH. The evolution of rest treatment of pulmonary tuberculosis. Ann Rev Tuberc. 1944;50:185-201.
46. Motus IY, Skorniakov SN, Sokolov VA, Egorov EA, Kildyusheva EI, Savel'ev AV, et al. Reviving an old idea: can artificial pneumothorax play a role in modern tuberculosis? Int J Tuberc Lung Dis. 2006;10(5):571-7.
47. Kumar A, Dilip D, Chandra A. Surgery for pleuropulmonary Tuberculosis. In: SK Sharma (Ed). Tuberculosis. 2009;55:798.
48. Steele JD. The surgical treatment of pulmonary tuberculosis. Ann Thorac Surg. 1968;6(5):484-502.
49. Alexander J. The collapse therapy of pulmonary tuberculosis. Springfield: Charles C Thomas; 1937.
50. Bertin F, Labrousse L, Gazaille V, Vincent F, Guerlin A, Laskar M. New modality of collapse therapy for pulmonary tuberculosis sequel; tissue expander. Ann Thorac Surg. 2007;84(3):1023-5.
51. Yim AP. The role of video-assisted thoracoscopic surgery in the management of pulmonary tuberculosis. Chest. 1996;110(3):829-32.
52. Kerti CA, Miron I, Cozma GV, Burlacu ON, Tunea CP, Voiculescu VT. The role of sugery in the management of pleuropulmonary tuberculosis - seven years' experience at a single institution. Interact Cardiovasc Thorac Surg. 2009;8(3):334-7.
53. Floyd RD, Hollister WF, Sealy WC. Complications in 430 consecutive pulmonary resections for tuberculosis. Surg Gynecol Obstet. 1959;109:467-72.
54. Pairolero PC, Trastek VF. Surgical management of chronic empyema: the role of thoracoplasty. Ann Thorac Surg. 1990;50(5):689-90.
55. Mani S, Mayekar R, Ramanavare R, Maniar D, Matthews Joseph J, Doshi A. Control of tubercular haemoptysis by bronchial artery embolization. Trop Doct. 1997;27(3):149-50.
56. Grebitekin C, Bayram AS, Akin S. Complex pulmonary aspergilloma treated with single stage cavernostomy and myoplasty. Eur J Cardiothorac Surg. 2005;27(5):737-40.
57. Faure E, Souilamas R, Riquet M, Chehab A, Le Pimpec-Barthes F, Manac'h D, et al. Cold abscess of the chest wall: a surgical entity? Ann Thorac Surg. 1998;66(4):1174-8.
58. Freixinet J, Varela A, Lopez Rivero L, Caminero JA, Rodríguez de Castro F, Serrano A. Surgical treatment of childhood mediastinal tuberculous lymphadenitis. Ann Thorac Surg. 1995;59(3):644-6.
59. Anthony RM, Nimmerjohn F, Ashline DJ, Reinhold VN, Paulson JC, Ravetch JV. Recapitulation of IVIG anti-inflammatory activity with a recombinant IgG Fc. Science. 2008;320(5874): 373-6.
60. Roy E, Stavropoulos E, Brennan J, Coade S, Grigorieva E, Walker B, et al. Therapeutic efficacy of high-dose intravenous immunoglobin in *Mycobacterium tuberculosis* infection in mice. Infect Immun. 2005;73(9):6101-9.
61. Stickney DR, Noveljic Z, Garsd A, Destiche DA, Frincke JM. Safety and activity of the immune modulator HE 2000 on the incidence of tuberculosis and other opportunistic infections in AIDS patients. Antimicrobial Agents Chemother. 2007;51(7):2639-41.
62. Dlugovitzky D, Fiorenza CT, Farroni M, Bogue C, Stanford C, Stanford J. Immunological consequences of three doses of heat-killed *Mycobacterium vaccae* in the immunotherapy of tuberculosis. Respir Med. 2006;100(6):1079-87.
63. Fan MM, Liu KW, Chen X, Wang X, Zhang ZZ, Li BH, et al. Adjuvant effect of *Mycobacterium vaccae* on the treatment of recurrent treated pulmonary tuberculosis; a meta-analysis. Chinese J Evidence Based Med. 2007;7(6):449-55.
64. Von Reyn CF, Arbeit RD, Mtri L. The Dar Dar prime-boost TB vaccine trial in HIV infection final results. Int J Tuber Lung Dis. 2008;12(11 suppl 2):s318-4.
65. Zuany-Amorin C, Sawicka E, Manlius C, Le Moine A, Brunet LR, Kemeny DM, et al. Suppression of airway eosinophilia by killed *Mycobacterium vaccae*-induced allergen-specific regulatory teels. Nat Med. 2002;8(6):625-9.
66. Lowrie DB, Tascon RE, Bonato VL, Lima VM, Faccioli LH, Stavropoulos E, et al. Therapy of tuberculosis in mice by DNA vaccination. Nature. 1999;400(6741):269-71.
67. Yu DH, Hu XD, Cai H. Efficient tuberculosis treatment in nice using chemotherapy and immunotherapy with the combined DNA vaccine encoding Ag85B, MPT-64 and MPT-83. Gene Ther. 2008;15(9):652-9.
68. Nikolaeva LG, Maystat TV, Pylypchuk VS, Volyanskii YL, Frolov VM, Kutsyna GA. Cytokine profiles of HIV patients with pulmonary tuberculosis resulting from adjunct immunotherapy with herbal phytoconcentrates Dzherelo and Anemia. Cytokine. 2008;44(3):392-6.
69. Prihoda ND, Arjanona OV, Yurchenko LV, Sokolenko NI, Frolov VM, Tarakanovskaya MG, et al. Adjunct immunotherapy of tuberculosis in drug resistant TB and TB/HIV coinfected patients. Int J Biomed Pharmacent Sci. 2008;2:59-64.
70. Cardona PJ, Amat I, Gordillo S, Arcos V, Guirado E, Díaz J, et al. Immunotherapy with fragmented *Mycobacterium tuberculosis* cells increases the effectiveness of chemotherapy against a chronical infection in murine model of tuberculosis. Vaccine. 2005;23(11):1393-8.
71. Cardona PJ. RUTI: a new chance to shorten the treatment of latent tuberculosis infection. Tuberculosis (Edinb). 2006;86(3-4):273-89.
72. Gottlieb AB, Strober B, Krueger JG, Rohane P, Zeldis JB, Hu CC, et al. An open-lable, single-arm pilot study in patients with severe plaque-type psoriasis treated with an oral anti-inflammatory agent, apremilast. Curr Med Res Opin. 2008;24(5):1529-38.
73. Kalamidas SA, Kuehnel MP, Peyron P, Rybin V, Rauch S, Kotoulas OB, et al. cAMP synthesis and degradation by phagosomes regulation actin assembly and fusion events: consequences for mycobacteria. J Cell Sci. 2006;119(Pt 17):3686-94.
74. Wallis RS, Kyambadde P, Johnson JL, Horter L, Kittle R, Pohle M, et al. A study of the safety, immunology, virology, and microbiology of adjunctive etanercept in HIV-1-associated tuberculosis. AIDS. 2004;18(2):257-64.
75. Mayanja-kizza H, Jones Lopez E, Okevera A, Wallis RS, Ellner JJ, Mugerwa RD, et al. Immunoadjuvant prednisolone therapy for HIV-associated tuberculosis: a phase 2 clinical trial in Uganda. J Infect Dis. 2005;191(6):856-65.
76. Raju B, Hashino Y, Kuwabara K, Belitskaya I, Prabhakar S, Canova A, et al. Aerosalized gamma interferon (IFN-gamma) induces expression of the genes encoding the IFN-gamma inducible 10-kilodalton protein but not inducible nitric oxide synthase in the lung during tuberculosis. Infect Immun. 2004;72(3):1275-83.
77. Johnson BJ, Bekker LG, Rickman R, Brown S, Lesser M, Ress S, et al. rhuIL-2 adjunctive therapy in multidrug resistant tuberculosis: a comparison of two treatment regimens and placebo. Tuber Lung Dis. 1997;78(3-4):195-203.
78. Johnson JL, Ssekasanvu E, Okwera A, Mayanja H, Hirsch CS, Nakibali JG, et al. Randomized trial of adjunctive interleukin-2 in adults with pulmonary tuberculosis. Am J Respir Crit Care Med. 2003;168(2):185-91.

79. Pedral-Sampair DB, Netto EM, Brites C, Bandeira AC, Guerra C, Barberin MG, et al. Use of Rhee-GM-CSF in pulmonary tuberculosis patients: results of a randomized clinical trial. Braz J Infect Dis. 2003;7(4):245-52.
80. Zhang M, Gong J, Iyer DV, Jones BE, Modlin RL, Barnes PF. T cell cytokine responses in persons with tuberculosis and human immunodeficiency virus infection. J Clin Invest. 1994;94(6):2435-42.
81. Fenton MJ, Vermeulen MW, Kim S, Burdick M, Strieter RM, Kornfeld H. Induction of gamma interferon production in human alveolar macrophages by *Mycobacterium tuberculosis*. Infect Immun. 1997;65(12):5149-56.
82. Hernandez-Pando R, Aguitar D, Garcia Herandez ML, Orozco H, Rook G. Pulmonary tuberculosis in BALB/c mice with non-fuctional IL-4 genes; changes in inflammatory effects of TNF-and in the regulation of fibrosis. Eur J Immunol. 2004;34(1):174-83.
83. Orellana C. Immune system stimulator shows promise against tuberculosis. Lancet Infect Dis. 2002;2(12):711.
84. Mohan VP, Scanga CA, Yu k, Scott HM, Tanaka KE, Tsang E, et al. Effects of tumor necrosis factor alpha on host immune response in chronic persistent tuberculosis: possible role for limiting pathology. Infect Immun. 2001;69(3):1847-55.
85. Lawrence HS, Borkowsky W. A new basis for immunoregulatory activities of transfer factor. Cell Immunol. 1983;82(1):102-16.
86. Gauss H. Nutrition and tuberculosis. Chest. 1936;2:20-4.
87. Karyadi E, Schultink W, Nelwan RH, Gross R, Amin Z, Dolmans WM, et al. Poor micronutrient status of active pulmonary tuberculosis patients in Indonesia. J Nutr. 2000;130(12):2953-8.
88. Sanyal MC. Nutritional factors in the prevention of tuberculosis as a mass disease. Ind J Tub. 1958;5(2):53-7.
89. Sirsi M. Studies on nutrition in experimental tuberculosis. Ind J Tub. 2:47-52.
90. Macallan DC. Malnutrition in tuberculosis. Diagn Microbiol Infect Dis. 1999;34(2):153-7.
91. WHO. Global tuberculosis control: surveillance, planning, financing: WHO Report. 2005. Geneva: World Health Organization; 2005.
92. Bakaev VV, Duntau AP. Ascorbic acid in blood serum of patients with pulmonary tuberculosis and pneumonia. Int J Tuberc Lung Dis. 2004;8(2):263-6.
93. Chandra RK. 1990 Mcollum Award lecture. Nutrition and immunity: lessons from the past and new insights into the future. Am J Clin Nutr. 1991;53(5):1087-101.
94. WFP. Getting started: WFP food assistance in the context of TBb care and treatment. Geneva. World Food Program. HIV/AIDS Service; 2005.
95. Chandra RK. Nutritional deficiency and susceptibility to infection. Bull World Health Organ. 1979;57(2):167-77.
96. Van Lettow M, Kumwenda JJ, Harries AD Whalen CC, Taha TE, Kumwenda N. Malnutrition and the severity of lung disease in adults with pulmonary tuberculosis in Malawi. Int J Tuberc Lung Dis. 2004;8(2):211-7.
97. Perronne C. Tuberculosis, HIV infection, and malnutrition: an infernal trio in central Africa. Nutrition. 1999;15(4):321-2.
98. Paton NI, Castello-Branco LR, Jennings G, Ortigao-de-Sampaio MB, Elia M, Costa S, et al. Impact of tuberculosis on the body composition of HIV-infected men in Brazil. J Acquir Immune Defic Syndr Hum Retrovirol. 1999;20(3):265-71.
99. Onwubalili JK. Malnutrition among tuberculosis patients in Harrow, England. Eur J Clin Nutr. 1988;42(4):363-6.
100. Paton NI, Chua YK, Earnest A, et al. Randomized controlled trial of nutritional supplementation in patients with newly diagnosed tuberculosis and wasting. Am J Clin Nutr. 2004;80(2):460-5.
101. Macallan DC, McNurlan MA, Kurpad AV, Souza G, Shetty PS, Calder AG, et al. Whole body protein metabolism in human pulmonary tuberculosis and undernutrition: evidence for anabolic block in tuberculosis. Clin Sci (Lond). 1998;94(3):321-31.
102. Tverdal A. Body mass index and incidence of tuberculosis. Eur J Respir Dis. 1986;69(5):355-62.
103. Cegielski JP, McMurray DN. The relationship between malnutrition and tuberculosis: evidence from studies in humans and experimental animals. Int J Tuberc Lung Dis. 2004;8(3):286-98.
104. Keusch GT. Micronutrients and susceptibility to infection. Ann NY Acad Sci. 1990;587:181-8.
105. Schwenk A, Hodgson L, Wright A, Ward LC, Rayner CF, Grubnic S, et al. Nutrient partitioning during treatment of tuberculosis: gain in body fat mass but not in protein mass. Am J Clin Nutr. 2004;79(6):1006-12.
106. Paton NI, Ng YM. Body composition studies in patients with wasting associated with tuberculosis. Nutrition. 2006;22(3):245-51.
107. Villamor E, Saathoff E, Mugusi F, Bosch RJ, Urassa W, Fawzi WW. Wasting and body composition of adults with pulmonary tuberculosis in relation to HIV-1 coinfection, socioeconomic status, and severity of tuberculosis. Eur J Clin Nutr. 2006;60(2):163-71.
108. Mugusi FM, Rusizoka O, Habib N, Fawzi W. Vitamin A status of patients presenting with pulmonary tuberculosis and asymptomatic HIV-infected individuals, Dar es Salaam, Tanzania. Int J Tuberc Lung Dis. 2003;7(8):804-7.
109. Chandra RK, Kumari S. Nutrition and immunity: an overview. J Nutr. 1994;124(8 Suppl):1433S-5S.
110. Fischer Walker C, Black RE. Zinc and the risk for infectious disease. Annu Rev Nutr. 2004;24:255-75.
111. Green JA, Lewin SR, Wightman F, Lee M, Ravindran TS, Paton NI. A randomized controlled trial of oral zinc on the immune response to tuberculosis in HIV-infected patients. Int J Tuberc Lung Dis. 2005;9(12):1378-84.
112. Ramachandran G, Santha T, Garg R, Baskaran D, Iliayas SA, Venkatesan P. Vitamin A levels in sputum-positive pulmonary tuerbculosis patients in comparison with household contacts and healthy 'normals'. Int J Tuberc Lung Dis. 2004;8(9):1130-3.
113. Egge K. Measuring the impact of targeted food assistance on HIV/AIDS-related beneficiary groups: with a specific focus on TB, ART, CI and PMYCT beneficiaries: C-SAFE Learning Spaces Initiative, 2005.
114. Treatment of tuberculosis: guidelines for national programmes. 3rd edition. Geneva: World Health Organization; 2003. p. 313.
115. Visser ME, Texeira-Swiegelaar C, Maartens G. The short-term effects of anti-tuberculosis therapy on plasma pyridoxine levels in patients with pulmonary tuberculosis. Int J Tuberc Lung Dis. 2004;8(2):260-2.
116. Zittermann A. Vitamin D in preventive medicine: are we ignoring the evidence? Br J Nutr. 2003;89(5):552-72.
117. Ustianowski A, Shaffer R, Collin S, Wilkinson RJ, Davidson RN. Prevalence and associations of vitamin D deficiency in foreign-born persons with tuberculosis in London. J Infect. 2005;50(5):432-7.

118. Paton NI, Ng YM, Chee CB, Persaud C, Jackson AA. Effects of tuberculosis and HIV infection on wholebody protein metabolism during feeding, measured by the glycine method. Am J Clin Nutr. 2003;78(2):319-25.
119. Van Lettow M, West CE, Van der Meer JW, Wieringa FT, Semba RD. Low plasma selenium concentrations, high plasma human immunodeficiency virus load and high interleukin-6 concentrations are risk factors associated with anemia in adults presenting with pulmonary tuberculosis in Zomba district, Malawi. Eur J Clin Nutr. 2005;59(4):526-32.
120. Das BS, Devi U, Mohan Rao C, Srivastava VK, Rath PK, Das BS. Effect of iron supplementation on mild to moderate anaemia in pulmonary tuberculosis. Br J Nutr. 2003;90(3):541-50.
121. Mookherji S. Food support to tuberculosis patients under DOTS: a case study of the collaboration between the World Food Program and the National TB Control Program in Cambodia. Arlington VA: Management Sciences for Health and Stop TB Partnership, 2005.
122. Macnee W. Chronic Bronchitis and Emphysema. In: Seaton A, Seaton D, Leitch AG (Eds). Crofton and Douglas's Respiratory Disease. United Kingdom: Blackwell Science; 2002. pp. 616-7.
123. Leitch AG. Pulmonary tuberculosis clinical features. In: Seaton A, Seaton D, Leitch AG (Eds). Crofton and Douglas's Respiratory Disease. United Kingdom: Blackwell Science; 2002. p. 523.
124. Hassan IS, Al-Jahdali HH. Obstructive airway disease in patients with significant post-tuberculosis scarring. Saudi Med J. 2005;26(7):1157-7.
125. Willcox PA, Ferguson AD. Chronic obstructive airway disease following treated pulmonary tuberculosis. Respir Med. 1989;83(3):195-8.
126. de Vallière S, Barker RD. Residual lung damage after completion of treatment for multidrug-resistant tuberculosis. Int J Tuberc Lung Dis. 2004;8(6):767-71.
127. Rajasekharan S, Savitri S, Jayaganesh D. Post-tuberculosis bronchial asthma. Ind J Tub. 2001;48:139.
128. Yasuda J, Okada O, Kuriyama T, Nagao K, Yamagishi F, Hashizume I, et al. Investigations of pulmonary hemodynamics and chest X-ray findings in patients pulmonary tuberculosis sequelae. Kekkaku. 1999;74(8):5-18.
129. Lee JH, Chang JH. Lung function in patients with chronic airflow obstruction due to tuberculosis destroyed lung. Respir Med. 2003;97(11):1237-42.

Prevention of Tuberculosis

Rajesh N Solanki, Jaydeep Odhwani, Kumar Utsav

INTRODUCTION

Tuberculosis (TB) is endemic in many countries, including in India. There are an estimated 490,000 new multidrug resistant (MDR) and 30,000 extensively-drug resistant (XDR) TB patients every year. Factors that worsen this trend include human immunodeficiency virus (HIV) infection, poverty, old age, overcrowding and poor sanitation. Unsuspected TB cases contribute to TB transmission because they go unsuspected for days or weeks. Unless TB is diagnosed (or at least suspected), proper treatment and infection control measures cannot be put in place. An untreated case of TB is responsible for about 10–12 new cases of TB. In a community or a group with a high burden of disease, it is the responsibility of the public health officials to put preventive measures in place to alleviate the burden. There are multiple levels of prevention that are crucial to decrease the mortality and morbidity of the disease, i.e. primordial, primary, secondary and tertiary prevention.[1] In case of TB, the community-based interventions were found to be most effective for prevention and control of TB in a large systematic evaluation of 41 studies on the subject.[2]

PRIMORDIAL PREVENTION

Adoption of proper lifestyle, especially in the early childhood is the basis of primordial prevention. For TB, it will involve the following measures:

- Nutritional interventions
- Environmental modifications (especially healthy housing and proper sanitation, improved socioeconomic status)
- Appropriate health education and behavioral changes.

PRIMARY PREVENTION

Primary prevention efforts aim at reducing an individual's susceptibility to the disease, illness or injury. Education, changes in lifestyle and behavior modification are components of primary prevention. TB is infectious when it occurs in the lungs or larynx. TB that occurs elsewhere in the body in isolation is usually not infectious. A person who has TB disease in his/her lungs or larynx, can release many tiny particles called droplet nuclei into the air by coughing or sneezing; smaller numbers of droplet nuclei are released during normal activities like talking or spontaneously during breathing. Approximately 5,000 droplets are produced while talking, which may increase fourfold or higher during coughing. These droplet nuclei particles of approximately 1–5μ microns in size, are invisible to the naked eyes. Droplet nuclei can remain airborne inside the room air for a long period of time, until they are removed by natural or mechanical ventilation or by exposure to direct sunlight, which kills the *Mycobacterium* very fast.

Comprehensive guidelines of the Central Tuberculosis Division of Government of India for prevention and control of airborne infections, in particular TB are available for further reading.[3]

ADMINISTRATIVE MEASURES

The first line of defense for preventing the spread of TB in health care settings is to apply administrative control measures, which have greater impact on preventing TB transmission in health care setting. The aim of administrative interventions in any health care facility that manages patients with suspected TB is to reduce the total time period that such a patient stays in the health care facility, reduce airborne transmission to other patients and healthcare workers (HCWs) in this limited time period, all rooms should require greater than 6–12 air changes per hour (ACH). Administration should also ensure rapid diagnostic evaluation, rapid initiation of treatment, limit employee and visitor exposure.

Outpatient Area

Patients of TB, like other patients, have to wait for long periods before they are actually examined by the physician. During this period, these patients are a constant source for airborne spread of disease to others. Reducing the overall stay of such patients in the health care facility is likely to prove the single-most effective measure of reducing airborne disease transmission in these areas. This can be achieved by fast-tracking these patients, which can be accomplished by several measures that are not mutually exclusive. Fast-tracking will also depend upon the type of health care facility. At a chest center/hospital, most patients are chest symptomatics where fast-tracking has no real application, but the process will be more useful for general hospitals. Implementation of key administrative intervention would vary from facility to facility.

- *Screening*: Screening for TB symptoms can be done at registration counter itself and those suspected of TB can be given priority. This screening can be performed by physicians, nurse, paramedical staff or volunteer specially deputed for this purpose.
- *Education on cough etiquette and respiratory hygiene*: This education can easily be imparted to patients through posters and other audiovisual means, as well as by actual discussion by paramedical staff or volunteers in the waiting area. Outpatient setting should make easy availability of tissue papers and bins with disinfectants for sputum disposal.
- *Patient segregation*: Segregation of patients with respiratory symptoms can be achieved by separate waiting areas for chest-symptomatics. Outpatient area should be well ventilated to reduce overall risk of airborne transmission.

Inpatient Care Facilities

- *Need-based hospitalization of TB patients:* One of the most effective means to reduce the risk of transmission of airborne pathogens, such as *Mycobacterium tuberculosis* in hospital settings is to manage such patients in the outpatient setting whenever possible. Many patients can be managed entirely as outpatients, thereby avoiding hospitalization and the risk of exposing other patients and staff.
- *Establish separate rooms, wards or areas within wards for patients with infectious respiratory diseases*: When hospitalization is required, TB patients should be physically separated from other patients so that others are not exposed to the infectious droplet nuclei that they generate. Policies on TB patients' separation inevitably generate concern about stigma. Appropriate measures, such as training and public posting of separation rules help to minimize stigma

  Administrative procedures should ensure that separation happens promptly, similar to the separation of men and women during inpatient admission. If sputum-smear microscopy or other relevant diagnostic tests are performed for patients with respiratory symptoms at the time of admission, then those who are smear-positive TB can be quickly identified for separation from other patients. Priorities for separation of TB patients are as follows:
  - Separation of sputum-smear positive TB patients from immune compromised patients
  - Separation of patients with known or suspected drug-resistant TB from immune compromised patients
  - Separation of patients with known or suspected TB from all other patients.

  The best choice for infectious or potentially infectious patients is to manage them in isolation rooms. Where such isolation rooms are not feasible, other options for physical separation include:
  - Having a few small "airborne precaution rooms" for patients with infectious respiratory disease patients
  - Having a separate ward designated for patients with infectious respiratory disease
  - Keeping a designated area with better ventilation available for the placement of potentially-infectious patients
  - When it is not possible to have a designated airborne precaution room, or area of a ward, there can at least be a designated area where TB inpatients can be preferentially placed.
- *Cough hygiene and adequate sputum disposal*: Tuberculosis or MDR-TB wards having infectious patients should display signboards in the ward demonstrating cough hygiene. All patients admitted in the ward/area should be issued surgical masks and counseled on their proper use. Adequate measures for safe collection and disposal of sputum should also be undertaken
  - *Establish safe radiology procedures for patients with infectious respiratory disease, including smear-positive TB cases or TB suspects*: When caring for an infectious TB case/suspect, the radiology departments should attempt to:
    - Schedule inpatient chest radiographs on infectious and suspect TB patients for non-busy times, such as the end of the afternoon
    - Provide coughing patients with a surgical mask to wear, or tissues or cloth to cover their mouths
    - Provide priority service to potentially infectious TB patients to minimize the length of time spent in the department
    - Restrict access to the radiology suite to patients and essential personnel only
    - Use the room with the best ventilation for taking images of potentially infectious TB patients.

Environmental Controls

Environmental control measures are the second-line of defense for preventing the spread of TB in health care settings. Environmental controls include ventilation (natural and mechanical), UV germicidal irradiation [Ultraviolet Germicidal Irradiation (UVGI)], filtration and other methods of air cleaning. Environmental controls work on the same

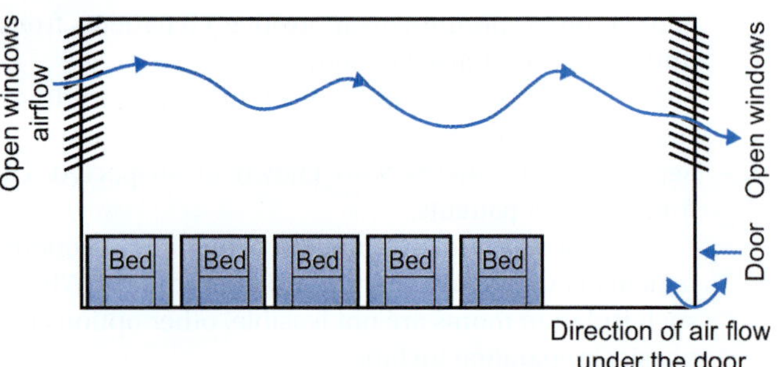

Fig. 1 Schema of a room with natural ventilation—fixed unrestricted openings on both sides allow for adequate air exchange

basic principle—dilution of infectious particles through real or "effective" air exchange. (One air change has occurred when the volume of air entering or exiting a room is equal to the volume of the room.)

Ventilation

In the case of ventilation, the dilution occurs through the introduction of fresh, uninfected air and removal of the infected air.

- *Natural ventilation*: It refers to fresh air that enters and leaves a room or other area through openings such as windows or doors **(Fig. 1)**. Natural ventilation is "controlled" when openings are fixed and unrestricted to maintain airflow at all times. Unrestricted openings (i.e. those that cannot be closed) on opposite sides of a room provide the most effective natural ventilation. In existing health care facilities that have natural ventilation, when possible, effective ventilation should be achieved by proper operation and maintenance of openings, and by regular checks to see that openings remain free of obstruction at all times.

  Simple natural ventilation can be optimized by maximizing the size of the windows, opening up fixed windowpanes, by locating windows on opposing walls, and by the use of propeller "mixing fans". Types of mixing fans include ceiling fans, stand/desk mounted fans, or window/exhaust fans located in open windows. Mixing of air can disperse the pockets of high concentrations, such as in the vicinity of patients. The total number of infectious particles in the room will not change with mixing; the concentration of particles near the source may be reduced, and the concentration in other parts of the room may increase. In other words, unless adequate ventilation is present the mixing fan will not be useful in reducing infectious particles and the risk of transmission.

  A common problem with reliance on natural ventilation is the closure of the windows during cold weather or at nights by patients or staff members. Further, there is likely to be variability of airflow patterns due to varying weather. In colder climates where rooms are closed to keep temperature adequately high especially in winter, natural ventilation can be implemented by airing via windows at frequent intervals. If natural ventilation of the room is inadequate, additional mechanical ventilation or other measures may be needed, especially in areas where risk of *M. tuberculosis* transmission is high.
- *Mechanical ventilation*: It uses fans to drive the airflow through a building. Mechanical ventilation can be fully-controlled and combined with air-conditioning and filtration systems as is normally done in some office buildings. Mechanical ventilation also includes "mixed mode ventilation", in which exhaust and/or supply fans are used in combination with natural ventilation to obtain adequate dilution when sufficient ventilation rate cannot be achieved by natural ventilation alone.

  The simplest form of mechanical ventilation is the use of "exhaust fans", placed for instance in windows to move air from inside a room to the outdoors. Exhaust fans also may be more acceptable to staff and patients than keeping windows consistently open. If exhaust fans are used, it is important to ensure that airflow is adequate, and air flows across the room (not in and out the same window or vent), and that exhaust fans and air intake (vents) should not be located side by side to avoid short-circuiting of air.

National Standards for Minimum Ventilation in Health Care Settings

Health care facilities should maintain a minimum amount of ventilation during all climatic conditions. This can be achieved by the fixed number of ACH. In settings relying on mechanical ventilation (either fan-assisted or closed systems) this can be calculated with the assistance of local engineers **(Table 1)**.

- *Where ACH is not possible to measure, as is usually the case in rooms with natural ventilation*: The following standards for ventilation should be followed to ensure that air exchange is safely greater than 12 ACH under all climactic conditions:
  - Natural ventilation should be "controlled", with fixed, unrestricted openings that are insensitive to climatic conditions
  - Openings should constitute greater than 20% of floor area
  - Openings should be there on both the sides, preferably on opposite sides. For example, a 100 square feet, room should have greater than 10 square feet fixed, unrestricted openings on both sides, total of 20 square feet.

Direction control of airflow is recommended in specific high-risk settings where infectious patients with drug resistant TB are managed. Natural ventilation would allow potentially infected air to cross HCWs.

With a "GOOD" seating arrangement the chance of such exposure is lessened.

Table 1 Minimum air changes per hour required for various health care settings

Type of health care setting	*Minimum air changes per hour (ACH)*	*Minimum hourly averaged ventilation rate (liters/second/patient)*
Registration areas	> 6 ACH*	> 40 L/s/patient
Outpatient departments and their waiting areas	> 6 ACH	> 40 L/s/patient
High-risk settings and their waiting areas ART centers	> 6 ACH	>40 L/s/patient
Bronchoscopy procedure rooms >12 ACH MDR-TB wards and clinics Airborne isolation rooms	> 12 ACH**	80–160 L/s/patient
*Equivalent to greater than 40 Litres/second (L/s) for a room-size of 24 m^3 i.e. 4 m × 2 m × 3 m. **Equivalent to greater than 80 L/s for a room-size of 24 m^3 i.e. 4 m × 2 m × 3 m.		

Ultraviolet Germicidal Irradiation

- *Mycobacterium tuberculosis* (MTB) is sensitive to germicidal radiation of ultraviolet (UV) rays found in the UV-C portion of the UV spectrum. The use of UVGI lamps is reserved for high-risk areas (laboratory, sputum collection area, poorly-ventilated spaces, etc.), where other environmental measures are not sufficient due to climatic or structural constraints.
- *Sputum collection area:* This area must be settled outside in open air where bacilli will naturally be dispersed by wind and killed by sun rather than in a closed room where the concentration of bacilli will be high. In cold regions, assign a specific room of small size (1 m) with one single glass door to opening outside. Keep the door largely open for 5 minutes between each patient. The small volume of air in this room facilitates rapid ventilation.
- *Constraints on the use of UV lamps:*
  - Monthly checking and daily maintenance (dusting).
  - Risk of mercury poisoning in case of broken or mishandled lamp; disposal of mercury from used lamps requires specific procedures.
  - May not work in humid areas.
    A UV lamp needs replacement after every 5,000 hours (as they begin to emit harmful wavelengths of light. A lamp working 8 hours per day must be replaced every six months). Use only lamp-type UVC-254 µm, made from mercury and quartz.
  - Use only indirect lamps (portable lamps or those mounted high up and directed toward the ceiling), to avoid possible burns to the conjunctiva or skin from direct exposure. Ensure that the airflow crosses in front of the lamp.
  - Use direct UV lamps in empty rooms only (they can be switched on at night).
- *Filtration [High-efficiency Particulate Air Filters]*
  Filtration is another option to remove infectious particles from the air. Situations where high-efficiency particulate air (HEPA) filter might be considered include the bronchoscopy suits, laboratories, individual TB patient room.
  If filters are chosen, then only true-HEPA membrane filters (rated to remove 99.97% of 1 µ particles) should be entertained. Other filtration mechanisms such as ionizer have not been adequately studied.

Personal Protection

- *Health staff:* Tuberculosis is transmitted mainly via the respiratory route. Only anti-inhalation masks (high-filtration masks, N95 masks) are capable of preventing inhalation of the bacilli.
  All members of the staff, whether caregiver or not must wear these masks under following conditions, when:
  - In contact with contagious patients
  - Collecting sputum samples and preparing slides
  - Collecting and disposing the sputum containers.
- *Patients and attendants:* Contagious patients must wear surgical masks (antiprojection mask) when they leave their rooms to go to another department or any other enclosed area (except outdoors). The mask is intended to prevent projection of *M. tuberculosis* by the carrier. Attendants and visitors must wear a high-filtration mask (like that worn by staff), when entering a contagious TB patient's room. Inform patients, visitors and attendants about the risk of TB transmission and how to avoid it, or protect themselves. Ask patients to cover their nose and mouth when they cough or sneeze, and to use a sputum container; explain why, when and how to use masks; display posters of protective measures inward, waiting rooms, etc.
- *Visitors and attendants' movement:* Inside the TB department, circulation of patients and attendants should be controlled as follows:
  - Limit the number of visits, duration of each visit, particularly for contagious patients
  - Encourage visits outside the building, in the open air
  - Before any visit, the nurse should provide information on the transmission risk.

In addition to wearing a mask, which is a specific protective measure, standard precautions (hand hygiene, gown, etc.) apply in TB wards, just as they do in any other hospital department.

Vaccines

The only vaccination for TB in the market is the bacillus Calmette-Guérin (BCG) vaccine.[4] It has poor efficacy ranging from 0% to 80%. The BCG vaccine is routinely given in India to the newborn after birth. It is not recommended in the United States because secondary prevention techniques are greatly hindered by the BCG vaccine, which can interfere with the management of persons who are possibly infected with *M. tuberculosis*.

Newer vaccines under investigations which have shown promising results in phase I and II trials, include recombinant BCG (rBCG and capsid) and fusion proteins (HyVac 4/AERAS 404, GSK M72). Their role in prevention of TB is somewhat remote at the present.

SECONDARY PREVENTION

Screening

Secondary prevention denotes the identification of people who have already developed a disease, at an early stage in the natural history. This is achieved through screening and early intervention.

Screening tests and preventive therapy accomplish secondary prevention efforts. This is particularly important for high-risk population groups such as the HCWs, prisoners and inmates of common living facilities.[5-7] Implementation of preventive therapy (treatment with antituberculosis drugs) reduces the risk that TB infection will progress to TB disease. Early identification and successful treatment of persons with TB disease remains the most effective means of preventing disease transmission.[8] Therefore, people who are likely to have infectious TB should be identified and provided treatment before they are able to widely transmit the *Mycobacteria*. Some of the screening methods applied for identification of high-risk group populations are as given below:

Symptomatic Screening

Whenever possible, HCWs should undergo the initial screening. During their initial medical screening, they should be asked about the history of TB disease or for the treatment for latent TB infection (LTBI) or TB disease, previously. Documentation of any such history should be obtained from medical records, if possible. They should be observed for the presence of a cough or evidence of significant weight loss. All new recruits/inmates should be immediately screened for symptoms of pulmonary TB.

The index of suspicion should be high when pulmonary symptoms are accompanied by general, systemic symptoms of TB (e.g. fever, chills, night sweats, easy fatigability, loss of appetite and weight loss). Individuals, who have symptoms suggestive of TB disease should immediately receive a thorough medical evaluation, including a tuberculin skin test (TST) or QuantiFERON-TB Gold (QFT-G) test, a chest radiograph, and if indicated, sputum examinations. Symptom screening alone is an unsatisfactory mechanism for TB, except in facilities with a minimal risk for TB transmission.

Chest Radiograph Screening

Screening with chest radiographs can be an effective means of detecting new cases of unsuspected TB disease. Radiographic screening requires fewer subsequent visits than a TST screening (i.e. only those with suspicious radiographs or TB symptoms require follow-up). However, such screening will not identify people with LTBI. Screening inmates with a chest radiograph doubled the TB case-finding rate and reduced the time from intake into the correctional facility to isolation substantially compared with TST testing (2.3 days and 7.5 days, respectively).[7] Digital radiographs (miniature or full size) provide enhanced imaging and improved storage and readability. A miniature radiograph can be performed in less than 1 minute and exposes the patient to approximately one-tenth the radiation dose of a conventional radiograph.

Screening with chest radiographs might be appropriate in certain jails and detention facilities that house substantial numbers of inmates for short periods and serve populations at high-risk for TB (e.g. those with high prevalence of HIV infection or history of injection-drug use and foreign-born persons from countries in which TB prevalence is high). Inmates who are infected with HIV might be anergic and consequently, might have false-negative TST results. Chest radiograph should be a part of the initial screening of HIV-infected patients and those who are at risk for HIV infection, but whose status is unknown. Persons who have radiographs suggestive of TB, should be isolated and evaluated further. Sputum-smear and culture examinations should be performed for inmates, whose chest radiographs are consistent with TB disease and it might be indicated at least for certain persons who are symptomatic, regardless of their TST, QFT-G or chest radiograph results.

Detection of Latent Tuberculosis Infection

The United States Centers for Disease Control and Prevention (CDC) recommends a strategy to identify those who have LTBI and, if indicated, the use of chemotherapy to prevent the latent infection from progressing to active TB disease. There are two tests that can be used to help detect LTBI.

- *Tuberculin skin test*: Skin testing using 0.1 mL of 5 tuberculin units (TU) of purified protein derivative (PPD), tuberculin, is the most common method of testing for TB infection. In this test tuberculin is injected intradermally to see if there is a reaction to the test. Persons who have a documented history of a positive TST result, a documented history of TB disease, or a reported history of a severe necrotic reaction to tuberculin should be exempted from a routine TST. The TST sensitivity ranges from 75% to 90%.[9,10] Despite this limitation, skin testing, along with symptom review, frequently constitutes the most practical approach to screening for the TB disease
- *QuantiFERON-TB Gold*: QFT-G is more sensitive than the TST. The test is highly specific and unaffected by BCG

vaccination status, a major cause of false-positive TST response.

Chemoprophylaxis

Chemoprophylaxis is most often the treatment for primary infection in order to sterilize the lesions and prevent the development of active TB. In the literal sense of the term, it is more a treatment than chemoprophylaxis. It may reduce the risk of developing TB by up to 90% in a patient with primary infection. It usually consists of daily administration of isoniazid (INH) 5 mg/kg (maximum 300 mg/day) for 6 months, in both children and adults. The effectiveness of isoniazid prophylaxis depends on the sensitivity to isoniazid. The use of isoniazid is contraindicated in patients with severe or chronic active hepatitis. It should be administered with caution to patients who regularly consume alcohol.

- *Chemoprophylaxis for newborn infant of sputum smear-positive mother:* In all the cases, where the mother is sputum smear-positive at birth of child, chemoprophylaxis is administered to the child for 6 months; BCG vaccination is done afterward (BCG vaccine should not be given during administration of isoniazid).

  If a child develops signs of TB immediately or subsequently (in general, only evident after approximately 2–8 weeks) e.g. arrested growth, splenohepatomegaly, jaundice, sometimes pneumonia, she/he should receive complete anti-TB treatment after exclusion of other possible medical causes.

  If a TST is possible, the approach is to administer isoniazid for 3 months, followed by a TST. If the TST is positive, isoniazid is continued for 3 more months. If the TST is negative, stop isoniazid and administer the BCG vaccine.
  - The child should not be separated from her/his mother unless she/he is severely ill. Breastfeeding should be continued. It is possible that isoniazid is not effective if primary resistance against this drug exists (varies according to the area) or if there is a problem of secondary resistance in the mother. The child must, therefore, be closely monitored in all cases
  - If a mother presents with TB during pregnancy or if the sputum becomes negative under treatment, it is sufficient to vaccinate the child at birth and to monitor him/her thereafter
- *Children under 5 years of age in contact with Mantoux positive patients:* If suspicion of TB exists before administering chemoprophylaxis it is imperative to rule out active TB. If TB is suspected, the child should undergo complete curative treatment. If not, prophylaxis should be administered for 6 months. If the child is healthy, administer chemoprophylaxis for 6 months, regardless of the vaccination status of the child. If it is not possible to administer the prophylaxis, vaccinate and monitor the child.

  The use of TST may help to better specify indications for prophylaxis. In practice, it is simpler and prudent to systematically administer prophylaxis, when indicated
- *Chemoprophylaxis in human immunodeficiency virus patient:* The use of antiretroviral therapy (ART) in HIV patients is the best TB prophylaxis, with up to 80% of risk reduction, without the use of isoniazid. The target population for chemoprophylaxis among HIV-seropositive includes all Mantoux (PPD) positive individuals who do not have active TB and could include PPD negative individuals living in high prevalence region for TB.

  The optimal duration of preventive therapy with single drug isoniazid, daily or twice weekly, should be greater than 6 months to provide the maximum degree of protection against TB. The effectiveness of preventive therapy should be evaluated at regular intervals by monitoring patients for drug adherence, drug toxicity and for the development of TB.

  Though the impact of preventive therapy on an individual basis may be rather small, widespread implementation would have substantial impact on morbidity due to TB and some impact on mortality. Preventive therapy should be offered at voluntary counseling and testing centers, as part of a package of care that includes prophylaxis and treatment of opportunistic infections, nutritional support and counseling.

  The CDC has recommended that preventive therapy for anergic HIV-infected persons should be considered if the patient has had known contact with an active TB case or belongs to a group in which the prevalence of TB infection is high.[11] In areas endemic for TB and HIV, purified protein derivative (PPD) or tuberculin test may not be helpful in identifying persons who could benefit from INH prophylaxis. Among TB patients with HIV infection, up to 40% could be anergic. This further complicates the issue of TB preventive therapy among individuals infected with HIV
  - *Chemoprophylaxis in tuberculin negative human immunodeficiency virus infected persons:* Tuberculin skin test negative, HIV infected persons from high-risk groups or from areas with a high prevalence of *M. tuberculosis* infection may be at increased risk of primary or reactivation TB. Combining the results of various studies on efficacy of preventive therapy in subjects with a negative PPD test, INH was found to be significantly better than placebo. Hence in HIV seropositive individuals, living in a high prevalence TB region, with negative PPD or in situations where tuberculin test cannot be performed, chemoprophylaxis with INH will reduce the risk of developing active TB in the short-term to around 60% of what it would have been without such a treatment
  - *Prerequisite to initiate preventive therapy:* Prior to starting an individual on preventive treatment for TB, it is essential to ensure that he/she does not have active TB.

This is done by a complete clinical examination along with a chest X-ray and sputum smear examination for acid-fast bacilli (AFB). It is advisable that chest X-ray is done for every individual before considering preventive therapy. Any HIV-infected patient with fever, cough or abnormal chest X-ray should not be given preventive treatment until a full evaluation is done to confirm that active TB disease is not present.

At times, it is difficult to exclude TB even when the chest radiograph is normal and two sputum smears are negative for AFB. Where mycobacterial culture facilities are available, sputum culture can be used to definitively diagnose TB. In general, it is safe to presume that completely asymptomatic individuals are unlikely to have TB.

- *Duration of preventive therapy:* A multicentric trial conducted in United States of America, Mexico, Brazil and Haiti, demonstrated that the magnitude of protection obtained from a regimen of isoniazid (H) administered daily for 12 months was similar to that obtained from a regimen of rifampicin (R) and pyrazinamide (Z) administered daily for 2 months.[12] Moreover, it was noted that persons taking R and Z for 2 months were significantly more likely (80%) to complete therapy than those taking H for 12 months (69%). However, due to several cases of fatal hepatotoxicity reported among HIV-negative individuals on the RZ regimen, it is no longer recommended for preventive therapy.

There is evidence to suggest that preventive therapy is efficacious in HIV positive persons with tuberculin reactions greater than 5 mm, and that optimal duration of isoniazid preventive therapy (using a single drug) should be greater than 6 months to provide the maximum degree of protection against TB. Although the American Thoracic Society has recommended that isoniazid therapy should be continued for 12 months in persons with HIV infection, there are only a few studies comparing the efficacy of this approach with that of either shorter or longer courses.[13] South Africa has now implemented the policy to administer isoniazid chemoprophylaxis for HIV positive patients for up to 36 months.[14]

- *Chemoprophylaxis in special situations:*
  - *Chemoprophylaxis in pregnancy:* Chemoprophylaxis for TB is recommended during pregnancy for HIV-infected women, who have a history of exposure to active TB or after active TB has been ruled out. INH with pyridoxine (to reduce the risk of neurotoxicity) is the prophylactic agent of choice.[15] Some may choose to initiate prophylaxis after the first trimester to avoid teratogenicity
  - *Chemoprophylaxis in children:* Infants born to HIV-infected mothers should have a Mantoux test (5-TU PPD or 1-TU PPD RT23 with Tween 80) at or before age of 9–12 months, should be retested at least every 2–3 years.[15] Children exposed to those with active TB, should be administered preventive therapy after active TB has been ruled out. However, there have been no clinical trials of preventive therapy in HIV-positive children.
- *Secondary prophylaxis:* The rate of recurrent TB is higher in HIV-1 positive individuals than in HIV-negative individuals with both reactivation and new infections contributing to recurrences.[16] It also showed that the absolute impact of secondary preventive therapy to reduce TB recurrence was highest among the individuals with low CD4 cell counts.
  - *Current recommendations for preventive therapy against TB in human immunodeficiency virus infected persons:*
    - ➢ *World Health Organization (WHO) recommendation:* Isoniazid is recommended drug (5 mg/kg to maximum 300 mg) to be taken daily, as self-administered therapy for 6 months. Individuals should be seen monthly and given only one month's supply of medication at each visit.
    - ➢ *CDC recommendation:* Isoniazid is chosen for prevention of TB in persons with HIV infection. It is recommended for 9 months rather than 6 months of rifampicin. Pyrazinamide may be offered daily for 2 months to contacts of patients with INH resistant, rifampicin susceptible TB.
    - ➢ *American Thoracic Society:* Isoniazid is recommended for 12 months as prophylaxis in person infected with HIV infection.[17]

- *Chemoprophylaxis and MDR-TB:* Among contacts of patients with MDR-TB, the use of INH is questionable.[18] Although alternative prophylaxis treatments have been suggested, there is no consensus regarding the choice of the drug(s) and the duration of treatment. Prompt treatment of MDR-TB is the most effective way of preventing the spread of infection to others. The following measures should be taken to prevent spread of MDR-TB disease:
  - Early diagnosis and appropriate treatment of MDR-TB cases
  - Screening of contacts as per revised National TB Control Programme (RNTCP) guidelines
  - Further research into effective and nontoxic chemoprophylaxis in areas of high MDR-TB prevalence.

TERTIARY PREVENTION

The treatment of people who have already developed a disease is often described as tertiary prevention. The final strategy used for preventing and controlling TB is the identification and treatment of patients with active TB. An individual with active TB is infectious. Special precautions or isolation may be necessary to avoid transmission to others. Once the individual begins treatment and continues to follow the prescribed regimen, the individual becomes usually noninfectious within days or weeks. As pilot project, drug sensitivity testing, of MDR suspects has been initiated at multiple centers, as is reaping high dividends under RNTCP.

REFERENCES

1. Central Tuberculosis Division. (2010) National Guidelines on Airborne Infection Control for health care and other settings. Directorate General of Health and Family Welfare Department, Government of India. [online] *Available from www.tbcindia.nic.in.* [Accessed January, 2016].
2. Arshad A, Salam RA, Lassi ZS, Das JK, Naqvi I, Bhutta ZA. Community based interventions for the prevention and control of tuberculosis. Infect Dis Poverty. 2014;3:27.
3. Guidelines on Airborne infection control in healthcare and other settings. (2010). Central Tuberculosis Division, Directorate General of Health Services, Ministry of Health and Family Welfare, Government of India. *[online] Available on www.tbcindia.nic.in.* [Accessed January, 2016].
4. Colditz GA, Brewer TF, Berkey CS, Wilson ME, Burdick E, Fineberg HV, et al. Efficacy of BCG vaccine in the prevention of tuberculosis. Meta-analysis of the published literature. JAMA. 1994;271(9):698-702.
5. White MC, Tulsky JP, Portillo CJ, Menendez E, Cruz E, Goldenson J, et al. Tuberculosis prevalence in an urban jail: 1994 and 1998. Int J Tuberc Lung Dis. 2001;5(5):400-4.
6. Salive ME, Vlahov D, Brewer TF. Coinfection with tuberculosis and HIV-1 in male prison inmates. Public Health Rep. 1990;105(3):307-10.
7. Puisis M, Feinglass J, Lidow E, Mansour M, et al. Radiographic screening for tuberculosis in a large urban county jail. Public Health Rep. 1996; 111(4):330-4.
8. Centers for Disease Control and Prevention (CDC). From the Centers for Disease Control and Prevention. Tuberculosis morbidity among U.S.-born and foreign-born populations—United States, 2000. MMWR Morb Mortal Wkly Rep. 2002; 51(5):101-4.
9. Huebner RE, Schein MF, Bass JB. The tuberculin skin test. Clin Infect Dis. 1993; 17(6):968-75.
10. Holden M, Dubin MR, Diamond PH. Frequency of negative intermediate-strength tuberculin sensitivity in patients with active tuberculosis. N Engl J Med. 1971; 285(27):1506-9.
11. Purified protein derivative (PPD)-tuberculin anergy and HIV infection: guidelines for anergy testing and management of anergic persons at risk of tuberculosis. MMWR Recomm Rep. 1991; 40(RR-5):27-32.
12. Gordin F, Chaisson RE, Matts JP, Miller C, de Lourdes Garcia M, et al. Rifampcin and pyrazinamide vs isoniazid for prevention of tuberculosis in HIV-infected persons: an international randomized trial. Terry Beirn Community Programs for Clinical Research on AIDS, the Adult AIDS Clinical Trials Group, the Pan American Health Organization and the Centers for Disease Control and Prevention Study Group. JAMA. 2000;283(11):1445-50.
13. Bass JB, Farer LS, Hopewell PC, et al. Treatment of tuberculosis and tuberculosis infection in adults and children. American Thoracic Society and the Centers for Disease Control and Prevention. Am J Respir Crit Care Med. 1994;149(5):1359-74.
14. Wood R, Bekker LG. Isoniazid preventive therapy for tuberculosis in South Africa: an assessment of the local evidence base. S Afr Med J. 2014;104(3):174-7.
15. Tripathy SP. Prophylaxis for tuberculosis in HIV infected persons. AIDS Res Rev. 1999;2:105-10.
16. Swaminathan S, Rajasekaran S, Shibichakravarthy K, Amarendran VA, Raja K, Hari L, et al. Multiple recurrences of tuberculosis in an HIV infected individual. J Assoc Physicians India. 2004;52:513-4.
17. Targeted tuberculin testing and treatment of latent tuberculosis infection. American Thoracic Society. MMWR Recomm Rep. 2000;49(RR-6):1-51.
18. Guidelines for PMDT in India. (2012). Central Tuberculosis Division, Directorate General of Health Services, Ministry of Health and Family Welfare, Government of India. [online] *Available on www.tbcindia.nic.in. [Accessed January, 2016].*

42 Chapter

Extrapulmonary Tuberculosis

Ashok K Janmeja, Prasanta R Mohapatra, Deepak Aggarwal

INTRODUCTION

According to the World Health Organization's (WHO's) Global Tuberculosis Report 2013, there were 8.6 million incident tuberculosis (TB) cases worldwide, while India contributed to 26% of the global TB burden.[1] Extrapulmonary TB (EPTB) constitutes about 15–20% of all TB cases, which rises to nearly 50% among human immunodeficiency virus (HIV)-TB coinfection.[2]

Tuberculosis is a disease, which can involve virtually any organ in the body. Whenever TB involves organs other than lungs, the disease is termed as extrapulmonary tuberculosis (EPTB). When EPTB patients have concomitant pulmonary disease, the entity is classified as pulmonary TB rather than EPTB. Around 80–85% of all TB cases are of pulmonary type and the remaining 15–20% are extrapulmonary TB cases.[3-13] As per recent WHO data, extrapulmonary TB comprised 20% of new cases of TB notified in 2012, in India.[14] The proportion of EPTB has shown an upward trend in the recent years both in the developed and developing countries. In countries like the United Kingdom and the United States of America, this surge is mainly due to the immigration of significant number of people from high-burden countries, while in developing countries of sub-Saharan Africa and South Asia, the increase is due to the impact of HIV coinfection.[6,7,15,16] In presence of HIV coinfection, lymph node or central nervous system TB (CNS-TB) is quite commonly seen.[17] The lymph node TB and the pleural TB together contribute to around 75% of the total pool of EPTB cases, followed by bone and joint TB, genitourinary TB (GUTB), tuberculous meningitis (TBM), abdominal and miliary TB. Other body organs involved in descending order are; skin, pericardium, brain parenchyma, larynx, liver, pancreas, eyes, ears, adrenals, pituitary and thyroid gland.

DIAGNOSIS

Diagnosis of EPTB is generally more difficult than that of pulmonary TB. Reasons for the same are multifold, such as the difficulties in obtaining the tissue, isolating causative mycobacteria from the pathological tissues, uneven distribution of disease, an insidious onset, atypical presentation and of course, limited clinical experience of individual experts from different disciplines. These problems are further compounded by the paucibacillary nature of disease, making it imperative to depend on investigations other than the gold standard for the diagnosis, i.e. demonstration of causative tubercle bacilli on microscopy. The classical constitutional clinical features like low-grade evening pyrexia, anorexia, weight loss, malaise and fatigue are also not regular manifestations. Sometimes, the disease may even present as the pyrexia of unknown origin.[18,19] However, clues specific to the involved organ are often available which help in reaching to the diagnosis. Nevertheless, physicians must be aware about various risk factors of EPTB for reaching to the accurate diagnosis in time.[20]

Extrapulmonary TB manifestations are nonspecific, not significantly different in the HIV-infected or the noninfected patients, however, extensive disease, inadequate or delayed treatment and HIV coinfection are the factors associated with increased mortality.[21] For the diagnosis of EPTB, all efforts must be exhausted to isolate of tubercle bacilli from the body fluids or the biopsy specimens. Role of adenosine deaminase (ADA) estimation in tuberculous fluid collections in various types of EPTB has been found helpful in reaching the diagnosis. Application of molecular methods, such as polymerase chain reaction (PCR), assay targeting IS6110, multiplex PCR and RT-PCR have also been reported useful in the diagnosis of EPTB, particularly where there is strong clinical suspicion, and conventional techniques are not conclusive.[22-24]

Neither tuberculin skin test (TST) nor interferon-gamma release assay (IGRA) are recommended for the diagnosis of tubercular disease as these tests depict the immune response against tubercular antigens and do not provide information on the presence of active TB disease.[25] The serological assays have shown unsatisfying diagnostic accuracies (low specificity and sensitivity) and their use has been banned by WHO.[26]

Amplification Cartridge Based Nucleic Acid Amplification Test

Cartridge based nucleic acid amplification like Xpert MTB/RIF is a fully automated, closed real-time PCR platform. Its capability to detect mutations conferring resistance to rifampicin extends its usefulness as a diagnostic test. In a recent meta-analysis, the Xpert pooled sensitivity in lymph node tissues or aspirates, was found to be 83.1%, in cerebrospinal fluid (CSF), 80.5% and in pleural fluid 46.4%.[27] The WHO now endorses Xpert over other conventional tests for the diagnosis of TB in lymph nodes and other tissues, and as the preferred initial test for diagnosis of TB meningitis.[27] However, the diagnostic utility of the assay in serosal fluids seems to be limited.[28]

LYMPH NODE TUBERCULOSIS

Lymph node TB caused by both typical and nontuberculous mycobacteria (NTM), is the most common type of EPTB encountered in the developing world, including India.[24,29,30] In the United States of America, NTM are responsible for lymph node disease in children lesser than 5 years of age; however, typical *Mycobacterium tuberculosis* remains the cause of tuberculous lymphadenitis in the higher age group.[31] Lymph node TB is more commonly seen in the Asian, Hispanic and African-American populations. Cervical, axillary, inguinal or chest wall nodes are the common involved sites.[32,33] About 10% cases may also have concomitant mediastinal lymph node disease, which may be due to the retrograde spread.[34,35] Hilar or mediastinal lymph nodes are frequently involved in primary TB and in HIV-infected patients particularly.

Pathogenesis

Lymph node TB is often a localized manifestation of systemic spread of tuberculous infection. Initially, at the time of primary infection, tubercle bacilli get into the lungs through inhalation and form a primary complex. During this stage, there occurs hematogenous and lymphatic spread of infection to the rest of the body, where they remain dormant in the majority of infected subjects. Later, whenever the host defense gets weakened due to systemic or local factors, the dormant foci get reactivated. The systemic nature of the disease is further substantiated by the fact that one-third of cervical lymph node TB cases are associated with current or past pulmonary TB. Sometimes, in primary cervical lymph node disease, the tubercle bacilli get entry through the tonsils, thereby reaching to cervical nodes resulting in lymphadenitis there. Contrary to the lymph node TB due to typical tubercle bacilli, the atypical mycobacterial lymphadenitis is a highly localized disease. In the atypical mycobacterial lymphadenitis, infection reaches the lymph nodes through tonsils, conjunctiva, gingival or oropharyngeal mucosa, hence, surgical excision is the modality of choice.

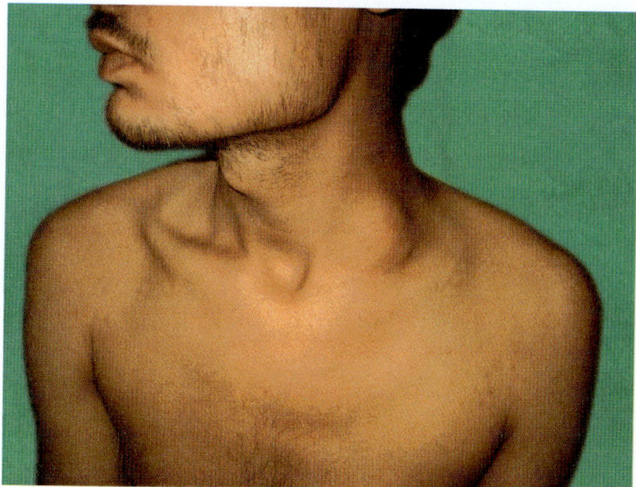

Fig. 1 A typical case of tuberculous cervical lymphadenitis

Often, the lymph nodes are small, discrete and grow very slowly, but occasionally they grow faster, become tender or painful **(Fig. 1)**. Subsequently, periadenitis develops, which causes matting and fixation of these lymph nodes. With the increasing size, there occurs caseation necrosis and liquefaction in the nodes. This leads to the perforation of deep fascia and formation of collar stud abscess. The absence of warmth and redness on overlying skin earns it a peculiar name, "cold abscess" which is almost synonymous with tuberculous etiology of the abscess. Sometimes, in an immunocompromised host or in HIV infection, the abscess grows very fast making the overlying skin warm, erythematous and painful, mimicking an acute pyogenic abscess. Such abscesses may burst and form chronic discharging sinuses or ulcers. Tuberculous sinuses characteristically have thin, bluish, undermined edges, while the discharge is usually watery **(Fig. 2)**.

Clinical Features

Lymph node TB is a disease of the children and young adults. In the developing countries with high TB burden, it is more commonly seen in children, while in developed countries its peak incidence is encountered in 20–40 years of age group. In immunocompetent subjects, only a single group of lymph nodes is involved in two-thirds cases and in remaining one-third cases multiple groups are affected, while around 90% of HIV-infected patients have involvement of multiple groups, simultaneously.

Also, concomitant pulmonary TB and intrathoracic or intra-abdominal lymph node involvement is more common in HIV-infected cases.[29,36-38] Apart from the classical symptoms of local visible swelling, the enlarged nodes may result in signs and symptoms due to obstruction or pressure on adjacent viscera, e.g. mediastinal lymphadenopathy can

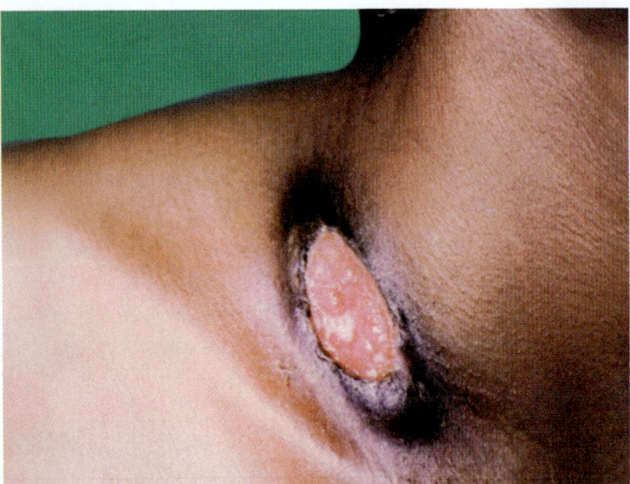

Fig. 2 Typical chronic tuberculous ulcer over right cervical region

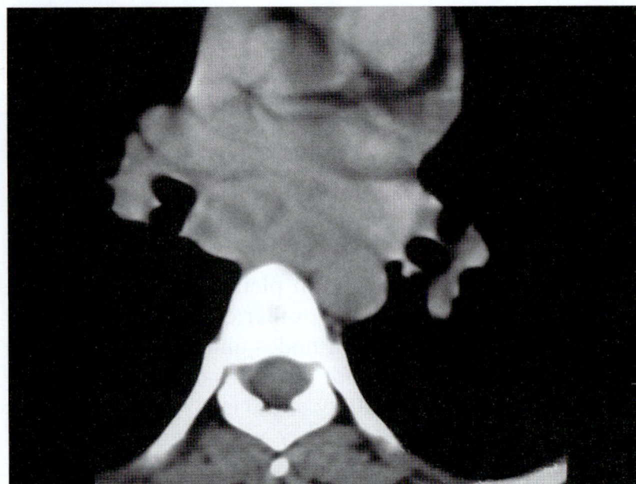

Fig. 3 Computed tomography (CT) imaging showing enlarged mediastinal lymph nodes with hypodense areas, peripheral rim enhancement and central necrosis

cause dysphagia, tracheoesophageal or esophagomediastinal fistula, etc. chylothorax, chyluria or chylous ascites may develop as a result of pressure on thoracic duct due to upper abdominal or mediastinal lymphadenopathy. Although rare, obstructive jaundice due to biliary duct compression by enlarged lymph nodes at porta hepatis has also been reported.[39]

Diagnosis

Lymph node TB usually presents as slowly enlarging swelling in cervical region without causing much pain or discomfort. Concomitant mediastinal and hilar nodal enlargement is seen in around 5–12% cases. The incidence of concomitant pulmonary TB is highly variable. Investigations like ultrasonography (USG), computed tomography (CT) scanning and magnetic resonance imaging (MRI) are helpful to delineate the extent of disease, whenever nodal involvement is suspected in mediastinum and abdomen. Enlarged nodes with hypodense areas, calcification, peripheral rim enhancement and central necrosis are the common imaging findings **(Fig. 3)**.

The gold standard for diagnosis of tuberculous lymphadenitis is the excision biopsy. Demonstration of tubercle bacilli in fine needle aspiration cytology (FNAC) or biopsy specimen or pus from the involved glands constitutes the most authentic diagnosis. Although, the tubercle bacilli positivity rate is not very impressive, larger biopsy sample may show positivity rate up to 50–70%.[39,40-43] Infrequent demonstration of bacilli on direct smear examination is basically due to the paucibacillary nature of the disease. In selected cases, endoscopic ultrasound-guided FNAC can also be used for assessing mediastinal and abdominal lymphadenopathy. It is a safe, minimally invasive, accurate, outpatient diagnostic modality and can be used early in suspected EPTB.[44] Recently, WHO has endorsed Xpert MTB/Rif over other conventional tests for diagnosis of TB in lymph nodes.[27]

Treatment

Anti-TB drug therapy alone is quite adequate to achieve cure in the majority of cases caused by typical tubercle bacilli. The recommended treatment for previously untreated lymph node TB comprises of short-course chemotherapy regimens of 6 months duration, in which four drugs, i.e. isoniazid (H), rifampicin (R), pyrazinamide (Z) and ethambutol (E) are given in the initial intensive phase of 2 months duration followed by two drugs (HR) for the next 4 months in the continuation phase. The Revised National TB Control Program (RNTCP) of the Government of India and several other similar national control programs elsewhere follow the WHO recommended directly observed therapy short course (DOTS) strategy under which drugs are administered intermittently thrice a week. As per the latest RNTCP recommendations, all EPTB cases including the lymph node TB, are treated using category-I regimen. Recent studies have demonstrated that the DOTS strategy is an effective treatment modality with treatment completion and success rate of 95–97%.[45,46]

While treating lymph node TB, a unique paradoxical phenomenon is encountered in some cases during the course drug therapy. There occurs further enlargement of already diseased nodes or even new lymph nodes might appear ipsilaterally or contralaterally in the same or different group of lymph nodes. Biopsy samples or aspirates from these nodes do not grow tubercle bacilli. This phenomenon in fact does not represent relapse or treatment failure. In fact, these lymph nodes tend to regress spontaneously on continuation of the same drug regimens without any alteration. Hence,

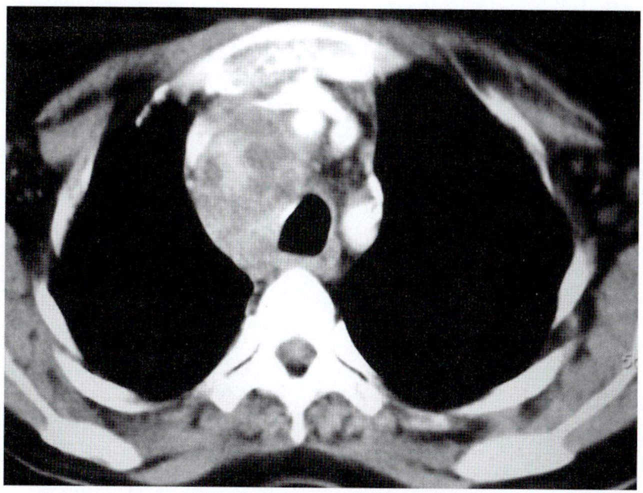

Fig. 4 Computed tomography (CT) image showing enlarged mediastinal lymph node compressing tracheobronchial tree

there is no need of changing the drug regimen in such situations. This phenomenon is mostly attributable to hypersensitivity toward tuberculous-proteins released due to the bactericidal action of drugs or the disrupted macrophages. The phenomenon of paradoxical response to TB chemotherapy is also termed as immune reconstitution inflammatory syndrome (IRIS).

Sometimes, the response is highly exaggerated when lymph nodes get significantly enlarged, become painful or lead to abscess formation. When located in the mediastinum, such enlarged nodes tend to mechanically press the esophagus or tracheobronchial tree, thereby causing dysphagia or respiratory difficulty respectively **(Fig. 4)**. In such situations, addition of a short course of corticosteroid is recommended, but only after ensuring the exclusion of other usual causes of treatment failure.[47]

PLEURAL EFFUSION

Tuberculous pleural effusion is the most common type of EPTB after lymph node disease. Nearly 20% of all EPTB cases both in HIV infected and noninfected patients are pleural effusion cases. Also, tuberculous pleural effusion is the most common cause of lymphocytic exudative type of effusion in TB high burden countries like India. Although, the fluid collection is intrathoracic in the pleural cavity intimately covering the lung, the entity is still classified as extrapulmonary disease.[39,48-51]

In most of the cases effusion is unilateral in nature occupying one-third to two-thirds of the hemithorax. Rupture of the parenchymal caseous focus, delayed hypersensitivity reactions and decreased pleural fluid clearance secondary to obstruction of pleural lymphatics are the likely pathogenetic mechanisms for the development of tuberculous pleural effusion. Usually it presents with acute or subacute onset of pleuritic chest pain and dry cough with or without constitutional symptoms.[52]

The diagnostic evaluation of tuberculous pleural effusion is initiated with the findings of lymphocytic predominant exudative pleural fluid **(Flow chart 1)**. Confirmation depends on the demonstration of tubercle bacilli in the pleural fluid or sputum or pleural biopsy specimens. However, diagnosis can be made to reasonable certainty by demonstrating elevated levels of ADA in pleural fluid. The most widely accepted cut-off value for pleural fluid ADA is 40 U/L. Higher the level, the greater is the chance of patient having TB etiology.[53]

TREATMENT

The recommendations for treatment are generally the same as for pulmonary and other forms of extrapulmonary TB. Six months regimen consisting of four first line antitubercular drugs is usually sufficient for treating most of the fresh cases of tuberculous pleural effusion. There is no indication for repeated aspiration of pleural fluid as a part of treatment unless it is massive in volume and causing significant breathlessness. Approximately 50% of patients will have some residual pleural thickening 6–12 months after the initiation of treatment.[54] The incidence of pleural thickening is slightly more in patients with low pleural fluid glucose and high pleural fluid LDH levels, as well as in those in which the pleural fluid is initially loculated.

The role of corticosteroids in the treatment of tuberculous pleurisy is controversial. The Cochrane review concluded that there is insufficient data to support evidence-based recommendations regarding the use of adjunctive corticosteroids in patients with tuberculous pleurisy.[55] However, a short course of steroids can be tried in cases of bilateral tuberculous pleural effusion as well as in patients who continue to have severe systemic symptoms (fever, pleuritic chest pain) despite therapeutic thoracocentesis and initiation of definitive therapy.

TUBERCULOUS EMPYEMA THORACIS

Tuberculous empyema represents a chronic, active infection of the pleural space resulting into the collection of frank pus loaded with large number of tubercle bacilli. The condition is less uncommon than tuberculous pleural effusion.[56] Tuberculous empyema commonly develops as a sequel to thoracoplasty, artificial pneumothorax or inadequately treated pleural effusion. The onset is usually gradual with the symptoms like mild fever, fatigue, weight loss, chest pain, dyspnea and cough. Chest X-ray (CXR) shows pleural effusion, but often with the thickening of pleura, pleural calcification, loculation or encystment of fluid in pleural cavity. Finger clubbing, intercostal narrowing with tenderness or empyema necessitatis may be observed on physical examination.

Treatment comprises of effective drainage of pleural pus and anti-TB chemotherapy. Problematic treatment issues

Flow chart 1 Algorithm for initial diagnostic evaluation of tuberculous pleural effusion

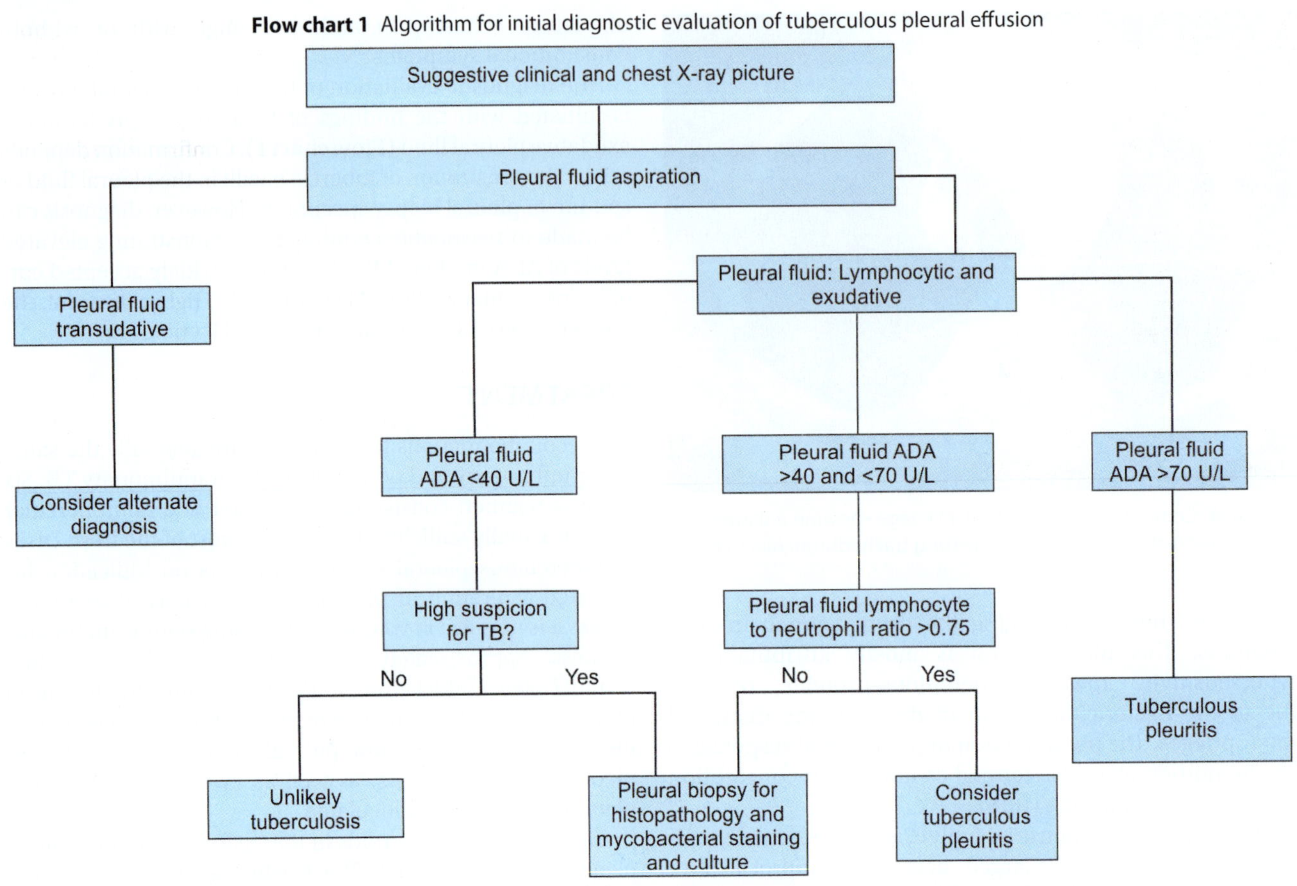

include the nonexpansion the trapped lung. Also, it is difficult to achieve therapeutic drug levels in pleural fluid which can lead to drug resistance. Such complications usually warrant decortication or thoracoplasty, should an adequate TB drug therapy coupled with repeated pleural tapping fails. Surgery should be undertaken by experienced thoracic surgeons.[56]

BONE AND JOINT TUBERCULOSIS

Spinal Tuberculosis (Pott's Disease)

Spinal TB is the most common type of osseous TB and nearly half of the bone and joint cases are due to spinal involvement. The next common site involved is the hip joint. Usually weight bearing joints are affected by TB.

Pathogenesis and Clinical Features

In spinal TB, lower thoracic and upper lumbar vertebrae are commonly affected, followed by middle thoracic and cervical region vertebrae. Usually, more than one adjacent vertebrae are involved and the body of the vertebra is predominantly affected rather than its other elements. The tubercle bacilli reach skeletal tissue as a result of hematogenous spread during primary tuberculous infection. Paradiskal, anterior and central vertebral lesions are commonly encountered. The disease originates in the cancellous area of bone close to the superior or the inferior end plates and extends into intervertebral disc after penetrating the subchondral bone plate and thence to the body of adjacent vertebra. With further progression, there occurs the demineralization of end plates and softening of body leading to vertebral collapse or anterior wedging **(Fig. 5)**. This is responsible for typical angulation or gibbus deformity in the spine seen in Pott's disease patients. The spread of disease may also follow subanterior longitudinal ligament route. The subligamentous downward spread of tuberculous abscess away from the primarily involved vertebrae can cause the destruction of anterior surface of other vertebral bodies.

The exudate tend to spread following the path of least resistance along with fascial planes, vasculature and nerves, and may present as cold abscesses elsewhere. Commonly, such abscesses are seen as a paravertebral abscess, psoas abscess in lumbar region, or abscess in iliac fossa **(Fig. 6)**, and some even gravitate below the inguinal ligament on medial side of thigh. Sometimes, it spreads laterally from the iliac fossa over the iliac crest. Rarely, it tracks with gluteal or femoral vessels to form gluteal or Scarpa's triangle abscess.[57]

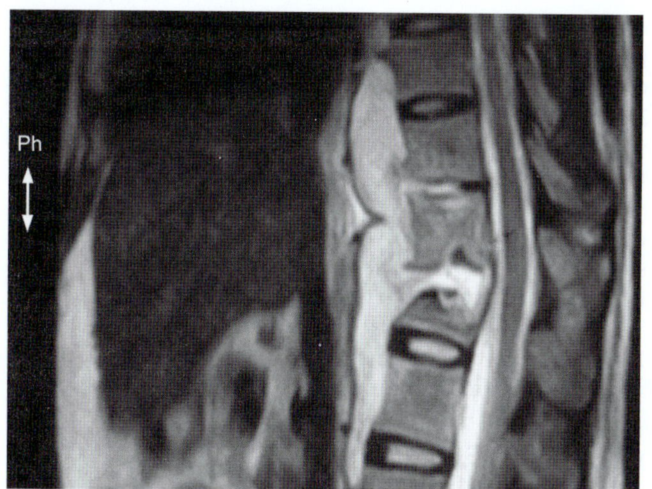

Fig. 5 Magnetic resonance image of young male suggests partial collapse of D12 vertebra with the involvement of intervening disks and prevertebral abscess suggesting spinal tuberculosis

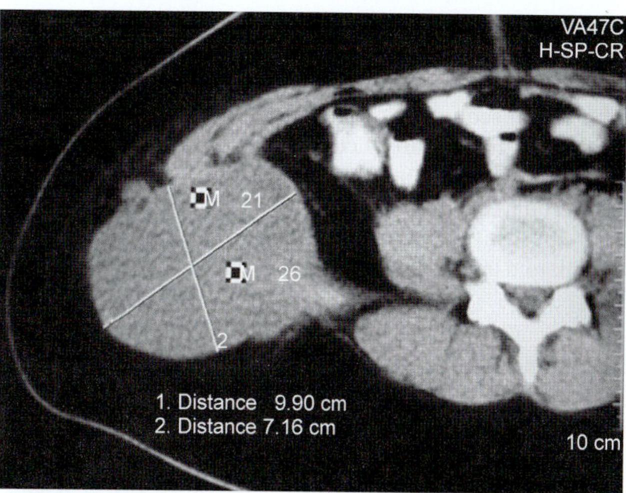

Fig. 6 Computed tomography (CT) scan pelvis reveals abscess in the right iliac fossa. There was pus collection both medial and lateral to right iliac bone. About 300 mL of pus was aspirated under ultrasound guidance and the pus was found positive for tubercle bacilli

If the cervical spine is involved with TB, the exudates track down in prevertebral area as a retropharyngeal abscess, which may mechanically cause deglutition and respiratory difficulty or hoarseness of voice. Accumulation of pus in the mediastinum may present as posterior mediastinal mass from where it can spread to the pleural cavity, esophagus or trachea.

Usual constitutional symptoms may be seen well before the localizing signs become actually perceivable in spinal TB. Often, local signs at the involved site or at the site of extended disease are more prominent. The characteristic clinical features include local pain, local tenderness, stiffness and spasm of the muscles progressing on to cold abscess and spinal deformity. The progression of disease is generally slow varying from few months to few years, average duration ranging from 4 months to 11 months. Neurological deficits are more common with the involvement of thoracic and cervical regions.

Paraplegia (Pott's paraplegia) develops in about 30% cases of Pott's disease.[57,58] Generally, it has been described as paraplegia of active disease (early onset paraplegia) and paraplegia of healed disease (late onset paraplegia). Early onset paraplegia develops during active disease due to mechanical pressure caused by formation of debris, pus and granulation tissue. Sometimes, nonmechanical causes are responsible for such neurological complications. Late onset paraplegia develops after a variable period in a patient with healed TB possibly due to the formation of a ridge of bone anterior to cord, fibrosis of dura mater or gliosis of cord, etc.[59]

Diagnosis

Plain radiography reveals narrowing or disappearance of disk space, area of destruction in the body and wedging or collapse of the vertebral bodies. The bony changes become perceivable on plain radiograph only about 5–6 months after the onset of pathology. However, CT and MRI scans may pick up such lesions quite early, also, the extent of associated complications is demarcated better with these investigations. The CT and MR imaging are particularly useful to study the status of the spinal cord or the canal and to pick up the involvement of posterior elements of vertebrae. Some of the complications, such as the prevertebral abscess in neck region and the typical fusiform abscess in the dorsal spine area, can also be appreciated better with such imaging techniques. CT scan is superior in detecting irregular lytic lesions, sclerosis, disc collapse, and disruption of bone circumference than the plain radiograph. MRI is the best diagnostic modality for Pott's spine.[60] Healed psoas abscess may show calcification too. Often, typical clinic-radiological or MR imagings are quite adequate to diagnose spinal TB. However, in atypical presentations, differentiation is necessary from conditions like pyogenic osteomyelitis, mycotic infection, syphilis, neoplasia, multiple myeloma, lymphoma, chondroma, metastasis, traumatic fracture or sarcoidosis, and others. In such situations, biopsy of the affected vertebra and culture of its contents would be necessary to clinch the diagnosis.

TUBERCULOUS ARTHRITIS

Tuberculous arthritis is typically a monoarticular disease, although multiple joint involvement has been described in literature.[57,61] About 15% of all skeletal TB cases are attributed by hip joint and about 10% cases by knee joint TB but shoulder joint is uncommonly involved. Involvement of joint may occur as a result of direct extension from adjacent tuberculous osteomyelitis or through hematogenous spread occurred during primary TB. Clinicopathological staging of joint TB usually decides the clinical features for that stage. Pain and circumferential limitation of joint movements are typical clinical features in such cases. Osteolytic areas, tuberculous sequestration along with the loss of the definition of articular margins are encountered in joint TB. In advanced stages, periarticular osteoporosis, peripheral bony erosions and gradual reduction in joint space constitute a radiological triad suggestive of joint TB. Often, pyogenic, fungal and rheumatoid arthritis may also need differentiation from joint TB.

Poncet's Disease

This is defined as parainfective polyarthritis in which active TB is located anywhere in the body, not necessarily in the affected joints and tubercle bacilli are never isolated from the involved joints. Commonly, the lymph node is the extra-articular site of active tuberculous disease.[61-63] This is basically a tuberculous hypersensitivity phenomenon, commonly accompanied by strongly positive TST or erythema nodosum. Mostly seen in children or young adults, it commonly involves knee, ankle, wrist, elbow, metacarpophalangeal and proximal interphalangeal joints. In addition to pain, swelling and tenderness of the involved joints, other constitutional features, fever, etc. are generally present. The joint synovial fluid is exudative type, sterile, negative for TB bacilli and even PCR is negative for *Mycobacterium* DNA. The condition responds very well to the standard drug treatment of primary tuberculous disease.

Tuberculosis Osteomyelitis

Osteomyelitis is usually seen in the bones of extremities involving small bones of hands and feet like phalanges, metacarpals and metatarsals. Although TB can involve any bone, the long bone disease is rare. The disease commonly presents with clinical features, such as pain, swelling with raised temperature, tenderness and boggy soft tissue at the involved site. An abscess or sinus may also be encountered over the involved bone. The condition often needs differentiation from chronic pyogenic osteomyelitis and neoplasia. The typical radiographic picture reveals honey combing, sequestration of diaphysis and subperiosteal new bone formation.

Treatment of Bone and Joint Tuberculosis

Overall consensus is that spinal TB without neurological involvement and without unsightly deformity is a medical condition. Combined management is the modality of choice, which comprises of orthopedic intervention by an orthopedician if necessary and TB drug therapy under supervision of a physician. The basic principles of TB drug therapy regimens essentially remain the same as for pulmonary TB. There have been some difference of opinion regarding the duration of therapy, the orthopedicians favored a longer duration 18–24 months of drug therapy in the past.[64,65] However, the evidence suggests that short-course chemotherapy of 9 months duration is quite adequate.[66,67] It is also recommended that 6-month short-course regimen with four drugs (HRZE) in the intensive 2 months phase and two drugs in the subsequent 4 months continuation phase is sufficient for the cure.[67] The latest WHO guidelines have also endorsed that pulmonary and EPTB should be treated with same regimens, but because there are technical difficulties in the assessment of treatment response of bone and joint TB, the 9-month treatment is recommended for such cases.[67] However, the duration of treatment can be prolonged according to clinical improvement on case to case basis.

CENTRAL NERVOUS SYSTEM TUBERCULOSIS

Although only about 5% of all EPTB cases are contributed by central nervous system-TB (CNS-TB), the latter has relatively high morbidity and mortality in comparison to other EPTB types. In developing countries, the prognosis of disease has been poor due to inadequate availability of diagnostic and treatment facilities in such cases. Human immunodeficiency virus has further compounded the risk for the development of CNS-TB. In one study its occurrence was found in up to 2 cases of 100 HIV-infected persons.[17]

Pathogenesis

Tubercle bacilli reach the brain parenchyma and the meninges during the stage of hematogenous spread of primary complex formation. Thereupon, these bacilli form tiny lesions prior to the development of delayed hypersensitivity or cell-mediated immunity. Consequent upon development of cell-mediated immunity, these lesions get resolved by natural healing in more than 95% cases. Later in life, such lesions may get reactivated and present with variety of different clinical forms of CNS-TB **(Table 1)**. Once reactivated, the foci may rupture into the subarachnoid space leading to arachnoiditis or grow intracranially as tuberculomas. Frequently, central nervous system-TB is the part of disseminated TB. Nearly, 20% of such patients have concomitant miliary TB. Occasionally, direct extension from TB of contiguous parts would lead to CNS-TB, like from skull bone TB, tuberculous otitis or spondylitis, etc. Rarely, extradural tuberculous abscess may occur with vault TB.[68] When tubercle bacilli enter the CSF, there occurs intense

Table 1 Different clinical forms of central nervous system (CNS) tuberculosis

- Meningitis—tuberculous brain abscess
- Tuberculoma—radiculomyelitis
- Arachnoiditis—behavioral abnormalities
- Encephalitis—demyelination
- Arteritis or vasculitis

inflammation of meninges, i.e. tuberculous meningitis and in TBM the meninges get covered with thick gelatinous gray exudate. The latter get extended to brainstem thereby affecting the cranial nerves. Cranial nerve palsies occur in 20–30% of patients and may be the presenting manifestation of TBM. The sixth cranial nerve is most commonly affected. Exudates further track down the spinal cord and spinal roots of the nerves. The thick gelatinous material also interferes with CSF drainage system, thereby causing hydrocephalus quite frequently.

Clinical Features

The TBM usually develops as a complication of primary TB, hence commonly seen in early childhood, but may occur at any age. The initial symptoms of disease are nonspecific in the form of loss of appetite, irritability, malaise, vomiting, headache, changed behavior, drowsiness or even convulsions. These features usually mark the prodromal stage of the disease, which may last for 2–8 weeks. Neck retraction or rigidity may be accompanied at this stage due to meningeal inflammation. In infants, fontanele may be found bulging on physical examination. Around 50% cases have papilledema, but usually without the loss of vision. Increasing hydrocephalus is responsible for decreasing consciousness and brain damage. Choroid tubercles may also be seen in some cases. Tuberculous meningitis patient can be classified in different clinical stages depending upon the level of consciousness and presence of neurological deficit **(Table 2)**.[69,70]

Diagnosis

Tuberculous meningitis often needs to be differentiated from other types of meningitis like bacterial, fungal, viral, carcinomatous or neurosyphilitic. The diagnosis is easy in the presence of suggestive clinical features and associated pulmonary or miliary TB, the conditions seen in more than half of such cases. The concomitant EPTB is more common in HIV-infected persons.

Cerebrospinal fluid findings play a vital role in the diagnosis of CNS-TB. Although CSF pressure is found elevated and papilledema is present, lumbar puncture can be performed safely because it is a chronic type of meningitis. White cell counts are raised with polymorph predominance initially, but lymphocytes take over in later stages. The counts are not elevated more than 500/mm^3. Usually, CSF is clear and its glucose level is less than 40% of the corresponding blood glucose level. Proteins in CSF are in the range of 100—200 mg/dL usually, although it may exceed 1 g/dL in the presence of spinal block due to coexisting spinal meningitis. If allowed to stand, one can see the cobweb formation in CSF. Chloride estimation in CSF is not helpful in differentiating TBM from viral or bacterial etiology. In about 5% of TBM cases, CSF may be normal also.

In the presence of HIV infection, CSF remains unremarkable and is not helpful in making of the diagnosis. Nevertheless, CSF must be sent in HIV-infected patients for acid-fast bacilli (AFB) culture, as it may come out to be positive in up to 50% cases. Sterile CSF culture for bacteria, fungi and negative gram staining are supportive of TBM diagnosis. A cut off level of more than 10 U/L, CSF-ADA has sensitivity of 92.5% and specificity of 97% for the diagnosis of TBM.[58] Values more than 8 U/L (sensitivity less than 59% and specificity greater than 96%) improve the diagnosis of TBM (p less than 0.001).[71] Polymerase chain reaction test for *M. tuberculosis* among Indian patients had sensitivity of 44.5% and specificity 92% in the most likely TBM cases.[72] The WHO has endorsed automated, heminested real-time PCR Xpert MTB/Rif over other conventional tests for diagnosis of TB meningitis.[27]

Computed tomography scan and MRI imaging often demonstrate findings in CNS-TB, such as thickening and enhancement of basal meninges, small granulomas, infarcts and basal exudates, hydrocephalus, periventricular edema, tuberculous abscess and tuberculoma **(Fig. 7)**. MRI images are particularly useful in differentiating TB from fungal, viral and bacterial disease. These are quite helpful in reaching the diagnosis as well as for following the progress of treatment. Serial CT scans performed for assessing the course may sometimes reveal new tuberculomas or accentuation of those pre-existing during TB drug therapy, the phenomenon commonly recognized as paradoxical response to TB drug therapy.[73,74] However, such accentuated lesions get resolved gradually with the continuation of the same chemotherapy. A substantial series has recently described the radiological features of paradoxical neurological TB-IRIS in HIV-infected patients with tuberculomas.[75]

Table 2 Contemporary criterion for staging of tuberculous meningitis (TBM)[70]

Stage	*Criterion*
I	Alert and oriented without focal neurological deficits
II	Glasgow coma score 14–11 or 15 with focal neurological deficits
III	Glasgow coma score 10 or less, with or without focal neurological deficits

Treatment

Tuberculous meningitis is a serious form of TB in the terms of morbidity and mortality, hence a better prognosis can only be anticipated if the disease is detected at an early stage and right treatment is initiated without wasting time. Isoniazid, pyrazinamide and ethionamide penetrate the blood-brain barrier (BBB) adequately; rifampicin enters poorly while streptomycin and ethambutol cross BBB adequately only when meninges are inflamed. Four drugs (HRZS/E) should be included in the intensive phase. Ethambutol is avoided

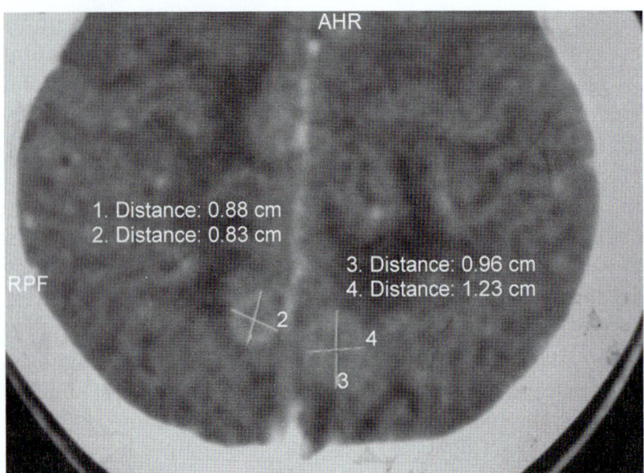

Fig. 7 Contrast-enhanced computed tomography (CECT) head showing hypodense lesions with rim shadow in a typical case of tuberculoma

in comatose patients because vision cannot be monitored. Therefore, streptomycin should be substituted for ethambutol accordingly. Intrathecal streptomycin is no longer used. The optimum duration of TB drug therapy in TBM is still debatable. Even in the absence of randomized controlled trials to compare the efficacy of 6 months verses 12 months regimens, the meta-analysis of available literature suggests that 6-month regimens are as affective as longer duration regimens provided the bacteria are fully susceptible to first line drugs.[76] However, chemotherapy for 9–12 months of treatment is recommended for TBM, because of the serious risk of mortality and morbidity.[76,77]

The use of corticosteroids is somewhat controversial. Although its use does not benefit stage I, but it improves prognosis in stage II and III disease. Therefore, if nothing is suggestive of drug resistance and fungal etiology is ruled out, corticosteroid should be used as adjuvant to TB drug therapy in stage II and III TBM.[77] In adults, dexamethasone 0.4 mg/kg/24 hours can be given, with a tapering course over 6–8 weeks. A recent Cochrane review supports the routine use of corticosteroids in HIV-negative patients with TBM to reduce mortality and disabling residual neurological deficits, however, adequate evidence is yet not available in favor or against a similar conclusion for those who are HIV-positive.[78] Surgery is sometimes necessary for the management of hydrocephalus, as an early drainage improves the outcome.[79] Surgical drainage of intracranial or extradural abscess will also be necessary.[80] Tuberculomas usually regress with chemotherapy; therefore, a trial of at least 2 months drug therapy must be given before surgery.

ABDOMINAL TUBERCULOSIS

Abdominal TB encompasses TB of gastrointestinal tract (GIT) anywhere from esophagus to anus, peritoneum, mesentery, omentum, mesenteric lymph nodes, hepatobiliary system, spleen and pancreas. The entity accounts for 3% of all EPTB cases. In abdominal TB concomitant pulmonary lesions are also found in about 25% of cases. As EPTB is more commonly encountered in HIV-infected cases in general, the incidence is expected to increase with an increase in the HIV incidence. A prechemotherapy era autopsy series of pulmonary TB cases had revealed intestinal involvement in 55–90% cases, and the disease was more common in the presence of extensive pulmonary involvement.

Pathogenesis

The tuberculous infection can reach the abdominal organs through hematogenous spread during its primary infection stage, due to swallowing of tubercle bacilli loaded sputum in pulmonary TB patients, through direct extension from adjacent organ harboring TB and occasionally by lymphatics spread. Transmission through milk from cattle suffering with bovine TB is not common these days due to the universal practice of pasteurization or boiling of milk before consumption. Further, the intestinal disease in India is primarily caused by *Mycobacterium tuberculosis* and not by *Mycobacterium bovis*.[81]

The most common site for abdominal TB is the ileocecal region possibly because of the abundance of lymphoid tissue in the Peyer's patches, physiological stasis and minimal digestive work undertaken in this part of intestine allowing more stagnation time to bacilli for invasion. The disease spreading from lymph nodes, intestine or from fallopian tubes usually leads to peritoneal TB. In about 30% cases, lymph node and peritoneal TB may be seen even without the intestinal disease.[82]

When TB bacilli reach intestine, they are trapped in the Peyer's patches and consequently granuloma formation takes place therein. These granulomas grow and get confluent with each other. The inflammation spreads to the submucosa, and then mucosa overlying the inflamed Peyer's patches ulcerate. These ulcers are superficial, do not penetrate beyond muscularis propria.[83] As the ulcers are transversely placed covering a ring of the intestinal mucosa and so, they are appropriately named as girdle ulcers. The ulcers may be single or multiple, the mucosa in between the girdle ulcers is quite healthy and termed as skip lesion. Subsequently stricture formation ensues when these ulcers heal by fibrosis. These strictures called "napkin ring strictures," are often responsible for intestinal obstruction. Other areas in intestine may show no granuloma formation, but for chronic inflammation. Sometimes, there occurs excessive inflammation and fibrosis causing adhesions of gut, mesentery and lymph nodes, altogether assuming a shape of a mass which may erroneously appear as neoplasm.

Grossly, intestinal TB is classified as ulcerative, ulcero-hyperplastic and hyperplastic type. While ulcerative and hyperplastic forms (stricture form) are seen in small intestine, ulcerohyperplastic form is found in colon and ileocecal region. Tuberculous peritonitis occurs in different forms; ascitic, encysted, fibrinous. It sometimes gives a feel as an abdominal mass comprising of a mesentery and thickened omentum. Gross examination on laparotomy or laparoscopy exhibits straw-colored fluid, multiple yellow-white tubercles scattered over peritoneum or greater omentum and the peritoneum lacks its usual shine and hyperemia.[84] The involved abdominal lymph nodes may be seen enlarged and matted with or without caseation. Granulomas are commonly found in the lymph nodes.

Clinical Features

Clinical presentation of abdominal TB is quite protean, may mimic many acute or chronic intestinal ailments. Nearly two-thirds cases of abdominal TB are young adults of 20–40 years of age with slight preponderance for female gender. The onset of symptoms may be acute, chronic or acute on chronic. Often, about one-third present as acute abdomen with pain in right iliac fossa mimicking acute appendicitis or as acute intestinal obstruction, while the remaining two-thirds have insidious onset with symptoms like pain in abdomen. Constitutional symptoms such as low grade fever, malaise, anorexia and weight loss are often present. Pain in abdomen is seen in around 80–95% cases, while alternate constipation and diarrhea are seen in about 9–20% cases. Other features like a moving ball of wind in abdomen, nausea, vomiting and malena may also be found. Features of malabsorption are also encountered in some cases.

No characteristic physical signs are described for abdominal TB, the popular classical "doughy" feel of the abdomen has only been observed in 6–11% cases in Indian series, however, not reported in some large series.[85] Right iliac tenderness like that in acute appendicitis or lump in this region mimicking carcinoma or appendicular abscess may be felt in these cases. The signs of acute or subacute small intestinal obstruction like abdominal distension, vomiting and absolute constipation with or without a palpable mass may be encountered as per the pathological stage of the disease. Many other clinical features ensue depending upon the involved organ or the site and type of involvement.

Diagnosis

Clinical presentation of abdominal TB is quite nonspecific and usually overlapping with malignant or inflammatory bowel diseases. Nevertheless, a high index of suspicion particularly arises in persons hailing from high-burden countries with suggestive constitutional symptoms and evidence of pulmonary or EPTB lesions. Anemia, reduced serum albumin (less than 3.5 g/dL) or raised C-reactive proteins and positive TST are usually detected, but not concluding investigations. Thus, the only disease site specific clinical features, radiological and USG findings, pathological lesions (both gross and microscopic) and isolation of mycobacteria, altogether are necessary for clinching the authentic diagnosis in majority of the cases. The following radio imaging techniques are substantially helpful in arriving at the diagnosis of abdominal TB.

- *Chest radiograph:* Concomitant pulmonary lesions either healed or active have been reported in 25–80% of abdominal TB cases.[83,86,87] There may be features suggestive of pulmonary TB, pleural effusion or mediastinal lymphadenopathy. In such situation, effort should be made to demonstrate tubercle bacilli in sputum, bronchoalveolar lavage (BAL) or gastric lavage samples in children. The presence of tuberculous lesion elsewhere in the body supports the diagnosis of abdominal TB.
- *Plain abdominal radiograph:* The presence of certain findings, such as multiple air fluid levels with distended bowel loops (intestinal obstruction), ascites, perforation or intussusception and calcified nodes indirectly support the diagnosis.
- *Small bowel barium study:* Hypersegmentation of barium column also called as chicken intestine, stiffened and thickened folds, luminal stenosis with smooth and stiff contours (hour glass stenosis), and multiple strictures with the segmental dilatation of intestinal loops are various suggestive signs. However, similar findings may also be encountered in Crohn's disease
- *Barium enema:* The thickened ileocecal valve gives a broad triangular picture having base toward cecum, popularly known as "inverted umbrella" sign. Extreme irritability due to ulceration results in rapid movement of barium, hence no barium contrast is visualized in inflamed segments of the ileum, cecum and ascending colon with normal column of barium on other side, also described as "Stierlin's sign". Whenever there is stenosis in the gut, a very narrow string of the contrast is visualized, known as "String sign". Both Stierlin's and String's signs may also be positive in Crohn's disease, hence are not specific for TB.
- *Ultrasonography:* Ultrasound is helpful in picking up the ascites (either loculated or free), thickened omentum and retroperitoneal or mesenteric lymphadenopathy. Ultrasonographic guidance for investigations like FNAC or fluid tapping always adds to the diagnostic yield.
- *CT scan:* It can show circumferential thickening of the wall of cecum and terminal ileum. Also, the ulceration and nodularity in terminal ileum along with narrowing and proximal dilatation may be visualized. Other abnormalities like obstruction, perforation and abscess can also be seen on CT scan. In tuberculous ascites, fluid density is usually very high, i.e. around 25–45 HU due to high protein content of the fluid. Peritoneal thickening and nodules may also be seen.

To confirm the diagnosis, we need to demonstrate TB bacilli in peritoneal fluid or typical histopathological picture in the biopsy taken through laparotomy. Blind percutaneous needle biopsy of peritoneum can also be performed. However, biopsy under direct visualization is always safer as it averts complication like gut perforation and gives a high diagnostic yield. Laparoscopy is the procedure of choice for biopsy, but minilaparotomy would be preferable in the presence of intense plastic peritonitis and extensive adhesions. Colonoscopic FNAC may be taken from the ileocecal lesions to improve its yield. Ascitic fluid is straw-colored, exudative with total cell count of around 150–4,000/mm^3 along with lymphocytes being more than 50%. Ascitic fluid TB bacilli positivity rate is usually less than 20%. The culture positivity could be improved up to 83%, when at least 1 liter fluid was centrifuged and subjected to culture for tubercle bacilli.[88] Ascitic fluid ADA level of more than 40 U/L is highly supportive of tuberculous etiology. High level of interferon gamma in ascitic fluid is also suggestive of tuberculous etiology. The role of immunological investigations for diagnosis of TB is still undefined.

Treatment

The treatment is essentially same as for pulmonary TB. All patients of abdominal TB should be treated with short-course chemotherapy for 6 months duration. The standard regimen includes four drugs (HRZE) in the initial 2-month intensive phase followed by two drugs (HR) in the 4-month continuation phase. 6 months short-course chemotherapy compared with 12 months chemotherapy regimen, achieved cure in 99% cases.[89] Six-month regimen is the standard regimen for the treatment of abdominal TB as per the recommendation of the Joint TB Committee of the British Thoracic Society.[67]

The routine use of adjuvant corticosteroid is not advisable in such cases.[85] Surgery in the form of intestinal resection and end-to-end anastomosis, is occasionally required, only if there is mechanical obstruction.[85,90,91] It is particularly indicated for strictures of longer than 12 cm with involvement at multiple sites. Obstructive intestinal lesions may respond to chemotherapy alone, without surgery. In one report, 91% patients had clinical improvement and 70% had complete radiological resolution while only 8% required surgery at the completion of chemotherapy.[92] Sometimes, the obstructive symptoms may increase initially, but only to regress ultimately. On an average, it takes around 6 months for the amelioration of obstructive symptoms.

GENITOURINARY TUBERCULOSIS

Genitourinary TB (GUTB) is a significant problem in the developing world and around 9% of all EPTB cases in India are estimated to be suffering from GUTB.[2] Often, the disease continues to progress late because of the delayed diagnosis.[18] Most GUTB patients present with renal failure, bladder and ureteric strictures, which could have been easily averted, had there been timely diagnosis and treatment there upon. Three to four percent cases of pulmonary TB also have concomitant GUTB commonly involving kidneys, bladder, urethra, and genital tract.[2]

Pathogenesis and Clinical Features of Urological Tuberculosis

The disease usually occurs during the second and fourth decade of life. Kidney is usually the primary organ infected in urinary disease, and other parts of the urinary tract become involved by direct extension of pathology. Epididymis in men and fallopian tubes in women are the primary sites of genital TB. The usual order of organ involvement is kidney, bladder, fallopian tube and scrotum.[93] The most common clinical presentation of urological TB is sterile pyuria and painless hematuria. Patient may present incidentally or with the symptoms of dysuria, hematuria, frank pyuria, fever and renal mass. These features are quite suggestive of urinary tract infection but for any isolation of common bacterial growth on culture.

The mycobacterial infection reaches kidneys and other urogenital organs during the stage of hematogenous spread of primary TB. These bacilli form tiny lesions as tubercles in the organs which heal either spontaneously or with treatment, only to get activated after the years of dormancy. The granulomas formed in the kidneys enlarge and rupture, leading on to bacilluria. The infection then spreads downward to the calyces, pelvis, ureter and bladder. The lesions in ureter may lead to ureteric stenosis particularly in distal region giving rise to obstructive uropathy, which ultimately results in tuberculous pyonephrosis. The bladder involvement causes features of cystitis and bladder wall fibrosis. The latter results in the marked reduction of bladder capacity commonly termed as thimble bladder deformity. The reduced bladder capacity is responsible for the frequency of micturition and nocturia.

Pathogenesis and Clinical Features of Gynecological Tuberculosis

Infertility, either primary or secondary is a common presentation of female genital TB. In India, one-third cases of tubal disease infertility are attributed to TB.[94] Alterations in menstrual pattern (menorrhagia, amenorrhea or postmenopausal bleeding, etc.) are common features in such patients. Female genital TB may sometime be mistaken for ovarian malignancy. The differentiation is further complicated by the presence of high levels of cancer antigen 125 (CA-125), which is also described in gynecological TB. Primary female genital TB is rare, usually seen when the male partner suffers from active genitourinary TB.[95,96] Mostly, genital TB is almost always secondary to TB elsewhere in the body. Commonly the infection spread directly from active abdominal tuberculous pathology.

Diagnosis

Sterile pyuria should raise the suspicion of GUTB. Urine culture for mycobacteria of particularly three consecutive early morning samples give better yield. The intravenous pyelography is an important investigation for the diagnosis of urological TB. The pyelogram may reveal abnormalities, such as the calyceal clubbing and pelviureteric junction stenosis with pelvic dilatation. Calcification in urinary tract and prostate may support the diagnosis of TB. Hydronephrosis and sometime small kidney may be seen on USG. Urinary tract and kidney abnormalities can also be picked on CT scanning. Sometimes, perinephric or psoas abscess may also be encountered. In males, the involvement of vas deferens will give a beaded feel on palpation and a draining scrotal sinus can also be found.

Diagnosis is confirmed by growing tubercle bacilli from urine or biopsy tissue culture. Urine for tubercle bacilli is usually not rewarding. Moreover, the positive microscopy may also raise the suspicion of contamination in laboratory reagents either by *Mycobacterium smegmatis*, a saprophytic mycobacteria or of environmental mycobacteria. Diagnosis of female genital TB is made with the help of multiple investigations, including the menstrual blood culture, FNAC, endometrial curettage and laparoscopic biopsy as per an algorithm defined for use in the developing countries.[73,97] Recently, PCR has also been shown as an important diagnostic tool.[98]

Treatment

Standard 6-month TB chemotherapy is advised, however controlled clinical trials are lacking for short-course chemotherapy in GUTB.[99] Adjuvant corticosteroids are recommended to avert ureteric stricture formation. Steroids have also been found helpful in the treatment of tuberculous interstitial nephritis.[100] Sometimes surgery such as nephrectomy is necessary for destroyed nonfunctioning kidney. Partial nephrectomy, ureteric stricture dilatation and bladder reconstruction may be required as per the indication in some cases. A full course of anti-TB chemotherapy is essential in addition to surgery. For female infertility, an early institution of antitubercular therapy based on diagnosis by PCR positivity alone has been recommended to prevent later sequelae.[101]

SKIN TUBERCULOSIS

Skin TB contributes 1–2.5% share of all skin disease cases and the ailment is more commonly found in poor socioeconomic strata of the society.[102,103] The skin may be involved by TB through different modes.

Clinical Features

There are three main types of skin TB determined by the presence of previous sensitization to tubercle bacilli, immune response of the host and route of inoculation by tubercle bacilli. In order of frequency, these are lupus vulgaris, TB verrucosa cutis and scrofuloderma. These three types are seen in persons who had previously been infected with tubercle bacilli and have delayed hypersensitivity to the tubercle bacilli. In absence of previous sensitization, the disease may occur in the form of tuberculous chancres and miliary TB of skin. Tuberculids are the hypersensitivity lesions of skin, which occur as a result of TB elsewhere in the body.

- *Lupus vulgaris:* It is the most common variety of skin TB, which is present with firm plaques that exhibit central clearing and activity at margins **(Fig. 8)**. The active margins show erythematous translucent papules, popularly described as apple-jelly nodules. Most often, the lesions are dry, but sometimes seropurulent discharge and crust formation may be seen. Long-standing lesions may occasionally get complicated with squamous cell carcinoma. Usually, the lesions are encountered over the face, buttocks and lower limbs. Sometimes, underlying TB in the deeper tissues may extend in the skin as lupus vulgaris.

  Bacillus Calmette-Guérin (BCG) vaccination may rarely get complicated as lupus vulgaris. Often, patients do not have constitutional symptoms and TST is usually positive in such cases. Typical clinical features, demonstration of *Mycobacterium* in the smear or biopsy, classical TB granuloma and response to the therapeutic trial authenticate the diagnosis. Skin TB can be adequately treated with standard 6-month short-course chemotherapy.[104]
- *Scrofuloderma:* It is the most common form in which TB involves the skin as a direct extension of the underlying tuberculous pathology of lymph nodes, bones or urogenital tract.[104-106]
- *Chancre:* This is a primary infection of skin, which occurs as a result of accidental inoculation of abraded or injured skin by tubercle bacilli. Commonly seen in children of the family having member suffering from sputum-positive pulmonary TB. The lesions are often seen over the limbs.

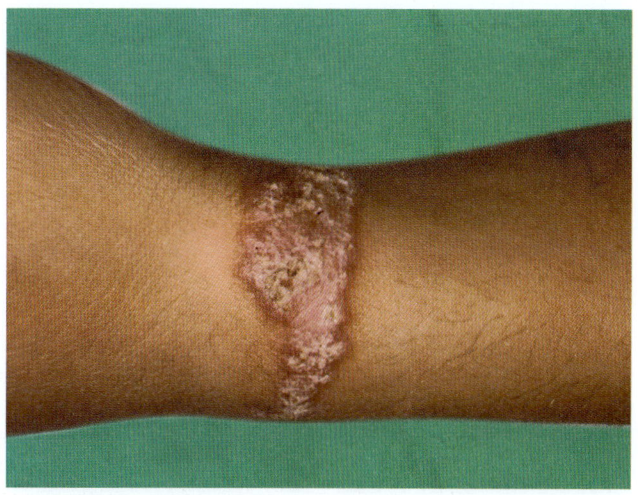

Fig. 8 Lupus vulgaris lesion showing central scarring and peripherally active lesion in upper limb just above the wrist

At the outset, a papilla or a nodule develops locally, which ulcerates subsequently. Simultaneously, there occurs enlargement of regional lymph nodes. This cutaneous lesion and regional lymphadenopathy together constitute the primary complex. Lesions usually heal spontaneously or may progress into lupus vulgaris. The biopsy from early lesions shows neutrophils and tubercle bacilli, however, typical tuberculous granulomas are seen later.

- *Miliary tuberculosis of skin:* Early skin lesions, consequent upon hematogenous spread of tubercle bacilli during primary infection, often go dormant or get healed with the development of immunity. These lesions get reactivated in the form of pustules and papules later in life whenever there occurs immunosuppression, e.g. during measles or viral infections. Usually, constitutional symptoms of TB are present along with such lesions.
- *Tuberculids:* Four diagnostic criteria must be fulfilled to qualify for the confirmed diagnosis of tuberculids—on biopsy, the lesion should have tuberculoid granuloma; *Mycobacterium* should not be seen in the lesion; Mantoux test is strongly positive; treatment of underlying TB should ameliorate the tuberculid skin lesions. There are four types of tuberculids described—lichen scrofulosorum, erythema induratum, papulonecrotic tuberculids and erythema nodosum with different morphological features **(Fig. 9)**.

MILIARY TUBERCULOSIS

Miliary tuberculosis is a disseminated form in which discrete millet seed size tuberculous foci are found homogeneously distributed in the lungs and other viscera.[19,107-109] Classical miliary mottling on chest radiograph is the familiar picture which supports the diagnosis. It is the cryptic variant, which poses a diagnostic dilemma even in the endemic area. Sometimes, the disease may present as acute respiratory distress syndrome (ARDS), therefore, the tuberculous etiology must be kept in mind, particularly when no obvious cause is available for the same.

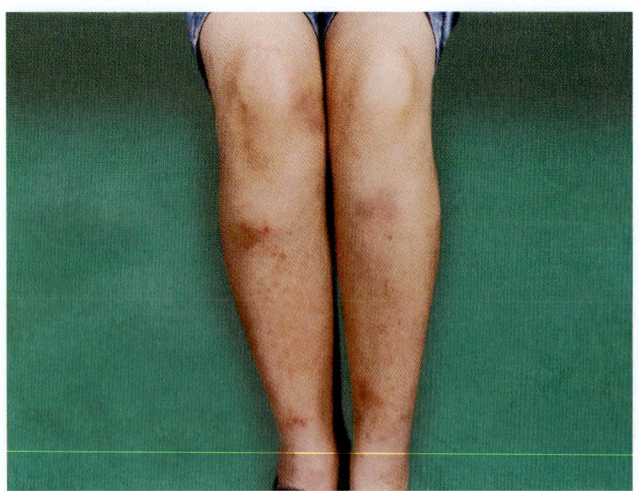

Fig. 9 Erythema nodosum over shin area in a 16-year-old girl suffering from tuberculous lymphadenitis

Pathogenesis

Commonly during the stage of hematogenous spread of primary TB, the tubercle bacilli get disseminated to various viscera particularly the highly vascularized organs like the lung, liver, spleen, bone marrow and brain. There upon, the bacilli develop discrete tuberculous foci in these organs. However, with development of immunity and delayed hypersensitivity, these foci heal in majority of the subjects. But in a few cases, healing fails and the disease progresses to acute miliary form of TB. In endemic areas, the miliary TB is seen in young children, however, in developed countries, majority of such patients are seen in the elderly population. Miliary TB can also come up later in life when healed primary foci, after getting reactivated with caseation necrosis, erode into the blood vessels. The erosion of active focus in blood vessel causes hematogenous embolization of tubercle bacilli giving rise to disseminated tuberculous foci all over the body. Microscopically, in an immunocompetent person, each focus represents a typical tubercle with caseation in the center comprising of Langhans type of giant cells, epithelioid cells, lymphocytes, fibrocytes and AFB. However, in immune-suppressed subjects or elderly persons, the appearance is often a nonreactive type lesion, which shows necrosis teaming with tubercle bacilli but without typical granuloma formation.

Clinical Features

The miliary TB has slight preponderance for male gender. Symptoms develop gradually and include generalized constitutional features along with spiky fever and chills. Nearly 6–8% of all EPTB cases are miliary TB cases. There are two main clinical variants of miliary TB, viz. acute miliary and cryptic miliary.

- *Acute miliary tuberculosis:* In addition to the usual constitutional features, headache may be encountered, possibly due to coexisting TBM, thus a lumbar puncture must be performed in patients with headache. Hemoptysis and dyspnea are not frequently seen in such cases. Hepatosplenomegaly and icterus may be present. Often, chest examination is unremarkable, but minimal pleural and pericardial effusions may be seen in some cases. Fundus should be looked for choroid tubercles. The latter seen as pale, grayish white, oblong patches and are frequently bilateral. These were encountered in 7.2% cases only in one series.

Demonstration of choroid tubercle is highly supportive of the diagnosis of miliary TB, however, the finding is more common in children. Tuberculomas may commonly complicate miliary TB. Adrenal insufficiency has also been

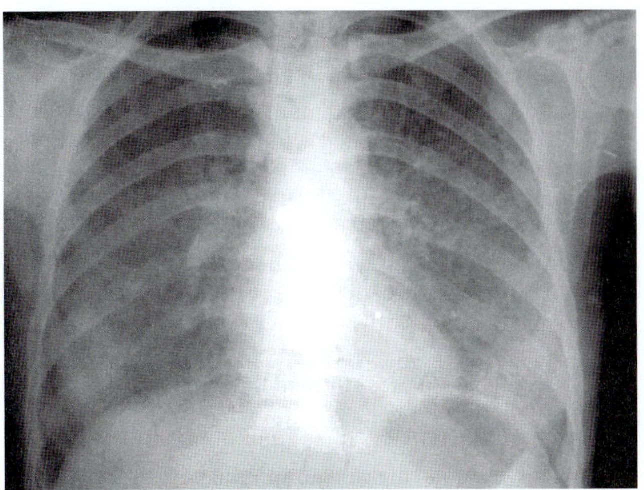

Fig. 10 The chest radiograph posterior-anterior view showing typical miliary tuberculosis in a young male

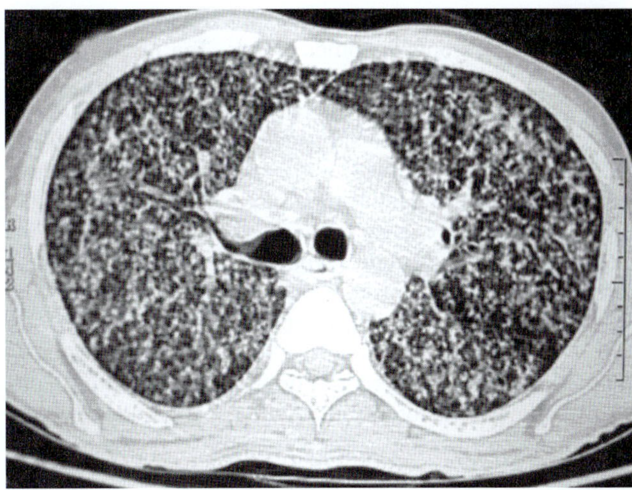

Fig. 11 High-resolution computed tomography (HRCT) thorax shows extensive miliary nodules in both lungs

commonly described in miliary TB. The chest radiograph reveals typical miliary pattern, i.e. homogeneously distributed discrete uniform size (1–2 mm) millet-shaped lesions in all lung zones **(Figs 10 and 11)**.

- *Cryptic miliary tuberculosis:* Cryptic is an atypical presentation of miliary TB in which chest radiograph does not reveal classical miliary mottling. The entity is usually encountered in elderly patients of over 60 years of age, but may be seen in the younger age group also, particularly in the endemic areas. The symptoms which usually appear insidiously, include weight loss, intermittent fever, malaise and mild hepatosplenomegaly. Meningitis and choroid tubercles are very uncommon features in this variant of miliary TB. A high index of suspicion in mind of the treating doctor is the only way for its timely diagnosis

Diagnosis

Classical miliary mottling on chest radiograph is most helpful finding for making the diagnosis of miliary TB, although the same may not be seen in early stages or in the cryptic miliary variant. In such situations, characteristic picture on high resolution computed tomography (HRCT) is very helpful. Sometimes, CXR picture just like that seen in ARDS or acute lung injury and shadows larger than usual miliary mottling may also be encountered. For confirmation of diagnosis, all efforts must be exhausted to isolate tubercle bacilli from various specimens such as sputum, pleural fluid, CSF, urine, BAL fluid, blood and histopathological samples. TST is often negative in these patients. In one series, tuberculin anergy was reported in 68% cases of miliary TB.[110]

Blood dyscrasias like pancytopenia and leukemoid reactions are commonly seen in the cryptic form of miliary TB. Sometimes, bone marrow examination is required, particularly in the presence of leukemoid reaction. Bone marrow aspiration may reveal granulomas or even *Mycobacterium tuberculosis*. Liver biopsy provides the highest yield, wherein granulomas have been reported in up to 75% cases. In unconfirmed cases, particularly when the patient is not willing for invasive procedure, therapeutic trial with anti-TB drugs must be given. Fever usually subsides within 7–10 days of starting anti-TB drugs but overall clinicoradiological improvement is appreciated only after 4–6 weeks of treatment. Early diagnosis is imperative for favorable outcome of treatment of miliary TB, which is uniformly fatal if untreated.[110,111]

Treatment

In principle, the standard 6-month treatment for pulmonary TB is adequate for miliary TB also. The standard regimens comprise of initial 2-month intensive phase of isoniazid, rifampicin, pyrazinamide and ethambutol (or streptomycin) followed by 4 months continuation phase of isoniazid plus rifampicin. 9-months regimen is recommended in infants and children.[112] Unequivocal evidence is lacking for the use of corticosteroid in the treatment of miliary TB.

PERICARDIAL TUBERCULOSIS

Tuberculous involvement of pericardium is usually secondary to TB elsewhere in the body. Nearly 1–8% of pulmonary TB patients have concomitant pericardial TB. Out of all acute pericarditis cases, about 4% in developed countries and 60–80% cases in the developing countries are due to tuberculous pathology.[113,114]

Pathogenesis

Direct extension from tuberculous mediastinal lymphadenitis is the most common route for the involvement of pericardium. The infection may also reach pericardium through lymphatic and hematogenous routes from tuberculous lesions of lungs, kidneys, bones or other organs. The pericardium is infrequently involved by breakdown and contiguous spread from a tuberculous lesion in the lung. Pericardial TB has following four pathological stages—(1) dry pericarditis; (2) effusive pericarditis; (3) absorptive and (4) constrictive pericarditis stage. Patient may present during any stage of the pathological progress. Invariably, the pericardial fluid is straw colored and exudative type; very rarely there could be frank pus in the pericardium due to intense inflammation. The pericardium may contain somewhere between 15 mL and 3500 mL of fluid. When the fluid collection occurs at very rapid rate, the patient may develop cardiac tamponade. Within a few weeks of development of pericardial effusion, there occurs thickening especially of the visceral pericardium resulting into effusive constrictive pericarditis. In the absence of effective anti-TB therapy, progressive fibrosis may lead to chronic constrictive pericarditis. Complete obliteration of pericardium due to fibrosis interferes with the proper cardiac functioning. Sometimes, the disease may involve the myocardium, ultimately leading to its myonecrosis and muscle atrophy. Around 15% of patients show pericardial calcification, but it is reported in around 75% in some studies.[115,116]

Clinical Features

The disease is usually seen during third to fifth decades of life. Gradual onset tuberculous toxemia with anorexia, weight loss, malaise, low-grade evening temperature, and early fatigability are usual presentations of pericardial TB. In around 20% cases, pericardial effusion may present as acute cardiac tamponade with tachycardia, high jugular venous pressure and feeling of retrosternal compression. Shortness of breath, chest pain and edema feet may be seen in around 40–70% cases.[117-119] Cardiac auscultation reveals muffled heart sounds and pericardial rub. Echocardiography is an important aid to confirm the diagnosis.

Effusive-constrictive pericarditis patients usually show cardiomegaly, edema feet and elevated jugular venous pressure. In chronic constrictive pericarditis, there occurs the impediment of venous return due to tough encasement of the heart; however, heart shape and size remain normal. This causes pulmonary and systemic congestion leading ultimately to shortness of breath, orthopnea with edema, ascites and pulsus paradoxus. Long-standing elevation of venous pressure may cause protein-losing enteropathy and resultant hypoproteinemia. Ascites is more prominent, called ascites praecox.[120]

Diagnosis

Idiopathic or viral pericarditis is a common condition, which needs to be distinguished from tuberculous pericarditis. The former conditions are usually acute in onset, have minimal or no effusion, and are self-limiting in 2–3 weeks. On the contrary, more prolonged course and large effusion are frequent in tuberculous pericarditis. Chest radiograph may reveal cardiomegaly, pericardial calcification and pulmonary disease. Whenever associated with pulmonary TB, sputum must be examined for tubercle bacilli. Electrocardiography changes of acute pericarditis such as ST elevation were seen in only 10% cases in some studies.[118,121] Echocardiography is a good test for detecting effusion and cardiac tamponade, although, not very accurate in picking up pericardial thickening. CT and MRI are other important adjuncts in helping the diagnosis.[122]

Pericardiocentesis is performed for diagnostic tests of the fluid as well as for therapeutic purpose in cardiac tamponade. Pericardiocentesis should preferably be done under echocardiography employing apical approach. Pericardial fluid characteristics are exactly the same as encountered in tuberculous pleural effusion as far as its physical, cellular, TB bacilli isolation, or ADA level, etc. are concerned, and the same diagnostic standards are applicable for both the conditions (**Table 3**).[123,124] Pericardial tissue taken by open biopsy may reveal typical granulomas with caseation necrosis in around 60% cases.

Treatment

If not treated, the disease is almost fatal and even with specific treatment the mortality is 3–14%. Medical treatment using standard 6-month short-course TB chemotherapy is successful in achieving the cure.[115,125] Addition of corticosteroids has been found associated with reduction in the frequency of pericardiocentesis and mortality.[115,125,126] Therefore, all patients of tuberculous pericarditis, barring contraindications should get 40–60 mg of prednisolone daily for 4–6 weeks with subsequent tapering over a 5-week period. Pericardiocentesis is life-saving in cardiac tamponade, but recurrent effusion may require pigtail catheter placement. Some cases may require pericardiotomy

Table 3 Proposed diagnostic criteria for tuberculous pericarditis[124]

Category and criteria
• *Definite tuberculous pericarditis* Tubercle bacilli are found in stained smear or culture of pericardial fluid; and/or Tubercle bacilli or caseating granuloma are found on histological examination of pericardium
• *Probable tuberculous pericarditis* Evidence of pericarditis in a patient with tuberculosis demonstrated elsewhere in the body; and/or Lymphocytic pericardial exudate with elevated ADA activity; and/or Good response to antituberculosis chemotherapy

and cardiopulmonary bypass may be necessary in cases with extensive calcification.[40]

HEPATIC TUBERCULOSIS

Hepatic TB is relatively uncommon form of extrapulmonary TB. It is secondary to pulmonary or gastrointestinal TB. Hepatic involvement has been reported in 10–15% of patients with pulmonary TB, and commonly found in patients with disseminated TB.[127] Hepatic TB generally occurs due to the reactivation of an old tuberculous focus, or on rare occasions as a result of a primary hepatic infection.[128,129] Tubercle bacilli reach the liver by way of hematogenous dissemination; the portal of entry in case of miliary TB is through the hepatic artery whereas in the case of focal liver TB, it is via the portal vein. The tuberculous liver abscess is an uncommon presentation in patients with hepatic TB.[128]

The clinical diagnosis of hepatic TB is difficult. Usually, symptoms and signs in this condition are nonspecific. Other than the constitutional symptoms, abdominal pain is present in 65–87% and jaundice in 20–35% patients. The jaundice may be caused by extra or intrahepatic biliary obstruction.[130] Hepatomegaly is frequently encountered. The laboratory investigations frequently reveal increase in alkaline phosphatase with normal transaminases.[131] USG finding of tuberculous liver abscess consists of a hypoechoic mass lesion in the liver, CT scan findings show a hypodense lesion with peripheral enhancement and central nonenhancing necrotic area.[127] The definitive diagnosis of tuberculous liver abscess needs microbiological and pathological examination of the specimen from the abscess. Aspiration of the liver lesion under the guidance of USG or CT can provide a precise specimen for confirmation.

Hepatic TB is treated with similar standard 6-month regimen (2HRZE/S, 4HR) as for other forms of TB. Drainage is occasionally required, especially for large abscess. Most of the lesions, including the abscess resolve with chemotherapy, provided an early treatment is instituted.

REFERENCES

1. Zumla A, George A, Sharma V, Herbert N, Baroness Masham of I. WHO's 2013 global report on tuberculosis: successes, threats, and opportunities. Lancet. 2013;382(9907):1765-7.
2. Sharma SK, Mohan A. Extrapulmonary tuberculosis. Indian J Med Res. 2004;120(4):316-53.
3. Fanning A. Tuberculosis: 6. Extrapulmonary disease. CMAJ. 1999;160(11):1597-603.
4. National survey of tuberculosis notifications in England and Wales in 1983: characteristics of disease. Report from the Medical Research Council Tuberculosis and Chest Diseases Unit. Tubercle. 1987;68(1):19-32.
5. National survey of notifications of tuberculosis in England and Wales in 1988. Medical Research Council Cardiothoracic Epidemiology Group. Thorax. 1992;47(10):770-5.
6. Weir MR, Thornton GF. Extrapulmonary tuberculosis. Experience of a community hospital and review of the literature. Am J Med. 1985;79(4):467-78.
7. Pitchenik AE, Fertel D, Bloch AB. Mycobacterial disease: epidemiology, diagnosis, treatment, and prevention. Clin Chest Med. 1988;9(3):425-41.
8. Snider DE, Roper WL. The new tuberculosis. N Engl J Med. 1992;326(10):703-5.
9. Diagnostic Standards and Classification of Tuberculosis in Adults and Children. This official statement of the American Thoracic Society and the Centers for Disease Control and Prevention was adopted by the ATS Board of Directors, July 1999. This statement was endorsed by the Council of the Infectious Disease Society of America, September 1999. Am J Respir Crit Care Med. 2000;161(4 Pt 1):1376-95.
10. Raviglione MC, Narain JP, Kochi A. HIV-associated tuberculosis in developing countries: clinical features, diagnosis, and treatment. Bull World Health Organ. 1992;70(4):515-26.
11. Theuer CP, Hopewell PC, Elias D, Schecter GF, Rutherford GW, Chaisson RE. Human immunodeficiency virus infection in tuberculosis patients. J Infect Dis. 1990;162(1):8-12.
12. Haas DW, Des Prez RM. Tuberculosis and acquired immunodeficiency syndrome: a historical perspective on recent developments. Am J Med. 1994;96(5):439-50.
13. Snider DE, Onorato M. Epidemiology. In: Rossman MD, MacGregor (Eds). Tuberculosis: clinical management and new challenges. New York: McGraw-Hill; 1995. pp. 3-17.
14. World Health Organization. (2014). WHO TB data. [online] Available from *https://extranet.who.int/sree/Reports?op=Repletandname=%2FWHO_HQ_Reports%2FG2%2FPROD%2FEXT%2FTBCountryProfileandISO2=INandLAN=ENandouttype=html.* [Accessed January, 2016].
15. Talbot EA, Moore M, McCray E, Binkin NJ. Tuberculosis among foreign-born persons in the United States, 1993-1998. JAMA. 2000;284(22):2894-900.
16. Corbett EL, Steketee RW, ter Kuile FO, Latif AS, Kamali A, Hayes RJ. HIV-1/AIDS and the control of other infectious diseases in Africa. Lancet. 2002;359:2177-87.
17. Berenguer J, Moreno S, Laguna F, Vicente T, Adrados M, Ortega A, et al. Tuberculous meningitis in patients infected with the human immunodeficiency virus. N Engl J Med. 1992;326(10):668-72.
18. Mesquita M, Libertalis M, Bakoto ES, Vandenhoute K, Damry N, Guillaume MP. Late diagnosis of extra-pulmonary tuberculosis leads to irreversible kidney failure in a non-immunocompromised patient. Int Urol Nephrol. 2010;42:227-32.
19. Yu YL, Chow WH, Humphries MJ, Wong RW, Gabriel M. Cryptic miliary tuberculosis. Q J Med. 1986;59(228):421-8.
20. Lin JN, Lai CH, Chen YH, Lee SS, Tsai SS, Huang CK, et al. Risk factors for extra-pulmonary tuberculosis compared to pulmonary tuberculosis. Int J Tuberc Lung Dis. 2009;13(5):620-5.
21. Kwara A, Roahen-Harrison S, Prystowsky E, Kissinger MR, Adams R, Mathison J, et al. Manifestations and outcome of extra-pulmonary tuberculosis: impact of human immunodeficiency virus co-infection. Int J Tuberc Lung Dis. 2005;9(5):485-93.
22. Sekar B, Selvaraj L, Alexis A, Ravi S, Arunagiri K, Rathinavel L. The utility of IS6110 sequence based polymerase chain reaction in comparison to conventional methods in the diagnosis of extra-pulmonary tuberculosis. Indian J Med Microbiol. 2008;26:352-5.
23. Bhigjee AI, Padayachee R, Paruk H, Hallwirth-Pillay KD, Marais S, Connoly C. Diagnosis of tuberculous meningitis: clinical and laboratory parameters. Int J Infect Dis. 2007;11:348-54.

24. Dandapat MC, Mishra BM, Dash SP, Kar PK. Peripheral lymph node tuberculosis: a review of 80 cases. Br J Surg. 1990;77:911-2.
25. Lange C, Sester M. TB or not TB: the role of immunodiagnosis. Eur J Immunol. 2012;42(11):2840-3.
26. Steingart KR, Flores LL, Dendukuri N, Schiller I, Laal S, Ramsay A, et al. Commercial serological tests for the diagnosis of active pulmonary and extrapulmonary tuberculosis: an updated systematic review and meta-analysis. PLoS Med. 2011;8:e1001062.
27. Denkinger CM, Schumacher SG, Boehme CC, Dendukuri N, Pai M, Steingart KR. Xpert MTB/RIF assay for the diagnosis of extrapulmonary tuberculosis: a systematic review and meta-analysis. Eur Respir J. 2014;44:435-46.
28. Sharma SK, Kohli M, Chaubey J, Yadav RN, Sharma R, Singh BK, et al. Evaluation of Xpert MTB/RIF assay performance in diagnosing extrapulmonary tuberculosis among adults in a tertiary care centre in India. Eur Respir J. 2014.
29. Subrahmanyam M. Role of surgery and chemotherapy for peripheral lymph node tuberculosis. Br J Surg. 1993;80:1547-8.
30. Jawahar MS, Sivasubramanian S, Vijayan VK, Ramakrishnan CV, Paramasivan CN, Selvakumar V, et al. Short course chemotherapy for tuberculous lymphadenitis in children. BMJ. 1990;301(6748):359-62.
31. Manolidis S, Frenkiel S, Yoskovitch A, Black M. Mycobacterial infections of the head and neck. Otolaryngol Head Neck Surg. 1993;109:427-33.
32. Lee KC, Tami TA, Lalwani AK, Schecter G. Contemporary management of cervical tuberculosis. Laryngoscope. 1992;102:60-4.
33. Cantrell RW, Jensen JH, Reid D. Diagnosis and management of tuberculous cervical adenitis. Arch Otolaryngol. 1975;101(1):53-7.
34. Rose AM, Watson JM, Graham C, Nunn AJ, Drobniewski F, Ormerod LP, et al. Tuberculosis at the end of the 20th century in England and Wales: results of a national survey in 1998. Thorax. 2001;56(3):173-9.
35. Kumar D, Watson JM, Charlett A, Nicholas S, Darbyshire JH. Tuberculosis in England and Wales in 1993: results of a national survey. Public Health Laboratory Service/British Thoracic Society/Department of Health Collaborative Group. Thorax. 1997;52:1060-7.
36. Thompson MM, Underwood MJ, Sayers RD, Dookeran KA, Bell PR. Peripheral tuberculous lymphadenopathy: a review of 67 cases. Br J Surg. 1992;79:763-4.
37. Powel DA. Tuberculous lymphadenitis. In: Schlossberg D, (Ed). Tuberculosis and nontuberculous mycobacterial infection. Philadelphia: WB Saunders Co; 1999. pp. 186-94.
38. Bem C. Human immunodeficiency virus-positive tuberculous lymphadenitis in Central Africa: clinical presentation of 157 cases. Int J Tuberc Lung Dis. 1997;1:215-9.
39. Valdes L, Pose A, San Jose E, Marti, nez Vazquez JM. Tuberculous pleural effusions. Eur J Intern Med. 2003;14:77-88.
40. Campbell IA, Ormerod LP, Friend JA, Jenkins PA, Prescott RJ. Six months versus nine months chemotherapy for tuberculosis of lymph nodes: final results. Respir Med. 1993;87:621-3.
41. Huhti E, Brander E, Paloheimo S, Sutinen S. Tuberculosis of the cervical lymph nodes: a clinical, pathological and bacteriological study. Tubercle. 1975;56:27-36.
42. Campbell IA, Dyson AJ. Lymph node tuberculosis: a comparison of various methods of treatment. Tubercle. 1977;58:171-9.
43. Short course chemotherapy for tuberculosis of lymph nodes: a controlled trial. British Thoracic Society Research Committee. Br Med J (Clin Res Ed). 1985;290(6475):1106-8.
44. Berzosa M, Tsukayama DT, Davies SF, Debol SM, Cen YY, Li R, et al. Endoscopic ultrasound-guided fine-needle aspiration for the diagnosis of extra-pulmonary tuberculosis. Int J Tuberc Lung Dis. 2010;14(5):578-84.
45. Jindal SK, Aggarwal AN, Gupta D, Ahmed Z, Gupta KB, Janmeja AK, et al. Tuberculous lymphadenopathy: a multicentre operational study of 6-month thrice weekly directly observed treatment. Int J Tuberc Lung Dis. 2013;17(2):234-9.
46. Indumathi CK, Prasanna KK, Dinakar C, Shet A, Lewin S. Intermittent short course therapy for pediatric tuberculosis. Indian Pediatr. 2010;47:93-6.
47. Janmeja AK, Das SK. Cervico-mediastinal lymphadenopathy as a paradoxical response to chemotherapy in pulmonary tuberculosis. A case report. Respiration. 2003;70(2):219-20.
48. Light RW. Management of pleural effusions. J Formos Med Assoc. 2000;99:523-31.
49. Ferrer J. Pleural tuberculosis. Eur Respir J. 1997;10:942-7.
50. Aggarwal AN, Gupta D, Jindal SK. Diagnosis of tuberculous pleural effusion. Indian J Chest Dis Allied Sci. 1999;41(2):89-100.
51. Sharma SK, Mitra DK, Balamurugan A, Pandey RM, Mehra NK. Cytokine polarization in miliary and pleural tuberculosis. J Clin Immunol. 2002;22:345-52.
52. Light RW. Update on tuberculous pleural effusion. Respirology (Carlton, Vic). 2010;15:451-8.
53. Porcel JM. Tuberculous pleural effusion. Lung. 2009;187:263-70.
54. Barbas CS, Cukier A, de Varvalho CR, Barbas Filho JV, Light RW. The relationship between pleural fluid findings and the development of pleural thickening in patients with pleural tuberculosis. Chest. 1991;100:1264-7.
55. Engel ME, Matchaba PT, Volmink J. Corticosteroids for tuberculous pleurisy. Cochrane Database Syst Rev. 2007.
56. Sahn SA, Iseman MD. Tuberculous empyema. Semin Respir Infect. 1999;14:82-7.
57. Malaviya AN, Kotwal PP. Arthritis associated with tuberculosis. Best Pract Res Clin Rheumatol. 2003;17:319-43.
58. Bhan S, Nag V. Skeletal tuberculosis. In: Sharma SK, Mohan A (Eds). Tuberculosis. New Delhi: Jaypee Brothers Medical Publishers (P) Ltd.; 2001.
59. Garg RK, Somvanshi DS. Spinal tuberculosis: a review. J Spinal Cord Med. 2011;34(5):440-54.
60. Ansari S, Amanullah MF, Ahmad K, Rauniyar RK. Pott's spine: Diagnostic imaging modalities and technology advancements. N Am J Med Sci. 2013;5(7):404-11.
61. Parkinson RW, Hodgson SP, Noble J. Tuberculosis of the elbow: a report of five cases. J Bone Joint Surg Br. 1990;72:523-4.
62. Janmeja AK, Mohapatra PR, Kaur R. Subungual erythema in lymph node tuberculosis with erythema nodosum. J Assoc Physicians India. 2005;53:903-5.
63. Arora VK, Verma V. Tuberculous rheumatism: Three case reports. Indian J Tuberc. 1991;38:229-31.
64. Hodgson AR, Stock FE, Fang HS, Ong GB. Anterior spinal fusion. The operative approach and pathological findings in 412 patients with Pott's disease of the spine. Br J Surg. 1960;48:172-8.
65. Valdazo JP, Perez-Ruiz F, Albarracin A, Sanchez-Nievas G, Perez-Benegas J, Gonzalez-Lanza M, et al. Tuberculous arthritis. Report of a case with multiple joint involvement and

periarticular tuberculous abscesses. J Rheumatol. 1990; 17(3):399-401.

66. Dutt AK, Moers D, Stead WW. Short-course chemotherapy for extrapulmonary tuberculosis. Nine years' experience. Ann Intern Med. 1986;104:7-12.
67. Chemotherapy and management of tuberculosis in the United Kingdom: recommendations 1998. Joint Tuberculosis Committee of the British Thoracic Society. Thorax. 1998;53(7):536-48.
68. Hodgson SP, Ormerod LP. Ten-year experience of bone and joint tuberculosis in Blackburn 1978-1987. J R Coll Surg Edinb. 1990;35:259-62.
69. Kennedy DH, Fallon RJ. Tuberculous meningitis. JAMA. 1979;241:264-8.
70. Thwaites GE, Tran TH. Tuberculous meningitis: many questions, too few answers. Lancet neurology. 2005;4:160-70.
71. Tuon FF, Higashino HR, Lopes MI, Litvoc MN, Atomiya AN, Antonangelo L, et al. Adenosine deaminase and tuberculous meningitis—a systematic review with meta-analysis. Scand J Infect Dis. 2010;42(3):198-207.
72. Rana SV, Chacko F, Lal V, Arora SK, Parbhakar S, Sharma SK, et al. To compare CSF adenosine deaminase levels and CSF-PCR for tuberculous meningitis. Clin Neurol Neurosurg. 2010;112(5):424-30.
73. Ravenscroft A, Schoeman JF, Donald PR. Tuberculous granulomas in childhood tuberculous meningitis: radiological features and course. J Trop Pediatr. 2001;47:5-12.
74. Chambers ST, Hendrickse WA, Record C, Rudge P, Smith H. Paradoxical expansion of intracranial tuberculomas during chemotherapy. Lancet. 1984;2:181-4.
75. Marais S, Scholtz P, Pepper DJ, Meintjes G, Wilkinson RJ, Candy S. Neuroradiological features of the tuberculosis-associated immune reconstitution inflammatory syndrome. Int J Tuberc Lung Dis. 2010;14:188-96.
76. van Loenhout-Rooyackers JH, Keyser A, Laheij RJ, Verbeek AL, van der Meer JW. Tuberculous meningitis: is a 6-month treatment regimen sufficient? Int J Tuberc Lung Dis. 2001;5:1028-35.
77. Caminero JA, de March P. Statements of ATS, CDC, and IDSA on treatment of tuberculosis. Am J Respir Crit Care Med. 2004;169:316-7.
78. Prasad K, Singh MB. Corticosteroids for managing tuberculous meningitis. Cochrane Database Syst Rev. 2008:CD002244.
79. Thwaites GE, Nguyen DB, Nguyen HD, Hoang TQ, Do TT, Nguyen TC, et al. Dexamethasone for the treatment of tuberculous meningitis in adolescents and adults. N Engl J Med. 2004;351(17):1741-51.
80. Peacock WJ, Deeny JE. Improving the outcome of tuberculous meningitis in childhood. S Afr Med J. 1984;66:597-8.
81. Wig KL, Chitkara NL, Gupta SP, Kishore K, Manchanda RL. Ileocecal tuberculosis with particular reference to isolation of Mycobacterium tuberculosis. With a note on its relation to regional ileitis (Crohn's disease). Am Rev Respir Dis. 1961;84:169-78.
82. Hoon JR, Dockerty MB, Pemberton Jde J. Ileocecal tuberculosis including a comparison of this disease with nonspecific regional enterocolitis and noncaseous tuberculated enterocolitis. Int Abstr Surg. 1950;91:417-40.
83. Tandon RK, Sarin SK, Bose SL, Berry M, Tandon BN. A clinico-radiological reappraisal of intestinal tuberculosis-changing profile? Gastroenterol Jpn. 1986;21(1):17-22.
84. Bhargava DK, Shriniwas, Chopra P, Nijhawan S, Dasarathy S, Kushwaha AK. Peritoneal tuberculosis: laparoscopic patterns and its diagnostic accuracy. Am J Gastroenterol. 1992;87: 109-12.
85. Klimach OE, Ormerod LP. Gastrointestinal tuberculosis: a retrospective review of 109 cases in a district general hospital. Q J Med. 1985;56:569-78.
86. Prakash A. Ulcero-constrictive tuberculosis of the bowel. Int Surg. 1978;63:23-9.
87. Kapoor VK, Chattopadhyay TK, Sharma LK. Radiology of abdominal tuberculosis. Australas Radiol. 1988;32:365-7.
88. Gulati MS, Sarma D, Paul SB. CT appearances in abdominal tuberculosis. A pictorial essay. Clin Imaging. 1999;23(1): 51-9.
89. Balasubramanian R, Nagarajan M, Balambal R, Tripathy SP, Sundararaman R, Venkatesan P, et al. Randomised controlled clinical trial of short course chemotherapy in abdominal tuberculosis: a five-year report. Int J Tuberc Lung Dis. 1997;1(1): 44-51.
90. Byrom HB, Mann CV. Clinical features and surgical management of ileocaecal tuberculosis. Proc R Soc Med. 1969;62: 1230-3.
91. Addison NV. Abdominal tuberculosis–a disease revived. Ann R Coll Surg Engl. 1983;65:105-11.
92. Anand BS, Nanda R, Sachdev GK. Response of tuberculous stricture to antituberculous treatment. Gut. 1988;29(1):62-9.
93. Balasubramanian R, Ramachandran R. Management of non-pulmonary forms of tuberculosis: review of TRC studies over two decades. Indian J Pediatr. 2000;67:S34-40.
94. Parikh FR, Nadkarni SG, Kamat SA, Naik N, Soonawala SB, Parikh RM. Genital tuberculosis–a major pelvic factor causing infertility in Indian women. Fertil Steril. 1997;67:497-500.
95. Bazaz-Malik G, Maheshwari B, Lal N. Tuberculous endometritis: a clinicopathological study of 1000 cases. Br J Obstet Gynaecol. 1983;90:84-6.
96. Siegler AM, Kontopoulos V. Female genital tuberculosis and the role of hysterosalpingography. Semin Roentgenol. 1979;14:295-304.
97. Jindal UN. An algorithmic approach to female genital tuberculosis causing infertility. Int J Tuberc Lung Dis. 2006;10:1045-50.
98. Jindal UN, Bala Y, Sodhi S, Verma S, Jindal S. Female genital tuberculosis: early diagnosis by laparoscopy and endometrial polymerase chain reaction. Int J Tuberc Lung Dis. 2010;14:1629-34.
99. Gow JG, Barbosa S. Genitourinary tuberculosis. A study of 1117 cases over a period of 34 years. Br J Urol. 1984;56:449-55.
100. Morgan SH, Eastwood JB, Baker LR. Tuberculous interstitial nephritis–the tip of an iceberg? Tubercle. 1990;71:5-6.
101. Jindal UN, Verma S, Bala Y. Favorable infertility outcomes following anti-tubercular treatment prescribed on the sole basis of a positive polymerase chain reaction test for endometrial tuberculosis. Hum Reprod. 2012;27(5):1368-74.
102. Kumar B, Muralidhar S. Cutaneous tuberculosis: a twenty-year prospective study. Int J Tuberc Lung Dis. 1999;3:494-500.
103. Ramesh V, Misra RS, Jain RK. Secondary tuberculosis of the skin. Clinical features and problems in laboratory diagnosis. Int J Dermatol. 1987;26:578-81.
104. Yates VM, Ormerod LP. Cutaneous tuberculosis in Blackburn district (U.K.): a 15-year prospective series, 1981-95. Br J Dermatol. 1997;136:483-9.

105. Kumar B, Rai R, Kaur I, Sahoo B, Muralidhar S, Radotra BD. Childhood cutaneous tuberculosis: a study over 25 years from northern India. Int J Dermatol. 2001;40:26-32.
106. Goldman SM, Fishman EK, Hartman DS, Kim YC, Siegelman SS. Computed tomography of renal tuberculosis and its pathological correlates. J Comput Assist Tomogr. 1985;9:771-6.
107. Mohan A, Sharma SK, Pande JN. Acute respiratory distress syndrome (ARDS) in miliary tuberculosis: a twelve years experience. Indian J Chest Dis Allied Sci. 1996;38:157-62.
108. Sharma SK, Mukhopadhyay S, Arora R, Varma K, Pande JN, Khilnani GC. Computed tomography in miliary tuberculosis: comparison with plain films, bronchoalveolar lavage, pulmonary functions and gas exchange. Australas Radiol. 1996;40:113-8.
109. Sharma SK, Mohan A, Pande JN, Prasad KL, Gupta AK, Khilnani GC. Clinical profile, laboratory characteristics and outcome in miliary tuberculosis. QJM. 1995;88(1):29-37.
110. Jacques J, Sloan JM. The changing pattern of miliary tuberculosis. Thorax. 1970;25:237-40.
111. Kim JH, Langston AA, Gallis HA. Miliary tuberculosis: epidemiology, clinical manifestations, diagnosis, and outcome. Rev Infect Dis. 1990;12:583-90.
112. American Academy of Pediatrics Committee on Infectious Diseases: Chemotherapy for tuberculosis in infants and children. Pediatrics. 1992;89(1):161-5.
113. Dalvi B. Tuberculous pericarditis. JAMA. 1992;267(7):931-2.
114. Strang JI. Tuberculous pericarditis in Transkei. Clin Cardiol. 1984;7:667-70.
115. Strang JI, Kakaza HH, Gibson DG, Girling DJ, Nunn AJ, Fox W. Controlled trial of prednisolone as adjuvant in treatment of tuberculous constrictive pericarditis in Transkei. Lancet. 1987;2:1418-22.
116. Talwar JR, Bhatia ML. Constrictive pericarditis. In: Ahuja MMS (Ed). Progress in Clinical Medicine in India. New Delhi: Arnold-Heinemann; 1981.
117. Bashi VV, John S, Ravikumar E, Jairaj PS, Shyamsunder K, Krishnaswami S. Early and late results of pericardiectomy in 118 cases of constrictive pericarditis. Thorax. 1988;43:637-41.
118. Fowler NO. Tuberculous pericarditis. JAMA. 1991;266:99-103.
119. Kothari SS, Juneja R. Tuberculosis and the heart. In: Sharma SK, Mohan A (Eds). Tuberculosis. New Delhi: Jaypee Brothers Medical Publishers (P) Ltd; 2001.
120. Rooney JJ, Crocco JA, Lyons HA. Tuberculous pericarditis. Ann Intern Med. 1970;72:73-81.
121. Permanyer-Miralda G, Sagrista-Sauleda J, Soler-Soler J. Primary acute pericardial disease: a prospective series of 231 consecutive patients. Am J Cardiol. 1985;56:623-30.
122. Sengupta PP, Eleid MF, Khandheria BK. Constrictive pericarditis. Circ J. 2008;72(10):1555-62.
123. Arroyo M, Soberman JE. Adenosine deaminase in the diagnosis of tuberculous pericardial effusion. Am J Med Sci. 2008;335:227-9.
124. Mayosi BM, Burgess LJ, Doubell AF. Tuberculous pericarditis. Circulation. 2005;112:3608-16.
125. Cohen H, Niedman L, Cohen A, Soto O, Castillo A, Brodsky M. Useful elements in the differential diagnosis of acute pericarditis of idiopathic purulent tuberculous origin. Rev Med Chil. 1969;97:517-22.
126. Fredriksen RT, Cohen LS, Mullins CB. Pericardial windows or pericardiocentesis for pericardial effusions. Am Heart J. 1971;82:158-62.
127. Hayashi M, Yamawaki I, Okajima K, Tomimatsu M, Ohkawa S. Tuberculous liver abscess not associated with lung involvement. Intern Med. 2004;43:521-3.
128. Patanakar T, Prasad S, Armao D, Mukherji SK. Tuberculous abscesses of the liver. AJR Am J Roentgenol. 2000;174:1166-7.
129. Mert A, Ozaras R, Tabak F, Ozturk R, Bilir M. Localized hepatic tuberculosis. Eur J Intern Med. 2003;14:511-2.
130. Balsarkar D, Joshi MA. Isolated tuberculous hepatic abscess in a non-immunocompromised patient. J Postgrad Med. 2000;46:108-9.
131. Huang WT, Wang CC, Chen WJ, Cheng YF, Eng HL. The nodular form of hepatic tuberculosis: a review with five additional new cases. J Clin Pathol. 2003;56:835-9.

Multidrug-resistant Tuberculosis

Surendra K Sharma, Dinkar Bhasin

INTRODUCTION

Tuberculosis (TB) despite being a curable infectious disease remains the leading cause of preventable death worldwide. Even with the advent of newer and better diagnostic tools for diagnosis of pulmonary as well as extrapulmonary TB, it is still a major global health concern. With over 1.5 million people dying in 2013 because of TB, the death toll for this disease is unacceptably high.[1] Globally, 3.5% of new TB cases and 20.5% of previously treated cases have been estimated to have multidrug-resistant TB (MDR-TB).[1] Of the reported MDR-TB cases, 9% were reported to have extensively drug-resistant TB (XDR-TB). Most of the XDR-TB cases in 2013 were reported from Ukraine, South Africa, India and Kazakhstan.[1] An estimated 13% of the total number of people who developed TB were human immunodeficiency virus (HIV) positive. The African region accounts for about every four out of the five HIV-TB cases and TB deaths among people who were HIV-positive.[1] Numerous efforts are being made globally to curb the disease; however, multidrug-resistant and extensively drug-resistant strains of tubercle bacilli have posed a major setback in controlling TB.

Drug-resistant TB (DR-TB) has emerged due to selection of mutant strains of the bacteria. The major cause can be attributed to improper administration of the antitubercular therapy and treatment regimen of the drug-susceptible patients and also failure to adherence to the treatment regimen.

DEFINITIONS

Multidrug-resistant TB is defined when the bacilli isolated from a clinical specimen are resistant to rifampicin and isoniazid with or without resistance to any other first-line antitubercular drug. Rifampicin, because of its rapid bactericidal activity, forms the backbone of any treatment regimen. Isolated resistance to rifampicin is quite rare without isoniazid resistance. Therefore, rifampicin is taken as a surrogate marker for MDR-TB and if the clinical specimen is resistant to rifampicin, the patient is put on MDR-TB treatment.

Microbiological isolates depicting resistance to isoniazid, rifampicin, one fluoroquinolone (ofloxacin, levofloxacin, or moxifloxacin) and a second-line injectable antitubercular drug (kanamycin, amikacin, or capreomycin) are labeled XDR-TB.[2]

Recently, TB bacilli have been isolated that have shown resistance to all know antitubercular drugs. These strains have been characterized as totally drug-resistant TB (TDR-TB) or XDR-TB, and have also been isolated from India.[3]

BASIS OF DRUG-RESISTANCE

Drug resistance can be classified as primary or acquired. Primary drug resistance refers to the cases, which have previously never received anti-TB treatment. Acquired drug resistance cases are those, which have previously been given anti-TB drugs in the past.[4]

From a molecular perspective, drug-resistant strains of *Mycobacterium tuberculosis* arise from spontaneous background chromosomal mutations occurring at low frequency.[5-7] Selection pressure that is caused by irrational use of anti-TB drugs like monotherapy or the addition of single drugs to failing regimens, results in the emergence of resistant mutants. Various genes are responsible for resistance to anti-TB drugs. These genes are enlisted in **Table 1**. Mutations in some genes are more common than the others. For instance, mutations in *katG* gene are majorly responsible for high level of isoniazid resistance. It has an important clinical implication that if the mutation pattern for the drug is known, respective dosage of the drug can be administered.[8] It needs to be emphasized that DR-TB occurs as a result of improper anti-TB therapy; hence, proper regimen, efficacious drugs and good adherence to treatment can help curb the problem of DR-TB. Causes of inappropriate treatment of DR-TB have been summarized in **Table 2**.

Mechanism of total drug-resistant (TDR) strains has been studied; it has been observed that the cell wall of these bacilli is thicker than the MDR-TB isolates.[9] The TDR strains are well adapted at the cellular level with pili-like structures protruding from the body of the bacillus.[10]

Table 1 Genes related to resistance of antitubercular drugs[11]

Drug	Genes involved in drug resistance
Isoniazid	Enoyl-acyl carrier protein (*acp*) reductase (*inhA*), catalase-peroxidase (*katG*)*, alkyl hydroperoxide reductase (*ahpC*), oxidative stress regulator (*oxyR*), β-ketoacyl-acyl carrier protein synthase (*kasA*)
Rifampicin	RNA polymerase subunit B (*rpoB*)
Pyrazinamide	Pyrazinamidase (*pncA*)
Streptomycin	Ribosomal protein subunit 12 (*rpsL*) 16s ribosomal RNA (*rrs*) Aminoglycoside phosphotransferase gene (*strA*)
Capreomycin	Hemolysin (*hlyA*)
Ethambutol	Arabinosyltransferase (*emb A, emb B* and *emb C*)
Fluoroquinolones	DNA gyrase (*gyr A* and *gyr B*)
Kanamycin	*rrs* A1401G mutation, aminoglycosideacetyltransferase encoding gene *(eis)*
Linezolid	Chloramphenicol-florfenicol resistance gene *(cfr)* methyltransferase
Bedaquiline	*atpE* gene
Cross resistance between clofazamine and bedaquiline	*rv068* gene
* katG gene is associated with high-level resistance	

Table 2 Causes of inappropriate treatment of drug-resistant tuberculosis[11]

Causes	*Description*
Patients: Inadequate drug intake	Poor adherence (or poor direct observation of treatment) Lack of information Lack of money (no free treatment available) Lack of transportation Side effects Social barriers Malabsorption of antituberculosis drugs Substance abuse disorders
Drugs: Inadequate supply/quality	Poor quality Unavailability of certain drugs (stockouts or delivery disruptions) Poor storage conditions Wrong dose or combination
Providers/Programs: Inadequate regimens	Absence of guidelines Inappropriate guidelines Noncompliance with available guidelines Poor training of the drug providers No monitoring of treatment Poorly organized or funded TB control programs
Abbreviation: TB, tuberculosis	

EPIDEMIOLOGY

According to the World Health Organization (WHO) Tuberculosis Report, 2013, there were 8.6 million incident TB cases globally with South-east Asia and Western Pacific regions contributing 58% of cases, India's share being 26%.[1] Globally, 3.5% of new and 20.5% of previously treated TB cases were estimated to have had MDR-TB in 2013.[1] This translates into an estimated 480,000 people having developed MDR-TB in 2013. On average, an estimated 9.0% of patients with MDR-TB had XDR-TB. India had an estimated 2.2% of new MDR-TB cases in the year 2013 and 15% retreatment cases with MDR-TB.[1]

The XDR-TB outbreak in KwaZulu-Natal, South Africa, in 2006 caught global attention on this deadly form of TB.[12] From the WHO Tuberculosis Report, 2013, 75 countries and five territories reported data about the proportion of MDR-TB cases, which had XDR-TB.[1] This is a grim situation as the facility for second-line drug susceptibility testing (DST) is available only in limited centers across the world and the real burden of XDR-TB is unknown. Various studies were conducted to determine the prevalence of MDR-TB in new cases and previously treated cases in India. **Tables 3 and 4** summarize the data of these studies.

In September 2014, the Health Minister of India launched a National Anti-Tuberculosis Drug Resistance Survey, India 2014–15 to provide information on drug resistance TB in new and patients undergoing treatment. The survey has been conducted on 5,214 patients across the country. It provides better management of DR-TB in the country and also keeps track of the defaulters.

DIAGNOSIS

Efficient and rapid diagnostic modalities are the cornerstone of any disease management. Detection of MDR and XDR-TB is purely based on laboratory diagnosis. The diagnosis of DR-TB requires isolation and culture of the tubercle

Table 3 Prevalence of multidrug-resistant tuberculosis among the new cases of pulmonary tuberculosis in India

Location	Period of study	No. of isolates	MDR-TB (%)
Bengaluru[13]	1980s	436	1.1
Wardha[14]	1982–89	323	5.3
North Arcot[15]	1985–89	2,779	1.6
Puducherry[15]	1985–91	1,841	0.8
Kolar[16]	1987–89	292	3.4
Jaipur[17]	1989–91	1,009	0.9
New Delhi[18]	1990–91	324	0.6
Pune[19]	1992–93	473	1.0
Tamil Nadu[20]	1997	384	3.4
North Arcot[21]	1999	282	2.8
Hyderabad[22]	2001–03	714	0.14
Ernakulam[23]	2004	305	2
Gujarat[24]	—	1,571	2.4
Delhi[25]	2008–09	177	1.1
Punjab[26]	2006–2010	121	9.9

Abbreviation: MDR-TB, multidrug-resistant tuberculosis

Table 4 Prevalence of multidrug-resistant tuberculosis among the previously treated cases of pulmonary tuberculosis in India

Location	Period of study	No. of isolates	MDR-TB (%)
Gujarat[27]	1983–86	1259	30.2
Delhi[18]	1990–91	81	33.3
Haryana[28]	1991–95	196	49
Tamil Nadu[29]	1996	162	20.3
Delhi[30]	1996–98	263	14
Bengaluru[31]	1999–2000	226	12.8
Ahmadabad[32]	2000-01	822	37
Delhi[33]	2006	2880	47.1
Delhi[25]	2005–08	196	20.4
Punjab[26]	2006–10	98	27.6
Hyderabad[34]	2010–11	100	28%

Abbreviation: MDR-TB, multidrug-resistant tuberculosis

bacilli followed by DST in a quality- assured, accredited laboratory. Limited resources and high burden of MDR-TB burden result in serious diagnostic challenges. Overdiagnosis may impose unnecessary financial burden on the health system and predispose the patient to potentially toxic drugs, whereas underdiagnosis or delayed diagnosis may lead to undertreatment of patients increasing the risk of further drug resistance, treatment failure and spread of resistant strains to others.

Diagnostic Modalities

Rapid detection is essential to control the growing problem of TB. Molecular DST or genotypic DST methods detect predetermined genetic mutations that are associated with phenotypic resistance. These include cartridge based nucleic acid amplification (CBNAAT) and line probe assay (LPA). CBNAAT or Xpert MTB/RIF assay is a heminested polymerase chain reaction (PCR) and has proven to be a rapid molecular test with high sensitivity and specificity for detecting TB cases with rifampicin resistance.[35] A study from India has shown that the test performs well even in cases with extrapulmonary TB cases where smear, conventional PCR, and LPA may not give satisfactory results.[36] The sensitivity and specificity of this technique are high which enable the detection of MDR-TB cases faster as compared to the conventional DST.

A previous study in Indian population reported that LPA had a sensitivity of 97% with 100% specificity for DR-TB detection in sputum-smear positive TB cases.[37] Though the test provides a better drug profile compared to Xpert MTB/RIF by providing DST for both rifampicin and isoniazid, it has its own limitations. It requires sophisticated laboratories and special training. The LPA can be done only in smear positive samples. **Table 5** describes the currently used diagnostic modalities, principle and their performance in diagnosing TB.

Taking into account the rapidity, good sensitivity and specificity of Xpert MTB/RIF assay, WHO strongly recommends it as the initial diagnostic test for adults and children suspected of MDR-TB or HIV-associated TB.[38] Though, Xpert MTB/RIF only gives data on rifampicin resistance, this is considered equivalent to MDR-TB, sufficient evidence to initiate treatment for the MDR-TB while awaiting conventional drug-susceptibility test results.

GenoType® MTBDR*sl* (MTBDR*sl*) is a new diagnostic tool which is at present the only rapid molecular test that detects resistance to second-line fluoroquinolone drugs and the second-line injectable drugs. Hence, this test can rapidly detect XDR-TB. The test can be done from culture isolate of the sample (indirect testing) and directly from the sample (direct testing). The pooled sensitivity of the test for second-line drugs is 70.9%, and specificity 98.8%.[39]

DISEASE MANAGEMENT

Patient Counseling

Counseling of patients is often an under-recognized aspect of disease management. Various issues need to be discussed, such as, the nature of the disease, the nature of treatment he/she is about to undergo, the duration of treatment, the possibility of adverse drug reactions (ADR), the need for strict adherence to treatment, the need for daily injections for at least 6–9 months and need for initial/subsequent hospitalization, if needed.

Table 5 Diagnostic modalities, principle and performance in diagnosing drug-resistant tuberculosis

	Principle	*Duration*	*Sensitivity*	*Specificity*	*PPV*	*NPV*
• *Phenotypic DST*						
Solid culture (LJ media) DST	Growth of *Mtb* on the media containing different ATT drugs	84 days	Gold standard			
Liquid culture DST[40]	Growth of *Mtb* in the media containing different ATT drugs	54 days	96%	97%	96%	97%
• *Genotypic DST*						
Line-probe assay[37]	Strip test which allows simultaneous molecular identification of *Mtb* and genetic mutations causing resistance to RIF and INH	72 hours	97%	100%	100%	99%
Xpert MTB/RIF[35,36]	Cartridge based nucleic acid amplification test, which is based on the principle of real-time PCR. It detects presence of *Mtb* and also RIF resistance.	2 hours				
		Pulmonary TB	96%	99%	99%	98%
		Extrapulmonary TB	71%	95%	83%	90%

Abbreviations: Mtb, Mycobacterium tuberculosis; PPV, positive predictive value; NPV, negative predictive value; DST, drug susceptibility testing; LJ media, Löwenstein-Jensen media; ATT, antitubercular treatment; RIF, rifampicin; INH, isoniazid; PCR, polymerase chain reaction; TB, tuberculosis

Pretreatment Evaluation

To ensure a good treatment outcome, a pretreatment evaluation (PTE) is mandatory. The rationale behind PTE is to identify the patients who are at high risk of developing ADR when put on MDR-TB treatment. It includes measurement of height, weight (to decide the drug dose according to appropriate weight band), total blood count, blood sugar levels (to rule-out diabetes), renal function tests, liver function tests, thyroid stimulation hormone, chest X-ray, pregnancy test for all women of reproductive age-group, electrocardiogram (to check the QT interval) and psychiatric evaluation.

TREATMENT

Three different strategies can be used in management of DR-TB, viz. (1) standardized treatment, (2) empirical treatment or (3) individualized treatment.

Standardized treatment refers to the use of a fixed combination of drugs for treating all patients. The regimen is usually based on the DST profile of population at large. Empirical treatment, on the other hand, uses those drugs to which the individual has not been previously exposed for less than 1 month and hence, presumed to be effective. Individualized treatment is based on individual DST results and uses only those drugs with proven in vitro susceptibility. Initiation of an empirical regimen till DST results are available and then switching over to an individualized regimen is probably the best strategy to achieve the highest cure rates.

World Health Organization recommends using a standardized treatment regimen.[2] The greatest advantage of a standardized treatment, when provided on a programmatic basis, is the easy availability, low cost and directly observed treatment ensuring regular and complete therapy. This is the most appropriate approach for a resource limited setting like India. Guidelines for programmatic management of MDR-TB [programmatic management of DR-TB, revised national tuberculosis control programme (RNTCP, 2012)] were formulated in 2012 on basis of WHO recommendations.[2,41] Standardized treatment regimen (STR), i.e. DOTS (directly observed treatment, short-course)-plus [programmatic management of drug-resistant TB (PMDT)] under the RNTCP program, comprises of 6 drugs (kanamycin, ofloxacin, ethionamide, pyrazinamide, ethambutol and cycloserine) during 6–9 months of the intensive phase and 4 drugs (ofloxacin, ethionamide, ethambutol and cycloserine) during the 18 months of the continuation phase.

Patients in whom subsequent cultures show resistance to other drugs as well, moxifloxacin can be replaced for isolates resistant to ofloxacin, and capreomycin for isolates resistant to kanamycin in addition to H and R. Isolates resistant to both ofloxacin and kanamycin in addition to H and R should be treated with XDR regimen. Para-aminosalicylic acid (PAS) is reserved as a substitute to patients not tolerating cycloserine or ethionamide. The recommended schedule for follow-up, sputum examination in the intensive phase is at 3rd, 4th, 5th, 6th and 7th month and in the continuation phase at 9th, 12th, 15th and 18th, 21st and 24th month. Duration of intensive phase is decided by prior culture results (smear conversion is not considered). Patient is shifted into continuation phase after at least 6 months of therapy and at least three consecutive negative culture results of sputum or other clinical specimen. If cultures remain positive, intensive phase can be extended for up to 9 months beyond which continuation phase is initiated irrespective of culture results. While all positive samples should be subjected to second-line DST, a high suspicion should be kept for patients who remain persistently culture positive.

The treatment regimen for XDR-TB treatment consists of the intensive phase of seven drugs (capreomycin, PAS, moxifloxacin, high-dose isoniazid, clofazimine, linezolid and amoxicillin/clavulanate) for 6–12 months and six drugs (PAS, moxifloxacin, high-dose isoniazid, clofazimine, linezolid, aamoxicillin/clavulanate) in the continuation phase for 18 months.

An aggressive regimen is an important predictor of MDR-TB treatment outcome.[42] An aggressive regimen has the following characteristics—at least five likely efficacious drugs, including a fluoroquinolone and injectable in the intensive phase; in the continuation phase, the requirement is at least four likely efficacious drugs, including a fluoroquinolone. A regimen that met all of these criteria was a robust predictor of successful MDR-TB treatment outcome in the face of all measured covariates.[42] In another study, it was reported that an aggressive regimen for at least 18 months was associated with a lower rate of recurrent TB.[43]

Drugs for Multidrug-resistant and Extensively Drug-resistant Tuberculosis

Table 6 lists the available drugs for the treatment of DR-TB. These second-line drugs are more likely to fail than the standard drug-susceptible treatment. Since the introduction of rifampicin, only a few anti-TB agents with new mechanism(s) of action have been developed in over 30 years, but many newer agents are under-development and some are already in clinical trials.

Bedaquiline (TMC207), which is a diarylquinoline, offers a novel mechanism of anti-TB action by inhibiting mycobacterial ATP synthase.[44] A recent phase II randomized placebo-controlled trial compared the efficacy and safety of this agent in combination with standard five-drug, second-line anti-TB regimen.[45] Adding TMC207 to standard MDR-TB therapy decreased the time to sputum conversion (negative sputum culture), when compared with placebo while increasing the proportion of patients with sputum conversion (48% versus 9%). Bedaquiline appears to be promising new anti-TB drug for the treatment of DR-TB cases.

Linezolid is an oxazolidinone antibiotic showing great promise based on studies of MDR-TB patients. The mode of action for the drug includes binding to the bacterial 23S ribosomal RNA of the 50S subunit.[46] This prevents the assembly of a functional 70S initiation complex, which is an essential component of the bacterial translation process. Some case series have reported good efficacy of linezolid against MDR and XDR-TB. Linezolid (600 mg twice daily in adults) is safe, generally well tolerated and cost effective for courses of therapy of less than 28 days, but long-duration treatment with linezolid has been associated with reversible hematopoietic suppression, primarily thrombocytopenia and neuropathy.[47,48] A daily dose of 300 mg linezolid is effective against MDR and XDR-TB with few neuropathic side effects.[49]

Delamanid (OPC-67683) is derived from the nitro-dihydro-imidazooxazole class of compounds that inhibits mycolic acid synthesis in the bacteria.[50] Findings of a randomized, placebo-controlled clinical trial suggest that treatment with delamanid was associated with an increase in sputum conversion at 2 months in patients with MDR-TB.[51]

PA-824, a nitroimidazole is a novel anti-TB drug, which is now in the late-phase clinical trials stage. PaMZ a new drug regimen consisting of PA-824, moxifloxacin and pyrazinamide is already in phase 3 clinical trial. The phase 2b trial of PaMZ delivered exciting results in South Africa and Tanzania. A recently published study describes about the safety and tolerability of this drug with the antiretroviral drugs to cure HIV-TB coinfected patients.[52]

With the upcoming of new novel anti-TB drugs, some studies are shifting to the basics of shortening the drug duration. A noninferiority, randomized, open-label, controlled trial was recently conducted where the course of treatment was reduced to 4 months and the regimen included gatifloxacin. Though the primary efficacy end point was not shown in the study, the study provided a strong base to conduct more studies to shorten the treatment duration.[53]

New Drug Delivery System

Newer drug delivery systems have been developed over the last few years, which include liposomes, microparticles and nanoparticles.[54] These drug delivery systems are more advantageous over the conventional drugs as they help in improving adherence of patients to anti-TB treatment, reduce the drug burden and also shorten the duration of anti-TB treatment. Nanoparticles help in a targeted drug delivery system, which can help in combating the TB bacillus in the body.[55] Appropriate clinical trials are required to completely understand these drug delivery modalities and their role in disease management.

Adverse Drug Reactions

Adverse drug reactions are an important cause of poor compliance and default **(Table 7)**. These reactions sometimes warrant stoppage of the offending drug and further curtail drug options. Even in short-course chemotherapy for drug-sensitive TB, side effects such as hepatitis, dyspepsia, skin reactions and arthralgia were responsible for the termination of therapy in up to 23% of patients during the intensive phase.[56] The side effects of TB chemotherapy get augmented in patients with concurrent HIV infection, prior history of hepatitis or in patients on second line TB drugs. The side effects may include anemia, thrombocytopenia, peripheral neuropathy, QT interval prolongation, and nausea.

Table 6 Drugs available for anti-tuberculosis treatment

Drug	*Daily dosage*	*Activity against TB*
• *Aminoglycosides*		
Streptomycin	15 mg/kg (750–1,000 mg)	Inhibit protein synthesis by irreversibly binding to 30S ribosomal subunit
Kanamycin	15 mg/kg (750–1,000 mg)	Inhibit protein synthesis by irreversibly binding to 30S ribosomal subunit
Amikacin	15 mg/kg (750–1,000 mg)	Inhibit protein synthesis through disruption of ribosomal function
Capreomycin	15 mg/kg (750–1,000 mg)	Has a different chemical structure from the aminoglycosides, but the mechanism of antibacterial activity is similar
• *Thioamides*		
Ethionamide	15–20 mg/kg (500–750 mg)	Inhibit mycolic acid synthesis
Pyrazinamide	20–30 mg/kg (1,200–1,600 mg)	Pyrazinamide diffuses into *M. tuberculosis*, where the enzyme pyrazinamidase converts pyrazinamide to the active form pyrazinoic acid. This acid binds to the ribosomal protein S1 and inhibits trans-translation
• *Fluoroquinolones*		
Ofloxacin	400 mg twice daily	Inhibits the A subunit of DNA gyrase (topoisomerase), which is essential in the reproduction of bacterial DNA
Levofloxacin	750 mg/mL	Inhibits the A subunit of DNA gyrase (topoisomerase), which is essential in the reproduction of bacterial DNA.
Ciprofloxacin	1,000–1,500 mg/day	Inhibits the A subunit of DNA gyrase (topoisomerase), which is essential in the reproduction of bacterial DNA
Moxifloxacin	400 mg	Inhibits the A subunit of DNA gyrase (topoisomerase), which is essential in the reproduction of bacterial DNA
Gatifloxacin	400 mg/day	Inhibits the A subunit of DNA gyrase (topoisomerase), which is essential in the reproduction of bacterial DNA
Cycloserine	10–15 mg/kg (maximum 1,000 mg)	Competitively blocks the enzyme that incorporates alanine into an alanyl-alanine dipeptide, an essential component of the mycobacterial cell wall
Terizodone	15–20 mg/kg (600 mg)	Bacteriostatic in nature
Para-aminosalicylic acid	150 mg/kg (10–12 g)	Is bacteriostatic in nature and distrupts folic acid metabolism
• *Adjuvant drugs*	Dosages not standardized	
Clofazamine		Clofazimine appears to bind preferentially to mycobacterial DNA (principally at base sequences containing guanine) and inhibit mycobacterial replication and growth
Rifamycin derivatives Rifapentine Rifabutin		Inhibition of bacterial DNA-dependent RNA synthesis
Macrolides		Protein synthesis inhibitor
Clarithromycin, telithromycin		Inhibits protein synthesis
Linezolid		Binds to the bacterial 23S ribosomal RNA of the 50S subunit thus inhibits translation
Bedaquiline		Inhibits mycobacterial ATP synthase
PA-824		Inhibition of cell wall mycolic acid biosynthesis
Delamanid		Inhibition of cell wall mycolic acid biosynthesis

Follow-up of Patients

Close follow-up and monitoring are mandatory for patients with MDR and XDR-TB to ensure strict compliance to the regime, prompt identification, management of ADR, early detection and treatment of treatment failure. Directly Observed Treatment (DOT) is integral for close follow- up and monitoring. Monitoring of patients on MDR- and XDR-TB treatment requires not only careful clinical examination, but also appropriate laboratory investigations like chest radiographs, renal and liver function tests, serum electrolytes and thyroid profile at appropriate time intervals for prompt

Table 7 Common adverse drug reactions of antituberculous drugs[11]

Drug	*Adverse event(s)*
Aminoglycosides (streptomycin, kanamycin, amikacin)	Pain at injection site, ototoxicity (vertigo and deafness), nephrotoxicity, hemolytic anemia, aplastic anemia, agranulocytosis, thrombocytopenia, and lupoid reactions
Capreomycin	Hypokalemia, hypocalcemia and hypomagnesemia, cutaneous reactions and occasionally hepatotoxicity
Thioamides (ethionamide, prothionamide)	Epigastric discomfort, anorexia, nausea, metallic taste and sulfurous belching, vomiting and excessive salivation; psychotic reactions including hallucinations and depression; hypoglycemia, hypothyroidism and goiter; hepatotoxicity; gynecomastia, menstrual disturbance, impotence, acne, headache and peripheral neuropathy; tolerance varies with ethnicity; usually well tolerated in Africa and Asia
Pyrazinamide	Hepatotoxicity, GI intolerance, hyperuricemia, and arthralgias
Fluoroquinolones (ofloxacin, levofloxacin, moxifloxacin)	Uncommon GI disturbance (e.g. anorexia, nausea, vomiting), CNS symptoms (e.g. dizziness, headache, mood changes and rarely convulsions), QT interval prolongation
Ethambutol	Dose-dependent optic neuritis and peripheral neuritis
Cycloserine	Dizziness, slurred speech and convulsions, confusion, depression, altered behavior, suicidal tendency, hypersensitivity reaction
Terizodone	Headache, tremor, insomnia, confusion, depression and altered behavior, suicide risk, generalized hypersensitivity reaction or hepatitis
Para-aminosalicylic acid	GI disturbance (e.g. anorexia, nausea, vomiting, abdominal discomfort and diarrhea), general skin or other hypersensitivity, and hepatic dysfunction, hypokalemia, hypothyroidism and goiter; best avoided in renal failure as it may exacerbate acidosis; sodium salt should not be given when a restricted sodium intake is indicated
Linezolid	Hematological (anemia, thrombocytopenia), peripheral neuropathy
TMC207	Nausea, QT interval prolongation
Abbreviations: GI, gastrointestinal; CNS, central nervous system	

identification of adverse reactions. Sputum smear should be examined at 30 days apart from 3rd to 7th month of treatment (i.e. at the end of the months 3rd, 4th, 5th, 6th and 7th) and at 3-month intervals from the 9th month onward till the completion of treatment (i.e. at the end of the months 9th, 12th, 15th, 18th, 21th and 24th).[41]

The importance of sputum examination during treatment needs to be emphasized since the most important objective evidence of improvement is the conversion of sputum smear and culture to negative. Patients will be considered culture converted after having two consecutive negative cultures taken at least 1 month apart. Patients who remain culture-positive despite 9 months of regular treatment are suspects of treatment failure; DST for second-line drugs should be done. An MDR-TB patient who has completed treatment and has been consistently culture negative with at least five consecutive negative results in the last 12–15 months is considered to be cured.

Regimen Reinforcement

A single agent should never be added to a failing regimen in patients with suspected DR-TB because of the risk of fostering further drug resistance. In patients who have persistent positive sputum microscopy after several months of treatment (e.g. 3 months), there is a need to incorporate additional agents in their treatment regimen, a concept called "regimen reinforcement." In this circumstance, there are no other viable four- or five-drug combination regimens that can be given. Thus, any remaining effective agents may be added, or current agents switched, based on the latest drug-resistance testing pattern.

Surgical Management of Drug-resistant Tuberculosis

Cavities in a destroyed lung of TB patients act as reservoirs for large bacillary load. These cavities actively replicate bacteria even in patients, which are sputum culture negative. The rationale behind surgery is to help in a significant decrease in the bacillary load. Various surgical procedures have been performed in patients with MDR-TB ranging from segmental resection to pleuropneumonectomy. A combined medical and surgical approach is increasingly being used to treat patients with MDR-TB. The cure rate with surgical resection as an adjunct to medical therapy approximates 83–93% in some published series.[57-59] It is important to note that at least 3 months of treatment should be given before surgery, if feasible. In cases of HIV-TB coinfection, it is important to wait for surgery until immunity is restored by antiretroviral therapy (ART) to withstand a major surgery.

Indications for surgery in patients include: (1) persistence of culture-positive MDR-TB despite extended drug treatment, (2) extensive patterns of drug resistance that are associated with treatment failure or additional resistance, (3) local cavitary, necrotic/destructive disease in a lobe or region of the lung that is amenable to resection without producing respiratory insufficiency and/or severe pulmonary hypertension.

Pre and postoperative care, specialized surgical facilities, safe blood transfusion services, and stringent infection control measures are additional considerations during surgical management.

TREATMENT OUTCOMES

According to the RNTCP guidelines, treatment outcome was categorized as cured, defaulted, failure and death. A patient can be declared cured after complete treatment for at least 24 months with last five cultures negative. However, patient having two or more of last five cultures positive is considered as treatment failure. A patient who interrupted treatment for 2 or more consecutive months can be considered as a defaulter.

The proportion of patients with successful outcome averaged to about 48% globally. Ethiopia, Kazakhstan, Myanmar, Pakistan and Viet Nam, all high MDR-TB burden countries achieved at least 70% treatment success in the 2011 cohort. In the 2011 cohort, treatment failure was highest in the European Region (15%), and the death rate was highest in South-east Asia (21%).[1] More efforts need to be made to improve the treatment outcomes especially in TB high-burden countries. **Table 8** summarizes the treatment outcomes in previously published studies.

Table 8 Treatment outcome in multidrug-resistant tuberculosis and extensively drug-resistant tuberculosis

Study, year of publication	*Type of DR-TB*	*Treatment outcome*
Goble et al., 1993	MDR-TB (n = 171)	Cured = 65%, treatment failure = 35%
Sharma et al., 1996	MDR-TB (n = 19)	Sputum smear conversion = 18/19 (94.7%)
Park et al., 1998	MDR-TB (n = 107)	Cured = 82.5%, treatment failure = 17.5%
Yew et al., 2000	MDR-TB (n = 63)	Cured = 81%, treatment failure = 14.3%
Kim et al., 2001	MDR-TB (n = 1,011)	Cured = 48%, treatment failure = 8.1%, default = 39%
Tahaoğlu et al., 2001	MDR-TB (n = 158)	Cured or completed treatment = 77%, treatment failure = 8%
Mitnick et al., 2003	MDR-TB (n = 75)	Cured = 83%, death = 8%
Nathanson et al., 2006	MDR-TB (n = 1,047)	Cured or completed treatment = 69.7%, treatment failure = 6.7%
Gandhi et al., 2006	XDR-TB (n = 53)	Death = 52/53 (98.1%), HIV positive = 44/44 tested
Sharma, 2007	MDR-TB (n = 172), XDR-TB (n = 1)	Cured = 41.6%, treatment failure = 38.7%
Dhingra et al., 2008	MDR-TB (n = 27)	Cured = 48%, default = 37%
Shean et al., 2008	MDR-TB (n = 491)	Cured or completed treatment = 49%, treatment failure = 5%, default = 29%
Masjedi et al., 2008	MDR-TB (n = 43)	Cured/completed treatment = 67.5%, death = 18.6%
Mitnick et al., 2008	XDR-TB (n = 48), MDR-TB (n = 603)	Cured or completed treatment = 60.4% of XDR-TB; Treatment failure = 10.4% of XDR-TB;cured or completed treatment = 66.3% of MDR-TB; treatment failure = 2.1% of MDR-TB
Bonilla et al., 2008	XDR-TB (n = 43)	Cured or completed treatment = 49%, death = 19%
Kwon et al., 2008	XDR-TB (n = 27), MDR-TB (n = 128)	Cured or completed treatment = 65% of XDR-TB, cured or completed treatment = 66% of MDR-TB, treatment failure = 14% overall
Banerjee et al., 2008	XDR-TB (n = 18), MDR-TB (n = 406)	Completed treatment = 41.2% XDR-TB, death = 29.4% XDR-TB
Keshavjee et al., 2008	XDR-TB (n = 29), MDR-TB (n = 579)	Cured or completed treatment = 48.3% of XDR-TB; Treatment failure = 31% of XDR-TB; cured or completed treatment = 66.7% of MDR-TB; treatment failure = 8.5% of MDR-TB
Anderson et al., 2013	MDR-TB (n = 204)	Cured or treatment completed = 70.6%, defaulter = 6.9%, died = 6.9%, loss to follow-up = 7.8%, relapsed cases= 0.5%
Jain K et al., 2014	MDR-TB (n = 130)	Cured or completed treatment = 44%, died = 19%, defaulter = 23%, treatment failure = 13%

Abbreviations: DR-TB, drug-resistant tuberculosis, MDR-TB, multidrug-resistant tuberculosis, XDR-TB, extensively drug-resistant tuberculosis

MULTIDRUG-RESISTANT TUBERCULOSIS IN SPECIAL CONDITIONS

Human Immunodeficiency Virus Tuberculosis Coinfection

It is estimated that in India, almost 50% of individuals with HIV will develop TB during their disease course making it the most common opportunistic infection.[60] HIV infection does not appear to predispose a person to MDR-TB. DR-TB, including MDR-TB is not more common among HIV-infected persons compared to the general population.[61,62] Despite this, theoretically speaking HIV-infected individuals have a greater chance of developing MDR-TB due to the following reasons: (1) increased susceptibility to TB, (2) increased risk of nosocomial transmission, (3) increased risk of treatment failure due to lack of compliance, drug interactions and malabsorption. Data in patients with drug-susceptible TB demonstrate that a low CD4 count is associated with high early mortality at the start of therapy and is most dramatic during the first 3 months of treatment.[63]

Pregnancy

All female patients of childbearing age should be tested for pregnancy on initial evaluation. Birth control is strongly recommended for all nonpregnant women receiving therapy for DR-TB. Hamedeh and Glassroth reviewed literature concerning over 2,000 pregnancies in mothers with TB and found no significant difference in side-effects compared with nonpregnant subjects and no higher incidence of fetal abnormalities.[64] TB in pregnancy poses special challenges due to three issues—first is the use of chest radiography for the diagnosis or follow-up risks of radiation exposure to the developing fetus; second, active TB can lead to adverse outcomes in both mother and fetus; third, the fetus is at risk of teratogenic effects. Since the majority of teratogenic effects occur in the first trimester, therapy may be delayed until the second trimester, considering the severity of the underlying disease. Aminoglycosides can be toxic to the developing fetal ear and should be avoided. Ethionamide has been shown to be teratogenic in animals and should be avoided.

Management of TB in pregnancy varies with the duration of pregnancy. If a woman is pregnant for less than 20 weeks, she can undergo medical termination of pregnancy (MTP) and then start or continue with category IV treatment. If the patient refuses for MTP, the treatment regimen should include a modified category IV treatment. If a woman is pregnant for less than 12 weeks, kanamycin, ethionamide and PAS are omitted from the regimen. When the fetus is for more than 12 weeks, kanamycin and ethionamide are omitted and PAS is added in the regimen. After delivery, PAS is replaced with kanamycin and continued till the end of intensive phase.

Breastfeeding

In lactating mothers on treatment, most anti-TB drugs will be found in the breast milk in concentrations that equalize only a small fraction of the therapeutic dose used in an infant. Any effects on infants of such exposure during the full course of MDR-TB treatment have not been established. Therefore, when resources and training are available, it is recommended to provide infant formula options as an alternative to breastfeeding. The mother and her baby should not be completely separated. If the mother is sputum smear-positive, the care of the infant should be left to family members until she becomes sputum smear-negative. In some settings, the mother may be offered the option of using a surgical mask or an N-95 respirator until she becomes sputum smear-negative.

In conclusion, the global TB epidemic has been complicated by the emergence of multidrug and extensively drug-resistant strains of TB and now, by TDR-TB. Indiscriminate use of second-line drugs for treating MDR-TB has already given rise to the development of XDR-TB. If this practice goes uncurbed, XDR-TB may soon emerge as the dominant TB strain throughout the world. Since drug resistance is a man-made phenomenon, every effort should be made to diagnose and treat drug-sensitive TB effectively at the grassroots level and prevent the development of drug resistance. MDR-TB or XDR-TB is a laboratory diagnosis and, therefore, requires quality laboratory support for timely and accurate results. Control of DR-TB requires a strong health infrastructure to ensure delivery of effective programmatic treatment coupled with surveillance and monitoring activities, for timely intervention to limit transmission and spread of the disease.

REFERENCES

1. WHO. (2014). Global tuberculosis report. [online] Geneva: World Health Organization. Available from *http://www.who.int/tb/publications/global_report/en/*. [Accessed January, 2016].
2. Guidelines for the Programmatic Management of Drug-Resistant Tuberculosis. (2011). [online] Geneva: World Health Organization. Available from *http://www.ncbi.nlm.nih.gov/books/NBK148644/*. [Accessed January, 2016].
3. Udwadia ZF, Amale RA, Ajbani KK, Rodrigues C. Totally drug-resistant tuberculosis in India. Clin Infect Dis. 2012;54(4):579-81.
4. WHO. (2000). Anti-tuberculosis drug resistance in the world. Report no. 2. Prevalence and trends. [online] Available from *http://www.who.int/csr/resources/publications/drugresist/WHO_CDS_TB_2000_278/en/*. [Accessed January, 2016].
5. David HL. Drug-resistance in M. tuberculosis and other mycobacteria. Clin Chest Med. 1980;1(2):227-30.
6. Ramaswamy S, Musser JM. Molecular genetic basis of antimicrobial agent resistance in Mycobacterium tuberculosis: 1998 update. Tuber Lung Dis. 1998;79(1):3-29.
7. Almeida Da Silva PE, Palomino JC. Molecular basis and mechanisms of drug resistance in Mycobacterium tuberculosis: classical and new drugs. J Antimicrob Chemother. 2011;66(7):1417-30.

8. Ando H, Kondo Y, Suetake T, Toyota E, Kato S, Mori T, et al. Identification of katG Mutations Associated with High-Level Isoniazid Resistance in Mycobacterium tuberculosis. Antimicrob Agents Chemother. 2010;54(5):1793-9.
9. Velayati AA, Farnia P, Ibrahim TA, Haroun RZ, Kuan HO, Ghanavi J, et al. Differences in cell wall thickness between resistant and nonresistant strains of Mycobacterium tuberculosis: using transmission electron microscopy. Chemotherapy. 2009;55(5):3037.
10. Velayati AA, Farnia P, Masjedi MR. Totally drug resistant tuberculosis (TDR-TB). Int J Clin Exp Med. 2013; 6(4): 307-9.
11. Sharma SK, Mohan A. Multidrug-resistant tuberculosis: a menace that threatens to destabilize tuberculosis control. Chest. 2006;130(1):261-72.
12. Gandhi NR, Moll A, Sturm AW, Pawinski R, Govender T, Lalloo U, et al. Extensively drug-resistant tuberculosis as a cause of death in patients co-infected with tuberculosis and HIV in a rural area of South Africa. Lancet. 2006;368(9547):1575-80.
13. Chandrasekaran S, Chauhan MM, Rajalakshmi R, Chaudhuri K, Mahadev B. Initial drug resistance to anti-tuberculosis drugs in patients attending an urban district tuberculosis centre. Indian J Tuberc. 1990;37:215-6.
14. Narang P, Nayyar S, Mendiratta DK, Tyagi NK, Jajoo U. Smear and culture positive cases of pulmonary tuberculosis found among symptomatics surveyed in Wardha district. Indian J Tuberc. 1992;39:159-63
15. Paramasivan CN, Chandrasekaran V, Santha T, Sudarsanam NM, Prabhakar R. Bacteriological investigations for short-course chemotherapy under the tuberculosis programme in two districts of India. Tuber Lung Dis. 1993;74(1):23-7.
16. Chandrasekaran S, Jagota P, Chaudhuri K. Initial drug resistance to antituberculosis drugs in urban and rural district tuberculosis programme. Ind J Tub. 1992;39:171-5.
17. Gupta PR, Singhal B, Sharma TN, Gupta RB. Prevalence of initial drug resistance in tuberculosis patients attending a chest hospital. Indian J Med Res. 1993;97:1027-3.
18. Jain NK, Chopra KK, Prasad G. Initial and acquired isoniazid and rifampicin resistance to M. tuberculosis and its implications for treatment. Paper presented at the 46th National conference on Tuberculosis and chest disease. [online]. 1991 Available from: *http://nitrd.nic.in/IJTB/Year%201992/April%201992/April%201992%20I.pdf.* [Accessed January, 2016].
19. Jena J, Panda BN, Nema SK, Ohri VC, Pahwa RS. Drug Resistance Pattern Of Mycobacterium Tuberculosis In A Chest Diseases Hospital Of Armed Forces. Lung India. 1995;13(2):56-9.
20. Paramasivan CN, Bhaskaran K, Venkataraman P, Chandrasekaran V, Narayanan PR. Surveillance of drug resistance in tuberculosis in the state of Tamil Nadu. Indian J Tuberc. 2000;47(1):27-33.
21. Paramasivan CN, Venkataraman P, Chandrasekaran V, Bhat S, Narayanan PR. Surveillance of drug resistance in tuberculosis in two districts of South India. Int J Tuberc Lung Dis. 2002;6(6):479-84.
22. Anuradha B, Aparna S, Hari Sai Priya V, Priya VHS, Vijaya Lakshmi V, Lakshmi VV, et al. Prevalence of drug resistance under the DOTS strategy in Hyderabad, South India, 2001-2003. Int J Tuberc Lung Dis. 2006;10(1):58-62.
23. Joseph MR, Shoby CT, Amma GR, Chauhan LS, Paramasivan CN. Surveillance of anti-tuberculosis drug resistance in Ernakulam District, Kerala State, South India. Int J Tuberc Lung Dis. 2007;11(4):443-9.
24. Ramachandran R, Nalini S, Chandrasekar V, Dave PV, Sanghvi AS, Wares F, et al. Surveillance of drug-resistant tuberculosis in the state of Gujarat, India. Int J Tuberc Lung Dis. 2009;13(9):1154-60.
25. Sharma SK, Kaushik G, Jha B, George N, Arora SK, Gupta D, et al. Prevalence of multidrug-resistant tuberculosis among newly diagnosed cases of sputum-positive pulmonary tuberculosis. Indian J Med Res. 2011;133:308-11.
26. Sethi S, Mewara A, Dhatwalia SK, Singh H, Yadav R, Singh K, et al. Prevalence of multidrug resistance in Mycobacterium tuberculosis isolates from HIV seropositive and seronegative patients with pulmonary tuberculosis in north India. BMC Infect Dis. 2013;13:137.
27. Trivedi SS, Desai SG. Primary antituberculosis drug resistance and acquired rifampicin resistance in Gujarat, India. Tubercle. 1988;69(1):37-42.
28. Janmeja AK, Raj B. Acquired drug resistance in tuberculosis in Harayana, India. J Assoc Physicians India. 1998;46(2):194-8.
29. Vasanthakumari R, Jagannath K. Multidrug Resistant Tuberculosis - A Tamilnadu Study. Lung India. 1997;15(4):178-80.
30. Dam T, Isa M, Bose M. Drug-sensitivity profile of clinical Mycobacterium tuberculosis isolates--a retrospective study from a chest-disease institute in India. J Med Microbiol. 2005;54(Pt 3):269-71.
31. Vijay Sophia, Balasangameshwara V H, Jagannatha P S, Kumar P. Initial Drug Resistance among tuberculosis patients under DOTS Program in Bangalore city. Indian Journal of Tuberculosis. 2004;51(1):17-22.
32. Shah AR, Agarwal SK, Shah KV. Study of drug resistance in previously treated tuberculosis patients in Gujarat, India. Int J Tuberc Lung Dis. 2002;6(12):1098-101.
33. Hanif M, Malik S, Dhingra VK. Acquired drug resistance pattern in tuberculosis cases at the State Tuberculosis Centre, Delhi, India. Int J Tuberc Lung Dis. 2009;13(1):74-8.
34. Kandi S, Kopuu D, Kondapaka K, Prasad S, Sagar Reddy Pn, Reddy VK, et al. Prevalence of multidrug resistance among retreatment pulmonary tuberculosis cases in a tertiary care hospital, Hyderabad, India. Lung India. 2013;30(4):277.
35. Boehme CC, Nabeta P, Hillemann D, Nicol MP, Shenai S, Krapp F, et al. Rapid Molecular Detection of Tuberculosis and Rifampin Resistance. N Engl J Med. 2010;363(11):1005-15.
36. Sharma SK, Kohli M, Chaubey J, Yadav RN, Sharma R, Singh BK, et al. Evaluation of Xpert MTB/RIF assay performance in diagnosing extrapulmonary tuberculosis among adults in a tertiary care centre in India. Eur Respir J. 2014.
37. Yadav RN, Singh BK, Sharma SK, Sharma R, Soneja M, Sreenivas V, et al. Comparative evaluation of GenoType MTBDRplus line probe assay with solid culture method in early diagnosis of multidrug resistant tuberculosis (MDR-TB) at a tertiary care centre in India. PloS One. 2013.
38. WHO. (2013) Information NC for B, Pike USNL of M 8600 R, MD B, USA 20894. [online] WHO's policy recommendations. Available from: *http://www.ncbi.nlm.nih.gov/books/NBK258597/*. [Accessed Jan 2016].
39. Theron G, Peter J, Richardson M, Barnard M, Donegan S, Warren R, et al. The diagnostic accuracy of the GenoType® MTBDR *sl* assay for the detection of resistance to second-line anti-tuberculosis drugs. In: The Cochrane Collaboration (Ed). Cochrane Database of Systematic Reviews Chichester. UK: John Wiley and Sons, Ltd; 2014.

40. Zhao P, Fang F, Yu Q, Guo J, Zhang J, Qu J, et al. Evaluation of BACTEC MGIT 960 System for Testing Susceptibility of Mycobacterium tuberculosis to First-Line Drugs in China. PLoS One. 2014.
41. RNTCP PMDT Guidelines: Central TB division, directorate general of health services, Ministry of health and family welfare, India. (2012). [online] Available from *http://tbcindia.nic.in/WriteReadData/l892s/8320929355Guidelines%20for%20PMDT%20in%20India%20-%20May%202012.pdf.* [Accessed January, 2016].
42. Mitnick CD, Franke MF, Rich ML, Alcantara Viru FA, Appleton SC, Atwood SS, et al. Aggressive regimens for multidrug-resistant tuberculosis decrease all-cause mortality. PloS One. 2013.
43. Franke MF, Appleton SC, Mitnick CD, Furin JJ, Bayona J, Chalco K, et al. Aggressive Regimens for Multidrug-Resistant Tuberculosis Reduce Recurrence. Clin Infect Dis. 2013;56(6):770-6.
44. Haagsma AC, Podasca I, Koul A, Andries K, Guillemont J, Lill H, et al. Probing the interaction of the diarylquinoline TMC207 with its target mycobacterial ATP synthase. PloS One. 2011.
45. Diacon AH, Pym A, Grobusch M, Patientia R, Rustomjee R, Page-Shipp L, et al. The Diarylquinoline TMC207 for Multidrug-Resistant Tuberculosis. N Engl J Med. 2009;360(23):2397-405.
46. Livermore DM. Linezolid in vitro: mechanism and antibacterial spectrum. J Antimicrob Chemother. 2003;51(Suppl 2):ii9-16.
47. Gerson SL, Kaplan SL, Bruss JB, Le V, Arellano FM, Hafkin B, et al. Hematologic Effects of Linezolid: Summary of Clinical Experience. Antimicrob Agents Chemother. 2002;46(8): 2723-6.
48. Frippiat F, Derue G. Causal relationship between neuropathy and prolonged linezolid use. Clin Infect Dis. 2004;39(3):439.
49. Koh WJ, Kang YR, Jeon K, Kwon OJ, Lyu J, Kim WS, et al. Daily 300 mg dose of linezolid for multidrug-resistant and extensively drug-resistant tuberculosis: updated analysis of 51 patients. J Antimicrob Chemother. 2012;67(6):1503-7.
50. Xavier A, Lakshmanan M. Delamanid: A new armor in combating drug-resistant tuberculosis. J Pharmacol Pharmacother. 2014;5(3):222.
51. Gler MT, Skripconoka V, Sanchez-Garavito E, Xiao H, Cabrera-Rivero JL, Vargas-Vasquez DE, et al. Delamanid for Multidrug-Resistant Pulmonary Tuberculosis. N Engl J Med. 2012;366(23):2151-60.
52. Dooley KE, Luetkemeyer AF, Park JG, Allen R, Cramer Y, Murray S, et al. Phase I safety, pharmacokinetics, and pharmacogenetics study of the antituberculosis drug PA-824 with concomitant lopinavir-ritonavir, efavirenz, or rifampin. Antimicrob Agents Chemother. 2014;58(9):5245-52.
53. Merle CS, Fielding K, Sow OB, Gninafon M, Lo MB, Mthiyane T, et al. A Four-Month Gatifloxacin-Containing Regimen for Treating Tuberculosis. N Engl J Med. 2014;371(17):1588-98.
54. Smith JP. Nanoparticle delivery of anti-tuberculosis chemotherapy as a potential mediator against drug-resistant tuberculosis. Yale J Biol Med. 2011;84(4):361-9.
55. Clemens DL, Lee BY, Xue M, Thomas CR, Meng H, Ferris D, et al. Targeted intracellular delivery of antituberculosis drugs to Mycobacterium tuberculosis-infected macrophages via functionalized mesoporous silica nanoparticles. Antimicrob Agents Chemother. 2012;56(5):2535-45.
56. Schaberg T, Rebhan K, Lode H. Risk factors for side-effects of isoniazid, rifampin and pyrazinamide in patients hospitalized for pulmonary tuberculosis. Eur Respir J. 1996;9(10):2026-30.
57. Shiraishi Y, Nakajima Y, Katsuragi N, Kurai M, Takahashi N. Resectional surgery combined with chemotherapy remains the treatment of choice for multidrug-resistant tuberculosis. J Thorac Cardiovasc Surg. 2004;128(4):523-8.
58. Somocurcio JG, Sotomayor A, Shin S, Portilla S, Valcarcel M, Guerra D, et al. Surgery for patients with drug-resistant tuberculosis: report of 121 cases receiving community-based treatment in Lima, Peru. Thorax. 2007;62(5):416-21.
59. Calligaro GL, Moodley L, Symons G, Dheda K. The medical and surgical treatment of drug-resistant tuberculosis. J Thorac Dis. 2014;6(3):186-95.
60. Narain JP, Raviglione MC, Kochi A. HIV-associated tuberculosis in developing countries: epidemiology and strategies for prevention. Tuber Lung Dis. 1992;73(6):311-21.
61. Spellman CW, Matty KJ, Weis SE. A survey of drug-resistant Mycobacterium tuberculosis and its relationship to HIV infection. AIDS Lond Engl. 1998;12(2):191-5.
62. Asch S, Knowles L, Rai A, Jones BE, Pogoda J, Barnes PF. Relationship of isoniazid resistance to human immunodeficiency virus infection in patients with tuberculosis. Am J Respir Crit Care Med. 1996;153(5):1708-10.
63. Lawn SD, Myer L, Orrell C, Bekker LG, Wood R. Early mortality among adults accessing a community-based antiretroviral service in South Africa: implications for programme design. AIDS. 2005;19(18):2141-8.
64. Hamadeh MA, Glassroth J. Tuberculosis and pregnancy. Chest. 1992;101(4):1114-20.

Treatment of Tuberculosis in Special Situations

Rajendra Prasad, Nikhil Gupta

INTRODUCTION

Treatment of tuberculosis (TB) poses a difficult clinical problem in special situations such as pregnancy, renal insufficiency and liver diseases. There are various concerns regarding dosage, toxicity and the method of administration of drugs. Prior to discussing the specific issues, it is important to know the important pharmacokinetic characteristics of individual antitubercular drugs.

PHARMACOKINETICS OF ANTITUBERCULAR DRUGS

Some antituberculosis drugs are metabolized in liver; while others are excreted either unchanged or in metabolized form, by the renal route. Their secretion in milk and ability to cross placenta is important in the situations of lactation and pregnancy, where there is concern of safety of the baby.

Isoniazid is rapidly absorbed from the gut, metabolized in liver by acetylation and the inactive metabolites are excreted in urine within 24 hours. Its half-life varies from one group of population to other, depending upon hepatic acetylation. Half-life is less than 1 hour in rapid acetylators, and more than three hours in slow acetylators. It is secreted in milk, but the amount is not sufficient to provide antitubercular chemoprophylaxis to infant. It is safe in pregnancy, but the risk of hepatitis may increase in the postpartum period.[1] Rifampicin is rapidly absorbed and widely distributed to tissues and bound to plasma protein. Its absorption is reduced if given with food (not of clinical significance), or if given along with para-aminosalicylic acid (PAS). It is extensively recycled by enterohepatic circulation, and the metabolites formed by deacetylation are excreted in feces. It is found to be safe in pregnancy, with some risk of postnatal hemorrhage.

Ethambutol is rapidly absorbed from the gut. It is predominantly excreted in urine in an unchanged form or an inactive hepatic metabolite (80%).[2] Only 20% is excreted in feces as unchanged drug.[3] Ethambutol is found to be safe in pregnancy and liver disease. Pyrazinamide is also rapidly absorbed from gut, metabolized in liver to its metabolites, pyrazinoic acid and 5-hydroxypyrazinoic acid, which are excreted largely by the renal route.[4] Its safety in pregnancy is somewhat controversial.[4] Streptomycin is largely concentrated in the extracellular fluid. In pregnant women, it may interfere with development of fetal ear.[5] Plasma half-life is prolonged in the newborn, elderly patients and in patients with renal failure. It is excreted unchanged in urine. Pharmacokinetics of amikacin, kanamycin or capreomycin are similar to those of streptomycin, and found unsafe in pregnancy, where they may cause fetal nephrotoxicity or congenital deafness.[5] They are considered safe in liver disease.

Ethionamide and prothionamide are toxic to liver and teratogenic in pregnant animals. Their safety in liver disease and pregnancy is doubtful, should not be used in pregnant women. They are considered relatively safe in mild renal disease. Cycloserine is about one-third metabolized, and the rest excreted in urine. It is not safe in patients with renal failure.

In alcoholics, it may lead to seizures. It crosses the placenta in pregnancy, its safety in this situation is not yet established. PAS is not safe in renal failure. About 80% of drug is excreted in urine, it should be avoided in severe renal insufficiency, where it may aggravate the problem of metabolic acidosis.[6] Old preparation of PAS interacted with rifampicin absorption, but new preparation of granules has no interaction.[7] There are no studies on its safety in pregnant women, but it has been safely used in pregnancy in the past. Fluoroquinolones are also not found safe, as they are found to inhibit the growing cartilages of bones in animal studies. About 80% of levofloxacin is cleared by kidney, its dose adjustment is recommended in the cases of renal insufficiency.[8] These drugs, except ciprofloxacin, which is metabolized in liver, are generally safe in the cases of liver disease.

Clofazimine is absorbed from the gastrointestinal tract in amounts varying from 45 to 70%. It is distributed to most organs, tissues and breast milk, crosses the placenta but not the blood-brain barrier. It is largely excreted unchanged in the feces, both as unabsorbed drug and via biliary excretion. Linezolid is rapidly and extensively absorbed after oral doses with maximum plasma concentration achieved after 1–2 hours. This drug has mainly renal route of excretion. Clarithromycin is rapidly absorbed from intestinal tract and undergoes extensive first-pass metabolism. It has biliary route of excretion predominantly whereas half-life is prolonged in renal impairment.

TREATMENT OF TUBERCULOSIS IN PREGNANCY AND LACTATION

Isoniazid is considered safe in pregnancy, except for some chance of postpartum hepatitis.[1] The American Thoracic Society (ATS) recommends supplementation with pyridoxine during pregnancy (25 mg/day).[4] Use of rifampicin and ethambutol is safe in pregnancy. Data regarding other rifamycins (rifabutin and rifapentine) is insufficient, and thus, they should be cautiously used. Safety regarding pyrazinamide cannot be assured, but when used for 6-month regimen, the benefits may outweigh the possible risk.[3]

Streptomycin may cause congenital deafness, as this drug interferes with the development of the ear.[5] Other injectables, like amikacin, kanamycin and capreomycin having pharmacokinetics similar to streptomycin, may also cause fetal nephrotoxicity and ototoxicity.[5] One study reported that 17% of babies born to women who received streptomycin during pregnancy, developed hearing loss.[9] Ethionamide and prothionamide are contraindicated in pregnancy, as they are found teratogenic in animal studies. Cycloserine crosses placenta, its safety in pregnancy is not established; it should be avoided, and used only if no other suitable alternatives are available.[5] The PAS has been used safely in pregnancy in the past. Since no well-designed study has been done to ascertain its safety in pregnancy, it should be used only in the absence of any other alternative.

Fluoroquinolones being toxic and inhibitor of growing cartilage in animals, should be avoided in pregnancy.[9] Animal studies demonstrated teratogenicity (retardation of fetal skull ossification) for clofazimine and crossing of placenta and excretion in milk. The World Health Organization (WHO) has approved this drug safe in pregnancy. Similarly, clarithromycin is not safe in pregnancy as higher dose has been associated with embryotoxicity. There are no adequate and well-controlled studies regarding teratogenicity of linezolid in pregnant women. It should be used during pregnancy only if the potential benefit justifies the potential risk to the fetus. Bedaqualine, a drug for extensively drug resistant TB (XDR-TB) has been recently approved. There are no data on its use in pregnancy, may be considered when other treatment options are limited.[10]

Treatment of TB in a pregnant woman is far less hazardous than leaving the disease untreated, both with regard to the baby and the mother. TB in pregnancy may lead to the birth of an underweight infant or to congenital TB.[11] Risk of miscarriage is much higher in active tuberculosis than the risk from the drug treatment, so standard treatment should be given. Treatment regimen for drug sensitive tuberculosis should include at least the three first-line drugs—rifampicin, isoniazid and ethambutol. Streptomycin should not be used. Opinion regarding the use of pyrazinamide is divided, but the WHO and International Union against Tuberculosis and Lung Disease (IUATLD) recommend its use.[3] The ATS does not confidently advocate its use.[4] According to the WHO, 6 months regimen based upon isoniazid, rifampicin and pyrazinamide should be used whenever possible, and ethambutol should be used only if a fourth drug is needed during the initial phase.[3] Contrary to this, ATS recommends that pyrazinamide should better be avoided in pregnancy, because of the lack of sufficient data for its safety.[4] If pyrazinamide is not used, duration of treatment should be prolonged to nine months. Although, isoniazid, rifampicin and ethambutol cross the placenta, they are not found to be teratogenic.[9]

Women taking first-line antituberculosis drugs should not be asked for termination of pregnancy, while those on reserve drugs should be counseled for possible adverse effects. Breastfeeding should not be discouraged, as the amount of drugs secreted in milk is insufficient to cause any toxic or therapeutic effect. Supplemental pyridoxine is recommended for both the nursing mother and her infant, even if no isoniazid is being given to the infant. All antituberculosis drugs can be used during lactation, except fluoroquinolones.[9] Baby of a woman who has taken rifampicin during pregnancy should receive vitamin K at birth, to avoid the risk of postnatal hemorrhage.[3] Rifampicin may induce metabolism of vitamin K and hamper hepatic synthesis of vitamin K dependent coagulation factors.

Women taking oral hormonal contraceptives should be counseled for possible contraceptive failure and occurrence of pregnancy. This is especially so in women on rifampicin containing antitubercular treatment regimen, because of the induction of metabolism of contraceptive drug by rifampicin.[12,13] Such women should be advised to use non-hormonal contraceptive measures during, and for 1 month after treatment with rifampicin containing regimen.[13,14] It is because of multiple problems of treatment and potential sequelae such as infertility that routine screening is advised for latent and active TB for high-risk populations.[15]

TREATMENT OF TUBERCULOSIS IN RENAL INSUFFICIENCY

Treatment of TB in renal insufficiency poses a difficult clinical problem because various anti-TB medications are cleared by kidney. On one hand, it raises the concern of drug-induced toxicity due to impaired excretion by the diseased kidney, while on the other hand, it raises the concern of undertreatment of TB. In later situation, adequate peak serum concentration is usually low, and not of therapeutic use.[4] Another issue of concern is the achievement of the therapeutic level of antituberculosis drugs in patients with end-stage renal disease, undergoing hemodialysis, which may alter/lower the serum drug levels.

The British Thoracic Society (BTS) advocates dose reduction for drugs, which are excreted by the renal route, while the ATS prefers increasing the dosing interval instead of decreasing the dose.[4,12] Administration of drugs, which are excreted by the kidneys should be changed by increasing the dosing interval, if creatinine clearance falls below 30 mL/min. There is paucity of data to guide the dosing recommendation if creatinine clearance is above 30 mL/min, when standard doses should be prescribed.[4] Rifampicin and isoniazid are eliminated by liver, and they could be given in the usual dosages.[16] Population with slow hepatic acetylation of isoniazid, could be given supplemental pyridoxine to prevent peripheral neuropathy.

Alteration in dose of ethambutol, which is 80% excreted by kidney,[2] should be made if creatinine clearance falls below 70 mL/min,[4] to the lowest possible dose, but if it falls below 30 mL/min, it should be given intermittently as three times a week in dose of 15–20 mg/kg body weight.[4] Pyrazinamide is metabolized in liver, but its metabolites, pyrazinoic acid and 5-hydroxypyrazinoic acid are excreted by kidneys.[17,18] Thus, the drug should be given three times a week, in dose of 25–35 mg/kg body weight, to avoid toxicity, if creatinine clearance falls below 30 mL/min.[4] The risk of developing hyperuricemia with pyrazinamide is also increased in the cases of renal insufficiency.

Since streptomycin is predominantly excreted by the renal route, and removed by hemodialysis to a significant extent (about 40%), it should be administered three times a week in dose of 12–15 mg/kg body weight in patients of renal insufficiency with creatinine clearance below 30 mL/min, and those on hemodialysis.[4,19] Since, pharmacokinetics of other aminoglycosides are similar to those of streptomycin, they need similar modifications of dosages.[4] Renal clearance of fluoroquinolones varies from drug to drug. It is greater for levofloxacin than moxifloxacin.[20] Dose adjustment for fluoroquinolones is recommended if creatinine clearance is less than 30 mL/min (750–1,000 mg, three times a week).[4]

Ethionamide needs no or little alteration of administration as it is not excreted by the kidney.[21] If creatinine clearance is less than 30 mL/min, dose of ethionamide should be reduced to 250–500 mg/day.[4] Dose of cycloserine should be modified if creatinine clearance falls below 30 mL/min or patient is on hemodialysis. It should be changed to 500 mg thrice a week or 250 mg daily.[4] Evidence for safety of 250 mg daily dose of cycloserine is not yet established with regard to neuropathy; 500 mg three times a week, is preferred. Serum concentrations of drug should be monitored. The PAS is not safe in renal disease and should only be given if no other alternative is available, as it may aggravate metabolic acidosis.[6] It should be given at a dose of 4 g/dose, twice daily.

Thiacetazone, also excreted in urine, should not be given to patients with renal disease.[22] The pharmacokinetics of the parent drug, linezolid, is not altered in patients with any degree of renal insufficiency; however, the two primary metabolites of linezolid may accumulate in patients with renal insufficiency, with the amount of accumulation increasing with the severity of renal dysfunction. The clinical significance of accumulation of these two metabolites has not been determined in patients with severe renal insufficiency. However, given the absence of information on the clinical significance of accumulation of the primary metabolites; use of linezolid in patients with renal insufficiency should be weighed against the potential risks of accumulation of these metabolites. Clofazimine is safe in patients having renal disease as excretion is mainly through biliary route. In patients with severe renal impairment dose of clarithromycin must be reduced. Imipenem is highly nephrotoxic but addition of cilastatin lessens its toxicity.

Hemodialysis may remove the drug before its therapeutic effect is established. If the drug is given sufficiently before hemodialysis, far less drug is likely to be removed. It therefore, gets time to be distributed throughout the body. Administration of drug after hemodialysis will avoid the premature removal of drug. This may also facilitate the directly observed treatment short-course (DOTS) strategy indirectly.[4] Premature removal of second-line drugs, by hemodialysis, may further aggravate the problem of drug resistance by exposing the tubercle bacillus to subtherapeutic drug concentrations. Rifampicin, isoniazid and ethambutol are removed to a much less by hemodialysis, but pyrazinamide is removed to a significant extent.[17] Thus, supplemental dosing is not needed with isoniazid, rifampicin and ethambutol, in patients of end-stage renal disease, undergoing hemodialysis. Similar to streptomycin, about 40% of drugs like kanamycin, amikacin and capreomycin are removed from blood, if they are given just before hemodialysis.[19] Fluoroquinolone and ethionamide are not cleared by hemodialysis and thus, their dose needs not be altered in this situation.[20,21] Usually, hemodialysis does not pose significant problem, if drugs are given after the procedure.

Ideally, it is important to monitor serum concentrations of drugs in persons with renal failure who are taking aminoglycosides, cycloserine or ethambutol to provide effective therapeutic drug concentrations and also to minimize dose-related toxicity. Patients with renal failure may have other comorbid conditions, like diabetes mellitus and gastroparesis, which may further complicate the pharmacokinetics of drugs. Presently, there is no data to guide administration of antituberculosis drugs in patients undergoing peritoneal dialysis. For this subset of patients, recommendations as of hemodialysis, are applicable. The safest regimen that is being advised in patients diagnosed as the new cases of tuberculosis with renal insufficiency, is rifampicin, isoniazid and pyrazinamide for 2 months followed by rifampicin and isoniazid for the next 4 months.[22]

Some of the anti-TB drugs, e.g. rifampicin are sometimes reported to induce acute kidney failure and hemolysis of immunological nature.[23,24] There is also an increased risk of TB in patients with chronic renal failure. Some of the Western Centres advocate TB screening for latent infection in patients with chronic renal failure undergoing dialysis.[25] Both *QuantiFERON-TB* Gold and tuberculin skin test show seasonal concordance for diagnosis of latent TB in such patients before kidney transplantation.[26]

TREATMENT OF TUBERCULOSIS IN LIVER DISEASE

Treatment of TB with deranged liver functions presents with two major clinical scenes. First is the issue of antitubercular drug-induced hepatotoxicity; and second, use of antitubercular drugs in persons with preexisting liver disease. Various antitubercular drugs are potentially hepatotoxic, and administration of these drugs may aggravate liver disease in a patient with compromised liver function. Drugs like ethambutol, streptomycin, kanamycin, amikacin and capreomycin are safe in liver disease as they are neither significantly metabolized, nor toxic to liver.[4]

Drug-induced Hepatotoxicity

It is found that, the period of latency between the start of drug regimen and the occurrence of drug-induced hepatitis is usually 4–9 days.[27] It must be known that about 10–30% of patients receiving antituberculosis therapy may normally have the transient rise of bilirubin and liver enzymes [serum glutaryl pyruvate transaminase (SGPT) and serum glutaryl oxalate transaminase (SGOT)], to about one to three times the normal, during the first-two months of therapy. The levels generally come down on continuation of treatment. It is of interest to note that about 10% of patients, who develop mild transaminase elevation (i.e. 1–2% of all treated adults), may have severe hepatitis and liver failure until the drug is discontinued. This clinical condition has the case fatality of approximately 10%. Drug-induced hepatitis is diagnosed, when serum level of SGPT or SGOT rises more than 150 IU/L on more than three occasions, or greater than 250 IU/L on one occasion, along with values of serum bilirubin of more than 34.2 μmol/L (2 mg%).[27]

The incidence of isoniazid-induced, clinical hepatitis is lesser than was previously thought. Hepatitis occurs in 0.6% patients, if isoniazid is given alone, but it is 1.6% if given with drugs, other than rifampicin.[28] With rifampicin, the incidence of hepatitis is 2.7%. Risk of drug-induced hepatitis increases with age, and it is 2% in persons aged 50–64 years. Rate of fatal hepatitis is 0.023%. If it is given to patient with preexisting liver disease, it may accumulate in body and further increase the risk of drug-induced hepatitis.[4] Frequent monitoring of serum level of hepatic transaminases is indicated in this clinical setting.[3]

Patients with alcoholic liver disease are at increased risk of peripheral neuropathy, and should be given pyridoxine prophylactically at a dose of 10 mg daily.[3] Rifampicin may cause normal transient hyperbilirubinemia in 0.6% patients. Incidence of hepatitis is 2.7% if it is given with isoniazid, and it is 1.1%, if given with a drug other than isoniazid.[28] Clearance of rifampicin may be impaired, causing serum levels to rise, if it is given to a patient with preexisting liver disease. Careful monitoring of liver functions is indicated in such patients.[3]

All the three first-line drugs—isoniazid, rifampicin and pyrazinamide—are associated with hepatotoxicity. Of the three, rifampicin is least likely to cause hepatocellular damage, although it is associated with cholestatic jaundice. Pyrazinamide is the most hepatotoxic of the three first-line drugs. Among the second-line drugs, ethionamide, prothionamide and PAS can also be hepatotoxic, although less so than any of the first-line drugs. Hepatitis occurs rarely with the fluoroquinolones.[29]

Chemical structure of ethionamide is similar to that of isoniazid. It can cause liver toxicity in about 2% patients, and should be cautiously used in the presence of preexisting liver disease. The PAS may cause clinical hepatitis in 0.3% cases. Since, pharmacokinetics of PAS are not significantly altered in liver disease, it could be used in usual doses and usual regimen.[6] Cycloserine can be safely used in liver disease, except in the case of alcohol-related hepatitis, where it increases the risk of seizures.[5] Thioacetazone is hepatotoxic, and it should be avoided. Fluoroquinolones except Ciprofloxacin, are safe for use in liver disease.[13]

Advanced age, female sex, poor nutritional status, preexisting liver disease, chronic alcoholism, Hepatitis B carrier state and slow acetylator status are considered risk factors for antitubercular drug-induced hepatitis.[27-31] Several studies have observed relation between serum markers for viral hepatitis and antituberculosis drug-induced hepatitis. It has been observed that viral hepatitis complicates treatment more frequently with regimen containing both rifampicin and isoniazid, than with regimen having only one or none of them.[27-31]

It is often difficult to find the culprit drug in a multidrug regimen causing drug-induced hepatitis. The rise in serum transaminase activity within 15 days of starting regimen is usually attributed to rifampicin, but if it occurs after 1 month, it is usually attributed to pyrazinamide.[32] Whether the toxicity occurs due to their additive effect, synergistic effect, hypersensitivity phenomenon or direct effect is not known. The Joint TB Committee of the (BTS) recommends that liver functions should be monitored weekly during the first-2 weeks, and then at 2 weekly intervals, in patients who have preexisting liver disease.[33] Recommendation for the frequency of monitoring liver functions, in patients with no known risk factors, is not clear.

If a patient on antituberculosis therapy develops mild and transient elevation of serum bilirubin or liver enzymes, treatment need not be stopped. They usually come down during the course of treatment. If, patient develops hepatitis related symptoms with the significant elevation of bilirubin and liver enzymes, treatment should be stopped and viral hepatitis should be ruled out by serology.[33] Drugs should be gradually reintroduced one by one starting from less hepatotoxic drug first, after liver functions come down to normal, with close monitoring for deterioration.

Antituberculosis Treatment with Preexisting Liver Disease

There are great concerns with antitubercular therapy in patients with chronic liver disease such as cirrhosis.[34,35] On the other hand, the frequency of TB is significantly increased in patients with cirrhosis.[34,36] In case of stable liver disease, all anti-TB drugs can be used with close observation for liver functions. In patients with unstable or advanced liver disease, liver function tests should be done at the start of treatment. If the serum SGPT level is more than three times normal before the initiation of treatment, lesser hepatotoxic regimens should be considered. The alternative regimens are devised on the premise that the more unstable or severe the liver disease is, the fewer the hepatotoxic drugs employed. Possible regimens include those that employ two hepatotoxic drugs (rather than three in the standard regimen): (a) 9 months of isoniazid and rifampicin, plus ethambutol (until or unless isoniazid susceptibility is documented); or (b) 2 months of isoniazid, rifampicin, streptomycin and ethambutol, followed by 6 months of isoniazid and rifampicin; or (c) 6–9 months of rifampicin, pyrazinamide and ethambutol is administered.[37]

When the liver disease is too serious to permit use of more than one hepatotoxic drug, a regimen comprising 2 months of isoniazid, ethambutol and streptomycin, followed by 10 months of isoniazid and ethambutol, are preferred.[30] In the extreme case of fulminant hepatic failure where antitubercular treatment is indispensable, a regimen devoid of any hepatotoxic drug is prescribed; such as 18–24 months of streptomycin, ethambutol and a fluoroquinolone.[37]

In conclusion, different options are used for the treatment of tuberculosis with deranged liver functions; mild derangements in liver enzymes require merely a close watch on the liver function without modifying the regimen while the progressively declining hepatic reserves prohibit the use of any potential hepatotoxic drug requiring a substantial revision of the antitubercular regimen. Expert consultation is hence desirable in treating patients with advanced liver disease.

REFERENCES

1. Franks AL, Binkin NJ, Sinder DE, Rokaw WM, Becker S. Isoniazid hepatitis among pregnant and postpartum Hispanic patients. Public Health Rep. 1989;104(2):151-5.
2. Strauss I, Erhardt F. Ethambutol absorption, excretion and dosage in patients with renal tuberculosis. Chemotherapy. 1970;15(3):148-57.
3. World Health Organization. Treatment of Tuberculosis. Guidelines for National Programmes. World Health Organization document. 2003;2:15-6.
4. Blumberg HM, Burman WJ, Chaisson RE, Daley CL, Etkind SC, Friedman LN, Fujiwara P, et al. American Thoracic Society/Centers for Disease Control and Prevention/Infectious Diseases Society of America: Treatment of Tuberculosis. Am J Respir Crit Care Med. 2003;167:603-62.
5. United States Pharmacopeial Dispensing Information. Drug Information for the Health Care Professional. Englewood, Colorado: Micromedex; 1999. pp. 69-1419.
6. Held H, Fried F. Elimination of para-aminosalicylic acid in patients with renal insufficiency. Chemotherapy. 1977;23(6):405-15.
7. Horne NW. Modern Drug Treatment of Tuberculosis, 7th edition. London: Chest, Heart and Stroke Association; 1990. pp. 24-9.
8. Lipsky BA, Baker CA. Fluoroquinolone toxicity profiles: a review focusing on newer agents. Clin Infect Dis. 1999;28(2):352-64.
9. Briggs GG, Freeman RK, Yaffe SJ. Drugs in Pregnancy and Lactation, 5th edition. Baltimore, Maryland: Williams and Wilkins; 1998. pp. 112-7.
10. Centre for Disease Control and Prevention. Provisional CDC guidelines for the use and safety monitoring of bedaquiline fumarate (Sirturo) for the treatment of multidrug-resistant tuberculosis. MMWR Recomm Rep. 2013;62(RR-09):1-22.
11. Jana N, Vasishta K, Jindal SK, Khunnu B, Ghosh K. Perinatal outcome in pregnancies complicated by pulmonary tuberculosis. Int J Gynaecol Obstet. 1994;44(2):119-24.
12. Ormerod P. Chemotherapy and management of tuberculosis in the United Kingdom: recommendations 1998. Thorax. 1998;53:536-648.
13. Skolnick JL, Stoler BS, Katz DB, Anderson WH. Rifampicin, oral contraceptive, and pregnancy. J Am Med Assoc. 1976;236(12): 1382.
14. Frieden T, Espinal M. What is the therapeutic effect and what is the toxicity of antituberculosis drugs? Toman's Tuberculosis. Case Detection, Treatment and Monitoring, 2nd edition. Geneva: World Health Organization; 2004. pp. 110-21.
15. Molina RL, Clouf X, Nour NM. Tuberculosis and the obstetrician-gynaecologist: a global perspective. Rev Obstet Gynecol. 2013;6:174-81.
16. Ellard GA. Chemotherapy of tuberculosis for patients with renal impairment. Nephron. 1993;64(2):169-81.
17. Malone RS, Fish DN, Spiegel DM, Childs JM, Peloquin CA. The effect of hemodialysis on isoniazid, rifampicin, pyrazinamide and ethambutol. Am J Respir Crit Care Med. 1999;159(5):1580-4.
18. Ellard GA. Absorption, metabolism and excretion of pyrazinamide in man. Tubercle. 1969;50(2):144-58.
19. Matzke GR, Halstenson CE, Keane WF. Hemodialysis elimination rates and clearance of gentamycin and tobramycin. Antimicrob Agents Chemother. 1984;25(1):128-30.
20. Fish DN, Chow AT. The clinical pharmacokinetics of levofloxacin. Clin Pharmacokinet. 1997;32(2):101-19.
21. Malone RS, Fish DN, Spiegel DM, Childs JM, Peloquin CA. The effect of hemodialysis on cycloserine, ethionamide, para-aminosalicylic acid and clofazimine. Chest. 1999;116(4):984-90.
22. Harries A. How does treatment of tuberculosis differ in patients with pregnancy, liver disease, or renal disease? Toman's Tuberculosis. Case Detection, Treatment and Monitoring, 2nd edition. Geneva: World Health Organization; 2004. pp. 166-8.
23. Chiba S, Tsuchiya K, Sakashita H, Ito E, Inase N. Rifampicin-induced acute kidney injury during the initial treatment for

pulmonary tuberculosis: a case report and literature review. Intern Med. 2013; 52(21):2457-60.
24. Manika K, Tasiopoulou K, Vlogiaris L, Lada M, Papaemmanouil S, Zarogoulidis K, et al. Rifampicin-associated acute renal failure and hemolysis: a rather uncommon but severe complication. Ren Fail. 2013; 35(8):1179-81.
25. Brij SO, Beck SC, Kleemann F, Jack AL, Wilkinson C, Enoch DA. Tuberculosis screening in a dialysis unit: detecting latent tuberculosis infection is only half the problem. J Hosp Infect. 2014; 87(4):241-4.
26. Kim JS, Cho JH, Park GY, Kang YJ, Kwon O, Choi JY, et al. Comparison of QuantiFERON-TB Gold with tuberculin skin test for detection of latent tuberculosis infection before kidney transplantation. Transplant Proc. 2013;45(8):2899-902.
27. Pande JN, Singh SPN, Khilnani GC, Khilnani S, Tandon RK. Risk factors for hepatoxicity from antituberculosis drugs: a case control study. Thorax. 1996;51(2):132-6.
28. Steele MA, Burk RF, DesPrez RM. Toxic hepatitis with isoniazid and rifampicin. Chest. 1991;99(2):465-71.
29. World Health Organization. Guidelines for the programmatic management of drug resistant tuberculosis. Emergency update. 2008;9:82-3.
30. Prasad R, Verma SK, Chaudhary SR, Chandra M. Predisposing factors in Hepatitis induced by antitubercular regimen containing isoniazid, rifampicin and pyrazinamide: A case control study. J Int Med India. 2006;9:73-8.
31. Kumar A, Misra PK, Mehrotra R, Govil YC, Rana GS. Hepatotoxicity of rifampicin and isoniazid. Is it all drug induced hepatitis? Am Rev Respir Dis. 1991;143:1350-2.
32. Devoto FM, Gonzalez C, Iannantuono R, Serra HA, Gonzalez CD, Saenz C. Risk factors for hepatotoxicity induced by antitubercular drugs. Acta Physiol Pharma Ther Latin Am. 1997;47(4):197-202.
33. Omerord LP, Skinner C, Wales J (on behalf of the Joint Tuberculosis Committee of the British Thoracic Society). Hepatotoxicity of antituberculosis drugs. Thorax. 1996;51:111-3.
34. Kumar N, Kedarisetty CK, Kumar S, Khillan V, Sarin SK. Antitubercular therapy in patients with cirrhosis: challenges and options. World J Gastroenterol. 2014;20(19):5760-72.
35. Shin HJ, Lee HS, Kim YI, Lim SC, Lung JP, Ko YC, et al. Hepatotoxicity of anti-tuberculosis chemotherapy in patients with liver cirrhosis. Int J Tuberc Lung Dis. 2014;18(3):347-51.
36. Lin YT, Wu PH, Lin CY, Lin MY, Chuang HY, Huang JF, et al. Cirrhosis as a risk factor for tuberculosis infection—a nationwide longitudinal study in Taiwan. Am J Epidemiol. 2014;180(1):103-10.
37. World Health Organization. WHO Treatment of Tuberculosis Guidelines, 4th edition. Geneva: World Health Organization. 2009;8:97-8.

Tuberculosis and Human Immunodeficiency Virus Infection

Aditya Jindal, SK Jindal

INTRODUCTION

The discovery of human immunodeficiency virus (HIV) infection followed upon a sequence of unusual events. The occurrence of at least 8 cases of Kaposi's sarcoma (KS) amongst gay men in New York in 1980–81 and of *Pneumocystis carinii* (*P. carinii*, now *P. jirovecii*) pneumonia in California and New York in 1981–82, led the Centre for Disease Control (CDC) in USA to form a task force on KS and opportunistic infection (KSOI). The condition was labeled as acquired immunodeficiency syndrome (AIDS) after the discovery of an immune-depressed state in these patients. Thereafter, several other opportunistic infections including tuberculosis (TB) were detected to occur more commonly in these individuals. The HIV infection was finally established as the root cause. In the short span of time elapsed since—about quarter of a century—the disease has made an enormously devastating impact on the global healthcare infrastructure.

In particular, it has worsened the scene of TB all over the world by adversely influencing its epidemiology, clinical outcomes and treatment-strategies. Both TB and HIV infections are deadlier together, TB causing one-fourth of AIDS-related deaths and HIV infecting at least 15% of patients with TB worldwide.[1] The HIV and TB coinfection has come to be known as a deadly duet, a difficult and frequently fatal combination. TB is the most common opportunistic infection in HIV infected persons in several countries, including in India.[2]

EPIDEMIOLOGY

There are an estimated 33.2 million persons infected with HIV, of whom about one-third are also infected with *Mycobacterium tuberculosis* (*M. tb*).[3] The TB incidence in HIV infected persons is about 100 fold more than in the general population. According to the WHO/UNAIDS estimates, up to half of the patients with HIV or AIDS develop TB. The estimated number of new cases of TB in HIV infected individuals rose by almost 100% from nearly 0.7 million in 2006 to 1.4 million in 2008; TB also accounted for 26% of AIDS related deaths.[2-4] In 2011 out of the 8.7 million new cases of TB, 1.1 million were among people living with HIV (PLHIV).

Most of the increase in HIV related TB, as well as the deaths from TB in patients of AIDS occurred in the developing countries. HIV infection was an important factor for the resurgence of TB in the United States and Europe around the turn of the millennium. However, the effective steps undertaken by these countries successfully contained the dual epidemic. A recent assessment of population based TB rates among HIV infected persons in the New York City (from 2001 to 2005) was made from the city's TB and HIV/AIDS surveillance registries; TB in HIV infected persons was 16 times the TB rate of a "non-HIV" population.[5] However, the decline was primarily limited to the US born and not to the foreign born HIV infected population.[5] As the majority of foreign born persons came from the developing countries, this clearly demonstrated the disparities in the prevalence of HIV-TB coinfection.

Although the HIV-TB scene in several countries is dismal, there is some evidence of a declining trend in India. The estimated number of people living with HIV/AIDS (PLWHA) in India has been revised to 2.5 million people from the earlier reported figure of 5.7 million.[6,7] The revised figures are also likely to reflect the reduced HIV-TB burden.

The HIV epidemic has greatly upset the TB control programs of several countries. TB has proven difficult to control in the high HIV prevalence zones.[8] Considering the observation that in some African countries, almost 80% of persons with TB have HIV infection, it was strongly felt that an integrated preventive strategy is essential for both TB and HIV infection.[8-10] Enhanced implementation of TB-HIV collaborative activities and a focused research agenda are critical to the success of control programs, especially in the resource-limited countries.[10,11] The World Health Organization (WHO) policy on TB/HIV activities initially released in 2004, was recently updated in 2012 **(Table 1)**. These activities aim at a comprehensive plan to contain the disease burden and strengthen the control services.

Table 1 World Health Organization (WHO) recommended collaborative tuberculosis (TB)/human immunodeficiency virus (HIV) activities

A. Establish and strengthen the mechanisms of delivering integrated TB and HIV services 1. Set up and strengthen a coordinating body for collaborative TB/HIV activities functional at all levels 2. Determine HIV prevalence among TB patients and TB prevalence among people living with HIV 3. Carry out joint TB/HIV planning to integrate the delivery of TB and HIV services 4. Monitor and evaluate collaborative TB/HIV activities
B. Reduce the burden of TB in people living with HIV and initiate early antiretroviral therapy (the Three I's for HIV/TB) 1. Intensify TB case-finding and ensure high quality antiTB treatment 2. Initiate TB prevention with isoniazid preventive therapy and early antiretroviral therapy 3. Ensure control of TB infection in healthcare facilities and congregate settings
C. Reduce the burden of HIV in patients with presumptive and diagnosed TB 1. Provide HIV testing and counseling to patients with presumptive and diagnosed TB 2. Provide HIV prevention interventions for patients with presumptive and diagnosed TB 3. Provide cotrimoxazole preventive therapy for TB patients living with HIV 4. Ensure HIV prevention interventions, treatment and care for TB patients living with HIV 5. Provide antiretroviral therapy for TB patients living with HIV

PATHOGENESIS

Both TB and HIV suppress the host's immune responses even though the mechanisms are not fully understood. There are many gaps in our understanding of mechanisms of interaction of these two pathogens.[12] There is evidence to suggest that the susceptibility to dual infection is also influenced by inborn errors of immunity, and genetic polymorphisms.[13]

There are several immunological defects in HIV infection, which predispose to TB and encourage HIV-TB coinfection **(Table 2)**. HIV infection is primarily responsible for impaired cell-mediated immunity (CMI) by causing a decline in the number and function of CD4++ subset of T-cells.[14] There is a diminished recruitment and activation of CD4++ cells. The other components of CMI, such as the macrophages and peripheral blood monocytes are also affected and their function impaired. There is resultant reduced production and activation of mediators, such as the cytokines and lymphokines. HIV infection also results in an increased secretion of TH-2 cytokines [interleukin-4 (IL-4) and IL-10] that are antagonist to cytokines [(IL-2, IL12 and interferon-gamma (IFNγ)], which mediate the immunity to tubercle bacilli. In addition, there is a failure of macrophage differentiation to epithelioid cells and formation of Langhans cells. This global impairment of the cellular arm of immunity seriously reduces the immune

Table 2 Immune alterations/defects in human immunodeficiency virus (HIV) infection, which predispose to tuberculosis (TB)

1. CD4++ T cells: Decline in number
i. Depletion ii. Functional impairment iii. Diminished recruitment and activation
2. Impairment of macrophages and peripheral blood monocytes
3. Increased secretion of TH-2 cytokines (IL-4 and IL-10) by the mononuclear cells
4. Failure of macrophage differentiation (to epithelioid cells)
5. Lack of formation of Langhans giant cells
6. Enhanced HIV replication by:
i. Increased production of TNF-α ii. *M.tb* and its cell wall components iii. Beta chemokine monocyte chemotactic protein iv. Downregulation of chemokines
Abbreviations: IL, interleukin; TNF-α, tumor necrotic factor-alpha; *M. tb., Mycobacterium tuberculosis*

defenses against several intracellular and other pathogens, especially the mycobacteria.

Factors additional to or other than CD4+ T-cell decline and impairment may also partly account for increased predisposition to TB.[15] Mycobacterium TB infection may induce nuclear factor binding to the nuclear factor-kappaB (NF-KB) sequences in the HIV replication. The increased HIV replication by *M. tb* sets a vicious cycle in both promoting growth of each other and therefore, the continuing damage to the host cells. TB can occur in patients with HIV infection at all levels, but the type, severity and manifestations depend on the CD4+ T-lymphocyte counts. The greater the degree of immunosuppression and the lower the CD4+ counts, more likely the atypical presentation.

As the immunosuppression progresses, there occurs increased likelihood of infection by atypical and opportunistic mycobacteria and decreased tuberculin reactivity. Granuloma formation is impaired while the lesions show high content of intracellular organisms. The absence of an inflammatory cellular response in the presence of a large number of organisms and "naked necrosis" is sometimes referred to as "nonreactive" form of TB.

TB in an HIV infected individual may develop either as reactivation of previous latent TB or as a new, acquired infection. HIV infected persons acquire TB infection more frequently when exposed to *M. tb.*[16] This phenomenon of increased susceptibility is now supported by the reports of explosive outbreaks of TB among HIV infected persons exposed to a patient with infectious TB—11 of 30 (37%) residents who were exposed to a patient with infectious TB living in a residential care facility for HIV infected persons in San Francisco, developed TB within 120 days.[17] It was also shown with the help of Restriction Fragment Length Polymorphism (RFLP) analysis that all 11 of those patients had TB caused by the same strain of *M. tb,* supporting the single source of origin of infection.

HIV infected patients with TB may be less infectious than those without HIV infection. TB in HIV infected patients is generally extrapulmonary or if pulmonary, paucibacillary, with fewer bacilli in the sputum.[18] This however, is not always true. There are other studies, which report the opposite findings.[19] In HIV infected communities with HIV-TB coinfection, the number of persons with communicable TB keeps on multiplying with increased transmission to other people regardless of their HIV status.[20]

HIV infection increases the rate of TB reactivation in a previously infected patient (latent TB). The annual risk of developing TB in a PLWHA, coinfected with *M. tb* is 5–15%.[21,22] Both reactivation of previous infection and exogenous reinfection are reported to occur in these patients.[23] Possibly, reactivation is the more likely mechanism in low prevalence Western countries with a lower level of exposure to patients with active disease, although the occurrence of new infection has been also shown with the help of RFLP analysis.[20,24,25] New infections from different strains are however, common in the high TB-burden countries.[26]

A recent study from Malawi explored differences in "clustering" (i.e. sharing of identical *M. tb* strains) in patients clustered by prior *M. tb* infection and HIV status. In HIV positive TB cases, clustering was similar in patients with previous *M. tb* infection and without prior infection.[26] It was thus concluded that the HIV infection also increased the risk of reinfection following exposure in patients with latent TB.[26]

CLINICAL FEATURES

The clinical features of TB in HIV infected patients depend upon the severity of immunosuppression **(Table 3)**.[27-30] The presentation in early HIV disease is almost similar to that observed in otherwise healthy individuals, in whom pulmonary disease with focal infiltration and cavities is more common, while extrapulmonary manifestations and other atypical features are common when the CD4+ counts are less than 200/mm.[3,4,31,32]

Table 3 Clinical features of human immunodeficiency virus (HIV)-tuberculosis (TB) coinfection

i. Clinical manifestations a. "Typical"- pulmonary b. "Atypical" pulmonary/pleural TB c. Extrapulmonary: Lymphadenopathy, meningitis, brain abscess, pericarditis, peritonitis, liver abscess (and others)
ii. Drug resistant TB a. Multidrug resistance b. Extensive drug resistance c. Poor treatment response d. Higher mortality rates
iii. Tuberculin skin sensitivity a. Diminished or absent

"Typical" pulmonary disease presenting with fever and other constitutional symptoms, cough, expectoration and hemoptysis is not uncommon. Several of these patients are diagnosed to have HIV coinfection only on serological tests. On the other hand, several series have emphasized the frequent presence of disseminated disease with extra-pulmonary organ involvement.[27,28,33-35] Lesions are more diffuse than granulomas in these patients with "systemic TB".[36] Lymphadenopathy, including mediastinal, hilar and peripheral is commonly described. Relatively uncommon sites for TB, such as the gastrointestinal (GIT), genitourinary, cardiac and central nervous system are more often involved in the presence of HIV infection. Disseminated disease is a common presentation in childhood TB. Night sweats, fatigue, diarrhea and hepatosplenomegaly are other common features in these patients.[36]

Both pleural and parenchymal pulmonary involvements are common in HIV-TB coinfection.[37] Pleural fluid in the presence of HIV infection may more often show the presence of acid-fast bacilli (AFB), on both smear and culture examinations.[38] These mycobacteria may also show the presence of drug resistance, similar to that seen in parenchymal TB.[38,39]

Occurrence of TB in an HIV infected patient in the previous 2 years is also used for HIV/AIDS staging. It is categorized as clinical stage 3 disease in case of pulmonary and stage 4 in case of extrapulmonary TB.[40] Systemic manifestations include the presence of associated/complicating illnesses attributed to HIV immunosuppression. Recurrent pneumonias, diarrhea, herpes zoster infection and mucosal (oral/genital/GIT) ulcerations are common. Weight loss of more than 10 kg or more than 20% of original weight loss is an important AIDS defining criterion.

Emergence of multidrug resistance (MDR) and extensive drug resistance (XDR) TB strains is a serious challenge all over the world.[41] As per 2008 WHO report, there were around 490,000 cases of MDR-TB with more than 110,000 deaths and 40,000 XDR-TB cases every year.[42] It was further assessed that only 7% of MDR-TB were identified and reported to WHO, of whom only one-fifth were noted according to WHO standards.[41] A recent systematic review and meta-analysis of published literature demonstrates an association of HIV infection with MDR-TB.[43] There is little doubt that the prevalence of both MDR-TB and XDR-TB have substantially increased, following the HIV epidemic.[44] The threat of an "untreatable TB", i.e. XDR-TB has particularly posed a global concern.[44]

The clinical and radiological manifestations of MDR-TB in HIV infected individuals are generally similar to those of MDR-TB in non-HIV infected patients, but pose greater problems of symptom and severity control due to poor treatment with pulmonary cavitary and/or disseminated disease. High mortality rates are reported in MDR-TB patients with than in those without HIV infection.[45] Transmission rate of MDR-TB in HIV infection is also high. The 98% mortality was reported in 53 patients of XDR-TB, of whom 44 were HIV infected with a median survival of only 16 days after the diagnosis was established.[46]

DIAGNOSIS

Diagnosis of TB in HIV infected patients is established on the same lines and methods as in non-HIV infected patients. However, diagnosis in the presence of HIV infection is somewhat difficult in view of the difficulties of AFB demonstration in cases of extrapulmonary and noncavitary pulmonary TB. There is lesser likelihood of sputum smear and culture positivity in the presence of HIV infection though this observation is not corroborated in some studies.[47,29] The lesser sensitivity and specificity of sputum microscopy is attributed to the presence of fewer bacilli in the sputum because of the diminished chances of cavitation from a disregulated cellular response and due to increased incidence of infection with nonTB mycobacteria.[48,49] Culture of *M. tb* from sputum and/or other pathological specimens and secretions is diagnostic of TB. The practical utility of mycobacterial culture is however limited, especially in control programs.

Radiological diagnosis of TB is nonspecific. This is especially so in the presence of HIV coinfection when the chest X-ray findings are generally atypical.[50] Moreover, the chest radiology is frequently negative in extrapulmonary manifestations of TB. There is some recent evidence to suggest the use of fluorodeoxyglucose-positron emission tomography (FDG/PET) and positron emission tomography-computed tomography (PET/CT) for early diagnosis, identification of extrapulmonary TB, staging of TB and assessment of response to therapy.[51] More importantly, one relies on cytological and/or histopathological examination for the demonstration of caseation, granuloma formation (which are ill formed and rare) and AFB. Investigational procedures, such as fine needle aspiration biopsy, pleural fluid aspiration, lumbar puncture, forceps biopsy, bronchoscopic or transbronchial biopsy and other methods are used to obtain the appropriate specimens for these examinations.

Interpretation of the tuberculin skin test (TST) in the presence of HIV infection for the diagnosis of TB is somewhat difficult, especially in the high TB prevalence countries. A positive TST is considered as suggestive of TB-infection or latent TB in any individual, more so in the presence of HIV infection in whom the test sensitivity is further reduced. In countries such as India, where there is presence of TB infection diagnosed by a positive TST in up to 40–50% of the normal healthy population, the positive test cannot be considered as an indication for treatment in non-HIV individuals.

However, in the presence of immunosuppression due to HIV infection, the positivity of TST can be considered as more valuable. The probability of a positive TST in these patients is significantly low,[52] therefore, a positive test may "strongly" suggest TB. It is for this reason that the cutoff values for positivity for TST are lower for HIV infected patients.[53,54] However, a lower "cutoff" may not necessarily differentiate between "infection" and "disease". In a retrospective medical record data-base review (1988–2007), the administration of TSTs to newly diagnosed HIV patients was inconsistent and different according to the country of birth, among other factors, resulting in "missed opportunities for TB prevention".[55]

The Interferon-Gamma Release Assays (IGRA) tests are now employed for the detection of latent TB with the help of QuantiFERON-TB Gold test and T-Spot tests.[56] These tests, like TST, are unable to differentiate between TB infection and active TB disease. We do not have figures on positive IGRA in otherwise healthy people, but the interpretation is somewhat similar to that of TST.[57] The updated guidelines for using IGRA in the United States suggest their use as aids in diagnosing TB infection in different populations.[58] It is not possible to make such a recommendation of their use to guide treatment in India.

Polymerase chain reaction tests such as Xpert *M.tb*/RIF assay from sputum and other samples have been recommended as point of care tests for rapid detection of mycobacteria, including in HIV positive patients.[59,60] The cost efficacy of the test in these settings is not yet established.[61]

MANAGEMENT

The greatest challenge in managing HIV-TB coinfection lies in the simultaneous treatment of both the infections and frequently of other concomitant opportunistic infections. The basic principles of treatment are similar as for TB treatment in non-HIV patients. There are however, several important issues related to the treatment **(Table 4)**. One needs to consider the HIV related problems, such as the compliance with the therapy, presence of drug resistance, the level of immunosuppression and presence of complicating or other coinfections. The outcomes of treatment in the presence of HIV infection are similar, if the basic principles are adequately

Table 4 Important issues in the treatment of tuberculosis (TB)-human immunodeficiency virus (HIV) coinfection

1. Antitubercular therapy
i. Choice of drugs ii. Choice of regimen iii. Optimum duration of therapy iv. Directly observed therapy short course (DOTS) v. Treatment for MDR-TB and XDR-TB vi. Prevention of recurrence of TB
2. Anti-HIV (retroviral) therapy
i. Polypharmacotherapy ii. Overlapping side effects of drugs iii. Drug-drug interaction iv. Immune reconstitution inflammatory syndrome (IRIS)
Abbreviations: MDR, multidrug resistance; XDR, extensive drug resistance

taken care of.[62-64] A recent report from Congo cites a four-times higher mortality in HIV-infected than noninfected children treated at primary care level.[65]

The four primary drugs, rifampicin (R), isoniazid (H), pyrazinamide (Z) and ethambutol (E) constitute the mainstay of treatment in drug-susceptible TB, administered as the standard two phase regimen: Initial intensive phase of 2 months of all the four drugs, followed by the maintenance phase of H and R for 4 months (2HRZE, 4HR).

Treatment of HIV-TB with *directly observed therapy* has been shown to prolong life,[66] prevent drug resistance and quickly render a TB patient noninfectious. It is the most effective method of promoting adherence to TB treatment, particularly in the presence of HIV coinfection.[67,68]

The issues related to intermittent versus daily regime and the optimum duration of therapy have remained somewhat debatable. Most of the studies of standard 6 month regimen (2 HRZE, 4 HR) have shown similar rates of treatment failure and relapse among HIV infected and non-HIV infected patients.[62,69,70] The current recommendation is to use standard 6 month regimen for all cases and to extend to 9 months for patients with delayed clinical (continued symptoms) or microbiological response (sputum culture positivity) at 2 months.[71,72]

Management of MDR-TB and XDR-TB in the HIV infected patients poses the biggest challenge. The choice of drugs and the duration of therapy for MDR-TB are variably recommended. Generally, the treatment duration is guided by AFB smear and culture reports. Most regimens contain 4–6 drugs, administered for at least 18 months after culture conversion, but extended to 24 months in patients with extensive pulmonary damage.[73-75] As per the Revised National TB Control Programme (RNTCP) recommendations, the regimen for MDR-TB comprises of 6 drugs (kanamycin, ofloxacin, ethionamide, pyrazinamide, ethambutol and cycloserine) during the 6–9 months of the intensive phase followed by four drugs (ofloxacin, ethionamide, cycloserine and ethambutol) for the 18 months of the continuation phase.[76]

Management of XDR-TB involves the use of toxic but less potent drugs with poorer outcomes than in MDR-TB cases.[77,78] The medication adherence is reported to be poorer for anti-TB drugs than the anti-HIV drugs in a prospective cohort of XDR-TB/HIV coinfected patients.[79]

A number of new drugs are in various phases of development with the aim of reduction in the number of drugs, as well duration of therapy.[80,81] No drug as yet has proven to achieve the goals. Linezolid, delamanid, bedaquiline and DA-824 are some of new anti-TB drugs for XDR-TB. There is a growing evidence to suggest the concurrent use of host-directed adjunctive therapies to enhance the role of pathogen directed therapy.[82] Immunotherapy, including the vaccines and vitamin D have also been used as adjunctive treatments.

Concurrent treatment of both TB and HIV infections has significantly improved the outcome of patients.[83-85] HIV treatment with highly active antiretroviral therapy (HAART) comprises a combination of at least three antiretroviral (ARV) drugs. *There are four major groups of antiviral drugs, which are currently available that include:*

1. Protease inhibitors
2. Reverse transcriptase inhibitors
3. Viral integrase enzyme inhibitors
4. Viral entry inhibitors.

ARV treatment does not completely cure the disease, but effectively suppresses the viral replication. ARV therapy (ART) is costly and required to be continued lifelong. The ARV drugs also have a high-toxicity profile. There are several important issues in the administration of ART, especially when used along with antitubercular treatment (ATT) **(Table 4)**. The WHO guidelines are generally followed in resource limited countries.[86]

The short-term risk of HIV disease progression in HIV related TB is related to the degree of immunosuppression (measured by CD4+ cell count or CD4+ cell percentage).[84,85] Patients with advanced immunosuppression (CD4+ T cell counts <100/µL) are likely to develop treatment failure, relapses and development of MDR-TB.

Combination of ART along with ATT has the potential of overlapping adverse effects of both the therapies. Moreover, the presence of other opportunistic infections adds further to the complication list. HIV related complications (e.g. thrombocytopenia) cause additional problems. Drug-drug interaction is an important problem, especially seen with the use of rifamycins, which increase the synthesis of a number of hepatic enzyme system. Rifampicin use results in a marked decrease in the concentrations of ARV agents, such as the protease inhibitors, which are metabolized by CYP3A. Rifabutin, with which the CYP3A expression is much less marked, is generally considered as an alternate drug. The dosages of these drugs, when used in combinations are therefore altered to maintain effective concentrations.[72,87-89] Thiacetazone should not be used in HIV-TB coinfection.

In view of the drug-drug interactions, the ART was withheld during the ATT administration in the past. WHO recommends that irrespective of the CD4+ count, all HIV-TB patients should be given ART. It is now believed that an early institution of ART helps in an early control of immunosuppression and improves mortality in patients with CD4+ T cell count of less than 200 cells/mm^3. In such patients, ART is started as soon as ATT is tolerated within the first 2 weeks to 2 months.[76] If the CD4+ T cell count is between 200 and 350 cells/mm^3, ART can start after the first 2 months of ATT. ART in patients with CD4+ counts of more than 350/mm^3 can be deferred until antitubercular therapy is completed.

In India, the integrated activities of the national programs (RNTCP and National AIDS Control Programme), facilitate the treatment of HIV-TB coinfection. The ARV treatment is provided through the Integrated Testing and Counseling Centres and ATT through the DOTS centers. The fewer number of ART centers however, is a limiting factor. The choice of regimens for ATT under RNTCP is made on the basis of standard categorization for different forms of tuberculosis irrespective of the HIV status.

Improvement in immunity following ARV therapy results in an increase in inflammatory response to mycobacteria in tuberculosis lesions. The worsening of clinical symptoms following institution of both ATT and ARV is termed as the immune reconstitution inflammatory syndrome (IRIS).[90-92] This paradoxical reaction is often noticed particularly with lymph node and pleural tuberculosis.

The common features of IRIS comprise of fever, increase in lymphadenopathy, effusion and pulmonary infiltrates.[93,94] Occasionally, there is worsening of meningeal, central nervous system, hepatopulmonary, soft tissue or other forms of tuberculosis when it can even be life threatening.[94] The tuberculin skin reaction may become positive in a few cases.

Immune reconstitution inflammatory syndrome generally develops in the presence of low baseline CD4+ cell counts, high viral load prior to ART initiation and a shorter interval between the start of ATT and HAART.[95] The presence of disseminated disease or a "better" response to treatment, i.e. a greater increase in the CD4+ cell count and a greater reduction in the viral load are other likely risk factors of IRIS.[96] Besides the "paradoxical" type of IRIS in which there is clinical worsening following ATT, an "unmasking" type of IRIS is also recognized in which the undiagnosed TB becomes apparent after the institution of HAART.[97] The pathogenesis of this unmasking is not clear, but it poses problems in management. Patients who develop IRIS were shown to have higher preART levels of tumor necrosis factor (TNF) and other inflammatory biomarkers.[98]

Most cases of IRIS are self-limiting. Treatment with anti-inflammatory drugs, (usually nonsteroidal) is generally adequate. ATT and ART should not be stopped, but for very severe reactions.[99] Corticosteroids are rarely required for severe and persistent IRIS. On an average, IRIS lasts for a period of six to eight weeks, but for the presence of lymph node enlargement, which may persist for longer periods.

Bacillus-Calmette-Guérin (BCG) vaccination in an HIV positive child is a cause of concern in view of the reports of local complications and disseminated BCG disease. The risk is not substantiated by the results of prospective studies in HIV infected and non-HIV infected infants. As per current recommendations, routine BCG vaccination in infants in the high HIV prevalence areas is not withheld, but it should not be given to known HIV infected individuals.[100,101]

REFERENCES

1. Harrington M. From HIV to tuberculosis and back again: a tale of activism in 2 pandemics. Clin Infect Dis. 2010;50(Suppl 3):S260-6.
2. WHO Report 2005. Global Tuberculosis Control: surveillance, planning, financing. Geneva: World Health Organization; 2005.
3. Getahun H, Gunneberg C, Granich R, Nunn P. HIV infection-associated tuberculosis: the epidemiology and the response. Clin Infect Dis. 2010;50(Suppl 3):S201-7.
4. Tripathy S, Paing M, Narain JP. Tuberculosis and human immunodeficiency virus infection. In: SK Sharma, Alladi Mohan (Eds.). Tuberculosis, 2nd edition. New Delhi: Jaypee Brothers Medical Publishers (P) Ltd; 2009. pp. 574-90.
5. Trieu L, Jiehui Li, Hanna DB, Harris TG. Tuberculosis rates among HIV infected persons in New York City, 2001-2005. Am J Public Health. 2001;100(6):1031-4.
6. Dandona L, Dandona R. Drop of HIV estimate for India to less than half. Lancet. 2007;370(9602):1811-3.
7. UNAIDS. (2006). Jointed United Nations Programme on HIV/AIDS, 2006 report on the global AIDS epidemic. [online] Available from: http://*www.unaids.org/en/HIV_data/2006GlobalReport/default.asp*. [Accessed January, 2016].
8. Bekker LG, Wood R. The changing natural history of tuberculosis and HIV coinfection in an urban area of hyperendemicity. Clin Infect Dis. 2010;50(Suppl 3):S208-14.
9. Granich R, Akolo C, Gunneberg C, Getahun H, Williams P, Williams B. Prevention of tuberculosis in people living with HIV. Clin Infect Dis. 2010;50(Suppl 3):S215-22.
10. Howard AA, El-Sadr WM. Integration of tuberculosis and HIV services in sub-Saharan Africa: lessons learned. Clin Infect Dis. 2010;50(Suppl 3):S238-44.
11. Chamie G, Luetkemeyer A, Charlebois E, Havlir DV. Tuberculosis as part of the natural history of HIV infection in developing countries. Clin Infect Dis. 2010;50(Suppl 3):S245-54.
12. Pawlowski A, Jansson M, Skold M, Rottenberg ME, Kallenius G. Tuberculosis and HIV coinfection. PLoS Pathog. 2012;8(2):e1002464.
13. Moller M, Hoal EG. Current findings, challenges and novel approaches in human genetic susceptibility to tuberculosis. Tuberculosis (Edinb). 2010;90(2):71-83.
14. Lawn SD, Butera ST, Shinnick TM. Tuberculosis unleashed: the impact of human immunodeficiency virus infection on the host granulomatous response to Mycobacterium tuberculosis. Microbes Infect. 2002;4(6):635-46.
15. Toossi Z. Virological and immunological impact of tuberculosis on human immunodeficiency virus type 1 disease. J Infect Dis. 2003;188(8):1146-55.
16. Nunn P, Mungai M, Nyamwaya J, Gicheha C, Brindle RJ, Dunn DT, et al. The effect of human immunodeficiency virus type-1 on the infectiousness of tuberculosis. Tuber Lung Dis. 1994;75(1):25-32.
17. Daley CL, Small PM, Schecter GF, Schoolnik GK, McAdam RA, Jacobs WR, et al. An outbreak of tuberculosis with accelerated progression among persons infected with the human immunodeficiency virus. An analysis using restriction-fragment-length polymorphisms. N Engl J Med. 1992;326(4):231-5.
18. Elliott AM, Hayes RJ, Halwiindi B, Luo N, Tembo G, Pobee JO, et al. The impact of HIV on infectiousness of pulmonary tuberculosis: a community study in Zambia. AIDS. 1993;7(7):981-7.
19. Theuer CP, Hopewell PC, Elias D, Schecter GF, Rutherford GW, Chaisson RE. Human immunodeficiency virus infection in tuberculosis patients. J Infect Dis. 1990;162(1):8-12.
20. Murray JF. Tuberculosis and HIV infection: a global perspective. Respiration. 1998;65(5):335-42.
21. Braun MM, Badi N, Ryder RW, Baende E, Mukadi Y, Nsuami M, et al. A retrospective cohort study of the risk of tuberculosis among women of child bearing age with HIV infection in Zaire. Am Rev Respir Dis. 1991;143(3):501-4.

22. Narain JP, Raviglione MC, Kochi A. HIV associated tuberculosis in developing countries: epidemiology and strategies for prevention. Tuber Lung Dis. 1992;73(6):311-21.
23. Sutherland I. The epidemiology of tuberculosis and AIDS. British Communicable Disease Report. 1990;90(10):3-4.
24. Small PM, Hopewell PC, Singh SP, Paz A, Parsonnet J, Ruston DC, et al. The epidemiology of tuberculosis in San Francisco: a population-based study using conventional and molecular methods. N Engl J Med. 1994;330(24):1703-9.
25. Alland D, Kalkut GE, Moss AR, McAdam RA, Hahn JA, Bosworth W, et al. Transmission of tuberculosis in New York City. An analysis by DNA fingerprinting and conventional epidemiologic methods. N Engl J Med. 1994;330(24):1710-6.
26. Houben RM, Glynn JR, Mallard K, Sichali L, Malema S, Fine PE, et al. Human immunodeficiency virus increases the risk of tuberculosis due to recent re-infection in individuals with latent infection. Int J Tuberc Lung Dis. 2010;14(7):909-15.
27. Sunderam G, McDonald RJ, Maniatis T, Oleske J, Kapila R, Reichman LB. Tuberculosis as a manifestation of the acquired immunodeficiency syndrome (AIDS). The Journal of the Ameri Medic Assoc. 1986;256(3):362-6.
28. Hopewell PC. Factors influencing transmission and infectivity of Mycobacterium tuberculosis: Implications for clinical and public health management. In: MA Sande, LD Hudson, RK Root (Eds). Respiratory Infections. New York: Churchill-Livingston; 1986. pp. 191-216.
29. Theuer CP, Hopewell PC, Elias D, Schecter GF, Rutherford GW, Chaisson RE. Human immunodeficiency virus infection in tuberculosis patients. J Infect Dis. 1990;162(1):8-12.
30. Batungwanayo J, Taelman H, Dhote R, Bogaerts J, Allen S, Van de Perre P. Pulmonary tuberculosis in Kigali, Rwanda: the impact of HIV infection on clinical and radiographic presentation. Am Rev Respir Dis. 1992;146(1):53-6.
31. Hopewell PC. Tuberculosis and infection with the human immunodeficiency virus. In: Reichman LB, Hershfield ES (Eds). Tuberculosis: a Comprehensive International Approach. New York: Marcel Dekker, Inc.; 1993. pp. 369-94.
32. Sharma SK, Mohan A, Kadhiravan T. HIV-TB coinfection: epidemiology, diagnosis and management. Indian J Med Res. 2005;121(4):550-67.
33. Chaisson RE, Schecter GF, Theuer CP, Rutherford GW, Echenberg DF, Hopewell PC. Tuberculosis in patients with the acquired immunodeficiency syndrome. Clinical features, response to therapy, and survival. Am Rev Respir Dis. 1987;136(3):570-4.
34. Nyandiko WM, Mwangi A, Ayaya SO, Nabakwe EC, Tenge CN, Gisore PM, et al. Characteristics of HIV infected children seen in Western Kenya. East Afr Med J. 2009;86(8):364-73.
35. de Noronha AL, Bafica A, Nogucira L, Barral A, Barral-Netto M. Lung granulomas from mycobacterium tuberculosis/HIV-I coinfected patients display decrease in situ TNF production. Pathol Res Pract. 2008;204(3):155-61.
36. Heyderman RS, Makunike R, Muza T, Odwee M, Kadzirange G, Manyemba J, et al. Pleural tuberculosis in Harare, Zimbabwe: the relationship between human immunodeficiency virus, CD4+ lymphocyte count, granuloma formation and disseminated disease. Trop Med Int Health. 1998;3(1):14-20.
37. Qiu L, Teeter LD, Liu Z, Ma X, Musser JM, Graviss EA. Diagnostic associations between pleural and pulmonary tuberculosis. J Infect. 2006;53(6):377-86.
38. Luzze H, Elliott AM, Joloba ML, Odida M, Oweka-Onyee J, Nakiyingi J, et al. Evaluation of suspected tuberculous pleurisy: clinical and diagnostic findings in HIV-1 positive and HIV-negative adults in Uganda. Int J Tuberc Lung Dis. 2001;5(8):746-53.
39. Baumann MH, Nolan R, Petrini M, Lee YC, Light RW, Schneider E. Pleural Tuberculosis in the United States: incidence and drug resistance. Chest. 2007;131(4):1125-32.
40. WHO. Interim WHO Clinical staging of HIV/AIDS and HIV/AIDS case definitions for surveillance. Geneva: WHO; 2005.
41. Gandhi NR, Nunn P, Dheda K, Schaaf HS, Zignol M, van Soolingen D, et al. Multidrug-resistant and extensively drug-resistant tuberculosis: a threat to global control of tuberculosis. Lancet. 2010;375(9728):1830-43.
42. WHO. Tuberculosis: MDR-TB and XDR-TB, the 2008 report. Geneva: WHO, the STOP TB Department; 2008.
43. Mesfin YM, Hailemariam D, Biadgilign S, Kibret KT. Association between HIV/AIDS and multi-drug resistance tuberculosis: a systematic review and meta-analysis. PLoS one. 2014:9(1):e82235.
44. Monedero I, Caminero JA. MDR-/XDR-TB management: what it was, current standards and what is ahead. Expert Rev Respir Med. 2009;3(2):133-45.
45. Wells CD, Cegielski JP, Nelson LJ, Laserson KF, Holtz TH, Finlay A, et al. HIV infection and multidrug resistant tuberculosis: the perfect storm. J Infect Dis. 2007;196(Suppl 1):S86-107.
46. Gandhi NR, Moll A, Sturm AW, Pawinski R, Govender T, Lalloo U, et al. Extensively drug-resistant tuberculosis as a cause of death in patients coinfected with tuberculosis and HIV in a rural area of South Africa. Lancet. 2006;368(9547):1575-80.
47. Havlir DV, Barnes PF. Tuberculosis in patients with human immunodeficiency virus infection. N Engl J Med. 1999;340(5):367-73.
48. Mendelson M. Diagnosing tuberculosis in HIV infected patients: challenges and future prospects. Br Med Bull. 2007;81-82:149-65.
49. Perkins MD, Cunningham J. Facing the crisis: improving the diagnosis of tuberculosis in the HIV era. J Infect Dis. 2007;196(Suppl 1):S15-27.
50. Getahun H, Harrington M, O'Brien R, Nunn P. Diagnosis of smear-negative pulmonary tuberculosis in people with HIV AIDS in resource-constrained settings: informing urgent policy changes. Lancet. 2007;369(9578):2042-9.
51. Vorster M, Sathekge MM, Bomanji J. Advances in imaging of tuberculosis: the role of 'F-FDG PET and PET/CT. Curr Opin Pulm Med. 2014;20(3):287-93.
52. Janis EM, Allen DW, Glesby MJ, Carey LA, Mundy LM, Gopalan R, et al. Tuberculin skin test reactivity, anergy and HIV infection in hospitalized patients. Longcope Firm of the Osler Medical Housestaff. Am J Med. 1996;100(2):186-92.
53. Long R, Houstan S, Hershfield E. Canadian Tuberculosis Committee of the Centre for Infectious Disease Prevention and Control, Population and Public Health Branch, Health Canada. Recommendations for screening and prevention of tuberculosis in patients with HIV and for screening for HIV in patients with tuberculosis and their contacts. CMAJ. 2003;169(8):789-91.
54. American Thoracic Society. Targeted tuberculin testing and treatment of latent tuberculosis infection. MMWR Recomm Rep. 2000;161:S221-S47.
55. Brassard P, Hottes TS, Lalonde RG, Klein MB. Tuberculosis screening and active tuberculosis among HIV infected persons in a Canadian tertiary care centre. Can J Infect Dis Med Microbiol. 2009;20(2):51-7.

56. Pai M, Riley LW, Colford JM. Interferon-gamma assays in the immunodiagnosis of tuberculosis: a systematic review. Lancet Infect Dis. 2004;4(12):761-76.
57. Dheda K, Udwadia ZF, Huggett JF, Johnson MA, Rook GA. Utility of the antigen-specific interferon-gamma assay for the management of tuberculosis. Curr Opin Pulm Med. 2005;11(3):195-202.
58. Mazurek M, Jereb J, Vernon A, LoBue P, Goldberg S, Castro K, et al. Updated guidelines for using interferon gamma release assays to detect Mycobacterium tuberculosis infection—United States, 2010. MMWR Recomm Rep. 2010;59(RR-5):1-25.
59. Moure R, Munoz L, Torres M, Santin M, Matin R, Alcaide F. Rapid detection of Mycobacterium tuberculosis complex and rifampin resistance in smear negative clinical samples by use of an integrated real time PCR method. J Clin Microbiol 2011;49(3):1137-9.
60. Feasey NA, Banada PP, Howson W, Sloan DJ, Mdolo A, Boehme C, et al. Evaluation of X-pert Mtb/Rif for detection of tuberculosis from blood samples of HIV infected adults confirm Mycobacterium tuberculosis bacteremia as an indicator of poor prognosis. J Clin Microbiol. 2013;51(7):2311-6.
61. Molicotti P, Bua A, Zanetti S. Cost-effectiveness in the diagnosis of tuberculosis: choices in developing countries. J Infect Dev Ctries. 2014;8(1):24-38.
62. Nettles RE, Mazo D, Alwood K, Gachuhi R, Maltas G, Wendel K, et al. Risk factors for relapse and acquired rifamycin resistance after directly observed tuberculosis treatment: a comparison by HIV serostatus and rifamycin use. Clin Infect Dis. 2004;38(5):731-6.
63. Kassim S, Sassan-Morokro M, Ackah A, Abouya LY, Digbeu H, Yesso G, et al. Two-year follow-up of persons with HIV-1 and HIV-2 associated pulmonary tuberculosis treated with short-course chemotherapy in West Africa. AIDS. 1995;9(10): 1185-91.
64. Chaisson RE, Clermont HC, Holt EA, Cantave M, Johnson MP, Atkinson J, et al. Six-month supervised intermittent tuberculosis therapy in Haitian patients with and without HIV infection. Am J Respir Crit Care Med. 1996;154(4 Pt 1):1034-8.
65. Henegar C, Behets F, Vanden Driessche K, Tabala M, Van Rie A. Impact of HIV on clinical presentation and outcomes of tuberculosis treatment at primary care level. Int J Tuberc Lung Dis. 2013;17(11):1411-3.
66. Perriens JH, St Louis ME, Mukadi YB, Brown C, Prignot J, Pouthier F, et al. Pulmonary tuberculosis in HIV infected patients in Zaire. A controlled trial of treatment for either 6 or 12 months. N Engl J Med. 1995;332(12):779-84.
67. Alwood K, Keruly J, Moore-Rice K, Stanton DL, Chaulk CP, Chaisson RE. Effectiveness of supervised, intermittent therapy for tuberculosis in HIV infected patients. AIDS. 1994;8(8): 1103-8.
68. Chaulk CP, Kazandjian VA. Directly observed therapy for treatment completion of pulmonary tuberculosis: consensus statement of the Public Health Tuberculosis Guidelines Panel. JAMA. 1998;279(12):943-8.
69. Connolly C, Reid A, Davies G, Sturm W, McAdam KP, Wilkinson D. Relapse and mortality among HIV infected and uninfected patients with tuberculosis successfully treated with twice weekly directly observed therapy in rural South Africa. AIDS. 1999;13(12):1543-7.
70. Sonnenberg P, Murray J, Glynn JR, Shearer S, Kambashi B, Godfrey-Faussett P. HIV-1 and recurrence, relapse and reinfection of tuberculosis after cure: a cohort study in South African mine-workers. Lancet. 2001;358(9294):1687-93.
71. Blumberg HM, Burman WJ, Chaisson RE, Daley CL, Etkind SC, Friedman LN, et al. American Thoracic Society/Centers for Disease Control and Prevention/Infectious Diseases Society of America: treatment of tuberculosis. Am J Respir Crit Care Med. 2003;167(4):603-62.
72. Burman WJ. Issues in the management of HIV-related tuberculosis. Clin Chest Med. 2005;26(2):283-94.
73. WHO. (2006). WHO Guidelines for the programmatic management of drug-resistant tuberculosis. World Health Organization, Geneva, Switzerland. [online] Available from http://*www.stoptb.org/resource_center/assets/documents/tb_guidelines.pdf*. [Accessed January, 2016].
74. Mitnick C, Bayona J, Palacios E, Shin S, Furin J, Alcántara F, et al. Community based therapy for multidrug resistant tuberculosis in Lima, Peru. N Engl J Med. 2003;348(2):119-28.
75. Mitnick C, Shin S, Seung KJ, Rich ML, Atwood SS, Furin JJ, et. al. Comprehensive treatment of extensively drug-resistant tuberculosis. N Engl J Med. 2008;359(6):563-74.
76. Government of India. (2008). RNTCP DOTS-plus Guidelines: Central TB division, directorate general of health services, Ministry of Health and Family Welfare, India. [online] Available from http://*www.tbcindia.org/pdfs/DOTS-Plus%20Guidelines%20Feb%2009.pdf*. [Accessed January, 2016].
77. Matteelli A, Roggi A, Carvalho AC. Extensively drug-resistant tuberculosis: epidemiology and management. Clin Epidemiol. 2014;6:111-8.
78. Pietersen E, Ignatius E, Streicher EM, Mastrapa B, Padanilam X, Pooran A, et al. Long-term outcomes of patients with extensively drug-resistant tuberculosis in South Africa: a cohort study. Lancet. 2014;383(9924):1230-9.
79. O'Donnell MR, Wolf A, Werner L, Horsburgh CR, Padayatchi N. Adherence in the treatment of patients with extensively drug-resistant tuberculosis and HIV in South Africa: A prospective cohort study. J Acquir Immune Defic Syndr. 2014;67(1): 22-9.
80. Lalloo UG, Ambaram A. New Antituberculous Drugs in Development. Curr HIV/AIDS Rep. 2010;7(3):143-51.
81. Nuermberger EL, Spigelman MK, Yew WW. Current development and future prospects in chemotherapy of tuberculosis. Respirology. 2010;15(5):764-78.
82. Ordonez AA, Maiga M, Gupta S, Weinstein EA, Bishai WR, Jain SK. Novel adjunctive therapies for the treatment of tuberculosis. Curr Mol Med. 2014;14(3):385-95.
83. Chaisson RE, Schecter GF, Theuer CP, Rutherford GW, Echenberg DF, Hopewell PC. Tuberculosis in patients with acquired immunodeficiency syndrome: clinical features, response to therapy, and survival. Am Rev Respir Dis. 1987;136(3):570-4.
84. el-Sadr WM, Perlman DC, Matts JP, Nelson ET, Cohn DL, Salomon N, et al. Evaluation of an intensive intermittent-induction regimen and short course duration of treatment for HIV-related pulmonary tuberculosis. Terry Beirn Community Programs for Clinical Research on AIDS (CPCRA) and the AIDS Clinical Trials Group (ACTG). Clin Infect Dis. 1998;26(5): 1148-58.
85. Murray J, Sonnenberg P, Shearer SC, Godfrey-Faussett P. Human immunodeficiency virus and the outcome of treatment for new and recurrent pulmonary tuberculosis in African patients. Am J Respir Crit Care Med. 1999;159(3):733-40.

86. World Health Organization. Scaling up antiretroviral therapy in resource-limited settings: treatment guidelines for a public health approach (2003 revision). Geneva: World Health Organization; 2004.
87. Centers for Disease Control and Prevention. Updated guidelines for the use of rifamycins for the treatment of tuberculosis among HIV infected patients taking protease inhibitors or non-nucleoside reverse transcriptase inhibitors. Atlanta: Centers for Disease Control and Prevention; 2004. Also Available from: *www.cdc.gov/nchstp/tb/TB_HIV_Drugs.* [Accessed January, 2016].
88. Kwara A, Flanigan TP, Carter EJ. Highly active antiretroviral therapy (HAART) in adults with tuberculosis: current status. Int J Tuberc Lung Dis. 2005;9(3):248-57.
89. Burman WJ, Jones BE. Treatment of HIV-related tuberculosis in the era of effective antiretroviral therapy. Am J Respir Crit Care Med. 2001;164(1):7-12.
90. French MA, Price P, Stone SF. Immune restoration disease after antiretroviral therapy. AIDS. 2004;18(12):1615-27.
91. Narita M, Ashkin D, Hollender ES, Pitchenik AE. Paradoxical worsening of tuberculosis following antiretroviral therapy in patients with AIDS. Am J Respir Crit Care Med. 1998;158(1):1 57-61.
92. Fishman JE, Saraf-Levi E, Narita M, Hollender ES, Ramsinghani R, Ashkin D. Pulmonary tuberculosis in AIDS patients: transient chest radiographic worsening after initiation of antiretroviral therapy. AJR Am J Roentgenol. 2000;174(1):43-9.
93. Meintjes G, Lawn SD, Scano F, Maartens G, French MA, Worodria W, et al. Tuberculosis-associated immune reconstitution inflammatory syndrome: case definitions for use in resource-limited settings. Lancet Infect Dis. 2008;8(8):516-23.
94. Shelburne SA, Hamill RJ, Rodriguez-Barradas MC, Greenberg SB, Atmar RL, Musher DW, et. al. Immune reconstitution inflammatory syndrome: emergency of a unique syndrome during highly active antiretroviral therapy. Medicine (Baltimore). 2002;81(3):213-27.
95. Breton G, Duval X, Estellat G, Poaletti X, Bonnet D, Mvondo D, et al. Determinants of immune reconstitution inflammatory syndrome in HIV-I infected patients with tuberculosis after initiation of antiretroviral therapy. Clin Infect Dis. 2004;39(11): 1709-12.
96. Valin N, Pacanowski J, Denoeud L, Lacombe K, Lalande V, Fonquernie L, et al. Risk factors for unmasking immune reconstitution inflammatory syndrome presentation of tuberculosis following combination antiretroviral therapy initiation in HIV infected patients. AIDS. 2010;24(10):1519-25.
97. Worodria W, Conesa-Botella A, Kisembo H, McAdam KP, Colebunders R. Coping with TB immune reconstitution inflammatory syndrome. Expert Rev Respir Med. 2009;3(2):147-52.
98. Boulware DR, Hullsiek KH, Puronen CE, Rupert A, Baker JV, French MA, et al. Higher levels of CRP, D-Dimer, IL-6 and hyaluronic acid before initiation of antiretroviral therapy: (ART) are associated with increased risk of AIDS or death. J Infect Dis. 2011;203(11):1637-46.
99. Jindal A, Duggal L, Jain N, Malhotra S. Immune reconstitution inflammatory syndrome in acquired immunodeficiency syndrome. Indian J Chest Dis Allied Sci. 2008;50(4):359-61.
100. Gopalan N, Andrade BB, Swaminathan S. Tuberculosis-immune reconstitution inflammatory syndrome in HIV: from pathogenesis to prediction. Expert Rev Clin Immunol. 2014;10(5):631-45.
101. Revised BCG vaccination guidelines for infants at risk for HIV infection. Wkly Epidemiol Res. 2007;82(21):193-6.

Nontuberculous Mycobacterial Diseases

PS Shankar, SK Jindal

INTRODUCTION

There are a large number of mycobacteria other than *Mycobacterium tuberculosis* which are now being increasingly recognized as a cause of human disease. Commonly referred to as nontuberculous mycobacteria (NTM), they are also known as atypical mycobacteria, anonymous mycobacteria, or mycobacteria other than tubercle bacilli (MOTT). They are weak pathogens and they are distinct from *M. tuberculosis* in their characteristics. The NTM are ubiquitously distributed in the environment, hence also called as environmental mycobacteria. Often, these organisms inhabit the respiratory passages as commensals. Pulmonary infection from NTM though rare, can cause disease similar to tuberculosis (TB). They more commonly infect the skin, soft tissue, lymph nodes, implant devices, wounds, bones and joints. Occasionally, the infection is disseminated systemically in patients who are immunosuppressed or who suffer from acquired immunodeficiency syndrome (AIDS).

CLASSIFICATION

Earnest Runyon classified small, rod-shaped, atypical mycobacteria into four groups based primarily on colony morphology, pigmentation and growth characteristics.[1]

Group I consists of photochromogens. *Mycobacterium kansasii* is an important pulmonary pathogen belonging to this group. It grows slowly over 2–4 weeks and becomes yellow on exposure to light. *Mycobacterium scrofulaceum* belongs to Group II and is a scotochromogen. It grows slowly over 2–4 weeks and produces yellow colonies even in darkness. It turns orange on exposure to light. *M. scrofulaceum* affects cervical lymph nodes. It occurs exclusively in children.

Nonchromogens belong to Group III. They grow slowly and produce white colonies that do not change color on exposure to light. *Mycobacterium avium* and *Mycobacterium intracellulare* [*Mycobacterium avium* complex (MAC) or *M. avium* and *M. intracellulare,* (MAI)] belong to this group of opportunistic pathogens, and are responsible for pulmonary lesions, or cervical lymphadenopathy, and occasionally cause a virulent disseminated disease. The organisms which belong to Group IV grow within 3–5 days on culture, hence referred as "rapid growers". They do not change color on exposure to light, hence nonchromogens. *Mycobacterium fortuitum, Mycobacterium chelonae and Mycobacterium smegmatus* are examples of this group. They often produce subcutaneous abscesses.

Recently, the mycobacterial species are classified on the basis of genetic differences, such as the sequence differences in the 16S ribosomal ribonucleic acid (RNA). The NTM species are divided into the slow (Group I, II, and III) and rapid (Group IV) growers. There is also an intermediate growing group that includes *M. marinum* and *M. gordonae.* They also vary in their nutritional requirements and grow on either the simple media or on the media supplemented with nutrients.

It is also considered appropriate to group the NTM based on the type of clinical disease they produce, such as pulmonary disease, lymphadenitis, cutaneous disease and disseminated disease.

HUMAN DISEASE

Though the NTM are widely distributed in the environment, the clinical infection is rare.[2] They may be falsely recovered from clinical specimens due to laboratory contamination or contamination of medical instruments. More than 90 species of NTM have been recognized. Of them, nearly one-third have been linked with disease in humans **(Table 1)**.[3,4] Unlike *M. tuberculosis,* NTM are not obligate pathogens.

Chronic pulmonary infection generally occurs in elderly persons by MAC and *M. kansasii.* Cervical lymphadenopathy occurs in children from *M. scrofulaceum* while skin and soft tissue infections may develop form *M. fortuitum, M. chelonei, M. xenopi* and *M. ulcerans*. Exposure of humans to NTM through bathing, swimming and drinking, especially through cuts and abrasions, is common. But risk of infection is generally less. Disseminated lesions are found in immunocompromised patients with infection from MAC. Sometimes, *M. chelonei* may cause very indolent pulmonary infection.

Table 1 Some of the important nontuberculous mycobacterial species linked with disease in humans

• *Mycobacterium avium*	• *M. xenopi*
• *M. intracellulare*	• *M. marinum*
• *M. kansassii*	• *M. malmoense*
• *M. paratuberculosis*	• *M. fortuitum*
• *M. scrofulaceum*	• *M. ulcerans*
• *M. simiae*	• *M. chelonaei*
• *M. habana*	• *M. smegmatis,*
• *M. interjectum*	• *M. xenopi*
• *M. genavense*	• *M. haemophilum*

EPIDEMIOLOGY

Nontuberculous mycobacteria (NTM) are widely distributed in the environment and commonly isolated from soil, water, and house dust except *M. kansasii* whose natural reservoir remains unidentified.[5] *Mycobacterium avium intracellular complex* (MAIC) is commonly recovered from residential bath rooms and showers.[6,7] Colonization of human body especially of upper airways, skin and gastrointestinal tract (GIT) by NTM is common without any evidence of disease. The pulmonary infection appears to result from inhalation of infectious droplets that have been aerosolized from the environmental sources. Ingestion of organism especially MAC by patients with AIDS infects the GIT tract and gets disseminated. Direct inoculation may result in infection of skin, soft tissue and joints. Human-to-human transmission is very unusual.[5] Familial clustering, however, is reported which suggests the role of genetic factors contributing to host susceptibility.[8]

The infection from NTM has been reported from different parts of the world especially United States, Europe and Japan. In the US, a rising prevalence of sensitization of one in six persons was reported in 1999–2000, up from one in nine persons in 1971–1972.[9] There was also an increase in NTM-related deaths between 1999 and 2010 in a population study.[10] The infection from NTM has been reported infrequently in India. However, the frequent occurrence of low-grade tuberculin reaction suggests a varying risk of human disease. NTM may be responsible for a significant proportion of mycobacterial infection in human immunodeficiency virus (HIV) seropositive patients. The higher endemicity of TB in India, the presence of NTM should be considered especially in immunocompromised HIV seropositive patients.[11]

There are isolated studies from different parts of India which report the variable rates of isolation of NTM species mostly from laboratory samples.[12-14] In an earlier report, atypical mycobacteria were grown in 13.7% of the sputum specimens from 6,829 patients diagnosed as "relapsed cases" of pulmonary TB or some other chronic respiratory disease.[15]

CLINICAL FEATURES

Infection in a healthy person from NTM (commonly *M. kansasii* and MAC) presents a picture of chronic pulmonary disease resembling TB. The lung infiltrates are more diffuse and nodular in appearance. Cavitary disease is common. Mediastinal lymph node involvement and pleural effusion are uncommon. The lymph nodes, skin, soft tissues, bones and joints are other important sites of NTM infection.[4]

PULMONARY DISEASE

The condition may present in one of the three different forms: a TB-like pattern; nodular bronchiectasis, and hypersensitivity pneumonitis.[16] The classical TB-like presentation commonly occurs in older male smokers frequently with underlying chronic obstructive pulmonary disease. It is more indolent than typical TB and presents with cough and expectoration. Though there can be fever, night sweats, weight loss, and hemoptysis occasionally, these constitutional symptoms are less severe. The progress of the disease is slow. These patients may have preexistent pulmonary diseases such as chronic obstructive pulmonary disease (COPD), bronchiectasis, cystic fibrosis, primary ciliary dyskinesia, silicosis and even prior pulmonary TB.[17] In such situations the features of infection from NTM may pose difficulty to distinguish them from those of underlying disease. The disease is commoner in persons with diabetes and a history of smoking.

An atypical form of illness has been described in postmenopausal, nonsmoker women. Though the condition has an insidious onset with chronic cough, it is not associated with any existing lung disease seen in "classical" form. The constitutional symptoms are rare.[6] This is a type of hypersensitivity pneumonitis which presents a typical episodic picture on exposure to bacteria such as MAC. This type of presentation commonly occurs in workers exposed to metal-working fluids and on exposure to aerosolizer MAC in association with indoor hot tub use.[18,19] MAC infection can present with any of the three different forms.[16,17]

There are variable clinical patterns of NTM infection in patients with immunosuppression, malignancies, solid organ transplantation and cystic fibrosis.[20-22] The disseminated infection may occur in patients with immunosuppression due to hematological malignancy or immunosuppressive agents.[20] Its incidence has shown an increase in patients with advanced stages of AIDS especially from MAC.[4,13] The condition presents with persistent fever, weight loss, anorexia and weakness. The pulmonary symptoms are infrequent and exhibit cough or dyspnea. There can be vomiting, diarrhea and abdominal pain. There is generalized lymphadenopathy, hepatomegaly, splenomegaly and nodular skin lesions. The condition is noted in children and young adults.

DIAGNOSIS

Diagnosis of NTM pulmonary disease is made on the basis of the presence of a variety of clinical, radiological and microbiological criteria, several of which may only suggest them to confirm the etiology **(Table 2)**. The joint guidelines

Table 2 Guidelines for making the diagnosis of nontuberculous mycobacteria (NTM)-pulmonary disease

1. Clinical features of an indolent, respiratory disease—cough, expectoration, fever and other constitutional symptoms.
2. Positive smear for acid-fast bacilli (AFB) and/or heavy growth of NTM on culture in respiratory specimens.
3. Histopathological features of mycobacterial/granulomatous disease or culture of NTM from biopsy specimens.
4. Radiological features of nodular infiltrates with or without cavitation and/or bronchiectatic lesions.
5. Underlying host condition: Immunosuppression, AIDS, alcoholism, COPD, cystic fibrosis, diabetes, malignancies, etc.
6. Absence of other causes of pulmonary lesions such as tuberculosis, aspergillosis, etc.
7. Persistence of AFB after antituberculosis treatment for 2 weeks or more.

Abbreviations: AIDS, acquired immunodeficiency syndrome; COPD, chronic obstructive pulmonary disease

of American Thoracic Society (ATS) and the Infectious Disease Society of America provide concise and standardized recommendations on diagnosis and management.[23]

Radiology

The radiographic appearance in "classic" form of NTM disease resembles chronic indolent TB, and is indistinguishable from those of TB. The most common radiological pattern is fibronodular infiltrates involving the upper lobes especially apical and posterior segments.[14,24] Unlike TB, the cavities are thin-walled with little surrounding infiltrate. The "non-classical" form of disease is characterized by multiple bilateral opacities, similar to those in bronchiectasis. The infiltrates are seen predominantly in middle lobe and lingula and are not associated with apical pattern resembling postprimary TB.[12]

The pleural involvement, especially effusion, is rare. *Computed tomography* (CT) of the chest defines the radiologic features precisely. Small nodular opacities are seen in the regions of maximal disease and also in areas away from the predominant site of the disease. Bronchiectasis changes are present adjacent to apical cavities in "classical" form. In non-classical form of disease, bronchiectasis is bilateral and widespread.

Disseminated form of disease may not show any radiologic abnormality or exhibit bilateral infiltrates. It may be associated with hilar or mediastinal adenoapthy and/or pleural effusion. The radiologic abnormalities are more likely produced by coexistent conditions in AIDS patients. On positron emission tomography (PET) scans, the nodular lesions of NTM show[18] F-fluorodeoxygenase (FDG) uptake.[25]

Bacteriology

Since NTM may colonize the respiratory tract of patients with preexisting lung disease, their isolation from sputum, bronchial washings or lung biopsy may not establish the infection. The appearance of NTM at microscopy is generally indistinguishable from that of *M. tuberculosis.* NTM are identified by their pattern of pigmentation, microscopic appearance, biochemical reactions and growth characteristics. In a study from Korea, only about a fourth of 794 patients from whom NTM was isolated from respiratory specimens were found to have clinically significant NTM lung infections.[26] Repeated sputum cultures demonstrating heavy growth of NTM are necessary to pin-point NTM as the etiologic agent, in a patient with a compatible clinical picture and radiograph. However, there is no need for repeated isolation of *M. kansasii* as it rarely occurs as a saprophyte. In disseminated form, blood culture demonstrates causative agent. The NTM are traditionally classified as rapid and slow growers on the basis of growth.

Other bacteriological investigations which are employed for identification include the biochemical tests and serotyping protein electrophoresis. The newer molecular methods such as the gene probes and gene amplification (polymerase chain reaction) are now available for the detection of NTM such as *M. avium, M. intracellulare* and some rapid growers. More advanced techniques such as DNA fingerprinting are sometimes used for characterization of NTM. DNA sequencing of variable genomic regions provides a rapid and accurate method to identify NTM.[27]

Histopathological dissection of granulomas with or without *acid-fast bacilli* (AFB) staining in biopsy specimens from lymph nodes, liver bone marrow or lungs may also help. However, NTM infections cannot be differentiated histopathologically from TB. Immunodiagnostic techniques such as the regions of difference (RD) antigens, encoded proteins have been used for the diagnosis of both latent and active TB. Some of these RD antigens are located in the genome of *M. tuberculosis, M. africanum* and *M. bovis,* but absent in many of NTM and Bacillus Calmette Guerin (BCG) substrains.[28] But their role in diagnosis or exclusion of NTM infection remains to be established.[28]

TREATMENT

The disease produced by NTM makes a slow progress, though it may remain stable for long periods. The disseminated form of disease has a rapid fatal course. NTM except *M. kansasii* exhibit a high degree of *in vitro* resistance to many of the standard anti-TB drugs.

Treatment of NTM infection is indicated only if the organism is responsible for the disease and is not simply a colonizer. Multiple antimicrobials are required for prolonged periods.[29,30] The infection from *M. kansasii* is treated with a combination of isoniazid, rifampicin and ethambutol (15 mg/kg) for 18 months.[31] Pyrazinamide is ineffective.

The treatment of infection due to MAC is difficult. Multiple drug therapy is indicated in those patients exhibiting a progressive course or those who are severely ill. Treatment

Table 3 Suggested drugs for treatment of infections with common nontuberculous mycobacteria (NTM)-isolates

NTM	*Suggested drugs*
1. *M. avium* intracellulare	H, R, E Aminoglycosides (Streptomycin, Amikacin) Quinolones (Ciprofloxacin/Ofloxacin) Clofazimine Macrolides (Clarithromycin / Azithromycin)
2. *M. fortuitum*-chelonae	Amikacin/Streptomycin Macrolides Doxycycline Cefoxitin Imipenem
3. *M. kansasii*	H, R, E
4. *M. ulcerans*	Surgery (with or without drugs as for *M. fortuitum*)
5. *M. scrofulaceum*	Surgical excision H, E, cycloserine Macrolide
Abbreviations: H, isoniazid; R, rifampicin; E, ethambutol	

consists of a macrolide, rifampicin and ethambutol given 3 times weekly for noncavitary disease and daily with or without an aminoglycoside for cavitary disease.[32] The choice of drugs depends upon the isolated NTM and the severity of manifestations **(Table 3)**. The success rate is low particularly in the AIDS patient as the organisms are usually resistant to most of the available anti-TB drugs including isoniazid.

Disseminated lesions due to MAC in AIDS patients may be treated with rifampicin, ethambutol, clofazamine and ciprofloxacin. Those exhibiting stable disease are observed and the underlying pulmonary disease is treated with bronchodilators, antibiotics if sputum is purulent, and smoking cessation. Mycobacterial disease may get eradicated without specific therapy. When specific treatment is initiated it consists of isoniazid, rifampicin and ethambutol (25 mg/kg for the first 2 months followed by 15 mg/kg) with an initial supplementation of streptomycin for 3–6 months.[31] Treatment has to be given for 18–24 months. Those exhibiting an extensive disease and those who fail to show sputum conversion on the four-drug regimen, cycloserine and ethionamide are to be added to the therapeutic regimen. Drug-drug interaction is an important treatment consideration especially in the elderly age group.[33] Inhaled amikacin has been used in some patients with treatment-refractory NTM disease.[34]

Surgical resection of the lesion may be undertaken in those having a localized disease. Some newer agents that may be active against NTM are rifabutin, clarithromycin, azithromycin and ofloxacin. *M. chelonae* is generally resistant to the anti-TB drugs and other conventional antibiotics. It shows susceptibility only to amikacin, cefoxitin and imipenem.

NONPULMONARY MANIFESTATIONS

Nonpulmonary features of NTM infection are more common than of TB. Infection of the extrapulmonary sites may occur through skin-contact, penetrating injuries, ingestion of contaminated water or aerosol inhalation. Hematogenous spread may be responsible for disseminated disease.

Lymphadenitis

Several NTM species are identified to cause cervical lymphadenitis in healthy individuals, especially in children. MAC group is the most common species in both the immunocompetent and the immunosuppressed patients.[32] Lymphadenitis is rare for children having BCG vaccine. Presence of cervical lymphadenopathy in an adult with HIV infection or with organ transplantation on immunosuppressive therapy should always arouse the strong suspicion of MAC infection. The other common organisms may include *M. scrofulaceum* and *M. malmoense.* Constitutional symptoms are generally absent. Poor response to standard antitubercular therapy or repeated appearance of lymph nodes in spite of therapy arouses the suspicion of NTM-lymphadenopathy. The lymph nodes may also undergo central caseation, cold development of sinuses or abscess formation. Surgery should be considered for treatment in addition to the antimicrobial therapy.

Skin and Subcutaneous Abscesses

Skin gets commonly infected following penetrating injury, inoculation or surgery with contaminated instruments. Clusters of cases of incisions and subcutaneous abscesses are reported following laparoscopic surgery especially when performed in Camps. A series of 145 laparoscopy post site infections were found in 35 patients following laparoscopy at a single hospital, the water used for washing chemically disinfected instruments.[35] The organism *M. chelonae* had survived and grown within the biofilm at the bottom of the disinfectant trays.

Inoculation superficial skin and subcutaneous infections as above, are commonly caused by the rapidly growing mycobacteria such as *M. fortuitum, M. chelonae, M. ulcerans, M. marinum* and *M. abscessus. M. fortuitum* and *M. chelonei* are sometimes responsible for deeper lesions as well as disseminated infections, for example, following the cardiac surgery. The rapid growers may occasionally cause superficial, intestinal ulceration, although the mere isolation from feces or colonoscopic specimens does not conclude a causal relationship with the GIT disease.

Treatment of infections with rapid growers consists of combined antibiotics therapy from amongst aminoglycosides, macrolide, doxycycline and fluoroquinolones. A prolonged course of 12–24 months treatment is generally required. Effective infection control measures and regulation of cosmetic procedures such as tattooing, mesotherapy (nonspecific surgical cosmetic medicine), liposunction, etc. are important for prevention of NTM infection.[36]

Disseminated Nontuberculous Mycobacteria Infection

Disseminated disease with NTM generally occurs in patients with HIV infection. Several other groups of diseases and clinical conditions are now described where NTM are recognized as responsible pathogens. Renal transplant recipients, patient underlying treatment for rheumatic disease, cystic fibrosis, lymphomas, leukemia and disseminated malignancies are particularly liable.[37-39] An increasing trend in non-HIV infected patients was reported from Thailand. Only 12% of 129 patients had any underlying disease.[40] The patient in this series reported with lymph node, skin, soft tissue and lung involvement, sometimes with coinfection from other opportunistic organisms.

Disseminated disease may present rarely with localized lesions in multiple lymph nodes, kidney, bones, joints, liver and central nervous system. Constitutional symptoms are common with multiple organ involvements. Involvement of multiple sites may sometimes mimic metastases on PET/CT scans.[41]

Nontuberculous Mycobacteria Infections in Children

Nontuberculous mycobacteria (NTM) infection is frequently recognized in children. A nationwide active surveillance network in Australian children, the NTM was isolated in 68 cases with MAC being the most frequent organism.[42] In children, the NTM infection is typically associated with lymphadenopathy, pulmonary involvement is rare in otherwise healthy children.[43]

Isolated pulmonary NTM disease is recognized more commonly in patients with cystic fibrosis.[39,44,45] Occasionally, pulmonary NTM infection, in otherwise healthy children, presenting with refractory stridor or wheezing with endobronchial lesions or hilar lymphadenopathy without association with recognized underlying immune deficiency or cystic fibrosis transmembrane conductance regulator (CFTR) mutations is also described.[43]

Miscellaneous Clinical Manifestations

Besides the pulmonary manifestations, lymphadenitis, skin and soft tissue infections, several other organs may also show isolated or disseminated NTM involvement. MAC disease, which commonly occurs in patients with HIV infection, may involve the eyes (corneal ulcers), heart (endocarditis), central nervous system (meningitis) and bones (osteomyelitis). Similar involvement may rarely occur with *M fortuitum, a chelonae* group of mycobacteria. Meningitis and hepatitis are known to occur with *M. scrofulaceum* and *M. gordonae* *M. smegmatis,* the first mycobacteria identified after *M. tuberculosis* is found to be associated with pneumonia, sternotomy wound infections and soft tissue infections.[45] *M. bovis* was commonly considered responsible for lymphadenitis and GIT manifestations due to ingestion of milk from infected cows before the pasteurization era. A report of 73 cases, seen during a 12-year period was described from San Diego.[46] More recently, the cases are reported to occur in patients with HIV infection and those working in cattle farms or slaughter houses.

In summary, an increased trend of NTM infections is recognized, especially in patients with HIV infection or with other causes of immunosuppression. Pulmonary manifestations and lymphadenitis are most common, while disseminated forms, skin and soft tissue involvement may also occur. Diagnosis is established on the basis of clinical features, radiological and microbiological investigations. Treatment is somewhat difficult requiring multiple drugs for prolonged periods. In view of the multiple and irreversible toxic effects of drugs used for prolonged periods with limited evidence, a patient-centered pragmatic approach has been recently advocated.[47] The approach is based on patient-reported outcome measures to make the clinical decisions.[47]

REFERENCES

1. Runyon EH. Anonymous mycobacteria in pulmonary disease. Med Clin North Amer. 1959:43(1);273-90.
2. Woods GL, Washington JA. Mycobacteria other than *Mycobacterium tuberculosis*: review of microbiology and clinical aspects. Rev Infect Dis. 1987;9(2):275-94.
3. Katoch VM. Infections due to non-tuberculous mycobacteria (NTM). Indian J Med Res. 2004(4);120:290-304.
4. Tortoli E. Clinical manifestations of nontuberculous mycobacteria infections. Clin Microbiol Infect. 2009;15(10):906-10.
5. O'Brien RJ. The epidemiology of non-tuberculous mycobacterial disease. Clin Chest Med. 1989;10:407-18.
6. Falkinham JO, Iseman MD, de Haas P, Van Soolingen D.*Mycobacterium avium* in a shower linked to pulmonary disease. J Water Health. 2008;6(2):209-13.
7. Nishiuchi Y, Maekura R, Kitada S, Tamaru A, Taguri T, Kira Y, et al. The recovery of *Mycobacterium avium*-intracellulare complex (MAC) from the residential bathrooms of patients with pulmonary MAC. Clin Infect Dis. 2007;45(3):347-51.
8. Colombo RE, Hill SC, Claypool RJ, Holland SM, Olivier KN. Familial clustering of pulmonary nontuberculous Mycobacterial disease. Chest. 2010;137(3):629-34.
9. Khan K, Wang J, Marras TK. Nontuberculous mycobacterial sensitization in the United States: national trends over three decades. Am J Respir Crit Care Med. 2007;176(3):306-13.
10. Mirsaeidi M, Machado RF, Garcia JG, Schraufnagel DE. Nontuberculous mycobacterial disease mortality in the United States, 1999-2010: a population-based comparative study. PLos One. 2014;9(3):e91879.
11. Khatter S, Singh UB, Arora J, Rana T, Seth P. Mycobacterial infections in human immunodeficiency virus seropositive patients: role of non-tuberculous mycobacteria. Indian J Tuberc. 2008;55(1):28-33

12. Parashar D, Das R, Chauhan DS, Sharma VD, Lavania M, Yadav VS, et al. Identification of environmental mycobacteria isolated from Agra, north India by conventional and molecular approaches. Ind J Med Res. 2009;129(4):424-31.
13. Sivasankari P, Khyriem AB. Venkatesh K, Parija SC. Atypical mycobacterial infection among HIV seronegative patients in Pondicherry. Indian J Chest Dis Allied Sci. 2006;48(2):107-9.
14. Kalita JB, Rahman H, Baruah KC. Delayed post-operative wound infections due to non-tuberculous Mycobacterium. Indian J Med Res. 2005;122(6):535-9.
15. Kotian M, Ganesan V, Sarvamangala JN, Shivananda PG, Achyutha KN. Pulmonary infections by atypical mycobacteria in a rural coastal region of Karnataka, India. Trop Geogr Med. 1981;33(2):117-21.
16. Glassroth J. Pulmonary Disease due to nontuberculous mycobacteria. Chest. 2008;133(1):243-51.
17. Johnson MM, Odell JA. Nontuberculous mycobacterial pulmonary infections. J Thorac Dis. 2014;6(3):210-20.
18. Laccase Y, Girard M, Cormier Y. Recent advances in hypersensitivity pneumonitis. Chest. 2012;142(1):208-17.
19. Rickman OB, Ryu JH, Fidler ME, Kalra S. Hypersensitivity pneumonitis associated with *Mycobacterium avium* complex and hot tub use. Mayo Clin Proc. 2002;77(11):1233-7.
20. Corti M, Palmero D, Eiguchi K. Respiratory infections in immunocompromised patients. Curr Opin Pulm Med. 2009;15(3):209-17.
21. Knoll BM. Update on nontuberculous mycobacterial infections in solid organ and hematopoietic stem cell transplant recipients. Curr Infect Dis Rep. 2014;16(9):421.
22. Qvist T, Pressler T, Høiby N, Katzenstein TL. Shifting paradigms of nontuberculous mycobacteria in cystic fibrosis. Respir Res. 2014;15:41-8.
23. Griffith DE, Aksamit T, Brown-Elliot BA, Catanzaro A, Daley C, Gordin F, et al. An official ATS/IDSA statement: diagnosis, treatment, and prevention of nontuberculous mycobacterial disease. Am J Respir Crit Care Med. 2007;175(4):367-416.
24. Patz EF, Swensen SJ, Erasmus J. Pulmonary manifestations of nontuberculous Mycobacterium. Radiol Clin North Am. 1995;33(4):719-29.
25. Bandoh S, Fujita J, Ueda Y, Tojo Y, Ishii T, Kubo A, et al. Uptake of fluorine-18 fluorodeoxyglucose in pulmonary *Mycobacterium avium* complex infection. Intern Med. 2003;42(8):726-9.
26. Koh WJ, Kwon OJ, Jeon K, Kim TS, Lee KS, Park YK, et al. Clinical significance of nontuberculous mycobacteria isolated from respiratory specimens in Korea. Chest. 2006;129(2):341-8.
27. Somoskovi A, Salfinger M. Nontuberculous mycobacteria in respiratory infections: advances in diagnosis and identification. Clin Lab Med. 2014;34(2):271-95.
28. Parkash O, Singh BP, Pai M. Regions of differences encoded antigens as targets for immunodiagnosis of tuberculosis in humans. Scand J Immunol. 2009;70(4):345-57.
29. Colombo RE, Olivier KN. Diagnosis and treatment of infections caused by rapidly growing mycobacteria. Semin Respir Crit Care Med. 2008;29(5):577-88.
30. Thomson RM, Yew WW. When and how to treat pulmonary and non-tuberculous mycobacterial diseases? Respirology. 2009;14(1):12-26.
31. Miller WT Jr, Miller WT Sr. Pulmonary infections with atypical mycobacteria in the normal host. Semin Roentgeonl. 1993;28(2):138-49
32. Kasperbauer SH, Daley CL. Diagnosis and treatment of infections due to *Mycobacterium avium* complex. Semin Respir Crit Care Med. 2008;29(5):569-76.
33. Mirsaeidi M, Farshidpour M, Ebrahimi G, Aliberti S, Falkinham J. Management of nontuberculous mycobacterial infection in the elderly. Eur J Intern Med. 2014;25(4):356-63.
34. Olivier KN, Shaw PA, Glaser TS, Bhattacharyya D, Fleshner M, Brewer CC, et al. Inhaled amikacin for treatment of refractory pulmonary nontuberculous mycobacterial disease. Ann Am Thorac Soc. 2014;11(1):30-5.
35. Vijayaraghavan R, Chandrashekhar R, Sujatha Y, Belagavi CS. Hospital outbreak of atypical mycobacterial infection of port sites after laparoscopic surgery. J Hosp Infect. 2006;64(4):344-7.
36. Atkins BL, Gottlieb T. Skin and soft tissue infections caused by nontuberculous mycobacteria. Curr Opin Infect Dis. 2014;27(2):137-45.
37. Ho TA, Rommelaere M, Coche E, Yombi JC, Kanaan N. Nontuberculous mycobacterial pulmonary infection in renal transplant recipients. Transpl Infect Dis. 2010;12(2):138-42.
38. Van Ingen J, Boeree MJ, Dekhuijzen PN, Van Soolingen D. Mycobacterial disease in patients with rheumatic disease. Nat Clin Pract Rhematol. 2008;4(12):649-56.
39. Whittaker LA, Teneback C. Atypical mycobacterial and fungal infections in cystic fibrosis. Semin Respir Crit Care Med. 2009;30(5):539-46.
40. Chetchotisakd P, Kiertiburanakul S, Mootsikapun P, Assanasen S, Chaiwarith R, Anunnatsiri S. Disseminated nontuberculous mycobacterial infection in patients who are not infected with HIV in Thailand. Clin Infect Dis. 2007;45(4):421-7.
41. Lin KH, Wang JH, Peng NJ. Disseminated nontuberculous mycobacterial infection mimic metastases on PET/CT scan. Clin Nucl Med. 2008;33(4):276-7.
42. Blyth C, Best EJ, Jones CA, Nourse C, Goldwater PN, Daley AJ, et al. Nontuberculous mycobacterial infection in children: a prospective national study. Pediatr Infect Dis J. 2009;28(9):801-5.
43. Freeman AF, Olivier KN, Rubio TT, Bartlett G, Ochi JW, Claypool RJ, et al. Intrathoracic nontuberculous mycobacterial infections in otherwise healthy children. Pediatr Pulmonol. 2009;44(11):1051-6.
44. Kim RD, Greenberg DE, Ehrmantraut ME, Guide SV, Ding L, Shea Y, et al. Pulmonary nontuberculous mycobacterial disease: prospective study of a distinct preexisting syndrome. Am J Respir Crit Care Med. 2008;178(10):1066-74.
45. Wallace RJ, Nash DR, Tsukamura M, Blacklock ZM, Silcox VA. Human disease due to *Mycobacterium smegmatis*. J Infect Dis. 1988;158(1):52-9.
46. Dankner WM, Waecker NJ, Essey MA, Moser K, Thompson M, Davis CE. *Mycobacterium bovis* infections in San Diego: a clinicoepidemiologic study of 73 patients and a historical review of a forgotten pathogen. Medicine. 1993;72(1):11-37.
47. Satta G, McHugh TD, Mountford J, Abubakar I, Lipman M. Managing pulmonary nontuberculous mycobacterial infection. Time for a patient-centered approach. Ann Am Thorac Soc. 2014;11(1):117-21.

Section 7

Nontuberculous Respiratory Infections

VK Vijayan, SK Jindal

Community-acquired Pneumonia

Charles Feldman, Ronald Anderson

INTRODUCTION

Community-acquired pneumonia (CAP) is described as a lung infection, acquired in the community, most commonly bacterial in nature, associated with the inflammation of the lung parenchyma, distal to the terminal bronchiole, with clinical and radiological evidence of consolidation of part or parts of one or both lungs. It is an extremely common infection that causes considerable morbidity and mortality, even in the modern world, especially among the very young, the elderly and patients with underlying comorbid disease.[1] The overall mortality of CAP varies from less than 1% in outpatients to approximately 14% in cases admitted to hospital and to 50% or more in patients requiring intensive care unit (ICU) admission.[1-3]

Community-acquired pneumonia puts an enormous burden on medical and economic resources, particularly if patients are hospitalized, since this is associated not only with direct hospital costs, but also with intensified laboratory investigation and broader empirical antimicrobial chemotherapy.[1,4] Studies from the United States,[1,5] Europe[4,6] the United Kingdom,[7,8] Latin America,[9] Middle East/ North Africa,[10] and the Asia-Pacific region,[11] attest to the considerable burden of disease that is associated with this infection in the developed world. Furthermore, most countries in Africa and Asia have two to ten times more pneumonia in children than in the United States. In the Asian region, the two most populous countries, namely China and India, contribute significantly to these numbers.[12] In developing countries like India, infectious diseases, including pneumonia are a leading cause of mortality, particularly among the lower social classes.[13] One review of the burden of pneumonia indicated that in children, pneumonia was estimated to be the cause of approximately 2 million deaths per year (20% of all childhood deaths), with 70% of these deaths occurring in Africa and Asia.[12]

EPIDEMIOLOGY

A number of studies have investigated in detail the global and regional burden of diseases in the world.[14-16] As early as 1990, the Global Burden of Disease Study using Disability-Adjusted Life-Years (DALYs) compared disease and death in different regions of the world.[14] Lower respiratory infections were the most common specific cause of global DALYs and the highest disease burdens were in sub-Saharan Africa (21.4%) and India (20.9%). In 2001, slightly more than 56 million people died.[15] Five of the ten leading causes of death in low- and middle-income countries were infectious diseases, including lower respiratory tract infections, which were the most common infectious cause, being even more common than human immunodeficiency virus (HIV)/acquired immunodeficiency syndrome (AIDS), diarrheal diseases, tuberculosis (TB) and malaria.

Similarly, in 2002, it was reported that slightly over 57 million people died in the world with lower respiratory tract infections, being the third leading cause of death (3.94 million deaths–6.9% of total deaths).[16] Lower respiratory tract infections were the second leading cause of burden of disease in low-and middle-income countries as measured by DALYs [92.2 DALYs (millions)–6.7% of total DALYs.][16] In sub-Saharan Africa, lower respiratory tract infections were the second leading cause of disease burden (second only to HIV/AIDS) [37.2 DALYs (millions)–10.0% of all DALYs].[16]

A more recent survey of causes of death for 20 age groups in 1990 and 2010 indicated that in 2010, there were 52.8 million deaths globally.[17] Decreases were noted in mortality from lower respiratory tract infections comparing 2010 with 1990; however, lower respiratory tract infections were still one of the leading causes of death in 2010. Lower respiratory tract infections were also one of the leading causes of years of life lost (YLLs) due to premature mortality in 2010. It is important to note that the survey revealed significant regional variations in leading causes of death.

With regard to infectious diseases themselves, one publication reviewing the impact of infections on global health indicated that of the estimated 58.5 million deaths per year, approximately 15 million (25.5%) are thought to be due to infectious diseases and of these respiratory tract infections are by far the most common.[18]

Although no proper field surveys have been conducted in India to generate concrete data for the epidemiology of CAP, it is likely that the situation in that country is not very different from the rest of the world.[19] Estimated deaths from lower respiratory tract infections in India in 2004 were estimated to be 113.6 per 100,000 population, in comparison with 25.3 in the United Kingdom (UK) and 11.7 in the United States of America (USA).[19] Furthermore, estimated DALYs due to lower respiratory tract infections in 2004 in India were 1,894 per 100,000 population versus 202 in the UK and 99 in the USA.[19]

One factor that has contributed significantly to the impact of CAP, particularly in patients in sub-Saharan Africa, has been the associated epidemic of HIV infection.[20] Worldwide, more than 40% of new HIV infections have occurred in adults aged 15–24 years, with 95% of these infections and associated deaths having occurred in developing countries. Sub-Saharan Africa is home to almost 64% of persons living with HIV and this burden is seen particularly among women.[20] However, a number of studies attest to the fact that the HIV epidemic is growing very rapidly in Asia, particularly in countries such as India and especially among the youth, such that an epidemic may be faced on the same scale as that in sub-Saharan Africa.[21-24] Pulmonary infections, including TB, opportunistic infections, but also CAP occur much more commonly in HIV-infected persons than in non-immunocompromised individuals and CAP is second among the pulmonary complications.[25,26] More recently, the subject of HIV-associated bacterial pneumonia has been extensively reviewed elsewhere.[27]

Table 1 Pathogens associated with community-acquired pneumonia

Relative frequency	*(%)*
• *Streptococcus pneumoniae*	35–80%
• *Haemophilus influenzae*	5–6%
• *Atypical pathogens*	
– *Legionella spp.**	2–15%
– *Mycoplasma pneumoniae*	2–14%
– *Chlamydophila spp.*†	4–15%
• *Staphylococcus aureus*‡	3%–14%
• Enteric Gram-negative bacilli§	6–12%
• *Pseudomonas aeruginosa*¶	4–9%
• *Coxiella burnetii*	2–4%
• *Moraxella catarrhalis*	<1%
• Influenza A virus	10–15%
• Other viruses»	5–10%
• *Mycobacterium tuberculosis*¥	Less than 1–5%
• Unknown	15–40%

*Vary in importance between countries; more than 95% are *L. pneumophila* serogroup 1; outbreaks are common.

†More than 99% due to *Chlamydophila pneumoniae* in adults.

‡Increasing in areas with high prevalence of community-acquired methicillin-resistant *S. aureus*.

§Main species associated with CAP are *Escherichia coli* and *Klebsiella pneumoniae*.

¶Risk factors include chronic steroid therapy, structural lung disease, previous hospitalization.

»Including respiratory syncytial virus, adenovirus, parainfluenza virus, metapneumovirus, varicella-zoster virus, measles and hanta virus.

¥Relative frequency varies considerably in different parts of the world.

(*Source:* **Reprinted with permission from Garau J, Calbo E. Community-acquired pneumonia. Lancet. 2008;371:455-8.)

MICROBIAL ETIOLOGY OF COMMUNITY-ACQUIRED PNEUMONIA

While CAP may be caused by a wide range of pathogens, in reality the majority of cases are caused by a relatively small number of predominantly bacterial pathogens, even among HIV-infected patients.[1] By far, the most common pathogen is *Streptococcus pneumoniae,* which accounts for some 20–80% of cases and remains the commonest pathogen even among cases requiring ICU admission.[1,3] In HIV-infected patients, as in non-immunocompromised cases, *S. pneumoniae* remains the most common pathogen in CAP.[25] Interestingly, on the basis of initial studies, it was commonly believed that *Pneumocystis carinii* (now called *Pneumocystis jirovecii*) was an uncommon cause of infection and/or death in patients in the developing world with HIV infection; however, this was probably as a consequence of the lack of recognition, and subsequent studies indicated its common occurrence in countries such as South Africa and India.[28-30]

Table 1 shows the prevalence of the common etiological agents of CAP.[3] A number of studies have been conducted in India with the aim of identifying the common bacterial pathogens associated with CAP. One study in Shimla (in India) using sputum, blood and pleural fluid culture, and serology for *Mycoplasma pneumoniae* identified 70 patients with CAP of whom 53 (75.5%) had an identifiable cause and 12 patients were noted to have mixed infections.[31] No cause was identified in 17 patients despite extensive investigation, including bronchoscopic aspiration of respiratory tract secretions. The most frequent pathogens were *S. pneumoniae* (19; 35.8%), *Klebsiella pneumoniae* (12; 22%), *Staphylococcus aureus* (9; 17%), *M. pneumoniae* (8; 15%), *Escherichia coli* (6; 11%), beta-hemolytic streptococci (4; 7.5%) and other Gram-negative bacilli (5; 9%). Another study from Srinagar in India investigated pathogens associated with CAP among patients requiring hospitalization and found a predominance of Gram-negative pathogens.[32] In that study there were very few pneumococcal infections.

One study from Kerala, India, documented *S. pneumoniae* as the most common pathogen, but also a high prevalence of Gram-negative infections.[33] A further study from Chennai, which noted that the prevalence of infection with *M. pneumoniae* was comparatively higher in HIV-infected persons when compared with HIV-noninfected adults, also documented *S. pneumoniae* as the most common cause of lower respiratory tract disease.[34] An additional study has also documented a high prevalence of *M. pneumoniae* infection in CAP in India (35%).[35] A study from New Delhi documented the serological evidence of *Legionella pneumophila* infection in 9 of 60 patients (15%) admitted to the All India Institute of Medical Sciences with CAP and the authors suggested that infection with *Legionella spp.*, may be a more frequent cause of CAP than previously recognized and recommended that empirical antibiotic therapy should include a combination of agents that cover both "atypical" and conventional bacterial pathogens.[36] One study has documented the occurrence of *Staphylococcus aureus* infections in a tertiary hospital in India, including cases with community-acquired respiratory tract infections.[37] Of the isolates 54% were methicillin-resistant and 16% carried the Panton-Valentine Leukocidin gene. The most recent study, which was a systematic review of adult CAP in Asia (including India), documented the importance of *S. pneumoniae, M. pneumoniae, Chlamydophila pneumoniae, Legionella spp.*, and *H. influenzae* as causes of CAP.[38] This study emphasized the relatively lesser importance of the *Pneumococcus* compared to other western studies and the greater importance of Gram-negative bacilli and *Mycobacterium tuberculosis.*

It is also becoming increasingly recognized that cases of CAP due to both seasonal and pandemic influenza may be complicated by secondary bacterial infections, most commonly due to the pneumococcus. In this regard it is interesting to note that during the occurrence of the recent H1N1 pandemic influenza infections, a substantial number of patients with CAP, particularly those requiring hospitalization or developing critically illness, were documented to have secondary bacterial infections.[39-42]

A number of studies have been undertaken in India in order to document the pneumococcal serotypes causing invasive disease and/or respiratory tract infections.[43-47] These studies have frequently documented serotypes 1, 6, 19, 7 and 5 to be the most common, with serotype 23 emerging in the later years. Among these isolates that were serotyped, resistance to co-trimoxazole, tetracycline and chloramphenicol was found to be common, whereas resistance to penicillin was infrequent and if present, was of intermediate resistance.[44,45,48] The prevalence of macrolide resistance in India has also been documented to be very low, as opposed to a number of other countries in Asia.[49]

A number of investigators throughout India and Asia are continuing to report the increase and spread of penicillin resistant and even multidrug resistant, invasive and colonizing, *S. pneumoniae* isolates.[50-55] One more recent study documented resistance to penicillin, erythromycin and ciprofloxacin of 5%, 20% and 23%, respectively.[46] Clearly, these investigators recommend that when choices of empirical antimicrobial therapy are made, they need to take into account local susceptibility patterns of the common infecting microorganisms. The subject of antibiotic resistance has been extensively reviewed elsewhere, including a discussion of the likely impact of antibiotic resistance, involving the different antibiotic classes, on the outcome of patients treated with the antibiotics commonly used for CAP.[56] Importantly, one recent study documented that the common serotypes causing invasive pneumococcal disease in Vellore, India, are included in the newer pneumococcal conjugate vaccines, such that the introduction of a program of childhood vaccination with these newer vaccines would be likely to be successful.[47]

RISK FACTORS FOR COMMUNITY-ACQUIRED PNEUMONIA

Risk factors for CAP are many and varied and include among many other factors, extremes of age (very young and the elderly), underlying comorbid conditions [in particular cardiovascular disease, chronic obstructive pulmonary disease (COPD) and HIV infection], lifestyle factors [including excessive alcohol consumption, cigarette smoking, and variations in body mass index (BMI) (malnutrition or obesity)], various medical treatments, and socioeconomic factors **(Table 2)**.[57-68] The exact mechanisms by which these conditions actually predispose to pneumonia is unclear, but in general terms they may predispose to an increase in bacterial colonization of the airway, and/or allow direct access of the bacteria to the lower respiratory tract, and/or be associated with impairment of normal host defenses and/or clearing mechanisms. In the case of the elderly, it appears that it may not be simple chronological age that is the important risk factor, but rather the underlying comorbid conditions that commonly exist in the aged. HIV infection itself is a risk factor for CAP, even in the era of highly active antiretroviral therapy (HAART), but the exact mechanisms are uncertain and are the subject of ongoing investigations. Many of the usual risk factors for pneumonia that exist in non-immunocompromised patients also act as risk factors in HIV-infected persons.[69,70]

Table 2 Risk factors for community-acquired pneumonia

- Extremes of age (very young and the elderly)
- Low socioeconomic status
- Lifestyle factors (cigarette smoking, excessive alcohol use, malnutrition or conversely high BMI)
- Underlying comorbid conditions (chronic cardiovascular, respiratory and renal disorders)
- HIV infection
- Other immunodeficiencies
- Medications

Abbreviations: HIV, human immunodeficiency virus; BMI, body mass index

(*Source:* *Reprinted with permission from Feldman C, Anderson R. New insights into pneumococcal disease. Respirology. 2009;14(2): 167-79.)

Many of the studies documented earlier, as well as several others, have clearly indicated the substantial role that cigarette smoking plays as a major risk factor for CAP, in both HIV-infected and -uninfected individuals.[58,67,68,71-77] The subject of cigarette smoking and the mechanisms of increased susceptibility to respiratory tract infections has been extensively reviewed elsewhere.[67] The exact mechanisms by which cigarette smoking predisposes to pneumonia are uncertain, but are almost certainly multifactorial and cigarette smoking has multiple effects on host defenses. Nasopharyngeal colonization by microorganisms, such as the pneumococcus is an essential first step in the pathogenesis of pneumococcal infections (see herein). Cigarette smoking and exposure to tobacco smoke has clearly been shown to increase pneumococcal carriage rates in both adults and children[78] and therefore, represents a major risk factor for pneumonia. The importance of cigarette smoking as a risk factor for nasopharyngeal colonization has been shown in south Indian infants, who experience high rates of pneumococcal carriage in the first 6 months of age, at least partly explaining their increased risk of pneumonia.[79] In that study, the odds of pneumococcal carriage were significantly increased in infants living in households in which 20 or more cigarettes were smoked each day. Interestingly, those same investigators documented that vitamin A supplementation at birth, delayed the onset of pneumococcal colonization.[80]

Cigarette smoking may also enhance the risk of CAP because of its association with COPD. The population prevalence of COPD is very high in India, the risk being related to the smoking of *bidis* and cigarettes, as well as environmental tobacco smoke exposure in nonsmokers.[81] In a study in Shimla (India), in addition to extremes of age, smoking and underlying COPD were significantly associated with the development of CAP.[31]

Even passive smoking plays a role in the risk of CAP and a recent population-based case-control study documented that passive smoking in the home is a risk factor for CAP in the elderly.[68] Most importantly in current smokers who have pneumococcal CAP, there is a greater risk of development of severe sepsis, the patients require hospitalization at a younger age with fewer underlying comorbid conditions, and there is an increased 30 days mortality independent of smoking-related or other comorbidity and age.[82]

PATHOGENESIS OF CAP WITH PARTICULAR REFERENCE TO THE *PNEUMOCOCCUS*

The section will focus on *S. pneumoniae,* the most common bacterial cause of CAP. Pneumococcal colonization of the airways is mostly asymptomatic, but is nevertheless the first step in the pathogenesis of invasive disease. This may be precipitated by infection with respiratory viruses, resulting in the increased expression of receptors for bacterial adhesins on airway epithelium.[83]

Prior to reviewing virulence factors, a brief consideration of the role of biofilm in microbial colonization/persistence is important, as this is a strategy utilized by the pneumococcus to evade host defenses.[84] Biofilm also restricts the penetration of antibiotics, favoring antibiotic resistance. Importantly, the pneumococcus, by the mechanisms described herein, adheres to and invades airway epithelium. Biofilm-encased bacterial aggregates attached to the epithelial surface, or sequestered intracellularly, therefore provide an effective mechanism for bacterial persistence.[84] Concealed in biofilm, in which it communicates by quorum sensing mechanisms, the pneumococcus can re-emerge at times when host defenses are transiently or irreversibly compromised, as may occur during infection with influenza virus/respiratory syncytial virus or HIV-1, respectively.

The polysaccharide capsule is generally recognized as being the major virulence factor of the pneumococcus, promoting resistance to entrapment by mucopolysaccharides present in mucus, as well as opsonophagocytosis. Other nonprotein virulence factors include hydrogen peroxide and phosphorylcholine. Hydrogen peroxide (H_2O_2) promotes structural damage to respiratory epithelium, interfering with the protective activities of the mucociliary escalator,[85] favoring attachment of the pneumococcus to epithelial cells via the interaction of phosphorylcholine with the platelet-activating factor (PAF) receptor.[86,87]

The pneumococcus also possesses an array of protein virulence factors, which contribute to evasion and/or suppression of host defenses. Some of these are recognized as potential vaccine candidates and include the choline binding proteins (Cbps), neuraminidase, hyaluronidase, zinc metalloproteinase, divalent metal-binding proteins, the pneumococcal lipoprotein surface adhesin A (PsaA) and the cholesterol-binding, pore-forming toxin, pneumolysin, generally recognized to be the most potent of the pneumococcal protein virulence factors. During colonization of the nasopharynx, virulence factors that neutralize both innate and adaptive host defenses enable bacterial adhesins to promote attachment of the pneumococcus to airway epithelium.

In addition to the polysaccharide capsule, the pneumococcus utilizes numerous strategies to subvert innate and adaptive host defenses. These include:

- Interference with the protective actions of the mucociliary escalator, primarily by pneumolysin acting in concert with H_2O_2 and hyaluronidase.[85,88]
- Interference by PspA and PspC (also known as CbpA) with activation of both the alternative and classical complement pathways.
- Pneumolysin-mediated depletion of complement via inappropriate activation of the classical pathway.
- Interference with neutrophil migration and the antimicrobial activity of phagocyte-derived reactive oxygen species and apolactoferrin, mediated by the zinc metalloproteinase, (ZmpC), the thioredoxin family proteins, Etrx1/2, and PspA respectively.
- Escape from neutrophil extracellular traps (NETs) mediated by endonuclease A.

- Cleavage of secretory IgA by the igA1 protease, a member of the Zmp family.[86,87,89-91]

Notwithstanding the proadhesive interactions between pneumococcal phosphorylcholine and the PAF receptor on airway epithelium, PspA and PspC also promote attachment via binding to the epithelial polymeric Ig receptor that normally transports secretory IgA, while E-cadherin, the cell-cell junction protein of respiratory epithelium is a receptor for PsaA.[86,92] In addition, some serotypes possess pilus-like structures that promote epithelial adhesion via interaction with uncharacterized receptors. A novel pneumococcal protein adhesin has been described recently. This is the 120 kDa plasminogen- and fibronectin-binding protein B (PfbB), which significantly increases the ability of the pneumococcus to adhere to epithelial cells.[93] Unmasking of these various pneumococcal adhesins necessitates a reduction in capsule size, with the accompanying risk of increased vulnerability to phagocytosis. This is apparently minimized by production of biofilm, a process in which bacterial neuraminidase[94] and possibly H_2O_2 participate. These aforementioned virulence mechanisms facilitate the translocation of the pneumococcus to the lower airways, while transcytosis of the pathogen across the epithelial barrier via the polymeric Ig receptor enables access to the bloodstream and invasion of the central nervous system.

Although nasopharyngeal colonization by the pneumococcus is the first stage in invasive disease, it may also protect against severe infection by activating host defences.[95] Innate and adaptive immune responses triggered by the aforementioned virulence factors, as well as cell wall components such as lipoteichoic acid (LTA) and proteoglycans, if efficiently mobilized, can control and eradicate pneumococcal colonization.

Interactions of LTA and pneumolysin with toll-like receptors (TLRs) -2 and -4, respectively, result in the mobilization of circulating neutrophils to the airways. These TLRs are the prototype pattern recognition molecules, which function as the sentinels of the innate immune system. Interaction of LTA and pneumolysin with TLRs on airway epithelium and other cells of the innate immune system in the airways, triggers a signaling cascade, which leads to the production of the cytokines, interleukin (IL)-1 beta, IL-6 and tumor necrosis factor (TNF), as well as the chemokine IL-8, all of which cooperate to promote transendothelial migration and the chemotaxis of neutrophils. In addition, nucleotide oligomerization (NOD)-like receptors also contribute to innate antipneumococcal host defenses. These are a specialized group of intracellular pattern recognition molecules, which like TLRs recognize highly conserved structures on bacterial pathogens. In the case of the pneumococcus, bacterial proteoglycans are recognized by epithelial NOD proteins, specifically NOD-2, resulting in the production of proinflammatory cytokines/chemokines and influx of neutrophils. This TLR/NOD-2-mediated inflammatory response contributes to the early control of colonization and also favors adaptive mucosal immunity by promoting the degradation of bacteria required for efficient delivery of pneumococcal antigens to nasal-associated lymphoid tissue.[96-99]

Immunoglobulin G and secretory IgA antibodies directed against the polysaccharide capsule of the pneumococcus are generally considered to be the primary determinants of immune-mediated type specific protection. Antibodies to pneumococcal proteins, particularly CbpA, PsaA and pneumolysin also confer protection, which although less efficient, are not serotype restricted.[100] Based on experimental animal and clinicoepidemiological studies, it is now evident that antibody independent, CD4+ T cell-mediated adaptive immune responses to pneumococcal protein antigens also contribute to the natural development of immunity to pneumococcal infection.[86,101,102] T-lymphocytes of the Th1 and Th17 subsets appear to be critically involved in these cell-mediated immune responses.[101,103,104] Protection mediated via Th1 cells may involve interferon-gamma-mediated enhancement of the antimicrobial activity of macrophages, especially mannose receptor-mediated phagocytosis.[105] In the case of Th17 cells, production of the cytokine IL-17A leads to the recruitment of neutrophils and increased pneumococcal killing by these cells.[101] Following initial partial control of colonization by innate neutrophil-mediated mechanisms, recent evidence favors a primary role for Th17 cells in the recruitment of monocytes/macrophages to mucosal surfaces, resulting in the clearance of primary bacterial colonization.[101,106]

In summary, entry of the *Pneumococcus* into the nasopharynx has several possible outcomes:

- Eradication by innate/adaptive host defenses.
- A carrier state in which the bacteria and host coexist in relative harmony.
- A state of persistence in which bacteria are encased in biofilm, either extracellularly or intracellularly following adherence to, and invasion of epithelial cells, enabling evasion of host defenses (this could also be considered as being a chronic infection).
- Acute infection. In the case of carrier and persistence states, the bacterial pathogen, seemingly subdued, may strike when host defenses are transiently compromised, as may occur during infection with influenza or other respiratory viruses.

DIAGNOSTIC TESTING

A vast number of studies have been undertaken over many years to assess the value of the various microbiological techniques, that are available for the diagnosis of likely microbial etiology in patients with CAP. Among more commonly used investigations currently available are sputum examination by Gram's stain and culture and pneumococcal antigen detection, blood for culture and serological testing, and urine for legionella and pneumococcal antigen detection.

Much less frequently used are invasive techniques such as fiberoptic bronchoscopy. While some studies have indicated that there is good diagnostic yield from many of these tests, including simple sputum examination,[107,108] others have suggested that routine initial sputum examination is of little value, particularly in nonseverely ill cases,[109] such that this investigation is frequently not used even in hospitalized cases.[110] One technique that has significantly improved the rapid sputum diagnosis of pneumococcal pneumonia is the real-time quantitative polymerase chain reaction (QRT-PCR), with detection of the *pneumolysin* (*ply*) gene appearing to be useful in patients who have already received antibiotics.[111] More recently, a modification of this procedure based on detection of the *pneumococcal autolysin* (*lytA*) gene in blood and/or sputum has been documented to be particularly useful, enabling measurement of bacterial load, an important indicator of both disease severity and outcome.[112,113]

Other recent innovations in CAP-related molecular diagnostics include multiplex PCR procedures which enable the simultaneous detection of a range of bacterial and viral pathogens in bronchoalveolar lavage, sputum, saliva and nasopharyngeal swab specimens. While isolation of microorganisms from blood culture is considered a "gold standard" for the diagnosis of likely etiology of CAP, a number of studies have indicated that there is a low yield from blood cultures and that even a positive result does not frequently result in a change in antibiotic management, or subsequent cost saving, particularly in nonseverely ill cases.[114-117] One study documented that the yield of blood cultures increased as the severity of infection increased, as measured by the *pneumonia severity index (PSI),* as did the likelihood of blood cultures changing antibiotic therapy. Rapid urine antigen tests for the detection of *S. pneumoniae* and *L. pneumophila* serogroup 1 infection are very useful for indicating these pathogens as likely cause of CAP in adults.[118] These tests have good sensitivity and specificity, but are expensive and in many guidelines, both in developed and developing countries, are not routinely recommended, but are reserved for special cases, such as severely ill patients requiring ICU admission.[119,120] Other serological testing for so-called atypical pathogens is not routinely recommended.[119] In HIV infected patients, additional microbiological testing for *P. jirovecii* and *M. tuberculosis* may need to be undertaken.[119]

There is considerable debate about the routine need for a chest radiograph in all patients with CAP, particularly in cases not apparently severe enough to require hospital admission. Some have suggested that it remains an "essential initial test" in the diagnosis of CAP that is recommended in most guidelines, certainly for hospitalized cases.[119-121] There are studies, however, indicating that the admission chest radiograph lacks sensitivity and that it may not demonstrate abnormalities initially in some 21% of patients.[122] The chest radiograph is unhelpful in suggesting likely microbial etiology and is performed in order to confirm the presence of pneumonia, to delineate the extent of the pulmonary involvement, as an indicator of the severity of infection, to delineate the presence of underlying disorders and to determine the presence of any complications.[119,120,123]

The assessment of oxygenation is recommended in both outpatients and inpatients and can be undertaken by pulse oximetry, particularly in outpatients or by arterial blood gas analysis.[124] Routine hematological and biochemical testing do not help to determine likely etiology, but will assist in the assessment of comorbid illness, and influence decisions regarding need for hospitalization, severity of infections and choice and dosage of initial, empiric antimicrobial therapy.[119] **Table 3** indicates the diagnostic testing that is commonly recommended in patients with CAP. These investigations are particularly recommended in high-risk cases, in those patients with underlying comorbid illnesses and in those with more severe infections.[119]

Table 3 Diagnostic testing recommended for more severely ill, hospitalized patients with community-acquired pneumonia

- Chest radiograph
- Sputum Gram stains and culture
- Blood cultures
- Blood gases (or assessment of oxygenation by pulse oximetry)
- Routine hematology and biochemistry
- Rapid urine antigen testing for *S. pneumoniae* and *Legionella spp.* serogroup 1
- Thoracentesis for pleural effusions.

PROGNOSIS

The outcome of CAP is influenced by a number of factors, including host factors, bacterial factors and antibiotic factors.[125] In a study of overall factors influencing the outcome of adult patients with CAP in New Delhi, India, factors such as old age, history of smoking, presence of COPD, high blood urea, low serum albumin and development of septic shock were associated with a higher risk of complications and a poorer prognosis.[126] In addition, older patients with a poor prognosis had a greater duration of symptoms and a poor neutrophil response to the infection.

Among the host factors, older age, the presence of underlying comorbid illness and various genetic characteristics of the host, all are potentially associated with the increased risk of pneumonia, as well as a worse outcome.[125] Severity of illness on its own may impact negatively on pneumonia outcome, even in the absence of any of these other risk factors.[3,125,127] Severity of illness assessment is therefore important not only because it gives an indication as to the likely outcome of the patient with CAP, but because it dictates the appropriate site of care of these patients, the extent of the microbiological workup needed and the choice of initial empirical antimicrobial chemotherapy.[3,125,127] A number of severity-of-illness indices and various scoring systems have been developed to assist in severity assessment, among which the PSI and the CURB-65 score [derived from the British Thoracic Society (BTS) Rules] are the most commonly used.[127]

The subject of severity of illness assessment and the various tools that are available, including the various scoring systems and the various biomarkers, are reviewed extensively elsewhere.[128-135] The PSI score comprises of 20 variables that include details of demographic characteristics, comorbidity, clinical features and results of laboratory and radiographic investigations.[136] The CURB-65 includes variables, indicative of severity including mental confusion (abbreviated mental test score ≤ 8), raised urea (>7 mmol/L), rapid respiratory rate (≥ 30 breaths/min), low blood pressure [systolic <90 mm Hg, and/or diastolic ≤60 mm Hg) and age ≥65 years].[137] The PSI was developed primarily to identify low risk patients who could safely be managed at home, whereas the CURB-65 score was developed to identify patients with severe CAP at high-risk of mortality.[138,139]

A modification of the latter score, the CRB-65 score has also been developed and studied with the advantage that it does not require the measurement of blood urea levels. It has been found to have similar accuracy to the CURB-65 score. A number of guidelines on the management of pneumonia, particularly from the developing world, have primarily recommended the use of the CURB-65 or CRB-65 as the severity scoring index of choice because of its simplicity, immediate applicability and ease of use, combined with an accuracy that is similar to that of more complicated systems such as the PSI.[119,120,140] The parameters that make up the CURB-65 score are indicated in **Table 4**. In a study in an Indian setting, both the PSI and the CURB-65 have been found to be equally sensitive in predicting death.[141] While the specificity of the CURB-65 was greater than the PSI, the PSI was more sensitive in predicting need for ICU admission.

Table 4 Parameters used to determine the CURB-65 severity of illness score

Symptom	*Points*
C = **C**onfusion	1
U = Raised **U**rea (> 7 mmol/L)	1
R = Rapid **R**espiratory rate (≥30 breaths/minute)	1
B = Low **B**lood pressure (systolic <90 mm Hg, and/or diastolic ≤60 mm Hg)	1
65 = Age ≥ 65 years	1

A point is assigned for each parameter, when present. Patients with a score of 0 or 1 have a mild pneumonia associated with a low mortality, those with a score of 2 have a moderate pneumonia with an intermediate mortality and those with a score of 3 or more have severe pneumonia associated with a high mortality.

Several other severity scores and indices have been developed and/or studied, particularly for use in predicting the outcome and need for ICU admission among severely ill cases,[139,142,143] as well as in the subset of patients with pneumococcal CAP.[144,145] It is important to remember that these scoring systems have a number of limitations, including lack of inclusion of certain social factors and other clinical conditions that may impact on outcome. Thus, while each scoring system has its own individual strengths and weaknesses, none of them is able to replace sound clinical judgment of the attending physician.[139]

There is also a myriad of biomarkers that have been studied with regard to their utility in the assessment of severity of CAP. These have been extensively reviewed elsewhere.[128-135] These biomarkers are probably more appropriate for use in the more severely ill, hospitalized patient with CAP and appear to be a promising area for future research. However, it is important to remember that neither severity of illness scoring systems, nor biomarkers can replace sound clinical judgment and should be seen as adjuncts to decision making.

Among the bacterial factors that may impact on the outcome of pneumonia, are the nature of the infecting microorganism, its associated virulence factors and its susceptibility to commonly prescribed antibiotics.[125] Significant consideration also needs to be given to the potential impact of antibiotic resistance, particularly pneumococcal resistance to beta-lactam agents on the outcome of pneumonia.[1,125,146-149] The subject of antibiotic resistance has recently been reviewed.[56] While much has been published on this subject, it does appear, overall, that the current levels of beta-lactam resistance among pneumococcal isolates are such that if appropriate beta-lactam agents are used in appropriate dosages, resistance should not impact negatively on the outcome of respiratory tract infections.[146,147,149] This is further supported by the fact that in January 2008, the Clinical and Laboratory Standards Institute (CLSI) revised its pneumococcal susceptibility breakpoints for penicillin for nonmeningeal infections being treated with parenteral antibiotics, supported by a careful consideration of microbiological, pharmacokinetic/pharmacodynamic and clinical data.[150] Breakpoints are now much higher with isolates with a minimum inhibitory concentration (MIC) of equal to or less than 2 µg/mL being considered susceptible, those with a MIC of 4 mg/mL being considered intermediately susceptible and those with a MIC equal to or greater than 8 mg/mL being considered resistant.

The situation is less clear-cut in the case of macrolide antibiotics, which have received much less attention, but it does appear that when these agents are used on their own, particularly in the presence of high-level macrolide resistance, failure of therapy, including breakthrough bacteremias might well occur.[125,151] With regard to pneumococcal fluoroquinolone resistance, while it is well recognized that phenotypic resistance with the presence of multiple mutations in the quinolone resistance-determining regions (QRDR) of *par*C and *gyr*A is known to be of clinical significance, what is not commonly appreciated is that first-step mutations in these regions, not producing MIC-defining phenotypic resistance, can easily mutate to the further levels of fluoroquinolone nonsusceptibility and lead to clinical failure.[151-153] However, the prevalence of such first-step mutants among populations of susceptible pneumococcal isolates is not reported and is therefore unknown in most parts of the world.

Of considerable concern internationally is the fact that there are very few new antibiotics in the developmental pipeline that would be available to combat infections due to highly resistant microorganisms, should these become more widespread, although some new ones have appeared.[154-157] While other adjunctive strategies are being studied for use, together with antibiotics, to improve the outcome of severely ill patients with CAP, it still remains true that the mainstay of therapy of such infections will always be effective antibiotic therapy.[127,158-160]

Among the antibiotic factors, choice of agent, dosage and duration of therapy and time to the initiation of antibiotics from the time of presentation of patients to hospital, all potentially play a role in the outcome of pneumonia.[3,156] Importantly, new strategies recommended for antibiotic management, for example, the use of combination antibiotic therapy in more severely ill hospitalized cases with pneumonia, including the subset of patients with bacteremic pneumococcal infections, have been said to have a positive impact on pneumonia outcomes.[64,125,128,161-165] The most commonly used combination therapy, which has been shown to be beneficial, is the addition of a macrolide to standard beta-lactam therapy, although benefit has also been shown with other combinations.[125,161] A number of questions still remain with regard to combination therapy, including an understanding of the reason(s) that some studies appear to indicate no beneficial effect of combination therapy on the pneumonia case-fatality rate.[166] Alternatively, should combination truly be shown to be beneficial, clarification is needed regarding which combination(s) are best,[167] as well as the exact mechanism(s) by which combination therapy may prove to be beneficial.[125,161]

One of the reasons suggested for the benefit of combination therapy is that it may be associated with the addition to the beta-lactam agent of an antibiotic effective against so called atypical pathogens (i.e. a macrolide, azalide, ketolide, tetracycline, or fluoroquinolone). Interestingly, a recent study investigated the outcome of bacteremic pneumonia in relationship to initial antibiotic therapy and although the investigation confirmed that the use of an agent active against atypical pathogens was independently associated with decreased 30-day mortality, further analysis suggested that this benefit was limited to the use of macrolides and not fluoroquinolones or tetracyclines.[168] Furthermore, an additional study documented that macrolide use was associated with a decreased mortality in patients with severe sepsis due to pneumonia, including the subset of patients infected with macrolide-resistant pathogens.[169] The role of macrolides in therapy is discussed further below (adjunctive therapy).

As a part of the global strategy, a number of national and international guidelines have been developed, including one from India, describing the optimal management of patients with CAP, with the intention of improving the care and outcome of these patients.[119,143,170-174] However, consensus on the optimal management of lower respiratory tract infections, particularly with regard to antibiotic therapy, has not been attained in the various guideline documents.[170] Part of the reason for the differences in the guideline recommendations may relate to local factors, such as different patient populations, causative microorganisms, antimicrobial resistance patterns and availability of resources, together with differences in the interpretation of existing data by the guideline committee members.[171] Certainly, until more recently, there has been a relative lack of a robust evidence base for several aspects of the guideline recommendations.[171] Many of the newer guidelines are being informed by the various studies of CAP and in particular, very large multicenter, international, collaborative studies of CAP being conducted currently, which are able to recruit large number of cases throughout the world.[175]

Yet another issue is whether there is general adherence to the guideline recommendations and/or whether adherence has any impact on the outcome of patients with CAP.[158,163,164,176-179] Some studies have suggested that compliance with guidelines may be associated with better outcome and lower costs of management in patients with CAP.[158,170,180,181] One recent study from Italy, conducted in three phases, documented an advantage for compliant versus noncompliant therapy, both in terms of failure rate [odds ratio (OR) 0.74: 95% confidence interval (CI) 0.60–0.90; p = 0.004] and mortality (OR 0.77: 95% CI 0.56–1.04; p = 0.082).[177] This was despite relatively low compliance with the national guideline recommendations, which did not increase substantially even after the guideline implementation phase of the study (from 33% to 44% compliance). These findings prompted the authors to suggest that there was need for a more aggressive and proactive approach to ensure guideline compliance. A single study from South Africa has documented very poor adherence to the local CAP Guideline, with the number of patients receiving compliant therapy being too low to confirm a clinical benefit from guideline adherence.[176]

One aspect of patient prognosis that requires special consideration is the presence of cardiac changes/complications as a consequence of all-cause CAP, as well as the subset of patients with pneumococcal CAP. While an initial publication in this area appeared in 1993,[182] this subject remained somewhat ignored until more recently. Renewed interest in this area has resulted in a number of studies and several reviews of the subject being published.[183-188] Mainly, what has been described in these studies and reviews is the frequent occurrence of cardiac failure, cardiac arrhythmias, and even myocardial infarction, as a complication of the pneumonia, even in patients with no previous underlying cardiac condition. These events tend to occur quite early in the course of the infection and are associated with an increased short-term mortality. Clinicians treating patients with CAP need to be wary of the likelihood of cardiac complications, particularly in patients not responding well to initial treatment, but their occurrence in patients with CAP also highlight the potential benefit of CAP prevention using pneumococcal and influenza vaccination.

Lastly, it is important for clinicians to be aware of the fact that while patients may survive their acute episode of CAP, the infection still has an impact on their prognosis for a number of years because of an ongoing long-term mortality.[189,190]

TREATMENT OF COMMUNITY-ACQUIRED PNEUMONIA

The mainstay of therapy for CAP is the use of antibiotics. Empirical antibiotic therapy should particularly take into consideration severity of illness, likely etiological agent, resistance patterns among commonly identified pathogens, especially *S. pneumoniae* and underlying comorbidities.[1] An additional consideration in the developing world is the cost of the individual drugs.[191] Antibiotic therapy should be commenced as soon as possible after diagnosis. With regard to outpatient therapy, a recent Cochrane review concluded that currently available evidence from randomized controlled trials was insufficient to make any evidence-based recommendations for antibiotic choice in the ambulatory setting.[192]

A number of guidelines, both in developed and developing worlds, recommend the use of oral therapy with amoxicillin for outpatients.[119,140] Macrolide monotherapy has been suggested as an alternative, particularly for patients allergic to penicillin, but this recommendation would need to take into consideration local susceptibility patterns to macrolides. Other oral agents, such as amoxicillin/clavulanate, second-generation cephalosporins and fluoroquinolones can be used, but are more expensive and are generally reserved for elderly patients, for those cases that are more severely ill and those that have underlying comorbid conditions, or that have failed initial therapy. The CAP guideline from India recommends the use of oral macrolides (e.g. azithromycin) or oral beta-lactams (e.g. amoxicillin) for outpatients without comorbidity and combined beta-lactam/macrolide for those with comorbidity, with the fluoroquinolones not being recommended for empiric use.[174]

For more severely ill, hospitalized cases, most guidelines recommend the use of a beta-lactam/macrolide combination or monotherapy with a respiratory fluoroquinolone.[119,140] The CAP guideline from India also recommends, in this setting, a beta-lactam/macrolide combination, with the use of fluoroquinolones as an alternative in the unusual scenario of hypersensitivity to beta-lactams and if TB is not a serious consideration.[174]

For cases requiring ICU admission, additional agents are recommended; for example, the addition of an aminoglycoside to a beta-lactam/macrolide combination to provide additional cover for suspected Gram-negative infection.[119,143] If a fluoroquinolone is used for an ICU patient, it is commonly recommended that it should be combined with another agent such as a beta-lactam.[119,143] The CAP guideline from India recommends, in this setting, the use of a beta-lactam/macrolide combination in patients not at risk of *Pseudomonas aeruginosa* with various recommendations for those with suspected *P. aeruginosa* infection.[174]

Caution must be exercised with the routine use of fluoroquinolone monotherapy for patients presenting with CAP in regions where TB is endemic, since such cases may actually be infected with *M. tuberculosis*, for which fluoroquinolones have excellent *in vitro* activity. Studies have indicated that in this situation, fluoroquinolone use may be associated with delays in the diagnosis of TB with the masking of this infection.[193,194] Consequent to this is the potential for patient morbidity and even mortality, as well as ongoing secondary transmission. Furthermore, there are additional concerns that fluoroquinolone monotherapy used in this situation may result in fluoroquinolone-resistant TB, although studies have suggested that this really only occurs in patients who have been exposed to multiple previous courses of fluoroquinolones.[195,196]

Adjunctive Therapy

General support for patients with CAP includes attention to nutrition and hydration, analgesia and supplemental oxygen. A number of adjunctive therapies have been studied, particularly in severely ill patients, including those in the ICU setting, in an attempt to further decrease the ongoing high mortality among these patients.[197] The two agents that appear to be most promising are the macrolide group of antibiotics and corticosteroids. The role of macrolides in the therapy of pneumonia has been fully described above (antibiotic factors). The reason they are included as possible adjunctive therapy is that many believe that the benefit of adding a macrolide to standard beta-lactam therapy may not be related to their antimicrobial activity, but rather to the considerable anti-inflammatory, immunomodulatory activities that the macrolide group of antibiotics possess, translating not only into beneficial effects in the human host, but also attenuation of the virulence factors of bacteria, such as the pneumococcus, even at low, sub-minimum inhibitory concentrations that do not kill the microorganisms.[90,162,198-202] A recently completed multicenter, prospective, randomized, controlled clinical trial, the results of which are awaited, has assessed the comparative efficacies of therapy of CAP with a beta-lactam alone or combined with a macrolide, and fluorquinolone monotherapy, using as an end-point all-cause mortality 90 days after hospital admission.[203]

With regard to corticosteroids, while two more recent systematic reviews[204,205] came to somewhat differing views as whether to recommend the routine use of corticosteroids in patients with CAP, there are clearly a number of studies documenting benefit of their use in hospitalized patients and/or cases with severe CAP[197,206-208] with some documenting a decrease in mortality and others a more rapid resolution of symptoms and a reduced duration of intravenous antibiotic therapy. There is also good scientific evidence to understand possible mechanisms by which corticosteroids may have benefit, considering their significant effects on inflammatory responses.[197] Corticosteroid use is most commonly recommended in patients with severe CAP in association with septic shock. Importantly, however, adjuvant therapy with corticosteroids proved disappointing in a recently completed large, randomised, prospective double-blinded, placebo-controlled clinical trial in adults with severe CAP,[209] with similar findings reported in another large retrospective study.[210] This issue continues to be addressed in 3 on going well-controlled clinical trials in the USA, Spain and Switzerland.[211-213] Thus, while some suggest that final recommendations regarding routine macrolide and/or corticosteroids use should await comprehensive randomized control trials, most clinicians would consider using them in severely ill cases with CAP.[160,161]

Interestingly, current statin use has been reported in a number of mainly small, retrospective studies to significantly reduce mortality in patients with CAP, including those with pneumococcal disease.[214,215] Although the role of current statin use in reducing CAP-associated mortality remains to be conclusively established, potential protective mechanisms include prevention of cardiovascular sequelae[216] and secondary anti-inflammatory activity.[214]

PREVENTION OF INFECTION—VACCINATION

An important aspect to consider in the overall control of CAP, and in particular pneumococcal pneumonia, is the prevention of infection using vaccination. Currently, two pneumococcal vaccines are commercially available, namely the polyvalent polysaccharide vaccine (PPV), used predominantly in adults and the pneumococcal conjugate vaccine (PCV), used predominantly in children.[217,218] While there remains considerable debate as to the efficacy of the PPV, meta-analysis certainly supports the evidence for its use in the prevention of invasive pneumococcal disease in adults.[218] Evidence is considered by some to be somewhat less compelling with respect to efficacy in adults with chronic illness and in its routine use to prevent all causes of pneumonia or reduce overall pneumonia mortality.[218] However, others have suggested that the evidence points to a lower, but not insignificant protective effect, even in nonbacteremic pneumonia, such that this should not preclude the more widespread use of the vaccine.[219] Furthermore, recent studies also point to a significant beneficial effect in preventing pneumococcal pneumonia and decreasing disease severity, even in the vaccinated elderly.[219] A lower overall rate of pneumonia and improved outcome have also been seen in HIV-infected adults who have received PPV previously.[220,221]

Even more compelling is the evidence for the use of the PCV in the safe prevention of pneumococcal infection in children in both low income and industrialized countries, including HIV-infected individuals, meeting international criteria of cost-effectiveness even for lower income countries.[217,222] For this reason, the vaccine is recommended by the World Health Organization for inclusion in National Vaccination Programs in countries such as South Africa and elsewhere. Interestingly, in some of the studies, the PCV has been effective in lowering the rate of invasive pneumococcal disease not only in vaccinated children, particularly those below the age of 2 years, but also in nonvaccinated children and even in adults and the elderly in the community.[223] As such the vaccine appears to have both direct immune benefits in those vaccinated, as well as indirect "herd immunity" effects.

PCVs have undergone progressive improvement, especially in respect of extended coverage against the most prevalent and virulent pneumococcal serotypes, with PCV13 the current leader. Acquisition of this vaccine together with an appreciation of the limitations of PPVs, of which PPV23 is the prototype, have resulted in updated immunization recommendations. In the case of infants and very young children, PCV13 has now been included in the National Immunization Programs of many developed and developing countries.[224] With respect to adults, PCV13 vaccination as a single dose is recommended by the Food and Drug Administration of the USA for adults aged more than or equal to 50 years, while in the case of those aged more than 19 years who have immunocompromising conditions, including HIV infection, a "prime-boost" strategy is recommended for vaccine-naïve recipients.[224] This is based on an initial dose of PCV13 followed at least 8 weeks later by a single dose of PPV23, with variations in schedules according to prior vaccination and/or the circulating $CD4^+$ T-cell count in the case of HIV infection.[224] Very recently, administration of PCV13 to adults aged more than or equal to 65 years has been found to confer significant protection against a first episode of vaccine-type CAP and invasive disease.[225] Current and pipeline pneumococcal vaccines have recently been extensively reviewed, including serotype-independent protein and whole cell vaccines.[91]

Influenza vaccination is also recommended in many CAP guidelines, even in the developing world.[119,120] While influenza vaccine may be administered to any individual wishing to reduce the risk of being infected with influenza, systematic annual vaccination is routinely recommended for individuals at high-risk of being infected with influenza and/or experiencing complications, such as pneumonia, from this infection.[120] It is also recommended that individuals that can transmit influenza to high-risk cases, such as healthcare workers, should be immunized yearly.[124]

CONCLUSION

It has been stated that the mortality of CAP remains substantial in both the developed and developing worlds, despite all recent advances in medicine, including the availability of potent antimicrobial therapy and even the establishment of ICU facilities. A number of questions and challenges still remain with regard to a full understanding of the nature of CAP and its optimal management that require continuing research.[138]

ACKNOWLEDGMENT

A significant portion of this chapter was derived from the introductory chapter of a DSc thesis submitted to the University of the Witwatersrand by Professor Charles Feldman.

REFERENCES

1. File TM. *Streptococcus pneumoniae* and community-acquired pneumonia: A cause for concern. Am J Med. 2004;117(Suppl 3A):39S-50S.
2. Woodhead M, Welch CA, Harrison DA, Bellingan G, Ayres JG. Community-acquired pneumonia on the intensive care unit: secondary analysis of 17,869 cases in the ICNARC Case Mix Programme Database. Critical Care. 2006;10(Suppl 2):S1.
3. Garau J, Calbo E. Community-acquired pneumonia. Lancet. 2008;371(9611):455-8.
4. Lode HM. Managing community-acquired pneumonia: A European perspective. Respir Med. 2007;101(9):1864-73.
5. File TM Jr, Marrie TJ. Burden of community-acquired pneumonia in North American Adults. Postgrad Med. 2010;122(2):130-41.
6. Welte T, Torres A, Nathwani D. Clinical and economic burden of community-acquired pneumonia among adults in Europe. Thorax. 2012;67(1):71-9.
7. Guest JF, Morris A. Community-acquired pneumonia: the annual cost to the National Health Service in the UK. Eur Respir J. 1997;10(7):1530-4.
8. Melegaro A, Edmunds WJ, Pebody R, Miller E, George R. The current burden of pneumococcal disease in England and Wales. J Infect. 2006;52(1):37-48.
9. Isturiz RE, Luna CM, Ramirez J. Clinical and economic burden of pneumonia among adults in Latin America. Int J Infect Dis. 2010;14(10):e852-6.
10. Shibl AM, Memish ZA, Ibrahim E, Kanj SS. Burden of adult community-acquired pneumonia in the Middle East/North Africa region. Rev Med Microbiol. 2009;21(1):11-20.
11. Song JH, Thamlikitkul V, Hsueh PR. Clinical and economic burden of community-acquired pneumonia amongst adults in the Asia-Pacific region. Int J Antimicrob Agents. 2011;38(2):108-17.
12. Singh V. The burden of pneumonia in children: an Asian perspective. Paediatr Respir Rev. 2005;6(2):88-93.
13. Singh RB, Singh V, Kulshrestha SK, Singh S, Gupta P, Kumar R. Social class and all-cause mortality in an urban population of North India. Acta Cardiol. 2005;60(6):611-7.
14. Murray CJ, Lopez AD. Global mortality, disability, and the contribution of risk factors: Global Burden of Disease Study. Lancet. 1997;349(9063):1436-42.
15. Lopez AD, Mathers CD, Ezzati M, Jamison DT, Murray CJ. Global and regional burden of disease and risk factors, 2001: systematic analysis of population health data. Lancet. 2006;367(9524):1747-57.
16. Lopez AD, Mathers CD. Measuring the global burden of disease and epidemiological transitions: 2002-2030. Ann Trop Med Parasitol. 2006;100(5-6):481-99.
17. Lozano R, Naghavi M, Foreman K, Lim S, Shibuya K, Aboyans V, et al. Global and regional mortality from 235 causes of death for 20 age groups in 1990 and 2010: a systematic analysis for the Global Burden of Disease Study 2010. Lancet. 2012;380(9859):2095-128.
18. Fauci AS, Morens DM. The perpetual challenge of infectious diseases. N Engl J Med. 2012;366(5):454-61.
19. Epidemiology of community-acquired pneumonia. J Assoc Physicians India. 2013;61(7 Suppl):7-8.
20. Merson MH. The HIV-AIDS pandemic at 25—the global response. N Engl J Med. 2006;354(23):2414-7.
21. India faces major AIDS burden by end of decade. AIDS Wkly Plus. 1995;18:24.
22. Dore GJ, Kaldor JM, Ungchusak K, Mertens TE. Epidemiology of HIV and AIDS in the Asia-Pacific region. Med J Aust. 1996;165(9):494-8.
23. Asia: fastest growing AIDS problem. Reprowatch. 1998;17(4):1-2.
24. Nath A. HIV/AIDS and Indian youth—a review of the literature (1980–2008). Sahara J. 2009;6(1):2-8.
25. Murray JF. Pulmonary complications of HIV-1 infection among adults living in sub-Saharan Africa. Int J Tuberc Lung Dis. 2005;9(8):826-35.
26. Swaminathan S, Narendran G. HIV and tuberculosis in India. J Biosci. 2008;33(4):527-37.
27. Feldman C, Anderson R. HIV-associated bacterial pneumonia. Clin Chest Med. 2013;34(2):205-16.
28. Abouya YL, Beaumel A, Lucas S, Dago-Akribi A, Coulibaly G, N'Dhatz M, et al. *Pneumocystis carinii* pneumonia. An uncommon cause of death in African patients with acquired immunodeficiency syndrome. Am Rev Respir Dis. 1992;145(3):617-20.
29. Mahomed AG, Murray J, Klempman S, Richards G, Feldman C, Levy NT, et al. *Pneumocystis carinii* pneumonia in HIV infected patients from South Africa. East Afr Med J. 1999;76(2):80-4.
30. Udwadia ZF, Doshi AV, Bhaduri AS. *Pneumocystis carinii* pneumonia in HIV infected patients from Mumbai. J Assoc Physicians India. 2005;53:437-40.
31. Bansal S, Kashyap S, Pal LS, Goel A. Clinical and bacteriological profile of community acquired pneumonia in Shimla, Himachal Pradesh. Indian J Chest Dis Allied Sci. 2004;46(1):17-22.
32. Shah BA, Singh G, Naik MA, Dhobi GN. Bacteriological and clinical profile of community acquired pneumonia in hospitalized patients. Lung India. 2010;27(2):54-7.
33. Menon RU, George AP, Menon UK. Etiology and anti-microbial sensitivity of organisms causing community acquired pneumonia: a single hospital study. J Family Med Prim Care. 2013;2(3):244-9.

34. Shankar EM, Kumarasamy N, Vignesh R, Balakrishnan P, Solomon SS, Murugavel KG, et al. Epidemiological studies on pulmonary pathogens in HIV-positive and negative subjects with or without community-acquired pneumonia with special emphasis on *Mycoplasma pneumoniae*. Jpn J Infect Dis. 2007;60(6):337-41.
35. Dey AB, Chaudhry R, Kumar P, Nisar N, Nagarkar KM. *Mycoplasma pneumoniae* and community-acquired pneumonia. Natl Med J India. 2000;13(2):66-70.
36. Chaudhry R, Dhawan B, Dey AB. The incidence of *Legionella pneumophila*: a prospective study in a tertiary care hospital in India. Trop Doct. 2000;30(4):197-200.
37. Eshwara VK, Munim F, Tellapragada C, Kamath A, Varma M, Lewis LE, et al. *Staphylococcus aureus* bacteremia in an Indian tertiary care hospital: observational study on clinical epidemiology, resistance characteristics, and carriage of the Panton-Valentine leukocidin gene. Int J Infect Dis. 2013;17(11):e1051-5.
38. Peto L, Nadjm B, Horby P, Ngan TT, van Doorn R, Van Kinh N. The bacterial aetiology of adult community-acquired pneumonia in Asia: a systematic review. Trans R Soc Trop Med Hyg. 2014;108(6):326-37.
39. Cillóniz C, Ewig S, Menéndez R, Ferrer M, Polverino E, Reyes S. Bacterial co-infection with H1N1 infection in patients admitted with community acquired pneumonia. J Infect. 2012;65(3): 223-30.
40. Martín-Loeches I, Sanchez-Corral A, Diaz E, Granada RM, Zaragoza R, Villavicencio C, et al. Community-acquired respiratory coinfection in critically ill patients with pandemic 2009 influenza A (H1N1) virus. Chest. 2011;139(3):555-62.
41. Rice TW, Rubinson L, Uyeki TM, Vaughn FL, John BB, Miller RR, et al. Critical illness from 2009 pandemic influenza A virus and bacterial coinfection in the United States. Crit Care Med. 2012;40(5):1487-98.
42. Muscedere J, Ofner M, Kumar A, Long J, Lamontagne F, Cook D, et al. The occurrence and impact of bacterial organisms complicating critical care illness associated with 2009 influenza A (H1N1) infection. Chest. 2013;144(1):39-47.
43. John TJ, Pai R, Lalitha MK, Jesudason MV, Brahmadathan KN, Sridharan G, et al. Prevalence of pneumococcal serotypes in invasive diseases in Southern India. Indian J Med Res. 1996;104:205-7.
44. Thomas K. Prospective multicentre hospital surveillance of *Streptococcus pneumoniae* disease in India. Invasive Bacterial Infection Surveillance (IBIS) Group, International Clinical Epidemiology Network (INCLEN). Lancet. 1999;353(9160):1216-21.
45. Kanungo R, Rajalakshmi B. Serotype distribution and antimicrobial resistance in *Streptococcus pneumoniae* causing invasive and other infections in South India. Indian J Med. 2001;114:127-32.
46. Shariff M, Choudhary J, Zahoor S, Deb M. Characterization of *Streptococcus pneumoniae* isolates from India with special reference to their sequence types. J Infect Dev Ctries. 2013;7(2):101-9.
47. Molander V, Elisson C, Balaji V, Backhaus E, John J, Vargheese R, et al. Invasive pneumococcal infections in Vellore, India: clinical characteristics and distribution of serotypes. BMC Infect Dis. 2013;13:532.
48. Shariff M, Thukral SS, Beall B. New multilocus sequence types of *Streptococcus pneumoniae* isolates from patients with respiratory infections in India. Indian J Med Res. 2007;126(2):161-4.
49. Song JH, Chang HH, Suh JY, Ko KS, Jung SI, Oh WS, et al. Macrolide resistance and genotypic characterization of *Streptococcus pneumoniae* in Asian countries: a study of the Asian Network for Surveillance of Resistant Pathogens (ANSORP). J Antimicrob Chemother. 2004;53(3):457-63.
50. Lalitha MK, Thomas K, Manoharan A, Song JH, Steinhoff MC. Changing trend in susceptibility pattern of *Streptococcus pneumoniae* to penicillin in India. Indian J Med Res. 1999;110:164-84.
51. Song J-H, Lee NY, Ichiyama S, Yoshida R, Hirakata Y, Fu W, et al. Spread of drug-resistant *Streptococcus pneumoniae* in Asian countries: Asian Network for Surveillance of Resistant Pathogens (ANSORP) study. Clin Infect Dis. 1999;28(6): 1206-11.
52. Lalitha MK, Pai R, Manohran A, Appelbaum PC. The CMCH Pneumococcal Study Group. Multidrug-resistant *Streptococcus pneumoniae* from India. Lancet. 2002;359(9304):445.
53. Goyal R, Singh NP, Kaur M, Talwar V. Antimicrobial resistance in invasive and colonising *Streptococcus pneumoniae* in North India. Indian J Med Microbiol. 2007;25(3):256-9.
54. Balaji V, Thomas K, Joshi HH, Beall B. Increasing invasive disease due to penicillin resistant *S. pneumoniae* in India. Indian J Med Sci. 2008;62(12):492-5.
55. Veeraraghavan B, Thomas K, Joshi HH, Beall B. Increasing invasive disease due to penicillin resistant *S. pneumoniae* in India. Indian J Med Sci. 2008;62:492-5.
56. Feldman C, Anderson R. Antibiotic resistance of pathogens causing community-acquired pneumonia. Semin Respir Crit Care Med. 2012;33(3):232-43.
57. Fernández-Solá J, Junqué A, Estruch R, Monforte R, Torres A, Urbano-Márquez A. High alcohol intake as a risk and prognostic factor for community-acquired pneumonia. Arch Intern Med. 1995;155(15):1649-54.
58. Almirall J, Bolibar I, Balanzó X, González CA. Risk factors for community-acquired pneumonia in adults: a population-based case-control study. Eur Respir J.1999;13(2):349-55.
59. Baik I, Curhan GC, Rimm EB, Bendich A, Willett WC, Fawzi WW. A prospective study of age and lifestyle factors in relation to community-acquired pneumonia in US men and women. Arch Intern Med. 2000;160(2):3082-8.
60. Farr BM, Bartlett CL, Wadsworth J, Miller DL. Risk factors for community-acquired pneumonia diagnosed upon hospital admission. British Thoracic Society Pneumonia Study Group. Respir Med. 2000;94(10):954-63.
61. Farr BM, Woodhead MA, MacFarlane JT, Bartlett CL, McCraken JS, Wadsworth J, et al. Risk factors for community-acquired pneumonia diagnosed by general practitioners in the community. Respir Med. 2000;94(5):422-7.
62. Johnstone J, Nerenberg K, Loeb M. Meta-analysis: proton pump inhibitor use and risk of community-acquired pneumonia. Aliment Pharmacol Ther. 2010;31(11):1165-77.
63. Almirall J, Bolibar I, Serra-Prat M, Roig J, Hospital I, Carandell E, et al. New evidence of risk factors for community-acquired pneumonia: a population-based study. Eur Respir J. 2008;31(6):1274-84.

64. Feldman C, Anderson R. New insights into pneumococcal disease. Respirology. 2009;14(2):167-79.
65. Sanz Herrero F, Blanquer Olivas J. Microbiology and risk factors for community-acquired pneumonia. Semin Respir Crit Care Med. 2012;33(3):220-31.
66. Torres A, Peetermans WE, Viegi G, Blasi F. Risk factors for community-acquired pneumonia in adults in Europe: a literature review. Thorax. 2013;68(11):1057-65.
67. Feldman C, Anderson R. Cigarette smoking and mechanisms of susceptibility to infections of the respiratory tract and other organ systems. J Infect. 2013;67(3):169-84.
68. Almirall J, Serra-Prat M, Bolibar I, Palomera E, Roig J, Hospital I, et al. Passive smoking at home is a risk factor for community-acquired pneumonia in older adults: a population-based case-control study. BMJ Open. 2014;4(6):e005133.
69. Hirschtick RE, Glassroth J, Jordan MC, Wilcosky TC, Wallace JM, Kvale PA, et al. Bacterial pneumonia in persons infected with the human immunodeficiency virus. Pulmonary Complications of HIV Infection Study Group. N Engl J Med. 1995;333(13):845-51.
70. Madeddu G, Porqueddu EM, Cambosu F, Saba F, Fois AG, Pirina P, et al. Bacterial community acquired pneumonia in HIV-infected inpatients in the highly active antiretroviral therapy era. Infection. 2008;36(3):231-6.
71. Almirall J, González CA, Balanzó X, Bolíbar I. Proportion of community-acquired pneumonia cases attributable to tobacco smoking. Chest. 1999;116(2):375-9.
72. Nuorti JP, Butler JC, Farley MM, Harrison LH, McGeer A, Kolczak MS, et al. Cigarette smoking and invasive pneumococcal disease. Active Bacterial Core Surveillance Team. N Engl J Med. 2000;342(10):732-4.
73. Miguez-Burbano MJ, Burbano X, Ashkin D, Pitchenik A, Allan R, Pineda L, et al. Impact of tobacco use on the development of opportunistic respiratory infections in HIV seropositive patients on antiretroviral therapy. Addict Biol. 2003;8(1):39-43.
74. Arcavi L, Benowitz NL. Cigarette smoking and infection. Arch Intern Med. 2004;164(20):2206-16.
75. Crothers K, Griffith TA, McGinnis KA, Barradas MC, Leaf DA, Weissman S, et al. The impact of cigarette smoking on mortality, quality of life, and comorbid illness among HIV-positive veterans. J Gen Intern Med. 2005;20(12):1142-5.
76. Miguez-Burbano MJ, Ashkin D, Rodriguez A, Duncan R, Pitchenik A, Quintero N, et al. Increased risk of *Pneumocystis carinii* and community-acquired pneumonia with tobacco use in HIV disease. Int J Infect Dis. 2005;9(4):208-17.
77. Jover F, Cuadrado J-M, Andreu L, Martínez S, Cañizares R, de la Tabla VO, et al. A comparative study of bacteremic and non-bacteremic pneumococcal pneumonia. Eur J Intern Med. 2008;19(1):15-21.
78. Greenberg D, Givon-Lavi N, Broides A, Blancovich I, Peled N, Dagan R. The contribution of smoking and exposure to tobacco smoke to *Streptococcus pneumoniae* and *Haemophilus influenzae* carriage in children and their mothers. Clin Infect Dis. 2006;42(7):897-903.
79. Coles CL, Kanungo R, Rahmathullah L, Thulasiraj RD, Katz J, Santosham M, et al. Pneumococcal nasopharyngeal colonization in young South Indian infants. Pediatr Infect Dis J. 2001;20(3):289-95.
80. Coles CL, Rahmathullah L, Kanungo R, Thulasiraj RD, Katz J, Santhosham M, et al. Vitamin A supplementation at birth delays pneumococcal colonization in South Indian infants. J Nutr. 2001;131(2):255-61.
81. Jindal SK, Aggarwal AN, Chaudhry K, Chhabra SK, D'Souza GA, Gupta D, et al. A multicentric study on epidemiology of chronic obstructive pulmonary disease and its relationship with tobacco smoking and environmental tobacco smoke exposure. Indian J Chest Dis Allied Sci. 2006;48(1):23-9.
82. Bello S, Menendez R, Torres A, Reyes S, Zalacain R, Capelastegui A, et al. Tobacco smoking increases the risk of death from pneumococcal pneumonia. Chest. 2014;146(4):1029-37.
83. Wang JH, Kwon HJ, Jang YJ. Rhinovirus enhances various bacterial adhesions to nasal epithelial cells simultaneously. Laryngoscope. 2009;119(7):1406-11.
84. Hall-Stoodley L, Stoodley P. Evolving concepts in biofilm infections. Cell Microbiol. 2009;11(7):1034-43.
85. Feldman C, Anderson R, Cockeran R, Mitchell T, Cole P, Wilson R, et al. The effects of pneumolysin and hydrogen peroxide, alone and in combination, on human ciliated epithelium *in vitro*. Respir Med. 2002;96(8):580-5.
86. Kadioglu A, Weiser JN, Paton JC, Andrew PW. The role of *Streptococcus pneumoniae* virulence factors in host respiratory colonization and disease. Nat Rev Microbiol. 2008;6(4):288-301.
87. Preston JA, Dockrell DH. Virulence factors in pneumococcal respiratory pathogenesis. Future Microbiol. 2008;3:205-21.
88. Feldman C, Cockeran R, Jedrzejas, Mitchell TJ, Anderson R. Hyaluronidase augments pneumolysin-mediated injury to human ciliated respiratory epithelium. Int J Infect Dis. 2007;11(1):11-5.
89. Lu L, Ma Z, Jokiranta TS, Whitney AR, DeLeo FR, Zhang JR. Species-specific interaction of *Streptococcus pneumoniae* with human complement factor H. J Immunol. 2008;181(10):7138-46.
90. Steel HC, Cockeran R, Anderson R, Feldman C. Overview of community-acquired pneumonia and the role of inflammatory mechanisms in the immunopathogenesis of severe pneumococcal disease. Mediators Inflamm. 2013;2013:490346.
91. Feldman C, Anderson R. Review: current and new generation pneumococcal vaccines. J Infect. 2014;69(4):309-25.
92. Rajam G, Anderton JM, Carlone GM, Sampson JS, Ades EW. Pneumococcal surface adhesin A (PsaA): a review. Crit Rev Microbiol. 2008;34(3-4):131-42.
93. Papasergi S, Garibaldi M, Tuscano G, Signorino G, Ricci S, Peppoloni S, et al. Plasminogen- and fibronectin-binding protein B is involved in the adherence of *Streptococcus pneumoniae* to human epithelial cells. J Biol Chem. 2010;285(10):7517-24.
94. Soong G, Muir A, Gomez MI, Waks J, Reddy B, Planet P, et al. Bacterial neuraminidase facilitates mucosal infection by participating in biofilm production. J Clin Invest. 2006;116(8):2297-2305.
95. Bogaert D, De Groot R, Hermans PW. *Streptococcus pneumoniae* colonisation: the key to pneumococcal disease. Lancet Infect Dis. 2004;4(3):144-154.
96. Malley R, Henneke P, Morse SC, Cieslewicz MJ, Lipsitch M, Thompson CM, et al. Recognition of pneumolysin by Toll-like receptor 4 confers resistance to pneumococcal infection. Proc Natl Acad Sci, USA. 2003;100(4):1966-71.
97. Matthias KA, Roche AM, Standish AJ, Shchepetov M, Weiser JN. Neutrophil-toxin interactions promote antigen delivery and mucosal clearance of *Streptococcus pneumoniae*. J Immunol. 2008;180(9):6246-54.
98. Dessing MC, Hirst RA, de Vos AF, van der Poll T. Role of Toll-like receptors 2 and 4 in pulmonary inflammation and injury

induced by pneumolysin in mice. PLoS One. 2009;4(11): e7993.

99. Franchi L, Warner N, Viani K, Nuñez G. Function of Nod-like receptors in microbial recognition and host defense. Immunol Rev. 2009;227(1):106-28.
100. Ogunniyi AD, Grabowicz M, Briles DE, Cook J, Paton JC. Development of a vaccine against invasive pneumococcal diseases based on combinations of virulence proteins of *Streptococcus pneumoniae*. Infect Immun. 2007;75(1):350-7.
101. Lu Y-J, Gross J, Bogaert D, Finn A, Bagrade L, Zhang Q, et al. Interleukin-17A mediates acquired immunity to pneumococcal colonization. PLoS Pathog. 2008;4(9):e1000159.
102. Malley R. Antibody and cell-mediated immunity to *Streptococcus pneumoniae*: implications for vaccine development. J Mol Med. 2010;88(2):135-42.
103. Van Rossum AM, Lysenko ES, Weiser JN. Host and bacterial factors contributing to the clearance of colonization by *Streptococcus pneumoniae* in a murine model. Infect Immun. 2005;73(11):7718-26.
104. Ferreira DM, Darrieux M, Silva DA, Leite LC, Ferreira JM Jr, Ho PL, et al. Characterization of protective mucosal and systemic immune responses elicited by pneumococcal surface protein PspA and PspC nasal vaccines against a respiratory pneumococcal challenge in mice. Clin Vaccine Immunol. 2009;16(5):636-45.
105. Raveh D, Kruskal BA, Farland J, Ezekowitz RA. Th1 and Th2 cytokines cooperate to stimulate mannose-receptor-mediated phagocytosis. J Leukoc Biol. 1998;64(1):108-13.
106. Zhang Z, Clarke TB, Weiser JN. Cellular effectors mediating Th17-dependent clearance of pneumococcal colonization in mice. J Clin Invest. 2009;119(7):1899-909.
107. Van der Eerden MM, Vlaspolder F, de Graaff CS, Jansen HM, Boersma WG. Value of intensive diagnostic microbiological investigation in low- and high-risk patients with community-acquired pneumonia. Eur J Clin Microbiol Infect Dis. 2005;24(4):241-9.
108. Miyashita N, Shimizu H, Ouchi K, Kawasaki K, Kawai Y, Obase Y, et al. Assessment of the usefulness of sputum Gram stain and culture for diagnosis of community-acquired pneumonia requiring hospitalization. Med Sci Monit. 2008;14(4):CR171-6.
109. Theerthakarai R, El-Halees W, Ismail M, Solis RA, Khan MA. Nonvalue of the initial microbiological studies in the management of nonsevere community-acquired pneumonia. Chest. 2001;119(1):181-4.
110. Signori LG, Ferreira MW, Vieira LC, Müller KR, Mattos WL. Sputum examination in the clinical management of community-acquired pneumonia. J Bras Pneumol. 2008;34(3):152-8.
111. Johansson N, Kalin M, Giske CG, Hedlund J. Quantitative detection of *Streptococcus pneumoniae* from sputum samples with real-time quantitative polymerase chain reaction for etiologic diagnosis of community-acquired pneumonia. Diagn Microbiol Infect Dis. 2008;60(3):255-61.
112. Werno AM, Anderson TP, Murdoch DR. Association between pneumococcal load and disease severity in adults with pneumonia. J Med Microbiol. 2012;61(Pt 8):1129-35.
113. Satzke C, Turner P, Virolainen-Julkunen A, Adrian PV, Antonio M, Hare KM, et al. Standard method for detecting upper respiratory carriage of *Streptococcus pneumoniae*: updated recommendations from the World Health Organization Pneumococcal Carriage Working Group. Vaccine. 2013;32(1): 165-79.
114. Waterer GW, Jennings SG, Wunderink RG. The impact of blood cultures on antibiotic therapy in pneumococcal pneumonia. Chest. 1999;116(5):1278-81.
115. Waterer GW, Wunderink RG. The influence of the severity of community-acquired pneumonia on the usefulness of blood cultures. Respir Med. 2001;95(1):78-82.
116. Corbo J, Friedman B, Bijur P, Gallagher EJ. Limited usefulness of initial blood cultures in community acquired pneumonia. Emerg Med J. 2004;21(4):446-8.
117. Ramanujam P, Rathlev NK. Blood cultures do not change management in hospitalized patients with community-acquired pneumonia. Acad Emerg Med. 2006;13(7):740-5.
118. Andreo F, Domínguez J, Ruiz J, Blanco S, Arellano E, Prat C, et al. Impact of rapid urine antigen tests to determine the etiology of community-acquired pneumonia in adults. Respir Med. 2006;100(5):884-91.
119. Working Group of the South African Thoracic Society. Management of community-acquired pneumonia in adults. S Afr Med J. 2007;97(12 pt 2):1296-306.
120. Corrêa Rde A, Lundgren FL, Pereira-Silva JL, Frare e Silva RL, Cardoso AP, Lemos AC, et al. Brazilian guidelines for community-acquired pneumonia in immunocompetent adults—2009. J Bras Pneumol. 2009;35(6):574-601.
121. Sharpe BA, Flanders SA. Community-acquired pneumonia: a practical approach to management for the hospitalist. J Hosp Med. 2006;1(3):177-90.
122. Hagaman JT, Rouan GW, Shipley RT, Panos RJ. Admission chest radiograph lacks sensitivity in the diagnosis of community-acquired pneumonia. Am J Med Sci. 2009;337(4):236-40.
123. Boersma WG, Daniels JM, Löwenberg A, Boeve WJ, van de Jagt EJ. Reliability of radiographic findings and the relation to etiologic agents in community-acquired pneumonia. Respir Med. 2006;100(5):926-32.
124. Laine C, Williams SV, Wilson JF. In the clinic: community-acquired pneumonia. Ann Intern Med. 2009;151:15-6.
125. Luján M, Gallego M, Rello J. Optimal therapy for severe pneumococcal community-acquired pneumonia. Intensive Care Med. 2006;32(7):971-80.
126. Dey AB, Nagarkar KM, Kumar V. Clinical presentation and predictors of outcome in adult patients with community-acquired pneumonia. Natl Med J India. 1997;10(4):169-72.
127. Valencia M, Sellares J, Torres A. Emergency treatment of community-acquired pneumonia. Eur Respir Monogr. 2006;36: 183-99.
128. Waterer GW, Rello J, Wunderink RG. Concise clinical review: Management of community-acquired pneumonia in adults. Am J Respir Crit Care Med. 2011;183(2):157-64.
129. Pereira JM, Paiva JA, Rello J. Assessing severity of patients with community-acquired pneumonia. Semin Respir Crit Care Med. 2012;33(3):272-83.
130. Importance of severity assessment: community-acquired pneumonia. J Assoc Physicians India. 2013;61(7 Suppl):14-9.
131. Sintes H, Sibila O, Waterer GW. Severity assessment tools in CAP. Eur Respir Monogr. 2014; 63:88-104.
132. Torres A, Ramirez P. Montull B, Menéndez R. Biomarkers and community-acquired pneumonia: tailoring management with biological data. Semin Respir Crit Care Med. 2012;33(3): 266-71.
133. Kolditz M, Ewig S, Höffken G. Management-based risk prediction in community-acquired pneumonia by scores and biomarkers. Eur Respir J. 2013;41(4):974-84.

134. Schuetz P, Litke A, Albrich WC, Mueller B. Blood biomarkers for personalized treatment and patient management decisions in community-acquired pneumonia. Curr Opin Infect Dis. 2013;26(2):159-67.
135. Lindstrom ST, Wong EKC. Procalcitonin, a valuable biomarker assisting clinical decision-making in the management of community-acquired pneumonia. Intern Med J. 2014;44(4):390-7.
136. Fine MJ, Auble TE, Yealy DM, Soto A, Gorordo I, García-Urbaneja M, et al. A prediction rule to identify low-risk patients with community-acquired pneumonia. N Engl J Med. 1997;336:243-50.
137. Lim WS, van der Eerden MM, Laing R, Boersma WG, Karalus N, Town GI, et al. Defining community acquired pneumonia severity on presentation to hospital: an international derivation and validation study. Thorax. 2003;58(5):377-82.
138. Niederman MS. Recent advances in community-acquired pneumonia: Inpatient and outpatient. Chest. 2007;131(4): 1205-15.
139. Niederman MS. Making sense of scoring systems in community acquired pneumonia. Respirology. 2009;14(3):327-35.
140. Lim WS, Baudouin SV, George RC, Hill AT, Jamieson C, Le Jeune I, et al. BTS guidelines for the management of community acquired pneumonia in adults: update 2009. Thorax. 2009;64 (Suppl 3):iii1-55.
141. Shah BA, Ahmed W, Dhobi GN, Shah NN, Khursheed SQ, Haq I. Validity of pneumonia severity index and CURB-65 severity scoring systems in community acquired pneumonia in an Indian setting. Indian J Chest Dis Allied Sci. 2010;52(1):9-17.
142. Niederman MS, Mandell LA, Anzueto A, Bass JB, Broughton WA, Campbell GD, et al. American Thoracic Society. Guidelines for the management of adults with community-acquired pneumonia. Diagnosis, assessment of severity, antimicrobial therapy and prevention. Am J Respir Crit Care Med. 2001;163(7):1730-54.
143. Mandell LA, Wunderink RG, Anzueto A, Bartlett JG, Campbell GD, Dean NC, et al. Infectious Diseases Society of America/American Thoracic Society consensus guidelines on the management of community-acquired pneumonia in adults. Clin Infect Dis. 2007;44(Suppl 2):S27-S71.
144. Ioachimescu OC, Ioachimescu AG, Iannini PB. Severity scoring in community-acquired pneumonia caused by *Streptococcus pneumoniae*: a 5-year experience. Int J Antimicrob Agents. 2004;24(5):485-90.
145. Spindler C, Ortqvist A. Prognostic score systems and community-acquired bacteremic pneumococcal pneumonia. Eur Respir J. 2006;28(4):816-23.
146. Metlay JP. Update on community-acquired pneumonia: impact of antibiotic resistance on clinical outcomes. Curr Opin Infect Dis. 2002;15(2):163-7.
147. Feldman C. Clinical relevance of antimicrobial resistance in the management of pneumococcal community-acquired pneumonia. J Lab Clin Med. 2004;143(5):269-83.
148. Metlay JP. Antibacterial drug resistance: implications for the treatment of patients with community-acquired pneumonia. Infect Dis Clin North Am. 2004;18(4):777-90.
149. Mufson MA, Chan G, Stanek RJ. Penicillin resistance not a factor in outcome from invasive *Streptococcus pneumoniae* community-acquired pneumonia in adults when appropriate empiric therapy is started. Am J Med Sci. 2007;333(3):161-7.
150. Weinstein MP, Klugman KP, Jones RN. Rationale for revised penicillin susceptibility breakpoints versus *Streptococcus pneumoniae*: coping with antimicrobial susceptibility in an era of resistance. Clin Infect Dis. 2009;48(11):1596-600.
151. Fuller JD, McGreer A, Low DE. Drug-resistant pneumococcal pneumonia: clinical relevance and approach to management. Eur J Clin Microbiol Infect Dis. 2005; 24(12):780-8.
152. Ambrose PG, Bast D, Doern GV, Iannini PB, Jones RN, Klugman KP, et al. Fluoroquinolone-resistant *Streptococcus pneumoniae*, an emerging but unrecognized public health concern: is it time to resight the goalposts? Clin Infect Dis. 2004;39(10):1554-6.
153. Richter SS, Heilmann KP, Beekmann SE, Miller NJ, Rice CL, Doern GV. The molecular epidemiology of *Streptococcus pneumoniae* with quinolone resistance mutations. Clin Infect Dis. 2005;40(2):225-35.
154. Wenzel RP. The antibiotic pipeline—challenges, costs, and values. N Engl J Med. 2004;351(6):523-6.
155. Norrby SR, Nord CE, Finch R. For the European Society of Clinical Microbiology and Infectious Diseases (ESCMID). Lack of development of new antimicrobial drugs: a potential serious threat to public health. Lancet Infect Dis. 2005;5(2):115-9.
156. Liapikou A, Torres A. Current treatment of community-acquired pneumonia. Expert Opin Pharmacother. 2013;14(10):1319-32.
157. Moran GJ, Rothman RE, Volturo GA. Emergency management of community-acquired bacterial pneumonia: what is new since the 2007 Infectious Diseases Society of America/American Thoracic Society guidelines. Am J Emerg Med. 2013;31(3):602-12.
158. Cazzola M, Centanni S, Blasi F. Have guidelines for the management of community-acquired pneumonia influenced outcome? Respir Med. 2003;97(3):205-11.
159. Cazzola M, Page CP, Matera MG. Alternative and/or integrative therapies for pneumonia under development. Curr Opin Pulm Med. 2004;10:204-10.
160. Rañó A, Agustí C, Sibila O, Torres A. Associated inflammatory response in pneumonia: role of adjunctive therapy with glucocorticoids. Curr Opin Infect Dis. 2006;19(2):179-84.
161. Waterer GW. Monotherapy versus combination antimicrobial therapy for pneumococcal pneumonia. Curr Opin Infect Dis. 2005;18(2):157-63.
162. Feldman C, Anderson R. Therapy for pneumococcal bacteremia: monotherapy or combination therapy? Curr Opin Infect Dis. 2009;22:137-42.
163. Asadi L, Eurich DT, Gamble J-M, Minhas-Sandhu JK, Marrie TJ, Majumdar SR. Guideline adherence and macrolides reduced mortality in outpatients with pneumonia. Respir Med. 2012;106(3):451-8.
164. Asadi L, Sligl WI, Eurich DT, Colmers IN, Tjosvold L, Marrie TJ, et al. Macrolide-based regimens and mortalilty in hospitalized patients with community-acquired pneumonia: a systematic review and meta-analysis. Clin Infect Dis. 2012;55(3):371-80.
165. Woodhead M, Noor M. Empirical antibiotic management of adult CAP. Eur Respir Monogr. 2014;63:140-54.
166. Dwyer R, Ortqvist A, Aufwerber E, Henriques Normark B, Marrie TJ, Mufson MA, et al. Addition of a macrolide to a beta-lactam in bacteremic pneumococcal pneumonia. Eur J Clin Microbiol Infect Dis. 2006;25(8):518-21.
167. Waterer GW, Rello J. Choosing the right combination in severe community-acquired pneumonia. Critical Care. 2006;10(1):115.
168. Metersky M, Ma A, Houck PM, Bratzler DW. Antibiotics for bacteremic pneumonia: improved outcomes with macrolides but not fluoroquinolones. Chest. 2007;131(2):466-73.

169. Restrepo MI, Mortensen EM, Waterer GW, Wunderink RG, Coalson JJ, Anzueto A. Impact of macrolide therapy on mortality for patients with severe sepsis due to pneumonia. Eur Respir J. 2009;33(1):153-9.
170. Dalhoff K. Worldwide guidelines for respiratory tract infections: community-acquired pneumonia. Int J Antimicrob Agents. 2001;18:S39-44.
171. Armitage K, Woodhead M. New guidelines for the management of adult community-acquired pneumonia. Curr Opin Infect Dis. 2007;20(2):170-6.
172. Niederman MS, Luna CM. Community-acquired pneumonia guidelines: a global perspective. Semin Respir Crit Care Med. 2012;33(3):298-310.
173. Dhar R. Pneumonia: review of guidelines. J Assoc Physicians India. 2012;60(Suppl):25-8.
174. Gupta D, Agarwal R, Aggarwal AN, Singh N, Mishra N, Khilnani GC, et al. Guidelines for diagnosis and management of community- and hospital-acquired pneumonia in adults: Joint ICS/NCCP(1) recommendations. Lung India. 2012;29(Suppl 2):S27-62.
175. Ramirez JA. Fostering international multicenter collaborative research: the CAPO Project. Int J Tuberc Lung Dis. 2007;11(10):1062-5.
176. Nyamande K, Lalloo UG. Poor adherence to South African guidelines for the management of community-acquired pneumonia. S Afr Med J. 2007;97(8):601-3.
177. Blasi F, Iori I, Bulfoni A, Corrao S, Costantino S, Legnani D. Can CAP guideline adherence improve patient outcome in Internal Medicine Departments? Eur Respir J. 2008;32(4):902-10.
178. Arnold FW, LaJoie S, Brock GN, Peyrani P, Rello J, Menéndez R, et al. Improving outcomes in elderly patients with community-acquired pneumonia by adhering to national guidelines. Community-acquired Pneumonia Organization International Cohort Study Results. Arch Intern Med. 2009;169(16):1515-24.
179. McCabe C, Kirchner C, Zhang H, Daley J, Fisman DN. Guideline-concordant therapy and reduced mortality and length of stay in adults with community-acquired pneumonia. Arch Intern Med. 2009;169(16):1525-31.
180. Menendéz R, Torres A, Zalacaín R, Aspa J, Martín-Villasclaras JJ, Borderías L. Guidelines for the treatment of community-acquired pneumonia: predictors of adherence and outcome. Am J Respir Crit Care Med. 2005;172(6):757-62.
181. Garau J, Baquero F, Pérez-Trallero E, Pérez JL, Martín-Sánchez AM, García-Rey C, et al. Factors impacting on length of stay and mortality of community-acquired pneumonia. Clin Microbiol Infect. 2008;14(4):322-9.
182. Seedat MA, Feldman C, Skoularigis J, Promnitz DA, Smith C, Zwi S. A study of acute community-acquired pneumonia, including details of cardiac changes. Q J Med. 1993;86(10):669-75.
183. Ramirez J, Aliberti S, Mirsaeidi M, Peyrani P, Filardo G, Amir A, et al. Acute myocardial infarction in hospitalized patients with community-acquired pneumonia. Clin Infect Dis. 2008;47(2):182-7.
184. Perry TW, Pugh MJV, Waterer GW, Nakashima B, Orihuela CJ, Copeland LA, et al. Incidence of cardiovascular events after hospital admission for pneumonia. Am J Med. 2011;124(3):244-51.
185. Corrales-Medina VF, Musher DM, Wells GA, Chirinos JA, Chen L, Fine MJ. Cardiac complications in patients with community-acquired pneumonia: incidence, timing, risk factors, and association with short-term mortality. Circulation. 2012;125(6):773-81.
186. Corrales-Medina VF, Musher DM, Shachkina S, Chirinos JA. Acute pneumonia and the cardiovascular system. Lancet. 2013;381(9865):496-505.
187. Viasus D, Garcia-Vidal C, Manresa F, Dorca J, Gudiol F, Carratalà J. Risk stratification and prognosis of acute cardiac events in hospitalized adults with community-acquired pneumonia. J Infect. 2013;66(1):27-33.
188. Krüger S, Frechen D. Cardiovascular complications and comorbidities in CAP. Eur Respir Monogr. 2014;63:256-65.
189. Mortensen EM, Metersky ML. Long-term mortality after pneumonia. Semin Respir Crit Care Med. 2012;33(3):319-24.
190. Restrepo MI, Faverio P, Anzueto A. Long-term prognosis in community-acquired pneumonia. Curr Opin Infect Dis. 2013;26(2):151-8.
191. Prabhudesai PP, Kuruvilla T, Tadvi S. Community-acquired pneumonia: need for a cost-effective approach to treatment. Chest. 1997;112(3):861-2.
192. Bjerre LM, Verheij TJM, Kochen MM. Antibiotics for community-acquired pneumonia in adult outpatients. Cochrane Database Syst Rev. 2009;4:CD002109.
193. Dooley KE, Golub J, Goes FS, Merz WG, Sterling TR. Empiric treatment of community-acquired pneumonia with fluoroquinolones, and delays in the treatment of tuberculosis. Clin Infect Dis. 2002;34(12):1607-12.
194. Chang KC, Leung CC, Yew WW, Lau TY, Leung WM, Tam CM, et al. Newer fluoroquinolones for treating respiratory infection: do they mask tuberculosis. Eur Respir J. 2010;35(3):606-13.
195. Long R, Chong H, Hoeppner V, Shanmuganathan H, Kowalewska-Grochowska K, Shandro C, et al. Empirical treatment of community-acquired pneumonia and the development of fluoroquinolone-resistant tuberculosis. Clin Infect Dis. 2009;48(10):1354-60.
196. Low DE. Fluoroquinolones for treatment of community-acquired pneumonia and tuberculosis: putting the risk of resistance into perspective. Clin Infect Dis. 2009;48(10):1361-3.
197. Sibila O, Agustí C, Torres A. Corticosteroids in severe pneumonia. Eur Respir J. 2008;32(2):259-64.
198. Kobayashi H. Biofilm disease: its clinical manifestation and therapeutic possibilities of macrolides. Am J Med. 1995;99(Suppl 6A):26S-30S.
199. Tamaoki J, Kadota J, Takizawa H. Clinical implications of the immunomodulatory effects of macrolides. Am J Med. 2004;117(Suppl 9A):5S-11S.
200. Tateda K, Standiford TJ, Pechere JC, Yamaguchi K. Regulatory effects of macrolides on bacterial virulence: potential role as quorum-sensing inhibitors. Curr Pharm Des. 2004;10(25):3055-65.
201. Amsden GW. Anti-inflammatory effects of macrolides - an underappreciated benefit in the treatment of community-acquired respiratory tract infections and chronic pulmonary conditions? J Antimicrob Chemother. 2005;55:10-21.
202. Steel HC, Theron AJ, Cockeran R, Anderson R, Feldman C. Pathogen- and host-directed anti-inflammatory activities of macrolide antibiotics. Mediators Inflamm. 2012;2012:584262.
203. Clinical Trials. (2014). CAP-START (Community-Acquired Pneumonia Study on the Initial Treatment with Antibiotics of Lower Respiratory Tract Infections). [online] Available from *http://clinicaltrials.gov/ct2/show/NCT01660204.* [Accessed January, 2016].

204. Salluh JIF, Povoa P, Soares M, Castro-Faria-Neto HC, Bozza FA, Bozza PT. The role of corticosteroids in severe community-acquired pneumonia: a systematic review. Critical Care. 2008;12:R76.
205. Siempos II, Vardakas KZ, Kopterides P, Falagas ME. Adjunctive therapies for community-acquired pneumonia: a systematic review. J Antimicrob Chemother. 2008;62:661-8.
206. Confalonieri M, Urbino R, Potena A, Piattella M, Parigi P, Puccio G, et al. Hydrocortisone infusion for severe community-acquired pneumonia. A preliminary randomized study. Am J Respir Crit Care Med. 2005;171:242-8.
207. Garcia-Vidal C, Calbo E, Pascual V, Ferrer C, Quintana S, Garau J. Effects of systemic steroids in patients with severe community-acquired pneumonia. Eur Respir J. 2007;30: 951-6.
208. Mikami K, Suzuki M, Kitagawa H, Kawakami M, Hirota N, Yamaguchi H, et al. Efficacy of corticosteroids in the treatment of community-acquired pneumonia requiring hospitalization. Lung. 2007;185(5):249-55.
209. Snijders D, Daniels JM, de Graaff CS, van der Werf TS, Boersma WG. Efficacy of corticosteroids in community-acquired pneumonia: a randomized double-blinded clinical trial. Am J Respir Crit Care Med. 2010;181(9):975-82.
210. Polverino E, Cillóniz C, Dambrava P, Gabarrús A, Ferrer M, Agustí C, et al. Systemic corticosteroids for community-acquired pneumonia: reasons for use and lack of benefit on outcome. Respirology. 2013;18(2):263-71.
211. ClinicalTrials. (2015). Extended Steroid in CAP(e) (ESCAPe). [Online] Available from *http://clinicaltrials.gov/show/NCT01283009.* [Accessed January, 2016].
212. Clinical Trials. (2013). Corticoids in Severe Community-Acquired Pneumonia (CAP). [Online] Available from *http://clinicaltrials.gov/show/NCT00908713.* [Accessed January, 2016].
213. Clinical Trials. (2015). Corticosteroid Treatment for Community-Acquired Pneumonia—The STEP Trial [online] Available from *http://clinicaltrials.gov/show/NCT00973154.* [Accessed January, 2016].
214. Troeman DP, Postma DF, van Werkhoven CH, Oosterheert JJ. The immunomodulatory effects of statins in community-acquired pneumonia: a systematic review. J Infect. 2013;67(2):93-101.
215. Doshi SM, Kulkarni PA, Liao JM, Rueda AM, Musher DM. The impact of statin and macrolide use on early survival in patients with pneumococcal pneumonia. Am J Med Sci. 2013;345(3):173-7.
216. Aliberti S, Ramirez JA. Cardiac diseases complicating community-acquired pneumonia. Curr Opin Infect Dis. 2014; 27(3):295-301.
217. Madhi SA, Levine OS, Hajjeh R, Mansoor OD, Cherian T. Vaccines to prevent pneumonia and improve child survival. Bull World Health Organ. 2008;86(5):365-72.
218. Moberley SA, Holden J, Tatham DP, Andrews RM. Vaccines for preventing pneumococcal infection in adults. Cochrane Database Syst Rev. 2008;(1):CD000422.
219. Vila-Corcoles A. Is the pneumococcal polysaccharide vaccine effective in preventing pneumonia? Lancet Infect Dis. 2008;8(7):405-6.
220. Teshale EH, Hanson D, Flannery B, Phares C, Wolfe M, Schuchat A, et al. Effectiveness of 23-valent polysaccharide pneumococcal vaccine on pneumonia in HIV-infected adults in the United States, 1998-2003. Vaccine. 2008;26(46):5830-4.
221. Imaz A, Falcó V, Peñaranda M, Jordano Q, Martínez X, Nadal C, et al. Impact of prior pneumococcal vaccination on clinical outcomes in HIV-infected adult patients hospitalized with invasive pneumococcal disease. HIV Med. 2009;10(6):356-63.
222. Zar HJ, Madhi SA. Pneumococcal conjugate vaccine—a health priority. S Afr Med J. 2008;98(6):463-7.
223. Whitney CG, Farley MM, Hadler J, Harrison LH, Bennett NM, Lynfield R, Decline in invasive pneumococcal disease after the introduction of protein-polysaccharide conjugate vaccine. N Engl J Med. 2003;348(18):1737-46.
224. Hibberd PL, Bartlett JG, Bloom A. Pneumococcal immunization in HIV-infected adults. UpToDate. 2014;11:1-8.
225. Medscape. Multispecialty. [Online] Available from *http://www.medscape.com/viewarticle/82019 print.* [Accessed January, 2016].

Pulmonary Fungal Infections

Arunaloke Chakrabarti

INTRODUCTION

Fungi, except dimorphic fungi, rarely cause respiratory tract infection in the general population. In contrast, fungal infections of the respiratory tract are important causes of morbidity and mortality in immunocompromised patients; the range of people at risk of these infections has been expanding for the last two decades with increased use of immunosuppressive agents in the treatment of malignancies, and autoimmune disorders, the growing number of transplant recipients, and the aging of the population.[1,2] Fortunately in some of those patients groups, a downwards trend of fungal infection-related mortality has been observed in the last decade with an improvement in medical care.[3,4] Parallel to this positive development, the spectrum of patients at risk for respiratory fungal infections is also expanding.[2,5] Pulmonary mycoses can either be the primary presentation of disease, or be a manifestation of disseminated fungal infections.

Table 1 Susceptible population for fungal respiratory tract infection

• *Classical risk groups* – Cytotoxic chemotherapy for neoplastic disease – Hematopoietic stem cell transplantation (HSCT) – Severe AIDS (CD4 cell count <100) – Immunosuppressive therapy in autoimmune diseases – Other transplantations – Aging population
• *Newly recognized risk groups* – Intensive care unit stay – Chronic obstructive lung disease – Recipients of low dose of steroids – Cirrhotic patients – Iron overload – Poorly controlled diabetic patients – Sepsis associated with immunoprophylaxis – Malnutrition – Moderate to severe renal or hepatic impairment
Abbreviation: AIDS, acquired immunodeficiency syndrome

EPIDEMIOLOGY

The susceptible population for pulmonary fungal infections can be divided in two groups: (1) classical and (2) newly recognized risk groups **(Table 1)**. The risk factors for pulmonary mycoses in developing countries appear similar to the developed world; though certain differences are observed due to local epidemiology including patient characteristics, cultural habitat, and patient care practices.[6-8] The developing countries have large number of poor population with little modern medical facilities at one end and rapidly developing prosperity and healthcare on the other end. Below optimum hospital care practice in the economically deprived groups, and modern medical intervention including transplantations in the prosperous groups, have led to an increase in number of invasive fungal respiratory tract infections in both the groups. Further, the large number of untrained healthcare providers and quacks, misuse of steroids, intravenous drug abuse, availability of spurious infusion sets, are possible additional risk factors for pulmonary mycoses in these countries. The number of persons at risk of pulmonary mycoses in developing countries is staggering.[6-8]

The growing incidence of pulmonary mycoses, which are linked to classical risk factors, is in the range of 3–56% **(Table 2)**.[9,10] The patients usually have significant neutropenia (<500 neutrophil/L for >10 days) as risk factor. The rise in number of pulmonary mycoses is partly due to increased indications of hematological transplantation procedures in recent years and evolving solid organ transplantation practices. Additionally, explosion in number of novel biological immunosuppressant agents and widespread use of antimicrobial prophylactic regimen including fluconazole prophylaxis render host at greater risk of fungal colonization and infection.[11] Other risk factors for those individuals include poor graft function, hepatic failure before transplantation, dialysis requirement, use of OKT3 antibodies, cytomegalovirus infection, and thrombocytopenia.[11] Among solid organ transplant recipients, lung and liver transplant recipients appear to have a higher incidence of pulmonary mycoses **(Table 2)**. In lung transplant, apart from immunosuppressant use, impairment of lymphatic drainage, blunted cough reflex, and defective mucociliary clearance

Table 2 Incidence of fungal pneumonias in classical risk factor groups (modified from Pound et al.)[9]

Population	*Incidence*	*Fungal pathogen*
HIV-infected patients	Not known (30–45% *Cryptococcus*)	*Cryptococcus, Aspergillus, Coccidioides, Histoplasma, Blastomyces*
Bone marrow transplant recipients		
Allogeneic	12–56%	*Aspergillus, Scedosoporium, Fusarium, Candida*
Autologous	Rare	
Solid organ transplant recipients		
Liver	~35%	*Aspergillus, Cryptococcus*
Lung	14–35%	*Aspergillus, Cryptococcus, Candida*
Heart	3–10%	*Aspergillus, Candida*
Kidney	Not known	*Cryptococcus, Aspergillus, Zygomycetes*
Abbreviation: HIV, human immunodeficiency virus		

contribute to fungal growth.[12] Among human immunodeficiency virus (HIV)-infected patients, pulmonary mycoses such as *Pneumocystis pneumonia* and cryptococcal infection are associated with peripheral CD4 count of less than 200 cells/µL. *Aspergillus* pneumonia in advanced HIV infection, is generally uncommon.[11]

Other than classical risk factors, prolonged stay in intensive care unit (ICU), corticosteroid (> 4 weeks) treatment, chronic obstructive pulmonary disease (COPD), liver cirrhosis, individuals with systemic inflammatory disease requiring immunosuppressive therapy, poorly controlled diabetes, iron overload **(Table 1)** are newly recognized risk factors for pulmonary mycoses.[13] The incidence of pulmonary mycoses in ICUs of developing countries is expected to be higher as cofactors (multiple intravenous lines, tracheostomy, endotracheal intubation, other invasive procedures, prolonged corticosteroid and antibiotic therapy) in ICUs are either higher in numbers or misused more due to suboptimal protocol adherence by ICU staff. The COPD is an emerging risk factor. In a recent review of 65 cases, invasive pulmonary aspergillosis was reported as a serious emerging infection in patients with COPD, majority of patients had advanced disease and/or on systemic corticosteroid therapy.[14] The reports of pulmonary mycoses in solid tumor are rare. In a large series from China, approximately 3% lung cancer patients had pulmonary aspergillosis.[15] On univariate analysis, chemotherapy, steroid use, and stage IV diseases were found to be the significant risk factors; while on multivariate analysis only stage IV disease was the significant risk factor; neutropenia and corticosteroid therapy correlated statistically with pulmonary aspergillosis in patients who died.[15]

TYPES OF FUNGI

Though many fungi can cause respiratory infections **(Table 3)**, aspergillosis is the greatest challenge in patients with prolonged neutropenia, recipients of hematopoietic stem cell or solid organ transplants, and patients with advanced acquired immunodeficiency syndrome (AIDS) or chronic granulomatous disease. Host factors govern both the risk and clinicopathological features of invasive aspergillosis.[16,17] Other filamentous fungi, such as *Fusarium spp., Pseudallescheria boydii, Zygomycetes* are reported with increasing frequency in patients with quantitative or qualitative defects in neutrophils.[2] Pulmonary mucormycosis is also reported in patients with uncontrolled diabetes.[18] The clinical presentation, radiological features, and histological appearance of pulmonary infections due to *Fusarium spp.* and *Pseudallescheria boydii* have marked resemblance to *Aspergillus* infections leading to frequent misidentification.[19] Other than these opportunistic fungal infections, endemic mycoses including those due to *Histoplasma capsulatum, Coccidioides immitis,* and *Penicillium marneffei* have increased in frequency in immunocompromised hosts in restricted geographic regions.[2] Rarely *Sporothrix schenckii* can also cause respiratory tract infection. A rare case of fatal pulmonary sporotrichosis caused *S. schenckii var. leurei* was reported from India.[20] *Pneumocystis jiroveci* infection

Table 3 Fungi causing respiratory tract infections

- *Aspergillus (most common)*
  - 10% of patients with leukemia
  - 30% of patients with solid organ transplantation
  - 10% of HSCT
- *Fusarium* and *Pseudallescheria*
- *Zygomycetes*
- Endemic mycotic agents (*H. capsulatum, Dermatitidis, C. immitis, P. marneffei,* rarely *S. schenckii*)
- *Pneumocystis jiroveci*
- Rarely yeasts (*Cryptococcus, Candida, Trichosporon*)
- Rarely black fungi (*Cladophialophora boppi*)

Abbreviation: HSCT, hematopoietic stem cell transplantation

had frequently been reported in patients with AIDS, but recent data showed a sharp decline in incidence after chemoprophylaxis and tridrug regimen in those patients.[21] Yeasts are rarely reported in respiratory tract infections.[2] Among yeasts, cryptococcal respiratory tract infections are seen more consistently. Though deep-seated infections due to black mycelial fungi are increasingly reported in recent years, they rarely cause pulmonary infections. A very rare case of pulmonary *Cladophialophora boppi* infection has been reported recently in lung transplant recipient.[22]

Aspergillosis

Pulmonary aspergillosis may be classified as allergic, saprophytic, and invasive diseases. The further subtype classification of each condition is presented in **Table 4**.

Allergic Alveolitis

The common epidemiological setting of extrinsic allergic alveolitis due to *Aspergillus* is repeated exposure in nonatopic workers to *Aspergillus* antigen in moldy hay or grain, hence the terms "farmer's lung" or "malt workers lung". Symptoms include cough, dyspnea, fever, chills and myalgias within 8 hours of exposure. A chest radiograph may reveal interstitial infiltrates. Relief of symptoms has been observed within 48 hours while away from exposure. Repeated exposure may lead to intractable pulmonary fibrosis.[2]

Allergic bronchopulmonary aspergillosis (ABPA): ABPA is an allergic pulmonary disorder caused by allergic response to *Aspergillus hyphae* without direct tissue invasion by the organism. It manifests as chronic asthma, recurrent pulmonary infiltrates, and bronchiectasis.[23,24] Bronchospasm in this process is thought to be mediated by an Immunoglobulin E (IgE) (type I reaction) mediated hypersensitivity, whereas the bronchial and peribronchial inflammation appears to be induced by immune complex formation (ICF) (Type III reaction), and eosinophil-rich inflammatory cell responses due to Type-IV hypersensitivity. Occasionally patients may develop a syndrome similar to ABPA, due to fungi other than *A. fumigatus* and is called allergic bronchopulmonary mycosis.

Table 4 Spectrum of *Aspergillus* pulmonary infections

- *Allergic*
  - Allergic alveolitis
  - Asthma
  - Allergic bronchopulmonary aspergillosis
  - Eosinophil-related sinusitis including allergic fungal rhinosinusitis
  - Sinobronchial allergic mycosis (SAM syndrome)
- *Colonizing*
  - Pulmonary aspergilloma
  - Chronic cavitary
  - Sinus aspergilloma (Fungal ball)
- *Invasive*
  - Acute invasive
  - Necrotizing tracheobronchitis
  - Local extension
  - Disseminated
  - Chronic necrotizing
  - Invasive rhinosinusitis
    - Acute invasive
    - Chronic granulomatous
    - Chronic invasive

The prevalence of ABPA is claimed as 1–2% in patients with asthma and 2–15% in patients with cystic fibrosis.[25] In the past two decades, there has been an increase in the number of cases of ABPA due to heightened physician awareness and improved laboratory facilities. The link between sensitization and infection with *Aspergillus* and asthma is a subject of study. In a recent study of patients attending chest clinic of a tertiary care center in north India, 27% of asthmatics met criteria for ABPA.[26]

Eosinophil-related fungal rhinosinusitis: Several types of sinus diseases have been attributed to the presence of fungal organisms in the nasal and sinus cavities. As the incidence of chronic rhinosinusitis (CRS) has increased over the last decade, fungal rhinosinusitis (FRS) has gained importance. Much confusion exists regarding classification of FRS. The most accepted classification divides FRS into invasive and noninvasive diseases based on histopathological evidence of tissue invasion by fungi. The invasive diseases include acute invasive, granulomatous invasive, and chronic invasive FRS. The noninvasive diseases include localized fungal colonization, fungal ball, and eosinophil-related FRS that includes allergic fungal rhinosinusitis (AFRS).[27]

The AFRS is considered as a nontissue invasive fungal process representing an allergic/hypersensitivity response to the presence of extramucosal fungi within the sinus cavity, possibly akin to ABPA.[28] In western world, dematiaceous fungi including *Alternaria alternata*, and in Middle East, Sudan and India *Aspergillus flavus* are commonly isolated from such patients.[27-29] It is believed that fungal allergens elicit IgE-mediated allergic and possibly type III-mediated mucosal inflammation in the absence of invasion in an atopic host. Moreover, when the sensitized individuals are exposed to an environment of high fungal content, symptoms of upper and/or lower airway hypersensitiveness increase significantly. Generalized sinonasal inflammation in combination with viscid allergic mucin effectively obstructs the normal drainage pathway. Fungi persist locally, stimulating locally destructive immune response. The process then extends to involve adjacent sinuses and may produce sinus expansion and bony erosion.[29] Although the presentation of disease is subtle, occasional dramatic presentations in form of acute visual loss, gross facial dysmorphia or complete nasal obstruction have been observed.

To diagnose AFRS, Bent and Kuhn proposed five diagnostic criteria: (1) type I hypersensitivity, (2) nasal polyposis, (3) characteristic findings on computed tomography (CT) scan,

(4) presence of fungi on direct microscopy or culture, and (5) allergic mucin containing fungal elements without tissue invasion.[30] Although the detection of fungi in allergic mucin is considered important, hyphae may be sparse in sinus content and may take considerable time to screen before identifying the fungus with commonly used stains. This has led to confusion in categorization of this entity, especially with description of eosinophilic mucin rhinosinusitis (EMRS).[31] Ferguson speculated that the EMRS is a systemic disease with dysregulation of immunological control where eosinophilic mucin could be present without the presence of fungi. The definition of AFRS has faced a greater challenge with the demonstration of fungi in eosinophilic mucin independently of Type-I hypersensitivity in most cases of CRS. Ponikau et al. proposed a new term for this condition, namely eosinophilic fungal rhinosinusitis (EFRS) to reflect the striking role of eosinophil.[32] It is proposed that high levels of major basic protein (MBP) is released from eosinophils in the mucus of patients with the CRS and postulated that MBP damages the nasal epithelium from the luminal side permitting secondary bacterial infections on the damaged epithelium.[33]

Saprophytic Aspergillosis

Saprophytic or colonizing forms of aspergillosis develop in an existing pulmonary cavity, caused by old tuberculosis (TB), emphysematous bullae or carcinoma. Children with cystic fibrosis and bronchiectasis may also have saprophytic involvement of airway due to *Aspergillus* spp. The mass of hyphae amidst a proteinaceous matrix is called as aspergilloma. The patient remains asymptomatic for a considerable period of time. Occasionally, aspergilloma may cause hemoptysis and may be fatal in rare situation. The radiographic appearance of a rounded density within a cavity partially surrounded by a radiolucent crescent halo (Monod's sign) is characteristic of an aspergilloma. Filamentous fungi other than *Aspergillus*, such as *Pseudoallescheria boydii* and *Zygomycetes*, may also cause intracavitary fungal balls and simulate an aspergilloma.[34]

Fungal ball is also described as the presence of noninvasive accumulation of dense conglomeration of fungal hyphae in a paranasal sinus cavity, usually maxillary sinus, although the disease may affect other sinuses or rarely multiple sinuses. Various terms, such as mycetoma, aspergilloma, and chronic noninvasive granuloma have been used interchangeably to designate sinus fungal balls.[27] The disease is defined by the following criteria: a dense conglomeration of noninvasive hyphae in cheesy or clay-like materials within the sinus, radiological evidence of sinus opacification with or without radiographic heterogeneity, nonspecific chronic inflammation of mucosa, nonpredominance of eosinophils or granuloma or allergic mucin, and absence of histopathological evidence of fungal invasion of mucosa.[34] The disease has been commonly found in middle-aged and elderly females of France.

Invasive Aspergillosis

Invasive aspergillosis occurs in patients with acquired (neoplastic diseases with persistent and profound neutropenia, receiving high doses of corticosteroids) or primary defects (chronic granulomatous disease and hyper-IgE syndrome) in neutrophil function. In recent years, even up to 41% of cases of invasive aspergillosis were diagnosed in non-neutropenic patients, especially patients with COPD, chronic liver disease, reactive airway disease, and rheumatoid arthritis.[35] Patients with HIV infection may develop invasive pulmonary aspergillosis when CD4 count falls less than 50 cells/mm^3. Invasive aspergillosis in patients with HIV infection remains restricted to only pulmonary involvement in majority of cases. The various clinical manifestations of invasive aspergillosis include pneumonia, hemoptysis, invasion of contiguous intrathoracic structures, and dissemination. These findings are reflection of angioinvasion, thrombosis, and infarction, not specific for aspergillosis but may be a manifestation of one of the several opportunistic angioinvasive fungi like *Zygomycetes, Pseudallescheria boydii, Fusarium* spp. Fever may be the earliest manifestation of pulmonary aspergillosis. The imaging modality of choice for early detection of invasive pulmonary aspergillosis is the high-resolution computed tomography (HRCT). The radiographic manifestations of invasive pulmonary aspergillosis include bronchopneumonia, nodules, halo sign, lobar consolidation, segmental pneumonia, crescent sign, and cavitary lesions.

Invasive pulmonary aspergillosis is highly prevalent in developing countries especially in patients with malignancies and transplant recipients.[36-40] In a series of invasive aspergillosis reported from a tertiary care hospital in Thailand,[41] lung was involved in 68% cases followed by sinuses (17%), eyes (8%), and brain (5%). In an autopsy study of childhood pneumonia from Bangladesh, pulmonary aspergillosis was diagnosed in 3% of all pneumonias and 10% of necrotizing pneumonias.[42] Other than classical manifestations of pulmonary aspergillosis, certain uncommon clinical presentations have been observed in developing countries. Some of these observations include development of invasive pulmonary aspergillosis in patients with colonizing aspergillosis (in a tubercular cavity),[43,44] ABPA or aspergilloma,[45,46] bronchial asthma.[15,43] Possibly long period of steroid therapy allowed fungal hyphae from cavitatory lesion or localized mass lesion to invade lung parenchyma. Invasive pulmonary aspergillosis was also found to be associated with antineutrophilic cytoplasmic antibodies positive vasculitis.[47,48] In a series of 157 patients with vasculitis, 7 (4.5%) developed invasive pulmonary aspergillosis, 2 had Wegener's granulomatosis, and 5 had microscopic polyangiitis. Invasive pulmonary aspergillosis developed within 2-13 weeks of immunosuppressive therapy.[48]

Tracheobronchial aspergillosis: The presence of *Aspergillus* spp. in the large airway may represent colonization or, rarely, tracheobronchitis. Isolated invasive *Aspergillus* tracheobronchitis is reported in patients with severely immunocompromised status due to transplantation or hematological malignancies or AIDS. However, 19 patients with isolated invasive *Aspergillus* tracheobronchitis from China had impaired airway structures or defense functions rather than severely immunocompromised status, only three (16%) patients had neutropenia, malignancy (13 cases of solid tumor, 1 case of lymphoma) was the most common underlying disease.[47] The disease could be classified into four different forms: (1) superficial infiltrative, (2) full layer involvement, (3) occlusion, and (4) mixed type.[49]

Chronic necrotizing pulmonary aspergillosis: It is another subset of pulmonary aspergillosis. This indolent infection has been reported in elderly patients with COPD, inactive TB, pneumoconiosis or sarcoidosis. Subtle defects in systemic host defense due to malnutrition, alcoholism, diabetes mellitus or low-dose corticosteroids may also be evident. It presents as a chronic refractory bronchopneumonia with fever, weight loss, cough, progressive infiltrates, and evidence of invasive aspergillosis on biopsy. The infection may progress to cavitation and formation of an aspergilloma or may develop from an aspergilloma as the initial focus.[2]

Invasive fungal rhinosinusitis: As mentioned earlier, invasive FRS includes acute invasive, granulomatous and chronic invasive FRS depending on host immune status and geographical region. Acute invasive FRS is described by a disease course of less than 4 weeks with predominant vascular invasion occurring in an immunocompromised patient. The histopathology demonstrates hyphal invasion of blood vessels, including carotid arteries and cavernous sinuses, vasculitis with thrombosis, hemorrhage, tissue infarction and acute neutrophilic infiltrates. Granulomatous invasive is described by a time course of more than 12 weeks with an enlarging mass in the cheek, orbit, nose, and paranasal sinuses in immunocompetent hosts. Proptosis is often a prominent feature. The disease is primarily seen in Sudan, India, Pakistan, and Saudi Arabia. The granulomatous response is seen with considerable fibrosis. Hyphae are usually scanty and *A. flavus* is the primary isolated agent. Chronic invasive FRS is a slowly destructive process with a time course of more than 12 weeks that commonly affects ethmoid and sphenoid sinuses, but may involve any paranasal sinus. In contrast to granulomatous invasive FRS, the entity is characterized as dense accumulation of hyphae, occasional presence of vascular invasion, and sparse inflammatory reaction in association with involvement of local structures. The disease is usually associated with AIDS, diabetes mellitus, and corticosteroid treatment. *A. fumigatus* is commonly isolated from such patients.[27,29]

Mucormycosis

It is an increasingly reported polymorphic disease caused by members of the class *Zygomycetes*. The common sites of mucormycosis are the rhinocerebral area (39%), lungs (24%), and skin (19%).[17] Pulmonary mucormycosis is most frequently observed in granulocytopenic and corticosteroid treated patients. Patients with advanced AIDS are also at risk. The epidemiology of mucormycosis seems to be different between developed and developing countries. In developed countries, the disease is a rare finding, usually seen in patients with hematological malignancies undergoing chemotherapy, in bone marrow transplant recipients, and as breakthrough infection in patients receiving voriconazole therapy or prophylaxis. In developing counties like India, the number of mucormycosis cases seems to be on the rise, occurring commonly in patients with uncontrolled diabetes. The number of cases with uncontrolled diabetes is so overwhelming that the other risk factors are overshadowed.[2,18,50,51] Most of the *Zygomycetes* causing respiratory infections in immunocompromised or debilitated hosts have a high propensity for thrombotic invasion of blood vessels, a rapidly evolving clinical course, high mortality, and a relative resistance to antifungal therapy.

Pulmonary mucormycosis may have a wide variety of disease manifestations including solitary nodular lesions, lobar involvement, cavitary or disseminated form. Infiltrates or mass lesions without any specific lobar predilectations are common findings. Pulmonary consolidation and cavitations are less frequent, though in a series from India, 23% had cavitary lesions.[52] Recently, two cases of pulmonary cavitary mucormycosis due to very rare species, *Rhizopus homothallicus* have been reported from India.[53] It is suggested that such cavities represent liquefaction of pulmonary infarcts. Antemortem diagnosis of pulmonary mucormycosis is difficult due to lack of specific symptoms and signs. Majority (44–100%) of cases are diagnosed postmortem, though increased awareness may improve the proportion of cases with antemortem diagnosis. Sputum or bronchoalveolar lavage (BAL) analysis is frequently employed, but rarely leads to confirmation of diagnosis. Bronchoscopic biopsy helps in early diagnosis of certain pulmonary mucormycosis cases. Open lung biopsy, surgical extirpation and needle aspiration under image guidance are the other improved modes of antemortem diagnosis.[52]

FUSARIUM AND SCEDOSPORIUM INFECTIONS

Over the past two decades, *Fusarium* spp. and *Scedosporium apiospermum* or *Pseudoallescheria boydii* (sexual stage) are emerging pathogens especially in patients with hematological malignancies undergoing chemotherapy and bone marrow transplants. The pulmonary infections caused by both agents are indistinguishable many times from that caused by *Aspergillus* spp. The organisms in tissue also resemble *Aspergillus* spp. having angular, septate dichotomously branching hyphae.[2,54,55]

F. solani, F. oxysporum, F. moniliforme, and *F. chlamydosporum* are commonly isolated agents from patients with invasive *Fusarium* infection. Though invasive *Fusarium* infections produce pulmonary disease similar to that of invasive aspergillosis, pulmonary infiltrates, cutaneous lesions, positive blood culture and sinusitis characterize *Fusarium* infection. Biopsy of cutaneous lesion and blood culture help in diagnosis of disseminated fusariosis.[54]

Scedosporium spp. cause sinusitis, pneumonia, and disseminated infections in immunocompromised hosts and fungal ball in immunocompetent patients. Pneumonia due to *S. apiospermum* is clinically indistinguishable from that due to *Aspergillus* spp. Other *Scedosporium* species, *S. prolificans* can also cause pneumonia in immunocompromised host and is considered to be mere virulent and resistant to amphotericin B. Diagnostic approaches are similar to aspergillosis or zygomycotic infections. The organism in tissue resembles *Aspergillus* spp. as angular, septate dichotomously branching hyphae. The definitive microbiologic diagnosis can be established by culture.[55] Blood culture may help in *S. prolificans* isolation.

RESPIRATORY INFECTIONS DUE TO DIMORPHIC FUNGI

Dimorphic fungi, including *Histoplasma capsulatum, Blastomyces dermatitidis, Coccidioides immitis, Paracoccidioides brasiliensis, Penicillium marneffei*, and rarely *Sporothrix schenckii* may cause respiratory tract infection. The dimorphic fungi do appear to follow a geographically defined endemic pattern of distribution. *Penicillium marneffei* causing penicilliosis has its environmental niche in Southeast Asia only.[56-58] Histoplasmosis, though considered uncommon in Asia-pacific region three decades back, is increasingly reported in many countries especially in patients with acquired immune deficiency syndrome.[59,60] Autochthonous cases of blastomycosis are occasionally reported from this region,[61] coccidioidomycois and paracoccidioidomycosis are rarely reported as imported disease.[62,63] Upon entry of the conidia of the dimorphic fungi into lower respiratory tract, the interaction of host defenses and various fungal factors determines the outcome of infection. The fungi are usually contained by alveolar macrophages, resulting in a localized granulomatous process for *H. capsulatum, P. marneffei*, and *P. brasiliensis*. A combined acute and chronic inflammatory response is observed in *C. immitis* and *B. dermatitidis* infections. Calcification develops at the site of resolving granulomatous foci of *H. capsulatum* infection.

Histoplasmosis usually presents as mild insignificant self-limiting respiratory disease in majority of patients from endemic areas. The clinical manifestations of histoplasmosis may be classified according to site (pulmonary, extrapulmonary or disseminated), duration of infection (acute, subacute, and chronic), and by pattern of infection (primary versus reactivation). Acute primary pulmonary histoplasmosis may develop in a normal, immunocompetent host when exposed to a heavy inoculum. Chronic cavitary pulmonary histoplasmosis is an indolent but progressive respiratory infection of patients with underlying COPD. Acute progressive disease is seen in immunosuppressed hosts. Though the number of cases of acute progressive disseminated histoplasmosis has steadily increased in Asia-Pacific region along with rise of AIDS population, a large number of cases are diagnosed from this region as chronic manifestations of disseminated histoplasmosis. These cases are easily diagnosed as the disease frequently presents with accessible mucocutaneous lesions that can be easily biopsied.[59,60] Few cases have been reported as adrenal histoplasmosis, misdiagnosed as adrenal tumor initially.

It is not clear whether blastomycosis is endemic in Asia-Pacific region as there are very few autochthonous cases reported from this region. Most of those cases were reported from India.[61] Though the fungus had been isolated from bats in Delhi, its soil source is not clearly known. The fungus was isolated from pulmonary, cutaneous, and cerebral lesions. The manifestations of *B. dermatitidis* infection are protean asymptomatic diseases, a brief influenza like illness, self-limited localized pneumonia in immune competent patients, subacute to chronic respiratory illness and fulminant infection with adult respiratory distress syndrome. The infiltrates of pulmonary blastomycosis are nonspecific and appear as bronchopneumonia or segmental consolidation.

The manifestations of pulmonary penicilliosis have striking resemblance to disseminated histoplasmosis in HIV-infected patients. Therefore, the recognition of penicilliosis is sometimes difficult especially in area where histoplasmosis is also endemic as both diseases present with fever, weight loss, cough, anemia, lymphadenopathy, hepatosplenomegaly. Skin lesions are more common (60–85%) in penicilliosis. In a hospital at Thailand when the medical records of patients with histoplasmosis and penicilliosis were compared, no statistical difference was observed in skin lesion between the two groups, though the rate of skin lesions was higher (53%) in patients with penicilliosis compared to 38% in histoplasmosis. Even laboratory findings were similar between the two groups except hyperbilirubinemia, which was more common in the penicilliosis group.[64] HIV-infected patients had a higher incidence of fungemia, higher antigen titer in *P. marneffei*-specific mannoprotein Mplp enzyme-linked immunosorbent assay, and low serum antibody level.[65] All those data indicate that only high degree of suspicion among clinicians treating HIV-infected patients may help in early diagnosis of penicilliosis especially when many diseases mimic similar clinical presentations. Further, biopsy of skin lesion can help in early diagnosis.

PULMONARY CRYPTOCOCCOSIS

The disease is frequently associated with disseminated infection especially in immunocompromised hosts. Cryptococcosis occurs in 0.3–5.3% (with a mean of 2.8%) of solid organ transplant recipients; 25–54% of transplant recipients with cryptococcosis have pulmonary disease, and the disease is limited to the lungs in 6–33% cases.[66] Fever, cough dyspnea, and pleural pain are common initial manifestations. Interstitial infiltrates, miliary nodules, ARDS, hilar lymphadenopathy and pleural effusion are typical radiographic features. Pulmonary cryptococcosis is relatively common and frequent finding in patients with AIDS. In an autopsy series of 8,421 South African Miners, with an estimated HIV prevalence of 24%, 589 cases (overall prevalence of 7%) of pulmonary cryptococcosis were identified. Antemortem diagnosis for cryptococcal meningitis was made in 47% of these cases, and pulmonary cryptococcosis in 1.2% cases. The remaining 52% of those cases had been misdiagnosed as pulmonary TB.[67]

PULMONARY CANDIDIASIS

Pulmonary candidiasis may be a secondary process arising from hematogenous dissemination or rarely a primary bronchopneumonia. Primary *Candida* bronchopneumonia may be observed in severely debilitated, neutropenic patients, and very low birth weight infants, is usually associated with aspiration of oropharyngeal content. The diagnosis of pulmonary candidiasis is difficult because of nonspecific clinical and radiological presentation. The presence of *Candida* in the sputum, tracheal aspiration or BAL mostly represents contamination from upper respiratory tract colonization. A definite diagnosis of *Candida* pneumonia requires histopathological proof of lung invasion. Children can also be affected by pulmonary allergic reaction due to *Candida* species.[68]

PNEUMOCYSTIS RESPIRATORY TRACT INFECTION

Pneumocystis jiroveci, formerly known as *Pneumocystis carinii* is a major cause of opportunistic infection in respiratory tract. Pneumonia caused by this organism is an AIDS defining illness having high morbidity and mortality. Though the infection rate has come down in HIV positive patients after antiretroviral therapy, patients with inherited or other acquired immune defects and those on immunosuppressive medications are vulnerable to *Pneumocystis* infection. Patients initially present with history of dry cough, fever, dyspnea, and difficulty in deep inspiration. Physical examination reveals varying degree of tachypnea, tachycardia, cyanosis, and rales. Chest radiographs often exhibit pathognomonic bilateral diffuse infiltrates with ground-glass appearance; focal infiltrates may be seen occasionally. Patients with AIDS and pneumocystis pneumonia have a significantly higher number of pneumocystis organisms and fewer neutrophils in their lungs than do patients with Pneumocystis pneumonia in absence of AIDS. The smaller number of neutrophils in patients with AIDS correlate with better oxygenation and survival as compared with pneumocystis pneumonia in patients without AIDS.[69,70]

Mortality rate in AIDS with pneumocystis pneumonia is 10–20% during the initial infection, though the rate increases substantially with the need for mechanical ventilation.[71] Mortality in patients with pneumocystis pneumonia in the absence of AIDS is 30–60% depending on the population at risk, with a greater risk of death among patients with cancer than among patients undergoing transplantation or those with connective tissue disease.[69] The gold standard for diagnosis is lung biopsy, though BAL fluid and induced sputum are also utilized for diagnosis. Gomori methenamine silver, and toluidine blue, calcofluor white stains, which stain pneumocystis cysts, are commonly used to identify *P. jiroveci* in those samples. Trophic forms can be detected with modified Papanicolaou, Wright-Giemsa, or Gram-Weigert stains. Monoclonal antibodies for detecting pneumocystis have a higher sensitivity and specificity in induced sputum samples than conventional stains, but the difference is much less in broncho-alveolar lavage fluid.[72,73] In patients with pneumocystis pneumonia, serum lactate dehydrogenase usually rises, but it may reflect underlying lung injury rather than any specific marker of disease. Lower level of plasma S-adenosyl methionine was observed in patients with pneumocystis pneumonia, but larger cohort study is required to prove its usefulness for diagnosis of pneumocystis infection.[70]

PULMONARY MYCOSES

With increase of opportunistic fungal respiratory tract infections in tertiary care centers especially with increase of susceptible population, the real challenge is to suspect and diagnose and treat these infections early, since these infections are associated with very high attributable mortality. Many centers recently reported unusually high incidence of opportunistic mycoses, including *Aspergillus* spp., *Fusarium* spp., *Scedosporium* spp., and *Zygomycetes.*[5] The time period between the first evidence of fungal infections and appearance of signs and symptoms represent a window of opportunity for early treatment. European Organization for Research and Treatment of Cancer-Mycosis Study Group (EORTC-MSG) has developed a diagnostic protocol for invasive fungal infections in immunocompromised patients as proven, probable, and possible infection depending on host, clinical and microbiological criteria.[74] Though it is developed for clinical research, majority clinicians handling immunosuppressed patients utilize the same criteria to diagnose their patients. The diagnosis of fungal infection depends on combination of all three instead of one criterion in isolation, though predictive value of the same may be high. Imaging helps to increase the suspicion of fungal disease. In an immunosuppressed patient, presence of a nodule, halo sign, air crescent sign, or reverse halo sign helps in suspecting fungal infections. In immunocompetent patients, such signs are not available. If the patient is in ICU, think of fungal infections even when infiltrative lesion is suspected. Mycological tools should always be used in conjunction with modern imaging techniques.[5]

Chest radiography is not a sensitive procedure for diagnosing pulmonary mold infections at an early stage. Chest CT scan helps to pick up the lesions. Classically these infections present as macronodular lesions or infiltrates. In neutropenic patients, approximately 80% of these nodular lesions will be surrounded by areas of lower attenuation or "halo sign" that represent areas of hemorrhagic inflammation.[5] The lesions may eventually cavitate during the course of therapy and following neutrophil recovery, creating what is commonly referred to as an "air crescent sign". These characteristics are neither highly sensitive nor fungal specific; other infections that elicit such inflammatory responses, including bacteria and viruses, can present with halo signs.[5,7]

Among mycological techniques, conventional procedures (direct microscopy, histopathology, and culture) are not sensitive and do not help in early diagnosis. Maximum attention has been drawn to find suitable serological or molecular diagnostic technique. Polymerase chain reaction (PCR) for detection of fungal nucleic acid in specimens, though holds promise, is awaiting further standardization and validation. The relative merits of diagnostic tests for detection of galactomannan and β-D-Glucan are being evaluated. In recent years, a lot of experience has been gained with the Platelia *Aspergillus* seroassay (Bio-Rad Laboratories). This sandwich enzyme immunoassay (EIA) detects galactofuranose-containing molecules (including galactomannan), cell wall components released by *Aspergillus* species during hyphal growth. Few other fungal organisms like *Penicillium* spp. share cross-reacting epitopes with *Aspergillus* species, but these pathogens are rare in patients at risk for fungal respiratory tract infections. The Platelia EIA is widely used as a screening tool for early detection of invasive aspergillosis in neutropenic patients, though sensitivity results varied in different studies.[5] The test with low cut-off of titer of 0.5 has good negative predictive value. A single positive assay serves as a microbiological criterion to define probable invasive aspergillosis in patients with appropriate radiographic abnormalities. Platelia EIA has been used to detect *Aspergillus* antigen not only in serum, but also in BAL and pleural fluid. Data from one major center demonstrated excellent sensitivity of Platelia EIA when used on BAL and pleural fluid.[75] It awaits corroboration from other centers treating similar patients. Of note, the use of Plasmalyte for performing BAL and the concomitant use of semisynthetic β-lactam antibiotics such as piperacillin-tazobactum may result in false-positive test result.

Glucans (1, 3)-β-D-linked polymers of glucose, are part of outer cell wall of most pathogenic fungi (except *Zygomycetes*, *Cryptococcus* species). D-Glucan can be detected by several commercial assays (Fungitell, Association of Cope Cod; Fungi Tec G, Seikagaku Kogyo Corporation, Japan; Wako-WB003, Wako Pure chemical Industries, Japan). The negative predictive value of glucan detection test by twice weekly sampling is 100%, and the sensitivity is 100% if one positive assay is considered as a positive result, though overall experience with this assay remains limited.[76] The test requires endotoxin-free and glucan-free glassware. A number of factors including the use of albumin or immunoglobulins, exposure to glucan containing gauze, and hemodialysis, may lead to false-positive readings in glucan detection test. The assay also cross-reacts with some antimicrobial preparations and can provide false-positive result in patients with Gram-positive bacteremia or *Pseudomonas aeruginosa* infections. None of these serological assays helps in diagnosis of other life-threatening fungal disease, invasive mucormycosis.[5,20,77,78]

In the absence of specific clinical symptoms and signs or radiological evidence, the big question is "Can we minimize the number of patients on empiric therapy in the high-risk patients groups?" Systemic antifungal therapy is toxic, expensive, and has many drug interactions. Emphasis should be made on preemptive therapy instead of empiric therapy **(Table 5)**. Though contradictory suggestions are available, at least in neutropenic patients with persistent or recrudescent fever with no other clinical or radiological evidence of fungal disease, the clinicians may withhold antifungal therapy when galactomannan and glucan tests are negative, as the serological tests have excellent negative predictive value. Conversely, in a patient population in which a positive serological test correlates with a high positive predictive value, positivity should trigger diagnostic work up, potentially leading to early therapy.[5] A highly suggestive CT scan and consecutive negative serological marker should trigger an aggressive diagnostic exploration (lung biopsy and imaging guided aspiration) for invasive mucormycosis especially in countries like India where mucormycosis rate is very high.[5,52,79] During recent years, fungal infections due to *Fusarium* spp. and *Scedosporium* spp. are on the rise. On histopathology, these fungi are indistinguishable from *Aspergillus* spp. As the therapy varies in these infections from aspergillosis, culture or molecular technique is essential for diagnosis.

The diagnosis of pulmonary infections due to dimorphic fungi largely depends on clinical suspicion, direct examination of respiratory specimens, histopathological examination of paraffin-embedded tissue, and culture of appropriate samples. Careful examination of fungal structure on direct microscopy helps in identification of fungus as each dimorphic fungus has distinctive morphology in tissue. In an immunocompetent host, serology for antibody detection helps in diagnosis of considerable number of cases. Conversely, in immunocompromised hosts, antigen detection would be a preferable alternative. Only in histoplasmosis, the detection of a carbohydrate antigen in serum or urine is found to be useful for diagnosis and therapeutic monitoring.[80]

Table 5 Paradigms for antifungal intervention

Intervention	*Setting*
1. Primary prophylaxis	Prevention use in patients at high risk. General principle—consider prophylaxis when fungal infection rate ≥10% (prophylaxis is not substitute to hospital care practice)
2. Empirical therapy	Preventive use in patients with prolonged (≥10 days) neutropenia (ANC ≤500/μL) with persistent or new fever despite adequate broad-spectrum antibacterial therapy (adequate period varies on experience of particular center)
3. Preemptive therapy	Preemptive use in patients at high risk (≥10%) of invasive fungal infections who have imaging findings (chest CT) and/or laboratory test results (positive for antigen or fungal specific markers) or specific score results consistent with invasive fungal infection by no conclusive evidence
4. Treatment—proven invasive fungal infections	Use in patients with direct microscopy or histopathological demonstration of fungal elements and/or microscopic documentation of a fungal organism in sterile body fluid or tissue
5. Secondary prophylaxis	Continuous use in patients who had a complete or partial response to treatment of an invasive fungal infection and need to undergo further intensive anticancer treatment or immunosuppression (till reversal of immunosuppression)
Abbreviation: CT, computed tomography	

Table 6 Spectrum of activity of antifungal agents

Organism	*AMB*	*FCZ*	*ITZ*	*PCZ*	*VCZ*	*CAS*	*ANID*	*MICA*	*5FC*
C. albicans	S	S	S	S	S	S	S	S	S
C. glabrata	S-I-R	SDD-R	S-I	S-I	S-I	S	S	S	S
C. parapsilosis	S	S	S	S	S	S-I	S-I	S-I	S
C. krusei	S-I-R	R	I-R	S-I-R	S-I-R	S	S	S	I-R
C. neoformans	S	S	S	S	S	R	R	R	S
A. fumigatus	S	R	S	S	S	S	S	S	R
A. flavus	S	R	S	S	S	S	S	S	R
Zygomycetes	S	R	I-R	S-I-R	I-R	R	R	R	R
Hyalohypho-mycetes	I-R	R	S-I-R	S-I-R	S-I-R	R	R	R	R
Phaeohypho-mycetes	S-I	R	S	S	S	I-R	I-R	I-R	S-R
Dimorphic fungi	S	S-R	S	S	S	-	-	-	S-R

Abbreviations: S, susceptible; SDD, susceptible dose-dependent; I, intermediate; R, resistant; AMB, amphotericin B; FCZ, fluconazole; ITZ, itraconazole; PCZ, posaconazole; VCZ, voriconazole; CAS, caspofungin; ANID, anidulafungin; MICA, micafungin; 5FC, 5-fluorocytosine

Therapy of Pulmonary Mycoses

For a long time, the available antifungal armamentarium consisted of amphotericin B deoxycholate (DAMB) and 5-fluorocytosine (SFC). The first therapeutic alternatives began to emerge with introduction of fluconazole and itraconazole in the late 1980s. In the past 10–15 years, expansion in antifungal drug research has led to the clinical development of lipid formulations of amphotericin B [amphotericin B colloidal dispersion (ABCD); amphotericin B lipid complex (ABLC); and liposomal amphotericin B (L-AMB)], a second generation of potent and broad-spectrum antifungal triazoles (posaconazole, voriconazole), and an entirely new class of antifungal agents, the echinocandins (caspofungin, anidulafungin, micafungin). The antifungal interventions may be in the different paradigms **(Table 5)**. The spectrum of activity of antifungal agents is provided in **Table 6**.

Presently, voriconazole is considered as the drug of choice for the first-line therapy of invasive aspergillosis. However, particular clinical conditions favor the use of a nonazole based primary treatment, including prior exposure to mold-active azoles, the concomitant use of prohibited medication (e.g. sirolimus), the risk of severe drug interaction, moderate to severe renal impairment, or the presence of mixed fungal infections (e.g. *Zygomycetes*).[5] Multiazole resistant *A. fumigatus* is also described.[81] Liposomal amphotericin B is considered alternative drug of choice for the first-line therapy of invasive aspergillosis. Data regarding the use of echinocandins in the primary therapy of invasive aspergillosis is scarce. Overall, up to 50% of the patients who fail first-line therapy can be salvaged with second-line use of caspofungin, posaconazole, or a lipid formulation of amphotericin B.[5,82] The Infectious Diseases Society of America (IDSA) guidelines recommend use of voriconazole (6 mg/kg IV every 12 hr for 1 day, followed by 4 mg/kg IV every 12 hr; oral dosage is 200 mg every 12 hr) as primary therapy in invasive pulmonary, invasive sinus, tracheobronchial, chronic necrotizing aspergillosis. L-AMB (3–5 mg/kg/day IV), ABLC (5 mg/kg/day IV), caspofungin (70 mg day 1 IV and 50 mg/day IV thereafter), micafungin (IV 100–150 mg/day; dose not established), posaconazole (200 mg QID initially, then 400 mg BID PO after stabilization of disease), itraconazole (dosage depends upon formulation) are recommended as alternative therapy in the above patients.[83]

Voriconazole and amphotericin B (preferably a lipid-based formulation) are also considered drugs of choice for treatment of *Fusarium* and *Scedosporium* infections, Posaconazole may be used as salvage therapy.[84-86] For mucormycosis, high dose of lipid-based formulations of amphotericin B (up to 10 mg/kg) remains the drug of choice for the first-line therapy, whereas posaconazole may be used in salvage or maintenance treatment. Surgical excision of infected lesions and reversal of underlying predisposing factors are also important in management of pulmonary mucormycosis and should complement antifungal therapy.[52,87]

Treatment of pulmonary mycoses due to dimorphic fungi depends on competency of the hosts and disease pattern. Self-limiting disease among immunocompetent hosts is managed with supportive care. Acute pulmonary histoplasmosis or blastomycosis is treated with itraconazole. Profoundly immunocompromised hosts or those with severe disease are treated with amphotericin B, preferably lipid formulations. Itraconazole or amphotericin B has been proven as effective also against penicilliosis.[88-91] In pulmonary cryptococcosis, if the patient is HIV infected, an initial course of amphotericin B with or without flucytosine, followed by maintenance therapy with fluconazole is recommended. Itraconazole may be used as alternative therapy in patients with mild disease of pulmonary cryptococcosis.[92,93]

In allergic fungal pulmonary diseases such as ABPA, corticosteroids are recommended. Early aggressive disease may slow down the irreversible fibrotic phase. Itraconazole may be added in resistant cases. In allergic fungal sinusitis, systemic steroids are found better than local steroids. Itraconazole may be effective in combination with corticosteroid. For fungal ball in sinuses and aspergilloma in lung, current therapeutic approaches include conservative management and surgical resection.[94-96]

REFERENCES

1. Segal BH. Aspergillosis. N Engl J Med. 2009;360(18):1870-84.
2. Donoghue M, Seibel NL, Fracis PS, Walsh TJ. Fungal infections of the respiratory tract. Anaissis EJ, McGinnis MR, Pfaller MA (Eds). Clinical Mycology, 2nd edition. New York: Churchill Livingston/Elsevier; 2009. pp. 561-89.
3. Pagano L, Caira M, Picardi M, Candoni A, Melillo L, Fianchi L, et al. Invasive Aspergillosis in patients with acute leukemia: update on morbidity and mortality—SEIFEM-C report. Clin Infect Dis. 2007;44(11):1524-5.
4. Upton A, Kirby KA, Carpenter P, Boeckh M, Marr KA. Invasive aspergillosis following hematopoietic cell transplantation: outcomes and prognostic factors associated with mortality. Clin Infect Dis. 2007;44(4):531-40.
5. Maertens J, Meersseman W, Van Bleyenbergh P. New therapies for fungal pneumonia. Curr Opin Infect Dis. 2009;22(2):183-90.
6. Chakrabarti A, Chatterjee SS, Shivaprakash MR. Overview of opportunistic fungal infections in India. Nippon Ishinkin Gakkai Zasshi. 2008;49(3):165-72.
7. Greene R. The radiological spectrum of pulmonary aspergillosis. Med Mycol. 2005;43(Suppl 1):S147-54.
8. Bassiri Jahromi S, Khaksar AA. Deep-seated fungal infections in immunocompromised patients in iran. Iran J Allergy Asthma Immunol. 2005;4(1):27-32.
9. Pound MW, Drew RH, Perfect JR. Recent advances in the epidemiology, prevention, diagnosis, and treatment of fungal pneumonia. Curr Opin Infect Dis. 2002;15(2):183-94.
10. Kubak BM. Fungal infection in lung transplantation. Transpl Infect Dis. 2002;4(Suppl 3):24-31.
11. Limper AH. The changing spectrum of fungal infections in pulmonary and critical care practice: clinical approach to diagnosis. Proc Am Thorac Soc. 2010;7(3):163-8.
12. Husain S. Unique characteristics of fungal infections in lung transplant recipients. Clin Chest Med. 2009;30(2):307-13.
13. Trof RJ, Beishuizen A, Debets-Ossenkopp YJ, Girbes AR, Groeneveld AB. Management of invasive pulmonary aspergillosis in non-neutropenic critically ill patients. Intensive Care Med. 2007;33(10):1694-703.
14. Samarakoon P, Soubani AO. Invasive pulmonary aspergillosis in patients with COPD: a report of five cases and systematic review of the literature. Chron Respir Dis. 2008;5(1):19-27.
15. Yan X, Li M, Jiang M, Zou LQ, Luo F, Jiang Y. Clinical characteristics of 45 patients with invasive pulmonary aspergillosis: retrospective analysis of 1711 lung cancer cases. Cancer. 2009;115(21):5018-25.
16. Segal BH, Walsh TJ. Current approaches to diagnosis and treatment of invasive aspergillosis. Am J Respir Crit Care Med. 2006;173(7):707-17.
17. Stergiopoulou T, Meletiadis J, Roilides E, Kleiner DE, Schaufele R, Roden M, et al. Host-dependent patterns of tissue injury in invasive pulmonary aspergillosis. Am J Clin Pathol. 2007;127(3):349-55.
18. Chakrabarti A, Das A, Mandal J, Shivaprakash MR, George VK, Tarai B, et al. The rising trend of invasive zygomycosis in patients with uncontrolled diabetes mellitus. Med Mycol 2006;44(4):335-42.
19. Al Refai M, Duhamel C, Le Rochais JP, Icard P. Lung scedosporiosis: a differential diagnosis of aspergillosis. Eur J Cardiothorac Surg. 2002;21(5):938-9.
20. Padhye AA, Kaufman L, Durry E, Banerjee CK, Jindal SK, Talwar P, et al. Fatal pulmonary sporotrichosis caused by *Sporothrix schenckii var. luriei* in India. J Clin Microbiol. 1992;30(9): 2492-4.

21. Antinori S, Nebuloni M, Magni C, Fasan M, Adorni F, Viola A, et al. Trends in the postmortem diagnosis of opportunistic invasive fungal infections in patients with AIDS: a retrospective study of 1,630 autopsies performed between 1984 and 2002. Am J Clin Pathol. 2009;132(2):221-7.
22. Lastoria C, Cascina A, Bini F, Matteo AD, Cavanna C, Farina C. Pulmonary *Cladophialophora boppi* infection in a lung transplant recipient: case report and literature review. J Heart Lung Transplant. 2009;28(6):635-7.
23. Agarwal R. Allergic bronchopulmonary aspergillosis. Chest. 2009;135(3):805-26.
24. Chakrabarti A, Sethi S, Raman DS, Behera D. Eight-year study of allergic bronchopulmonary aspergillosis in an Indian teaching hospital. Mycoses. 2002;45(8):295-9.
25. Greenberger PA. Clinical aspects of allergic bronchopulmonary aspergillosis. Front Biosci. 2003;8:S119-27.
26. Agarwal R, Gupta D, Aggarwal AN, Behera D, Jindal SK. Allergic bronchopulmonary aspergillosis: lessons from 126 patients attending a chest clinic in north India. Chest. 2006;130(2):442-8.
27. Chakrabarti A, Das A, Panda NK. Controversies surrounding the categorization of fungal sinusitis. Med Mycol. 2009;47(Suppl 1):S299-308.
28. Robson JM, Hogan PG, Benn RA, Gatenby PA. Allergic fungal sinusitis presenting as a paranasal sinus tumour. Aust NZJ Med. 1989;19(4):351-3.
29. Chakrabarti A, Denning DW, Ferguson BJ, Ponikau J, Buzina W, Kita H, et al. Fungal rhinosinusitis: a categorization and definitional schema addressing current controversies. Laryngoscope. 2009;119(9):1809-18.
30. Bent JP, Kuhn FA. Diagnosis of allergic fungal sinusitis. Otolaryngol Head Neck Surg. 1994;111(5):580-8.
31. Ferguson BJ. Eosinophilic mucin rhinosinusitis: a distinct clinicopathological entity. Laryngoscope. 2000;110(5 Pt 1):799-813.
32. Ponikau JU, Sherris DA, Kern EB, Homburger HA, Frigas E, Gaffey TA, et al. The diagnosis and incidence of allergic fungal sinusitis. Mayo Clin Proc. 1999;74(9):877-84.
33. Ponikau JU, Sherris DA, Kephart GM, Kern EB, Congdon DJ, Adolphson CR, et al. Striking deposition of toxic eosinophil major basic protein in mucus: implications for chronic rhinosinusitis. J Allergy Clin Immunol. 2005;116(2):362-9.
34. Hope WW, Walsh TJ, Denning DW. The invasive and saprophytic syndromes due to *Aspergillus* spp. Med Mycol. 2005;43(Suppl 1):S207-38.
35. Cornillet A, Camus C, Nimubona S, Gandemer V, Tattevin P, Belleguic C, et al. Comparison of epidemiological, clinical, and biological features of invasive aspergillosis in neutropenic and non-neutropenic patients: a 6-year survey. Clin Infect Dis. 2006;43(5):577-84.
36. Sinko J, Csomor J, Nikolova R, Lueff S, Kriván G, Reményi P, et al. Invasive fungal disease in allogeneic hematopoietic stem cell transplant recipients: an autopsy-driven survey. Transpl Infect Dis. 2008;10(2):106-9.
37. George B, Mathews V, Srivastava A, Chandy M. Infections among allogeneic bone marrow transplant recipients in India. Bone Marrow Transplant. 2004;33(3):311-5.
38. Sridhar H, Jayshree RS, Bapsy PP, Appaji L, Navin Kumar M, Shafiulla M, et al. Invasive aspergillosis in cancer. Mycoses. 2002;45(9-10):358-63.
39. Carvalho-Dias VM, Sola CB, Cunha CA, Shimakura SE, Pasquini R, Queiroz-Telles F. Invasive aspergillosis in hematopoietic stem cell transplant recipients: a retrospective analysis. Braz J Infect Dis. 2008;12(5):385-9.
40. Ozcan D, Gulec AT, Haberal M. Multiple subcutaneous nodules leading to the diagnosis of pulmonary aspergillosis in a renal transplant recipient. Clin Transplant. 2008;22(1):120-3.
41. Kiertiburanakul S, Thibbadee C, Santanirand P. Invasive aspergillosis in a tertiary-care hospital in Thailand. J Med Assoc Thai. 2007;90(5):895-902.
42. Tomashefski JF, Butler T, Islam M. Histopathology and etiology of childhood pneumonia: an autopsy study of 93 patients in Bangladesh. Pathology. 1989;21(2):71-8.
43. Vaideeswar P, Prasad S, Deshpande, Pandit SP. Invasive pulmonary aspergillosis: a study of 39 cases at autopsy. J Postgrad Med. 2004;50(1):21-6.
44. Kumar AA, Shantha GP, Jeyachandran V, Rajkumar K, Natesan S, Srinivasan D, et al. Multidrug resistant tuberculosis co-existing with aspergilloma and invasive aspergillosis in a 50- year old diabetic woman: a case report. Cases J. 2008; 1(1):303.
45. Kuruvilla S, Saldanha R, Joseph LD. Recurrent respiratory papillomatosis complicated by aspergillosis: a case report with review of literature. J Postgrad Med. 2008;54(1):32-4.
46. Martinez R, Castro G, Machado AA, Moya MJ. Primary aspergilloma and subacute invasive aspergillosis in two AIDS patients. Rev Inst Med Trop Sao Paulo. 2009;51(1):49-52.
47. Rojas-Serrano J, Pedroza J, Regalado J, Robledo J, Reyes E, Sifuentes-Osornio J, et al. High prevalence of infections in patients with systemic lupus erythematosus and pulmonary haemorrhage. Lupus. 2008;17(4):295-9.
48. Su T, Li HC, Chen M, Gao L, Zhou FD, Wang RG, et al. Invasive pulmonary aspergillosis in patients with antineutrophil cytoplasmic antibody associated vasculitis. J Clin Rheumatol. 2009;15(8):380-2.
49. Wu N, Huang Y, Li Q, Bai C, Huang HD, Yao XP. Isolated invasive Aspergillus tracheobronchitis: a clinical study of 19 cases. Clin Microbiol Infect. 2010;16(6):689-95.
50. Chakrabarti A, Das A, Sharma A, Panda N, Das S, Gupta KL, et al. Ten years' experience in zygomycosis at a tertiary care centre in India. J Infect. 2001;42(4):261-6.
51. Meis JF, Chakrabarti A. Changing epidemiology of an emerging infection: zygomycosis. Clin Microbiol Infect. 2009;15(Suppl 5):10-4.
52. Chakrabarti A, Chatterjee SS, Das A, Panda N, Shivaprakash MR, Kaur A, et al. Invasive zygomycosis in India: experience in a tertiary care hospital. Postgrad Med J. 2009;85(1009):573-81.
53. Chakrabarti A, Marak RS, Shivaprakash MR, Gupta S, Garg R, Sakhuja V, et al. Cavitary pulmonary zygomycosis caused by *Rhizopus homothallicus*. J Clin Microbiol. 2010;48(5):1965-9.
54. Martino P, Gastaldi R, Raccah R, Girmenia C. Clinical patterns of Fusarium infections in immunocompromised patients. J Infect. 1994;28(Suppl 1):7-15.
55. Cortez KJ, Roilides E, Quiroz-Telles F, Meletiadis J, Antachopoulos C, Knudsen T, et al. Infections caused by *Scedosporium* spp. Clin Microbiol Rev. 2008;21(1):157-97.
56. Ranjana KH, Priyokumar K, Singh TJ, Gupta ChC, Sharmila L, Singh PN, et al. Disseminated *Penicillium marneffei* infection among HIV-infected patients in Manipur state, India. J Infect. 2002;45(4):268-71.

57. Duong TA. Infection due to *Penicillium marneffei*, an emerging pathogen: review of 155 reported cases. Clin Infect Dis. 1996;23(1):125-30.
58. Supparatpinyo K, Khamwan C, Baosoung V, Nelson KE, Sirisanthana T. Disseminated *Penicillium marneffei* infection in southeast Asia. Lancet. 1994;344(8915):110-3.
59. Randhawa HS, Khan ZU. Histoplasmosis in India: current status. Indian J Chest Dis Allied Sci. 1994;36(4):193-213.
60. Wang TL, Cheah JS, Holmberg K. Case report and review of disseminated histoplasmosis in South-East Asia: clinical and epidemiological implications. Trop Med Int Health. 1996;1(1):35-42.
61. Randhawa HS, Khan ZU, Gaur SN. *Blastomyces dermatitidis* in India: first report of its isolation from clinical material. Sabouraudia. 1983;21(3):215-21.
62. Bharucha NE, Ramamoorthy K, Sorabjee J, Kuruvilla T. All that caseates is not tuberculosis. Lancet. 1996;348(9037):1313.
63. Kamei K, Sano A, Kikuchi K, Makimura K, Niimi M, Suzuki K, et al. The trend of imported mycoses in Japan. J Infect Chemother. 2003;9(1):16-20.
64. Mootsikapun P, Srikulbutr S. Histoplasmosis and penicilliosis: comparison of clinical features, laboratory findings and outcome. Int J Infect Dis. 2006;10(1):66-71.
65. Wong SS, Wong KH, Hui WT, Lee SS, Lo JY, Cao L, et al. Differences in clinical and laboratory diagnostic characteristics of *Penicilliosis marneffei* in human immunodeficiency virus (HIV)- and non-HIV-infected patients. J Clin Microbiol. 2001;39(12):4535-40.
66. Singh N, Alexander BD, Lortholary O, Dromer F, Gupta KL, John GT, et al. Pulmonary cryptococcosis in solid organ transplant recipients: clinical relevance of serum cryptococcal antigen. Clin Infect Dis. 2008;46(2):e12-8.
67. Wong ML, Back P, Candy G, Nelson G, Murray J. Cryptococcal pneumonia in African miners at autopsy. Int J Tuberc Lung Dis. 2007;11(5):528-33.
68. Pasqualotto AC. *Candida* and the paediatric lung. Paediatr Respir Rev. 2009;10(4):186-91.
69. Limper AH, Offord KP, Smith TF, Martin WJ. *Pneumocystis carinii* pneumonia. Differences in lung parasite number and inflammation in patients with and without AIDS. Am Rev Respir Dis. 1989;140(5):1204-9.
70. Thomas CF, Limper AH. *Pneumocystis pneumonia.* N Engl J Med. 2004;350(24):2487-98.
71. Curtis JR, Yarnold PR, Schwartz DN, Weinstein RA, Bennett CL. Improvements in outcomes of acute respiratory failure for patients with human immunodeficiency virus-related *Pneumocystis carinii* pneumonia. Am J Respir Crit Care Med. 2000;162(2 Pt 1):393-8.
72. Kovacs JA, Ng VL, Masur H, Leoung G, Hadley WK, Evans G, et al. Diagnosis of *Pneumocystis carinii* pneumonia: improved detection in sputum with use of monoclonal antibodies. N Engl J Med. 1988;318(10):589-93.
73. Armbruster C, Pokieser L, Hassl A. Diagnosis of *Pneumocystis carinii* pneumonia by bronchoalveolar lavage in AIDS patients. Comparison of Diff-Quik, fungifluor stain, direct immunofluorescence test and polymerase chain reaction. Acta Cytol. 1995;39(6):1089-93.
74. De Pauw B, Walsh TJ, Donnelly JP, Stevens DA, Edwards JE, Calandra T, et al. Revised definitions of invasive fungal disease from the European Organization for Research and Treatment of Cancer/Invasive Fungal Infections Cooperative Group and the National Institute of Allergy and Infectious Diseases Mycoses Study Group (EORTC/MSG) Consensus Group. Clin Infect Dis. 2008;46(12):1813-21.
75. Meersseman W, Lagrou K, Maertens J, Wilmer A, Hermans G, Vanderschueren S, et al. Galactomannan in bronchoalveolar lavage fluid: a tool for diagnosing aspergillosis in intensive care unit patients. Am J Respir Crit Care Med. 2008;177(1):27-34.
76. Senn L, Robinson JO, Schmidt S, Knaup M, Asahi N, Satomura S, et al. 1,3-Beta-D-glucan antigenemia for early diagnosis of invasive fungal infections in neutropenic patients with acute leukemia. Clin Infect Dis. 2008;46(6):878-85.
77. Mennink-Kersten MA, Warris A, Verweij PE. 1,3-beta-D-glucan in patients receiving intravenous amoxicillin-clavulanic acid. N Engl J Med. 2006;354(26):2834-5.
78. Pickering JW, Sant HW, Bowles CA, Roberts WL, Woods GL. Evaluation of a (1→3)-beta-D-glucan assay for diagnosis of invasive fungal infections. J Clin Microbiol. 2005;43(12):5957-62.
79. Lass-Florl C, Resch G, Nachbaur D, Mayr A, Gastl G, Auberger J, et al The value of computed tomography-guided percutaneous lung biopsy for diagnosis of invasive fungal infection in immunocompromised patients. Clin Infect Dis. 2007;45(7):e101-4.
80. Wheat LJ, Kohler RB, Tewari RP. Diagnosis of disseminated histoplasmosis by detection of Histoplasma capsulatum antigen in serum and urine specimens. N Engl J Med. 1986;314(2):83-8.
81. Snelders E, van der Lee HA, Kuijpers J, Rijs AJ, Varga J, Samson RA, et al. Emergence of azole resistance in *Aspergillus fumigatus* and spread of a single resistance mechanism. PLoS Med. 2008;5(11):e219.
82. Cornely OA, Maertens J, Bresnik M, Ebrahimi R, Ullmann AJ, Bouza E, et al. Liposomal amphotericin B as initial therapy for invasive mold infection: a randomized trial comparing a high-loading dose regimen with standard dosing (AmBiLoad trial). Clin Infect Dis. 2007;44(10):1289-97.
83. Walsh TJ, Anaissie EJ, Denning DW, Herbrecht R, Kontoyiannis DP, Marr KA, et al. Treatment of aspergillosis: clinical practice guidelines of the Infectious Diseases Society of America. Clin Infect Dis. 2008;46(3):327-60.
84. Perfect JR, Marr KA, Walsh TJ, Greenberg RN, DuPont B, de la Torre-Cisneros J, et al. Voriconazole treatment for less-common, emerging, or refractory fungal infections. Clin Infect Dis. 2003;36(9):1122-31.
85. Gonzalez GM, Tijerina R, Najvar LK, Bocanegra R, Rinaldi MG, Loebenberg D, et al. Activity of posaconazole against *Pseudallescheria boydii:* in vitro and in vivo assays. Antimicrob Agents Chemother. 2003;47(4):1436-8.
86. Raad, II, Hachem RY, Herbrecht R, Graybill JR, Hare R, Corcoran G, et al. Posaconazole as salvage treatment for invasive fusariosis in patients with underlying hematologic malignancy and other conditions. Clin Infect Dis. 2006;42(10):1398-403.
87. Petrikkos G, Skiada A. Recent advances in antifungal chemotherapy. Int J Antimicrob Agents. 2007;30(2):108-17.
88. Tucker RM, Williams PL, Arathoon EG, Stevens DA. Treatment of mycoses with itraconazole. Ann N Y Acad Sci. 1988;544:451-70.
89. Kauffman CA. Histoplasmosis: a clinical and laboratory update. Clin Microbiol Rev. 2007;20(1):115-32.
90. Dismukes WE, Bradsher RW, Cloud GC, Kauffman CA, Chapman SW, George RB, et al. Itraconazole therapy for

blastomycosis and histoplasmosis. NIAID Mycoses Study Group. Am J Med. 1992;93(5):489-97.

91. Sirisanthana T, Supparatpinyo K, Perriens J, Nelson KE. Amphotericin B and itraconazole for treatment of disseminated *Penicillium marneffei* infection in human immunodeficiency virus-infected patients. Clin Infect Dis. 1998;26(5):1107-10.
92. Yamada H, Kotaki H, Takahashi T. Recommendations for the treatment of fungal pneumonias. Expert Opin Pharmacother. 2003;4(8):1241-58.
93. Powderly WG, Saag MS, Cloud GA, Robinson P, Meyer RD, Jacobson JM, et al. A controlled trial of fluconazole or amphotericin B to prevent relapse of cryptococcal meningitis in patients with the acquired immunodeficiency syndrome. The NIAID AIDS Clinical Trials Group and Mycoses Study Group. N Engl J Med. 1992;326(12):793-8.
94. Rains BM, Mineck CW. Treatment of allergic fungal sinusitis with high-dose itraconazole. Am J Rhinol. 2003;17(1):1-8.
95. Chen JC, Chang YL, Luh SP, Lee JM, Lee YC. Surgical treatment for pulmonary aspergilloma: a 28-year experience. Thorax. 1997;52(9):810-3.
96. Rupa V, Jacob M, Mathews MS, Seshadri MS. A prospective, randomised, placebo-controlled trial of postoperative oral steroid in allergic fungal sinusitis. Eur Arch Otorhinolaryngol. 2010;267(2):233-8.

49

Chapter

Pulmonary Mycetoma

Alladi Mohan, B Vijayalakshmi Devi, Abha Chandra

INTRODUCTION

The genus *Aspergillus* includes saprophytic, ubiquitous, soil-dwelling organisms that are found in organic debris, dust, compost, foods, and damp areas such as basements.[1] While there are close to 200 species of *Aspergillus*, only a few are known to cause disease in humans. Among these, *Aspergillus fumigatus* is responsible for nearly 90% of all human infections. Several other important species that cause human disease include *Aspergillus flavus*, and *Aspergillus niger*. Rarely, species such as, *Aspergillus terreus*, *Aspergillus clavatus*, *Aspergillus niveus*, *Aspergillus nidulans*, among others, have been implicated in the causation of human disease.[2-5]

PATHOGENESIS

Aspergillus grows at 15–53 °C and can thrive in the human respiratory tract. It is a spore-forming fungus with septate dichotomous branching hyphae. These hyphae branch at an acute angle and contain conidiophores which harbor hundreds of conidia or spores. The spores are easily dispersed by air currents or physical contact.[1-3,6]

Aspergillus infection is usually acquired from an inanimate reservoir by the inhalation of airborne spores and these spores are common inhabitants of the airway. Even though humans may daily inhale hundreds of spores, only some develop disease from *Aspergillus* manifesting as a variety of clinical syndromes. In immunocompetent individuals, inhalation of conidia rarely has any adverse effect as the conidia are eliminated efficiently by innate immune mechanisms. Inhalation of airborne spores by immunocompromised hosts may cause fatal life-threatening infection. Clinically, aspergillosis has been classically defined as invasive, saprophytic, or allergic.[2] In saprophytic aspergillosis, the fungus, without invading normal pulmonary tissue, can remain quiescent and grow for months or even years.

The various manifestations of saprophytic aspergillosis include airway colonization; pulmonary mycetoma; and invasion of necrotic tissue. Pulmonary mycetoma (aspergilloma), a saprophytic manifestation of aspergillosis, usually develops in a pre-existing cavity in the lung and is the most common and best recognized form of pulmonary involvement due to *Aspergillus*. Impairment or absence of normal mucociliary clearance mechanisms in a cavity may facilitate adherence and germination of fungal conidia resulting in the formation of a pulmonary mycetoma. Some workers have also postulated that inflammatory reaction in the cavity and the ensuing secretion of toxins, enzymes and other mediators of inflammation may facilitate creation or advancement of a cavity.[7]

Pulmonary mycetomas have been most commonly reported in cavities of pulmonary tuberculosis. They have also been described in other lung diseases associated with cavity formation **(Table 1)**.[2-5,8-14] There have been case reports from India of pulmonary aspergilloma occurring in a hydatid cavity[15] and in patients with cavitary sarcoidosis.[16]

Table 1 Cavitary lung diseases complicated by pulmonary mycetoma[2,5,8-14]

- *Infections:*
  - Tuberculosis
  - Sarcoidosis
  - Bronchiectasis
  - Suppurative lung disease (lung abscess)
  - Hydatid cyst
  - Paragonimiasis
  - *Pneumocystis jiroveci* pneumonia
  - Cavities of other fungal infections
- *Cystic lung disease:*
  - Lung sequestration
  - Bronchial cysts
  - Bullous lung disease
- *Others:*
  - Pulmonary neoplasms
  - Ankylosing spondylitis
  - Cystic fibrosis

Table 2 Comparison of characteristics of simple aspergilloma and chronic cavitary pulmonary aspergillosis

Variable	*Simple pulmonary aspergilloma*	*Chronic cavitary pulmonary aspergillosis (complex aspergilloma)*
Clinical symptoms	None or minimal	Significant pulmonary and systemic symptoms
Host immunity	Not immunocompromised	Not immunocompromised or the immunocompromised state has remitted or is trivial
Radiographic findings	Single pulmonary cavity containing a fungal ball	One or more pulmonary cavities which may or may not contain a fungal ball
Serological/microbiological evidence of infection with *Aspergillus* species	Yes	Yes
Progression of disease	No radiological Progression over at least 3 months of observation	Radiological progression (new cavities, increasing pericavity infiltrates or increasing fibrosis) is evident over at least 3 months of observation. Hyphae are found in the cavity, but the wall of the cavity is composed of chronic inflammatory cells and fibrosis, but not tissue invasion. In some patients, a strong pleural/pulmonary fibrosis may result in chronic fibrosing pulmonary aspergillosis

Source: Denning DW, Riniotis K, Dobrashian R, Sambatakou H. Chronic cavitary and fibrosing pulmonary and pleural aspergillosis: case series, proposed nomenclature change, and review. Clin Infect Dis. 2003;37(Suppl 3):S265-80.

PATHOLOGY

Pulmonary mycetomas grow in areas of devitalized lung, such as a cavity, damaged bronchial tree, or a pulmonary cyst. Aspergillomas have been described in cavities in the lung parenchyma, bronchi and pleura. They consist of masses of living and dead fungal mycelia, inflammatory cells, fibrin, mucus, other blood products and tissue debris, are solid fragmented only with force.[2-5] Tissue invasion by the fungus does not occur in pulmonary mycetoma. Inadequate drainage is thought to facilitate the growth of *Aspergillus* on the walls of these cavities.[2]

Earlier, aspergillomas were classified as "simple" and "complex" aspergillomas.[17] "Simple aspergillomas" develop in isolated thin-walled cysts of bronchial origin, there is little or no abnormality in the surrounding lung and the cyst wall itself is usually lined by ciliated epithelium. "Complex aspergillomas" develop in cavities with gross disease in the surrounding lung tissue.[17]

Recently, aspergillomas have been classified as "simple" and "chronic cavitary pulmonary aspergillosis."[18] "Simple aspergillomas" are encased by thin-walled cysts with little surrounding parenchymal disease. "Chronic cavitary pulmonary aspergillosis" is associated with thick walls, multiple cavities (that may or may not contain fungal balls), and surrounding parenchymal changes **(Table 2)**.[18]

Natural History

In the majority of cases, the aspergilloma remains stable, but in up to 10% of cases the lesion may decrease in size or resolve spontaneously without treatment.[2,3,19] Rarely, progressive enlargement of a single thin-walled cavity may occur slowly over months or rapidly within weeks. These patients have minor or moderate degrees of immune dysfunction, such as, diabetes mellitus or corticosteroid use. This entity has been called "chronic necrotizing pulmonary aspergillosis (subacute invasive aspergillosis)".[18] Although aspergillomas are often thought of as benign saprophytic colonizations of the lung with *Aspergillus*, invasive pulmonary aspergillosis may develop from an aspergilloma and may be often fatal.[20]

Table 3 Causes of hemoptysis in patients with aspergilloma

- Mechanical friction of the blood vessels in the cavity wall by the moving fungal ball
- Local invasion of blood vessels lining the cavity
- Endotoxins released by the fungus with hemolytic properties
- Release of trypsin like proteolytic enzymes
- Type III (antigen-antibody) hypersensitivity reaction resulting in injury to cavity wall and hemorrhage

CLINICAL PRESENTATION

Patients may remain asymptomatic for several years, and the pulmonary mycetoma may be evident as an incidental finding on radiographic studies carried out for some other purpose.[2-5] Symptomatic patients with simple pulmonary aspergilloma commonly present with hemoptysis. The source of hemoptysis is usually the bronchial artery;[2,3] rarely anastomotic plexus between pulmonary and bronchial arteries[21] has been implicated. The various causes of hemoptysis in patients with pulmonary mycetoma are listed in **Table 3**. Hemoptysis is described in 69% to 91% of patients in some of the recently published studies.[11,22,23] In a series published from India,[21,24,25] this figure ranged from 65% to

Table 4 Clinical presentation and radiological features in pulmonary aspergilloma documented in studies from India

Variable	*Akbari, et al.*[24]	*Pratap, et al.*[25]	*Shah, et al.*[21]
• Place of study	Thiruvananthapuram, Kerala	New Delhi	Mumbai, Maharashtra
• Year of publication	2005	2007	2008
• No. of patients	60	72	41
• Male: female	36:24	47:25	25:16
• Age (years)	Mean 42.7 ± 11.8	Mean 32	Range 16–65*
• Predisposing conditions (%)			
– Tuberculosis	45	85	76
– Bronchiectasis	28	13	15
– Lung abscess	12	02	07
– No associated pathology	08	ND	02
• Others	05†	ND	ND
• Salient clinical manifestations (%)			
– Hemoptysis	93	65	85
– Dyspnea	22	11	32
– Cough	60	24	68
– Chest pain	07	11	12
– Weight loss	07	ND	05
– Fever	ND	11	24
• Type of aspergilloma (%)			
– Simple aspergilloma	23	11	02
– Complex aspergilloma	77	89	98
• Radiological manifestations			
– Location (%)			
– Right upper lobe	50		ND
– Left upper lobe	35		ND
– Right middle lobe	03		ND
– Right lower lobe	05		ND
– Destroyed right lung	ND		ND
– Destroyed left lung	ND		ND
• Multiple	07		ND
• Other findings (%)	Cavity(40) Opacity (37) Infiltrate (05) Cyst (07) Nodule (02) Mass (10)	Cavity with aspergilloma (58) Destroyed one lung (29) Localized bronchiectasis (13)	Cavity with aspergilloma (54)‡ Only cavity (09)‡ Destroyed one lung (09)‡ Bronchiectasis (09)‡ Mass (03)‡

All values corrected to the nearest round figure.
*21 patients were in 4th decade of life.
†Acute lymphatic leukemia, chronic infiltrates, carcinoma in situ in 1 patient each.
‡Described in 32 patients.
Abbreviation: ND, not described

93% **(Table 4)**. The severity of hemoptysis may range from mild to massive and life-threatening. In the series from India, massive hemoptysis requiring bronchial artery embolization/surgery was observed to be 7% to 18% patients.[21,24,25]

Other symptoms include chronic cough and breathlessness **(Table 4)**. These symptoms may probably be due to the underlying lung disease. Expectoration of blackish-brown sputum (melanoptysis) has also been documented in patients with pulmonary aspergilloma.[26,27] Occasionally, fever and weight loss may be present which usually signify secondary bacterial infection.

Rare Manifestations

Coexistence of active pulmonary tuberculosis is uncommon in patients with pulmonary aspergilloma, but has rarely been documented.[28] The occurrence of pulmonary aspergilloma in patients with allergic bronchopulmonary aspergillosis is also uncommon.[29,30] Clinical presentation with pneumothorax has also been reported.[31]

Pulmonary Mycetoma in Special Situations

Human Immunodeficiency Virus Seropositive Individuals

Apart from occasional case reports of aspergilloma in HIV-infected individuals,[32-35] there have been few publications on pulmonary mycetoma in human immunodeficiency virus (HIV) seropositive individuals. In one series, 10 of the 25 patients with pulmonary aspergilloma were HIV-seropositive, 7 of the 10 HIV-seropositive patients had a history of pulmonary tuberculosis and 3 of them had a history of *Pneumocystis jiroveci* pneumonia (PCP).[12] Severe hemoptysis (>150 mL/day) occurred in 5 of 15 (33%) in the HIV-seronegative group compared with 1 of 10 (10%) of the HIV-seropositive group. Compared with HIV-seronegative individuals, disease progression occurred more frequently among the HIV-seropositive individuals with a CD4+ T-lymphocyte count <100/mm^3 (4/8, 50% vs 1/13, 8%; p = 0.05). Mortality was also higher among HIV-infected individuals (4/8, 50% vs 1/13,8%; p = 0.05).

Lung Transplant Recipients

Aspergillomas have been reported in two single-lung transplant recipients both of whom presented with hemoptysis.[36]

Neutropenic Patients

While invasive pulmonary aspergillosis has frequently been described in patients with neutropenia, the occurrence of pulmonary mycetoma has also been occasionally described.[37] Acute myeloid leukemia was the most common underlying diagnosis in these patients (17 of the 38 patients, 45%), hemoptysis occurred in nearly 50% of patients and the mortality was approximately 25%. As these pulmonary mycetomas did not develop in pre-existing lung cavities, but developed in necrotic lung tissue due to fungal invasion, the term "mycotic lung sequestration" was suggested for this condition.[36]

Considering the potential for progression of disease, immunosuppressed patients who have aspergilloma should be monitored closely for this complication.

DIAGNOSIS

The diagnosis of pulmonary mycetoma is usually established based on the clinical presentation and radiographic features, combined with serological or microbiologic evidence of infection with *Aspergillus* species.[6,38] In patients with past history of pulmonary tuberculosis presenting with hemoptysis, the possible differential diagnosis includes relapse, reactivation/reinfection tuberculosis, aspergilloma and scar carcinoma. The diagnostic work-up should include testing for ruling-out these causes.

Chest Radiograph

The chest radiograph is useful in demonstrating the presence of a pulmonary mycetoma. In a chest radiograph, aspergilloma appears as a mobile, spherical intracavitary mass that is separated from the cavity by an airspace that appears as an "air-crescent" in the periphery (*ball-in-hole appearance*) **(Figs 1A and B)**.[2-5,39] As these lesions usually develop in a pre-existing pulmonary tuberculosis cavity, the lesions are frequently found in the upper lobes.[40] After moving the patient from supine to prone position, a change in the position of the fungus ball can be demonstrated.[2-5,39] If the lesion is peripherally located, pleural fibrosis is frequently evident. The chest radiograph may also reveal the sequelae of the pre-existing lung disease.

Computed Tomography

Computed tomography (CT) is increasingly being used for the evaluation of patients with pulmonary mycetoma. The CT offers the advantages of facilitating better delineation of fungal ball and the air crescent and documenting the change in the position of the fungal ball **(Figs 2 and 3)**. The CT also facilitates detection of fungal balls that may not be discernible on chest radiograph. Coexistent lung disease, sequelae of previous lung disease can also be appreciated better on CT.[2-5]

DIFFERENTIAL DIAGNOSIS

Radiologically, aspergillomas must be differentiated from other causes like coccidioidal fungal ball seen in cavitary pulmonary disease due to coccidioidomycosis, pulmonary actinomycosis, nocardiosis, candidiasis, scedosporiosis [caused by the asexual (*Scedosporium apiospermum*) and/or sexual (*Pseudallescheria boydii*) forms] presenting as a fungal ball; hematoma; abscess; hydatid cyst; retained intrathoracic surgical swab (gossypiboma) and granulomatosis with polyangiitis [Wegener's granulomatosis]. However, aspergilloma may coexist with any of these conditions.[41-45] Rarely, lung cancer mimicking aspergilloma with the air-crescent sign, occurrence of aspergilloma within a malignant cavity have been documented. In one study,[43] the mural nodules within cavitating lung cancer were more enhanced and showed a nondependent location more frequently than those of intracavitary aspergillomas. The cavitary walls were significantly thicker in cavitating lung cancer (mean thickness 5.8 mm) than those in intracavitary aspergillomas (mean thickness 2.6 mm). Adjacent bronchiectasis and volume decrease of the involved lobe were observed more frequently in intracavitary aspergillomas than in cavitating lung cancers.

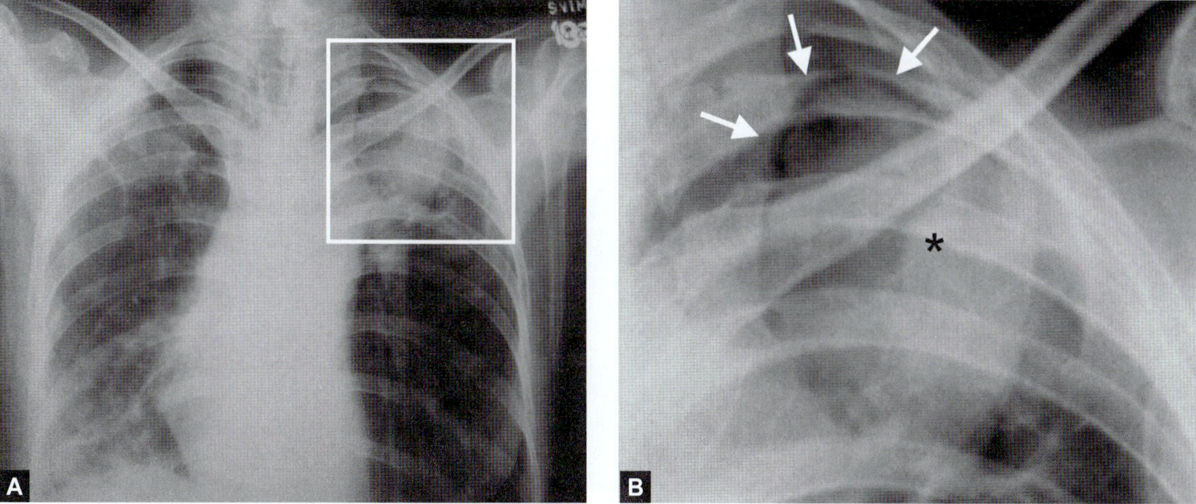

Figs 1A and B Chest radiograph (posteroanterior view) (A) of a patient with past history of pulmonary tuberculosis who presented with hemoptysis showing parenchymal infiltrates in both upper zones, fibrotic changes in right lower zone. In the left upper zone, a spherical intracavitary fungal ball that is separated from the cavity by an airspace that appears as an "air-crescent" in the periphery (square) can also be seen. Close-up view of the same (B) showing a intracavitary fungal ball (asterisk) that is separated from the cavity by an airspace that appears as an "air-crescent" in the periphery (arrows)

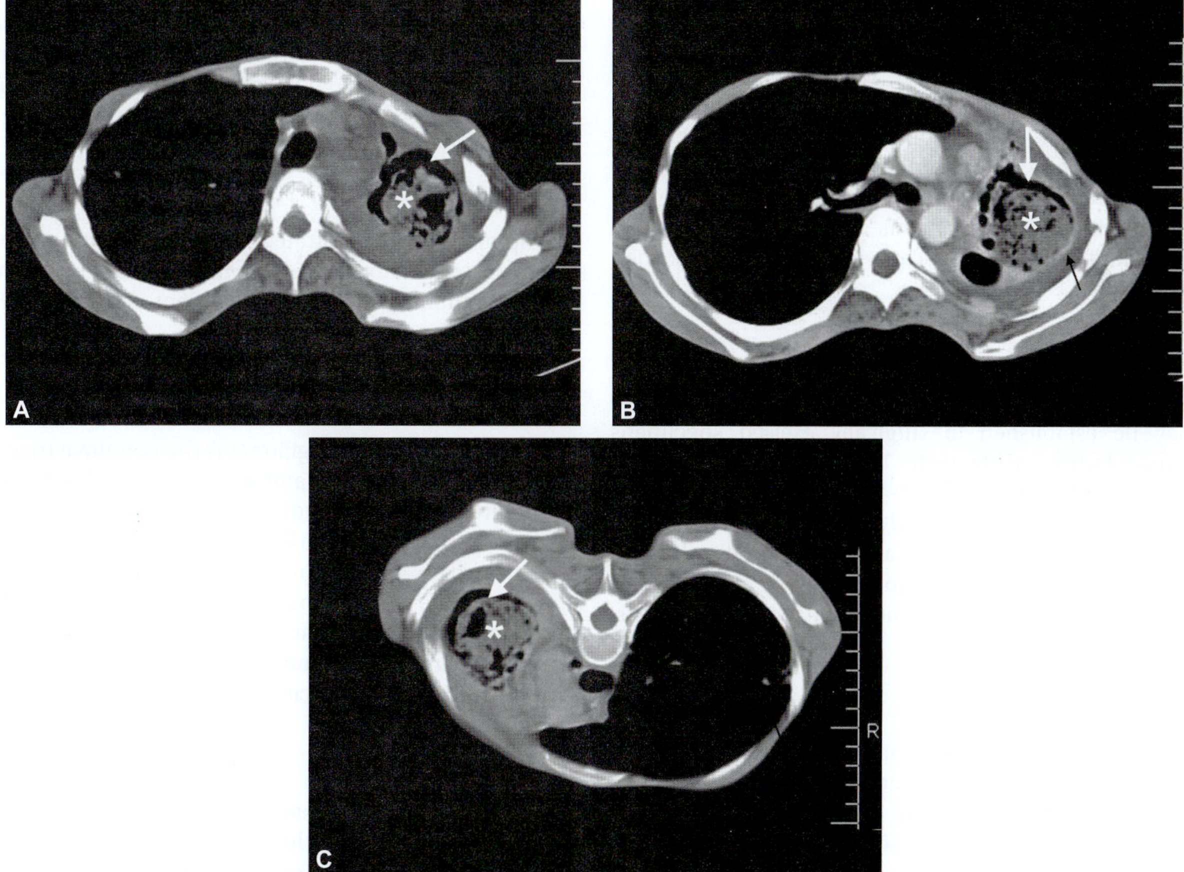

Figs 2A to C Computed tomography of the chest (plain study, mediastinal window) (A) and contrast-enhanced study (lung-window) (B) showing an intracavitary fungal ball (asterisk) that is separated from the cavity by an airspace that appears as an "air-crescent" in the periphery (white arrow); thickened pleura is also evident (black arrow). Contrast-enhanced computed tomography chest obtained after moving the patient from supine to prone position (C) shows a change in the position of the fungus ball (asterisk) and the air-crescent (arrow)

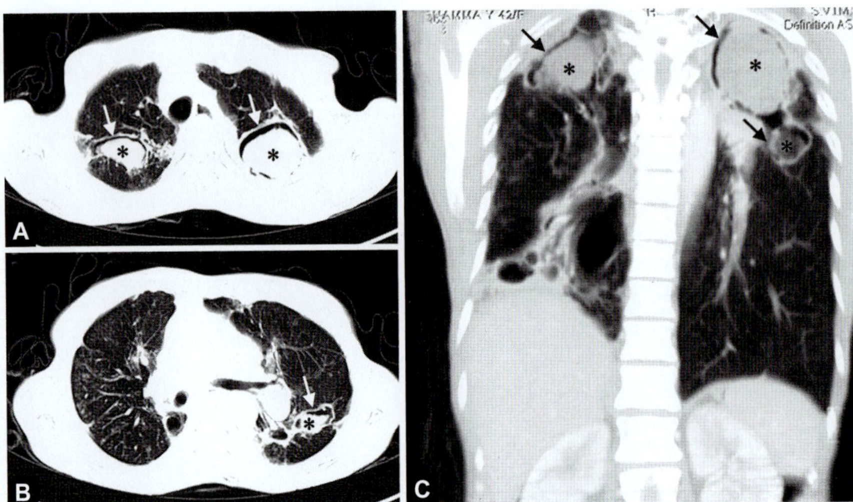

Figs 3A to C Contrast-enhanced computed tomography of the chest (A) of the same patient shown in Figure 1 showing complex pulmonary aspergillomas (asterisk) in both upper lobes and another aspergilloma in the left upper lobe; (B) air-crescent sign (arrow) is also evident. Coronal reconstruction (C) reveals the aspergillomas (asterisk), air-crescent sign (arrow) and fibrocavitary disease. The computed tomography was helpful in revealing several other details that were not discernible in the chest radiograph (Fig. 1)

Serological and Microbiological Methods

Sputum, bronchoalveolar lavage (BAL) fluid culture may reveal the presence of *Aspergillus* species in 50% of patients with pulmonary aspergilloma.[6,38] Serum precipitins [immunoglobulin G (IgG) antibodies] against *A. fumigatus* are usually positive in almost all cases; false-negative reports have been described in patients receiving corticosteroid treatment and in mycetomas caused by species other than *A. fumigatus*.[6,38]

Histopathology

Histopathological evidence of aspergilloma **(Figs 4A to C)** may be established in surgically excised specimens by demonstrating acute-angle branching, septate, non-pigmented hyphae measuring 2–4 μ in width that are best demonstrated with best detected by Gomori methenamine silver and periodic acid-Schiff stains.[6,38] *Aspergillus* hyphae are histopathologically difficult to distinguish from those of Fusarium species, *P. boydii,* agents of phaeohyphomycosis, among others.

Molecular Methods

Polymerase chain reaction (PCR) has been used for the diagnosis of pulmonary aspergilloma. The PCR amplification of Asp fl (18 kDa) and alkaline protease (33 kDa) antigens derived from *A. fumigatus* and implicated as possible virulence factors in the pathogenesis of *Aspergillus*-induced diseases has been found to be useful for the diagnosis of pulmonary aspergilloma.[46] In another study,[47] TacMAN-MGB probes, which covered the loci Gly54, Leu98, Gly138, and Met220 of the enzyme CYP51A coded by the gene CYP51A, as well as the 34-bp tandem repeated sequence in the promoter region (–288 and –322 from the start codon) of this gene, was useful in detecting itraconazole-resistant strains of *A. fumigatus*. These protocols need to be evaluated in the field setting.

TREATMENT

The optimal treatment strategy for patients with pulmonary mycetoma is unknown, there is no consensus regarding the choice or timing of therapy. Treatment aims at preventing life-threatening hemoptysis.

Surgery

Surgical removal of aspergilloma is the definitive treatment. In view of the morbidity and mortality associated with the procedure, it has to be used judiciously. As per the Infectious Disease Society of America (IDSA) guidelines[38] surgery is indicated as the definitive treatment in patients with episodes of life-threatening hemoptysis, and those who are at risk for such a complication, like patients with underlying sarcoidosis, immunocompromised patients, and those with increasing *Aspergillus* specific IgG titers.

Morbidity

Commonly observed postoperative complications include hemorrhage, incomplete lung re-expansion, prolonged air leak, empyema, and respiratory failure, wound infection, respiratory insufficiency, and chylothorax.[11,48-53] Various surgical procedures used in the treatment of pulmonary aspergilloma in two studies from India[24,25] and associated morbidity are shown in **Table 5**.

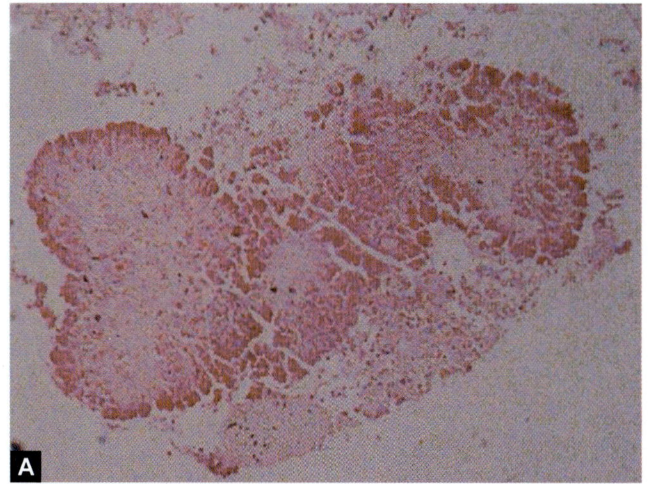

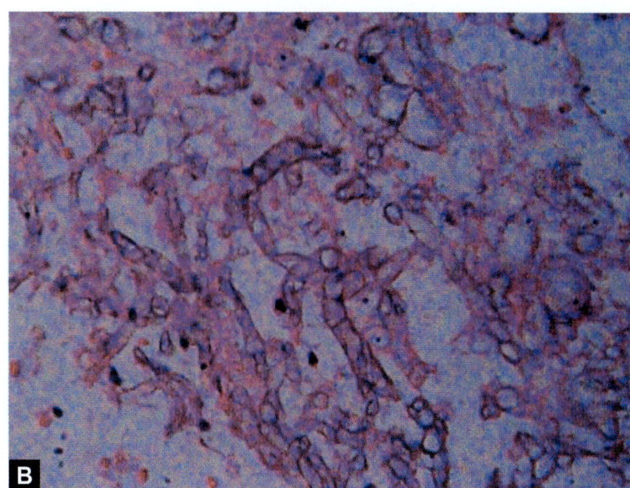

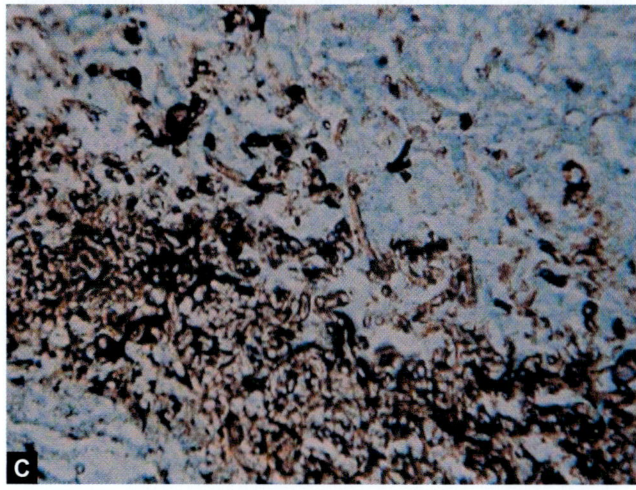

Figs 4A to C (A) Photomicrograph of a surgically excised specimen showing an aspergilloma (Hematoxylin and eosin × 100); (B) under high power view acute-angle branching, septate, nonpigmented hyphae measuring 2–4 μ can be seen (hematoxylin and eosin × 400); (C) the fungal hyphae are better appreciated on Gomori-Methenamine silver staining (× 400)

Source: *Dr KV Sreedhar Babu, Department of Pathology, Sri Venkateswara Institute of Medical Sciences, Tirupati*

Table 5 Surgical treatment, complications and mortality documented in studies from India

Variable	*Akbari, et al.*[24]	*Pratap, et al.*[25]
Place of study	Thiruvananthapuram, Kerala	New Delhi
Year of publication	2005	2007
No. of patients	60	72
Treatment	Lobectomy (n = 55), pneumonectomy (n = 02), segmental resection (n = 02), and cavernoplasty (n = 02). One patient underwent bilateral lobectomy at 14 months interval	Pneumonectomy (n = 21); lobectomy (n = 51). In 10 of the right upper lobe lesions, bilobectomies were done by removing both the right upper and middle lobes, due to presence of adhesions
Morbidity*	12/46 complex aspergilloma patients (26%)	22/64 complex aspergilloma patients (34%)
Major complications*	Air-leak (>10 days) (n = 4), bleeding (n = 2), empyema (n = 4), respiratory problems (n = 1), wound dehiscence (n = 1)	Air-leak (>10 days) (n = 5), massive hemorrhage (n = 5), persistent pleural space (n = 3)
Mortality in complex pulmonary aspergilloma	02/46 (4%)	02/64 (3%)
Overall mortality (%)	02/60 (3%)	02/72 (3%)

All values corrected to the nearest round figure.
* Morbidity and mortality were observed only in patients with complex aspergilloma. Surgery was uneventful in patients with simple aspergilloma.

Mortality

Surgery for pulmonary aspergilloma was associated with a high mortality rate, ranging from 7% to 23% in earlier studies.[11,48-53] More recent data from nine published studies[54-61] (n = 456) reveal a cumulative mortality rate of 2.3%.[4] Surgical mortality has been reported to be less than 1% for simple aspergilloma.[2-5] In two large Indian studies, the overall mortality rate was 3% **(Table 4)**.[24,25] All deaths had occurred in patients with complex aspergilloma, the mortality ranged from 3% to 4% in this group of patients **(Table 4)**.

Aspergillomas do not result in life-threatening hemoptysis in a majority of the patients, the morbidity and the expense involved in the treatment must be weighed against the clinical benefits.[62] Asymptomatic patients with pulmonary mycetoma should be carefully followed for their life time as they have a potential for developing hemoptysis.

Bronchial Artery Embolization

Patients with life-threatening hemoptysis who require surgery would need to have adequate pulmonary function to undergo the operation. Several patients are sick and may not be fit to undergo major surgery. In this situation, bronchial artery embolization may be useful as a temporary life-saving procedure in patients with life-threatening hemoptysis. Unlike several other conditions where bronchial artery embolization produces more favorable outcome, the results have not been as promising for patients with aspergilloma.[63] In one study (n = 118), the only significant factor associated with re-bleeding 1 year after bronchial artery embolization was the presence of an aspergilloma (n = 32).[64] Presently, bronchial artery embolization is not considered to be a replacement for surgery, but, is recommended by the IDSA guidelines[38] as a short-term therapy to stabilize patients for more definitive treatment, including surgery.

Medical Treatment

The role of intravenously administered amphotericin B failed to show benefit in patients with aspergilloma.[65] Inhaled, intracavitary, and endobronchial instillation of antifungal agents has been tried with limited success for the treatment.[22,66,67] Percutaneous transthoracic intracavitary administration of amphotericin B under CT guidance has been found to be useful in patients with massive hemoptysis, with resolution of hemoptysis occurring within few days. While the results have been promising in some of the studies[62,68-70] simliar success was not documented in others.[71,72]

Itraconazole has a high tissue penetration, and significant itraconazole levels have been demonstrated within the cavity containing aspergilloma.[73] Oral itraconazole has been used with promising results with symptomatic and radiographic improvement being evident in half to two-thirds of patients; and a complete response in the occasional patient.[69-71,74] However, itraconazole works slowly and may not be useful in patients presenting with life-threatening hemoptysis.

According to the IDSA guidelines,[38] for patients with pulmonary aspergilloma, voriconazole [6 mg/kg intravenous (IV) every 12 hours for 1 day, followed by 4 mg/kg IV every 12 hours; oral dosage is 200 mg every 12 hours], or itraconazole (oral dosage 600 mg/day for 3 days, followed by 400 mg/day; parenteral dosage 200 mg every 12 hours IV for 2 days, followed by 200 mg daily thereafter) are advocated as the alternatives to surgery, advocated as the primary therapeutic strategy. For chronic cavitary pulmonary aspergilloma, these guidelines[38] indicate voriconazole and itraconazole as the primary therapy. Potential utility of therapy with interferon-gamma in pulmonary aspergilloma has occasionally been documented[18,38] and merits further study.

PROGNOSTIC FACTORS

Factors associated with poor prognosis in patients with aspergilloma include severe underlying lung disease, increasing size or number of lesions on imaging, presence of immunosuppression (including corticosteroid treatment), increasing *Aspergillus*-specific IgG titers, recurrent large-volume hemoptysis, and underlying sarcoidosis or HIV infection.[6]

OVERALL MORTALITY

Mortality in patients who have pulmonary aspergillomas has been reported as 5% to 6% per year.[4] In a retrospective study of 85 cases over 24 years, overall mortality over 10 years was 56%, with 10 deaths directly attributable to aspergillomas.[75] The age of the patients and underlying comorbid lung disease also seem to have a bearing on the mortality.

CONCLUSION

Pulmonary mycetomas most often develop in old tuberculosis cavities. Majority of patients with pulmonary mycetomas remain asymptomatic, the lesions may be picked up on a routine chest radiograph. Pulmonary aspergillomas are often noticed when patients present with life-threatening hemoptysis. Surgery is the preferred treatment of choice in fit patients. Bronchial artery embolization may be used to control bleeding as a temporary measure. Therapy with voriconazole and itraconazole appear to be useful. Asymptomatic patients should be carefully followed periodically for their lifetime, they have potential for developing life-threatening hemoptysis.

REFERENCES

1. Godet C, Philippe B, Laurent F, Cadranel J. Chronic pulmonary aspergillosis: an update on diagnosis and treatment. Respiration. 2014;88:162-74.
2. Kousha M, Tadi R, Soubani AO. Pulmonary aspergillosis: a clinical review. Eur Respir Rev. 2011;20:156-74.

3. Izumikawa K. Recent advances in chronic pulmonary aspergillosis. Respir Investig. 2016;54:85-91.
4. Passera E, Rizzi A, Robustellini M, Rossi G, Della Pona C, Massera F, et al. Pulmonary aspergilloma: clinical aspects and surgical treatment outcome. Thorac Surg Clin. 2012;22:345-61.
5. Daly P, Kavanagh K. Pulmonary aspergillosis: clinical presentation, diagnosis and therapy. Br J Biomed Sci. 2001;58:197-205.
6. Stevens DA, Kan VL, Judson MA, Morrison VA, Dummer S, Denning DW, et al. Practice guidelines for diseases caused by Aspergillus. Infectious Diseases Society of America. Clin Infect Dis. 2000;30:696-709.
7. Fraser RS. Pulmonary aspergillosis: pathologic and pathogenetic features. Pathol Annu. 1993;28 Pt 1:231-77.
8. Hours S, Nunes H, Kambouchner M, Uzunhan Y, Brauner MW, Valeyre D, et al. Pulmonary cavitary sarcoidosis: clinico-radiologic characteristics and natural history of a rare form of sarcoidosis. Medicine (Baltimore). 2008;87:142-51.
9. Sarosi GA, Silberfarb PM, Saliba NA, Huggin PM, Tosh FE. Aspergillomas occurring in blastomycotic cavities. Am Rev Respir Dis. 1971;104:581-4.
10. Kawamura S, Maesaki S, Tomono K, Tashiro T, Kohno S. Clinical evaluation of 61 patients with pulmonary aspergilloma. Intern Med. 2000;39:209-12.
11. Chen JC, Chang YL, Luh SP, Lee JM, Lee YC. Surgical treatment for pulmonary aspergilloma: a 28-year experience. Thorax. 1997;52:810-3.
12. Addrizzo-Harris DJ, Harkin TJ, McGuinness G, Naidich DP, Rom WN. Pulmonary aspergilloma and AIDS. A comparison of HIV-infected and HIV-negative individuals. Chest 1997;111:612-8.
13. Maguire CP, Hayes JP, Hayes M, Masterson J, FitzGerald MX. Three cases of pulmonary aspergilloma in adult patients with cystic fibrosis. Thorax. 1995;50:805-6.
14. Logan M, McLoughlin R, Gibney RG. Aspergilloma complicating cystic fibrosis. AJR Am J Roentgenol. 1993;161:674-5.
15. John BV, Jacob M, Abraham OC, Thomas S, Thankachan R, Shukla V. Aspergilloma in a hydatid cavity. Trop Doct. 2007;37:112-4.
16. Hede J, Bahot R, Shah JR. Aspergilloma in sarcoidosis. Lung India. 2009;26:127-9.
17. Belcher JR, Plummer NS. Surgery in bronchopulmonary aspergillosis. Br J Dis Chest. 1960;54:335-41.
18. Denning DW, Riniotis K, Dobrashian R, Sambatakou H. Chronic cavitary and fibrosing pulmonary and pleural aspergillosis: case series, proposed nomenclature change, and review. Clin Infect Dis. 2003;37(Suppl 3):S265-80.
19. Gefter WB. The spectrum of pulmonary aspergillosis. J Thorac Imaging. 1992;7:56-74.
20. Tomee J, VanDerWerf T, Latge J, Koeter G, Dubois A, Kauffman H. Serologic monitoring of disease and treatment in a patient with pulmonary aspergilloma. Am J Respir Crit Care Med. 1995;151:199-204.
21. Shah R, Vaideeswar P, Pandit SP. Pathology of pulmonary aspergillomas. Indian J Pathol Microbiol. 2008;51:342-5.
22. Jewkes J, Kay PH, Paneth M, Citron KM. Pulmonary aspergilloma: analysis of prognosis in relation to haemoptysis and survey of treatment. Thorax 1983;38:572-8.
23. Aspergilloma and residual tuberculous cavities—the results of a resurvey. Tubercle. 1970;51:227-45.
24. Akbari JG, Varma PK, Neema PK, Menon MU, Neelakandhan KS. Clinical profile and surgical outcome for pulmonary aspergilloma: a single center experience. Ann Thorac Surg 2005;80:1067-72.
25. Pratap H, Dewan RK, Singh L, Gill S, Vaddadi S. Surgical treatment of pulmonary aspergilloma: a series of 72 cases. Indian J Chest Dis Allied Sci. 2007;49:23-7.
26. Haro M, Nuñez A, González G, Vizcaya M. Black sputum and progressive cavitary lung lesion in a coal miner. Chest. 1997; 111:808-9.
27. Korzeniowska-Koseła M, Halweg H, Bestry I, Podsiadło B, Krakówka P. Pulmonary aspergilloma caused by *Aspergillus niger*. Pneumonol Pol. 1990;58:328-33.
28. Kumar AA, Shantha GP, Jeyachandran V, Rajkumar K, Natesan S, Srinivasan D, et al. Multidrug resistant tuberculosis co-existing with aspergilloma and invasive aspergillosis in a 50-year-old diabetic woman: a case report. Cases J. 2008;1:303.
29. Agarwal AK, Bhagat R, Panchal N, Shah A. Allergic bronchopulmonary aspergillosis with aspergilloma mimicking fibrocavitary pulmonary tuberculosis. Asian Pac J Allergy Immunol. 1996;14:5-8.
30. Shah A, Khan ZU, Chaturvedi S, Ramchandran S, Randhawa HS, Jaggi OP. Allergic bronchopulmonary aspergillosis with coexistent aspergilloma: a long-term followup. J Asthma. 1989;26:109-15.
31. Baradkar VP, Mathur M, Kumar S. Uncommon presentation of pulmonary aspergilloma. Indian J Med Microbiol. 2009;27: 270-2.
32. Lombardo GT, Anandarao N, Lin CS, Abbate A, Becker WH. Fatal hemoptysis in a patient with AIDS-related complex and pulmonary aspergilloma. N Y State J Med. 1987;87:306-8.
33. Torrents C, Alvarez-Castells A, de Vera PV, Coll S, Solduga C, Puy R. Postpneumocystis aspergilloma in AIDS: CT features. J Comput Assist Tomogr. 1991;15:304-7.
34. Höhler T, Schnütgen M, Mayet WJ, Meyer zum Büschenfelde KH. Pulmonary aspergilloma in a patient with AIDS. Thorax 1995;50(3):312-3.
35. Keating JJ, Rogers T, Petrou M, Cartledge JD, Woodrow D, Nelson M, et al. Management of pulmonary aspergillosis in AIDS: an emerging clinical problem. J Clin Pathol. 1994;47: 805-9.
36. Westney GE, Kesten S, De Hoyos A, Chapparro C, Winton T, Maurer JR. Aspergillus infection in single and double lung transplant recipients. Transplantation. 1996;61:915-9.
37. Kibbler CC, Milkins SR, Bhamra A, Spiteri MA, Noone P, Prentice HG. Apparent pulmonary mycetoma following invasive aspergillosis in neutropenic patients. Thorax. 1988;43:108-12.
38. Walsh TJ, Anaissie EJ, Denning DW, Herbrecht R, Kontoyiannis DP, Marr KA, et al. Infectious Diseases Society of America. Treatment of aspergillosis: clinical practice guidelines of the Infectious Diseases Society of America. Clin Infect Dis. 2008;46:327-60.
39. Sharma SK, Mohan A. Case track series 1. Case report collection series. Pulmonary tuberculosis: Typical and atypical cases. Mumbai: Merind Ltd.; 1997.
40. Behera D. Complications of pulmonary tuberculosis. In: Sharma SK, Mohan A (Eds). Tuberculosis. 2nd edition. New Delhi: Jaypee Brothers Medical Publishers; 2009. p. 519-31.
41. Bandoh S, Fujita J, Fukunaga Y, Yokota K, Ueda Y, Okada H, et al. Cavitary lung cancer with an aspergilloma-like shadow. Lung Cancer. 1999;26:195-8.
42. Le Thi Huong D, Wechsler B, Chamuzeau JP, Bisson A, Godeau P. Pulmonary aspergilloma complicating Wegener's granulomatosis. Scand J Rheumatol. 1995;24:260.

43. Park Y, Kim TS, Yi CA, Cho EY, Kim H, Choi YS. Pulmonary cavitary mass containing a mural nodule: differential diagnosis between intracavitary aspergilloma and cavitating lung cancer on contrast-enhanced computed tomography. Clin Radiol. 2007;62:227-32.
44. Mir R, Singh VP. Retained intrathoracic surgical pack mimicking as recurrent aspergilloma. J Clin Diagn Res. 2012;6:1775-7.
45. Gazzoni FF, Severo LC, Marchiori E, Guimarães MD, Garcia TS, Irion KL, et al. Pulmonary diseases with imaging findings mimicking aspergilloma. Lung. 2014;192:347-57.
46. Urata T, Kobayashi M, Imamura J, Tanaka Y, Muneishi H, Iwahara Y, et al. Polymerase chain reaction amplification of Asp f I and alkaline protease genes from fungus balls: clinical application in pulmonary aspergillosis. Intern Med 1997;36:19-27.
47. Xu H, Chen W, Li L, Wan Z, Li R, Liu W. Clinical itraconazole-resistant strains of *Aspergillus fumigatus*, isolated serially from a lung aspergilloma patient with pulmonary tuberculosis, can be detected with real-time PCR method. Mycopathologia. 2010;169:193-9.
48. Aslam PA, Eastridge CE, Hughes FA. Aspergillosis of the lung—an eighteen-year experience. Chest. 1971;59:28-32.
49. Garvey J, Crastnopol P, Weisz D, Khan F. The surgical treatment of pulmonary aspergillomas. J Thorac Cardiovasc Surg. 1977;74:542-7.
50. Daly RC, Pairolero PC, Piehler JM, Trastek VF, Payne WS, Bernatz PE. Pulmonary aspergilloma. Results of surgical treatment. J Thorac Cardiovasc Surg. 1986;92:981-8.
51. Soltanzadeh H, Wychulis AR, Sadr F, Bolanowski PJ, Neville WE. Surgical treatment of pulmonary aspergilloma. Ann Surg. 1977;186:13-6.
52. Massard G, Roeslin N, Wihlm JM, Dumont P, Witz JP, Morand G. Pleuropulmonary aspergilloma: clinical spectrum and results of surgical treatment. Ann Thorac Surg. 1992;54:1159-64.
53. Kilman JW, Ahn C, Andrews NC, Klassen K. Surgery for pulmonary aspergillosis. J Thorac Cardiovasc Surg. 1969;57:642-7.
54. Brik A, Salem AM, Kamal AR, Abdel-Sadek M, Essa M, El Sharawy M, et al. Surgical outcome of pulmonary aspergilloma. Eur J Cardiothorac Surg. 2008;34:882-5.
55. Okubo K, Kobayashi M, Morikawa H, Hayatsu E, Ueno Y. Favorable acute and long-term outcomes after the resection of pulmonary aspergillomas. Thorac Cardiovasc Surg. 2007;55:108-11.
56. Endo S, Otani S, Tezuka Y, Tetsuka K, Tsubochi H, Hasegawa T, et al. Predictors of postoperative complications after radical resection for pulmonary aspergillosis. Surg Today. 2006;36:499-503.
57. Shiraishi Y, Katsuragi N, Nakajima Y, Hashizume M, Takahashi N, Miyasaka Y. Pneumonectomy for complex aspergilloma: is it still dangerous? Eur J Cardiothorac Surg. 2006;29:9-13.
58. Kim YT, Kang MC, Sung SW, Kim JH. Good long-term outcomes after surgical treatment of simple and complex pulmonary aspergilloma. Ann Thorac Surg. 2005;79:294-8.
59. Park CK, Jheon S. Results of surgical treatment for pulmonary aspergilloma. Eur J Cardiothorac Surg. 2002;21:918-23.
60. Babatasi G, Massetti M, Chapelier A, Fadel E, Macchiarini P, Khayat A, et al. Surgical treatment of pulmonary aspergilloma: current outcome. J Thorac Cardiovasc Surg. 2000;119:906-12.
61. Regnard JF, Icard P, Nicolosi M, Spagiarri L, Magdeleinat P, Jauffret B, et al. Aspergilloma: a series of 89 surgical cases. Ann Thorac Surg. 2000;69:898-903.
62. Moodley L, Pillay J, Dheda K. Aspergilloma and the surgeon. J Thorac Dis. 2014;6:202-9.
63. Kato A, Kudo S, Matsumoto K, Fukahori T, Shimizu T, Uchino A, et al. Bronchial artery embolization for hemoptysis due to benign diseases: immediate and long-term results. Cardiovasc Intervent Radiol. 2000;23:351-7.
64. Kim YG, Yoon HK, Ko GY, Lim CM, Kim WD, Koh Y. Long-term effect of bronchial artery embolization in Korean patients with haemoptysis. Respirology. 2006;11:776-81.
65. Hammerman KJ, Sarosi GA, Tosh FE. Amphotericin B in the treatment of saprophytic forms of pulmonary aspergillosis. Am Rev Respir Dis. 1974;109:57-62.
66. Yamada H, Kohno S, Koga H, Maesaki S, Kaku M. Topical treatment of pulmonary aspergilloma by antifungals. Relationship between duration of the disease and efficacy of therapy. Chest. 1993;103:1421-5.
67. Munk PL, Vellet AD, Rankin RN, Müller NL, Ahmad D. Intracavitary aspergilloma: transthoracic percutaneous injection of amphotericin gelatin solution. Radiology. 1993;188:821-3.
68. Klein JS, Fang K, Chang MC. Percutaneous transcatheter treatment of an intracavitary aspergilloma. Cardiovasc Intervent Radiol. 1993;16:321-4.
69. Campbell JH, Winter JH, Richardson MD, Shankland GS, Banham SW. Treatment of pulmonary aspergilloma with itraconazole. Thorax. 1991;46:839-41.
70. Dupont B. Itraconazole therapy in aspergillosis: study in 49 patients. J Am Acad Dermatol. 1990;23:607-14.
71. Impens N, De Greve J, De Beule K, Meysman M, De Beuckelaere S, Schandevyl W. Oral treatment with itraconazole of aspergilloma in cavitary lung cancer. Eur Respir J. 1990;3:837-9.
72. Caras WE, Pluss JL. Chronic necrotizing pulmonary aspergillosis: pathologic outcome after itraconazole therapy. Mayo Clin Proc. 1996;71:25-30.
73. Tsubura E. Multicenter clinical trial of itraconazole in the treatment of pulmonary aspergilloma. Pulmonary Aspergilloma Study Group. Kekkaku. 1997;72:557-64.
74. Agarwal R, Vishwanath G, Aggarwal AN, Garg M, Gupta D, Chakrabarti A. Itraconazole in chronic cavitary pulmonary aspergillosis: a randomised controlled trial and systematic review of literature. Mycoses. 2013;56:559-70.
75. Jewkes J, Kay PH, Paneth M, Citron KM. Pulmonary aspergilloma: analysis of prognosis in relation to haemoptysis and survey of treatment. Thorax. 1983;38:572-8.

Nosocomial Pneumonia

Vishwanath Gella, SK Jindal

INTRODUCTION

Nosocomial pneumonia is a significant problem worldwide. It is responsible for an increased mortality, morbidity, hospital stay and healthcare costs. Hospital-acquired pneumonia (HAP) is the second most common form of nosocomial infection. The burden of HAP is estimated at around 5–10 cases per 1,000 hospital admissions with a 6–20-fold increased risk of acquiring HAP/ventilator associated pneumonia (VAP) in the mechanically ventilated patients. The incidence of VAP in Indian studies ranges from 16% to 53.9% of hospitalized patients. Gram-negative organisms are the most common cause of VAP/HAP, whereas in the West, infections due to Methicillin-resistant *Staphylococcus aureus* (MRSA) are increasing. Common aerobic Gram-negative bacilli include *Pseudomonas aeruginosa, Escherichia coli, Klebsiella pneumoniae,* and *Acinetobacter* species.[1]

Definitions According to the American Thoracic Society/Infectious Diseases Society of America Guidelines[2]

Nosocomial pneumonia which includes HAP and VAP has been defined as an infection of the lung parenchyma that was neither present nor incubating at the time of hospital admission.

- *Hospital-acquired pneumonia:* It is defined as pneumonia occurring 48 hours after admission which is neither present nor incubating at the time of admission
- *Ventilator-associated pneumonia:* It is defined as pneumonia occurring 48–72 hours after endotracheal intubation or tracheostomy
- *Healthcare associated pneumonia:* It is defined as pneumonia occurring in patients in the nonhospital settings but who have got extensive healthcare contact; it excludes HAP, VAP and community-acquired pneumonia (CAP). HCAP is associated with the following risk factors:
  - Hospitalization for more than two days in preceding 90 days
  - Residence in a nursing home or extended care facility
  - Home infusion therapy
  - Patients receiving chronic dialysis or home wound care.

There is a lot of controversy surrounding the definition of HCAP. It is not as well standardized as HAP or VAP. There is a lot of heterogeneity in HCAP definitions provided in various studies and guidelines regarding duration of preceding hospitalization (ranging from 30 to 360 days).[3] Nursing homes in the West provide long-term care whereas in the Indian settings, they represent small hospitals with lesser infrastructure. The recently published Indian guidelines on pneumonia[1] chose not to use the term HCAP in its guideline document and suggested an individualized risk stratification approach regarding acquisition of multidrug resistant (MDR) pathogen rather than using an umbrella definition of HCAP.

PATHOGENESIS

Nosocomial pneumonia develops when microorganisms reach the lung and overcome the lung host defenses. The main mechanism involved in the pathogenesis of nosocomial pneumonia is the colonization of oropharynx with pathogenic microorganisms and subsequent microaspiration of these contents. Colonization can occur in almost 75% of the hospitalized patients within 48 hours either through exogenous or endogenous sources. Predominant exogenous sources include breach of normal mucosal integrity (with numerous devices–nasogastric tube, endotracheal tube), contact through health-care personnel, colonization of endotracheal tube biofilm. Endogenous factors that lead to increase in the gastric pH like acute illness, drugs [like proton-pump inhibitors (PPIs)] can disrupt the sterility of the stomach and upper gastrointestinal tract, and lead to gastrointestinal colonization. The presence of nasogastric tube and supine position in critically ill patients allow the intragastric microorganisms to reach the oropharynx.[4]

There are multiple reasons for aspiration such as the altered level of consciousness, depressed gag reflex, impaired swallowing and altered gastrointestinal motility. Though endotracheal tube may prevent macroaspiration, it does not prevent microaspiration around the cuff of the tube. Sometimes, the microorganisms inhabiting the biofilm of the endotracheal tube can get dislodged and reach the lower respiratory tract. Further, it depends on the number and virulence of microorganisms, and host defenses whether VAP develops or not. Rarely, hematogenous spread can occur leading to VAP.

PREVENTION OF HOSPITAL-ACQUIRED PNEUMONIA AND VENTILATOR-ASSOCIATED PNEUMONIA

There are multiple risk factors for VAP which are amenable to intervention by nonpharmacological measures. All the methods which aim at preventing HAP decrease the colonization of the upper respiratory tract, oral cavity and digestive tract, thereby preventing infection.

Decontamination with Antimicrobials

- *Chlorhexidine:* Oral decontamination with chlorhexidine (2%) solution (15 mL four times daily) till after extubation has been shown to be effective in preventing VAP.[5] The principle for this effect lies in the cidal action of chlorhexidine for the microbes residing the dental and gingival plaques. Popovich and colleagues[6] studied the role of whole body chlorhexidine cleansing on the rates of nosocomial infections and concluded that the procedure leads to reduction of catheter-related bloodstream infections and blood culture contamination, but did not lead to reduction in the rates of VAP
- Selective decontamination of the digestive tract (SDD) with topical and systemic antibiotics has been shown to be of modest benefit in preventing VAP, but not favored by all in view of the emergence of the resistant organisms.[7]

Hand Hygiene

Healthcare personnel should do hand wash before and after contact with patients with alcohol-based solutions to prevent cross-infection between patients. Peter Pronovost has introduced a simple checklist which has significantly reduced the incidence of central line associated infections and deaths.[8] This checklist includes the five things to be adhered to before each central line insertion—wash your hands; clean the patient's skin; put on a cap, gown and mask; avoid placing the catheter on groin; and take out lines when you do not need them. This checklist has saved more lives than any other scientific work has been done in the recent years. Some of these measures are true for HAP as well.

Airway

The care of the airway is important in preventing VAP. In a cost-efficacy analysis,[9] silver-coated endotracheal tubes have been shown to be effective in preventing VAP. Others which have shown to be effective are continuous aspiration of subglottic secretions (CASS); which is effective in reducing the incidence of VAP to as much as half especially in patients requiring mechanical ventilation for greater than 72 hours.[10] The most commonly used CASS device is Hi-Lo Evac. This device is costlier than routine endotracheal tubes and the cost-effectiveness has not been adequately assessed.

Cuff Pressure

Endotracheal tube cuff pressure should be maintained between 20 cm to 30 cm H_2O to prevent aspiration of gastric and oropharyngeal contents directly into the trachea. Excessive pressures more than that recommended lead to tracheal mucosal injury.

Ventilatory Circuit

The whole circuit which connects ventilator to the patient including devices like nebulizers which are included in the circuit. Regular changes of ventilator circuits have not shown to decrease the incidence of VAP,[11] are not recommended as a measure to prevent VAP. Care-taker should avoid flushing of the condensate into the lower airway and should be emptied regularly. Passive humidifiers [heat and moisture exchanger (HME) filters] are not superior to active humidifiers as shown in a large systematic review.[12] Closed suctioning system has not been shown to be superior to open system.[13] It seems logical to use closed systems to avoid the risk of spraying the condensate and secretions into the intensive care unit (ICU) environment.

Use of metered dose inhalers (MDI) for delivering aerosolized medication may reduce the risk of VAP since nebulizers get contaminated rapidly. Heated circuits are not superior to unheated circuits. Heated circuits decrease the amount of condensate; at the same time, excessive heating of inspired air can lead to drying of tracheal secretions with impending risk of endotracheal tube blockade with secretions.

Positioning

Semi-recumbent position at 45° is effective in preventing VAP compared to supine position. Semi-recumbent position prevents aspiration and decreases the odds of developing VAP. A randomized controlled trial comparing the rates of VAP in semi-recumbent and supine position was terminated early when it was found that the rates of VAP were significantly lower in patients in semi-recumbent position.[14]

Regular suctioning of respiratory secretions after instilling 8 mL of normal saline showed a reduction of VAP, compared to suctioning without instilling normal saline.[15]

Role of Proton Pump Inhibitor and H2 Receptor Blockers

Proton-pump inhibitors and H2 receptor blockers have been shown to increase the gastric colonization and odds of VAP and HAP by increasing gastric pH.[16] They should be replaced by sucralfate and antacids which do not alter the gastric pH in noncritically ill patients but the risks of stress ulcer bleed needs to be considered when stopping these agents as the risk of gastric bleeding increases with sucralfate though not significant.

Nasogastric and nasoduodenal tubes should be removed immediately when not required in hospitalized patients. Nasoduodenal tube feeding group has been shown to have lower incidence of VAP and achieved nutritional goals earlier compared to nasogastric tube group.

Preventing intubation, re-intubation and decreasing the duration of mechanical ventilation and using noninvasive ventilation, wherever possible, can help prevent VAP.

Certain components of ventilator bundles like sedation, vacation and assessment of ability to wean daily have been shown to decrease the incidence of VAP. However, ventilator bundle should be hospital-specific, tailored according to the available facilities.

DIAGNOSIS

Diagnosis of HAP/HCAP is predominantly based on clinical, radiological and sputum evaluation. The data on HAP/HCAP are mainly extrapolated from studies from VAP. VAP should be suspected in all intubated patients who develop new onset fever, respiratory symptoms, new chest infiltrates. In patients on ventilator, VAP is suspected from increased respiratory rate, increased minute volume, decreased tidal volume and increasing oxygen requirement. There are two different strategies to diagnose VAP, i.e. the clinical approach and quantitative bacteriological approach.[2]

Clinical Approach

Clinical approach combines clinical features with semi-quantitative cultures of endotracheal aspirate or sputum. In this approach, diagnosis of VAP/HAP is based on presence of new radiographic infiltrate, and presence of the following clinical criteria—fever, leukocytosis or leukopenia, purulent lower respiratory secretions, abnormal respiratory system examination, worsening oxygenation. The above constellation of clinicoradiological criteria has been comprehensively included in modified centers for disease control and prevention (CDC) algorithm for "clinically defined pneumonia" for diagnosis of HAP/VAP.[17]

The specificity of clinical criteria is increased by addition of tracheal aspirate, microscopic examination and semiquantitative cultures. Microscopic examination of the tracheal aspirate for gram stain and white blood cells will guide empirical therapy and prevent inappropriate therapy. A negative tracheal aspirate for gram stain, inflammatory cells and semiquantitative cultures in the absence of recent change in antibiotic therapy within 72 hours has a strong negative predictive value (94%) for VAP;[18] suggest the need to rule out other noninfectious causes of pulmonary infiltrates.

Semiquantitative cultures are reported as light, moderate or heavy growth. These cultures are highly sensitive with low specificity and cannot differentiate colonization from infection. However, combined with clinical criteria, their specificity increases. Cultures of blood and of other clinical specimens (like pleural fluid) wherever feasible, have to be sent. Isolation of the same microorganism from different sites clinches the diagnosis with very high accuracy.

Clinical pulmonary infection score (CPIS)[19] has been devised by Pugin et al. to increase the specificity of clinical diagnosis. It incorporates clinical, radiological, physiological (PaO_2/FiO_2 ratio) and microbiological data into a single numerical value. When CPIS score exceeded 6, a good correlation was found with pneumonia diagnosed by quantitative cultures of samples obtained by bronchoscopic and nonbronchoscopic methods. A CPIS score of less than/equal to 6 at 72 hours[20] has been used to stop antibiotics without adversely affecting mortality and ICU stay, thereby preventing inappropriate use of antibiotics.

Clinical response after 48–72 hours in combination with semiquantitative cultures are taken into consideration to decide the further course of action regarding antibiotics. Later studies did not show good sensitivity and specificity of CPIS for diagnosis of VAP.[21] A meta-analysis of 13 studies[22] concluded that the diagnostic accuracy of CPIS for ventilator-associated pneumonia is moderate with sensitivity and specificity of 65% and 64% respectively.

Clinical pulmonary infection score is simple and easy to perform at bedside. It is a useful tool not only in diagnosing VAP with modest sensitivity and specificity but also in evaluating the clinical response to treatment and determining the appropriate duration of treatment.[23]

Clinical approach hinges on the fact that failure to initiate treatment in cases of VAP as soon as the diagnosis is suspected will lead to increased mortality. All the patients suspected to have VAP will receive broad-spectrum antibiotics according to risk factors and local microbiological epidemiology after lower respiratory tract secretions are sent for culture. The initiation of antibiotics should not be delayed for obtaining cultures especially in hemodynamically unstable patients. Other mimics of pulmonary infection like atelectasis, pulmonary thromboembolism (PTE), hemorrhage and congestive heart failure which can present with similar clinical manifestations should be ruled out before considering a diagnosis of VAP/HAP. Clinical approach may sometimes lead to excessive antibiotic treatment if other mimics are not ruled out before labeling a patient as having VAP.

Bacteriological Approach

In this approach, patients are only treated after culture results arrive, and if cultures of the respiratory samples show growth above a threshold level. The Achilles heel of this approach lies in avoiding over-treatment and thereby preventing resistance to antibiotics. Quantitative cultures on the other hand are more specific with variable sensitivity and differentiate colonization from infection when a specific threshold is taken for diagnosis of VAP. The growth of the bacteria in the respiratory samples above the threshold indicates infection, and growth below the threshold indicates colonization. These samples can be collected bronchoscopically or nonbronchoscopically (blindly). The more distal the sampling from the lower respiratory tract, the more specific and less sensitive it is. The lower respiratory tract secretions obtained through bronchoscopic bronchoalveolar lavage (BAL) and protected specimen brushing (PSB) are highly specific. Mini-BAL and blind endotracheal aspirate (nonbronchoscopic) quantitative cultures have high sensitivity and low specificity retaining the diagnostic accuracy.

Bronchoscopic sampling and quantitative culture techniques as compared to nonbronchoscopic samples and nonquantitative cultures do not improve mortality, length of hospital stay, duration of mechanical ventilation, or length of ICU stay but may lead to narrower spectrum of antimicrobial therapy and early de-escalation of antibiotics.[24,25] VAP is a patchy process and not all samples for cultures are taken from areas involved with pneumonia so the sensitivity of bronchoscopic techniques is highly variable from 38% to 100% with poor reliability and reproducibility. There is also a lot of variability between different operators and different centers.

The threshold varies depending on the site from which the sample has been taken. A threshold of 10^6, 10^4 to 10^5 and 10^3 cfu/mL has been taken as cut-off for blind endotracheal aspirate, BAL and PSB respectively. Patients are treated only if the quantitative cultures exceed the threshold. The main disadvantage of this approach is failure to treat a patient with false-negative culture report and lack of immediate availability of the culture report. It is now a well-known fact that outcomes of patient with VAP depends very much on the initial appropriateness of treatment. To overcome, the clinician can take clues from the Giemsa or Gram-stain of the endotracheal aspirates to guide the initial appropriate therapy. False-negative cultures can occur in cases of specific fastidious pathogen, or cultures taken after starting antibiotics. Threshold for diagnosis may be lowered in such cases to increase the sensitivity.

A combined approach shown in the algorithm **(Flow chart 1)** is better in view of the shortcomings of both the approaches and will address most of the issues.

Response to Therapy

Response to therapy occurs in 48–72 hours in most (75%) of the patients. Response can be assessed by the improvement in fever, oxygen requirement, tracheal secretions, leukocytosis and radiological picture. Most importantly, fever and oxygen requirements improve after 48–72 hours, other things may take time to improve. Radiological resolution generally lags behind, although there may be initial deterioration in radiological picture. Radiological resolution depends on the age and the associated comorbidity [e.g. chronic obstructive pulmonary disease (COPD)]. Resolution is slower in elderly, patients with COPD and patients with associated

Flow chart 1 Algorithm of a combined approach for VAP management

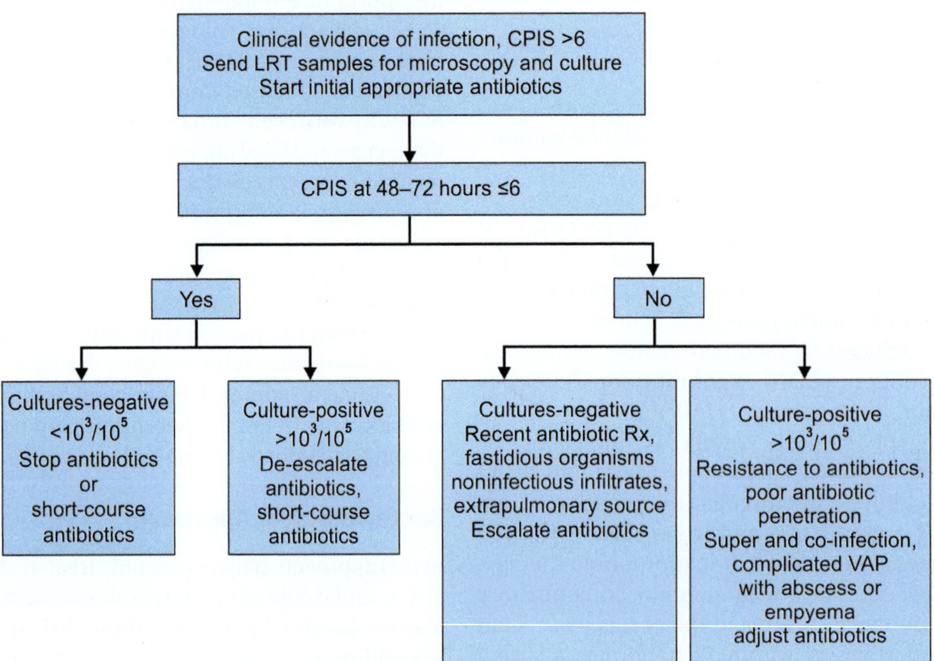

Abbreviations: CPIS, clinical pulmonary infection score; LRT, lower respiratory tract; VAP, ventilator-associated pneumonia

endobronchial obstruction. The presence of the following radiological features indicates rapid deterioration:
- Multilobar involvement
- >50% increase in infiltrates in 48 hours
- Development of cavitary or necrotizing pneumonia
- Development of large pleural effusion.

Antibiotics should not be changed in the initial 48–72 hours unless there is evidence of progressive deterioration.

Tools to Assess Clinical Response

- Combined clinical and microbiological approach (repeating quantitative cultures)
- CPIS has been used to assess the improvement of VAP

Absence of clinical response in patients with VAP requires to be evaluated aggressively. *The following factors need to be considered in case of nonresponse:*
- Wrong organism/resistant organism—consider mycobacteria, fungus, coexisting acquired immunodeficiency syndrome (AIDS) and other viral infection
- *Wrong diagnosis:* Noninfectious mimics of pneumonia—pulmonary embolism with infarct, pulmonary hemorrhage, atelectasis, acute respiratory distress syndrome (ARDS) or presence of neoplasm
- *Complications:* Empyema, lung abscess, extrapulmonary infection (e.g. catheter-related bloodstream infection (CRBSI), sinusitis, *Clostridium difficile* colitis)

Therapy needs to be escalated to cover resistant organisms in nonresponding patients. Some clinicians wait for the response after changing treatment whereas others proceed with additional investigations. Fiberoptic bronchoscopy (FOB), open lung biopsy may need to be considered in a subset of nonresponding patients.

RISK STRATIFICATION OF PATIENTS WITH VENTILATOR-ASSOCIATED PNEUMONIA

Presently, there is no score to assess the severity of VAP at the time of diagnosis. APACHE II has not been shown to be a good modality for risk stratifying these patients as shown in a matched cohort study.[26] Experts have come up with a concept called PIRO. This is based on predisposition (P), insult/infection (I), host response (R) and organ dysfunction (O). This concept was built upon a system of IRO during the 2001 International Sepsis Definitions Conference which discussed the weaknesses of systemic inflammatory response syndrome (SIRS) and sepsis definitions.[27] By mixing the PIRO concept with VAP, a VAP-PIRO score was created which was based on the study of 441 patients.[28] On multivariate analysis, four variables were associated with mortality: presence of comorbidities—COPD, immunocompromise, heart failure, cirrhosis, or chronic renal failure (predisposition-P); bacteremia (infection/insult-I), systolic blood pressure below 90 mm Hg or need of vasopressors to maintain blood pressure (response-R) and ARDS (organ dysfunction-O). These results were converted into a four variable PIRO score with one point assigned to each variable, with score ranging from 0 to 4. The mortality increased significantly as the score increased. **Table 1** shows the categorization and mortality according to the VAP-PIRO score.

TREATMENT

Appropriate and early antibiotic therapy improves survival. Inappropriate initial therapy has been shown to increase the mortality in patients with severe sepsis and VAP. The most important factor for initial inappropriate therapy is the presence of MDR pathogens in culture reports obtained subsequently after admission; the mortality risk does not decrease even if antibiotics are changed subsequently. So the most important step in treatment of VAP is to identify patients at risk of MDR pathogens and treat them appropriately from the beginning itself. Initial broad-spectrum empirical therapy has been advocated for use in patients with risk factors **(Table 2)**.

Recent literature[29] outlines the specific risk factors for specific pathogens (e.g. MRSA in hemodialysis patients), also describes that the distribution of MDR pathogens is very heterogeneous and may not be present in all patients who qualify the definition of HCAP. Local epidemiological studies need to be done to identify infecting microorganisms in specific settings **(Table 3)**.

Initial, empiric antibiotic treatment should be based on the individual risk factors, comorbidities, local microbiological epidemiology and should be patient specific. Broad-spectrum empiric antimicrobial regimen should be started in patients with MDR risk factor/s **(Table 4)**.

Table 1 Risk categorization and mortality based on VAP-PIRO scoring

Risk category	*Score*	*Mortality*
Mild risk	0–1 point	9.8–17%
High risk	2 points	52.9%
Very high risk	3–4 points	76.5–93.3%

Table 2 Risk factors for multidrug resistant pathogens as per 2005 American Thoracic Society/Infectious Diseases Society of America guidelines

Risk factors for MDR pathogens:
• Infection occurring 5 days after hospitalization • High antibiotic resistance in the community/hospital • Presence of pulmonary comorbidities, immunosuppressive therapy or disease • Antibiotic therapy in the preceding 90 days • Hospitalization >2 days in preceding 90 days • Residence in nursing home or extended care facility • Home infusion therapy including antibiotics, recent chemotherapy • Attending hemodialysis clinic.
Abbreviation: MDR, multidrug resistant

Table 3 Some important multidrug resistant and nonmultidrug resistant pathogens

Non-MDR pathogens	*MDR pathogens*
Streptococcus pneumoniae	Methicillin-resistant *Staphylococcus aureus* (MRSA)
Haemophilus influenzae	*Pseudomonas aeruginosa*
Methicillin sensitive *Staphylococcus aureus* (MSSA)	*Klebsiella pneumoniae*
Antibiotic sensitive GNB	*Acinetobacter baumannii* complex
Escherichia coli	*Legionella pneumophila*
Klebsiella pneumoniae	
Enterobacter, Serratia	
Proteus spp.	
Abbreviations: MDR, multidrug resistant; non-MDR, nonmultidrug resistant	

Table 4 Drugs which are commonly employed for nonmultidrug resistant pathogens

Drugs and their dosages for non-MDR pathogens: • Ceftriaxone 2 g IV 12 hourly • Ampicillin-sulbactam 3 g IV 6 hourly • Piperacillin-tazobactam 4.5 g IV 6 hourly • Levofloxacin 750 mg IV OD • Moxifloxacin 400 mg IV OD • Ertapenem 1g IV OD
Abbreviations: Non-MDR, nonmultidrug resistant; IV, intravenous

Drug Regimen for Nonmultidrug Resistant Pathogens (Table 5)

A combination regimen containing at least 3 drugs has to be given for patients with late onset VAP/HAP and HCAP (all cases) so as to provide a broad-spectrum antimicrobial cover which should include 2 broad-spectrum drugs with antipseudomonas cover and 1 drug with MRSA cover.

1. *Antipseudomonas agents:*
   - Carbapenems—meropenem, doripenem, imipenem
   - Third generation cephalosporin—cefoperazone-sulbactam, cefepime, ceftazidime
   - Beta-lactam antibiotics—piperacillin-tazobactam, ticarcillin-clavulanic acid.
2. *Antipseudomonas agent:* It can be used either a fluoroquinolone/aminoglycoside—
   - *Fluoroquinolone*: Levofloxacin, ciprofloxacin
   - *Aminoglycoside:* Gentamicin, tobramycin, amikacin
3. *Anti-MRSA agent:*
   - Vancomycin/linezolid

Newer drugs for MRSA such as oritavancin, dalbavancin and telavancin have been developed which need to be studied in larger cohort of patients. Colistin has been used for treating MDR pathogens.

Recent evidence does not advocate combination drug therapy for all patients with HCAP.[30] Patients should be treated for MDR pathogens if 2 out of 3 risk factors are present, i.e. [severe illness (requiring mechanical ventilation or ICU care)], prior antibiotic therapy (for 3 days in the preceding 6 months) and poor functional status [activities of daily living (ADL) score >12.5)]. Limited spectrum therapy for non-MDR pathogens will suffice if these risk factors are not present. These guidelines are based mainly on consensus as there is no sufficient evidence as to whether combination therapy/monotherapy is effective. Most importantly, antimicrobial therapy has to be tailored according to local microbiological flora and their antibiotic susceptibility. Each ICU/hospital should have a protocol according to this data.

Till date, no regimen has been shown to be superior over the other. A recent meta-analysis showed no difference in mortality and treatment failure in single versus combination therapy group concluding that single agent therapy is not inferior to combination therapy.[31] In places with high risk of *Pseudomonas aeruginosa* and other Gram-negative bacilli, local microbiological bacterial susceptibility pattern should be taken into consideration before starting empirical regimen. Institution specific guidelines should be developed taking all these factors into account.

In a broader view, for patients with early onset VAP/HAP at places where there is no increased incidence of early onset MDR pathogens, treatmemt cover should be provided for *Streptococcus pneumoniae, Haemophilus influenzae,* MSSA and the usual community-acquired pathogens with beta-lactam and beta-lactamase inhibitor combinations (piperacillin-tazobactam, ampicillin-sulbactam), ceftriaxone, fluoroquinolones (levofloxacin moxifloxacin) and doripenem.

For patients with late onset VAP-HAP, combination therapy is preferable. Proposed benefits of combination therapy include prevention of emergence of antimicrobial resistance, synergism of antibiotics and to provide a broader cover for all MDR pathogens.

Treatment Failure

In addition to the appropriateness of the antibiotic therapy, there are various other host and antibiotic factors which can lead to treatment failure.[32]

Table 5 Drugs for multidrug resistant pathogens

		Group	*Drug and dosage*
Anti-pseudomonas drugs	1.	Carbapenem or	Imipenem 0.5 g 6 hourly or 1.0 g IV 8 hourly
			Meropenem 1g IV 8 hourly
			Doripenem 0.5 g IV 8 hourly
		Third generation cephalosporin or	Cefoperazone-sulbactam 2 g IV 8–12 hourly
			Cefipime 1–2 g IV 8–12 hourly
			Ceftazidime 2 g IV 8–12 hourly
		Beta-lactam antibiotics	Piperacillin-tazobactam 4.5 g IV 6–8 hourly
			Ticarcillin-clavulanic acid 3.2 g IV 6 hourly
	2.	Fluoroquinolone or	Ciprofloxacin 400 mg IV 8 hourly
			Levofloxacin 750 mg IV OD
		Aminoglycosides	Amikacin 20 mg/kg weight IV OD
			Gentamicin 7 mg/kg IV OD
			Tobramycin 7 mg/kg IV OD
MRSA	3.	Glycopeptides	Vancomycin 15–20 mg/kg actual body weight BD (maximum 30 mg/kg as loading dose)
		Streptogramins	Linezolid 600 mg IV 12 hourly
	4.	Polymyxins	Colistimethate sodium (CMS) 3 million units IV 8th hourly or 4.5 million units IV 12th hourly
Abbreviations: IV, intravenous			

Host Factors

Many of the critically ill patients have increased third space volume secondary to hypoalbuminemia and excessive fluids which these patients receive to correct their hypotension. The consequence of the increased third space volume is a decrease in plasma drug concentration. Hypoalbuminemia also leads to increased free drug levels which can lead to accelerated clearance of the drug thereby decreasing the drug $t_{1/2}$.

Antibiotic Factors (Table 6)

Time-dependent antibiotics are best administered in multiple doses and as continuous infusions. These antibiotics require serum concentrations to be greater than minimum inhibitory concentration (MIC) for certain time period between doses which usually range from 40–50% of interdose time interval for their best action. It varies for different antibiotics, e.g. 30–40% for carbapenems, 50–70% for cephalosporins. On the other hand, concentration-dependent antibiotics are best administered as single daily dosage. These antibiotics require attainment of the peak concentration many times higher than the MIC for their microbiological action and they have prolonged postantibiotic effect (PAE) which makes them effective even after their drug concentration falls below MIC.

Table 6 Time and concentration-dependent antibiotics

Time-dependent antibiotics	*Concentration-dependent antibiotics*
Penicillins	Fluoroquinolones-levofloxacin
Cephalosporins	Aminoglycosides
Carbapenems	
Vancomycin, linezolid	

Treatment of Ventilator-associated Pneumonia Caused by Multidrug Resistant Gram-negative Bacilli

In the past few years, the emergence of MDR Gram-negative bacteria and lack of new antibiotics has led to increased interest in an old class of drugs, "Polymyxins". These drugs have been abandoned for clinical use nearly 20 years ago after serious reports of nephrotoxicity and neurotoxicity (mostly paresthesias).[33] Recent studies have shown that these antibiotics have considerable effectiveness and less toxicity. Polymyxins are an old class of cationic, cyclic polypeptide antibiotics which consist of polymyxin B and polymyxin E (popularly known as colistin). Colistin is available as colistin sulfate (for oral use) and colistimethate sodium

(CMS) for parenteral use. CMS acts by binding to anionic lipopolysaccharide cell membrane of Gram-negative bacilli leading to permeability changes in the cell envelope, leakage of cell content, and cell death. CMS has been the most commonly and widely used polymyxin. CMS is active against aerobic Gram-negative bacilli—*Acinetobacter, Pseudomonas, Klebsiella* and enterobacter species, MDR Gram-negative bacilli.[34] Nephrotoxicity is the most important side effect of CMS. It is dose-dependent and reversible. The incidence of acute kidney injury from intravenous CMS has been reported to be around 10%, and increases with coadministration of other nephrotoxic drugs.[35] Renal functions should be closely monitored for patients receiving CMS.

Colistin and other antimicrobials have been tried in combination in clinical practice with a view of increasing efficacy and overcoming resistance. Most notable among them are colistin-rifampicin, colistin-carbapenems and ampicillin-sulbactam. Microbiological studies have shown synergy for *Acinetobacter* infection with colistin-rifampicin and colistin-carbapenem combinations. In clinical studies, these combination therapies were noninferior to monotherapy.[36] Reasonably good clinical outcomes have been reported with sulbactam alone and in combination with ampicillin for treatment of nosocomial infections including VAP caused by *Acinetobacter*.[37,38] Sulbactam has intrinsic bacteriostatic or cidal action against *A. baumannii* and is the most active agent beta-lactamase inhibitors.[39]

Finally, it should be kept in mind that the nosocomial pneumonias are occasionally caused by fungi viruses or other microorganisms such as *Mycobacterium tuberculosis*.[40]

(The diagnosis and management of these conditions are discussed in individual chapters in this book).

The strategies to identify risk factors and choice of drugs for initial therapy for individual patients depend on the most recent guidelines practiced in the country. An analysis of guidelines of several different societies reveals that the correct choice of initial intravenous antibiotic treatment as per most current treatment guideline recommendations affect the costs as well as the clinical outcomes.[41]

Antibiotic Stewardship

The antibiotic resistance has posed a major threat to treatment practices for infections. The World Health Organization (WHO) along with most other international bodies, has issued messages of concern to warn against this problem. It has been even said that there is a real risk of increased number of deaths from even common infections and minor injuries in the postantibiotic era in the 21st century.[42] Antibiotic stewardship programs have been advocated to contain the risk of antibiotic resistance. These programs are meant to optimize and monitor the antibiotic use (or misuse) and minimize the adverse effects with the help of coordinated, multidisciplinary practices in the hospitals.[43] Several examples of these programs are already available which demonstrate the efficacy and success in preventing antibiotic resistance.[44]

REFERENCES

1. Gupta D, Agarwal R, Aggarwal AN, Singh N, Mishra N, Khilnani GC, et al. Guidelines for diagnosis and management of community-and hospital-acquired pneumonia in adults: Joint ICS/NCCP(I) recommendations. Lung India. 2012;29(Suppl 2):S27-62.
2. Guidelines for the management of adults with hospital-acquired, ventilator-associated, and healthcare-associated pneumonia. Am J Respir Crit Care Med. 2005;171(4):388-416.
3. Falcone M, Venditti M, Shindo Y, Kollef MH. Healthcare-associated pneumonia: diagnostic criteria and distinction from community-acquired pneumonia. Int J Infect Dis. 2011;15(8):e545-50.
4. Wunderink RD, Rello J. Ventilator-associated pneumonia. Berlin: Springer; 2001.
5. Tantipong H, Morkchareonpong C, Jaiyindee S, Thamlikitkul V. Randomized controlled trial and meta-analysis of oral decontamination with 2% chlorhexidine solution for the prevention of ventilator-associated pneumonia. Infect Control Hosp Epidemiol. 2008;29(2):131-6.
6. Popovich KJ, Hota B, Hayes R, Weinstein RA, Hayden MK. Effectiveness of routine patient cleansing with chlorhexidine gluconate for infection prevention in the medical intensive care unit. Infect Control Hosp Epidemiol. 2009;30(10):959-63.
7. de Smet AM, Kluytmans JA, Cooper BS, Mascini EM, Benus RF, van der Werf TS, et al. Decontamination of the digestive tract and oropharynx in ICU patients. N Engl J Med. 2009;360(1):20-31.
8. Berenholtz SM, Pronovost PJ, Lipsett PA, Hobson D, Earsing K, Farley JE, et al. Eliminating catheter-related bloodstream infections in the intensive care unit. Crit Care Med. 2004;32(10):2014-20.
9. Shorr AF, Zilberberg MD, Kollef M. Cost-effectiveness analysis of a silver-coated endotracheal tube to reduce the incidence of ventilator-associated pneumonia. Infect Control Hosp Epidemiol. 2009;30(8):759-63.
10. Dezfulian C, Shojania K, Collard HR, Kim HM, Matthay MA, Saint S. Subglottic secretion drainage for preventing ventilator-associated pneumonia: a meta-analysis. Am J Med. 2005;118(1):11-8.
11. Hess D, Burns E, Romagnoli D, Kacmarek RM. Weekly ventilator circuit changes. A strategy to reduce costs without affecting pneumonia rates. Anesthesiology. 1995;82(4):903-11.
12. Siempos II, Vardakas KZ, Kopterides P, Falagas ME. Impact of passive humidification on clinical outcomes of mechanically ventilated patients: a meta-analysis of randomized controlled trials. Crit Care Med. 2007;35(12):2843-51.
13. Siempos II, Vardakas KZ, Falagas ME. Closed tracheal suction systems for prevention of ventilator-associated pneumonia. Br J Anaesth. 2008;100(3):299-306.
14. Drakulovic MB, Torres A, Bauer TT, Nicolas JM, Nogué S, Ferrer M. Supine body position as a risk factor for nosocomial pneumonia in mechanically ventilated patients: a randomised trial. Lancet. 1999;354(9193):1851-8.
15. Caruso P, Denari S, Ruiz SA, Demarzo SE, Deheinzelin D. Saline instillation before tracheal suctioning decreases the incidence of ventilator-associated pneumonia. Crit Care Med. 2009;37(1):32-8.

16. Prod'hom G, Leuenberger P, Koerfer J, Blum A, Chiolero R, Schaller MD, et al. Nosocomial pneumonia in mechanically ventilated patients receiving antacid, ranitidine, or sucralfate as prophylaxis for stress ulcer. A randomized controlled trial. Ann Intern Med. 1994;20(8):653-62.
17. Horan TC, Andrus M, Dudeck MA. CDC/NHSN surveillance definition of health care-associated infection and criteria for specific types of infections in the acute care setting. Am J Infect Control. 2008;36(5):309-32.
18. Blot F, Raynard B, Chachaty E, Tancrède C, Antoun S, Nitenberg G. Value of gram stain examination of lower respiratory tract secretions for early diagnosis of nosocomial pneumonia. Am J Respir Crit Care Med. 2000;162(5):1731-7.
19. Pugin J, Auckenthaler R, Mili N, Janssens JP, Lew PD, Suter PM. Diagnosis of ventilator-associated pneumonia by bacteriologic analysis of bronchoscopic and nonbronchoscopic "blind" bronchoalveolar lavage fluid. Am Rev Respir Dis. 1991;143(5 Pt 1):1121-9.
20. Singh N, Rogers P, Atwood CW, Wagener MM, Yu VL. Short-course empiric antibiotic therapy for patients with pulmonary infiltrates in the intensive care unit. A proposed solution for indiscriminate antibiotic prescription. Am J Respir Crit Care Med. 2000;162(2 Pt 1):505-11.
21. Schurink CA, Van Nieuwenhoven CA, Jacobs JA, Rozenberg-Arska M, Joore HC, Buskens E, et al. Clinical pulmonary infection score for ventilator-associated pneumonia: accuracy and inter-observer variability. Intensive Care Med. 2004;30(2):217-24.
22. Shan J, Chen HL, Zhu JH. Diagnostic accuracy of clinical pulmonary infection score for ventilator-associated pneumonia: a meta-analysis. Respir Care. 2011;56(8):1087-94.
23. Luna CM, Blanzaco D, Niederman MS, Matarucco W, Baredes NC, Desmery P, et al. Resolution of ventilator-associated pneumonia: prospective evaluation of the clinical pulmonary infection score as an early clinical predictor of outcome. Crit Care Med. 2003;31(3):676-82.
24. Canadian Critical Care Trials Group. A randomized trial of diagnostic techniques for ventilator-associated pneumonia. N Engl J Med. 2006;355(25):2619-30.
25. Shorr AF, Sherner JH, Jackson WL, Kollef MH. Invasive approaches to the diagnosis of ventilator-associated pneumonia: a meta-analysis. Crit Care Med. 2005;33(1):46-53.
26. Rello J, Sole-Violan J, Sa-Borges M, Garnacho-Montero J, Muñoz E, Sirgo G, et al. Pneumonia caused by oxacillin-resistant *Staphylococcus aureus* treated with glycopeptides. Crit Care Med. 2005;33(9):1983-7.
27. Levy MM, Fink MP, Marshall JC, Abraham E, Angus D, Cook D, et al. 2001 SCCM/ESICM/ACCP/ATS/SIS International Sepsis Definitions Conference. Crit Care Med. 2003;31(4):1250-6.
28. Lisboa T, Diaz E, Sa-Borges M, Socias A, Sole-Violan J, Rodríguez A, et al. The ventilator-associated pneumonia PIRO score: a tool for predicting ICU mortality and health-care resources use in ventilator-associated pneumonia. Chest. 2008;134(6):1208-16.
29. Poch DS, Ost DE. What are the important risk factors for healthcare-associated pneumonia? Semin Respir Crit Care Med. 2009;30(1):26-35.
30. Kollef MH, Morrow LE, Baughman RP, Craven DE, McGowan JE, Micek ST., et al. Healthcare-associated pneumonia (HCAP): a critical appraisal to improve identification, management, and outcomes--proceedings of the HCAP Summit. Clin Infect Dis. 2008;46 Suppl 4:S296-334.
31. Aarts MA, Hancock JN, Heyland D, McLeod RS, Marshall JC. Empiric antibiotic therapy for suspected ventilator-associated pneumonia: a systematic review and meta-analysis of randomized trials. Crit Care Med. 2008;36(1):108-17.
32. Diaz E, Ulldemolins M, Lisboa T, Rello J. Management of ventilator-associated pneumonia. Infect Dis Clin North Am. 2009;23(3):521-33.
33. Munoz-Price LS, Weinstein RA. Acinetobacter infection. N Engl J Med. 2008;358(12):1271-81.
34. Biswas S, Brunel JM, Dubus JC, Reynaud-Gaubert M, Rolain JM. Colistin: an update on the antibiotic of the 21st century. Expert Rev Anti Infect Ther. 2012;10(8):917-34.
35. Falagas ME, Rafailidis PI, Ioannidou E, Alexiou VG, Matthaiou DK, Karageorgopoulos DE, et al. Colistin therapy for microbiologically documented multidrug-resistant Gram-negative bacterial infections: a retrospective cohort study of 258 patients. Int. J. Antimicrob Agents. 2010;35(2):194-9.
36. Petrosillo N, Ioannidou E, Falagas ME. Colistin monotherapy vs. combination therapy: evidence from microbiological, animal and clinical studies. Clin. Microbiol. Infect. 2008;14(9):816-27.
37. Betrosian AP, Frantzeskaki F, Xanthaki A, Douzinas EE., et al. Efficacy and safety of high-dose ampicillin/sulbactam vs. colistin as monotherapy for the treatment of multidrug resistant *Acinetobacter baumannii* ventilator-associated pneumonia. J Infect. 2008;56(6):432-6.
38. Corbella X, Ariza J, Ardanuy C, Vuelta M, Tubau F, Sora M, et al. Efficacy of sulbactam alone and in combination with ampicillin in nosocomial infections caused by multiresistant *Acinetobacter baumannii.* J Antimicrob Chemother. 1998;42(6):793-802.
39. Karageorgopoulos DE, Falagas ME. Current control and treatment of multidrug-resistant *Acinetobacter baumannii* infections. Lancet Infect Dis. 2008;8(12):751-62.
40. Luyt CE, Bréchot N, Chastre J. What role do viruses play in nosocomial pneumonia? Curr Opin Infect Dis. 2014;27(2):194-9.
41. Wilke M, Grube R. Update on management options in the treatment of nosocomial and ventilator assisted pneumonia: review of actual guidelines and economic aspects of therapy. Infect Drug Resist. 2013;7:1-7.
42. Pulcini C, Mainardi JL. Antimicrobial stewardship: an international emergency. Clin Microbiol Infect. 2014; 20(10):947-8.
43. Pollack LA, Srinivasan A. Core elements of hospital antibiotic stewardship programs from the centers for disease control and prevention. Clin Infect Dis. 2014;59 Suppl 3:S97-S100.
44. Huttner B, Harbarth S, Nathwani D; ESCMID Study Group for Antibiotic Policies (ESGAP). Success stories of implementation of antimicrobial stewardship: a narrative review. Clin Microbiol Infect. 2014;20(10):954-62.

51

Chapter

Viral Pneumonias

Arjun Srinivasan, Ritesh Agarwal

INTRODUCTION

Community-acquired pneumonia (CAP) is an important cause of morbidity and mortality throughout the world in all age groups. A clear understanding of the etiology is essential for the adequate management, more importantly to prevent the use of inappropriate antibiotics which promote the emergence of multidrug resistant organisms. It is also imperative to recognize viral pneumonias since antibiotics have no effect and antivirals are few with the rapid onset of resistance, if misused. Viruses, especially respiratory syncytial virus (RSV), influenza A and B viruses, parainfluenza viruses and adenoviruses, are recognized as important causes of CAP in children. In adults, viral causes of CAP are not well-characterized, specific recommendations about the assessment and management of viral CAP are sparse. Studies are handicapped by the difficulty in isolating the viruses and due to the presence of large number of viruses with a potential to cause pneumonia. Most studies have utilized antibody detection to confirm the etiology, hence may have compromised the ability to detect viruses as the cause of pneumonia. Most reports cite an incidence of 9–29% viral pneumonias among all CAPs, influenza being the most common.[1,2]

RESPIRATORY VIRUSES

Viruses of importance in the respiratory tract infection include primary respiratory viruses, whose replication is generally restricted to the respiratory tract, and others whose respiratory involvement is a part of systemic involvement.

Classification of viruses is dependent on the type of nucleic acid core, family of the virus, protein configuration and the lipid envelope. Postinfection immunity depends on the number of antigenic subtypes in the viral family with more effective protection amongst families with multiple immunotypes like the rhinovirus or adenovirus. Immunity is also dictated by the stability of the viral antigens, the best example is that of influenza A, which undergoes periodic minor, as well as major changes in its surface antigens leading to susceptibility to reinfection as the acquired immunity is no longer effective. Pulmonary and systemic complications of seasonal influenza contribute to the morbidity and the mortality, especially among the vulnerable subset of extremes of age and immunocompromise.

Resurgence of interest among the medical community in viral pneumonias has been catapulted by the outbreak of severe acute respiratory syndrome (SARS) in 2003, the pandemic of novel swine origin H1N1 influenza 2009 and the more recent middle east respiratory syndrome (MERS). On the other end of the spectrum lie the viruses with the potential to cause a pandemic with even higher mortality than H1N1 2009, like the avian influenza (H5N1). Viruses like cytomegalovirus (CMV), which were considered to affect only the immunocompromised hosts are being identified in healthy individuals with pneumonias. Cases with dramatic presentation like sporadic hantavirus pulmonary syndrome (HPS) and ebola virus hemorrhagic fever are geographically restricted but should be considered in this era of unrestricted globetrotting.

Individual viruses **(Table 1)** will be dealt with in greater details after an overview of the common characteristics of viral pneumonias, including similarities in clinical presentations, radiological manifestations and pathogenesis.

Table 1 Important respiratory viral infections

- Varicella pneumonia
- Cytomegalovirus pneumonia
- Corona virus respiratory illness
  - Severe acute respiratory syndrome (SARS)
  - Middle east respiratory syndrome (MERS)
- Hantavirus pulmonary syndrome
- Adenovirus pneumonia
- Influenza
  - Seasonal influenza A pneumonia
  - Avian influenza A (H5N1)
  - Swine origin influenza (H1N1) 2009.

PRESENTING FEATURES

Pneumonia is usually a complication of descending infection from the upper respiratory tract, and hence, patients may give history of upper respiratory tract infection, conjunctivitis or myalgia and malaise at the onset of illness or may harbor telltale signs of the same on examination. Among patients who are not overtly immunocompromised, viral pneumonias are common among the children, elderly, pregnant women, patients with chronic obstructive pulmonary disease (COPD) and cardiovascular disease.

Viral pneumonia in adults is usually associated with nonproductive cough, although production of frothy, blood-tinged sputum is seen in some severely ill individuals. Cyanosis, tachypnea and use of accessory muscles are red flag signs indicating respiratory failure on examination. Tracheal tenderness may be present in case of associated tracheitis. Chest examination may reveal only occasional rales and wheeze despite extensive respiratory involvement. The clinical features of sporadic cases of viral pneumonia are usually not sufficiently characteristic to permit specific viral diagnosis or differentiation from bacterial pneumonias on clinical grounds alone. Exceptions include measles and varicella pneumonia, in which the associated rash establishes the diagnosis.

The damage to the host respiratory tract is the result of direct injury by the invading virus, unregulated immune response with the release of inflammatory cytokines and blunting of local protective mechanisms like mucociliary clearance and phagocytosis. Viruses are also known to disturb the bacterial flora of the upper respiratory tract thus promoting better adhesion and increasing the chances of secondary bacterial infection in the immediate post-viral period. Secondary bacterial pneumonias typically occur after 5–7 days of the initial onset of symptoms with usually a period of apparent improvement whereas progressive viral pneumonias have a continuous downhill course. The associated bacteria are the same as in community-acquired pneumonia (CAP) *Streptococcus pneumoniae*, mycoplasma and *Haemophilus influenzae* being the most common. Interestingly, community-acquired methicillin resistant *Staphylococcus aureus* (CA-MRSA) is increasingly being isolated in the post-viral setting.

Interstitial infiltrates rather than lobar consolidation are common but findings are not specific to help differentiation based on chest radiograph alone. The severity of viral CAP in normal hosts is directly related to the degree and duration of hypoxemia. The magnitude of oxygen diffusion defect caused by viral involvement of lung interstitium in severe viral CAPs is best assessed by the alveolar-arterial (A-a) gradient. Patients presenting with severe viral CAP typically have increased A-a gradients of more than 35 cm H_2O. The degree of hypoxemia is related to the degree of oxygen diffusion defect caused by interstitial pathogens. Studies in patients of proven viral pneumonias have identified certain patterns in high resolution computerized tomography (HRCT), which may help differentiate viral from bacterial pneumonias. These include multifocal consolidation, multifocal ground-glass and tree-in-bud opacities, and widespread bronchial wall thickening.[3-5]

Varicella Pneumonia

Varicella-zoster virus (VZV) causes two distinct clinical entities—varicella (chickenpox) and herpes zoster (shingles). Chickenpox, a ubiquitous and extremely contagious infection, is usually a benign illness of childhood characterized by an exanthematous vesicular rash. Less than 20% of all cases of VZV infection occur in adults.[6] Varicella pneumonia, the most serious complication following chickenpox, develops more commonly in adults (up to 20% of cases) than in children and is particularly severe in pregnant women. Pneumonia due to VZV usually has its onset 3–5 days into the illness and is associated with tachypnea, cough, dyspnea and fever. Varicella-zoster virus pneumonia (VZVP) has a reported mortality of between 2.15% and 20% in the general population, but in pregnancy, it may be as high as 41%.[7,8]

Diagnosis

Early clues to the diagnosis of pneumonia in subjects at risk are continued eruption of new lesions, persistent fever and new onset cough. The development of VZVP in the absence of fever and after the cessation of new lesion formation is exceedingly rare. Chest radiographs of VZVP typically show ill-defined nodular or reticular densities scattered in bilateral lung fields. Initially, the nodules are 2–5 mm in diameter and are best visualized in the periphery of the lung. With progressive disease, the nodules enlarge and coalesce, forming extensive infiltrates, especially near the hila and in the lung bases.[9,10] In the milder cases, the infiltrates may resolve in 3–5 days. However, in widespread severe disease, the radiographic abnormalities may persist for several weeks or months. In a few patients, the lesions calcify and remain indefinitely as numerous well-defined, randomly scattered, 2–3 mm dense calcifications in otherwise normal lung.[9,10]

Treatment

Any adult with varicella should be closely monitored for signs of respiratory difficulty; should it occur, chest radiographs and arterial blood gases should be obtained. Early institution of intravenous acyclovir in a dosage of 10 mg/kg three times a day for 5–10 days is effective for VZVP or other complications in adults and children. Patients who develop respiratory failure will require invasive mechanical ventilation with protective lung ventilation strategy. Adjunctive therapy with corticosteroids was associated with decrease in duration of mechanical ventilation and accelerated physiological recovery in a retrospective analysis of 19 patients receiving mechanical ventilation in a single center.[11] A multicenter prospective study is needed before the same can be recommended for routine management.

Cytomegalovirus Pneumonia

Cytomegalovirus (CMV) DNA viruses are of the murine and human variety. Cytomegaloviruses are DNA viruses with an icosahedral capsid with 162 capsomeres and the viral particles have a diameter of 120–200 nm. Cytomegaloviruses are members of the herpesviridae family, which consists of eight human herpes viruses (HHVs). Morphologically, CMV resembles other herpes viruses, particularly HSV, with important cytopathic differences. Although both HSV and CMV produce intranuclear inclusions, only CMV produces cytoplasmic inclusions (dense bodies).[12] Because only CMV produces perinuclear cytoplasmic inclusions, cytopathologic diagnosis is possible. Cytopathologic changes in host tissue indicate active infection. *Pneumocystis jerovecii* and CMVs are recognized pathogens in compromised hosts, for example, those who undergo transplants and those on immunosuppressive drugs or steroids. CMV, influenza (human, avian, swine) and adenovirus are the three most common causes of severe viral CAP in immunocompetent adults.

Cytomegalovirus CAP in immunocompetent hosts is uncommon but is now being recognized more frequently, particularly when presenting as severe viral CAP. As with any respiratory virus, the severity of the disease in immunocompetent individuals varies from mild flu to acute respiratory distress syndrome, requiring mechanical ventilation. Severe CMV pneumonia may initially show minimal or no pulmonary infiltrates on chest radiograph but is accompanied by varying degree of hypoxemia. Cytomegalovirus CAP has no distinct radiologic findings on chest radiograph. It usually is necessary to rule out other causes of respiratory failure like lobar consolidation in bacterial pneumonias or other mimics of CAP. Cytomegalovirus should be included in the differential diagnosis when there are other clinical features to suggest CMV rather than other causes of severe viral CAP. Other systemic involvement, including liver, gastrointestinal tract, central nervous system and bone marrow favors CMV. The immunomodulatory effects of CMV may precipitate a flare of underlying connective tissue disease or may be the cause of deterioration thereby making management difficult.

Diagnosis

Diagnosis is established most commonly by serologic testing. The diagnosis of recent CMV infection depends on demonstrating either a single elevated CMV immunoglobulin M (IgM) titer or a four-fold increase in CMV immunoglobulin G (IgG) titers. False positive or negative serologic results can occur in the presence of other reacting antibodies like rheumatoid factor (RF) or antibodies against Epstein-Barr virus (EBV). Cytomegalovirus semiquantitative antigenemia assay is a sensitive/specific and rapid method to detect CMV activation in lymphocytes. Cytomegalovirus polymerase chain reaction (CMV PCR) is very sensitive and indicates reactivation of CMV in lymphocytes.

The main difficulty in using CMV PCR is that it does not distinguish between asymptomatic or latent and active infection. Because PCR is so sensitive, serial qualitative PCR, as with semiquantitative CMV antigen levels, may be clinically more useful. Importantly, in immunocompetent hosts with primary CMV pneumonia, CMV PCR is usually negative. Virus can be isolated in human fibroblast cultures, but as the cytopathic changes are slow to occur, cultures need to be maintained for up to 3 weeks before they can be declared negative. The typical cytopathic change is classically described as "owl's eye" appearance and may be identified directly in tissue specimens or in cultures.

Treatment

Treatment is the only hope for cure in immunocompromised individuals, but in immunocompetent patients the decision to treat depends on the severity of infection. Patients with hypoxemia should be treated with antivirals, but prolonged therapy usually is not required. Although acyclovir is active against other herpes viruses, it is ineffective against CMV. The mainstay of anti-CMV therapy is ganciclovir 5 mg/kg (intravenous) every 12 hours for the duration of infection.

The oral equivalent of parenteral ganciclovir is valganciclovir, which is metabolized to ganciclovir and is as effective as parenteral ganciclovir. Oral valganciclovir may be used to complete therapy after the initial ganciclovir therapy or may be used for the entire duration of therapy. The dosage of oral valganciclovir for induction therapy is 900 mg (by mouth) every 12 hours for 21 days. In immunocompetent hosts, a complete course of therapy with ganciclovir/valganciclovir is usually not necessary, patients usually improve after 1–2 weeks of therapy. In such patients, anti-CMV therapy is often continued for an additional week to prevent potential relapse. Foscarnet is an alternative CMV therapy, but has to be administered intravenously and is nephrotoxic. Unlike immunocompromised host, prognosis of CMV pneumonia in normal hosts is often good.[12]

Corona Virus-associated Respiratory Illnesses

Severe Acute Respiratory Syndrome

From November 2002 to July 2003, SARS quickly spread from Foshan (Shunde district), Guangdong Province in the People's Republic of China to 33 other countries or regions on 5 continents.[13,14] There were 8,447 cases, 21% occurring in healthcare workers (HCWs) and 813 deaths (9.6% overall mortality) by the time SARS was contained in July 2003. The case-fatality rate in 2003 was estimated at 13.2% for patients younger than 60 years and 50% for patients of more than 60 years of age. 50% of patients with acute respiratory distress syndrome (ARDS) had died.[13,14]

The pathogen, the human coronavirus (CoV) group 2b, SARS-CoV, is of animal origin. The SARS-like-CoV (SL-CoV) virus from animal hosts has a nucleotide homology greater than 99% with SARS-CoV. From virus sequence data, it seems that the masked (Himalayan) palm civet (*Paguma larvata*) acted as an amplification host. The epidemic strains (including SARS-Urbani) evolved because of civet-human interaction in Chinese animal markets. Serologic evidence of natural SL-CoV infection is also found in the Chinese ferret-badger (*Melogale moschata*).[15]

The World Health Organization case definition for probable SARS includes:

- Fever greater than 38°C or history of fever in the preceding 48 hours
- New infiltrates on chest radiograph consistent with pneumonia
- Chills or cough or malaise or myalgia or history of exposure
- One or more positive tests for SARS-CoV.

As with all epidemics, during an outbreak, these points are useful in screening individuals, but outside the setting suggest only presence of common flu.

During the last epidemic, most patients presented with flu-like symptoms (fever, chills, cough and malaise) and two-thirds of them developed dyspnea and recurrent or persistent fever. 30% patients significantly improved within 1 week. Advanced age, high admission neutrophil count and initial elevated lactic dehydrogenase (LDH) were independent correlates of an adverse outcome. Watery diarrhea was present in more than a third of patients and was the most common extrapulmonary symptom correlated in autopsy studies by the isolation of maximum concentrations of the virus in small bowel, next only to the lungs. Cardiovascular complications in the form of hypotension and unexplained tachycardia were common. Reactive hepatitis was in 24% of the patients with up to 69% developing transient elevation of liver enzymes during their course of illness. Overall subclinical infections were very few and far apart.

Post-traumatic stress disorder and other psychiatric manifestations have been reported in survivors of intensive care. Approximately one-fifth of patients presented with a normal chest radiograph, but developed infiltrates within 7 days (median 3 days) of onset of fever. Of the 78.3% who presented with opacities on the chest radiographs, 54.6% were unilateral. The involvement of more than one lung zone and bilateral versus unilateral disease were associated with a higher risk of intensive care unit (ICU) admission and death.[16]

Diagnosis: Sensitivity of RT-PCR collected in the first 3 days of the illness was inadequate. For the emergency screening of febrile patients as per protocol, the sensitivity and specificity were 92.6% and 71.6%, respectively. Confirmation of infection was made by identifying the SARS-CoV nucleocapsid (N) protein in the serum by N antigen-capture enzyme-linked immunosorbent assay (ELISA) and N antigen-capture chemiluminescent immunoassay. Generally, in the first 4–5 days of illness, nasopharyngeal aspirates and throat swabs are more useful in detecting virus, whereas stool specimens are more valuable after 5 days of illness (20% sensitivity).

Treatment: Suspected patients were immediately isolated using contact, droplet and airborne isolation precautions in a negative-pressure single room. Treatment is largely based on the results of uncontrolled trials as randomized controlled trials evaluating treatment regimens are not available. Early positive outcomes using ribavirin and steroids led to widespread use of that combination. In a study of 71 cases (97% laboratory confirmed); antibiotics, ribavirin plus a 3-week step-down steroid therapy and pulse methylprednisolone "rescue" resulted in 3.4% mortality, all in patients older than 65 years.[17] Various agents like indomethacin, lopinavir/ritonavir have shown in vitro activity against the virus. A review in 2006 of SARS therapy administered during the epidemic revealed that finding clear-cut treatment benefits was elusive. There were 26 reports of inconclusive benefits and 4 reports of possible harm related to ribavirin therapy, 25 inconclusive reports and 4 reports of possible harm from steroid therapy, and inconclusive reports for lopinavir-ritonavir therapy[2], IFN-α therapy[3] and convalescent plasma or immunoglobulin therapy.[7,18]

Middle East Respiratory Syndrome

Approximately a decade after the SARS epidemic, first index case of severe viral pneumonia caused by a novel corona virus was reported in June 2012 from Saudi Arabia. This has subsequently been named Middle-East Respiratory Syndrome (MERS). Most of the cases have been reported from the Arabian Peninsula with few travel related cases from Europe and the United states. Dromedary camels are the zoonotic vector and possible reservoir with bats as alternate possible vectors for human transmission. Despite both MERS and SARS being caused by corona viruses, the disease pattern appears very different with MERS having higher mortality rate (35–50%) and ineffective human transmission as compared to SARS which had efficient human transmission and relatively low mortality.

The median period of incubation for person to person transmission is around 5 days, and median time to progression to pneumonia after onset of infection, approximately 7 days. Patients typically present with influenza like illness (ILI). Concomitant symptoms are typical of any viral illness, include sore throat, myalgias and diarrhea. Radiological involvement is again nonspecific though unilateral basal lobar infiltrate are more common initially than in other viral pneumonias, making it difficult to differentiate from bacterial pneumonia. Infiltrates progress rapidly to involve both sides in a diffuse interstitial pattern, consolidations may occur but cavitation is uncommon. Bacterial co-infection is rare and clinical progression to ARDS with severe hypoxemia and death from acute refractory hypoxemia is typically rapid. Mortality of patients admitted to ICU is around 58%.

Non-specific laboratory abnormalities include leukopenia, relative lymphocytosis and thrombocytopenia. Elevation of liver enzymes is frequent with most hospitalized patients demonstrating significant transaminitis. Definite diagnosis is made by demonstration of MERS-CoV in lower respiratory tract secretions by RT PCR, though virus is present in blood, feces and urine as well. Without evaluation in an epidemic setting or history of travel to endemic region, the presentation of MERS cannot be differentiated from that of any other severe respiratory viral pneumonia.

Treatment: Treatment of MERS is largely supportive with early institution of mechanical ventilation and extracorporeal membrane oxygenation (ECMO) in cases with refractory hypoxemia. Interferon-α 2b and ribavirin have shown promise in experimental studies in monkeys with reduction of corona virus replication and moderating hosts immune response but have no definite role in humans.

Hantavirus Pulmonary Syndrome

The hantaviruses are an enveloped genus of the family bunyaviridae. Virions are spherical and encapsulated by a bilayered phospholipid membrane. Vascular endothelial cells are the principal target, but also infect alveolar macrophages and follicular dendritic cells. Renal tubular epithelium can also be a site for infection. Genus consists of multiple viruses, which are known to cause HPS in humans. Rodents act as reservoirs, but the virus is not pathogenic to them. Transmission largely occurs through inhalation of aerosolized urine, feces, or saliva of the rodent host. HPS is most often acquired indoors as captured animals tend to have higher rates of active infection than wild ones (25% vs 10%), and humans are more likely to encounter rodent excreta in a closed environment rather than open. Most cases reported till now have been isolated cases or clusters, in contrast to other epidemic viruses.

The disease has four recognized clinical phases—prodrome, pulmonary edema and shock, diuresis and convalescence.[19] Prodrome lasts for 3-6 days, in which phase the onset of pulmonary edema and shock is abrupt. The second phase also lasts for 3-6 days with maximum mortality occurring within the first 24 hours after the onset of shock. Patients who survive this phase enter a diuretic phase with urine output ranging from 300-500 mL/hour, and this is associated with rapid resolution of respiratory symptoms. Patients then enter a phase of convalescence, which may last a few weeks to several months before complete recovery takes place. A trio of hematologic findings, including thrombocytopenia, leukocytosis with a left shift and circulating immunoblastoid lymphocytes, is unique to HPS in the United States.

Treatment

Careful history, recognizing typical phases and a high index of suspicion are essential to achieve a diagnosis in HPS. Commercial laboratories can serologically confirm or rule out the diagnosis of HPS within 24 hours; IgM antibodies to nucleocapsid antigen are universally present in symptomatic patients and IgG antibodies are present in the most. There are no specific antiviral therapies for the management of HPS as of now and the management is supportive. Patients need admission to an intensive care unit with continuous monitoring of hemodynamic status, inotropic support and invasive mechanical ventilation with protective lung ventilatory strategy. A subset of patients may benefit from extracorporeal membrane oxygenation (ECMO) in centers where it is available though there are no controlled trials in the setting of HPS.

Adenovirus Pneumonia

Adenoviruses are common causes of CAP. Clinically, adenovirus pneumonia cannot be differentiated from other viral pneumonias. It was first recognized to cause pneumonia among military recruits. Subsequently, outbreaks have been reported from institutionalized populations. The severity of disease ranges from mild to severe requiring hospitalization and ventilatory support. In fatal cases, there has been extensive pulmonary damage, with death occurring 2-3 weeks into the illness. Intravascular coagulopathy has also been a late feature of some cases and a septic shock picture has been described. Bacterial superinfection, especially secondary to *Neisseria meningitidis* may complicate the course of the disease. There is no specific therapy which involves only supportive care.

Influenza

Influenza viruses belong to the family of orthomyxoviridae, which are lipid-enveloped, single-stranded, negative-sense, eight-segmented RNA viruses. Serotype A and B are the frequent cause of clinical disease, serotype A has multiple subtypes based on various combination of 16 known hemagglutinin (HA) and 9 neuraminidase (NA) genes that code for these viral envelope or surface proteins whereas B has only a single subtype. So far, only 3 subtypes of HA (H1, H2, H3) and 2 subtypes of NA (N1, N2) have caused pandemics in humans.

Traditional pandemic surveillance has focused on monitoring the antigenic shift, the reassortment of HA and/or NA genes between human and zoonotic influenza A viruses during rare events of dual infections in a human or an intermediate host. For the surveillance of currently circulating seasonal influenza viruses, most recently the A (H3N2) and A (H1N1) viruses, viral isolates are collected throughout the year to determine the most appropriate seasonal/influenza vaccine composition for the coming influenza seasons.[20] The influenza virus-associated pneumonias will be reviewed in the following sections as seasonal influenza A, avian influenza and H1N1 2009 pandemic-associated pneumonias.

Seasonal Influenza A Pneumonia

Seasonal influenza results in 200,000 admissions and over 40,000 deaths yearly in the United States alone. Influenza activity is generally seasonal—activity increases during the cooler months and peaks from December to March. Virus invades and attaches to the respiratory epithelial cells of the upper respiratory tract. Dissemination occurs due to the generation of droplets ranging in size from 1-5 micron when the patient coughs or sneezes.

Incubation period is usually 1-2 days, but may be up to four days. Presentation is usually with fever, myalgias and rhinitis consistent with symptoms of flu. Most cases of influenza are restricted to the upper respiratory tract and have a self-limited, benign clinical course. Severe disease with primary influenza pneumonia is more common in patients older than 65 years of age, those with underlying health conditions and young children.[2] Bilateral diffuse interstitial/alveolar infiltrates are seen as the most common radiographic abnormality (52%), followed by right lower lobe consolidation (35%).

Diagnosis: Primary influenza pneumonias are difficult to distinguish from other viral, bacterial or atypical pneumonias based on clinical, radiologic or laboratory features alone. The duration of shedding depends on the severity of illness, and age; generally virus can be isolated from throat and nasopharyngeal swabs obtained within 2 days of the onset of illness. There are several modalities to document influenza infection. These include direct viral detection (antigen tests, PCR, immunofluorescence and culture) or serologic tests. Rapid viral detection in the secretions can be achieved by commercially available antigen detection kits. Viral culture is the gold standard for detection of virus, but takes up to 48 hours to achieve diagnosis. Serologic testing requires demonstration of fourfold rise in titer and are helpful for research purposes rather than in patient management.

Treatment: Neuraminidase inhibitors (NAI), such as oseltamivir and zanamivir have shown to decrease the duration and severity of illness, if given within 36 hours of the onset of symptoms. In complicated influenza with primary pneumonia, studies showing efficacy of antivirals in decreasing mortality or duration of illness are less convincing. In spite of this, there is a tendency to use oral oseltamivir in patients with pneumonia and ARDS. Another member of the NAI group, peramivir, is still in clinical trials. Peramivir has an advantage over oseltamivir (taken orally) and zanamivir (taken by inhalation) as it can be given intravenously. Management is usually supportive with mechanical ventilation for respiratory failure and surveillance for the evidence of secondary bacterial pneumonia and early institution of appropriate antibiotics. Yearly vaccination has shown to decrease the incidence and severity of influenza and should be encouraged in patients over 65 years of age or in the presence of comorbid conditions.

Avian Influenza A (H5N1)

A zoonotic virus, avian influenza A (H5N1) emerged for the first time in Hong Kong in 1997 from chickens to infect humans, infecting 18 people and killing 6 of them, a high mortality rate of more than 30%.[21] As of 2009, the WHO has reported 440 cases of sporadic H5N1 human infection, of which 262 were lethal (a 60% case-fatality rate).[22] Different viral subtypes have varied ability to cause disease in human population. Though the cases of H5N1 have been sporadic and infective potential low, fear stems from the high mortality rate among infected individuals and demonstration of certain strains of low infectivity can rapidly mutate (within 6-9 months) to become highly virulent, if allowed to circulate freely among poultry. The incubation period for this virus has been estimated to be up to 7 days, but is more commonly 2-5 days after the last known exposure to sick or dead poultry. In cases where human-to-human transmission was suspected, the incubation period was estimated to be between 2-10 days.

Diagnosis: Common laboratory findings in patients with A (H5N1) infection at the time of hospital admission include leukopenia, lymphopenia and mild-to-moderate thrombocytopenia. No distinct radiological findings help to differentiate it from other viral infections. Acute respiratory distress syndrome complicated 76.5% (13 in 17) of cases in Thailand and 44.4% (8 in 18) of cases in Hong Kong.[23] Multiple organ failure, with signs of renal dysfunction and sometimes cardiac compromise, was often noted. In fatal cases, the median time from onset to death was 9 days.[24]

Treatment: High degree of resistance to amantadine has made it obsolete, NAI have been used for the treatment. Antivirals should be started within the first 48 hours before the efficacy declines. The mainstay and most effective approach to treating the disease is similar to most viral pneumonias and involves good supportive care. Intensive care during critical period of multiorgan dysfunction goes a long way in improving outcome. Adjuvant therapy with corticosteroids is not proven to improve outcome and hence is not routinely recommended.

Swine Origin Influenza (H1N1) 2009

The world witnessed an influenza pandemic in 2009, with an outbreak in Mexico which soon spread to engulf the whole world to nearly all countries by early 2010. By the WHO estimates, more than 17,700 deaths among laboratory-confirmed cases were reported by March 2010. As with any pandemic, the reported cases may have formed merely the tip of the iceberg with many subclinical cases which were never reported to the healthcare providers.

The pandemic A (H1N1) virus originated from the triple-reassortment swine influenza (H1) virus circulating in North American pigs.[25,26] Complete genome sequencing has shown that the known molecular markers of pathogenicity (PB1-F2 and nonstructural-1 proteins) are not expressed in the pandemic A (H1N1) virus.[27] Animal studies have shown that the novel influenza virus caused increased morbidity, replicated to higher titers in lung tissue, and was recovered from the intestinal tract of intranasally inoculated ferrets, in contrast to seasonal influenza H1N1 virus. This may explain why the novel virus is relatively more pathogenic than seasonal influenza viruses in its capacity to invade the lower respiratory tract and cause rapidly progressive pneumonia in humans because of our lack of background immunity to the former.

RISK FACTORS AND FEATURES OF SEVERE DISEASE

Unlike the seasonal flu, up to 40% of patients who required hospitalization or died were previously healthy. Surprisingly, the elderly (>65 years) are less frequently infected by the novel virus, probably because of some pre-existing cross-reactive immunity against the virus due to their past exposure to previous circulating seasonal influenza A (H1N1) strains, similar to the current pandemic A (H1N1) virus. Whether the components of vaccine against seasonal flu confer any cross immunity against the pandemic strain is unclear. The risk factors for severe disease include obesity, diabetes mellitus, and chronic respiratory, cardiovascular and kidney diseases, as well as diseases related to smoking, pregnancy, immunosuppression and delay in diagnosis. Diffuse alveolar damage, necrotizing bronchiolitis and diffuse alveolar damage with intense alveolar hemorrhage have been the distinct pathologic findings observed in patients who had died from H1N1 pandemic.[28]

Secondary bacterial infections were documented in 14–29% of patients with severe disease and required early detection with appropriate management.[29,30] The principal clinical syndrome leading to hospitalization and intensive care is diffuse viral pneumonitis associated with severe hypoxemia, ARDS, and sometimes shock and renal failure. This syndrome has accounted for approximately 49–72% of ICU admissions for 2009 H1N1 virus infection.[31] Rapid progression is common, typically starting on day 4–5 after the onset of illness and intubation is often necessary within 24 hours after admission. Median duration of ICU care was 7 days and mechanical ventilation 8 days.[32]

Radiographic findings commonly included diffused mixed interstitial and alveolar infiltrates, although lobar and multilobar distributions occur, particularly in patients with bacterial coinfection **(Fig. 1)**. Chest computed tomography has shown multiple areas of ground-glass opacities, air bronchograms and alveolar consolidation, particularly in the lower lobes **(Fig. 2)**.

Pulmonary thromboembolism has been reported in critically ill patients in spite of prophylaxis. Laboratory findings at presentation in patients with severe disease typically include normal or low-normal leukocyte counts with lymphocytopenia and elevations in the levels of

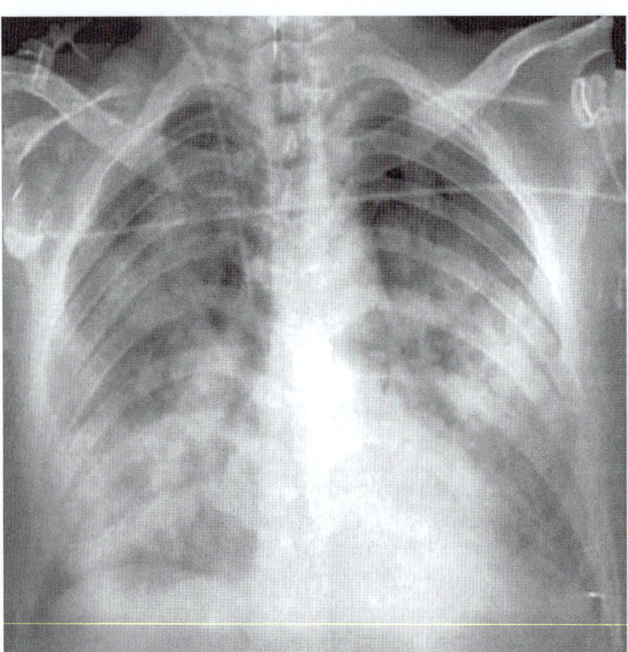

Fig. 1 Chest radiograph of a patient with proven severe H1N1 infection presenting with acute respiratory distress syndrome

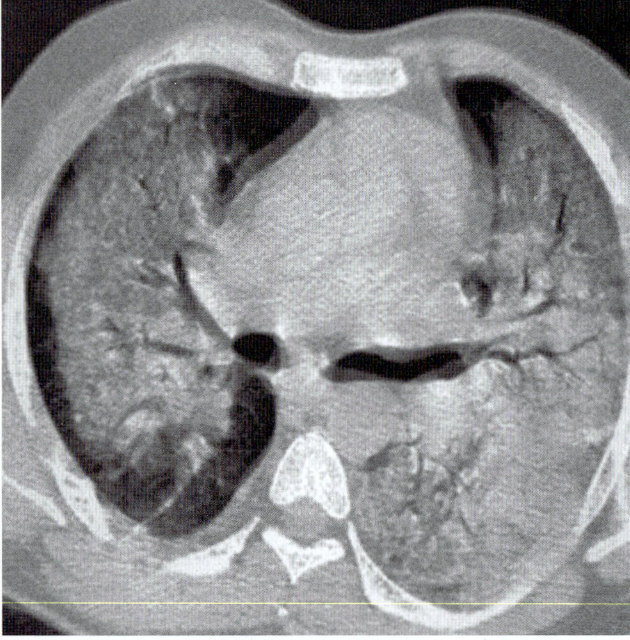

Fig. 2 Computed tomography scan of the same patient showing extensive areas of consolidation

serum aminotransferases, lactate dehydrogenase (LDH), creatine kinase and creatinine. Elevated creatine kinase, LDH, creatinine, metabolic acidosis and thrombocytopenia portend poor prognosis.[33] A few cases of encephalitis and myocarditis have been reported.

RESPIRATORY PROTECTION FOR HEALTHCARE PROFESSIONALS

Standard and droplet precautions are considered adequate to control the transmission of influenza in most healthcare settings. Vaccination of healthcare staff against seasonal and pandemic influenza strains is an essential protective strategy, but may be difficult to incorporate in practice as even with seasonal influenza the compliance among healthcare professionals for vaccination is only about 40%. Management principles include—performance of hand hygiene measures before and after every patient contact or with the patient environment, disinfection of the patient environment; early identification and isolation of patients with suspected or proven influenza; adoption of a greater minimum distance of patient separation (2 meters) than previously recommended; use of a surgical mask and eye protection for personal protection on entry to infectious areas or within 2 meters of an infectious patient.[34]

The center for disease control (CDC) recommends the use of N95 respirators for people involved in aerosol generating procedures like suctioning or bronchoscopy. Prophylactic antivirals should be restricted to individuals with sustained and heavy exposure. In high aerosol-risk settings, use of particulate mask, eye protection, impervious long-sleeved gown and gloves donned in that sequence (and removed in reverse sequence) avoiding self-contamination should be practiced. Symptomatic staff should be excluded from discharging duties till such time criteria for noninfectivity are met. These simple precautions go a long way in conferring protection, especially in a resource-constrained setting.

Diagnosis

Viral RNA detection by conventional or real-time reverse-transcriptase-polymerase-chain-reaction (RT PCR) assay remains the best method for the initial diagnosis of 2009 H1N1 virus infection. Nasopharyngeal aspirates or swabs taken early after the onset of symptoms are suitable samples, but endotracheal or bronchoscopic aspirates have higher yields in patients with lower respiratory tract illness. Consequently, negative results in single respiratory specimens do not rule out 2009 H1N1 virus infection and repeated collection of multiple respiratory specimen types is recommended when clinical suspicion is high. Commercially available rapid influenza detection kits have poor sensitivity and cannot differentiate H1N1 2009 from seasonal influenza. Virus can be isolated in various cell cultures, but usually takes several days for diagnosis.

Antiviral Therapy

H1N1 2009 is susceptible to neuraminidase inhibitors, such as oseltamivir and zanamivir, but is almost universally resistant to amantadine and rimantadine. Early institution of oseltamivir results in the reduction of duration, illness-severity and clearance of virus from the upper respiratory tract. Progression of disease and death can occur despite early therapy. Administration of oseltamivir within 48 hours of the onset of symptoms has been associated with reduced mortality among hospitalized patients. One should not wait for test results for starting antivirals. Even if negative, should be continued on oseltamivir until an alternate diagnosis is achieved. In severely ill patients, viral RNA may be detectable in endotracheal aspirates for several weeks after the initiation of oseltamivir therapy. An increased dose of the drug (e.g. 150 mg twice daily in adults) and particularly an increased duration of therapy (e.g. a total of 10 days) without treatment interruptions are reasonable in patients with pneumonia or evidence of clinical progression.

A His275Tyr mutation in viral neuraminidase confers high-level resistance to oseltamivir, but not to zanamivir. Most oseltamivir-resistant 2009 H1N1 viruses have been sporadic isolates from treated patients, particularly those with immunosuppression who have received prolonged oseltamivir therapy or those in whom postexposure oseltamivir chemoprophylaxis failed. A few cases of de novo resistance have been reported, which is a cause for concern.[35] Inhaled zanamivir has not been adequately studied in influenza, but it is the only drug that can be used in oseltamivir resistance.

Intravenous peramivir and zanamivir have shown good efficacy in seasonal influenza, but His275Tyr mutation also confers resistance to peramivir. Intravenous zanamivir is the drug of choice in the presence of oseltamivir resistance. Food and Drug Administration (FDA) recently approved intravenous peramivir for emergency use in hospitalized patients.

MANAGEMENT OF CRITICALLY ILL PATIENTS WITH H1N1 INFLUENZA 2009 (TABLE 2)

Severe respiratory insufficiency necessitating mechanical ventilation was encountered in 10–30% of hospitalized patients with H1N1 influenza 2009.[36] Noninvasive positive pressure ventilation (NPPV) relieves hypoxemia, decreases work of breathing and therefore tachypnea, but does not alter the course of illness. As with other cases of ARDS, NPPV is not routinely recommended for the management of hypoxemic individuals as it may delay intubation and inadvertently increase mortality. NPPV may be used under controlled circumstances, with the knowledge that most people would require invasive ventilation and early decision to intubate, if no improvement occurs in the first hour.

Table 2 Management of critically ill H1N1 influenza 2009 patients

• Definite benefit in all critically ill patients	Benefit in subgroup of patients not responding to standard care	Potential or unproven benefit
• Oseltamivir, zanamivir		Pooled hyperimmune serum
• Low tidal volume ventilatory strategy and conservative fluid management	ECMO, high frequency oscillatory ventilation, prone ventilation	Noninvasive positive pressure ventilation (NPPV)
• DVT and stress ulcer prophylaxis	Recruitment maneuvers	IVIG, statins and N-acetyl-L cysteine
• Corticosteroids in shock and persistent ARDS	Corticosteroids upfront in the absence of shock	
Abbreviations: ECMO, extracorporeal membrane oxygenation; DVT, deep vein thrombosis; IVIG, intravenous immunoglobulin; ARDS, acute respiratory distress syndrome		

Table 3 Priority groups for vaccination against H1N1 influenza

- Healthcare professionals and paramedical staff
- Pregnant women
- Individuals between 6 months to 24 years of age
- Those above 25 years of age with underlying cardiopulmonary disease, diabetes mellitus and renal disease
- Household contacts of infants younger than 6 months of age.

The WHO interim guidelines on the prevention and control of acute respiratory diseases in health care have included NPPV among those aerosol generating procedures in which there is possibly increased risk of respiratory pathogen transmission. Invasive mechanical ventilation (IMV) should be given with low tidal volume [6 mL/kg ideal body weight (IBW)], lung protective ventilation (plateau pressures <30 cm H_2O)[37] and conservative fluid strategy.[38] In ICUs where the infrastructure is available, ECMO has been shown to improve survival in patients with refractory hypoxemia.[31,39]

H1N1 Influenza 2009 Monovalent Vaccine

Efficacy of monovalent vaccine against H1N1 influenza 2009 has been established in two separate trials. There has been ambiguity regarding the dosage of vaccine (15 vs 7.5 microgram) and whether one or two doses are needed for adequate immune response. Based on the pandemic proportion of the current influenza, time needed for eliciting immune response and on need versus availability of vaccine, it is recommended that a single dose of 15 microgram of monovalent vaccine should elicit seroprotective levels of antibodies in at least 80% of recipients. The CDC recommends vaccination for the defined groups of individuals **(Table 3)**.[40]

REFERENCES

1. Jennings LC, Anderson TP, Beynon KA, Chua A, Laing RT, Werno AM, et al. Incidence and characteristics of viral community-acquired pneumonia in adults. Thorax. 2008; 63(1):42-8.
2. de Roux A, Marcos MA, Garcia E, Mensa J, Ewig S, Lode H, et al. Viral community-acquired pneumonia in nonimmunocompromised adults. Chest. 2004;125(4):1343-51.
3. Shiley KT, Van Deerlin VM, Miller WT. Chest CT features of community-acquired respiratory viral infections in adult inpatients with lower respiratory tract infections. J Thorac Imaging. 2010;25(1):68-75.
4. Gasparetto EL, Escuissato DL, Marchiori E, Ono S, Frare e Silva RL, Müller NL. High-resolution CT findings of respiratory syncytial virus pneumonia after bone marrow transplantation. AJR Am J Roentgenol. 2004;182(5):1133-7.
5. Franquet T, Rodriguez S, Martino R, Giménez A, Salinas T, Hidalgo A. Thin-section CT findings in hematopoietic stem cell transplantation recipients with respiratory virus pneumonia. AJR Am J Roentgenol. 2006;187(4):1085-90.
6. I'iller E, Marshall R, Vurdien J. Epidemiology, outcome and control of varicella-zoster infection. Rev Med Microbiol. 1993;4:222-30.
7. El-Daher N, Magnussen R, Betts RF. Varicella pneumonitis: clinical presentation and experience with acyclovir treatment in immunocompetent adults. Int J Infect Dis. 1998;2(3):147-51.
8. Davidson RN, Lynn W, Savage P, Wansbrough-Jones MH. Chickenpox pneumonia: experience with antiviral treatment. Thorax. 1988;43(8):627-30.
9. Triebwasser JH, Harris RE, Bryant RE, Rhoades ER. Varicella pneumonia in adults. Report of seven cases and a review of literature. Medicine (Baltimore). 1967;46(5):409-23.
10. Feldman S. Varicella-zoster virus pneumonitis. Chest. 1994;106(1 Suppl):22S-27S.
11. Adhami N, Arabi Y, Raees A, Al-Shimemeri A, Ur-Rahman M, Memish ZA. Effect of corticosteroids on adult varicella pneumonia: cohort study and literature review. Respirology. 2006;11(4):437-41.
12. Cunha BA. Cytomegalovirus pneumonia: community-acquired pneumonia in immunocompetent hosts. Infect Dis Clin North Am. 2010;24(1):147-58.
13. Christian MD, Poutanen SM, Loutfy MR, Muller MP, Low DE. Severe acute respiratory syndrome. Clin Infect Dis. 2004;38(10):1420-7.
14. Gillim-Ross L, Subbarao K. Emerging respiratory viruses: challenges and vaccine strategies. Clin Microbiol Rev. 2006;19(4):614-36.
15. Hui DS, Chan PK. Severe acute respiratory syndrome and coronavirus. Infect Dis Clin North Am. 2010;24(3):619-38.

16. Hui DS, Wong KT, Antonio GE, Lee N, Wu A, Wong V, et al. Severe acute respiratory syndrome: correlation between clinical outcome and radiologic features. Radiology. 2004;233(2):579-85.
17. Lau AC, So LK, Miu FP, Yung RW, Poon E, Cheung TM, et al. Outcome of coronavirus-associated severe acute respiratory syndrome using a standard treatment protocol. Respirology. 2004;9(2):173-83.
18. Stockman LJ, Bellamy R, Garner P. SARS: systematic review of treatment effects. PLoS Med. 2006;3(9):e343.
19. Levy H, Simpson SQ. Hantavirus pulmonary syndrome. Am J Respir Crit Care Med. 1994;149(6):1710-3.
20. Tang JW, Shetty N, Lam TT, Hon KL. Emerging, novel, and known influenza virus infections in humans. Infect Dis Clin North Am. 2010;24(3):603-17.
21. Subbarao K, Klimov A, Katz J, Regnery H, Lim W, Hall H, et al. Characterization of an avian influenza A (H5N1) virus isolated from a child with a fatal respiratory illness. Science. 1998;279(5349):393-6.
22. World Health Organization. Cumulative number of confirmed human cases for avian influenza A(H5N1). [online] Available from *http://www.who.int/influenza/human_animal_interface/EN_GIP_201503031cumulativeNumberH5N1cases.pdf.* [Accessed March 2016].
23. Uyeki TM. Human infection with highly pathogenic avian influenza A (H5N1) virus: review of clinical issues. Clin Infect Dis. 2009;49(2):279-90.
24. Tran TH, Nguyen TL, Nguyen TD, Luong TS, Pham PM, Nguyen vV, et al. Avian influenza A (H5N1) in 10 patients in Vietnam. N Engl J Med. 2004;350(12):1179-88.
25. Trifonov V, Khiabanian H, Rabadan R. Geographic dependence, surveillance, and origins of the 2009 influenza A (H1N1) virus. N Engl J Med. 2009;361(2):115-9.
26. Shinde V, Bridges CB , Uyeki TM , Shu B, Balish A, Xu X, et al. Triple-reassortant swine influenza A (H1) in humans in the United States, 2005-2009. N Engl J Med. 2009;360(25):2616-25.
27. Garten RJ, Davis CT, Russell CA, Shu B, Lindstrom S, Balish A, et al. Antigenic and genetic characteristics of swine-origin 2009 A(H1N1) influenza viruses circulating in humans. Science. 2009;325 (5937):197-201.
28. Mauad T, Hajjar LA, Callegari GD, da Silva LF, Schout D, Galas FR, et al. Lung pathology in fatal novel human influenza A (H1N1) infection. Am J Respir Crit Care Med. 2010;181(1):72-9.
29. Centers for Disease Control and Prevention (CDC). Intensive care patients with severe novel influenza A (H1N1) virus infection-Michigan, June 2009. MMWR Morb Mortal Wkly Rep. 2009;58(27):749-52.
30. Centers for Disease Control and Prevention (CDC). Bacterial coinfections in lung tissue specimens from fatal cases of 2009 pandemic influenza A (H1N1)-United States, May-August 2009. MMWR Morb Mortal Wkly Rep. 2009;58(38):1071-4.
31. ANZIC Influenza Investigators, Webb SA, Pettilä V, Seppelt I, Bellomo R, Bailey M, et al. Critical care services and 2009 H1N1 influenza in Australia and New Zealand. N Engl J Med. 2009;36(20):1925-34.
32. Dominguez-Cherit G, Lapinsky SE, Macias AE, Pinto R, Espinosa-Perez L, de la Torre A, et al. Critically ill patients with 2009 influenza A (H1N1) in Mexico. JAMA. 2009;302(17):1880-7.
33. Perez-Padilla R, de la Rosa-Zamboni D, Ponce de Leon S, Hernandez M, Quiñones-Falconi F, Bautista E, et al. Pneumonia and respiratory failure from swine-origin influenza A (H1N1) in Mexico. N Engl J Med. 2009;361(7):680-9.
34. Stuart RL, Cheng AC, Marshall CL, Ferguson JK. Healthcare infection control special interest group of the Australian Society for Infectious Diseases. ASID (HIC SIG) position statement: infection control guidelines for patients with influenza-like illnesses, including pandemic (H1N1) influenza 2009, in Australian health care facilities. Med J Aust. 2009;191(8):454-8.
35. Writing Committee of the WHO Consultation on Clinical Aspects of Pandemic (H1N1) 2009 Influenza, Bautista E, Chotpitayasunondh T, Gao Z, Harper SA, Shaw M, et al. Clinical aspects of pandemic 2009 influenza A (H1N1) virus infection. N Engl J Med. 2009;362(18):1708-19.
36. World Health Organization. Clinical management of human infection with pandemic (H1N1) 2009: revised guidance. [online] Available from *http://www.who.int/csr/resources/publications/swineflu/clinical_management_h1n1.pdf.* [Accessed March 2016].
37. de Durante G, del Turco M, Rustichini L, Cosimini P, Giunta F, Hudson LD, et al. ARDSNet lower tidal volume ventilatory strategy may generate intrinsic positive end-expiratory pressure in patients with acute respiratory distress syndrome. Am J Respir Crit Care Med. 2002;165(9): 1271-4.
38. National Heart, Lung, and Blood Institute Acute Respiratory Distress Syndrome (ARDS) Clinical Trials Network1, Wiedemann HP, Wheeler AP, Bernard GR, Thompson BT, Hayden D, et al. Comparison of two fluid-management strategies in acute lung injury. N Engl J Med. 2006;354(24):2564-75.
39. Australia and New Zealand Extracorporeal Membrane Oxygenation (ANZ ECMO) Influenza Investigators, Davies A, Jones D, Bailey M, Beca J, Bellomo R, et al. Extracorporeal Membrane Oxygenation for 2009 Influenza A(H1N1) Acute Respiratory Distress Syndrome. JAMA. 2009;302(17):1888-95.
40. National Center for Immunization and Respiratory Diseases. CDC; Centers for Disease Control and Prevention (CDC). Use of influenza A (H1N1) 2009 monovalent vaccine: recommendations of the Advisory Committee on Immunization Practices (ACIP), 2009. MMWR Recomm Rep. 2009; 58(RR-10):1-8.

Pulmonary Manifestations of Human Immunodeficiency Virus Infection

Jai B Mullerpattan, Zarir F Udwadia

INTRODUCTION

Ever since the first description of human immunodeficiency virus (HIV) infection, lung has been the most commonly affected organ. Early autopsy studies in the mid-80s showed that there was pulmonary involvement in 90% of acquired immunodeficiency syndrome (AIDS) patients with a wide-spectrum of infectious and noninfectious complications. Both HIV1 and HIV2 have been isolated from the lung, it is clear that the lungs are an important organ of viral replication. There is a wide spectrum of pulmonary problems encountered in HIV **(Table 1)**. The type of complication depends upon several factors related to the host, the organisms and the environment **(Box 1 and Table 2)**.

(Details of individual problems are available in the respective chapters on the subjects).

HUMAN IMMUNODEFICIENCY VIRUS AND THE LUNG

Evidence for pulmonary tissue-level effects of HIV is conflicting. Alveolar macrophages and dendritic cells within the lung are targets for HIV infection.[1] Infection of human alveolar macrophages occurs preferentially via the CCR5 coreceptor.[2] Alveolar macrophages become increasingly infected as HIV infection progresses.[3] HIV-infected individuals may also have increased infiltration of CD8 T-lymphocytes within the interstitium and alveoli.[4] Lymphocytic alveolitis falls within the spectrum of lymphocytic infiltrative disorders, most common of which is lymphocytic interstitial pneumonitis in children.[5] Lymphocytic alveolitis is relatively common in HIV-infected adults, and can be seen in patients with no evidence of respiratory symptoms.[5] The infiltration of CD8 cytotoxic cells may represent an immune response to HIV-infected cells, and appears to correlate with high viral load burden within the lung.[6] B-cell abnormalities may lead to altered production of immunoglobulins (Igs). Bronchoalveolar lavage (BAL) from asymptomatic patients with HIV demonstrated decreased concentration of IgG compared to uninfected control subjects in one study,[7,8] but BAL immunoglobulin levels were not found to differ when patients were receiving ARV therapy. Impaired local and systemic host defenses due to the effects of HIV replication on immune function serve to provide an explanation for the frequency of serious pulmonary infections in this population.

Indian Epidemiology

Data from India on pulmonary complications in HIV patients are limited. An early autopsy study showed that tuberculosis accounted for 61% of all pulmonary diseases while bacterial pneumonias featured second at 18% in the terms of frequency.[9] In this study, *Pneumocystis jiroveci* pneumonia (PJP) infection accounted for only 5% of all cases. A more recent study of all hospitalizations for HIV in a tertiary center in Mumbai for over 2 years (2002–2003), which looked at 300 consecutive HIV-positive admissions revealed that the lungs were most commonly affected (120 of 300 admissions, 40%). In this study, tuberculosis (pulmonary and extrapulmonary) was the most common pulmonary cause of admissions (40%). The novel information emerged from this study that *Pneumocystis carinii* pneumonia (PCP), previously considered rare in the Indian context, ranked second in importance (30%), bacterial infections (pneumonia) ranked third with 30 cases (25%), while malignancies and miscellaneous conditions accounted for 4% each.[10]

PNEUMOCYSTIS JIROVECII (CARINII) PNEUMONIA

The long-standing controversy whether to place PCP in the parasitic or fungal families was finally settled by elegant gene sequencing studies by Edman incontrovertibly linking PCP to the fungal family.[11] The term PCP was subsequently changed to PJP after the name of Czech parasitologist, Otto Jírovec. The new name first proposed by Frenkel, has now been accepted by the Centers for Disease Control and Prevention (CDC) and the National Institutes of Health (NIH) since 2002 onward.

Table 1 Important pulmonary complications observed in HIV-infected patients

Respiratory infections caused by
• Bacterial
M. tuberculosis *S. pneumoniae* *H. influenzae* *S. aureus* *Nocardia spp* *Listeria* *Klebsiella spp* *Pseudomonas spp* *Rhodococcus equi*
• Fungal
Pneumocystis jirovecii *Cryptococcus neoformans* *Histoplasma capsulatum* *Candida albicans* *Coccidioides immitis* *Aspergillus spp*
• Parasitic
Toxoplasma gondii *Cryptosporidium spp* *Microsporidium spp* *Leishmania spp* *Strongyloides spp*
• Viral
Cytomegalovirus *Herpes simplex virus* *Varicella zoster virus* *Epstein-Barr virus* *Human herpesvirus 6 (HHV-6)* *JC virus* *Respiratory syncytial virus (RSV)* *Human herpesvirus 8 (HHV-8) (KSAHV)*
Malignancies
• Kaposi's sarcoma • B-cell lymphoma • Bronchogenic carcinoma
Idiopathic
• Interstitial lung disease (Lymphocytic interstitial pneumonia, nonspecific interstitial pneumonia) • Airway disease; bronchiolitis, emphysema • Diffuse infiltrative CD8 lymphocytosis • Sarcoidosis • Organizing pneumonia • Primary pulmonary hypertension • Alveolar hemorrhage

Globally, PJP accounted for about two-thirds of AIDS index diagnoses in the first decade of the HIV pandemic. It still remains the most prevalent opportunistic infection (OI) in patients with HIV. Considered rare in the Indian, Asian and African subcontinent, it was probably being underdiagnosed in the developing world due to lack of a wider availability of special diagnostic facilities like high resolution computed tomography (HRCT) scanning, bronchoscopy and BAL studies and special immunofluorescence staining.[12] This study not only showed it to be common when diligently searched for, but also revealed that almost half of all cases (49%) would have been missed without access to the sophisticated diagnostic techniques.[12] Earlier deaths from diseases caused by more pathogenic organisms may also have been partly responsible for less prevalence reported from Africa and India. In this series, PJP infection occurred at a low mean count of 96 of CD4 cells.

Whilst PJP remains one of the common opportunistic infections in the developed world, the incidence is declining

Table 2 CD4 cell count ranges for selected HIV-related and non-HIV-related respiratory illnesses

• *Any CD4 cell count* – Upper respiratory tract illness - Upper respiratory tract infection - Sinusitis - Pharyngitis – Acute bronchitis – Obstructive airway disease – Bacterial pneumonia – Tuberculosis – Non-Hodgkin lymphoma – Pulmonary embolus – Bronchogenic carcinoma
• *CD4 count ≤ 500 cells/μL* – Bacterial pneumonia (recurrent) – Pulmonary mycobacterial pneumonia
• *CD4 count ≤ 200 cells/μL* – *Pneumocystis pneumonia* – *Cryptococcus neoformans* pneumonia/pneumonitis – Bacterial pneumonia (associated with bacteremia/sepsis) – Disseminated or extrapulmonary tuberculosis.
• *CD4 count ≤ 100 cells/μL* – Pulmonary Kaposi sarcoma – Bacterial pneumonia (Gram-negative bacilli and *Staphylococcus aureus* increased) – *Toxoplasma pneumonitis*
• *CD4 count ≤ 50 cells/μL* – Disseminated *Histoplasma capsulatum* – Disseminated *Coccidioides immitis* – Cytomegalovirus pneumonitis – Disseminated *Mycobacterium avium* complex – Disseminated mycobacterium (nontuberculous) infection – *Aspergillus spp* pneumonia

BOX 1 Factors on which the type of pulmonary disease in the HIV-positive patient depends

- Geographical distribution
- Severity of immunocompromised
- Use of disease (such as *Pneumocystis jirovecii*) prophylaxis
- Use of antiretrovirals (ARVs)

in the West. There are two reasons for this decline in the West: Firstly, effective trimethoprim-sulfamethoxazole (TMP-SMX) prophylaxis used in almost all patients with CD4 counts less than 200 who are otherwise nine times more likely to develop PCP; secondly, the widespread availability of ARV therapy. PJP, however, retains its importance in HIV and continues to develop in patients who are unaware of their HIV status, in those with no access to care, and those who are unwilling or unable to adhere to therapy, nonresponders or in failures with ARV therapy.

Clinical Features

Dyspnea and cough are the most common symptoms while tachypnea is the most common sign. A study from Zimbabwe established that a respiratory rate more than 40/min is the single best clinical predictor of PJP infection in HIV-positive patients.[13] Crackles and rhonchi are infrequent. Whilst hypoxia is common, it is by no means universal. In our series from Hinduja Hospital, Mumbai, 50% of patients had a normal SaO_2 at rest and 15% had completely normal clinical examination. The mean duration from the onset of symptoms to final diagnosis averaged as long as 30 days. In fact, the rapid onset of symptoms, high fever and rigors, which are commonly encountered in pyogenic infections, are all rare in PJP.

Radiology

In the early stages, bilateral mid-zone interstitial shadows are seen. These are often subtle, normal chest radiographs have been reported in 5–34% of series. In our own series, 10% of patients had normal radiographs. HRCT greatly increases the diagnostic rate. The commonest CT pattern consists of bilateral patchy areas of ground glass density, which are centrally located. Air-filled cysts or pneumatoceles may be seen in upper lobes in approximately 10% of cases. A variety of atypical radiographic features has been reported, which include upper lobe infiltrates (especially in patients on nebulized pentamidine prophylaxis), cystic changes, pneumothorax, pleural effusions, focal nodular lesions, cavitation and adenopathy. It may be pointed out that effusions, upper lobe infiltrates and adenopathy are all more often secondary to TB than to PJP especially in India and other countries where TB prevalence is high.

Of importance is the fact that whilst the evolution of shadows is often rapid, they are slow to resolve. In an earlier report on 104 PJP patients, 35% of patients' radiographs had actually improved at 3 weeks, complete resolution had occurred in only 43% at 5 months.[14]

Of other diagnostic tests, lactate dehydrogenase (LDH) estimation and desaturation with exercise are both sensitive, but not specific for PJP infection. Microbiology is crucial to make a diagnosis. Sputum is often not produced, hence induced by nebulization with hypertonic saline. The yield can be improved by examination of BAL fluid. A transbronchial biopsy is seldom performed, but further increases diagnostic yield. The organisms are best seen on staining with Gomori methenamine, Calcofluor white and immunofluorescence staining, which are sensitive and highly specific for identifying trophic and cystic forms.

Treatment

Trimethoprim-sulfamethoxazole remains the treatment of choice. Unfortunately, side effects are common at the high doses required for PJP infection. As many as 50% of patients develop major side effects, which demand temporary or permanent discontinuation of treatment.

Clindamycin plus primaquine is a reasonable alternative that is better tolerated. A large multicenter study, which compared clindamycin plus primaquine with TMP-SMX in 87 patients found it better tolerated with similar success rates.[15] Other drugs which are used include nebulized and intravenous pentamidine, dapsone and atovaquone.

Role of steroids: Steroids are unequivocally useful in moderate to severe PJP. Their use should be reserved for PJP patients who are hypoxic (PaO_2 <70 mm Hg). Steroids are shown to reduce the rate of worsening respiratory failure and death by as much as 50% in some series. They are most effective when given within 72 hours of onset of disease. They act by blunting the inflammatory response when used in a dose of oral prednisolone 20 mg twice daily or 40 mg once daily for five days, or 20 mg once daily for 11 days.

Antiretroviral therapy: The timing of ARV in relation to PJP is controversial. Whilst it was earlier felt best to complete the TMP-SMX therapy before commencing ARV therapy, evidence from the Adult/Adolescent Spectrum of HIV Disease Project showed that the concurrent prescription of ARV was associated with improved early survival.[16]

Outcome: There is little doubt that the outcome of PJP has improved. In the Adult/Adolescent Spectrum of HIV Disease Project, which looked at 4,412 patients with 5,222 episodes of PJP infection, survival at one-year improved from 40% in 1992 to 63% in 1998, despite the emergence of antibiotic resistant PJP strains.[16] This improvement in survival is attributable to widespread use of steroids, better ICU care of these patients and earlier introduction of ARV therapy.

COMMUNITY-ACQUIRED PNEUMONIAS

Bacterial pneumonia remains one of the most common causes of pulmonary infection, and a cause of considerable morbidity and mortality worldwide.[17,18] Etiologically, *Streptococcus pneumoniae* predominates followed by *Haemophilus influenzae*, in the developed and developing world settings.[19-21] *Staphylococcus aureus* and *Pseudomonas aeruginosa* account for about 5% of cases each.[20,22]

Pre-highly active antiretroviral therapy (HAART) rates of pneumonia in the developed world were significantly higher than in uninfected individuals, similar to rates seen in resource-limited settings. In a prospective study[17] in North America, rates of pneumonia in HIV-infected individuals in the period between 1988 and 1990 were 5.5 per 100 person-years compared to 0.9 per 100 person-years in uninfected individuals. More recently, a large cohort of HIV-infected women revealed rates of 8.5 per 100 person-years compared to 0.7 per 100 person-years during 1993 to 2000. Risk of pneumonia was clearly associated with decreasing CD4 counts, rates were as high as 10.8 per 100 person-years, and 17.9 per 100 person-years for patients with CD4 counts of 200 cells/L.[17,23] Rates of pneumonia were similarly high in a large cohort of HIV-infected miners in South Africa and even higher at 33 cases per 100 person-years in a cohort of postpartum women in Kenya.[24,25] In both settings, risk of pneumonia increased as CD4 cell counts decreased to 200 cells/L.[24,25]

Bacteremia associated with *S. pneumoniae* contributes significantly to morbidity in HIV-infected individuals worldwide. Rates of invasive pneumococcal disease have been seen to climb in parallel with the emerging HIV epidemic in the pre-HAART era in North America and similarly in Africa.[26-29]

Impact of HIV-related Interventions and HAART on Bacterial Pneumonia

Prior to the advent of HAART, interventions such as antimicrobial prophylaxis had been shown to decrease overall rates for bacterial pneumonias. TMP-SMX use was associated with a 67% reduction in rates of pneumonia in a large US retrospective cohort study.[22] Similarly, it was found to be protective in the prospective US women's cohort (the HIV Epidemiologic Research Study).[23] Of note, the protective effect of TMP-SMX was no longer detectable in another cohort study[30] conducted during the HAART era in which reductions in bacterial pneumonia rates were associated with ARV use.

The efficacy of the 23-valent pneumococcal polysaccharide vaccine is less clear. Studies[22,30,31] in the developed world have suggested that pneumococcal vaccine may prevent invasive disease; however, a randomized clinical trial[31] conducted in Uganda failed to confirm a protective effect. Nonetheless, the vaccine continues to be recommended, particularly for patients with higher CD4 cell counts. Multiple studies[23,29,32,33] from sites within the United States and Europe have now demonstrated reduction in rates of bacterial pneumonia after introduction of HAART.

The HIV Epidemiologic Research Study found that each month of HAART decreased risk of bacterial pneumonia by 10% in those not receiving TMP-SMX prophylaxis.

Malignancies

Lymphomas, Kaposi's sarcoma (KS) and bronchial carcinoma are the malignancies, which are more frequently reported in patients who are HIV positive.

1. *Kaposi's sarcoma:* KS was one of the initial pulmonary complications. It is now known to be associated with human herpesvirus type 8 (HHV-8) infection. HIV is believed to activate this virus, which lies dormant in the endothelial cells, acts as the trigger for angiogenesis, which results in the development and proliferation of this vascular tumor.[34] KS becomes more prevalent as the CD4 declines. In the United States, it is strikingly more common in homosexual population. The prevalence has dropped dramatically in the Western world after the introduction of ARV therapy. KS is considered rare in India apart from a few, scattered case reports. Typical radiographic features of KS include nodules and pleural effusions. In the setting of the typical KS skin lesions, the diagnosis is often presumptive. The diagnosis can be made more definitely, if similar raised purple plaques are seen on bronchoscopic examination. These lesions are highly vascular and distinctive, they are best not biopsied for the fear of bleeding. Treatment involves the combination of ARVs and chemotherapy in systemic disease.

2. *Non-Hodgkin lymphoma (NHL):* HIV-positive individuals are almost 500 times more at the risk of developing NHL compared to the normal population. NHL too occurs with an increasing frequency as the CD4 counts reduce. Epstein-Barr-Virus (EBV) may be implicated in the pathogenesis of many cases.[35] In the HIV-infected patients, NHL is aggressive and usually stage 4 at presentation. The outlook, despite aggressive chemotherapy, is poor. ARV therapy is responsible for the reducing prevalence of NHL in the developed world. ARV combined with chemotherapy has been responsible for an improved survival, which is now reported.

3. *Bronchogenic carcinoma:* HIV-positive patients are at the greater risk of developing lung cancer. Some studies suggest that adenocarcinomas are more frequent. As in NHLs, lung cancers in the HIV-positive population tend to be present in more aggressive and advanced forms. Unlike with NHL or KS, the CD4 counts tend to be well-preserved in patients with HIV-associated lung cancer.[36]

Immune Reconstitution Inflammatory Syndrome

Reconstitution of a functional immune system due to suppression of HIV replication by HAART has led to unusual clinical presentations with features of an exaggerated inflammatory response to newly recognized antigens. This phenomenon has been named immune reconstitution inflammatory syndrome (IRIS). Proposed criteria include documented viral load decreases in addition to new or worsening symptoms of an infectious or inflammatory condition after initiation of HAART.[37] Currently the severity of the inflammatory syndrome is thought to be due to the interactions between the degree of immune recovery, previously unrecognized (subclinical or residual) antigenic burden and possible host genetic factors.[38] Pulmonary manifestations of IRIS have been well-described with both *P. jirovecii* infection and *M. tuberculosis*. IRIS in the setting of tuberculosis can present either as a paradoxical worsening of tuberculosis symptoms in otherwise clinically improving patients who initiate ARV therapy sometime after tuberculosis therapy, or as an unmasking of unrecognized tuberculosis when ARVs are initiated.[39,40]

Most of the reported cases of tuberculosis-IRIS have been observed among patients whose tuberculosis diagnosis preceded the initiation of HAART.[41] The reported incidence of IRIS in this setting ranges from 7% to 45% in retrospective reviews.[39,40] Clinical manifestations include increased respiratory symptoms, fever and lymphadenopathy. Worsening of radiologic findings is common, with increasing infiltrates, lymphadenopathy or pleural effusions.[42] IRIS occurs usually within 6–8 weeks after initiation of HAART, and has been associated with lower CD4 cell counts at the time of initiation, higher viral loads at baseline and shorter duration of TB therapy before HAART initiation.[39-41] In addition, degree of CD4 cell count or HIV viral response has also been identified as a risk factor. Despite worsening symptoms, mortality is low. *Mycobacterium avium* complex IRIS includes a pulmonary-thoracic presentation in 29% of cases. Aside from constitutional symptoms, cough or wheeze (93%) and dyspnea (47%) are the most frequent respiratory symptoms. The imaging and bronchoscopy findings most often include mediastinal and/or hilar lymphadenopathy, endobronchial nodular lesions, cavities, pleural-based lesions or pulmonary infiltrates.[43] Clinical management usually includes therapy with nonsteroidal anti-inflammatories or corticosteroids, and HAART is continued unless life-threatening features are present.[38]

Miscellaneous Nonmalignant Conditions

Chronic Obstructive Pulmonary Disease

HIV-infected patients in the developed world have higher rates of smoking than the general population. Almost 75% of patients report a smoking history and 40–50% are current smokers.[44,45] Smoking history in conjunction with pulmonary effects of prior opportunistic lung infections and drug use-related lung damage, combine to place patients with HIV at risk for development of emphysema, airway disease and chronic obstructive pulmonary disease (COPD).[45] Furthermore, there is growing evidence that HIV itself may be a risk factor for the development of COPD. The management of COPD in the setting of HIV infection follows the same principles as in other patient populations.[45] It is now clear that there is a significant drug interaction between commonly used inhaled corticosteroids and the protease inhibitor (PI) ritonavir (even when used at low "boosting" doses). This has proven to be clinically problematic, as current HAART guidelines favor the use of ritonavir boosting when PI-based HAART is used.

Pulmonary hypertension: HIV is a rare cause of pulmonary arterial hypertension (PAH). The prevalence before the HAART era was estimated at around 0.5% in HIV-infected patients.[46] Most recently, a study in 2008 revealed that the prevalence has remained at 0.5% in the modern era of HIV therapy, suggesting that HAART has not had a dramatic impact on the prevention of HIV-related PAH.[47] In a retrospective chart review of patients with HIV infection, the incidence of PAH was higher in individuals who received HAART compared with those individuals who only received nucleoside analog reverse-transcriptase inhibitors (NRTIs).[48] This result may have arisen from differences in the cohort populations: the HAART cohort may have had more progressed HIV disease as it was defined as individuals with a CD4 count of less than 300 cells/µL and a viral load of more than 30,000 copies/mL, whereas the NRTI cohort was defined as individuals with stage C2 (CD4 count between 200 cells/µL and 499 cells/µL and AIDS-defining illness) or greater disease. The reason that HAART does not favorably impact the prevalence of HIV-related PAH is unclear at the present time. We do know from studies that HIV does not directly infect vascular endothelial cells or smooth muscle cells.[49] Hence, the association between HIV and PAH may not be related to viral load or immune status, partially explaining why HAART does not prevent PAH.

Prognosis is guarded and treatment is administered as for any other patient with pulmonary hypertension, though interactions between sildenafil and PIs should be borne in mind.[50]

Lymphocytic interstitial pneumonia (LIP): LIP, may be EB virus related, is more common in children with HIV infection. It is now increasingly encountered in adults as well. The CT appearance with interstitial shadowing may be confused with PJP infection; however, the symptoms are more insidious. Thoracoscopic biopsy is usually needed to make a definitive diagnosis. Treatment consists of a combination of ARVs and steroids.

Sarcoidosis: Sarcoidosis and HIV are both known to cause peripheral CD4 cell depletion. HIV does so by destruction of the cells while in sarcoidosis, they are concentrated in the granulomas. HIV has been known to attenuate the clinical effects of sarcoidosis, which reappear after immune reconstitution. There have been case reports of sarcoidosis in patients with HIV, but in all cases, the CD4 count was above 200 cells/µL.[51]

Bronchiolitis obliterans and organizing pneumonia (BOOP): All reported HIV-infected patients with BOOP had a far-advanced disease with the highest reported CD4 count being 168 cells/µL. Cough, dyspnea and fever are the most common clinical findings. Chest radiographs in BOOP usually show bilateral patchy infiltrates. Definitive evaluation in these patients is often not done because of reluctance to perform open lung biopsy in patients not suspected of having an acute, potentially reversible respiratory infection. This may account for why BOOP has not been previously recognized in patients with HIV infection since the more commonly performed transbronchial biopsy generally does not yield enough tissue to adequately identify the intrabronchiolar granulation tissue polyps and BAL findings are not specific for bronchiolitis obliterans. PCP because of compatible clinical and radiologic manifestations, and response to anti-pneumocystis drugs and steroids might, in fact, have BOOP. This diagnosis should be considered in patients with respiratory symptoms and abnormal chest radiographs in whom a microbiological diagnosis is not available.[52,53]

Abacavir hypersensitivity: A hypersensitivity reaction occurs in association with initiation of abacavir therapy as part of combination ARV therapy in approximately 3.7% of patients. The reaction is possibly the result of a combination of altered drug metabolism and immune dysfunction, which is poorly understood. The abacavir hypersensitivity reaction as a multiorgan process manifested by a sign or symptom from at least two of the following groups: (1) Fever, (2) rash, (3) gastrointestinal, (4) constitutional or (5) respiratory. The Whites appear to be at higher risk while patients of African descent have a lower risk of abacavir hypersensitivity. Clinical management involves supportive measures and discontinuation of abacavir therapy. Rechallenge with abacavir in a hypersensitive patient should be avoided because it might precipitate a life-threatening reaction. Studies have shown HLA-B*5701 serves as an excellent predictor of abacavir hypersensitivity syndrome.[54,55]

REFERENCES

1. Beck JM. The immunocompromised host: HIV infection. Proc Am Thorac Soc. 2005;2:423-7.
2. Park IW, Koziel H, Hatch W, Li X, Du B, Groopman JE. CD4 receptor-dependent entry of human immunodeficiency virus type-1 env-pseudotypes into CCR5-, CCR3-, and CXCR4-expressing human alveolar macrophages is preferentially mediated by the CCR5 co-receptor. Am J Respir Cell Mol Biol. 1999;20:864-71.
3. Sierra-Madero JG, Toossi Z, Hom DL, Finegan CK, Hoenig E, Rich EA. Relationship between load of virus in alveolar macrophages from human immunodeficiency virus type 1-infected persons, production of cytokines, and clinical status. J Infect Dis. 1994;169:18-27.
4. Semenzato G, Agostini C. HIV-related interstitial lung disease. Curr Opin Pulm Med. 1995;1:383-91.
5. Das S, Miller RF. Lymphocytic interstitial pneumonitis in HIV infected adults. Sex Transm Infect. 2003;79:88-93.
6. Twigg HL, Soliman DM, Day RB, Knox KS, Anderson RJ, Wilkes DS, et al. Lymphocytic alveolitis, bronchoalveolar lavage viral load, and outcome in human immunodeficiency virus infection. Am J Respir Crit Care Med. 1999;159:1439-44.
7. Twigg HL III, Spain BA, Soliman DM, Bowen LK, Heidler KM, Wilkes DS. Impaired IgG production in the lungs of HIV-infected individuals. Cell Immunol. 1996;170:127-33.
8. Fahy RJ, Diaz PT, Hart J, Wewers MD. BAL and serum IgG levels in healthy asymptomatic HIV-infected patients. Chest. 2001;119:196-203.
9. Hira SK, Shroff HJ, Lanjewar DN, Dholkia YN, Bhatia VP, Dupont H. The natural history of HIV infection amongst adults in Mumbai. Natl Med J India. 2003;16(3):126-31.
10. Udwadia ZF, Doshi A, Bhaduri AS. *Pneumocystis carinii* pneumonia in HIV-infected patients from Mumbai. J Assoc Physicians India. 2005;53:437-40.
11. Edman J, Kovacs J, Masur H, Santi DV, Elwood HJ, Sogin ML. Ribosomal RNA sequence shows *Pneumocystis carinii* to be a member of the fungi. Nature. 1988;334(6182):519-21.
12. Udwadia ZF, Doshi A, Bhaduri AS. Pneumocystis pneumonia. New Engl J Med. 2004;351(12):1262-3.
13. Malin AS, Gawanzura LK, Klein S, Robertson VJ, Musvaire P, Mason PR. *Pneumocystis carinii* pneumonia in Zimbabwe. Lancet. 1995;346(8985):1258-61.
14. DeLorenzo LJ, Huang CT, Maguire GP. Roentgenographic patterns of *Pneumocystis carinii* pneumonia in 104 patients with AIDS. Chest. 1987;91(3):332-7.
15. Toma E, Thorne A, Singer J, Raboud J, Lemieux C, Trottier S, et al. Clindamycin with primaquine vs Trimethoprim-sulfamethoxazole therapy for mild and moderately severe PCP in patients with AIDS: a multicenter, double-blind, randomized trial (CTN 004). CTN-PCP Study Group. Clin Infect Dis. 1998;27(3):524-30.
16. Farizo KM, Buehler JW, Chamberland ME, Whyte BM, Froelicher ES, Hopkins SG, et al. Spectrum of disease in persons with human immunodeficiency virus infection in the United States. JAMA. 1992;267(13):1798-805.
17. Hirschtick RE, Glassroth J, Jordan MC, Wilcosky TC, Wallace JM, Kvale PA, et al. Bacterial pneumonia in persons infected with the human immunodeficiency virus: Pulmonary Complications of HIV Infection Study Group. N Engl J Med. 1995;333:845-51.
18. Mayaud C, Parrot A, Cadranel J. Pyogenic bacterial lower respiratory tract infection in human immunodeficiency virus-infected patients. Eur Respir J Suppl. 2002;36:28s-39s.
19. Park DR, Sherbin VL, Goodman MS, Pacifico AD, Rubenfeld GD, Polissar NL, et al. The etiology of community-acquired pneumonia at an urban public hospital: influence of human immunodeficiency virus infection and initial severity of illness. J Infect Dis. 2001;184:268-77.
20. Rimland D, Navin TR, Lennox JL, Jernigan JA, Kaplan J, Erdman D, et al. Prospective study of etiologic agents of community-acquired pneumonia in patients with HIV infection. AIDS. 2002;16:85-95.
21. Scott JA, Hall AJ, Muyodi C, Lowe B, Ross M, Chohan B, et al. Aetiology, outcome, and risk factors for mortality among adults with acute pneumonia in Kenya. Lancet. 2000;355:1225-30.
22. Feikin DR, Feldman C, Schuchat A, Janoff EN. Global strategies to prevent bacterial pneumonia in adults with HIV disease. Lancet Infect Dis. 2004;4:445-55.
23. Kohli R, Lo Y, Homel P, Flanigan TP, Gardner LI, Howard AA, et al. Bacterial pneumonia, HIV therapy, and disease progression among HIV-infected women in the HIV epidemiologic research (HER) study. Clin Infect Dis. 2006;43:90-8.
24. Corbett EL, Churchyard GJ, Charalambos S, Samb B, Moloi V, Clayton TC, et al. Morbidity and mortality in South African gold miners: impact of untreated disease due to human immunodeficiency virus. Clin Infect Dis. 2002;34:1251-8.

25. Walson JL, Brown ER, Otieno PA, Mbori-Ngacha DA, Wariua G, Obimbo EM, et al. Morbidity among HIV-1-infected mothers in Kenya: prevalence and correlates of illness during 2-year postpartum follow-up. J Acquir Immune Defic Syndr. 2007;46:208-15.
26. Plouffe JF, Breiman RF, Facklam RR. Bacteremia with *Streptococcus pneumoniae*: implications for therapy and prevention; Franklin County Pneumonia Study Group. JAMA. 1996;275:194-8.
27. Gilks CF, Ojoo SA, Ojoo JC, Brindle RJ, Paul J, Batchelor BI, et al. Invasive pneumococcal disease in a cohort of predominantly HIV-1 infected female sex-workers in Nairobi, Kenya. Lancet. 1996;347:718-23.
28. Jones N, Huebner R, Khoosal M, Crewe-Brown H, Klugman K. The impact of HIV on *Streptococcus pneumoniae* bacteraemia in a South African population. AIDS. 1998;12:2177-84.
29. Sullivan JH, Moore RD, Keruly JC, Chaisson RE. Effect of antiretroviral therapy on the incidence of bacterial pneumonia in patients with advanced HIV infection. Am J Respir Crit Care Med. 2000;162:64-7.
30. Dworkin MS, Ward JW, Hanson DL, Jones JL, Kaplan JE. Adult and Adolescent Spectrum of HIV Disease Project. Pneumococcal disease among human immunodeficiency virus-infected persons: incidence, risk factors, and impact of vaccination. Clin Infect Dis. 2001;32:794-800.
31. French N, Nakiyingi J, Carpenter LM, Lugada E, Watera C, Moi K, et al. 23-valent pneumococcal polysaccharide vaccine in HIV-1-infected Ugandan adults: double-blind, randomised and placebo controlled trial. Lancet. 2000;355:2106-11.
32. Heffernan RT, Barrett NL, Gallagher KM, Hadler JL, Harrison LH, Reingold AL, et al. Declining incidence of invasive *Streptococcus pneumoniae* infections among persons with AIDS in an era of highly active antiretroviral therapy, 1995-2000. J Infect Dis. 2005;191:2038-45.
33. Grau I, Pallares R, Tubau F, Schulze MH, Llopis F, Podzamczer D, et al. Epidemiologic changes in bacteremic pneumococcal disease in patients with human immunodeficiency virus in the era of highly active antiretroviral therapy. Arch Intern Med. 2005;165:1533-40.
34. Ziegler JL, Newton R, Katongole-Mbidde E, Mbulataiye S, De Cock K, Wabinga H, et al. Risk factors for Kaposi's sarcoma in HIV-positive subjects in Uganda. AIDS. 1997;11(13):1619-26.
35. Hernandez AM, Shibata D. Epstein-Barr virus-associated non-Hodgkins lymphoma in HIV-infected patients. Leuk Lymphoma. 1995;16:217-21.
36. Bazot M, Cadranel J, Khalil A. Computed tomographic diagnosis of Bronchogenic carcinoma in HIV-infected patients. Lung Cancer. 2000;28(3):203-9.
37. Robertson J, Meier M, Wall J, Ying J, Fichtenbaum CJ. Immune reconstitution syndrome in HIV: validating a case definition and identifying clinical predictors in persons initiating antiretroviral therapy. Clin Infect Dis. 2006;42:1639-46.
38. French MA, Price P, Stone SF. Immune restoration disease after antiretroviral therapy. AIDS. 2004;18:1615-27.
39. McIlleron H, Meintjes G, Burman WJ, Maartens G. Complications of antiretroviral therapy in patients with tuberculosis: drug interactions, toxicity, and immune reconstitution inflammatory syndrome. J Infect Dis. 2007;196(Suppl 1):S63-75.
40. Murdoch DM, Venter WD, Van Rie A, Feldman C. Immune reconstitution inflammatory syndrome (IRIS): review of common infectious manifestations and treatment options. AIDS Res Ther. 2007;4:9.
41. Lawn SD, Bekker LG, Miller RF. Immune reconstitution disease associated with mycobacterial infections in HIV-infected individuals receiving antiretrovirals. Lancet Infect Dis. 2005;5:361-73.
42. Fishman JE, Saraf-Lavi E, Narita M, Hollender ES, Ramsinghani R, Ashkin D. Pulmonary tuberculosis in AIDS patients: transient chest radiographic worsening after initiation of antiretroviral therapy. AJR Am J Roentgenol. 2000;174:43-9.
43. Phillips P, Bonner S, Gataric N, Bai T, Wilcox P, Hogg R, et al. Non-tuberculous mycobacterial immune reconstitution syndrome in HIV-infected patients: spectrum of disease and long-term follow-up. Clin Infect Dis. 2005;41:1483-97.
44. Niaura R, Shadel WG, Morrow K, Tashima K, Flanigan T, Abrams DB. Human immunodeficiency virus infection, AIDS, and smoking cessation: the time is now. Clin Infect Dis. 2000;31:808-12.
45. Crothers K. Chronic obstructive pulmonary disease in patients who have HIV infection. Clin Chest Med.2007;28:575-87.
46. Opravil M, Pechere M, Speich R, Joller-Jemelka HI, Jenni R, Russi EW, et al. HIV-associated primary pulmonary hypertension. A case control study. Swiss HIV Cohort Study. Am J Respir Crit Care Med. 1997;155:990-5.
47. Sitbon O, Lascoux-Combe C, Delfraissy JF, Yeni PG, Raffi F, De Zuttere D, et al. Prevalence of HIV-related pulmonary arterial hypertension in the current antiretroviral therapy era. Am J Respir Crit Care Med. 2008;177:108-13.
48. Pugliese A, Isnardi D, Saini A, Scarabelli T, Raddino R, Torre D. Impact of highly active antiretroviral therapy in HIV-positive patients with cardiac involvement. J Infect. 2000;40:282-4.
49. Mette SA, Palevsky HI, Pietra GG, Williams TM, Bruder E, Prestipino AJ, et al. Primary pulmonary hypertension in association with human immunodeficiency virus infection. A possible viral etiology for some forms of hypertensive pulmonary arteriopathy. Am Rev Respir Dis. 1992;145:1196-1200.
50. Pellicelli AM, Barbaro G, Palmieri F, Girardi E, D'Ambrosio C, Rianda A, et al. Primary pulmonary hypertension in HIV patients: a systematic review. Angiology. 2001;52(1):31-41.
51. Gomez V, Smith PR, Burack J, Daley R, Rosa U. Sarcoidosis after antiretroviral therapy in a patient with acquired immunodeficiency syndrome. Clin Infect Dis. 2000;31:1278-80.
52. Diaz F, Collazos J, Martinez E, Mayo J. Bronchiolitis obliterans in a patient with HIV infection. Respir Med. 1997;91:171-3.
53. Allen JN, Wewers MD. HIV-associated bronchiolitis obliterans organizing pneumonia. Chest. 1989;96:197-8.
54. Hetherington S, McGuirk S, Powell G, Cutrell A, Naderer O, Spreen B, et al. Hypersensitivity reactions during therapy with the nucleoside reverse transcriptase inhibitor abacavir. Clin Ther. 2001;23:1603-14.
55. Hewitt RG. Abacavir hypersensitivity reaction. Clin Infect Dis. 2002;34:1137-42.

Lung Abscess

C Ravindran, Jyothy E

DEFINITION

Latin word "abscessus" means collection of pus that has accumulated in a cavity. Lung abscess is defined as localized suppurative infection in the substance of the lung, associated with necrotic cavity formation.[1] The lesion is usually surrounded by a fibrous tissue forming the abscess wall. Failure to recognize and treat lung abscess is associated with poor clinical outcome. The formation of multiple small (< 2 cm) abscesses is occasionally referred to as necrotizing pneumonia or lung gangrene. Both lung abscess and necrotizing pneumonia are the manifestations of a similar pathologic process. In the last two decades, the increasing use of corticosteroids, immunosuppressive agents and chemotherapeutic drugs has changed the natural milieu of the oropharyngeal cavity and contributed to the mounting frequency of opportunistic lung abscesses.

EPIDEMIOLOGY

Lung abscesses are uncommon in the West with an incidence of 4–5 cases per 10,000 hospital admissions. But, lung abscess continues to pose a major problem in the developing countries. In a retrospective study of 1,150 consecutive patients with thoracic and cardiovascular diseases, 75 (16%) had lung abscess, 53 of whom were treated medically with 8 deaths, while 22 had emergency resection for massive hemoptysis with 9 deaths. The mortality from lung abscesses also has decreased, but remains between 2% and 10% for community-acquired lung abscess and 60% for hospital-acquired lung abscess.[2] Majority of patients with primary lung abscess improve with antibiotics, with cure rates documented at 90–95%. Host factors associated with a poor prognosis include an advanced age, debilitation, malnutrition, human immunodeficiency virus (HIV) infection, or other forms of immunosuppression, malignancy and duration of symptoms of more than 8 weeks.[3,4] The mortality rate for patients with underlying immunodeficiency or bronchial obstruction who develop lung abscess may be as high as 75%.[5] A retrospective study reported the overall mortality rate of lung abscesses caused by the mixed Gram-positive and Gram-negative bacteria at approximately 20%.[4] One-hundred eighty-four patients with lung abscess admitted to the hospital of the University of Mississippi between 1960 and 1982 were studied and data from the different decades show a mortality rate of 22% in the 1960s, 25% in the 1970s and 28% in 1980–1982.[6]

CLASSIFICATION

Lung abscess is considered acute if the duration of symptoms at the time of presentation is less than 6 weeks and chronic if it exceeds 6 weeks.[7] Primary abscess is infectious in origin, caused by aspiration or pneumonia in the healthy host; secondary abscess is caused by a pre-existing condition causing obstruction, spread from an extrapulmonary site, bronchiectasis, and/or an immuno-compromised state **(Table 1)**.[8] In a retrospective review of 23 children with documented lung abscess, 11 cases were of primary and 12 of secondary lung abscess.[9]

ETIOLOGY

Lung abscesses have numerous infectious causes[10-22] **(Table 2)**. Anaerobic bacteria continue to account for most cases.[10] Aspiration lung abscesses are mostly caused by anaerobic bacteria. In one report from India, the anaerobes accounted for about 38% of 198 cultures from 100 patients of pleuropulmonary infections, of whom all the 13 patients of lung abscess had anaerobic infection either in isolation or along with aerobic bacteria.[11] These bacteria predominate in the upper respiratory tract and are heavily concentrated in the areas of oral-gingival disease.

Other bacteria involved in lung abscesses are aerobic Gram-positive and Gram-negative organisms.[12-15] Among the aerobic organisms, *Staphylococcus aureus, Klebsiella pneumoniae, E. coli* and Type III *Streptococcus pneumoniae* are frequently associated with lung abscess formation.[12-15] Complicated pneumococcal pneumonia especially with lung abscess formation was found to be a rare but important cause of lung abscess.[16]

Table 1 Factors contributing to the development of lung abscess

- Oral cavity disease
  - Periodontal disease
  - Gingivitis
- Altered consciousness
  - Alcoholism
  - Coma
  - Drug abuse
  - Anesthesia
  - Seizures
- Immunocompromised host
  - Steroid therapy
  - Chemotherapy
  - Malnutrition
  - Multiple trauma
- Esophageal disease
  - Achalasia
  - Reflux disease
  - Esophageal obstruction
- Bronchial obstruction
  - Tumor
  - Foreign body
  - Stricture
- Generalized sepsis

Nonbacterial and atypical bacterial pathogens may also cause lung abscesses, usually in the immune-compromised host. These microorganisms include *Mycobacterium* species, parasites (e.g. *Paragonimus* and *Entamoeba* species), fungi (e.g. *Aspergillus, Cryptococcus, Histoplasma, Blastomyces, Coccidioides* species and *Basidiobolus ranarum*) **(Figs 1A to C)**.[17-22] The organisms are aspirated to lower respiratory tract due to many factors, which may be local or general **(Table 1)**. Other routes of the spread of infection to lungs include infected chest wall foci, infradiaphragmatic abscesses and hematogenous spread.

PATHOGENESIS

Aspiration of infectious material is the most frequent etiologic mechanism in the development of pyogenic lung abscess.[23] Aspiration due to dysphagia (e.g. achalasia) or compromised consciousness (e.g. alcoholism, seizures, cerebrovascular accident, head trauma) appears as important predisposing factors. Poor oral hygiene, dental infections and gingival disease are also common in these patients. Patients with alcoholism and those with chronic illnesses frequently have oropharyngeal colonization with Gram-negative bacteria, especially when they undergo prolonged endotracheal intubation and are administered agents that neutralize gastric acidity. A pyogenic lung abscess can also develop from the aspiration of infectious material from the oropharynx into the lung when the cough reflex is suppressed in a patient with gingivodental disease.

Table 2 Microorganisms responsible for lung abscess

Group	*Organism*
Aerobic organisms	*Klebsiella pneumoniae* *Nocardia* sp. *Pseudomonas aeruginosa* *Staphylococcus aureus* *Burkholderia pseudomallei*[19-21] **(Fig. 2)** *Pasteurella multocida*[22] *Streptococcus milleri* Other streptococci[11]
Anaerobic organisms	*Bacteroides* sp. *Fusobacterium* sp. *Clostridium* sp. *Peptostreptococcus* sp. *Actinomyces* sp. *Prevotella* sp.
Fungi	*Aspergillus* sp. (aspergillosis) *Blastomyces dermatitidis* (blastomycosis) *Coccidioides immitis* (coccidioidomycosis) *Cryptococcus neoformans* (cryptococcosis) *Histoplasma capsulatum (histoplasmosis)* *Pneumocystis jirovecii* *Rhizomucor* (mucormycosis) *Rhizopus* sp. (mucormycosis) *Sporothrix schenckii* (sporotrichosis) *Basidiobolus* sp.
Mycobacteria	*Mycobacterium avium-intracellulare* *Mycobacterium kansasii* *Mycobacterium tuberculosis*
Parasites	*Entamoeba histolytica* (amebiasis) *Echinococcus granulosus* (echinococcosis) *Echinococcus multilocularis* (echinococcosis) *Paragonimus westermani* (paragonimiasis)

PATHOLOGY

Aspiration and abscess formation most often occur in the dependent regions of the lungs. In the supine position, these are most often located in the posterior segment of the upper lobes and superior segment of the lower lobes. In the more upright position, materials flow into the basal segments of the lower lobes. When a person is in the lateral decubitus position, the axillary branches of the subsegments of apical and posterior upper lobe bronchi are favored.[24] Lung abscess that occurs as a part of hematogenous spread may be found in any part of lung. Initially, the aspirated material settles in the distal bronchial system and develops into a localized pneumonitis. Within 24–48 hours, a large area of inflammation results, consisting of exudate, blood and necrotic lung tissue. Multiple areas of liquefactive necrosis ("cross-country" pattern) [24] can occur secondary to bacterial proliferation.

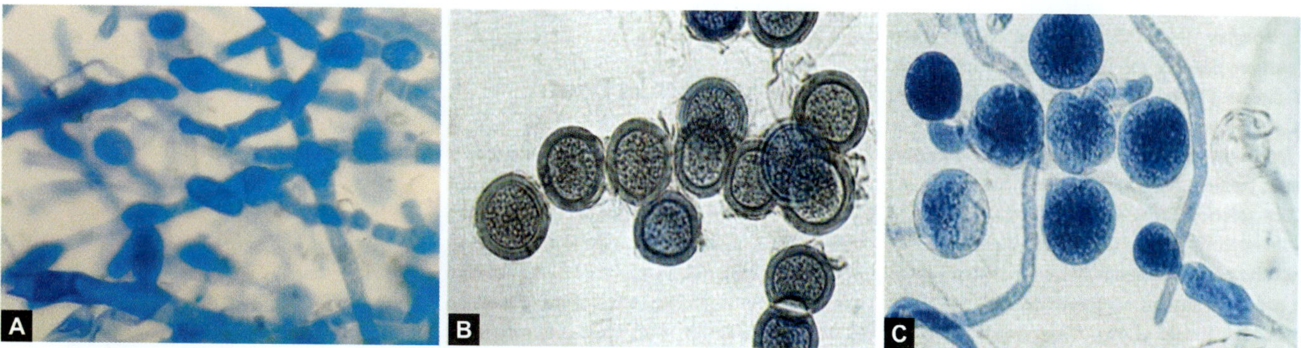

Figs 1A to C Basidiobolus

This type of necrosis involves destruction of lung parenchyma, bronchi and arteries. In contrast, cavities that are more chronic and more slowly formed, such as the tuberculous cavities, often have remnants of fibrotic bronchopulmonary bands coursing through the cavity.[24] The abscess frequently connects with a bronchus allowing drainage of the necrotic material leaving an empty or partially empty cavity with or without fluid level. The infection may extend into the pleural space and produce an empyema without rupture of the abscess cavity. The infectious process can also extend to the hilar and mediastinal lymph nodes, and these too may suppurate.

Sometimes, septic emboli may reach the lungs from right-sided bacterial endocarditis, which commonly complicates intravenous drug abuse, the usual organism being *Staphylococcus aureus*. Septic emboli may arise from the infected intravenous cannulae or from thrombophlebitis of the deep veins of the legs or pelvis or in relation to superficial cutaneous cellulitis. Gram-negative sepsis elsewhere, such as the urinary tract, the abdominal or the pelvic cavities may also contribute to the development of abscess. Alternatively, an abscess may develop as an infectious complication of a pre-existing bulla or lung cyst or secondary to carcinoma of the bronchus.

CLINICAL FEATURES

Symptoms

Onset of symptoms in lung abscess is often insidious. This is more acute following pneumonia, where it begins with spiking temperature, rigors and night sweats followed by cough with sputum production. The expectorated sputum characteristically is foul smelling and bad tasting and often blood stained. Abscesses due to organisms other than anaerobes (e.g. *Mycobacteria* or *Nocardia*) do not demonstrate putrid respiratory secretions. There will be associated pleuritic chest pain and breathlessness.[25] In a series of 252 consecutive patients studied by Moreira and associates,[26] 70.2% were alcoholic. Cough, expectoration, fever and overall poor health were observed in 97% of patients, chest pain was reported by 64%, digital clubbing in 30.2%; dental disease in 82.5%; lost consciousness at least once in 78.6% and foul smelling sputum in 67.5%.[26]

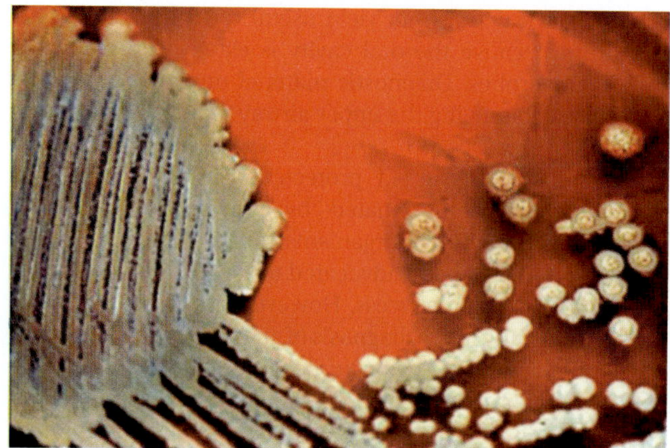

Fig. 2 Dry wrinkled colonies with metallic sheen of *Burkholderia pseudomallei* in blood agar

Signs

There are no specific signs for lung abscess. Patients usually have signs of periodontal disease or a condition causing impaired consciousness. Patients are often febrile and tachypneic. Those with an abrupt onset lung abscess are often sick. Clubbing of fingers may be present, which may develop within a few weeks and this is reversible as the abscess resolves. If the abscess is localized, there will be crackles on auscultation. If it is secondary to pneumonia, it is associated with dullness on percussion, bronchial breathing, egophony and crackles. There will be dullness on percussion and reduced breath sound if associated with pleural effusion. Primary lung abscesses that occur following staphylococcal suppurative pneumonia in infants and children tend to be abrupt and more life threatening.[27]

Laboratory Diagnosis

A large number of conditions may present with a cavitary lung lesion **(Box 1)**. Several different laboratory investigations are therefore, required for the differential diagnosis of a lung abscess.

Hematological Diagnosis

A complete and differential white blood cell count will reveal leukocytosis and a left shift.

Microbiological Diagnosis

- *Sputum for Gram stain, culture and sensitivity*: Expectorated sputum and other methods of sampling, the upper airway does not yield useful results for anaerobic culture because the oral cavity is extensively colonized with anaerobes. Diagnostic material uncontaminated by bacteria colonizing the upper airway may be obtained for culture **(Box 2)**.[28-30]
- Bronchoscopy using a protected brush[30] to obtain a specimen uncontaminated by the upper airway or quantitative culture of organisms from the bronchoalveolar lavage fluid has been advocated to establish bacteriologic diagnosis of lung abscess. However, the experience with this technique in the diagnosis of anaerobic lung infections is limited and the diagnostic yield is uncertain.[31] But more importantly, cultures obtained by any of these methods are unlikely to be positive after the initiation of antibiotics.
- *Blood culture*: Blood cultures are infrequently positive in patients with lung abscess. If tuberculosis is suspected, acid-fast bacilli staining and mycobacterial culture are also required. Obtain sputum for ova and parasite whenever a parasitic cause for lung abscess is suspected.

BOX 1 Differential diagnosis of a cavitary lung lesion

- Cavitating lung cancer
- Localized empyema
- Infected bulla containing a fluid level
- Infected bronchogenic cyst or sequestration
- Pulmonary hematoma
- Cavitating pneumoconiosis
- Hiatus hernia
- Lung parasites (e.g. hydatid cyst, *Paragonimus* infection)
- Actinomycosis
- Wegener's granulomatosis and other vasculitides
- Cavitating lung infarcts
- Cavitating sarcoidosis

BOX 2 Uncontaminated pulmonary samples for microbiological demonstration and culture

- Transtracheal aspirate[28,29]
- Transthoracic pulmonary aspirate
- Fiberoptic bronchoscopy with protected specimen brush[30]
- Bronchoalveolar lavage fluid for quantitative culture
- Surgical specimens
- Pleural fluid (if empyema present)

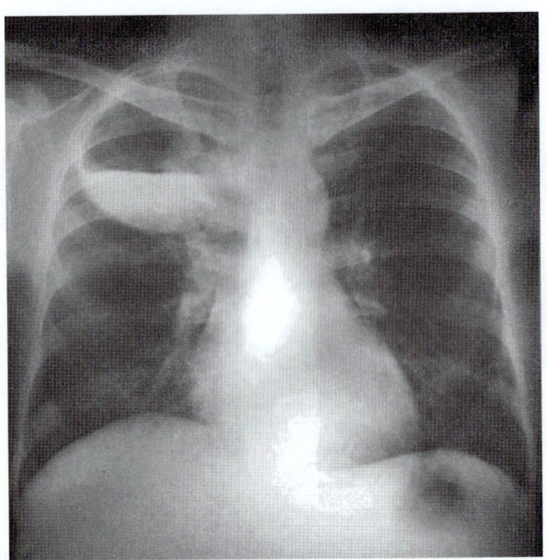

Fig. 3 X-ray chest PA showing lung abscess right upper zone

Imaging Studies

Chest radiograph: A typical chest radiographic appearance of a lung abscess is an irregularly-shaped cavity with an air-fluid level inside.[32] Lung abscesses as a result of aspiration most frequently occur in the posterior segments of the upper lobes or in the superior segments of the lower lobes **(Fig. 3)**. *Klebsiella* lung abscess usually develops in the right upper lobe and is characterized by the bulging fissure sign. Lung abscesses due to *Staphylococcus* species are often multiple and bilateral.

The wall thickness of a lung abscess progresses from thick to thin as it evolves. The cavity wall can be smooth or ragged, but is less commonly nodular, which raises the possibility of cavitating carcinoma. The extent of the air-fluid level within a lung abscess is often the same in posteroanterior and lateral views.[32] The abscess may extend to the pleural surface, in which case it forms acute angles with the pleural surface.[33]

Anaerobic infection is suggested by cavitation within a dense segmental consolidation in the dependent lung zones **(Figs 4 and 5)**.[34] Lung infection with a virulent organism results in more widespread tissue necrosis, which facilitates progression of the underlying infection to pulmonary gangrene. Up to one-third of lung, abscesses may be accompanied by an empyema.

Computed tomography (CT): CT scanning of the lungs may help visualize the anatomy better than the chest radiography.[32] CT scanning is very useful in the identification of concomitant empyema or lung infarction.[32] On CT scan, an

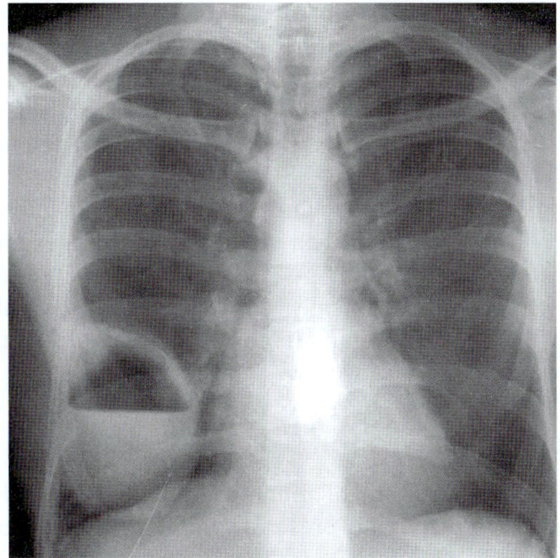

Fig. 4 X-ray chest PA showing lung abscess right lower lobe

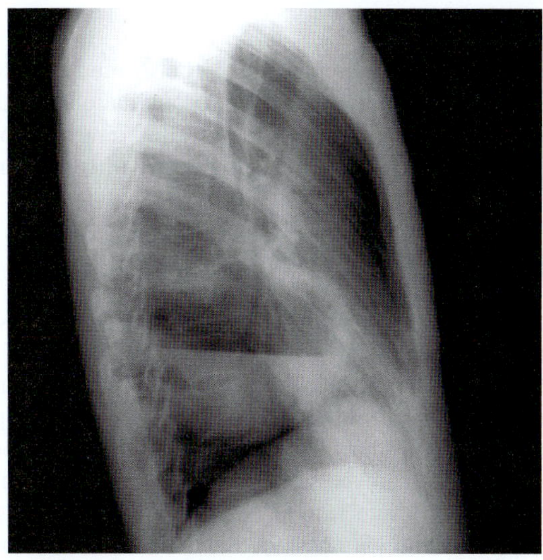

Fig. 5 X-ray chest right lateral showing lung abscess right lower lobe

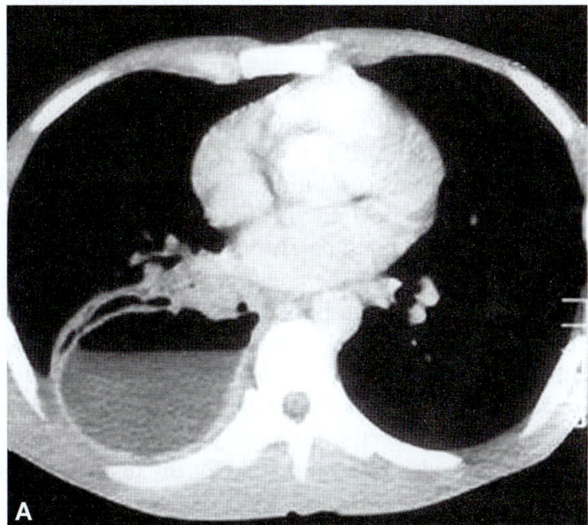

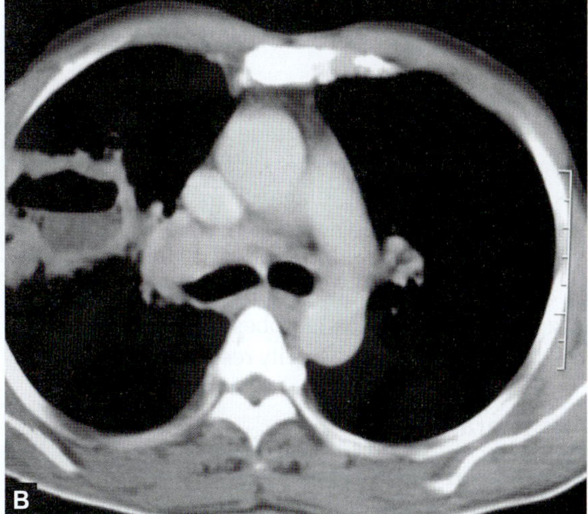

Figs 6A and B CT thorax showing lung abscess

abscess often is a rounded radiolucent lesion with a thick wall with ill-defined irregular margins **(Fig. 6A)**. Abscess walls are typically irregular in width and have regular luminal margins and exterior surfaces **(Fig. 6B)**. Infected bullae may mimic an abscess especially when there is adjacent pneumonia; however, a smooth luminal margin on plain film[35] or CT suggests the correct diagnosis. The vessels and bronchi are not displaced by the lesion, as they are by an empyema.[33] The lung abscess is located within the parenchyma compared with loculated empyema, which may be difficult to distinguish on chest radiographs.[33,36] The lesion forms acute angles with the pleural surface of chest wall.

Ultrasound (US) examination: Ultrasound and ultrasound-guided transthoracic aspiration is an alternative method for CT thorax and guided aspiration. In a case series of 35 patients, 33 of the abscesses (94%) were demonstrated at ultrasound, while two lesions were not depicted. On ultrasound examination, lung abscesses were depicted as hypoechoic lesions with irregular outer margins and an abscess cavity that was manifested as a hyperechoic ring. Ultrasound-guided transthoracic needle aspiration of fluid from the abscess cavity was performed successfully in 31 of 33 patients (94%). A total of 65 pathogens were isolated from 31 aspirates (41 anaerobes and 24 aerobes).[37]

Bronchoscopy

Flexible fiberoptic bronchoscopy is performed to exclude bronchogenic carcinoma whenever bronchial obstruction is suspected or less commonly, to identify and remove a foreign body.[38] Bronchoscopy also helps to retrieve uncontaminated specimen for culture, as well as to remove pus.

COMPLICATIONS

Lung abscess if not diagnosed and treated early is met with few complications. Approximately one-third of lung abscesses are complicated by empyema. This may be observed with or without bronchopleural fistula. Hemoptysis is a common complication of lung abscess. Occasionally, the hemoptysis can be massive, thus requiring urgent surgery. Spread of infection to other parts of same lung and to the opposite lung is possible. Bacteremia and metastatic abscesses including brain abscess may also occur in patients who receive inadequate treatment. Metastatic brain abscess most frequently involve temporal lobe and cerebellum. Rarely, it may rupture into the mediastinum causing acute mediastinitis. Poor treatment response may lead on to bacteremia and septicemia.

TREATMENT

Treatment of lung abscess is guided by the available microbiology and knowledge of the underlying or associated conditions. Once the clinical diagnosis of lung abscess is made and the respiratory secretions sent for culture and drug sensitivity tests, patient should be initiated on broad-spectrum antibiotics. Antibiotics with a spectrum covering Gram-negative aerobes and anaerobes are preferred. This may be modified once drug sensitivity results are available.

Antibiotic Therapy

Most patients, even with necrotizing pneumonia, respond well to high-dose penicillin[39] and show clinical improvement within a week to 10 days. Clindamycin is preferred in the cases of severe underlying disease or when penicillin fails to yield signs of recovery.[40,41] The presence of empyema not only increases the duration of therapy, but also carries a higher mortality rate (20% vs. 5%).[42] Standard treatment of an anaerobic lung infection is clindamycin (600 mg IV q8h followed by 150–300 mg PO qid). This regimen has been shown to be superior to parenteral penicillin. Several anaerobes may produce beta-lactamase (e.g. various species of *Bacteroides* and *Fusobacterium*) and therefore, develop resistance to penicillin.[43]

Although, metronidazole is an effective drug against anaerobic bacteria,[44,45] the experience with metronidazole in treating lung abscess has been rather disappointing because these infections are generally polymicrobial. A failure rate of 50% has been reported in the past.[44,45] Necrotizing pneumonia and pulmonary abscess that develop in the nursing home or in the hospital setting require a more aggressive diagnostic approach and broad-spectrum antibiotic coverage. In spite of these measures and appropriate antibiotic selection, nosocomial-acquired disease carries a mortality rate of 30–50%.[42]

Ampicillin plus sulbactam is well tolerated and is as effective as clindamycin with or without a cephalosporin in the treatment of aspiration pneumonia and lung abscess.[46]

Moxifloxacin is clinically effective and is as safe as ampicillin plus sulbactam in the treatment of aspiration pneumonia and lung abscess.[47]

Duration of Therapy

Although the duration of therapy is not well established, most clinicians generally prescribe antibiotic therapy for 4–6 weeks.

It generally suggests that antibiotic treatment should be continued until the chest radiograph has shown either the resolution of lung abscess or the presence of a small stable lesion. The extended treatment is recommended since there is a risk of relapse with a shorter antibiotic regimen.

Response to Therapy

Patients with lung abscesses usually show clinical improvement within 3–4 days of initiating the antibiotic therapy. Clinical resolution is expected in 7–10 days. Persistent fever beyond this time indicates a therapeutic failure, and these patients should undergo further diagnostic studies to determine the cause of failure. Considerations in patients with poor response to antibiotic therapy include bronchial obstruction with a foreign body, a neoplasm or an infection with resistant bacteria, mycobacteria or fungi. Large cavity size (> 6 cm in diameter) usually requires prolonged therapy.[48] The infection of a pre-existing sequestration, cyst or bulla may also be responsible for the delayed response to antibiotics.[49]

Physiotherapy

Physiotherapy is useful in helping the patient to clear the purulent material. Postural drainage can be given keeping the affected pulmonary segments uppermost. However, chest physical therapy and postural drainage are not widely recommended because of the fear of spillage and extension of infection.

Surgical Care

Surgery is very rarely required for patients with uncomplicated lung abscesses. The usual indications for surgery are failure to respond to medical management, suspected neoplasm or congenital lung malformation.[50] The surgical procedure is either lobectomy or pneumonectomy. When surgery is necessary, lobectomy is the most common procedure; segmental resection may suffice for small lesions (< 6 cm diameter cavity). Pneumonectomy may become necessary for multiple abscesses or for pulmonary gangrene, unresponsive to drug therapy.

Percutaneous Drainage

Percutaneous drainage of a complicated abscess (i.e. one associated with fever and signs of sepsis) is beneficial in selected patients who do not respond to adequate medical therapy.[15] They are ventilator-dependent patients who are not candidates for extensive thoracic procedures. Other indications for drainage include ongoing sepsis despite adequate antimicrobial therapy, a progressively enlarging lung abscess in imminent danger of rupture, failure to wean from mechanical ventilation and contamination of the opposite lung. Results achieved with percutaneous drainage show it to be safe and effective method when compared with surgery. Percutaneous drainage is rarely complicated by empyema, hemorrhage or bronchopleural fistula.[51] Although, a few patients who undergo percutaneous drainage develop bronchopleural fistula, and most of these fistulae close spontaneously with the resolution of the abscess cavity. Percutaneous drainage may be used to stabilize and prepare critically-ill patients for surgery. Percutaneous or surgical drainage of lung abscesses is necessary in roughly 10% of patients.[52] Aggressive interventional therapy can be diagnostic and therapeutic in the infected lung abscess.[53] But interventional therapy can be harmful in the case of postinfectious necrotizing pneumonia.[54]

In current practice, most of the lung abscesses are drained under CT guidance. CT allows optimal placement of catheter and hence enables the safe and effective percutaneous evacuation of lung abscess. After catheter insertion, once the cavity is evacuated, gentle irrigation with normal saline can be done. A small intercostal drainage tube of size 10–14 F is usually adequate to drain pus. The morbidity and mortality of patients with percutaneous catheter drainage is lower than that with surgical resection.[55] Hence, CT-guided drainage should be considered the first therapeutic choice in most patients of lung abscess who do not respond to medical therapy. However, percutaneous drainage may be avoided if the abscess is completely surrounded by normal lung parenchyma, as this increases the risk of empyema and bronchopleural fistula.

Endoscopic lung abscess drainage is considered in selected patients when antibiotic treatment fails. Success of this treatment represents an additional option other than percutaneous catheter drainage or surgical resection.[56-59] Earlier rigid bronchoscope was used to pass angiography catheter into the abscess cavity to facilitate bacteriologic diagnosis and drainage of the cavity. Now fiberoptic bronchoscope is used for endoscopic drainage of lung abscess. For endoscopic drainage, a guidewire is introduced into the abscess cavity through fiberoptic bronchoscope under fluoroscopic guidance. Then a pigtail catheter of at least 7 F is introduced over the guidewire and it is secured at the nose. The abscess cavity can be flushed with normal saline.[56,59] Endobronchial catheters with the use of laser appear to be relatively safe and effective for the treatment of lung abscess in selected patients in whom the abscess is adjacent to the central airway. Dekel Shlomi[60] has reported three cases in which laser was used to perforate the abscess wall through the airway and provide a pathway for catheter insertion. Here, laser was used to perforate the bulging airway adjacent to the abscess cavity in patients where the abscess was not communicating with the airway. In all these patients, there was clinical and radiological improvement after catheter insertion. In a series of 42 patients with lung abscess, Herth[56] reported 38 patients being successfully treated by bronchoscopic pigtail catheter insertion.

PROGNOSIS

The prognosis of patients with lung abscesses depends on the underlying or predisposing pathologic event, and the speed with which appropriate therapy is established. Negative prognostic factors include a large cavity (>6 cm), necrotizing pneumonia, multiple abscesses, immunocompromised state, age extremes, associated bronchial obstruction and aerobic bacterial pneumonia.[3] The prognosis associated with amebic lung abscess is good when treatment is prompt.

REFERENCES

1. Alexander JC, Wolfe WG. Lung abscess and empyema of the thorax. Surg Clin North Am. 1980;60(4):835-49.
2. Adebonojo SA, Grillo IA, Osinowo O, Adebo OA. Suppurative diseases of the lung and pleura: a continuing challenge in developing countries. Ann Thorac Surg. 1982;33(1):40-7.
3. Mwandumba HC, Beeching NJ. Pyogenic lung infections: factors for predicting clinical outcome of lung abscess and thoracic empyema. Curr Opin Pulm Med. 2000;6(3):234-9.
4. Hirshberg B, Sklair-Levi M, Nir-Paz R, Ben-Sira L, Krivoruk V, Kramer MR. Factors predicting mortality of patients with lung abscess. Chest. 1999;115(3):746-50.
5. Pohlson EC, McNamara JJ, Char C, Kurata L. Lung abscess: a changing pattern of the disease. Am J Surg. 1985;150(1):97-101.
6. Hagan JL, Hardy JD. Lung abscess revisited. A survey of 184 cases. Ann Surg. 1983;197(6):755-62.
7. Perlman LV, Lerner E, D'Esopo N. Clinical classification and analysis of 97 cases of lung abscess. Am Rev Respir Dis. 1969;99(3):390-8.
8. Mansharamani NG, Koziel H. Chronic lung sepsis: lung abscess, bronchiectasis, and empyema. Curr Opin Pulm Med. 2003;9(3):181-5.
9. Yen CC, Tang RB, Chen SJ, Chin TW. Pediatric lung abscess: a retrospective review of 23 cases. J Microbiol Immunol Infect. 2004;37(1):45-9.
10. Bartlett JG. The role of anaerobic bacteria in lung abscess. Clin Infect Dis. 2005;40(1):923-5.

11. De A, Varaiya A, Mathur M. Anaerobes in pleuropulmonary infections. Indian J Med Microbiol. 2002;20(3):150-2.
12. Nicolini A, Cilloniz C, Senarega R, Ferraiopi G, Barlascini C. Lung abscess due to *Streptococcus pneumoniae*: a case series and brief review of literature. Pneumonol Alergol Pol. 2014;82:276-85.
13. Williams DM, Krick JA, Remington JS. Pulmonary infections in the compromised host: part I. Am Rev Respir Dis. 1976;114(2):359-94.
14. Wang JL, Chen KY, Fang CT, Hsueh PR, Yang PC, Chang SC. Changing bacteriology of adult community-acquired lung abscess in Taiwan: *Klebsiella pneumoniae* versus anaerobes. Clin Infect Dis. 2005;40(7):915-22.
15. Leatherman JW, Iber C, Davies SF. Cavitation in bacteremic pneumococcal pneumonia. Causal role of mixed infection with anaerobic bacteria. Am Rev Respir Dis. 1984;129(2):317-21.
16. Fletcher MA, Schmitt HJ, Synrochkina M, Sylvester G. Pneumococcal empyema and complicated pneumonia: global trends in incidence, prevalence and serotype epidemiology. Eur J Clin Mibrobial Infect Dis. 2014;33:879-910.
17. Ravindran C, Sarma MSD, Suraj KP, Jyothi E, Mohammed S, Philomina BJ, et al. Basidiobolus: An unusual cause of lung abscess. Lung India. 2010;27:89-92.
18. Bigliazzi C, Poletti V, Dell'Amore D, Saragoni L, Colby TV. Disseminated basidiobolomycosis in an immunocompetent woman. J Clin Microbiol. 2004;42(3):1367-9.
19. Dworzack DL, Pollack AS, Hodges GR, Barnes WG, Ajello L, Padhye A. Zygomycosis of the maxillary sinus and palate caused by Basidobolus haptosporus. Arch Intern Med. 1978;138(8):1274-6.
20. Chierakul W, Winothai W, Wattanawaitunechai C, Wuthiekanun V, Rugtaengan T, Rattanalertnavee J, et al. Melioidosis in 6 Tsunami survivors in southern Thailand. Clin Infect Dis. 2005;41(7):982-90.
21. Peetermans WE, Van Wijngaerden E, Van Eldere J, Verhaegen J. Melioidosis brain and lung abscess after travel to Sri Lanka. Clin Infect Dis. 1999;28(4):921-2.
22. Umemori Y, Hiraki A, Murakami T, Aoe K, Matsuda E, Makihara S, et al. Chronic lung abscess with *Pasteurella multocida* infection. Intern Med. 2005;44(7):754-6.
23. Prather AD, Smith TR, Poletto DM, Tavora F, Chung JH, Nallamshetty L, et al. Aspiration-related lung diseases. J Thorac Imaging. 2014;29:304-9.
24. Joseph F, Tomashefski, David H Dail. Aspiration, bronchial obstruction, bronchiectasis and related disorders in Dail and Hammar's Pulmonary Pathology, Volume 1, 3rd edition. Non-Neoplastic Lung Diseases. Springer; 2008. pp. 94-8.
25. Schweppe HI, Knowles JH, Kane L. Lung abscess. An analysis of the Massachusetts General Hospital cases from 1943 through 1956. N Engl J Med. 1961;265:1039-43.
26. Moreira Jda S, Camargo Jde J, Felicetti JC, Goldenfun PR, Moreira AL, Porto Nda S. Lung abscess: analysis of 252 consecutive cases diagnosed between 1968 and 2004. J Bras Pneumol. 2006;32(2):136-43.
27. Gillet Y, Issartel B, Vanhems P, Fournet JC, Lina G, Bes M, et al. Association between *Staphylococcus aureus* strains carrying gene for Panton-Valentine leukocidin and highly lethal necrotising pneumonia in young immunocompetent patients. Lancet. 2002;359(9308):753-9.
28. Bartlett JG. Diagnostic accuracy of transtracheal aspiration bacteriology. Am Rev Respir Dis. 1977;115(5):777-82.
29. Bartlett JG. The technique of transtracheal aspiration. J Crit Illn. 1986;1:43.
30. Wimberley NW, Bass JB, Boyd BW, Kirkpatrick MB, Serio RA, Pollock HM. Use of a bronchoscopic protected catheter brush for the diagnosis of pulmonary infections. Chest. 1982;81(5):556-62.
31. Bartlett JG. Anaerobic bacterial infections of the lung. Chest. 1987;91(6):901-9.
32. Stark DD, Federle MP, Goodman PC, Podrasky AE, Webb WR. Differentiating lung abscess and empyema: radiography and computed tomography. AJR Am J Roentgenol. 1983;141(1): 163-7.
33. Williford ME, Godwin JD. Computed tomography of lung abscess and empyema. Radiol Clin North Am. 1983;21(3):575-83.
34. Landay MJ, Christensen EE, Bynum LJ, Goodman C. Anaerobic pleural and pulmonary infections. AJR Am J Roentgenol. 1980;134(2):233-40.
35. Stark P, Gadziala N, Greene R. Fluid accumulation in preexisting pulmonary air spaces. AJR Am J Roentgenol. 1980;134(4): 701-6.
36. Mayer T, Matlak ME, Condon V, Shasha I, Glasgow L. Computed tomographic findings of neonatal lung abscess. Am J Dis Child. 1982;136(1):39-41.
37. Yang PC, Luh KT, Lee YC, Chang DB, Yu CJ, Wu HD, et al. Lung abscesses: US examination and US-guided transthoracic aspiration. Radiology. 1991;180(1):171-5.
38. Sosenko A, Glassroth J. Fiberoptic bronchoscopy in the evaluation of lung abscesses. Chest. 1985;87(4):489-94.
39. Weiss W, Cherniack NS. Acute nonspecific lung abscess: A controlled study comparing orally and parenterally administered penicillin G. Chest. 1974;66(4):348-51.
40. Levison ME, Mangura CT, Lorber B, Abrutyn E, Pesanti EL, Levy RS, et al. Clindamycin compared with penicillin for the treatment of anaerobic lung abscess. Ann Intern Med. 1983;98(4):466-71.
41. Gudiol F, Manresa F, Pallares R, Dorca J, Rufi G, Boada J, et al. Clindamycin vs penicillin for anaerobic lung infections. High rate of penicillin failures associated with penicillin-resistant *Bacteroides melaninogenicus*. Arch Intern Med. 1990;150(12):2525-9.
42. Pennza PT. Aspiration pneumonia, necrotizing pneumonia, and lung abscess. Emerg Med Clin North Am. 1989;7(2):279-307.
43. Appelbaum PC, Spangler SK, Jacobs MR. Beta-lactamase production and susceptibilities to amoxicillin, amoxicillin clavulanate, ticarcillin, ticarcillin-clavulanate, cefoxitin, imipenem, and metronidazole of 320 non-*Bacteroides fragilis* Bacteroides isolates and 129 fusobacteria from 28 U.S. centers. Antimicrob Agents Chemother. 1990;34(8):1546-50.
44. Perlino CA. Metronidazole vs clindamycin treatment of anaerobic pulmonary infection. Failure of metronidazole therapy. Arch Intern Med. 1981;141(11):1424-7.
45. Sanders CV, Hanna BJ, Lewis AC. Metronidazole in the treatment of anaerobic infections. Am Rev Respir Dis. 1979;120(2):337-43.
46. Allewelt M, Schüler P, Bölcskei PL, Mauch H, Lode H. Study Group on Aspiration Pneumonia. Ampicillin + sulbactam vs clindamycin +/- cephalosporin for the treatment of aspiration pneumonia and primary lung abscess. Clin Microbiol Infect. 2004;10(2):163-70.

47. Ott SR, Allewelt M, Lorenz J, Reimnitz P, Lode H. German Lung Abscess Study Group. Moxifloxacin vs ampicillin/sulbactam in aspiration pneumonia and primary lung abscess. Infection. 2008;36(1):23-30.
48. Weiss W. Cavity behavior in acute, primary, nonspecific lung abscess. Am Rev Respir Dis. 1973;108(5):1273-5.
49. Smith DT. Medical treatment of acute and chronic pulmonary abscesses. J Thorac Surg. 1948;17(1):72-90.
50. Allen CI, Blackman JF. Treatment of lung abscess with report of 100 consecutive cases. J Thorac Surg. 1936;6:156.
51. Weissberg D. Percutaneous drainage of lung abscess. J Thorac Cardiovasc Surg. 1984;87(2):308-12.
52. Wali SO, Shugaeri A, Samman YS, Abdelaziz M. Percutaneous drainage of pyogenic lung abscess. Scand J Infect Dis. 2002;34(9):673-9.
53. Taniguchi M, Morita S, Ueno E, Hayashi M, Ishikawa M, Mae M. Percutaneous transhepatic drainage of lung abscess through a diaphragmatic fistula caused by a penetrating liver abscess. Jpn J Radiol. 2011;29(9):663-6.
54. Hoffer FA, Bloom DA, Colin AA, Fishman SJ. Lung abscess versus necrotizing pneumonia: implications for interventional therapy. Pediatr Radiol. 1999;29(2):87-91.
55. Parker LA, Melton JW, Delany DJ, Yankaskas BC. Percutaneous small bore catheter drainage in the management of lung abscesses. Chest. 1987;92(2):213-8.
56. Herth F, Ernst A, Becker HD. Endoscopic drainage of lung abscesses: technique and outcome. Chest. 2005;127(4):1378-81.
57. Schmitt GS, Ohar JM, Kanter KR, Naunheim KS. Indwelling transbronchial catheter drainage of pulmonary abscess. Ann Thorac Surg. 1988;45(1):43-7.
58. Rowe LD, Keane WM, Jafek BW, Atkins JP Jr. Transbronchial drainage of pulmonary abscesses with the flexible fiberoptic bronchoscope. Laryngoscope. 1979;89(1):122-8.
59. Connors JP, Roper CL, Ferguson TB. Transbronchial catheterization of pulmonary abscesses. Ann Thorac Surg. 1975;19(3):254-60.
60. Shlomi D, Kramer MR, Fuks L, Peled N, Shitrit D. Endobronchial drainage of lung abscess: the use of laser. Scand J Infect Dis. 2010;42(1):65-8.

54
Chapter

Bronchiectasis and Cystic Fibrosis

David Honeybourne

Bronchiectasis

INTRODUCTION

Bronchiectasis is a chronic condition with a variable clinical course that may include acute exacerbations and also chronic deterioration in some cases. Bronchiectasis was first described by Laënnec in 1812. Clinical features in a patient with bronchiectasis include the presence of a frequent productive cough often accompanied with shortness of breath on effort. The prevalence of bronchiectasis in populations has been found to be very variable and many older studies were carried out before high-resolution computed tomography (HRCT) thoracic scans were available. Prevalence figures have varied from 4 per 100,000 population and 272 per 100,000 population partly dependent upon the age range studied.[1,2] There are sparse data on the prevalence of bronchiectasis in the Indian subcontinent.

Bronchiectasis is not infrequently misdiagnosed as chronic bronchitis and/or chronic obstructive pulmonary disease (COPD) with 15–30% of patients diagnosed with COPD having the evidence of bronchiectasis on HRCT lung scans.[3,4]

There is some evidence that in populations with poor access to health care and high rates of lower respiratory tract infections, particularly during childhood, there may be a higher prevalence of bronchiectasis.[5]

PATHOLOGY

Until recently, the original definition of bronchiectasis was based on the pathological findings. Pathologically, bronchiectasis is defined as permanent dilatation of the bronchi.[6] Further, morphological definition has classified bronchiectasis as cylindrical or tubular, which involves dilatation of the airways and also varicose bronchiectasis. There are, in addition, focal areas of narrowing within the dilated airways. A further type is saccular or cystic bronchiectasis, which is characterized by progressive dilatation of the bronchi with collection of large clusters of cysts **(Fig. 1)**. However, morphological subtyping of bronchiectasis is of little practical value in terms of patient management.

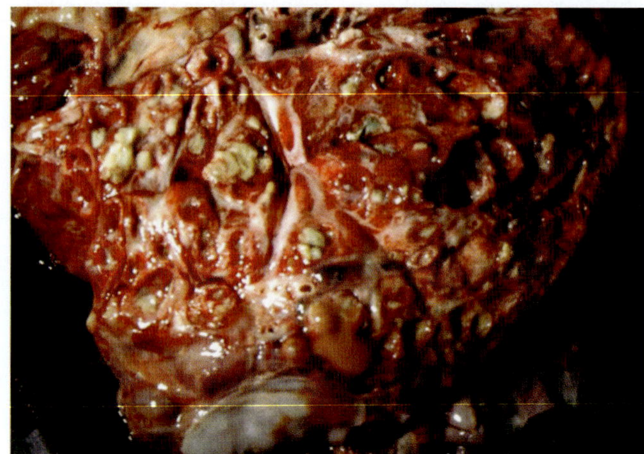

Fig. 1 Extensive advanced bronchiectasis

The airways in bronchiectasis show evidence of chronic inflammatory changes with high sputum concentrations of substances such as elastase, interleukin-8 and other proinflammatory agents. It is thought that an increase in the levels of these agents is driven by recurrent bacterial infections.

PHYSIOLOGY

Classically, patients with bronchiectasis show evidence of airflow obstruction. Around 40% of cases may show significant improvement in forced expiratory volume in one second (FEV_1) after using a beta-2 bronchodilator.[7] Also, a significant number of patients show evidence of bronchial hyper-reactivity.[8] Patients may also have a restrictive defect due to fibrotic changes associated with bronchiectasis.

ETIOLOGY

Childhood viral or bacterial infections particularly in malnourished children are known to predispose to lung damage within the growing lung and lead to the emergence of bronchiectasis **(Box 1)**. The increasing use of immunization against whooping cough (*Bordetella pertussis*) and measles has led to a reduction in such cases. In countries where there is a high incidence of pulmonary tuberculosis, there are also likely to be many cases of patients with subsequent bronchiectasis secondary to fibrotic damage caused by tuberculosis. Other bacterial infections are known to be involved in both the early and later stages of bronchiectasis, e.g. *Pseudomonas aeruginosa* and *Haemophilus influenzae*. There is likely an inverse relationship of *P. aeruginosa* abundance with that of *H. influenzae* bacterial community.[9]

Atypical mycobacteria are being increasingly recognized in patients with bronchiectasis and infection with these atypical organisms may initiate bronchiectasis or colonization may occur and further tissue damage is a consequence in patients with pre-existing bronchiectasis.

Aspergillus fumigatus is commonly found in the environment and in susceptible patients may cause an allergic reaction, causing the clinical condition allergic bronchopulmonary aspergillosis (ABPA). Allergic reactions to the fungus in the airways may cause inflammation and collateral damage to the airway walls as a result. Occasionally, invasive aspergillosis may also occur. Chronic pulmonary aspergillosis along with *Mycobacterium avium* complex infection in patients with bronchiectasis is a strong predictor of mortality.[10] Patients who are human immunodeficiency virus (HIV) positive may also develop bronchiectasis related to their reduced immunity.

Genetic and congenital conditions may lead to bronchiectasis. These include cystic fibrosis (CF) (see later part of this chapter for further description) and primary ciliary dyskinesia. Primary ciliary dyskinesia is an inherited autosomal recessive condition with a birth frequency of approximately 1 in 30,000. In this condition, bronchial cilia are unable to beat normally. This is due to an absent or shortened dynein arm within the cilia. Some of these patients also have Kartagener's syndrome where there is bronchiectasis, situs inversus and chronic sinusitis. This condition causes a lack of correct rotation of organs in the fetus and hence there is often association with situs inversus and dextrocardia. Some progress has recently been made in identifying the underlying genetic mutations. Another uncommon condition is Mounier-Kuhn syndrome, which causes tracheobronchomegaly. Bronchiectasis has also been reported to be found in associated with alpha-1 antitrypsin deficiency and Marfan's syndrome.

It is important to think of the possibility of an underlying immune deficiency causing an increased risk of lung infections leading on to the development of bronchiectasis. Such immunodeficiency disorders include X-linked agammaglobulinemia, IgA deficiency, severe combined immunodeficiency of childhood (SCID) and common variable immunodeficiency (CVID).

BOX 1 The etiology of bronchiectasis

- Postinfectious, e.g. tuberculosis, whooping cough, pneumonia
- Cystic fibrosis
- Connective tissue diseases, e.g. systemic lupus erythematosus (SLE), rheumatoid arthritis,
- SLE, Sjögren's syndrome, relapsing polychondritis
- Allergic bronchopulmonary aspergillosis
- Ciliary defects, e.g. primary ciliary dyskinesia, Young's syndrome, Kartagener's syndrome
- Immune deficiency, e.g. IgA deficiency, X-linked agammaglobulinemia, common variable immunodeficiency, secondary to chronic lymphatic leukemia
- Congenital defects, e.g. tracheobronchomegaly (Mounier-Kuhn syndrome), pulmonary sequestration
- Secondary to inhalation or aspiration, e.g. due to a foreign body
- Inflammatory bowel disease, e.g. ulcerative colitis.

In some subjects with bronchiectasis, there may be a history of aspiration of a foreign body, such as a peanut during childhood. Aspiration of food may cause a foreign body to be lodged in an airway, which may then gradually result in the development of bronchiectasis over a long period of time. Aspiration will typically, but not invariably involve the right middle or right lower lobe.

Bronchiectasis may be associated with connective tissue diseases, especially rheumatoid arthritis, but also systemic sclerosis, systemic lupus erythematosus or ankylosing spondylitis. It is also an important manifestation of Sjögren syndrome.[11]

Clinical evidence of bronchiectasis has been reported in around 3% of patients with rheumatoid arthritis. More detailed investigations including HRCT scanning have reported much higher levels.[12,13] There is an association between inflammatory bowel disease and bronchiectasis particularly in patients with chronic ulcerative colitis.[14] Airway inflammation may be exacerbated by effector lymphocytes. Sometimes immune modulating drugs may result in an exacerbation of lung symptoms. It is interesting that in some patients, who have a bowel resection for ulcerative colitis, the respiratory symptoms may increase postoperatively.

The proportion of bronchiectasis patients with underlying disorders **(Box 1)** will vary according to the population studied. Clearly in a population, where there is a high prevalence of pulmonary TB, postinfectious bronchiectasis will be relatively common. Also, the availability of complex immune testing may be limited in some countries and, therefore, this cause may remain underdiagnosed. However, in many published series, around 50% of patients with bronchiectasis will have no definite identified cause.

Bronchiectasis is often diffuse, but sometimes may be local. A good example of local bronchiectasis is the one, which occurs after an inhaled foreign body and may lodge in the right middle or right lower lobe.

Cases of bronchiectasis may be identified in association with nail dystrophy often with yellow discoloration called "yellow nail syndrome" and is usually associated with sinusitis, pleural effusions and primary lymphedema. Young's syndrome is a combination of bronchiectasis, obstructive azoospermia and chronic sinusitis.

There is some emerging evidence that there may be an association between asthma and bronchiectasis. A history of asthma usually occurs first and then evidence of bronchiectasis occasionally emerges many years later. Some of these cases may be related to ABPA.

SYMPTOMS AND SIGNS

Recurrent cough with sputum production may be an indication of underlying bronchiectasis in children. There should also be a high index of suspicion for underlying bronchiectasis in children with chronic respiratory symptoms. Furthermore, the finding of persisting inspiratory crackles over the lungs should raise the possibility of bronchiectasis.

In adults, similar symptoms to those in children, i.e. a chronic productive cough with shortness of breath and occasionally wheezing may occur. Also, the patient may have recurrent hemoptysis and fever at times of acute infective exacerbations. Pleuritic chest pain may also occur occasionally. Frequent respiratory infections may be associated with weight loss. Based on appearance, sputum can be classified into mucoid, mucopurulent or purulent types. A higher proportion of patients with varicose or cystic bronchiectasis have purulent sputum compared to those with tubular bronchiectasis as assessed by HRCT lung scans.[4]

Dyspnea correlates with the degree of impairment of FEV_1, sputum volume and extent of changes seen on HRCT scans. Dyspnea occurs in around 72% of cases.[15] Chest pains, usually nonpleuritic the may occur in around one-third of patients. Hemoptysis occurs in around half of cases, may be massive and life-threatening in a small proportion of cases. There is a form of bronchiectasis in adults where the cough is nonproductive. The absence of purulent sputum production does not exclude the possibility of underlying bronchiectasis.

A full assessment of symptoms should include an estimated or measured 24-hour sputum volume when clinically stable, a record of the number of infective exacerbations that the patient has per year, the extent of the use of antibiotics and also assessment of the effects of the symptoms on activities of daily living. The St. George's respiratory questionnaire has been used to assess the quality of life in the adult patients with bronchiectasis.[16]

A classical sign on examination is the presence of coarse inspiratory crackles over the affected lungs especially in the lower zones, which may be present in about 70% of patients. Crackles may often extend into expiration. Coughing may temporarily lessen the crackles. Wheezing may be heard in around 45% of cases. Finger clubbing has been reported to occur in around 40% cases, although this has been less frequent in some reports.[15]

DIAGNOSIS

Prior to CT lung scanning, bronchograms were the definitive way of diagnosing and delineating the extent of bronchiectasis. The advent of HRCT lung scanning has revolutionized the diagnosis of bronchiectasis.[17] CT scanning has been shown to be the most sensitive and specific way of diagnosing the condition. In particular, the HRCT is superior to a plain chest X-ray. CT scan appearances **(Fig. 2)** may include ring-like shadows where airways are seen in cross-section or a tramline appearance where airways are seen in longitudinal section. Modern HRCT scanners can produce 3-D reconstruction of affected areas **(Fig. 3)**.

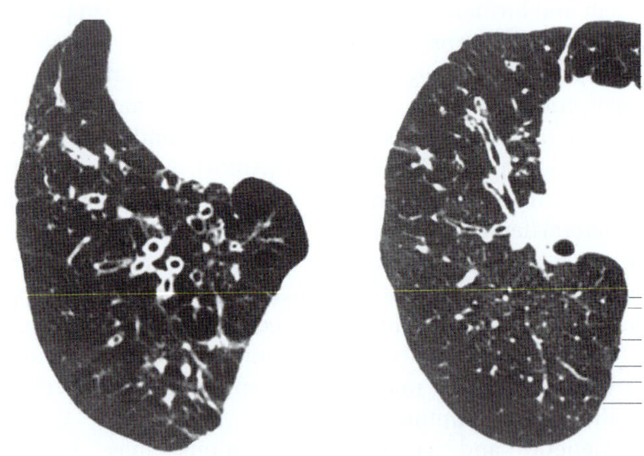

Fig. 2 High-resolution CT scans showing the signs of signet ring shadowing and tramline changes typical of bronchiectasis

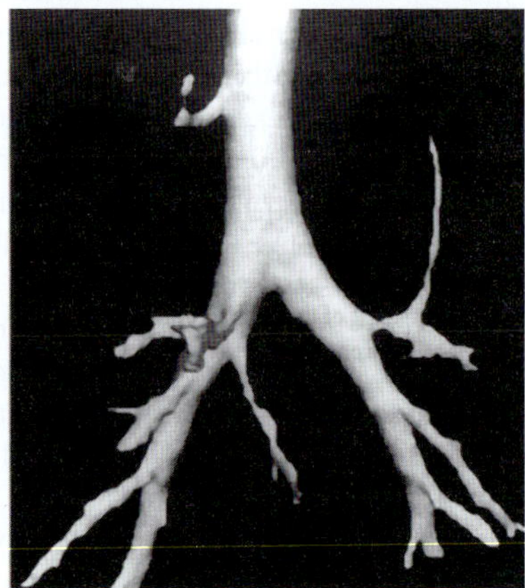

Fig. 3 Three-dimensional reconstruction from a CT scan showing bronchiectasis

Nonspecific findings include focal pneumonitis or areas of atelectasis. CT scanning may also visualize varicose constrictions. The distribution of abnormalities seen on the CT scan may occasionally give some clue as to the underlying etiology. For instance, localized bronchiectasis in the right middle or right lower lobe suggests a foreign body aspiration; CF and ABPA tend to have an initial predilection for the upper lobes.

Other investigations (after taking a careful history and performing a thorough examination) include assessment of sputum samples for bacterial, mycobacterial and fungal infections such as *Aspergillus*. The possibility of ABPA should be investigated by measuring the total serum IgE and looking for specific IgE and IgG to *Aspergillus fumigatus*. Immune deficiency may be detected by looking at serum IgG, IgA and IgM levels, IgG subclasses and also an assessment of functional antibody levels, particularly against *Haemophilus influenzae* and *Streptococcus pneumoniae*. In some cases, investigations for possible underlying CF may be appropriate (see later in this chapter). In selected patients, studies of cilial function will be appropriate particularly for primary ciliary dyskinesia. They will usually require referral to a specialist center where mucosal biopsies are examined by ultramicroscopy. Also, investigations should look for the possibility of an associated underlying connective tissue disease.

MICROBIOLOGY

Patients with established bronchiectasis may have a wide range of respiratory pathogens in the sputum. Common causes of bacterial exacerbation in bronchiectasis include *Haemophilus influenzae*, *Staphylococcus aureus*, Methicillin-resistant *Staphylococcus aureus* (MRSA), *Streptococcus pneumoniae*, coliforms (e.g. *Klebsiella*, *Enterobacter*) or *Pseudomonas aeruginosa*. Assessment of sputum samples, over the course of weeks or months often provides invaluable information. Patients' airways may eventually become colonized by one or more organisms and occasionally the numbers of those organisms increase and initiate an acute exacerbation requiring antibiotics. In particular, *Pseudomonas aeruginosa* is likely to cause chronic colonization in more severe cases and may lead to progressive lung damage as part of a "vicious circle" of recurrent infection, tissue damage, predilection to further infection and then further tissue damage.

Specific sputum testing for mycobacteria should be carried out, firstly to exclude the possibility of tuberculosis, and secondly to look for colonization and possible infection with atypical mycobacteria such as *Mycobacterium avium-intracellulare, Mycobacterium kansasii or Mycobacterium abscessus*. The finding of atypical mycobacteria on two samples of sputum will then indicate the need for prolonged multiple antibiotic therapy.[18]

TREATMENT

Treatment comprises two broad components: firstly for an exacerbation of bronchiectasis and secondly for long-term maintenance treatment.

An exacerbation causes the patient to have symptoms of one or more symptoms such as increasing frequency of cough, sputum volume and sputum purulence. Initially the treatment depends partly on the previous microbiology results. If the patient is colonized with *Pseudomonas aeruginosa*, the treatment can be done with an oral agent, such as ciprofloxacin 500 mg twice a day; for more severe exacerbations, intravenous antibiotics may be more effective. The use of two different types of intravenous antibiotics at the same time will help in reducing the risk for emergence of antibiotic resistance. Intravenous therapy is indicated if there is a failure of improvement on oral treatment. There are currently very few oral agents available, which are effective against *Pseudomonas aeruginosa*. Ciprofloxacin is often the first choice of oral agent. Infection due to other bacterial agents such as *Streptococcus pneumoniae, Haemophilus influenzae, Moraxella catarrhalis* or *Staphylococcus aureus*, may be treated with an oral agent, or alternatively, a single intravenous agent may be used. If the exacerbation is caused by MRSA, then two antibiotics are often recommended, either orally or intravenously **(Table 1)**.

Due to difficulties with antibiotic penetration into the damaged lung and airways,[19] a prolonged course of antibiotics is often required. The optimum duration of such a course is unclear, however if there is a clinical improvement with a fall of serum inflammatory markers, such as C-reactive protein, then this would indicate improvement and often such a course of antibiotics would last for 10–14 days.

There has been some recent evidence, which suggests that physiotherapy is effective in acute exacerbations.[20] Patients may also benefit from nebulized bronchodilators during an exacerbation. It is unclear whether a course of steroids given

Table 1 Recommendation of antibiotics to be used for these infections

Bacterial infection	*First choice*	*Second-line treatment*
Haemophilus influenzae or Moraxella catarrhalis	Co-amoxiclav	Doxycycline, ciprofloxacin
Streptococcus pneumoniae	Amoxicillin	Clarithromycin
Methicillin-resistant Staphylococcus aureus (MRSA)	Rifampicin and trimethoprim	Rifampicin and doxycycline or linezolid
	or IV vancomycin or teicoplanin	
Pseudomonas aeruginosa	Ciprofloxacin	Ceftazidime and tobramycin or colistin

at the same time as the course of antibiotics has any beneficial effect. Theoretically, it may reduce the inflammatory response in the lung, but the possibility of side effects also needs to be considered.

The choice of intravenous agents for an exacerbation due to *Pseudomonas aeruginosa* includes ceftazidime, aztreonam, tazobactam, meropenem, colistin, and aminoglycosides such as tobramycin or gentamicin. Availability of these drugs will vary between different countries. If intravenous aminoglycosides are used, then monitoring of blood levels is essential to reduce the risk of renal or auditory side effects. If tobramycin is given two or three times per day, predose and postdose levels should be measured to assess the trough and peak levels. If a single daily dose of aminoglycoside is used,[21] e.g. a 30-minute infusion of tobramycin, monitoring of trough levels may be sufficient.

It is of utmost importance to address general issues such as maintaining adequate hydration and oxygen saturation. Noninvasive ventilation may be useful for those patients who slip into type 2 respiratory failure.[22]

Long-term Management of Stable Disease

The general advice about stopping smoking and improving nutrition applies to bronchiectasis patient. Annual vaccination against seasonal influenza is advised as is pneumococcal vaccination, approximately every 10 years. Patients with significant bronchiectasis should receive instructions from a respiratory physiotherapist about the choice of different airway clearance techniques and should be strongly advised to carry out home physiotherapy regularly. There is currently no good evidence to use nebulized recombinant human DNase as a mucolytic agent, although larger studies are required.[23] There have been some studies recently looking at nebulized hypertonic saline[24] and inhaled mannitol[25] as agents to help sputum production. There is some evidence to suggest the beneficial effects of inhaled hyperosmolar agents to reduce exacerbations.[26] Lung function tests should be carried out before and after bronchodilators use to look for evidence of reversibility of airflow obstruction with both inhaled β-agonists and anticholinergic agents. Sometimes exercise tolerance and symptoms may improve with these agents despite there being no significant improvement in lung function measurements.

The evidence base for using inhaled corticosteroids is limited.[27,28] There have been some studies that have shown a reduction in sputum volume and an improvement in quality of life measurements without any obvious effects on lung function or exacerbation rates. Some patients may benefit from a trial of inhaled steroids for several months. Adrenal insufficiency is common in patients of bronchiectasis but this was not associated with use of inhaled steroids.[29]

In patients who are colonized with *Pseudomonas aeruginosa*, the use of long-term nebulized antibiotics may be helpful in reducing the bacterial load in the airways. This, in turn, may reduce chronic inflammation and hence reduce lung damage. The inhaled antibiotics, however, have the drawback of being expensive, sometimes, may cause wheezing even after predosing with inhaled β-2 agonists. There is some limited evidence in the literature of benefit from long-term nebulized antibiotics in patients with more severe bronchiectasis colonized with pseudomonas.[30,31] On first isolation of *Pseudomonas aeruginosa* in the sputum, attempts should be made to eradicate the infection to try and stop chronic colonization.

In a small number of patients with very localized bronchiectasis, the possibility of surgery should be considered.[32] They apply for instance to those patients who have localized bronchiectasis following aspiration of a foreign body or related to previous localized tuberculosis. Surgery with localized lung resection may benefit selected patients with hemoptysis, chronic debilitating cough or a lung abscess unresponsive to antibiotic treatment.[33] Lung transplantation may also be considered for advanced disease.

The role of long-term oral antibiotics in bronchiectasis, perhaps given as a rotation of different antibiotics, is uncertain. However, there is some evidence in the literature regarding benefit of such an approach in patients with severe bronchiectasis in terms of reduced sputum volume, number of days absent from work due to ill-health and reduction in exacerbation frequency. Recently, there has been some evidence of the potential benefit of reducing exacerbation frequency by using long-term oral azithromycin as an anti-inflammatory agent in bronchiectasis.[34]

Noninvasive ventilation can improve quality of life in some patients with chronic type 2 respiratory failure due to bronchiectasis.[35]

Complications

Acute respiratory exacerbations are common and important cause of morbidity and decline in lung function.[36] Maintenance therapy with macrolide antibiotics has been shown to be safe and effective to reduce exacerbations.[37] Hemoptysis is a rare, but potentially a life-threatening complication of bronchiectasis. Severe hemoptysis (defined as more than 300 mL) of blood coughed up per 24 hours may occur. Whenever possible, the bleeding site should be identified by a combination of tests such as bronchoscopy, CT lung scanning and angiography. Often, bleeding occurs from a bronchial artery and an interventional radiologist may be able to embolize the vessel.[38] Occasionally, surgery may be necessary in a patient with severe hemoptysis. The risk of hemoptysis is shown to increase with the use of inhalers especially of β-2 agonist agents.[39]

Amyloidosis is an occasional complication of chronic, advanced bronchiectasis. A lung abscess may develop due to bronchiectasis and this may be refractory to prolonged antibiotic therapy.

Prognosis

The prognosis of bronchiectasis is very variable, depending upon any underlying cause, particularly immunodeficiency, the extent of the bronchiectasis and also the type of bacterial colonization. Generally, colonization with *Pseudomonas aeruginosa* is linked to a worse prognosis.

Cystic Fibrosis

EPIDEMIOLOGY

Cystic fibrosis is a disease caused by an autosomal recessive mutation on chromosome 7. In European populations, CF affects approximately 1 in 2,500 live births. In some countries, there is now a national screening program to detect such cases soon after birth. Again in European populations, approximately 1 in 25 live births carries 1 mutation. There is some speculation in the literature that heterozygotes may possibly have a survival advantage when faced with other gastrointestinal infections such as cholera or typhoid. This may explain why the disease has not become gradually rarer over the centuries. However in the Indian subcontinent, CF is less common. The exact incidence and prevalence figures are unknown. However, in European countries like the United Kingdom with significant number of immigrants from the Indian subcontinent, there are a substantial number of CF patients that are now being recognized.

The prevalence of CF in Asian immigrants in Britain has been estimated at around 1 in 10,000 and the clinical course tends to be more severe than in matched, non-Asian controls.[40]

Genetics and Cellular Dysfunction

The CF mutation on chromosome 7 leads to an abnormality in a protein that is called cystic fibrosis transmembrane regulator (CFTR). This defective protein leads to the disruption of ion transport in epithelial lined organs, particularly the airways, but can also involve the sweat ducts, pancreatic ducts, bile ducts and the intestine. The genetic abnormality was isolated on chromosome 7.[41] This led to a great hope that gene therapy would eventually become a cure. Since 1989, more than a 1,000 different mutations have been identified, any of which may produce the CF phenotype. Some of these mutations are extremely rare, however. The commonest mutation in the UK is deletion of phenylalanine (delta F508). This mutation has also been reported in 19–56% Indian patients.[42,43]

Patients who are homozygous for delta F508 tend to have severe respiratory and pancreatic involvement although occasionally exceptions may occur. Indeed there is sometimes a discrepancy between the known genotype and the phenotype. There is increasing evidence of influence of other genes on different chromosomes, so called "modifying genes" and extensive research work is currently being carried out to identify such genes with potential implications for treatment. Potential modifying genes include mannose-binding lectin, transforming growth factor beta and protease inhibitors.

The CFTR is a 1,480 amino acid product coded for the long arm on chromosome 7. It is a glycoprotein and its function is to mediate ATP-related chloride conductance. Deficiency of the CFTR causes reduced chloride conductance and consequent changes in sodium absorption by the cells. In the airways, excess sodium and water is absorbed across the cell membrane into the cell and this leads to a concentration of macromolecules and mucus in the airways. This, in turn, acts as a magnet for pathogens such as *Pseudomonas aeruginosa*. There is also some evidence that the defective CFTR may also be proinflammatory leading to airway damage in early childhood.

The CFTR mutations have been divided into five groups:

1. No synthesis, e.g. the nonsense mutation G542X
2. A block in processing, e.g. delta F508
3. A block in regulation, e.g. missense G551D
4. Altered conductance, e.g. missense R117H
5. Reduced synthesis, e.g. missense 455E.

Generally, groups 4 and 5 are associated with a mild phenotype. Some of these mild phenotypes may present only in adult life; in males, they may be first diagnosed in the infertility clinics.

DIAGNOSIS

Diagnosis is usually made in early childhood either by neonatal screening or by the development of symptoms such as failure to thrive or intestinal obstruction in neonates.

The diagnosis of CF depends upon a positive sweat test, gene analysis and also the clinical picture. Sweat testing classically involves pilocarpine iontophoresis, which is applied to the skin to stimulate sweat production, usually on the forearm. A 5 millivolt electric charge is then applied to the skin for 10 minutes and sweat is collected on a tiny piece of gauze. The chloride content of the gauze is then analyzed together with the difference in weights before and after sweat simulation.

Normally, sweat chloride levels are less than 30 millimoles/liter. The diagnostic level for classical CF is a chloride level of 60 or more millimoles/liter. The sodium content will also increase, although usually not to quite such a high level as the sweat chloride level. If an abnormal sweat test is recorded, it is usual to repeat the test to ensure accuracy. A small number of individuals will have a borderline sweat test between 30 millimoles/liter and 59 millimoles/liter, and this may be associated with the condition called "atypical CF." These tend to be patients, who have mild symptoms and who are often diagnosed in late childhood or as adults. Patients with atypical CF are less likely than classical CF patients to have pancreatic insufficiency.

CLINICAL FEATURES

Cystic fibrosis is a multiorgan disease. The lungs bear the brunt of the disorder with eventual recurrent severe respiratory infections leading to bronchiectasis. However, 85% of CF patients have pancreatic insufficiency and around 5–10% have significant CF-related liver disease. Deficiency of micronutrients such as vitamin A, D and E, iron, copper and zinc has been demonstrated in Indian CF children.[44] The liver disease occurs due to chronic inflammation of the bile ducts, which may eventually lead to biliary cirrhosis. Many patients with CF have a low bone mass, partly due to the effects of chronic infection, but partly due to the presence of the CFTR mutation itself. The sweat glands function abnormally and paradoxically produce a rise in sweat chloride and sodium levels, which is used (as detailed above) to diagnose the condition. Male patients are usually infertile due to inability of sperm to pass through the blocked vas deferens. With modern fertility treatments, sperm may be aspirated from the testes of such patients and in vitro fertilization may be possible. Generally, females with CF are fertile. Patients with CF are at increased risk of pneumothoraces **(Fig. 4)**.

The CFTR abnormality leads to the development of thick and highly viscous sputum in the airways, which is very difficult for the patient to expectorate and also is an ideal area for bacterial colonization. The bacteria involved in respiratory infections in CF patients vary according to age. *Haemophilus influenzae* and *Staphylococcus aureus* are typical bacterial infections in earlier childhood. As the patient grows older, it is more likely that *Pseudomonas aeruginosa* will become the predominant pathogen and by late teens, over 50% of patients will be colonized with this organism. Chronic colonization may then lead to intermittent acute exacerbations leading to increasing shortness of breath and increased purulent sputum volume.

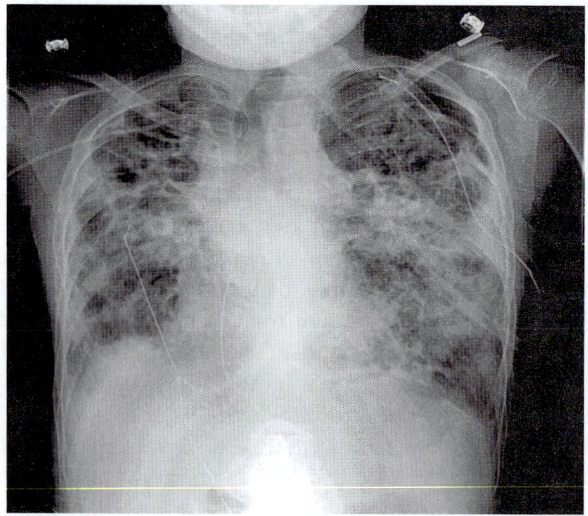

Fig. 4 Chest X-ray showing extensive bronchiectasis changes in a patient with cystic fibrosis. Intercostal tubes following a pneumothorax

INFECTIONS AND TREATMENT

The cornerstone of treatment is to reduce the viscosity of sputum, improve airway clearance, treat lung infections vigorously and use anti-inflammatory agents. There is a considerable amount of research currently underway looking at the possibility of gene therapy and also drugs to influence ion transport.

An essential part of treatment is to modify and improve the nutrition of CF patients. Pancreatic insufficiency leads to poor fat absorption, which in turn, leads to abdominal symptoms of distension, diarrhea and malabsorption. Consequently, malnutrition leads to a stunting of growth and increased risk of severe lung infections.

In the early 1970s, a radical change in approach was made initially in Toronto, Canada, when a combination of high fat, high-energy diets were used in combination with pancreatic enzyme supplements. Nowadays, this is the norm for managing such patients. This is extremely important because poor nutrition leads to an energy deficit with weight loss, poor respiratory muscle strength, increased pulmonary infection with increased lung damage and a vicious cycle of further lung infections.

Some patients with more advanced disease are helped by nasogastric feeding or feeding through a percutaneous endoscopic gastrostomy (PEG) tube.

Other pathogens in CF, which are less common than *Pseudomonas aeruginosa*, include the *Burkholderia cepacia* complex. These include over 14 different species or genovars. Genovars 2 and 3 are particularly infectious and damaging to the lung. Genovar 3 is called *B. cenocepacia* and this tends to be associated with the worst prognosis of patients infected with this complex. The *Burkholderia* complex is highly infectious and damaging to lung tissues and patients may deteriorate rapidly once they acquire this infection. Other Gram-negative organisms, which may be isolated from the sputum, include *Stenotrophomonas maltophilia, Acinetobacter* and *Pandorea* species. Some of these relatively rare Gram-negative organisms may emerge due to the long-term effects of antibiotic pressure caused by the need for recurrent courses of intravenous antibiotics in CF patients. *Aspergillus fumigatus* may cause a direct necrotizing infection in the lungs, but more commonly, some patients with CF may develop allergic bronchopulmonary aspergillosis.

An increasing problem in CF patients is the appearance of atypical nontuberculous mycobacteria especially *Mycobacterium abscessus*, but also occasionally *Mycobacterium avium-intracellulare* and *Mycobacterium kansasii*. These nontuberculous mycobacteria are usually difficult to eradicate. The presence of such infection, particularly *Mycobacterium abscessus*, may be a relative contraindication to patients subsequently being accepted for lung transplantation.

Cystic fibrosis patients have no detectable immune deficiency and bacteremia is uncommon. The altered airway secretions lead to increased sputum viscosity and then colonization with bacteria. There is a defect in the mucociliary escalator due to highly viscous sputum. Chronic infection causes collateral damage to lung tissue. The sputum itself consists of a large amount of bacterial DNA and phagocytic debris.

Exacerbations of lung infection in CF are diagnosed partly on a clinical basis in the terms of symptoms and signs, but also on evidence of a reduction in lung function particularly the FEV1% predicted, sputum bacteriology, sometimes, including bacterial counts and also X-ray or CT lung scan evidence.

Specific treatments of known bacterial infections in CF are as follows:

- *Staphylococcus aureus* is usually treated with drugs such as flucloxacillin or fusidic acid. Some patients acquire MRSA and may require intravenous vancomycin, teicoplanin or oral/IV linezolid.
- *Haemophilus influenzae* is often treated with co-amoxiclav. *Pseudomonas aeruginosa* may be sensitive to oral ciprofloxacin and in some countries oral chloramphenicol is used (although there are concerns about its side effect of aplastic anemia). Often, *Pseudomonas aeruginosa* treatment requires intravenous antibiotics. The usual practice is to give at least two intravenous antibiotics together to reduce the risk of emergence of bacterial resistance.

High doses of intravenous antibiotics are often required in CF because of increased renal clearance of some antibiotics and also concerns about antibiotic penetration into the mucoid forms of *Pseudomonas aeruginosa* often with associated biofilms. Typical combinations for IV antibiotic use in CF include ceftazidime plus tobramycin or ceftazidime plus colomycin/colistin. Alternatives to ceftazidime include meropenem, tazocin or aztreonam. If tobramycin or gentamicin is used, it is essential to check blood levels particularly the trough levels, to make sure that excessive doses do not lead to accumulation in the blood, which may lead to toxicity to the inner ear and/or the kidneys.

Increasingly, long-term nebulized antibiotics are used in CF patients who are colonized with *Pseudomonas aeruginosa*. The aim is to reduce the bacterial load in the lungs and delay tissue damage. Typical examples of nebulized antibiotics that are currently in use include tobramycin and colistin. Other nebulized forms of antibiotics are currently being assessed, e.g. aztreonam, meropenem and ciprofloxacin. The local pulmonary administration of drugs seems ideal, though the clinical outcomes depend upon the drug concentrations and the ability of the drug to overcome the local barriers.[45]

Duration of IV antibiotic treatment is often around 14 days for pseudomonal infections. The dose and frequency of dosing with antibiotics depends partly on the type of antibiotic used. Some antibiotic effects are concentration dependent, i.e. the higher the peak blood level, the more effective it is, e.g. tobramycin. The idea here is to give high infrequent doses. Recently, single daily doses of tobramycin have become the norm rather than dosing two or three times per day. Other beneficial antibiotic effects depend upon the time above the minimum inhibitory concentration of that antibiotic for a particular bacterial infection. An example of this is ceftazidime. In this case, it is better to give frequent doses or even a continuous infusion rather than a single daily dose.

Lung function testing in CF usually occurs at each outpatient visit. Spirometry is the usual measurement made. As the disease progresses, the FEV1% predicted progressively deteriorates. A decline in FVC is less rapid. It is important to recognize and to treat lung infections at an early age in children to try and delay airway colonization and to delay the rate of lung function decline with age.

The commonest way to assess pancreatic dysfunction is to measure fecal pancreatic elastase-1 levels in a small sample of feces rather than carrying out three-or five-day fecal fat collection. The more advanced the pancreatic disease, the lower the fecal elastase-1 level becomes. Nutrition in CF usually aims for a high calorie, high-fat diet often with additional food supplements. Sometimes, in addition, nasogastric or gastrostomy feeding is used. It is important to give oral fat-soluble vitamin supplements to patients with CF-related pancreatic deficiency, i.e. vitamins A, D, E and K.

Some older children and adults may develop abdominal distension and blockage due to distal intestinal obstruction syndrome (DIOS) previously called meconium ileus equivalent. Clinically, the patient complains of abdominal pain, bloating, vomiting or constipation. On examination, there may be a palpable lump in the right iliac fossa and a plain abdominal X-ray may show fecal loading and sometimes fluid levels. Treatment involves the use of bowel cleansing solutions.

Cystic fibrosis-related liver disease can lead in severe cases to biliary cirrhosis, which may then lead to portal hypertension. There are lung complications associated with severe liver diseases, including intrapulmonary shunting, pulmonary hypertension and respiratory muscle weakness due to poor nutrition. Hepatomegaly may cause the right diaphragm to be raised and low blood albumin levels may lead to the onset of ascites and/or pleural effusions. Treatment includes the daily use of oral ursodeoxycholic acid. In severe cases, liver transplantation may be indicated.

The management of CF is based around a multidisciplinary team approach. This patient-centered approach promotes optimal treatment and improved life outcomes.[46] The CF team consists of doctors, nurses, physiotherapists, dieticians and clinical psychologists with additional input from specialists in diabetes, liver disease, infertility, etc.

Chest physiotherapy is essential to help the patient clear the airways and there are a variety of physical maneuvers and mechanical devices, which aid sputum production. Nebulized bronchodilators are often used to help as well. Many patients use nebulized DNase (Dornase alfa), which is a drug that acts by cleaving bacterial DNA in the sputum, making it less viscous. The usual dose in adults is 2.5 mg nebulized once daily.

Other Treatments

There has been considerable interest in the development of anti-inflammatory drugs. Ibuprofen was used in the past but a significant number of patients suffered from side effects from this medication. More recently, the macrolide antibiotic azithromycin has been used in a single daily dose of 250 mg in adults for its anti-inflammatory effects. Several studies have shown an improvement in lung function, quality of life and fewer infective exacerbations. Oral steroids may also have a beneficial effect in some patients, but of course, this needs to be weighed against the problems of long-term side effects, particularly osteoporosis.

Cross infection between CF patients is a serious problem. This was first recognized with *Burkholderia cepacia* infections, but more recently epidemic forms of *Pseudomonas aeruginosa* have been described and some of these epidemic forms may be more pathogenic than sporadic forms. Therefore, in outpatient clinics, both special and temporal separation of patients is required.

Lung transplantation should be considered when the patient's lung function has declined with an FEV_1% predicted of 30% or less.[47] When patients reach that level of lung function, the two-year survival is around 50% and the potential advantages of lung transplantation should then be discussed with the patient.

Gene therapy is being investigated in research trials at the moment. The main problem has been finding a suitable vector, which enables sufficient epithelial cells to become transfected with subsequent incorporation of the normal gene into the host's genome. Initial results appear very promising.

Prognosis

The median survival for CF has shown a remarkable improvement over the past few decades. For instance in the United States in 1985, the median survival was 25.5 years and in 2001, it was around 37 years. Generally, survival is better in patients who are pancreatic sufficient. Median survival is slightly better in males in comparison to female patients and is better in patients who have group 4 or group 5 CF mutations. There is also a close correlation between survival and poor nutritional status. Around 40% of adults with CF have CF-related diabetes. There is some evidence that raised airway glucose concentrations may increase the likelihood of frequent and more severe respiratory infections.

Finally, the story of the unraveling of the pathogenesis of CF and subsequent development of effective treatments has been one of medicine's great success stories during the past few decades. The management of the condition also serves as a model for multidisciplinary team working.

REFERENCES

1. Weycker D, Edelsberg J, Oster G, Tino G. Prevalence and economic burden of bronchiectasis. Clin Pulm Med. 2005;12:205-9.
2. Twiss J, Metcalfe R, Edwards E, Byrnes C. New Zealand national incidence of bronchiectasis "too high" for a developed country. Arch Dis Chest. 2005;90(7):737-40.
3. Patel IS, Vlahos I, Wilkinson TM, Lloyd-Owen SJ, Donaldson GC, Wilks M, et al. Bronchiectasis, exacerbation indices and inflammation in chronic obstructive pulmonary disease. Am J Respir Crit Care Med. 2004;170(4):400-7.
4. O'Brien C, Guest PJ, Hill SL, Stockley RA. Physiological and radiological characterisation of patients diagnosed with chronic obstructive pulmonary disease in primary care. Thorax. 2000;55(8):635-42.
5. Singleton R, Morris A, Redding G, Poll J, Holck P, Martinez P, et al. Bronchiectasis in Alaska native children: causes and clinical courses. Pediatr Pulmonol. 2000;29(3):182-7.
6. Reid LM. Reduction in bronchial subdivision in bronchiectasis. Thorax. 1950;5(3):233-47.
7. Murphy MB, Reen DJ, Fitzgerald MX. Atopy, immunological changes and respiratory function in bronchiectasis. Thorax. 1984;39(3):179-84.
8. Pang J, Chan HS, Sung JY. Prevalence of asthma, atopy and bronchial hyperreactivity in bronchiectasis: a controlled study. Thorax. 1989;44(11):948-51.
9. Purcell P, Jary H, Perry A, Perry JD, Stewart CJ, Nelson A, et al. Polymicrobial airway bacterial communities in adult bronchiectasis patients. BMC Microbiol. 2014;14(1):130.
10. Zoumot Z, Boutou AK, Gill SS, Van Zeller M, Hansell DM, Wells AU, et al. *Mycobacterium avium* complex infection in non-cystic fibrosis bronchiectasis. Respirology. 2014;19(5):714-22.
11. Kreider M, Highland K. Pulmonary involvement in Sjögren syndrome. Semin Respir Crit Care Med. 2014;35:255-64.
12. McMahon MJ, Swinson DR, Shettar S, Wolstenholme R, Chattopadhyay C, Smith P, et al. Bronchiectasis and rheumatoid arthritis: a clinical study. Ann Rheum Dis. 1993;52(11):776-9.
13. Hassan WU, Keaney NP, Holland CD, Kelly CA. High resolution computed tomography of the lung in lifetime non-smoking patients with rheumatoid arthritis. Ann Rheum Dis. 1995;54(4):308-10.
14. Camus P, Colby TV. The lung in inflammatory bowel disease. Eur Respir J. 2000;15(1):5-10.
15. Nicotra MB, Rivera M, Dale AM, Shepherd R, Carter R. Clinical, pathophysiologic, and microbiologic characterization of bronchiectasis in an aging cohort. Chest. 1995;108(4):955-61.
16. Wilson CB, Jones PW, O'Leary CJ, Cole PJ, Wilson R. Validation of the St. George's Respiratory Questionnaire in bronchiectasis. Am J Respir Crit Care Med. 1997;156(2 Pt 1):536-41.
17. Hansell DM. Bronchiectasis. Radiol Clin North Am. 1998;36(1):107-28.
18. Griffith DE, Aksamit T, Brown-Elliott A; ATS Mycobacterial Diseases Subcommittee; American Thoracic Society; Infectious Disease Society of America, et al. An official ATS/IDSA statement: Diagnosis, treatment, and prevention of nontuberculous mycobacterial diseases. Am J Respir Crit Care Med. 2007;175(4):367-416.
19. Honeybourne D. Antibiotic penetration in the respiratory tract and implications for the selection of antimicrobial therapy. Curr Opin Pulm Med. 1997;3(2):170-4.

20. Murray MP, Pentland JL, Hill AT. A randomised crossover trial of chest physiotherapy in non-cystic fibrosis bronchiectasis. Eur Respir J. 2009;34(5):1086-92.
21. Barza M, Ioannidis JP, Cappelleri JC, Lau J. Single or multiple daily doses of aminoglycosides: a meta-analysis. BMJ. 1996;312(7027):338-45.
22. Dupont M, Gacouin A, Lena H, Lavoué S, Brinchault G, Delaval P, et al. Survival of patients with bronchiectasis after the first ICU stay for respiratory failure. Chest. 2004;125(5):1815-20.
23. Wilkinson M, Sugumar K, Milan SJ, Hart A, Crockett A, Crossingham I. Mycolytics for bronchiectasis. Cochrane Database Syst Rev. 2014;5:CD001289.
24. Kellett F, Redfern J, Niven RM. Evaluation of nebulised hypertonic saline (7%) as an adjunct to physiotherapy in patients with stable bronchiectasis. Respir Med. 2005;99(1):27-31.
25. Daviskas E, Anderson SD, Eberl S, Young IH. Effect of increasing doses of mannitol on mucus clearance in patients with bronchiectasis. Eur Respir J. 2008;31(4):765-72.
26. Hart A, Sugumar K, Milan SJ, Fowler SJ, Crossingham I. Inhaled hyperosmolar agents for bronchiectasis. Cochrane Database Syst Rev. 2014;5:CD002996.
27. Kapur N, Bell S, Kolbe J, Chang AB. Inhaled steroids for bronchiectasis. Cochrane Database Syst Rev. 2009;(1):CD000996.
28. Martínez-García MA, Perpiñá-Tordera M, Román-Sánchez P, Soler-Cataluña JJ. Inhaled steroids improve quality of life in patients with steady state bronchiectasis. Respir Med. 2006;100(9):1623-32.
29. Gokdemir Y, Hamzah A, Erdem E, Cimsit C, Ersu R, Karakoc F, et al. Quality of life in children with non-cystic fibrosis bronchiectasis. Respiration. 2014;88(1):46-51.
30. Orriols R, Roig J, Ferrer J, et al. Inhaled antibiotic therapy in non-cystic fibrosis patients with bronchiectasis and chronic bronchial infection by *Pseudomonas aeruginosa*. Respir Med. 1999; 93(7):476-80.
31. Haworth CS, Foweraker JE, Wilkinson P, Kenyon RF, Bilton D. Inhaled colistin in patients with bronchiectasis and chronic *Pseudomonas aeruginosa* infection. Am J Respir Crit Care Med. 2014;189(8):975-82.
32. Ashour M, Al-Kattan K, Rafay MA, Saja KF, Hajjar W, Al-Fraye AR. Current surgical therapy for bronchiectasis. World J Surg. 1999;23(11):1096-104.
33. Schneiter D, Meyer N, Lardinois D, Korom S, Kestenholz P, Weder W. Surgery for non-localized bronchiectasis. Br J Surg. 2005;92(7):836-9.
34. Cymbala AA, Edmonds LC, Bauer MA, Jederlinic PJ, May JJ, Victory JM, et al. The disease-modifying effects of twice-weekly oral azithromycin in patients with bronchiectasis. Treat Respir Med. 2005;4(2):117-22.
35. Simonds AK, Elliott MW. Outcome of domiciliary nasal intermittent positive pressure ventilation in restrictive and obstructive disorders. Thorax. 1995;50(6):604-9.
36. Redding GJ, Singleton RJ, Valery PC, Williams H, Grimwood K, Morris PS, et al. Respiratory exacerbations in indigenous children from two countries with non-cystic fibrosis chronic suppurative lung disease/bronchiectasis. Chest. 2014;146(3):762-74.
37. Gao YH, Guan WJ, Xu G, Tang Y, Gao Y, Lin ZY, et al. Macrolide therapy in adults and children with non-cystic fibrosis bronchiectasis : a systematic review and meta-analysis. PLoS One. 2014;9(3):e90047.
38. Sharma S, Kothari SS, Bhargava AD, Dey J, Wali JP, Wasir HS. Transcatheter indigeneous coil embolization in recurrent massive hemoptysis secondary to post-tubercular bronchiectasis. J Assoc Physicians India. 1995;43(2):127-9.
39. Lee JK, Lee J, Park SS, Heo EY, Park YS, Lee CH, et al. Effect of inhalers on the development of hemoptysis in patients with non-cystic fibrosis bronchiectasis. Int J Tuberc Lung Dis. 2014;18(3):363-70.
40. Callaghan BD, Hoo AF, Dinwiddie R, Balfour-Lynn IM, Carr SB. Growth and lung function in Asian patients with cystic fibrosis. Arch Dis Child. 2005;90(10):1029-32.
41. Kerem B, Rommens JM, Buchanan JA, Markiewicz D, Cox TK, Chakravarti A, et al. Identification of the cystic fibrosis gene: genetic analysis. Science. 1989;245(4922):1073-80.
42. Shastri SS, Kabra M, Kabra SK, Pandey RM, Menon PS. Characterisation of mutations and genotype-phenotype correlation in cystic fibrosis: experience from India. J Cyst Fibros. 2008;7(2):110-5.
43. Ashavaid TF, Raghavan R, Dhairyawan P, Bhawalkar S. Cystic fibrosis in India: a systematic review. J Assoc Physicians India. 2012;60:39-41.
44. Yadav K, Singh M, Angurana SK, Attri SV, Sharma G, Tageja M, et al. Evaluation of micronutrient profile of North Indian children with cystic fibrosis; a case control study. Pediatr Res. 2014;75(6):762-76.
45. d'Angelo I, Conte C, La Rotonda MI, Miro A, Quaglia F, Ungaro F. Improving the efficacy of inhaled drugs in cystic fibrosis: challenges and emerging drug delivery strategies. Adv Drug Deliv Rev. 2014;75:92-111.
46. Jamieson N, Fitzgerald D, Singh-Grewal D, Hanson CS, Craig JC, Tong A. Children's experiences of cystic fibrosis: A systematic review of qualitative studies. Pediatrics. 2014;133:e1683-97.
47. Kerem E, Reisman J, Corey M, Canny GJ, Levison H. Prediction of mortality in patients with cystic fibrosis. N Engl J Med. 1992;326(18):1187-91.

Rare Respiratory Infections

Mohankumar Thekkinkattil

INTRODUCTION

There is an increased recognition of new and rare respiratory infections in clinical practice. These are attributed to the emergence of new pathogens, especially in the immunocompromised patients.[1]

VIRAL INFECTIONS

Several viruses complicate the course of chronic obstructive pulmonary disease (COPD), bronchial asthma and in patients in the intensive respiratory care unit (IRCU). Respiratory syncytial virus (RSV) and influenza virus are the most prevalent, but corona virus, parainfluenza, adenovirus, bocavirus and others are sometimes detected in these patients during exacerbation episodes.[2] Immunosuppressed patients are susceptible to infections from cytomegalovirus, herpes viruses, adenoviruses and paramyxoviruses. Infections from hantaviruses, human metapneumoviruses (hMPV), avian influenza A viruses, and viruses of severe acute respiratory syndrome (SARS) and their mutations have been reported in the recent years. Upper respiratory tract infections due to viruses present with well-defined clinical syndromes according to the virulence and the dose of the viruses, and the resistance of the host.[3,4]

Human Metapneumovirus

Human metapneumovirus is a negative single stranded ribonucleic acid (RNS) virus of the family *Paramyxoviridae* and is closely related to avian metapneumovirus (AMPV) subgroup c. The genomic organization of hMPV is analogous to RSV, but lacks nonstructural genes. Diagnosis is made by detection of antigens in nasopharyngeal secretion by immunofluorescent antibody test, immunofluorescence staining with monoclonal antibodies and use of polyclonal antibodies and direct isolation in cultured cells. HMPV is a human pathogen, which resembles RSV, causes respiratory illness in all age groups.[5-7] hMPV was detected in 2.78% of 1,728 patients of acute exacerbations of COPD from 19 studies.[2] hMPV infection in children often exists with other respiratory virus infections, especially the RSV. Maximum number of cases occurs during winter.[8,9] Clinical presentations vary from very mild to severe bronchiolitis and pneumonitis. The clinical features are often mistaken as RSV infection in children. It is common to have bronchiolitis, wheezing and severe hypoxemia, in children who are hospitalized. Nasal secretion levels of the virus chemokine's RANTES are reported as suppressed whereas level of Interleukin 8 (IL-8) are increased.[10]

Hantavirus Pulmonary Disease

Hantavirus pulmonary disease or hantavirus hemorrhagic fever is an endemic zoonosis, which affects both adults and children in Europe and Asia. It has been also reported from India.[11] The causative agents belong to the genus hantavirus, of family *Bunyaviridae*.[11,12] It is carried by specific rodent host species, but host switches have been reported.[13] The clinical picture varies from place-to-place with the type of infection. Hemorrhagic complications like disseminated intravascular coagulopathy, severe thrombocytopenia, shock, oliguric renal failure, pleural effusion, ascites, and neurological complications like hemiparesis, epilepsy and seizures are possible in this virus infection.[14-16.] These infections are usually diagnosed by using IgM capture test and/or real time polymerase chain reaction (RT-PCR) detection of viral RNA. Neutralization tests and gene sequencing are required for genotyping and serotyping. Immunofluorescence immunoassay (IFA) or enzyme-linked immunosorbent assay (ELISA) is also done in some cases.

Bocavirus

Bocavirus is a member of family of *Parvoviridae* virus that is small (20 nm), nonenveloped virus with single-stranded DNA. There are three strains: (i) Human Boca virus (HB01), (ii) $HBoV_2$ and (iii) $HBoV_3$. It is often detected in patients with other viral infections and also in children with pneumonia or diarrhea. There is no evidence that this causes infection or disease. There are no diagnostic tests or medical treatment, or vaccines. They are seen in upper respiratory tract.

BACTERIAL INFECTIONS

Streptococci in rare cases produce severe bacteremia, high fever and toxic shock syndrome in adults.[16] High fever and tonsillopharyngitis are often observed. *Streptococcus pneumoniae* can occasionally present with lung abscess formation.[17]

Hemolytic-uremic syndrome in streptococcal pneumonia is mainly seen in the young children; the morbidity and mortality are high. Pneumonia, disseminated intravascular coagulopathy, chronic renal and respiratory failure are important clinical features.[18] Lemierre's syndrome can rarely produce complications like septic arthritis, sternoclavicular joint sepsis and cavitating pneumonia.[19] The clinical features include fever, myalgia, tachypnea and tachycardia.

Sometimes, *Salmonella* can also involve the lungs. *Salmonella* infections, apart from the usual pneumonitis, can also produce myocarditis. Multiple organ failure in a previously healthy adult with or without fever, diarrhea, and shortness of breath, altered sensorium, acute pulmonary edema and respiratory failure should warrant a differential diagnosis of *Salmonella* infection. In some patients, hepatic and muscular enzymatic surge, rhabdomyolysis and disseminated intravascular coagulation have been reported.[20]

Mycoplasma hominis infection in the lungs is mainly seen in immunocompromised patients especially in organ transplant patients, cardiac or sternotomy patients.[21]

RARE FORMS OF TUBERCULOUS INFECTIONS

Human tuberculosis, typically caused by *Mycobacterium tuberculosis* complex, can rarely occur due to rare genetic variants such as *Mycobacterium canetti, Mycobacterium microti* and *Mycobacterium pinnipedii.* The natural reservoir, mode of transmission and host factors are not well studied. So far, there is no drug resistance and the species are susceptible to rifampicin, pyrazinamide and ethambutol. Delayed growth on the solid media, contact with animals and special phenotypic pictures should be borne in mind for the diagnosis of this forms.[22]

Mycobacterium asiaticum was reported first in 1982. Chronic lung disease was a risk factor for pulmonary infection. It can produce both pulmonary and extrapulmonary disease.[23] It responds well to standard anti-TB regimens.[24]

Mycobacterium szulgai comes under nontuberculosis mycobacteria in the nonhuman immunodeficiency virus (HIV) infected population. The clinical presentation is with cough with purulent sputum, fever, fatigue, and weight loss. Chest radiography usually shows poorly defined opacities mimicking pulmonary tuberculosis. Diagnosis is by culture and gas chromatography. Usually a 6-month regimen of rifampicin, isoniazid and pyrazinamide is used.[25]

Mycobacterium celatum is another rare cause of disseminated disease in immunosuppressed patients, but can also occur in the immunocompetent individuals in whom the lungs and lymph node involvement has been reported.[26]

ATYPICAL BACTERIAL INFECTIONS

Chlamydia psittaci is an intracellular Gram-negative bacterium, which causes psittacosis. It has seven genotypes, A to F, which can be transmitted to humans from the bird's feces. The incidence seems to increase in the Western world. Clinical presentation varies from febrile episodes to the occurrence of severe pneumonia.[27] Pleuritic pain and dyspnea are common. Chest radiography shows ground-glass opacity with small areas of radiolucency. Hilar lymph nodes are involved in most of the cases.

Nocardia asteroides, an aerobic nonspore-forming bacterium, can produce pulmonary nocardiosis. Pulmonary nocardiosis can also occur in the immunocompetent patients, especially if an underlying lung disease is present.[28] Clinical features include the presence of cough, increased sputum production, pleural pain and microabscess. X-ray findings show air space consolidation and multilobar, nonsegmental nodules. True infection may involve the pleural space with effusions and empyema. The prognosis is good with treatment.[29]

Pulmonary actinomycosis is a relatively rare disease caused by *Actinomyces israelii.* Though they are Gram-positive bacteria, the characteristic branching filaments clustered with neutrophils (sulfur granules) usually require special stain to diagnose. Coinfection with *Staphylococcus aureus* increases the pathogenicity. It usually presents with pneumonia; mass-like consolidation will mimic malignancy. Airway obstruction is common.[30] Penicillin is the mainstay of treatment. Periodic therapeutic bronchoscopy may felicitate medical treatment.

Melioidosis (Whitmore's Disease)

Melioidosis is caused by *Burkholderia pseudomallei,* a bacterium. It is an infectious disease seen in humans, as well as in animals such as sheep, goats, horses, cattle, dogs and cats. Humans with underlying chronic illnesses are more at risk of acquiring the infection through direct contact with the contaminated soil and water in endemic areas. Pulmonary melioidosis may present as an acute or a chronic suppurative form. In acute pulmonary infection, the onset is associated with high-grade fever, headache, anorexia, chest pain, generalized myalgia, and productive cough with normal sputum production or with nonproductive cough.[31]

Patient may present with the symptoms of mild bronchitis to those of severe pneumonia. Lung abscess and empyema may also occur. Melioidosis is diagnosed from the blood, sputum or skin lesions by serology or by isolating *B. pseudomallei.* Radiological investigations, like chest X-ray and computed tomography (CT) thorax, may show features of pneumonia. Treatment with antibacterials should be started as early as possible to prevent the progression. Drugs like penicillin, doxycycline, amoxicillin-clavulanic acid, imipenem, aztreonam or ceftriaxone are given intravenously for treatment.

Tularemia (Rabbit Fever)

Francisella tularensis is a Gram-negative facultative intracellular bacterium, which causes tularemia in animals. The organism that spreads by aerosol transmission is highly virulent. Tularemia can be transmitted to humans by contact with infected animals or blood sucking arthropods like ticks, deer flies and mosquitoes. Pneumonic tularemia follows inhalation of *F. tularensis* during lawn mowing or bush cutting, which disturbs the carcasses and facilitates the release of bacterial aerosols. Patients present with cough, dyspnea, fever, chills, headache and pleurisy.[32] Chest X-ray shows bronchopneumonia, hilar node enlargement with or without pleural effusion. Treatment with streptomycin or gentamicin subsides the symptoms.

Rhodococcus Equi

Formerly recognized as *Corynebacterium equi*; it is an opportunistic pathogen which was commonly found in animals such as horses and cattle. In immunocompromised patients, *R. equi* causes pulmonary manifestations without any animal contact. In immunocompetent individuals, exposure to animals or soil contaminated with the animal waste is important to cause rhodococcus disease. Patients usually present with the symptoms of pneumonia. Erythromycin, rifampicin and fluoroquinolones are recommended for treatment.

Moraxella Catarhalis

Moraxella catarhalis was initially recognized as a commensal of pharynx. In recent years, it is shown to have significant pathogenicity in humans. *M. catarhalis* requires iron for its growth in tissues. This organism utilizes hemoglobin as the sources of iron.[33] Expression of type IV pilli, which in turn is affected by iron deficiency, is required for natural persistent colonization of *M. catarhalis* on mucosal surface.[34] The iron deficiency or inadequate heme component of hemoglobin is the vital factor for *M. catarhalis* to become invasive.[35]

Meningococcal Pneumonia

Neisseria meningitidis colonizes the nasopharyngeal mucosa in 5–10% patients, but invasive disease is rare. A preceding viral respiratory infection facilitates the invasion by meningococci. Patients present with fever, chills, productive cough and pleuritic pain. Radiographic picture shows focal pneumonia. Rarely, *N. meningitidis* may cause interstitial pneumonitis, and the clinical picture resembles that of viral pneumonia. Histopathologically, the lung shows diffuse generalized, inflammation of the alveolar septa with intra-alveolar edema. The bacteremia results in lodging of the organisms and of meningococcal antigens in the interstitial capillaries of the lung. Diagnosis is made by immunohistochemical analysis and RT-PCR assays. Antibiotics of penicillin group and cephalosporin's are used for treatment. Immunoprophylaxis is advisable for high-risk grousp.[36-38]

PARASITIC INFECTIONS

Balantidium coli, a ciliated protozoan, commonly cause intestinal infection. There are some rare cases of lung involvement. Thick-walled upper lobe cavity in a farmer with exposure to pig manure was reported with the disease.[39] Bronchoalveolar lavage fluid showed trophozoites of *B. coli*. Doxycycline is the drug of choice.

Parasitic Pneumonias

Parasitic pneumonias are seen in many protozoan and helminthic infections.[40] During the larval stage, the parasite passes through pulmonary circulation, gets sequestered resulting in pneumonia. Sometimes, pneumonia may result from direct extension from the contiguous sites. If left untreated, it may result in life-threatening problems.[36-39]

Due to the wide travel across continents and globalization, the parasitic diseases are now reported from all over the world, not only from the tropical and the subtropical regions. Parasitic pneumonias can be caused by protozoa, trematodes, cestodes and nematodes. *Leishmania donovani* causes pulmonary leishmaniasis in lung transplant patients and in other immunocompromised patients. *Entamoeba histolytica* infection results pulmonary amebiasis.

Tropical pulmonary eosinophilia presents as chronic mild interstitial lung disease is caused by *Wuchereria bancrofti* and *Brugia malayi*. Pulmonary dirofilariasis is caused by *Dirofilaria immitis* and *Dirofilaria repens*.

Plasmodium falciparum, as well as *Plasmodium vivax* can cause pulmonary manifestations, in the severe forms of malaria. There is no typical malarial pneumonitis, and it may occur due to secondary bacterial or viral infections. The clinical symptoms consist of fever, cough and respiratory distress. Noncardiogenic pulmonary edema and pleural effusion are important radiological findings. Treatment for severe malaria consists of injectable artemisinin, parenteral chloroquine, quinidine gluconate, and quinine hydrochloride. In severe respiratory distress conditions, mechanical ventilation is recommended.

RARE FUNGAL INFECTIONS

Hyalohyphomycosis is an infection in the lung of heterogeneous fungi.[41,42] These molds appear like hyaline (color less or lightly pigmented) septate, filamentous branching fungi, sometimes indistinguishable from aspergillosis. There are five specific molds of this type, viz. *S. Fusarium, P Varitoli, Paecilomyes, Acremonium* and *Trichoderma.* These are isolated from water, soil, sewage, manure, from farm animals, polluted water, etc. Fusariosis can occur in immunocompetent patients with severe burns, hematological malignancy. Rarely, mucormycosis presents with pleuropulmonary manifestations.[43]

Definite diagnosis of fungal infections is made by culture of the fungus. Newer triazoles such as voriconazole appear to be effective. Amphotericin B is effective in some cases like in *P. Varitoli, Trichoderma.*

ZOONOTIC BACTERIAL PNEUMONIAS

Yersinia enterocolitica of Enterobacteriaceae, commonly results in gastroenteritis. It can rarely cause pneumonias in immunocompromised individuals. Bacteremia causes spontaneous pleural empyema. Children and adults are equally affected. Treatment consists of third-generation cephalosporins, quinolones and chloramphenicol. Management of empyema may also require intercostal tube drainage and intrapleural fibrinolysis.[44]

Pasteurella multocida may cause infection in humans following animal bite, scratch or lick, but may occur even without animal contact. Upper respiratory tracts are colonized by the *P. multocida* as commensals in cats and dogs, poultry, and domestic pet animals. *P. multocida* infection may occur in healthy, as well as immunocompromised persons. It affects all age groups, but more commonly in young children who have contact with pet animals. Elaborate history is needed to elicit exposure to animals. Skin manifestations, following animals bite, mimic *Streptococcus pyogenes* infection. Pulmonary manifestations consist of sinusitis, otitis media, pharyngitis, mastoiditis, epiglottitis and Ludwig's angina.

In cases with pre-existing chronic pulmonary disease, *P. multocida* may cause pneumonia, tracheobronchitis, lung abscess and empyema.[45] COPD increases the mortality by 30%. The clinical presentation consists of hoarseness of voice, sinus tenderness and pharyngeal erythema. In addition to routine wound care for animal bite and vaccination prophylaxis, empirical antibiotic therapy is recommended for treatment. Oral antimicrobials like amoxicillin, amoxicillin-clavulanic acid combination, second-generation cephalosporins, carbapenems and fluoroquinolones are effective. In severe infections, parenteral antibiotics are recommended.

Yersinia pestis, a rod-shaped (safety pin appearance) facultative Gram-negative anaerobe, can infect both humans and animals, commonly rodents are the reservoir host for *Y. pestis.* In human plague outbreaks, fleas from other mammals may also have some role. The vector, fleas acquires *Y. pestis* during feeding on an infected rodent. Transmission of *Y. pestis* infection from rodents to humans occurs by skin contact. Human-to-human infection spreads by sneezing, coughing or through direct contact with the infected tissue. *Y. pestis* infection may clinically present in three forms: (i) bubonic plague, (ii) septicemic plague and (iii) pneumonic plague.

In pneumonic plague, the symptoms of the other two types are not always seen. Patients are present with various symptoms such as cough, dyspnea, fever, chills, chest pain, hemoptysis, hypotension, lethargy and shock. During severe bacteremia, several organs are affected resulting in disseminated intravascular coagulation and bleeding. Necrosis of skin and soft tissue increases the mortality by over 20%. Early diagnosis of plague is difficult since the initial symptoms may mimic many other diseases. Treatment is given with intravenous antibiotics for pneumonic plague. Streptomycin, gentamicin, chloramphenicol and fluoroquinolones are the first-line drugs used for the treatment.

In conclusion, the diagnosis of rare respiratory diseases requires taking a good clinical history, awareness of these diseases and appropriate diagnostic procedures. The list is not complete. The emergence of new pathogens, with modified lifecycles, newer genetic transformations, and mutations make rare infections a difficult proposition in the terms of diagnosis and treatment. There also exists the possibility of multiple infections which has to be evaluated.[46]

REFERENCES

1. Mohankumar T. Pulmonary infection in immunocompromised patients. Chest (India Edition) 2010;2(6):313-15.
2. Zwaans WA, Mallia P, Van vinden ME, Rohde GG. The relevance of respiratory tract viral infections in the exacerbations of chronic obstructive pulmonary disease—a systematic review. J Clin Virol 2014; July 4. [Epub ahead of print].
3. Denny FW. The clinical impact of human respiratory virus infections. Am J Respir Crit Care Med. 1995;152(4 Pt 2):S4-S12.
4. Andersen P. Pathogenesis of lower respiratory tract infections due to Chlamydia, Mycoplasma, Legionella and viruses. Thorax. 1998;53:302-7.
5. Van den Hoogen BG, de Jong JC, Groen J, et al. A newly discovered human pneumovirus isolated from young children children with respiratory tract disease. Nat Med. 2001;7(6):719-24.
6. Davies DE, Wicks J, Powell RM, et al. Airway remodelling in asthma, new insights. J Allergy Clin Immunol. 2003;111(2): 215-25.
7. Evans MJ, Fanucchi MV, Baker GL, et al. Atypical development of the tracheal basement membrane zone of infant rhesus monkey exposed to ozone and allergen. AM J Physiol Lung Cell Mol Biol Physiol. 2003;285(4):L931-9.
8. Williams JV, Aarris PA, Tollefson SJ, et al. Human metapneumovirus and lower respiratory tract disease in otherwise healthy infants and children. N Engl J Med. 2004; 350(5):443-50.
9. Greensill J, McNamara PS, Dove W, et al. Human metapneumovirus in severe respiratory syncytial virus bronchiolitis. Emerg Infect Dis. 2003;9(3):372-5.
10. Jatti T, van den Hoogen B, Garofalo RP, et al. Metapneumovirus and acute wheezing in children. Lancet. 2002;360(9343): 1393-4.

11. Chandy S, Mitra S, Sathish N, et al. A pilot study for serological evidence of hantavirus infection in human population in South India. Indian J Med Res. 2005;122(3):211-5.
12. Khaiboullina SF, Morzunov SP, St Jeor SC. Hantaviruses: molecular biology, evoluation and pathogenesis. Curr Mol Med. 2005;5(8):773-90.
13. Plyusnin A, Vapalahti O, Vaheri A. Hantaviruses: genone structure, expression and evolution. J Gen Virol. 1996;77(pt 11):2677-87.
14. Avsic-Zupanc T, Petrovec M, Furlan P, et al. Hemorrhagic fever with renal syndrome in the Dolenjska region of Slovenia-a 10 years survey. Clin Infect Dis. 1999;28(4):860-5.
15. Markotiae A, Nichol ST, Kuzman I, et al. Charecteristics of Puumala and Dobrava infections in Croatia. J Med Virol. 2002; 66(4):542-51.
16. Papa A, Bojovic B, Antoniadis A. Hantaviruses in Serbia and Montenegro. Emerg Infect Dis. 2006;12(6):1015-8.
17. Nicolini A, Cilloniz C, Senarega R, Ferraioli G, Barlascini C. Lung abscess due to *Streptococcus pneumonia*: a case series and brief review of the literature. Pneumonol Alergol Pol. 2014;82:275-85.
18. Copelovitch L, Kapaln BS. *Streptococcus pneumonia*-associated hemolytic uremic syndrome: classification and emergence of serotype 19A. Pediatrics 2010;125(1):174-82.
19. Cinquetti G, Banal F, Mohamed S, et al. Rare complications of Lemmier's syndrome: septic sternoclavicular joint arthritis and cavitating pneumonia. Rev Med Interne. 2009;30(12):1061-3.
20. Al-Aqeedi RF, Kamha A, Al-Aani FK, et al. Salmonella myocarditis in a young patient presenting with acute pulmonary edema, rhabdomyolysis, and multi-organ failure. J Cardiol. 2009;54(3):475-9.
21. Mufson MA. *Mycoplasma Hominis*: A review of its role as a respiratory tract pathogen of humans. Sex Trasm Dis. 1983;10:335-40.
22. Katoch VM, Mohankumar. T. Textbook of tuberculosis. Surendra K Sharma (Ed). Non tuberculosis mycobacterial infections. 2009. pp. 665-81.
23. Grech M, Carter R, Thomson R. Clinical significance of *Mycobacterium asiaticum* isolates in Queensland. J Clin Microbiol. 2010;48(1):162-7.
24. Mc Sweeney FG, O' Bnien ME, Sheehan S, Plant B, Corcoran G. Ir Med J. 2012;105(8):275-7.
25. Maloney JM, Gegg CR, David S, Stephens FA, Manian DR. Infections caused by *Mycobacterium Szulgai* in humans. Clin Inf Dis. 1987;9(6):1120-6.
26. Patsche CB, Svensson E, Wejse C. Disseminated *Mycobacterium celatum* disease with prolonged pulmonary involvement. Int J Infect Dis. 2014;26c:88-90.
27. Vam Berkel M, Dik H, Vander Meer JW, et al. Acute respiratory insufficiency from psittacosis. Br Med J (Clin Res Ed). 1985; 290(6480):1503-4.
28. Kurahara Y, Tachiibana K, Tsuyuguchi K, Akira M, Suzuki K, Hayashi S. Pulmonary nocardiosis: a clinical analysis of 59 cases. Respir Investig. 2014;52:160-6.
29. Feigin DS. Norcardiosis of the lung: radiographic findings in 21 cases. Radiology. 1986;159(1):9-14.
30. El Ghannam H, Bai C, Qiao R. Pulmonary actinomycosis presenting as a mass-like consolidation. South Med J. 2010; 103(1):81-3.
31. White NJ. Melioidosis. Lancet. 2003;361(9370):1715-22.
32. Ryan KJ, Ray CG. Sherris Medical Microbiology, 4th edition. McGraw Hill; 2004. pp. 488-90.
33. Furano K, Luke NR, Howlett AJ, et al. Identification of a conserved *Moraxella catarrhalis* haemoglobin-utilization protein, MhuA. Microbiology. 2005;151(Pt 4):1151-8.
34. Luke NR, Howlett AJ, Shao J, et al. Expression of type IV pilli by *Moraxella catarrhalis* is essential for natural competence and is affected by iron limitation. Infect Immun. 2004;72(112):6262-70.
35. Furano K, Campagnari AA. Identificatin of a hemin utilization protein of *Moraxella catarrhalis* (HumA). Infect Immun. 2004;72(11):6426-32.
36. Rosenstein NE, Perkins BA, Stephens DS, et al. Meningococcal disease. N Engl J Med. 2001;344(18):1378-88.
37. Van Deuren M, Brandtzaeg P, van der Meer JW. Update on meningococcal disease with pathogenesis and clinical management. Clin Infect Dis. 2000;30:87-94.
38. WinsteadJ, McKinsey DS, Tasker S, et al. Meningococcal pneumonia: characterization and review of cases seen over the past 25 years. Clin Infect Dis. 2000;30:87-94.
39. Sharms S, Harding G. Necrotizing lung infection caused by protozoan *Balantidium coli*. Can J Infect Dis. 2003;14(3): 163-6.
40. Vijayan VK. How to diagnose and manage common parasitic pneumonias. Curr Opin Pulm Med. 2007;13(3):218-24.
41. Nucci M, Anaissie E. Emerging fungi. Inf Dis Clin North Am. 2006;20;563-79.
42. Walsh T, Groll R, Hiemenez, et al. Infections due to emerging and uncommon medically important fungal pathogens. Clin Microbiol Infect. 2004;10(Supp 1):48-66.
43. Jha VK, Borpujari PJ, Shenoy G, Bhargav S. Empyema with pleuro-pulmonary mucormycosis. J Ass Phy India. 2013;61: 665-7.
44. Prentice MB, Rashalision L. Plague. Lancet. 2007;369 (9568): 1196-207.
45. Dryden MS, Dalgliesh D. Pasteurella multocida from a dog causing Ludwig's angina. Lancet. 1996;347(8994):123.
46. Puneetha M, Mohankumar T. A case study of polymicrobial pneumonia: Indian Journal of Respiratory Care 2014;3(1): 408.

Parasitic Lung Diseases

VK Vijayan

INTRODUCTION

Lung diseases due to parasitic infestations are common in tropical regions of the world.[1] However, these diseases are being increasingly reported from many parts of the world due to globalization and travel across the continents.[2] The emergence of human immunodeficiency virus (HIV) infection/acquired immunodeficiency syndrome (AIDS), the frequent use of immunosuppressive drugs in many diseases and organ transplantations have also resulted in resurgence of parasitic lung infestations.[3] Though many parasitic infestations have a benign course, a large number of parasitic infestations will cause considerable morbidity and mortality.[4] The important pulmonary diseases that can occur due to parasitic infestations are listed in **Table 1**. There is an overall decline in the number of patients in the past few decades but a number of new human parasites have aroused further interest in the subject.[5]

Diagnosis of parasitic infestations remains a challenge in an unsuspected patient. It is chiefly based in the presence of epidemiological suspicion. The definitive diagnosis is established on demonstration of causative organism and/or serological investigations. Radiological findings are frequently helpful and sometimes diagnostic.[6,7] Treatment essentially comprises antiparasitic treatment along with symptomatic and supportive management of clinical manifestations.

PULMONARY AMOEBIASIS

Amoebiasis is one of the most common infections in the world. It has been estimated that approximately 50 million cases of invasive amoebiasis occur worldwide each year with up to 100,000 deaths. Ingestion of mature *Entamoeba histolytica* cysts in fecally contaminated food, water or hands causes infection. The trophozoites released in the intestine pass through the bloodstream to reach extraintestinal sites such as liver, brain and lungs resulting in pathological lesions. Pulmonary amoebiasis occurs primarily due to extension of the amoebic liver abscess.[8] Pleuropulmonary amoebiasis may also occur following hematogenous spread of organisms to the lungs or lymphatic spread from the liver to the diaphragm. The main manifestations of pleuropulmonary amoebiasis consist of fever, right upper quadrant abdominal pain, chest pain and cough. Hemoptysis and expectoration of "anchovy sauce-like" pus indicate amoebiasis.

The diagnostic findings in pleuropulmonary amoebiasis consist of elevated hemidiaphragm, tender hepatomegaly, pleural effusion and basal pulmonary involvement. Active trophozoites of *E. histolytica* can be demonstrated in sputum or pleural pus. Microscopic examination of stool samples may reveal cysts or trophozoites of amoebae. The presence of amoeba in the stool does not signify that the disease is due to *E. histolytica* as two non-pathogenic species found in humans (*E. dispar* and *E. moshkovskii*) are indistinguishable morphologically. Other diagnostic tests include culture of *E. histolytica* and serological tests [indirect hemagglutination test, enzyme-linked immunosorbent assay (ELISA) and indirect fluorescent antibody test].

Nitroimidazoles (metronidazole or tinidazole) are the main drugs in the treatment of invasive amoebiasis.[9] Metronidazole is given in a dosage of 750 mg orally three times a day for 7–10 days. Tinidazole can be prescribed in a dosage of 800 mg orally three times a day for 10 days. Treatment with nitroimidazole should be followed by treatment with a luminal amoebicidal drug (paromomycin or diloxanide furoate) to cure intestinal luminal infection. Paromomycin is given as 25–35 mg/kg per day in three divided doses for 7 days or diloxanide furoate is given in a dosage of 500 mg orally three times a day for 10 days. Lactoferrin and lactoferricins have been found to kill *E. histolytica*, and it has been suggested that lactoferrin and lactoferricin can be coadministered with a low dose of metronidazole to reduce toxicity of metronidazole. Surgical treatment of pulmonary amoebiasis may be required when there is direct pulmonary involvement or spread to pleura.

PULMONARY LEISHMANIASIS

The important protozoan parasites that cause leishmaniasis are *Leishmania donovani, Leishmania tropica, Leishmania major* and *Leishmania infantum.*[10] Various species of female

Table 1 Pulmonary diseases caused by parasitic infections

Diseases	*Parasites*
I. *Protozoa*	
1. Pulmonary amoebiasis	*Entamoeba histolytica*
2. Pulmonary leishmaniasis	*Leishmania donovani*
3. Pulmonary malaria	*Plasmodium vivax*
	Plasmodium falciparum
	Plasmodium malariae
	Plasmodium ovale
	Plasmodium knowlesi
4. Pulmonary babesiosis	*Babesia microti*
	Babesia divergens
5. Pulmonary toxoplasmosis	*Toxoplasma gondii*
II. *Helminths*	
a. *Cestodes*	
1. Pulmonary cystic hydatidosis	*Echinococcus granulosus*
2. Pulmonary alveolar echinococcosis	*Echinococcus multilocularis*
b. *Trematodes*	
1. Pulmonary schistosomiasis	*Schistosoma haematobium*
	Schistosoma mansoni
	Schistosoma japonicum
2. Pulmonary paragonimiasis	*Paragonimus westermani*
c. Nematodes	
1. Pulmonary ascariasis	*Ascaris lumbricoides*
2. Pulmonary ancylostomiasis	*Ancylostoma duodenale*
	Necator americanus
	Ancylostoma ceylanicum
3. Pulmonary strongyloidiasis	*Strongyloides stercoralis*
4. Tropical pulmonary eosinophilia	*Wuchereria bancrofti*
(Filarial infection)	*Brugia malayi*
5. Pulmonary dirofilariasis	*Dirofilaria immitis*
	Dirofilaria repens
6. Visceral larva migrans	*Toxocara canis*
	Toxocara cati
7. Pulmonary trichinellosis	*Trichinella spiralis*
Source: Vijayan VK. Parasitic lung infections. Curr Opin Pulm Med. 2009;15(3):274-82, with permission.	

Phlebotomus (the sandfly) transmits infection to man.[11] Leishmaniasis is endemic in Asia, Africa, Central and South America and the Mediterranean area. Leishmaniasis and HIV infections coexist in a deadly synergy and leishmaniasis accelerates the onset of AIDS in persons infected with HIV.[12] Visceral leishmaniasis is characterized by irregular fever, persistent dry cough, hemoptysis, weight loss, enlargement of liver and spleen and anemia. Pneumonitis, septal fibrosis, pleural effusion and mediastinal adenopathy are reported in patients coinfected with HIV. Pleural effusion has also been reported in immunocompetent individuals.

Leishmaniasis has also been reported in lung transplant patients.[13] *Leishmania* amastigotes can be found in the alveoli, pulmonary septa and bronchoalveolar lavage (BAL) fluid. Diagnosis of leishmaniasis is by the demonstration of the parasites in bone marrow aspirates and by the demonstration of specific DNA sequences in tissues by molecular biology techniques. The treatment of leishmaniasis includes amphotericin B especially the liposome formulations and pentavalent antimonials.[14] Liposomal amphotericin B is prescribed in a dosage of 3 mg/kg/day intravenously on days 1–5, 15 and 21. Sodium stibogluconate is given in a dosage of 20 mg/kg daily intravenously or intramuscularly for 28 days.[8] Miltefosine, the first oral drug for the treatment of visceral leishmaniasis, is prescribed in a dosage of 2.5 mg/kg daily orally for 28 days and the maximum daily dose is 150 mg.[15] A single infusion of liposomal amphotericin B (at a dose of 10 mg/kg body weight) was found to be as effective as conventional therapy with amphotericin B deoxycholate.[16]

PULMONARY MALARIA

The malarial parasites that infect man are *P. vivax, P. falciparum, P. malariae, P. ovale* and *P. knowlesi* and are transmitted primarily by the bite of an infected female *Anopheles* mosquito. Falciparum malaria is the most deadly type of malaria infection.[17] The pulmonary manifestations range from cough to severe and rapidly fatal noncardiogenic pulmonary edema like acute respiratory distress syndrome (ARDS). Acute lung injury and ARDS have also been reported to occur in 3–30% of patients with severe malaria and have been described with *falciparum, vivax, ovale* and *knowlesi* malaria.[18] Acute lung injury and ARDS usually occur a few days in the disease course even after initial response to antimalarial treatment and clearance of parasitemia.

Pulmonary manifestations are common in children, pregnant women and travelers with malaria.[19] Pneumonia in malaria is due to secondary bacterial infection. Pleural effusion is rarely reported in malaria. Cardiovascular involvement (circulatory failure, congestive cardiac failure and pulmonary edema) is also reported in *vivax* and *falciparum* malaria. Light microscopy of stained thick and thin blood smears is the gold standards for the diagnosis of malaria. Thin smears allow identification of malaria species. Radiological findings in severe *falciparum* malaria include lobar consolidation, diffuse interstitial edema, pulmonary edema and pleural effusion.

The drugs used for treatment of severe malaria are quinine dihydrochloride, quinidine gluconate and injectable artemisinin derivatives. Artemisinin-based combination therapies (artesunate and sulfadoxine-pyrimethamine, artesunate and amodiaquine, artesunate and mefloquine or artemether and lumefantrine) are the best antimalarial drugs.[20] Quinine dihydrochloride is given intravenously (IV) as a loading dose of 20 mg salt/kg body weight (bw) diluted in 10 mL/kg bw of 5% dextrose or dextrose saline over 4 hours followed 8 hours later by the maintenance dose of 10 mg/kg salt diluted in 10 mL/kg bw of 5% dextrose saline IV over 4 hours repeated every 8 hours until the patient can swallow. Then prescribe quinine tablets 10 mg salt/kg bw every 8 hours in combination with doxycycline or clindamycin to complete 7 days treatment.

Quinidine gluconate reconstituted in normal saline is infused IV in a dose of 10 mg/kg bw over 1–2 hours followed by the maintenance dose of 0.02 mg/kg per minute continuous infusion at least 24 hours followed by oral medication. Artesunate is given as a loading dose of 2.4 mg/kg IV bolus at 0, 12 and 24 hours followed by the maintenance dose of 2.4 mg/kg daily for 7 days. Artesunate is dispensed as a powder of artesunic acid and this is dissolved in 5% sodium bicarbonate to form sodium artesunate. The solution is then diluted in 5 mL of 5% dextrose, which is given by IV injection. Once the patient can tolerate oral therapy, parenteral therapy is switched to a complete treatment course of an artemisinin-based combination therapy (ACT). Artemether is given as a loading dose of 3.2 mg/kg IM followed by the maintenance dose of 1.6 mg/kg IM daily.

The patients presenting with ARDS require invasive mechanical ventilation with intensive care management.[21] Early positive-pressure ventilation with lung-protective strategy using low tidal volumes and appropriate positive end expiratory pressure (PEEP) in volume assist control mode help prevent the high mortality associated with ARDS in severe malaria. Extracorporeal membrane oxygenation (ECMO) support has been shown to allow adequate oxygenation and correction of hypercapnia under lung protective ventilation reducing ventilator-induced lung injury. It has therefore been suggested to use ECMO early in malaria complicated by severe ARDS refractory to conventional treatment.

PULMONARY BABESIOSIS

Babesiosis is caused by hemoprotozoan parasites, *Babesia microti* and *Babesia divergens*.[22] Man gets the infection by the bite of an infected tick, *Ixodes scapularis* and can also be infected from a contaminated blood transfusion. The parasites attack the red blood cells and can be misdiagnosed as *Plasmodium*. The parasites are pear-shaped, oval or round. Their ring form and peripheral location in the erythrocyte frequently lead to their being mistaken for *Plasmodium falciparum*. The risk factors for systemic infection are immunosuppression, advanced age and splenectomy. The symptoms are fever, drenching sweats, cough, tiredness, and loss of appetite, myalgia and headache.

Acute respiratory distress syndrome occurring a few days after initiation of medical therapy is the important pulmonary manifestation.[23] Chest radiological features include bilateral infiltrates with an alveolar pattern and thickening of the septa. Specific diagnosis is made by examination of a Giemsa-stained thin blood smear, DNA amplification using polymerase chain reaction (PCR) or detection of specific antibody. The peripheral blood smears may show, in addition to ring forms, tetrads inside the red blood cells. These tetrads known as Maltese cross formations are pathognomonic of babesiosis since they are not seen in malaria.[24] Treatment is with a combination of clindamycin (600 mg every 6 hours) and quinine (650 mg every 8 hours) for 7–10 days or atovaquone (750 mg every 12 hours) and azithromycin (500–600 mg on first day and 250–600 mg on subsequent days) for 7–10 days.[25]

PULMONARY TOXOPLASMOSIS

Toxoplasmosis is caused by the protozoan parasite *Toxoplasma gondii*. Cats are the primary carriers of the organism.[26] Man gets the infection by eating parasitic cyst-contaminated raw or undercooked meat, vegetables or milk products. The symptoms of toxoplasmosis are flu-like syndrome, enlarged lymph nodes or myalgia. Pulmonary toxoplasmosis has been reported with increasing frequency in patients with HIV infection. Toxoplasma pneumonia can manifest as interstitial pneumonia/diffuse alveolar damage or necrotizing pneumonia. Diagnosis of toxoplasmosis is based on the detection of the protozoa in body tissues. A real-time PCR-based assay in BAL fluid has been reported in HIV-positive patients.[27,28] Toxoplasmosis can be treated with a combination of pyrimethamine (25–100 mg per day orally) and sulfadiazine (1–1.5 g four times a day orally) for 3–4 weeks.[10]

Rare Pulmonary Protozoal Infections

Free-living *Acanthamoeba* species can cause systemic disease with pulmonary manifestations of nodular infiltrates, pneumonitis and respiratory failure in immunocompromised patients.[29] *Cryptosporidium parvum* infection has been reported to produce interstitial pulmonary infiltrates and focal areas of consolidation in AIDS patients.[30] Recurrent aspiration secondary to mega esophagus can lead to pneumonitis, lung abscess and bronchiectasis in *Trypanosoma cruzi* infection (Chagas disease). Cardiogenic pulmonary edema and pulmonary hypertension secondary to cardiac failure and dilatory cardiomyopathy have also been reported in Chagas disease.[31] East African trypanosomiasis due to *Trypanosoma brucei rhodesiense* has been reported to cause non-cardiogenic pulmonary edema and ARDS in acute stage. Other rare pulmonary protozoal infections that have been reported in immunocompromised individuals are listed in **Table 2**.[10]

Table 2 Rare pulmonary protozoal infections in immunocompromised individuals

Diseases	*Parasites*
1. Pulmonary acanthamoebiasis	*Acanthamoeba castellanii*
	Acanthamoeba polyphaga
2. Pulmonary balamuthiasis	*Balamuthia mandrillaris*
3. Pulmonary naegleriasis	*Naegleria fowleri*
4. Pulmonary trichomoniasis	*Trichomonas vaginalis*
	Trichomonas tenax
	Trichomonas hominis
5. Pulmonary lophomoniasis	*Lophomonas blattarum*
6. Pulmonary trypanosomiasis	*Trypanosoma cruzi*
	Trypanosoma brucei gambiense
	Trypanosoma brucei rhodesiense
7. Pulmonary cryptosporidiosis	*Cryptosporidium parvum*
	Cryptosporidium hominis
	Cryptosporidium meleagridis
8. Pulmonary cyclosporiasis	*Cyclospora cayetanensis*
9. Pulmonary encephalitozoonosis	*Encephalitozoon cuniculi*
	Encephalitozoon hellem
	Encephalitozoon intestinalis
10. Pulmonary entercytozoonosis	*Enterocytozoon bieneusi*
11. Pulmonary balantidiasis	*Balantidium coli*
Source: Vijayan VK. Parasitic lung infections. Curr Opin Pulm Med. 2009;15(3):274-82, with permission.	

PULMONARY CYSTIC HYDATIDOSIS

Cystic hydatidosis or hydatid cyst caused by *Echinococcus granulosus* is a serious health problem in most parts of the world particularly in sheep-raising areas of the Mediterranean countries, Middle East, the Balkan, South America, Australia and New Zealand. Dogs are the definitive hosts and sheep the main intermediate host. The eggs shed in dog feces contaminate food sources of intermediate hosts (sheep, cattle, horses and man). Humans get infection after eating food contaminated with eggs and the ingested eggs hatch, releasing larvae, which migrate from the gastrointestinal tract to the circulation. The eggs travel to the liver or lungs and slowly develop into hydatid cysts. The liver is the primary location followed by the lungs.[32]

Occasionally, lung cysts are formed after trans-diaphragmatic spread of parasites following the rupture of liver cysts. Typically, the larvae that pass through or bypass the liver filter is trapped in pulmonary arterial capillaries. The entrapped larvae develop into hydatid cyst that grows gradually and often complicate by rupturing in the airway or less commonly in the pleural space. Secondary pulmonary hydatidosis may occur by rupture of a liver cyst in vena caval circulation or a heart cyst in the right ventricular cavity or primary lung cyst in the bronchi; and then seeding the protoscolices along the bronchial tree. In the majority of cases, primary lung hydatidosis is single. Multiple hydatidosis may be unilateral or bilateral. Patients are asymptomatic in the initial stages of infection. Chest pain, hemoptysis, dyspnea or allergic reaction may appear subsequently. Bronchial rupture of the cyst can result in vomiting of contents of hydatid cysts. Intrapleural rupture may be acute leading to hydropneumothorax or empyema, or insidious with delayed development of secondary pleural hydatidosis.

Secondary metastatic hydatidosis is often associated with obstruction of pulmonary artery branches resulting in chronic hydatid cor pulmonale. Vomiting of small or entire hydatids is a specific sign called "hydatidosis". Diagnosis of pulmonary hydatid cyst is still based on radiography and noncomplicated cyst presents as well-defined homogeneous hydrous round (cannon ball) opacity that may be lobulated by contiguous bronchovascular axes. Fissured or ruptured cyst in the bronchi may have the characteristic findings of "air crescent", pneumocyst, floating membrane, ring within a ring or completely empty cavity images. Thoracic ultrasonography may be useful if the cyst is accessible to ultrasound examination. It may confirm the cystic structure showing the characteristic double contour aspect (the pericyst and the parasite membrane endocyst) in nonruptured cysts. Detached or retracted membrane may be observed in ruptured cysts. Collapsed laminated membrane may float in the cyst cavity, producing the "water lily" sign. Daughter cysts are diagnostic in lung hydatidosis.

Liver and abdomen ultrasound study is generally systematically performed to search for associated abdominal hydatid cysts. CT is helpful in doubtful cases as it can analyze the internal structure of the cyst and measures the density; evaluate the state of the neighboring parenchyma, the whole thorax and abdomen for associated cystic lesions or anomalies **(Fig. 1)**.[33] Laboratory tests are complementary to clinical and imaging investigations. Eosinophils can be slightly increased in complicated cysts. Serological tests are less sensitive in patients with lung hydatidosis (65%) than in those localized in liver (80–94%).[34]

Surgery is the main treatment for pulmonary hydatidosis and aims to remove the parasite and treat associated parenchymal, bronchial or pleural disease.[35] During surgery, spillage of hydatid fluid must be avoided to prevent secondary hydatidosis. Relapse rates up to 11.3% have been reported. Surgery must be as conservative as possible and resection is necessary in case of severe and irremediable lung damage. Bilateral lung hydatidosis, present in 4–26% of operated cases, may be treated in one-stage or two-stage surgery either by bilateral thoracotomy or sternotomy. Video-assisted thoracoscopic surgical (VATS) approach can be safely used in selected cases with the same surgical rules as in open surgery.[36]

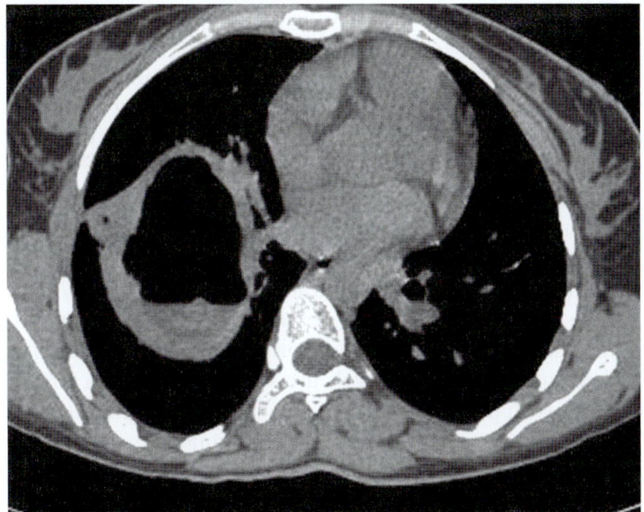

Fig. 1 Thoracic CT scan in a patient with cystic hydatid disease
Source: Vijayan VK. Parasitic lung infections. Curr Opin Pulm Med. 2009;15(3):274-82, with permission.

Long-term treatment with benzimidazole carbamates (albendazole or mebendazole) has not been found to be very effective in lung hydatidosis. Treatment with benzimidazole has been suggested to prevent recurrences, though there is no evidence of their efficacy.[37,38] Treatment with these drugs has also been found to be associated with alopecia and hepatic and hematologic toxicity. Therefore, the medical therapy must be reserved to inoperable or complex cases. Percutaneous treatment by puncture-aspiration-injection-reaspiration (PAIR) or percutaneous thermal ablation is used in hepatic hydatidosis. PAIR has been rarely used for lung hydatidosis because of the risk of anaphylactic shock, pneumothorax with pleural spillage and bronchopleural fistulae. PAIR is contraindicated for lung cysts as per the World Health Organization guidelines.

PULMONARY ALVEOLAR ECHINOCOCCOSIS

Alveolar echinococcosis caused by *Echinococcus multilocularis* is a rare but severe, highly pathogenic and potentially fatal form of echinococcosis. Wild canines especially the foxes are the definitive hosts and other hosts are dogs, cats, wolves. Small animals mainly rodents are the intermediate hosts. Alveolar echinococcosis is restricted to northern hemisphere (Europe, North America, some regions of China and Japan).[39] The liver is the first target of the parasite with a silent and long incubation period (5–15 years). Exogenous proliferation causes infiltration of adjacent tissues and pressure necrosis. It can metastasize to distant organs mainly lungs, brain and bones. Lung involvement results from metastatic dissemination or direct extension through the diaphragm of hepatic echinococcosis with intrathoracic rupture into bronchial tree, pleural cavity or mediastinum. Direct extension to the right atrium through the inferior vena cava with recurrent episodes of pulmonary embolism has also been reported. Imaging studies with radiography, ultrasonography, CT and magnetic resonance imaging (MRI) may help in the diagnosis of metastatic lung disease. Biopsy may be needed to confirm the diagnosis.[40,41]

Serologic tests, ELISA and indirect hemagglutination assay (IHA), are available and are of great value for early detection in endemic areas to confirm diagnosis and to plan early surgery.[41] Radical resection of localized lesions is the only curative way for alveolar echinococcosis but it is rarely possible in invasive and disseminated disease. Medical treatment is with mebendazole 40–50 mg/kg/day in three divided doses or with albendazole 10–15 mg/kg/day orally in two divided doses for a long period (minimum of 2 years) after radical surgery or lifetime treatment for nonresectable or incompletely resected lesions.[38]

PULMONARY SCHISTOSOMIASIS

The schistosomes that cause human disease are *Schistosoma haematobium, Schistosoma mansoni* and *Schistosoma japonicum*. The adult trematode worms are found in the vesical plexus (*S. haematobium*) or in the mesenteric veins (*S. mansoni* and *S. japonicum*). The schistosome eggs are passed in urine (*S. haematobium*) or in feces (*S. mansoni* and *S. japonicum*) by the infected humans. The eggs released in fresh water are ingested by snails (intermediate host) in which the eggs hatch and develop into cercariae. The infective cercariae are excreted into the water and these cercariae penetrate human skin or are ingested to penetrate the gut. Pulmonary schistosomiasis can manifest clinically as an acute form and a chronic form. The acute form, also known as Katayama syndrome, present with fever, chills, weight loss, diarrhea, abdominal pain, myalgia, urticaria, shortness of breath, wheezing and dry cough and is seen in nonimmune patients.[42]

Diffuse pulmonary infiltrates are seen radiologically in Katayama syndrome and almost all patients have eosinophilia.[43] Pulmonary nodules and pleural effusions have been reported in acute phase of infection with *Schistosoma mansoni.*[44] Chest radiography and CT show small ill-defined nodular lesions, reticulonodular lesions or diffuse ground glass opacity. Chronic pulmonary schistosomiasis results from granulomatous reaction to eggs and/or worms embolized from pelvic veins in small pulmonary vessels through inferior vena cava for *S. haematobium* or from mesenteric veins through portacaval anastomosis in patients with portal hypertension (*S. mansoni* and *S. japonicum*).

The commonest symptoms in the chronic stage are dyspnea, reduced exercise tolerance and chest pain. Patients with chronic schistosomiasis present with features of pulmonary hypertension and cor pulmonale.[45] Severe hypoxemia such as digital clubbing may be seen in chronic cases. The chronic form may also cause pulmonary arteriovenous fistulas. Chest X-rays in chronic cases may show features resembling granulomatous disease or tuberculosis. CT scan of the thorax may show nodular changes and ground glass opacification. Peripheral blood eosinophilia is present in more than 65% of patients. Diagnosis of chronic schistosomiasis is based on the demonstration of eggs in stool, urine, sputum or BAL fluid by direct microscopy or rectal/bladder biopsy. IgG antibodies to *Schistosoma* egg antigen are detectable 6–12 weeks following infection and can be measured by ELISA.

Acute schistosomiasis can be treated with praziquantel 40 mg/kg for three days (for *S. mansoni* or *S. haematobium*) and 60 mg/kg for 6 days (for *S. japonicum*) with or without steroids.[10,43] Praziquantel can be repeated several weeks later to eradicate the adult flukes. Treatment may cause a reactive pneumonitis to dying eggs or worms. Acute pneumonia can be observed 2 weeks after treatment, which is thought to be related to lung embolization by detached adult worms in pelvic veins. Artemisinin has been found to be useful in the early stage after exposure, as the drug has been found to act on juvenile forms of the schistosomes and may reduce the risk of the Katayama syndrome.[46] Chronic schistosomiasis can also be treated with praziquantel with the same dosage, but less beneficial. Patients with pulmonary arterial hypertension are treated with specific pulmonary artery hypertension treatment along with antiparasitic medication.

PULMONARY PARAGONIMIASIS

Ninety percent of the cases occur in Asia where nearly 20 million people are infected.[47,48] Paragonimiasis is caused by infection with *Paragonimus* species and manifest as subacute or chronic inflammation of the lung. The main species that cause paragonimiasis in man is *Paragonimus westermani.* Adult worms live in the lungs and the unembryonated eggs of *Paragonimus westermani* are excreted in the sputum, or they can be swallowed and passed with stool. The eggs become embryonated in the external environment and miracidia are produced. The miracidia penetrates the soft tissues of the first intermediate host, a snail and go through several developmental stages inside the snail forming free-swimming cercariae. Many cercariae then emerge from the snail and invade the second intermediate host, a crustacean such as a crab or crayfish. Cercariae encyst and produce metacercariae, which are the infective stage for the mammalian host.

The man gets infection when raw or undercooked crabs or crayfish infected with infective metacercariae are ingested. The metacercariae excyst in the duodenum penetrate through the intestinal wall into the peritoneal cavity, then through the abdominal wall and diaphragm into the lungs. In the lungs, they become encapsulated and develop into adults. Pulmonary manifestations include fever, chest pain, chronic cough with blood tinged sputum or hemoptysis that may mimic tuberculosis. Pleural effusion or pneumothorax may be the first manifestation during intrapleural migration of the juvenile worms.[47,48] Chest radiography or CT may show patchy airspace consolidation due to exudative or hemorrhagic pneumonia that may cavitate. Worm cysts may be seen as solitary or multiple nodules or gas-filled cysts with ring shadows and crescent-shaped areas within the cyst that represent worms attached to the wall of the cavity.[49,50] Adult worms are seen in pulmonary cysts usually in pairs. Diagnosis is confirmed by the detection of characteristic operculated eggs in the sputum samples, feces, BAL fluid or lung biopsy specimens. Fine needle aspiration biopsy of pulmonary nodule has been found to be useful in the diagnosis of pulmonary paragonimiasis.[51,52] Peripheral blood eosinophilia and elevated serum IgE levels are seen in more than 80% of patients with paragonimiasis. Specific IgG and IgM antibody testing may be useful when paragonimiasis is suspected. Differentiation of paragonimiasis from tuberculosis may be difficult. Paragonimiasis can be treated with praziquantel (75 mg/kg/day for 3 days), bithionol (30–40 mg/kg in 10 days on alternate days), niclofolan (2 mg/kg as a single dose) or triclabendazole (20 mg/kg in two equal doses).

PULMONARY ASCARIASIS

Ascaris lumbricoides is the most common intestinal helminthic infestation. The fertilized eggs passed in the feces and released in the soil to embryonate within 2–4 weeks and become infectious depending on the environmental conditions (moist, warm and shaded soil). Infection occurs through soil contamination of hands or food with eggs and then swallowed. The eggs hatch into larvae in the small intestine. These first-stage larvae moult into second-stage larvae in the lumen of the small intestine. The second-stage larvae penetrate the wall of the intestine and travel via capillaries and lymphatics to the hepatic circulation and to the right side of the heart and then reach the lungs. The second-stage larvae moult twice more in the alveoli to produce third and fourth-stage larvae. The fourth-stage larvae are formed 14 days after ingestion, travel up to the trachea and are then swallowed to reach back the small intestine.

Respiratory symptoms are due to larval pulmonary migration, airway hyperreactivity and bronchospasm. Symptomatic pulmonary disease may range from mild cough to a Loffler's syndrome. Loffler's syndrome is a self-limiting inflammation of the lungs and is associated with blood and lung eosinophilia. This syndrome can occur as a result of parasitic infestations (especially ascariasis in children) and exposure to various drugs. Patients may present with general symptoms of malaise, loss of appetite, fever lasting 2–3 days, headache and myalgia. The respiratory symptoms include chest pain, cough with mucoid sputum, hemoptysis, shortness of breath and wheezing. There may be rapid respiratory rate and crackles can be heard on auscultation. Leukocytosis, particularly eosinophilia, is an important laboratory finding. Chest radiographs demonstrate unilateral or bilateral, transient, migratory and non-segmental opacities of various sizes.

These opacities are often peripherally situated and appear to be pleural based.

A diagnosis of pulmonary disease due to ascariasis can be made in an endemic region in a patient who presents with dyspnea, dry cough, fever and eosinophilia. Total serum IgE may be elevated. Eosinophils and larvae may be found in sputum. Sputum may show Charcot-Leyden crystals and the chest radiograph may reveal fleeting pulmonary infiltrates. Because of the occurrence of respiratory symptoms during larval pulmonary migration, stool examination usually does not show *Ascaris* eggs and stool samples may be negative until 2–3 months after respiratory symptoms occur unless the patient was previously infected. Larvae can sometimes be demonstrated in respiratory or gastric secretions.

Pulmonary disease due to ascariasis usually does not require any treatment as it is a self-limiting disease. However, the persistence of gastrointestinal ascariasis may result in repeated respiratory symptoms due to larval migration. In order to eradicate *Ascaris lumbricoides* from the intestine, specific antihelminthic treatment is given. Mebendazole and albendazole are equally effective in the treatment of ascariasis.[53] Mebendazole is given in a dose of 100 mg twice a day for 3 days. It can also be given as a single-dose of 500 mg. Albendazole is given as a single-dose of 400 mg. The safety of mebendazole and albendazole during pregnancy has not been established. A single-dose of pyrantel pamoate (11 mg/kg, maximum dose 1 g) and piperazine citrate (50–75 mg/kg/day for 2 days) are also useful in the treatment. Pediatric dose is same as adult dose. Ivermectin has also been found to be useful.[54]

PULMONARY ANCYLOSTOMIASIS

Ancylostomiasis or hookworm disease is caused by three parasite species; *Ancylostoma duodenale, Necator americanus* and *Ancylostoma ceylanicum*. Man is the only definitive host. The eggs containing segmented ova with four blastomeres are passed out in the feces. A rhabditiform larva develops from each egg in the soil and this larva moults twice and develops into a filariform larva, which is infective to man. The filariform larva penetrates through the intact skin. *N. americanus* larvae can infect man only through the skin whereas *A. duodenale* larvae can enter the human host via the oral route in addition to the entry through the skin.[55] These larvae reach pulmonary circulation through the lymphatics and venules. The larvae then pierce the alveolar walls and ascend the bronchi, trachea, larynx and pharynx and are ultimately swallowed to reach the upper part of small intestine. The interval between the time of skin penetration and laying of eggs by adult worms is about 6 weeks.

Ancylostoma dermatitis, which manifests as intense pruritus, erythema and rash (ground itch), occurs at the site of skin penetration. During pulmonary larval migration, patients may present with fever, cough, wheezing and transient pulmonary infiltrates in chest radiographs. This is associated with blood and pulmonary eosinophilia. The other characteristic feature is iron-deficiency anemia due to chronic blood loss. During massive infection from oral ingestion of hookworm larvae, patients can present with nausea, vomiting, cough, dyspnea and eosinophilia and this condition is termed as Wakana disease. Prominent gastrointestinal symptoms in hookworm disease are abdominal pain, nausea, anorexia and diarrhea.

A direct microscopical examination of stool demonstrates the presence of characteristic hookworm eggs. Concentration method may be used when the infection is light. Eosinophilia in the peripheral blood is a prominent finding. A peripheral blood smear examination will reveal microcytic hypochromic anemia. A PCR to differentiate between *A. duodenale* and *N. americanus* has been developed.[56] Both mebendazole and albendazole are useful in the treatment of hookworm. Mebendazole is given as 100 mg twice daily for 3 days and albendazole is given as a single dose of 400 mg. Pyrantel pamoate at a dose of 11 mg/kg orally (maximum 1 g) as a single dose has also been found to be useful. Ivermectin can also be used in the treatment of hookworm infections. Anemia can be treated with oral ferrous sulfate tablets.

PULMONARY STRONGYLOIDIASIS

Strongyloides stercoralis is seen worldwide, but common in South America, South East Asia, sub-Saharan Africa and the Appalachian region of the United States of America. The parasitic females live in the wall (mucous membrane) of the small intestine of man and lay the eggs. The rhabditiform larvae emanating from the eggs pierce the mucous membrane and reach the lumen of the intestine. These larvae are then passed with the feces and eggs are, therefore, not found in the feces. The rhabditiform larvae can metamorphose into filariform larvae in the lumen of the bowel. These filariform larvae can penetrate the intestinal epithelium or perianal skin without leaving the host. This is responsible for autoinfection and for persistence of infection for 20–30 years in persons who have left the endemic areas.[57] The unique feature of the life cycle of *S. stercoralis* is that it can complete its life cycle either in the human host or in the soil. The rhabditiform larvae that are voided with the feces can undergo two distinct cycles in the soil: direct (host-soil-host) and indirect cycle. In direct cycle, the rhabditiform larvae directly metamorphose into filariform larvae and can infect man through skin. In indirect cycle, the rhabditiform larvae mature into free-living sexual forms (males and females). A second generation of rhabditiform larvae is then produced and these are then transformed into filariform larvae. The filariform larvae can penetrate directly through the skin, invade the tissues, penetrate into the venous or lymphatic channels and are carried by the blood stream to the heart and then to the lungs. They pierce the pulmonary capillaries and enter the alveoli. These larvae then migrate to the bronchi, trachea, larynx and epiglottis and are swallowed back into the intestine. In the duodenum and jejunum, they develop into sexual forms to continue the life cycle.

The cutaneous reaction as a result of the penetration of the skin by the filariform larvae may be due to immediate hypersensitivity reaction. The cell-mediated immunity that develops following primary infection prevents reinfection.[58] As a result, the larvae and adult worms remain confined to the intestine and the tissue invasion is prevented in immunocompetent individuals. When there is immunosuppression, autoinfection is exaggerated and leads to hyperinfection. In this situation, the number of migrating larvae increases tremendously and disseminate into many organs including lungs, meninges, brain, lymph nodes and kidneys. The parasite can produce hyperinfection syndrome in individuals with deficient cell-mediated immunity as seen in patients with immunosuppressive therapy (especially corticosteroids) and other immune-deficient states (malnutrition, lymphoma, leukemia, etc.). Human immunodeficiency virus (HIV)-infected patients are at a higher risk of dissemination and this may occur without elevations of IgE or eosinophils.[59]

During migration of filariform larvae through the lungs, bronchopneumonia and hemorrhages in the alveoli can occur. These areas are infiltrated with eosinophils. This is associated with elevated IgE and eosinophilia in the blood. As the larvae penetrate the intestinal mucosa, Gram-negative bacteria from the gut are carried by the larvae on their cuticle. In addition, small breaks in the mucous membrane as the larvae penetrate the intestine also facilitate the entry of enteric bacteria into the blood stream. The inflammation that follows such invasion of larvae leads to disseminated strongyloidiasis and this is usually fatal. As a result of invasion of bacteria along with larvae, diffuse and patchy bronchopneumonia and pulmonary abscess can occur. In the lung, massive pulmonary bleeding can occur due to alveolar microhemorrhages.

Pulmonary signs and symptoms include cough, shortness of breath, wheezing and hemoptysis.[60] In patients at high risk for strongyloidiasis, adult respiratory distress syndrome and septicemia due to intestinal transmural migration of bacteria can occur. In addition, acute anemia, acute renal failure and systemic inflammatory response syndrome are also reported.[61] In immunocompetent patients with strongyloidiasis, the parasite load is usually low and the larval output is irregular. As a result, the diagnosis of strongyloidiasis by examination of a single stool specimen using conventional techniques usually fails to detect larvae in up to 70% of cases. The diagnostic yield can be increased by examination of several stool specimens on consecutive days. In disseminated disease, larvae and adult parasites can be seen in sputum, urine, BAL fluid and other body fluids. Ivermectin, thiabendazole or albendazole can be used for treatment of strongyloidiasis in immunocompetent individuals without complications. Ivermectin is given in a dosage of 200 μg/kg orally for 1 or 2 days. Thiabendazole is given orally as 25 mg/kg twice a day for 2 days. Albendazole 400 mg twice a day for 5 days has been found to be useful in the treatment of strongyloidiasis. In immunocompromised individuals with disseminated strongyloidiasis, the dose of thiabendazole has to be doubled and the duration of treatment may be several weeks. Corticosteroids should not be prescribed to prevent life-threatening hyperinfection syndrome.

TROPICAL PULMONARY EOSINOPHILIA

Immunologic hyper-responsiveness to human filarial parasites, *Wuchereria bancrofti* and *Brugia malayi* results in an occult form of filariasis termed as tropical pulmonary eosinophilia (TPE).[62] The evidences for filarial etiology of TPE are the close epidemiological relationship between filarial infection and TPE, a positive filarial complement fixation test and a positive immediate reaction to intradermal skin tests with *Dirofilaria immitis* antigens, histopathological demonstration of microfilariae of *Wuchereria bancrofti* in the lungs, liver and lymph nodes of patients, the usefulness of diethylcarbamazine citrate (DEC), an antifilarial drug, in the treatment, the elevated levels of filarial specific IgG and IgE antibodies and the ultrasonographic demonstration of living adult *Wuchereria bancrofti* in the lymphatic vessels of the spermatic cord of patients with TPE. The demonstration that basophils from patients with TPE released greater amounts of histamine when cells were challenged with *Brugia* or *Wuchereria* antigens than with *Dirofilaria* antigen suggested that TPE resulted from immunologic hyper-responsiveness to human filarial parasites.[63-68] Histopathological examination of lung biopsy specimens has shown acute eosinophilic infiltrations of interstitial, peribronchial and perivascular tissues leading to the formation of eosinophilic abscesses and eosinophilic bronchopneumonia in the acute stage and in untreated cases, fibrosing alveolitis with honey combing.[63]

Bronchoalveolar lavage studies have demonstrated that TPE is characterized by intense eosinophilic inflammatory process in the lower respiratory tract.[69] Electron microscopic examination of lung eosinophils shows severe degranulation with loss of both the cores and the peripheral portions of the granules suggesting that the eosinophils are in an activated state.[68,69] A major IgE-inducing antigen (Bm23-25) of the filarial parasite *Brugia malayi* has been identified and this antigen has been found to be the homolog of the enzyme gamma-glutamyl transpeptidase (GGTP) light chain subunit[66,70] and expresses mainly in the infective L3 larvae.[71] In addition, *Brugia malayi* GGTP can induce IgG1 and IgE antibody production in patients with TPE.[72] BAL fluid from patients with TPE contains IgE antibodies that recognize *Brugia malayi* antigen Bm23-25.[66] There is a molecular mimicry between the parasite GGTP and the human GGTP present on the surface of pulmonary epithelium. Thus, the profound antibody response to filarial infection especially to filarial GGTP observed in the lungs of patients with TPE plays an important role in the pathogenesis of tropical eosinophilia.

Tropical pulmonary eosinophilia is a systemic disease involving mainly the lungs, but other organs such as liver, spleen, lymph nodes, brain, gastrointestinal tract, etc. may also be involved. The disease occurs predominantly in males, with a male to female ratio of 4:1, and is mainly seen in older children and young adults between the ages 15–40 years.[63] The systemic symptoms are fever, weight loss and fatigue. Respiratory symptoms include paroxysmal cough, breathlessness, and wheeze and chest pain. The symptoms occur predominantly at night, but can persist during the day. Sputum is usually scanty, viscous and mucoid. The sputum often shows clumps of eosinophils; and rarely Charcot-Leyden crystals are seen. On examination, patients are often breathless. Bilateral scattered rhonchi and crackles may be heard on auscultation.

Leukocytosis with an absolute increase in eosinophils in the peripheral blood is the hallmark of TPE. Absolute eosinophil counts are usually more than 3,000 cells/mm^3 and may range from 5,000 to 80,000.[73] As patients with TPE especially from endemic areas can be simultaneously infected with other helminthic parasites, stool examination may reveal ova or larvae of other helminths (*Ascaris*, *Ancylostoma*, whipworm and *Strongyloides*) in 20% of patients with TPE. This observation does not deter the physician from making a diagnosis of TPE, if other conditions for diagnosis are fulfilled.

The chest radiological features of TPE include reticulonodular shadows predominantly seen in mid and lower zones and miliary mottling of 1–3 mm in diameter often indistinguishable from miliary tuberculosis. Twenty percent of patients have a normal chest radiograph.[63] Lung function tests reveal mainly a restrictive ventilation defect with superimposed airways obstruction.[74,75] Single breath carbon monoxide transfer factor (T_{LCO}) is reduced in 88% of untreated patients with TPE.[76] The reduction in T_{LCO} is due to reduced pulmonary membrane diffusing capacity (Dm).[77] Most of the patients had mild arterial hypoxemia. Following 3 weeks treatment with DEC, pulmonary function parameters including TLCO continued to be significantly lower than the control subjects.[74] Till a diagnostic test that can differentiate filarial TPE from other TPE-like syndrome due to other helminthic infections is available. *The following diagnostic criteria can be used for the diagnosis of TPE:*

- Appropriate exposure history (mosquito bite) in an endemic area of filariasis,
- A history of paroxysmal nocturnal cough and breathlessness,
- Chest radiographic evidence of pulmonary infiltrations,
- Leukocytosis in blood,
- Peripheral blood eosinophils more than 3,000 cells/mm^3,
- Elevated serum IgE levels,
- Elevated serum antifilarial antibodies (IgG and/or IgE) and
- A clinical response to DEC.

The treatment is with oral DEC (6 mg/kg per day) for 3 weeks.[78] Relapses following treatment occur in 20% of patients followed up for 5 years.[63] Though most patients had shown marked symptomatic improvement, there was an incomplete reversal of clinical, hematological, radiological and physiological changes in TPE one month after a 3-week course of DEC.[74,79] Thus, a chronic mild interstitial lung disease has been found to persist in TPE despite treatment.[80]

PULMONARY DIROFILARIASIS

Pulmonary dirofilariasis is a zoonotic infection caused by filarial nematodes, *Dirofilaria immitis* and *Dirofilaria repens.* Humans are accidental hosts of this parasite, which is transmitted to man by the mosquito. The parasite, which is a vascular parasite,[81] is usually seen in the pulmonary artery where they produce a pulmonary nodule or "coin lesion."[82] Nearly 50% of subjects infected with dirofilariasis are asymptomatic. Clinical symptoms are chest pain, cough, fever, hemoptysis and dyspnea. CT scan may show a well-defined nodule with smooth margin connected to an arterial branch.[83] Rarely cavity formation in the lung has also been reported. A PCR-based diagnosis of *D. repens* in human pulmonary dirofilariasis is available. A definitive histopathological diagnosis of pulmonary dirofilariasis can be made in tissue specimens obtained by wedge biopsy, video-assisted thoracoscopy or rarely by fine needle biopsy. There is no specific treatment for human dirofilariasis.

PULMONARY TOXOCARIASIS (VISCERAL LARVA MIGRANS)

Certain nematode parasites when enter into an unnatural host (e.g. man) may not be able to complete their life cycle and their progress is arrested in the "unnatural host". If the entry of such parasitic larvae is through skin penetration, it causes cutaneous larva migrans (creeping eruption). If the entry is via oral route, it causes visceral larva migrans (VLM). Cutaneous larva migrans is caused by the parasite, *Ancylostoma braziliense,* which is a parasite of dogs and cats. The common parasites that cause VLM and eosinophilic lung disease in man are a dog ascarid *(Toxocara canis)* and less commonly a cat ascarid (*Toxocara cati*). Adult *Toxocara canis* and *Toxocara cati* live in the intestines of juvenile dogs and cats respectively. Animals acquire infection by ingestion of eggs of the parasites from contaminated soil. The life cycle is then completed in definitive hosts, dogs and cats and the eggs are passed by the animals in the feces and embryonate in the soil. Fresh animal feces are not infectious as the eggs require 2–3 weeks to embryonate in the soil.

The embryonated toxocara eggs, when ingested by an intermediate host (e.g. man), hatch into infective larvae in the intestine. The infective larvae penetrate the intestinal wall and are carried by the circulation to many organs including liver, lungs, muscles, central nervous system and eye. The progress of the larvae is arrested in these sites of the intermediate host by the formation of a granulomatous lesion. In man, the larvae never develop into adult worms. Therefore, infected man never excretes toxocara eggs in the feces. The larvae can get encapsulated within the granuloma where they are either destroyed or persist for many years in a viable state. Larval antigens can cross-react with human A and B blood group antigens.[84]

The main symptoms in patients with VLM are fever, cough, wheezing, seizures, anemia and fatigue. Pulmonary manifestations are reported in 80% of cases and patients may present with severe asthma. Scattered crackles and rhonchi are heard on auscultation. VLM is characterized by leukocytosis and eosinophilia. Skiagram of the chest may reveal focal patchy infiltrates. In some cases, severe eosinophilic pneumonia may lead to respiratory distress.[85] Other clinical features include generalized lymph node enlargement, hepatomegaly and splenomegaly. VLM is usually reported in young children with a history of pica. A history of exposure to puppies or dogs supports the diagnosis of VLM. Serological tests by ELISA method using excretory-secretory proteins obtained from cultured *T. canis* may be useful in the diagnosis. Histopathological examination of lung or liver biopsy specimens may demonstrate granulomas with eosinophils, multinucleated giant cells and fibrosis. Since man is not the definitive host of *Toxocara* spp., eggs or larvae cannot be demonstrated in the feces.

Visceral larva migrans is a self-limiting disease and there may be spontaneous resolution. Therefore, mild-to-moderately symptomatic patients need not require any drug therapy. Patients with severe VLM can be treated with thiabendazole, mebendazole or DEC. Treatment with antihelminthic treatment may exacerbate the inflammatory reactions in the tissues due to the killing of larvae. It is, therefore, advised to combine antihelminthic treatment with corticosteroids. DEC can be given in a dose of 6 mg/kg/day for 21 days. Mebendazole is prescribed in a dose of 20–25 mg/kg/day for 21 days.[86] Albendazole 10 mg/kg/day for 5 days has been shown to have a moderate effect compared to thiabendazole.

PULMONARY TRICHINELLOSIS

Human trichinellosis is an important food-borne zoonosis. Five species of *Trichinella* (*T. spiralis, T. nativa, T. nelsoni, T. britovi* and *T. pseudospiralis*) can infect man.[87] The most important species that infect man is *Trichinella spiralis*. The parasite has a direct life cycle with complete development is one host (pig, rat or man). However, two hosts are required to complete the life cycle and for the preservation of the species from extinction. Man gets infection from raw and partially cooked pork when infected pig's muscle containing larval trichinellae is eaten by man. The infective larvae in the muscle are surrounded by a host capsule, which is a modified striated muscle known as "nurse" cell. In the stomach, the "nurse" cell is digested and the free larva is liberated. The larvae develop into adults (males and females) in the duodenum and jejunum. The newborn larvae produced by female parasites pass through the lymphatics or blood vessels to reach the striated muscles.[88] The larvae undergo encystment in the muscle and a host capsule develops around the larvae. Later on, it may get calcified. The life cycle is completed when infected muscle is ingested by a suitable host.

The common symptoms of trichinellosis are muscle pain, periorbital edema, fever and diarrhea.[89] Pulmonary symptoms include dyspnea, cough and pulmonary infiltrates. Dyspnea may be due to the involvement of diaphragm. Leukocytosis, eosinophilia and elevated levels of serum muscle enzymes (creatine phosphokinase, lactate dehydrogenase, aldolase and aminotransferase) are important laboratory findings. An ELISA for detection of anti-*Trichinella* antibodies using excretory-secretary antigens may be useful in the diagnosis. A definitive diagnosis can be made by muscle biopsy (usually deltoid muscle) that may demonstrate larvae of *T. spiralis*.[90] Symptomatic treatment of trichinellosis includes analgesics and corticosteroids. Specific treatment is with mebendazole 200–400 mg three times a day for 3 days followed by 400–500 mg three times a day for 10 days. Albendazole can be given in a dosage of 400 mg per day for 3 days followed by 800 mg per day for 15 days. Trichinellosis can be prevented by consuming properly cooked pork.

REFERENCES

1. Vijayan VK. Tropical parasitic lung diseases. Indian J Chest Dis Allied Dis. 2008;50:49-66.
2. Vijayan VK. Parasitic lung infections. Curr Opin Pulm Med. 2009;15:274-82.
3. Vijayan VK. Is the incidence of parasitic lung diseases increasing, and how this affects modern respiratory medicine? Expert Rev Respir Med. 2009;3:339-44.
4. Vijayan VK. How to diagnose and manage common parasitic pneumonias? Curr Opin Pulm Med. 2007;13:218-24.
5. Cheepsattayakorn A, Cheepsattayakorn R. Parasitic pneumonia and lung involvement. Biomed Res Int. 2014;2014:874021.
6. Henry TS, Cummings KW. Role of imaging in the diagnosis and management of parasitic infections. Curr Opin Pulm Med. 2013;19:310-7.
7. Hur JH, Lee IJ, Kim JH, Kim DG, Hwang HJ, Koh SH, et al. Chest CT findings of toxocariasis: correlation with laboratory results. Clin Radiol. 2014;69:e285-90.
8. Shamsuzzaman SM, Hashiguchi Y. Thoracic amoebiasis. Clin Chest Med. 2002;23:479-92.
9. Haque R, Huston CD, Hughes M, Houpt E, Petri WA Jr. Amoebiasis. N Engl J Med. 2003;348:1565-73.
10. Martinez-Giron R, Estiban JG, Ribas A, Doganci L. Protozoa in respiratory pathology: a review. Eur Respir J. 2008;32:1354-70.
11. Piscopo TV, Mallia AC. Leishmaniasis. Postgrad Med J. 2006;82:649-57.
12. Desjeux P, Alvar J. Leishmania/HIV co-infection: Epidemiology in Europe. Ann Trop Med Parasitol. 2003;97(Suppl 1):3-15.
13. Antinori S, Cascio A, Parravicini C, Bianchi R, Corbellino M. Leishmaniasis among organ transplant recipients. Lancet Infect Dis. 2008;8:191-9.
14. Sunder S, Rai M. Treatment of visceral leishmaniasis. Expert Opin Pharmacother. 2005;6:2821-9.

15. Jha TK, Sunder S, Thakur CP, Bachmann P, Karbwang J, Fischer C, et al. Miltefosine, an oral agent, for the treatment of Indian visceral leishmaniasis. N Engl J Med. 1999;341:1795-800.
16. Sunder S, Chakravarty J, Agarwal D, Rai M, Murray HW. Single-dose liposomal amphotericin B for visceral leishmaniasis in India. N Engl J Med. 2010;362:504-12.
17. Taylor WR, Hanson J, Turner GD, White NJ, Dondorp AM. Respiratory manifestations of malaria. Chest. 2012;142(2):492-505.
18. Tan LK, Yacoub S, Scott S, Bhagani S, Jacobs M. Acute lung injury and other serious complications of *Plasmodium vivax* malaria. Lancet Infect Dis. 2008;8:449-54.
19. Freedman DO. Clinical practice: Malaria prevention in short-term travelers. New Engl J Med. 2008;359:603-12.
20. World Health Organisation, Geneva. Guidelines for the treatment of malaria, 2006; 1-266.
21. Talwar A, Fein AM, Ahluwalia G. Pulmonary and critical care aspects of severe malaria. In: Om P Sharma (Ed). Lung Biology in Health and Disease: Tropical Lung Diseases, 2nd edition. New York: Taylor & Francis Group; 2006. pp. 255-77.
22. Vannier E, Gewurz BE, Krause PJ. Human babesiosis. Infect Dis Clin North Am. 2008;22:469-88.
23. Boustani MR, Lepore TJ, Gelfand JA, Lazarus DS. Acute respiratory failure in patients treated for babesiosis. Am J Respir Crit Care Med. 1994;149:1689-91.
24. Noskoviak K, Broome E. Babesiosis. N Engl J Med. 2008;358:e19.
25. Krause PJ. Babesiosis: diagnosis and treatment. Vector-borne Zoonotic Dis. 2003;3:45-51.
26. Dodds EM. Toxoplasmosis. Curr Opin Ophthalmol. 2006;17:557-61.
27. Petersen E, Edvinsson B, Lundgren B, Benfield T, Evengård B. Diagnosis of pulmonary infection with *Toxoplasma gondii* in immunocompromised HIV-positive patients by real-time PCR. Eur J Clin Microbiol Infect Dis. 2006;25:401-4.
28. Contini C. Clinical and diagnostic management of toxoplasmosis in the immunocompromised patient. Parasitologia. 2008;50:45-50.
29. Duarte AG, Sattar F, Granwehr B, Aronson JF, Wang Z, Lick S. Disseminated acanthamebiasis after lung transplantation. J Heart Lung Transplant. 2006;25:237-40.
30. Corti M, Villafane MF, Muzzio E, Bava J, Abuín JC, Palmieri OJ. Pulmonary cryptosporidiosis in AIDS patients. Rev Argent Microbiol. 2008:40:106-08.
31. Lemle A. Chaga's disease. Chest. 1999;115:906.
32. Kilani T, El Hammami S. Pulmonary hydatid and other lung parasitic infections. Curr Opin Pulm Med. 2002;8:218-23.
33. Ben Miled-M'rad K, Bouricha A, Hantous S, Zidi A, Mestiri I, El Hammami S, et al. Ultrasonographic, CT and MRI findings of chest wall hydatidosis. J Radiol. 2003;84(2 Pt 1):143-6.
34. Eckert J, Deplazes P. Biological, epidemiological, and clinical aspects of echinococcosis, a zoonosis of increasing concern. Clin Microbiol Rev. 2004;17:107-35.
35. Ghoshal AG, Sarkar S, Saha K, Sarkar U, Kundu S, Chatterjee S, et al. Hydatid lung disease: an analysis of five years cumulative data from Kolkata. J Assoc Phys India. 2012;60:12-6.
36. Shehatha J, Alizzi A, Alward M, Konstantinov I. Thoracic hydatid disease: A review of 763 cases. Heart Lung Circ. 2008;17:502-4.
37. Junghanns T, Menezes Da Silva A, Horton J, et al. Clinical management of cystic echinococcosis: state of the art, problems and perspectives. Am J Trop Med Hyg 2008;79: 301-311
38. World Health Organisation Informal Working Group on Echinococcosis. Guidelines for treatment of cystic and alveolar echinococcosis in humans. Bull World Health Organ. 1996;74:231-42.
39. Craig P. Echinococcus multilocularis. Curr Opin Infect Dis. 2003;16:437-44.
40. Ozkok A, Gul E, Okumus G, Yekeler E, Gulluoglu MG, Kiyan E, et al. Disseminated alveolar echinococcosis mimicking a metastatic malignancy. Inter Med. 2008;47:1495-7.
41. Carmena D, Benito A, Eraso E. The immunodiagnosis of *Echinococcus multilocularis* infection. Clin Microbiol Infect. 2007;13:460-75.
42. Doherty JF, Moody AH, Wright SG. Katayama fever; an acute manifestation of schistosomiasis. Br Med J. 1996;313:1071-2.
43. Ross AG, Vickers D, Olds GR, Shah SM, McManus DP. Katayama syndrome. Lancet Infect Dis. 2007;7:218-24.
44. Lambertucci JR, Silva LC, de Queiroz LC. Pulmonary nodules and pleural effusion in the acute phase of schistosomiasis mansonii. Rev Soc Bras Med Trop. 2007;40:374-5.
45. Lapa MS, Ferreira EV, Jardim C, Martins Bdo C, Arakaki JS, Souza R. Clinical characteristics of pulmonary hypertension patients in two reference centres in the city of Sao Paulo. Rev Assoc Med Bras. 2006;52:139-43.
46. Utzinger J, Xiao SH, Tanner M, Keiser J. Artemisinins for schistosomiasis and beyond. Curr Opin Investig Drugs. 2007;8:105-16.
47. Liu Q, Wei F, Liu W, Yang S, Zhang X. Paragonimiasis: an important food-borne zoonosis in China. Trends Parasitol. 2008;24:318-23.
48. Doanh PN, Horii Y, Nawa Y. Paragonimus and paragonimiasis in Vietnam: an update. Korean J Parasitol. 2013;51:621-7.
49. Strobel M, Veasna D, Saykham M, Wei Z, Tran DS, Valy K, et al. Pleuro-pulmonary paragonimiasis. Med Mal Inf. 2005;35:476-81.
50. Im JG, Whang HY, Kim WS, Han MC, Shim YS, Cho SY. Pleuropulmonary paragonimiasis: radiologic findings in 71 patients. AJR Am J Roentgenol. 1992;159:39-43.
51. Kim TS, Han J, Shim SS, Jeon K, Koh WJ, Lee I, et al. Pleuropulmonary paragonimiasis: CT findings in 31 patients. AJR Am J Roentgenol. 2005;185:616-21.
52. Zarrin-Khameh N, Citron DR, Stager CE, Laucirica R. Pulmonary paragonimiasis diagnosed by fine-needle aspiration biopsy. J Clin Microbiol. 2008;46:2137-40.
53. St Georgie V. Pharmacotherapy of ascariasis. Expert Opin Pharmacother. 2001;2:223-39.
54. Belizaro VY, Amarillo ME, de Leon WU, de los Reyes AE, Bugayong MG, Macatangay BJ. A comparison of the efficacy of single dose of albendazole, ivermectin and diethylcarbamazine alone or in combination against *Ascaris* and *Trichuris* spp. Bull World Health Organ. 2003;81:35-42.
55. Hoagland KE, Schad GA. *Necator americanus* and *Ancylostoma duodenale*. Life history parameters and epidemiological implications of two sympatric hookworms on humans. Exp Parasitol. 1978;44:36-49.
56. Howdon JM. Differentiation between the human hookworm *Ancylostoma duodenale* and *Necator americanus* using PCR-RFLP. J Parasitol. 1996;82:642-7.
57. Scowden EB, Schaffner W, Stone WJ. Overwhelming strongyloidiasis: an unappreciated opportunistic infection. Medicine (Baltimore). 1978;57:527-44.
58. Neva FA. Biology and immunology of human strongyloidiasis. J Infect Dis. 1986;153:397-406.

59. Lessman KD, Can S, Talavera W. Disseminated *Strongyloides stercoralis* in human immunodeficiency virus-infected patients: Treatment failure and review of literature. Chest. 1993;104:119-22.
60. Nwokolo C, Imohiosen E. Strongyloidiasis of respiratory tract presenting as "asthma". Br Med J. 1973;2:153-4.
61. Casati A, Cornero G, Muttini S, Tresoldi M, Gallioli G, Torri G. Hyperacute pneumonitis in a patient with overwhelming *Strongyloides stercoralis* infection. Eur J Anesthesiol. 1996;13:498-501.
62. Vijayan VK. Immunopathogenesis and treatment of eosinophilic lung diseases in the tropics. In: Sharma OP (Ed). Tropical Lung Disease (Lung Biology in Health and Disease). New York: Marcel Dekker Inc; 2006. pp. 195-239.
63. Udwadia FE. Tropical eosinophilia. In: Herzog H (Ed). Pulmonary Eosinophilia: Progress in Respiration Research. Basel: S. Karger; 1975. pp. 35-155.
64. Ottesen EA, Nutman TB. Tropical pulmonary eosinophilia. Ann Rev Med. 1992;43:417-24.
65. Vijayan VK. Tropical pulmonary eosinophilia. Curr Opin Pulm Med. 2007;13:428-33.
66. Lobos E, Ondo A, Ottesen EA, Nutman TB. Biochemical and immunologic characterization of a major IgE-inducing filarial antigen of *Brugia malayi* and implications for the pathogenesis of tropical pulmonary eosinophilia. J Immunol. 1992;149:3029-34.
67. O'Bryan L, Pinkston P, Kumaraswamy V, Vijayan VK, Yenokida G, Rosenberg HF, et al. Localized eosinophil degranulation mediates disease in tropical pulmonary eosinophilia. Infect Immun. 2003;71:1337-42.
68. Nutman TB, Vijayan VK, Pinkston P, Steel R, Crystal RG, Ottesen EA. Tropical pulmonary eosinophilia: analysis of antifilarial antibody localized to the lung. J Infect Dis. 1989;160: 1042-50.
69. Pinkston P, Vijayan VK, Nutman TB, Rom WN, O'Donnell KM, Cornelius MJ, et al. Acute tropical pulmonary eosinophilia: characterization of the lower respiratory tract inflammation and its response to therapy. J Clin Invest. 1987;80:216-25.
70. Lobos E, Zahn R, Weiss N, Nutman TB. A major allergen of lymphatic filarial nematodes is a parasite homolog of the gamma-glutaryl transpeptidase. Mol Med. 1996;2:712-24.
71. Lobos E, Nutman TB, Hothersall JS, Moncada S. Elevated immunoglobulin E against recombinant *Brugia malayi* gamma-glutaryl transpeptidase in patients with bancroftian filariasis: association with tropical pulmonary eosinophilia or putative immunity. Infect Immun. 2003;71:747-53.
72. Gounni AS, Spanel-Borowski K, Palacios M, Heusser C, Moncada S, Lobos E. Pulmonary inflammation induced by a recombinant *Brugia malayi* gamma-glutaryl transpeptidase homolog: involvement of human autoimmune process. Mol Med. 2001;7:344-54.
73. Cooray JH, Ismail MM. Re-examination of the diagnostic criteria of tropical pulmonary eosinophilia. Respir Med. 1999;93:655-9.
74. Vijayan VK, Kuppurao KV, Sankaran K, Venkatesan P, Prabhakar R. Tropical eosinophilia: clinical and physiological response to diethylcarbamazine. Respir Med. 1991;85:17-20.
75. Poh SC. The course of lung function in treated tropical eosinophilia. Thorax. 1974;29:710-2.
76. Vijayan VK, Kuppurao KV, Sankaran K, Venkatesan P, Prabhakar R. Diffusing capacity in acute untreated tropical eosinophilia. Indian J Chest Dis Allied Sci. 1988;30:71-7.
77. Vijayan VK, Kuppurao KV, Sankaran K, Venkatesan P, Prabhakar R. Pulmonary membrane diffusing capacity and capillary blood volume in tropical eosinophilia. Chest. 1990;97:1386-9.
78. Final report. Joint WPRO/SEARO working group on Brugian filariasis. Manila: WHO 1979;1-47.
79. Vijayan VK, Sankaran K, Venkatesan P, Prabhakar R. Effect of diethylcarbamazine on the alveolitis of tropical eosinophilia. Respiration. 1991;58:255-9.
80. Rom WN, Vijayan VK, Cornelius MJ, Kumaraswamy V, Prabhakar R, Ottesen EA, et al. Persistent lower respiratory tract inflammation associated with interstitial lung disease in patients with tropical pulmonary eosinophilia following treatment with diethylcarbamazine. Am Rev Respir Dis. 1990;142:1088-92.
81. Theis JH. Public health aspects of dirofilariasis in the United States. Vet Parasitol. 2005;133(2-3):157-80.
82. Miyoshi T, Tsubouchi H, Iwasaki A, Shiraishi T, Nabeshima K, Shirakusa T. Human pulmonary dirofilariasis: a case report and review of the recent Japanese literature. Respirology. 2006;11:343-7.
83. Oshiro Y, Murayama S, Sunagawa U, Nakamoto A, Owan I, Kuba M, et al. Pulmonary dirofilariasis: computed tomographic findings and correlation with pathologic features. J Comput Assist Tomogr. 2004;28:796-800.
84. Smith HV, Kusel JR, Girdwood RW. The productions by human A and B blood group like substances by *in vitro* maintained second stage *Toxocara canis* larvae. Their presence on the outer larval surfaces and in their excretions/secretions. Clin Exp Immunol. 1983;54:625-33.
85. Bartelink AK, Kortbeek LM, Huidekoper HJ, Meulenubelt J, Van Knapen F. Acute respiratory failure due to toxocara infections. Lancet. 1993;342:1234.
86. Magnaval JF. Comparative efficacy of diethylcarbamazine and mebendazole for the treatment of human toxocariasis. Parasitology. 1995;110:529-33.
87. Pozio E, La Rosa G, Murrell KD, Lichtenfels JR. Taxonomic revision of the genus *Trichinella*. J Parasitol. 1992;78:654-9.
88. Despommier DD. How does *Trichinella spiralis* make itself at home? Parasitol Today. 1998;14:318-23.
89. Capo V, Despommier DD. Clinical aspects of infections with *Trichinella* spp. Clin Microbiol Rev. 1996;9:47-54.
90. Bruschi F, Murrell K. Trichinellosis. In: Guerrant RL, Walker DH, Weller PF (Eds). Tropical Infectious Diseases: Principles, Pathogens and Practice, Volume II, (Elsevier Science Health Science Div.) Philadelphia: Churchill Livingstone; 1999. pp. 917-25.

Anaerobic Bacterial Infections of Lungs and Pleura

Ashok Shah, Chandramani Panjabi

INTRODUCTION

The role of anaerobes in causing an infective disease has been appreciated for more than a century, but anaerobic bacterial infections of the respiratory system continue to remain in the subconscious domain of the pulmonologist. Anaerobes, as the cause of respiratory infection, are infrequently recognized and rarely established. More often than not these infections are caused by endogenous organisms that predominantly are commensals of the upper respiratory tract. Disruption of the harmonious relationship between the host and the bacteria lead to various clinic-pathologic processes that occur with anaerobic pleuropulmonary infections **(Table 1)**.

HISTORY

In 1860, Antonie van Leeuwenhoek, the inventor of the microscope, discovered some "animalcules" which survived in the absence of air.[1] Almost at same time Louis Pasteur coined the term "anaerobies" and recognized the phenomenon of anaerobiosis.[2] A few years later, Veillon identified anaerobic cocci in four patients.[3]

Anaerobic pleuropulmonary infections were first described in greater detail a little more than a century ago by Rendu and Rist in 1899.[4] A few years later, Guillemont and coworkers[5] published 13 cases of putrid "empyema". Subsequently, during the next 2 decades infections caused by the synergy of fusiform bacilli and spirochetes were documented.[6-8] These "fusospirochetal" bacteria were first described by Willoughby Miller, a dentist, in 1883;[9] while ulcerative gingivitis due to these bacilli was reported in detail by Vincent.[10] These microbes, popularly known as "Miller-Vincent" organisms, were chiefly responsible for pulmonary spirochetosis.

Table 1 Clinical categories of anaerobic pleuropulmonary infections

- Acute pneumonia (consolidation)
  - Aspiration pneumonia
  - Community-acquired pneumonia
  - Nosocomial pneumonia
- Chronic anaerobic pneumonitis (pulmonary infiltrates without cavitations)
- Lung abscess (usually single, greater than 2 cm)
- Necrotizing pneumonia (bilateral lung infiltrates with multiple cavitations less than 1 cm)
- Pleural empyema
- Septic emboli.

During the late 1920s, elegant work done by David Smith[11] on lung abscess revealed the resemblance of bacteria seen in the walls of abscesses on autopsy to the organisms present in the gingival crevice of healthy individuals. This led to the postulation that lung abscesses commonly occurred due to aspiration of oral microbial flora. Experimental animal studies[12-14] to prove this hypothesis demonstrated that four anaerobic bacteria which included (1) an anaerobic spirochete, (2) *Fusobacterium nucleatum*, (3) *Peptostreptococcus* species and (4) a fastidious Gram-negative anaerobe (possibly *Bacteroides fragilis*) were collectively responsible for the development of typical pulmonary abscess. This was a classic demonstration of bacterial synergy since no single microorganism was able to cause this disease.

The euphoria caused by the discovery of antibiotics resulted in anaerobes being largely ignored. There were hardly any samples that were not contaminated, and cultures for these microbes were rarely performed. Most lung abscesses were labeled as "nonspecific" because no pathogen could routinely be cultured from the sputum.[15] The decade of the 1970s was described by Bartlett[16] as the "renaissance" of anaerobic pleuropulmonary infections. It was during this period that specific sampling methods for anaerobic organisms evolved. Simultaneously, culture methods too improved and bacteriologic confirmation became easy. Furthermore, the placement of different anaerobic microbes into an organized taxonomic order also helped in generating further interest in this field.

PATHOPHYSIOLOGY

Aspiration

Anaerobic infections of the lungs and their suppurative complications are mainly caused by aspiration of bacteria that constitute the normal flora of the oral cavity. In the gingival crevice, the anaerobic microbes outnumber the aerobes by a 1,000:1 ratio.[17] The concentration of anaerobes here approaches geometric limits up to 10^{12}/gram.[17-19] It is well-known that edentulous subjects have a lower risk of acquiring anaerobic lung infections. Although aspiration especially during deep sleep occurs in 45% of healthy individuals,[20] this does not usually cause any disease. Normal bronchopulmonary defenses aid in clearing these aspirates. Any breach in protective mechanisms facilitates an inflammatory process thereby leading to disease. The frequency, volume and virulence of anaerobic organisms in the aspirated inoculums are decisive in determining the pathology.

Aspiration is likely to occur in patients undergoing general anesthesia or having altered consciousness. At one point in time, aspiration was observed in one out of every six patients receiving general anesthesia.[21] The presence of artificial airways impairs glottic closure and makes the patient more vulnerable to aspiration. When aspiration is due to esophageal dysfunction or intestinal obstruction, the gastrointestinal tract is the likely source of the causative bacteria.[22,23] Several other conditions that predispose to clinically significant aspiration are responsible for anaerobic infections **(Table 2)**.

Anaerobic Lung Infections and Dental Disorders

Persons with poor dental hygiene are prone to develop anaerobic infections of respiratory tract. Suppurative periodontitis predisposes to aspiration as it harbors a potentially large quantity of anaerobic bacteria.[24] Any kind of anesthesia in the oropharynx given for dental purposes is also associated with a high chance of aspiration. Tooth extraction and scaling lead to a breach in the normal mucosal barrier, thereby further increasing the risk of aspiration.[25] It would be prudent for a pulmonologist to carefully extract a detailed dental history and also to examine the oral cavity for evidence of any inflammatory or suppurative disease while dealing with respiratory infections in order to evaluate for the presence of anaerobes.

Table 2 Predisposing conditions

- Aspiration
  - Alcoholism
  - General anesthesia
  - Altered consciousness
    - Cerebrovascular accident
    - Drug overdose
    - Epilepsy
    - Smoke inhalation
    - Head trauma
  - Dental disorders
    - Periodontal disease
      - Gingivitis
      - Pyorrhea
    - Tooth extraction
  - Esophageal dysfunction or intestinal obstruction
- Local underlying conditions
  - Pulmonary infarction
  - Bronchogenic carcinoma
  - Bronchiectasis
  - Foreign body
- Systemic underlying conditions
  - Diabetes mellitus
  - Extrapulmonary malignancy
  - Corticosteroids and other immunosuppressants
  - Preceding antimicrobial therapy.

Source: Modified from Reference No. 57.

Other Predisposing Factors

Anaerobic lung infections can also occur following dissemination from preexisting extrapulmonary infections.[26-28] The classical example of this is Lemierre's syndrome,[26,29] which is almost always accompanied by secondary seeding, most commonly in the lungs. Subsequent to the introduction of effective antibiotics, the natural history of bacterial spread was interrupted and the incidence of such an infection reduced to a great extent. In the early 1970s, lung involvement was observed in 20–30% of patients with *Bacteroides* bacteremia.[30,31] This could have been due to penicillin-resistant strains of the genus *Bacteroides*, a phenomenon which was discovered a few years later.

Necrosis of the lung tissue due to stasis is also associated with anaerobic infections. This commonly occurs in bronchiectasis, pulmonary infarction and postobstructive pneumonitis secondary to bronchogenic carcinoma or a foreign body. The other mechanisms that can cause anaerobic infections in the lungs and the pleural spaces include hematogenous and lymphatic spread and diaphragmatic translocation from subphrenic collections. Infection via the blood stream is noted in patients with septic thrombophlebitis of the jugular or pelvic veins.

NATURAL HISTORY AND CLINICAL CLASSIFICATION

The distinct clinical categories of anaerobic respiratory infections include pneumonitis, lung abscess, necrotizing pneumonia and pleural empyema. These different pathologic entities **(Flow chart 1)** are believed to be the manifestations of different stages in the natural history of infection. By and large, the predisposing event in most anaerobic lung infections is aspiration of normal upper respiratory tract flora seen in up to 90% of patients.[16] The dependent portions of the lungs are most commonly involved. In the supine position, either the posterior segments of the upper lobes or the superior (apical) segments of the lower lobes are involved. When aspiration occurs in the semirecumbent posture, the basal segments of the lower lobes are chiefly affected. The right lung is twice as commonly affected as the left since the right main bronchus is more aligned with the trachea.[32,33]

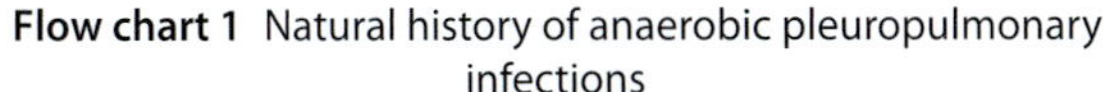
Flow chart 1 Natural history of anaerobic pleuropulmonary infections

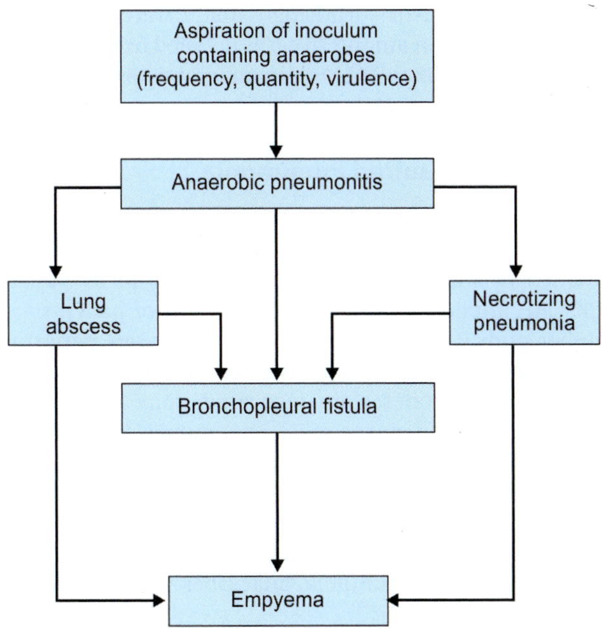

Acute Anaerobic Pneumonia

The earliest manifestation of anaerobic lung disease is pneumonia. The anaerobic etiology may not always be established due to similarities with acute bacterial pneumonias. Involvement of dependent segments could provide the initial hint. With appropriate therapy, the pathogenesis is arrested at this stage and the disease does not progress further toward suppuration.

Lung Abscess

Approximately 10–14 days later, necrosis and liquefaction in an area of anaerobic pneumonitis leads to the formation of a lung abscess.[34] A thick-walled cavity greater than 1 cm in diameter, often with an air-fluid level, develops within the pneumonic infiltrate.

Necrotizing Pneumonia

Necrotizing pneumonia is characterized by suppurative lung infiltrates with necrotic areas leading to multiple small cavities (<1 cm in diameter). In comparison to a lung abscess, a greater number of pulmonary segments are involved. Such lesions first described in 1905[35] and labeled as "pulmonary gangrene"[8] were often rapidly spreading and culminated in fatal lung destruction. Even though the incidence of necrotizing pneumonia reduced drastically after the introduction of antibiotics, the clinical response was unsatisfactory and mortality remained high.

Empyema

Empyemas are defined as the collection of pus in the pleural cavity. They result after either an ensuing bronchopulmonary fistula or as a direct extension from subpleural segmental pneumonitis. All the three clinical entities described above can be complicated by empyema. Spread from infradiaphragmatic and subphrenic collections can also lead to the formation of empyema.

Chronic Anaerobic Pneumonitis

The term chronic anaerobic pneumonitis is used when there is no evidence of either parenchymal necrosis or pleural involvement. Histopathologic examination of such lesions reveals an intra-alveolar or an interstitial infiltrate.[36] Inability to procure an appropriate sample for identifying the causative bacteria renders this entity to be relatively uncommon.

Septic Emboli

Another rarely encountered disease process is the occurrence of septic emboli. Like necrotizing pneumonias diffuse and discrete infiltrates that appeared due to embolization from anaerobic thrombophlebitis were documented mainly in the first half of the previous century.[37]

ANAEROBES AND UPPER RESPIRATORY SYNDROMES

Lemierre's Syndrome[29,38]

This disease, also known as postanginal sepsis and human necrobacillosis, is a form of thrombophlebitis of the internal jugular vein predominantly caused by *Fusobacterium necrophorum*. An acute oropharyngeal infection leading to a putrid peritonsillar abscess is most often the trigger factor for this potentially destructive disease. Septicemic spread occurs primarily to the lungs and also to bones and joints. A triad of pharyngitis, neck swelling/tenderness and noncavitating lung infiltrates is described.[39]

Ludwig's Angina[40]

This is a periodontal infection arising from the tissues surrounding the lower third molar teeth. Although Ludwig's angina is most commonly caused by *Streptococcus*, polymicrobial infections with anaerobes have been noted in up to 40% of cases.[41] The key features include marked local swelling over the floor of the mouth, which is usually associated with pain and trismus. Submandibular cellulitis ensues leading to impairment in swallowing. In cases of glottis obstruction leading to respiratory distress, tracheotomy may be life-saving.

Vincent's Angina[42,43]

This is also termed as "trench mouth", and it is heralded by an acute and sudden gingivitis. This progresses to ulceration of the interdental papillae and necrosis of the gingivae. The most common pathogen is *Prevotella intermedia*. The acute necrotizing ulcerative gingivitis may spread occasionally to cause destruction of buccal mucosa, teeth and jawbones.

INCIDENCE

For reasons more than one, it is not easy to calculate the true incidence of anaerobic lung infections. Sample collection techniques are difficult and appropriate culture methods may not be available in all laboratories. In addition, many patients respond to the initial empiric antibiotics even before specimens are obtained for confirmation.

Lung Abscess

Lung abscess and empyema are the two most frequently encountered forms of anaerobic pleuropulmonary infections. Prior to 1940s, almost all chronic pulmonary abscesses were either tuberculous or due to anaerobic bacteria. In three different case series, culture of abscess material obtained during surgical drainage or excision of the nontuberculous abscesses yielded anaerobic bacteria in 100% of patients.[44-46] Landmark studies conducted during the 1970s showed that anaerobes still accounted for more than 90% of all lung abscesses.[47]

Empyema

During the preantibiotic era, approximately two-thirds of all empyemas were caused by *Streptococcus pneumoniae*, while putrid fluid was aspirated in only 5–7% of patients.[48] With the advent of antibiotics, in addition to a marked reduction in the incidence of empyemas, there was a significant alteration in the microbiological profile. During the decades of 1960s and 1970s, anaerobic microorganisms accounted for up to 40% of all patients with empyema.[49-55] A very high yield of 76% in one particular study was attributed to diligent case finding and processing of samples in dedicated anaerobic research laboratories.[51]

Aspiration Pneumonia

In a prospective study on community and hospital-acquired cases of aspiration pneumonia, the community-acquired cases were caused mainly by anaerobic organisms while approximately two-thirds of hospital-acquired diseases were due to aerobic bacteria.[56] Bartlett and Finegold[57] extensively reviewed available literature on anaerobic pleuropulmonary infections and found that necrotizing pneumonias occurred in approximately a quarter of patients during the preantibiotic era and in only 13.7% among cases studied thereafter. Septic emboli were documented in 21% of patients reported prior to circa 1944 and in only 7.6% after effective antibiotics were prescribed. Not surprisingly, there were no cases of septic embolization among 70 cases detailed over a period of 14 years (from 1958 to 1971) at an anaerobic research center in California, USA.

Community-acquired Pneumonia

The incidence of anaerobic infections in community-acquired pneumonia (CAP) has not been studied in detail. Samples obtained by transtracheal aspiration (TTA) in 89 patients with CAP implicated anaerobes in a third of patients.[58] In another study wherein quantitative cultures were performed on fiberoptic bronchoscopy-guided protected catheter specimens, anaerobes were recovered from 16 (22%) out of 74 patients.[59] In nosocomial pneumonia, it is not easy to establish anaerobes as the chief cause since patients are already receiving broad spectrum antibiotics before sample collection. When appropriate specimens were processed prior to empiric antibiotic therapy in 159 patients with hospital-acquired pneumonia, anaerobes were identified in 56 (35%) of 159 patients.[60]

Ventilator-associated Pneumonia

The role of anaerobes as a cause of nosocomial pneumonia, particularly ventilator-associated pneumonia (VAP), is now well-documented. In 130 patients with VAP, diagnosed by quantitative protective specimen brush cultures, anaerobic bacteria were grown in 30 (23%) patients.[61] Among these 30 subjects, aerobic organisms were isolated in 26 patients while only four had a pure growth of anaerobic strains. The authors found that patients with impaired consciousness, more severe illness and initial admission to the medical ICU, had a higher chance of developing VAP due to anaerobes. Although the adequacy of empiric antibiotics prescribed for VAP in these 130 patients was not assessed, another study[62] demonstrated that the outcome was superior in those patients who had received adequate empiric anaerobic cover for VAP. Appropriate measures to minimize the chances of VAP should be advocated.

Colonization in Artificial Airways

Anaerobic bacteria, which are present in abundance in the oral flora, frequently colonize the lower respiratory tract in hospitalized patients, particularly those on mechanical ventilation.[63] This poses a significant risk for the development of life-threatening nosocomial pneumonias. In a study focusing on bacterial colonization in the lower airways in intubated patients, it was observed that approximately one-fourth of patients harbored anaerobic organisms during the first 24 hours of intubation. When analyzed over time, anaerobes were cultured from samples taken from the bronchial tree in 40–100% of patients requiring prolonged ventilation. The common anaerobic bacteria isolated were *Peptostreptococcus, Prevotella, Eubacterium, Veillonella* and *Fusobacterium*.[64]

MICROBIOLOGY

The phenomenon of bacterial synergy, initially described by Smith in the 1920s, was repeatedly demonstrated in many studies on anaerobic lung infections. Way back in 1932,[45] bacteriological cultures performed on thoracotomy aspirates of 16 patients with lung abscess grew anaerobic streptococci and anaerobic diphtheroids from all patients and *Bacteroides melaninogenicus* from 14 (88%). The other organisms identified included *Fusobacterium* species *Bacteroides fragilis* and *Sphaerophorus necrophorus*. In subsequent large series[16,57,65] of anaerobic lung infections, the common microorganisms identified were peptostreptococci, *Bacteroides melaninogenicus* (now reclassified as *Prevotella melaninogenicus*) and *F. nucleatum*. Given their predominance, this triplet is often referred to as the "Big Three" of anaerobic lung infections.[16] It was also noted that approximately a third to half of patients had mixed infections with potential pathogenic aerobes or facultative anaerobes as well. Another key pathogen is *B. fragilis* because of its inherent resistance to many of the commonly prescribed broad-spectrum antibiotics. This organism was consistently cultured in up to 20% of adults and children with anaerobic lung infections.[16] This assumes clinical importance since *B. fragilis* is not a normal commensal in the oral cavity.

It is also well-documented that the same bacteria can be recovered from patients with different clinical expressions viz. pneumonitis, lung abscess, necrotizing pneumonia and empyema. The clinical course and subsequent development of suppurative complications is not determined by a specific anaerobe but by other nonmicrobiologic factors.

As more anaerobes were identified, the taxonomy of anaerobic bacteria was revised during the last few decades. Many anaerobic streptococci and the genus *Peptococcus* were omitted in the current classification. Almost all clinically relevant species of *Peptococcus*, barring *Peptococcus niger*, were reassigned as *Peptostreptococcus*.[66] Based on lactic acid production, most peptostreptococci were grouped under the genus *Streptococcus*.[67] Many bacteria largely identified as *B. fragilis* were found to be other penicillin-resistant species of *Bacteroides*. Different bacteria grouped as *B. melaninogenicus* were reclassified as either *Prevotella* or *Porphyromonas*. Most of these species produced the enzyme penicillinase. The clinically important organisms that cause pleuropulmonary infections are highlighted in **Table 3**.

Table 3 Important anaerobic bacteria

Anaerobic bacteria
Anaerobic Gram-negative bacilli • *Prevotella* • *Porphyromonas* • *Fusobacterium* • *Bacteroides* • *Capnocytophaga* • *Leptotrichia* • *Campylobacter* • *Selenomonas*
Anaerobic Gram-negative cocci • *Veillonella*
Anaerobic Gram-positive cocci • *Peptostreptococcus* • *Streptococcus* • *Clostridium*
Anaerobic Gram-positive bacilli • *Eubacterium*

CLINICAL FEATURES

The clinical spectrum of anaerobic pleuropulmonary infections ranges from an acute pneumonic process to a chronic indolent disease.[68] Based on duration of symptoms and the disease pathology, the presentation can be divided into acute, subacute and chronic.

In patients with acute anaerobic pneumonitis without any associated suppuration, the clinical findings and radiologic picture mimic acute pneumococcal pneumonia. When 46 patients with anaerobic pneumonitis were compared with other 46 with *Streptococcus pneumoniae* pneumonia, the key differentiating features included an absence of rigors, presence of conditions that predisposed to aspiration and longer mean duration of presenting symptoms in those with anaerobic infections.[68] The common features included a febrile respiratory illness, peripheral leukocytosis and absence of bacteremia. Since the natural history of cavity formation and subsequent tissue necrosis take about 7–14 days, the presentation of lung abscess and empyema is subacute and the median duration of symptoms is around 2 weeks.

Foul Smell

The association of anaerobes and putrid odor dates way back to 1893 when Veillon[69] observed foul smell in a pure culture of an "anaerobic" organism. Ever since the classical study of Altemeier[70] in 1938, foul smell is considered to be pathognomonic of anaerobic infections. The putridity is believed to be due to volatile short chain fatty acids, which are the end-products of anaerobic metabolism. Some anaerobic cocci do not produce these volatile fatty acids.

While this characteristic feature is noted in approximately 50–60% of patients with lung abscess, necrotizing pneumonia and empyema, the incidence of putrid sputum is only 5–18% in patients with acute anaerobic pneumonitis.[33] The absence of putridness does not exclude the possibility of anaerobic lung infections.

Chronic Anaerobic Pneumonitis

Chronic anaerobic pneumonitis is an uncommon clinical entity. Although this form was produced in experimental animals,[13] there was hardly any documented report. During the last two decades, we have so far documented four patients (three adults and a child) with chronic anaerobic pneumonitis.[71-74] As is evident from the paucity of such a presentation, this chronic clinical category is yet to receive the recognition that it deserves.

Patients with chronic anaerobic pneumonitis usually present as an indolent disease with a protracted course. The mean duration of illness is usually weeks to months rather than a few days. Recurrent low-grade fever and weight loss are observed. Foul smell is usually not a feature of the chronic form as is evidenced by the fact that none of the reported patients[71-74] had foul smelling sputum. Three of these four patients received antituberculous treatment for prolonged duration prior to establishment of the diagnosis. Chronic anaerobic pneumonitis can easily be mistaken for pulmonary tuberculosis in high tuberculous prevalent areas.

In all the four documented patients,[71-74] a small number of anaerobic pathogens were isolated in the cultures. In none of these patients, any aerobic organism was grown. It is quite possible that the chronicity is due to selective but paucibacillary presence of anaerobes, in contrast to other forms of anaerobic pleuropulmonary infections where there is associated polymicrobial aerobic growth. The clinical features and different anaerobic organisms isolated are detailed in **Table 4**.

LABORATORY DIAGNOSIS

Since the anaerobes have an inherent property of inability to survive in the atmosphere, it is not easy to obtain specimens for microbiologic examination. In order to establish the diagnosis, a strong coordination is needed between the clinician and the microbiologist. Appropriate specimens that have been collected stringently in order to avoid contamination should be expeditiously sent in an appropriate transport medium to the anaerobic laboratory for specific anaerobic cultures.

Sampling Techniques

The collection of specimens for diagnosing anaerobic pleuropulmonary infections is based on the premise that the normal tracheobronchial tree is sterile below the level of the larynx. Expectorated sputum, nasopharyngeal aspirate, endotracheal or tracheostomy tube aspirates, and

Table 4 Characteristics of patients with chronic anaerobic pneumonitis

Patient no.	*Year and reference*	*Age and gender*	*Symptoms*	*Duration of illness*	*Whether received ATT*	*Radiological involvement*	*Mode for obtaining culture material*	*Anaerobic organisms cultured*	*Treatment*	*Outcome*
1	1990[71]	44 years, male	Hemoptysis, cough, low-grade fever, expectoration	1 year	No	Left upper lobe	Transtracheal aspirate	*Bacteroides*, *Fusobacterium* and *Peptostreptococcus*	Metronidazole for 12 weeks	Hemoptysis abolished, radiological improvement after 6 weeks
2	1998[72]	7 years, female	Wheezing dyspnea, cough, fever, expectoration	4 years	Yes	Right middle and lower lobes	Ultrasonographic-guided transthoracic fine needle aspiration	*Peptostreptococcus*, *Bacteroides*	Phenoxymethyl penicillin and metronidazole for 6 weeks	Asymptomatic, radiological clearance
3	2000[73]	45 years, male	Cough, low-grade fever, hemoptysis, precordial chest pain	2 years	Yes	Apical segment of left lower lobe	Transtracheal aspirate	*Fusobacterium*, *Bacteroides*	Phenoxymethyl penicillin and metronidazole for 6 weeks	No further hemoptysis, radiological clearance
4	2008[74]	44 years, male	Cough, low-grade fever, hemoptysis, sneezing, rhinorrhea	7 months	Yes	Right upper lobe	CT-guided transthoracic aspirate	*Veillonella* and *Fusobacterium*	Clindamycin for 8 weeks	Cessation of hemoptysis, radiological clearance at 2 weeks

BOX 1 Respiratory specimens valid for culture of anaerobes

- Transtracheal aspirate
- Percutaneous transthoracic needle aspirate (under imaging guidance)
- Empyema/pleural fluid
- Protected fiberoptic bronchoscopic catheter brushing
- Thoracotomy (open lung biopsy) specimen

Note: To be collected immediately in an anaerobic transport medium.

unprotected bronchoscopic aspirates are rendered unsuitable for subjecting to culture methods as these specimens contain a significant amount of commensal anaerobic microbes. Pleural fluid and tissue samples collected during surgical procedures like thoracotomy and thoracoscopy are by and large uncontaminated but difficult to obtain. In order to procure an ideal and valid sample **(Box 1)** that is free of the anaerobic-rich oral flora, various specialized techniques were described to procure the specimen directly from the lower respiratory passages and beyond.

Transtracheal Aspiration

As the name suggests this technique involves collection of the specimen directly from the trachea. In doing so, the upper respiratory tract is bypassed thereby avoiding contamination of the sample. First employed in the 1960s,[75-77] this soon became the procedure of choice in patients with pneumonia.[78] The task of procuring a reliable specimen was made easier and recovery of anaerobes by this method was consistently demonstrated in many studies.[16,33,57] Now, TTA is no longer in vogue as this technique is fraught with complications and samples are rarely obtained prior to initiating empiric antibiotic therapy for "pneumonia".

Percutaneous Transthoracic Needle Aspiration

Transthoracic needle aspiration is another means of obtaining an uncontaminated specimen.[79] The best use of this technique was described from France in 1965[49] where culture of the aspirated material grew anaerobic bacteria in 22 out of 26 patients with lung abscesses. Although there are no large trials with this investigative modality, the advent of modern imaging techniques has resulted in this method being adopted as the procedure of choice in patients suspected to have anaerobic lung infections, including pleural collections. The authors employed this method under image guidance to establish the anaerobic etiology in two of their four documented patients with chronic anaerobic pneumonitis.[72,74]

Bronchoscopic-protected Catheter Brush

The use of bronchoscopic-protected catheter brush for the diagnosis of anaerobic lung infections was also advocated.[80-82] To further improve the bacteriologic yield, local anesthetic agents were restricted and lignocaine preparations without antibacterial additives were preferred.[83,84] The limitation of this procedure is that it may not be feasible to perform before initiating antibiotic therapy. Moreover, quantitative cultures may not be readily available.

Specimen Transport and Processing

Given the anaerobic nature of the organisms, it is essential to exercise extra caution while collecting and transporting specimens. The samples should immediately be transferred into the tubes, which are free from oxygen.[85] Once the specimens reach the anaerobic laboratory, recovery of pathogenic bacteria should be ensured by appropriate processing. As expected, the yield of anaerobes was much higher when the specimens were analyzed in dedicated anaerobic research laboratories. When 25 specimens were simultaneously examined in a routine clinical microbiology laboratory and an anaerobic research laboratory, the etiologic bacteria were identified in all 25 specimens by the research laboratory and in only four by the routine laboratory.[57] Furthermore, in specimens of these four subjects, a total of 14 anaerobes (i.e. 3.5 anaerobes per patient) were grown by the research laboratory while the clinical laboratory recovered only one organism per patient. A negative culture of a potential specimen containing anaerobic organisms can occur due to several factors **(Box 2)**.

Gram's Staining and Culture Methods

Gram's staining of the specimens gives a rapid clue about the class of anaerobic bacteria responsible for disease. Even staining of expectorated sputum, which is a far from ideal sample for diagnosing anaerobic infections, would help in determining whether anaerobes are the causative organisms. The microscopic appearances of some of the common anaerobes as visualized after Gram staining are quite characteristic **(Table 5)**.

Cultures performed on invariably "contaminated" samples containing dense anaerobic flora of upper respiratory tract are usually futile. Growth of normal oral commensals may be an indication of anaerobic lung infection. The specimens

BOX 2 Causes of failure to culture anaerobes from potential specimens

- Prolonged air exposure during collection, transport and processing
- Failure to perform Gram staining so as to obtain the initial clue
- Failure to utilize satisfactory selective and differential culture media
- Overdependence on fluid thioglycollate medium
- Failure to hold anaerobic cultures for a prolonged time

Source: Adapted from reference no. 57.

Table 5 Appearance on Gram's stain

P. melaninogenicus	Pale staining Gram-negative coccobacillus
B. fragilis	Pale, somewhat pleomorphic Gram-negative bacillus
F. nucleatum	Pale, Gram-negative bacillus with pointed ends
Peptostreptococcus	Small Gram-positive cocci, usually in chains
Veillonella	Very small Gram-negative cocci in clumps, pairs or short chains

should be inoculated on at least three different culture media to get a definitive growth of anaerobic bacteria. Quantitative cultures are applied to achieve an etiologic diagnosis in as many of the specimens thus obtained.[86-88] Newer techniques like gas liquid chromatography have helped in detecting the metabolic end-products of anaerobic bacteria.

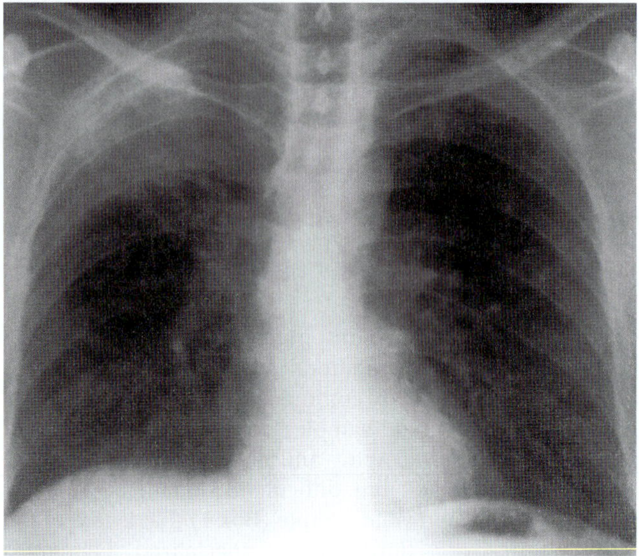

Fig. 1 Chest roentgenogram showing nonhomogeneous opacity in the right upper lobe in a patient with chronic anaerobic pneumonitis[74]

RADIOLOGICAL MANIFESTATIONS

The radiological findings depend on the stage of involvement during the natural history of the disease. Patterns of pneumonia can range from subsegmental infiltrates to bilateral multilobar consolidation. A review of the radiological features in patients with anaerobic pulmonary and pleural infections reveal that approximately 50% of patients had lung parenchymal involvement while the other 30% had pleural empyemas without lung disease and the remaining 20% had combined parenchymal and pleural shadowing.[89] Half of the lung parenchymal abnormalities were consolidation while the other 50% were either lung abscesses or necrotizing pneumonias. Radiologic worsening was noted in all patients during the initial 3 days and in a third of the cases during the first week.

In our four documented patients with chronic anaerobic pneumonitis,[71-74] right lung involvement **(Fig. 1)** was noted in two patients and the left lung was affected in the other two. Radiological progression from pneumonitis to lung abscess after initiation of therapy was noted in 20–30% of patients.[68,89] Mediastinal and hilar lymphadenopathy have been reported in a patient with anaerobic lung abscess.[90] Gas producing organisms can cause pyopneumothorax.[91]

TREATMENT

During the first half of the previous century, when antibiotics were yet to be discovered, the therapeutic measures included postural drainage of lung abscesses and surgical management of empyemas. The main drugs used were arsenicals[92-94] and sulphonamides.[95,96] This was supplemented with adequate rest and proper nutrition.[97]

Subsequent to the advent of antibiotics, the prognosis improved significantly. During the initial few decades, penicillin G was the treatment of choice for more than half of the cases. Phenoxymethyl penicillin was often used during the follow-up period. Alternative antibiotics included lincomycin, chloramphenicol, tetracycline and erythromycin.[98,99] The clinical category of anaerobic lung infections was the deciding factor for usage of combinations as well as dosage and duration of treatment. Since necrotic lung tissue is relatively avascular, a lower than the required dose would probably result in progressive damage. This could lead to suppurative complications and metastasis to other organs, e.g. cerebral abscess. Insufficient duration of therapy was responsible for a high relapse rate and distant seeding.[100]

Metronidazole too showed good bactericidal activity in vitro against anaerobes and initial results were encouraging.[101,102] Other advantages of this drug included 100% oral bioavailability and a substantially lower cost of therapy. After initial promising results, studies with metronidazole were discouraging. Collective data on 28 patients from three studies revealed therapeutic failures in 12 (43%) cases.[103-105] This poor performance was due to the fact that aerobic and microaerophilic streptococci are resistant to metronidazole. In another study[106] spanning 6 years, clinical success was noted when metronidazole was used in combination with penicillin or amoxicillin.

During the same period, better clinical efficacy of clindamycin in comparison to lincomycin was demonstrated.[107] In 1983, Levison and colleagues[108] published the first large scale prospective trial wherein clindamycin (1,800 mg/day) was compared with penicillin G (6 million units/day). There were no failures with clindamycin, while one in every five patients treated with penicillin did not show a satisfactory response. The mean durations of foul smelling sputum and fever were significantly lower in the clindamycin group. In patients with anaerobic pleuropulmonary infections, these studies led to the endorsement of three different regimes in circa 1984 by the consultants of the "Medical Letter," which included[109]: (1) penicillin G, (2) clindamycin, and (3) metronidazole + penicillin. Subsequently, a randomized controlled trial[110] comparing clindamycin versus penicillin in 37 patients with anaerobic lung infections confirmed the efficacy of clindamycin when a failure rate of 44% with penicillin and only 5.3% with clindamycin was demonstrated. The specimens of nine patients eventually grew penicillin-resistant strains of the genus *Bacteroides*, five of whom had been randomized to the penicillin arm. The authors concluded that clindamycin should be the initial choice for empiric treatment. The authors have documented the occurrence of isolates from a patient with anaerobic lung abscess that were resistant to penicillin and metronidazole.[111]

In recent times, although efficacy of several new antibiotics has been demonstrated in community-acquired pneumonia, the role of these drugs in bacteriologically confirmed lung abscess and empyema has not been systematically studied. Most of these agents show excellent activity against common aerobic respiratory pathogens including the trio of "atypical" organisms. Amongst the fluoroquinolones, moxifloxacin and gemifloxacin have good in vitro activity against anaerobic organisms.[112,113] Although ticarcillin and piperacillin, the semisynthetic penicillins, possess substantial antianaerobic properties,[114,115] up to 30% of β-lactamase producing anaerobic Gram-negative bacilli, especially *B. fragilis*, are resistant to this group of drugs.[116] Imipenem, which belongs to the carbapenem group, is highly effective against β-lactamase producing *B.* fragilis.[117] The suggested dosages of common antianaerobic drugs are given in **Table 6**. Antibiotics should be continued until symptoms have subsided, any fluid collection has resolved or stabilized and there is appreciable radiological clearing.[118] A minimum duration of 2–3 weeks is recommended.[119]

Table 6 Suggested antianaerobic drugs and dosage

Antimicrobial agents	*Dosages (per day)*
Penicillin G	10–20 million units (IV/IM)
Metronidazole	400 mg 3 times a day (oral)
Clindamycin	600 mg 3–4 times a day (oral)
Chloramphenicol	500–1,000 mg 4 times a day (oral)
Amoxicillin + clavulanate	500 mg + 125 mg 3 times a day (oral)
Ticarcillin + clavulanate	3 g + 100 mg 3–4 times a day (IV)
Piperacillin + tazobactam	4 g + 500 mg 3 times a day (IV)
Imipenem	500 mg 3–4 times a day (IV)
Note: Dosages to be adjusted as per the patients' profile.	

Surgery

Surgical drainage is the cornerstone for management of patients with empyema. The frequency of surgery for lung abscess reduced drastically once effective antibiotics became available. In comparison to approximately half of the patients requiring surgical treatment for pulmonary abscess during the preantibiotic era,[120] only 10–14% patients needed intervention 40 years later.[121-123] In patients with lung abscess and necrotizing pneumonia without pleural involvement, the indications for surgery include failure of antibiotics and life-threatening hemoptysis. Lobectomy may also be indicated if an underlying malignancy is suspected. When surgery is contraindicated due to comorbid conditions, percutaneous catheter drainage is helpful in alleviating the symptoms.[124]

PROGNOSIS

After the introduction of antibiotics, most patients have had a favorable outcome with the overall mortality rate reducing from 34% to 10% over time.[16] Fatal diseases like necrotizing pneumonia and septic emboli are rarely seen. A delayed clinical response is noted in subjects with empyema and cavitary disease, especially if the cavity is greater than 6 cm in diameter. Morbidity in such patients does not improve until drainage of fluid is achieved or cavitary closure occurs over time. Other factors responsible for a poor prognosis include chronic presentation beyond two months, elderly age group, bronchial obstruction, nosocomial aspiration and associated serious comorbidities. In the largest series of 193 patients,[16] mortality directly due to the anaerobic infection was observed in 4% while in other 7%, the disease triggered a downhill course that eventually culminated in death.

CONCLUSION

The bacterial flora of the oral cavity is predominantly anaerobic. These commensal organisms have the propensity to cause disease in persons prone to aspiration. Unfortunately, anaerobes as a key cause of pleuropulmonary infections are largely overlooked. The clinical and radiological features are often mistaken which increases morbidity. In a patient with poor orodental hygiene and history suggestive of aspiration, along with radiological picture compatible with involvement of the dependent pulmonary segments, pulmonologists must exclude anaerobic lung infections. An indolent course of illness along with foul-smelling sputum would strengthen the case for anaerobes.[125]

REFERENCES

1. Finegold SM. A century of anaerobes: a look backward and a call to arms. Clin Infect Dis. 1993;16(Suppl 4):S453-7.
2. Pasteur L. Motile microbes ("animalcules infusoires") living without free oxygen and causing fermentation [in French]. C R Acad Sci. 1861;52:344-7.

3. Veillon A, Zuber A. Sur quelques microbes strictement anaérobies et leur role dans la pathologie humaine. C R Soc Biol. 1897;49:253-5.
4. Rendu M, Rist ME. Etude clinique et bacteriologique de trois cas de pleurésie putride. Bull et Mém Soc Med Hôp Paris. 1899;16:133-50.
5. Gullimont L, Halle J, Rist E. Recherches bacteriologiques et experimentales sur les pleuresies putrides. Arch Méd Expt et Anat Path (Paris). 1904;16:571-640.
6. Castellani A. Note on a peculiar form of haemoptysis with presence of numerous spirochetes in the expectoration. Lancet. 1906;1:1384.
7. Castellani A. Bronchial spirochaetosis. Brit Med J. 1909;2:782.
8. Pilot I, Davis DJ. Studies in fusiform bacilli and spirochetes. IX. Their role in pulmonary abscess, gangrene and bronchiectasis. Arch Intern Med. 1924;34:313-54.
9. Miller WD. The microorganisms of the human mouth. In: SS White (Ed). Philadelphia: Dental Mfg Co; 1890. p. 80.
10. Jackson C. Ulcerative bronchitis due to "Vincent's organisms." JAMA. 1924;83:1845.
11. Smith DT. Fusospirochetal disease of the lungs. Tubercle. 1928;9:420.
12. Smith DT. Experimental aspiratory abscess. Arch Surg. 1927;14:231-9.
13. Smith DT. Fusospirochetal disease of the lungs: its bacteriology, pathology and experimental reproduction. Am Rev Tuberc. 1927;16:584.
14. Smith DT. Fusospirochetal disease of the lungs produced with cultures from Vincent's angina. J Infect Dis. 1930;46:303.
15. Weiss W. Delayed cavity closure in acute nonspecific primary lung abscess. Am J Med Sci. 1968;255:313-9.
16. Bartlett JG. Anaerobic bacterial infections of the lung. Chest. 1987;91:901-9.
17. Hirsch RS, Clarke NG. Infection and periodontal diseases. Rev Infect Dis. 1989;11(5):707-15.
18. Slots J. Microflora in the healthy gingival sulcus in man. Scand J Dent Res. 1977;85(4):247-54.
19. Neiders ME, Chen PB, Suido H, Reynolds HS, Zambon JJ, Shlossman M, et al. Heterogeneity of virulence among strains of *Bacteroides gingivalis*. J Periodontal Res. 1989;24:192-8.
20. Huxley EJ, Viroslav J, Gray WR, Pierce AK. Pharyngeal aspiration in normal adults and patients with depressed consciousness. Am J Med. 1978;64(4):564-8.
21. Culver GA, Makel HP, Beecher HK. Frequency of aspiration of gastric contents by lungs during anesthesia and surgery. Ann Surg. 1951;133(3):289-92.
22. Bailey AS, Dotter CT, Steinberg I. Pulmonary complications of cardiospasm. N Engl J Med. 1951;245:441-7.
23. Lake RA. Pulmonary changes related to cardiospasm. Ann Intern Med. 1951;35(3):593-9.
24. Rosenow EC, Tunnicliff R. Pyemia due to an anaerobic polymorphic bacillus, probably *Bacillus fusiformis*. J Infect Dis. 1912;10:1.
25. Stern L. Etiologic factors in pathogenesis of putrid abscess of the lung. J Thorac Surg. 1936;6:202.
26. Lemierre A. On certain septicemias due to anaerobic organisms. Lancet. 1936;1:701-3.
27. Reid JD, Snider GE, Toone EC, Howe JS. Anaerobic septicemia, report of 6 cases with clinical, bacteriologic and pathologic studies. Am J Med Sci. 1945;209:296-306.
28. Tynes BS, Utz JP. Fusobacterium septicemia. Am J Med. 1960;29:879-87.
29. O'Brien WT Sr, Lattin GE Jr, Thompson AK. Lemierre syndrome: an all-but-forgotten disease. AJR Am J Roentgenol. 2006;187(3):W324.
30. Felner JM, Dowell VR Jr. *Bacteroides* bacteremia. Am J Med. 1971;50:787-96.
31. Marcoux JA, Zabransky RJ, Washington JA, Wellman WE, Martin WJ. *Bacteroides* bacteremia. Minn Med. 1970;53(11):1169-76.
32. Bartlett JG, Gorbach SL, Finegold SM. The bacteriology of aspiration pneumonia. Am J Med. 1974;56(2):202-7.
33. Bartlett JG, Finegold SM. Anaerobic infections of the lung and pleural space. Am Rev Respir Dis. 1974;110(1):56-77.
34. Neuhof H, Wessler H. Putrid lung abscess - its etiology, pathology, clinical manifestations, diagnosis and treatment. J Thorac Surg. 1931;32:637.
35. Rona S. Plaut-Vinccentschen Angina, der stomakace, der Stomatitis gangraenosa idiopathica, beziehungsweise der Noma, der stomatitis mercurialis gangraenosa und der Lungengangren. Arch f Dermat u Syph. 1905;74:171.
36. Tillotson JR, Lerner AM. *Bacteroides pneumonias*. Characteristics of cases with empyaema. Ann Intern Med. 1968;68:308-17.
37. Thompson L. Bacteremia due to anaerobic Gram-negative organisms *(Bacteroides)*. Mayo Clin Proc. 1931;6:372.
38. Karkos PD, Asrani S, Karkos CD, Leong SC, Theochari EG, Alexopoulou TD, et al. Lemierre's syndrome: A systematic review. Laryngoscope. 2009;119(8):1552-9.
39. Chirinos JA, Lichtstein DM, Garcia J, Tamariz LJ. The evolution of Lemierre syndrome: report of 2 cases and review of the literature. Medicine (Baltimore). 2002;81(6):458-65.
40. Srirompotong S, Art-Smart T. Ludwig's angina: a clinical review. Eur Arch Otorhinolaryngol. 2003;260(7):401-3.
41. Har-El G, Aroesty JH, Shaha A, Lucente FE. Changing trends in deep neck abscess. A retrospective study of 110 patients. Oral Surg Oral Med Oral Pathol. 1994;77(5):446-50.
42. Waring JJ, Ryan JG, Thompson R, Spencer FR. *Bacteroides* septicemia, report of a case with recovery. The Laryngoscope. 1943;53:717-23.
43. Berthold P. Noma: a forgotten disease. Dent Clin North Am. 2003;47:559-74.
44. Lambert AVS, Miller JA. Abscess of lung. Arch Surg. 1924;8:446-56.
45. Cohen J. The bacteriology of abscess of the lung and methods for its study. Arch Surg. 1932;24:171-88.
46. Varney PL. Bacterial flora of abscesses of the lung. Arch Surg. 1920;19:1602-14.
47. Bartlett JG. The role of anaerobic bacteria in lung abscess. Clin Infect Dis. 2005;40(7):923-5.
48. Ehler AA. Non-tuberculous thoracic empyema: collective review of literature from 1934 to 1939. International Abstracts in Surgery. 1941;72:17-38.
49. Beerens H, Tahon-Castel M. Infections humaines à bactéries anaérobies non toxigènes. Brussels: Presses Académiques Européennes;1965. pp. 91-114.
50. Sullivan KM, O'Toole RD, Fisher RH, Sullivan KN. Anaerobic empyema thoracis. The role of anaerobes in 226 cases of culture-proven empyemas. Arch Intern Med. 1973;131:521-7.
51. Bartlett JG, Gorbach SL, Thadepalli H, Finegold SM. Bacteriology of empyema. Lancet. 1974;1(7853):338-40.
52. Varkey B, Rose HD, Kutty CP, Politis J. Empyema thoracis during a ten-year period: analysis of 72 cases and comparison to a previous study (1952 to 1967). Arch Intern Med. 1981;141(13):1771-6.

53. Mavroudis C, Symmonds JB, Minagi H, Thomas AN. Improved survival in management of empyema thoracis. J Thorac Cardiovasc Surg. 1981;82(1):49-57.
54. Grant DR, Finley RJ. Empyema: analysis of treatment techniques. Can J Surg. 1985;28(5):449-51.
55. Lemmer JH, Botham MJ, Orringer MB. Modern management of adult thoracic empyema. J Thorac Cardiovasc Surg. 1985;90(6):849-55.
56. Lorber B, Swenson RM. Bacteriology of aspiration pneumonia, a prospective study of community and hospital-acquired cases. Ann Intern Med. 1974;81(3):329-31.
57. Bartlett JG, Finegold SM. Anaerobic pleuropulmonary infections. Medicine (Baltimore). 1972;51(6):413-50.
58. Ries K, Levison ME, Kaye D. Transtracheal aspiration in pulmonary infection. Arch Intern Med. 1974;133(3):453-8.
59. Pollock HM, Hawkins EL, Bonner JR, Sparkman T, Bass JB Jr. Diagnosis of bacterial pulmonary infections with quantitative protected catheter cultures obtained during bronchoscopy. J Clin Microbiol. 1983;17(2):255-9.
60. Bartlett JG, O'Keefe P, Tally FP, Louie TJ, Gorbach SL. Bacteriology of hospital-acquired pneumonia. Arch Intern Med. 1986;146(5):868-71.
61. Doré P, Robert R, Grollier G, Rouffineau J, Lanquetot H, Charrière JM, et al. Incidence of anaerobes in ventilator-associated pneumonia with use of a protected specimen brush. Am J Respir Crit Care Med. 1996;153(4):1292-8.
62. Robert R, Grollier G, Doré P, Hira M, Ferrand E, Fauchère JL. Nosocomial pneumonia with isolation of anaerobic bacteria in ICU patients: therapeutic considerations and outcome. J Crit Care.1999;14(3):114-9.
63. Robert R, Grollier G, Frat JP, Godet C, Adoun M, Fauchère JL, et al. Colonization of lower respiratory tract with anaerobic bacteria in mechanically ventilated patients. Intensive Care Med. 2003;29(7):1062-8.
64. Agvald-Ohman C, Wernerman J, Nord CE, Edlund C. Anaerobic bacteria commonly colonize the lower airways of intubated ICU patients. Clin Microbiol Infect. 2003;9(5):397-405.
65. Finegold SM, George WL, Mulligan ME. Anaerobic infections. Dis Month. 1985;31(11):8-77.
66. Ezaki T, Yamamoto N, Ninomiya K, Suzuki S, Yabuuchi E. Transfer of *Peptococcus indolicus, Peptococcus asaccharolyticus, Peptococcus prevotii,* and *Peptococcus magnus* to the genus *Peptostreptococcus* and proposal of *Peptostreptococcus tetradius* sp. nov. Int J Syst Bacteriol. 1983;33:683-98.
67. Cato EP. Transfer of *Peptostreptococcus parvulus* (Weinberg, Nativelle, and Prévot 1937) Smith 1957 to the genus *Streptococcus: Streptococcus parvulus* (Weinberg, Nativelle, and Prévot 1937) comb. nov. nom. rev. emend. Int J Syst Bacteriol. 1983;33:82-4.
68. Bartlett JG. Anaerobic bacterial pneumonitis. Am Rev Respir Dis. 1979;119(1):19-23.
69. Veillon A. Sur un microcoque anaerobe trouvé dans suppurations fétides. C R Soc Biol. 1893;5:807.
70. Altemeier WA. The cause of the putrid odor of perforated appendicitis with peritonitis. Ann Surg. 1938;107:634-6.
71. Shah A, Bhagat R, Chokhani R, Pant K, Thukral SS. Chronic anaerobic pneumonitis. Indian J Chest Dis Allied Sci. 1990;32(2):117-20.
72. Agarwal AK, Bhagat R, Panchal N, Thukral SS, Shah A. Chronic anaerobic pneumonitis in a seven-year-old girl. Pediatr Pulmonol. 1998;26(2):135-7.
73. Guptan A, Agarwal AK, Thukral SS, Shah A. Chronic anaerobic pneumonitis presenting as a pseudohilar opacity. Indian J Chest Dis Allied Sci. 2000;42(1):27-9.
74. Shah A, Panjabi C, Nair V, Chaudhry R, Thukral SS. *Veillonella* as a cause of chronic anaerobic pneumonitis. Int J Infect Dis. 2008;12(6):e115-7.
75. Pecora DV, Kohl M. Transtracheal aspiration in the diagnosis of acute lower respiratory tract infection. Am Rev Respir Dis. 1962;86:755-8.
76. Pecora DV. A comparison of transtracheal aspiration with other methods of determining the bacterial flora of the lower respiratory tract. N Engl J Med. 1963;269:664-6.
77. Kalinske RW, Parker RH, Brandt D, Hoeprich PD. Diagnostic usefulness and safety of transtracheal aspiration. N Engl J Med. 1967;276(11):604-8.
78. Bartlett JG. Diagnostic accuracy of transtracheal aspiration bacteriologic studies. Am Rev Respir Dis. 1977;115(5):777-82.
79. Gherman CR, Simon HJ. Pneumonia complicating severe underlying disease. A current appraisal of transthoracic lung puncture. Dis Chest. 1965;48(3):297-304.
80. Wimberley N, Faling LJ, Bartlett JG. A fiberoptic bronchoscopy technique to obtain uncontaminated lower airway secretions for bacterial culture. Am Rev Respir Dis. 1979;119(3):337-43.
81. Wimberley NW, Bass JB Jr, Boyd BW, Kirkpatrick MB, Serio RA, Pollock HM. Use of a bronchoscopic protected catheter brush for the diagnosis of pulmonary infections. Chest. 1982;81(5):556-62.
82. Marquette CH, Ramon P, Courcol R, Wallaert B, Tonnel AB, Voisin C. Bronchoscopic protected catheter brush for the diagnosis of pulmonary infections. Chest. 1988;93:746-50.
83. Bartlett JG, Alexander J, Mayhew J, et al. Should fiberoptic bronchoscopy aspirates be cultured? Am Rev Respir Dis. 1976;114(1):73-8.
84. Wimberley N, Willey S, Sullivan N, Bartlett JG. Antibacterial properties of lidocaine. Chest. 1979;76(1):37-40.
85. Attebery HR, Finegold SM. Combined screw-cap and rubber-stopper closure for Hungate tubes (pre-reduced anaerobically sterilized roll tubes and liquid media). Appl Microbiol. 1969;18(4):558-61.
86. Bartlett JG, Finegold SM. Bacteriology of expectorated sputum with quantitative culture and wash technique compared to transtracheal aspirates. Am Rev Respir Dis. 1978;117(6):1019-27.
87. Bartlett JG, Faling LJ, Willey S. Quantitative tracheal bacteriologic and cytologic studies in patients with long-term tracheostomies. Chest. 1978;74(6):635-9.
88. Teague RB, Wallace RJ Jr, Awe RJ. The use of quantitative sterile brush culture and Gram stain analysis in the diagnosis of lower respiratory tract infection. Chest. 1981;79(2):157-61.
89. Landay MJ, Christensen EE, Bynum LJ, Goodman C. Anaerobic pleural and pulmonary infections. AJR Am J Roentgenol. 1980;134(2):233-40.
90. Rohlfing BM, White EA, Webb WR, Goodman PC. Hilar and mediastinal adenopathy caused by bacterial abscess of the lung. Radiology. 1978;128(2):289-93.
91. Raff MJ, Johnson JD, Nagar D, Ferris FZ, McCormick ML. Spontaneous clostridial empyema and pyopneumothorax. Rev Infect Dis. 1984;6(5):715-9.
92. Allen CI, Blackman JF. Treatment of lung abscess with report of 100 consecutive cases. J Thorac Surg. 1936;6:156.
93. Kline BS, Berger SS. Spirochetal pulmonary gangrene treated with arsphenamines. JAMA. 1925;85:1452.

94. Sweet RH. Lung abscess: an analysis of the Massachusetts General Hospital cases from 1933 through 1937. Surg Gynecol Obstet. 1940;70:1011-21.
95. D'Ingianni U. Non-tuberculous lung abscess; survey of 417 cases. Am J Surg. 1944;65:46.
96. Martin WB. Human infection with *B. necrophorum*. Am J Clin Path. 1940;10:567.
97. Smith DT. Medical treatment of acute and chronic pulmonary abscesses. J Thorac Surg. 1948;17(1):72-90.
98. Finegold SM, Harada NE, Miller LG. Lincomycin: activity against anaerobes and effect on normal human fecal flora. Antimicrob Agents Chemother. 1965;5:659-67.
99. Finegold SM, Harada NE, Miller LG. Antibiotic susceptibility patterns as an aid in classification and characterization of Gram-negative anaerobic bacilli. J Bacteriol. 1967;94(5):1443-50.
100. Sandler BP. The prevention of cerebral abscess secondary to pulmonary suppuration. Dis Chest. 1965;48:32-6.
101. Davies AH, McFadzean JA, Squires S. Treatment of Vincent's stomatitis with metronidazole. Br Med J. 1964;1(5391):1149-50.
102. Glenwright HD, Sidaway DA. The use of metronidazole in the treatment of acute ulcerative gingivitis. Br Dent J. 1966;121(4):174-7.
103. Tally FP, Sutter VL, Finegold SM. Treatment of anaerobic infections with metronidazole. Antimicrob Agents Chemother. 1975;7(5):672-5.
104. Sanders CV, Hanna BJ, Lewis AC. Metronidazole in the treatment of anaerobic infections. Am Rev Respir Dis. 1979;120(2):337-43.
105. Perlino CA. Metronidazole vs clindamycin treatment of anaerobic pulmonary infection. Failure of metronidazole therapy. Arch Intern Med. 1981;141(11):1424-7.
106. Eykyn SJ. The therapeutic use of metronidazole in anaerobic infection: six years' experience in a London hospital. Surgery. 1983;93(1 Pt 2):209-14.
107. Finegold SM, Bartlett JG, Sutter VL. New antimicrobial drugs for anaerobic infections. Clin Res. 1972;20:165.
108. Levison ME, Mangura CT, Lorber B, Abrutyn E, Pesanti EL, Levy RS, et al. Clindamycin compared with penicillin for the treatment of anaerobic lung abscess. Ann Intern Med. 1983;98(4):466-71.
109. Drugs for anaerobic infections. Med Lett Drugs Ther. 1984;26:87-9.
110. Gudiol F, Manresa F, Pallares R, Dorca J, Rufi G, Boada J, et al. Clindamycin vs penicillin for anaerobic lung infections. High rate of penicillin failures associated with penicillin-resistant *Bacteroides melaninogenicus*. Arch Intern Med. 1990;150(12):2525-9.
111. Shah A, Sircar M, Bhagat R, Jaiswal A, Thukral SS. Clindamycin in the treatment of anaerobic lung abscess. Indian J Chest Dis Allied Sci. 1991;33(1):25-9.
112. Goldstein EJ. Review of the in vitro activity of gemifloxacin against Gram-positive and Gram-negative anaerobic pathogens. J Antimicrob Chemother. 2000;45 (Suppl 1):55-65.
113. Ackerman G, Schaumann R, Pless B, Claros MC, Goldstein EJ, Rodloff AC. Comparative activity of moxifloxacin in vitro against obligately anaerobic bacteria. Eur J Clin Microbiol Infect Dis. 2000;19(3):228-32.
114. Sutter VL, Finegold SM. Susceptibility of anaerobic bacteria to 23 antimicrobial agents. Antimicrob Agents Chemother. 1976;10(4):736-52.
115. Finegold SM. Anaerobic Bacteria in Human Disease. New York: Academic Press; 1977.
116. Finegold SM. In vitro efficacy of beta-lactam/beta-lactamase inhibitor combinations against bacteria involved in mixed infections. Int J Antimicrob Agents. 1999;12 (Suppl 1):S9-14.
117. Brook I. Treatment of anaerobic infection. Expert Rev Anti Infect Ther. 2007;5(6):991-1006.
118. Bartlett JG. Anaerobic bacterial infections of the lung and pleural space. Clin Infect Dis. 1993;16 (Suppl 4):S248-55.
119. Fishman A. Aspiration empyema, lung abscess, and anaerobic infections. In: Fishman's Pulmonary Diseases and Disorders, 4th edition. New York: McGraw hill; 2008. pp. 2141-60.
120. Bartlett JG. Clinical conferences at the Johns Hopkins Hospital: Lung abscess. Johns Hopkins Med J. 1982;150:141-7.
121. Harber P, Terry PB. Fatal lung abscesses: review of 11 years' experience. South Med J. 1981;74:281-7.
122. Hagan JL, Hardy JD. Lung abscess revisited. A survey of 184 cases. Ann Surg. 1983;197(6):755-62.
123. Pohlson EC, McNamara JJ, Char C, Kurata L. Lung abscess: a changing pattern of the disease. Am J Surg. 1985;150(1):97-101.
124. Weissberg D. Percutaneous drainage of lung abscess. J Thorac Cardiovasc Surg. 1984;87(2):308-12.
125. Bartlett JG. How important are anaerobic bacteria in aspiration pneumonia: when should they be treated and what is optimal therapy? Infect Dis Clin North Am. 2013;27(1):149-55.

Section 8

Asthma

SK Jindal, Inderpaul Singh Sehgal

Bronchial Asthma: Epidemiology

SK Jindal

INTRODUCTION

Asthma, although known since antiquity, remains a disease of unclear etiology, wide heterogeneity and marked variability. There is no uniform agreement on its definition in spite of the fact that the problem is recognized and appreciated by even the lay, all over the world. For a clinician, it is characterized by episodic wheezing, breathlessness and/or cough. Functionally, there is widespread narrowing of the intrapulmonary airways and demonstrable, reversible obstruction. Pathologically, it is a chronic inflammatory disorder of the airways.

The definition of asthma has been revised in last Global Initiative for Asthma (GINA) Update (2014)[1] as follows:

"Asthma is a heterogeneous disease, usually characterized by chronic inflammation. It is defined by the history of respiratory symptoms such as wheeze, shortness of breath, chest tightness and cough that vary over time and in intensity, together with variable airflow limitation."

The operational definition as above is fairly broad and comprehensive, but lacks precision. This is particularly difficult from an epidemiological point of view for the assessment of burden and comparative analysis. More recently, asthma is described as a syndrome consisting of many disease entities because of the presence of a wide clinical heterogeneity and overlap syndromes **(Table 1)**.[2,3] Further, asthma is recognized to present with a large number of systemic manifestations and other associations. Factually asthma is now considered as a syndrome of a number of different diseases.[4] These features make it even more difficult to define the disease and its epidemiology.

EPIDEMIOLOGY

There is a marked variability in the global prevalence. It is reported to involve from about 1% to over 20% individuals in different populations.[1,5,6] An overall global asthma burden of about 300 million patients had been previously estimated based on the then prevalence figures.

Table 1 Overlap syndromes and disease entities of asthma

A. *Overlap syndromes and associations*
• Asthma-COPD overlap
• Remodeled asthma
• Asthma–obstructive sleep apnea overlap
• Metabolic syndrome and asthma
B. *Specific asthma entities*
• Allergic bronchopulmonary aspergillosis
• Aspirin exacerbated asthma (Samter's triad)
• Exercise induced asthma
• Churg-Strauss syndrome
• Good's syndrome
• Irritant-induced work place asthma
• Schnitzler syndrome

These variations can be attributed to the differences in the environmental and climatic risk factors, the genetic predisposition and the inheritance patterns. Other important reasons, which can be counted for the difference include the differences in the definitions used for the diagnosis of asthma, the type of sample selection and the methodologies employed in different studies.[7,8] Frequently, the episodes of upper respiratory tract catarrh (especially when recurrent), chronic bronchitis, bronchiectasis and miscellaneous causes of cough, breathlessness and other respiratory symptoms are also inadvertently misdiagnosed as asthma. The prevalence rates and burden will also differ if one employs the definitions of "ever-asthma" or "current asthma", "symptomatic asthma" or "asthma, including bronchial hyperresponsiveness (BHR)".

Several of the global estimates of "current asthma" point to variable rates from 1.2% to 3.7% in Belgium to as high as 25.5% in Australia.[7] The prevalence figures are also different if one uses the definition of "diagnosed asthma," "recent wheeze" or "airway hyperresponsiveness (AHR)".

The mean prevalence of clinical asthma for Southern Asia (Bangladesh, Bhutan, India, Nepal, Seychelles and Sri Lanka) was assessed to be 3.5% for a total population of 1.21 billions,[1,7] but several of these estimates, based on limited data from a particular region, do not truly represent the overall population prevalence.

From India, the prevalence as high as over 10% among school children were reported in some studies. The field prevalence of diagnosed asthma was about 5% in children and about 3% in adults **(Table 2)**.[5,9-19] The average population prevalence was 2.4% amongst 73,605 adults of over 15 years of age, studied at four different centers in Phase I of the Indian Multicentric Study on Epidemiology of Asthma, Respiratory Symptoms and Chronic Bronchitis in Adults (INSEARCH) when a validated questionnaire and a relatively stringent definition of "ever-asthma" were used.[11]

The most recent Phase II of the INSEARCH study conducted at 12 different centers in a population sample of 169,575 individuals has reported a mean prevalence of 2.05% of current asthma.[20] Another cross-sectional survey around the same period reported the prevalence of self-reported asthma as 1.8% among men and 1.9% among women.[21] This reflected an enormous overall burden of asthma in India. For a total population of 1.028 billion (including children and adults) as per Census of India (2001), the minimum burden of asthma is about 21 millions for all age groups.

The total number of patients could actually be higher considering the higher prevalence rates in children. If one uses more sensitive criteria, such as the "wheeze alone" or the presence of BHR, the estimates are likely to rise. The prevalence in India, although somewhat lower than that described from the West, is similar to prevalence in other Asian countries.[22] Some of the possible explanations, which have been advocated for a lower prevalence of asthma, may include the presumably protective influence of a higher incidence of childhood respiratory infections and ambient atmospheric pollution, which may partially suppress the allergic immune responses. A higher likelihood of breastfeeding in the Asian children may also be partially protective. The increasing trends in asthma prevalence, also in Asian countries may suggest a rise in asthma burden in the near future.[22]

Allergic bronchopulmonary aspergillosis (ABPA) is frequently recognized in about 10–15% of asthmatic individuals in India.[23] This is an important cause of difficult or poorly controlled asthma. At the primary health care levels, more than half of the ABPA patients are known to have received antitubercular treatment because of the similarities in the clinical and the radiological findings before the diagnosis is established.

DISEASE BURDEN

Asthma is responsible for a significant disease morbidity. In children, the frequent absenteeism from school due to illness episodes constitutes an important cause of poor scholastic performance. Poor control may also result in irreversibility of airway obstruction and impairment of lung function later in adulthood. In adults, it results in poor work efficiency and loss of days of productive work.

Table 2 Summary of the important population studies from India on prevalence of asthma

Author	*Region*	*Type of study*	*Number*	*Age (years)*	*Percentage (%)*
Adults					
Chowgule (1998)[10]	Mumbai	Field	2,313	20–44	3.5
Aggarwal (2006)[11]	Multicentric	Field	73,605	>15	2.4
Jindal SK (2012)[20]	Multicentric	Field	169,575	>15	2.04
Agrawal S (2013)[21]	Data from NFHS*		109,041	>15	Men 1.8, Women 1.9
Children					
Chhabra (1998)[12]	North	Schools	2,609	4–17	11.6
Shah (2000)[13]	Multicentric	Schools	37,171	13–14	3.7
			31,697	6–7	4.5
Gupta (2001)[14]	North	Schools	9,090	9–20	2.3
Paramesh (2002)[15]	South	Schools	6,550	6–15	16.6
Chakravarthy (2002)[16]	South	Field	855	<12	5
Mistry (2004)[17]	North	Schools	575	13–14	12.5
Awasthi (2004)[18]	Lucknow	Schools	3,000	13–14	3.3
				6–7	2.3
Pakhale (2008)[19]	West	Schools	3,668	13–14	7.3
Lai (2009)[5]	West	Schools		6–7	2.4

*India's Third National Family Health Survey (NFHS-3, 2005–6)

There is also a huge economic burden of asthma. The burden is related to the direct and indirect costs of management. Moreover, there are fiscal losses due to work absenteeism. The costs of "not treating" or mistreating asthma are even higher.[24]

The data available on economic burden from India are rather sparse. An attempt at assessment was made on the basis of prevalence rates available in different studies.[25] The estimated total annual cost of about ₹ 32 billion for patients with chronic asthma with additional costs of about ₹ 5 billion for acute asthma (for the year 2011) is an enormous burden for the health care infrastructure of a developing country.

RISK FACTORS OF ASTHMA

The prevalence of asthma is influenced by several risk factors, which can be broadly categorized into the host and the environmental factors **(Table 3)**. The development is largely determined by host factors, while the triggering is mostly caused by environmental exposures. Some of the factors from both the host and the environmental groups may also overlap in their roles and cause asthma development, as well as the trigging of symptoms.

Host Factors

Age and sex: On an average, asthma occurs with equal frequency in both sexes. There is a male predominance in children, asthma is twice as common in boys as in girls before 14 years of age. The sex difference disappears as the age advances, to a higher incidence in women in adults.

Asthma is more common in children in the 5–14 years age groups. The cumulative prevalence of asthma increases as the age advances. The earlier belief that "children often grow out of asthma" is not factually true. Although from about a third to half of the children may become asymptomatic as they grow, the disease cannot be labeled as "eliminated." A large number of these children develop symptoms later in life.

Table 3 Important risk factors that influence the development of asthma

A. *Host factors*
• Age and sex • Socioeconomic status • Racial and ethnic factors • Genetic polymorphisms • Other atopic conditions • Obesity
B. *Environmental factors*

• Aeroallergens
• Infections (? Protective role)
• Occupational exposures
• Environmental pollutants
• Outdoor air pollution?
• Indoor pollution
  – Environmental tobacco smoke/In utero exposure to smoke
  – Solid fuel combustion
• *Diet:* Processed foods
  Breastfeeding (Protective role)

Genetic factors: There is a strong genetic predisposition of asthma. The presence of a family history of asthma and other allergies in the first degree relatives of patients, indicates the role of genetic factors. Identical twins were found to have a very high relative risk (17.9) of asthma in a study on cumulative incidence of asthma in twins.[26] The evidence was strongly considered in favor of the genetic predisposition.

No single gene defect is identifiable in asthmatic patients. However, multiple genetic polymorphisms associated with clinical asthma and/or BHR have been identified, some of which may actually affect the bronchodilator responsiveness.[27] Various other genes are found to modify the treatment response to antiasthma drugs, including the bronchodilators, corticosteroids and leukotriene modifiers.[28-30]

Genetic factors are important determinants of susceptibility to allergic diseases and asthma. Recent studies have highlighted their role in determining the in utero development and early life susceptibility to allergies.[31] This has resulted in better endophenotying, prognostication and prediction of treatment responses.[31] It can be therefore, anticipated that the gene polymorphism may play an important role in future in planning and improving the management of asthma.[29-32]

Childhood asthma in European children is also shown to relate to a younger gestational age at birth and higher infant weight gain.[33]

Other host factors: Asthma is known to differ in prevalence in different racial and ethnic populations. Some of these differences could actually be attributed to different genetic polymorphisms. Common environmental exposures may also influence the prevalence differences.

Presence of nasal (allergic rhinitis) and skin (atopic dermatitis) atopies, sinusitis and nasal polyposis is frequently associated with asthma. They possibly share a common genotyping and pathogenesis. Nasal allergy in particular is said to exist with asthma as an essential companion—"one airway-one disease".

Presence of obesity is also a recognized risk factor. Obesity is partly genetic and partly environmental in origin. In obesity, nonatopic mechanisms are more relevant in causing asthma.[34,35]

Environmental Factors

Several environmental exposures, such as aeroallergens, occupational agents, tobacco smoke, outdoor and indoor air pollutants and possibly infectious agents have been implicated in the development of asthma. Some of these agents may also act as "precipitating" or "aggravating" factors (triggers) for clinical symptoms of asthma.

Residence in the urban areas and lower socioeconomic status are other important factors likely to increase the occurrence of asthma. Tobacco smoking of all types, including the cigarettes, "*bidis*" and "*hukkah*," as well as the passive exposure to environmental tobacco smoke (ETS) form other important factors, which may provoke asthma.[36,37] Both "in utero" and childhood smoking exposure may also have an important role in the causation of asthma and BHR in children, as well as in adults. Indoor exposure at home to pollutants from solid fuel or fossil fuel combustion may act in a similar fashion as the tobacco smoke. Their role in causing asthma, as well as in producing exacerbations has been described in the past, as well as in the INSEARCH study.[20,38,39]

Allergens: The role of allergens in asthma development is not entirely clear. House dust mites, contact with domestic pets and exposure to a number of aeroallergens can precipitate and manifest asthma. Pollens of several plants, such as prosopis, ricinus, argemone, amaranthus, cannabis, parthenium, etc. have been implicated in the causation of asthma in India. Many airborne pollens, fungal spores, home dust mite, insect debris, cat and dog dander have been implicated as independent risk factors for asthma.[40-43] Early exposure to cat and dog dander has been reported as protective against allergen sensitization in some studies, while others suggest that it increases the risk.[43-45]

Infections: Infections are important triggers of asthma symptoms. Respiratory syncytial virus (RSV) and parainfleunza virus infections are known to cause asthma in children.[46] On the other hand, early childhood infections are reported to protect from asthma (hygiene hypothesis),[47] possibly explaining the lower asthma prevalence in the developing countries, including in India, attributable to higher occurrence of childhood infections. The "hygiene hypothesis" is based on the concept that exposure to airway infections and allergens early in life causes maturation of T helper 1 (Th1) lymphocytes over Th2 lymphocytes, thereby decreasing the risk of allergies.[48] The theory has been further supported by some studies, but not by others.[49] The issue remains unresolved. Genetic susceptibility of an individual may also contribute to this development of asthma.

The common organisms, which have been cultured from bronchoalveolar lavage samples are the viruses (adenovirus, parainfluenza, RSV and influenza), Mycoplasma and Chlamydia. They may have important role in asthma development, airway inflammation and remodeling.[50] Of various parasites, only hook worm infestations have been shown to reduce the risk.[51]

Occupational exposures: Exposure to chemical vapors, irritant gases, metal fumes and other exhausts amongst persons engaged in different occupations may cause airway sensitization and increased production of immunoglobulin E (IgE), which commonly manifest as occupational asthma.[52,53] Occupational sensitization is also responsible for both the development and precipitation of asthma.

Occupational asthma occurs mostly in adults, generally after an exposure period of month to years in sensitized individuals. Both IgE- and cell-mediated immunological reactions are involved.[54]

Environmental pollution and smoking: Exposure to environmental air pollutants in both outdoor and indoor conditions is an important cause of respiratory morbidity and increased asthma exacerbations.[39] Domestic combustion of solid fuel for cooking and heating is an important cause of indoor air pollution in India as well as in several third world countries.[55] Combustion exhausts are responsible for increased respiratory infections as well as lung function impairment in children. However, the role of environmental pollutants in the development of asthma remains debatable.[56]

Passive exposure to tobacco smoking, an important source of indoor air pollution ETS, is another important cause of increased asthma morbidity amongst both children and adults.[37] There is no good evidence to attribute the development of asthma to ETS exposure. However, in utero exposure of the fetus to smoking from a smoker mother is reported to influence the lung development. In utero tobacco smoke exposure is also shown to be responsible for persistent wheezing problems in children in the first year of life.[57]

Diet: Foods are commonly blamed to aggravate asthma, but scientific evidence is somewhat inadequate.[58,59] There are very few types of foods which can be definitely identified as triggers. Fish, eggs, certain types of mushrooms, bananas and some beans have been listed as triggers in some studies. There are some data to suggest the role of processed foods, contributing to the increased incidence of asthma. Breast milk fed infants have been shown to have lower incidence than those fed with formula milk or soy proteins.

The presence of gastroesophageal reflux (GER) is considered as an important trigger especially in patients with nocturnal asthma, though the relationship of GER with asthma has recently been disputed. It was shown in a large double-blind trial that silent GER was not a likely cause of poorly controlled asthma.

In summary, asthma involves a complex interplay of different mechanisms, which result in a common clinical presentation of widespread airway obstruction. There are large epidemiological and clinical variations in the disease spectrum. Several of these differences are perhaps based on different inflammatory phenotypes, which are now unfolding.[60,61]

REFERENCES

1. Global Initiative for Asthma. (2014). Global Strategy for Asthma Management and Prevention, 2014. [online] *www.ginasthma.org* [Accessed Februrary, 2016].
2. Lotvall J, Akdis CA, Bacharier LB, Biermer L, Casale TB, Custovic A, et al. Asthma endotypes: a new approach to classification of disease entities within the asthma syndrome. J Allergy Clin Immunol. 2011;127:355-60.

3. Nakawah MO, Hawkins C, Barbandi F. Asthma, chronic obstructive pulmonary disease (COPD) and the overlap syndrome. J Am Board Fam Med. 2013;26(4):470-77.
4. Borish L, Culp JA. Asthma: a syndrome composed of heterogenous diseases. Ann Allergy Asthma Immunolo. 2008;101(1):1-8.
5. Lai CK, Beasley R, Crane J, Foliaki S, Shah J, Weiland S, et al. Global variation in the prevalence and severity of asthma symptoms: phase three of the International Study of Asthma and Allergies in Childhood (ISAAC). Thorax. 2009;64(6):476-83.
6. Bousquet J, Dahl R, Khaltaev N. Global alliance against chronic respiratory disease. Eur Respir J. 2007;29(2):233-9.
7. Global initiative for asthma. NHLBI/WHO Workshop Report: Global Strategy for Asthma. N.I.H. Publication No. 02-3659 Revised 2007-8.
8. Torén K, Brisman J, Jarvholm B. Asthma and asthma-like symptoms in adults assessed by questionnaire. A literature review. Chest. 1993;104(2):600-8.
9. Jindal SK. Bronchial asthma: the Indian scene. Curr Opin Pulm Med. 2007;13(1):8-12.
10. Chowgule RV, Shetye VM, Parmar JR, Bhosale AM, Khandagale MR, Phalnitkar SV, et al. Prevalence of respiratory symptoms, bronchial hyperreactivity, and asthma in a megacity. Results of the European community respiratory health survey in Mumbai (Bombay). Am J Respir Crit Care Med. 1998;158(2):547-54.
11. Aggarwal AN, Chaudhry K, Chhabra S, D'Souza GA, Gupta D, Jindal SK, et al. Prevalence and risk factors for bronchial asthma in Indian adults: A multicentre study. Indian J Chest Dis Allied Sci. 2006;48(1):13-22.
12. Chhabra SK, Gupta CK, Chhabra P, Rajpal S. Prevalence of bronchial asthma in schoolchildren in Delhi. J Asthma. 1998;35(3):291-6.
13. Shah JR, Amdekar YK, Mathur RS. Nationwide variation in prevalence of bronchial asthma. Indian J Med Sci. 2000;6:213-20.
14. Gupta D, Aggarwal AN, Kumar R, Jindal SK. Prevalence of bronchial asthma and association with environmental tobacco smoke exposure in adolescent school children in Chandigarh, North India. J Asthma. 2001;38(6):501-7.
15. Paramesh H. Epidemiology of asthma in India. Indian J Pediatr. 2002;69(4):309-12.
16. Chakravarthy S, Singh RB, Swaminathan S, Venkatesan P. Prevalence of asthma in urban and rural children in Tamil Nadu. Natl Med J India. 2002;15(5):260-3.
17. Mistry R, Wickramasingha N, Ogston S, Singh M, Devasiri V, Mukhopadhyay S. Wheeze and urban variation in South Asia. Eur J Pediatr. 2004;163(3):145-7.
18. Awasthi S, Kalra E, Roy S, Awasthi S. Prevalence and risk factors of asthma and wheeze in school-going children in Lucknow, North India. Indian Pediatr. 2004;41(12):1205-10.
19. Pakhale S, Wooldrage K, Manfreda J, Anthonisen N. Prevalence of asthma symptoms in 7th and 8th grade school children in a rural region in India. J Asthma. 2008;45(2):117-22.
20. Jindal SK, Aggarwal AN, Gupta D, Agarwal R, Kumar R, Kaur T, et al. Indian study on epidemiology of asthma, respiratory symptoms and chronic bronchitis in adults (INSEARCH). Int J Tuberc Lung Dis. 2012;16:1270-77.
21. Agrawal S, Pearce N, Ebrahim S. Prevalence and risk factors for self-reported asthma in an adult Indian population: a cross-sectional survey. Int J Tuberc Lung Dis. 2013;17:275-82.
22. Song WJ, Kang MG, Chang YS, Chox SH. Epidemiology of adult asthma in Asia: toward a better understanding. Asia Pac Allergy. 2014;4:75-85.
23. Agarwal R. Allergic bronchopulmonary aspergillosis. Chest. 2009;135(3):805-26.
24. Accordini S, Bugiani M, Arossa W, Gerzeli S, Marinoni A, Olivieri M, et al. Poor control increases the economic cost of asthma. A multicentre population-based study. Int Arch Allergy Immunol. 2006;141(2):189-98.
25. Murthy KJR, Sastery JG. Economic burden of asthma: NCMH Report- Background paper. [online] Available from *www.whoindia.org/non-communicable diseases.* [Accessed Februrary 2016].
26. Holloway JW, Beghé B, Holgate ST. The genetic basis of atopic asthma. Clin Exp Allergy. 1999;29(8):1023-32.
27. Israel E, Chinchilli VM, Ford JG, Boushey HA, Cherniack R, Craig TJ, et al. Use of regulatory scheduled albuterol treatment in asthma: genotype-stratified, randomized, placebo-controlled crossover trial. Lancet. 2004;364 (9444):1505-12.
28. Ito K, Chung KF, Adcock IM. Update on glucocorticoid action and resistance. J Allergy Clin Immunol. 2006;117(3):522-43.
29. Drazen J, Weiss ST. Genetics: inherit the wheeze. Nature. 2002;418(6896):383-4.
30. Tattersfield AE, Hall IP. Are beta2-adrenoceptor polymorphisms important in asthma—an unravelling story. Lancet. 2004;364(9444):1464-6.
31. Holloway JW, Yang IA, Holgate ST. Genetics of allergic disease. J Allergy Clin Immunol. 2010;125 (2 Suppl 2):S81-94.
32. Howard TD, Postma DS, Jongepier H, Moore WC, Koppelman GH, Zheng SL, et al. Association of a disintegrin and metalloprotease 33 (ADAM33) gene with asthma in ethnically diverse populations. J Allergy Clin Immunol. 2003;112(4):717-22.
33. Sonnenschein-van der Voort AM, Arends LR, de Jongste JC, Annesi-Maesano I, Arshad SH, Barros H, et al. Preterm birth, infant weight gain, and childhood asthma risk: a meta-analysis of 147,000 European children. J allergy Clin Immunol. 2014;133:1317-29.
34. Beuther DA, Weiss ST, Sutherland ER. Obesity and asthma. Am J Respir Crit Care Med. 2006;174(2):112-9.
35. Sutherland ER. Linking obesity and asthma. Ann N Y Acad Sci. 2014;1311:31-41.
36. Jindal SK. Effects of smoking on asthma. J Ass Phy India (Suppl.). 2014;62:32-7.
37. Siroux V, Pin I, Oryszczyn MP, Le Moual N, Kauffmann F. Relationships of active smoking to asthma and asthma severity in the EGEA study. Epidemiological study on the Genetics and Environment of Asthma. Eur Respir J. 2000;15(3):470-7.
38. US Environmental Protection Agency. Respiratory health effects of passive smoking: lung cancer and other disorders. Office of Research and Development: Washington DC; 1992. EPA/600/ 6-90/006F.
39. De Koning HW, Smith KR, Last JM. Biomass fuel combustion and health. Bull World Health Organ. 1985;63(1):11-26.
40. Wahn U, Lau S, Bergmann R, Kulig M, Forster J, Bergmann K, et al. Indoor allergen exposure is a risk factor for sensitization during the first three years of life. J Allergy Clin Immunol. 1997;99 (6 Pt 1):763-9.
41. Sporik R, Holgate ST, Platts-Mills TA, Cogswell JJ. Exposure to house-dust mite allergen (Der p 1) and the development of asthma in childhood. A prospective study. N Engl J Med. 1990;323(8):502-7.

42. Sears MR, Greene JM, Willan AR, Wiecek EM, Taylor DR, Flannery EM, et al. A longitudinal, population-based, cohort study of childhood asthma followed to adulthood. N Engl J Med. 2003;349(15):1414-22.
43. Ownby DR, Johnson CC, Peterson EL. Exposure to dogs and cats in the first year of life and risk of allergic sensitization at 6 to 7 years of age. JAMA. 2002;288(8):963-72.
44. Gern JE, Reardon CL, Hoffjan S, Nicolae D, Li Z, Roberg KA, et al. Effects of dog ownership and genotype on immune development and atopy in infancy. J Allergy Clin Immunol. 2004;113(2):307-14.
45. Almqvist C, Egmar AC, Van Hage-Hamsten M, Berglind N, Pershagen G, Nordvall SL, et al. Heredity, pet ownership, and confounding control in a population-based birth cohort. J Allergy Clin Immunol. 2003;111(4):800-6.
46. Gern JE, Busse WW. Relationship of viral infections to wheezing illnesses and asthma. Nat Rev Immunol. 2002;2(2):132-8.
47. Strachan DP. Hay fever, hygiene, and household size. BMJ. 1989;299(6710):1259-60.
48. McDonnell WF, Abbey DE, Nishino N, Lebowitz MD. Long-term ambient ozone concentration and the incidence of asthma in nonsmoking adults: the AHSMOG Study. Environ Res. 1999;80(2 Pt 1):110-21.
49. Kraft M. The role of bacterial infections in asthma. Clin Chest Med. 2000;21(2):301-13.
50. Martin RJ, Kraft M, Chu HW, Berns EA, Cassell GH. A link between chronic asthma and chronic infection. J Allergy Clin Immunol. 2001;107(4):595-601.
51. Leonardi-Bee J, Pritchard D, Britton J. Asthma and current intestinal parasite infection: systematic review and meta-analysis. Am J Respir Crit Care Med. 2006;174(5):514-23.
52. Malo JL, Lemiere C, Gautrin D, Labrecque M. Occupational asthma. Curr Opin Pulm Med. 2004;10(1):57-61.
53. Sastre J, Vandenplas O, Park HS. Pathogenesis of occupational asthma. Eur Respir J. 2003;22(2):364-73.
54. Tarlo SM, Lemiere C. Occupational asthma. N Engl J Med. 2014;370:640-9.
55. Trevor J, Antony V, Jindal SK. The effect of biomass fuel exposure on the prevalence of asthma in adults in India–review of current evidence. J Asthma. 2014;51:136-41.
56. American Thoracic Society. What constitutes an adverse health effect of air pollution? Official statement of the American Thoracic Society. Am J Respir Crit Care Med. 2000;161 (2 Pt 1):665-73.
57. Dezateux C, Stocks J, Dundas I, Fletcher ME. Impaired airway function and wheezing in infancy: the influence of maternal smoking and a genetic predisposition to asthma. Am J Respir Crit Care Med. 1999;159(2):403-10.
58. Agarkhedkar SR, Bapat HB, Bapat BN. Avoidance of food allergens in childhood asthma. Indian Pediatr. 2005;42(4):362-6.
59. Jain P, Kant S, Mishra R. Perception of dietary food items as food allergens in asthmatic individuals in north Indian population. J Am Coll Nutr. 2011;30:274-83.
60. Gibson PG. Inflammatory phenotypes in adult asthma: clinical applications. Clin Respir J. 2009;3(4):198-206.
61. Lemanske RF, Busse WW. Asthma: clinical expression and molecular mechanisms. J Allergy Clin Immunol. 2010;125(2 Suppl 2):S95-102.

Allergic Rhinitis, Asthma and Comorbidities

Ruby Pawankar, Satoko Kimura, Sachiko Mori, Yukiko Yokoyama, Miyuki Hayashi, Shingo Yamanishi

INTRODUCTION

The prevalence of both allergic rhinitis (AR) and asthma are rising to epidemic proportions, especially in children who bear the greatest brunt of these diseases.[1-4] While AR is an immunoglobin E (IgE)-mediated inflammation of the nasal mucosa, IgE-mediated inflammation of the airways can manifest as AR and also as asthma or both. Approximately 80% of patients with asthma have AR, and rhinitis is a major independent risk factor for asthma in cross-sectional and longitudinal studies.[5-7] Moreover, AR is the strongest predictor as risk for asthma[8] and serum IgE levels have been shown to be associated with persistent wheeze in preschool children.[9]

While the temporal relation of AR and asthma diagnosis may be variable, AR often precedes asthma. Moreover, AR is linked to other comorbid conditions like chronic hyperplastic eosinophilic sinusitis, nasal polyposis, otitis media with effusion and sleep disorders. Also, children with AR have been shown to have increased number of respiratory tract infections and longer durations of each infection.[10]

Over 400 million patients worldwide suffer from AR and 300 million people suffer from asthma. Both AR and asthma are chronic inflammatory diseases of the airways and their inflammatory mechanisms are characterized by an inflammatory infiltrate made up of eosinophils, T cells and mast cells that release several mediators, chemokines and cytokines, local and systemic IgE synthesis, and a systemic link via the bone marrow. Studies have shown that patients with AR exhibit bronchial hyperresponsiveness (BHR) and increase in inflammatory cells, and that nasal allergen challenge further increases this hyperreactivity.[11,12] This potential link may be due to crosstalk between the upper and lower airway, the direct impact of inflammatory mediators released locally and to the systemic link between the two.

Although there are cardinal structural differences between the upper and lower airways, the relationships between rhinitis and asthma can be viewed under the concept that the two conditions may be the manifestations of one syndrome, the "chronic allergic respiratory syndrome." Moreover, the impact on costs, frequency of emergency room visits, hospitalization and quality of life is greater, if AR is associated with asthma as compared to asthma alone[13,14] and treating AR in patients with asthma, and comorbid AR has shown to reduce hospitalization by 61%.[15]

INFLAMMATION IN ALLERGIC RHINITIS

Upon allergen exposure, sensitized mast cells degranulate within minutes to release preformed and newly synthesized mediators that include histamine, proteases, cysteinyl leukotrienes (CysLTs), prostaglandins and cytokines; some of which induce the characteristic early phase symptoms of AR, while others orchestrate the late phase response via the infiltration of inflammatory cells, like eosinophils, basophils and T cells, into the nasal mucosa.[16,17] This infiltration of inflammatory cells can also be orchestrated by T-helper type 2 (Th2) cells within the local microenvironment. The subsequent release of additional mediators from these inflammatory cells, including histamine and CysLTs, sustains the inflammatory characteristic of the late phase reaction. In chronic ongoing allergen inflammation, mast cells exhibit increased histamine releasability consequent to the enhanced FcεRI expression (increased numbers of IgE receptors) and surface-bound IgE, as well as the enhancement of signal transduction pathways.[17-21] While these processes together induce the phenomenon of priming, mast cells in patients with AR also express increased levels of β1 integrins and activation via the integrin receptors results in an enhanced release of inflammatory mediators even in the presence of lower amounts of allergen.[14-18] This process may, in part, contribute to the phenomenon of nasal hyperresponsiveness.

LINK BETWEEN ALLERGIC RHINITIS AND ASTHMA

Epidemiology and Trigger Factors

Allergic rhinitis and asthma are closely linked based on a variety of parameters ranging from epidemiologic, immunologic and clinical evidences.[22] Epidemiologically, up to 40% patients with AR have comorbid asthma and up to 80% of patients with asthma experience nasal symptoms. Furthermore, in a study assessing the burden of AR in children, the prevalence of asthma was 3-fold higher in those children who had AR at baseline.[23] The trigger factors of AR, like indoor and outdoor allergens, can also cause asthma.

Inflammation and Pathomechanisms

Both AR and asthma are inflammatory diseases and their inflammatory mechanisms are similar in a way that they are characterized by an inflammatory infiltrate made up of eosinophils, T cells and mast cells that release several mediators, chemokines and cytokines, local and systemic IgE synthesis, and a systemic link via the bone marrow. Typical early- and late-phase responses are also common features to both rhinitis and asthma. Studies have shown that patients with AR exhibit BHR and increased number of inflammatory cells in their bronchial mucosa.[8,9] This increase in bronchial inflammation in response to allergen-induced rhinitis might contribute to the exacerbations of asthma frequently seen in individuals with underlying AR. Experimental studies in patients with seasonal allergic rhinitis (SAR) without asthma have demonstrated an upregulation of adhesion molecule expression, eosinophil infiltration in both the upper and lower airways, after nasal allergen challenge and increased bronchial hyperreactivity.[24] These results demonstrate that an allergic nasal reaction produces systemic inflammatory changes.

Systemic Inflammation in Allergic Rhinitis

Allergic rhinitis is not associated with just localized inflammation of the nasal mucosa but also has a systemic component to it. This may explain in a significant way the mechanisms underlying the rhinitis-asthma link. Thus, in patients with AR, allergen exposure results in the activation of immune cells, including Th2 lymphocytes. Some of these Th2 cells migrate to the bone marrow, where they stimulate the bone marrow to produce and recruit inflammatory cells, i.e. basophils, eosinophils and mast cell precursors to the inflamed target tissues. The selective recruitment of inflammatory cells into the lower airways can occur only in those individuals, with at least subclinical inflammation in the lower airways, in whom specific adhesion molecules, such as vascular cell adhesion molecule 1 and chemoattractants, such as thymus and activation-regulated chemokine (TARC) and eotaxin, are already upregulated. This parallel relationship is influenced by many interactions between the nose and the lower airways in that the nose plays a major homeostatic role by conditioning inhaled air, but perhaps even more important is the bidirectional interaction that results from the systemic inflammation that is produced after local allergic reactions.

Therapeutic Outcomes of Treating Allergic Rhinitis in Asthma

Several studies have shown that treating comorbid AR results in a lowered risk of asthma-related resource utilizations and hospitalizations.[15] For patients with asthma, the presence of comorbid AR is associated with higher total annual medical costs as well as increased likelihood of asthma-related hospital admissions and emergency visits.[13,14] Thus, there is a clear evidence that comorbid AR can be an indicator marker for more difficult-to-control asthma or poor asthma outcomes. In a recent international survey on the impact of concomitant AR and asthma on patient health and quality of life, the presence of AR in children with asthma disrupted their lives by limiting their ability to get a good night sleep, concentrate at work/school or enjoy social activities and that when AR symptoms flared up, asthma symptoms worsened.[25] Corren et al. reported that nasal symptoms of subjects exposed to a "cat room" were more severe if they had concomitant asthma than if they had rhinitis alone.[26]

In a recent web-based national survey in Japan looking at asthma control in children, comorbid allergic diseases, specially rhinitis were a significant risk of uncontrolled asthma (adjusted or for severe rhinitis: 3.88, 95% CI 2.50–6.00) and the severity of rhinitis symptoms was inversely correlated with the Childhood Asthma Control Test (C-ACT) score.[27] In another study in adults, data from this large nationwide analysis provided evidence that AR along with gastroesophageal disease and acetylsalicylic acid exacerbated respiratory disease (AERD) are all common comorbidities.[28] More interestingly, severe eczema was associated with a higher prevalence of comorbid chronic health disorders, including asthma, hay fever and food allergies.[29] These findings highlight the potential for improving asthma outcomes by treating comorbid AR.

Yet there are individuals who suffer only from rhinitis, but not asthma. The precise reason for this is not completely known, but can be presumed that these patients might have a milder form of the disease. Therefore, the relationships between rhinitis and asthma can be viewed under the concept that the two conditions are manifestations of one syndrome, the chronic allergic respiratory syndrome, in two parts of the respiratory tract. At the low end of the syndrome's severity spectrum, rhinitis appears to be the sole manifestation, although pathologic abnormalities in the lower airways are already present. At the higher end, rhinitis is worse and the lower airways disease becomes clinically evident. Once manifested, the two conditions track in parallel in the terms of severity.[30]

However, AR is often underdiagnosed and poorly managed due to the lack of appreciation of the disease burden and its impact on the quality of life, socially at school and in the workplace and its huge economic burden. Thus, there was clearly a need for a global evidence-based document that would highlight the interactions between the upper and lower airways, including diagnosis, epidemiology, common risk factors, management and prevention. The allergic rhinitis and its impact on asthma (ARIA) document was first published in 2001 as a state-of-the-art document for the specialist, the general practitioner and other health care professionals.[31]

ALLERGIC RHINITIS AND ITS IMPACT ON ASTHMA

In 1999, during the ARIA, WHO workshop, an evidence-based document was produced using an extensive review of the literature available up to December 1999. The statements of evidence for the development of ARIA followed WHO rules and were based on Shekelle findings.[32]

The ARIA document was intended to be a state-of-the-art review for the specialist as well as for the general practitioner and other health care professionals:

- To update their knowledge of AR
- To highlight the impact of AR on asthma
- To provide an evidence-based documented revision on the diagnosis methods
- To provide an evidence-based revision on the treatments available
- To propose a stepwise approach to the management of the disease.

The ARIA Classification of Allergic Rhinitis

Allergic rhinitis was previously classified into seasonal, perennial and occupational. Perennial AR is usually caused by indoor allergens such as dust mites, molds, insects (cockroaches) and animal danders. SAR is related to a wide variety of outdoor allergens such as pollens or molds.

However, from a therapeutic point of view, it is often difficult to differentiate between seasonal and perennial symptoms. Some seasonal allergens cause perennial symptoms, some perennial allergens may cause symptoms only during certain periods of the year and the majority of patients are now polysensitized to seasonal and perennial allergens. Therefore, a new classification to provide a better description of AR has been proposed by the ARIA as "intermittent" or "persistent" rhinitis **(Fig. 1)**.[31] The severity of AR on the other hand can be classified as "mild" or "moderate-severe" on the basis of symptoms as well as the quality of life of the patient. Several studies have now validated this classification.[33,34]

Allergic Rhinitis and its Impact on Asthma Update

The pharmacological treatment of AR proposed by ARIA is an evidence-based and stepwise approach depending on the classification of the symptoms and comprises of patient education, allergen avoidance, pharmacotherapy and validated allergen-specific immunotherapy. Nonsedating, second-generation antihistamines are the mainstay in mild-to-moderate intermittent and persistent AR. As a step up, intranasal corticosteroids (INCS) may be added. INCS is the first-line in moderate-severe persistent AR. However, subsequent research and increasing knowledge have resulted in the ARIA 2008 update which includes new information on existing therapies as well as newer therapies like anti-IgE mAb and antileukotrienes with a new level of evidence for pharmacotherapy and increasing information on the link between the upper and lower airways. Most importantly ARIA emphasizes that successful management of both rhinitis and asthma requires an integrated view of the airways and an integrated approach of treatment.

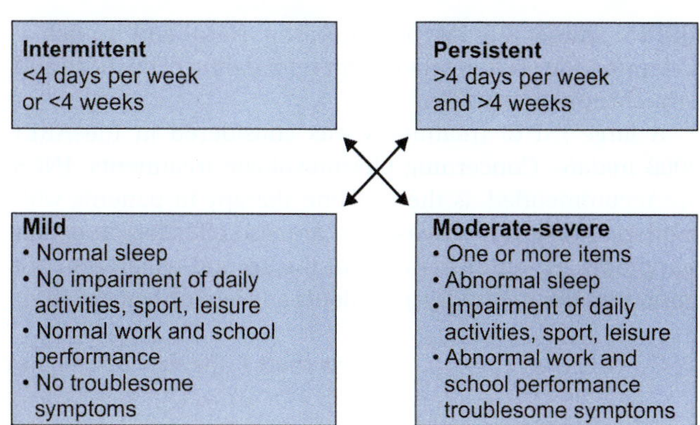

Fig. 1 The new ARIA classification

The ARIA update was commenced in 2004. Several chapters of ARIA were extensively reviewed using the Shekelle evidence-based model and papers were published in peer reviewed journals: Tertiary prevention of allergy, complementary and alternative medicine, pharmacotherapy and anti-IgE treatment, allergen-specific immunotherapy, links between rhinitis and asthma and mechanisms of rhinitis. There was then a need for a global document that would highlight the interactions between the upper and lower airways, including diagnosis, epidemiology, common risk factors, management and prevention. Moreover, the allergy perspective should also be targeted toward developing countries. Thus, the ARIA 2008 update was published.[35-39]

One important aspect of the ARIA update was to consider the comorbidities of AR and in particular, asthma. Epidemiologic studies have consistently shown that asthma and rhinitis often coexist in the same patients in every region of the world. The vast majority of patients with asthma have rhinitis, but the prevalence of asthma in rhinitis patients still needs to be assessed. Adults and children with asthma and documented concomitant AR experience more asthma-related hospitalizations and physician visits and incur higher asthma drug costs than adults with asthma alone. These patients also experience more frequent absence from work and decreased productivity. However, some studies have not shown such an association.

Many patients with AR have an increased bronchial reactivity to methacholine or histamine, especially during and sometime after the pollen season. Nasal and bronchial inflammation is often related, but remodeling of the nose and bronchi appears to differ.

A large list of treatments was considered in the ARIA 2008 update. Concerning pharmacologic treatments, INCS are recommended as the first-line therapy in patients with moderate-to-severe disease and are also effective on ocular symptoms, H_1-antihistamines of the second-generation are important treatments for all patients and leukotriene receptor antagonists are particularly important for patients with rhinitis and asthma. On the other hand, tertiary prevention of allergy is still a matter of debate since clinical trials do not usually show any efficacy of single allergen avoidance measures. Allergen-specific immunotherapy in patients with AR has a prolonged preventive effect on the development of asthma when stopped. Sublingual allergen-specific immunotherapy has proven to be a safe and effective treatment,[40] but clinical trials need to be standardized.

Flow chart 1 The algorithm for the treatment of AR recommended by ARIA

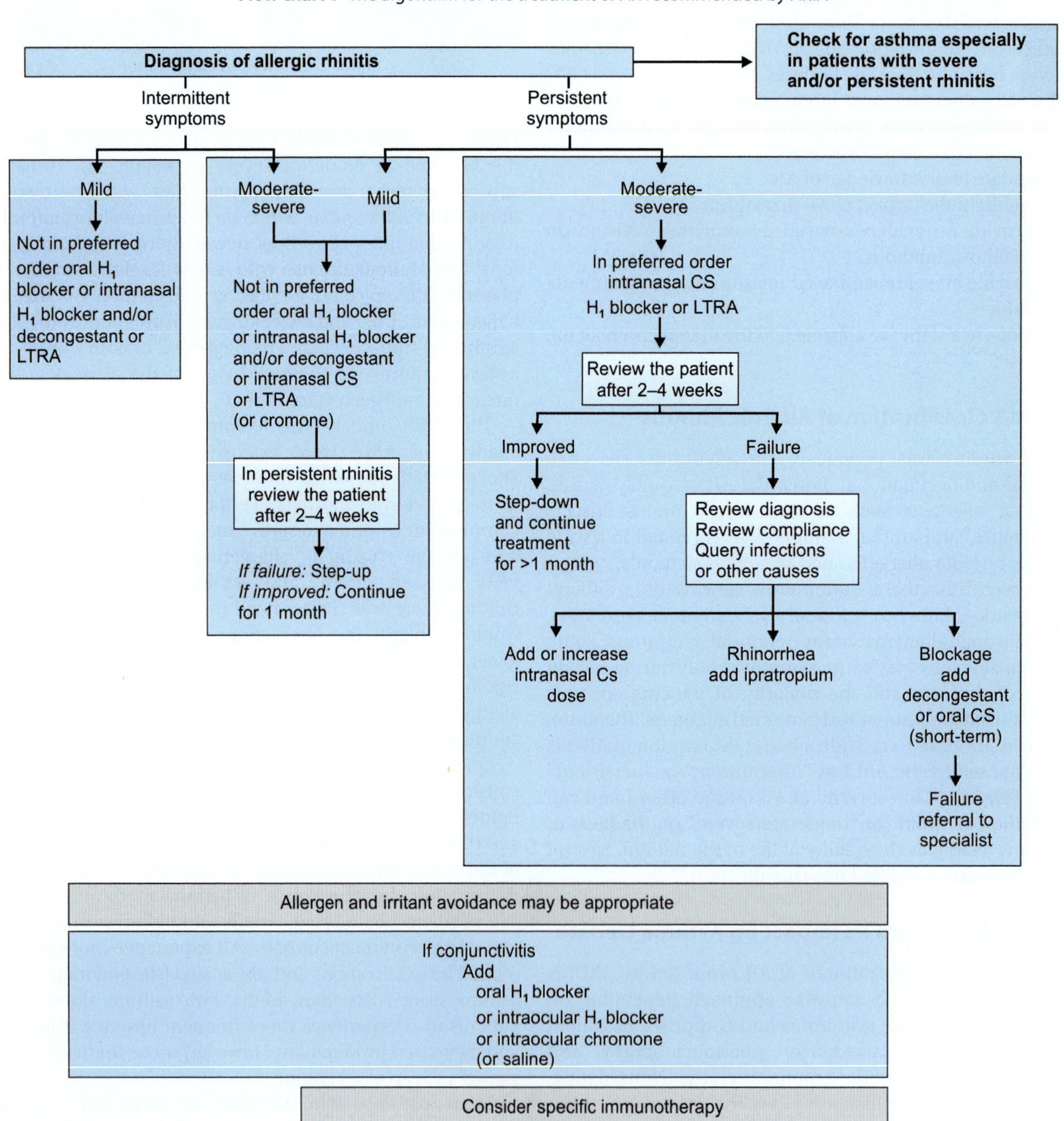

Abbreviations: CS, corticosteroids; LTRA, leukotriene receptor antagonist

Mechanistic studies have repeatedly demonstrated that sublingual swallow immunotherapy (SLIT) is able to affect the T response by modulating some of the activities of T regulatory cells. Recent studies have shown the dose-dependency of the clinical effects of SLIT and the magnitude of the effect over placebo largely exceeded the 20% suggested threshold, required for defining an immunotherapy as clinically effective and that SLIT has been formally shown the capability of reducing both the direct and indirect costs of the disease. A new World Allergy Organization (WAO) consensus document on SLIT has summarized the state-of-the-art on SLIT with relevant recommendations.[41] Specific immunotherapy, allergen avoidance and pharmacotherapy have come to be the recommended form of treatment for allergic diseases, both in adults and children. An algorithm of the management of AR is provided **(Flow chart 1)**. The ARIA guidelines was then updated in 2010 and recommendations were made based on the GRADE (Grading of Recommendations Assessment, Development and Evaluation) level of evidence base approach.[42]

OTHER COMORBIDITIES OF ALLERGIC RHINITIS

Allergic rhinitis (AR) is linked to other comorbid conditions like rhinosinusitis, nasal polyps, sleep disturbances like obstructive sleep apnea (OSA) and otitis media with effusion **(Fig. 2)**. As many as 70% of patients with AR reported suffer from nasal and ocular symptoms. Acute sinusitis is found to be more common in patients with AR and eustachian tube obstruction has been shown to increase in the peak season in patients with SAR. AR interferes with sleep and leads to increased daytime sleepiness. AR patients reported difficulty falling asleep, nocturnal awakening, early awakening, nonrestorative sleep, lack of sleep and snoring.

The socioeconomic burden via annual costs of treating asthma and AR—both direct costs (hospitalization, medications) and indirect costs (time lost from work, premature death)—are substantial and represent an even heavier burden in societies with emerging economies. In eight countries in

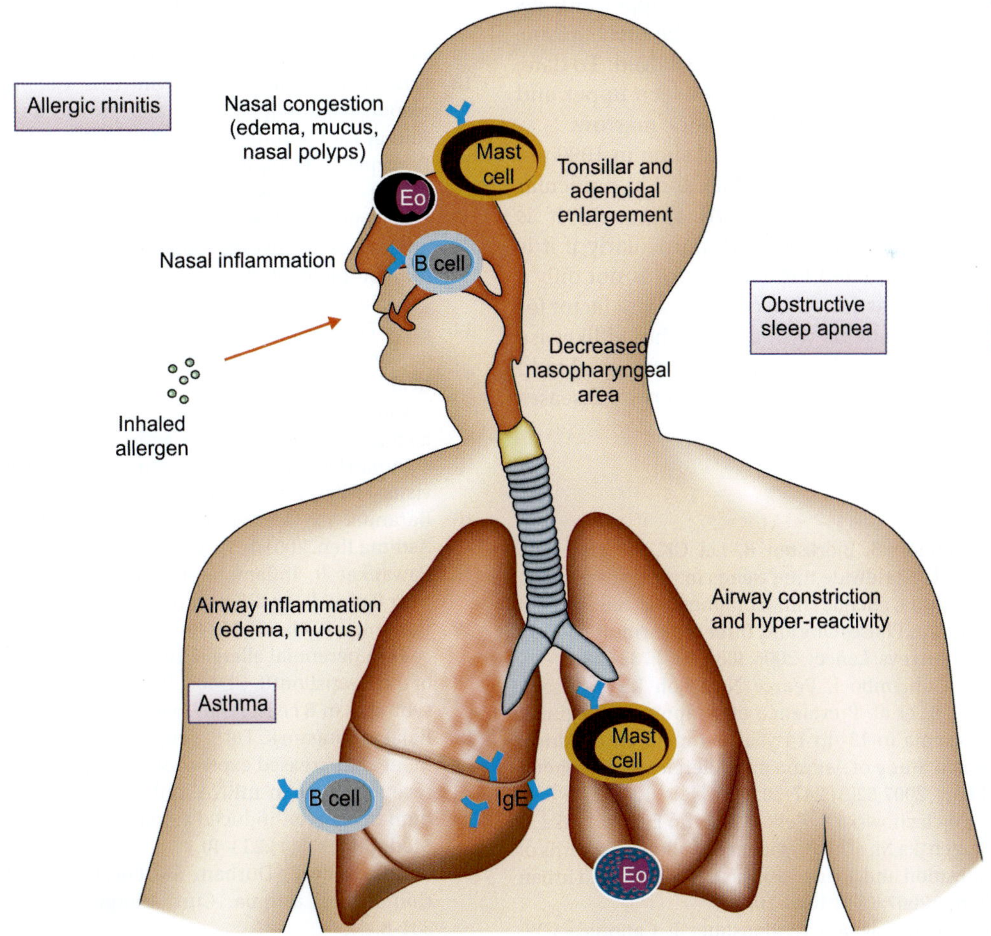

Fig. 2 Chronic allergic respiratory syndrome

Source: Stokes JR, Casale TB. Allergic rhinitis, asthma and obstructive sleep apnea: The link. In: Pawankar R, Holgate ST, Rosenwasser LJ (Eds). Allergy Frontiers Epigenetics to Future Perspective. Springer Science and Business Media; 2009.

the Asia-Pacific, the annual per patient direct costs ranged from US $108 to US $1,010, total per patient costs, including productivity costs, ranged from US $184 to US $1,189.[43] The treatment of AR is shown to improve coexisting conditions, including conjunctivitis, asthma, rhinosinusitis, otitis media with effusion and sleep disorders.

CONCLUSION

Asthma and AR are the most common manifestations of the atopic syndrome followed by atopic eczema and food allergy. Epidemiologic, experimental and clinical data highlight the importance of this link. Although the diseases commonly occur together, it is still unclear why some allergic patients develop only asthma and others only rhinitis. The reason for the variety in clinical expression of allergic airway disease is not known. Besides a genetic predisposition, environmental factors contribute to the development of the allergic phenotype. Local and systemic inflammatory processes also seem to be involved. However, their exact contribution to the clinical picture of airway allergy still remains to be elucidated. Although it is clear that the condition of the upper airways has an impact on lower airway physiology, the mechanisms underlying this relation are far from being resolved. To date, most data point toward a systemic link between upper and lower airways involving bloodstream and bone marrow.

The recommendations of the ARIA workshop in 1999 are still valid with respect to the ARIA update and in particular the ARIA 2010 update by the GRADE approach, it is recommended that all patients with AR, particularly if it is persistent, should be evaluated for asthma. AR is not only a risk factor for underlying asthma, but could be a risk factor for asthma exacerbations. Patients with asthma should likewise be evaluated for rhinitis and a combined strategy should ideally be used to treat the upper and lower airway diseases in the terms of efficacy and safety.

REFERENCES

1. Asher MI, Montefort S, Bjorksten B, Lai CK, Strachan DP, Weiland SK, et al. Worldwide time trends in the prevalence of symptoms of asthma, allergic rhinoconjunctivitis, and eczema in childhood: ISAAC Phases One and Three repeat multicountry cross-sectional surveys. Lancet. 2006;368(9537):733-43.
2. Ait-Khaled N, Odhiambo J, Pearce N, Adjoh KS, Maesano IA, Benhabyles B, et al. Prevalence of symptoms of asthma, rhinitis and eczema in 13- to 14-year-old children in Africa: the International Study of Asthma and Allergies in Childhood Phase III. Allergy. 2007;62(3):247-58.
3. Majkowska-Wojciechowska B, Pelka J, Korzon L, Kozłowska A, Kaczała M, Jarzebska M, et al. Prevalence of allergy, patterns of allergic sensitization and allergy risk factors in rural and urban children. Allergy. 2007;62(9):1044-50.
4. Pawankar R, Baena-Cagnani C, Bousquet J, Canonica GW, Cruz AA, Kaliner MA, et al. State of world allergy report 2008: allergy and chronic respiratory diseases. World Allergy Organ J. 2008;1(6):S4-17.
5. Linneberg A, Henrik Nielsen N, Frølund L, Madsen F, Dirksen A, Jørgensen T, et al. The link between allergic rhinitis and allergic asthma: a prospective population-based study. The Copenhagen Allergy Study. Allergy. 2002;57(11):1048-52.
6. Leynaert B, Neukirch C, Kony S, Guénégou A, Bousquet J, Aubier M, et al. Association between asthma and rhinitis according to atopic sensitization in a population-based study. J Allergy Clin Immunol. 2004;113(1):86-93.
7. Downie SR, Andersson M, Rimmer J, Leuppi JD, Xuan W, Akerlund A, et al. Association between nasal and bronchial symptoms in subjects with persistent allergic rhinitis. Allergy. 2004;59(3):320-6.
8. Shaaban R, Zureik M, Soussan D, Neukirch C, Heinrich J, Sunyer J, et al. Rhinitis and onset of asthma: a longitudinal population-based study. Lancet. 2008;372(9643):1049-57.
9. Simpson A, Soderstrom L, Ahlstedt S, Murray CS, Woodcock A, Custovic A. IgE antibody quantification and the probability of wheeze in preschool children. J Allergy Clin Immunol. 2005;116(4):744-9
10. Ciprandi G, Tosca MA, Fasce L. Allergic children have more numerous and severe respiratory infections than non-allergic children. Pediatr Allergy Immunol. 2006;17(5):389-91.
11. Chakir J, Laviolette M, Turcotte H, Boutet M, Boulet LP. Cytokine expression in the lower airways of nonasthmatic subjects with allergic rhinitis: influence of natural allergen exposure. J Allergy Clin Immunol. 2000;106(5):904-10.
12. Corren J, Adinoff AD, Irvin CG. Changes in bronchial responsiveness following nasal provocation with allergen. J Allergy Clin Immunol. 1992;89(2):611-8.
13. Bousquet J, Gaugris S, Kocevar VS, Zhang Q, Yin DD, Polos PG, et al. Increased risk of asthma attacks and emergency visits among asthma patients with allergic rhinitis: a subgroup analysis of the investigation of montelukast as a partner agent for complementary therapy [corrected]. Clin Exp Allergy. 2005;35(6):723-7.
14. Price D, Zhang Q, Kocevar VS, Yin DD, Thomas M. Effect of a concomitant diagnosis of allergic rhinitis on asthma-related health care use by adults. Clin Exp Allergy. 2005;35(3):282-7.
15. Crystal-Peters J, Neslusan C, Crown WH, Torres A. Treating allergic rhinitis in patients with comorbid asthma: the risk of asthma-related hospitalizations and emergency department visits. J Allergy Clin Immunol. 2002;109(1):57-62.
16. Baraniuk JN. Mechanisms of allergic rhinitis. Curr Allergy Asthma Rep. 2001;1(3):207-17.
17. Pawankar R. Inflammatory mechanisms in allergic rhinitis. Curr Opin Allergy Clin Immunol. 2007;7(1):1-4.
18. Pawankar R, Okuda M, Yssel H, Okumura K, Ra C. Nasal mast cells in perennial allergic rhinitis exhibit increased expression of the Fc epsilonRI, CD40L, IL-4, and IL-13, and can induce IgE synthesis in B cells. J Clin Invest. 1997;99(7):1492-9.
19. Rajakulasingam K, Till S, Ying S, Humbert M, Barkans J, Sullivan M, et al. Increased expression of high affinity Ig (FcεpsilonRI) receptor-α chain mRNA and protein-bearing eosinophils in human allergen-induced atopic asthma. Am J Respir Crit Care Med. 1998;158(1):233-40.
20. Smurthwaite L, Durham SR. Local IgE synthesis in allergic rhinitis and asthma. Curr Allergy Asthma Rep. 2002;2(3):231-8.
21. Pawankar R, Yamagishi S, Yagi T. Revisiting the roles of mast cells in allergic rhinitis and its relation to local IgE synthesis. Am J Rhinol. 2000;14(5):309-17.

22. Corren J. Allergic rhinitis and asthma: how important is the link? J Allergy Clin Immunol. 1997;99(2):S781-6.
23. Meltzer EO, Blaiss MS, Derebery MJ, Mahr TA, Gordon BR, Sheth KK, et al. Burden of allergic rhinitis: results from the Pediatric Allergies in America survey. J Allergy Clin Immunol. 2009;124(Suppl 3):S43-70.
24. Braunstahl GJ, Overbeek SE, Kleinjan A, Prins JB, Hoogsteden HC, Fokkens WJ. Nasal allergen provocation induces adhesion molecule expression and tissue eosinophilia in upper and lower airways. J Allergy Clin Immunol. 2001;107(3):469-76.
25. Valovirta E, Pawankar R. Survey on the impact of comorbid allergic rhinitis in patients with asthma. BMC Pulm Med. 2006;6(Suppl 1):S3.
26. Corren J, Spector S, Fuller L, Minkwitz M, Mezzanotte W. Effects of zafirlukast upon clinical, physiologic, and inflammatory responses to natural cat allergen exposure. Ann Allergy Asthma Immunol. 2001;87(3):211-7.
27. Sasaki M, Yoshida K, Adachi Y, Furukawa M, Itazawa T, Odajima H, et al. Factors associated with asthma control in children: findings from a national web-based survey. Pediatr Allergy Immunol. 2014;25(8):804-9.
28. Steppuhn H, Langen U, Scheidt-Nave C, Keil T. Major comorbid conditions in asthma and association with asthma-related hospitalizations and emergency department admissions in adults: results from the German National Health Telephone Interview Survey (GEDA) 2010. BMC Pulm Med. 2013;13:46.
29. Silverberg JI, Simpson EL. Association between severe eczema in children and multiple comorbid conditions and increased healthcare utilization. Pediatr Allergy Immunol. 2013;24(5):476-86.
30. Togias A. Rhinitis and asthma: evidence for respiratory system integration. J Allergy Clin Immunol. 2003;111(6):1171-83.
31. Bousquet J, Van Cauwenberge P, Khaltaev N. Aria Workshop Group; World Health Organization. Allergic rhinitis and its impact on asthma. J Allergy Clin Immunol. 2001;108(Suppl 5):S147-334.
32. Shekelle PG, Woolf SH, Eccles M, Grimshaw J. Clinical guidelines: developing guidelines. BMJ. 1999;318(7183):593-6.
33. Demoly P, Allaert FA, Lecasble M, Bousquet J. PRAGMA. Validation of the classification of ARIA (allergic rhinitis and its impact on asthma). Allergy. 2003;58(7):672-5.
34. Van Hoecke H, Vastesaeger N, Dewulf L, De Bacquer D, van Cauwenberge PB. Is the allergic rhinitis and its impact on asthma classification useful in daily primary care practice? J Allergy Clin Immunol. 2006;118(3):758-9.
35. Passalacqua G, Bousquet PJ, Carlsen KH, Kemp J, Lockey RF, Niggemann B, et al. ARIA update: I—Systematic review of complementary and alternative medicine for rhinitis and asthma. J Allergy Clin Immunol. 2006;117(5):1054-62.
36. Bonini S, Bonini M, Bousquet J, Brusasco V, Canonica GW, Carlsen KH, et al. Rhinitis and asthma in athletes: an ARIA document in collaboration with GA2LEN. Allergy. 2006;61(6):681-92.
37. Bousquet J, van Cauwenberge P, Ait Khaled N, Bachert C, Baena-Cagnani CE, Bouchard J, et al. Pharmacologic and anti-IgE treatment of allergic rhinitis ARIA update (in collaboration with GALEN). Allergy. 2006;61(9):1086-96.
38. Passalacqua G, Durham SR. Allergic rhinitis and its impact on asthma update: allergen immunotherapy. J Allergy Clin Immunol. 2007;119(4):881-91.
39. Cruz AA, Popov T, Pawankar R, Annesi-Maesano I, Fokkens W, Kemp J, et al. Common characteristics of upper and lower airways in rhinitis and asthma: ARIA update, in collaboration with GA(2)LEN. Allergy. 2007;62 (Suppl 84):1-41.
40. Passalacqua G, Pawankar R, Baena-Cagnani CE, Canonica GW. Sublingual immunotherapy: where do we stand? Present and future. Curr Opin Allergy Clin Immunol. 2009;9(1):1-3.
41. Canonica GW, Bousquet J, Casale T, Lockey RF, Baena-Cagnani CE, Pawankar R, et al. Sub-lingual immunotherapy: World Allergy Organization Position Paper 2009. Allergy. 2009;64(Suppl 91):1-59.
42. Brozek JL, Bousquet J, Baena-Cagnani CE, Bonini S, Canonica GW, Casale TB, et al. Allergic Rhinitis and its Impact on Asthma (ARIA) guidelines: 2010 revision. J Allergy Clin Immunol. 2010; 126(3):466-76.
43. Lai CK, Kim YY, Kuo SH, Spencer M, Williams AE. Cost of asthma in the Asia-Pacific region. Eur Respir Rev. 2006;98:10-6.

Asthma Diagnosis

Liesel D'silva, Parameswaran Nair

INTRODUCTION

Correct diagnosis of asthma is the first step towards achieving disease control. To establish a diagnosis of asthma, the clinician should determine that episodic symptoms of airflow obstruction or airway hyperresponsiveness are present; airflow obstruction is at least partially reversible; and alternative diagnoses are excluded. The guidelines recommend the use of a detailed medical history, a physical examination and spirometry.[1,2] Additional pulmonary function studies, bronchoprovocation tests, measures of allergic status, chest radiography and specific blood tests are not routinely necessary but may be useful when considering alternative diagnoses. Over the last 15 years, there has been increasing interest in the noninvasive biomarkers of airway inflammation as an adjunct to the assessment of clinical asthma control.

CLINICAL DIAGNOSIS

Asthma is heterogeneous in character, may manifest with different clinical phenotypes. The criteria for diagnosis may vary depending upon the phenotype with which a patient may present.

Medical History

A detailed medical history of the new patient who is known or thought to have asthma should address the following items listed in **Table 1**.[1-3]

Physical Examination

Physical examination may reveal findings **(Table 2)** that increase the probability of asthma, but the absence of these findings does not rule out asthma because asthma symptoms are variable. Therefore, examination of the respiratory system may be normal during asymptomatic periods.[1]

TESTS FOR DIAGNOSIS AND MONITORING

In 1891, Lord Kelvin (Kelvin L, 1883) emphasized the importance of measurements by stating that "When you can measure what you are speaking about and express it in numbers, you know something about it; but when you cannot measure it, when you cannot express it in numbers, your knowledge is of a meager and unsatisfactory kind".

Symptoms are nonspecific and can result from variable airflow limitation, inflammation, moderate or severe chronic airflow limitation or other respiratory and nonrespiratory conditions. There are poor correlations between symptoms and airway function or airway inflammation and between airway function and inflammation. Reliance on symptoms alone could lead to misdiagnosis and under- or overtreatment. Therefore, measurements are critical to understanding and individually treating airway disease such as asthma.[6]

Measurements of Lung Function

Although the diagnosis of asthma is usually based on the presence of characteristic symptoms, patients with asthma frequently have poor recognition of their symptoms. If their asthma is long standing they also have poor perception of symptom severity.[7] Physicians may also be inaccurate in their assessment of symptoms such as dyspnea and wheezing.[8,9] Therefore, measurement of lung function provides an objective confirmation of the diagnosis of asthma, measures severity of airflow limitation, its reversibility and variability.

Of the various methods available to assess airflow limitation, spirometry, particularly the measurement of forced expiratory volume in 1 second (FEV1), and forced vital capacity (FVC) and peak expiratory flow (PEF) measurement are widely accepted for use in patients over 5 years of age.[1]

Predicted values of FEV1, FVC and PEF based on age, sex and height have been obtained from population studies. With the exception of PEF for which the range of predicted values is too large, they are useful to assess whether a given value

Table 1 Medical history in asthma

- Symptoms that occur or worsen in the presence of precipitating factors
  - Recurrent cough
  - Wheezing
  - Shortness of breath
  - Chest tightness
  - Sputum production
- Pattern of symptoms
  - Perennial, seasonal or both
  - Continual, episodic or both
  - Onset, duration, frequency (number of days or nights, per week or month)
  - Diurnal variations, especially nocturnal and on awakening in early morning
  - Colds go to the chest or take more than 10 days to clear up
  - Symptoms improve by appropriate asthma treatment
- Precipitating and/or aggravating factors
  - Viral respiratory infections
  - Environmental allergens, indoor (e.g. mold, house-dust mite, cockroach, animal dander, mosquito repellants such as Type I synthetic pyrethroids) and outdoor (e.g. pollens, congress grass)
  - Characteristics of home including age, air conditioning system, wood-burning stove, carpeting, over concrete, presence of molds or mildew, presence of pets with fur, characteristics of rooms where patient spends time (e.g. bedroom and living-room with attention to upholstery)
  - Smoking, environmental tobacco smoke
  - Exercise
  - Occupational chemicals or allergens
  - Environmental change (e.g. moving to new home; going on vacation; and/or alterations in workplace, work processes or materials used)
  - Irritants (e.g. tobacco smoke, strong odors, air pollutants, occupational chemicals, dusts and particulates, vapors, gases and aerosols)
  - Emotions (e.g. fear, anger, frustration, hard crying or laughing)
  - Stress (e.g. fear, anger, frustration)
  - Drugs (e.g. aspirin, and other nonsteroidal anti-inflammatory drugs, beta-blockers including eyedrops, others)
  - Food (e.g. black gram), food additives, and preservatives (e.g. sulfites)
  - Changes in weather, exposure to cold air
  - Endocrine factors (e.g. menses, pregnancy, thyroid disease)
  - Comorbid conditions [e.g. sinusitis, rhinitis, nasal polyposis, gastroesophageal reflux disease, obesity, pulmonary tuberculosis*, allergic bronchopulmonary aspergillosis, obstructive sleep apnea, Churg-Strauss syndrome (very rare)]
- Development of disease and treatment
  - Age of onset and diagnosis
  - History of early-life injury to airways (e.g. bronchopulmonary dysplasia, pneumonia, parental smoking)
  - Progression of disease (whether the disease has got better or worse)
  - Present management and response to therapy, including management of exacerbations
  - Frequency of using short-acting β2 agonist (SABA)
  - Need for oral corticosteroids including dose and frequency of use
- Family history
  - History of asthma, allergy, sinusitis, rhinitis, eczema, or nasal polyps in close relatives
- Social history
  - Social factors that interfere with adherence:
    - Substance abuse
    - Social network
    - Level of literacy
    - Ability to afford the medication
    - Employment status
- History of exacerbations
  - Usual prodromal signs and symptoms
  - Rapidity of onset
  - Duration
  - Frequency
  - Severity [need for urgent care, hospitalization, intensive care unit (ICU) admission]
  - Life-threatening exacerbations (e.g. intubation, ICU admission)
  - Number and severity of exacerbations in the past year
  - Usual management (what has worked in the past to treat the exacerbation)

Contd...

Contd...

• Impact of asthma on patient and family – Episodes of unscheduled care (emergency department visits, urgent care, hospitalization) – Number of days missed from school/work – Limitation of activity, especially sports and strenuous work – History of nocturnal awakening – Effect on growth, development, behavior, school or work performance and lifestyle – Impact on family routines or activities – Economic impact • Assessment of patient's and family's perceptions of disease – Patient's, parent's and spouse's knowledge of asthma and belief in the chronicity of asthma and in the efficacy of treatment – Patient's perception and beliefs regarding use and long-term effects of medications especially inhaled corticosteroids – Ability of patient, parents or spouse to cope with the disease – Level of family support and patient's, parent's or spouse's capacity to recognize severity of an exacerbation – Economic resources – Sociocultural beliefs
*Presence of additional symptoms of fever, expectoration or chest pain should raise the suspicion of pulmonary tuberculosis. Any patient who presents with cough of more than 3 weeks duration should have the sputum examined for pulmonary tuberculosis.[4,5]

Table 2 Physical examination in asthma

System	*Physical examination findings*
Upper respiratory tract	Increased nasal secretion, mucosal swelling, deviated nasal septum, nasal polyp, tenderness over sinuses, ear discharge, oral candidiasis (because of inhaled corticosteroid therapy)
Chest	– Wheezing, wheezing during prolonged phase of forced exhalation – In severe asthma exacerbations: ▪ Wheezing may be absent, cyanosis, drowsiness, difficulty in speaking, tachycardia, hyperinflated chest, use of accessory muscles, intercostal retraction – Chronicity of asthma could lead to appearance of hunched shoulders, chest deformity
Skin	Atopic dermatitis, eczema

is abnormal or not. Caucasian prediction equations are most commonly used for the interpretation of the results of routine spirometry in India; however a study[10] was undertaken to assess the interchangeability of Caucasian and north Indian prediction equations while interpreting routine spirometric data. The use of Caucasian prediction equations resulted in poor agreement with Indian equation in most height and age categories among both men and women. One of the reasons suggested was that the lung volumes in Indian subjects are approximately 10% smaller than corresponding values in Caucasians.[11] Therefore, one needs to assess the most appropriate prediction equation for use in one's own clinical practice after considering ethnic differences in spirometric values.

Spirometry

Forced expiratory volume in 1 second and FVC are measured during a forced expiratory maneuver using a spirometer. Variable airflow limitation of asthma is recognized objectively by the presence of SABA reversibility of FEV1, i.e. greater than or equal to 12% and greater than equal to 200 mL from the prebronchodilator value;[12] however many asthma patients may not exhibit this reversibility at each assessment especially if they are on treatment. It is advisable to repeat the test at different visits. As spirometry is effort-dependent, proper instructions on how to perform the forced expiratory maneuver must be given to the patients and the highest of the three recordings selected. Spirometry should be accurately performed on appropriate equipment by trained personnel with monitoring of quality control.[12]

Spirometry with FEV1 and vital capacity (VC) values is an initial requirement and is better than PEF because it is more sensitive and discriminates between obstructive and nonobstructive ventilatory defects. FEV1/FVC ratio less than 0.75 to 0.80 in adults and less than 0.90 in children suggests airflow limitation.[12]

Normal spirometry does not rule out asthma in a patient with a history of asthma-like symptoms or in a patient taking asthma controller medications.[13] Spirometry is often useful for excluding the possibility of chronic obstructive pulmonary disease (COPD)[14] and spirometry may reveal that asthma is more poorly controlled (i.e. a low FEV1) than suggested by the frequency of symptoms and use of a rescue inhaler reported by the patient.[15] A low FEV1 is also a strong predictor of a subsequent asthma exacerbation particularly in children.[16] FEV1 can be measured accurately even during acute asthma attacks and helps to determine the need for hospitalization.[12,17]

Some of the common reasons for limited widespread use of spirometry include the lack of availability, a false belief that the test does not reveal additional information; "too time consuming" in a busy clinical practice or difficulty in interpretation of the test. General practitioners should be encouraged to use spirometry in their clinical practice.[18,19]

Peak Expiratory Flow

Although spirometry is the preferred method of documenting airflow limitation, PEF monitoring is valuable to confirm the diagnosis of asthma and to monitor the disease particularly in patients who are poor perceivers of symptoms, and to identify occupational causes of asthma symptoms.[20] There are different methods of calculation for within-day variability and between-day variability in PEF, which may be documented in patient diaries.[20,21]

One of the most common methods for calculation of "within-day variability" is the following:

$$\frac{\text{Day's highest PEF value - Day's lowest PEF value}}{\text{Mean PEF}}$$

A diurnal variability of more than 8% suggests a diagnosis of asthma.

One of the most common methods for calculation of "between-day variability" is the following:

$$\frac{\text{Lowest morning PEF over 1–2 weeks}}{\text{Highest PEF}}$$

This index increases as PEF variation decreases.

Peak expiratory flow measurements are made with peak flow meters, which are relatively inexpensive, portable, plastic instruments that can be used by patients at home. However, PEF measurements are not interchangeable with FEV1[22,23] and can underestimate the degree of airflow limitation. As the range of predicted values for PEF is too wide when measured with different peak flow meters, PEF measurements should be compared to the patient's own previous best measurements using his/her own peak flow meter.[24] PEF measurements are effort dependent and careful instruction is required to reliably measure PEF.

Key Recommendations for Clinical Practice

Encourage patients to record and monitor their lung function in a diary for the diagnosis of asthma. The upper limit of normal for diurnal variability in PEF is 8% and not the traditionally believed cut-point of 15–20%. Normal lung function does not exclude a diagnosis of asthma. Perform lung function measures accurately, on appropriate (calibrated) equipment, by trained personnel, and monitor quality control. Enter actual values of lung function in the medical records (not just normal or abnormal). Use the same peak flow meter on each occasion to compare PEF measurements within the same patient.

Measurements of Airway Responsiveness

When patients have symptoms consistent with asthma, but normal lung function, measurements of airway responsiveness to direct or indirect bronchoprovocation challenges are frequently used to establish a diagnosis of asthma; however bronchoprovocation challenge tests are not readily available in clinical practice. The direct bronchoconstrictors act on the airway smooth muscle receptors to induce bronchoconstriction. The indirect bronchoconstrictors involve an intermediate pathway, such as osmotic or nonosmotic mediator release from inflammatory cells, sensory nerve stimulation, and perhaps others and include exercise and eucapnic voluntary hyperpnea (EVH), hypertonic saline, distilled water, adenosine monophosphate and the newest challenge test which is dry powder mannitol.[25] Direct airway responsiveness has been measured primarily by histamine and methacholine. Histamine and methacholine produce near identical responses on a milligram for milligram or millimole for millimole basis;[26] however, histamine is now used infrequently because of a greater prevalence of adverse effects, such as cough, flushing and occasional syncope.[25]

Direct Challenges

Methacholine challenge is a highly sensitive test. Two of the most commonly used methods are the tidal breathing method and the dosimeter method.[27] Doubling concentrations of methacholine up to 16 mg/mL (higher for research purposes) are inhaled at 5-minute intervals from the start of one inhalation to the start of the next. Single measurements of FEV1 are made at 30 and 90 seconds. The percent reduction in FEV1 is compared with post saline FEV1, and the test is continued until there has been a 20% or more decrease in FEV1 or until the maximum concentration has been administered. The results are expressed as the provocation concentration causing a 20% FEV1 decrease (PC20 for the tidal breathing method and PD20 for the dosimeter method). A sigmoid log dose-response curve is recorded. The normal range of PC20 is greater than or equal to 8 mg/mL,[28] while that for PD20 is greater than or equal to 7.8 µmol.[29]

A positive methacholine challenge is consistent with, but not diagnostic of asthma. When a patient has current symptoms, a negative methacholine challenge result excludes asthma with reasonable certainty.[25] Methacholine challenge is of limited value in guiding treatment in patients with isolated cough because a positive methacholine challenge result does not predict response to asthma therapy,[30] and a negative methacholine challenge result fails to identify individuals with eosinophilic bronchitis and does not predict nonresponse to asthma therapy.[31] Serial monitoring of methacholine challenge may serve as a useful guide in asthma therapy,[32] but is valuable as a guide to diagnose occupational asthma.[33]

Indirect Challenges

Indirect airway challenges[34] such as exercise and EVH, hypertonic saline and dry powder mannitol create a hyperosmolar airway milieu, leading to the release of inflammatory cell mediators from mast cells and basophils. Ultrasonic nebulized distilled water is a hypoosmolar stimulus that also causes mediator release but is infrequently used. Adenosine monophosphate (AMP) results in inflammatory cell mediator release by nonosmotic mechanisms.

In contrast to the direct challenges, the indirect challenges are more specific and thus more valuable for confirming a diagnosis of asthma. Indirect challenges may be preferred for the diagnosis of occupational asthma; however this needs further study.[25] Although the indirect challenges are not sensitive enough to exclude a diagnosis of asthma, the utility of the mannitol challenge test in this area requires further study. Indirect challenge tests are the challenges of choice to evaluate individuals who may have exercise-induced bronchoconstriction and as a guide to monitor asthma treatment. A normal mannitol challenge result in a treated asthmatic patient should be taken as an indication to consider tapering of treatment. On the other hand, a persistent positive mannitol challenge result would indicate that treatment should not be tapered and might even suggest that treatment could be increased.[35] Normalization of the mannitol challenge result with inhaled corticosteroids has the potential to become a treatment goal.[36]

Key Recommendations for Clinical Practice

Histamine and methacholine challenge tests should be made more available to general practitioners through hospitals or other pulmonary function test laboratories. It is important to increase the availability of methacholine inhalation tests in general practice because this is where milder disease occurs; patient presents with symptoms but spirometry is normal, which could commonly result in misdiagnosis. A normal histamine or methacholine challenge test only reflects the current status of the patient. Normal results do not exclude past asthma which might have been reversed completely by the avoidance of allergen or occupational sensitizer, the clearing of infection or by corticosteroid treatment. In this situation, if current symptoms are present, they are of another cause than asthma.

Noninvasive Markers of Airway Inflammation

Airway inflammation (bronchitis) is an important component of all diseases of the airways of the lungs, including asthma. The inflammation has various causes (inhaled allergens, occupational chemical sensitizers, reduction of corticosteroid treatment, cigarette smoking, air pollution, bacterial or viral infections).[37] These different causes result in different types of inflammation which cause different clinical presentations and respond differently to the treatment. The use of traditional methods to indirectly assess airway inflammation from symptoms, use of reliever medication, peripheral blood eosinophilia and spirometry is problematic and, even among specialists, is frequently inaccurate.[38] Hence its measurement is beneficial, especially in specialist practice where disease is often more severe, complicated and difficult to control.

A number of noninvasive measures (in sputum, blood, urine, exhaled air) have been evaluated in clinical trials, of which only exhaled nitric oxide and quantitative sputum cell counts have reached clinical practice.[39] Use of these markers in practice is supported by published data, the GINA guidelines (since 2008) and Canadian asthma treatment guidelines (since 2007). Therefore, we will focus on these two markers in this chapter.

Although included in recent treatment guidelines, quantitative sputum cell counts and exhaled nitric oxide are available only at a few centers around the world. They are not more widely available because the introduction of new procedures into practice is difficult and physicians cannot appreciate the need for them when they are not available to use. Also, there is a perceived unpleasantness of sputum induction and skepticism related to patient and physician satisfaction with the results of cell counts.

Quantitative Sputum Cell Counts

Spontaneous or induced quantitative sputum cell counts provide the most valid, reliable, reproducible, comprehensive and specific measure of airway inflammation.[40] Sputum induction is safe,[41] has a success rate of more than 80% in adults;[42] however the success rate is somewhat lower in children, and induced sputum may not be possible in children of less than 8 years.[43] Low lung function (FEV1 less than 1 L) is a relative contraindication.[44]

Two methods have been used to induce sputum with an aerosol of hypertonic saline from an ultrasonic nebulizer. In one, the subject is pretreated with inhaled salbutamol to protect against airway constriction that could be caused by inhalation of hypertonic saline.[45] The concentration of saline and duration of inhalation is either 3% for up to 20–21 minutes or 3%, followed by 4%, followed by 5% each for 7 minutes. In the other method,[46] 4.5% hypertonic saline is given without pretreatment and inhaled for doubling times from 30 seconds to 8 minutes. Sputum plug or whole sputum can be processed with the aid of a mucolytic dithiothreitol.[47] A stained cytospin is examined to obtain a differential inflammatory (eosinophils, neutrophils, macrophages, lymphocytes and epithelial cells, expressed as a percentage based on a manual count of 400 cells) and total inflammatory cell count, cell viability and squamous cell contamination. The induced sputum supernatant can be used to assay molecular markers of inflammation and has contributed significantly to our understanding of the mechanisms of airway disease.[44] Spontaneous or induced sputum may be collected and have generally shown no differences in total or differential cell counts or concentrations of inflammatory mediators.[48] Fifty-one to eighty-two percentage of spontaneous samples have an adequate cellular viability of more than 40%.[42]

The procedure is not difficult. Sputum can be induced by a pulmonary function technologist. A dedicated hematologically or cytologically trained technologist can process and examine quantitative sputum cell counts. Sputum induction takes about 30 minutes; the results take 1.5 hour to obtain and involve 1 hour of the technologist's time.[39] A questionnaire survey demonstrated that induced sputum cell counts was well accepted by patients and physicians,[49] which further supports the need for their implementation into routine clinical practice, particularly for specialists. Normal values for total and differential cell counts (total cell count of less than 9.7 million cells/g of sputum and proportion of neutrophils less than 64% and eosinophils less than 1.1%) have been well established in healthy subjects.[50]

Sputum cell counts identify different inflammatory subtypes of bronchitis such as eosinophilic (usually normal total cell count, percentage of sputum eosinophils ≥1.1%), neutrophilic (total cell count of ≥9.7 million cells/g of sputum and proportion of neutrophils ≥64%), mixed granulocytic (total cell count ≥9.7 million cells/g of sputum and proportion of eosinophils and neutrophils ≥1.1% and ≥64% respectively) and trivial neutrophilia of unknown significance (an isolated rise in total cell count of ≥9.7 million cells/g of sputum or proportion of sputum neutrophils ≥64%).[42]

Bronchitis can be heterogeneous during stable (eosinophilic 36%, neutrophilic 14%, mixed granulocytic 6%, trivial neutrophilia 16%, normal cell counts 28%) and exacerbated asthma (eosinophilic 35%, neutrophilic 21%, mixed granulocytic 13%, trivial neutrophilia 16%, normal cell counts 15%).[42] In approximately 50% of the patients, quantitative sputum cell counts can change during successive exacerbations in the same patient.[51]

Eosinophilic bronchitis is usually noninfective. There is strong evidence that sputum eosinophilia (>3%) is a predictor of clinical improvement with corticosteroid treatment.[52] Monitoring sputum eosinophils benefited patients with moderate to severe asthma by reducing the number of eosinophilic exacerbations and decreasing the severity of all exacerbations without increasing the total inhaled corticosteroid dose.[53] In contrast, neutrophilic bronchitis is usually infective in nature; however the intensity of neutrophilia tends to differ from the trivial neutrophilia of cigarette smoking or pollutants to mild/modest and intense neutrophilia usually associated with viral and bacterial infections respectively.[39,54] When we do not have sputum cell counts to identify the type of bronchitis, it is standard practice to treat presumed infective exacerbations of asthma with both additional antibiotic and corticosteroid treatment. However most infective exacerbations are considered to be viral and will be unresponsive to antibiotic. Also corticosteroid treatment will only be expected to improve eosinophilic and not noneosinophilic exacerbations.[55]

Sputum cell counts should be examined at least twice a year in stable disease and during exacerbations; quantitative cell counts should be repeated after treatment of an exacerbation with additional corticosteroid and/or antibiotic treatment. Determining the inflammatory subtypes of bronchitis with quantitative sputum cell counts will avoid the inappropriate use of antibiotics (and reduce possible antibiotic resistance) or corticosteroids (and reduce their side effects including the potentiation of infection) and eventually lead to better management of asthma, reduce the overall cost of therapy[56] and improve the quality of life of these patients.

Exhaled Nitric Oxide

Nitric oxide is a biological mediator that plays many important physiological and pathological roles. It is synthesized from the amino acid L-arginine by the enzyme nitric oxide synthase (NOS). There are three different isoforms of NOS in the human body, of which the calcium-independent, cytokine-inducible NOS (iNOS), is the predominant isoform involved in the production of nitric oxide in the airways. Inducible NOS is present in airway epithelial and inflammatory cells of asthma patients and has been implicated in the pathogenesis of asthma. There is an upregulation of iNOS in the airways of asthmatics as part of the inflammatory response. This increased iNOS activity is responsible for an increase in exhaled nitric oxide.[57]

Fractional concentration of exhaled nitric oxide (FeNO) is best measured before spirometric maneuvers at an exhaled rate of 50 mL/second maintained within 10% for more than 6 seconds and with an oral pressure of 5–20 cm H_2O to ensure velum closure. The results are expressed as NO concentration in ppb based on the mean of two to three values within 10%.[58]

The exact relationship between FeNO and the underlying pathology in asthma remains unclear.[59] Although there is an increasing use of FeNO as a surrogate marker for the presence of clinically relevant airway eosinophilia,[60] there is a scope for both false positives and false negatives.[61] FeNO does not reliably identify noneosinophilic bronchitis which is also frequently seen in asthma.

The upper limit of normal FeNO is widely variable (12.7–22.8 ppb in children, 24–54 ppb in adults).[62,63] Additionally, FeNO levels are affected by a number of other factors. It is often higher in atopic subjects,[64] higher levels with increasing age in children aged 17 years or less,[65] higher in males and lower in current smokers.[66] FeNO is increased by about 60% during the late allergic response in atopic asthma[67] and is reduced two to four fold by corticosteroids in asthma between 3 days to 8 weeks.[68,69] A dose-response effect is observed with low-dose treatment but no additional benefit is seen above a budesonide dose of 400 µg/day.[70]

Four studies have shown that a raised FeNO is predictive of loss of asthma control[71-74] but two other studies were less convincing.[75,76] Management strategies based on monitoring FeNO level resulted in lowering of ICS dose[77] and improved airway hyperresponsiveness (AHR).[78] However, in contrast with the use of sputum cell counts to guide ICS treatment, exhaled nitric oxide was unable to reduce exacerbations in asthma patients.[79] Measurement of FeNO requires expensive equipment and is currently available in a few specialist laboratories. Although cheaper portable FeNO analyzers are now becoming available, there are concerns that absolute values may differ between different analyzers and stability over time needs to be established.[80,81] These factors may have implications in clinical practice.

Although there is some evidence that FeNO is useful in the diagnosis of asthma, in the prediction of asthma exacerbations and tailoring of asthma therapy, yet many ambiguities still remain. The variability of FeNO measurements in populations and within individuals needs to be more clearly defined, and specific cutoff points for FeNO values need to be more firmly established. Further studies are needed to address its exact role in guiding asthma management.

Key Recommendations for Clinical Practice

Noninvasive biomarkers of airway inflammation should be used to identify the bronchitic component of asthma that is otherwise not available to the clinician. The only clinical comprehensive measurement currently available to assess airway inflammation is quantitative sputum cell counts. It is imperative to introduce quantitative sputum cell counts in specialist practice to manage moderate to severe asthma. Identification of eosinophils or neutrophils in the airway does not diagnose asthma. They help to predict the response to anti-inflammatory treatment and guide appropriate treatment.

In contrast to traditional clinical management, the use of induced sputum has been shown to be cost-effective in a specialist setting. FeNO measurements may be used as a surrogate marker for airway eosinophilia, may be used to predict response to corticosteroid therapy, low values may be of use to aid reduction in corticosteroid dose or to determine that ongoing respiratory symptoms are less likely to be due to eosinophilic airway inflammation. Further studies with FeNO are needed to address outstanding questions about its exact role in guiding asthma management.

Exhaled Breath Condensate

A more recent noninvasive tool to assess airway inflammation is exhaled breath condensate (EBC) measurements. The warm breath of subjects is collected on to cooled tubes so that the moisture condenses and the condensate can be collected. This condensate can then be analyzed for airway pH and various inflammatory markers (e.g. hydrogen peroxide, isoprostanes and cytokines).[20,82] Although the technique is noninvasive, allowing repeated samples to be collected and can be used even with small children, there are several unresolved problems with this methodology.[83] Currently the technique remains a promising research tool, with the potential for monitoring the inflammatory state in the airways and the effect of the novel therapeutic agents; however, more sensitive methods for measuring analytes and standardization of the collection methodology are needed.[20]

Measures of Allergic Status

Physicians commonly encounter patients with symptoms consistent with allergy. It can be difficult to determine which allergen is causing symptoms from the patient's history alone. Allergy tests yield information on sensitization, which is not always equivalent to clinical allergy; thus, interpretation in the context of clinical history is important. The two main allergy tests that are available to assist the physician to make an allergy diagnosis include the allergy skin tests and the measurements of allergen specific immunoglobulin E (IgE) (serum s-IgE) in addition to a thorough clinical history. However, it is very important for the clinician to understand which allergy diagnostic tests to order, how to interpret the results of these tests and how to use the information obtained from the allergy evaluation to develop an appropriate treatment plan.

Medical History and Physical Examination

A history of allergic symptoms, seasonal variation, rapidity of onset and age of onset will help the clinician to determine if the patient's presentation is likely from an allergic cause. Physical examination findings such as allergic shiners, nasal crease, boggy nasal turbinates and pharyngeal cobblestones may further guide the physician.[84] If you suspect IgE-mediated allergic disease, always request and interpret skin tests and s-IgE tests in context of the clinical history. Positive test results provide objective confirmation of IgE sensitization, which will support a history of symptoms on exposure to a particular allergen. A negative test makes allergy to a suspected allergen unlikely. Avoid indiscriminate use of allergy tests as they may be commonly associated with false-positive results. Skin and serum IgE tests should never be used as a substitute for a careful clinical history.

Allergen skin tests: In clinical practice, the prick or puncture test is the preferred initial technique because it is relatively nontraumatic, elicits reproducible results when placed on specific areas such as arms or back and has better overall predictability. The reliability of prick/puncture tests depends on the skill of the tester, the test instrument, color of the skin, skin reactivity on the day of the test, potency and stability of test reagents. Sensitivity tends to be higher among pollens, certain foods, dust mite and fungi, compared with drugs and chemicals.[84,85] The number of skin tests and the allergens selected for skin testing should be determined from the patient's age, history, environment and living conditions, occupation, and activities. A routine use of large number of skin tests without a definite clinical indication is not justified.[84]

Serum s-IgE: Multiple methods have been used to measure serum allergen s-IgE including radioallergosorbent test (RAST), Turbo RAST (Agilent Technologies Co, Santa Clara, California), Immulite (Siemens Medical Solutions Diagnostics, Tarrytown, New York) and ImmunoCAP (Phadia, Uppsala, Sweden). ImmunoCAP is the assay that has been most extensively studied.[86]

If the clinical history is positive and the serum s-IgE test result is negative, allergy skin testing should be considered. Serum s-IgE testing is preferred to prick or puncture testing when the patient has severe skin disease, is receiving medications that may suppress skin tests and cannot be removed from them, for uncooperative patients, or if the history suggests a risk of anaphylaxis from the testing.[84]

Levels of total and *Aspergillus fumigatus* specific IgE also help to differentiate allergic bronchopulmonary aspergillosis from asthma.[87] It is important in serum s-IgE tests and skin tests that results correlate with the history, physical examination findings, and in some cases timing of natural exposure to allergen. Therefore, it is often inappropriate to choose immunotherapy from remote laboratories based on history alone.

DIAGNOSTIC CHALLENGES

Preschool Children

Diagnosis of asthma in children aged 5 years and younger may be difficult because episodic respiratory symptoms such as wheezing and cough are also common in children who do not have asthma, particularly in those younger than 3 years.[87,88] It is further complicated by the difficulty in obtaining lung function in this age group. Alternative causes that can lead to respiratory symptoms of wheeze, cough and breathlessness must be excluded before making an asthma diagnosis. These include recurrent respiratory infections, allergic rhinitis, sinusitis, tuberculosis, foreign body in trachea or bronchus, vocal cord dysfunction, enlarged lymph nodes or tumor that may compress the large airways, recurrent aspiration due to dysfunction of swallowing reflex or gastroesophageal reflux and congenital problems such as tracheomalacia, tracheal stenosis, bronchostenosis, cystic fibrosis, bronchopulmonary dysplasia, congenital malformation of intrathoracic airways, primary ciliary dyskinesia syndrome, immune deficiency and congenital heart disease.[89]

Nevertheless, a diagnosis of asthma in young children can often be made based on symptom patterns, family history (first degree relatives, especially the mother) and physical findings. The presence of atopy (atopic dermatitis, food allergy and/or allergic rhinitis) increases the likelihood that a wheezing child will have asthma. It is important to avoid under diagnosing asthma, and thereby missing the opportunity to treat a child, by using such labels as "wheezy bronchitis", "recurrent pneumonia", or "reactive airway disease".

Symptoms

Wheeze, cough, breathlessness and nocturnal symptoms/ awakenings may indicate a diagnosis of asthma.

- *Wheeze*: Not all wheezing indicates asthma. The ERS Task Group[90] has described two wheezing phenotypes (episodic wheeze and multiple trigger wheeze), whereas the US cohort study[91] has identified three wheezing phenotypes (transient wheeze, persistent wheeze, late-onset wheeze). The "episodic wheeze" is the wheeze that occurs during discrete time periods, often in association with a common cold, with absence of wheeze between episodes. A "multiple trigger wheeze" occurs as episodic exacerbations but also with symptoms including cough and wheeze occurring between these episodes, during sleep or with triggers such as activity, laughing, or crying. In "transient wheeze", symptoms begin and end before the age of 3 years; in "persistent wheeze", symptoms begin before the age of 3 years and continue beyond the age of 6 years; and in "late-onset wheeze", symptoms begin after the age of 3 years. The clinical usefulness of these phenotypes remains a subject of much debate. Asthma occurs much more rarely in the episodic wheeze and transient wheeze phenotypes compared to the other phenotypes.

  Based on data from the Tucson (USA) Respiratory Study,[92] the asthma predictive index (API) is recommended to predict the development of asthma in children with four or more wheezing episodes in a year.[93] A child with a positive API has a 4–10 fold greater chance of developing asthma between the ages of 6 years and 13 years, while 95% of children with a negative API remained free of asthma.[93] The applicability and validation of the API in clinical practice is awaited.[89]

  Since many young children may wheeze with viral infections (respiratory syncytial virus and rhinovirus), it is challenging to differentiate whether the presence of wheeze with infections is truly an initial or recurrent clinical presentation of childhood asthma.[94]
- *Cough*: Cough due to asthma is recurrent and/or persistent, and is usually accompanied by some wheezing and breathing difficulties. Nocturnal cough or cough occurring with exercise, laughing or crying in the absence of an apparent respiratory infection, strongly supports a diagnosis of asthma.
- *Breathlessness*: Very often, parents describe this symptom as difficult breathing, heavy breathing or shortness of breath. Breathlessness that occurs during exercise, laughing and crying and is recurrent increases the likelihood of asthma.

Tests for Diagnosis and Monitoring

There is no test that will diagnose asthma with certainty in young children, but the following may be useful in making a diagnosis:[89]

- *Therapeutic trial*: A marked clinical improvement in daytime and nocturnal symptoms and frequency of exacerbations during a trial of treatment with short-acting bronchodilators and inhaled glucocorticosteroids for at least 8–12 weeks and deterioration when it is stopped supports a diagnosis of asthma. A therapeutic trial may need to be repeated more than once to confirm the diagnosis of asthma.
- *Tests for atopy*: Sensitization to allergens can be assessed using either skin testing or antigen-specific IgE antibody. Skin prick testing is less reliable for confirming atopy in infants.
- *Chest radiograph*: If there is doubt about the diagnosis of asthma in a wheezing child, a plain chest radiograph may help to exclude infection (e.g. tuberculosis), congenital malformations of the airway such as congenital lobar emphysema or other diagnoses.
- *Other tests*: Lung function testing, bronchial challenge tests and other physiological tests do not have a major role in the diagnosis of asthma in children of 5 years and younger because children in this age group do not perform reproducible expiratory maneuvers. Such tests are only possible in specialized centers, and are undertaken mainly for research purposes.
- *Exhaled nitric oxide*: High exhaled nitric oxide levels have been used to differentiate preschool wheezers with a high and low risk of developing asthma from preschool coughers.[95] However, there is still no evidence to show whether exhaled nitric oxide levels can be used to differentiate persistent wheezers who are likely to develop asthma from other wheezy phenotypes.[89]

Older Children and Adults

In most cases, a careful history and physical examination together with the demonstration of reversible and variable airflow limitation by spirometry will confirm the diagnosis of asthma. Other causes of airway obstruction leading to wheeze should be considered both in the initial diagnosis and if the patient does not respond to initial therapy. These conditions may coexist with asthma or complicate the diagnosis and management of asthma. Common diagnostic challenges include the following:

Cough-variant Asthma

Cough-variant asthma (CVA) is a distinct subset of asthma in which the main respiratory symptom is chronic cough associated with bronchial hyperresponsiveness and airway eosinophilia.[96] It can be encountered in both children and adults. In some patients, the cough may be associated with wheezing, chest tightness and various degrees of airflow obstruction, whereas in others cough could be the only presenting symptom with normal pulmonary function.[97] Higher sensitivities of cough reflex could explain the predominance in females.[98] In both adults and children, CVA may be a precursor of typical asthma; adults developed typical asthma after a period ranging from 1.5 year to 9 years.[96]

The predictors of progression to typical asthma include increased airway hyperresponsiveness,[99] eosinophilic airway inflammation,[100] blood eosinophilia,[101] longer duration of coughing,[102] age of onset[103] and no use of inhaled corticosteroids.[101,104] Typical asthma developed in 7.4% of patients taking inhaled corticosteroids and in 35.7% patients not taking inhaled corticosteroids.[101] Monitoring of PEF or bronchoprovocation may be helpful. Diagnosis is confirmed by a positive response to asthma medications.[96]

Vocal Cord Dysfunction

Vocal cord dysfunction (VCD) can mimic asthma, but it is a distinct disorder that is caused by abnormal adduction of the vocal cords during inspiration causing extrathoracic airway obstruction resulting in episodic dyspnea and wheeze.[105,106] In addition to severe asthma, VCD frequently occurs in mild-to-moderate asthma (72%).[106] Although physicians commonly refer patients with "classic" symptoms of stridor or hoarseness for VCD testing, a recent study[106] reports the lack of classic VCD symptoms among asthmatics. In fact, patients with both VCD and asthma present with nonspecific symptoms such as dyspnea, cough and wheeze, highlighting the need for a high index of suspicion for VCD in patients with asthma. The high prevalence of gastroesophageal reflux disease (GERD) (56.8%) raises the question of the role of acid reflux in the pathogenesis of VCD in asthmatics.[106]

Diagnosing vocal cord dysfunction requires a high index of suspicion. There is variable flattening of the inspiratory flow loop on spirometry; however, a normal flow-volume loop should not influence the decision to perform a laryngoscopy.[107] Access to specialized videolaryngostroboscopy (VLS) testing is required to definitively document VCD. The laryngeal movements during the entire procedure are digitally recorded. In order to be diagnosed as VCD, the patient must demonstrate abnormal constriction during the respiratory cycle and also normal complete abduction during some portion of the examination;[106] however false-negative tests can occur because VCD is paroxysmal.[105,108] Therefore, provocation with exercise or noxious stimuli is important to increase the likelihood of capturing an episode of VCD during VLS testing.[106]

It is yet unknown whether diagnosis and treatment of VCD has any impact on asthma control. Future prospective studies are needed to establish the impact of the diagnosis and treatment of VCD on asthma control.[106]

Gastroesophageal Reflux Disease

Although 80% of asthmatic patients with positive pH probes have typical GERD symptoms such as heartburn,[109] approximately 40% have asymptomatic or silent GERD.[110]

Gastroesophageal reflux disease may induce asthma symptoms either by direct bronchospasm and increased airway hyperresponsiveness[111] or indirectly via microaspiration-induced airway inflammation.[112] Asthma patients have hyperinflated chests. Descent of the diaphragm in hyperinflated lungs increases the pressure gradient between the abdomen and chest and may cause the lower esophageal sphincter (LES) to herniate into the chest where its barrier function is impaired.[113,114] Asthma medications such as β2 agonists and methylxanthine bronchodilators may decrease LES tone and may promote acid reflux.[113]

The use of pH probe findings is considered the most sensitive diagnostic test for GERD; however it does not reliably identify a subgroup of asthmatic patients who is likely to benefit from GERD treatment.[106]

Other Differential Diagnosis

Other differential diagnostic possibilities for asthma include congestive heart failure, pulmonary embolism, mechanical obstruction of the airways (benign and malignant tumors), pulmonary infiltration with eosinophilia, cough secondary to drugs [e.g. angiotensin converting enzyme (ACE) inhibitors].[1]

Elderly

The diagnosis of asthma in the elderly is based mainly on clinical history and demonstration of reversible airflow obstruction with pulmonary function testing, but there are unique diagnostic challenges in older patients.

Medical History

Shortness of breath, chest tightness, usually dry cough, recurrent wheezing, nocturnal symptoms, worsening of disease at night, precipitation of symptoms following exposure to cold air, exercise or allergens support a diagnosis of asthma in the elderly.[115]

Pulmonary Function Testing

Many older patients will have difficulty in performing PFT. Performing PFT has been shown to be feasible in up to 88% of outpatients aged 65 and older.[116] Older adults may find it difficult to perform effective PFT because of the following reasons:[115]

- Inability to perform efficient forced expiration.
- Unable to follow instructions from the PFT technician because of cognitive impairment, sensory deficits (e.g. deafness, cataract) and/or impaired coordination (e.g. stroke).
- Poor postbronchodilator reversibility with β2 agonists.
- Fatigue and associated comorbidities (e.g. cardiovascular disease).
- Mouth or dental problems (e.g. ulcers, dentures), which may affect the ability to hold onto the mouthpiece.

Difficulties Faced by a Clinician during Interpretation of PFT Reports

An obstructive pattern alone on spirometry in the absence of symptoms may reflect age-related pulmonary change such as decreased vital capacity, increased residual volume and functional residual capacity and not necessarily asthma.[117]

The predicted values of FEV1 and FVC in normal elderly patients are based on data that is extrapolated from younger patients and therefore, tend to over predict values.[118] There is an accelerated decline in FEV1 and FVC with advancing age, which is more rapid in men than women.[117] The clinician should consider these factors while making a diagnosis of asthma.

Age-dependent changes in pulmonary function and fixed obstruction (unchanged FEV1 and FEV1/FVC values pre- and postbronchodilator administration), which develops subsequent to airway remodeling makes it difficult for clinicians to differentiate between long-standing asthma and COPD.[119] Although bronchodilator reversibility will aid in distinguishing between asthma and COPD, a low diffusion capacity of carbon monoxide (DLCO) may tilt the diagnosis toward COPD and not asthma.[115] Beta-adrenergic dysfunction may be implicated in older patients.[120] Therefore, with the absence of a detectable change in the reversibility of airflow obstruction with SABAs, the test may be repeated with an anticholinergic agent. In some individuals, PFT does not demonstrate postbronchodilator reversibility, but an improvement is seen after systemic corticosteroid. The explanation of this phenomenon is based on the anti-inflammatory effect of corticosteroids. A 2-week trial of oral corticosteroid should be considered before repeating spirometry to detect an improvement in airflow obstruction which will aid in diagnosing asthma in difficult cases.[121] Nonetheless, asthma and COPD can both coexist in the same patient.[122]

Alternative Assessments

- *Peak flow rates*: The use of peak flow variability to diagnose asthma in the elderly patients is not recommended because peak flow declines with age and peak flow variability becomes less reliable.[123] It is useful in detecting poorly controlled asthma, but it may not be fully reliable even in these circumstances.
- *Relaxed vital capacity*: Since older patients find it difficult to perform efficient forced expiratory maneuvers, a suitable alternative test is relaxed VC because it will be more discriminatory in older patients. The ratio of FEV:relaxed VC may be used to determine whether obstructive airway disease is present; however assessment of relaxed VC is more time consuming and requires technical expertise to perform the test correctly.[115]
- *Airway resistance*: As measurement of airway resistance or impedance using impulse oscillometry[124] and

plethysmography[125] do not rely on maximal expiratory efforts, these methods have been proposed as a measure of airflow obstruction in older patients. Impulse oscillometry was successfully used to assess and quantify the airway obstruction in patients with dementia.[124] Further clinical studies need to address the validity and feasibility of these methods to assess airflow obstruction in the elderly.

Occupational Asthma

It is first necessary to establish a diagnosis of asthma in a patient and then identify occupational asthma (OA). A thorough medical history and objective work-related testing usually provides a reliable diagnosis of occupational asthma. A detailed history for suspected OA include chronological work history, job duties, exposures at work, onset and timing of symptoms, use of protective devices, presence of respiratory disease in coworkers, medication use and past lung function.[126]

The 2008 ACCP guidelines[127] recommend that the physician needs to address the following questions related to the onset and timing of the symptoms:

- Whether there were changes in work processes preceding the onset of symptoms
- Whether there was unusual exposure to sensitizers at work within 24 hours before the onset of symptoms
- Whether there is a temporal relationship of symptoms to periods while at and away from work (e.g. weekends, holidays)
- Whether symptoms of allergic rhinitis and /or conjunctivitis get worse with work.

It would be very helpful to have up-to-date material safety data sheet (MSDS) in place for every chemical or material that may pose an occupational hazard for patients. MSDS contains information that will help to identify the suspect agent in the workplace.[128]

Objective Testing

- *Peak expiratory flow rates*: Current guidelines[127] recommend that peak expiratory flow rates (PEFR) should be recorded at the workplace for a minimum period of 4 weeks including at least 1 week away from work. These PEFR readings should be performed in triplicate at least four times a day (e.g. preshift, midshift, postshift and bedtime, with similar times on days off work). Careful patient instruction is required because PEFRs are effort dependent. A typical pattern of OA is for patients to have better peak flow rates when they return to work after a weekend (e.g. on a Monday) or after holidays and get worse as the week progresses. PEF assessment has a sensitivity of 64% and 77% specificity.[129]
- *Airway hyperresponsiveness*: A methacholine or histamine challenge test should be performed at the end of a work week. The patient should remain away from work for at least 10–14 days, following which the challenge test should be repeated. A worsening of PC20 at work versus off work (greater than or equal to 4 fold change) further supports a diagnosis of OA.[127] A methacholine challenge test can revert to normal when a patient is away from occupational exposure.[130]
- *Specific inhalation challenge*: Specific inhalation challenge (SIC) exposes a worker to a specific suspect OA sensitizer in a controlled setting to demonstrate a direct relationship between exposure to the test agent and an asthmatic response. SIC may be associated with significant risk and should be performed in a specialized center under close supervision. This test is performed at limited centers in the world.[126]
- *Immunologic testing*: A negative skin test to a validated occupational protein allergen can reliably exclude occupational asthma.[127,131] Low molecular weight (LMW) sensitizers (e.g. metals, organic chemicals) may be associated with specific IgE antibody but limited in vitro tests are available for specific IgE to LMW agents and commercial tests have not been validated. Although these tests are not very sensitive, when positive they can support a diagnosis of OA.[132]
- *Workplace challenge*: Workplace challenge testing is used when a specific agent cannot be identified as a potential cause for sensitizer induced OA or SIC is not available. The patient's spirometry is monitored at the workplace suspected to cause sensitizer induced OA.[133] For the purpose of comparison, the workplace challenge testing should be preceded by a control spirometry performed away from work.
- *Induced sputum cell counts*: Induced sputum analysis may assist in diagnosis of OA even before the development of respiratory symptoms and pulmonary function changes.[134] Although majority of subjects with OA show an eosinophilic airway inflammation after exposure to occupational agents during SIC,[135,136] neutrophilic inflammation has also been reported following exposure to isocyanates[137] and metal working fluid.[138] If there is an isolated increase in sputum eosinophil count of at least 2% without functional changes, the physician should pursue further investigation by increasing the duration of exposure to the suspected occupational agent.[139]
- *Exhaled nitric oxide*: There have been few studies examining work related changes of exhaled nitric oxide. Some studies have reported a higher exhaled nitric oxide in patients with OA[140,141] while others do not report a clear relationship.[142]
- *Exhaled breath condensate*: Exhaled breath condensate (EBC) collection is a noninvasive and repeatable tool to assess oxidative stress, acidification and inflammation in the airways.[143] The EBC concentration of hydrogen peroxide was increased in asymptomatic welders.[144] EBC pH was lower in welders exposed to cadmium, chromium, iron, lead, and nickel, than those exposed to aluminum

and iron at the workplace. EBC analysis may be useful in occupational studies on a group level and in individuals who serve as their own controls. Based on methodological limitations, lack of standardization and difficulties in the interpretation of the data, EBC collection and analysis are primarily research tools and not yet suitable for implementation into clinical practice.[145]

Differential Diagnosis

Other conditions that may mimic occupational asthma include vocal cord dysfunction, upper respiratory tract infection, hypersensitivity pneumonitis, rhinosinusitis, byssinosis, popcorn worker's disease, flock worker's disease, eosinophilic bronchitis and psychogenic factors.[126]

Asthma and COPD

Guideline-recommended definitions for asthma and COPD are useful but limited because they do not fully depict the spectrum of obstructive airway disease that we see in clinical practice. There is a need to revaluate the concept of asthma and COPD as separate conditions. The various components of airway disease include symptoms, variable airflow limitation (asthma), chronic airflow limitation (COPD), airway hyperresponsiveness and airway inflammation. They can exist in various combinations, and bronchitis or airway inflammation is the central component. When considered in this way, asthma and COPD are physiological components of airway disease and bronchitis is the inflammatory component.[146] An asthma patient may or may not have eosinophilic bronchitis, COPD can occur in a nonsmoker. A smoker with COPD may have an eosinophilic bronchitis. A neutrophilic bronchitis can occur in asthma or COPD. Hence, the diseases are not mutually exclusive and can overlap (overlap syndrome). Combinations commonly occur and can vary from one patient to another.

Why is the Overlap Syndrome Important?

With increasing age, there is a greater increase in the proportion of patients (55%) with the overlap syndrome and fewer (19%) older patients have the classical phenotypes of emphysema alone or chronic bronchitis alone.[147]

Patients with the overlap syndrome are excluded from randomized controlled clinical trials and therefore, data on the efficacy of treatment may not be relevant in this population.[148] Studies on the efficacy of inhaled corticosteroids in asthma excluded smokers with asthma despite the fact that up to 32% of asthma patients are smokers.[149] As a result extrapolation of efficacy results for corticosteroids in nonsmokers to smokers with asthma is flawed and we know that smokers with asthma have a relative corticosteroid resistance.[150] Overlap syndrome of asthma and COPD need to be included in drug evaluation programs.

Clinicians are often confused as to how to differentiate between asthma and COPD and use extended nonuniform diagnostic labels for obstructive airway disease (e.g. asthma with chronic bronchitis, asthmatic bronchitis).[151] Recognition of the overlap syndrome may help identify shared risk factors such as increasing age and smoking,[152] bronchial hyperresponsiveness[153] and exacerbations,[154] which will help to understand and modify the accelerated decline in lung function that leads to COPD.

Clinical Recognition of the Overlap Syndrome

The clinical recognition of both asthma and COPD requires assessment of symptoms and physiological function abnormalities.[148] Patients with asthma, COPD and overlap syndrome can all present with symptoms; however there is a difference in the physiological function abnormalities. Patients with the overlap syndrome have incomplete reversible airflow obstruction [FEV1/FVC <70%, FEV1% Pred (postbronchodilator) <80%] but also have increased bronchial hyperresponsiveness (PD15 of hypertonic saline that induces a 15% fall in FEV1 is less than 12 mL).

Patient groups that have features of both asthma and COPD include smokers with asthma, asthma patients who develop COPD and nonsmokers who develop COPD.[148] Long-standing asthma patients who develop COPD tend to be older (44 years), more often males and have a long duration of disease (25 years).[155,156] Sixteen percent of patients with asthma developed COPD after 21–33 years of follow-up.[157] In a recent study[148] only 16% and 21% patients could be reported definitely as asthma and COPD respectively. Majority (65%) of the patients had the overlap syndrome of asthma and COPD. The rate of atopy was intermediate (64%) in the overlap syndrome. Airway complications resembled COPD rather than asthma.

Inflammatory Features of the Overlap Syndrome

The pattern of airway inflammation associated with both asthma and COPD is heterogeneous but is more likely to resemble COPD rather than asthma with increased sputum neutrophils. Smokers with asthma are less likely to have eosinophilic inflammation[158] and more likely to have airway neutrophilia.[159] In our retrospective survey of 2,443 patients with airway disease,[42] 9% had asthma with COPD. In stable disease, eosinophilic bronchitis was more frequently seen (35%) whereas neutrophilic inflammation was more common during exacerbations (33%). Induced sputum biomarkers such as IL-12, IL-13 and IFN-gamma were predominant in patients with both asthma and COPD, whereas IL-9, IL-17, monocyte chemotactic protein 1, and regulated upon activation, normal T cell expressed and secreted (RANTES) were dominant in those with asthma without chronic airflow obstruction.[160]

Airway Remodeling in Overlap Syndrome

Subjects with severe asthma and chronic persistent obstruction have increased airway smooth muscle (15.65%) versus that (8.96%) seen in patients without chronic airflow obstruction; however, airway measurements on high-resolution computed tomographic scans revealed no differences between the groups.[160]

The overlap syndrome of asthma and COPD is supported by the Dutch Hypothesis,[161] which states that the different types of airway diseases should not be considered as separate conditions but as one disease entity with different components. The presence of different components (asthma, COPD) is influenced by host and environmental factors. We need to evaluate the components of the disease in order to individualize and optimize treatment to achieve the best effect with the least side effects and cost to the patient.

CONCLUSION

The clinical diagnosis of asthma is usually based on an accurate medical history, supported by physical examination and demonstration of variable airflow obstruction. This would involve demonstration of bronchodilator reversibility in patients with baseline airflow obstruction or bronchial hyperresponsiveness in patients without baseline airflow obstruction. An alternative would be demonstration of natural variability in airflow obstruction using home peak flow recording. Although this is less sensitive than demonstration of bronchial hyperresponsiveness to diagnose asthma, new statistical methods to analyze peak flow recording such as autocorrelation and coefficient of variation of measurements[162] may prove increasingly useful. Objective assessment of airway inflammation especially quantitative sputum cell counts needs to be implemented into specialist practice to identify the bronchitis component of asthma. They do not help to diagnose asthma. A referral to a specialist center that has expertise to perform bronchial provocation tests, evaluation of allergy and measurement of airway inflammometry is appropriate in patients with uncertain diagnosis, particularly, those who do not seem to improve with conventional treatment for asthma.

REFERENCES

1. NHLBI Guidelines for the Diagnosis and Management of Asthma. National Institutes of Health and the US Department of Health and Human Services. 2007.
2. Global Initiative for Asthma. Global Strategy for Asthma Management and Prevention 2014. Available from *www.ginathma.org*. [Accessed February 2016].
3. Jindal SK. Bronchial asthma: the Indian scene. Curr Opin Pulm Med. 2007;13(1):8-12.
4. Agarwal R, Dhooria S, Aggarwal AN, Maturu VN, Sehgal IS, Muthu V, et al. Guidelines for diagnosis and management of bronchial asthma: Joint ICP/NCCP (India) recommendations. Lung India. 2015;32(Suppl 1):S3-S42.
5. Prasad R, Nautiyal RG, Mukherji PK, Jain A, Singh K, Ahuja RC, et al. Diagnostic evaluation of pulmonary tuberculosis: what do doctors of modern medicine do in India? Int J Tuberc Lung Dis. 2003;7(1):52-7.
6. Hargreave FE, Nair P. The definition and diagnosis of asthma. Clin Exp Allergy. 2009;39(11):1652-8.
7. Kendrick AH, Higgs CM, Whitfield MJ, Laszlo G. Accuracy of perception of severity of asthma: patients treated in general practice. BMJ. 1993;307(6901):422-4.
8. Adelroth E, Hargreave FE, Ramsdale EH. Do physicians need objective measurements to diagnose asthma? Am Rev Respir Dis. 1986;134(4):704-7.
9. LindenSmith J, Morrison D, Deveau C, Hernandez P. Overdiagnosis of asthma in the community. Can Respir J. 2004; 11(2):111-6.
10. Aggarwal AN, Gupta D, Behera D, Jindal SK. Applicability of commonly used Caucasian prediction equations for spirometry interpretation in India. Indian J Med Res. 2005;122(2):153-64.
11. Lung function throughout life: determinants and reference values. In: Cotes JE (Ed). Lung Function. Assessment and Application in Medicine, 5th edition. Oxford: Blackwell Scientific Publications; 1993. pp. 445-513.
12. GINA Report, Global Strategy for Asthma Management and Prevention. 2009.
13. McCormack MC, Enright PL. Making the diagnosis of asthma. Respir Care. 2008;53(5):583-90.
14. GOLD Report, Global Strategy for Diagnosis, Management, and Prevention of COPD. 2009.
15. Stout JW, Visness CM, Enright P, Lamm C, Shapiro G, Gan VN, et al. Classification of asthma severity in children: the contribution of pulmonary function testing. Arch Pediatr Adolesc Med. 2006;160(8):844-50.
16. Tantisira KG, Fuhlbrigge AL, Tonascia J, Van Natta M, Zeiger RS, Strunk RC, et al. Bronchodilation and bronchoconstriction: predictors of future lung function in childhood asthma. J Allergy Clin Immunol. 2006;117(6):1264-71.
17. Silverman RA, Flaster E, Enright PL, Simonson SG. FEV1 performance among patients with acute asthma: results from a multicenter clinical trial. Chest. 2007;131(1):164-71.
18. Derom E, van Weel C, Liistro G, Buffels J, Schermer T, Lammers E, et al. Primary care spirometry. Eur Respir J. 2008;31(1):197-203.
19. Enright P. The use and abuse of office spirometry. Prim Care Respir J. 2008;17(4):238-42.
20. Reddel HK, Taylor DR, Bateman ED, Boulet LP, Boushey HA, Busse WW, et al. An official American Thoracic Society/European Respiratory Society statement: asthma control and exacerbations: standardizing endpoints for clinical asthma trials and clinical practice. Am J Respir Crit Care Med. 2009;180(1):59-99.
21. Boezen HM, Schouten JP, Postma DS, Rijcken B. Distribution of peak expiratory flow variability by age, gender and smoking habits in a random population sample aged 20-70 yrs. Eur Respir J. 1994;7(10):1814-20.
22. Sawyer G, Miles J, Lewis S, Fitzharris P, Pearce N, Beasley R. Classification of asthma severity: should the international guidelines be changed? Clin Exp Allergy. 1998;28(12):1565-70.
23. Eid N, Yandell B, Howell L, Eddy M, Sheikh S. Can peak expiratory flow predict airflow obstruction in children with asthma? Pediatrics. 2000;105(2):354-8.
24. Reddel HK, Marks GB, Jenkins CR. When can personal best peak flow be determined for asthma action plans? Thorax. 2004;59(11):922-4.

25. Cockcroft D, Davis B. Direct and indirect challenges in the clinical assessment of asthma. Ann Allergy Asthma Immunol. 2009;103(5):363-9.
26. Juniper EF, Cockcroft DW, Hargreave FE. Histamine and Methacholine Inhalation Tests. In: Tidal Breathing Method: Laboratory Procedure and Standardisation, 2nd edition. Sweden: AB Draco; 1994.
27. Cockcroft DW, Davis BE. Lack of tachyphylaxis to methacholine at 24 h. Chest. 2005;128(3):1248-51.
28. Hargreave FE, Ryan G, Thomson NC, O'Byrne PM, Latimer K, Juniper EF, et al. Bronchial responsiveness to histamine or methacholine in asthma: measurement and clinical significance. J Allergy Clin Immunol. 1981;68(5):347-55.
29. Jayet PY, Schindler C, Künzli N, Zellweger JP, Brändli O, Perruchoud AP, et al. Reference values for methacholine reactivity (SAPALDIA study). Respir Res. 2005;6:131.
30. Irwin RS, French CT, Smyrnios NA, Curley FJ. Interpretation of positive results of a methacholine inhalation challenge and 1 week of inhaled bronchodilator use in diagnosing and treating cough-variant asthma. Arch Intern Med. 1997;157(17):1981-7.
31. Gibson PG, Dolovich J, Denburg J, Ramsdale EH, Hargreave FE. Chronic cough: eosinophilic bronchitis without asthma. Lancet. 1989;1(8651):1346-8.
32. Sont JK, Willems LN, Bel EH, van Krieken JH, Vandenbroucke JP, Sterk PJ, et al. Clinical control and histopathologic outcome of asthma when using airway hyperresponsiveness as an additional guide to long-term treatment. The AMPUL Study Group. Am J Respir Crit Care Med. 1999;159(4 Pt 1):1043-51.
33. Cartier A, Pineau L, Malo JL. Monitoring of maximum expiratory peak flow rates and histamine inhalation tests in the investigation of occupational asthma. Clin Allergy. 1984;14(2):193-6.
34. Joos GF. Bronchial hyperresponsiveness: too complex to be useful? Curr Opin Pharmacol. 2003;3(3):233-8.
35. Leuppi JD, Salome CM, Jenkins CR, Anderson SD, Xuan W, Marks GB, et al. Predictive markers of asthma exacerbation during stepwise dose reduction of inhaled corticosteroids. Am J Respir Crit Care Med. 2001;163(2):406-12.
36. Brannan JD, Koskela H, Anderson SD, Chan HK. Budesonide reduces sensitivity and reactivity to inhaled mannitol in asthmatic subjects. Respirology. 2002;7(1):37-44.
37. Simpson JL, Scott R, Boyle MJ, Gibson PG. Inflammatory subtypes in asthma: assessment and identification using induced sputum. Respirology. 2006;11(1):54-61.
38. Parameswaran K, Pizzichini E, Pizzichini MM, Hussack P, Efthimiadis A, Hargreave FE. Clinical judgement of airway inflammation versus sputum cell counts in patients with asthma. Eur Respir J. 2000;15(3):486-90.
39. Hargreave FE. Quantitative sputum cell counts as a marker of airway inflammation in clinical practice. Curr Opin Allergy Clin Immunol. 2007;7(1):102-6.
40. Pizzichini E, Pizzichini MM, Efthimiadis A, Evans S, Morris MM, Squillace D, et al. Indices of airway inflammation in induced sputum: reproducibility and validity of cell and fluid-phase measurements. Am J Respir Crit Care Med. 1996;154(2 Pt 1):308-17.
41. Pizzichini E, Pizzichini MM, Leigh R, Djukanović R, Sterk PJ, et al. Safety of sputum induction. Eur Respir J Suppl. 2002;37:9s-18s.
42. D'silva L, Hassan N, Wang HY, Kjarsgaard M, Efthimiadis A, Hargreave FE, et al. Heterogeneity of bronchitis in airway diseases in tertiary care clinical practice. Can Respir J. 2011;18(3):144-8.
43. Covar RA, Spahn JD, Martin RJ, Silkoff PE, Sundstrom DA, Murphy J, et al. Safety and application of induced sputum analysis in childhood asthma. J Allerg Clin Immunol. 2004;114(3):575-82.
44. Pavord ID, Pizzichini MM, Pizzichini E, Hargreave FE. The use of induced sputum to investigate airway inflammation. Thorax. 1997;52(6):498-501.
45. Djukanoviæ R, Sterk PJ, Fahy JV, Hargreave FE. Standardised methodology of sputum induction and processing. Eur Respir J Suppl. 2002;37:1s-2s.
46. Kips JC, Fahy JV, Hargreave FE, Ind PW, in't Veen JC. Methods for sputum induction and analysis of induced sputum: a method for assessing airway inflammation in asthma. Eur Respir J Suppl. 1998;26:9S-12S.
47. Belda J, Parameswaran K, Hargreave FE. Comparison of two methods of processing induced sputum: selected versus entire sputum. Am J Respir Crit Care Med. 1998;158(2):680-2.
48. Pizzichini MM, Popov TA, Efthimiadis A, Hussack P, Evans S, Pizzichini E, et al. Spontaneous and induced sputum to measure indices of airway inflammation in asthma. Am J Respir Crit Care Med. 1996;154 (4 Pt 1):866-9.
49. Firestone Institute for Respiratory Health. 2008; Unpublished data.
50. Belda J, Leigh R, Parameswaran K, O'Byrne PM, Sears MR, Hargreave FE. Induced sputum cell counts in healthy adults. Am J Respir Crit Care Med. 2000;161(2 Pt 1):475-8.
51. D'Silva L, Cook RJ, Allen CJ, Hargreave FE, Parameswaran K. Changing pattern of sputum cell counts during successive exacerbations of airway disease. Respir Med. 2007;101(10):2217-20.
52. Bacci E, Cianchetti S, Bartoli M, Dente FL, Di Franco A, Vagaggini B, et al. Low sputum eosinophils predict the lack of response to beclomethasone in symptomatic asthmatic patients. Chest. 2006;129(3):565-72.
53. Jayaram L, Pizzichini MM, Cook RJ, Boulet LP, Lemière C, Pizzichini E, et al. Determining asthma treatment by monitoring sputum cell counts: effect on exacerbations. Eur Respir J. 2006;27(3):483-94.
54. Pallan S, Mahony JB, O'Byrne PM, Nair P. Asthma management by monitoring sputum neutrophil count. Chest. 2008;134(3):628-30.
55. Green RH, Brightling CE, Woltmann G, Parker D, Wardlaw AJ, Pavord ID, et al. Analysis of induced sputum in adults with asthma: identification of subgroup with isolated sputum neutrophilia and poor response to inhaled corticosteroids. Thorax. 2002;57(10):875-9.
56. D'Silva L, Gafni A, Thabane L, Jayaram L, Hassack P, Hargreave FE, et al. Cost analysis of monitoring asthma treatment using sputum cell counts. Can Respir J. 2008;15(7):370-4.
57. Lane C, Knight D, Burgess S, Franklin P, Horak F, Legg J, et al. Epithelial inducible nitric oxide synthase activity is the major determinant of nitric oxide concentration in exhaled breath. Thorax. 2004;59(9):757-60.
58. Kharitonov SA, Gonio F, Kelly C, Meah S, Barnes PJ. Reproducibility of exhaled nitric oxide measurements in healthy and asthmatic adults and children. Eur Respir J. 2003;21(3):433-8.
59. Ricciardolo FL, Sterk PJ, Gaston B, Folkerts G. Nitric oxide in health and disease of the respiratory system. Physiol Rev. 2004;84(3):731-65.

60. Taylor DR, Pijnenburg MW, Smith AD, De Jongste JC. Exhaled nitric oxide measurements: clinical application and interpretation. Thorax. 2006;61(9):817-27.
61. Berry MA, Shaw DE, Green RH, Brightling CE, Wardlaw AJ, Pavord ID, et al. The use of exhaled nitric oxide concentration to identify eosinophilic airway inflammation: an observational study in adults with asthma. Clin Exp Allergy. 2005;35(9):1175-9.
62. Kovesi T, Kulka R, Dales R. Exhaled nitric oxide concentration is affected by age, height, and race in healthy 9- to 12-year-old children. Chest. 2008;133(1):169-75.
63. Olin AC, Bake B, Toren K. Fraction of exhaled nitric oxide at 50 mL/s: reference values for adult lifelong never-smokers. Chest. 2007;131(6):1852-6.
64. Gratziou C, Lignos M, Dassiou M, Roussos C. Influence of atopy on exhaled nitric oxide in patients with stable asthma and rhinitis. Eur Respir J. 1999;14(4):897-901.
65. Buchvald F, Baraldi E, Carraro S, Gaston B, De Jongste J, Pijnenburg MW, et al. Measurements of exhaled nitric oxide in healthy subjects age 4 to 17 years. J Allergy Clin Immunol. 2005;115(6):1130-6.
66. Dressel H, de la Motte D, Reichert J, Ochmann U, Petru R, Angerer P, et al. Exhaled nitric oxide: independent effects of atopy, smoking, respiratory tract infection, gender and height. Respir Med. 2008;102(7):962-9.
67. Kharitonov SA, O'Connor BJ, Evans DJ, Barnes PJ. Allergen-induced late asthmatic reactions are associated with elevation of exhaled nitric oxide. Am J Respir Crit Care Med. 1995;151(6):1894-9.
68. Massaro AF, Gaston B, Kita D, Fanta C, Stamler JS, Drazen JM. Expired nitric oxide levels during treatment of acute asthma. Am J Respir Crit Care Med. 1995;152(2):800-3.
69. Kharitonov SA, Donnelly LE, Montuschi P, Corradi M, Collins JV, Barnes PJ. Dose-dependent onset and cessation of action of inhaled budesonide on exhaled nitric oxide and symptoms in mild asthma. Thorax. 2002;57(10):889-96.
70. Wilson AM, Lipworth BJ. Dose-response evaluation of the therapeutic index for inhaled budesonide in patients with mild-to-moderate asthma. Am J Med. 2000;108(4):269-75.
71. Jones SL, Kittelson J, Cowan JO, Flannery EM, Hancox RJ, McLachlan CR, et al. The predictive value of exhaled nitric oxide measurements in assessing changes in asthma control. Am J Respir Crit Care Med. 2001;164(5):738-43.
72. Pijnenburg MW, Hofhuis W, Hop WC, De Jongste JC. Exhaled nitric oxide predicts asthma relapse in children with clinical asthma remission. Thorax. 2005;60(3):215-8.
73. Zacharasiewicz A, Wilson N, Lex C, Erin EM, Li AM, Hansel T. Clinical use of noninvasive measurements of airway inflammation in steroid reduction in children. Am J Respir Crit Care Med. 2005;171(10):1077-82.
74. Michils A, Baldassarre S, Van Muylem A. Exhaled nitric oxide and asthma control: a longitudinal study in unselected patients. Eur Respir J. 2008;31(3):539-46.
75. Leuppi JD, Salome CM, Jenkins CR, Koskela H, Brannan JD, Anderson SD, et al. Markers of airway inflammation and airway hyperresponsiveness in patients with well-controlled asthma. Eur Respir J. 2001;18(3):444-50.
76. Deykin A, Lazarus SC, Fahy JV, Wechsler ME, Boushey HA, Chinchilli VM, et al. Sputum eosinophil counts predict asthma control after discontinuation of inhaled corticosteroids. J Allergy Clin Immunol. 2005;115(4):720-7.
77. Smith AD, Cowan JO, Brassett KP, Herbison GP, Taylor DR. Use of exhaled nitric oxide measurements to guide treatment in chronic asthma. N Engl J Med. 2005;352(21):2163-73.
78. Pijnenburg MW, Bakker EM, Hop WC, De Jongste JC. Titrating steroids on exhaled nitric oxide in children with asthma: a randomized controlled trial. Am J Respir Crit Care Med. 2005;172(7):831-6.
79. Shaw DE, Berry MA, Thomas M, Green RH, Brightling CE, Wardlaw AJ, et al. The use of exhaled nitric oxide to guide asthma management: a randomized controlled trial. Am J Respir Crit Care Med. 2007;176(3):231-7.
80. Muller KC, Jorres RA, Magnussen H, Holz O. Comparison of exhaled nitric oxide analysers. Respir Med. 2005;99(5):631-7.
81. Borrill Z, Clough D, Truman N, Morris J, Langley S, Singh D. A comparison of exhaled nitric oxide measurements performed using three different analysers. Respir Med. 2006;100(8):1392-6.
82. Kostikas K, Koutsokera A, Papiris S, Gourgoulianis KI, Loukides S. Exhaled breath condensate in patients with asthma: implications for application in clinical practice. Clin Exp Allergy. 2008;38(4):557-65.
83. Horvath I, Hunt J, Barnes PJ, Alving K, Antczak A, Baraldi E, et al. Exhaled breath condensate: methodological recommendations and unresolved questions. Eur Respir J. 2005;26(3):523-48.
84. Cox L, Williams B, Sicherer S, Oppenheimer J, Sher L, Hamilton R, et al. Pearls and pitfalls of allergy diagnostic testing: report from the American College of Allergy, Asthma and Immunology/American Academy of Allergy, Asthma and Immunology Specific IgE Test Task Force. Ann Allergy Asthma Immunol. 2008;101(6):580-92.
85. Bernstein IL, Li JT, Bernstein DI, Hamilton R, Spector SL, Tan R. Allergy diagnostic testing: an updated practice parameter. Ann Allergy Asthma Immunol. 2008;100(3 Suppl 3):S1-148.
86. Wood RA, Segall N, Ahlstedt S, Williams PB. Accuracy of IgE antibody laboratory results. Ann Allergy Asthma Immunol. 2007;99(1):34-41.
87. Agarwal R, Aggarwal AN, Garg M, Saikia B, Chakrabarti A. Cut-off values of serum IgE (total and A. fumigatus -specific) and eosinophil count in differentiating allergic bronchopulmonary aspergillosis from asthma. Mycoses. 2014;57(11):659-63.
88. Pedersen S. Preschool asthma—not so easy to diagnose. Prim Care Respir J. 2007;16(1):4-6.
89. Piacentini GL, Peroni DG, Bodini A, Bonafiglia E, Rigotti E, Baraldi E, et al. Childhood Asthma Control Test and airway inflammation evaluation in asthmatic children. Allergy. 2009;64(12):1753-7.
90. Brand PL, Baraldi E, Bisgaard H, Boner AL, Castro-Rodriguez JA, Custovic A, et al. Definition, assessment and treatment of wheezing disorders in preschool children: an evidence-based approach. Eur Respir J. 2008;32(4):1096-110.
91. Martinez FD, Wright AL, Taussig LM, Holberg CJ, Halonen M, Morgan WJ. Asthma and wheezing in the first six years of life. The Group Health Medical Associates. N Engl J Med. 1995;332(3):133-8.
92. Taussig LM, Wright AL, Holberg CJ, Halonen M, Morgan WJ, Martinez FD. Tucson Children's Respiratory Study: 1980 to present. J Allergy Clinical Immunol. 2003;111(4):661-75.
93. Castro-Rodriguez JA, Holberg CJ, Wright AL, Martinez FD. A clinical index to define risk of asthma in young children with recurrent wheezing. Am J Respir Crit Care Med. 2000;162(4 Pt 1):1403-6.

94. Martinez FD. Respiratory syncytial virus bronchiolitis and the pathogenesis of childhood asthma. Pediatr Infect Dis J. 2003;22(2 Suppl):S76-82.
95. Moeller A, Diefenbacher C, Lehmann A, Rochat M, Brooks-Wildhaber J, Hall GL, et al. Exhaled nitric oxide distinguishes between subgroups of preschool children with respiratory symptoms. J Allergy Clin Immunol. 2008;121(3):705-9.
96. Antoniu SA, Mihaescu T, Donner CF. Pharmacotherapy of cough-variant asthma. Expert Opin Pharmacother. 2007;8(17): 3021-8.
97. Cough variant asthma. In: Redington A, Morice AH (Eds). Acute and Chronic Cough. London: Taylor and Francis Group; 2005. pp. 303-22.
98. Kastelik JA, Thompson RH, Aziz I, Ojoo JC, Redington AE, Morice AH. Sex-related differences in cough reflex sensitivity in patients with chronic cough. Am J Respir Crit Care Med. 2002;166(7):961-4.
99. Koh YY, Park Y, Kim CK. Maximal airway response in adolescents with long-term asthma remission and persisting airway hypersensitivity: its profile and the effect of inhaled corticosteroids. Chest. 2002;122(4):1214-21.
100. Kim CK, Kim JT, Kang H, Yoo Y, Koh YY. Sputum eosinophilia in cough-variant asthma as a predictor of the subsequent development of classic asthma. Clin Exp Allergy. 2003;33(10):1409-14.
101. Fujimura M, Nishizawa Y, Nishitsuji M, Nomura S, Abo M, Ogawa H. Predictors for typical asthma onset from cough variant asthma. J Asthma. 2005;42(2):107-11.
102. Nakajima T, Nishimura Y, Nishiuma T, Kotani Y, Funada Y, Nakata H, et al. Characteristics of patients with chronic cough who developed classic asthma during the course of cough variant asthma: a longitudinal study. Respiration. 2005;72(6):606-11.
103. Todokoro M, Mochizuki H, Tokuyama K, Morikawa A. Childhood cough variant asthma and its relationship to classic asthma. Ann Allergy Asthma Immunol. 2003;90(6):652-9.
104. Matsumoto H, Niimi A, Takemura M, Ueda T, Tabuena R, Yamaguchi M, et al. Prognosis of cough variant asthma: a retrospective analysis. J Asthma. 2006;43(2):131-5.
105. Newman KB, Mason UG, Schmaling KB. Clinical features of vocal cord dysfunction. Am J Respir Crit Care Med. 1995;152(4 Pt 1):1382-6.
106. Parsons JP, Benninger C, Hawley MP, Philips G, Forrest LA, Mastronarde JG, et al. Vocal cord dysfunction: beyond severe asthma. Respir Med. 2010;104(4):504-9.
107. Watson MA, King CS, Holley AB, Greenburg DL, Mikita JA. Clinical and lung-function variables associated with vocal cord dysfunction. Respir Care. 2009;54(4):467-73.
108. Ibrahim WH, Gheriani HA, Almohamed AA, Raza T. Paradoxical vocal cord motion disorder: past, present and future. Postgrad Med J. 2007;83(977):164-72.
109. Sontag SJ, O'Connell S, Khandelwal S, Miller T, Nemchausky B, Schnell TG, et al. Most asthmatics have gastroesophageal reflux with or without bronchodilator therapy. Gastroenterology. 1990;99(3):613-20.
110. Mastronarde JG, Anthonisen NR, Castro M, Holbrook JT, Leone FT, Teague WG, et al. Efficacy of esomeprazole for treatment of poorly controlled asthma. N Engl J Med. 2009;360(15):1487-99.
111. Wu DN, Tanifuji Y, Kobayashi H, Yamauchi K, Kato C, Suzuki K, et al. Effects of esophageal acid perfusion on airway hyperresponsiveness in patients with bronchial asthma. Chest. 2000;118(6):1553-6.
112. Jack CI, Calverley PM, Donnelly RJ, Tran J, Russell G, Hind CR, et al. Simultaneous tracheal and oesophageal pH measurements in asthmatic patients with gastro-oesophageal reflux. Thorax. 1995;50(2):201-4.
113. Choy D, Leung R. Gastro-oesophageal reflux disease and asthma. Respirology. 1997;2(3):163-8.
114. Zerbib F, Guisset O, Lamouliatte H, Quinton A, Galmiche JP, Tunon-De-Lara JM, et al. Effects of bronchial obstruction on lower esophageal sphincter motility and gastroesophageal reflux in patients with asthma. Am J Respir Crit Care Med. 2002;166(9):1206-11.
115. Chotirmall SH, Watts M, Branagan P, Donegan CF, Moore A, McElvaney NG, et al. Diagnosis and management of asthma in older adults. J Am Geriatr Soc. 2009;57(5):901-9.
116. Sherman CB, Kern D, Richardson ER, Hubert M, Fogel BS. Cognitive function and spirometry performance in the elderly. Am Rev Respir Dis. 1993;148(1):123-6.
117. Janssens JP, Pache JC, Nicod LP. Physiological changes in respiratory function associated with ageing. Eur Respir J. 1999;13(1):197-205.
118. Milne JS, Williamson J. Respiratory function tests in older people. Clin Sci. 1972;42(3):371-81.
119. Ten Hacken NH, Postma DS, Timens W. Airway remodeling and long-term decline in lung function in asthma. Curr Opin Pulm Med. 2003;9(1):9-14.
120. Connolly MJ, Crowley JJ, Nielson CP, Charan NB, Vestal RE, et al. Peripheral mononuclear leucocyte beta adrenoceptors and non-specific bronchial responsiveness to methacholine in young and elderly normal subjects and asthmatic patients. Thorax. 1994;49(1):26-32.
121. Brodde OE, Howe U, Egerszegi S, Konietzko N, Michel MC. Effect of prednisolone and ketotifen on beta 2-adrenoceptors in asthmatic patients receiving beta 2-bronchodilators. Eur J Clin Pharmacol. 1988;34(2):145-50.
122. Soriano JB, Davis KJ, Coleman B, Visick G, Mannino D, Pride NB. The proportional Venn diagram of obstructive lung disease: two approximations from the United States and the United Kingdom. Chest. 2003;124(2):474-81.
123. Enright PL, Burchette RJ, Peters JA, Lebowitz MD, McDonnell WF, Abbey DE. Peak flow lability: association with asthma and spirometry in an older cohort. Chest. 1997;112(4):895-901.
124. Carvalhaes-Neto N, Lorino H, Gallinari C, Escolano S, Mallet A, Zerah F, et al. Cognitive function and assessment of lung function in the elderly. Am J Respir Crit Care Med. 1995;152(5 Pt 1):1611-5.
125. Gimeno F, Postma DS, van Altena R. Plethysmographic parameters in the assessment of reversibility of airways obs truction in patients with clinical emphysema. Chest. 1993; 104(2):467-70.
126. Dykewicz MS. Occupational asthma: current concepts in pathogenesis, diagnosis, and management. J Allergy Clin Immunol. 2009;123(3):519-28.
127. Tarlo SM, Balmes J, Balkissoon R, Beach J, Beckett W, Bernstein D, et al. Diagnosis and management of work-related asthma: American College Of Chest Physicians Consensus Statement. Chest. 2008;134(3 Suppl):1S-41S.
128. Bernstein JA. Material safety data sheets: are they reliable in identifying human hazards? J Allergy Clin Immunol. 2002;110(1):35-8.
129. Beach J, Rowe BH, Blitz S, Crumley E, Hooton N, Russell K, et al. Diagnosis and management of work-related asthma. Evid Rep Technol Assess (Summ). 2005;(129):1-8.

130. Mapp CE, Dal Vecchio L, Boschetto P, De Marzo N, Fabbri LM, et al. Toluene diisocyanate-induced asthma without airway hyperresponsiveness. Eur J Respir Dis. 1986;68(2):89-95.
131. Vandenplas O, Binard-Van Cangh F, Brumagne A, Caroyer JM, Thimpont J, Sohy C, et al. Occupational asthma in symptomatic workers exposed to natural rubber latex: evaluation of diagnostic procedures. J Allergy Clin Immunol. 2001;107(3): 542-7.
132. Beach J, Russell K, Blitz S, Hooton N, Spooner C, Lemiere C, et al. A systematic review of the diagnosis of occupational asthma. Chest. 2007;131(2):569-78.
133. Rioux JP, Malo JL, L'Archeveque J, Rabhi K, Labrecque M, et al. Workplace-specific challenges as a contribution to the diagnosis of occupational asthma. Eur Respir J. 2008;32(4):997-1003.
134. Chan-Yeung M, Obata H, Dittrick M, Chan H, Abboud R. Airway inflammation, exhaled nitric oxide, and severity of asthma in patients with western red cedar asthma. Am J Respir Crit Care Med. 1999;159(5 Pt 1):1434-8.
135. Maestrelli P, Calcagni PG, Saetta M, Di Stefano A, Hosselet JJ, Santonastaso A, et al. Sputum eosinophilia after asthmatic responses induced by isocyanates in sensitized subjects. Clin Exp Allergy. 1994;24(1):29-34.
136. Lemiere C, Chaboillez S, Malo JL, Cartier A. Changes in sputum cell counts after exposure to occupational agents: what do they mean? J Allergy Clin Immunol. 2001;107(6):1063-8.
137. Lemiere C, Romeo P, Chaboillez S, Tremblay C, Malo JL. Airway inflammation and functional changes after exposure to different concentrations of isocyanates. J Allergy Clin Immunol. 2002;110(4):641-6.
138. Leigh R, Hargreave FE. Occupational neutrophilic asthma. Can Respir J. 1999;6(2):194-6.
139. Quirce S. Eosinophilic bronchitis in the workplace. Curr Opin Allergy Clin Immunol. 2004;4(2):87-91.
140. Swierczynska-Machura D, Krakowiak A, Wiszniewska M, Dudek W, Walusiak J, Pałczynski C, et al. Exhaled nitric oxide levels after specific inahalatory challenge test in subjects with diagnosed occupational asthma. Int J Occup Med Environ Health. 2008;21(3):219-25.
141. Allmers H, Chen Z, Barbinova L, et al. Challenge from methacholine, natural rubber latex, or 4,4-diphenylmethane diisocyanate in workers with suspected sensitization affects exhaled nitric oxide [change in exhaled NO levels after allergen challenges]. Int Arch Occup Environ Health. 2000;73(3):181-6.
142. Obata H, Dittrick M, Chan H, Chan-Yeung M. Sputum eosinophils and exhaled nitric oxide during late asthmatic reaction in patients with western red cedar asthma. Eur Respir J. 1999;13(3):489-95.
143. Hoffmeyer F, Raulf-Heimsoth M, Bruning T. Exhaled breath condensate and airway inflammation. Curr Opin Allergy Clin Immunol. 2009;9(1):16-22.
144. Fireman E, Lerman Y, Stark M, Schwartz Y, Ganor E, Grinberg N, et al. Detection of occult lung impairment in welders by induced sputum particles and breath oxidation. Am J Ind Med. 2008;51(7):503-11.
145. Koutsokera A, Loukides S, Gourgoulianis KI, Kostikas K. Biomarkers in the exhaled breath condensate of healthy adults: mapping the path towards reference values. Curr Med Chem. 2008;15(6):620-30.
146. Hargreave FE, Parameswaran K. Asthma, COPD and bronchitis are just components of airway disease. Eur Respir J. 2006;28(2):264-7.
147. Marsh SE, Travers J, Weatherall M, Williams MV, Aldington S, Shirtcliffe PM, et al. Proportional classifications of COPD phenotypes. Thorax. 2008;63(9):761-7.
148. Gibson PG, Simpson JL. The overlap syndrome of asthma and COPD: what are its features and how important is it? Thorax. 2009;64(8):728-35.
149. de Granda-Orive JI, Escobar JA, Gutierrez T, Albiach JM, Sáez R, Rodero A, et al. Smoking-related attitudes, characteristics, and opinions in a group of young men with asthma. Mil Med. 2001;166(11):959-65.
150. Chaudhuri R, Livingston E, McMahon AD, Thomson L, Borland W, Thomson NC, et al. Cigarette smoking impairs the therapeutic response to oral corticosteroids in chronic asthma. Am J Respir Crit Care Med. 2003;168(11):1308-11.
151. Pride NB, Vermeire P, Allegra L. Diagnostic labels applied to model case histories of chronic airflow obstruction. Responses to a questionnaire in 11 North American and Western European countries. Eur Respir J. 1989;2(8):702-9.
152. James AL, Palmer LJ, Kicic E, Maxwell PS, Lagan SE, Ryan GF, et al. Decline in lung function in the Busselton Health Study: the effects of asthma and cigarette smoking. Am J Respir Crit Care Med. 2005;171(2):109-14.
153. Brutsche MH, Downs SH, Schindler C, Gerbase MW, Schwartz J, Frey M, et al. Bronchial hyperresponsiveness and the development of asthma and COPD in asymptomatic individuals: SAPALDIA cohort study. Thorax. 2006;61(8):671-7.
154. ten Brinke A. Risk factors associated with irreversible airflow limitation in asthma. Curr Opin Allergy Clin Immunol. 2008;8(1):63-9.
155. Bumbacea D, Campbell D, Nguyen L, Carr D, Barnes PJ, Robinson D, et al. Parameters associated with persistent airflow obstruction in chronic severe asthma. Eur Respir J. 2004;24(1):122-8.
156. Panizza JA, James AL, Ryan G, de Klerk N, Finucane KE. Mortality and airflow obstruction in asthma: a 17-year follow-up study. Intern Med J. 2006;36(12):773-80.
157. Vonk JM, Jongepier H, Panhuysen CI, Schouten JP, Bleecker ER, Postma DS. Risk factors associated with the presence of irreversible airflow limitation and reduced transfer coefficient in patients with asthma after 26 years of follow up. Thorax. 2003;58(4):322-7.
158. Chalmers GW, MacLeod KJ, Thomson L, Little SA, McSharry C, Thomson NC. Smoking and airway inflammation in patients with mild asthma. Chest. 2001;120(6):1917-22.
159. Boulet LP, Lemiere C, Archambault F, Carrier G, Descary MC, Deschesnes F. Smoking and asthma: clinical and radiologic features, lung function, and airway inflammation. Chest. 2006;129(3):661-8.
160. Kaminska M, Foley S, Maghni K, Storness-Bliss C, Coxson H, Ghezzo H, et al. Airway remodeling in subjects with severe asthma with or without chronic persistent airflow obstruction. J Allergy Clin Immunol. 2009;124(1):45-51.e1-4.
161. Orie NG. Second International Symposium. Assen, Royal Van Gorcum; 1964.
162. Frey U, Brodbeck T, Majumdar A, Taylor DR, Town GI, Silverman M, et al. Risk of severe asthma episodes predicted from fluctuation analysis of airway function. Nature. 2005; 438(7068):667-70.

61 Chapter

Airway Inflammation and Remodeling

Ruby Pawankar, Shu Hashimoto, Miyuki Hayashi, Shingo Yamanishi, Manabu Nonaka

INTRODUCTION

Allergic rhinitis (AR) and asthma are considered as part of a chronic respiratory allergic syndrome, based on the unifying concept of "One airway–One disease". The AR is a chronic inflammation of the nose, characterized by symptoms of sneezing, rhinorrhea, nasal itching and nasal obstruction. Asthma is a chronic, inflammatory condition of the lower airways characterized by reversible airflow obstruction, airway hyper-responsiveness, and episodic respiratory symptoms, including wheezing, productive cough breathlessness and chest tightness.[1]

Clinically, AR is an immunoglobulin E (IgE)-mediated, T helper cell 2-type (Th2-type) inflammatory disease whereas asthma may be divided into allergic and nonallergic asthma, distinguished by the presence or absence of IgE antibodies to common environmental allergens. About 80% of childhood and 50% of adult asthma is allergic (i.e. IgE associated). In the latter, the triggers are not well-known, but are probably microbes or microbial components. Both forms of asthma are characterized by Th2-type inflammation, stimulation of inflammatory cell (like mast cells) causing eosinophilia, leukocytosis, and enhanced B-cell IgE production, leading to airway hyperresponsiveness and tissue remodeling. The determinants for an individual to develop an asthmatic phenotype require both exposure to appropriate stimuli and a genetic predisposition.[2,3]

Airway remodeling involves structural changes in the airway wall characterized by epithelial alterations (epithelial shedding or denudation as a result of toxic proteins released especially by eosinophils), goblet cell metaplasia (their numbers increase first), bronchial mucus gland enlargement (excess production of mucus), subepithelial fibrosis and extracellular matrix (ECM) deposition, increased smooth muscle mass and increased vascularization.[2] Chronic inflammation causes tissue injury, which is partly repaired between inflammatory exacerbations. Airway remodeling is associated with poorly-reversible or nonreversible airway narrowing, more severe airflow limitation and airway hyperresponsiveness in all the components of adult severe asthma.[4] These changes involve both large and small airways, but the individual variations are large. Airway secretions also contribute to airflow limitation in asthma. Increase in amount and viscosity of secretions play a crucial role in acute, life-threatening exacerbations.[5] Based on the current knowledge, the characteristic structural changes seen in remodeling are not a feature of AR.

Although much more is known in terms of the inflammatory mechanisms underlying AR and asthma, there is still a gap in our understanding of the cellular and molecular pathways involved in remodeling. Both inflammation and remodeling occur in the tracheobronchial tree of patients with asthma. Persistent, eosinophilic inflammation seems to be a prerequisite for the development of remodeling.[6] Increased vascularity and expression of vascular endothelial growth factor (VEGF) are features of the asthmatic airways, but little is known about their contribution to airway remodeling. Vascular remodeling is a feature of asthma, inversely correlated with post-bronchodilator forced expiratory volume in one second (FEV_1) indicating a role in airflow obstruction.[7]

Until recently, airway remodeling was considered as a secondary phenomenon, developing later in the disease process as a consequence of persistent inflammation. The presence of airway inflammation and remodeling in children with asthma indicates that the process of remodeling begins early in the disease process of asthma synchronously with ongoing and repeated airway inflammation rather than as a consequence of airway inflammation.[8] Structural changes of the airways are already present and maximal in severely asthmatic school children, indicating that the changes begin early in life between the ages of 1 and 3 years; and in good association with tissue eosinophilia and reticular basement membrane thickening.[9,10] This gives a window of opportunity for early intervention that can possibly modify the natural history of asthma.[11]

CHRONIC INFLAMMATION IN ALLERGIC RHINITIS AND ASTHMA (FIGS 1 AND 2)

Inflammatory Response

The upper and lower airways have a similar mucosal structure, exhibit similar inflammatory reactions to irritants

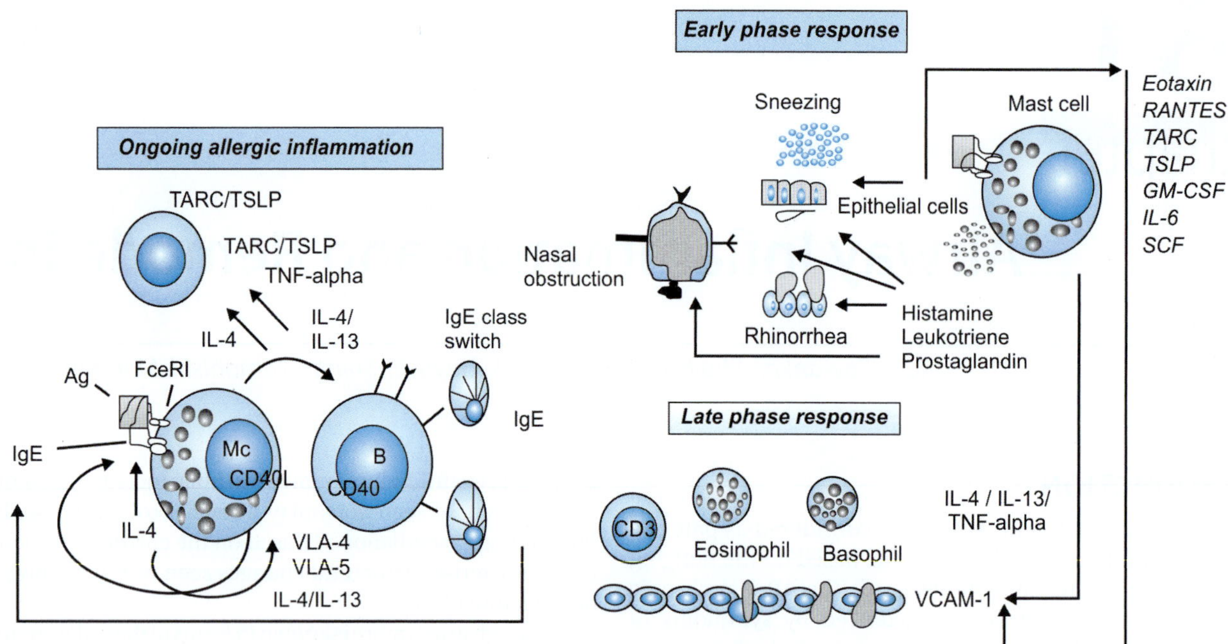

Fig. 1 Inflammatory mechanisms in allergic rhinitis (AR)
[Modified from Pawankar et al. AR pathomechanisms. Ed Kurup et al.]

Abbreviations: TARC, thymus and activation-regulated chemokine; TSLP, thymic stromal lymphopoietin; TNF, tumor necrosis factor; IgE, immunoglobulin E; GM-CSF, granulocyte-macrophage colony-stimulating factor; RANTES, regulated upon activation, normal T-cell expressed and secreted; IL, interleukin; Ag, antigen; FceRI, *fragment crystallizable* IgE receptor; Mc, macrophage; CD40L, cluster of differentiation 40 ligand; CD, cluster of differentiation; VLA, very late activation antigen; VCAM, vascular cell adhesion molecule; SCF, stem cell factor

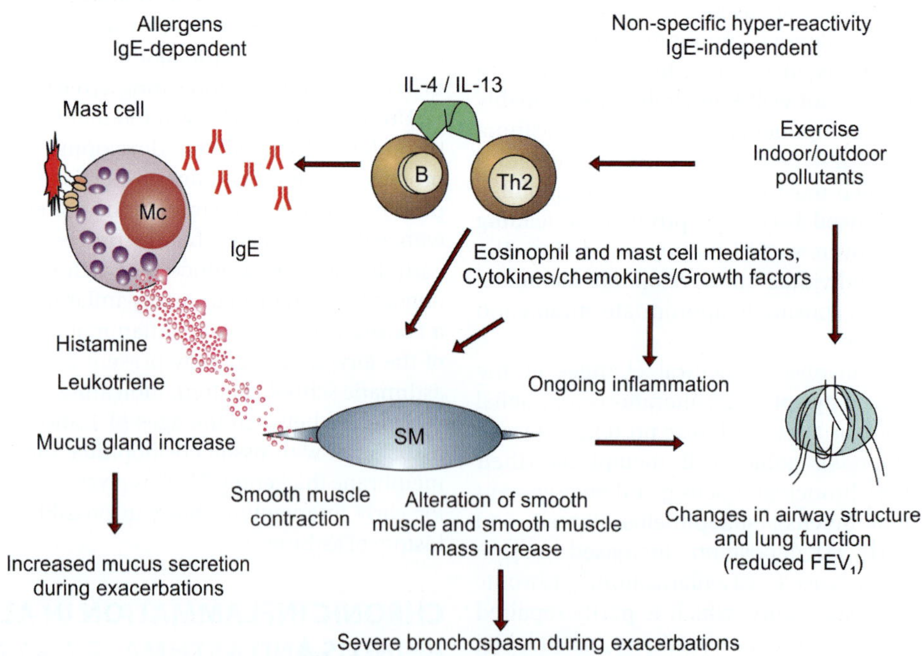

Fig. 2 Pathophysiology of asthma

Abbreviations: FEV_1, forced expiratory volume in one second; IgE, immunoglobulin E; Th, T helper cell

and allergens. Increasing evidence indicates that there is marked similarity in the degree of cell infiltration or cytokine expression during allergic inflammation between the nasal and bronchial mucosa.[12,13] There are minimal structural changes of the nasal mucosa in AR unlike that in asthma.

In allergic asthma and AR, inhaled allergens penetrate the mucociliary lining and enter the airway epithelium either via the tight junctions that surround the apical zone of epithelial cells or by direct uptake by the cells per se. Allergens are presented to T-cells that then react by forming a pool of Th2 (IL-4, IL-5 and IL-13 secreting T-cells) that drive the production of IgE via interaction with B-cells. Subsequently, the IgE binds to the high affinity IgE receptor on mast cells. Cross-linking of allergen specific IgE on the surface of mast cells by allergens causes the activation of mast cells and release of mediators such as histamine and leukotrienes. They increase vascular permeability and initiate a cascade of recruitment of more inflammatory cells responsible for further release of proinflammatory mediators.

Effector Cells of Inflammation

Mast Cells and Basophils

Mast cells are critical in mediating the early phase of inflammatory response in AR and asthma. More recently, it is known that mast cells are not only effector cells of the immediate phase response, but also play a role in ongoing allergic inflammation. They store and produce Th2-type cytokines, chemokines, induce IgE synthesis in B cells, express cysteinyl leukotriene-1 (CysLT1) receptor, glucocorticoid (GR) receptor, SAF-2, and upregulate the production of cytokines/chemokines in epithelial cells and fibroblasts.[14-19]

Accumulation of mast cells into the nasal and bronchial epithelium, a feature of AR and atopic asthma is also reported in idiopathic rhinitis.[20] Regulated upon activation, normal T-cell expressed and secreted (RANTES) and transforming growth factor (TGF-β) are implicated in the intraepithelial migration of mast cells. Increase in mast cells and basophils occur within 1 hour of nasal allergen challenge (NAC).[19,21,22] Patients with AR, with or without asthma, have similar number of intraepithelial mast cells.[23] Segmental bronchial challenge (SBC) induces an increase in basophils and eosinophils predominate in nasal and bronchoalveolar lavage (BAL).[24-27]

Airway mast cells stimulated via the *fragment crystallizable* receptor (FcRI) are an important source of Th2 cytokines, proinflammatory cytokines like tumor necrosis factor (TNF)-α (preformed in mast cells) and chemokines like thymus and activation-regulated chemokine (TARC), as well as the IL-7 like cytokine thymic stromal lymphopoietin (TSLP).[28,29] FcRI-mediated TSLP production from mast cells is further enhanced in an autocrine manner by IL-4.[30] Moreover, mast cells can interact with structural cells, like epithelial cells to enhance the production of cytokines and chemokines from epithelial cells. TNF-α in concert with IL-4 and IL-13 enhances the production of TARC, TSLP and eotaxin from epithelial cells.[19] These result in increased infiltration of Th2 cells, eosinophils and differentiation of dendritic cells. Moreover, tryptase and chymase from mast cells can upregulate RANTES and granulocyte-macrophage colony-stimulating factor (GM-CSF) production from epithelial cells.[19] TNF-α also promotes antigen and Th17 cell-dependent neutrophilia after allergenic stimulation and induces dendritic cell migration.[31,32] Murine mast cells have been shown to induce $CD4^+$T-cell migration in vitro, but downregulate FcRI expression in T regulatory (T reg) cells, while activated T reg cells suppress mast cell FcRI expression.

Mast cells can induce IgE synthesis in B-cells and local IgE synthesis has been demonstrated in the nasal mucosa of patients with AR.[33,34] IL-4 and IgE upregulate *FcRI* expression in mast cells suggesting a crucial role for the mast cell-IgE-IgE receptor cascade in ongoing inflammation in AR and asthma.[34] A role for mast cells in antigen presentation is also suggested.[35]

While classically, mast cell activation occurs following the allergen crosslinking of FcRI-bound, allergen-specific IgE, they may also be activated through multiple other mechanisms, such as the complement receptors, FcRI and via toll-like receptors (TLRs) even in the absence of FcRI stimulation.[36-40]

Other novel mechanisms of mast cell activation, independent of IgE, are via the protein S100A12 and the receptors CD200R3/CD200R, whereas IL-33, a member of the IL-1 cytokine family, has demonstrated the ability to activate mast cells, even in the absence of FcεR1 stimulation.[36-40]

Basophils are increased in the nasal secretions and BAL of patients with AR and asthma. Like mast cells, basophils can also initiate allergic inflammation through the binding of allergen-specific IgE antibodies to the FcR1 on basophil cell surface.[41] Basophils also drive Th2 cell differentiation of activated naive $CD4^+$T cells via production of IL-4 and direct cell-cell contact.[42] Basophils in AR and atopic asthmatics also express high levels of the FcRI.[43] Downregulation of FcRI in basophils and mast cells comprises one of the target mechanisms of the efficacy of anti-IgE monoclonal antibody (Omalizumab).

Eosinophils

Eosinophils increase in both the early and late phase of AR, correlate with nasal flow, IL-4, IL-5, IL-8 and IFN-γ, spirometric values, methacholine test positivity, percentage of predicted FEV_1 and bronchial hyper-reactivity (BHR).[44-54] Eosinophils are increased in symptomatic ectopics and increase in nasal as well as bronchial epithelium and lamina propria after NAC.[22,55-57] Eosinophils are a major source of migration inhibitory factor (MIF) and nerve growth factor (NGF), express 5-lipoxygenase (5-LO), the function of 5-lipoxygenase activating protein (FLAP) and leukotriene C(4) synthase (LTC4S), and $CysLT_1$ and $CysLT_2$ receptors, are involved in the loss of epithelial integrity and are also seen in the esophageal mucosa of symptomatic patients with respiratory allergy.[58-62]

Interleukin-5 (IL-5) has a key role modulating eosinophil differentiation and survival. Targeting IL-5 as a therapeutic strategy for allergic asthma with anti-IL-5 therapy has demonstrated marked reduction of peripheral blood eosinophils, but only partial abrogation of the pulmonary eosinophilic response and with minimal impact on clinical outcomes.[63,64] In selected patients with refractory, eosinophilic asthma, anti-IL-5 monoclonal antibody (mepolizumab) reduced both peripheral blood and sputum eosinophil levels, asthma exacerbations, and resulted in a reduction in oral corticosteroid dose.[65,66] These results indicate that at least in a subset of patients with asthma, eosinophils are critical effector cells in persistent asthma and severe exacerbations.

Eosinophil chemoattractants include eotaxin, macrophage/monocyte chemotactic protein-4 (MCP4), RANTES, and CysLTs among others.[67,68] They act on distinct cell surface receptors [e.g. CC chemokine receptor 3 (CCR3) and $cysLT_1$] present on the eosinophil, but not exclusively so. Challenge with leukotriene E_4 (LTE_4) or leukotriene D_4 (LTD_4) results in increased nasal secretion and nasal obstruction in AR and greatly increased numbers of eosinophils in the bronchial wall.[67,68] $CysLT_1$ receptor is expressed on a variety of nasal and bronchial inflammatory cells, including eosinophils, neutrophils, mast cells, macrophages, B lymphocytes and plasma cells.[69] These numbers of inflammatory cells expressing the $cysLT_1$ receptor are also increased in AR and asthma. There is a further, significant increase among patients experiencing a severe exacerbation of asthma leading to hospitalization.[70]

Activated eosinophils release highly toxic granules, the evolutionary function of which has probably been killing the potentially dangerous invader. Especially in asthma, eosinophil derivatives damage the surface epithelial cells, loosening their attachments and resulting in the shedding of cells into the airway lumen, where they admix with eosinophils, neutrophils and mucus.

T Lymphocytes

In PAR patients, $CD3^+$, $CD25^+$ (activated) and $CD45RA^+$ (naïve) T-lymphocytes are increased in the nasal mucosa. In PAR, memory T-cells and in idiopathic rhinitis, CD8+ T-cells correlate with mucosal mast cells.[71] While CD86 is expressed on CD19; CD1a, CD14 and CD3 T-cells in PAR; CD80, CD28 and CD152 are expressed after NAC.[72] Moreover, CCR4+ CD4 cells are increased in AR.[73] Besides, Th2 cytokines and chemokines, T-cells in AR express IL-16, CXCR1 and CX(3)CR(1).[74-76] Mucosal $\delta\gamma$ T-cells in PAR and asthma are increased, induce IgE synthesis in B-cells and induce proliferation of $\alpha\beta$ T-cells.[77] $CD23^+$ B-cells increase in PAR, but do not correlate with the mucosal Th2 cells.[73]

Although conventionally, both AR and allergic asthma have been considered to be due to a disruption in the normal Th1/Th2 balance, there is new evidence on the emerging roles of Th17 cells, which are a distinct subpopulation of CD4+ T-cells that produce IL-17A, IL-17F, IL-22, TNF-α, and IL-21.[78] Th17 cells were found in the nasal mucosa of AR patients and in bronchial biopsies of asthmatics.[79,80] IL-17 induces the release of proinflammatory cytokines/chemokines from a variety of cell types, is linked to the development of airway neutrophilia, and its presence in the asthmatic airway, correlates with increased severity of disease.[79] T reg cells play roles in the determination of self-tolerance and the regulation of immune responses. Th17 and T reg cells have opposing actions, and T reg cells secrete IL-10 and TGF-β and are increased in patients after immunotherapy.

Neutrophils

Although neutrophils are predominantly increased in nonallergic infective rhinitis and chronic rhinosinusitis, the increased expression of activation markers on neutrophils and myeloperoxidase (MPO) levels in AR and increase in neutrophils in BAL after NAC suggests roles for neutrophils in AR.[25,81] In acute, severe exacerbations of asthma, there are increased eosinophils and neutrophils within the airway, and the increase in neutrophils is proportionately greater.[82] Inhaled corticosteroids reduce airway eosinophils, but increase airway neutrophils and neutrophil chemoattractant IL-8, with loss of asthma control.[83]

Epithelial Cells

Conventionally, epithelial cells placed at the interface between the external environment and the host have been considered to play a role as a defense barrier against environmental agents. Over the past several years, the roles of epithelial cells as effector cells has become more evident, directly via the action of inflammatory mediators, as well as via cell-cell interaction with immune cells. Moreover, its pivotal position in orchestrating airway remodeling and fibroblast proliferation is also crucial.[84]

Airway epithelial cells are an important source of a variety of inflammatory mediators, including multifunctional cytokines and chemokines like IL-1, IL-6, IL-8, TNF-α, GM-CSF, RANTES, Eotaxin and TARC, leading to their crucial role in the migration and activation of immune cells like eosinophils, basophils and Th2 cells.[85,86] More recently, TSLP derived from epithelial cells is increased in the nasal mucosa of AR patients and in the asthmatic airway.[87] TSLP can activate dendritic cells, promote Th2 responses and activate mast cells.[30] Epithelial cells also express costimulatory molecules like CD86 and HLA-DR, CD86 and the FcRI can present antigen to T-cells.[88,89] Particulate matter like diesel exhaust particles (DEP) can induce the release of proinflammatory mediators and enhance the expression of costimulatory molecules on epithelial cells.

Innate Lymphoid Cells

Previous studies have demonstrated a crucial role for innate lymphoid cells (ILC2s) in the development of lung inflammation from alternaria species and airway hyperreactivity caused by influenza, and allergic sensitization from dust mite and peanut.[90-93]

In an animal model study performed to elucidate factors contributing to the persistence of asthma, although T cells contributed to the severity of chronic asthma, they were reported to be redundant in maintaining airway hyperreactivity and remodeling. A critical network of feedback and feed-forward interactions between epithelial cells and ILC2s was found to be involved in maintaining chronic asthma.[94]

Minimal Persistent Inflammation

Even when symptoms are absent in chronic inflammatory diseases like AR and asthma, a minimal level of persistent inflammation may persist. To prevent unexpected exacerbations, the treatment strategy may need to include its management. Immunotherapy and antihistamines reduce persistent inflammation by decreasing intercellular adhesion molecule 1 (ICAM-1) expression in epithelial cells and eosinophil cationic protein in patients with mite-induced AR.

REMODELING IN ASTHMA (FIG. 3)

Remodeling is defined as a change in structure that is inappropriate to maintain the normal airway function.[95,96] Some features of remodeling are evident, even in newly diagnosed or mild asthmatics and is characterized by epithelial fragility and reticular basement membrane thickening. With increasing severity of asthma, the changes are more pronounced and clear: increase of airway smooth muscle mass, vascularity, numbers of fibroblasts, and interstitial collagen, as well as mucus gland hypertrophy.[97] These changes appear to be the greatest in the larger, more proximal airways. Thickening of the reticular basement membrane occurs early in asthma, even before diagnosis, and is detected in children with mild asthma. In school children between the ages of 6 and 16 with severe asthma there is already maximally thickening, but with no relation to the age or symptom duration.[9] These changes appear in preschool wheezy children by the age of 29 months.[7] Reticular basement thickness is shown to be the hallmark of severe asthma, but not of mild asthma or chronic obstructive pulmonary disease (COPD).[98]

Airway smooth muscle surrounds the airways as two opposing helices, i.e. a geodesic pattern. As the muscle shortens, it constricts and also tends to shorten the airway against an elastic load. Airway smooth muscle mass is increased in the asthmatic airway.[99] Airway smooth muscle cells can secrete mediators that may promote mast cell chemotaxis, proliferation and survival, while cell-cell interaction between airway smooth muscle cells and mast cells enhances activated complement-induced mast cell degranulation.[100-102] Human lung mast cells migrate towards Th2 cytokine-stimulated airway smooth muscle cells from

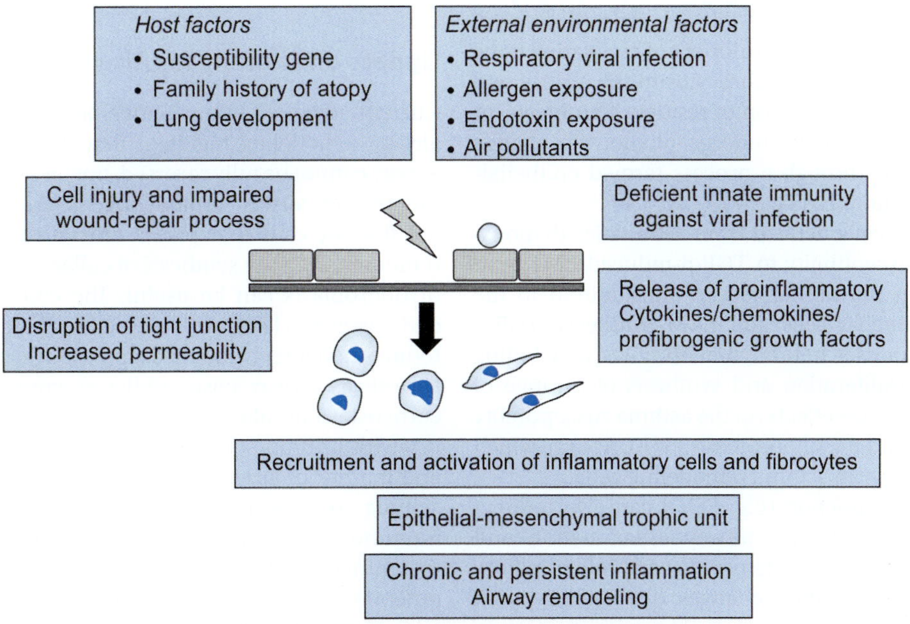

Fig. 3 Airway inflammation and remodeling in asthma [Modified from Hashimoto et al. ACII., 2002]

asthmatics, while supernatants obtained from airway smooth muscle cell cultures of nonasthmatics inhibit this chemotaxis.[103] Large numbers of mast cells are found located within the bronchial smooth muscle of asthmatics and mast cell mediators, such as tryptase and cytokines can modulate airway smooth muscle cell function. Mast cells also express matrix metallopeptidase 9 (MMP-9) and contribute to multiple features of chronic asthma tissue remodeling.[19]

Bronchial epithelial cell experiments have demonstrated a role for TLR signaling in the activation of epidermal growth factor receptor, suggesting a role for TLRs in potentiating remodeling.[104] In the asthmatic airway, there are increased numbers of subepithelial myofibroblasts, and allergen challenge in people with asthma leads to the increased accumulation of myofibroblasts in the airway mucosa.[84,105] In genetically susceptible individuals, impaired epithelial barrier function renders the airways vulnerable to early life virus infection. This, in turn, provides the stimulus to prime immature dendritic cells toward directing a Th2 response and local allergen sensitization. Continued environmental insults due to viral, allergen, and pollutant exposure and impaired repair responses lead to asthma persistence and provide the mediator and growth factor microenvironment for persistence of inflammation and airway wall remodeling. There is also increased deposition of matrix in the epithelial lamina reticularis and physical distortion of the epithelium consequent upon repeated bronchoconstriction enhances inflammation and remodeling.[106]

Histamine can induce the transition from fibroblasts to myofibroblasts (as measured by α-smooth muscle actin expression), and induce connective tissue growth factor expression in fibroblasts, suggesting the ability to participate in the process of remodeling.[107,108] Fibroblastic infiltration of lung may be secondary to the recruitment of circulating bone marrow-derived progenitors of fibrocytes to the airway and to the proliferation and expansion of resident fibroblasts, or possibly, epithelial cells may undergo phenotypic change to effector fibroblasts through a process termed epithelial-mesenchymal transition (EMT).

Airway epithelial cells derived from asthmatics demonstrated increased susceptibility to TGF-β-induced EMT than those derived from normal subjects.[109] In addition to the stimulation of epithelial cells and ECM synthesis, TGF-β can elicit other responses in bronchial fibroblasts, including stimulating their proliferation and synthesis of a range of growth factors. It also has effects on the asthma susceptibility gene, a disintegrin and metalloprotease 33 (ADAM33), which has been implicated as an asthma remodeling gene.

Measuring airway function (e.g. FEV_1) can give indirect information on the long-term airway inflammation and structural changes, but cannot detect the early inflammatory processes. Such inflammatory changes can exist even in patients with normal lung function, but with symptoms indicative of asthma.[110] On the other hand, symptomatic infants, who have reversible airflow obstruction may not have bronchial mucosal eosinophilia or remodeling.[8]

How Early can Remodeling Start?

Airway biopsy studies in children suggest that pathological changes, such as epithelial loss, basement membrane thickening and angiogenesis occur early in the asthmatic airways. In children with difficult asthma (mean age of 13, age range of 6–16) recruited to investigate whether the thickening of reticular basement membrane could occur in childhood asthma have shown that the thickening of reticular basement membrane was seen in the airway.[9] Barbato A et al. had examined the biopsy specimens of airway in nine children with asthma (age of 4–12 years), six children with atopic without asthma (age of 4–12 years), and in eight control children without asthma or atopic to elucidate whether airway inflammation and remodeling could occur even in mild childhood asthma.[97] It was nicely demonstrated that airway eosinophilia and basement membrane thickness were present in children with mild asthma, even in children with atopic without asthma.[97] This indicates the following:

- Airway inflammation shown by airway eosinophilia occurs even in mild as well as difficult asthma
- Airway inflammation occurs before episodic wheezing, although asthma symptoms are difficult to establish in children
- The presence of both airway inflammation and remodeling indicates that remodeling process begins early and occurs synchronously with ongoing and repeated airway inflammation rather than as a subsequent event of airway inflammation.

Update on Therapy for Airway Remodeling

Current advances in our understanding of the treatment for airway remodeling highlight that the remodeled asthmatic airway cannot be fully reversed, but targeting therapy reduces the risk of airway remodeling, is crucial. Myofibroblasts are the key cells that play a crucial role in the process of remodeling via the synthesis of collagen. Therefore, targeting myofibroblasts can be useful. The combination of inhaled corticosteroids (ICS) with long-acting beta 2-agonists (LABA) reduce the allergen-induced increase in airway myofibroblasts as well as airway eosinophilia as compared with inhaled corticosteroids alone, indicating that the combination of ICS with LABA is superior for reducing airway inflammation and the risk of airway remodeling.[111] For difficult-to-control asthma or severe corticosteroid-refractory asthma, an immunomodulator like the anti-IgE mAb (Omalizumab) is recommended. Bronchial thermoplasty is another novel and potentially effective therapy with growing evidence on its clinical effectiveness. More evidence is needed on the long-term benefits of thermoplasty.[112]

SUMMARY

The development of AR and asthma requires an interaction between the environment, immune system and genetic susceptibility. While pollen-induced rhinitis is the most characteristic IgE-mediated allergic disease; in perennial AR the allergic triggers are more continuous and lead to an ongoing inflammation. Several cells and mediators orchestrate and maintain this inflammation. Although histamine is still one of the major mediators of the allergic reaction, many other mediators produced by different cell types are involved. The intricate interactions amongst these mediators, cytokines, chemokines, neuropeptides, adhesion molecules and various cells in the form of a complex network lead to the development of specific symptoms and nonspecific hyper-reactivity of AR.

Asthma is characterized by variable degrees of chronic inflammation and structural alterations in the airways, which include epithelial denudation, goblet cell metaplasia, subepithelial thickening, increased airway smooth muscle mass, bronchial gland enlargement, angiogenesis, and alterations in ECM components, involving large and small airways. Chronic inflammation is thought to initiate and perpetuate cycles of tissue injury and repair in asthma, although remodeling may also occur in parallel with inflammation. While AR and asthma share several similarities in the inflammatory cell and mediator profiles and responses, remodeling as seen in asthma is not characteristic of AR. A variety of inflammatory cells and structural cells play a role in orchestrating the inflammation and structural changes in asthma. Increased airway responsiveness is a surrogate marker of inflammation, may reflect the development of structural changes in the airways. Such persistently increased bronchial responsiveness indicates remodeling, which is partly resistant to therapy.

With the increasing evidence on the links between AR and asthma from epidemiological, immunological and clinical studies, early intervention and downregulation of inflammation are the keys for better control of both AR and asthma. New modes of immunomodulatory therapies are under trials or at different stages of development for both AR and asthma. Anti-IgE and anti-TNF-α therapies hold more promising outcomes, but their effect on halting airway remodeling in severe asthma is not known. Among the new approaches are anti-IL-5 mAb, anti-IL-13mAb, anti-IL 4 antagonist, TLR agonists, and transcription factor modulators targeting syk kinase, peroxisome proliferator-activated receptor gamma, and nuclear factor kappa B. One has to also look at their efficacy, safety, cost efficacy as well as their utility in multiorgan diseases like asthma, rhinitis and eczema, urticaria, etc. Their disease modifying effects, especially in the long term. Given the similarity that exists between the patterns of inflammation in asthma and AR and the impact of AR on asthma, treatment should focus on a global approach to treat both the upper and lower airways for better outcomes.

REFERENCES

1. Bousquet J, Jeffery PK, Busse WW, Johnson M, Vignola AM. Asthma. From bronchoconstriction to airways inflammation and remodeling. Am J Respir Crit Care Med. 2000;161(5):1720-45.
2. Kabesch M, Schedel M, Carr D, Woitsch B, Fritzsch C, Weiland SK, et al. IL-4/IL-13 pathway genetics strongly influence serum IgE levels and childhood asthma. J Allergy Clin Immunol. 2006;117(2):269-74.
3. Loza MJ, Chang BL. Association between Q551R IL4R genetic variants and atopic asthma risk demonstrated by meta-analysis. J Allergy Clin Immunol. 2007;120(3):578-85.
4. Holgate ST, Polosa R. The mechanisms diagnosis, and management of severe asthma in adults. Lancet. 2006;368 (9537):780-93.
5. Bai TR, Cooper J, Koelmeyer T, Paré PD, Weir TD. The effect of age and duration of disease on airway structure in fatal asthma. Am J Respir Crit Care Med. 2000;162(2 Pt 1):663-9.
6. Humbles AA, Lloyd CM, McMillan SJ, Friend DS, Xanthou G, McKenna EE, et al. A critical role for eosinophils in allergic airways remodeling. Science. 2004;305(5691):1776-9.
7. Siddiqui S, Sutcliffe A, Shikotra A, Woodman L, Doe C, McKenna S, et al. Vascular remodeling is a feature of asthma and nonasthmatic eosinophilic bronchitis. J Allergy Clin Immunol. 2007;120(4):813-9.
8. Saglani S, Malmström K, Pelkonen AS, Malmberg LP, Lindahl H, Kajosaari M, et al. Airway remodeling and inflammation in symptomatic infants with reversible airflow obstruction. Am J Respir Crit Care Med. 2005;171(7):722-7.
9. Payne DN, Rogers AV, Adelroth E, Bandi V, Guntupalli KK, Bush A, et al. Early thickening of the reticular basement membrane in children with difficult asthma. Am J Respir Crit Care Med. 2003;167(1):78-82.
10. Saglani S, Payne DN, Nicholson AG. Thickening of the epithelial reticular basement membrane in preschool children with troublesome wheeze. Am Thorac Soc. 2005;2005:A515.
11. Saglani S, Payne DN, Zhu J, Wang Z, Nicholson AG, Bush A, et al. Early detection of airway remodeling and eosinophilic inflammation in preschool wheezers. Am J Respir Crit Care Med. 2007;176(9):858-64.
12. Pawankar R. Allergic rhinitis and asthma: are they manifestations of one syndrome? Clin Exp Allergy. 2006;36(1):1-4.
13. Cruz AA, Popov T, Pawankar R, Annesi-Maesano I, Fokkens WJ, Kemp J. ARIA Initiative Scientific Committee. Common characteristics of upper and lower airways in rhinitis and asthma: ARIA update, in collaboration with GA(2)LEN. Allergy. 2007;62(Suppl 84):1-41.
14. Wilson AM, Duong M, Crawford L, Denburg J. An evaluation of peripheral blood eosinophil/basophil progenitors following nasal allergen challenge in patients with allergic rhinitis. Clin Exp Allergy. 2005;35(1):39-44.
15. Pawankar R, Yamagishi S, Yagi T. Revisiting the roles of mast cells in allergic rhinitis and its relation to local IgE synthesis. Am J Rhinol. 2000;14(5):309-17.
16. Shirasaki H, Kanaizumi E, Watanabe K, Matsui T, Sato J, Narita S, et al. Expression and localization of the cysteinyl leukotriene 1 receptor in human nasal mucosa. Clin Exp Allergy. 2002;32(7):1007-12.
17. Shirasaki H, Watanabe K, Kanaizumi E, Konno N, Sato J, Narita S, et al. Expression and localization of steroid receptors in human nasal mucosa. Acta Otolaryngol. 2004;124(8):958-63.

18. Kikly KK, Bochner BS, Freeman SD, Tan KB, Gallagher KT, D'alessio KJ, et al. Identification of SAF-2, a novel siglec expressed on eosinophils, mast cells, and basophils. J Allergy Clin Immunol. 2000;105(6 Pt 1):1093-100.
19. Pawankar R. Mast cells in allergic airway disease and chronic rhinosinusitis. Chem Immunol Allergy. 2005;87:111-29.
20. Powe DG, Hiskisson RS, Carney AS, Jenkins D, Jones NS. Idiopathic and allergic rhinitis show a similar inflammatory response. Clin Otolaryngol Allied Sci. 2000;25(6):570-6.
21. Salib RJ, Kumar S, Wilson SJ, Howarth PH. Nasal mucosal immunoexpression of the mast cell chemoattractants TGF-beta, eotaxin, and stem cell factor and their receptors in allergic rhinitis. J Allergy Clin Immunol. 2004;114(4):799-806.
22. KleinJan A, McEuen AR, Dijkstra MD, Buckley MG, Walls AF, Fokkens WJ. Basophil and eosinophil accumulation and mast cell degranulation in the nasal mucosa of patients with hay fever after local allergen provocation. J Allergy Clin Immunol. 2000;106(4):677-86.
23. Braunstahl GJ, Fokkens WJ, Overbeek SE, KleinJan A, Hoogsteden HC, Prins JB. Mucosal and systemic inflammatory changes in allergic rhinitis and asthma: a comparison between upper and lower airways. Clin Exp Allergy. 2003;33(5):579-87.
24. Braunstahl GJ, Overbeek SE, Fokkens WJ, Kleinjan A, McEuen AR, Walls AF, et al. Segmental bronchoprovocation in allergic rhinitis patients affects mast cell and basophil numbers in nasal and bronchial mucosa. Am J Respir Crit Care Med. 2001;164(5):858-65.
25. Gorski P, Krakowiak A, Ruta U. Nasal and bronchial responses to flour-inhalation in subjects with occupationally induced allergy affecting the airway. Int Arch Occup Environ Health. 2000;73(7):488-97.
26. Krakowiak A, Ruta U, Gorski P, Kowalska S, Pałczyński C. Nasal lavage fluid examination and rhinomanometry in the diagnostics of occupational airway allergy to laboratory animals. Int J Occup Med Environ Health. 2003;16(2):125-32.
27. Pałczyński C, Walusiak J, Krakowiak A, Szymczak W, Wittczak T, Ruta U, et al. Nasal lavage fluid examination in diagnostics of occupational allergy to chloramine. Int J Occup Med Environ Health. 2003;16(3):231-40.
28. Bradding P, Holgate ST. The mast cell as a source of cytokines in asthma. Ann N Y Acad Sci. 1996;796:272-81.
29. Pawankar R, Okuda M, Hasegawa S, Suzuki K, Yssel H, Okubo K, et al. Interleukin-13 expression in the nasal mucosa of perennial allergic rhinitis. Am J Respir Crit Care Med. 1995;152(6 Pt 1):2059-67.
30. Okayama Y, Okumura S, Sagara H, Yuki K, Sasaki T, Watanabe N, et al. FcepsilonRI-mediated thymic stromal lymphopoietin production by interleukin-4-primed human mast cells. Eur Respir J. 2009;34(2):425-35.
31. Nakae S, Suto H, Berry GJ, Galli SJ. Mast cell-derived TNF can promote Th17 cell-dependent neutrophil recruitment in ovalbumin-challenged OTII mice. Blood. 2007;109(9):3640-8.
32. Suto H, Nakae S, Kakurai M, Sedgwick JD, Tsai M, Galli SJ. Mast cell-associated TNF promotes dendritic cell migration. J Immunol. 2006;176(7):4102-12.
33. Pawankar R, Okuda M, Yssel H, Okumura K, Ra C. Nasal mast cells in perennial allergic rhinitics exhibit increased expression of the Fc epsilonRI, CD40L, IL-4, and IL-13, and can induce IgE synthesis in B cells. J Clin Invest. 1997;99(7):1492-9.
34. Smurthwaite L, Durham SR. Local IgE synthesis in allergic rhinitis and asthma. Curr Allergy Asthma Rep. 2002;2(3):231-8.
35. Kambayashi T, Baranski JD, Baker RG, Zou T, Allenspach EJ, Shoag JE, et al. Indirect involvement of allergen-captured mast cells in antigen presentation. Blood. 2008;111(3):1489-96.
36. Yang Z, Yan WX, Cai H, Tedla N, Armishaw C, Di Girolamo, et al. N S100A12 provokes mast cell activation: a potential amplification pathway in asthma and innate immunity. J Allergy Clin Immunol. 2007;119(1):106-14.
37. Kojima T, Obata K, Mukai K, Sato S, Takai T, Minegishi Y, et al. Mast cells and basophils are selectively activated in vitro and in vivo through CD200R3 in an IgE-independent manner. J Immunol. 2007;179(10):7093-100.
38. Ho LH, Ohno T, Oboki K, Kajiwara N, Suto H, Iikura M, et al. IL-33 induces IL-13 production by mouse mast cells independently of IgE-FcepsilonRI signals. J Leukoc Biol. 2007;82(6):1481-90.
39. Iikura M, Suto H, Kajiwara N, Oboki K, Ohno T, Okayama Y, et al. IL-33 can promote survival, adhesion and cytokine production in human mast cells. Lab Invest. 2007;87(10):971-8.
40. Allakhverdi Z, Smith DE, Comeau MR, Delespesse G. Cutting edge: the ST2 ligand IL-33 potently activates and drives maturation of human mast cells. J Immunol. 2007;179(4):2051-4.
41. Obata K, Mukai K, Tsujimura Y, Ishiwata K, Kawano Y, Minegishi Y, et al. Basophils are essential initiators of a novel type of chronic allergic inflammation. Blood. 2007;110(3):913-20.
42. Oh K, Shen T, Le Gros G, Min B. Induction of Th2 type immunity in a mouse system reveals a novel immunoregulatory role of basophils. Blood. 2007;109(7):2921-7.
43. MacGlashan D. IgE and FcepsilonRI regulation. Clin Rev Allergy Immunol. 2005;29(1):49-60.
44. Milanese M, Ricca V, Canonica GW, Ciprandi G. Eosinophils, specific hyper-reactivity and occurrence of late phase reaction in allergic rhinitis. Eur Ann Allergy Clin Immunol. 2005;37(1):7-10.
45. Ciprandi G, Vizzaccaro A, Cirillo I, Tosca M, Massolo A, Passalacqua G. Nasal eosinophils display the best correlation with symptoms, pulmonary function and inflammation in allergic rhinitis. Int Arch Allergy Immunol. 2005;136(3):266-72.
46. Ciprandi G, Marseglia GL, Klersy C, Tosca MA. Relationships between allergic inflammation and nasal airflow in children with persistent allergic rhinitis due to mite sensitization. Allergy. 2005;60(7):957-60.
47. Ciprandi G, Cirillo I, Vizzaccaro A, Milanese M, Tosca MA. Nasal obstruction in patients with seasonal allergic rhinitis: relationships between allergic inflammation and nasal airflow. Int Arch Allergy Immunol. 2004;134(1):34-40.
48. Kurt E, Bavbek S, Aksu O, Erekul S, Misirligil Z The effect of natural pollen exposure on eosinophil apoptosis and its relationship to bronchial hyperresponsiveness in patients with seasonal allergic rhinitis. Ann Allergy Asthma Immunol. 2005;95(1):72-8.
49. Di Lorenzo G, Pacor ML, Mansueto P, Esposito Pellitteri M, Lo Bianco C, Ditta V, et al. Determinants of bronchial hyper-responsiveness in subjects with rhinitis. Int J Immunopathol Pharmacol. 2005;18(4):715-22.
50. Sale R, Silvestri M, Battistini E, Defilippi AC, Sabatini F, Pecora S, et al. Nasal inflammation and bronchial reactivity to methacholine in atopic children with respiratory symptoms. Allergy. 2003;58(11):1171-5.
51. Jang AS. Nasal eosinophilic inflammation contributes to bronchial hyperresponsiveness in patients with allergic rhinitis. J Korean Med Sci. 2002;17(6):761-4.

52. Silvestri M, Battistini E, Defilippi AC, Sabatini F, Sale R, Pecora S, et al. Early decrease in nasal eosinophil proportion after nasal allergen challenge correlates with baseline bronchial reactivity to methacholine in children sensitized to house dust mites. J Investig Allergol Clin Immunol. 2005;15(4):266-76.
53. Ciprandi G, Cirillo I, Vizzaccaro A, Milanese M, Tosca MA Correlation of nasal inflammation and nasal airflow with forced expiratory volume in 1 second in patients with perennial allergic rhinitis and asthma. Ann Allergy Asthma Immunol. 2004;93(6):575-80.
54. Ciprandi G, Cirillo I, Vizzaccaro A, Milanese M, Tosca MA. Airway function and nasal inflammation in seasonal allergic rhinitis and asthma. Clin Exp Allergy. 2004;34(6):891-6.
55. Tatar M, Petriskova J, Zucha J, Pecova R, Hutka Z, Raffajova J, et al. Induced sputum eosinophils, bronchial reactivity, and cough sensitivity in subjects with allergic rhinitis. J Physiol Pharmacol. 2005;56(Suppl 4):227-36.
56. Braunstahl GJ, Overbeek SE, Kleinjan A, Prins JB, Hoogsteden HC, Fokkens WJ. Nasal allergen provocation induces adhesion molecule expression and tissue eosinophilia in upper and lower airways. J Allergy Clin Immunol. 2001;107(3):469-76.
57. Braunstahl GJ, Kleinjan A, Overbeek SE, Prins JB, Hoogsteden HC, Fokkens WJ Segmental bronchial provocation induces nasal inflammation in allergic rhinitis patients. Am J Respir Crit Care Med. 2000;161(6):2051-7.
58. Nakamaru Y, Oridate N, Nishihira J, Takagi D, Furuta Y, Fukuda S. Macrophage migration inhibitory factor in allergic rhinitis: its identification in eosinophils at the site of inflammation. Ann Otol Rhinol Laryngol. 2004;113(3 Pt 1):205-9.
59. Kobayashi H, Gleich GJ, Butterfield JH, Kita H. Human eosinophils produce neurotrophins and secrete nerve growth factor on immunologic stimuli. Blood. 2002;99(6):2214-20.
60. Figueroa DJ, Borish L, Baramki D, Philip G, Austin CP, Evans JF. Expression of cysteinyl leukotriene synthetic and signalling proteins in inflammatory cells in active seasonal allergic rhinitis. Clin Exp Allergy. 2003;33(10):1380-8.
61. Amin K, Rinne J, Haahtela T, Simola M, Peterson CG, Roomans GM, et al. Inflammatory cell and epithelial characteristics of perennial allergic and nonallergic rhinitis with a symptom history of 1 to 3 years' duration. J Allergy Clin Immunol. 2001;107(2):249-57.
62. Onbasi K, Sin AZ, Doganavsargil B, Onder GF, Bor S, Sebik F. Eosinophil infiltration of the oesophageal mucosa in patients with pollen allergy during the season. Clin Exp Allergy. 2005;35(11):1423-31.
63. Flood-Page P, Swenson C, Faiferman I, Matthews J, Williams M, Brannick L et al. International Mepolizumab Study Group. A study to evaluate safety and efficacy of mepolizumab in patients with moderate persistent asthma. Am J Respir Crit Care Med. 2007;176(11):1062-71.
64. Flood-Page PT, Menzies-Gow AN, Kay AB, Robinson DS. Eosinophil's role remains uncertain as anti-interleukin-5 only partially depletes numbers in asthmatic airway. Am J Respir Crit Care Med. 2003;167(2):199-204.
65. Haldar P, Brightling CE, Hargadon B, Gupta S, Monteiro W, Sousa A, et al. Mepolizumab and exacerbations of refractory eosinophilic asthma. N Engl J Med. 2009;360(10):973-84.
66. Nair P, Pizzichini MM, Kjarsgaard M, Inman MD, Efthimiadis A, Pizzichini E, et al. Mepolizumab for prednisone-dependent asthma with sputum eosinophilia. N Engl J Med. 2009;360(10):985-93.
67. Pawankar R. Inflammatory mechanisms in allergic rhinitis. Curr Opin Allergy Clin Immunol. 2007;7(1):1-4.
68. Nonaka M, Pawankar R, Fukumoto A, Ogihara N, Sakanushi A, Yagi T. Induction of eotaxin production by interleukin-4, interleukin-13 and lipopolysaccharide by nasal fibroblasts. Clin Exp Allergy. 2004;34(5):804-11.
69. Parnes SM. Targeting cysteinyl leukotrienes in patients with rhinitis, sinusitis and paranasal polyps. Am J Respir Med. 2002;1(6):403-8.
70. Zhu J, Qiu YS, Figueroa DJ, Bandi V, Galczenski H, Hamada K, et al. Localization and upregulation of cysteinyl leukotriene-1 receptor in asthmatic bronchial mucosa. Am J Respir Cell Mol Biol. 2005;33(6):531-40.
71. Powe DG, Huskisson RS, Carney AS, Jenkins D, McEuen AR, Walls AF, et al. Mucosal T-cell phenotypes in persistent atopic and nonatopic rhinitis show an association with mast cells. Allergy. 2004;59(2):204-12.
72. Hattori H, Okano M, Yoshino T, Akagi T, Nakayama E, Saito C, et al. Expression of costimulatory CD80/CD86-CD28/CD152 molecules in nasal mucosa of patients with perennial allergic rhinitis. Clin Exp Allergy. 2001;31(8):1242-9.
73. Horiguchi S, Okamoto Y, Chazono H, Sakurai D, Kobayashi K. Expression of membrane-bound CD23 in nasal mucosal B cells from patients with perennial allergic rhinitis. Ann Allergy Asthma Immunol. 2005;94(2):286-91.
74. Karaki M, Dobashi H, Kobayashi R, Tokuda M, Ishida T, Mori N. Expression of interleukin-16 in allergic rhinitis. Int Arch Allergy Immunol. 2005;138(1):67-72.
75. Francis JN, Jacobson MR, Lloyd CM, Sabroe I, Durham SR, Till SJ. CXCR1+CD4+ T cells in human allergic disease. J Immunol. 2004;172(1):268-73.
76. Rimaniol AC, Till SJ, Garcia G, Capel F, Godot V, Balabanian K, et al. The CX3C chemokine fractalkine in allergic asthma and rhinitis. J Allergy Clin Immunol. 2003;112(6):1139-46.
77. Pawankar R. gammadelta T cells in allergic airway diseases. Clin Exp Allergy. 2000;30(3):318-23.
78. Miossec P, Korn T, Kuchroo VK. Interleukin-17 and type 17 helper T cells. N Engl J Med. 2009;361(9):888-98.
79. Han D, Wang C, Lou W, Gu Y, Wang Y, Zhang L Allergen-specific IL-10-secreting type I T regulatory cells, but not CD4(+) CD25(+)Foxp3(+) T cells, are decreased in peripheral blood of patients with persistent allergic rhinitis. Clin Immunol. 2010;136(2):292-301.
80. Pène J, Chevalier S, Preisser L, Vénéreau E, Guilleux MH, Ghannam S, et al. Chronically inflamed human tissues are infiltrated by highly differentiated Th17 lymphocytes. J Immunol. 2008;180(11):7423-30.
81. Kinhult J, Egesten A, Benson M, Uddman R, Cardell LO. Increased expression of surface activation markers on neutrophils following migration into the nasal lumen. Clin Exp Allergy. 2003;33(8):1141-6.
82. Qiu Y, Zhu J, Bandi V, Guntupalli KK, Jeffery PK. Bronchial mucosal inflammation and upregulation of CXC chemoattractants and receptors in severe exacerbations of asthma. Thorax. 2007;62(6):475-82.
83. Maneechotesuwan K, Essilfie-Quaye S, Kharitonov SA, Adcock IM, Barnes PJ. Loss of control of asthma following inhaled corticosteroid withdrawal is associated with increased sputum interleukin-8 and neutrophils. Chest. 2007;132(1):98-105.
84. Holgate ST. Epithelium dysfunction in asthma. J Allergy Clin Immunol. 2007;120(6):1233-44.

85. Takizawa H. Bronchial epithelial cells in allergic reactions. Curr Drug Targets Inflamm Allergy. 2005;4(3):305-11.
86. Pawankar R. Epithelial cells as immunoregulators in allergic airway diseases. Curr Opin Allergy Clin Immunol. 2002;2(1): 1-5.
87. Ying S, O'Connor B, Ratoff J, Meng Q, Fang C, Cousins D, et al. Expression and cellular provenance of thymic stromal lymphopoietin and chemokines in patients with severe asthma and chronic obstructive pulmonary disease. J Immunol. 2008;181(4):2790-8.
88. Gereke M, Jung S, Buer J, Bruder D. Alveolar type II epithelial cells present antigen to CD4(+) T cells and induce Foxp3(+) regulatory T cells. Am J Respir Crit Care Med. 2009;179(5):344-55.
89. Takizawa R, Pawankar R, Yamagishi S, Takenaka H, Yagi T. Increased expression of HLA-DR and CD86 in nasal epithelial cells in allergic rhinitics: antigen presentation to T cells and upregulation by diesel exhaust particles. Clin Exp Allergy. 2007;37(3):420-33.
90. Doherty TA, Khorram N, Chang JE, Kim HK, Rosenthal P, Croft M, et al. STAT6 regulates natural helper cell proliferation during lung inflammation initiated by Alternaria. Am J Physiol Lung Cell Mol Physiol. 2012;303:L577-88.
91. Halim TY, Krauss RH, Sun AC, Takei F. Lung natural helper cells are a critical source of Th2 cell-type cytokines in protease allergen-induced airway inflammation. Immunity. 2012;36: 451-63.
92. Chu DK, Llop-Guevara A, Walker TD, Flader K, Goncharova S, Boudreau JE, et al. IL-33, but not thymic stromal lymphopoietin or IL-25, is central to mite and peanut allergic sensitization. J Allergy Clin Immunol. 2013;131:187-200, e181-8.
93. Chang YJ, Kim HY, Albacker LA, Baumgarth N, McKenzie AN, Smith DE, et al. Innate lymphoid cells mediate influenza-induced airway hyper-reactivity independently of adaptive immunity. Nat Immunol 2011;12:631-8.
94. Christianson CA, Goplen NP, Zafar I, Irvin C, Good JT Jr, Rollins DR, Gorentla B, Liu W, Gorska MM, Chu H, Martin RJ, Alam R. Persistence of asthma requires multiple feedback circuits involving type 2 innate lymphoid cells and IL-33. J Allergy Clin Immunol. 2015 Jan 21. pii: S0091-6749(14)01740-0.
95. Mauad T, Bel EH, Sterk PJ. Asthma therapy and airway remodeling. J Allergy Clin Immunol. 2007;120(5):997-109.
96. Jeffery PK. Remodeling and inflammation of bronchi in asthma and chronic obstructive pulmonary disease. Proc Am Thorac Soc. 2004;1(3):176-83.
97. Barbato A, Turato G, Baraldo S, Bazzan E, Calabrese F, Tura M Airway inflammation in childhood asthma. Am J Respir Crit Care Med. 2003;168(7):798-803.
98. Bourdin A, Neveu D, Vachier I, Paganin F, Godard P, Chanez P. Specificity of basement membrane thickening in severe asthma. J Allergy Clin Immunol. 2007;119(6):1367-74.
99. Panettieri RA, Kotlikoff MI, Gerthoffer WT, Hershenson MB, Woodruff PG, Hall IP, et al. Airway smooth muscle in bronchial tone, inflammation, and remodeling: basic knowledge to clinical relevance. Am J Respir Crit Care Med. 2008;177(3): 248-52.
100. El-Shazly A, Berger P, Girodet PO, Ousova O, Fayon M, Vernejoux JM, et al. Fraktalkine produced by airway smooth muscle cells contributes to mast cell recruitment in asthma. J Immunol. 2006;176(3):1860-8.
101. Hollins F, Kaur D, Yang W, Cruse G, Saunders R, Sutcliffe A, et al. Human airway smooth muscle promotes human lung mast cell survival, proliferation, and constitutive activation: cooperative roles for CADM1, stem cell factor, and IL-6. J Immunol. 2008;181(4):2772-80.
102. Thangam EB, Venkatesha RT, Zaidi AK, Jordan-Sciutto KL, Goncharov DA, Krymskaya VP, et al. Airway smooth muscle cells enhance C3a-induced mast cell degranulation following cell-cell contact. FASEB J. 2005;19(7):798-800.
103. Sutcliffe A, Kaur D, Page S, Woodman L, Armour CL, Baraket M, et al. Mast cell migration to Th2 stimulated airway smooth muscle from asthmatics. Thorax. 2006;61(8):657-62.
104. Koff JL, Shao MX, Ueki IF, Nadel JA. Multiple TLRs activate EGFR via a signaling cascade to produce innate immune responses in airway epithelium. Am J Physiol Lung Cell Mol Physiol. 2008;294(6):L1068-75.
105. Schmidt M, Sun G, Stacey MA, Mori L, Mattoli S. Identification of circulating fibrocytes as precursors of bronchial myofibroblasts in asthma. J Immunol. 2003;171(1):380-9.
106. Holgate ST. The sentinel role of the airway epithelium in asthma pathogenesis. Immunol Rev. 2011;242(1):205-19.
107. Vancheri C, Gili E, Failla M, Mastruzzo C, Salinaro ET, Lofurno D, et al. Bradykinin differentiates human lung fibroblasts to a myofibroblast phenotype via the B2 receptor. J Allergy Clin Immunol. 2005;116(6):1242-8.
108. Kunzmann S, Schmidt-Weber C, Zingg JM, Azzi A, Kramer BW, Blaser K, et al. Connective tissue growth factor expression is regulated by histamine in lung fibroblasts: potential role of histamine in airway remodeling. J Allergy Clin Immunol. 2007;119(6):1398-407.
109. Hackett TL, Warner SM, Stefanowicz D, Shaheen F, Pechkovsky DV, Murray LA, et al. Induction of epithelial—mesenchymal transition in primary airway epithelial cells from patients with asthma by transforming growth factor-beta1. Am J Respir Crit Care Med. 2009;180(2):122-33.
110. Rytila P, Metso T, Heikkinen K, Saarelainen P, Helenius IJ, Haahtela T. Airway inflammation in patients with symptoms suggesting asthma but with normal lung function. Eur Respir J. 2000;16(5):824-30.
111. Kelly MM, O'Connor TM, Leigh R, Otis J, Gwozd C, Gauvreau GM, et al. Effects of budesonide and formoterol on allergen-induced airway responses, inflammation, and airway remodeling in asthma. J Allergy Clin Immunol. 2010;125(2):349-56.
112. Castro M, Rubin AS, Laviolette M, Fiterman J, De Andrade Lima M, Shah PL, et al. Effectiveness and safety of bronchial thermoplasty in the treatment of severe asthma: a multicenter, randomized, double-blind, sham-controlled clinical trial. Am J Respir Crit Care Med. 2010;181(2):116-24.

Control and Management of Stable Asthma

Sidney S Braman, Gwen S Skloot

INTRODUCTION

Treatment protocols for the management of stable asthma have undergone considerable change over the past 60 years. During the mid-20th century there was an effort made to improve currently available bronchodilator medications. Selective inhaled short-acting adrenoceptor agonists became available in 1969. They offered fewer cardiostimulatory effects than were experienced with commonly used drugs like racemic epinephrine and isoproterenol. Ephedrine, a drug used for centuries as a Chinese herbal remedy, *Ma Huang*, was eliminated in some countries as an asthma treatment because of the potential for cardiovascular and central nervous system (CNS) stimulatory effects and the use as a recreational drug. Anhydrous theophylline was commonly used but side effects and drug-drug interactions lead to significant toxicity and mortality. While its use has declined in recent years, theophylline still plays a role in asthma care as a third or fourth-line agent and when less expensive alternatives are required. The end of the 20th century introduced a dramatic new approach to asthma care as the disease became recognized as a chronic inflammatory disease of the airways. It is the inflammation that causes the recurring symptoms, episodes of wheezing, breathlessness, chest tightness, and cough, symptoms that are especially problematic at night and/or in the early morning. Asthma symptoms are the result of widespread but variable airflow obstruction that is at least partially reversible in most individuals, either spontaneously or as a result of treatment. The inflammation of asthma is also associated with an increase in airway responsiveness to a variety of stimuli such as cold air, exercise and respiratory irritants.

While sudden, unexpected asthma symptoms can be relieved with "rescue" inhaled bronchodilator treatment, the long-term goal of asthma treatment is directed at reducing airway inflammation. Medications labeled "controller therapy" are used for this purpose. In 1974, inhaled glucocorticoids became available to treat asthma and since that time they have become the mainstay of controller therapy for persistent asthma symptoms. Proinflammatory mediators called leukotrienes are also important in the pathogenesis of asthma. Agents that are capable of inhibiting the synthesis or action of leukotrienes were introduced in the 1990s as controller treatment for asthma.

There is a growing consensus that asthma is not a single disease, but rather an umbrella term for multiple diseases with different phenotypes (i.e. observable characteristics) and different endotypes, each with its own unique mechanism of inflammation.[1-3] Due to our increased understanding of the heterogeneity of asthma, attention has been directed to targeted therapy that addresses these differences. With new insights into the pathogenesis of asthma and new and safer medications to control the disease, there is reason for optimism in terms of asthma management. National and international asthma guidelines have provided a roadmap for asthma care, including evidence-based protocols to lead clinicians to successful outcomes for their patients.[4-8]

GOALS OF ASTHMA TREATMENT

There are both short-term and long-term therapeutic objectives for every asthmatic patient **(Box 1)**. The short-term objectives are to control immediate symptoms and respond to falling lung function measurements (peak flow-rates, spirometry). Long-term objectives are those directed at disease prevention of exacerbations, since there are now well-proven strategies to avoid serious acute bronchospasm

BOX 1 Goals of asthma treatment

- Limit symptoms of dyspnea, wheeze, chest tightness and cough, day and night
- Provide normal daily activity level; no absenteeism from work or school
- Maintain normal or near-normal lung function
- Reduce or eliminate asthma exacerbations; avoid emergency visits and hospitalizations
- Minimize use of rescue medication and use lowest dose and fewest medications possible
- Avoid side effects of medications

that may lead to emergency care, hospitalization and asthma mortality. In order to meet these therapeutic objectives, four components of asthma care should be addressed **(Box 2)**. First, measures should be taken to avoid exposure to respiratory allergens and irritants, or other "triggers" of asthma that can cause the worsening of symptoms **(Fig. 1)**. This includes the avoidance of outdoor and indoor allergens and irritants that can be found in the household or work environment and treatment of asthma comorbidities such as gastroesophageal reflux. Second, the optimal management of asthma depends on a careful assessment of the patient's symptoms, including the use of objective measures of asthma control with questionnaires and physiologic testing. Third, the treatment of asthma with bronchodilator and anti-inflammatory medications is tailored to the patient's needs in a step-up and step-down manner. This approach begins with a staging system that is based on the patient's symptoms and objective measures of lung function and relies on an assessment of the control of asthma symptoms for ongoing care. Fourth, patient education can be a powerful tool in asthma control. Family members can be helpful, especially with children and elderly adults. Active participation by a patient in monitoring lung function, avoiding provocative agents and making decisions regarding therapy provide asthma management skills that give that patient the confidence to control his or her own disease.

BOX 2 Essential components of successful asthma care

- *Avoidance:* Eliminate asthma "triggers" such as allergen exposure and home/workplace irritants
- *Monitoring:* Use of self-assessment questionnaires, peak flow measures, spirometry
- *Treatment:* Anti-inflammatory therapy is the foundation of successful treatment for persistent asthma; short-acting bronchodilators for rescue therapy
- *Patient education:* Provide the necessary tools for self-management including an action plan for exacerbation of symptoms

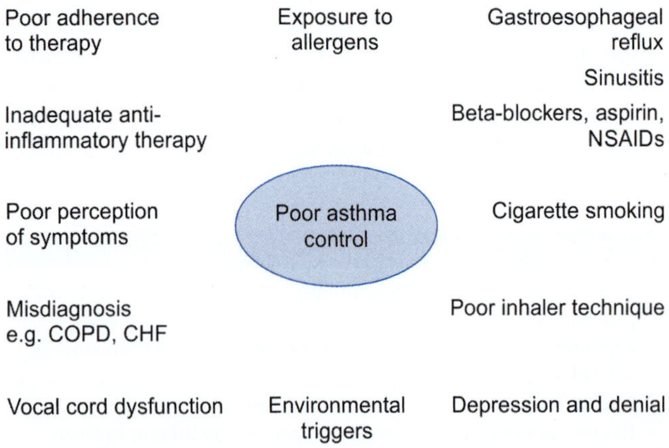

Fig. 1 Triggers of asthma leading to poor control
Abbreviations: COPD, chronic obstructive pulmonary disease; CHF, congestive heart failure; NSAIDs, nonsteroidal anti-inflammatory drugs

ESSENTIAL COMPONENTS OF ASTHMA CARE

Avoidance

In developing regions of the world (Africa, Central and South America, Asia and the Pacific), asthma prevalence rose sharply with increasing urbanization and westernization.[9] The reason for this increased prevalence remains largely unknown, but it has been noted to be associated with a parallel rise in atopic sensitization and increase in other allergic conditions (e.g. eczema and rhinitis). While there is unquestionably a genetic component to asthma, it is possible that changing patterns of environmental influences, such as exposure to microorganisms, pollutants, indoor and outdoor allergens exert a strong influence on the development of the disease in susceptible individuals.

Allergens and occupational factors are considered to be the most important triggers of asthma. For successful long-term management of asthma these triggers must be identified and prevention of exposures should be the first-line of defense.[10,11] This is a foundation of national and international guidelines.[4,5]

Several epidemiologic studies have shown a correlation between allergen exposure and the risk of developing asthma.[12-14] For example, there is a dose response relationship between levels of house dust mite allergen found in the beds of infants of atopic parents at age of 2–3 months and asthma at school age.[15] Symptoms and need for medication correlate with the level of household exposure of known allergens in susceptible individuals.[14,16] Improvement of asthma symptoms occurs when allergen exposure is reduced.[17-20]

The important allergens for children and adults appear to be those that are inhaled. Important indoor allergens include a number of domestic factors: house dust mites, cockroach allergen, fungi (*Alternaria, Aspergillus, Cladosporium* and *Candida*); and warm-blooded animals (cats, dogs and rodents). Rodents are problematic as they excrete urine, feces, saliva and dander that can be highly allergenic. Removal of a pet from the home of a sensitized patient is encouraged but it may require several months before allergen levels decrease.[21,22] These antigens have also been identified in locations where no pets reside including homes, schools, daycare centers and work environments. Controlled trials of animal dander avoidance have been reported to be successful in schools and homes without an animal.[23] House dust has been shown to be composed of several organic and inorganic compounds including insects and insect feces, mold spores, mammalian danders, pollen grains, fibers, mites, and mite feces. In poor and inner city locations, mouse and rat allergen exposure and sensitization are common in children who have asthma.[24] Rodent exposure is also common in underdeveloped regions of the world and must be considered in asthma control in these populations.

Single-intervention efforts to improve environmental allergen control in the home are not likely to improve asthma control. For example, a study using allergen-impermeable mattress covers failed to show significant differences between intervention and control populations.[19] Single-interventions are likely to be unhelpful because most patients are sensitized to more than one allergen. Multiple-intervention environmental control studies have been conducted in high-risk urban asthmatic children with comprehensive allergen reduction methods. They have demonstrated positive outcomes.[19,25,26] Successful interventions included construction remediation aimed at moisture sources within homes with a documented mold problem, and home visits by community health workers who promote dust mite and cockroach control.[26] Home visits have stressed behavioral changes such as smoking cessation, and offer an individualized approach to address pressing concerns, including asthma-related questions and social issues (e.g. poor housing, inadequate income). Multiple visits are required to encourage completion of asthma action plans and deliver resources to reduce exposures. These have included allergy control pillow and mattress encasements, low-emission vacuums, commercial-quality doormats, cleaning kits, roach bait, and rodent traps. Such multiple intervention programs have advocated for improved housing conditions and provided much needed education and social support. Overall, targeted home-based environmental interventions can improve health and reduce healthcare costs for poorly controlled asthmatics who live in resource poor communities.[27] A list of effective measures of environmental control is listed in **Box 3**.

BOX 3 Avoiding asthma triggers

Effective environmental control:

- Stop smoking and avoid exposure to second-hand smoke
- Use insecticides to eliminate cockroaches from the house (if the patient can stay away for some time)
- Shake mattresses, pillows, bedspreads and blankets and expose them to the sun as often as possible
- Remove carpets from the bedroom; minimize number of stuffed toys for children and wash them weekly
- Avoid piling up books, toys, clothes, shoes and other items that accumulate dust in the bedroom
- When cleaning the house: sprinkle the floor with water before sweeping to avoid raising dust; clean furniture with a damp cloth
- Wash the sheets and blankets on the patient's bed weekly in hot water
- A temperature of more than 130°F is necessary for killing house-dust mites (but will not remove the allergen). Cold water and detergent/bleach wash also acceptable
- If available, encase pillow and mattress with allergen-impermeable cover.

  Avoid, if possible, exposure to gas stoves and appliances that are not vented to the outside, fumes from wood-burning appliances or fireplaces, sprays, or strong odor.

Outdoor allergens include pollens (mainly from trees, weeds, and grasses), fungi molds, and pollens have been especially associated with seasonal asthma symptoms.[28] Food allergens while an important cause of anaphylaxis are not a common precipitant of asthma symptoms.

Both outdoor and indoor pollutants contribute to worsening asthma symptoms.[29-31] They may directly trigger bronchoconstriction and act indirectly to worsen asthma by increasing bronchial hyperresponsiveness. This will further enhance responses to inhaled aeroallergens as well as other provoking agents. The two main outdoor pollutants are (1) industrial smog (sulfur dioxide particulate complex); and (2) photochemical smog (ozone and nitrogen oxides). Whether long-term exposure is injurious is not clear. It is advisable to recommend to asthmatic patients to avoid, to the extent possible, exertion or exercise outside when levels of air pollution are high.

Indoor pollutants include cooking and heating fuel exhausts as well as insulating products, paints and varnishes. Modern construction techniques have been suspected of causing greater indoor air pollution. In energy-efficient buildings, there is 50% less turnover of fresh air. Formaldehyde and volatile organic compounds such as isocyanates have been implicated as potential risk factors for the onset of asthma and wheezing.[29-33] Clinicians should advise patients to be aware of the potential irritating effects of newly installed furnishings and finishes which can arise from new linoleum flooring, synthetic carpeting, particleboard, wall coverings, furniture and fresh paint.

The use of poorly vented gas stoves and appliances results in increased indoor levels of nitrogen dioxide (NO_2) and this has been associated with increased respiratory symptoms.[34,35] Installing nonpolluting, more effective heating in the homes of children with asthma does not significantly improve lung function but can reduce symptoms of asthma, days off from school and healthcare utilization.[36] Also, fumes from wood burning appliances or fireplaces, commonly used for heating and cooking in poor, underserved regions of the world, can precipitate symptoms in persons who have asthma.[37] Sprays and strong odors, particularly perfumes, can also irritate the lungs and precipitate asthma symptoms.

In asthmatics, active smoking is a cause of worsening symptoms and deterioration of lung function and also reduces the efficacy of inhaled and systemic corticosteroids in treating asthma.[38,39] Long-term passive cigarette smoke exposure has been linked to new-onset asthma in children and adults as well as worsening asthma symptoms, decreased lung function, and greater use of health services in those with preexisting asthma.[40] Children are more likely to be affected when the mother smokes rather than others in the household.[41] Tobacco smoke exposure in adults with asthma may be more likely to occur in the work environment.[42]

Estimates of the prevalence of occupational asthma vary.[43-45] It has been reported that 2–15% of all cases of adult-onset asthma arise from workplace exposure. Taking an occupational history can be very rewarding and can lead to primary prevention and avoidance of the offending environment. Patients should be questioned about exposure to animals, shellfish, fish, and arthropods. They may cause asthma in farmers, laboratory workers, grain handlers, and poultry workers. Exposure to wood, plants and vegetables can cause asthma in woodworkers, carpenters, grain handlers, bakers and tobacco workers. Exposure to enzymes and pharmaceuticals should be questioned in pharmaceutical workers, pharmacists, and detergent industry workers. Solderers, spray painters, chemical manufacturers, polyurethane manufacturers, and electronics workers are another susceptible group. Electroplaters, hard metal workers, polishers, and solderers may have asthma caused by metals and metal salts such as aluminum, chromium, cobalt, nickel and platinum fumes.

While there is no compelling evidence that shows that emotional stress is a cause of asthma onset, there is some evidence in children and adolescents that psychological problems of the child and the caregivers can contribute to a worsening course of asthma. Interventions to reduce psychological burdens should be considered as they may improve the quality of life of patients with asthma.

Monitoring Asthma: Use Objective Measures of Asthma

Objective measurements of pulmonary function are important in patients with asthma to confirm the diagnosis and to assess disease activity control at various time intervals. While there is a poor correlation between the airway inflammation and lung function, physiological measurements are extremely important in the management of asthma.[46,47] The symptoms of asthma are nonspecific and can be confused with or coexist with other pulmonary conditions such as chronic obstructive pulmonary disease (COPD), tracheobronchial tumors and inflammatory lung diseases. Congestive heart failure and gastroesophageal reflux disease are two other common conditions that can mimic the symptoms of asthma. Functional disorders such as psychogenic dyspnea are also on the differential diagnosis and must be considered. Physiologic testing can demonstrate the major diagnostic features of asthma such as airflow obstruction, reversibility of airflow obstruction and bronchial hyperresponsiveness, and therefore can be useful in confirming or excluding the diagnosis. The following four tests of pulmonary function are extremely useful for establishing the diagnosis of asthma and/or for following the clinical course of the patient once the diagnosis has been made:

1. Spirometry
2. Peak expiratory flow rate (PEFR) measurements
3. Bronchoprovocation testing
4. Exhaled levels of nitric oxide (NO)

These physiologic tests are also important tools to assess the degree of control of asthma. The perception of asthma symptoms by the patient is often poor, especially in the elderly or if the patient has had long-standing asthma.[48-51] Also, the physician's findings on physical examination may either overestimate or underestimate the severity of the airflow obstruction. Although measurements of lung function do not correlate that well with patient's reported symptoms, they do add an objective measure to the assessment of how well the disease is controlled and have been proven to be important tools in the management and control of asthma.[52,53]

- *Spirometry:* It is useful for the diagnosis of asthma and for following clinical outcomes.[54] Airflow obstruction, a classic feature of asthma can be demonstrated on spirometry using the timed vital capacity maneuver. The test provides a quantitative assessment of asthma and can be used in children who are 5 years of age and older. The forced vital capacity (FVC), which is the total amount of volume exhaled and the forced expiratory volume in the one second (FEV_1), which is the volume exhaled in the first second of expiration are measured. The patient's results are compared with reference values based on age, height, sex and race.[55] A reduced FEV_1 and ratio of FEV_1/FVC show the presence of airflow obstruction. In younger children who cannot perform acceptable spirometry, impulse oscillometry can serve as an alternative test of lung function. This test is done during quiet breathing and can measure resistance in both large and small airways.

A brisk improvement in spirometry (postbronchodilator FEV_1 increases more than 12% and 200 mL) 10–20 minutes after the inhalation of a short-acting β-agonist can demonstrate the second cardinal feature of asthma, reversibility.[56,57] Some patients with asthma never meet the reversibility criteria after repetitive testing with a short-acting bronchodilator. In such patients, after vigorous treatment, the FEV_1 may show significant improvement on a subsequent clinic visit and this would strongly support a diagnosis of asthma. A single postbronchodilator test, therefore, cannot be used to exclude the diagnosis of asthma.

Regular monitoring of pulmonary function is important for asthma patients. It is helpful after treatment has been initiated to document improvement and also during periods of worsening symptoms to offer an objective assessment of airflow obstruction. Spirometry has been advised at least every 1 or 2 years to monitor lung function.[4] Physicians have a poor ability to assess the degree of airflow[58] and patients too often cannot perceive the severity of their disease.[52,53,58] One study reported that one-third of the children who had moderate-to-severe asthma based on symptoms were reclassified to a more severe asthma category when pulmonary function was considered.[59] This is especially important in patients with poor lung function, as a low FEV_1 is associated with an increased risk of severe asthma exacerbations.[60,61] On the other hand, another study showed that a majority of children who had mild-to-moderate asthma classified by symptoms had normal FEV_1.[62] Reversibility to following an inhaled short-acting bronchodilator correlates with the degree of airway inflammation and can also offer an assessment of future risk.[63] A pronounced increase in FEV_1 after a bronchodilator is a strong marker of subsequent risk of death from asthma. One study showed that asthmatics with a 25–49% reversibility and those with more than 50% reversibility; had a 2.7 and 7.0 higher risk of death from asthma, respectively.[64] In addition, those patients who have the greatest degree of reversibility in response to a short-acting bronchodilator may be at the greatest risk of developing fixed airflow obstruction and have the greatest loss of future lung function.[64]

- *Peak expiratory flow rate:* Short-term home monitoring with the peak flow meter can detect early signs of deterioration when symptoms change. Long-term monitoring is useful for those with severe brittle asthma and for those who have a poor perception of asthma symptoms. Spirometry, however, is the preferred method for measuring lung function to classify asthma severity as peak flow measures may underestimate airflow obstruction, particularly with more severe disease.[65,66] Peak flow measurements ideally should be done 10–20 minutes after inhaling a β-agonist. A zone system has been developed for patient ease, as follows: green is more than 80% of the personal best and shows good control; yellow is 50–80% of the personal best and signals caution that asthma is not under sufficient control; and red is less than 50% of personal best and signifies danger and the need for immediate physician intervention.

  A diurnal variation in PEFR of greater than 20% is diagnostic of asthma. The magnitude of peak flow variability is in general proportional to the severity of the disease. A high degree of variability signals unstable asthma and poor outcomes that demands increased medication.
- *Inhalation challenge testing:* It is useful in some patients when the diagnosis of asthma is questionable.[67] This occurs when the patient has normal peak flow rates and spirometry findings yet typical asthma symptoms are present. Increasing concentrations of an agonist such as methacholine are inhaled and if the FEV_1 drops 20% below baseline at a dose less than 16 mg/mL, the test result is positive. The test is better at excluding asthma than ruling it in since there are false positives with the test. Bronchoprovocation testing can also be done using alternative challenges such as with histamine, mannitol cold air and exercise.[68-70]
- *Measures of inflammation:* The presence and quantification of various inflammatory cells and mediators in sputum and body fluids have been used to reflect the disease. These biomarkers, such as sputum eosinophil counts, have been used mainly for clinical investigation. Elevated levels of NO have been detected in the exhaled air of asthmatic subjects. Exhaled NO is well-established as a marker of eosinophilic airway inflammation. A standardized method of measurement must be carefully followed to prevent spurious results.[71]The American Thoracic Society (ATS) in 2011 recommended the use of fractional exhaled nitric oxide (FeNO) testing and concluded that it offers added advantages for patient care including, (1) detecting of eosinophilic airway inflammation, (2) determining the likelihood of corticosteroid responsiveness, (3) monitoring of airway inflammation to determine the potential need for corticosteroid, and (4) unmasking of otherwise unsuspected nonadherence to corticosteroid therapy. When levels of FeNO are below 25 ppb (20 ppb in children), eosinophilic inflammation and response to inhaled corticosteroid (ICS) is very unlikely. Levels over 50 ppb (35 ppb in children) predict responsiveness to ICS while levels between these extremes must be put in clinical context.[72]

  Unfortunately, exhaled NO levels do not correlate with disease severity, but serial measurements may aid in monitoring disease activity. It has shown promise, for example, in identifying pending exacerbations of asthma.[73] The availability of a low cost hand-held analyzer may lead to future use in resource-poor regions.

Treatment of Stable Asthma

Asthma Pharmacotherapy

β-2-adrenoceptor agonists: Selective inhaled β-2-adrenoceptor agonists are the main bronchodilating agents for the treatment of asthma, through their rapid and potent effects in relaxing airway smooth muscle. They are classified based on the duration of action into short- and long-acting. They produce bronchodilation by direct stimulation of the airway smooth muscle leading to relaxation via the activation of the adenylate cyclase pathway. Inhaled agents are preferred and they can be delivered by metered-dose inhaler, dry powder capsules, and compressor-driven nebulizers. Corticosteroids upregulate the expression of β-2 adrenoreceptors by increasing transcription of the genes.

Short-acting β-agonists (SABAs): Short-acting β-agonists such as salbutamol are widely used due to their acute (4–6 hours) bronchodilator effects and for the ability to protect against various triggers such as cold air, exercise and allergen. They are generally well-tolerated, even with frequent use. Frequency of use is a measure of the level of symptom control. Anti-inflammatory treatment should be given when use of SABAs exceeds two times a week.

Long-acting β-agonists (LABAs): Long-acting β-agonists, mainly salmeterol and formoterol provide bronchodilation and improve bronchial responsiveness for up to 12 hours. Like SABAs, they also inhibit the acute early allergic response, but in addition, they inhibit the late phase response and airway hyperresponsiveness lasting up to 24–34 hours after allergen challenge.[74] The use of LABAs as monotherapy should be avoided in the stable asthmatic. Conclusions from a large randomized study were that LABA monotherapy may increase asthma-related deaths and hospitalizations, especially in certain ethnic groups.[75] A large meta-analysis showed that concomitant use of inhaled steroids appears to modify this effect and prospective studies will be reported to confirm this finding.[76] Side effects are generally uncommon with inhaled LABAs therapy **(Table 1)**.

Anticholinergic agents: Anticholinergic agents, traditionally have not been part of asthma treatment plans since the short-acting agent, ipratropium, did not have the rapid onset as a reliever and was not as effective as a short-acting beta agonist. In poorly controlled asthmatics, adding tiotropium, a long-acting once a day anticholinergic, to a low to medium dose of ICS is as effective as adding salmeterol or doubling the dose of the ICS on top of ICS/LABAs combination in moderate-severe asthmatic patients.[77] Also, long-term studies of severe asthmatics uncontrolled with an ICS/LABAs combination have shown that tiotropium can improve lung function and increase the time to the first severe asthma exacerbation. Tiotropium is now considered a valid therapeutic option for asthma.[78]

Inhaled corticosteroids: Since their introduction in the early 1970s, ICS have become the mainstay of treatment in persistent asthma. This is because of its proven efficacy, superior to other class of asthma therapy and also its lower potential for systemic side effects compared to oral glucocorticosteroids. It exerts its anti-inflammatory activity via the glucocorticoid receptor complex that regulates gene transcription of proteins that inhibit proinflammatory cytokines. ICS have highly lipophilic compounds that have much higher binding affinity compared to hydrocortisone and also a highly efficient first-pass hepatic metabolism, resulting in lower systemic absorption. Clinically, they improve airway inflammation, hyperresponsiveness, airflow obstruction and symptoms in asthmatics. In the stable asthmatic with persistent symptoms, adherence to ICS treatment is of paramount importance as it has been associated with decreased risk of near fatal and fatal asthma **(Fig. 2)**.[79]

Establishing dose-response relationship characteristics of ICS have been challenging. These characteristics vary between patients. The impetus for discovering the lowest effective dose in any patient is to minimize the potential systemic side effects especially when used over many years. In patients with mild to moderate asthma, most of the therapeutic benefit of budesonide is achieved at 200–400 µg/day and its maximum effect at 1,000 µg/day.[80] Similar dose-response curves have been seen to plateau at lower doses (100–200 µg) of fluticasone.[81] For patients with asthma who require ICS, initial moderate ICS dose appears to be more effective than initial low ICS dose.[82] Beginning with a moderate dose ICS has no advantages to commencing with a high dose ICS and down-titrating.[82]

There is an emerging evidence that higher doses of inhaled glucocorticosteroid might be effective for preventing progression to severe exacerbation patients who quadruple their dose of inhaled glucocorticosteroid after a fall in peak flow rate has been shown to be significantly less likely to require oral glucocorticosteroids.[83,84] Another strategy that has been shown to be effective has been the use of budesonide or formoterol combination for maintenance and relief (called "single-inhaler therapy" or "symbicort for maintenance and relief"). This has been shown to offer significantly longer time to first exacerbation and reduction in the number of exacerbations.[85] Side effects of ICS are both local and systemic **(Table 1)**. They are generally well tolerated especially, at lower doses. The use of higher doses for self-management of asthma exacerbations must be balanced against the potential for side effects.

Theophylline: The xanthines, particularly theophylline, have been a widely prescribed oral therapy for maintenance of stable asthma worldwide. In the 1980s, the introduction of the slow release preparation that provided more steady plasma levels was a large reason of its widespread use. The weak bronchodilator effect of theophylline on the airways can be demonstrated in vitro on human airway tissues and it may result from inhibition of phosphodiesterases especially, type III and IV.[86] Phosphodiesterase inhibitors also have anti-inflammatory effects that block the late phase response to allergen challenge and improve the symptoms of nocturnal asthma when used in a chronotherapeutic manner (i.e. choosing the time of medication administration to have the most efficacious outcome).[87,88] The guidelines recommend that theophylline may be considered for use as add-on therapy in patients not well-controlled on low dose ICS but recommend LABAs as more effective with fewer adverse events.[89] For the patient with uncontrolled asthma, low dose inhaled budesonide with theophylline compared to high-dose inhaled budesonide produced similar benefits and this may be achieved at theophylline concentrations below the recommended therapeutic range of 5–15 mg/dL.[90]

Despite its attractiveness, side effects are the main limitation to its use **(Table 1)**. This is especially pronounced in the elderly where polypharmacy and potential drug-to-drug interaction are becoming more frequent. Theophylline has a rather narrow therapeutic window and unwanted effects are usually seen at plasma levels above 20 mg/dL. To avoid untoward effects, it is advisable to monitor blood theophylline levels.

Leukotriene pathway modifiers: Substantial evidence exists for involvement of the cysteinyl leukotrienes in the pathophysiology of asthma. They exert a number of important pharmacologic actions that contribute to airflow obstruction in asthma: airway smooth-muscle contraction, edema formation, and mucus secretion. Numerous studies have shown that leukotriene modifiers have protective effects against bronchoprovocative challenges and ease bronchial obstruction in asthma patients.

Table 1 Pharmacological agents for stable asthma

Pharmacological agents	*Potential adverse effects*	*Therapeutic considerations*
Corticosteroids (glucocorticoids)		
	Cough, dysphonia, oral candidiasis	The use of chamber devices and mouth-washing after inhalation decrease local side effects
Inhaled:		
Beclomethasone dipropionate, budesonide, flunisolide, fluticasone propionate,	In high doses systemic effects may occur. Although studies are not conclusive, and clinical significance of these effects has not been established since not studied for long periods (e.g., adrenal suppression, osteoporosis, growth suppression, and skin thinning and easy bruising)	The risk-benefit ratio of uncontrolled asthma to the limited risks of inhaled corticosteroids (ICS) should be considered
Systemic:		
Methylprednisolone, prednisolone, prednisone	Short-term use: Reversible hyperglycemia, increased appetite, fluid retention, psychological alterations, hypertension, gastric ulcer, and rarely aseptic necrosis of femur	Use at lowest effective dose. For long-term use, alternate-day a.m. dosing may produce less adverse effects
	Long-term use: adrenal axis suppression, growth retardation, dermal thinning, hypertension, diabetes, Cushing's syndrome, cataracts, muscle weakness	
Nedocromil		
	15–20% of patients complain of an altered or unpleasant taste from nedocromil	Therapeutic response to nedocromil often requires a 4–6 weeks trial to determine response clinically
		Safety is the main advantage of these agents
Long-acting β-2-Agonists		
	Tachycardia, muscle tremor, hypokalemia, prolongation of QT interval in overdose	Not for monotherapy or clinical asthma exacerbations
Inhaled:		
Salmeterol formoterol	Tolerance may occur within 1 week of chronic therapy	Clinical significance of potentially developing tachyphylaxis is uncertain
Oral:		
Albuterol, sustained-release		Inhaled long-acting β_2-agonists are preferred because they have fewer adverse reactions than oral agents
Methylxanthines		
Theophylline, sustained-release tablets and capsules	Dose-related acute toxicities: tachycardia, nausea and vomiting, arrhythmias, headache, seizures, hematemesis, hyperglycemia, and hypokalemia	Routine serum concentration monitoring is essential due to significant toxicities, narrow therapeutic range, individual differences in metabolic clearance and drug-drug interactions as well
Leukotriene Modifiers Zafirlukast, Montelukast Pranlukast		
	Well tolerated overall. One reported case of reversible hepatitis and hyperbilirubinemia; high concentrations may develop in patients with underlying hepatic disease	Administration with meals decreases bioavailability
Zafirlukast	Limited case reports of reversible hepatitis	Zafirlukast can inhibit the metabolism of terfenadine, warfarin, and theophylline

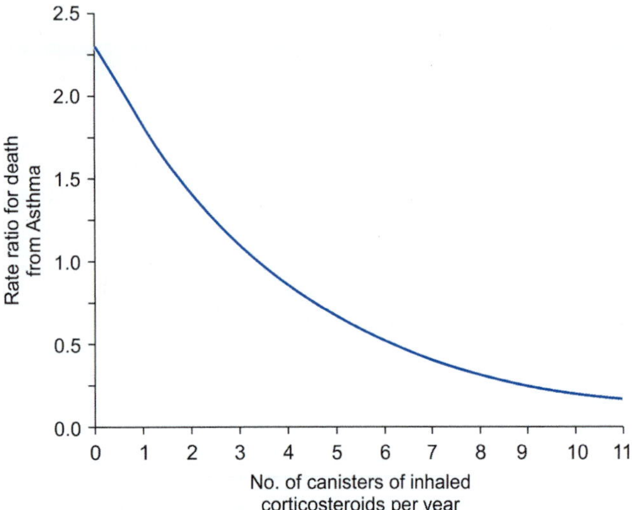

Fig. 2 The regular use of low-dose inhaled corticosteroids is associated with a decreased risk of death from asthma

The anti-leukotrienes may be used as first-line therapy when anti-inflammatory therapy is needed but they are generally less effective than ICS. They also have less effect compared to LABA as add-on therapy to ICS.[91] They may however, have a special role in the aspirin sensitive asthmatic.[92] If one is chosen, a therapeutic trial of 4–6 weeks should be allowed to determine its effectiveness. There is currently no evidence that supports its use beyond this time if there is no symptomatic improvement. The leukotriene modifiers may have an additive effect to ICS and inhaled β-2 agonist in the severe asthmatic when step-up care is needed.[93,94] There is little data to suggest a role for the leukotriene modifiers for acute asthma.

Antileukotrienes are generally well tolerated. In a safety study over 3,000 patients, 4.5% developed reversible elevations of transaminases with zileuton after a few months of therapy.[95] Reports of Churg-Strauss syndrome after initiation of zafirlukast and montelukast have also emerged, but it is likely that this has occurred as a result of systemic steroid withdrawal.

Oral corticosteroids: Systemic administration of corticosteroids are generally reserved for patients with severe asthma, or as trial of therapy to attempt to optimize lung function in patients with a component of fixed airflow obstruction despite conventional asthma therapies. Corticosteroids such as prednisolone and methylprednisolone are rapidly absorbed across the gastrointestinal tract. Because of the side effects of systemic corticosteroids they should be avoided if possible in the routine treatment of chronic stable asthma even at lower doses.

A summary of the therapeutic agents used for chronic stable asthma is listed in **Table 1**.

Other Approaches to Asthma Treatment

Antibiotics: The role of *Chlamydia pneumoniae* and *Mycoplasma pneumoniae* in the pathogenesis of asthma symptoms and exacerbations has been suggested.[96] As macrolides have both anti-inflammatory and antimicrobial effects that could target these organisms, a number of randomized, double-blind, placebo-controlled trials have been conducted to assess their effects in chronic asthma. Results have been contradictory and trials have been underpowered. One relatively small but well-conducted study showed no evidence of benefit from the addition of clarithromycin to adults with mild to moderately severe asthma on low dose inhaled glucocorticosteroids.[97] A meta-analysis of 12 clinical studies concluded that there is no improvement in FEV_1, but significant improvements in peak expiratory flow (PEF), symptoms, and quality of life can be seen.[98] There is evidence to suggest that macrolides may be more beneficial in subgroups of patients with noneosinophilic asthma (i.e., neutrophil predominant).[99] This emphasizes the fact that asthma therapy is best targeted to the underlying mechanism of disease. The long-term safety and efficacy of macrolides for asthma care needs further study.

Biological therapies: Biological therapies are the newest treatments available for asthma and offer a personalized approach that can optimize outcomes and minimize adverse effects. Immunoglobulin E (IgE) is recognized as a key component of atopic asthma pathophysiology. Omalizumab is an IgE monoclonal antibody that binds free IgE and decreases circulating IgE. It, therefore, decreases allergen-driven cell degranulation and reduces the release of preformed proinflammatory mediators and newly synthesized cytokines.[100] This agent is used in difficult to control asthmatics who are not responding to conventional therapy. Multiple other biologic agents that target Th2 cytokines such as IL-5 and IL-13 will likely become available to treat targeted asthmatics.

Allergen immunotherapy: Allergen specific immunotherapy is the practice of administering gradual quantities of an allergen extract to a patient to ameliorate symptoms from subsequent exposures. Clinical evidence suggests that immunotherapy is effective to treat seasonal or perennial allergic rhinitis and asthma. It should be considered when conventional pharmacotherapy is not able to control asthma symptoms in an allergic individual. It has been shown to reduce symptoms and medication use and to improve overall asthma control, often without concomitant changes in lung function.[101] It has also been shown to reduce the development of asthma in children with seasonal rhinoconjunctivitis.[102] Subcutaneous administration has generally been used and it is highly effective when the optimal dose of high quality vaccine is administered. An important limitation of this route is the risk of potential side effects, which include systemic allergic reactions, occasional anaphylaxis and even, fatalities.[103] As a

Table 2 Allergen immunotherapy

Consider allergy immunotherapy: • IgE mediated disease • Continuous symptoms and exacerbations despite adherence to adequate pharmacotherapy • Unable to avoid allergens that provoke symptoms • Positive skin tests or RAST tests to relevant allergens • Limited spectrum of allergies • Specific high-quality allergen extracts are available • Patient consents to risks and benefits
Relative contraindications to initiating allergy immunotherapy • Severe uncontrolled asthma • Known malignancy • Autoimmune disease present • Patients taking beta-blockers • Children less than 5 years • Pregnancy (may be continued during pregnancy) • Noncompliant patient
Abbreviations: IgE, immunoglobulin E; RAST, radioallergosorbent test

result, safer approaches, such as sublingual immunotherapy, have been used to induce tolerance to inhaled antigens.[104] The sublingual route is better tolerated and does not seem to be inferior with respect to effectiveness. Allergen immunotherapy should always be combined with appropriate allergen avoidance strategies. The mechanisms of immunotherapy are based on a restored balance between Th2 and Th1 cells inducing a reduction of inflammation in the target organ. Clinical indications and relative contraindications based on the World Health Organization (WHO) position paper and recommendations from the European Academy of Allergy and Immunology and the European Union (EU)-funded Global Allergy and Asthma European Network (GA2LEN) taskforce are seen in **Table 2.**[105,106]

Antifungal therapy: Air-borne exposure to fungi is a common phenomenon worldwide. Fungal sensitization is uncommon but in some asthmatics, it can greatly affect the course of their disease.[107] There are three main recognized syndromes related to fungal sensitization and asthma: (1) allergic bronchopulmonary aspergillosis (ABPA); (2) allergic bronchopulmonary mycosis (ABPM); and (3) trichophyton asthma. While antifungal therapy cannot eliminate the exposure to fungal elements, it can be effective in these syndromes. Antifungal therapy is effective adjunct therapy in the treatment of ABPA with oral corticosteroids.[108] Although antifungal agents are not recommended as standard of care for ABPM, in severe asthmatics with this endotype, they have been reported to improve quality of life measures, peak flows and IgE levels.[109] In all patients with uncontrolled asthma who are sensitized to fungal antigens shown by a radioallergosorbent test (RAST) testing and have evidence of colonization by culture, antifungal therapy should be considered.[110]

Diet and asthma: The relationship between dietary nutrients and asthma has been suspected but evidence from prospective and randomized trials is lacking.[111] For example, although there is an epidemiological association between low serum levels of vitamin D and the development of asthma, asthma severity and recurrent exacerbations, results from a randomized, double-blind, parallel, placebo-controlled trial in which adults with symptomatic asthma and low vitamin D3 levels received supplementation were disappointing in terms of asthma outcomes.[112,113] Recommendations cannot be made for vitamin D supplementation based on the evidence available to date. General advice for patients with stable asthma is intuitive: eat a balanced diet comprised of natural, nonprocessed foods with ample fruits and vegetables.

There is an association between obesity and risk for the development of asthma and in addition, asthmatic patients with obesity generally have more severe disease with poorer control and decreased response to conventional treatment such as ICS therapy.[114]

Patient Education

Asthma management plans have become popular, especially with high-risk patients.[115-118] They are designed to give patients the skills for routine management of their disease and the ability to recognize and control exacerbations of symptoms. They are usually offered by physicians and nurses but also can be taught by lay educators who have been shown to provide comparable outcomes when compared to nurse educators.[119] An effective plan starts with good communication between the patient or family member (in the case of children or the frail elderly) and the healthcare provider **(Table 3)**. Evidence is now abundant that asthma self-management education is effective in improving outcomes of chronic asthma and can be delivered in many settings: doctor's offices, outpatient clinics, hospitals, emergency departments and schools.[120-126] In addition to person to person sessions, internet based home monitoring mobile phones and computerized reminder devices have also been used successfully to improve asthma control.[127-130] Real time reminders from the pharmacy can also be effective using informational pharmacy technology to reinforce self-management skills.[131]

Benefits from self-management education include reduction in symptoms, less limitation of activity, improvement in quality of life and perceived control of asthma and improved medication adherence.[132-138] Also, death from asthma can be reduced. The use of a peak flow meter, a written action plan and oral glucocorticoids prior to a severe attack can impact mortality.

A written action plan should include instructions for daily management, including what medications to use and how to avoid specific triggers relevant to the patient, and techniques for recognizing and handling worsening asthma. Patients should be taught how to recognize the signs and symptoms of worsening asthma and how peak-flow measurements can be used to recognize an attack. It should also include what medications to take in response to these signs, what symptoms and peak flow measurements indicate the need for urgent medical attention, and how to obtain the required urgent medical care. Written action plans are particularly recommended for patients who have moderate or severe persistent asthma, who have difficulty perceiving the signs of worsening asthma and for those with a history of severe exacerbations or poorly controlled asthma. It has been shown that key components of a written action plan should include the use of 2–4 action points, advice on both inhaled and oral corticosteroids and use of personal best PEF measurements rather than percentage predicted PEF.[139] Similarly, telehealthcare follow-up of patients should be directed to those with more severe disease as it has been shown to have little impact in those with milder asthma.[140] Optimal management outcomes can be best assured when the patient develops the confidence to act on the skills learned from a congenial patient-provider partnership.

Table 3 Essential elements of asthma self-management program

- Develop active partnership with patient and family
  - Provide an open two-way communication
  - Establish realistic goals of successful therapy
  - Discuss treatment preferences
  - Explore barriers to successful treatment
- Offer basic knowledge of asthma causes and how to avoid triggers
  - Identify potential environmental allergens
  - Discuss occupational triggers
  - Avoid outside exposure on high pollution days
- Give pharmacy-based education
  - Difference between controller and rescue medications
  - Role of each medication prescribed
    - Proper inhaler technique
    - MDI (with holding chamber or spacer)
    - Dry powder inhalers (DPIs)
- Provide patient with action plan for
  - Daily control
  - Recognition of acute exacerbations of symptoms
  - Management of exacerbation: how to increase medication and for how long
  - Where and when to seek help
- Explain how to measure asthma control
  - Peak flow meter use
  - Home diary or asthma control tests
- Offer, when available, computer and internet programs for asthma care

Abbreviation: MDI, metered-dose inhaler

TREATMENT PROTOCOLS FOR ASTHMA

Asthma is generally an episodic disease and the clinical presentation and natural history is highly variable from patient to patient. Some patients have persistent symptoms and exacerbations from time to time. Others show long periods of remission, with sudden worsening after exposure to asthma triggers **(Fig. 1)**. Treatment protocols use a step-up care pharmacologic approach based on the intensity of the asthma over time **(Fig. 3)**.[4,5] As symptoms and lung function worsen, step-up or add-on therapy is given. As symptoms improve, therapy can be "stepped down".

It has been challenging for clinicians to quantify the degree of asthma for any given patient and to make decisions based on that assessment regarding treatment. Lung function was often used as the primary endpoint but because of the poor correlation between lung function and patient symptoms and outcomes, a composite of measures are suggested by international asthma guidelines. Initially, they were based on

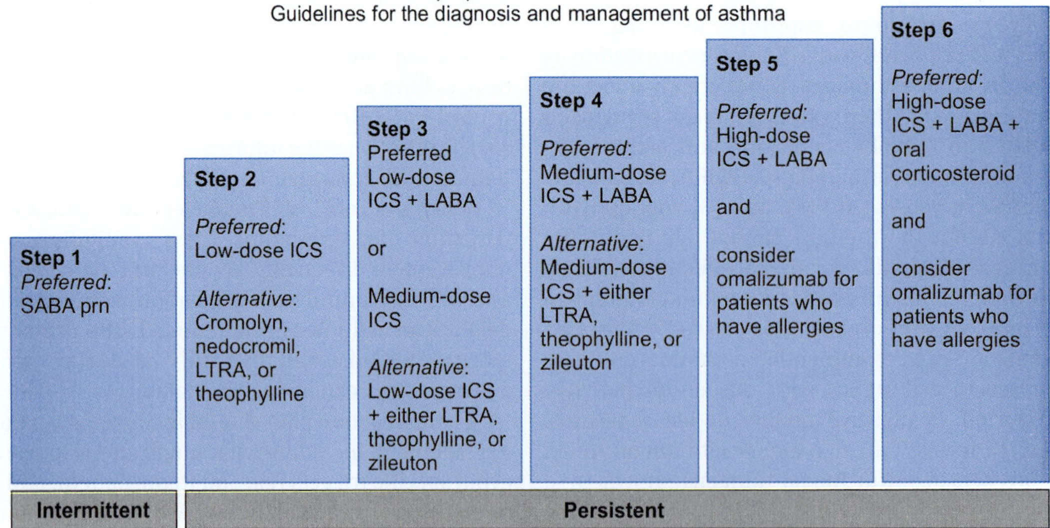

Fig. 3 Guidelines for the step-up treatment of asthma

Abbreviations: SABA, short-acting beta2-agonist; ICS, inhaled corticosteroid; LTRA, leukotriene receptor antagonist; LABA, long-acting beta 2-agonist

a scale of disease severity.[4,5] The asthma severity scale reflects the intensity of the disease. It is advocated for and can be used when a patient is not receiving long-term control therapy. The components of impairment include daily symptoms, night-time awakenings, need of quick relief rescue therapy, work or school days missed, interference with normal daily activities, and lung function, measured by spirometry **(Table 4)**.

When symptoms occur more often than two times per week, nocturnal symptoms are more than twice per month or FEV_1 is less than 80% of predicted, regular treatment with anti-inflammatory therapy (ICS) is recommended and the patient is considered to have "persistent" asthma. The response to therapy, that is how the manifestations of asthma have been reduced or eliminated, is referred to as the degree of asthma control. Asthma control has two components: (1) the level of clinical asthma control (symptoms and quality of life) and (2) the risk of future adverse events (exacerbations of asthma, loss of lung function, side effects of the therapy). At each visit the patient should be assessed for the level of asthma control, adherence to the recommended treatment and for potential side effects of the drugs used. A simplified scheme to identify patients who are controlled, partly controlled and poorly controlled has been developed **(Table 5)**.[4,5] Several composite measures of asthma control have been developed to help the clinician assess asthma control.[141-146] Step-up therapy is advised for patients not well-controlled according to guideline recommendations. There are no hard and fast rules on stepping down asthma care, but at least 3 months of stability is recommended until a reduction in medication is tried. The lowest dose of medication to maintain stability is offered. At each step, reliever medication with a SABA is used for breakthrough symptoms, but increased use implies poor control and need for step-up therapy.

Helpful guidelines for the use of asthma medications are given in **Box 4**.

ASTHMA CONTROL IN DEVELOPING COUNTRIES

More than 300 million people worldwide suffer with asthma and many live in developing countries or in deprived populations. They have received insufficient attention from the healthcare community, government officials, media, patients and families.[147] While the value of asthma disease management interventions has been well-documented, they are expensive and difficult to implement, especially in developing countries where the infrastructure for the diagnosis and management of chronic diseases, such as asthma, is either not available or is viewed as low priority on the public-health agenda. While asthma has the same prevalence in low and middle income countries as more economically advanced counrtries, poor asthma control has resulted in greater severity of disease [148] In addition, surveillance systems and diagnostic services are often poorly developed, and the true burden of diseases such as asthma and occupational lung disease is largely unknown. The Global Asthma Report in 2011 showed that the tools to manage asthma are not reaching many of the 235 million people affected. It is evident that asthma is underdiagnosed and undertreated (in particular in children), causing a high morbidity and a significant mortality. For example, in the Asthma Insights and Reality in Latin America (AIRLA), study between 5% and 15% of patients had severe symptoms and between 40% and 77% needed hospital medical assistance.[149]

In 2000, the WHO adopted a resolution for a global strategy for the prevention and control of chronic diseases such as asthma, with special emphasis on developing

Table 4 Classification of asthma severity adults not on controller therapy

Components of severity	*Classification of asthma severity**			
	Intermittent	*Persistent*		
		Mild	*Moderate*	*Severe*
Impairment				
Symptoms	≤2 days/week	>2 days/week but not daily	Daily	Throughout day
Night-time awakening	0	1–2x/month	3–4x/month	>1x/week
Short-acting (β_2 not for EIBa)	≤2 days/week	>2 days/week, not daily	Daily	Several times per day
Interference with normal activity	None	Minor limitation	Some limitation	Extremely limited
Lung function	FEV_1 >80% of predicted FEV_1/FVC normal	FEV_1 >80% of predicted FEV_1/FVC normal	FEV_1 >60% <80% of predicted	FEV_1 <60% of predicted
Risk of exacerbations	>1/year with oral corticosteroid	>2/year with oral corticosteroid	>2/year with oral corticosteroid	>2/year with oral corticosteroid

Abbreviations: FEV_1, forced expiratory volume in one second; FVC, forced vital capacity
*(*Source:* Adapted from NAEPP, NHLBI, NIH. Expert Panel Report 3: Guidelines for the Diagnosis and Management of Asthma. 2007)

Table 5 Classification of asthma control youth is greater than 12 years and adults*

Characteristics of impairment	*Controlled (All of the following)*	*Not well-controlled (Any measure present in any week)*	*Very poorly controlled*
Daytime symptoms	Note (d ≤2/week)	>2 times/week	Throughout day
Interference with normal activities	None	Any	Extremely limited
Nocturnal symptoms/awakening	<2 times/month	1–3 times/week	>4 times/week
Need for short-acting beta agoinst (rescue treatment)	None (d ≤2/week)	>2 times/week	Several times a day
Lung function (PEFR or FEV_1)	>80% predicted or personal best	60–80% predicted or personal best	<60 predicted or personal best
Validated Questionnaire (e.g. ACT score)	>20	16–19	15 or less

* Adapted from NAEPP, NHLBI, NIH. Expert Panel Report 3: Guidelines for the Diagnosis and Management of Asthma, 2007.[3]
Abbreviations: PEFR, peak expiratory flow rate; FEV_1, forced expiratory volume in one second; ACT, asthma control test
*(Source: Adapted from NAEPP, NHLBI, NIH. Expert Panel Report 3: Guidelines for the Diagnosis and Management of Asthma, 2007)

BOX 4 Principles of asthma treatment

- Use rescue medication (SABA) for symptoms of dyspnea, wheezing and chest tightness at any stage
- Begin anti-inflammatory medication (medium dose inhaled ICS preferred) when symptoms and need for rescue medication occurs two or more times a week
- Do not use LABA bronchodilators continuously as solo treatment
- LABA is the preferred add-on to ICS when step-up therapy is needed
- High dose ICS may be necessary to control persistent symptoms, but this risks more systemic absorption
- Sustained-released theophylline is a bronchodilator with weak anti-inflammatory properties and frequent side effects; may be helpful for nocturnal asthma
- Spacer devices are recommended when MDI canisters are used to reduce oropharyngeal deposition and systemic absorption; consider the use of single or multidose DPIs. They are easier to use correctly than MDI
- Systemic corticosteroids have many side effects. They may be necessary for severe asthma; oral use is preferred over intramuscular or intravenous delivery

Abbreviations: SABA, short-acting β-agonists; ICS, inhaled corticosteroid; LABA, long-acting β-agonists; MDI, metered-dose inhaler; DPI, dry powder inhalers

countries.[150] To assess the progress of this effort, a survey was done in 2005-2006 and compared to one done in 2000-2001. Between surveys from 118 countries great progress was made in tobacco control legislation (from 59% to 84% of countries) and in legislation and ministerial decrees on nutrition related to chronic diseases. Models were developed like the WHO Practical Approach to Lung Health (PAL).[151,152] This is an initiative for low-and middle-income countries that is focused on improving the management of patients with respiratory symptoms in the primary care setting and improving the efficiency of the delivery of respiratory services within a district health care system, with a focus on coordination and integration of respiratory case management. The program uses standardized clinical practice guidelines that have been developed to suit the local needs. Key components are: providing guidance, technical support and assistance with funding, assuring access to essential diagnostics and drugs; and education for healthcare workers in these activities. A follow-up WHO assessment was completed by the Global Alliance against Chronic Respiratory Diseases (GARD), a group that contributes to the WHO's work to prevent and control chronic respiratory diseases. A 2007 document "Global surveillance, prevention and control of chronic respiratory diseases: a comprehensive approach" will raise awareness of diseases like asthma and the need for comprehensive programs country by country.

Using a PAL educational outreach program for the integrated case, management of chronic respiratory diseases has been used in poor, underdeveloped regions such as South Africa.[152,153] Combining educational outreach delivered to nurse practitioners by health department trainers and integrated case management has provided a promising model for disease prevention and improved care for respiratory diseases such as asthma. With local adaptations of international asthma guidelines, success with asthma control in resource-poor areas have been also reported from Latin America.[154,155] Important suggestions for asthma control of patients in low and middle-income countries are suggested by the WHO in the "Practical Approach to Lung Disease Handbook".

In the majority of developing countries, diagnostic tests like spirometry that are required for the diagnosis and assessment of severity of asthma are not readily available, resulting in incorrect assessment and under-diagnosis of asthma. Most asthmatics who live in developing countries and in deprived areas often have limited access to essential drugs as they are either not available or not affordable.[156]

The asthma drug facility has been proposed by the International Union to address this issue and make good quality essential asthma drugs available to all patients who live in low and middle income countries.[157] Steps have been taken by the Union to insure a transparent, straightforward and efficient distribution.[158-161]

CONCLUSION

The approach to the patient with asthma has undergone a great transition in recent years. Successful outcomes can be expected for most patients. International guidelines have underscored the importance of controlling the underlying inflammation that drives the manifestations of the disease. A step-up approach has been advocated beginning with a short-acting β-agonist for infrequent symptoms. For persistent symptoms, ICS are recommended as first-line therapy. Monitoring with objective measures of disease activity, including pulmonary function and symptom questionnaires, have been advised and patient education programs can lead to self-reliance, better adherence to therapy and improved outcomes. The challenges in asthma control faced by underdeveloped countries can be overcome with educational outreach programs adapted to local needs and resources.

REFERENCES

1. Anderson GP. Endotyping asthma: new insights into key pathogenic mechanisms in a complex, heterogeneous disease. Lancet. 2008;372:1107-19.
2. Moore WC, Meyers DA, Wenzel SE, Teague WG, Li H, Li X, et al. Identification of asthma phenotypes using cluster analysis in the Severe Asthma Research Program. Am J Respir Crit Care Med. 2010;181:315-23.
3. Travers J, Weatherall M, Fingleton J, Beasley R. Towards individualised medicine for airways disease: identifying clinical phenotype groups. Eur Respir J. 2012;39:1033-48.
4. Global Initiative for Asthma (GINA).(2012). Global strategy for asthma management and prevention. [Online]. Available from http://www.ginasthma.org. [Accessed 6 April 2016].
5. National Heart, Lung and Blood Institute (NHLBI). National Asthma Education and Prevention Program (NAEPP) (2007). Expert Panel Report 3 (EPR3): Guidelines for the diagnosis and management of asthma. [online]. Available from http://www.nhlbi.nih.gov/guidelines/asthma/asthgdln.pdf. [Accessed 06 April 2016].
6. Bacharier LB, Boner A, Carlsen KH, Eigenmann PA, Frischer T, Götz M, et al. Diagnosis and treatment of asthma in childhood: a PRACTALL consensus report. Allergy. 2008;63:5-34.
7. Jindal SK, Gupta D, Aggarwal AN, Agarwal R. Gidelines for management of asthma at primary and secondary levels of health care in India. Indian J Chest Dis Allied Sci. 2005;47:309-43.
8. Guidelines Network (SIGN). British guideline on the management of asthma. A national clinical guideline. (SIGN publication no. 101). [online]. http://www.sign.ac.uk/guidelines/fulltext/101/index.html. [Accessed 06 April 2016].
9. Braman SS. The Global Burden of asthma. Chest. 2006;130:4S-12S.
10. Ashrad SH. Primary prevention of asthma and allergy. J Allergy Clin Immunol. 2005;116:3-14.
11. Gaffin JM, Phipatanakul W. The role of indoor allergens in the development of asthma. Curr Opin Allergy Clin Immunol. 2009;9:128-35.
12. Halonen M, Stern DA, Wright AL, Taussig LM, Martinez FD. Alternaria as a major allergen for asthma in children raised in a desert environment. Am J Respir Crit Care Med. 1997;155:1356-61.
13. Sears MR, Burrows B, Herbison GP, Holdaway MD, Flannery EM. Atopy in childhood. II. Relationship to airway responsiveness, hay fever and asthma. Clin Exp Allergy. 1993;23:949-56.
14. Sporik R, Holgate ST, Platts-Mills TA, Cogswell JJ. Exposure to house-dust mite allergen (Der p I) and the development of asthma in childhood. A prospective study. N Engl J Med. 1990;323:502-7.
15. Celedon JC, Milton DK, Ramsey CD, Litonjua AA, Ryan L, Platts-Mills TA, et al. Exposure to dust mite allergen and endotoxin in early life and asthma and atopy in childhood. J. Allergy Clin. Immunol. 2007;120:144-9.
16. Vervloet D, Charpin D, Haddi E, N'guyen A, Birnbaum J, Soler M, et al. Medication requirements and house dust mite exposure in mite-sensitive asthmatics. Allergy 1991;46:554-8.
17. Piacentini GL, Martinati L, Fornari A, Comis A, Carcereri L, Boccagni P, et al. Antigen avoidance in a mountain environment: influence on basophil releasability in children with allergic asthma. J Allergy Clin Immunol. 1993;92:644-50.
18. Simon HU, Grotzer M, Nikolaizik WH, Blaser K, Schöni MH. High altitude climate therapy reduces peripheral blood T lymphocyte activation, eosinophilia, and bronchial obstruction in children with house dust mite allergic asthma. Pediatr Pulmonol. 1994;17:304-11.
19. Morgan WJ, Crain EF, Gruchalla RS, O'Connor GT, Kattan M, Evans R, et al. Results of a home-based environmental intervention among urban children with asthma. N Engl J Med. 2004;351:1068-80.
20. Peroni DG, Piacentini GL, Costella S, Pietrobelli A, Bodini A, Loiacono A, et al. Mite avoidance can reduce air trapping and airway inflammation in allergic asthmatic children. Clin Exp Allergy. 2002;32:850-5.
21. Wood RA, Chapman MD, Adkinson NF, Eggleston PA. The effect of cat removal on allergen content in household-dust samples. J Allergy Clin Immunol. 1998;83:730-4.
22. Popplewell EJ, Innes VA, Lloyd-Hughes S, Jenkins EL, Khdir K, Bryant TN. The effect of high-efficiency and standard vacuum-cleaners on mite, cat and dog allergen levels and clinical progress. Pediatr Allergy Immunol. 2000;11:142-8.
23. Phipatanakul W, Cronin B, Wood RA, Eggleston PA, Shih MC, Song L, et al. Effect of environmental intervention on mouse allergen levels in homes of inner-city Boston children with asthma. Ann Allergy Asthma Immunol. 2004;92:420-5.
24. Woodcock A, Forster L, Matthews E, Martin J, Letley L, Vickers M, et al. Control of exposure to mite allergen and allergen impermeable bed covers for adults with asthma. N Engl J Med. 2003;349:225-36.
25. Krieger JW, Takaro TK, Song L, Weaver M. The Seattle-King County Healthy Homes Project: a randomized, controlled trial of a community health worker intervention to decrease exposure to indoor asthma triggers. Am J Public Health. 2005;95:652-9.
26. Kercsmar CM, Dearborn DG, Schluchter M, Xue L, Kirchner HL, Sobolewski J, et al. Reduction in asthma morbidity in

children as a result of home remediation aimed at moisture sources. Environ Health Perspect. 2006;114:1574-80.
27. Kattan M, Stearns SC, Crain EF, Stout JW, Gergen PJ, Evans R, et al. Cost-effectiveness of a home-based environmental intervention for inner-city children with asthma. J Allergy Clin Immunol. 2005;116:1058-63.
28. Sears MR, Herbison GP, Holdaway MD, Hewitt CJ, Flannery EM, Silva PA. The relative risks of sensitivity to grass pollen, house dust mite and cat dander in the development of childhood asthma. Clin Exp Allergy. 1989;19:419-24.
29. Reid MJ, Moss RB, Hsu YP, Kwasnicki JM, Commerford TM, Nelson BL. Seasonal asthma in northern California: allergic causes and efficacy of immunotherapy. J Allergy Clin Immunol. 1986;78:590-600.
30. Creticos PS, Reed CE, Norman PS, Khoury J, Adkinson NF, Buncher CR, et al. Ragweed immunotherapy in adult asthma. N Engl J Med. 1996;334:501-6.
31. Abbey DE, Petersen F, Mills PK, Beeson WL. Long-term ambient concentrations of total suspended particulates, ozone, and sulfur dioxide and respiratory symptoms in a nonsmoking population. Arch Environ Health. 1993;48:33-46.
32. Moseholm L, Taudorf E, Frosig A. Pulmonary function changes in asthmatics associated with low-level SO_2 and NO_2 air pollution, weather, and medicine intake. An 8-month prospective study analyzed by neural networks. Allergy. 1993;48:334-44.
33. Garrett MH, Hooper MA, Hooper BM, Rayment PR, Abramson MJ. Increased risk of allergy in children due to formaldehyde exposure in homes. Allergy. 1999;54:330-7.
34. Jaakkola JJ, Parise H, Kislitsin V, Lebedeva NI, Spengler JD. Asthma, wheezing, and allergies in Russian school children in relation to new surface materials in the home. Am J Public Health. 2004;94:560-2.
35. Rumchev K, Spickett J, Bulsara M, Phillips M, Stick S. Association of domestic exposure to volatile organic compounds with asthma in young children. Thorax. 2004;59:746-51.
36. Garrett MH, Hooper MA, Hooper BM, Abramson MJ. Respiratory symptoms in children and indoor exposure to nitrogen dioxide and gas stoves. Am J Respir Crit Care Med. 1998;158:891-5.
37. Withers NJ, Low L, Holgate ST, Clough JB. The natural history of respiratory symptoms in a cohort of adolescents. Am J Respir Crit Care Med. 1998;158:352-7.
38. Howden-Chapman P, Pierse N, Nicholls S, Gillespie-Bennett J, Viggers H, Cunningham M, et al. Effects of improved home heating on asthma in community dwelling children: randomised controlled trial. BMJ. 2008;337:469-76.
39. Ostro BD, Lipsett MJ, Mann JK, Wiener MB, Selner J. Indoor air pollution and asthma. Results from a panel study. Am J Respir Crit Care Med. 1994;149:1400-6.
40. Chaudhuri R, Livingston E, McMahon AD, Lafferty J, Fraser I, Spears M, et al. Effects of smoking cessation on lung function and airway inflammation in smokers with asthma. Am J Respir Crit Care Med. 2006;174:127-33.
41. Chalmers GW, Macleod KJ, Little SA, Thomson LJ, McSharry CP, Thomson NC. et al. Influence of cigarette smoking on inhaled corticosteroid treatment in mild asthma. Thorax. 2002;57:226-30.
42. Sippel JM, Pedula KL, Vollmer WM, Buist AS, Osborne ML. Associations of smoking with hospital-based care and quality of life in patients with obstructive airway disease. Chest. 1999;115(3):691-6.
43. Ehrlich R, Jordaan E, Du TD, Potter P, Volmink J, Zwarenstein M, et al. Household smoking and bronchial hyperresponsiveness in children with asthma. J Asthma. 2001;38:239-51.
44. Radon K, Busching K, Heinrich J, Wichmann HE, Jörres RA, Magnussen H, et al. Passive smoking exposure: a risk factor for chronic bronchitis and asthma in adults? Chest. 2002;122:1086-90.
45. Malo JL, Lemiere C, Gautrin D, Labrecque M. Occupational asthma. Curr Opin Pulm Med. 2004;10:57-61.
46. Tarlo SM, Balmes J, Balkissoon R, Beach J, Beckett W, Bernstein D, et al. Diagnosis and management of work-related asthma: American College of Chest Physicians Consensus Statement. Chest. 2008;134(3):1S-41S.
47. Tibosch MM, Verhaak CM, Merkus PJ. Psychological characteristics associated with the onset and course of asthma in children and adolescents: a systematic review of longitudinal effects. Patient Educ Couns. 2011;82:11-9.
48. Rosi E, Ronchi MC, Grazzini M, Duranti R, Scano G. Sputum analysis, bronchial hyperresponsiveness, and airway function in asthma: results of a factor analysis. J Allergy Clin Immunol. 1999;103:232-7.
49. Crimi E, Spanevello A, Neri M, Ind PW, Rossi GA, Brusasco V. Dissociation between airway inflammation and airway hyperresponsiveness in allergic asthma. Am J Respir Crit Care Med. 1998;157:4-9.
50. Kendrick AH, Higgs CM, Whitfield MJ, Laszlo G. Accuracy of perception of severity of asthma: patients treated in general practice. BMJ. 1993;307:422-4.
51. Killian KJ, Watson R, Otis J, St Amand TA, O'Byrne PM. Symptom perception during acute bronchoconstriction. Am J Respir Crit Care Med. 2000;162:490-6.
52. Connolly MJ, Crowley JJ, Charan NB, Nielson CP, Vestal RE. Reduced subjective awareness of bronchoconstriction provoked by methacholine in elderly asthmatic and normal subjects as measured on a simple awareness scale. Thorax. 1992;47:410-3.
53. Ekici M, Apan A, Ekici A, Erdemoğlu AK. Perception of bronchoconstriction in elderly asthmatics. J Asthma. 2001;38:691-6.
54. Kerstjens HA, Brand PL, de Jong PM, Koëter GH, Postma DS. Influence of treatment on peak expiratory flow and its relation to airway hyperresponsiveness and symptoms. The Dutch CNSLD Study Group. Thorax. 1994;49:1109-15.
55. Brand PL, Duiverman EJ, Waalkens HJ, van Essen-Zandvliet EE, Kerrebijn KF. Peak flow variation in childhood asthma: correlation with symptoms, airways obstruction, and hyperresponsiveness during long-term treatment with inhaled corticosteroids. Dutch CNSLD Study Group. Thorax. 1999;54:103-7.
56. Smith HR, Irvin CG, Cherniack RM. The utility of spirometry in the diagnosis of reversible airways obstruction. Chest. 1992;101:1577-81.
57. American Thoracic Society Statement. Lung function testing: Selection of reference values and interpretive strategies. Am Rev Respir Dis. 1991;144:1202-18.
58. Pellegrino R, Viegi G, Brusasco V, Crapo RO, Burgos F, Casaburi R, et al. Interpretative strategies for lung function tests. Eur Respir J. 2005;26:948-68.
59. Nair SJ, Daigle KL, DeCuir P, Lapin CD, Schramm CM. The influence of pulmonary function testing on the management of asthma in children. J Pediatr. 2005;147:797-801.

60. Aburuz S, McElnay J, Gamble J, Millership J, Heaney L. Relationship between lung function and asthma symptoms in patients with difficult to control asthma. J Asthma. 2005;42:859-64.
61. Stout JW, Visness CM, Enright P, Lamm C, Shapiro G, Gan VN. Classification of asthma severity in children: the contribution of pulmonary function testing. Arch Pediatr Adolesc Med. 2006;160:844-50.
62. Fuhlbrigge AL, Kitch BT, Paltiel AD, Kuntz KM, Neumann PJ, Dockery DW, et al. FEV(1) is associated with risk of asthma attacks in a pediatric population. J Allergy Clin Immunol. 2001;107:61-7.
63. Adams RJ, Smith BJ, Ruffin RE. Factors associated with hospital admissions and repeat emergency department visits for adults with asthma. Thorax. 2000;55:566-73.
64. Bacharier LB, Strunk RC, Mauger D, White D, Lemanske RF, Sorkness CA. Classifying asthma severity in children: mismatch between symptoms, medication use, and lung function. Am J Respir Crit Care Med. 2004;170:426-32.
65. Covar RA, Spahn JD, Martin RJ, Silkoff PE, Sundstrom DA, Murphy J, et al. Safety and application of induced sputum analysis in childhood asthma. J Allergy Clin Immunol. 2004;114:575-82.
66. Urlik CS, Frederiksen J. Mortality and markers of risk of asthma death among 1,075 outpatients with asthma. Chest. 1995;108:10-5.
67. Ulrik CS, Backer V. Nonreversible airflow obstruction in life-long nonsmokers with moderate to severe asthma. Eur Respir J. 1999;14:892-6.
68. Eid N, Yandell B, Howell L, Eddy M, Sheikh S. Can peak expiratory flow predict airflow obstruction in children with asthma? Pediatrics. 2000;105:354-8.
69. Llewellin P, Sawyer G, Lewis S, Cheng S, Weatherall M, Fitzharris P, et al. The relationship between FEV_1 and PEF in the assessment of the severity of airways obstruction. Respirology. 2002;7:333-7.
70. Cain H. Bronchoprovocation testing. Cllin Chest Med. 2001;22:651-9.
71. Parkerson J, Ledford D. Mannitol as an indirect bronchoprovocation test for the 21st century. Ann Allergy Asthma Immunol. 2011;106:91-6.
72. Holley AB, Cohee B, Walter RJ, Shah AA, King CS, Roop S. Eucapnic voluntary hyperventilation is superior to methacholine challenge testing for detecting airway hyperreactivity in nonathletes. J Asthma. 2012;49:614-9.
73. Parsons JP. Current concepts in the diagnosis and management of exercise-induced bronchospasm. Phys Sportsmed. 2010;38:48-53.
74. Silkoff PE. Recommendations for standardized procedures for the online and off-line measurement of exhaled lower respiratory nitric oxide and nasal nitric oxide in adults and children—1999. Am J Respir Crit Care Med. 1999;160:2104-17.
75. Dweik RA, Boggs PB, Erzurum SC, Irvin CG, Leigh MW, Lundberg JO, et al. An official ATS clinical practice guideline: interpretation of exhaled nitric oxide levels (FENO) for clinical applications. Am J Respir Crit Care Med. 2011;184:602-15.
76. Donohue JF, Jain N. Exhaled nitric oxide to predict corticosteroid responsiveness and reduce asthma exacerbation rates. Respir Med. 2013;107:943-52.
77. Weersink EJ, Aalbers R, Koeter GH, Kauffman HF, De Monchy JG. Postma DS. Partial inhibition of the early and late asthmatic response by a single dose of salmeterol. Am J Respir Crit Care Med. 1994;150:1262-7.
78. Nelson HS, Weiss ST, Bleecker ER, Yancey SW, Dorinsky PM; SMART Study Group. The Salmeterol Multicenter Asthma Research Trial: a comparison of usual pharmacotherapy for asthma or usual pharmacotherapy plus salmeterol. Chest. 2006;129:15-26.
79. Jaeschke R, O'Byrne PM, Mezja F, Nair P, Leśniak W, Brożek J, et al. The safety of long-acting β2-agonists among patients with asthma using inhaled corticosteroids: systematic review and meta-analysis. Am J Respir Crit Care Med. 2008:178:1009-16.
80. Peters SP, Kunselman SJ, Icitovic N, Moore WC, Pascual R, Ameredes BT, et al. Tiotropium bromide step-up therapy for adults with uncontrolled asthma. N Engl J Med 2010;363:1715-26.
81. Novelli F, Costa F, Latorre M, Malagrinò L, Celi A, Vagaggini B, et al. Tiotropium: a new therapeutic option in asthma. Monaldi Arch Chest Dis. 2013;79:109-15.
82. Suissa S, Ernst P, Benayoun S. Baltzan M, Cai B. Low-Dose Inhaled Corticosteroids and the Prevention of Death from Asthma. NEJM. 2000;343:332-6.
83. Masoli M, Holt S, Weatherall M, Beasley R. Dose-response relationship of inhaled budesonide in adult asthma: a meta-analysis. Eur Respir J. 2004;23:552-8.
84. Holt S, Suder A, Weatherall M, Cheng S, Shirtcliffe P, Beasley R. Dose-response relation of inhaled fluticasone propionate in adolescents and adults with asthma: meta-analysis. BMJ. 2001;323:1-8.
85. Powell H, Gibson PG. High dose versus low dose inhaled corticosteroid as initial starting dose for asthma in adults and children. Cochrane Database Syst Rev. 2004:CD004109.
86. Reddel HK, Barnes DJ. Pharmacological strategies for self-management of asthma exacerbations. Eur Respir J. 2006;28:182-99.
87. Oborne J, Mortimer K, Hubbard RB, Tattersfield AE, Harrison TW. Quadrupling the dose of inhaled corticosteroid to prevent asthma exacerbations: a randomized, double-blind, placebo-controlled, parallel-group clinical trial. Am J Respir Crit Care Med. 2009;180:598-602.
88. Scicchitano R, Aalbers R, Ukena D, Manjra A, Fouquert L, Centanni S, et al. Efficacy and safety of budesonide/formoterol single inhaler therapy versus a higher dose of budesonide in moderate to severe asthma. Curr Med Res Opin. 2004;20:1403-18.
89. Giembycz MA. Could isoenzyme-selective phosphodiesterase inhibitors render bronchodilator therapy redundant in the treatment of bronchial asthma? Biochem Pharmacol. 1992;43:2041-51.
90. Pauwels R, Van Renterghem D, Van Der Straeten M, Johannesson N, Persson CG. The effect of theophylline and enprofylline on allergen-induced bronchoconstriction. J Allergy Clin Immunol. 1985;76:583-90.
91. Skloot GS. Nocturnal asthma: mechanisms and management. Mt Sinai J Med. 2002;69:140-7.
92. Tee AK, Koh MS, Gibson PG, Lasserson TJ, Wilson AJ, Irving LB. Long-acting beta 2-agonists versus theophylline for maintenance treatment of asthma. Cochrane Database Syst Rev. 2007;18:CD001281.
93. Evans DJ, Taylor DA, Zetterstrom O, Chung KF, O'Connor BJ, Barnes PJ. A Comparison of Low-Dose Inhaled Budesonide

plus Theophylline and High-Dose Inhaled Budesonide for Moderate Asthma. NEJM. 1997;337:1412-19.

94. Nelson HS, Busse WW, Kerwin E, Church N, Emmett A, Rickard K, et al. Fluticasone propionate/salmeterol combination provides more effective asthma control than low-dose inhaled corticosteroid plus Montelukast. J Allergy Clin Immunol. 2000;106:1088-95.
95. Dahlén B, Nizankowska E, Szczeklik A, Zetterström O, Bochenek G, Kumlin M, et al. Benefits from adding the 5-lipoxygenase inhibitor zileuton to conventional therapy in aspirin-intolerant asthmatics. Am J Respir Crit Care Med. 1998;157:1187-94.
96. Hui KP, Barnes NC. Lung function improvement in asthma with a cysteinyl-leukotriene receptor antagonist. Lancet. 1991;337(8749):1062-3.
97. Lofdahl C-G, Reiss TF, Leff JA, Israel E, Noonan MJ, Finn AF, et al. Randomised, placebo controlled trial of effect of a leukotriene receptor antagonist, montelukast, on tapering inhaled corticosteroids in asthmatic patients. BMJ. 1999;319:87-90.
98. Israel E, Cohn J, Dube L, Drazen JM. Effect of treatment with zileuton, a 5-lipoxygenase inhibitor, in patients with asthma. A randomized controlled trial. Zileuton Clinical Trial Group. J Am Med Assoc. 1996;275:931-6.
99. Martin RJ, Kraft M, Chu HW, Berns EA, Cassell GH. A link between chronic asthma and chronic infection. J Allergy Clin Immunol. 2001;107:595-601.
100. Sutherland ER, King TS, Icitovic N, Ameredes BT, Bleecker E, Boushey HA, et al. A trial of clarithromycin for the treatment of suboptimally controlled asthma. J Allergy Clin Immunol. 2010;126:747-53.
101. Reiter J, Demirel N, Mendy A, Gasana J, Vieira ER, Colin AA, et al. Macrolides for the long-term management of asthma: a meta-analysis of randomized clinical trials. Allergy. 2013;68:1040-9.
102. Brusselle GG, VanderStichele C, Jordens P, Deman R, Slabbynck H, Ringoet V, et al. Azithromycin for prevention of exacerbations in severe asthma (AZISAST): a multicentre randomized double-blind placebo-controlled trial. Thorax. 2013;68:322-9.
103. Fahy JV. Anti-IgE: lessons learned from effects on airway inflammation and asthma exacerbation. J Allergy Clin Immunol. 2006;117:1230-2.
104. Flood-Page P, Swenson C, Faiferman I, Matthews J, Williams M, Brannick L, et al. A study to evaluate safety and efficacy of mepolizumab in patients with moderate persistent asthma. Am J Respir Crit Care Med. 2007;176:1062-71.
105. Compalati E, Braido F, Canonica GW. An update on allergen immunotherapy and asthma. Curr Opin Pulm Med. 2014;20:109-17.
106. Jacobsen L, Niggemann B, Dreborg S, Ferdousi HA, Halken S, Høst A, et al. Specific immunotherapy has long-term preventive effect of seasonal and perennial asthma: 10-year follow-up on the PAT study. Allergy. 2007;62:943-8.
107. Reid MJ, Lockey RF, Turkeltaub PC, Platts-Mills TA. Survey of fatalities from skin testing and immunotherapy 1985-1998. J Allergy Clin Immunol. 1993;92:6-15.
108. Broide DH. Immunomodulation of allergic disease. Annu Rev Med. 2009;60:279-91.
109. Bousquet J, Lockey RF, Malling HJ. Position Paper. Allergen immunotherapy: therapeutic vaccines for allergic diseases. A WHO position paper. Allergy. 1998;53(Suppl 44):1-42.
110. Zuberbier T, Bachert C, Bousquet PJ, Passalacqua G, Walter Canonica G, Merk H, et al. GA^2 LEN/EAACI pocket guide for allergen-specific immunotherapy for allergic rhinitis and asthma. Allergy. 2010;65:1525-30.
111. Denning DW, O'Driscoll BR, Hogaboam CM, Bowyer P, Niven RM. The link between fungi and severe asthma: a summary of the evidence. Eur Respir J. 2006;27:615-26.
112. Moreira AS, Silva D, Ferreira AR, Delgado L. Antifungal treatment in allergic bronchopulmonary aspergillosis with and without cystic fibrosis: a systematic review. Clin Exp Allergy. 2014;44:1210-27.
113. Denning DW, O'Driscoll BR, Powell G, Chew F, Atherton GT, Vyas A, et al. Randomized controlled trial of oral antifungal treatment for severe asthma with fungal sensitization: the fungal asthma sensitization trial (fast) study. Am J Respir Crit Care Med. 2009;179:11-8.
114. Platts-Mills TAE, Woodfolk JA. Trichophyton Asthma. Chest. 2009;135:887-8.
115. McKeever TM, Britton J. Diet and Asthma. Am J Resp Crit Care. 2004;170:725-9.
116. Rajabbik MH, Lotfi T, Alkhaled L, Fares M, El-Hajj Fuleihan G, Mroueh S, et al. Association between low vitamin D levels and the diagnosis of asthma in children: a systematic review of cohort studies. Allergy Asthma Clin Immunol. 2014;10:31.
117. Castro M, King TS, Kunselman SJ, Cabana MD3, Denlinger L4, Holguin F, et al. Effect of vitamin D3 on asthma treatment failures in adults with symptomatic asthma and lower vitamin D levels: the VIDA randomized clinical trial. J Am Med Assoc. 2014;311:2083-91.
118. Dixon AE, Holguin F, Sood A, Salome CM, Pratley RE, Beuther DA, et al. An official American Thoracic Society Workshop report: obesity and asthma. Proc Am Thorac Soc. 2010;7:325-35.
119. Jones KP, Mullee MA, Middleton M, Chapman E, Holgate ST. Peak flow based asthma self-management: a randomised controlled study in general practice. British Thoracic Society Research Committee. Thorax. 1995;50:851-7.
120. Sommaruga M, Spanevello A, Migliori GB, Neri M, Callegari S, Majani G. The effects of a cognitive behavioural intervention in asthmatic patients. Monaldi Arch Chest Dis. 1995;50:398-402.
121. Cote J, Cartier A, Robichaud P, Boutin H, Malo JL, Rouleau M, et al. Influence on asthma morbidity of asthma education programs based on self- management plans following treatment optimization. Am J Respir Crit Care Med. 1997;155:1509-14.
122. Turner MO, Taylor D, Bennett R, Fitzgerald JM. A randomized trial comparing peak expiratory flow and symptom self-management plans for patients with asthma attending a primary care clinic. Am J Respir Crit Care Med. 1998;157:540-6.
123. Partridge MR, Caress AL, Brown C, Hennings J, Luker K, Woodcock A, et al. Can lay people deliver asthma self-management education as effectively as primary care based practice nurses? Thorax. 2008;63:778-83.
124. Bartholomew LK, Gold RS, Parcel GS, Czyzewski DI, Sockrider MM, Fernandez M, et al. Watch, Discover, Think, and Act: evaluation of computer-assisted instruction to improve asthma self-management in inner-city children. Patient Educ Couns. 2000;39:269-80.
125. Cicutto L, Murphy S, Coutts D, O'Rourke J, Lang G, Chapman C, et al. Breaking the access barrier: evaluating an asthma center's efforts to provide education to children with asthma in schools. Chest. 2005;128:1928-35.
126. Cordina M, McElnay JC, Hughes CM. Assessment of a community pharmacy-based program for patients with asthma. Pharmacotherapy. 2001;21:1196-203.

127. Guevara JP, Wolf FM, Grum CM, Clark NM. Effects of educational interventions for self-management of asthma in children and adolescents: systematic review and meta-analysis. BMJ. 2003;326:1308-9.
128. Teach SJ, Crain EF, Quint DM, Hylan ML, Joseph JG. Improved asthma outcomes in a high-morbidity pediatric population: results of an emergency department-based randomized clinical trial. Arch Pediatr Adolesc Med. 2006;160:535-41.
129. Cowie RL, Revitt SG, Underwood MF, Field SK. The effect of a peak flow-based action plan in the prevention of exacerbations of asthma. Chest. 1997;112:1534-8.
130. Bruzzese JM, Sheares BJ, Vincent EJ, Du Y, Sadeghi H, Levison MJ, et al. Effects of a school-based intervention for urban adolescents with asthma. A controlled trial. Am J Respir Crit Care Med. 2011;183:998-1006.
131. Chan DS, Callahan CW, Hatch-Pigott VB, Lawless A, Proffitt HL, Manning NE, et al. Internet-based home monitoring and education of children with asthma is comparable to ideal office-based care: results of a 1-year asthma in-home monitoring trial. Pediatrics. 2007;119:569-78.
132. Van der Meer V, Bakker MJ, van den Hout WB, Rabe KF, Sterk PJ, Kievit J, et al. Internet-based self-management plus education compared with usual care in asthma: a randomized trial. Ann Intern Med. 2009;151:110-20.
133. Liu WT, Huang CD, Wang CH, Lee KY, Lin SM, Kuo HP. A mobile telephone-based interactive self-care system improves asthma control. Eur Respir J. 2011;37:310-7.
134. Foster JM, Usherwood T, Smith L, Sawyer SM, Xuan W, Rand CS, et al. Inhaler reminders improve adherence with controller treatment in primary care patients with asthma. J Allergy Clin Immunol. 2014;134:1260-8.
135. Zeiger RS, Schatz M, Li Q, Solari PG, Zazzali JL, Chen W, et al. Real-Time Asthma Outreach Reduces Excessive Short-acting β2-Agonist Use: A Randomized Study. J Allergy Clin Immunol Pract. 2014;2:445-56.
136. Bonner S, Zimmerman BJ, Evans D, Irigoyen M, Resnick D, Mellins RB. An individualized intervention to improve asthma management among urban Latino and African-American families. J Asthma. 2002;39:167-79.
137. Clark NM, Brown R, Joseph CL, Anderson EW, Liu M, Valerio MA. Effects of a comprehensive school-based asthma program on symptoms, parent management, grades, and absenteeism. Chest. 2004;125:1674-9.
138. Janson SL, Fahy JV, Covington JK, Paul SM, Gold WM, Boushey HA. Effects of individual self-management education on clinical, biological, and adherence outcomes in asthma. Am J Med. 2003;115:620-6.
139. McLean W, Gillis J, Waller R. The Community Pharmacy Asthma Study: a study of clinical, economic and holistic outcomes influenced by an asthma care protocol provided by specially trained community pharmacists in British Columbia. Can Respir J. 2003;10:195-202.
140. Perneger TV, Sudre P, Muntner P, Uldry C, Courteheuse C, Naef AF, et al. Effect of patient education on self-management skills and health status in patients with asthma: a randomized trial. Am J Med. 2002;113:7-14.
141. Saini B, Krass I, Armour C. Development, implementation, and evaluation of a community pharmacy-based asthma care model. Ann Pharmacother. 2004;38:1954-60.
142. Thoonen BP, Schermer TR, Van Den Boom G, Molema J, Folgering H, Akkermans RP, et al. Self-management of asthma in general practice, asthma control and quality of life: a randomised controlled trial. Thorax. 2003;58:30-6.
143. Gibson PG, Powell H. Written action plans for asthma: an evidence-based review of the key components. Thorax. 2004;59:94-9.
144. McLean S, Chandler D, Nurmatov U, Liu J, Pagliari C, Car J, et al. Telehealthcare for asthma. Cochrane Database Syst Rev. 2010:CD007717.
145. Juniper EF, Guyatt GH, Feeny DH, Ferrie PJ, Griffith LE. Townsend M. Measuring quality of life in children with asthma. Qual Life Res. 1996;5:35-46.
146. Juniper EF, O'Byrne PM, Guyatt GH, Ferrie PJ, King DR. Development and validation of a questionnaire to measure asthma control. Eur Respir J. 1999;14:902-7.
147. Bayliss MS, Espindle DM, Buchner D, Blaiss MS, Ware JE. A new tool for monitoring asthma outcomes: the ITG Asthma Short Form. Qual Life Res. 2000;9:451-66.
148. Marks GB, Dunn SM, Woolcock AJ. An evaluation of an asthma quality of life questionnaire as a measure of change in adults with asthma. J Clin Epidemiol. 1993;46:1103-11.
149. Nathan RA, Sorkness CA, Kosinski M, Schatz M, Li JT, Marcus P, et al. Development of the Asthma Control Test: a survey for assessing asthma control. J Allergy Clin Immunol. 2004;113:59-65.
150. Bousquet J, Dahl R, Khaltaev N. Global Alliance against Chronic Respiratory Diseases. Eur Respir J. 2007;29:233-9.
151. Sánchez-Borges M, Capriles-Hulett A, Caballero-Fonseca F. Asthma care in resource-poor settings. World Allergy Organ J. 2011;4:68-72.
152. Neffen H, Fritscher C, Schacht FC, Levy G, Chiarella P, Soriano JB, et al. Asthma control in Latin America: the Asthma Insights and Reality in Latin America (AIRLA) Survey. Rev Panam Salud Pública. 2005;4:191-7.
153. World Health Organization. (2005) Preventing chronic diseases: a vital investment. WHO global report. [online]. Available from *http://www.who.int/chp/chronic_disease_report/en/. [Accessed February, 2016].*
154. Murray JR, Pio A, Ottman P, PAL. A new and practical approach to lung health. Int J Tuberc Lung Dis. 2006;10:1188-91.
155. World Health Organization. A primary health care strategy for the integrated management of respiratory conditions in people of five years of age and over. WHO/HTM/TB/2005.351. Geneva;WHO:2005.
156. Fairall LR, Zwarenstein M, Bateman ED, Bachmann M, Lombard C, Majara BP, et al. Effect of educational outreach to nurses on tuberculosis case detection and primary care of respiratory illness: pragmatic cluster randomised controlled trial. BMJ. 2005;331:750-4.
157. Fischer GB, Camargos PA, Mocelin HT. The burden of asthma in children: a Latin American perspective. Paediatr Respir Rev. 2005;6:8-13.
158. Cabral ALB. Carvalho WAF, Chinen MC. Are International Asthma Guidelines effective for low-income Brazilian children with asthma? Eur Respir J. 1998;12:35-40.
159. Bilo N. Do we need an Asthma Drug Facility? Int J Tuberc Lung Dis. 2006;8:391.
160. Tan WC, Aït-Khaled N. Dissemination and implementation of guidelines for the treatment of asthma. Int J Tuberc Lung Dis. 2006;10:710-6.
161. The Asthma Drug Facility (ADF) [online]. Available from *http://www.globaladf.org. [Accessed 06 April, 2016].*

Acute Asthma Exacerbations

Aditya Jindal

INTRODUCTION

An asthma exacerbation is defined as an acute or subacute worsening of symptoms and signs of disease in a patient with preexisting asthma necessitating a change in treatment.[1] Sometimes a patient may present simply with an acute episode for the first time, or after a long period of months or years. Such an attack does not generally qualify as an exacerbated attack. An exacerbation is sometimes labeled as an attack or an episode of asthma. It also incorporates the other commonly employed terms such as acute severe asthma or status asthmaticus to distinguish patients who require more intensive therapy, sometimes in a critical care unit.

Several investigators now prefer to use an umbrella term critical asthma syndrome (CAS) to include patients with acute severe asthma, status asthmaticus, refractory asthma and near-fatal asthma.[2,3] Several of these forms may represent different clinical phenotypes of severe asthma. Almost all the patients with CAS require hospitalization and management in an intensive care unit (ICU). Even patients with mild to moderate asthma may develop a severe exacerbation, thus requiring ICU management.[4]

TRIGGERS CAUSING EXACERBATIONS

There are a large number of environmental exposures and/or other factors which are known to trigger acute exacerbations **(Table 1)**. Not infrequently, the actual precipitating factor may remain unidentified. In some situations, more than one trigger may be responsible for an acute attack. Importantly, the frequently cited triggers across different regions and countries were similar as assessed from 85 articles published between 2002 and 2012 from six continents.[5] It has been also reported that patients with more severe asthma attacks had higher trigger burden.[6]

Table 1 Common types of triggers which precipitate an acute asthma exacerbation

- Respiratory tract infections
  - Viral infections (respiratory syncytial virus, influenza, rhinovirus)
  - Mycoplasma pneumonia
- Environmental allergens
  - Pollen
  - Molds
  - House dust mites
- Pet dander
- Tobacco smoke
- Air pollutants and particulates
- Exercise
- Foods and drinks

- *Infections*: An acute respiratory infection is the most commonly identifiable trigger. Both viruses and bacteria have been blamed though respiratory viruses have emerged as the most common triggers.[7] An upper respiratory tract infection is most likely to precede an acute exacerbation. The viruses which are usually responsible include respiratory syncytial virus (RSV), influenza and rhinovirus while Mycoplasma pneumonia is the most common bacterial infection. Pyogenic bacterial infections are not usually responsible.
- *Allergen exposure*: Exposure to different environmental allergens is responsible for over 90% of childhood asthma and around 50% of adult asthma.
  - *Pollens*: Pollen grains of different grasses and plants are the common recognized triggers for acute episodes. A retrospective review of emergency visits of adult asthma patients for acute exacerbations revealed a positive correlation of visit with tree pollen exposure and humidity.[8] Pollens of grasses and weeds are important for nasobronchial allergies. In Australia, an analysis of a large database of hospital readmissions for asthma in children showed increased risk in boys during the grass pollen season.[9] Pollen exposure precipitated attacks of allergic rhinitis and asthma.

    Pollination of plants occurs during the same season each year; therefore, asthma attacks are somewhat predictable in each individual patient. The atmospheric pollen load however varies depending upon the climatic conditions such as the temperature, humidity, occurrence of rain and wind conditions. The presence of insects also influences the pollen counts. Worldwide, grass pollens of the temperate subfamily and subtropical subfamilies of grasses are major sources of aero allergens.[10]

- *Fungal spores*: Fungal spores are smaller in size than pollen, therefore do not generally cause rhinitis. *Aspergillus, Cladosporium, Basidiomycetes, Alternaria* and *Fusarium* species are some of commonly identified spore producing fungi in asthma.[11] Dampness in dwelling units, compost heaps and rotting wood promote fungus growth and high spore burden.
- *House dust and mites*: House dust is an important source of respiratory allergies and asthma attacks. The indoor atmosphere with exposure to mites, mice, cockroaches, molds and endotoxins is especially important in case of children with asthma.[12] Fecal pellets of the mites, *Dermatophagoides* species, *Euroglyphus* species and *Tyrophagus* species are some of the important house dust allergens.[13] They rapidly breed in the dust in blankets, mattresses, pillows, curtains and carpets. Poor cleaning conditions cause further increase in their concentration. Animal dander and feathers are some of other allergenic material present in the house dust.
- *Pet animals*: Almost a quarter of atopic asthmatics are sensitized to pet animals such as cats, dogs, horses and guinea pigs and birds. Sensitization to animals may also occur from indirect exposures through ownership. There is an increased tendency these days to live with exotic pets like rodents, amphibians, fish and birds that are also allergenic.[14] Exposure of a sensitized individual to a pet animal is likely to result in an acute attack.

- *Air pollution*: Ambient air pollution is known to increase asthma morbidity and mortality. Epidemiological studies in the past have shown an association of asthma exacerbations with episodes of air pollution especially with ozone and particulate matter.[15] Significant association of asthma exacerbations has been also shown with traffic related pollution in children born to atopic parents and in those suffering from recurrent wheezing or asthma.[16] There is also evidence to support the association of household air pollution due to domestic solid fuel combustion with increased risk of asthma symptoms in children and asthma exacerbations.[17,18]
- *Smoking*: Both active smoking and passive exposure to environmental tobacco smoke are associated with increase in asthma symptoms and other morbidity indices.[19] However, the exact role in causing acute exacerbations remains controversial.
- *Miscellaneous factors*: There are a number of other asthma triggers known to precipitate symptoms of asthma. Foods like eggs, fish, cereals, nuts and chocolates and drugs like aspirin, nonsteroidal anti-inflammatory drugs and beta-blockers have been blamed in different reports. Cold and dry weather, exercise and gastroesophageal reflux are other important factors. Psychological stresses such as bereavement or excitement and sometimes fear may precipitate an asthma attack. Hyperventilation induced by anxiety or laughter may cause an asthmatic reaction.

Occupational asthma is a separate entity in itself although work related factors may also prove an attack in asthmatic individuals. Most of these factors may not be solely responsible for severe exacerbations. Nonetheless, the acute precipitation of asthma symptoms may frequently create panic which will require immediate attention and adequate treatment.

Finally, an exacerbation is more likely to occur in a patient with history of similar episodes in the recent past.[20] It has been suggested that frequent exacerbators may constitute a distinct subphenotype of asthma with specific characteristics[21] of 104 exacerbations in severe and 18 in mild to moderate asthma patients in a study, the frequent exacerbators had higher use of inhaled and oral glucocorticoids, worse asthma control, poorer quality of life scores, higher sputum eosinophil counts and showed a rapid decline in lung function; they also had higher exhaled nitric oxide and significant history of smoking.[20] An analysis of data from the National Health and Nutrition Examination Survey had also shown that patients (both children and adults) with higher blood eosinophil counts had suffered from more asthma attacks than those with lower counts.[22]

Besides the listed asthma triggers, a number of risk factors are also identified in patients with asthma exacerbations **(Table 2)**; these include uncontrolled symptoms, poor adherence to treatment with inhalational corticosteroids (ICS), comorbidites such as obesity, rhinosinusitis or food allergy, pregnancy, low FEV1 and presence of major psychiatric disorders. Some of these factors are also recognized to be associated with increased risk of asthma related deaths, for example the nonuse or stopping of ICS, overuse of short-acting β-agonists (SABAs), history of near fatal asthma, previous hospitalization, emergency care visits, intubation and mechanical ventilation and presence of comorbidities.

Table 2 Risk factors associated with acute severe exacerbations

- Uncontrolled symptoms
- Poor adherence to inhalational corticosteroids
- Over use of short-acting beta-agonists
- History of recent exacerbations, hospitalization, emergency room visits, intubation and mechanical ventilation
- Pregnancy
- *Comorbidities:* Obesity, major psychiatric disorder, food allergy, rhinosinusitis
- Poor lung function
- *Environmental exposures*: Smoking, allergens
- Sputum or blood eosinophilia
- Socioeconomic problems

Diagnosis and Evaluation of Severity

An attack may sometimes happen suddenly though more frequently it progressively develops over a few hours or days. Diagnosis is primarily made from the history of uncontrolled symptoms in spite of an increase in therapy. Characteristically, the patient complains of increasing breathlessness, cough, chest tightness, wheezing and limitation in exercise capacity. There may be symptoms of respiratory tract infection such as fever, sore throat, increased cough and sputum production. Nasal symptoms of excessive sneezing, rhinorrhea and nasal blockade may also be present. Nocturnal symptoms may cause disturbance in sleep.

Physical signs may demonstrate tachypnea, tachycardia, presence of prolonged expiration and wheezing sounds on auscultation. A severe case may present with the picture of life-threatening respiratory failure—cyanosis, headache, increased sweating and confusion.[23] Examination in such a case shows paradoxical pulse, low blood pressure, hyperinflated thorax and diminished breath sounds; wheezing sounds may not be audible in such a case.

Only urgent and essential investigations are required during an attack. Acute management should not be kept pending while waiting for the tests. Lung functions such as forced expiratory volume in the first second (FEV1) or peak expiratory flow (PEF) show sharp decline from the previous values. Chest roentgenography is done to look for a lung infection and/or complications such as pneumothorax and pneumomediastinum. Electrocardiogram is important to diagnosis cardiac arrhythmias. Blood gas and acid-base assessment is essential, especially for severer exacerbations. It generally shows hypoxemia, hypocapnia and respiratory alkalosis. Normocapnia in the presence of tachypnea during an exacerbation points to a state of carbon dioxide retention, while hypercapnia and respiratory acidosis occur late in the course of severe exacerbations. Lactic acidosis is also described due to combined effects of both acute severe asthma and treatment related effects.[24]

It is important to assess the degree of severity to decide the site of management **(Table 3)**. A nonsevere attack which does not fulfill the criteria for severe asthma may be managed in the outpatient setting, while others require admission in the emergency ward or in ICU.[25]

The diagnosis of an acute attack may sometimes be difficult, especially in case a patient presents in the emergency for the first time. A number of conditions may present with acute breathlessness **(Table 4)** which can be excluded with the help of clinical findings and appropriate investigations.

MANAGEMENT

Management of an exacerbation depends upon the severity of an attack, the status of the preexisting functional status and the level of asthma control. The goals of management should be stratified as immediate, early and long term **(Table 5)** and action initiated accordingly. The broad principles of management for different levels of care as per guidelines recommended in the Global Initiative for Asthma are briefly summarized here:[25]

Guided Self-management

A mild exacerbation or early worsening of asthma can be recognized at home with help of guided self-management education. A written asthma plan includes specific instructions about changes and addition of asthma drugs under

Table 3 Assessment of the severity of acute asthma exacerbation

Severity	*Symptoms*	*Signs/investigations*
Nonsevere: Outpatient management	Not fulfilling the criteria for severe or life-threatening asthma	
Severe: Management in emergency room/ward	Inability to complete sentences, agitation	• Use of accessory muscles • Respiratory rate >30/minute • Heart rate >110/minute • Pulsus paradoxus >25 mm Hg • Silent chest • PEF < 60% of predicted or personal best • PaO_2 < 60 mm Hg or $SpO_2 \leq 92\%$*
Life-threatening: ICU management	Alteration in mental status, orthopnea	• Cyanosis • Paradoxical breathing • $PaCO_2$ >40 mm Hg with worsening pH • Heart rate <60/minute (excluding drug related bradycardia#)

Note:
*Presence of this parameter qualifies as severe asthma irrespective of other signs
#Drugs like verapamil, diltiazem and beta-blockers
Abbreviations: PaO_2, partial pressure of O_2 in arterial blood; SpO_2, blood oxygen saturation level; $PaCO_2$, partial pressure of CO_2 in arterial blood.
Source: Aggarwal AN. (2014). Global Initiative for Asthma by Global Strategy for Asthma Management and Prevention. [online]. Available from *www.ginasthma.org*. [Accessed May 2014] with permission.

Table 4 Differential diagnosis of acute severe exacerbation of asthma

- Acute exacerbation of chronic obstructive pulmonary disease (COPD)
- Acute left heart failure
- Pneumothorax
- Pulmonary thromboembolism
- Fluid retention
- Renal failure
- Foreign body inhalation
- Vocal cord dysfunction
- Drug hypersensitivity
- Panic attack–hyperventilation

Table 5 Goals of management of an acute exacerbation

- Immediate
  - Resuscitation
  - Adequate oxygenation
- Early
  - Relief of symptoms
  - Reversal of airway obstruction
  - Removal/treatment of aggravating factor/s
  - Prevention of next episode of worsening
- Long-term
  - Recovery from wheezing
  - Normalization of pulmonary mechanics and lung function
  - Return to the baseline activity after the acute episode

appropriate medical guidance.[26] The plan is generally helpful to abort a severe exacerbation.

Management in Primary Care

An acute exacerbation in a primary care set up should be immediately managed. A severe exacerbation requires repetitive administration of SABAs, systemic corticosteroids and controlled flow oxygen supplementation.[27] While a mild exacerbation can usually be treated appropriately, a severe case requires transfer to a specialty/acute care setting.

Management in the Emergency Room/Hospital Ward

A severe exacerbation is characterized by two or more of the symptoms and signs listed in **(Table 3)**. There is a serious threat of such patients worsening and entering into a life-threatening situation. Management is done according to the following principles:

Clinical Assessment

Besides the history of aggravating factors and essential vital signs, the objective parameters generally include the measurement of oxygen saturation, lung function tests (e.g. PEF or FEV1), chest X-ray and arterial blood gas assessment. However, management should not be delayed for any of the investigation.

Oxygen Administration

It is important to achieve and maintain normal arterial saturation (SaO_2 between 93% and 95%). Higher oxygen concentration of 100% may prove to be harmful and cause significant carbon dioxide retention.[28] Oxygen is generally provided with the help of nasal cannulae or masks. Nonavailability of pulse oximetry/arterial blood analysis should not deter from oxygen administration. The treatment should be weaned off once the attack subsides, guided with the help of pulse oximetry.

Short Acting Bronchodilators

Bronchodilator administration is important to relieve airway obstruction and improve lung mechanics.[29] SABAs are the first line drugs due to the rapidity of their action. SABAs are administered either with the help of a pressurized metered dose inhaler (PMDI) with spacer or through nebulization. It is generally recommended that continuous therapy with nebulization be given for the initial period followed by intermittent on-demand administration. Salbutamol, levo-salbutamol (racemic salbutamol) or formoterol are commonly employed. There is no significant difference in the outcomes seen with the use of any of the SABAs.

There is no advantage of parenteral (intravenous) administration of SABA.[30] A recent study of retrospective data of 42 patients who received continuous terbutaline infusion was shown to reduce hospitalization for severe unstable asthma, but was associated with significant side effects.[31]

Corticosteroids

Systemic corticosteroids should be administered at the earliest within the first hour in all except mild exacerbations.[32] Oral administration is preferred over the intravenous route. A 5–7 day course of oral steroids is fairly effective to terminate the acute episode; different dosage schedules recommended in different reports **(Table 6)** have been found to be equally effective.[33]

There is no additional benefit of ICS along with systemic use. Patients on ICS prior to the exacerbation should not stop taking inhalational treatment. A recent study reports the additional benefit with use of nebulized high-dose budesonide in children with moderate to severe acute exacerbation on nebulized SABAs.[34]

Other Bronchodilators

- *Anticholinergic agents*: Use of a short acting anticholinergic (ipratropium) along with a SABA (salbutamol) causes greater improvement in PEF and FEV1.[35] There is a

Table 6 Different dosage schedules of corticosteroids reported as equally efficacious in hospitalized patients[34]

- Low dose steroids
  - ≤80 mg/day methyl prednisolone, or
  - ≤400 mg/day hydrocortisone, or
  - ≤100 mg/day prednisolone; or
- Medium dose
  - 80 mg ≤360 mg/day methyl prednisolone, or
  - 400 ≤1800 mg/day hydrocortisone, or
  - 100 mg ≤450 mg/day prednisolone; or
- High dose
  - 360 mg/day methyl prednisolone, or
  - 1800 mg/day hydrocortisone or
  - 450 mg/day prednisolone

significant reduction in the number of hospitalization in both children and adults. However, other studies have shown no additional benefit over SABAs and systemic corticosteroids.

- *Aminophylline and theophylline*: Intravenous aminophylline continues to be widely used in several developing countries. A meta-analysis of several studies has shown an increase in arrhythmias and vomiting with its use without any demonstrable benefit.[36] The Indian guidelines recommend use only in exceptional circumstances such as brittle asthma or in patients on mechanical ventilation with intense bronchospasm causing ineffective delivery of nebulized drugs.[25]
- *Combined use of ICS and long-acting beta-agonists (LABAs)*: There is no clear indication to use an ICS plus LABA combination for an acute attack. In one report, the use of high dose inhaled budesonide and formoterol in patients who had received prednisolone showed similar efficacy as with SABA.[37]

Magnesium Sulfate

There is some evidence to support the use of nebulized or intravenous magnesium sulfate ($MgSO_4$) in acute severe asthma. Intravenous infusion of 1.2 or 2 g over 15–20 minutes has been shown to reduce hospital admission in adults who fail to respond to initial treatment and persist with hypoxemia.[38] In a large study, there was no benefit of nebulized $MgSO_4$ in adults though a limited role was reported for intravenous $MgSO_4$.[39] Considering its safety and cost benefit profile, some investigators justify the use of either inhaled or intravenous $MgSO_4$ in all children with acute severe asthma.[40]

Antibiotics

Antibiotics for acute asthma are used only in the presence of evidence of lung infection. There was no demonstrable role in two studies on their use in reducing symptoms or length of stay in acute asthma.[41]

Leukotriene Antagonists

There is no significant clinical benefit with the use of either oral or intravenous leukotriene antagonists.

Heliox Therapy

Heliox, the mixture of helium and oxygen has lower density and higher viscosity than air oxygen mixture. Heliox inhalation thereby reduces the work of breathing. As per recent review, there is a mild benefit with its use in both children and adults.[42]

Noninvasive Ventilation

Noninvasive ventilation has no significant benefit except to reduce the dose of inhaled bronchodilators.[43] A few studies suggest a beneficial role to reduce the need for more invasive treatments, justifying the need for well conducted studies.[44] Noninvasive ventilation should always be administered under close supervision and continuous monitoring and should not be tried in agitated patients.

Sedatives

Use of sedation should be strictly avoided because of the fear of respiratory depression, which can occasionally prove to be fatal.

Hospital Discharge

The patient is fit for discharge when there is return to the previous state of health and clinical stability for at least 24 hours, i.e. patient is able to eat and lie flat. He should go back to the previous inhalers and other medication.

Management in the ICU

A patient who deteriorates in spite of the intensive therapy in the ward should be shifted to the ICU or to a place where facilities are available for intubation and ventilation. Patient may require mechanical ventilation in the presence of refractoriness to initial treatment and other signs of persistent hypoxemia **(Table 7)**.

Timely intervention helps in early recovery from the life threatening episode. The principles of ventilatory support remain similar to ventilation in other conditions. Use of

Table 7 Indications for mechanical ventilation in acute severe asthma

- Cardiorespiratory arrest
- Coma
- Refractory hypoxemia
- Refractory to initial management
- Drowsy, somnolent patient
- Cardiovascular compromise
- Failure of noninvasive ventilation

Table 8 Initial ventilator settings in patients with acute asthma

Setting	*Recommendation*
Mode	Volume assist control mode ventilation
Rate	8–12/minute
Tidal volume	4–6 mL/kg predicted body weight
I:E ratio	1:4 and higher, avoid inspiratory plateau except to measure plateau pressure
Waveform	Square waveform
Inspiratory flow	100–120 L/minute
FiO_2	Titrate to maintain $PaO_2 \geq 60$ mm Hg or $SpO_2 \geq 89\%$. Avoid hyperoxia
PEEP	Up to 5 cm H_2O
Plateau pressure	<30 cm H_2O
pH	≥7.1 in young adults; ≥7.2 in elderly

higher flow rates and prolonged expiratory time may be needed **(Table 8)**.

REFERENCES

1. Reddel HK, Taylor DR, Bateman ED, Boulet LP, Boushey HA, Busse WW, et al. An official American Thoracic Society/European Respiratory Society statement: asthma control and exacerbations: standardizing endpoints for clinical asthma trials and clinical practice. Am J Respir Crit Care Med. 2009;180(1):59-99.
2. Kenyon N, Zeki AA, Albertson TE, Louie S. Definition of critical asthma syndromes. Clin Rev Allergy Immunol. 2015;48(1):1-6.
3. Schivo M, Phan C, Louie S, Harper RW. Critical Asthma Syndrome in the ICU. Clin Rev Allergy Immunol. 2013;[Epub ahead of print].
4. Pauwels RA, Pedersen S, Busse WW, Tan WC, Chen YZ, Ohlsson SV, et al. Early intervention with budesonide in mild persistent asthma: a randomized, double-blind trial. Lancet. 2003;361(9363):1071-6.
5. Vernon MK, Wiklund I, Bell JA, Dale P, Chapman KR. What do we know about asthma triggers? A review of the literature. J Asthma. 2012;49(10):991-8.
6. Price D, Dale P, Elder E, Chapman KR. Types, frequency and impact of asthma triggers on patients' lives: a quantitative study in five European countries. J Asthma. 2014;51(2):127-35.
7. Jackson DJ, Sykes A, Mallia P, Johyinston SL. Asthma exacerbations: origin, effect, and prevention. J Allergy Clin Immunol. 2011;128(6):1165-74.
8. May L, Carim M, Yadav K. Adult asthma exacerbations and environmental triggers: a retrospective review of ED visits using an electronic medical record. Am J Emerg Med. 2011;29(9):1074-82.
9. Vicendese D, Abramson MJ, Dharmage SC, Tang ML, Allen KJ, Erbas B. Trends in asthma readmissions among children and adolescents over time by age, gender and season. J Asthma 2014;51(10):1055-60.
10. Davies JM. Grass pollen allergens globally: the contribution of subtropical grasses to burden of allergic respiratory diseases. Clin Exp Allergy. 2014;44(6):790-801.
11. Chen CH, Chao HJ, Chan CC, Chen BY, Guo YL. Current asthma in school children is related to fungal spores in classrooms. Chest. 2014;146(1):123-34.
12. Pingitore G, Pinter E. Environmental interventions for mite-induced asthma: a journey between systematic reviews, contrasting evidence and clinical practice. Eur Ann Allergy Clin Immunol. 2013;45(3):74-7.
13. Fernández-Caldas E, Puerta L, Caraballo L. Mites and allergy. Chem Immunol Allergy. 2014;100:234-42.
14. Díaz-Perales A, González-de-Olano D, Pérez-Gordo M, Pastor-Vargas C. Allergy to uncommon pets: new allergies but the same allergens. Front Immunol. 2013;4:492.
15. Devalia JL, Rusznak C, Davies RJ. Air pollution in the 1990s-cause of increased respiratory disease? Respir Med. 1994;88(4):241-4.
16. Esposito S, Galeone C, Lelii M, Longhi B, Ascolese B, Senatore L, et al. Impact of air pollution on respiratory diseases in children with recurrent wheezing or asthma. BMC Pulm Med. 2014;14:130.
17. Wong GW, Brunekreef B, Ellwood P, Anderson HR, Asher MI, Crane J, et al. Cooking fuels and prevalence of asthma: a global analysis of phase three of the International Study of Asthma and Allergies in Childhood (ISAAC). Lancet Respir Med. 2013;1(5):386-94.
18. Trevor J, Antony V, Jindal SK. The effect of biomass fuel exposure on the prevalence of asthma in adults in India-review of current evidence. J Asthma. 2014;51(2):136-41.
19. Jindal SK. Effects of smoking on asthma. J Ass Phy India. 2014;62(Suppl):32-7.
20. Miller MK, Lee JH, Miller DP, Wenzel SE. TENOR Study Group. Recent asthma exacerbations: a key predictor of future exacerbations. Respir Med. 2007;104:481-9.
21. Kupczyk M, ten Brinke A, Sterk PJ, Bel EH, Papi A, Chanez P, et al. Frequent exacertations-a distinct phenotype of severe asthma. Clin Exp Allergy. 2014;44(2):212-21.
22. Tran TN, Khatry DB, Ke X, Ward CK, Gossage D. High blood eosinophil count is associated with more frequent asthma attacks in asthma patients. Ann Allergy Asthma Immunol. 2014;113(1):19-24.
23. McFadden ER Jr. Acute severe asthma. Am J Respir Crit Care Med. 2003;168:740-59.
24. Raimondi GA, Gonzalez S, Zaltsman J, Menga G, Adrogue HJ. Acid-base patterns in acute severe asthma. J Asthma. 2013;50(10):1062-8.
25. Aggarwal AN. (2014). Global Initiative for Asthma by Global Strategy for Asthma Management and Prevention. [online]. Available from *www.ginasthma.org*. [Accessed May 2014].
26. Gibson PG, Powell H, Coughian J, Wilson AJ, Abramson M, Haywood P, et al. Self-management education and regular practitioner review for adults with asthma. Cochrane Database Syst Rev. 2003;(1):CD001117.
27. FitzGerald JM, Grunfeld A. Status asthmaticus. In: Lichtenstein LM, Fauci AS (Eds). Current therapy in allergy, immunology and rheumatology, 5th edition. St Louis MO: Mosby; 1996. pp. 63-7.
28. Rodrigo GJ, Rodriquez Verde M, Peregalli V, Rodrigo C. Effects of short-term 28% and 100% oxygen on PaCO2 and peak expiratory flow rate in acute asthma: a randomized trial. Chest. 2003;124(4):1312-7.
29. Emerman CL, Cydulla RK, McFadden ER. Comparison of 2.5 vs 7.5 mg of inhaled albuterol in the treatment of acute asthma. Chest. 1999;115(1):92-6.

30. Travers AH, Rowe BH, Barker S, Jones A, Camargo CA Jr. The effectiveness of IV beta-agonists in treating patients with acute asthma in the emergency department: a meta-analysis. Chest. 2002;122(4):1200-7.
31. Mansur AH, Afridi L, Sullivan J, Ayres JG, Wilson D. Continuous terbutaline infusion in severe asthma in adults: a retrospective study of long term efficacy and safety. J Asthma. 2014;51(10):1076-82.
32. Rowe BH, Spooner C, Ducharme FM, Bretzlaff JA, Bota GW. Early emergency department treatment of acute asthma with systemic corticosteroids. Cochrane Database Syst Rev. 2001;(1):CD002178.
33. Manser R, Reid D, Abramson M. Corticosteroids for acute severe asthma in hospitalized patients. Cochrane Database Syst Rev. 2001;(1):CD001740.
34. Chen AH, Zeng GQ, Chen RC, Zhan JY, Sun LH, Huang SK, et al. Effects of nebulized high-dose budesonide on moderate-to-severe acute exacerbation of asthma in children: a randomized, double-blind, placebo-controlled study. Respirology. 2013;18 (Suppl 3):47-52.
35. Rodrigo GJ, Castro-Rodriguez JA. Anticholinergics in the treatment of children and adults with acute asthma: a systematic review with meta-analysis. Thorax. 2005;60(9):740-6.
36. Nair P, Milan SJ, Rowe BH. Addition of intravenous aminophylline to inhaled beta(2)-agonists in adults with acute asthma. Cochrane Database Syst Rev. 2012;12:CD002742.
37. Balang VM, Yunus F, Yang PC, Jorup C. Efficacy and safety of budesonide/formoterol compared with salbutamol in the treatment of acute asthma. Pulm Pharmacol Ther. 2006;19(2):139-47.
38. Kew KM, Kirtchuk L, Michell CI. Intravenous magnesium sulfate for treating adults with acute asthma in the emergency department. Cochrane Database Syst Rev. 2014;5:CD010909.
39. Goodacre S, Cohen J, Bradburn M, Gray A, Benger J, Coats T, et al. Intravenous or nebulized magnesium sulphate versus standard therapy for severe acute asthma (3Mg trial): a double-blind randomised controlled trial. Lancet Respir Med. 2013;1(4):293-300.
40. Ohn M, Jacobe S. Magnesium should be given to all children presenting to hospital with acute severe asthma. Paediatr Respir Rev. 2014;15(4):319-21.
41. Graham V, Lasserson T, Rowe BH. Antibiotics for acute asthma. Cochrane Database Syst Rev. 2001;(3):CD002741.
42. Rodrigo GJ, Castro-Rodriguez JA. Heliox-driven β2-agonists nebulization for children and adults with acute asthma: a systematic review with meta-analysis. Ann Allergy Asthma Immunol. 2014;112(1):29-34.
43. Gupta D, Nath A, Agarwal R, Behera D. A prospective randomized controlled trial on the efficacy of noninvasive ventilation in severe acute asthma. Respir Care. 2010;55(5):536-43.
44. Carson KV, Usmani ZA, Smith BJ. Noninvasive ventilation in acute severe asthma: current evidence and future perspectives. Curr Opin Pulm Med. 2014;20(1):118-23.

Immunotherapy and Immunomodulators for Allergic Rhinitis and Asthma

Ruby Pawankar, Giovanni Passalacqua, Miyuki Hayashi, Shingo Yamanishi, Toru Igarashi

INTRODUCTION

Allergies occur as a result of aberrant immune reactivity against common harmless environmental proteins called allergens. A key component of the pathomechanisms of allergic diseases is the production of Th2 cytokines, generation of allergen-specific immunoglobulin E (IgE), crosslinking of IgE molecules by allergen, activation of mast cells with the release of potent mediators which, in turn, elicit the acute allergic reactions and initiate the development of chronic inflammation. Most therapeutic approaches for allergic diseases focus primarily on symptom control and suppression of inflammation. Nevertheless, none of the available drugs are capable of modifying the immune response; their effects vanish within a few hours or days after discontinuation. Allergen specific immunotherapy (SIT) is the only disease—modifying treatment for allergic rhinitis and asthma; benefits may persist years after treatment is discontinued.

Allergen immunotherapy has been used for almost a century as a desensitizing therapy for allergic diseases. It was introduced in 1911, based on the empiric concept that administering the substances, which produce clinical manifestations in the allergic subject, would result in a sort of vaccination with consequent clinical benefit. Despite the rationale being wrong, the results were favorable. With a better knowledge of the mechanisms of specific immunotherapy **(Fig. 1)**, the development of improved allergen extracts and the studies done using these, there has been a marked improvement in our understanding of immunotherapy. Furthermore, the standardization of allergenic extracts allowed the availability of vaccines of high quality and safety. The World Health Organization (WHO) published a position paper on SIT in 1998;[1] further, recommendations for the use of immunotherapy were reported in the allergic rhinitis and its impact on asthma (ARIA).[2]

The standard modality of administration of SIT is the subcutaneous route, but in recent years, the sublingual route has achieved credibility and is now considered a viable alternative to subcutaneous immunotherapy (SCIT). Specific immunotherapy, both subcutaneous and sublingual, is

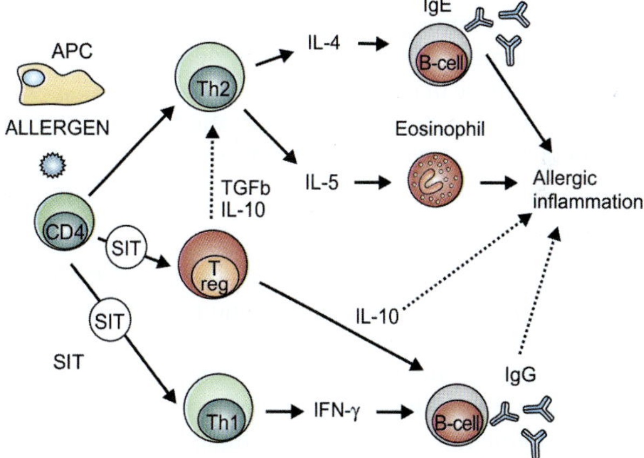

Fig. 1 Mechanisms of immunotherapy
Abbreviations: SIT, specific immunotherapy; Th, T helper cell; IFN, interferon; IL, interleukin; TGF, transforming growth factor; CD, cluster of differentiation; APC, antigen presenting cell.

currently indicated for respiratory allergy (rhinitis/asthma); whereas for hymenoptera venom allergy, only SCIT is used.

SUBCUTANEOUS IMMUNOTHERAPY

Subcutaneous immunotherapy is an allergen-specific therapy that induces long-term remission of allergic rhinitis and allergic asthma. In contrast to pharmacotherapy, SCIT prevents the onset of new sensitizations,[3,4] and reduces the progression of disease from allergic rhinitis to allergic asthma.[5] Such responses involve immunological memory and therefore direct and/or indirect effects on T- and/or B-lymphocytes.

Indications

- In ascertained IgE-mediated respiratory diseases (supported by a positive SPT/RAST) and when the causal role of the allergen(s) is well established

- In patients with clinical symptoms due to a single or limited spectrum of allergies
- In patients inadequately responding to drug treatment
- In patients unwilling to use medication
- In patients in whom pharmacotherapy induces undesirable side effects.

Contraindications

- Coexistent uncontrolled asthma/severe asthma
- Patients taking beta-blockers
- Patients with other medical/immunological diseases, including major cardiovascular disease, cancer or chronic infections
- Small children less than five years (relative contraindication)
- Pregnancy (maintenance injections may be continued during pregnancy, but it is recommended not to start induction phase in pregnancy)
- Patients unable to comply with the immunotherapy protocol or with psychiatric disorders.

Efficacy

The clinical efficacy of SCIT is well established, both for rhinitis and asthma. A review of 43 double-blind placebo-controlled (DBPC) trials has confirmed an efficacy (improvement of symptoms greater than 30% as compared to placebo) in 75–80% of studies.[6] This clinical efficacy is associated with a marked reduction in the use of antiallergic medications during the pollen season and with an improvement in patients quality of life. In some studies, it was shown that the efficacy is dose dependant.[7-24] SCIT is also effective in allergic asthma. A Cochrane meta-analysis of 62 randomized controlled trials performed between 1954 and 1998 demonstrated a significant improvement in symptoms, reduction in the use of rescue medication and improvement in both allergen-specific and nonspecific bronchial hyperresponsiveness.[25] The results were consistent across the trials, although the methodological quality of the studies was, on average, low. An updated grading of the strength of the experimental evidence for SCIT and sublingual immunotherapy (SLIT) is provided in **Table 1**.

Table 1 Grading of the strength of the experimental evidence for SCIT and SLIT

	SCIT	*SLIT*
Clinical efficacy: Rhinitis	Ib	Ia
Clinical efficacy: Asthma	Ia	Ia
Clinical efficacy: Children (rhinitis)	Ib	Ia
Prevention of new sensitizations	IIb	III
Long-term effect	Ib	IIa
Prevention of asthma	IIb	IIb

Note:
Ia Evidence from meta-analysis of randomized controlled trials
Ib Evidence from at least one randomized controlled trial
IIa Evidence from at least one controlled trial without randomization
IIb Evidence from at least one other type of quasi experimental trial
III Evidence from nonexperimental descriptive studies (comparative, correlation, case-control)
IV Evidence from panels of experts or clinical experience or authorities.
Abbreviations: SCIT, subcutaneous immunotherapy; SLIT, sublingual immunotherapy

Long-term Benefit (Carry-over Effect)

Allergen immunotherapy has been shown in several studies to maintain a long-term benefit after discontinuation. In one DBPC withdrawal study, 3–4 years grass pollen immunotherapy was shown to result in sustained reduction in symptoms and rescue medication for at least 3 years following discontinuation.[26] Other studies have confirmed long-term benefit in relation to cat allergy, ragweed, tree pollen and venom allergy. Immunotherapy has been also shown to reduce the onset of new allergen sensitivities in children.[3,4] In a prospective randomized controlled trial of pollen immunotherapy in children with seasonal allergic rhinitis, development of asthma was followed over a period of 5 years. Two years following cessation of immunotherapy, there was a marked reduction in the risk of development of physician-diagnosed asthma (odds ratio 2.7, 95% confidence intervals 1.3–5.6) as compared to controls.[5] Taken together, these studies emphasize the important prophylactic value of injection immunotherapy, which is in contrast to pharmacotherapy where relapse of symptoms occurs immediately following discontinuation.

Safety

The major drawback of SCIT is the risk of potential side effects, like systemic allergic reactions, occasional anaphylaxis and even, fatalities. Risk factors for systemic reactions include extremely high sensitivity, coseasonal allergen exposure, history of previous systemic reactions and most importantly, the presence of uncontrolled bronchial asthma.[1,2]

Immunotherapy must be performed only under the supervision of a qualified physician/specialist with a trained staff and adequate available facilities[1] with an appropriate observation area, facilities for vaccine storage at 4°C and access to the resuscitation facilities.[1,2] Immunotherapy protocols, in general, involve an updosing (induction) phase with weekly injections for 8–16 weeks, followed by a monthly maintenance injection (empirically this interval has been extended in some centers to 6–8 weeks). The maintenance phase should last 3–5 years. At each immunotherapy visit, it is recommended to record the date, dose and volume of allergen vaccine given. Adrenaline should always be available immediately. The patient should be observed for at least 30 minutes following injections.

Injections should be postponed in the presence of a respiratory infection, intercurrent illness, current asthma or symptoms due to concomitant allergen exposure. Dosage reduction, according to standard guidelines, should be performed in relation to previous systemic or large local reactions, during increased allergen exposure, and if there is an extended time interval since the previous injections. In a randomized DBPC study with grass and birch vaccines, systemic mild reactions with SCIT occurred in 3.3% of injections with grass and in 0.7% of injections with birch,[27] but no specific predictor could be identified. A postmarketing surveillance study reported a rate of mild-to-moderate level systemic reactions of 0.9% of the total doses given in 3.7% of patients.[28] Another survey on grass pollen SCIT reports an occurrence of systemic reactions in 2% of patients,[29] with no life-threatening side effects. In a survey of more than 500 subjects, an occurrence of severe reactions was reported in 5.2% of patients and 0.1% of doses.[30] A retrospective study[31] in 65 patients receiving multiple vaccines and rush immunotherapy reported a 38% rate of systemic reactions with one severe episode. An e-mail survey involving more than 17,000 physicians reports a high rate of errors in administration (wrong patient or wrong dose),[32] which confirms the importance of careful administration of SCIT as recommended by international guidelines.[1,2,33] In general, according to USA surveys, fatality occurs in less than 1 case per 2,000,000 injections.[1]

Management of Adverse Events

Local swelling following injections is common and no treatment is required other than reassurance, occasional use of an antihistamine may be indicated. According to recommended guidelines, systemic reactions should be recognized and treated promptly. A grading system for systemic adverse reactions has been recently developed by World Allergy Organization (WAO), American Academy of Allergy, Asthma and Immunology (AAAAI) and American College of Allergy, Asthma and Immunology (ACAAI).[34] In general, mild rhinitis or wheezing is treated by an antihistamine or bronchodilator, prolonging the observation period. More severe reactions, including moderate asthma, urticaria or angioedema require intravenous hydrocortisone and antihistamine. Adrenaline, 0.5 mg by intramuscular route, is indicated in rapidly evolving systemic reactions which do not respond to these measures and in all patients where there is associated moderate/severe respiratory impairment or hypotension. In general, if in doubt, give adrenaline which is more effective when administered early during a systemic reaction. Delayed systemic reactions are almost always mild, involving mild urticaria or asthma and respond to antihistamines and/or inhaled bronchodilator therapy.

SUBLINGUAL ROUTE

Starting from the beginning of 1900s, SIT was administered only subcutaneously, although various mucosal routes of administration were anecdotally proposed. When serious concerns about the safety of immunotherapy were raised, clinical research with noninjection routes developed rapidly. Since its introduction in 1986, SLIT was regarded as a favorite alternative candidate to SCIT, especially due to its optimal safety profile.

After more than 20 years of clinical trials, postmarketing surveys and mechanistic studies, SLIT is nowadays considered a real step forward in the management of respiratory allergy. It currently represents the only realistic alternative to the traditional injection route **(Table 2)**.[35] The clinical efficacy (in term of symptom improvement) has been

Table 2 Main characteristics of SLIT

Mechanisms	It is an allergen-specific immunomodulatory treatment which affects the Th2/Th1 balance and induces regulatory cytokines.
Association with drugs	SLIT does not replace drugs but must be used in association.
	In the long term, it reduces the need for rescue medications.
Additional effects	Sustained efficacy after discontinuation, prevention of asthma onset.
Indications	Respiratory allergy (mite, grass, birch, olive, paritaria and cat)
Pharmaceutical forms	Available as drops, predosed dispensers, monodose vials and tablets.
Use	To be taken in the morning before breakfast. Keep under the tongue for 1–2 minutes, and then swallow. The first dose must be given under medical supervision.
Regimens	Updosing phase 10–30 days. Maintenance for 3–5 years daily or on alternate days as per manufacturer instructions. Can be used also without an updosing phase. Preseasonal (stop at the beginning of the pollen season); coseasonal (start at the beginning of the pollen season); precoseasonal (start before the pollen season and stop at the end).
Side effects	Itching/swelling of the oral mucosa or tongue. Usually self-limiting in few days. Nausea or abdominal pain is rarer. Systemic side effects are also rare. Only six cases of anaphylaxis described in 25 years.
Starting and Duration	At least 4 weeks before the pollen season. For mites can be started in every period of the year. Duration 3–5 years.

Abbreviations: SLIT, sublingual immunotherapy; Th, T helper cells

demonstrated for the most common allergens in more than 60 clinical trials,[36] confirmed in meta-analyses in adult and pediatric populations.[37,38] Although meta-analyses have serious limitations, essentially due to the great heterogeneity of the clinical trials, so far they are the only instrument available for attempting to achieve an overall evaluation of the results of numerous trials according to evidence-based principles. Some concerns about SLIT still remain including the extent or magnitude of the clinical efficacy and the optimal maintenance dose to be used.

Due to the large variability of the doses of allergen employed in many clinical trials[39] and various schedules of administration, SLIT is less rigidly formalized than SCIT. On the other hand, the recent large clinical trials conducted with grass tablets[40,41] have consistently shown the dose dependency of the clinical effects of SLIT. This fact strongly increases the proof of efficacy, according to the GRADE recommendations.[42] Of note, in both those clinical trials, the magnitude of the effect over placebo largely exceeded the 20% suggested threshold, required for defining immunotherapy as clinically effective.[43] Finally, taking into account the economic aspects, which are of relevance in the case of AR, SLIT has been formally shown capable of reducing both the direct and indirect costs of disease.[44-46]

It is also important to consider the effects of SLIT in a broader sense. The clinical data demonstrate the preventive effects of SLIT, in particular, in reducing the risk of inception of asthma in children with allergic rhinitis.[47,48] The most recent open controlled study[48] on this aspect, conducted in more than 200 children, receiving either SLIT or pharmacotherapy only for 3 years, showed a 40% reduction of the onset of persistent asthma in the SLIT-treated subjects, associated with a significant decrease of the onset of new sensitizations. Concerning the safety, the most common side effects are local (oral itching/swelling or nausea), but they are mild and self-resolving in few days. The satisfactory safety profile (only six cases of anaphylaxis in 20 years) has suggested the possibility of avoiding the induction phase. In fact, the more recent large trials used a no up dosing regimen. The good safety profile of SLIT in children, even below the age of 5 years, gives the window of opportunity to use this treatment, taking advantage of the preventative effects.[49,50]

Despite the optimistic results of studies so far conducted, some important points need to be addressed, including the optimal dose for each allergen and the optimal duration of a SLIT course needed to achieve the maximum benefits and the longest duration of the effects. In this context, recent large trials have started to provide some valuable information, at least for grass allergens, suggesting that an 8-week preseasonal treatment achieves the best benefits.[51] The preliminary results of a 15-year follow-up study reported that the optimal duration of a SLIT course should be 4 years.[52]

Mechanisms of SCIT and SLIT

Subcutaneous Immunotherapy

Subcutaneous immunotherapy is associated with a transient increase in allergen-specific IgE followed by blunting of seasonal increases in IgE. These effects are accompanied by increases in allergen-specific IgG4 antibodies.[53-56] Studies confirm and extend these observations to include measurements of the biological effects of IgG. These include the IgG-dependent ability of postimmunotherapy serum to inhibit allergen-IgE complexes to B cells, the blocking of subsequent IgE-facilitated allergen presentation and activation of allergen-specific T lymphocytes and prevention of allergen-IgE dependent activation of peripheral basophils.[57-59] SCIT is accompanied by inhibition of the recruitment and/or activation of effector cells including mast cells and eosinophils. Studies before and after SCIT confirm the reduction of the numbers of nasal mucosal eosinophils, basophils and mast cells during the pollen season,[60-64] a reduction in mucosal expression of the vascular adhesion molecule (VAM) and decrease in IL-4 and IL-13.[65]

There is blunting of allergen-driven Th2 responses with reductions in IL-4, IL-13, IL-5 and IL-9[64,66-71] and an immune deviation to Th1 responses with overproduction of IFN-γ and/or the emergence of a population of regulatory T-lymphocytes which produce the inhibitory cytokines IL-10 and/or TGF-β.[53-57,72] It is hypothesized that these regulatory T-cells act directly to suppress allergen-specific Th2 responses. Alternatively IL-10 is a known switch factor for IgG4 production,[73] whereas TGF-β favors IgA.[56]

Sublingual Immunotherapy

Sublingual immunotherapy is associated with qualitatively similar events to SCIT including modest increase in IgG, a transient increase in IgE and suppression of eosinophil recruitment and activation in target organs.[74-78] On the contrary, other studies failed to demonstrate changes in systemic T-cell and cytokine response[79,80] or local changes in T-cells or effector cells within the sublingual mucosa. Some studies report an increase in IL-10 production[81,82] and another shows suppression of allergen-specific T cell responses after 12 months of grass therapy.[83,84] A recent study shows *in vitro* that SLIT reduces the expression of IL-5 and enhances the expression of IL-10 in peripheral blood mononuclear cell (PBMC) stimulated with the allergen.[85] Further studies are needed to determine whether the same or alternative mechanisms are important for the effects of SLIT.

The oral mucosa is a natural site of immune tolerance [Langerhans cells, FcR1, IL-10, IDO (indoleamine 2,3-dioxygenase)]. Therefore, SLIT in optimal doses is effective and may induce remission after discontinuation and prevent new sensitizations, features consistent with induction of tolerance. SLIT induces modest systemic changes consistent with SCIT and is associated with early increases in antigen-specific IgE, and blunting of seasonal IgE, persistent increases in antigen-specific IgG4 and IgE blocking activity that parallel long-term clinical benefits of SLIT, inhibition of eosinophils, reduction of adhesion molecules in target organ and an early increase in peripheral $CD25^+$,$FOXP^+$ phenotypic T regulatory cells and delayed (6–12 months) immune deviation in favor of Th1 responses.

Molecular diagnosis of IgE sensitivities will aid patient selection for immunotherapy. Serum IgG-associated functional blocking activity and basophil activation tests merit further study.[86]

SAFETY OF SUBLINGUAL IMMUNOTHERAPY

- Sublingual immunotherapy appears to be better tolerated than SCIT
- Sublingual immunotherapy should only be prescribed by physicians with appropriate allergy training and expertise
- Specific instructions should be provided to patients regarding the management of adverse reactions, unplanned interruptions in treatment and situations when SLIT should be withheld
- The majority of SLIT adverse events are local reactions (e.g. oromucosal pruritus) that occur during the beginning of treatment and resolve within a few days or weeks without any medical intervention (e.g. dose adjustment, medication)
- A few cases of SLIT-related anaphylaxis but no fatalities have been reported
- Risk factors for the occurrence of SLIT severe adverse events have not yet been established. There is some suggestion that there may be increased risk in patients who have had prior SCIT systemic reactions
- There is a need for a generally accepted system of reporting AIT adverse reactions that is applicable to both clinical practice and research. A uniform classification system for grading for AIT systemic reactions has been developed
- A classification system for grading SLIT local reactions has been also developed consistent use of the systemic reaction and SLIT local reaction grading systems is recommended.

Impact of Sublingual Immunotherapy on the Natural History of Respiratory Allergy

Allergen specific immunotherapy may alter the natural history of respiratory allergy by preventing the onset of new skin sensitizations and/or reducing the risk of asthma onset.

Three DBPC-RCT studies for grass pollen rhino-conjunctivitis confirm the persistence of clinical effects of sublingual immunotherapy for at least 1–2 years after treatment discontinuation.

There are two randomized open controlled studies suggesting that SLIT reduces the risk of asthma onset in children with rhinitis.

Sublingual Immunotherapy in Children

Grass-pollen SLIT is effective in seasonal allergic rhinitis in children more than or equal to 5 years of age. Grass or house dust mite (HDM) SLIT can be used for allergic rhinitis in children with asthma. Pre-coseasonal SLIT with grass pollen in children might be as effective as continuous treatment. SLIT must not be suggested as monotherapy for treating asthma. There is not enough evidence to recommend *Alternaria* SLIT in children.

FUTURE DEVELOPMENTS OF IMMUNOTHERAPY

The more and more detailed immunological knowledge and the concerns on the possible side effects of SCIT have prompted the development of new routes of administration and of modified vaccines. There is preliminary evidence that both intralymphatic and epicutaneous delivery of vaccines is effective and could represent an additional therapeutic option.[87,88] The introduction of recombinant allergens undoubtedly would allow a better standardization of allergen extracts, envisages the possibility of a tailored treatment according to individual sensitizations. At present, the few published trials of recombinant allergens for immunotherapy suggest that their clinical efficacy is not superior to that of traditional extracts.[89,90]

Another possible approach is the use of adjuvants to enhance TH1 lymphocyte responses. Alum is the traditional adjuvant widely used in Europe. Alum has the effect of delaying absorption and in contrast to murine studies, downregulates Th2 responses in humans, shown in both *in vitro* and *in vivo* studies. Bacterial adjuvants include lipopolysaccharide and deoxyribonucleic acid (DNA) oligonucleotides. Monophosphoryl lipid A (MPLA), derived from the bacterial wall of *Salmonella*, is widely used as an adjuvant in prophylactic vaccines for infectious diseases and induces preferential Th1 responses. An immunotherapy product with MPLA adjuvant was proven to be effective and is currently commercialized in Europe.[91] Bacterial DNA oligonucleotides containing an abundance of CPG motifs were shown to promote Th1 responses and also induce IL-10, possibly by inducing T-regulatory cells.[19] Preliminary data in humans from controlled trials support the use of these adjuvants in allergen extracts for treating respiratory allergy, but further studies are required, especially to rule out possible side effects.

The use of allergen-derived peptides for immunotherapy has the potential to stimulate protective Th1 and/or T-regulatory responses whilst avoiding systemic side effects associated with crosslinking of IgE on mast cells and basophils, which are the risk associated with conventional whole allergen extracts. Initial studies for cat allergy are encouraging, although, further studies are required.

IMMUNOMODULATORS AND BIOLOGICS

Immunomodulators with broad upstream actions might have therapeutic utility, but higher risks for adverse events limit their clinical application. Most recent therapeutic developments include agents like anti-IgE monoclonal antibody (mAb), omalizumab in patients with severe asthma, and several others are at various stages of clinical trials. Anti-IgE has been shown to improve forced expired volume in one second (FEV_1), downregulates inflammatory markers, reduces the symptoms and severe exacerbations as well as the emergency room visits. Among these new approaches are anti-IL-5 mAb, anti-IL-13 mAb, anti-IL-4 Rα antagonist, toll-like receptor agonists, and transcription factor modulators targeting SYK kinase, peroxisome proliferator-activated receptor gamma, and nuclear factor kappa B (NF-KB).[92-94] One has to also look at their efficacy, safety, cost efficacy as well as their utility in multiorgan diseases like asthma, rhinitis, eczema and urticaria and their disease modifying effects, especially in the long-term.

CONCLUSION

Immunotherapy is an effective treatment for respiratory allergy. Since the 2001 allergic rhinitis and its Impact on asthma (ARIA) document, new studies have enhanced the knowledge about this form of therapy. Subcutaneous immunotherapy (SCIT) acts by either inducing immune deviation of T-lymphocyte responses in favor of Th1 responses to allergens and/or by the downregulation of Th2 responses probably via regulatory T cells. IgG antibodies are also involved and have functional significance. The clinical efficacy of SCIT in allergic rhinitis and allergic asthma has been confirmed for most of the relevant allergens (grasses, trees, weeds, cats and mites).

Subcutaneous immunotherapy is safe, provided that recommendations to minimize/manage adverse reactions are followed. Several studies show the long-term efficacy of SCIT and the preventive effect on the onset of sensitization to additional allergens as assessed by skin testing. SCIT in children with pollen-sensitive rhinitis may reduce the risk of progression from allergic rhinitis to asthma.

Sublingual immunotherapy (SLIT) is effective in allergic rhinitis in adults and children.[83] One meta-analysis confirmed the efficacy also in asthma. Current data indicate that SLIT is safe and the rate of adverse reactions is not greater in children below 5 years of age. Further, SLIT studies are needed to identify the optimal maintenance dose for all the relevant allergens and to elucidate the mechanism of action. Novel approaches for various other forms of allergen immunotherapy currently under evaluation include the use of adjuvants, peptides, recombinant/engineered allergens and DNA-conjugated allergens. A plethora of immunomodulators are currently at different stages of clinical development for the therapy of asthma and allergic diseases. Agents that are very specific for a particular molecule might not be effective in all patients because of the redundancy in the immune system and the heterogeneity of the diseases.

REFERENCES

1. Bousquet J, Lockey R, Malling HJ, Alvarez-Cuesta E, Canonica GW, Chapman MD, et al. Allergen immunotherapy: therapeutic vaccines for allergic diseases. World Health Organization. American Academy of Allergy, Asthma and Immunology. Ann Allergy Asthma Immunol. 1998;81(5):401-5.
2. Bousquet J, Van Cauwenberge P, Khaltaev N, Aria Workshop Group, World Health Organization. Allergic rhinitis and its impact on asthma. J Allergy Clin Immunol. 2001;108(5 Suppl):S147-334.
3. Pajno GB, Barberio G, De Luca F, Morabito L, Parmiani S. Prevention of new sensitizations in asthmatic children monosensitized to house dust mite by specific immunotherapy. A six-year follow-up study. Clin Exp Allergy. 2001;31(9):1392-7.
4. Purello-D'Ambrosio F, Gangemi S, Merendino RA, Isola S, Puccinelli P, Parmiani S, et al. Prevention of new sensitizations in monosensitized subjects submitted to specific immunotherapy or not: a retrospective study. Clin Exp Allergy. 2001;31(8):1295-302.
5. Möller C, Dreborg S, Ferdousi HA, Halken S, Høst A, Jacobsen L, et al. Pollen immunotherapy reduces the development of asthma in children with seasonal rhinoconjunctivitis (the PAT-study). J Allergy Clin Immunol. 2002;109(2):251-6.
6. Wilson DR, Torres LI, Durham SR. Sublingual immunotherapy for allergic rhinitis. Cochrane Database Syst Rev. 2003;(2):CD002893.
7. Arvidsson MB, Lowhagen O, Rak S. Allergen specific immunotherapy attenuates early and late phase reactions in lower airways of birch pollen asthmatic patients: a double-blind placebo-controlled study. Allergy. 2004;59(1):74-80.
8. Winther L, Malling HJ, Moseholm L, Mosbech H. Allergen-specific immunotherapy in birch-and grass-pollen-allergic rhinitis. I. Efficacy estimated by a model reducing the bias of annual differences in pollen counts. Allergy. 2000;55(9):818-26.
9. Leynadier F, Banoun L, Dollois B, Terrier P, Epstein M, Guinnepain MT, et al. Immunotherapy with a calcium phosphate-adsorbed five-grass-pollen extract in seasonal rhinoconjunctivitis: a double-blind, placebo-controlled study. Clin Exp Allergy. 2001;31(7):988-96.
10. Corrigan CJ, Kettner J, Doemer C, Cromwell O, Narkus A, Study group. Efficacy and safety of preseasonal-specific immunotherapy with an aluminium-adsorbed six-grass pollen allergoid. Allergy. 2005;60(6):801-7.
11. Frew AJ, Powell RJ, Corrigan CJ, Durham SR: UK Immunotherapy Study Group. Efficacy and safety of specific immunotherapy with SQ allergen extract in treatment-resistant seasonal allergic rhinoconjunctivitis. J Allergy Clin Immunol. 2006;117(2):319-25.
12. Walker SM, Pajno G, Lima MT, Wilson DR, Durham SR. Grass pollen immunotherapy for seasonal rhinitis and asthma:

a randomized, controlled trial. J Allergy Clin Immunol. 2001;107(1):87-93.

13. Rak S, Heinrich C, Jacobsen L, Scheynius A, Venge P. A double-blinded, comparative study of the effects of short preseason specific immunotherapy and topical steroids in patients with allergic rhinoconjunctivitis and asthma. J Allergy Clin Immunol. 2001;108(6):921-8.
14. Bødtger U, Poulsen LK, Jacobi HH, Malling HJ. The safety and efficacy of subcutaneous birch pollen immunotherapy: a one-year, randomised, double-blind, placebo-controlled study. Allergy. 2002;57(4):297-305.
15. Polosa R, Li Gotti F, Mangano G, Paolino G, Mastruzzo C, Vancheri C, et al. Effect of immunotherapy on asthma progression, BHR and sputum eosinophils in allergic rhinitis. Allergy. 2004;59(11):1224-8.
16. Polosa R, Li Gotti F, Mangano G, Mastruzzo C, Pistorio MP, Crimi N. Monitoring of seasonal variability in bronchial hyper-responsiveness and sputum cell counts in non-asthmatic subjects with rhinitis and effect of specific immunotherapy. Clin Exp Allergy. 2003;33(7):873-81.
17. Grembiale RD, Camporota L, Naty S, Tranfa CM, Djukanovic R, Marsico SA. Effects of specific immunotherapy in allergic rhinitic individuals with bronchial hyperresponsiveness. Am J Respir Crit Care Med. 2000;162(6):2048-52.
18. Pifferi M, Baldini G, Marrazzini G, Baldini M, Ragazzo V, Pietrobelli A, et al. Benefits of immunotherapy with a standardized Dermatophagoides pteronyssinus extract in asthmatic children: a three-year prospective study. Allergy. 2002;57(9):785-90.
19. Pichler CE, Helbling A, Pichler WJ. Three years of specific immunotherapy with house-dust-mite extracts in patients with rhinitis and asthma: significant improvement of allergen-specific parameters and of nonspecific bronchial hyperreactivity. Allergy. 2001;56(4):301-6.
20. Varney VA, Tabbah K, Mavroleon G, Frew AJ. Usefulness of specific immunotherapy in patients with severe perennial allergic rhinitis induced by house dust mite: a double-blind, randomized, placebo-controlled trial. Clin Exp Allergy. 2003;33(8):1076-82.
21. Maestrelli P, Zanolla L, Pozzan M, Fabbri LM, Regione Veneto Study Group on the "Effect of immunotherapy in allergic asthma". Effect of specific immunotherapy added to pharmacologic treatment and allergen avoidance in asthmatic patients allergic to house dust mite. J Allergy Clin Immunol. 2004;113(4):643-9.
22. Alvarez-Cuesta E, Aragoneses-Gilsanz E, Martín-Garcia C, Berges-Gimeno P, Gonzalez-Mancebo E, Cuesta-Herranz J. Immunotherapy with depigmented glutaraldehyde-polymerized extracts: changes in quality of life. Clin Exp Allergy. 2005;35(5):572-8.
23. Ameal A, Vega-Chicote JM, Fernández S, Miranda A, Carmona MJ, Rondón MC, et al. Double-blind and placebo-controlled study to assess efficacy and safety of a modified allergen extract of Dermatophagoides pteronyssinus in allergic asthma. Allergy. 2005;60(9):1178-83.
24. Nanda A, O'connor M, Anand M, Dreskin SC, Zhang L, Hines B, et al. Dose dependence and time course of the immunologic response to administration of standardized cat allergen extract. J Allergy Clin Immunol. 2004;114(6):1339-44.
25. Abramson MJ, Puy RM, Weiner JM. Allergen immunotherapy for asthma. Cochrane Database Syst Rev. 2003;(4):CD 001186.
26. Durham SR, Walker SM, Varga EM, Jacobson MR, O'Brien F, Noble W, et al. Long-term clinical efficacy of grass-pollen immunotherapy. N Engl J Med. 1999;341(7):468-75.
27. Winther L, Malling HJ, Mosbech H. Allergen-specific immunotherapy in birch- and grass-pollen-allergic rhinitis. II. Side-effects. Allergy. 2000;55(9):827-35.
28. Moreno C, Cuesta-Herraz J, Fernandez-Tavora L, Alvarez-Cuesta E. Immunotherapy Committee, Sociedad Española de Alergología e Inmunología Clínica. Immunotherapy safety: a prospective multi-centric monitoring study of biologically standardized therapeutic vaccines for allergic diseases. Clin Exp Allergy. 2004;34(4):527-31.
29. Arifhodzic N, Behbehani N, Duwaisan AR, Al-Mosawi M, Khan M. Safety of subcutaneous specific immunotherapy with pollen allergen extracts for respiratory allergy. Int Arch Allergy Immunol. 2003;132(3):258-62.
30. Nettis E, Giordano D, Pannofino A, Ferrannini A, Tursi A. Safety of inhalant allergen immunotherapy with mass units-standardized extracts. Clin Exp Allergy. 2002;32(12):1745-9.
31. Harvey SM, Laurie S, Hilton K, Khan DA. Safety of rush immunotherapy to multiple aeroallergens in an adult population. Ann Allergy Asthma Immunol. 2004;92(4):414-9.
32. Aaronson DW, Gandhi TK. Incorrect allergy injections: allergists' experiences and recommendations for prevention. J Allergy Clin Immunol. 2004;113(6):1117-21.
33. Lockey RF, Nicoara-Kasti GL, Theodoropoulos DS, Bukantz SC. Systemic reactions and fatalities associated with allergen immunotherapy. Ann Allergy Asthma Immunol. 2001;87(1 Suppl 1):47-55.
34. Cox L, Larenas Linneman D, Lockey RF, Passalacqua G. Speaking the same language: The World Allergy Organization Subcutaneous Immunotherapy Systemic Reaction Grading System. J Allergy Clin Immunol. 2010;125(3):569-74.
35. Bousquet J, Kaltaev N, Cruz AA, Denburg J, Fokkens WJ, Togias A, et al. Allergic Rhinitis and its impact on asthma (ARIA) 2008 update (in collaboration with the World Health Organization, GA(2)LEN and Allergen). Allergy. 2008;63(Suppl 86):8-160.
36. Canonica GW, Bousquet J, Casale T, Lockey RF, Baena-Cagnani CE, Pawankar R, et al. Sub-lingual immunotherapy: World Allergy Organization Position Paper 2009. Allergy. 2009;64(Suppl 91):1-59.
37. Cox LS, Larenas Linnemann D, Nolte H, Weldon D, Finegold I, Nelson HS. Sublingual immunotherapy: a comprehensive review. J Allergy Clin Immunol. 2006;117(5):1021-35.
38. Penagos M, Compalati E, Tarantini F, Baena-Cagnani R, Huerta J, Passalacqua G, et al. Efficacy of sublingual immunotherapy in the treatment of allergic rhinitis in pediatric patients 3 to 18 years of age: a meta-analysis of randomized, placebo-controlled, double-blind trials. Ann Allergy Asthma Immunol. 2006;97(2):141-8.
39. Röder E, Berger MY, de Groot H, van Wijk RG. Immunotherapy in children and adolescents with allergic rhinoconjunctivitis: a systematic review. Pediatr Allergy Immunol. 2008;19(3):197-207.
40. Durham SR, Yang WH, Pedersen MR, Johansen N, Rak S. Sublingual immunotherapy with once-daily grass allergen tablets: a randomized controlled trial in seasonal allergic rhinoconjunctivitis. J Allergy Clin Immunol. 2006;117(4):802-9.
41. Didier A, Malling HJ, Worm M, Horak F, Jäger S, Montagut A, et al. Optimal dose, efficacy, and safety of once-daily sublingual immunotherapy with a 5-grass pollen tablet for seasonal allergic rhinitis. J Allergy Clin Immunol. 2007;120(6):1338-45.

42. Brozek JL, Baena-Cagnani C, Bonini S, Canonica GW, Rasi G, van Wijk RG, et al. Methodology for development of the allergic Rhinitis and its Impact on Asthma guideline 2008 update. Allergy. 2008;63(1):38-46.
43. Canonica GW, Baena-Cagnani CE, Bousquet J, Bousquet PJ, Lockey RF, Malling HJ, et al. Recommendations for standardization of clinical trials with allergen specific immunotherapy for respiratory allergy: a statement of a World Allergy Organization (WAO) taskforce. Allergy. 2007;62(3):317-24.
44. Berto P, Passalacqua G, Crimi N, Frati F, Ortolani C, Senna G, et al. Economic evaluation of sublingual immunotherapy vs symptomatic treatment in adults with pollen-induced respiratory allergy: the Sublingual Immunotherapy Pollen Allergy Italy (SPAI) study. Ann Allergy Asthma Immunol. 2006;97(5):615-21.
45. Bachert C, Vestenbaek U, Christensen J, Griffiths UK, Poulsen PB. Cost-effectiveness of grass allergen tablet (GRAZAX) for the prevention of seasonal grass pollen induced rhinoconjunctivitis: a Northern European perspective. Clin Exp Allergy. 2007;37(5):772-9.
46. Canonica GW, Poulsen PB, Vestenbaek U. Cost-effectiveness of GRAZAX for prevention of grass pollen induced rhinoconjunctivitis in Southern Europe. Respir Med. 2007;101(9):1885-94.
47. Novembre E, Galli E, Landi F, Caffarelli C, Pifferi M, De Marco E, et al. Coseasonal sublingual immunotherapy reduces the development of asthma in children with allergic rhinoconjunctivitis. J Allergy Clin Immunol. 2004;114(4):851-7.
48. Marogna M, Tomassetti D, Bernasconi A, Colombo F, Massolo A, Businco AD, et al. Preventive effects of sublingual immunotherapy in childhood: an open randomized controlled study. Ann Allergy Asthma Immunol. 2008;101(2):206-11.
49. Rienzo VD, Minelli M, Musarra A, Sambugaro R, Pecora S, Canonica WG, et al. Post-marketing survey on the safety of sublingual immunotherapy in children below the age of 5 years. Clin Exp Allergy. 2005;35(5):560-4.
50. Jacobsen L, Valovirta E. How strong is the evidence that immunotherapy in children prevents the progression of allergy and asthma? Curr Opin Allergy Clin Immunol. 2007;7(6):556-60.
51. Calderon MA, Birk AO, Andersen JS, Durham SR. Prolonged preseasonal treatment phase with Grazax sublingual immunotherapy increases clinical efficacy. Allergy. 2007;62(8):958-61.
52. Marogna M, Spadolini I, Massolo A, Canonica GW, Passalacqua G. Long-lasting effects of sublingual immunotherapy according to its duration: a 15-year prospective study. J Allergy Clin Immunol. 2010;126(5):969-75.
53. Nouri-Aria KT, Wachholz PA, Francis JN, Jacobson MR, Walker SM, Wilcock LK, et al. Grass pollen immunotherapy induces mucosal and peripheral IL-10 responses and blocking IgG activity. J Immunol. 2004;172(5):3252-9.
54. Francis JN, Till SJ, Durham SR. Induction of IL-10+CD4+CD25+ T cells by grass pollen immunotherapy. J Allergy Clin Immunol. 2003;111(6):1255-61.
55. Jeannin P, Lecoanet S, Delneste Y, Gauchat JF, Bonnefoy JY. IgE versus IgG4 production can be differentially regulated by IL-10. J Immunol. 1998;160(7):3555-61.
56. Zan H, Cerutti A, Dramitinos P, Schaffer A, Casali P. CD40 engagement triggers switching to IgA1 and IgA2 in human B cells through induction of endogenous TGF-beta: evidence for TGF-beta but not IL-10-dependent direct S mu->S alpha and sequential S mu->S gamma, S gamma->S alpha DNA recombination. J Immunol. 1998;161(10):5217-25.
57. García BE, Sanz ML, Gato JJ, Fernández J, Oehling A. IgG4 blocking effect on the release of antigen-specific histamine. J Investig Allergol Clin Immunol. 1993;3(1):26-33.
58. Van Neerven RJ, Wikborg T, Lund G, Jacobsen B, Brinch-Nielsen A, Arnved J, et al. Blocking antibodies induced by specific allergy vaccination prevent the activation of CD4+ T cells by inhibiting serum-IgE-facilitated allergen presentation. J Immunol. 1999;163(5):2944-52.
59. Wachholz PA, Soni NK, Till SJ, Durham SR. Inhibition of allergen-IgE binding to B cells by IgG antibodies after grass pollen immunotherapy. J Allergy Clin Immunol. 2003;112(5):915-22.
60. Durham SR, Varney VA, Gaga M, Jacobson MR, Varga EM, Frew AJ, et al. Grass pollen immunotherapy decreases the number of mast cells in the skin. Clin Exp Allergy. 1999;29(11):1490-6.
61. Wilson DR, Nouri-Aria KT, Walker SM, Pajno GB, O'Brien F, Jacobson MR, et al. Grass pollen immunotherapy: symptomatic improvement correlates with reductions in eosinophils and IL-5 mRNA expression in the nasal mucosa during the pollen season. J Allergy Clin Immunol. 2001;107(6):971-6.
62. Tulic MK, Fiset PO, Christodoulopoulos P, Vaillancourt P, Desrosiers M, Lavigne F, et al. Amb a 1-immunostimulatory oligodeoxynucleotide conjugate immunotherapy decreases the nasal inflammatory response. J Allergy Clin Immunol. 2004;113(2):235-41.
63. Arvidsson MB, Löwhagen O, Rak S. Allergen specific immunotherapy attenuates early and late phase reactions in lower airways of birch pollen asthmatic patients: a double blind placebo-controlled study. Allergy. 2004;59(1):74-80.
64. Nouri-Aria KT, Pilette C, Jacobson MR, Watanabe H, Durham SR. IL-9 and c-Kit+ mast cells in allergic rhinitis during seasonal allergen exposure: effect of immunotherapy. J Allergy Clin Immunol. 2005;116(1):73-9.
65. Watanabe H, Nouri-Aria KT, Wilson DR, Walker SM, Jacobson MR, Durham SR. Inhibition of nasal mucosal eosinophils after immunotherapy is associated with a decrease in interleukin-13 mRNA and vascular cell adhesion molecule-1 expression. Allergology International. 2004;53(3):255-64.
66. Varney VA, Hamid QA, Gaga M, Ying S, Jacobson M, Frew AJ, et al. Influence of grass pollen immunotherapy on cellular infiltration and cytokine mRNA expression during allergen-induced late-phase cutaneous responses. J Clin Invest. 1993;92(2):644-51.
67. Durham SR, Ying S, Varney VA, Jacobson MR, Sudderick RM, Mackay IS, et al. Grass pollen immunotherapy inhibits allergen-induced infiltration of CD4+ T lymphocytes and eosinophils in the nasal mucosa and increases the number of cells expressing messenger RNA for interferon-gamma. J Allergy Clin Immunol. 1996;97(6):1356-65.
68. Jutel M, Pichler WJ, Skrbic D, Urwyler A, Dahinden C, Müller UR. Bee venom immunotherapy results in decrease of IL-4 and IL-5 and increase of IFN-gamma secretion in specific allergen-stimulated T cell cultures. J Immunol. 1995;154(8):4187-94.
69. Ebner C, Siemann U, Bohle B, Willheim M, Wiedermann U, Schenk S, et al. Immunological changes during specific immunotherapy of grass pollen allergy: reduced lymphoproliferative responses to allergen and shift from TH2

to TH1 in T-cell clones specific for Phl p 1, a major grass pollen allergen. Clin Exp Allergy. 1997;27(9):1007-15.

70. Klimek L, Dormann D, Jarman ER, Cromwell O, Riechelmann H, Reske-Kunz AB. Short-term preseasonal birch pollen allergoid immunotherapy influences symptoms, specific nasal provocation and cytokine levels in nasal secretions, but not peripheral T-cell responses, in patients with allergic rhinitis. Clin Exp Allergy. 1999;29(10):1326-35.
71. Wachholz PA, Nouri-Aria KT, Wilson DR, Walker SM, Verhoef A, Till SJ, et al. Grass pollen immunotherapy for hayfever is associated with increases in local nasal but not peripheral Th1:Th2 cytokine ratios. Immunology. 2002;105(1):56-62.
72. Jutel M, Akdis M, Budak F, Aebischer-Casaulta C, Wrzyszcz M, Blaser K, et al. IL-10 and TGF-beta cooperate in the regulatory T cell response to mucosal allergens in normal immunity and specific immunotherapy. Eur J Immunol. 2003;33(5):1205-14.
73. Jeannin P, Lecoanet S, Delneste Y, Gauchat JF, Bonnefoy JY. IgE versus IgG4 production can be differentially regulated by IL-10. J Immunol. 1998;160(7):3555-61.
74. Lima MT, Wilson D, Pitkin L, Roberts A, Nouri-Aria K, Jacobson M, et al. Grass pollen sublingual immunotherapy for seasonal rhinoconjunctivitis: a randomized controlled trial. Clin Exp Allergy. 2002;32(4):507-14.
75. Bufe A, Ziegler-Kirbach E, Stoeckmann E, Heidemann P, Gehlhar K, Holland-Letz T, et al. Efficacy of sublingual swallow immunotherapy in children with severe grass pollen allergic symptoms: a double-blind placebo-controlled study. Allergy. 2004;59(5):498-504.
76. Enrique E, Pineda F, Malek T, Bartra J, Basagaña M, Tella R, et al. Sublingual immunotherapy for hazelnut food allergy: a randomized, double-blind, placebo-controlled study with a standardized hazelnut extract. J Allergy Clin Immunol. 2005;116(5):1073-9.
77. Bahceciler NN, Arikan C, Taylor A, Akdis M, Blaser K, Barlan IB, et al. Impact of sublingual immunotherapy on specific antibody levels in asthmatic children allergic to house dust mites. Int Arch Allergy Immunol. 2005;136(3):287-94.
78. Marcucci F, Sensi L, Di Cara G, Salvatori S, Bernini M, Pecora S, et al. Three-year follow-up of clinical and inflammation parameters in children monosensitized to mites undergoing sub-lingual immunotherapy. Pediatr Allergy Immunol. 2005;16(6):519-26.
79. Rolinck-Werninghaus C, Kopp M, Liebke C, Lange J, Wahn U, Niggemann B. Lack of detectable alterations in immune responses during sublingual immunotherapy in children with seasonal allergic rhinoconjunctivitis to grass pollen. Int Arch Allergy Immunol. 2005;136(2):134-41.
80. Dehlink E, Eiwegger T, Gerstmayr M, Kampl E, Bohle B, Chen KW, et al. Absence of systemic immunologic changes during dose build-up phase and early maintenance period in effective specific sublingual immunotherapy in children. Clin Exp Allergy. 2006;36(1):32-9.
81. Cosmi L, Santarlasci V, Angeli R, Liotta F, Maggi L, Frosali F, et al. Sublingual immunotherapy with Dermatophagoides monomeric allergoid down-regulates allergen-specific immunoglobulin E and increases both interferon-gamma- and interleukin-10-production. Clin Exp Allergy. 2006;36(3): 261-72.
82. Ciprandi G, Fenoglio D, Cirillo I, Vizzaccaro A, Ferrera A, Tosca MA, et al. Induction of interleukin 10 by sublingual immunotherapy for house dust mites: a preliminary report. Ann Allergy Asthma Immunol. 2005;95(1):38-44.
83. Fanta C, Bohle B, Hirt W, Siemann U, Horak F, Kraft D, et al. Systemic immunological changes induced by administration of grass pollen allergens via the oral mucosa during sublingual immunotherapy. Int Arch Allergy Immunol. 1999;120(3): 218-24.
84. Bohle B, Kinaciyan T, Gerstmayr M, Radakovics A, Jahn-Schmid B, Ebner C. Sublingual immunotherapy induces IL-10-producing T regulatory cells, allergen-specific T-cell tolerance, and immune deviation. J Allergy Clin Immunol. 2007;120(3):707-13.
85. Savolainen J, Jacobsen L, Valovirta E. Sublingual immunotherapy in children modulates allergen-induced in vitro expression of cytokine mRNA in PBMC. Allergy. 2006;61(10):1184-90.
86. Canonica GW, Cox L, Pawankar R, Baena-Cagnani CE, Blaiss M, Bonini S, et al. Sublingual immunotherapy: World Allergy Organization position paper 2013 update. World Allergy Organ J. 2014;7(1):6.
87. Senti G, Graf N, Haug S, Rüedi N, von Moos S, Sonderegger T, et al. Epicutaneous allergen administration as a novel method of allergen-specific immunotherapy. J Allergy Clin Immunol. 2009;124(5):997-1002.
88. Senti G, Prinz Vavricka BM, Erdmann I, Diaz MI, Markus R, McCormack SJ, et al. Intralymphatic allergen administration renders specific immunotherapy faster and safer: a randomized controlled trial. Proc Natl Acad Sci USA. 2008;105(46): 17908-12.
89. Pauli G, Larsen TH, Rak S, Horak F, Pastorello E, Valenta R, et al. Efficacy of recombinant birch pollen vaccine for the treatment of birch-allergic rhinoconjunctivitis. J Allergy Clin Immunol. 2008;122(5):951-60.
90. Jutel M, Jaeger L, Suck R, Meyer H, Fiebig H, Cromwell O. Allergen-specific immunotherapy with recombinant grass pollen allergens. J Allergy Clin Immunol. 2005;116(3):608-13.
91. Drachenberg KJ, Wheeler AW, Stuebner P, Horak F. A well-tolerated grass pollen-specific allergy vaccine containing a novel adjuvant, monophosphoryl lipid A, reduces allergic symptoms after only four preseasonal injections. Allergy. 2001;56(6):498-505.
92. Casale TB, Stokes JR. Immunomodulators for allergic respiratory disorders. J Allergy Clin Immunol. 2008;121(2): 288-96.
93. Holgate ST, Polosa R. Treatment strategies for allergy and asthma. Nat Rev Immunol. 2008;8(3):218-30.
94. Fanta CH. Asthma. N Engl J Med. 2009;360(10):1002-14.

Allergen Desensitization

Vikram Jaggi

INTRODUCTION

The three main modalities of treatment of allergic diseases are avoidance, pharmacotherapy and immunotherapy. Avoidance of common allergens is at best difficult and at worst impossible. It has been often said that "asthma is neither curable nor preventable".[1] Pharmacotherapy is highly effective and predictable in most patients, but only for as long as it is being taken. Immunotherapy fills the gaps left by avoidance and pharmacotherapy. It is the only treatment modality that has been shown to alter the natural history of asthma. It is often effective for years after stopping treatment. This has also been shown to prevent the development of asthma in patients with allergic rhinitis and to prevent the development of new sensitizations in patients with asthma. However, it is neither highly effective nor predictably effective in all patients.

DEFINITION

Allergen immunotherapy is the repeated administration of specific allergens to patients with immunoglobulin E (IgE)-mediated conditions, to protect against the allergic symptoms and inflammatory reactions associated with natural exposure to these allergens.[2] Other terms used for allergen immunotherapy include desensitization (which is almost never achieved), hyposensitization (which lacks specificity) and the lay terms "allergy shots" or "allergy injections". The currently preferred term is allergen immunotherapy. From a humble beginning in 1911, when crude pollen extracts were employed to treat seasonal allergic rhinitis (or hay fever),[3,4] it has come a long way and is now recognized as a scientific method to both treat the patients with allergy and to prevent the progression of "allergic-march". Allergen immunotherapy today would merit consideration in allergic rhinitis (both seasonal and perennial), allergic asthma, insect sting allergy (hymenoptera hypersensitivity) and in certain drug allergies.

To paraphrase William Osler, the father of American Medicine, allergen immunotherapy is "an art based on science". The last decade has seen a vast accumulation of scientific evidence to support its use.

HISTORICAL BACKGROUND

There are accounts of "Vish-Kanyas" (poisonous girls) in the ancient Indian scripts, the courtesan girls were given minute, but increasing doses of poison to render them immune to the lethal effects of the poison. Native American Indians were known to chew poison ivy to prevent severe skin rash or anaphylaxis. These were practices based on observations; there was no scientific understanding or proof of how or why it worked. It was during 1910 and 1920 that immunotherapy found its roots in clinical practice. It was used first in allergic rhinitis and later in allergic asthma. It was thought at that time that subanaphylactic doses lead to "using up" or "exhausting" the antibodies responsible for causing allergy; IgE was unknown at that time. IgE, discovered in 1965–1966, was later characterized and its role in type I hypersensitivity elucidated.

In the last 15 years, there has been a vast accumulation of scientific evidence on the mechanisms and efficacy of allergen immunotherapy. The publication of the World Health Organization (WHO) position paper on allergen immunotherapy[5] in 1998 reaffirmed scientific faith in this time-tested treatment modality. Later, the preventing allergy treatment (PAT) study[6] showed that allergen immunotherapy could prevent the development of asthma in patients with allergic rhinitis. PAT was an important prospective, long-term (10 years) study in children with allergic rhinitis: 205 allergic rhinitis patients in five European countries were given 3 years of subcutaneous immunotherapy and followed for a further period of 7 years; 45% of children with allergic rhinitis not treated with immunotherapy developed asthma. The risk of developing asthma decreased by approximately 50% in the group of vaccinated children. This confirmed a long-held scientific belief that allergy vaccination early in the disease development could reduce the risk of the development of asthma in children suffering from allergic rhinitis.

MECHANISMS OF ALLERGEN IMMUNOTHERAPY

Asthma is a complex disease in which many cells and cellular elements play a role. Allergen-specific immunotherapy, which for the present is the only etiology-based disease modifying treatment induces rapid desensitization and long-term allergic-specific immune tolerance.[7] The immune responses in asthma are skewed towards the abnormal Th2 type responses and away from the normal Th1 type of response. Immunotherapy is shown to lead to the complex series of changes in the cellular, cytokine and chemokine profile to steer the immune system away from the Th2 response towards a Th1 type of response.[8] The following changes in cells and mediators have been noted with successful immunotherapy.

Allergen-specific IgE: In patients who receive allergen immunotherapy, initially there is an increase in specific IgE antibody levels followed by a gradual and sustained reduction in IgE levels.[9] Immunotherapy also blunts the seasonal increase in specific IgE levels that normally occurs due to seasonal exposure to the aeroallergens.[10] Consequent to the reduction in serum IgE levels, histamine release from the basophils and the mast cells is reduced.[11]

Acute and late phase reactants: Allergen immunotherapy is shown to block both immediate- and late-phase allergic response.[12] It reduces the recruitment of mast cells, basophils and eosinophils in the skin, nose, eye and bronchial mucosa after provocation and after natural exposure to allergens.[13]

Blocking antibodies: In successful immunotherapy, there is an increase in allergen specific IgA and IgG levels (particularly the IgG4 isotype). Allergen specific IgG induced by immunotherapy has been shown to "block" IgE-dependent histamine release and subsequent IgE-mediated antigen presentation to T cells.[14] However, there is a poor correlation between the rise in specific IgG levels and clinical improvement.[15]

Interleukins: There is an increased production of IL-12, a strong inducer of TH1 response.[16]

IL-10 is also increased. IL-10 reduces beta cell antigen specific IgE and increases the IgG4 levels, reduces proinflammatory cytokine release from mast cells, eosinophils and T-cells.[17]

Although the changes mentioned above are clinically measurable, the correlation between these changes and clinical response is not consistent or strong. At present, these changes cannot be used to clinically monitor immunotherapy or its efficacy.[15]

Indications

There are three main indications for allergen immunotherapy **(Table 1)**: (1) allergic rhinitis (both seasonal and perennial), (2) allergic asthma, and (3) hymenoptera allergy. Randomized, prospective, double-blind, placebo-controlled studies have shown the effectiveness of allergen immunotherapy in allergic rhinitis and allergic asthma.[18,19]

Table 1 Indications and contraindications of immunotherapy

• Usual indications – Allergic rhinitis – Allergic asthma – Sting allergy
• Usually not indicated – Food allergy – Chronic idiopathic urticaria – Angioedema atopic dermatitis
• Caution required – Severe coronary artery disease – Unstable angina – Cancer unstable asthma – Uncooperative patients – Use of beta-blockers

Allergen immunotherapy will merit consideration in any patient who has natural aeroallergen exposure with the symptoms of upper and/or lower respiratory allergy symptoms with demonstrable evidence of specific IgE antibodies to the clinically relevant allergen(s). Allergen immunotherapy is recommended for patients who are unable to avoid the allergens (pollens or house dust mites for instance), have an inadequate response to avoidance and pharmacotherapy, have unacceptable side-effects of medicines or who do not wish to take noncurative medication indefinitely. The ideal candidate for allergen immunotherapy is the patient with moderate-to-severe rhinitis and mild-to-moderate asthma induced by a few selected seasonal or perennial allergens. In allergic rhinitis, the more severe the allergic rhinitis, the stronger is the reason to consider allergen immunotherapy. In asthma, on the other hand, severity is generally a reason not to consider allergen immunotherapy. Allergen immunotherapy in asthmatics should not be initiated unless the patient's asthma is stable with pharmacotherapy. Patients with severe or uncontrolled asthma are at an increased risk for systemic reactions to immunotherapy.[20]

Selection of Allergens for Immunotherapy

A carefully taken history, knowledge of local and regional aerobiology and corroboration with a properly performed skin prick test (SPT) will guide the physician to select the relevant allergens to be included in the immunotherapy vaccine for a given patient. SPT information is to be interpreted judiciously with caution. The results are not to be taken at their face value. For most patients, it is possible to find out less than four or five important relevant allergens. If more than one pollen from the same family has tested positive, inclusion of only the representative, one of them would suffice. Cockroach and fungal antigens have the ability to cause proteolytic degradation of other allergens, particularly the pollens.[21,22]

BOX 1 Prescription requirements of a good, allergy vaccine

- The relevant and confirmed allergens (not more than five usually; the lesser the better)
- The starting dose (which is usually 0.1 mL of 1:5,000 dilution w/v)
- The projected therapeutic dose
- The frequency of injections (usually once or twice in a week initially in the build-up phase, then fortnightly or monthly in the maintenance phase).

BOX 2 Conditions which require a gradual doing schedule

- The SPT has caused significant reactions
- There is a history of anaphylaxis
- There is a history of allergic reaction to allergen immunotherapy
- More severe forms of asthma
- In the natural pollen season.

Abbreviation: SPT, skin prick test

Hence, these should not be mixed. House dust mite antigen does not seem to have a similar deleterious effect on pollens, hence can be mixed with pollens.[23] A good allergy vaccine prescription should include comprehensive information **(Box 1)**.

Schedule

The general principle is to start a dilute dose, which is gradually built up in concentration to the dose that is maximally tolerated or which gives adequate clinical response (build-up phase). This dose is then continued initially weekly, then fortnightly and finally on a monthly basis for the maintenance phase. Certain patients would require a departure from this usual dosing schedule in that a more dilute dose is used initially and the increase in dose is more gradual **(Box 2)**.

Place for Allergen Immunotherapy

The ideal venue for the allergen immunotherapy injections is the doctor's clinic. The doctor should be available at all times when the injections are being given. The staff giving injections should be suitably trained. A written informed consent of the patient should be obtained. The facility to store the vials at 4°C should exist. A standardized color code and marking system of vials of different concentrations with the name of the patient should be clearly printed on it.

Measurement of peak expiratory flow (PEF) should be done before the injection. A policy should be in place to either reduce or withhold the dose in case there is a significant (20–30%) fall in the PEF reading. Patient should be observed for 20–30 minutes after the injections. Resuscitation equipment, including adrenaline and oxygen should be available.

For the sake of convenience, the patient may take the injections from another physician near his home. This has been shown to be safe, provided all the prerequisites of safe immunotherapy mentioned above are met and are available there as well.[24] It is not advisable to take immunotherapy injections at the patient's residence.

Technique of Injections

The injections are given in the posterior portion of the upper one-third of the arm where the deltoid meets the triceps muscle. Here, the subcutaneous tissue is maximum. It is given subcutaneously (not intradermally or intramuscularly). The injections can be alternated between the two arms. After the injection, heavy exercise is to be avoided for 1 hour for this can lead to rapid absorption, which may precipitate a systemic allergic reaction.

Duration of Allergen Immunotherapy

Most patients, who show response to aeroallergen immunotherapy, demonstrate clinical improvement once the maintenance dose is reached in 6–9 month time. The response is maintained during immunotherapy. To prevent the relapse of symptoms on stopping allergen immunotherapy, it should be continued for 3 years in most patients.

After discontinuation, some patients experience sustained clinical remission while some relapse. At present, there are no reliable or specific tests to predict as to which patient will relapse and which will maintain long-term remission after discontinuing effective immunotherapy. In a prospective controlled study, designed to look for the immunotherapy relapse rate during the 3 years period after discontinuation of immunotherapy, 55% of 40 asthmatic patients who were treated with immunotherapy for 12–96 months, relapsed. The relapse rate was 62% in the group treated for less than 35 months as compared to 48% in the group treated for greater than 36 months.[25]

At the end of 3 years of effective immunotherapy, a decision has to be made whether allergen immunotherapy should be continued or stopped. The doctor and the patient should jointly decide keeping in mind the benefits and risks associated with continuing or discontinuing immunotherapy. Reasons to favor continuing immunotherapy are: a good response to allergen immunotherapy; a maintenance dose of monthly injections; asthma rather than allergic rhinitis; and no major inconvenience to the patient of a monthly injection. Most patients who have benefited prefer to continue monthly immunotherapy. Reasons favoring a trial to stop allergen immunotherapy to see if remission is maintained are allergic rhinitis rather than asthma; less than optimum response to immunotherapy and a major inconvenience of injections.

Efficacy

Many double-blind, placebo controlled, randomized clinical trials demonstrate a beneficial effect of allergen immunotherapy in the treatment of allergic rhinitis, allergic asthma and stinging insect hypersensitivity, it is effective in both children and adults.[18,19,26,27] The inconsistency in the assessment of "primary" and "secondary" outcomes of allergen, immunotherapy has affected the comparison of efficacy of different interventions.[28]

Allergic Rhinitis

The efficacy of allergen immunotherapy in allergic rhinitis has been clearly demonstrated in a large number of trials. These studies have shown significant improvements in symptoms, quality of life, medication use and in immunological parameters. Allergen immunotherapy is also shown to be beneficial for up to 3-6 years or more after completion of treatment. Allergen immunotherapy is shown to prevent the development of asthma in allergic rhinitis patients who receive immunotherapy.

Asthma

A Cochrane review of 75 trials with 3,188 patients revealed a significant reduction in symptoms and medication use and an improvement in bronchial hyper-reactivity after immunotherapy.[19] As per the current evidence, allergen immunotherapy can be used in asthma associated with rhinitis provided the asthma is stable with pharmacotherapy.[29] Allergen immunotherapy also prevents the development of new allergen sensitization in monosensitized patients.[30] It may also be effective in house-dust mite induced allergic rhinitis and asthma; rigorous clinical trials are, however, required.[31]

Bee Sting Allergy

Bee sting allergy is a "pure" reflection of a type I hypersensitivity reaction where allergy is demonstrated unequivocally to a single unambiguous allergen. Once the maintenance dose is achieved for venom immunotherapy, 80–98% of the individuals will be protected from a systemic reaction upon sting challenge. Allergen immunotherapy is generally given for 5 years for this indication. After discontinuation of allergen immunotherapy, the risk of a systemic reaction to sting is very low—about 10%.[26] The very high efficacy of allergen immunotherapy in bee sting allergy and its continued benefits even after stopping immunotherapy are good proof of the power of allergen immunotherapy per se, provided allergy is clearly demonstrated, a single allergen is incriminated and the vaccine is made using that single relevant allergen. This enhances confidence on the innate ability of allergen immunotherapy to be effective.

Side Effects and Risks

There can be local and systemic side effects. Local reactions at the injection site, such as itching, redness and swelling are quite common. The patients, in fact, welcome such reactions as an additional proof of allergy to that substance. They are generally less than 2–3 cm in diameter and subside on their own in a day. If troublesome, these can be managed by the local application of ice or with an oral antihistaminic. Such reactions generally do not require any reduction in the dose. Large reactions (>2.5 cm) that occur repeatedly or after a day, may predict a more serious systemic reaction; a dose reduction to the previously tolerated dose may be required.

Systemic reactions in the form of increased upper or lower respiratory allergy symptoms, urticaria/angioedema or hypotension can also occur rarely. A majority of such reactions occur within 30 minutes of the injection; hence the mandatory 30 minute waiting period in the clinic. Most of the reasons responsible for systemic reactions are predictable and avoidable **(Box 3)**.

Very rarely, a severe reaction may occur in spite of all due diligence, due to the inherent high degree of allergic sensitivity. The physician must be prepared and equipped to handle these reactions. Systemic reactions are managed in the usual way with adrenaline, injectable antihistamine and steroid administration. Volume replacement is also required.

Fatalities during allergen immunotherapy, although extremely rare, are reported. There is no reliable data from India. The fatality rate in the United States of America was one death per 2.5 million injections or an average of 3.4 deaths per year.[32] This has been constant on a per decade rate for the last 3 decades. More recently, the surveillance study between the years 2008 and 2012 has shown decline.[33] Near fatal reactions, hypotension or respiratory arrest or both, are 2.5 times more common than fatal reactions.

Special Considerations in Various Patient Groups

Children Under 5 Years of Age

There have been reports of the efficacy of allergen immunotherapy in children of less than 5 years of age.[34] In children with allergic rhinitis, allergen immunotherapy might prevent the development of asthma.[35] Yet, most allergists hesitate to prescribe allergen immunotherapy to small children or toddlers for the following, very valid, reasons:

Small children often outgrow their allergic symptoms on their own, as they grow older.

Older Children

Allergen immunotherapy in older children is effective and well tolerated. In general, the clinical indications are

BOX 3 Important reasons responsible for systemic reactions with immunotherapy

- Wrong dose or wrong injection
- Injection given at the height of the natural pollen season
- Uncontrolled asthma (FEV_1 < 70% of predicted)
- Patient on beta-blockers
- Patient having a natural exacerbation
- Injection from a new vial

similar for adults and children. Recently, studies in children receiving allergen immunotherapy have shown improvement **(Box 4)**. Most allergists agree that the response to allergen immunotherapy is better in children and young adults than in older adults.

Elderly Patients

Elderly patients generally respond less favorably to allergen immunotherapy. Further, presence of certain comorbid conditions like hypertension, coronary artery disease or cerebrovascular disease make them more prone to the risks of allergen immunotherapy. The fact that they may be taking beta-blockers may make resuscitation difficult if an allergic or anaphylactic reaction were to occur. However, elderly patients may also benefit therefore, age alone should not be the reason to deny allergen immunotherapy.[38]

Pregnancy

Allergen immunotherapy is effective in pregnancy. However, if an allergic or anaphylactic reaction occurs in pregnancy due to allergen immunotherapy, it could have serious consequences on the continuation of pregnancy. For these reasons, the general policy is:

- Allergen immunotherapy is not initiated in pregnancy
- If allergen immunotherapy is being given and is well-tolerated, it is not discontinued in pregnancy
- If maintenance dose has already been reached, it is continued at the same dose
- If maintenance dose has not been reached, dose escalation is generally not done during pregnancy.

Autoimmune Disorders

There are concerns regarding allergen immunotherapy aggravating autoimmune disorders by their uncertain effects on various parameters of immune modulation. These concerns are largely theoretical without any substantial evidence that such treatment is harmful in these diseases. Most allergists hesitate to prescribe allergen immunotherapy to patients with autoimmune diseases for the simple practical reason that the blame of even a spontaneous flare up, not uncommon in these diseases, would fall on immunotherapy if it happens during this period.

BOX 4 Improvement in children following immunotherapy

- Improvement in symptom control for asthma and allergic rhinitis[35]
- Increased PC_{20} to histamine[36]
- Decreased risk of development of asthma[35]
- Decreased development of new sensitizations[37]
  - The diagnosis of asthma sometimes cannot be made with confidence in a young wheezy child
  - Injections are traumatic to small children
  - Compliance with scheduled injections is not guaranteed in small children
  - Children may find it difficult to communicate the symptoms of impending allergic or anaphylactic reaction to allergen immunotherapy.

Sublingual Immunotherapy

The conventional route of immunotherapy has been through subcutaneous administration. Reports of an alternate (and a more convenient and safe) route, i.e. the sublingual route, appeared in the literature, mostly from Europe, after 1985. This came to be called sublingual immunotherapy (SLIT), as opposed to conventional subcutaneous immunotherapy (SCIT). It is now being approved in the United States after satisfactory results of trials with single allergen immunotherapy.[39]

Effectiveness of SLIT has been shown in both the children and adults for both allergic rhinitis and asthma. It is effective against pollens (particularly grass pollen), house dust mites and cat antigens. It generally takes longer (1–2 years) before there is improvement in symptoms.[40] There is good theoretical support for the sublingual route for immunotherapy. The dendritic cells in the oral mucosa are different from the dendritic cells of the skin in that the oral dendritic cells have an increased expression of certain major histocompatibility complexes and costimulatory molecules, which make these cells particularly adept at antigen presentation. This may play an important role in directing subsequent immune effects.[41]

Both SCIT and SLIT are effective though the SCIT has more often provided better clinical and immunological results.[42] SLIT appears to a have a favorable safety profile as compared to SCIT. Local symptoms like itching and burning in the lips, tongue and mouth are common. Mild gastrointestinal symptoms are also commonly seen. Rarely, aggravation of rhinitis, or even more rarely of asthma symptoms may occur. Anaphylaxis is reported, but is extremely rare. No deaths have been reported so far.

Sublingual immunotherapy is being widely used in Europe. There are a few questions, which remain to be answered before it is widely used: the optimum dose and dosage schedules for each allergen need to be clearly defined. Moreover, trials with mixtures of antigens are required and long-term efficacy compared to SCIT remains to be seen. With growing experience, this has the potential for greater use in allergic rhinitis and asthma. Its major advantages are the obviously ease of administration (by the patient at the home), no waiting period in the doctor's clinic, very low incidence of side effects and lower costs. There are many instances of poorly practiced immunotherapy, which need to improve **(Box 5)**.

FUTURE DIRECTIONS

Advances and improvements in allergen immunotherapy continue to occur. The sublingual route of allergen immunotherapy is promising, likely to be more widely

BOX 5 Poor practices in allergen immunotherapy

- Allergen immunotherapy being practiced by untrained or poorly trained physicians
- Immunotherapy being prescribed on the basis of serum specific IgE results without any correlation to clinical history
- Inclusion of too many antigens in the immunotherapy vaccine (many of them unnecessary or irrelevant)
- Inclusion of more than one pollen of the same family where only one representative allergen would suffice
- Use of nonstandardized allergens for allergy testing and vaccine preparation
- Allergens with ability to cause proteolytic degradation of other allergens (fungal spores and cockroach) being mixed with other allergens
- Maintenance dose that is too weak to give a full therapeutic response
- Immunotherapy, indiscriminately used in severe or chronic asthma with chronic airflow limitation where not much benefit is to be expected, but the risk of serious side effects is more
- Immunotherapy being used in conditions with no proven role: urticaria, angioedema, atopic dermatitis, or food allergy.

Abbreviation: IgE, immunoglobulin E

used.[43] Other methods of administration (epicutaneous, intranasal, intralymphatic and oral) are also being studied.[44] The existing practices of allergen immunotherapy need to be optimized. The extracts to be used require standardization, at present only a few extracts are standardized. Today, it is possible to identify and monitor the chemical and cellular changes that occur with immunotherapy. The challenge lies in transforming this information into a clinically effective method of monitoring immunotherapy. Several approaches to modify immunotherapy have been tested, such as the use of allergoids, alum precipitates and most recently of peptides.[44] Recombinant technology has provided a powerful technique both for sequencing proteins and producing allergens in commercial quantities. To reduce the risk of allergic reactions, recombinant protein can be modified so as to decrease the reactivity with IgE antibody while maintaining reactivity with "T" cells.

REFERENCES

1. Holgate S, Bisgaard H, Bjermer L, Haahtela T, Haughney J, Horne R, et al. The Brussels Declaration: the need for change in asthma management. Eur Respir J. 2008;32(6):1433-42.
2. Practice parameters for allergen immunotherapy. Joint Task Force on Practice Parameters, representing the American Academy of Allergy, Asthma and Immunology, and the Joint Council of Allergy, Asthma and Immunology. J Allergy Clin Immunol. 1996;98(6 Pt 1):1001-11.
3. Noon L. Prophylactic inoculation against hay fever. Lancet. 1911;1:1572-3.
4. Freeman J. Further observations of the treatment of hay fever by hypodermic inoculations of pollen vaccine. Historical document. Ann Allergy. 1960;18:427-34.
5. Bousquet J, Lockey R, Malling HJ, Alvarez-Cuesta E, Canonica GW, Chapman MD. Allergen immunotherapy: therapeutic vaccines for allergic diseases. World Health Organization. American Academy of Allergy, Asthma and Immunology. Ann Allergy Asthma Immunol. 1998;81(5):401-5.
6. Möller C, Dreborg S, Ferdousi HA, Halken S, Høst A, Jacobsen L, et al. Pollen immunotherapy reduces the development of asthma in children with seasonal rhinoconjunctivitis (the PAT-study). J Allergy Clin Immunol. 2002;109(2):251-6.
7. Jutel M. Allergen-specific immunotherapy in asthma. Curr Treat Options Allergy. 2014;1:213-19.
8. Bousquet J, Braquemond P, Feinberg J, Guerin B, Maasch H, Michel FB, et al. Specific IgE response before and after rush immunotherapy with a standardized allergen or allergoid in grass pollen allergy. Ann Allergy. 1986;56(6):456-9.
9. Gleich GJ, Zimmermann EM, Henderson LL, Unginger JW. Effect of immunotherapy on immunoglobulin E and immunoglobulin G antibodies to ragweed antigens: a six-year prospective study. J Allergy Clin Immunol. 1982;70(4):261-71.
10. Lichtenstein LM, Ishizaka K, Norman PS, Sobotka AK, Hill BM. IgE antibody measurement in ragweed hay fever. Relationship to clinical severity and results of immunotherapy. J Clin Invest. 1973;52(2):472-82.
11. Verney VA, Hamid QA, Gaga M, Ying S, Jacobson M, Frew AJ, et al. Influence of grass pollen immunotherapy on cellular infiltration and cytokine mRNA expression during allergen-induced late phase cutaneous responses. J Clin Invest. 1993;92(2):644-51.
12. Durham SR, Verney VA, Gaga M, Jacobson MR, Varga EM, Frew AJ, et al. Grass pollen immunotherapy decreases the number of mast cells in the skin. Clin Exp Allergy. 1999;29(11):1490-6.
13. Moingeon P, Batard T, Fadel R, Frati F, Sieber J, Van Overtvelt L. Immune mechanisms of allergen-specific sublingual immunotherapy. Allergy. 2006;61(2):151-65.
14. Wachholz PA, Soni NK, Till SJ, Durham SR. Inhibition of allergen-IgE binding to B cells by IgG antibodies after grass pollen immunotherapy. J Allergy Clin Immunol. 2003;112(5):915-22.
15. Ewan PW, Deighton J, Wilson AB, Lachmann PJ. Venom-specific IgG antibody in bee and wasp allergy; lack of correlation with protection from stings. Clin Exp Allergy. 1993;23(8):647-60.
16. Hamid QA, Schotman E, Jacobson MR, Walker SM, Durham SR. Increase in IL-12 messenger RNA+ cells accompany inhibition of allergen-induced late skin responses after successful grass pollen immunotherapy. J Allergy Clin Immunol. 1997;99(2):254-60.
17. Blaser K, Akdis CA. Interleukin-10, T regulatory cells and specific allergy treatment. Clin Exp Allergy. 2004;34(3):328-31.
18. Ross RN, Nelson HS, Finegold I. Effectiveness of specific immunotherapy in the treatment of allergic rhinitis: an analysis of randomized, prospective, single-or double-blind, placebo-controlled studies. Clin Ther. 2000;22(3):342-50.
19. Abramson MJ, Puy RM, Weiner JM. Allergen immunotherapy for asthma. Cochrane Database Syst Rev. 2003;(4):CD001186.
20. Lockey RF, Nicoara-Kasti GL, Theodoropoulos DS, Bukantz SC. Systemic reactions and fatalities associated with allergen immunotherapy. Ann Allergy Astma Immunol. 2001;87(1 Suppl 1):47-55.
21. Kosdash TR, Amend MJ, Williamson SL, Jones JK, Plunkett GA. Effect of mixing allergenic extracts containing Helminthosporium, D. farinae, and cockroach with perennial ryegrass. Ann Allergy. 1993;71(3):240-6.

22. Nelson HS, Iklé D, Buchmeier A. Studies of allergen extract stability: the effects of dilution and mixing. J Allergy Clin Immunol. 1996;98(2):382-8.
23. Esch RE. Role of proteases on the stability of allergenic extracts. Arb Paul Ehrlich Inst Bundesamt Sera Impfstoffe Frankf A M. 1992;(85):171-7.
24. Position statement on the administration of immunotherapy outside of the prescribing allergist facility. Drug and Anaphylaxis Committee of the American College of Allergy, Asthma and Immunology. Ann Allergy Asthma Immunol. 1998;81(2):101-2.
25. Des Roches A, Paradis L, Knani J, Hejjaoui A, Dhivert H, Chanez P, et al. Immunotherapy with a standardized Dermatophagoides pteronyssinus extract.V. Duration of the efficacy of immunotherapy after its cessation. Allergy. 1996;51(6):430-3.
26. Ross RN, Nelson HS, Finegold I. Effectiveness of specific immunotherapy in the treatment of hymenoptera venom hypersensitivity: a meta-analysis. Clin Ther. 2000;22(3):351-8.
27. Partnoy JM. Immunotherapy for allergic diseases. Clin Rev Allergy Immunol. 2001;21(2-3):241-59.
28. Makatsori M, Pfaar O, Calderon MA. Allergen immunotherapy: clinical outcomes assessment. J Allergy Clin Immunol Pract. 2014;2(2):123-9.
29. Passalacqua G. Specific immunotherapy in asthma: a comprehensive review. J Asthma. 2014;51(1):29-33.
30. Purello_D'Ambrosio F, Gangemi S, Merindino RA, Isola S, Puccinelli P, Parmiani S, et al. Prevention of new sensitizations in monosensitized subjects submitted to specific immunotherapy or not. A retrospective study. Clin Exp Allergy. 2001;31(8):1295-302.
31. Calderon MA, Casale TB, Nelson HS, Demoly P. An evidence-based analysis of house dust mite allergen immunotherapy: a call for more rigorous clinical studies. J Allergy Clin Immunol. 2013;132(6):1322-36.
32. Lockey RF, Nicoara-Kasti GL, Theodoropoulos DS, Bukantz SC. Systemic reactions and fatalities associated with allergen immunotherapy. Ann Allergy Asthma Immunol. 2001;87(1 Suppl 1):47-55.
33. Epstein TG, Liss GM, Murphy-Berendts K, Bernstein DI. AAAAI/ACAAI surveillance study of subcutaneous immunotherapy, years 2008-2012: an update on fatal and nonfatal systemic allergic reactions. J Allergy Clin Immunol Pract. 2014;2(2):161-7.
34. Cantani A, Arcese G, Lucenti P, Gagliesi D, Bartolucci M. A three-year prospective study of specific immunotherapy to inhalant allergens: evidence of safety and efficacy in 300 children with allergic asthma. J Investiq Allergol Clin Immunol. 1997;7(2):90-7.
35. Jacobsen L. Preventive aspects of immunotherapy: prevention for children at risk of developing asthma. Ann Allergy Asthma Immunol. 2001;87(1 Suppl 1):43-6.
36. Hedlin G, Wille S, Browwaldh L, Hildebrand H, Holmgren D, Lindfors A, et al. Immunotherapy in children with allergic asthma: effect on bronchial hyper-reactivity and pharmacotherapy. J Allergy Clin Immunol. 1999;103(4):609-14.
37. Pajno GB, Barbero G, De Luca F, Morabito L, Parmiani S. Prevention of new sensitizations in asthmatic children monosensitized to house dust mite by specific immunotherapy. A six-year follow-up study. Clin Exp Allergy. 2001;31(9):1392-7.
38. Asero R. Efficacy of injection immunotherapy with ragweed and birch pollen in elderly patients. Int Arch Allergy Immunol. 2004;135(4):332-5.
39. Nelson HS. Sublingual immunotherapy: the U.S. experience. Curr Opin Allergy Clin Immunol. 2013;13(6):663-8.
40. Wilson DR, Lima MT, Durham SR. Sublingual immunotherapy for allergic rhinitis: systematic review and meta-analysis. Allergy. 2005;60(1):4-12.
41. Ciprandi G, Fenoglio D, Cirillo I, Vizzaccaro A, Ferrera A, Tosca MA, et al. Induction of interleukin 10 by sublingual immunotherapy for house dust mites: a preliminary report. Ann Allergy Asthma Immunol. 2005;95(1):38-44.
42. Nelson HS. Subcutaneous immunotherapy versus sublingual immunotherapy: which is more effective? J Allergy Clin Immunol Pract. 2014;2(2):144-9.
43. Canonica GW, Bousquet J, Casale T, Lockey RF, Baena-Cagnani CE, Pawankar R, et al. Sub-lingual immunotherapy: World Allergy Organization Position Paper 2009. Allergy. 2009;64 Suppl 91:1-59.
44. Casale TB, Stokes JR. Immunotherapy: what lies beyond? J Allergy Clin Immunol. 2014;133(3):612-9.

Patient Education in Asthma

Bharat Bhushan Sharma, Virendra Singh

INTRODUCTION

With the availability of inhaled and modern means of therapy now, we have effective treatment options to reduce agony of asthmatic patients. In spite of effective therapy for diseases such as asthma, many patients still suffer due to ignorance, lack of understanding and faulty perception of the disease. Patient education is the only means, which can impart skills to enable a patient to use modern therapy and to remove wrong notions. Patient education is an integral part of the treatment in almost all respiratory diseases, but its efficacy in evidence-based medicine is proved mainly in asthma. Patient education is also important for risk factor reduction, especially for the quit-tobacco plan. It is an essential component of respiratory rehabilitation, for example, in patients with chronic obstructive pulmonary disease (COPD).

Recent guidelines have contributed significantly in the elucidation of this question in the terms of sound evidence base.[1,2] In patients with COPD, rehabilitation has been recognized as an established modality of treatment as it can increase functional capacity, lead to improvement in dyspnea and quality of life.[1] The role of rehabilitation in other respiratory disorders is gradually being scrutinized, however, further evidence is needed to have clear guidelines (see chapter on Rehabilitation for more details).

Patients must become effective partners in their own care, for the treatment of a chronic respiratory disorder to become successful. Patient education in asthma is well supported by evidence based documents almost similar to the effectiveness of respiratory rehabilitation in COPD patients.[3] Asthma is one disease which starts in childhood and continues throughout life with marked fluctuations in severity. When a patient is sick, even to take a breath becomes a mounting task. In contrast, during symptom-free period, a patient considers himself as fit as a normal person. Patients must make day-to-day or even moment-to-moment decisions, in response to such fluctuations, mainly regarding self-medication or to ask for medical help. Factors like patient motivation, literacy and socioeconomic setup markedly influence such decisions.

Education need of the asthmatic patient, which often remains neglected by health care providers, is no less important than that of patients with coronary artery disease or diabetes mellitus. Asthma education is commonly practiced in the western countries, but there are hardly any organized asthma education programs in India except for the availability of some expert documents and reports on efficacy of asthma education.[4-7]

GOALS OF ASTHMA EDUCATION PROGRAMS

The primary aim of asthma education is to keep the patient well and to impart ability to adjust the doses of the medicines according to an action plan. Reducing the costs is the primary aim for the health care services. The Global Initiative for Asthma (GINA) treatment has recommended the following issues for discussion with a patient:[3]

- Asthma is a continuous disease
- Patient's expectation from treatment
- Patient's fears and apprehensions about asthma.

To achieve these goals, specific information with a practical goal should be given to change behavior. Teaching over several days, covering many general topics may not be as useful as regular review of basic principles. Frequent verification of understanding and application of learned behavior are important.

BENEFITS OF ASTHMA EDUCATION PROGRAMS

One of the earliest published, randomized clinical trial of an education program for patients with asthma was a study in 1973 which included adult, inner-city residents. Members of the treatment group participated in a single, small-group session. This project had led to conclusions, which have now become the mainstay of planning and evaluation in patient education and health promotion.[8] The model recognizes three sets of variables that must be considered in determining the type of educational interventions:

1. *Predisposing factors:* The knowledge, attitudes, beliefs, and perceptions make up a baseline on which an action can take place.
2. *Enabling factors:* Skills and resources required to be able to enact a motivated behavior.
3. *Reinforcing factors:* Make the behavior more or less likely to be repeated or sustained over time. This has led to popular concept of precede-proceed framework.[9]

Some of more recent studies underline the importance of behavioral change over education alone.[10] However, the main drawback of systematic reviews in the asthma education is the variability between the study interventions and their insufficient documentation, which requires a more uniform and standard approach in these studies.[11,12]

The National Asthma Education and Prevention Program (NAEPP) guidelines gave an evidence grade of A to the recommendation for asthma self-management education.[13] Asthma education should be provided to every patient encounter by all providers and at all points of care (evidence grade B). The guidelines also recommend written action plans that include specific treatments and actions to respond to changes in symptoms, especially for patients with moderate-to-severe asthma (evidence grade B).[14,15]

Several adult asthma education programs have also reported better correlation between knowledge and outcome. A Cochrane review of 36 trials that compared usual care to self-management plus regular review and an action plan found more regular physician visits, fewer emergency department visits, slightly better lung function and peak flow measurements, need of fewer drugs and rescue medication in later group.[16] Studies that involved less intensive interaction and monitoring, had less effect, while written action plans had better outcomes.[17]

METHODS AND SETTINGS

Methods

No single teaching method or medium will work for all patients in all settings **(Table 1)**. Many factors will influence the selection of methods. Written material allows the patients to understand information at their ease, and is on hand for future reference. Interactive computer programs are somehow individualized in approach and many are available on the internet.[18] Videotapes are attractive for patients, but have the limitation of not being individualized. Utility of videotapes and other material ultimately depends upon individualized counseling, either in a one-on-one or group setting.

Table 1 Methods and benefits of asthma education[3,13]

Methods	*Improvements*
Small group sessions	Knowledge of asthma
Individual teaching	Feelings of control
Large group lectures	Positive attitudes
Problem-solving sessions	Physical activity
Booklets	Inhaler technique
Diaries	Use of peak flow meters
Computer games	Peak flow rates
Promotion of peak flow	Asthma severity
Monitoring use	Reduction of school absenteeism
Repeated audits	Health care costs
Checklists	Emergency room visits/ hospitalizations

Settings

There is evidence of positive asthma-education outcomes in multiple settings.[19] Settings that provide follow-up visits, education-reinforcement and continuing asthma monitoring are associated with better asthma control. The NAEPP guidelines recommend asthma education at all points of care, so that the patient has multiple chances to learn about asthma and build up self-management skills.[13] It is quite interesting that the clinic setting would allow the best opportunity for an ongoing collaborative relationship between the patient and the provider, and better outcomes (evidence grade A).

Asthma education in the school is important because of the potential for reaching a large number of children. Comprehensive school-based asthma programs can improve symptom control and reduce acute-care utilization.[20,21] Home-based education programs can significantly impact allergen control (evidence grade A).[13] Decreasing allergen exposure reduces exacerbations, and should be a component of asthma education when allergens are an important trigger.

ASTHMA EDUCATION PROGRAM COMPONENTS

The written action plan is the single most important strategy of asthma education. Patients who recognize asthma symptoms, understand peak flow measurements and how to respond appropriately are more likely to maintain asthma control. The NAEPP guidelines include example action plans.[13]

What should be the Content of Asthma Education?

Patient is educated to impart skills in following aspects of asthma:

- Diagnosis
- Inhaler medicines
- Difference between reliever and controller drugs
- Potential side effects of medicines
- Control of symptoms
- Early detection of exacerbation
- Monitoring control of asthma
- How and when to take medical assistance?

The two main components of asthma, i.e. inflammation and bronchoconstriction should be made clear to the patients. The differences between smooth muscle contraction and the inflammatory components should be explained with the use of figures. The patient must be able to distinguish between reliever (bronchodilators) and controller (anti-inflammatory) agents. They also should know that reliever act rapidly, but controller-steroids work more slowly. Importantly, patients must understand that the controller drugs will allow asthma control to be achieved and must be taken regularly instead of "on demand" basis.

The use of beta2-agonists before exercise, exposure to irritants and cold air, should be suggested. Inhaler technique should be demonstrated and checked regularly, as should the use of spacer devices or dry powder inhalers. The key to achieving asthma control is the patient's understanding of what are the criteria of control or of loss of control of asthma, and how to monitor severity according to symptoms and expiratory peak flow rates.[22] Peak expiratory flow (PEF) monitoring may be beneficial because of the learning and reinforcement value of self-monitoring and the greater sense of control and self-efficacy that comes with self-monitoring.[23]

After establishing the goals of therapy, corresponding symptom and peak flow end points, patients must know how to adjust medication and when to seek medical care according to the symptoms and PEF, using their action plans instead of relying solely on their physicians. Action plans have been developed and seem to reduce morbidity significantly, although it is difficult to dissociate their effects from treatment adjustments and other aspects of the education program.

Asthmatic patient should also receive general counseling about nutrition, sleeping habits and relaxation methods, and they must have an opportunity to ask questions of general relevance to asthma management.

How to Assess Adequacy of Teaching and Understanding?

Evaluation can be made immediately after the teaching session by a questionnaire incorporating key issues. The level of confidence of the patient does not necessarily mean level of understanding of asthma management. The level of the control of asthma achieved, health services use (emergency visits, hospitalizations), quality of life evaluation of the asthmatic, and the level of airflow obstruction are useful parameters to determine long-term benefits of asthma education.[24] Overall assessment may be repeated after a few weeks, and then at intervals of 3–6 months.

PATIENT EDUCATION: PROBLEMS

Among the barriers to effective asthma education, one must include the limited time available for teaching in the physician's office, the use by physicians of terms that the patient does not understand, the tendency of medical personnel to concentrate on acute treatment instead of long-term control, and until recently, the fact that treatment emphasized symptomatic relief and not prolonged control of airway inflammation. Patients often report that it is difficult to discuss their illness during a hurried medical consultation, they may be embarrassed to ask questions, and likely to forget or confuse multiple recommendations if they are not written **(Box 1)**.

BOX 1 The barriers to effective asthma education[6,13]

Physician related

- Limited time available for teaching patients
- Use of terms that the patient will not understand
- Tendency to concentrate on acute treatment instead of long-term control.

Patients related

- Difficult to discuss their illness—hurried consultation, embarrassed to ask questions
- Likely to forget or confuse multiple recommendations if they are not written
- Problems with acceptance and understanding of asthma
- Misunderstanding the fundamental principles
  - Inadequate perception of symptoms, leading to nonapplication or delay in the application of principles taught
  - Inadequate perception of signs, e.g. misinterpretation of changes in peak flow
- False expectations and a desire to be "cured"
- Abrupt cessation of the medication. The patient should be advised stepping down instead of stopping suddenly
- Preconceived assumptions, fears and concerns, e.g. fear of steroids.

Other problems relate to the acceptance and the understanding of asthma. As with other chronic diseases, there is often an initial denial of the problem; efforts should be made to help the asthmatic accept his condition, a prerequisite to effective control. False expectations are frequent. A desire to be cured may push patients to try different forms of treatment that offer a miraculous cure (e.g. popular Fish therapy of South India). The importance of regular treatment, even when asthma is apparently controlled, is often not understood, leading to gross undertreatment.[25] Preconceived assumptions, fears and concerns, e.g. fear of steroids, and inadequate counseling from misinformed sources may also interfere with teaching.

CONCLUSION

Effective respiratory rehabilitation incorporates exercise schedules and patient education comprehensively to encompass treatment and other aspects needed to make any individual patient recover gradually from the deterioration of the condition and to remain in a fully functional state as far as possible. Patient education is one of the major components of asthma treatment and prevention. A variety of teaching programs have been developed to improve self-management skills. An action plan that incorporates objective measurements like peak flow has been more successful in improving control and reducing morbidity than that based on the improvement of only knowledge. Such measures are aimed at specifically preventing needless delays in treating exacerbations and improving compliance with preventive measures.

REFERENCES

1. Nici L, Donner C, Wouters E, Zuwallack R, Ambrosino N, Bourbeau J, et al. American Thoracic Society/European Respiratory Society statement on pulmonary rehabilitation. Am J Respir Crit Care Med. 2006;173(12):1390-413.
2. Global initiative for chronic obstructive pulmonary disease. (2016). Global strategy for the diagnosis, management and prevention of chronic obstructive pulmonary disease. *www.goldcopd.org* [Accessed March 2016].
3. Global initiative for asthma. (2015). The global strategy for asthma management and prevention. *www.ginasthma.org* [Accessed March 2016].
4. Jindal SK, Gupta D, Aggarwal AN, Agarwal R; World Health Organization; Government of India. Guidelines for management of asthma at primary and secondary levels of health care in India (2005). Indian J Chest Dis Allied Sci. 2005;47(4):309-43.
5. Singh V, Khandelwal R, Bohra S, Gupta R, Gupta BS. Evaluation of communication skills of physicians about asthma. J Assoc Physicians India. 2002;50:1266-9.
6. Bedi RS. Patient education programme for asthmatics: Indian perspective. Indian J Chest Dis Allied Sci. 2007;49:93-7.
7. Ghosh CS, Ravindran P, Joshi M, Stearns SC. Reductions in hospital use from self management training for chronic asthmatics. Soc Sci Med. 1998;46(8):1087-93.
8. Boulet LP, Chapman KR, Green LW, FitzGerald JM. Asthma education. Chest. 1994;106(4 Suppl):184S-96S.
9. Green LW, Frankish CJ. Theories and principles of health education applied to asthma. Chest. 1994;106(4 Suppl):219S-30S.
10. Kolbe J, Vamos M, Fergusson W, Elkind G, Garrett J. Differential influences on asthma self-management knowledge and self-management behavior in acute severe asthma. Chest. 1996;100(6):1463-8.
11. Sudre P, Jacquemet S, Uldry C, Perneger TV. Objectives, methods and content of patient education programmes for adults with asthma: systematic review of studies published between 1979 and 1998. Thorax. 1999;54(8):681-7.
12. Fink JB. Identifying asthma patient education materials that support National Heart, Lung and Blood Institute guidelines. Chest. 1999;116(4 Suppl 1):195S-6S.
13. National Heart, Lung, and Blood, Institute National Asthma Education and Prevention Program. (2015). Needs assessment report for potential update of the expert panel report-3: Guidelines for the diagnosis and management of asthma. *www.nhlbi.nih.gov/sites/www.nhlbi.nih.gov/files/Asthma-Needs-Assessment-Report.pdf.* [Accessed March 2016].
14. Song WS, Mullon J, Regan NA, Roth BJ. Instruction of hospitalized patients by respiratory therapists on metered-dose inhaler use leads to decrease in patient errors. Respir Care. 2005;50(8):1040-5.
15. Armour C, Bosnic-Anticevich S, Brillant M, Burton D, Emmerton L, Krass I, et al. Pharmacy Asthma Care Program (PACP) improves outcomes for patients in the community. Thorax. 2007;62(6):496-502.
16. Gibson PG, Powell H. Written action plans for asthma: an evidence based review of the key components. Thorax. 2004;59(2):94-9.
17. Adams RJ, Appleton S, Wilson DH, Ruffin RE. Participatory decision making, asthma action plans, and use of asthma medication: a population survey. J Asthma. 2005;42(8):673-8.
18. Cabana MD, Le TT. Challenges in asthma patient education. J Allerg Clin Immunol. 2005;115(6):1225-7.
19. Jones MA. Asthma self-management patient education. Respir Care. 2008;53(6):778-84; discussion 784-6.
20. Butz A, Pham L, Lewis L, Lewis C, Hill K, Walker J, et al. Rural children with asthma: impact of a parent and child asthma education program. J Asthma. 2005;42(10):813-21.
21. Cicutto L, Murphy S, Coutts D, O'Rourke J, Lang G, Chapman C, et al. Breaking the access barrier: evaluating an asthma center's efforts to provide education to children with asthma in schools. Chest. 2005;128(4):1928-35.
22. Hargreave FE, Dolovich J, Newhouse MT. The assessment and treatment of asthma: a conference report. J Allergy Clin Immunol. 1990;85(6):1098-111.
23. Beasley R, Cushley M, Holgate ST. A self-management plan in the treatment of adult asthma. Thorax. 1989;44(3):200-4.
24. Wilson SR, Scamagas P, German DF, Hughes GW, Lulla S, Coss S, et al. A controlled trial of two forms of self-management education for adults with asthma. Am J Med. 1993;94(6):564-76.
25. Singh V, Sinha HV, Gupta R. Barriers in the management of asthma and attitudes towards complementary medicine. Resp Med. 2002;96(10):835-40.

Pharmacotherapy of Bronchial Asthma

Nusrat Shafiq, Samir Malhotra

Two groups of drugs—controllers and relievers—are used to manage asthma. In general, the controller drugs, primarily the anti-inflammatory agents, are used for maintenance therapy. Reliever drugs, i.e. bronchodilators are used for symptomatic relief from acute episodes. Most of the antiasthma drugs are preferred through inhalational route.

ANTI-INFLAMMATORY AGENTS

The major role of this class of drugs is for long-term control of asthma, these agents are not indicated when rapid bronchodilation is needed. Short-acting beta agonists (SABAs) are used for quick relief.

Corticosteroids

Corticosteroids are amongst the most universal anti-inflammatory agents thereby reducing airway inflammation and hyper-responsiveness. Therefore, they form the cornerstone of asthma management. Both inhalational and systemic routes of administration are used in the management of asthma. Inhalational therapy is highly suitable for maintenance therapy, it needs lower doses and delivers the drug directly to the site of action minimizing the systemic adverse effects associated with corticosteroids. A large number of steroids are available for inhalational therapy, their main differences are in pharmacokinetics, potency (budesonide > beclomethasone > flunisolide), dosing frequency and adverse effects, although most evidences suggest that they do not differ in the terms of efficacy **(Table 1)**. Systemic steroids are indicated when inhaled therapy does not work due to severe spasm during acute exacerbations, and also in chronic severe asthma. Dose should not be a deterrent, high dose must be used, usually needed only for 5–7 days. Prolonged use of systemic steroids requires to be tapered.

Mechanism of Action

Their major actions **(Flow chart 1)** include, but are not limited to:

- Suppression of inflammatory proteins (panel 1) caused by the inhibition of genes that encode these proteins. Key among these are inflammatory cytokines (interleukins, TNF-α), chemokines (IL-8, rantes, MIP-1 α, MCP-1, MCP-3, MCP-4, exotoxins), adhesion molecules (ICAM-1, VCAM-1, E-selectin), enzymes (nitric oxide synthetase and cyclooxygenase and cytoplasmic phospholipase A2) receptors (tachykinin NK-1 and NK-2, bradykinin B2) and peptides (endothelin-1)
- Inhibition of accumulation of mast cells, basophils, eosinophils, dendritic and other cells in the mucosa and submucosa of the lung tissue
- Reduced goblet cell hyperplasia
- Decreased epithelial cell injury
- Decreased vascularity and vascular permeability.

Flow chart 1 Transcription of genes during chronic inflammation

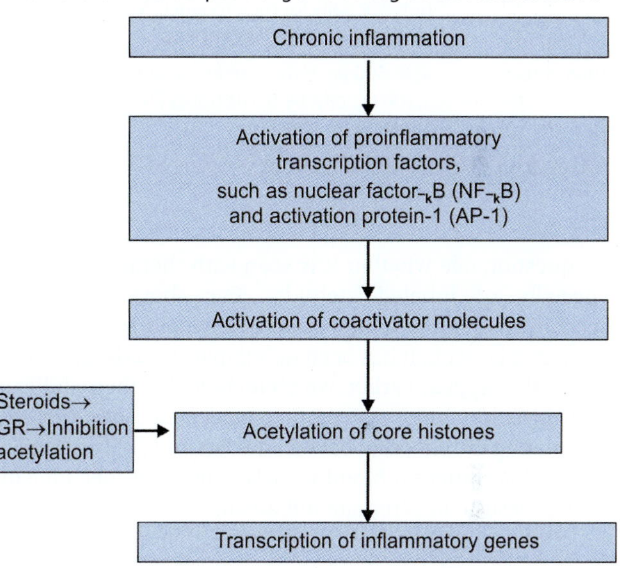

Abbreviation: GR, glucocorticoid receptor

Besides suppressing inflammatory genes, steroids also switch on anti-inflammatory genes like annexin-1 (lipocortin-1), secretory leukocyte protease inhibitor (SLPI), interleukin-10 (IL-10) and the inhibitor of NF-κB (IκB-α). Although, this effect occurs at high concentrations,

Table 1 Some commonly used inhaled corticosteroids

Steroids	*Doses*	*Remarks*
Beclomethasone	400 µg/day in two to four divided doses; Maximum initial dose may go up to 1 mg/day; Pediatric dose is 50–100 µg/day	Higher doses may be needed if asthma is severe or if usual dose is inadequate
Budesonide	400 µg/day in two divided doses. Maximum initial dose may go up to 2 mg/day. Pediatric dose is 50–400 µg/day	Metabolized by CYP3A4
Ciclesonide	160 µg/day once daily as starting dose, decreased to 80 µg once daily as maintenance dose	Not used in children
Flunisolide	1 mg/day into divided doses. Maximum dose 2 mg/day. Maximum pediatric dose 500 µg twice daily	Dose is lesser (160 µg twice daily) for CFC free inhaler, maximum dose 320 µg twice daily. Pediatric dose 80 µg twice (maximum 160 µg twice daily)
Fluticasone	200–500 µg/day in two divided doses; Maximum dose 2 mg/day for severe cases; Pediatric dose 100–200 µg/day, maximum dose 400 µg	Most commonly used doses are 0.5–1 mg twice daily
Mometasone	400 µg inhaled once daily initial dose followed by 200 µg once or twice daily for maintenance. Maximum dose 800 µg/day and pediatric dose 110 µg once daily	The drug should be given in the evening
Triamcinolone	450–600 µg in three to four divided doses up to a maximum of 1,200 µg/day. Pediatric doses 75 or 150 µg three to four times up to a maximum of 900 µg	Also available for oral and parenteral use

Abbreviation: CFC, chlorofluorocarbons

it is questionable whether it is seen with therapeutic doses, especially of inhaled steroids. The above mentioned mechanisms require a lag period of few days before steroid effects can be seen. It has been noted that steroids have other actions that appear earlier, which include: (A) their ability to resensitize adrenergic receptors to catecholamines, thereby, potentiating the effects of beta-2 agonists and (B) contraction of bronchial mucosal blood vessels. The exact mechanisms behind these actions remain unknown.

Pharmacokinetics

Corticosteroids are lipid soluble drugs, therefore, rapidly absorbed from the gastrointestinal tract (GIT), as well through inhalation and get widely distributed across the body tissues. They, especially the natural steroids, are the highly protein (globulin, albumin and transcortin) bound drugs. Their metabolism occurs mainly in the liver and they are excreted by the kidneys. Natural steroids are metabolized faster than the synthetic steroids, thus, have shorter half-lives, which coupled with their higher affinity for plasma proteins makes them less potent than the synthetic preparations. Many steroids have high first-pass metabolism leading to very low systemic bioavailability, for instance 10% for budesonide, 20% for fluticasone and just 1% for flunisolide.

Systemic steroids are needed for emergency management of asthma, but frequently misused for maintenance therapy. Prednisone is commonly used in asthma (30-60 mg/day) orally in the morning or methylprednisolone 4 mg/kg/day intravenously in four divided doses for severe cases. Hydrocortisone is cheaper than methylprednisolone, but also has mineralocorticoid activity. Once symptoms improve, the doses can be reduced. Some authorities recommend late afternoon administration, if nocturnal asthma is a major problem. A Cochrane review[1] of pooled data from six trials had shown that oral prednisolone (7.5-12 mg/day) was as effective as inhaled steroid (300-2,000 µg/day), but was associated with more adverse effects.

Dissociated Steroids

There are several problems of steroid therapy in asthma **(Table 2)**.

There have been attempts to discover novel steroids that lack the adverse effect potential of currently available steroids; such steroids are called dissociated steroids.[4] The concept of dissociated steroids was an attempt to dissociate side effects, which are presumably caused by deoxyribonucleic acid (DNA) binding and gene activation (transactivation or cis repression) from therapeutic anti-inflammatory effects, which are probably due to the inhibition of inflammatory gene expression by NF-κB and other proinflammatory transcription factors through a non-DNA binding mechanism (transrepression).[5,6] It is hoped that this novel class of "dissociated" steroids will have the property for transrepression with relatively little transactivation and, therefore, lesser incidence of adverse effects.

Adverse Effects of Steroids

Corticosteroids are life-saving drugs with an excellent risk benefit ratio in asthma. However, they have potential to cause a large number of adverse effects, some of which can

Table 2: Major drawbacks of steroid therapy for asthma

• Systemic adverse effects even with inhaled drugs
• Local adverse effects and dislike of inhaled steroids
• Poor patient adherence with inhaled steroids seen in 30–60% of patients[2]
• Lack of rapid symptom relief
• Complicated treatment regimens[3]
• Inability to properly use inhaler devices, especially in children and elderly

Table 3 Potential adverse effects associated with inhaled steroids[7]

Adverse effect	*Risk*
• Hypothalamic-pituitary-adrenal axis suppression	No significant risk until dosages of budesonide or beclomethasone increased to >1,500 µg/day in adults or >400 µg/day in children
• Bone resorption	Modest but significant effects at doses possibly as low as 500 µg/day
• Carbohydrate and lipid metabolism	Minor, clinically insignificant changes occur with dosages of beclomethasone >1,000 µg/day
• Cataracts	Anecdotal reports, risk unproven
• Skin thinning	Dosage-related effect with beclomethasone dipropionate over a range of 400–2,000 µg/day
• Purpura	Dosage-related increase in occurrence with beclomethasone over a range of 400–2,000 µg/day
• Dysphonia	Usually of little consequence; Decreased by mouth rinsing after every inhalation
• Candidiasis	Incidence <5%, reduced by use of spacer device and mouth rinsing after every inhalation
• Growth retardation	Difficult to separate effect of disease from effect of treatment, but no discernible effects on growth when all studies are considered and normal predicted height is seldom affected

be severe and others serious. The adverse effect potential of inhaled steroids is lesser, but may be significant **(Table 3)**. It is important to appreciate that while the dose-response curve of inhaled steroids plateaus at higher doses, the dose-systemic absorption curve is linear and continues to rise even at the high doses of inhaled steroids, with the result that even as the therapeutic effects plateau at a dose equivalent to 1,600 µg/day of beclomethasone, the probability of systemic adverse effects continues to rise with the rising doses.

Systemic corticosteroid therapy is known to cause a vast number of adverse effects **(Table 4)**, their incidence and severity are directly proportional to dose (<7.5 mg/day of prednisolone is usually considered physiological) and duration of treatment, but are not dependent on the type of steroid used. The long history of their use has shown that short-course treatment (<5–10 days) even at high doses does not cause much toxicity. On the other hand, long duration of treatment even at relatively low doses is likely to cause adverse effects. The most common adverse effects during a brief course as is used during asthma exacerbations are mood disturbances, increased appetite, impaired glucose control in diabetics and candidiasis.

Steroid Withdrawal

There are two main risks of abrupt steroid withdrawal—adrenocortical insufficiency and relapse of disease for which a steroid was being given. It is generally recommended to gradually taper the dose. The United Kingdom committee on safety of medicines (CSMs) recommends that moderate dosage with corticosteroids (up to 40 mg daily of prednisolone or equivalent), for up to 3 weeks, may be stopped without tapering provided that the original disease is unlikely to relapse, although prophylactic cover may be required for any stress within a week of finishing the course.[8] In practice, there is a large variation in how steroids are tapered from 1 mg monthly to more practical, 2.5 to 5 mg every two to 7 days. It must be kept in mind that although gradual withdrawal leads to the normalization of adrenal function, it is not sufficient for conditions associated with stress, such as infection, surgery or trauma, when patients must be given supplementary steroids. It is recommended to withdraw steroids and gradually even if patient had received a shorter course of therapy, if (A) higher doses were being given, (B) patient had risk factors for adrenocortical insufficiency, (C) patient had received repeated courses, and (D) patient was taking his or her doses in the evening.

Drug Interactions

Enzyme inducers like barbiturates, carbamazepine, phenytoin, primidone, or rifampicin increase their metabolism, leading to decrease in their effects. An increased risk of hypokalemia occurs with concomitant use of potassium-depleting diuretics, amphotericin B, xanthenes and beta-2 agonists. Concurrent administration with nonsteroidal anti-inflammatory drugs (NSAIDs) leads to increased incidence of gastrointestinal (GI) bleed and peptic ulcers. Reduced efficacy of antidiabetics and antihypertensives may need dose adjustment. There was a case report of severe peripheral edema caused by a synergistic effect of montelukast and prednisone on sodium and water retention in a patient, which did not recur when either drug was used alone.[9]

In asthma, inhaled steroids are the drugs of first choice for prophylaxis and maintenance treatment in patients whose symptoms need regular use of beta-2 agonists. Their regular

Table 4 Adverse effects associated with systemic steroids

Adverse effects	*Risk and prevention*
Hypothalamic-pituitary-adrenal axis suppression	The most feared complication of steroid therapy, usually occurs with supraphysiological doses used for >3 weeks and may last for a year or more. The incidence is less when a single morning dose is used, even lesser if used on alternate day
Bone/joints	Avascular necrosis of bone, may occur with short courses of high-dose treatment (even with inhaled) although relatively uncommon. Osteoporosis is almost universal, if steroids are used for sufficiently long duration, and is greatest in spine, hip, distal radius, pelvis and ribs. Intermittent therapy (alternate day, twice a week) does not appear to reduce the risk. All patients on steroids should be prescribed calcium and vitamin D, advised to exercise regularly and quit smoking and limit alcohol. There are case reports of rupture of tendons (achilles and patellar) as well
Carbohydrate, protein and lipid metabolism	Systemic steroids induce glucose intolerance although diabetic control may be worsened even with inhaled therapy (high doses). Steroids can also cause a catabolic state with protein loss. Besides hyperglycemia, steroids also lead to hypertension, hyperlipidemia and obesity all of which are established coronary risk factors. Along with this, steroids cause body fat redistribution leading to typical Cushingoid features with moon face and buffalo hump
Immunity	Steroids are potent immunosuppressant drugs, their use can lead to increased susceptibility to infection, aggravation of existing infection and activation of latent infection. This increased susceptibility to infection coupled with the masking of symptoms can lead to disseminated, often fatal infections (for instance, fungal) with unusual organisms at unusual sites
Neuropsychiatric	Mood disorders (depression, mania, euphoria), delirium; in children, psychosis, insomnia and hyperactivity. Memory loss has been reported with parenteral methylprednisolone, which is reversible
Eye	Cataract, rarely and retinal detachment
Gastrointestinal tract (GIT)	It is widely believed that steroids cause peptic ulcers although not all studies have shown increased risk. There also are reports of steroid-induced gastrointestinal perforation with the additional hazard of masking of symptoms due to their anti-inflammatory actions, which can cause delay in the diagnosis
Skin	Dermatological adverse effects include striae and skin thinning, acne ("steroid acne"), bruising and purpura
Hypersensitivity	Paradoxically, steroids have been associated with Stevens-Johnson syndrome, hypersensitivity and anaphylaxis
Growth in children	Systemic steroids can impair growth in children and may be used intermittently to reduce this adverse effect

use decreases bronchial reactivity, provides symptomatic relief, reduces the requirement for inhaled beta-2 agonist "rescue" and also has "systemic steroid sparing effect". Their effects are apparent within a few days to a week, but maximum effects need months of use. Despite these advantages, they cannot be considered as curative drugs; however, there is clinical trial evidence to show that discontinuation of steroids leads to disease exacerbation.

Fixed dose combinations: Fixed dose combinations of steroids with long-acting beta-2 adrenergic agonists are also available, for instance budesonide plus formoterol and fluticasone plus salmeterol. The combination has been shown to be synergistic and provides several advantages; the molecular mechanisms for the same have now been elucidated. It has been shown inhaled beta-2 agonists lead to the increased localization of steroid receptors in the nucleus and provide the additive suppression of release of inflammatory mediators.[10] Steroids, in turn, increase the expression of beta-2 receptors by increasing gene transcription and prevent their desensitization by restoring coupling of G-proteins with beta-2 receptors.[11,12]

Leukotriene Receptor Antagonists

Leukotrienes, the products of arachidonic acid metabolism have important role in bronchial asthma **(Flow chart 2)**. They are highly potent bronchoconstrictors, the action is primarily mediated via LT1 receptors. While montelukast, zafirlukast and pranlukast are cys-LT1 receptor antagonists, zileuton is lipoxygenase inhibitor; both the approaches are effective in asthma with decreased frequency of exacerbations (as effective as steroids) and improved asthma control seen in randomized trials. They have been shown to reduce symptoms, increase airway caliber, improve bronchial reactivity and decrease airway inflammation, but to a lesser degree than steroids. The response to therapy is less homogeneous as compared with other antiasthma drugs and patients can be classified into responders and nonresponders; only in responders can these drugs be considered as alternatives to steroids. There are no parameters that can help to predict, which patients will respond. They are taken orally, which leads to a better compliance amongst patients unable to handle inhalers well such as children. However, combination of antileukotriene drugs with inhaled corticosteroids (ICS)

Flow chart 2 Arachidonic acid metabolism and bronchial asthma

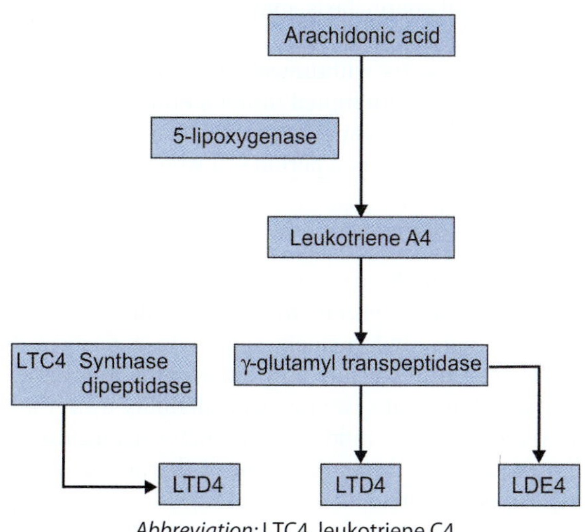

Abbreviation: LTC4, leukotriene C4

may not be as efficacious as a combination of the steroids with long-acting beta agonists (LABAs). Theoretically, zileuton provides several additional advantages over and above LT1 receptor antagonists. Firstly, it inhibits LTB4 synthesis, which is a potent chemotactic autacoid; secondly it inhibits the formation of other 5-lipoxygenase products, which also have a role in the pathogenesis of asthma; and lastly, it inhibits cys-LT effects that are not mediated via LT1 receptors.[13]

- *Zafirlukast*: A selective, competitive antagonist of the LTC4, D4 and E4 receptors, this was the first marketed compound of this class. Its peak plasma concentrations occur in 3 hours; food reduces its bioavailability (by 40%) with reduction in both the rate and the extent of absorption. It is highly (99%) proteins bound, extensively metabolized in liver by CYP2C9, and excreted primarily (90%) by the GIT, the rest in urine, as metabolites. The most common adverse effects seen in 1–2% of patients include were headache, rash, abdominal pain, malaise and GI disturbances (nausea, diarrhea and dyspepsia). An increased incidence of respiratory tract infection and depression may occur. Less common are fever, malaise, abdominal and joint/muscle pains, insomnia, dizziness and elevations in liver function tests. Frank hepatitis is rare, but fatalities have been seen. Hypersensitivity reactions (rash, pruritus, urticaria and angioedema), agranulocytosis and bleeding are uncommon.

There are case reports of Churg-Strauss syndrome (systemic eosinophilia) with its use. It is recommended to discontinue treatment, although the causality has remained questionable.[14] In some patients it had occurred after steroid withdrawal, which had led to speculation that asthma might have been a part of some undiagnosed vasculitis, which got unmasked by steroid withdrawal. Others have contended that Churg-Strauss syndrome may have been a precursor of severe asthma. Lastly, similar systemic eosinophilias have been observed in patients taking fluticasone and cromoglycate, a finding that points towards a nondrug cause. On the contrary, Churg-Strauss syndrome has been seen with other leukotriene antagonists, montelukast and pranlukast as well, which points towards a class effect.[15] Therefore, it is now recommended to monitor erythrocyte sedimentation rate (ESR), C-reactive protein (CRP) and total leukocyte count (TLC) (particularly eosinophils) if the introduction of a leukotriene antagonist allows the physicians to reduce the dose of oral steroids.[16]

Zafirlukast is metabolized by CYP2C9 and inhibits CYP2C9 and CYP3A4. Therefore, use with drugs that are metabolized by these cytochromes may lead to the possibility of increases in plasma concentrations. Patients on warfarin may need dose adjustment as the prolongation of the prothrombin time can occur. Inducers of CYP29 may lead to reduction in plasma concentrations of zafirlukast. Zafirlukast has rarely been reported to increase plasma theophylline concentrations while the concentration of zafirlukast may be increased by aspirin (high dose).

- *Montelukast*: Montelukast is probably the most commonly used compound of this class. It reaches peak plasma concentration in 3–4 hours after oral dose, has an oral bioavailability of more than 60%, is more than 99% bound to plasma proteins, metabolized by CYP3A4, CYP2A6 and CYP2C9 and excreted by the GIT. It is similar to zafirlukast in most aspects, but has a longer duration of action. It is also licensed for use in children in reduced doses. These drugs have been tried with varied success in several other indications, such as in rhinitis, bronchiolitis, cystic fibrosis, eczema, eosinophilic esophagitis, graft-versus-host disease, mastocytosis, sleep-disordered breathing and urticaria. The adverse effect profile is similar to that of zafirlukast. Suspected postmarketing adverse effects reported to the regulatory agencies include edema, agitation and restlessness, allergy (anaphylaxis, angioedema and urticaria), chest pain, tremor, dry mouth, vertigo, arthralgia, depression, suicidality and anxiousness.[17,18]
- *Zileuton*: Zileuton is an orally active 5-lipoxygenase inhibitor for use as an alternative adjuvant to long-acting beta agonist and corticosteroids in chronic management of asthma. It is well-absorbed from the GIT, the peak levels are seen in 2 hours. It is highly proteins (93%) bound, metabolized by CYP1A2, CYP2C9 and CYP3A4 and inactive metabolites are eliminated renally. The most common adverse effects are headache, pharyngolaryngeal pain, GI disturbances, myalgia and sinusitis. Rarely, hypersensitivity, urticaria, rash and leukopenia have occurred. Elevated liver enzymes and severe hepatic injury may rarely occur. It is, therefore, advisable to monitor liver function once monthly particularly in the first 3 months of therapy. It may increase the plasma levels (leading to toxicity) of warfarin, propranolol and theophylline.

Leukotriene inhibitors inhibit early and late bronchoconstrictor responses to antigens, not suitable for the acute attacks of asthma. Recently, it has been shown in a randomized trial in adults with acute asthma that intravenous (IV) montelukast plus standard treatment produced significant relief of airway obstruction forced expiratory volume 1 second (FEV_1) with an early (10 minutes) onset of action.[19] These drugs are particularly useful for asthma induced by NSAIDs, cold air and exercise. They can be used along with inhaled steroids in patients with moderate persistent asthma and may have a steroid-sparing. Montelukast has been shown to improve both asthma control and asthma-related quality of life in patients insufficiently controlled with inhaled steroids or inhaled steroids plus long-acting beta agonists (LABAs).[20]

Mast Cell Stabilizers

Two drugs in this category—cromolyn and nedocromil probably act by several mechanisms: inhibition of the release of mediators from mast cells, inhibition of white blood cell trafficking in airways, reversal of increased leukocyte activation, antagonism of substance P, inhibition of the effects of platelet-activating factor (PAF) and suppression of the effects of chemotactic peptides on blood cells. There is enough clinical evidence to show that pretreatment with these agents blocks allergen-induced bronchoconstriction making them suitable for use before exercise or allergen exposure. Moreover, their long-term use reduces the severity of symptoms and the need for bronchodilators. They are not as effective as inhaled steroids, but combination with steroids improves asthma control. Like anticholinergics, an n-of-1 trial for 4 weeks can help identify individual patients that respond best (or do not respond) to this class of drugs.

Cromolyn

The first agent in this class, cromolyn is available in inhalational forms, administered in a dose of 2 mg four times daily. The dose may be increased to six or eight times daily, if poor control is a problem. Besides prophylaxis of asthma, cromolyn is also used, with variable success, in prophylaxis and treatment of seasonal and perennial allergic rhinitis, acute and chronic allergic conjunctivitis, vernal keratoconjunctivitis, prevention of food allergies (orally), mastocytosis, Cogan's syndrome, cough associated with angiotensin-converting enzyme (ACE) inhibitor therapy, nonspecific cough in children and moderately severe atopic dermatitis (in children).

Poor systemic bioavailability implies fewer incidences of systemic adverse effects. Local adverse effects, such as irritation in the throat, cough, dryness of mouth, bad taste, nasal congestion, tightness of chest, transient bronchospasm and wheezing (aggravation of existing asthma) may occur. Serious adverse effects are uncommon; dermatitis, myositis, joint pain and swelling or gastroenteritis (<2%), dysuria, urinary frequency, rarely pulmonary infiltration with eosinophilia and anaphylaxis, may occur.

Cromolyn is not indicated for the treatment of acute asthmatic attacks. Its withdrawal may lead to recurrence, should therefore be attempted under steroid cover if steroid doses were reduced because of its use. Also, the dose should be gradually tapered over a period of 1 week.

Nedocromil Sodium

It is similar to cromolyn in most aspects, generally considered to be its alternative except that its duration of action is somewhat longer. It is usually started in a dose of 4 mg (inhaled) four times a day. The other uses are similar to cromolyn. It has poor systemic bioavailability from the GIT. The adverse effects are mild, infrequent, mostly transient and do not require the discontinuation of therapy. Paradoxical bronchospasm is rare.

The major indication for the use of mast cell stabilizers is to prevent asthmatic attacks in patients with mild-to-moderate asthma. Nedocromil is not approved for use in patients less than 12 years of age while cromolyn is approved for use in adults as well as children.

Anti-immunoglobulin E Monoclonal Antibodies

Monoclonal antibodies, which bind to the site on IgE antibody to prevent its binding to receptors (FCεR1 and FCεR2) present on mast cells and other inflammatory cells, are a new class of drugs approved for use in certain cases of asthma. Omalizumab is the prototype of this class of "biological drugs".

Omalizumab: It is a recombinant humanized monoclonal antibody targeted against IgE. Once it binds to IgE receptors on inflammatory cells, it prevents interaction of IgE with these inflammatory cells and prevents their release. It is produced in Chinese hamster ovary (CHO) cells in cell culture. It is approved for prophylactic use as add-on therapy to standard treatment in adult patients with moderate to severe, persistent, allergic, IgE-induced asthma.[20] It decreases exacerbations, improves quality of life and reduces steroid requirements.[21] It does not have a bronchodilator effect, has no role during acute exacerbations.

The dose is variable, ranging from 75 mg to 300 mg every 4 weeks to 225 mg to 375 mg every 2 weeks. The dose depends on the patient's body weight and pretreatment serum IgE concentrations. It is administered subcutaneously, it is not recommended to give more than 150 mg at one site. Injection site reactions, including erythema, stinging, bruising and induration are the most common adverse effects. Generalized pain, fatigue, arthralgia, dizziness, earache, GI disturbances, headache and alopecia are some other adverse effects. Flu-like syndrome and an increased incidence of infections (parasitic, viral) has been seen. Rarely, Churg-Strauss syndrome, hypersensitivity reactions, including urticaria, dermatitis, pruritus and anaphylaxis are reported. The temporal relation of anaphylactic reactions to omalizumab is unpredictable. The side effects may occur after the first dose or within a few days after a dose, or even more than 1 year after a patient is on regular therapy. Severe, thrombocytopenia and an increased incidence of cancer are two other potentially serious adverse effects with its use.

Miscellaneous Drugs

Mepolizumab

Mepolizumab, a monoclonal antibody against IL-5 has received an orphan drug status for the management of hypereosinophilic syndrome. When given as an infusion to patients with refractory eosinophilic asthma with a history of recurrent exacerbations, mepolizumab reduced the number of blood and sputum eosinophils, had steroid-sparing effect in patients who had asthma with sputum eosinophilia despite prednisone treatment.[22]

Magnesium Sulfate

Magnesium is known to reduce smooth muscle contraction, decrease histamine release from mast cells and inhibit acetylcholine release. In a study in pediatric patients with acute severe exacerbation, unresponsive to standard treatment, $MgSO_4$ in a dose of 40 mg/kg IV bolus, led to symptomatic improvement within a few minutes that lasted for about 2 hours.[23] Similarly, in adult patients with severe, acute asthma, it caused improvement in pulmonary function when used in a dose of 2 g IV, as an adjunct to standard therapy.[24] Nebulized magnesium may also improve symptoms over and above the effects of standard inhaled drugs, the most severely ill derive the most benefit.[25] However, some recent evidence is contradictory (see later).

Nebulized Lidocaine

The safety and efficacy of nebulized lidocaine was evaluated in a randomized, placebo-controlled trial in 50 patients with mild-to-moderate asthma.[26] Nebulized lignocaine improved the various indicators of asthma severity, such as the FEV_1, night-time awakenings, clinical symptoms, bronchodilator use and blood eosinophil counts.

Inhaled Heparin

In a small study in 12 patients with exercise-induced asthma, nebulized heparin (1,000 U/kg) prevented exercise-induced asthma without influencing histamine-induced bronchoconstriction.[27] This nonanticoagulant action of heparin is more likely to relate to the modulation of mediator release than to a direct effect on smooth muscle.

Beta-adrenergic Blockers

Some recent studies have suggested a role of beta-blockers in the management of asthma. This paradox has been likened to the beta-blocker paradox in heart failure. In a preliminary study, the safety and efficacy of escalating doses of the beta-blocker, nadolol (an inverse agonist), administered over 9 weeks to 10 subjects with mild asthma was evaluated.[28] A dose-dependent decrease in airway hyperresponsiveness to methacholine was seen in eight out of the 10 patients after 9 weeks of nadolol treatment. Clearly, more data are needed before any conclusions can be drawn.

Steroid Sparing Anti-inflammatory Agents

There are various steroid sparing-agents, like azathioprine that have been evaluated. There is a lack of larger, well designed studies to provide evidence for its use. It cannot be recommended for clinical practice as of now.[29] Cyclosporine is another drug that has been evaluated for its steroid-sparing effect. A Cochrane review of 98 patients with severe asthma treated with cyclosporine showed a small, but significant treatment effect for cyclosporine in the terms of steroid dose reduction.[30] It is a drug with a large number of side effects, not recommended for routine use. A Cochrane review of small clinical trials showed a small, but significant treatment effect for gold in the terms of steroid dose reduction.[31] It should not be routinely used because of the adverse effects concern.

Colchicine and dapsone are two other steroid-sparing drugs. There is no reliable evidence to recommend the use of either of them in the management of steroid-dependent asthmatic patients.

BRONCHODILATORS

Treatment of asthma with bronchodilatory drugs has a long, fascinating history. Ancient Ayurvedic texts recommended inhaled therapy particularly with steam, cinnamon, castor oil and herbs such as *Atropa belladonna, Datura stramonium* or mixtures containing anticholinergic compounds (like atropine, hyoscyamine and scopolamine). These compounds were also used by the ancient Greeks with the help of specially made inhaler devices. The first evidence for use of sympathomimetics drugs is available from the traditional Chinese medicine (Ma huang, from the plant *Ephedra sinica* containing ephedrine). Some of the other remedies tried before the modern era that might or might not have been effective include owl's blood in wine, opium-induced vomiting and chicken soup.

The treatment of asthma achieved a landmark in 1897 when John Abel was able to prepare crude adrenal extract (*epinephrine*). Subsequently, in 1920s and 1930s, many epinephrine analogs were synthesized, including isoproterenol. However, its beta selectivity was not known. Its use became widespread only in the middle part of the 20th century. Development of isoprenaline in inhalational form was a big step, but tragically caused thousands of deaths during the 1960s. The discovery by lands and coworkers of β_1 and β_2 receptors led to the development of salbutamol in 1967.

It is safe to assume that most of the world population consumes (and has consumed for 100 of years) either tea or coffee/cocoa or cola drinks. Tea leaves (*Thea sinensis*) contain theophylline (small amount), caffeine and theobromine; cocoa and chocolate seeds (*Theobroma cacao*) contain theobromine and some caffeine; coffee fruit (*Coffea arabica*) and the nuts of *cola acuminata* contain caffeine. All these plant alkaloids are known to possess mood elevating, stimulant and bronchodilating properties. Although, theophylline was first extracted in the 19th century, its use as bronchodilator was first described only in 1922.[32]

The next paradigm shift in the treatment of asthma came in the 1960s with the use of anti-inflammatory drugs. Khellin, a naturally occurring chromone (*Ammi visnaga* extract) had been used in Egypt and the Eastern mediterranean countries for centuries in the treatment of respiratory diseases. The synthesis of *Cromolyn* (Roger Altounyan) in 1965 was an attempt to improve the bronchodilator activity and reduce the adverse effects of khellin. The Nobel Prize winning discovery of kendall, Reichstein and Hench "relating to the hormones of the adrenal cortex", was soon followed by observations that adrenocorticotropic hormone and cortisol helped in asthma. As the use of corticosteroids in bronchial asthma was appreciated, the physicians started becoming more aware of their adverse effects, need for topical preparation was realized and inhaled steroids were introduced in 1972.

Bronchodilators are broadly classified as below:

- *Beta-2 adrenergic agonists:* Short-acting, long-acting and ultra-long-acting
- Methylxanthines
- Anticholinergic agents.

Beta-2 Adrenergic Agonists

Beta-2 adrenergic agonists are the most efficacious and the most widely used bronchodilators. They can be used by inhalation or systemically, provide excellent smooth muscle relaxation and rapid bronchodilation with relatively few side effects, thus providing excellent risk-benefit ratio. The most preferred route when using these drugs is inhalational because the mast cells are located close to the airway lumen and more easily accessible to this route. However, less than 10% of the inhaled drug reaches the site of action, the remainder is swallowed. In order to reduce systemic adverse effects, the stress is on developing drugs that have low systemic bioavailability (poor absorption from the GIT or high first-pass hepatic metabolism). Another strategy is to increase the drug delivery to lungs and simultaneously decrease the amount of drug reaching the GIT; for example, by attaching a spacer to the metered-dose inhaler (MDI).

Mechanism of action: Human lungs contain both alpha and beta adrenergic receptors; alpha receptors are not known to play any significant role in the regulation of the airway smooth muscle (ASM) tone. On the other hand, beta adrenergic receptors, subtype-2, are the most important regulators of ASM tone. Traditionally, the mechanism of action of beta-2 adrenergic agonists has concentrated on ASM relaxation mediated through elevated cAMP levels **(Flow chart 3)**. Beta-2 agonists act through heterotrimeric G-proteins leading to the stimulation of adenylyl cyclase. This, in turn, leads to the elevation of cAMP levels. Elevated cAMP activates protein kinase A (PKA). Activated PKA, in turn, phosphorylates myosin light chain kinase, thereby preventing ASM contraction. While this concept still holds, several other mechanisms have been elucidated.[33] PKA may also bring about the activation of potassium channels leading to potassium efflux, which in turn, causes hyperpolarization of ASM. Cross activation of protein kinase G (PKG) may also lead to the relaxation of ASM.

Flow chart 3 Molecular mechanism of action of beta-2 adrenergic agonists

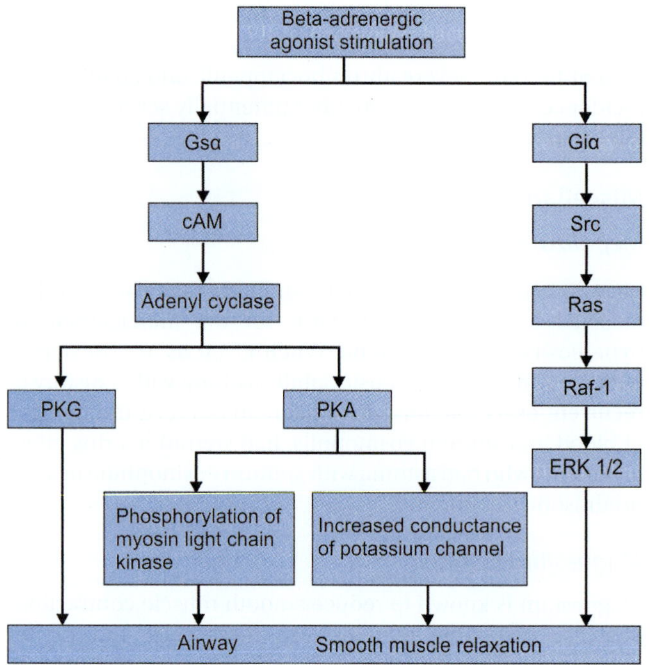

Abbreviations: ERK, extracellular signal-regulated kinase; PKA, protein kinase A

Additionally, beta-2 adrenoceptors are expressed in inflammatory cells like mast cells, macrophages, neutrophils, eosinophils, as well as in type I and II alveolar cells. Activation of beta-2 adrenoceptors leads to the inhibition of these cells. This may additionally contribute to the benefits obtained with beta-2 adrenergic agonists.

Short-acting Beta-2 Agonists

The agents of this group are used by inhalational route mainly. They are considered the most effective agents for relieving acute bronchospasm (level A evidence). They are also indicated for preventing exercise-induced bronchospasm. Two epidemics of asthma deaths in the 1960s and 1970s in United Kingdom and New Zealand were attributed to the use of SABAs. Subsequently, the results of mild asthma trial evaluated regular versus "as needed" albuterol in 255 patients with mild asthma.[34] Patients were randomized to 16 weeks treatment of "as needed" or regular use albuterol. Peak expiratory flow (PEF) variability, FEV_1, number of puffs of albuterol or symptoms were not different in the two groups. It was thus concluded that "as needed" therapy was preferable for the regular inhalation of bronchodilators. In a Cochrane review,[35] data from 31 outcomes were analyzable. There was little difference between the treatments for nearly all outcomes. In cross-over studies, evening peak flow was better with regular treatment. Bronchial hyperreactivity was slightly better in the "as needed" group. It was thus concluded that there was little advantage in using SABAs regularly.

If SABAs are needed more than twice per week, it is considered to indicate the inadequate control of bronchial asthma. Use of more than one SABA canister for quick relief of bronchospasm in a period of one month indicates an increased possibility of emergency department visit. Pharmacogenomics have thrown some light on the variability in propensity to deterioration of lung function while taking SABAs, albuterol in particular.[36] Polymorphism of beta-2 adrenoceptor gene may explain some of this variability. Patients homozygous for arginine at position 16 are more likely to experience the worsening of lung functions than those who are either Arg/Gly or Gly/Gly genotype at the same locus.

Salbutamol: Salbutamol (albuterol) is the prototype SABA. It is given by inhalation, orally and parenterally (but not in all countries). The preferred route of administration is inhalation, even though only 10–20% of the administered dose reaches the site of action while the rest is swallowed or left behind in the device.[37] Salbutamol, unintentionally, but invariably swallowed from the inhaler device or taken orally as tablet, is readily absorbed from the GIT. Peak plasma levels (C_{max}) are seen considerably earlier with inhaled formulation (T_{max} 0.2 hour) as compared to oral administration (T_{max} 1.8 hour).[38] Salbutamol undergoes considerable first-pass metabolism in the liver and gut wall, but not in the lung and has no active metabolites. Its plasma half-life is 4–6 hours as it is rapidly excreted, primarily in the urine. Its metabolism is stereoselective and levosalbutamol [*R*(–)-enantiomer] is metabolized about eight times more rapidly than the S(+)-enantiomer (also has no bronchodilator effect).[39] This property has been utilized to develop and market levosalbutamol as a novel drug (approved by the food and drug administration in 1999), with some evidence of fewer adverse effects.

Adverse drug reactions: Tremors and nervousness are the most common adverse effects, they are dose-dependent and seen in up to 20% of patients. Headache (7%), palpitations, tachycardia (5%), muscle cramps (3%), elevated blood pressure, insomnia, restlessness, weakness, nausea, dizziness, and chest discomfort/heartburn are also observed. Throat irritation or sore throat and nosebleeds can also occur. Other rare adverse effects, which are occasionally seen are: allergic reactions, rash, hives, throat irritation itching; difficulty in breathing; tightness in the chest; swelling of the mouth, face, lips or tongue; chest pain; ear pain; fast or irregular heartbeat; new or worsened troubled breathing; pounding in the chest; red, swollen, blistered or peeling skin; severe headache or dizziness; unusual hoarseness; and wheezing, swelling, bronchospasm or anaphylaxis (shock). Worsening of diabetes and lowering of potassium have been also reported. In a rare patient, inhaled salbutamol can paradoxically precipitate life-threatening bronchospasm.

Salbutamol should be given with caution in hyperthyroidism, myocardial insufficiency, arrhythmias, susceptibility to QT-interval prolongation, hypertension and diabetes mellitus. Hypokalemia should be kept in mind in severe asthma as the hypoxia associated with the condition and the concomitant drugs used in the situation may exacerbate hypokalemia. There are reports of abuse of salbutamol among both asthmatic and nonasthmatic (especially) young persons.

Drug interactions: Though pharmacokinetic interactions are not remarkable, pharmacodynamic interactions may be of concern. Concomitant use with other beta-2 agonists, corticosteroids, diuretics and xanthines may cause increased risk of hypokalemia. A propensity to cause hypokalemia increases the predisposition to digitalis induced arrhythmias. There may be adverse cardiovascular additive effects such as hypertension and tachycardia (if combined with tricyclic antidepressants or monoamine oxidase inhibitors). Similar interaction can occur with other stimulant sympathomimetic drugs, especially in patients with underlying coronary heart disease. Beta-blockers (especially nonselective) block salbutamol effects and bronchospasm may occur.

Use in asthma: For the relief of acute bronchospasm, one or two inhalations of salbutamol 100 μg may be given from a conventional metered-dose aerosol as required, up to four times daily. Two inhalations may also be given just before the exertion for the prophylaxis of exercise-induced bronchospasm. Due to environmental concerns with the use of chlorofluorocarbons (CFC), CFC-free aerosols have been developed. These contain hydrofluoroalkanes (HFA). These are also available as dry powder inhalers. A dose, double to that of conventional aerosol is often required when the drug is administered in the powder forms. Long-term use of beta adrenergic agonists is known to reduce the efficacy of the agents. This has been attributed mainly to the process of receptor desensitization. Uncoupling of the receptor from Gs, receptor internalization, upregulation of cyclic adenosine monophosphate (cAMP) phosphodiesterase and downregulation of Gs are some of the reasons for receptor desensitization.

Bitolterol: A long-acting beta-adrenergic agonist, it is the prodrug of colterol—a long-acting beta-adrenergic agonist synthesized mainly in the lungs. Although, it has a long duration of action (>5 hours), unlike other long-acting beta-adrenergic agonists, it can be given for acute exacerbations of bronchospasm because of its rapid onset of action (about 2 minutes).

Orciprenaline: Also known as metaproterenol, it is less selective for beta-2 receptors than salbutamol, therefore causes more adverse effects. When given by inhalation, its onset of action is 30 minutes and duration 1–5 hours. Because of its nonselective action, it has been used orally or by slow IV infusion in the treatment of bradycardia (like isoprenaline).

Pirbuterol: It is a selective beta-adrenergic agonist with properties similar to that of salbutamol. The onset occurs in 10 minutes and the action lasts for 5 hours.

Terbutaline: Terbutaline is similar to salbutamol in most aspects except that its half-life is longer (16–20 hours). It is given mainly for the relief of acute exacerbations. It is available for inhalational, parenteral and oral administration.

Fenoterol: It has a rapid onset (5 minutes) after inhalation. It was implicated in the asthma-related epidemic (increased morbidity and mortality) in New Zealand in 1970s and 1980s with similar reports from Canada and Japan. Subsequently, a meta-analysis concluded that the increase in asthma-related mortality associated with beta-adrenergic agonist was only slight.[40] Moreover, the link between asthma-related deaths and fenoterol remained controversial as it was proposed that patients who used the drug had more severe disease.

Oral beta agonists: Oral preparations of beta-2 agonists have the disadvantage of a worse side-effect profile compared to inhaled preparations. A brief course of albuterol or metaproterenol syrup may be considered in the children of less than 5 years of age who cannot manipulate metered-dose inhalers (MDIs) and yet have occasional wheezing. In occasional patients with severe asthma exacerbations, in whom the aerosol delivery causes worsening of cough and bronchospasm; oral forms of albuterol, metaproterenol or terbutaline may still be effective.

Long-acting Beta-2 Adrenergic Agonists

Long-acting beta-2 adrenergic agonists as well as ultra long-acting agents are used for the maintenance therapy of asthma. The mechanism of action is similar to that of SABAs.

- *Salmeterol:* This LABA (duration of action 12 hours) is used for maintenance therapy in conjunction with corticosteroids. The onset occurs at 10–20 minutes, but the peak effect is delayed making it unsuitable for the treatment of acute spasm. Publication of the results of interim analysis of Salmeterol Multicenter Asthma Research Trial (SMART) showed a small and significant increase in asthma-related deaths with the use of salmeterol, mainly in African-Americans.[41] A meta-analysis of 19 trials showed a similar increased propensity to cause asthma-related deaths, increased incidence of hospitalization due to asthma exacerbations and life-threatening asthma attacks in those treated with salmeterol.[42] Therefore, the current practice in chronic asthma is not to use salmeterol as a substitute to inhaled steroids, but to add it to ICS rather than increasing the dose of ICS.
- *Formoterol:* Formoterol is a partial agonist, touted for lesser propensity to desensitization of the beta-agonist activity. Experimental studies, however, have demonstrated that at equally effective doses, all beta-2 agonists may be equally susceptible to desensitization.[43] Like salmeterol, it has to be used in conjunction with corticosteroids. Addition of long-acting beta-adrenergic agonist to low or high dose of ICS reduces the risk of asthma exacerbation compared to ICS given alone. Inhaled formoterol is rapidly absorbed after inhalation. The plasma half-life of the drug after administration is around 10 hours. Due to its rapid onset and long duration of action it is used both as a reliever and as a controller (in combination with corticosteroids).
- *Bambuterol:* Bambuterol metabolizes to terbutaline, the active metabolite. As a result of slow metabolism, its approximate duration of action is around 24 hours. It may cause an increase in nonfatal heart failure in elderly patients.
- *Clenbuterol:* It is used in the dose of 20 mcg twice daily, by inhalation. It is being widely abused by sportsperson for improving performance and also by farmers for improving the muscle mass of livestock. These effects remain unproven.

Ultra (Very) Long-acting Beta-2 Adrenergic Agonists

Attempts to further increase the duration of action of beta-2 agonists have been made so as to get compounds suitable for once daily administration, which by improving compliance, may also improve the outcomes. Most of these compounds are R, R-enantiomers of existing drugs since it is likely that these isomers will have less desensitization. Arformoterol, the R, R-isomer of formoterol, has been shown to have duration of action of 24 hours. However, studies have also indicated that clinically important difference may not exist between the duration of action of formoterol and arformoterol. Carmoterol is another ultralong-acting beta-agonist with the structural elements of both formoterol and procaterol. In clinical trials, it has been shown to be as effective as formoterol, but is not yet approved. Clinical trials have also demonstrated safety and efficacy of another ultra long-acting beta2-adrenoceptor agonists (ULABA), indacaterol. It has, in addition to prolonged duration of action, a quick onset of action. Some of these agents are likely to be marketed soon. Many of the beta-2 adrenergic agonists are available as fixed dose combinations with ICS while some are available as fixed-dose combinations with once-daily long-acting muscarinic antagonists (LAMAs).

Besides asthma, LABAs and ULABAs are being evaluated in chronic obstructive pulmonary disease (COPD) as well. It is an issue of concern whether LABAs may increase the mortality in COPD, in view of the result of the increased mortality seen in the SMART.[44] On the other hand, the landmark trial, towards a revolution in COPD Health (TORCH)[45] showed that there was a 17% relative risk reduction (amounting to 2.6% absolute reduction); in all-cause mortality. However, a combination of inhaled steroid (fluticasone) and a long-acting agent (salmeterol) was used in this large (> 6,000 patients), multinational (42 countries), randomized trial. The combination improved lung function, reduced the total number of exacerbations and reduced the yearly rate of decline in FEV_1 more than the two individual drugs. Importantly, monotherapy with salmeterol had better survival than placebo, although statistical significance was not achieved.

Methylxanthines (Xanthines)

Theophylline, theobromine and caffeine are three important methylxanthines (some nonmethylated xanthines are under development). Aminophylline (theophylline-diamine) is a commonly used derivative of theophylline. The exact mode of action of xanthines is not known. The primary action (although at high concentrations, in vitro) is through inhibition of phosphodiesterases group of enzymes (PDEs), which in turn, prevent breakdown of cAMP and cyclic guanosine monophosphate (cGMP), leading to their accumulation and effects such as relaxation of smooth muscle, stimulation of cardiac function and inhibition of release of cytokines and chemokines (TNF alpha, leukotrienes).

Although, xanthines are nonselective inhibitors of PDEs (of which at least five types are known), the enzyme most likely responsible for their action is PDE4 (to a lesser extent, PDE5), located on bronchial smooth muscle and inflammatory cells. Attempts to make selective PDE4 inhibitors ("designer xanthines") have not been successful, the development of at least three selective PDE4 inhibitors (roflumilast, cilomilast and tofimilast) have been stopped due to various toxicities seen at low doses.

The second important mechanism of action of xanthines is through competitive inhibition of adenosine receptors. Adenosine can modulate adenyl cyclase activity, cause bronchial smooth muscle contraction and histamine release leading to bronchoconstriction. Although, considered important by some, it must be mentioned that enprofylline (xanthine without adenosine antagonistic action) also has bronchodilator effect. Deacetylation of histones by xanthines may decrease the recruitment of histone deacetylases by corticosteroids to areas where the transcription of pro-inflammatory genes occurs. This can actually lead to synergism between steroids and xanthines, a theoretical interaction that now has some clinical evidence since theophylline was able to restore responsiveness to steroids in (smoker) asthmatics. In conclusion, xanthines have both bronchodilatory and anti-inflammatory effects, but which one is more important remains unclear.

The other effects of xanthines include central nervous system (CNS) stimulation (especially with caffeine), positive chronotropic and inotropic effects on heart, stimulation of gastric acid and intestinal enzyme secretion, mild diuretic effect (especially with theophylline) and stimulation of skeletal muscle (including the diaphragm) contraction.

Theophylline

It is the prototype drug of the class available for oral and parenteral administration. Dosage of modified release formulations should be titrated for an individual patient. Parenteral preparations are seldom used. Elimination is primarily hepatic, the metabolites as well as the unchanged drug (10%) are excreted in urine except in neonates (50% excreted unchanged). Its half-life in healthy, nonsmoking adults is 7–9 hours, and 3–5 hours in children and smokers, but higher (10–30 hours) in neonates, premature infants, elderly nonsmokers and in patients with liver disease or heart failure.

Solutions or uncoated tablets of theophylline produce maximal concentration in plasma within 2 hours. Sustained release preparations have marked interpatient variability in their bioavailabilities and may warrant careful dose titration. Food-drug interactions are also highly variable. These agents are widely distributed, may cross placenta and pass into breast milk. Allopurinol, macrolides, quinolones, oral contraceptives and albendazole are known to decrease the clearance of theophylline, thus its dose needs to be reduced. On the other hand phenytoin, ritonavir, rifampicin and sulfinpyrazone may increase its clearance.

Therapeutic drug monitoring (TDM) may be needed with its use, it being a narrow therapeutic index drug and having multiple interactions. An optimum therapeutic concentration is generally considered to be between 10 μg/mL and 30 μg/mL. Toxicity has been seen with the rapid IV administration of therapeutic doses of aminophylline resulting in cardiac arrhythmias.

The adverse effects commonly encountered with theophylline and xanthine derivatives irrespective of the route are GI irritation and stimulation of the CNS. Serum concentrations of greater than 20 μg/mL are associated with an increased risk of adverse effects. Overdosage may also cause agitation, diuresis, repeated vomiting, cardiac arrhythmias, hypotension, electrolyte disturbances (such as hypokalemia, hyperglycemia and hypomagnesemia), metabolic acidosis, rhabdomyolysis, convulsions and death.

Aminophylline

It is a prodrug of theophylline (joined with ethylenediamine), releases theophylline in vivo. It is given slowly intravenously by slow injection (or infusion) in acute severe bronchospasm, at a rate greater than 25 mg/minute. It is important to elicit drug history of the patients before the administration of IV aminophylline. In patients already on xanthine medication, it is safe to omit the loading dose or if possible, serum concentration estimated and the required dose calculated. It is also administered orally and rarely, rectally absorption from the latter route is erratic. Besides asthma, it is also used in the management of COPD, neonatal apnea and erectile dysfunction (local application). It has been also tried in motor neuron disease, methotrexate-induced neurotoxicity and for removal of fat (locally).

Diprophylline

Unlike theophylline, diprophylline is largely cleared unchanged renally (half-life 2 hours) and does not need dose modification in patients with hepatic dysfunction. Unlike theophylline, drug interactions are uncommon. It is used in doses of 15 mg/kg, three to four times a day.

Caffeine

Caffeine is a xanthine that is more widely acknowledged as a CNS stimulant. It increases alertness and reduces sleep. In doses of 5–10 mg/kg, it has a bronchodilator action that is weaker (40%) compared to theophylline, which is why it is hardly used in asthma.

Xanthines (particularly theophylline and aminophylline) were used as first-line bronchodilators in the past, but their position was taken by steroids and beta-2 agonists. Xanthines are less efficacious and have greater potential for adverse effects. There has been a resurgence of their use for their anti-inflammatory properties and because of the availability of slow-release preparations for nocturnal control.

Anticholinergic Agents

Airway smooth muscles express both M2 and M3 muscarinic receptors. Besides in ASM, muscarinic receptors are also present in glandular and surface epithelial cells, endothelial cells and various inflammatory cells in the airway. Acetylcholine produces bronchoconstriction predominantly by acting through M3 muscarinic receptors. Activation of these receptors leads to the activation of phospholipase C (PLC) resulting in the formation of IP3 and diacylglycerol (DAG). Additionally, M2 receptors augment the contractile response mediated by M3 receptors. This is achieved by limiting adrenergic relaxation and inhibitory effects on calcium-activated potassium channels. M3 receptors are also involved in the stimulation of mucus secretion from submucosal glands and goblet cells.

There are several reviews on the usefulness of anticholinergics in acute and chronic bronchial asthma in children and adults. Mostly, it is shown that while the agents are useful in acute asthma, there is insufficient evidence for their role in chronic asthma.[45-48] Specifically, they were shown to cause significant reductions in hospital admissions with favorable symptom scores, particularly in the respect of daytime dyspnea and daily peak flow measurements. For the latter, the clinical significance was small and in terms of peak flow measurements, equated to approximately a modest 7% increase over placebo. The more clinically relevant comparison of a combination of anticholinergic plus SABA versus SABA alone gave no evidence in respect of symptom scores or peak flow rates of any significant differences between the two regimes. Thus, these drugs may be used to provide additive benefit to SABA in moderate-to-severe asthma exacerbations or may be used as alternative bronchodilators for patients who do not tolerate SABA.

Ipratropium Bromide

It is a quaternary ammonium antimuscarinic agent. When given by inhalation, it causes direct bronchodilatation. Ipratropium bromide provides additive benefit to SABAs in moderate-to-severe asthma exacerbations, leads to somewhat higher and prolonged effect compared to either agent used alone. It may also be used as an alternative bronchodilator for patients who do not tolerate SABAs. When ipratropium is used alone, the bronchodilation by onset is slower, the magnitude is lesser and more variable as compared to SABAs. The exact cause of variability in response to ipratropium is not known, may be related to the intrinsic parasympathetic tone in a particular patient as well as the contribution of parasympathetic system in causing bronchoconstriction.

Ipratropium is used by the inhalational route; 10–30% of the drug is deposited in the lungs, very small amount reaches the systemic circulation as it is not absorbed from the GIT. It is available as metered-dose inhalers (alone and in combination with beta-2 agonists), dry powder capsules and as nebulizer solution. The usual dose from an MDI is one or two inhalations (20–40 µg) three or four times daily, but the total daily dose should not exceed 12 inhalations. Inhaled antimuscarinics have greater usefulness in COPD. Intranasal ipratropium is also used in the management of rhinitis (reduces rhinorrhea and sneezing).

Being an anticholinergic, it is associated with the dryness of mouth, constipation (rarely paralytic ileus), tachycardia, palpitations and arrhythmias. Rarely, it can cause urinary retention (especially in the presence of prostatic hyperplasia) and precipitation of angle closure glaucoma. Patients with glaucoma should be advised to be careful while using these agents to avoid the mist entering the eyes. Antimuscarinics cause impaired drainage of aqueous humor while beta-2 agonists increase the production of aqueous humor; their concomitant use (which is routinely done) may be potentially harmful in susceptible patients. Rarely, paradoxical bronchospasm (seen also with other bronchodilators, may be attributable to some preservative) and hypersensitivity reactions (urticaria, angioedema, rash and anaphylaxis) have been reported. There is some evidence of increased mortality in COPD seen with ipratropium while not seen in others.[49-51]

Tiotropium Bromide

It is a long-acting quaternary ammonium anticholinergic agent (duration of action 24 hours) available for aerosol administration. About one-fifth reaches systemic circulation after dry powder inhalation and about one-third after inhalation of the solution. Its half-life is 5–6 days, excreted by the kidneys and, therefore, its use in patients with renal impairment, especially if creatinine clearance is less than 50 mL/minute, should be avoided.

It should not be used for the initial treatment of acute bronchospasm, primarily used in the maintenance treatment of COPD, as well as of asthma. It is used once daily as two inhalations of 2.5 μg from the MDI. Besides the adverse effects seen with other antimuscarinics, pharyngitis, sinusitis, rhinitis and epistaxis have been reported. Recently, a small increase in the risk of stroke (8 per 1,000 patients treated for 1 year compared with 6 per 1,000 patients on placebo) has been seen.[52] There have been case reports of dermatological adverse reactions such as cutaneous lupus and photosensitive lichenoid eruption.

Recent advances in anticholinergics have focused on the development of agents with lower systemic absorption and thereby having lesser adverse drug reactions, as well as on oral formulations. Aclidinium bromide is a long-acting anticholinergic agent selective for M3 receptors. The drug is being evaluated mainly for COPD and was shown to have bronchodilator effect lasting for 24 hours in healthy volunteers challenged with methacholine.[53] With better efficacy observed when anticholinergics are used in conjunction with beta-adrenergic agonists, certain fixed-dose combinations have been recently approved, several others, particularly with tiotropium, are under development.

NOVEL APPROACHES IN CLINICAL TRIALS

The role of thymic stromal lymphopoietin (TSLP), which is an epithelial-cell-derived cytokine that may be important in initiating allergic inflammation, was investigated in a small double-blind, placebo-controlled study in which AMG 157 (human anti-TSLP monoclonal immunoglobulin) was used. AMG 157 was found to reduce measures of allergen-induced early and late asthmatic responses as well as indexes of airway inflammation.[54]

In a series of exploratory studies, the efficacy and safety of a novel inhaled dual phosphodiesterase 3 (PDE3) and PDE4 inhibitor RPL554 was evaluated for its bronchodilator and anti-inflammatory properties in patients with severe disease that respond poorly to a combination of an inhaled bronchodilator and glucocorticosteroid.[55] In these studies, inhaled RPL554 was found to be effective and well-tolerated bronchodilator and anti-inflammatory drug.

Although, previous studies have shown some efficacy for IV or nebulized magnesium sulphate in patients with acute asthma, a recent multicentric, double-blind, placebo-controlled trial from United Kingdom, which evaluated whether IV or nebulized magnesium sulphate will improve breathlessness and reduce the need for hospital admission in adults with severe acute asthma, showed that nebulized magnesium sulphate was not effective whereas IV magnesium sulphate had a limited role.[56] Similarly, nebulized isotonic magnesium sulphate was assessed in acute severe asthma in children and found to lead to a statistically nonsignificant improvement in asthma severity scores except in those with more severe attacks (SaO_2<92%) at presentation and those with symptoms lasting less than 6 hour.[57]

Despite the association of IL-13 with asthma pathology, GSK679586, a humanized mAb that inhibits IL-13 binding to both IL-13 receptor α1 and α2, did not show improvements in asthma control, pulmonary function, or exacerbations in patients with severe asthma.[58] Similarly, although IL-17 signaling is also implicated in asthma, a human anti-IL-17 receptor A monoclonal antibody brodalumab failed to show a beneficial effect in subjects with inadequately controlled moderate to severe asthma taking regular ICS.[59]

Another strategy that did not show desirable efficacy was addition of a 5-lipoxygenase-activating protein (FLAP) inhibitor to an ICS or an ICS/long-acting beta-2 agonist combination.[60] FLAP is a nuclear membrane protein necessary for the synthesis of leukotrienes.[4] It is an integral within the FLAP is necessary in synthesis of leukotrienes.[61]

An interesting recent study questioned the role of SABA in exercise-induced bronchoconstriction and showed that combination of budesonide and formoterol on demand was superior to terbutaline on demand in improving asthma control and was similar to regular budesonide use despite using lower doses of steroid.[62]

REFERENCES

1. Williams LK, Pladevall M, Xi H, Peterson EL, Joseph C, Lafata JE, et al. Relationship between adherence to inhaled corticosteroids and poor outcomes among adults with asthma. J Allergy Clin Immunol. 2004;114(6):1288-93.
2. Van der Palen J, Klein JJ, van Herwaarden CL, Zielhuis GA, Seydel ER. Multiple inhalers confuse asthma patients. Eur Respir J. 1999;14(5):1034-7.
3. Brown TJ, Belvisi MG, Foster ML. Dissociated steroids. Prog Respir Res. 31st Volume. 2001. pp. 98-101.
4. Schäcke H, Schottelius A, Döcke WD, Strehlke P, Jaroch S, Schmees N, et al. Dissociation of transactivation from transrepression by a selective glucocorticoid receptor agonist leads to separation of therapeutic effects from side effects. Proc Natl Acad Sci USA. 2004;101(1):227-32.

5. Miner JN, Hong MH, Negro-Vilar A. New and improved glucocorticoid receptor ligands. Expert Opin Investig Drugs. 2005;14(12):1527-45.
6. Undem BJ. Pharmacotherapy of asthma. In: Brunton LL, Lazo JS, Parker KL (Eds). Goodman and Gilman's: The Pharmacologic Basis of Therapeutics; 2006.
7. CSM/MCA. Withdrawal of systemic corticosteroids. Current Problems. 1998;24:5-7.
8. Geller M. Marked peripheral edema associated with montelukast and prednisone. Ann Intern Med. 2000; 132(11):924.
9. Roth M, Johnson PR, Rudiger JJ, King GG, Ge Q, Burgess JK, et al. Interaction between glucocorticoids and beta-2 agonists on bronchial airway smooth muscle cells through synchronized cellular signalling. Lancet. 2002;360(9342):1293-9.
10. Adcock IM, Maneechotesuwan K, Usmani O. Molecular interactions between glucocorticoids and long-acting beta-2 agonists. J Allergy Clin Immunol. 2002;110(Suppl 6):S261-8.
11. Mak JC, Hisada T, Salmon M, Barnes PJ, Chung KF. Glucocorticoids reverse IL-1beta-induced impairment of beta-adrenoceptor-mediated relaxation and upregulation of G-protein-coupled receptor kinases. Br J Pharmacol. 2002;135(4):987-96.
12. Pedersen KE, Bochner BS, Undem BJ. Cysteinyl leukotrienes induce P-selectin expression in human endothelial cells via a non-CysLT1 receptor-mediated mechanism. J Pharmacol Exp Ther. 1997;281(2):655-62.
13. Keogh KA. Leukotriene receptor antagonists and Churg-Strauss syndrome: cause, trigger or merely an association? Drug Saf. 2007;30(10):837-43.
14. Green RL, Vayonis AG. Churg-Strauss syndrome after zafirlukast in two patients not receiving systemic steroid treatment. Lancet. 1999;353(9154):725-6.
15. D'Cruz DP, Barnes NC, Lockwood CM. Difficult asthma or Churg-Strauss syndrome? BMJ. 1999;318(7182):475-6.
16. Committee on Safety of Medicines. Leukotriene antagonists: a new class of asthma treatment. Current Problems in Pharmacovigilance. 1998;24:14.
17. Food and Drug Administration (FDA). Early communication about an ongoing safety review of montelukast (Singulair). [online]. Available from *http://www.fda.gov/cder/drug/early_comm/montelukast.htm*. [Accessed 27 March, 2008].
18. Camargo CA, Gurner DM, Smithline HA, Chapela R, Fabbri LM, Green SA, et al. A randomized placebo-controlled study of intravenous montelukast for the treatment of acute asthma. J Allergy Clin Immunol. 2010;125(2):374-80.
19. Virchow JC, Mehta A, Ljungblad L, Mitfessel H. Add-on montelukast in inadequately controlled asthma patients in a 6-month open-label study: the MONtelukast In Chronic Asthma (MONICA) study. Respir Med. 2010;104(5):644-51.
20. Busse W, Corren J, Lanier BQ, McAlary M, Fowler-Taylor A, Cioppa GD, et al. Omalizumab, anti-IgE recombinant humanized monoclonal antibody, for the treatment of severe allergic asthma. J Allergy Clin Immunol. 2001;108(2):184-90.
21. Soler M, Matz J, Townley R, Buhl R, O'Brien J, Fox H, et al. The anti-IgE antibody omalizumab reduces exacerbations and steroid requirement in allergic asthmatics. Eur Respir J. 2001;18(2):254-61.
22. Nair P, Pizzichini MM, Kjarsgaard M, Inman MD, Efthimiadis A, Pizzichini E, et al. Mepolizumab for prednisone-dependent asthma with sputum eosinophilia. N Engl J Med. 2009;360(10):985-93.
23. Ciarallo L, Brousseau D, Reinert S. Higher dose intravenous magnesium therapy for children with moderate to severe acute asthma. Arch Pediatr Adolesc Med. 2000;154(10):978-83.
24. Silverman RA, Osborn H, Runge J, Gallagher EJ, Chiang W, Feldman J, et al. IV magnesium sulfate in the treatment of acute severe asthma: a multicenter randomized controlled trial. Chest. 2002;122(2):489-97.
25. Hughes R, Goldkorn A, Masoli M, Weatherall M, Burgess C, Beasley R. Use of isotonic nebulised magnesium sulphate as an adjuvant to salbutamol in treatment of severe asthma in adults: randomised placebo-controlled trial. Lancet. 2003;361(9375):2114-7.
26. Hunt LW, Frigas E, Butterfield JH, Kita H, Blomgren J, Dunnette SL, et al. Treatment of asthma with nebulized lidocaine: a randomized, placebo-controlled study. J Allergy Clin Immunol. 2004;113(5):853-9.
27. Ahmed T, Garrigo J, Danta I. Preventing bronchoconstriction in exercise-induced asthma with inhaled heparin. N Engl J Med. 1993;329(2):90-5.
28. Hanania NA, Singh S, El-Wali R, Flashner M, Franklin AE, Garner WJ, et al. The safety and effects of the beta-blocker, nadolol, in mild asthma: an open-label pilot study. Pulm Pharmacol Ther. 2008;21(1):134-41.
29. Dean T, Dewey A, Bara A, Lasserson TJ, Walters EH. Azathioprine as an oral corticosteroid sparing agent for asthma. Cochrane Database Syst Rev. 2004;(1):CD003270.
30. Evans DJ, Cullinan P, Geddes DM. Cyclosporine as an oral corticosteroid sparing agent in stable asthma. Cochrane Database Syst Rev. 2001;(2):CD002993.
31. Evans DJ, Cullinan P, Geddes DM. Gold as an oral corticosteroid sparing agent in stable asthma. Cochrane Database Syst Rev. 2001;(2):CD002985.
32. Schultze-Werninghaus G, Meier-Sydow J. The clinical and pharmacological history of theophylline: first report on the bronchospasmolytic action in man by S. R. Hirsch in Frankfurt (Main) 1922. Clin Allergy. 1982;12(2):211-5.
33. Giembycz MA, Newton R. Beyond the dogma: novel beta-2-adrenoceptor signalling in the airways. Eur Respir J. 2006;27(6):1286-306.
34. Drazen JM, Israel E, Boushey HA, Chinchilli VM, Fahy JV, Fish JE, et al. Comparison of regularly scheduled with as-needed use of albuterol in mild asthma. Asthma Clinical Research Network. N Engl J Med. 1996;335(12):841-7.
35. Walters EH, Walters J. Inhaled short acting beta-2-agonist use in asthma: regular vs as needed treatment. Cochrane Database Syst Rev. 2000;(4):CD001285.
36. Ortega VE, Hawkins GA, Peters SP, Bleecker ER. Pharmacogenetics of the beta 2-adrenergic receptor gene. Immunol Allergy Clin North Am. 2007;27(4):665-84.
37. Walker SR, Evans ME, Richards AJ, Paterson JW. The clinical pharmacology of oral and inhaled salbutamol. Clin Pharmacol Ther. 1972;13(6):861-7.
38. Du XL, Zhu Z, Fu Q, Li DK, Xu WB. Pharmacokinetics and relative bioavailability of salbutamol metered-dose inhaler in healthy volunteers. Acta Pharmacol Sin. 2002;23(7):663-6.
39. Boulton DW, Fawcett JP. Enantioselective disposition of salbutamol in man following oral and intravenous administration. Br J Clin Pharmacol. 1996;41(1):35-40.
40. Bateman E, Nelson H, Bousquet J, Kral K, Sutton L, Ortega H, et al. Meta-analysis: effects of adding salmeterol to inhaled corticosteroids on serious asthma-related events. Ann Intern Med. 2008;149(1):33-42.

41. Nelson HS, Weiss ST, Bleecker ER, Yancey SW, Dorinsky PM. The Salmeterol Multicenter Asthma Research Trial: a comparison of usual pharmacotherapy for asthma or usual pharmacotherapy plus salmeterol. Chest. 2006;129(1):15-26.
42. Salpeter SR, Buckley NS, Ormiston TM, Salpeter EE. Meta-analysis: effect of long-acting beta-agonists on severe asthma exacerbations and asthma-related deaths. Ann Intern Med. 2006;144(12):904-12.
43. Düringer C, Grundström G, Gürcan E, Dainty IA, Lawson M, Korn SH, et al. Agonist-specific patterns of beta-2-adrenoceptor responses in human airway cells during prolonged exposure. Br J Pharmacol. 2009;158(1):169-79.
44. Calverley PM, Anderson JA, Celli B, Ferguson GT, Jenkins C, Jones PW, et al. Salmeterol and fluticasone propionate and survival in chronic obstructive pulmonary disease. N Engl J Med. 2007;356(8):775-89.
45. Westby MJ, Benson MK, Gibson PG. Anticholinergic agents for chronic asthma in adults. Cochrane Database of Systematic Reviews. 2004;(3):CD003269.
46. Rodrigo GJ, Castro-Rodriguez JA. Anticholinergics in the treatment of children and adults with acute asthma: a systematic review with meta-analysis. Thorax. 2005;60(9):740-4.
47. McDonald NJ, Bara AI. Anticholinergic therapy for chronic asthma in children over 2 years of age. Cochrane Database Syst Rev. 2003;(3):CD003535.
48. Guite HF, Dundas R, Burney PG. Risk factors for death from asthma, chronic obstructive pulmonary disease, and cardiovascular disease after a hospital admission for asthma. Thorax. 1999;54(4):301-7.
49. Ringbæk T, Viskum K. Is there any association between inhaled ipratropium and mortality in patients with COPD and asthma? Respir Med. 2003;97(3):264-72.
50. Sin DD, Tu JV. Lack of association between ipratropium bromide and mortality in elderly patients with chronic obstructive airway disease. Thorax. 2000;55(3):194-7.
51. Food and Drug Administration. Tiotropium. [online] Available from *http://www.fda.gov/cder/drug/early_comm/tiotropium.htm.* [Accessed April, 2016].
52. Jansat JM, Lamarca R, Garcia Gil E, Ferrer P. Safety and pharmacokinetics of single doses of aclidinium bromide, a novel long-acting, inhaled antimuscarinic, in healthy subjects. Int J Clin Pharmacol Ther. 2009;47(7):460-8.
53. Mash BR, Bheekie A, Jones P. (2001). Inhaled versus oral steroids for adults with chronic asthma. [online] *http://www2.cochrane.org/reviews/en/ab002160.html.* [Accessed 25 March, 2010].
54. Gauvreau GM, O'Byrne PM, Boulet LP, Wang Y, Cockcroft D, Bigler J, et al. Effects of an anti-TSLP antibody on allergen-induced asthmatic responses. N Engl J Med. 2014;370(22):2102-10.
55. Franciosi LG, Diamant Z, Banner KH, Zuiker R, Morelli N, Kamerling IM, et al. Efficacy and safety of RPL554, a dual PDE3 and PDE4 inhibitor, in healthy volunteers and in patients with asthma or chronic obstructive pulmonary disease: findings from four clinical trials. Lancet Respir Med. 2013;1(9):714-27.
56. Goodacre S, Cohen J, Bradburn M, Gray A, Benger J, Coats T, et al. Intravenous or nebulised magnesium sulphate versus standard therapy for severe acute asthma (3Mg trial): a double-blind, randomised controlled trial. Lancet Respir Med. 2013;1(4):293-300.
57. Powell C, Kolamunnage-Dona R, Lowe J, Boland A, Petrou S, Doull I, et al. Magnesium sulphate in acute severe asthma in children (MAGNETIC): a randomised, placebo-controlled trial. Lancet Respir Med. 2013;1(4):301-8.
58. De Boever EH, Ashman C, Cahn AP, Locantore NW, Overend P, Pouliquen IJ, et al. Efficacy and safety of an anti-IL-13 mAb in patients with severe asthma: a randomized trial. J Allergy Clin Immunol. 2014;133(4):989-96.
59. Busse WW, Holgate S, Kerwin E, Chon Y, Feng J, Lin J, et al. Randomized, double-blind, placebo-controlled study of brodalumab, a human anti-IL-17 receptor monoclonal antibody, in moderate to severe asthma. Am J Respir Crit Care Med. 2013;188(11):1294-302.
60. Snowise NG, Clements D, Ho SY, Follows RM. Addition of a 5-lipoxygenase-activating protein inhibitor to an inhaled corticosteroid (ICS) or an ICS/long-acting beta-2-agonist combination in subjects with asthma. Curr Med Res Opin. 2013;29(12):1663-74.
61. Peters-Golden M, Brock TG. 5-lipoxygenase and FLAP. Prostaglandins Leukot Essent Fatty Acids. 2003;69(2-3):99-109.
62. Lazarinis N, Jørgensen L, Ekström T, Bjermer L, Dahlén B, Pullerits T, et al. Combination of budesonide/formoterol on demand improves asthma control by reducing exercise-induced bronchoconstriction. Thorax. 2014;69(2):130-6.

Childhood Asthma

Meenu Singh, Amit Agarwal, Anil Chauhan

EPIDEMIOLOGY

Bronchial asthma is the most common chronic disease of childhood, affecting an estimated 6 million children. The burden of asthma affects the patients, their families, and the society in terms of loss of work and school days, poorer quality of life, avoidable emergency department visits, hospitalizations and deaths. Improved scientific understanding of asthma has led to significant improvements in asthma care. The International Study of Asthma and Allergies in Children (ISAAC) study noted a significant variation in its prevalence in different parts of India with a range of 0.5–18% in a 12-month prevalence of self-reported asthma symptoms with a written questionnaire.[1] A 20–60 fold difference in prevalence of symptoms was found between various centers involved in this study.

Although prevalence data of allergic disease in India is scarce, the little data that is available suggests that the patterns differ in different areas.[1-4] A study of 271 children from rural areas of Tamil Nadu reported a prevalence of breathing difficulty at any time in the past in 9% of children.[4] In a study from rural areas of North India, the prevalence of chronic cough among children aged 1–15 years (n = 2,275) was 1.06%, two-thirds were due to asthma.[3] Such variable patterns also exist across urban regions. Prevalence rates ranging from 1.9% to 15.7% have been reported. Such national variation, with almost 10–15-fold difference in the prevalence of allergic disorders, is probably unique to India. In a recently conducted study at our center under the aegis of the Asthma Task Force of the Indian Council of Medical Research, a survey was conducted on 10,028 school children (10–15 years of age) belonging to 39 randomly selected schools for the diagnosis of asthma and other atopic disease in Chandigarh. A total of 536 children were found to have a current clinical diagnosis of asthma, allergic rhinitis or eczema with a 3.3% prevalence of asthma. These findings were similar to those of ISAAC surveys conducted earlier at our center.

The comparative prevalence of wheeze in 13–14-year-olds between the two South Asian cities (Galle, Sri Lanka and Chandigarh, India) representing each of the above archetypes has been studied.[5] The validated one page ISAAC questionnaire for 13–14-year-olds was used for the study. Crude prevalence rates and odds ratios [with 95% two sides confidence intervals (CIs) for comparison of prevalence rates] were calculated. The prevalence rate for wheezing in Galle (28.7%) was higher than that in Chandigarh (12.5%). The odd ratios (ORs) for prevalence for Galle versus Chandigarh were: 2.3 (95% CI 1.8–2.9) for lifetime wheezing; 2.1 (95% CI 1.6–2.7) for wheezing in the previous year; 4.8 (95% CI 3.5–6.7) for exercise-related wheeze; and 1.7 (95% CI 1.2–2.3) for physician diagnosed wheeze, thus demonstrating significant differences in wheeze prevalence between the two cities ($p < 0.05$). The numbers of 13–14-year-olds experiencing less than 12 wheezing episodes per year or sleep disturbance due to wheeze of less than one night per week were also significantly higher for Galle. Hence, a higher prevalence of wheeze was noticed in 13–14-year-old children living in an old-fashioned, congested city (Galle) than in a clean city, Chandigarh.

DEFINITION

Clinically, asthma is a complex disorder characterized by variable and recurring symptoms, airflow obstruction, bronchial hyperresponsiveness and an underlying inflammation. The interaction of these features determines clinical manifestations, severity of asthma and the response to treatment.[6,7] Asthma is a chronic inflammatory disorder of airways in which many cells and cellular elements play a role: mast cells, eosinophils, neutrophils, T lymphocytes, macrophages and epithelial cells. In susceptible individuals, this inflammation causes recurrent episodes of cough, particularly at night or early in the morning, wheezing, breathlessness and chest tightness. These episodes are usually associated with widespread, but variable airflow obstruction that is often reversible, either spontaneously or with treatment.

PATHOPHYSIOLOGY

Airway Narrowing

Airway narrowing is the final common pathway leading to symptoms and physiological changes in asthma; with airway narrowing itself likely to be an additional stimulus for remodeling. Several factors contributing to the development of airway narrowing in asthma are listed as under:

- *Airway smooth muscle contraction:* Occurs in response to multiple bronchoconstrictor mediators and neurotransmitters, the predominant mechanism of airway narrowing. It is largely reversed by bronchodilators.
- *Airway edema*: Due to increased microvascular leakage in response to inflammatory mediators. Airway edema may be particularly important during acute exacerbations.
- *Airway thickening*: Results from structural changes, often termed 'remodeling'. Airway thickening is not fully reversible using current therapies, may be important in more severe disease.
- *Mucus hypersecretion*: A product of increased mucus secretion and inflammatory exudates, mucus hypersecretion may lead to luminal occlusion ('mucus plugging').

Airway Hyperresponsiveness

Airway hyperresponsiveness (AHR), a characteristic functional abnormality of asthma, results in airway narrowing in a patient with asthma in response to a stimulus that would be innocuous in a healthy person. This airway narrowing leads to variable airflow limitation and intermittent symptoms. AHR is linked to both inflammation and to repair of airways, and is partially reversible with therapy. The mechanisms of AHR is incompletely understood but includes the following:

- *Excessive contraction of airway smooth muscle*: Results from increased volume and/or contractility of airway smooth muscle cells.
- *Uncoupling of airway contraction*: A result of inflammatory changes in the airway wall that may lead to excessive narrowing of the airways, and a loss of the maximum plateau of contraction that is found in normal airways when bronchoconstrictor substances are inhaled.
- *Thickening of the airway wall*: Edema and structural changes amplify airway narrowing due to contraction of airway smooth muscle for geometric reasons.
- *Sensory nerves*: These may be sensitized by inflammation, leading to exaggerated bronchoconstriction in response to sensory stimuli.

Immunobiology of Asthma

Airway obstruction in asthma is mediated by hyper-responsive bronchial smooth muscle, secreted airway glycoproteins, and inflammatory debris produced by airway goblet cells and other cells, as well as edema or swelling of airway wall. Development of asthma involves the interplay between the host factors and the environmental exposures that occur at a crucial time in the development of immune system. Genetic susceptibility also plays a crucial role in this interaction. A definitive cause of inflammatory process leading to asthma is not yet established.

a. *Innate Immunity*
   Numerous factors may affect the balance between Th1-type and Th2-type cytokine responses in early life and downregulate the Th1 immune response that fights infection. Instead there is dominance of Th2 cells leading to expression of allergic diseases and asthma. This is known as the "hygiene hypothesis", which postulates that certain infections early in life; exposure to other children (e.g. presence of older siblings and early enrolment in childcare, which have greater likelihood of exposure to respiratory infection); less frequent use of antibiotics, and "country living" are associated with a dominant Th1 response and lower incidence of asthma. On the other hand, the absence of these factors is associated with a persistent Th2 response and higher rates of asthma.
b. *Genetic Factors*
   Asthma has an inheritance component, but the genetic factors, which are involved, remain complex. As the linkage of genetic factors to different asthma phenotypes becomes clearer, treatment approaches may become more directed to specific patient phenotypes and genotypes.
c. *Environmental Factors*
   The two major factors that are important in the development, persistence and possibly the severity of asthma are:
   1. Airborne allergens (particularly sensitization and exposure to house dust-mite and *Alternaria*), and
   2. Viral respiratory infections [including respiratory syncytial virus (RSV) and rhinovirus].

Other environmental factors under study are:

- Tobacco smoke (exposure *"in utero"* is associated with an increased risk of wheezing, but it is not certain that this is linked to subsequent development of asthma)
- Air pollution (ozone and particulate matter)
- Diet (obesity or low intake of antioxidants and omega-3 fatty acids).

The association of these factors with the onset of asthma has not been clearly defined. A number of clinical trials have investigated dietary and environmental manipulations, but the trials have not been sufficiently conclusive to permit recommendations.

Knowledge of the importance of inflammation central to pathogenesis of asthma continues to expand and underscores inflammation as the primary target of treatment. Numerous studies indicate that current therapeutic approaches are effective in controlling symptoms, reducing airflow limitation and preventing exacerbations, but currently available treatments do not appear to prevent the progression of asthma in children. As the various phenotypes of asthma are defined and inflammatory and genetic factors become more apparent, new therapeutic approaches will be developed that may allow more specific treatments to the individual patient's needs and circumstances.

DIAGNOSIS

To establish a diagnosis of asthma, the clinician should determine that symptoms of recurrent episodes of airflow obstruction or AHR are present; airflow obstruction is at least partially reversible; and alternative diagnoses are excluded.[6]

Key Symptom Indicators for Considering a Diagnosis of Asthma

The presence of multiple key indicators increases the probability of asthma:

- Wheezing is a high-pitched whistling sound that comes out while breathing out, especially in children. A lack of wheezing and a normal chest examination do not exclude asthma.
- History of any of the following:
  - Cough (worse, particularly at night)
  - Recurrent wheeze
  - Recurrent difficulty in breathing
  - Recurrent chest tightness.
- Symptoms occur or worsen in the presence of:
  - Exercise
  - Viral infection
  - Inhalant allergens (e.g. animals with fur or hair, house dust-mites, mold, pollen)
  - Irritants (tobacco or wood smoke, airborne chemicals)
  - Changes in weather
  - Strong emotional expression (laughing or crying hard)
  - Stress
  - Menstrual cycles
- Symptoms occur or worsen at night, awakening the patient.

Recommended Methods to Establish the Diagnosis According to Expert Panel Report III

- Detailed medical history.
- *Physical examination*: It may reveal findings that increase the probability of asthma, but the absence of these findings does not rule out asthma because the disease is variable and signs may be absent between episodes. The examination focuses on:
  - Upper respiratory tract (increased nasal secretion, mucosal swelling, and/or nasal polyps)
  - Chest (sounds of wheezing during normal breathing or prolonged phase of forced exhalation, hyperexpansion of the thorax, use of accessory muscles, appearance of hunched shoulders, chest deformity); and skin (atopic dermatitis, eczema).
- Spirometry can demonstrate obstruction and assess reversibility in patients of more than 5 years of age. Patients' perceptions of airflow obstruction are highly variable. Spirometry is an essential objective measure to establish the diagnosis of asthma, the medical history and physical examination are not reliable means of excluding other diagnoses or of assessing lung status. Spirometry is generally recommended, rather than measurements by a peak flow meter, due to wide variability in peak flow meters and reference values. Peak flow meters are designed for monitoring, not as diagnostic tools.

A differential diagnosis of asthma should be considered. Recurrent episodes of cough and wheezing most often are due to asthma in both children and adults; other significant causes of airway obstruction leading to wheeze must be considered both in the initial diagnosis and if there is no clear response to initial therapy.

- Additional studies are not routinely necessary, but may be useful when considering alternative diagnoses
- Additional pulmonary function studies, such as diffusing capacity, measures of lung volumes and evaluation of inspiratory flow-volume loops will help if there are questions about other diseases such as a restrictive defect, vocal cord dysfunction or bullous lung diseases

Bronchoprovocation with methacholine, histamine, cold air or exercise challenge may be useful when asthma is suspected and spirometry is normal or near normal. For safety reasons, bronchoprovocation should be carried out only by a trained individual. A positive test for AHR, which is a characteristic feature of asthma is diagnostic, but can also be present in other conditions. Thus, a positive test is consistent with asthma, but a negative test may be more helpful to rule out asthma.

- Chest X-ray may be needed to exclude other diagnoses
- Biomarkers of inflammation are currently being evaluated for their usefulness in the diagnosis and assessment of asthma. Biomarkers include total and differential cell count and mediator assays in sputum, blood, urine and exhaled air.

Common Diagnostic Challenges

- *Cough variant asthma*: Cough can be the principal or only manifestation of asthma, especially in young children. Monitoring of peak expiratory flow (PEF) or bronchoprovocation may be helpful. Diagnosis is confirmed by a positive response to asthma medications.
- Vocal cord dysfunction (VCD), which is seen commonly in adolescent girls, can mimic asthma, but it is a distinct disorder. Vocal cord dysfunction may coexist with asthma. Asthma medications typically do little to relieve VCD symptoms. Variable flattening of inspiratory flow loop on spirometry is strongly suggestive of VCD. Diagnosis of VCD is made from indirect or direct vocal cord visualization

during an episode, during which the abnormal adduction can be documented. VCD should be considered in difficult-to-treat, atypical asthma patients and in athletes who have exercise-related breathlessness unresponsive to asthma medication.

- Gastroesophageal reflux disease (GERD), obstructive sleep apnea (OSA) and allergic bronchopulmonary aspergillosis (ABPA) may coexist with asthma and complicate diagnosis. Children in the age group of 0–4 years pose particularly a challenge. Diagnosis in infants and young children is elusive, complicated by the difficulty in obtaining objective measurements of lung function in this age group. Caution is needed to avoid giving inappropriate, prolonged asthma therapy. It is important to avoid under-diagnosing asthma by using such labels as "wheezy bronchitis", "recurrent pneumonia", or "reactive airway disease (RAD)", thereby missing the opportunity to treat a child. The chronic airway inflammatory response and structural changes that are characteristic of asthma can develop in the preschool years, and appropriate asthma treatment will reduce the morbidity.

GUIDELINE-BASED MANAGEMENT OF ASTHMA

National Asthma Education and Prevention Program (NAEPP) is dedicated to translating research findings into clinical practice.[7] The first NAEPP guidelines were published in 1991, and updates were made in 1997, 2002 and 2007. Important gains have been made in reducing morbidity and mortality rates due to asthma; however, challenges remain. Several guidelines have been made in India for adults as well as for children.

The goal of NAEPP, EPR3 2007 guideline,[7] is to help people with asthma control their disease so that they are active all day and sleep well at night. New focus of management is on monitoring asthma control as the goal for asthma therapy and distinguishing between classifying asthma severity and monitoring asthma control **(Fig. 1)**. The impairment and the risk are the two key domains of assessment of severity and control. The domains represent different manifestations of asthma, they may not correlate with each other, and may respond differentially to treatment. Impairment represents the frequency and intensity of symptoms and functional limitations, the patient is experiencing currently or has recently experienced. Risk represents the likelihood of either asthma exacerbations, progressive decline in lung function or for children, lung growth; or risk of adverse effects from medication. Modifications have been made in stepwise approach to managing long-term asthma.

Treatment recommendations are presented for three age groups (0–4 years of age, 5–11 years of age, and youths more than 12 years of age and adults) because of several different reasons:

- The course of the disease may change over time;
- The relevance of different measures of impairment or risk and potential short- and long-term impact of medications may be age-related; and
- Varied levels of scientific evidence are available for these three age groups.

The stepwise approach expands to six steps to simplify actions within each step **(Fig. 2)**. Previous guidelines had several progressive actions within different steps; these are now separated into different steps. Medications also have been repositioned within the six steps of care. The new emphasis is made on multifaceted approaches to patient education and to the control of environmental factors or comorbid conditions that affect asthma. Modifications to treatment strategies for managing asthma exacerbations have also been improvised.

Management

Goal of Therapy: Control of Asthma

a. *Reduce impairment*
   - Prevent chronic and troublesome symptoms (e.g. coughing or breathlessness in daytime, in the night, or after exertion)
   - Require infrequent use (≤2 days a week) of inhaled short-acting beta agonists (SABA) for quick relief of symptoms [not including prevention of exercise-induced bronchospasm (EIB)]
   - Maintain (near) normal pulmonary function
   - Maintain normal activity levels (including exercise and other physical activity and attendance at school or work)
   - Meet patients' and families' expectations of and satisfaction with asthma care.

b. *Reduce risk*
   - Prevent recurrent exacerbations of asthma and minimize the need for emergency department visits or hospitalizations
   - Prevent loss of lung function; for children, prevent reduced lung growth
   - Provide optimal pharmacotherapy with minimal or no adverse effects of therapy.

ROUTE OF ADMINISTRATION

Inhaled administration delivers drugs directly into the airways, producing higher local concentrations with significantly less risk of systemic side effects. However, mishandling of inhalers is the most common cause of poor control of asthma.[8] Inhaled medications for asthma are available as pressurized metered-dose inhalers (pMDIs), breath-actuated pMDIs, dry powder inhalers (DPIs), soft mist inhalers and nebulized or "wet" aerosols. Inhaler devices differ in their efficiency of drug delivery to the lower respiratory tract, depending on

Components of severity		Assessing asthma control and adjusting therapy in children					
		Well-controlled		Not well-controlled		Very poorly controlled	
		Ages 0–5	Ages 5–11	Ages 0–5	Ages 5–11	Ages 0–5	Ages 5–11
Impairment	Symptoms	≤2 days/week. But not more than once on each day		2 days/week or multiple times on <2 days/week		Throughout the day	
	Night-time awakenings	≤1x/month		>1x/month	≥2x/month	>1x/week	≥2x/week
	Interference with normal activity	None		Some limitation		Extremely limited	
	Short-acting beta-2 agonist use for symptom control (Prevention for EBI)	≤2 days/week		>2 days/week		Several times per day	
	Lung function • FEV_1 predicted or peak flow (Personal best)	N/A	>80%	N/A	60–80%	N/A	<60%
	• FEV_1/FVC		>80%		75–80%		<80%
Risk	Exacerbations requiring oral systemic corticosteroids	0–1x/year		>2–3 x/year	>2x/year	>3x/year	≥2x/year
	Reduce in lung growth	N/A	Requires long-term follow-ups	N/A		N/A	
	Treatment-related adverse effects	Medication side effects can vary in intensity from none to very troublesome and worrisome. The level of intensity does not correlate to specific levels of control but should be considered in the overall assessment of risk.					
Recommended action for treatment (see "Stepwise Approach for Managing Asthma" for treated steps) The stepwise approach is meant to assist, not replace the clinical decision making required to meet individual patient needs.		• Maintain current step • Regular follow-up every 1–6 months • Consider step down if well-controlled for at least 3 months.		Step up 1 step	Step up at least 1 step	• Consider short course of oral systemic corticosteroids • Step up 1–2 steps.	
				• Before step up: Review adherence to medication, inhaler technique and environmental control. If alternative treatment was used, discontinue it and use preferred treatment for that step. • Re-evaluate the level of asthma control in 2–6 months to achieve control, every 1–6 months to maintain control. *Children 0–4 years old:* If no clear benefit is observed in 4–6 weeks, consider alternative diagnoses or adjusting therapy. *Children 5–11 years old:* Adjust therapy accordingly. • For side effects, consider alternative treatment options.			

Contd...

Contd...

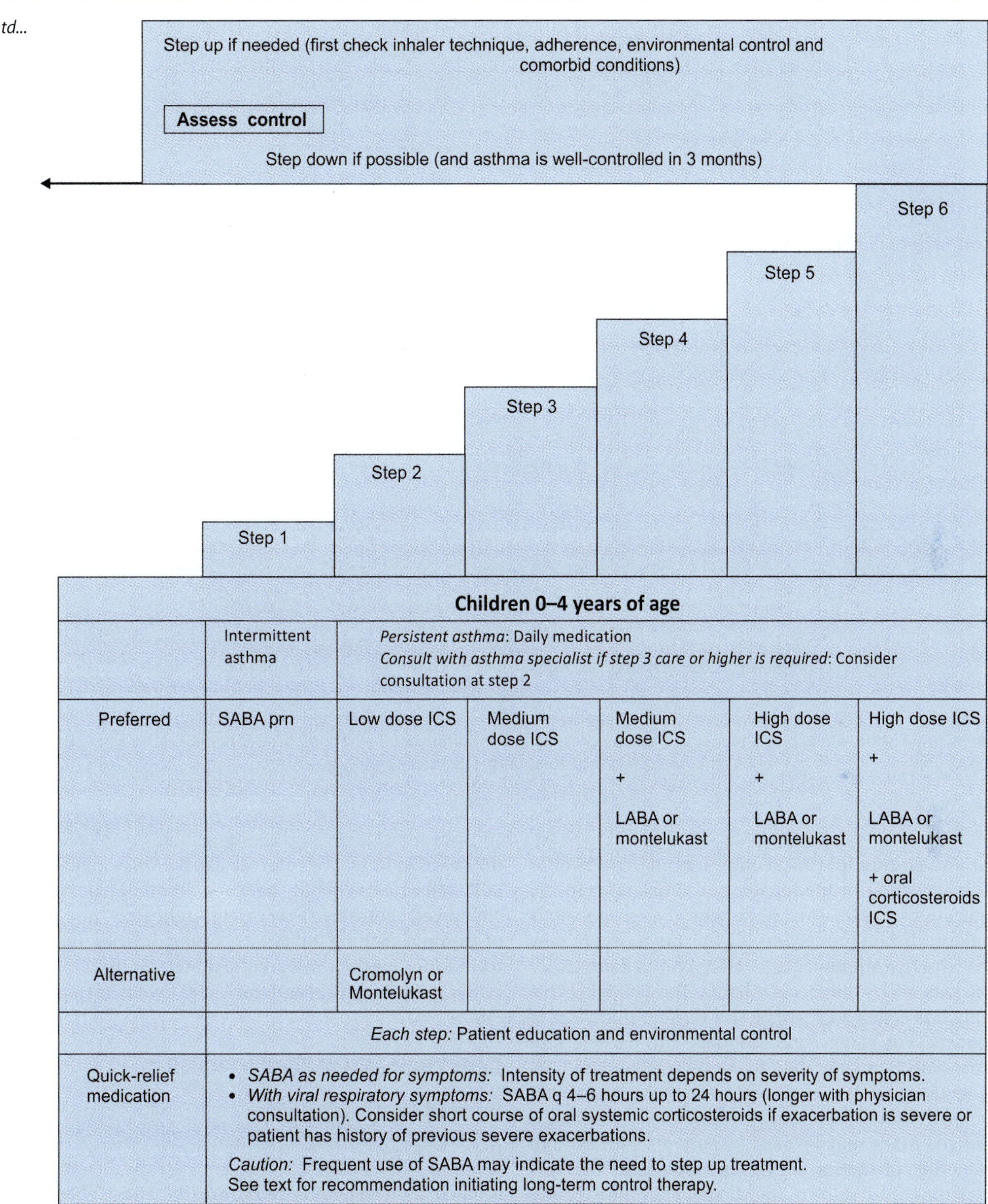

Children 0–4 years of age						
	Intermittent asthma	*Persistent asthma*: Daily medication *Consult with asthma specialist if step 3 care or higher is required*: Consider consultation at step 2				
Preferred	SABA prn	Low dose ICS	Medium dose ICS	Medium dose ICS + LABA or montelukast	High dose ICS + LABA or montelukast	High dose ICS + LABA or montelukast + oral corticosteroids ICS
Alternative		Cromolyn or Montelukast				
	Each step: Patient education and environmental control					
Quick-relief medication	• *SABA as needed for symptoms:* Intensity of treatment depends on severity of symptoms. • *With viral respiratory symptoms:* SABA q 4–6 hours up to 24 hours (longer with physician consultation). Consider short course of oral systemic corticosteroids if exacerbation is severe or patient has history of previous severe exacerbations. *Caution:* Frequent use of SABA may indicate the need to step up treatment. See text for recommendation initiating long-term control therapy.					

Fig. 1 Assessing asthma control and adjusting therapy in children
Source: Adapted from Expert Panel Report-3 (EPR-3) guidelines for asthma[7]

the form of device, formulation of medication, particle size, velocity of the aerosol cloud or plume (where applicable), and ease with which the device can be used by the majority of patients. Individual patient preference, convenience, and ease of use may influence not only the efficiency of drug delivery but also patient adherence to treatment. Problems with incorrect inhaler technique are common in community-based studies, regardless of device, and are associated with

Children 5–11 years of age						
	Intermittent asthma	*Persistent asthma:* Daily medication *Consult with asthma specialist if step 3 care or higher is required:* Consider consultation at step 2				
Preferred	SABA prn	Low dose ICS	Low dose ICS + LABA, LTRA or Therapy line	Medium dose ICS + LABA	High dose ICS + LABA	High dose ICS + LABA + oral corticosteroids
Alternative		Cromolyn LTRA Nedocromil or Therapy line	Medium dose ICS	Medium dose ICS + LTRA or Therapy line	High dose ICS + LTRA or Therapy line	High dose ICS + LTRA + oral corticosteroids
	Each step: Patient education and environmental control and management of comorbidities *Step 2–4:* Consider subcutaneous allergen immunotherapy for patients who have persistent, allergic asthma					
Quick-relief medication	• *SABA as needed for symptoms:* Intensity of treatment depends on severity of symptoms: up to 3 treatments at 20-minutes intervals as needed. Short course of oral systemic corticosteroids may be needed. Exacerbation is severe or patient has history of previous severe exacerbations. *Caution:* Increase use of SABA or use >2 days a week for symptoms relief (no prevention of EIB) generally indicates inadequate control and the need to step up treatment.					

Fig. 2 Stepwise approach for managing asthma in children, 0–4 years and 5–11 years of age
Abbreviations: SABA, short-acting beta agonists; prn, when necessary (*pro re nata*); ICS, inhaled corticosteroids; LABA, long-acting beta agonist; LTRA, leukotriene receptor antagonist; EIB, exercise-induced asthma

worse asthma control. pMDIs require training and skill to coordinate activation of the inhaler and inhalation. In the past, medications in pMDIs were dispensed as suspensions in chlorofluorocarbon propellants (CFCs), but most are now dispensed with hydrofluoroalkane (HFAs) propellant, either as suspensions or as solutions in ethanol. The aerosol plume of HFA inhalers is generally softer and warmer than that of CFC products. For some corticosteroids, the particle size for HFA aerosols is smaller than for the corresponding CFC product, resulting in less oral deposition (with associated reduction in oral side effects), and greater lung deposition.

Pressurized MDIs may be used by patients with asthma of any severity, including during exacerbations. Patients require training and skill to coordinate activation of the inhaler and inhalation, and this is often easier with use of a valved spacer. Breath-actuated aerosols may be helpful for patients who have difficulty using conventional pMDIs. Dry powder inhalers are generally easier to use than pMDIs, but sufficient inspiratory flow (which varies between different DPI devices) is required to disaggregate the powder, and this may prove difficult for some patients to generate. DPIs differ with respect to the fraction of ex-actuator dose delivered to lung. For some drugs, the dose may need to be adjusted when switching between different types of devices. Nebulized aerosols are rarely indicated for treatment of chronic asthma in adults. Some inhaler devices and techniques for their use are illustrated on the GINA website (www.ginasthma.org) and the ADMIT website *(www.admit-online.info)*.

CONTROLLER MEDICATIONS

Inhaled Corticosteroids

Role in Therapy

Inhaled corticosteroids (ICS) are the most effective anti-inflammatory medications for the treatment of persistent asthma. Studies have demonstrated their efficacy in reducing asthma symptoms, improving quality of life, improving lung function, reducing the frequency and severity of exacerbations and reducing asthma mortality, as well as decreasing AHR and controlling airway inflammation. They do not cure asthma, and when discontinued, approximately 25% of patients experience an exacerbation within 6 months.

Patients not receiving ICS appear to be at increased risk of airway remodeling and loss of lung function. ICS differ in their potency and bioavailability, but because of relatively flat dose-response relationships in asthma relatively few studies have been able to confirm the clinical relevance of these differences.

ICS/LABA Combinations

Role in Therapy

When a medium dose of ICS alone fails to achieve good control of asthma, addition of LABA is the preferred option, preferably as a combination ICS/LABA inhaler. The addition of LABA to ICS improves clinical asthma outcomes and reduces the number of exacerbations, does not increase the risk of asthma-related hospitalizations, and achieves clinical control of asthma in more patients, more rapidly, and at a lower dose of ICS than with ICS given alone.[6] Controlled studies have shown that delivering ICS and LABA in a combination inhaler is as effective as giving each drug separately. Fixed combination inhalers are more convenient for patients, may increase adherence compared with using separate inhalers, and ensure that the LABA is always accompanied by ICS.[8]

Adverse Effects

Therapy with LABAs may be associated with headache or cramps, but systemic adverse effects such as cardiovascular stimulation, skeletal muscle tremor and hypokalemia, are less common than with oral beta-agonist therapy. The regular use of beta-2-agonists in both short- and long-acting forms may lead to relative refractoriness to beta-2-agonists. Based on data indicating a possible increased risk of asthma-related death associated with use of salmeterol in a small number of individuals, and increased risk of exacerbations when LABA is used regularly as monotherapy, LABAs should never be used as a substitute for inhaled or oral corticosteroids. LABAs are used only in combination with an appropriate dose of ICS as determined by a physician.

Achieving and Maintaining Asthma Control Requires Four Components of Care

1. Assessment and monitoring.
2. Education for a partnership in care.
3. Control of environmental factors and comorbid conditions.
4. Medications.

A stepwise approach to asthma management incorporates these four components, emphasizing that pharmacologic therapy is initiated based on asthma severity and adjusted (stepped up or down) based on the level of asthma control. Special considerations of therapeutic options within the stepwise approach may be necessary for situations such as EIB, surgery and others. This approach is used for assessing a patient's overall asthma severity, once the most optimal asthma control is achieved and maintained, or for population-based evaluations.

REFERENCES

1. Worldwide variations in the prevalence of asthma symptoms: the International Study of Asthma and Allergies in Childhood (ISAAC). Eur Respir J. 1998;12(2):315-35.
2. Chakravarthy S, Singh RB, Swaminathan S, Venkatesan P. Prevalence of asthma in urban and rural children in Tamil Nadu. Natl Med J India. 2002;15(5):260-3.
3. Singh D, Arora V, Sobti PC. Chronic recurrent cough in rural children in Ludhiana, Punjab. Ind Pediatr. 2002;39(1):23-9.
4. Paramesh H. Epidemiology of asthma in India. Ind J Pediatr. 2002;69(4):309-12.
5. Mistry R, Wickramasingha N, Ogston S, Singh M, Devasiri V, Mukhopadhyay S. Wheeze and urban variation in South Asia. Eur J Pediatr. 2004;163(3):145-7.
6. Global Initiative for Asthma. (2014). Global strategy for asthma management and prevention. [online] Available from *www.ginaasthma.com*. [Accessed March 2016].
7. National Asthma Education and Prevention Programme. (2007). EPR III Guidelines. [online] Available from *www.nhlbi.nih.gov*. [Accessed March 2016].
8. Melani AS, Bonavia M, Cilenti V, Cinti C, Lodi M, Martucci P, et al. Inhaler mishandling remains common in real life and is associated with reduced disease control. Respir Med. 2011;105:930-8.

Allergic Bronchopulmonary Aspergillosis

Ritesh Agarwal

INTRODUCTION

Aspergillus spp. can cause several noninfective pulmonary disorders including allergic bronchopulmonary aspergillosis (ABPA), severe asthma with fungal sensitization and others **(Table 1)**.[1] ABPA is a complex immunological pulmonary disorder caused by hypersensitivity to antigenic products released by *Aspergillus fumigatus* colonizing the tracheobronchial tree of patients with bronchial asthma and cystic fibrosis (CF), with resultant systemic immune activation.[2-4] This may clinically manifest as chronic asthma, recurrent pulmonary infiltrates and bronchiectasis.[5] The disease remains underdiagnosed in many countries; as many as one-third of all cases are initially misdiagnosed as pulmonary tuberculosis in the developing countries.[6-9] The disorder was first described by Hinson et al. in 1952 in the United Kingdom,[10] in 1957 from Australia,[11] and in 1958 from the United States.[12] From India, the first case was described in 1971.[13] More than 6 decades have elapsed since the first description of ABPA, yet the condition remains poorly understood.[14] The International Society of Human and Animal Mycology (ISHAM) has also formed a working group on "ABPA in asthmatics" to enable collaborative research on this subject. The working group has laid down new criteria for diagnosis and classification of ABPA.[15] This will hopefully facilitate early diagnosis and better stratification of the disease for future studies and drug trials.

Table 1 Noninfective allergic pulmonary syndromes caused by *Aspergillus* species

• *Aspergillus*-sensitized asthma	• Bronchial asthma (nonsevere) • *Aspergillus* sensitization • IgE <500 IU/mL
• Severe asthma with fungal sensitization	• Bronchial asthma (severe) • *Aspergillus* sensitization • IgE <1,000 IU/mL • No evidence of ABPA
• Allergic bronchopulmonary aspergillosis (ABPA)	• Bronchial asthma • IgE >1,000 IU/mL • Bronchiectasis • Raised specific IgE, eosinophil count
• Serologic ABPA (ABPA-s)	• ABPA • No evidence of lung damage in the form of bronchiectasis
• ABPA with bronchiectasis	• ABPA • Evidence of lung damage in the form of bronchiectasis
• Hypersensitivity pneumonitis	• Acute to subacute exposure to *Aspergillus* • Centrilobular nodules with ground glass opacities on computed tomography of the chest

The disease presents with varied clinical and radiological manifestations ranging from an asymptomatic patient with or without pulmonary infiltrates to severe uncontrolled asthma with or without central bronchiectasis (CB) and pulmonary fibrosis.[16-23] A lung biopsy is generally not required, and the diagnosis can often be made on clinical, radiologic and serologic grounds.[24] An early diagnosis is not difficult in the presence of an increased clinical suspicion. However, there are reports of mean diagnostic latency of as long as 10 years between the occurrence of first symptoms and the diagnosis.[25] In the past 2 decades, there has been an increase in the number of cases possibly due to the heightened physician awareness and availability of serologic assays for the diagnosis of ABPA.[6-8,26,27] This chapter summarizes the current concepts in pathogenesis, diagnosis and management of this complex entity.

CHARACTERIZATION OF *ASPERGILLUS* SPECIES

Aspergillus was first catalogued in 1729 by the Italian biologist Pietro Antonio Micheli and the species *A. fumigatus* was described in 1863 by Johann Baptist Georg Wolfgang Fresenius. There are approximately 250 species of *Aspergillus* but only a few are known to be pathogenic for humans.[28] *A. fumigatus*, *A. flavus* and *A. niger* are the most commonly encountered pathogenic species.[29] It is of interest to note that only pathogenic species (e.g. *A. fumigatus, A. flavus* and others) can grow at body temperature. *Aspergillus* is a ubiquitous mold found in organic debris, dust, compost, foods, spices and rotted plants. It is also one of the most common indoor molds especially in the attics and basements, bedding, curtains, floor mats and house dust. Worldwide surveys have found that *Aspergillus* species represent between 0.1% and 22% of the total sampled air spores.[30] *Aspergillus* species are thermotolerant and capable of growing at a wide range of temperatures. These fungi can be cultured using Sabouraud's agar medium at 37°C in contrast to many other fungi whose growth is inhibited beyond 35°C. The spores of *A. fumigatus* (2–3.5 µm in size) are in the respirable range, can thus easily enter the airways. In susceptible persons, spores germinate into hyphae which colonize the bronchi. *Aspergillus* is recognized by its filamentous, septate hyphae appearance, approximately 3–7 µm wide with Y-shaped branching in tissue preparations.

The clinical, radiological and histological manifestations of bronchopulmonary aspergillosis are due to a complex interplay between the number and virulence of the organisms and the patient's immune response.[31] Depending on the host immunity and the organism virulence, *Aspergillus* can cause a variety of respiratory diseases, which include simple colonization, aspergilloma, hypersensitivity pneumonitis, *Aspergillus*-sensitized asthma, severe asthma with fungal sensitization, ABPA, chronic pulmonary aspergillosis (CPA), invasive airway aspergillosis and invasive pulmonary aspergillosis.[32-35] ABPA is the best recognized manifestation of *Aspergillus*-associated hypersensitivity disorders. An ABPA like syndrome can also be caused by numerous fungi other than *A. fumigatus*, and is known as allergic bronchopulmonary mycosis (ABPM).[36]

EPIDEMIOLOGY OF ALLERGIC BRONCHOPULMONARY ASPERGILLOSIS

Aspergillus sensitization (AS), also known as *Aspergillus* hypersensitivity (AH) is defined by the presence of an increase in *Aspergillus* specific immunoglobulin E (IgE) levels or an immediate-type cutaneous hypersensitivity to commercial (or an indigenously prepared) extracts of *Aspergillus*.[37-39] ABPA can be conceptualized as an exaggerated form of AS and AS is currently considered as the first step in the development of ABPA.[40] Only a small proportion of patients with AS develop the complete clinical picture of ABPA.[7-9,40] Despite numerous published case series on ABPA, the exact prevalence of AS and/or ABPA in bronchial asthma remain speculative because of the lack of population-based data for this purpose.[41] The National Health and Nutrition Examination Survey (NHANES) conducted in the United States provides the only available population based data for AS, where the prevalence of AS was found to be 6.4% using *A. fumigatus* specific IgE levels.[42] The prevalence of AS/ABPA is likely to be higher in special clinics than in the community, and may vary by the risk factor (bronchial asthma or CF), ethnicity and exposure risk. The prevalence of AS will also vary depending on the type of skin tests (intracutaneous vs prick tests) and the antigens (commercial vs locally prepared) employed for the performance of these skin tests.[41,43] Hence, future studies should utilize specific IgE levels for the purpose of estimating AS.

The population prevalence of ABPA is generally stated about 1–2% in patients with bronchial asthma and 2–15% in patients with CF.[3,23,44,45] This estimate is based on the inference of only three studies and may not be entirely correct.[46,47] In the only peer-reviewed study, 14 patients with ABPM were identified from a total of 1,390 new referrals in a catchment area population of around half a million, estimating a period prevalence of just above 1%.[46] In a questionnaire-based study carried out in 2.4 million people (orange county, California), there were 143 cases of ABPA under the care of pulmonary and allergy specialists.[47] In another analysis conducted in 1991, the ABPA committee of the American Academy of Allergy, Asthma and Immunology performed a survey among the members of academy to find the number of ABPA cases under their treatment. Of the 33% respondents, it was observed that 703 patients with ABPA were under current care and other physicians shared 49% of them. If the same case rate is assumed amongst nonrespondents, this figure might increase to 2 thousand. Both the above surveys from the United States projected the maximum number of ABPA patients as around 11 thousand, which in 1991 (in the 260 million United States population), represented 1% of the estimated 12 million asthma patients in the United States.

In a scoping review, Denning et al. assumed the prevalence of ABPA of about 2.5% in secondary care cohorts. The global burden of ABPA was then estimated at about 4.8 million (range 1.4–6.8) patients in a worldwide asthma population of 193 million.[48] The prevalence of ABPA in asthma is likely to be much higher than currently believed. In a systematic review, we demonstrated a pooled prevalence of AS and ABPA of 28% (95% CI, 24–34) and 12.9% (95% CI, 7.9–18.9), respectively.[41] The only limitation of this analysis was that all studies were performed in specialized chest or asthma clinics, which could represent a selection bias as only the most symptomatic patients were likely to reach these clinics, thus may not represent the true population prevalence of ABPA.

The prevalence of ABPA involving asthma from India, is generally higher than that reported from other centers. The prevalence of ABPA in bronchial asthma reported in 10 large studies in the last decade **(Table 2)**[8,9,27,49-55] shows a significantly higher prevalence in the Indian studies compared to studies published from other countries [292/1,855 (15.7%) vs 24/707 (3.3%); p <0.00001]. The prevalence of AS and ABPA is even higher in patients with severe acute asthma. In a study conducted in 57 patients with severe acute asthma admitted to a respiratory intensive care unit (ICU), we found the prevalence of AS and ABPA of around 51% and 39%,

Table 2 Studies describing the prevalence of *Aspergillus* sensitization (AS) and/or allergic bronchopulmonary aspergillosis in patients with bronchial asthma over the last decade

Study	*Country*	*Type of study*	*Criteria used for diagnosis of ABPA*§	*Prevalence of AH in asthma (n/N)*	*Prevalence of ABPA in asthma (n/N)*
Eaton et al.[49]	New Zealand	Prospective	5 major	47/255	9/243
Kumar et al.[50]	India	Prospective	5 major	47/200	32/200
Al-Mobeireek et al.[27]	Saudi Arabia	Prospective	5 major	12/53	7/264*
Maurya et al.[51]	India	Prospective	8 major	30/105	8/105
Agarwal et al.[8]	India	Prospective	5 major	291/755	155/755
Prasad et al.[52]	India	Prospective	5 major	74/244	18/244
Agarwal et al.[9]	India	Prospective	5 major	87/242	54/242
Ghosh et al. (2010)[53]	India	Prospective	5 major, 1 minor	54/215	15/215
Sarkar et al. (2010)[54]	India	Prospective	4 of (A/T/I/C/S)	40/126	10/126*
Ma et al. (2011)[55]	China	Prospective	–	11/200	5/200

§*Criteria for ABPA*: Major (A-asthma, R-radiologic opacities, T-immediate positive skin test, E-eosinophilia, P-precipitins to *A. fumigatus*, I-IgE elevated, C-central bronchiectasis, S-specific IgG/IgE to *A. fumigatus*); Minor (C-sputum cultures of *A. fumigatus*, S-type III skin test positivity, B-brownish black mucus plugs);
*Allergic bronchopulmonary mycosis
Abbreviations: ABPA, allergic bronchopulmonary aspergillosis; AH, *Aspergillus* hypersensitivity

respectively in severe acute asthma compared to the AS and ABPA prevalence of 39% and 21%, respectively in the outpatient bronchial asthma.[56] With the best assumption of the population prevalence of ABPA complicating asthma of about 5% in India, the burden of ABPA was estimated as about 1.38 million in adult asthmatic population of about 27.7 million.[57]

PATHOGENESIS OF ALLERGIC BRONCHOPULMONARY ASPERGILLOSIS

The reason why only a minority of asthmatics develop ABPA is not fully understood.[4] Exposure to high concentrations of *A. fumigatus* spores from garbage dump sites, agricultural conditions, bird droppings and smoking moldy marijuana have been reported to cause ABPA.[10,58-61] Environmental factors are currently not considered as the main pathogenetic factors in causation of ABPA because not all asthmatics develop ABPA despite being exposed to the same environment.[62] Fungal conidia do not elicit any immunological reaction because the surface hydrophobin prevents immune recognition of the spores.[63] In patients with asthma and CF, inhaled conidia of *A. fumigatus* and occasionally other fungi, due to defective clearance, are able to germinate leading to the growth of hyphae in mucus plugs. In healthy individuals, *Aspergillus* is rapidly cleared by alveolar macrophages utilizing oxidase-dependent killing mechanisms, with the immune reaction to *Aspergillus* being a Th1 CD4+ T cell response.[64]

Table 3 Genetic factors associated with allergic bronchopulmonary aspergillosis

• Presence of HLA-DR-2 and DR-5; absence of HLA-DQ2 sequences[66,75,76,91]
• Mannose-binding lectin polymorphisms[81,85,90]
• Surfactant protein A gene polymorphisms[79,85]
• Toll-like receptor 9 gene polymorphisms[86]
• Interleukin-4 receptor-α polymorphisms[83]
• Interleukin-10 promoter polymorphisms[80,84]
• Interleukin-13 polymorphisms[82]
• Transforming growth factor-β polymorphisms[84]
• Tumor necrosis factor-α polymorphisms[84]
• CFTR gene mutation[74,77,78,88,89]
• Chitotriosidase gene polymorphisms[87]
Abbreviations: HLA, human leukocyte antigen; CFTR, cystic fibrosis transmembrane conductance regulator

The immune response in AS/ABPA is not only a Th2 CD4+ T cell response,[65-69] but is also quantitatively greater in ABPA than AS.[65,70-72] This aberrant response is currently believed due to a genetically susceptibility to the disorder,[73] and several defects have been described in innate and adaptive immunity **(Table 3)**.[66,74-91] Familial occurrence of about 5% has been documented in ABPA.[92]

The fungi release antigens and exoproteases that compromise mucociliary clearance, stimulate and breach the airway epithelial barrier, and activate the innate immune system of the lung, including the epithelial and the alveolar production of several inflammatory cytokines.[93-96] This leads to influx of inflammatory cells including the neutrophils and the eosinophils with resultant early and late-phase inflammatory reactions.[97,98] The antigens are further processed by the antigen presenting cells and presented to T-cells. There is activation of both Th1 and Th2 responses, but heavily skewed towards a Th2 CD4+ T-cell response with release of IL-4, IL-5 and IL-13.[66-69] The Th2 cytokines lead to total and *A. fumigatus* specific IgE synthesis, mast cell degranulation and promotion of a strong eosinophilic response. The inflammatory cells (partly contributed by fungal proteases) lead to tissue injury and the characteristic pathology of ABPA. Animal models suggest the necessity of both IgE and IgG anti-*Aspergillus* antibodies in the pathogenesis of the disease.[99,100]

PATHOLOGY OF ALLERGIC BRONCHOPULMONARY ASPERGILLOSIS

The pathology of ABPA varies from patient to patient **(Table 4)** and is different in different areas of the lung in the same patient.[101] Although, the clinical picture of ABPA is well documented, detailed information is not available on its pathology, which reflects the fact that the diagnosis is primarily based on immunological investigations and only a minority of patients require lung biopsy. The finding of proximal bronchiectasis, i.e. involvement of segmental and subsegmental bronchi with sparing of the distal branches is typical of ABPA.[102] The bronchi are filled with thick tenacious mucus plugs of dense eosinophilic material with many cells and granular debris. Histopathological examination reveals the presence of mucus, fibrin, Curschmann's spirals, Charcot-Leyden crystals and inflammatory cells. Scanty hyphae can often be demonstrated in the bronchiectatic cavities. The bronchial wall in ABPA is usually infiltrated by inflammatory cells, primarily the eosinophils.[102] The peribronchial parenchyma contains a mixed chronic inflammatory response, often with conspicuous eosinophilia.

Table 4 Pathologic findings encountered in allergic bronchopulmonary aspergillosis

• Bronchiectasis involving segmental and subsegmental bronchi with sparing of distal bronchi
• Eosinophilic pneumonia
• Eosinophilic bronchitis
• Granulomatous bronchiolitis or bronchocentric granulomatosis
• Bronchiolitis obliterans with organizing pneumonia
• Localized tissue invasion by *A. fumigatus* without vascular invasion.

Recurrent or transient parenchymal opacities are generally the result of eosinophilic pneumonia. Occasionally, fungal growth in the lung parenchyma can occur in some patients with ABPA.[103] Patients can also demonstrate a pattern similar to that of bronchiolitis obliterans with organizing pneumonia.[104] A prominent feature is the presence of noncaseating granulomatous inflammation containing eosinophils and multinucleated giant cells centered on the airways, referred to as bronchocentric granulomatosis.[105,106] Fungal hyphas may be identified in the centers of some granulomas in the peribronchial tissue. The pathologic appearance is quite distinct from that of necrotizing pneumonia with vascular invasion described in patients with invasive aspergillosis. In patients with ABPA and localized tissue invasion, the host response seems to be able to limit the growth of the fungus and severe tissue destruction does not occur. Rarely, cases of invasive aspergillosis complicating the course of ABPA have been described in the literature.[107-112]

Clinical Features

Most patients are diagnosed in the 3rd–4th decades and there is no gender predilection.[113] Although, the initial descriptions involved mainly the adults, an increasing awareness of the disorder has led to recognition of the disease in infancy[114] and early childhood.[115] The clinical features of ABPA encountered in three large series published from the author's institute are summarized in **Table 5**.[6,8,9] The most common clinical presentation is that of poorly controlled asthma.[116,117] Patients may also be symptomatic with low grade fever, wheezing, bronchial hyper-reactivity, hemoptysis or productive cough. Expectoration of brownish black mucus plugs believed to a characteristic symptom is seen in 31–69% of patients.[6,8,50] Presence of hemoptysis, expectoration of brownish-black mucus plugs, history of pulmonary opacities all points towards the diagnosis of ABPA. However, patients with ABPA can be surprisingly asymptomatic.[7,8,49] In a series of 155 cases of ABPA, almost 19% of patients with ABPA had well controlled asthma.[7,8] Thus, ABPA should be suspected in all asthmatics whatever the severity, especially in asthma and chest clinics.

There are no characteristic findings on physical examination. Physical examination can be normal or may reveal findings of polyphonic wheeze. Clubbing is seen in only 16% of patients, usually in those with long standing bronchiectasis.[7] On auscultation, coarse crackles can be heard in about 15% of patients.[8] Wheeze on physical examination and pulmonary opacities on chest radiograph may suggest ABPA. Physical examination also detects complications of ABPA such as pulmonary hypertension and/or respiratory failure. During exacerbations of ABPA, localized findings of consolidation (localized crackles, bronchial breath sounds) and atelectasis (diminished breath sounds) can occur and needs to be differentiated from other pulmonary diseases. It is often difficult to differentiate these conditions based on

Table 5 Clinical features encountered in three large case series of allergic bronchopulmonary aspergillosis published from the author's institute

	Chakrabarti et al.[6]	*Agarwal et al.*[8]	*Agarwal et al.*[9]
• Number of patients	89	155	54
• Male:Female	53:35	79:76	29:25
• Mean age (years)	36.4	33.4	34.3
• Mean duration of asthma (years)	12.1	8.9	10.9
• History of asthma	90%	100%	100%
• Expectoration of sputum plugs	69%	46.5%	27.8%
• Mean eosinophil count (per µL)	–	1,264	1,146
• AEC more than 500/µL (%)	100%	76%	74%
• Fleeting shadows	74%	40%	35%
• History of intake of antituberculous drugs	29%	45%	33%
• Skin test against *Aspergillus*			
– Type 1	85%	100%	100%
– Type 3	16.9%	83.2%	70.4%
• Mean IgE levels (mean)	Not done	6,434	7,829
• Elevated *Aspergillus*-specific IgE/IgG	Not done	100%	100%
• Serum precipitins against *Aspergillus*	71.9%	86.5%	78%
• Central bronchiectasis	69%	76%	82%

Abbreviations: AEC, absolute eosinophil count; IgE, immunoglobulin E

clinical assessment alone and in this situation immunological investigations are of great value in differential diagnosis.

Laboratory Findings

Aspergillus skin test: An immediate cutaneous hypersensitivity to *A. fumigatus* antigens is a hallmark of ABPA. The test can be performed using either a skin prick test (SPT) or by intradermal injection of the antigen. A positive reaction is characterized by development of a wheal and erythema within 1 minute which reaches a maximum after 10–20 minutes, and resolves within 1–2 hours. A positive test result is found in majority of patients with ABPA and the reported sensitivity of a positive result in diagnosis of ABPA is about 90%.[118] However, almost 40% of asthmatic patients without ABPA can also demonstrate immediate skin reactivity to *Aspergillus* antigen.[119] Although theoretically, both the intradermal and SPTs should perform in a similar manner, it has been shown that intradermal tests are generally more sensitive than SPTs.[120,121] The higher prevalence of AS with intradermal testing compared to prick test has been previously described in patients with ABPA.[120] In a meta-analysis, we had observed that the prevalence of AS in bronchial asthma was higher with an intradermal test versus SPT (28.7% vs 24.8%). The intradermal test is also believed to be associated with a higher complication rate than SPT. In our experience of more than 5,000 intradermal tests, we have not encountered any complication.[6-9,26,56,122] Thus, if technically feasible, a prick test should be performed for *Aspergillus* skin testing, and if the prick test is negative it should be confirmed by an intradermal test.

Total serum immunoglobulin E levels: The total serum IgE level is an important test in diagnosis of ABPA and is currently the most useful investigation in the follow-up of ABPA patients. A normal serum IgE level excludes ABPA as the cause of patient's current symptoms, if the patient is not taking glucocorticoids. There is a controversy on what should be the cut-off value of IgE level that should be used for the diagnosis of ABPA, further compounded by reporting of IgE in different units [1 kilo unit of antibody (kUA) of IgE/L is equivalent to 1 IU/mL and in turn is equal to 2.42 ng/mL].[123,124] An elevated IgE in allergic aspergillosis was described in 1970 wherein the study reported IgE values in a semiquantitative fashion (>0.8 µg/mL).[125] The Patterson group (Northwestern University allergy-immunology group) initially suggested a cutoff value of more than 2,500 ng/mL (>1,042 IU/mL).[18,126] Subsequently, they proposed various cutoffs namely less than 1,000 ng/mL for "ABPA probably excluded" and more than 2,000 ng/mL (833 IU/mL) for "further serologic studies required".[19] Over the years, the IgE cutoff has been cited as more than 1,000 ng/mL by several studies without any clear explanation.[3,45,127,128] Thus, some studies have used a cutoff value of 1,000 IU/mL,[7,8,18,19,126,129-131] while others employ a value of 1,000 IU/mL.[3,45,49,50,132]

We believe that a cut-off of 500 IU/mL will lead to overdiagnosis of ABPA as these levels are often seen in patients with AS without ABPA.[38,39] As this will lead to unwarranted steroid therapy, hence we use a cut-off value of 1,000 IU/mL. This cut-off was also agreed upon by the ISHAM-ABPA working group.[15] Recently, we have also proposed cut-off values for total IgE (>2,347 IU/mL) based on analysis of our population of ABPA in asthma.[133] The results of this finding further suggests that 1,000 IU/mL is likely to be better than 500 IU/mL. After treatment with glucocorticoids, the serum IgE level starts declining but in most patients, the level does not reach normal value. A 25% decline in IgE levels is taken as a criteria for response.[9,15,134] Repeated measurements of IgE levels need to be performed to determine the "new" baseline value for an individual patient during remission. The serum IgE also represents an important clinical tool in follow-up of patients. Increase in IgE by 50% of the patient's base-line value along with clinical or radiological worsening signifies exacerbation of the disease.

Serum IgE antibodies specific to A. fumigatus: An elevated level of specific antibodies to *A. fumigatus* is considered the hallmark of disease and is usually measured by fluorescent enzyme immunoassay (FEIA) tests.[7] A cut-off value of *A. fumigatus* specific IgE more than twice the pooled serum samples from patients with *Aspergillus*-hypersensitive asthma has been proposed to differentiate ABPA from patients with asthma and AS.[126] In our opinion, this is difficult to establish and hence we currently use a cut-off of 0.35 kUA/L of *A. fumigatus* specific IgE (manufacturer specified cut-off). In the past, immediate cutaneous hyper-reactivity to *Aspergillus* antigens has been recommended as the preferred test for screening asthmatic patients for ABPA.[132,135] However, a positive skin test is probably not the gold standard screening test in the context of ABPA. In a recent study using latent class analysis, we found that *Aspergillus* skin test (intradermal, indigenous antigen) had sensitivity ranging between 88% and 94% (with different assumptions) for the diagnosis of ABPA in asthmatics whereas the sensitivity was 100% for *A. fumigatus* specific IgE.[118] This implies that one in 10 asthmatic patients with ABPA can be potentially missed if *Aspergillus* skin test is used as the screening test for ABPA. Hence, we believe that *A. fumigatus* specific IgE should be used as a screening test for ABPA in asthma. An *Aspergillus* skin test may be performed if specific IgE assay is not available, with the caveat that 6–12% of patients can be potentially missed with this screening approach.[118]

Radiological investigations: A wide spectrum of radiographic abnormalities is encountered in ABPA although there are no unique roentgenographic findings to define a particular stage **(Table 6)**.[136,137] The most common chest radiographic findings of ABPA is considered to be transient or fixed pulmonary opacities which are often described as consolidation **(Fig. 1)**.[138,139] This observation is from the time when computed tomography (CT) was not available. In a recent study, we found that mucoid impaction presenting as "finger in glove" opacities and not consolidation was the most common finding.[140] Other findings include the presence of tramline shadows, finger-in-glove opacities and tooth paste shadows.[139,141-143] On prolonged follow-up of these patients, there can be fibrosis and collapse mainly affecting the upper lobes, which may be considered as development of CPA.[48,143] High-resolution computed tomography (HRCT) of the chest (1-1.5 × 5-15 mm) has a sensitivity and specificity of 96–98% and 93–99%, respectively compared to bronchography for the diagnosis of bronchiectasis.[144,145] Moreover, it detects abnormalities that are not visualized on chest radiograph and allows better delineation of the extent and type (cylindrical,

Table 6 Radiologic findings (in order of frequency) encountered in patients with allergic bronchopulmonary aspergillosis

Chest radiographic findings
Radiologic infiltrates—"toothpaste" and "gloved finger" shadows due to mucoid impaction in dilated bronchi, collapse—lobar or segmental, parallel-line shadows representing bronchial widening, ring-shadows representing dilated bronchi en face, patchy areas of consolidation fibrotic scarred upper lobes with cavitation, bronchial wall thickening—"tramline" shadows, air-fluid levels from dilated central bronchi filled with fluid, perihilar infiltrates simulating adenopathy, massive consolidation—unilateral or bilateral, small nodules, pleural effusions, pleural thickening
High-resolution computed tomographic findings
Central bronchiectasis, mucus plugging with bronchoceles, consolidation, centrilobular nodules with tree-in-bud opacities, bronchial wall thickening, areas of atelectasis, mosaic perfusion with air-trapping on expiration, high-attenuation mucus (HAM) (finding most helpful in differential diagnosis), pleural involvement, randomly scattered nodular opacities.

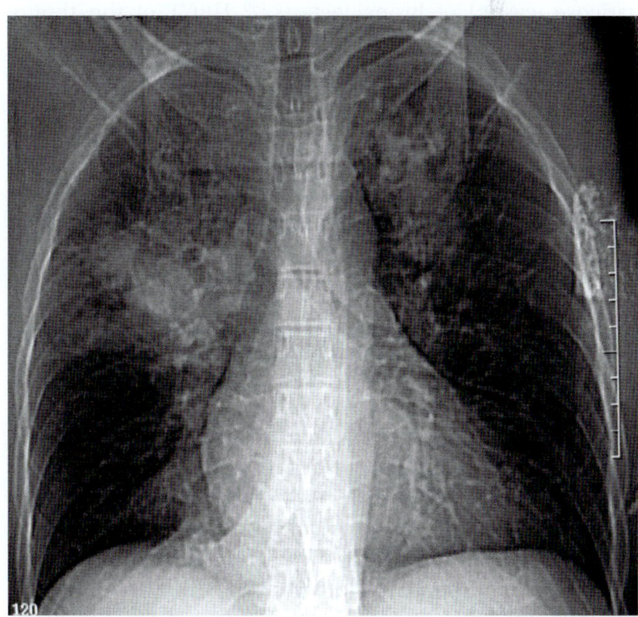

Fig. 1 Chest radiograph showing multifocal areas of consolidation

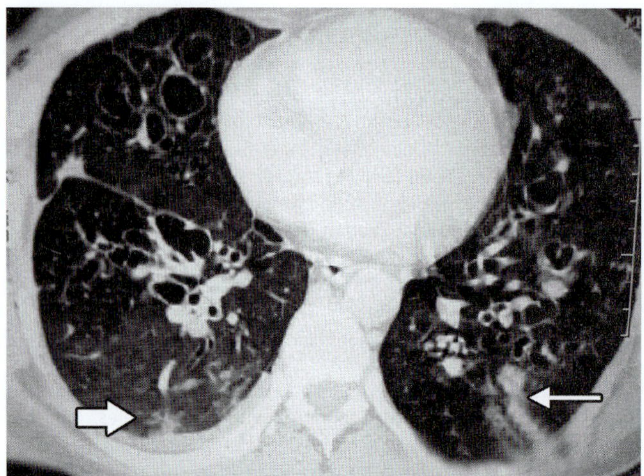

Fig. 2 High-resolution computed tomographic image of a patient with allergic bronchopulmonary aspergillosis showing bilateral central bronchiectasis with centrilobular nodules (bold arrow) and mucus plugging (thin arrow)

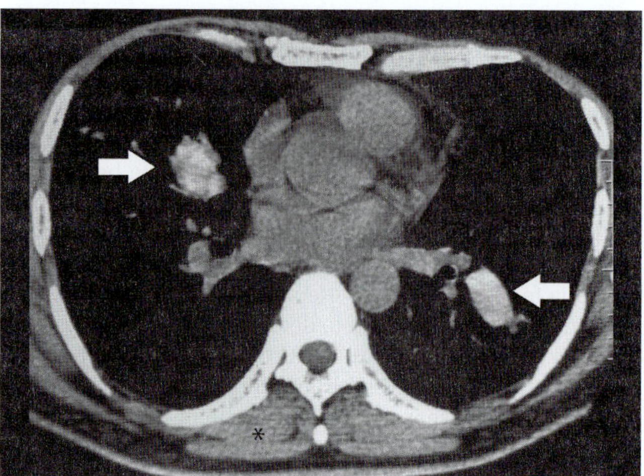

Fig. 3 Computed tomographic image of high-attenuation mucoid impaction (bold arrows). The mucoid impaction is visually denser than the paraspinal skeletal muscle (asterisk)

varicose, cystic) of bronchiectasis.[146] HRCT of the thorax has thus replaced bronchography as the imaging modality of choice for the diagnosis of ABPA.[147] Findings on HRCT include the presence of bronchiectasis, mucoid impaction, mosaic attenuation, presence of centrilobular nodules and tree-in-bud opacities **(Fig. 2)**.[148,149] Bronchiectasis in ABPA has been described as being "central", radiologically defined when confined to the medial two-thirds or medial half of the lung, at a point midway between the hilum and the chest wall.[150] CB with peripheral tapering of bronchi is believed to be a *sine qua non* for the diagnosis of ABPA.[151] Bronchiectasis in ABPA extends to the periphery in up to 40% of the lobes involved by bronchiectasis.[7,149] The prevalence of peripheral bronchiectasis also varies depending on the criteria used for defining CB (medial two-thirds vs medial half). In a recent study, we found that bronchiectasis extended to the periphery in 33–43% with different definitions.[140] Bronchiectasis can be seen on HRCT in patients with bronchial asthma,[152,153] although, the findings of bronchiectasis affecting three or more lobes, centrilobular nodules, and mucoid impaction are suggestive of ABPA,[154] a recent study noted all these findings in patients with AS without ABPA.[155] Thus, the significance of CB as a specific finding for ABPA is uncertain.[7,149,156] Finally, in one study, the sensitivity of CB was only 37% for the diagnosis of ABPA.[157] The ABPA working group has thus removed central from the bronchiectasis in ABPA. Further, bronchiectasis has been considered a complication and not a diagnostic criterion of ABPA.[15]

Mucoid impaction is one of the most common findings in ABPA. Mucus plugs in ABPA can be normo, hypo or hyperdense; hyperdense mucus is seen in up to 20% of patients.[7-9,158] High-attenuation mucus (HAM), radiologically defined when the mucus is visually denser than the paraspinal skeletal muscle, is a pathognomonic finding in patients with ABPA **(Fig. 3)**.[8,159-165] In a recent study, the presence of HAM was shown to have 100% specificity for diagnosis of ABPA.[118] Thus, the presence of HAM confirms ABPA as the cause of underlying bronchiectasis.[165] The identification of HAM also has prognostic implications. HAM is not only associated with an immunologically severe disorder but is also a marker of recurrent relapses.[7-9,158] The uncommon radiologic manifestations described in ABPA include miliary nodular opacities,[166-168] perihilar opacities simulating hilar lymphadenopathy,[115,139,169] pleural effusions,[170-173] pulmonary masses [174-179] and whole lung collapse.[180]

Many patients with ABPA require repeated chest CTs for monitoring the efficacy of treatment or for exclusion of other causes. Recently, we have shown that magnetic resonance imaging (MRI) of chest can be a useful modality in imaging of ABPA.[181] MRI will be especially useful in population at high-risk for potential effect of cumulative radiation leading to malignancy such as children and during pregnancy.

Serum precipitins (or immunoglobulin G antibodies) against A. fumigatus: The precipitating IgG antibodies are elicited from crude extracts of *A. fumigatus* and other fungi and can be demonstrated using ouchterlony double gel diffusion techniques of Longbottom and Pepys,[182] enzyme-linked immunosorbent assay (ELISA), FEIA or other methods.[183] In a recent study, two commercial assays [immunoCap and platelia *Aspergillus* IgG enzyme immunoassays (EIA)] were demonstrated to have higher sensitivity in detection of *Aspergillus* IgG antibodies compared with the traditional counter immunoelectrophoresis.[184] The immunoCap method was found to have better reproducibility and thus may be more useful for monitoring IgG levels following treatment.[184]

Present in almost 69–90% of patients with ABPA,[8,116,182,185,186] they probably indicate the continued growth of fungus in bronchi or body tissues.[128] These precipitins are however not specific as they are also present in 1–10% of normal subjects, hospitalized patients, and other pulmonary disorders including asthma, severe asthma with fungal sensitizations (SAFS) and CPA.[128,182,187] Thus, they represent supportive, not diagnostic evidence for ABPA. Increasing titers in ABPA, with evidence of persistent or progressive pleural fibrosis or pulmonary cavitation, may represent the interval development of CPA.[188-190]

Peripheral eosinophilia: A peripheral blood total eosinophil count greater than 1,000 cells/μL is considered as a major criterion for the diagnosis of ABPA. However, a low eosinophil count does not exclude ABPA as there is little correlation between pulmonary eosinophilia (almost universal) compared to peripheral blood eosinophil count.[191,192] We have recently shown that only 40% of patients with ABPA had eosinophil count more than 1,000 cells/μL at diagnosis.[193] Not only elevated eosinophil counts are common in many other disorders such as parasitic infestations and others, but also patients receiving oral steroids can have lower or normal eosinophil levels. To overcome this difficulty, the recent working group has suggested that the limit for eosinophil count be decreased from 1,000 cells/μL to 500 cells/μL as this level is seen in about 75% of cases.[193]

Sputum cultures for A. fumigatus: Growth of *A. fumigatus* in the sputum supports the diagnosis of ABPA. Because of the ubiquitous nature of the fungus, it can be isolated in normal subjects as well as in other pulmonary diseases.[185] The rates of culture positivity in ABPA ranges from 39% to 60%, mainly depending on the number of specimens examined.[6,186] It is interesting to note that the vast majority of culture-negative ABPA patients have detectable *A. fumigatus* DNA in their sputum.[194] It has been suggested that routine processing procedures for isolating filamentous fungi from respiratory sputum samples have actually underestimated fungal prevalence. In a recent study, a significantly higher growth was demonstrated using a different sputum processing method wherein the sputum plugs were separated from saliva and aliquots of approximately 150 mg were inoculated directly onto potato dextrose agar.[195] The other important utility of sputum cultures is in the investigation of azole susceptibility in *A. fumigatus.*[194] Thus, it may be valuable if cultures are obtained before starting antifungal therapy and susceptibility testing and/or real-time molecular testing for resistance of any isolates, are performed.[196] Sputum cultures are not required in routine care, if they are solely being employed for the diagnosis of ABPA.

Pulmonary function tests: These tests have no diagnostic value in ABPA. In fact, pulmonary function tests can be normal in ABPA and should not constitute the basis for screening.[7] They are however extremely beneficial in monitoring the patient. Spirometry is used in categorizing the severity of asthma and/or the underlying lung disease. The pulmonary function tests generally show obstructive physiology with varying severity and reduction in diffusion capacity.[116,117,197] In the past, bronchial provocation testing with *Aspergillus* antigens have been used for diagnosis of ABPA; but, they are generally not advisable as they can cause severe bronchospasm.[186]

Role of specific Aspergillus antigens: Patients with ABPA are mostly evaluated with crude extracts from *Aspergillus.* These antigens lack reproducibility and consistency and frequently cross react with other antigens.[198] Advances in molecular techniques have enabled detection of almost 20 specific *Aspergillus* antigens with diverse biochemical nature and function. In fact, a number of allergens from *A. fumigatus* have been cloned and highly purified proteins have been synthesized from complementary deoxyribonucleic acid (cDNA) libraries of *A. fumigatus.* These recombinant proteins have the potential of significantly improving the diagnostic specificity and reproducibility compared to crude extracts.[199] A number of these antigens have also been evaluated for diagnosis of ABPA both in patients with asthma and CF.[200] The recombinant allergens secreted ribotoxin (rAsp f1), unknown function (rAsp f2), peroxisomal protei (rAsp f3), unknown function (rAsp f4) and cellular manganese superoxide dismutase (rAsp f6) have been evaluated in ABPA for their diagnostic performance both in asthmatic patients,[201-204] and in CF.[200,203,205,206] Preliminary data suggest a promising role of these antigens for diagnosis of ABPA. The results from these studies suggest that rAsp f4 and f6 represent specific markers for ABPA, and allow differentiation of ABPA from *Aspergillus* sensitized asthma.[200,201] The recombinant proteins rAsp f4 and f6 are intracellular nonsecreted proteins,[203] and it is proposed that only patients suffering from ABPA are exposed to these antigens due to fungal damage resulting from cellular defense mechanisms.[202] On the other hand, *A. fumigatus* sensitized asthmatics mount IgE responses only to secreted proteins (rAsp f1 and f3) that are produced shortly after spore germination.[207] Thus, a combination of these antigens is more useful in contrast to the use of a single antigen.[208,209] One study suggested that serial IgE responses to rAsp f3 provides improved distinction between flares and response in contrast to IgE measure against crude *Aspergillus* extract.[210] Commercial automated assays for determination of IgE levels against recombinant *A. fumigatus* antigens are available.[204,209,211] Although detection of IgE response to recombinant *Aspergillus* proteins looks promising, in one study the responses were different when performed in different centers.[201,212] Further studies performed in larger samples are required before incorporation of this test into routine clinical practice.[213]

Recent developments in investigations for ABPA: In a recent study, serum galactomannan (GM) was found to have limited role for the initial diagnosis of ABPA.[214] Thymus- and activation- regulated chemokine (TARC)/CCL17 is a chemoattractant to Th2 type of cells acting through CCR4 and CCR8 receptors present on these cells and has been evaluated in

ABPA.[96] TARC was shown to have a better diagnostic accuracy than specific IgE (to crude or recombinant *A. fumigatus* antigens) with sensitivity of 100% and a specificity of 97.2% for diagnosis of ABPA in CF.[215] Serial determination of TARC may have better accuracy than IgE levels for diagnosis of ABPA exacerbations.[216] Patients with CF complicated by ABPA display increase in blood basophil CD203c levels identified by fluorescence activated cell sorting (FACS) at baseline (and following in vitro stimulation with an allergenic extract of *A. fumigatus*) compared to patients with CF alone and in CF colonized with *A. fumigatus*.[217] More studies are required to evaluate the role of TARC and FACS CD203c basophil assay in the diagnosis and follow-up of ABPA complicating asthma.

Diagnosis and Diagnostic Criteria

The Rosenberg-Patterson criteria, which are a constellation of clinical, radiological and immunological features, are most often used for diagnosis of ABPA **(Table 7)**.[16] There are also a set of minimal diagnostic criteria for ABPA using which the diagnosis of ABPA may be secured, possibly at an earlier stage.[49,218] The criteria continue to be challenged and modified.[4,7] The Patterson criteria have several limitations. They lay equal weightage to all parameters while some elements of the criteria are more important than others. For example, the specificity of *Aspergillus* IgG for ABPA as opposed to other forms of aspergillosis, especially ABPA remains unknown. Also, *Aspergillus* IgE is likely to be more sensitive than total eosinophil count. Moreover, there is no agreement on the optimum cut-off values for IgE levels and eosinophil count due to the lack of receiver operator curve (ROC) analysis. Importantly, there is no consensus on the number of major or minor criteria required to make the diagnosis and most studies have used five criteria **(Table 2)**.[7,8,50,53]

Recently, we have shown that six Patterson criteria offer the best diagnostic performance in identification of ABPA.[118] There is a decline in specificity if five criteria are employed and fall in sensitivity if seven criteria are employed. The differentiation of patients with ABPA from AS can also be problematic. Serum precipitins to *A. fumigatus* are present in 69–90% of patients with ABPA[8,116,182,185,186] but also in 9% of asthmatics.[182] CB can be seen in patients with asthma without ABPA.[152-154] The total IgE levels are elevated in the sera in all patients with ABPA, and reflect disease activity,[219,220] however, a moderate rise in IgE levels is also noted in patients with asthma without ABPA.[221]

The ISHAM-ABPA working group has recently proposed new criteria so as to simplify the diagnosis of ABPA **(Table 7)**.[15] Patients who meet some but not all of these criteria may be labeled as "ABPA-at risk" and require close monitoring and follow-up. The new criteria are simpler, more objective and thus beneficial in clinical research studies as they will facilitate a uniform diagnosis across centers. The new criteria will need validation and the proposed cut-off values will need to be

Table 7 Criteria used for the diagnosis of allergic bronchopulmonary aspergillosis (ABPA)

Rosenberg-Patterson criteria[16,19]
Major criteria • Bronchial asthma • Immediate cutaneous hyper-reactivity to *Aspergillus* antigen • Elevated serum IgE levels • Elevated levels of *A. fumigatus* specific IgG and/or IgE in serum • Central bronchiectasis • Fleeting pulmonary opacities on chest radiograph • Peripheral blood eosinophilia • Elevated serum precipitins against *Aspergillus* *Minor criteria* • Expectoration of brownish-black mucus plugs • Delayed cutaneous hypersensitivity to *Aspergillus* antigen • Presence of *Aspergillus* in sputum
ISHAM-ABPA working group criteria[15] Predisposing conditions • Bronchial asthma • Cystic fibrosis *Obligatory criteria* • Elevated IgE levels against *A. fumigatus* (>0.35 kUA/L) or immediate cutaneous hypersensitivity to *Aspergillus* antigen • Elevated total IgE levels (1,000 IU/mL)
Other criteria (at least three of five) • Presence of serum precipitating antibodies against *A. fumigatus* • Radiographic pulmonary opacities (fixed/transient) • Absolute eosinophil count >500 cells/μL
Abbreviations: ISHAM, International Society of Human and Animal Mycology; ABPA, allergic bronchopulmonary aspergillosis

verified. Bronchiectasis has been removed from the diagnostic criteria. The minor criteria do not offer any additional value in diagnosis and hence have also been removed. We found total IgE, *A. fumigatus* specific IgE and eosinophil count at values of 2,347 IU/mL, 1.91 kUA/L and 507 cells/μL, respectively offered 70% sensitivity and 100% specificity in diagnosis of ABPA. In clinical practice, many patients will fall short of these cut-off values and an algorithmic approach proposed below will allow accurate diagnosis.

While investigating a patient with asthma, we first perform an *A. fumigatus* specific IgE. If the value is more than 0.35 kUA/L, total serum IgE are then measured **(Flow chart 1)**.[222] If the total IgE is more than 1,000 IU/mL, then total eosinophil count is assayed. If the patient meets the afore mentioned cut-offs, a diagnosis of ABPA is confirmed. In clinical practice, many patients will fall short of these cut-offs. In these situations, other investigations including serum precipitins or IgG against *A. fumigatus*, *Aspergillus* skin test and HRCT of the chest need to be done. An occasional patient will fulfill all other criteria but the IgE would be less than 1,000 IU/mL. In such situations a diagnosis of ABPA can be made. Patients with "ABPA at-risk" should be followed with IgE levels. If there is a rising trend with clinical/radiologic deterioration, then treatment is started.

Natural History

The natural history of ABPA is currently not well characterized and is often difficult to predict because spontaneous improvement of symptoms and pulmonary opacities characterize an important aspect of disease.[19,129,223-226] ABPA is most often a nonacute respiratory syndrome that lingers on for years without diagnosis. Rarely, the condition presents in an acute fashion.[180,227,228] If the disease is not recognized, the chronic inflammatory process can progress relentlessly and result in irreversible pulmonary dysfunction due to bronchiectasis and/or pulmonary fibrosis, ultimately culminating in respiratory failure and cor pulmonale.[22] Thus, an early diagnosis and initiation of therapy is essential for prevention of bronchiectasis and/or pulmonary fibrosis.[229] The natural history of ABPA is characterized by recurrent episodes of remissions and relapses. It can be best understood if we appreciate the clinical **(Table 8)** and radiological **(Table 9)** classification schemes of ABPA.

Clinical staging of allergic bronchopulmonary aspergillosis: Although, ABPA has been classified into five stages by Patterson **(Table 8)**,[18] there is lack of precise definitions of these stages leading to considerable ambiguity. The ISHAM-ABPA working group has laid down new staging criteria

Flow chart 1 Algorithm for investigating asthmatic patients for allergic bronchopulmonary aspergillosis

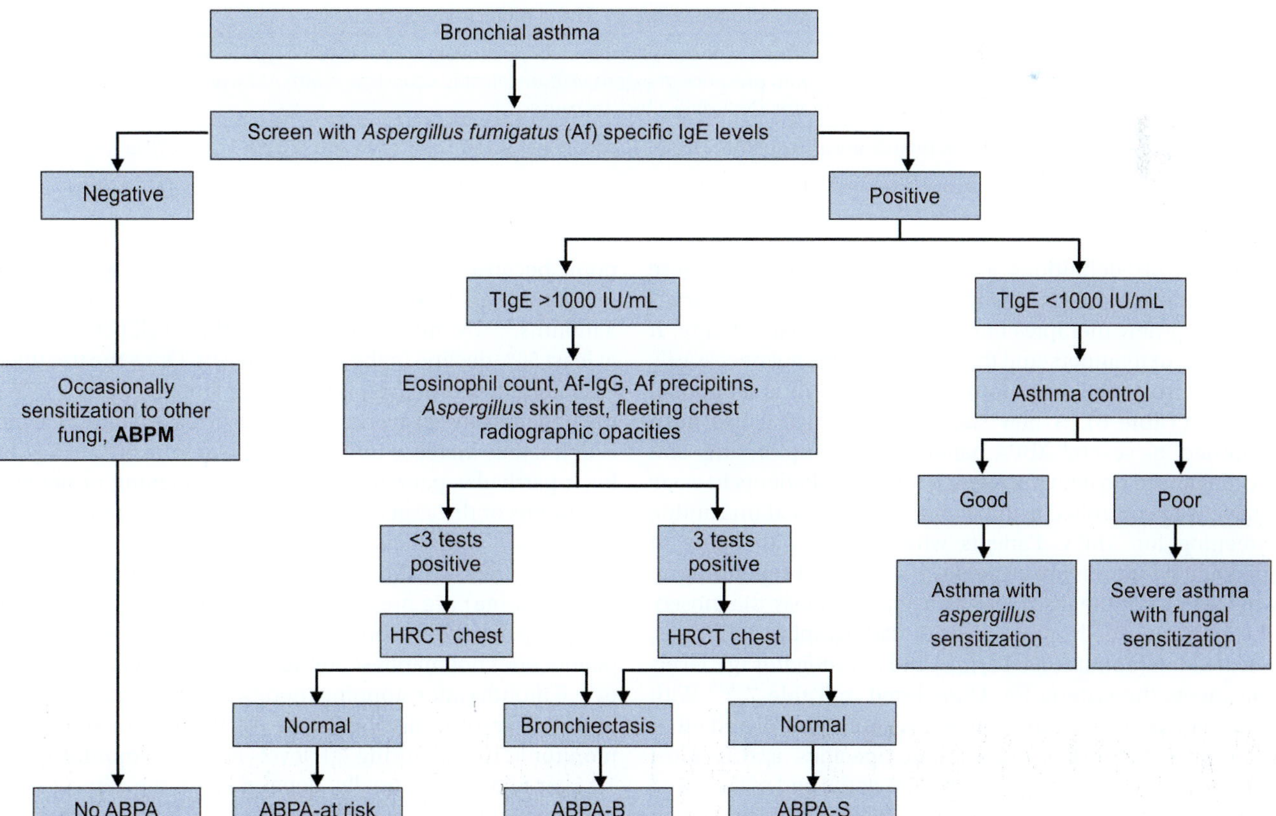

Table 8 Clinical staging of allergic bronchopulmonary aspergillosis

Patterson et al.[18]	
I	Acute phase
II	Remission
III	Exacerbation
IV	Glucocorticoid-dependent ABPA
V	End-stage (fibrotic) ABPA
ISHAM-ABPA working group criteria[15]	
0 (asymptomatic)	Never diagnosed to have ABPA in the past; presentation with controlled asthma (according to GINA guidelines), and meeting the diagnostic criteria of ABPA (Table 1)
1 (acute)	Never diagnosed to have ABPA in the past; presentation with uncontrolled asthma/ constitutional symptoms, and meeting the diagnostic criteria of ABPA
1a (with mucoid impaction)	Mucoid impaction on thoracic imaging or bronchoscopy
1b (without mucoid impaction)	No mucoid impaction on thoracic imaging or bronchoscopy
2 (response)	Clinical and/or radiological improvement and fall in IgE by ≥25% of baseline at 8 weeks
3 (exacerbation)	Clinical and/or radiological worsening accompanied by an increase in IgE by ≥50% from the previous baseline
4 (remission)	Sustained clinicoradiological improvement with IgE levels remaining at or below baseline (or increase by <50%) for ≥6 months off therapy with oral steroids
5a (treatment-dependent ABPA)	Two or more consecutive relapses within 6 months of stopping treatment or deterioration in clinical and/or radiological condition and/or immunological worsening on tapering oral steroids/azoles
5b (glucocorticoid-dependent asthma)	Systemic corticosteroids required for asthma control while the ABPA activity is controlled (as indicated by IgE levels and thoracic imaging)
6 (advanced ABPA)	Presence of complications (cor pulmonale and/or chronic type II respiratory failure) along with presence of extensive bronchiectasis consistent with ABPA on thoracic radiology after excluding alternate causes.

Abbreviations: ABPA, allergic bronchopulmonary aspergillosis; ISHAM, International Society of Human and Animal Mycology; GINA, global initiative for asthma

with rigorous definitions for each stage **(Table 8)**. These modifications would not only be beneficial in clinical trials evaluating new therapies but also in routine patient care. It is important to understand that a patient does not necessarily progress from one stage to the other stage in a sequential fashion **(Table 8)**. A new stage namely stage 0 has been proposed, as several ABPA patients are asymptomatic, and are diagnosed on active screening for ABPA. Patients in stage 0 have well controlled asthma and are diagnosed on routine screening for ABPA. Patients who present with acute to subacute symptoms are generally in stage 1 or 3 depending on whether or not the disorder has been previously diagnosed. The patient usually presents with radiographic infiltrates, elevated IgE (about 5,000 IU/mL) and *A. fumigatus* IgE levels and meets the criteria for ABPA listed in **Table 7**.[8,15] With treatment, there is improvement in asthma control and other symptoms, clearing of radiographic opacities, and in most patients, there is decline of IgE by 25% at the end of 8 weeks.[9] This is classified as response (stage 2). This is an important point because the aim of therapy is not the achievement of normal IgE levels but a 25–50% decline by 6 weeks to 3 months.[134] By the end of 3 months almost all patients show at least 50% decline in the total IgE levels. Once the treatment (usually glucocorticoids) is tapered or stopped, almost 50% of the patients have exacerbation of the disease (stage 3), which is defined as increase in IgE levels by at least 50% of last IgE for a particular patient usually with worsening of patient's symptoms or the appearance of radiologic infiltrates.[7,18,19]

Certain radiological markers such as extensive bronchiectasis, HAM and the presence of fungal ball (aspergilloma) are predictors of recurrent relapses and this subgroup of patients should be monitored closely.[158,230] If the patient does not manifest any additional ABPA exacerbations over 6 months after stopping therapy, the patient has entered into a stage of remission (stage 4). Patients in stage 4 are monitored by measuring IgE levels every 3–6 months for the 1st year and then annually, depending on the clinical status of the patient. Even in patients who have achieved complete

Table 9 Radiologic staging of allergic bronchopulmonary aspergillosis

Patterson et al.[19]	
Seropositive ABPA (ABPA-S)	All the diagnostic features of ABPA but no evidence of central bronchiectasis (CB) on high-resolution computed tomographic (HRCT). Patients with ABPA-S may be classified as Patterson stages I to IV. These patients may have recurrent exacerbations and may also be classified as stage III
ABPA with central bronchiectasis (ABPA-CB)	All findings of ABPA including CB on HRCT. Patients with ABPA-CB may belong to any of the Patterson stages
Kumar et al.[236]	
ABPA-S	ABPA without CB
ABPA-CB	ABPA with CB
ABPA-CB-other radiologic findings (ABPA-CB-ORF)	ABPA with CB other radiologic features such as pulmonary fibrosis, bleb, bullae, pneumothorax, parenchymal scarring, emphysematous change, multiple cyst, fibro-cavitary lesions, aspergilloma, ground-glass appearance, collapse, mediastinal lymph node, pleural effusion and pleural thickening
Agarwal et al.[158]	
ABPA-S	ABPA without CB
ABPA-CB	ABPA with CB
ABPA-CB-high attenuation mucus (ABPA-CB-HAM)	ABPA with CB and high attenuation mucus
ISHAM-ABPA working group criteria[15]	
ABPA-S (serological ABPA)	Fulfils the diagnostic criteria of ABPA **(Table 7)** with absence of any radiological finding of ABPA on HRCT of the thorax
ABPA-B (ABPA with bronchiectasis)	Satisfies the diagnostic requirements of ABPA along with presence of bronchiectasis
ABPA-HAM (ABPA with high attenuation mucus)	ABPA along with presence of high attenuation mucus on HRCT of the thorax
ABPA-CPF (ABPA with chronic pleuropulmonary fibrosis)	Fulfils the diagnostic criteria of ABPA with at least two radiological features suggestive of fibrosis (fibrocavitary lesions, pulmonary fibrosis, pleural thickening and others) without presence of mucoid impaction (or HAM)
Abbreviations: ABPA, allergic bronchopulmonary aspergillosis; HAM, high attenuation mucus; ISHAM, International Society of Human and Animal Mycology; CB, central bronchiectasis; HRCT, high-resolution computed tomographic	

remission, the IgE levels do not return to normal values.[223] Some patients in stage 4 may enter into prolonged or even a permanent remission. A prolonged remission, however, is not synonymous with cure as exacerbations of the disease have been documented for as long as 7 years after remission.[225] Remission can be sustained with low-dose glucocorticoids, itraconazole, monthly methylprednisolone pulses and nebulized amphotericin B.[1,231-233]

Patients in stage 5 are difficult to treat ABPA and can be divided into 2 types. (1) The first group (treatment-dependent ABPA) includes patients who require recurrent courses of oral glucocorticoids or azoles. They are characterized by clinicoradiological worsening and IgE levels rise once treatment is tapered. (2) The other group (glucocorticoid-dependent asthma) requires steroids for control of asthma but do not have radiological worsening or rise in IgE levels.[7,20] Patients in stage six are those with widespread bronchiectasis and varying degrees of pulmonary dysfunction with type two respiratory failure and/or cor pulmonale. It is important to remember that the IgE levels decline to below 1,000 IU/mL in only a minority (<10–15%) of patients with stages II and V.[129,223] Even in stage V ABPA, the disease can be clinically as well as immunologically active, and long-term glucocorticoid therapy may be required for control of asthma and/or ABPA.[226,234]

Radiological staging of allergic bronchopulmonary aspergillosis: Depending on the absence or presence of bronchiectasis, ABPA was classified as ABPA-S or ABPA-CB, respectively **(Table 9)**.[19] It was believed that patients with ABPA-S would have a milder clinical course and less severe immunologic findings when compared to ABPA-CB as it represented the earliest stage of the disorder.[22,235,236] In the largest of these three studies (76 patients), which was also the first study that suggested that ABPA-S is less severe immunologically, only the *A. fumigatus* specific IgG levels were higher in patients with ABPA-CB compared to ABPA-S. Other immunologic parameters were not significantly different between the two groups.[22] ABPA has also been classified into three groups namely, (1) ABPA-S (mild), (2) ABPA-CB (moderate) and (3) ABPA-CB-other radiologic findings (ORF). However, this was a single study and included only 18 patients.[236] Also, the findings included in the categorization of ABPA-CB-ORF were pulmonary fibrosis, bleb, bullae, pneumothorax, parenchymal scarring, emphysematous change, multiple cyst, fibrocavitary lesions and pleural thickening; all changes representing the fibrotic stage. In one of the largest studies in ABPA published from our center (126 patients), we have shown that the clinical, spirometric and immunologic findings were not significantly different either classifying ABPA into two groups (1) ABPA-S and (2) ABPA-CB or the above mentioned three categories (1)ABPA-S, (2) ABPA-CB and (3) ABPA-CB-ORF.[7] In ABPA-S there is active ongoing inflammation with progressive immunologic damage, and understandably the immunologic findings will not be very different from those in ABPA-CB.

Recently, we have re-evaluated the clinical and serological severity of both these classifications using data from a large set of patients (234 subjects).[158] The classification scheme by Patterson et al. showed immunological severity in some parameters (eosinophil count and *A. fumigatus* specific IgE levels) but not in others (total IgE levels). Moreover, on excluding patients with HAM, the immunological severity was restricted only to eosinophil counts. Interestingly, in the Kumar classification, the immunological markers were most severe in patients with ABPA-CB and not ABPA-CB-ORF. This suggests that ORF does not determine serological severity and probably represents the burnt out phase of the disease. In addition to evaluating these two classifications, we proposed a new classification based on HAM. High-attenuation mucus is a CT sign of mucus impaction,[142,165] which in turn is a marker of active inflammation.[101] The HAM-based classification was most consistently associated with immunological severity.[101] The ABPA-ISHAM working group has proposed a new classification, which incorporates all previous radiological classifications. Radiologically, ABPA has been classified into four major categories **(Table 9)**, (1) namely, serological ABPA (ABPA-S), (2) ABPA with bronchiectasis (ABPA-B), (3) ABPA with high-attenuation mucus (ABPA-HAM) and (4) ABPA with chronic pleuropulmonary fibrosis (ABPA-CPF).

The course of patients with ABPA-S is likely to be less severe when compared to those with ABPA-B. In two separate multivariate analyses of 155 and 54 patients with ABPA, we demonstrated that the severity of bronchiectasis, and presence of HAM on HRCT predicted relapses of ABPA and the severity of bronchiectasis was an independent predictor of failure to achieve remission.[8,9] This suggests that an early diagnosis of ABPA is essential because one not only prevents permanent lung damage but also improves the likelihood of a smoother course of this relapsing-remitting disorder. Thus, it remains prudent to diagnose and treat ABPA early so as to prevent the development of bronchiectasis.

Management

The management of ABPA includes two important aspects namely initiation of immunosuppressive therapy (primarily glucocorticoids) to control the immunologic activity, and the use of antifungal agents to reduce the fungal burden secondary, to the fungal colonization in the airways. The goals of therapy include asthma control, prevention and treatment of ABPA exacerbations and prevention of the onset/progression of bronchiectasis and thus CPA.

Systemic glucocorticoid therapy: Oral corticosteroids are currently considered the treatment of choice for ABPA despite lack of well-designed trials, based on large clinical experience across several centers.[7-9,140,158,230,237,238] They not only suppress the immune hyperfunction but are also anti-inflammatory thereby controlling the activity of both asthma and ABPA. There is no robust data to guide the dose and duration of glucocorticoids, and different regimens of glucocorticoids have been used **(Table 10)**. The use of lower doses of glucocorticoids (regime 1 in **Table 10**) is associated with higher occurrence of recurrent relapses or glucocorticoid dependence (45%).[19] A higher dosage of glucocorticoids (regime 2 in **Table 10**) was shown to be associated with higher remission rates and a lower prevalence of glucocorticoid-dependent ABPA (13.5%).[7] Whether a higher dose and prolonged duration of corticosteroid therapy is associated with better outcomes remains unclear in the absence of direct comparison between the two regimens. Currently, the choice between the two regimens is a matter of institutional preference. A randomized controlled trial on the efficacy and safety of the above mentioned two glucocorticoid dose regimens in ABPA has been completed (clinicaltrials.gov; NCT00974766). Hopefully, the results of this trial will contribute in choosing a particular dose of glucocorticoid in ABPA.

The clinical effectiveness of steroid therapy is reflected by clinicoradiological improvement and decrease in patient's total serum IgE levels. There does not seem to be any correlation between serum levels of *A. fumigatus* specific IgE levels and disease activity.[239] The goal of therapy is not to attempt normalization of IgE levels but to decrease by 25% which in most cases is associated with complete clinical and radiographic improvement. Repeated measurements of IgE are also required to establish baseline serum level of total IgE during the stable disease, which serves as a guide to future detection of relapse and helps in follow-up of the patient.

Inhaled corticosteroids: Inhaled steroids achieve high concentrations in the tracheobronchial tree and are associated with minimal systemic side-effects, and thus have been evaluated in ABPA as systemic steroid-sparing therapy. Numerous case series have reported the use of ICS in ABPA.[240-246] These studies are not only limited by their small sample size but also in using varying doses of ICS. Moreover, many patients were continued on lower doses of oral steroids while receiving ICS. Several studies were not methodologically robust and only clinical or radiological and spirometric criteria were used to define response, and IgE levels were not measured. This makes it difficult to analyze whether the beneficial effects were solely due to ICS. Currently, there is no role of ICS in the management of ABPA. We use ICS only for

Table 10 Glucocorticoid protocols for the management of allergic bronchopulmonary aspergillosis (ABPA)

Regime 1[3]
Prednisolone 0.5 mg/kg/day for 1–2 weeks, then on alternate days for 6–8 weeks. Then taper by 5–10 mg every 2 weeks and discontinue. Repeat total serum IgE levels and chest X-ray every 6–8 weeks to determine the baseline IgE concentrations
Regime 2[7,128]
Prednisolone, 0.75 mg/kg for 6 weeks, 0.5 mg/kg for 6 weeks, then tapered by 5 mg every 6 weeks to continue for a total duration of at least 6–12 months. The total IgE levels are repeated every 6–8 weeks for 1 year to determine the baseline IgE concentrations

control of asthma once the oral prednisolone dose is reduced to below 10 mg/day.

Oral azoles: Systemic steroids are highly efficacious, but 50% of patients experience exacerbations when steroids are tapered and almost 20–45% become glucocorticoid-dependent.[7,19] Further, many patients also develop adverse effects related to chronic steroid therapy.[247,248] Hence, there is a dire need of steroid-sparing agents. The use of specific antifungal agents in ABPA is based on the principle that removal or reduction of fungal burden and thus the antigenic stimulus would mitigate the immune response.

Ketoconazole has been tried in the past,[249] but has been replaced by the less toxic and more effective agent, itraconazole.[131,239,250-262] Two randomized controlled studies (84 patients) have evaluated the efficacy of itraconazole in ABPA.[131,258] In one study, 55 "glucocorticoid-dependent" ABPA patients were randomized to receive either itraconazole 200 mg twice a day versus placebo. While the difference between the two groups was significant in terms of overall response [reduction in the dose of corticosteroid by 50% or more; and, decrease in the total IgE concentration by 25% or more; and, at least one of the following (increase in exercise tolerance by at least 25%, improvement by 25% in results of the pulmonary function tests, resolution of pulmonary infiltrates), it failed to reach statistical significance when each of the outcomes were examined separately.[258] The other study included 29 "clinically stable" ABPA patients randomized to receive itraconazole or placebo. Majority of the patients did not receive glucocorticoids in this study. There were significant decline in sputum inflammatory markers and serum IgE levels. The study also demonstrated a decrease in the number of exacerbations warranting glucocorticoid usage.[131]

Pooled analysis showed that itraconazole could significantly decrease the IgE levels by 25% or more when compared to placebo but did not cause significant improvement in lung function.[263] A major limitation was that neither of the study reported outcomes more than 8 months in terms of relapses of ABPA. Itraconazole has been also used as monotherapy in acute stages of ABPA.[131,255] However, more data is required to confirm this approach. A randomized controlled trial comparing monotherapy of itraconazole versus prednisolone in ABPA (MIPA study; clinicaltrials.gov; NCT01321827) is underway, which aims to answer this question.

We currently use itraconazole in the first relapse of ABPA or in patients with glucocorticoid-dependent ABPA.[7] Because of erratic gastrointestinal absorption and interaction with several other drugs, itraconazole therapy should generally be monitored by drug levels to ensure adequate bioavailability.[264,265] Suboptimal blood levels of the drug have been correlated with clinical failure and possible development of azole resistance in *A. fumigatus*.[264,266] There is data on reduction of itraconazole adverse reactions if blood levels are maintained in a therapeutic range.[267] Newer antifungal agents including voriconazole,[268-276] and posaconazole[277,278] have also been shown to be efficacious. Without more data, these drugs are indicated in those intolerant to itraconazole or in itraconazole failures.[231,279] A randomized controlled trial comparing monotherapy of voriconazole versus prednisolone in ABPA (clinicaltrials.gov; NCT01621321) has been completed and the results of this study would likely clarify the role of voriconazole monotherapy in ABPA.

Therapy with azoles have numerous adverse effects including skin cancer with long-term voriconazole therapy.[247,248,278,280-286] In a study of 189 patients treated with itraconazole (average, 400 mg/day), adverse effects occurred in almost 39% of patients.[280] There are also numerous drug interactions with the use of itraconazole. Most notably it may inhibit the hepatic metabolism of terfenadine, astemizole, and cisapride, prolonging the electrocardiographic QT interval thus increasing the risk for cardiac arrhythmia. Caution should also be exercised when treating concomitantly with glucocorticoids. Itraconazole inhibits the metabolism of methyl prednisolone (but not prednisolone) and can lead to increased frequency of side-effects of steroids including profound adrenal insufficiency.[281] Adrenal suppression has also been reported with the concomitant use of itraconazole and inhaled budesonide.[282,283]

Other therapies: Numerous other therapies have been tried in ABPA. They can be tried in individual patients such as those with treatment-dependent ABPA who develop drug-related adverse reactions, but should be not be used a routine measure. There are several reports of ABPA treated with nebulized amphotericin and inhaled steroids.[232,287-290] A randomized trial is evaluating the efficacy of nebulized amphotericin in maintaining remissions in ABPA (clinicaltrials.gov; NCT01857479). Omalizumab a humanized monoclonal antibody against IgE, could be a potential therapeutic approach since ABPA is associated with elevated IgE levels. The use of omalizumab in ABPA has been associated with improvement in symptoms, reduction in exacerbations and asthma hospitalizations, improvement in lung function and reduction in dose of oral steroids.[228,275,291-305] Pulse doses of intravenous methyl prednisolone have also been used for treatment of severe exacerbations of ABPA or as a steroid-sparing agent.[227,228,233,277,306-308] We also use methotrexate as steroid-sparing agent in patients with steroid-dependent ABPA or in patients where steroids are absolutely contraindicated such as cystoid macular edema, a potentially sight-threatening condition.

Future therapies: Vitamin D has been shown to down regulate the Th2 pathway through OX40 ligand-dependent process in ABPA complicating CF.[309] Vitamin D supplementation may have a beneficial role in the treatment of ABPA, and is the focus of a recent trial in patients with CF and ABPA (clinicaltrials.gov; NCT01222273). In the last few years, several trials of monoclonal antibodies directed against the Th2 cytokine IL-5 have been demonstrated to have clinical benefit in patients with severe asthma and sputum eosinophilia,[310-312] while a monoclonal antibody against IL-13 has been found effective in asthmatic patients with a high Th2 endotype.[313] These "anti-Th2" therapies may also be investigated for their efficacy in patients with ABPA.[314,315]

Treatment Protocol

All therapies used in ABPA are associated with adverse reactions and most patients with ABPA require long-term treatment. It is not known whether treatment with steroids or itraconazole will improve long-term outcomes, in particular prevent (or reverse) bronchiectasis and CPA. Hence, any treatment strategy should be judiciously chosen in patients with ABPA. Whether ABPA patients in stage 0 can be followed without any treatment or should be treated is also not clear. If a decision is made not to follow the patient without treatment, then he/she should be closely monitored, and any considerable worsening in clinical, radiological or immunological status should prompt treatment. The choice of a particular therapy (glucocorticoid monotherapy, azole monotherapy and steroid and azole combination) in different clinical phenotypes of ABPA is not known. Patients of ABPA with mucoid impaction and/or significant deterioration of lung function attributed to worsening asthma or ABPA (and not intercurrent infection) generally benefit from treatment with glucocorticoids. Failure of response of mucoid impaction and proximal collapse after 3 weeks of treatment should prompt therapeutic bronchoscopy. In those with recurrent exacerbations, one should consider itraconazole therapy.

Azoles are effective in preventing ABPA exacerbations and can be used either as recurrent short courses (4–6 months) or as long-term therapy. One drawback of prolonged treatment with azoles is the development of resistance.[194,316] Whatever the treatment approach, it should provide greatest benefit to the patient with the least possible adverse reactions. Inhaled steroids should either be continued for asthma control or initiated once the oral prednisolone dose is reduced to below 10 mg/day. Clinicians should also be aware of the profound interaction between inhaled steroids (especially budesonide) and itraconazole in some patients leading to cushingoid effects and long-term adrenal failure, if dose of inhaled corticosteroids (ICS) is not significantly reduced. In the author's experience, the interaction is least with fluticasone. Itraconazole also increases drug levels of methyl prednisolone but not prednisolone and thus the latter should be used if combination therapy is preferred. A treatment protocol based on current evidence is shown in **Flow chart 2**.

Follow-up of patients on treatment: Patients should initially be followed every 8 weeks with clinical symptomatology, serum IgE levels, chest radiograph and lung function test. The clinical response is measured by decline in patient's total serum IgE levels along with symptomatic and radiologic improvement. As stated earlier, the goal of therapy is not normalization of IgE levels but decrease in the IgE levels by 25%, which in most cases is associated with clinical and radiographic improvement.[9] One should establish serum level of total IgE during stable phase of the disease, which serves as a baseline to future detection of exacerbation. Chest radiographs need not be performed once they have normalized or returned to the patient's baseline. Subsequent, chest radiographs need to be done only if there is significant clinical worsening.

Differential Diagnosis

The diagnosis of the condition rests on clinical suspicion and performance of serological and radiological tests including high-resolution CT of the chest. Occasionally, the disorder needs to be differentiated from the following conditions: pulmonary tuberculosis in endemic areas, community-acquired pneumonia (especially acute presentations of ABPA), and other inflammatory pulmonary disorders such

Flow chart 2 Suggested treatment algorithm for management of allergic bronchopulmonary aspergillosis

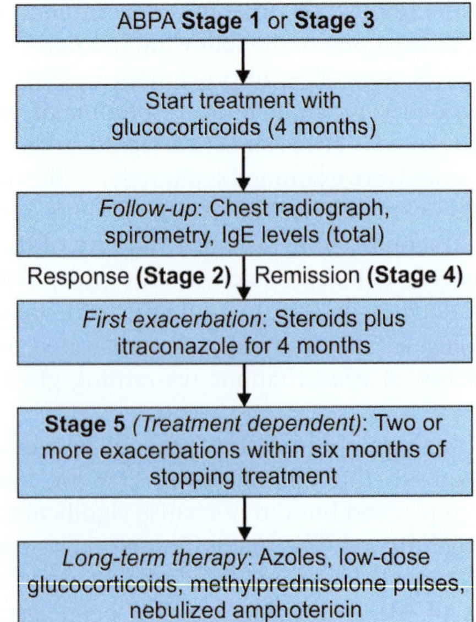

as eosinophilic pneumonia, bronchocentric granulomatosis and Churg-Strauss syndrome.

Complications

The complications of ABPA include recurrent asthma exacerbations, and if untreated development of bronchiectasis with occurrence of pulmonary hypertension and type 2 respiratory failure.[317] Patients can occasionally present with large airway collapse and acute hypoxemic respiratory failure although, this is an uncommon occurrence.[318] In these patients, therapeutic bronchoscopy (either fiberoptic or rigid) is indicated depending on the severity of respiratory failure. Some patients with ABPA develop CPA,[319] manifesting with upper lobe pulmonary fibrosis and shrinkage,[143,320] pulmonary cavitation,[138,143,149,320,321] lobar collapse[138,143] and pleural fibrosis.[143,149] CPA progresses at a variable rate, but may be arrested by successful therapy with azoles.[322] We have also encountered a patient who has developed secondary amyloidosis due to bronchiectasis associated with ABPA. All these complications are likely to be prevented by early diagnosis and treatment. In fact, this is the reason why routine screening is recommended in bronchial asthma to prevent the afore mentioned complications.

Allergic Bronchopulmonary Aspergillosis without Bronchial Asthma

Allergic bronchopulmonary aspergillosis is most commonly known to complicate the course of pre-existing bronchial asthma. It may occasionally develop in an individual without pre-existing bronchial asthma. In a systematic review for the occurrence of ABPA without bronchial asthma, we found 36 cases reported across the globe.[166] Two cases demonstrated bronchodilator reversibility,[323] and one showed airway hyperresponsiveness to methacholine challenge.[324] Majority of the cases demonstrated hypersensitivity to *A. fumigatus* but three showed hypersensitivity to *Helminthosporium*,[323] and one case to *A. niger*.[325,326] Because of absence of bronchial asthma these cases are often mistaken initially for other pulmonary disorders like bronchogenic carcinoma [326-328] or pulmonary tuberculosis.

Allergic Bronchopulmonary Aspergillosis in Cystic Fibrosis

The association of ABPA and CF was first reported in 1965 by Mearns et al. who reported two cases.[329] ABPA is now recognized as a potential complication in patients with CF.[330] The pathogenesis is similar to that of bronchial asthma, and a key element in the immunopathogenesis may be exposure of bronchial lymphoid tissue to high levels of *Aspergillus* allergens, perhaps because of abnormal mucus and immunologic properties resulting from the CF transmembrane conductance regulator mutations.[331-336] Unlike asthma, the recognition of ABPA in CF is difficult as ABPA shares many clinical characteristics with poorly controlled CF lung disease. Presence of wheezing (due to intercurrent infections), transient pulmonary infiltrates, bronchiectasis and mucus plugging are common manifestations of CF-related pulmonary disease with or without ABPA.[337]

Numerous studies have described the prevalence of AH and/or ABPA in patients with CF.[255,338-364] A meta-analysis of these studies suggest the prevalence of AH in CF of 34% (95% CI, 27–41) and the prevalence of ABPA of 7.8% (95% CI, 5.8–10).[2] There was however, no uniformity in the diagnostic criteria with varying criteria used for diagnosis of AH and ABPA in different studies. This fact was also reported in a questionnaire-based study, which revealed a considerable variability in the criteria used for the diagnosis of ABPA in CF.[365] Therefore, prospective reporting of cases with uniform criteria would be the only way to reliably identify the true prevalence of ABPA in CF, and it is likely that database surveys may have overestimated the true prevalence. Atopy seems to be an important risk factor for ABPA in CF. In CF, ABPA was seen in 22% of atopic patients and only 2% of nonatopic patients.[255,353,355,360]

A number of patients with CF develop sensitization to *A. fumigatus* with an increase in total and *A. fumigatus* specific IgE levels; the surprising aspect is that many a patient demonstrate a spontaneous decrease in many immunologic parameters including IgE levels.[349] Thus, the diagnosis of ABPA in CF should not be based solely on serology and skin test results as patients with CF may demonstrate variable responses to *A. fumigatus* and prolonged testing might be required to make a definite diagnosis **(Table 11)**.[330] It is important to identify the development of ABPA in patients with CF as it has been shown that deterioration of lung function is most strikingly pronounced in patients with ABPA compared with a control group of CF patients not sensitized to *A. fumigatus*.[255,362,366] Also, patients with ABPA and CF were demonstrated to have higher rates of microbial colonization, pneumothorax, massive hemoptysis and poorer nutritional status.[357]

Recently, Baxter et al. have proposed a novel immunological classification of aspergillosis in adult CF based on immunoCap total IgE, *A. fumigatus* specific IgE, *A. fumigatus* specific IgG, sputum real-time *Aspergillus* polymerase chain reaction (PCR) and sputum GM.[367] Patients have been classified into four groups: (1) nondiseased group— patients with or without positive RT-PCR but no immunologic response to *A. fumigatus* and negative GM; (2) ABPA-S— patients with positive RT-PCR, elevated total and specific *A. fumigatus* IgE/IgG, and positive GM; (3) *Aspergillus* sensitization— patients with or without positive RT-PCR, elevated *A. fumigatus* IgE (not IgG), and negative GM; and (4) *Aspergillus* bronchitis— patients with positive RT-PCR, elevated *A. fumigatus* IgG (not IgE), and positive GM. It is likely that this classification will allow better clinical phenotyping, pathogenesis studies and management evaluation.

Table 11 Consensus conference proposed diagnostic and screening criteria for allergic bronchopulmonary aspergillosis (ABPA) in cystic fibrosis (CF)[330]

Classic diagnostic criteria
• Acute or subacute clinical deterioration (cough, wheeze and other pulmonary symptoms) not explained by another etiology • Serum total IgE levels >1,000 IU/mL • Immediate cutaneous reactivity to *Aspergillus* or presence of serum IgE antibody to *A. fumigatus* • Precipitating antibodies to *A. fumigatus* or serum IgG antibody to *A. fumigatus* • New or recent abnormalities on chest radiography or chest CT that have not cleared with antibiotics and standard physiotherapy
Minimal diagnostic criteria
• Acute or subacute clinical deterioration (cough, wheeze and other pulmonary symptoms) not explained by another etiology • Total serum IgE levels >500 IU/mL. If total IgE level is 200–500 IU/mL, repeat testing in 1–3 months is recommended • Immediate cutaneous reactivity to *Aspergillus* or presence of serum IgE antibody to *A. fumigatus* • *One of the following*: (A) precipitins to *A. fumigatus* or demonstration of IgG antibody to *A. fumigatus*; or (B) new or recent abnormalities on chest radiography (on chest radiography or chest CT that have not cleared with antibiotics and standard physiotherapy
Screening for ABPA in CF
• Maintain a high level of suspicion for ABPA in patients with CF • Determine the total serum IgE levels annually. If the total serum IgE levels is >500 IU/mL perform *A. fumigatus* skin test or use an IgE antibody to *A. fumigatus*. If results are positive, consider diagnosis on the basis of minimal criteria • If the total serum IgE levels is 200–500 IU/mL, repeat the measurement, if there is increased suspicion for ABPA and perform further diagnostic tests (immediate skin test reactivity to *A. fumigatus*, IgE antibody to *A. fumigatus*, *A. fumigatus* precipitins, or serum IgG antibody to *A. fumigatus*, and chest radiography)
Abbreviations: ABPA, allergic bronchopulmonary aspergillosis; CF, cystic fibrosis; CT, computed tomography

The treatment of ABPA in CF is not very different from that of ABPA in bronchial asthma except that it is more complex as itraconazole capsules are poorly absorbed. Voriconazole may be more successful but often leads to photosensitivity in caucasians, and corticosteroids often induce diabetes mellitus, with its serious consequences in CF.[330]

Coexistence of Allergic Bronchopulmonary Aspergillosis and Aspergilloma

The concurrent presentation of ABPA and aspergilloma in the initial stages of disease represents an immunologically severe form of ABPA with chances of recurrent relapses.[230] In this situation, administration of glucocorticoids alleviates asthma, thus decreasing sputum production.[368] The immunological findings of ABPA have also been reported in patients with pre-existing aspergilloma[368-378] and chronic necrotizing pulmonary aspergillosis.[189] This ABPA-like syndrome can be true hypersensitivity reaction consequent to colonization of *Aspergillus* in long-standing pulmonary cavities of pulmonary diseases like tuberculosis or sarcoidosis.[368,369] Probably, there is a continuous release of *Aspergillus* antigens which leads to immunologic activation in a genetically predisposed individual, thus leading to serological manifestations of ABPA. On the other hand, it can also represent saprophytic *Aspergillus* colonization and subsequent aspergilloma formation in bronchiectatic cavities of ABPA.[377,378] Whatever the predisposing cause, patients with fungal ball and IgE responses show brisk response to glucocorticoids.[368-371,378] Antifungal therapy (with or without steroids) is also helpful in stabilizing the disease and decrease the occurrence of relapses.

Allergic Bronchopulmonary Mycosis

Allergic bronchopulmonary mycosis is the occurrence of ABPA-like syndrome due to non-*A. fumigatus* fungal organisms.[36] A variety of fungal agents **(Table 12)** have been reported to cause this syndrome but the frequency is far less when compared to ABPA.[372,379-394] The diagnostic criteria are similar to that for ABPA except sensitization to the specific fungi needs to be documented.

Allergic Bronchopulmonary Aspergillosis Complicating Other Conditions

Allergic bronchopulmonary aspergillosis is mainly described in patients with bronchial asthma or CF. Occasionally, ABPA has been reported to complicate other lung diseases like idiopathic bronchiectasis,[395] post-tubercular bronchiectasis,[396,397] bronchiectasis secondary to Kartagener's syndrome,[398] chronic obstructive pulmonary disease,[122,399-401] patients with chronic granulomatous disease and hyper IgE syndrome.[402] Most of these are examples comprise of single

Table 12 Fungi implicated in the causation of allergic bronchopulmonary mycosis

- *Aspergillus niger*[372]
- *Helminthosporium* spp.[379]
- *Penicillium* spp.[380]
- *Aspergillus ochraceus*[381]
- *Stemphylium* spp.[382]
- *Aspergillus terreus*[383]
- *Drechslera* spp.[384]
- *Torulopsis* spp.[385]
- *Mucor-like* spp.[386]
- *Candida* spp.[387]
- *Pseudallescheria* spp.[388]
- *Bipolaris* spp.[389]
- *Curvularia* spp.[389]
- *Schizophyllum* spp.[390]
- *Fusarium* spp.[391]
- *Cladosporium* spp.[392]
- *Saccharomyces* spp.[393]
- *Alternaria* spp.[394]

case reports or small case studies; larger observations are required to definitely establish an association.

Sinobronchial Allergic Mycosis Syndrome

The presence of concomitant allergic fungal sinusitis and ABPM in the same patient represents an expression of the same process of fungal hypersensitivity involving the upper and lower airways called the sinobronchial allergic mycosis (SAM) syndrome.[41] Allergic aspergillus sinusitis (AAS), is an entity in which mucoid impaction similar to ABPA occurs in the paranasal sinuses.[403] The pathogenesis is similar to ABPA and represents an allergic hypersensitivity response to the presence of fungi within the sinus cavity.[404] It can also be regarded as the upper airway analogue of ABPA. The patient can be asymptomatic or manifest with symptoms of nasal obstruction, rhinorrhea, headache and epistaxis. In clinical practice, it may not be possible to confirm the diagnosis of AAS in many patients as they decline to undergo the invasive procedures required to establish the diagnosis.[404,405]

The ISHAM-ABPA working group has suggested that patients with ABPA can be labeled as having concomitant AAS if there is combination of hyperattenuating mucus and/or bony erosion on a paranasal CT scan. Treatment is initiated for ABPA with patients receiving additional intranasal glucocorticoids. If the symptoms persist or are troublesome, surgical management may be required for management. Occasionally, the inflammatory mass (fungocele) from the sinus may extend into adjacent spaces such as orbit and manifest as proptosis.[406] Histopathological examination can show findings of branching septate fungi interspersed with eosinophilic mucin and Charcot-Leyden crystals without fungal invasion of soft tissue, with intracranial extension.[407] It is important to differentiate this entity from invasive rhinocerebral aspergillosis as many patients are inadvertently treated with intravenous amphotericin when in fact they should be treated with minimally invasive surgery and glucocorticoid therapy (with or without concomitant azole therapy).[407]

CONCLUSION

A high index of suspicion for ABPA should be maintained while managing any patient with bronchial asthma whatever the severity or the level of control. Host immunologic responses are central to pathogenesis and are the primary determinants of clinical, biological, pathological and radiological features of this disorder. ABPA may precede the clinical recognition of the disorder for many years or even decades, and is often misdiagnosed for a variety of pulmonary diseases. As a patient with ABPA can be minimally symptomatic or asymptomatic, all patients with bronchial asthma should be routinely screened with *A. fumigatus* specific IgE levels. In patients with *Aspergillus* sensitization, further immunologic studies are warranted to diagnose ABPA before the development of bronchiectasis.

REFERENCES

1. Agarwal R, Chakrabarti A. Allergic bronchopulmonary aspergillosis in asthma: epidemiological, clinical and therapeutic issues. Future Microbiol. 2013;8(11):1463-74.
2. Agarwal R. Allergic bronchopulmonary aspergillosis. Chest. 2009;135(3):805-26.
3. Greenberger PA. Allergic bronchopulmonary aspergillosis. J Allergy Clin Immunol. 2002;110(5):685-92.
4. Agarwal R. Controversies in allergic bronchopulmonary aspergillosis. Int J Respir Care. 2010;6(2):53-4, 6-63.
5. Hogan C, Denning DW. Allergic bronchopulmonary aspergillosis and related allergic syndromes. Semin Respir Crit Care Med. 2011;32(6):682-92.
6. Chakrabarti A, Sethi S, Raman DS, Behera D. Eight-year study of allergic bronchopulmonary aspergillosis in an Indian teaching hospital. Mycoses. 2002;45(8):295-9.
7. Agarwal R, Gupta D, Aggarwal AN, Behera D, Jindal SK. Allergic bronchopulmonary aspergillosis: lessons from 126 patients attending a chest clinic in north India. Chest. 2006;130(2): 442-8.
8. Agarwal R, Gupta D, Aggarwal AN, Saxena AK, Chakrabarti A, Jindal SK. Clinical significance of hyperattenuating mucoid impaction in allergic bronchopulmonary aspergillosis: an analysis of 155 patients. Chest. 2007;132(4):1183-90.
9. Agarwal R, Gupta D, Aggarwal AN, Saxena AK, Saikia B, Chakrabarti A, et al. Clinical significance of decline in serum IgE levels in allergic bronchopulmonary aspergillosis. Respir Med. 2010;104(2):204-10.
10. Hinson KF, Moon AJ, Plummer NS. Broncho-pulmonary aspergillosis; a review and a report of eight new cases. Thorax. 1952;7(4):317-33.
11. Elder JL, Smith JT. Allergic bronchopulmonary aspergillosis. Med J Aust. 1967;1:231-3.
12. Patterson R, Golbert TM. Hypersensitivity disease of the lung. Univ Mich Med Cent J. 1968;34(1):8-11.
13. Shah JR. Allergic bronchopulmonary aspergillosis. J Assoc Physicians India. 1971;19(12):835-41.
14. Agarwal R. Burden and distinctive character of allergic bronchopulmonary aspergillosis in India. Mycopathologia. 2014;178(5-6):447-56.
15. Agarwal R, Chakrabarti A, Shah A, Gupta D, Meis JF, Guleria R, et al. Allergic bronchopulmonary aspergillosis: review of literature and proposal of new diagnostic and classification criteria. Clin Exp Allergy. 2013;43(8):850-73.
16. Rosenberg M, Patterson R, Mintzer R, Cooper BJ, Roberts M, Harris KE. Clinical and immunologic criteria for the diagnosis of allergic bronchopulmonary aspergillosis. Ann Intern Med. 1977;86(4):405-14.
17. Greenberger PA, Patterson R, Ghory A, Arkins JA, Walsh T, Graves T, et al. Late sequelae of allergic bronchopulmonary aspergillosis. J Allergy Clin Immunol. 1980;66(4):327-35.
18. Patterson R, Greenberger PA, Radin RC, Roberts M. Allergic bronchopulmonary aspergillosis: staging as an aid to management. Ann Intern Med. 1982;96(3):286-91.
19. Patterson R, Greenberger PA, Halwig JM, Liotta JL, Roberts M. Allergic bronchopulmonary aspergillosis. Natural history and classification of early disease by serologic and roentgenographic studies. Arch Intern Med. 1986;146(5):916-8.
20. Patterson R, Greenberger PA, Lee TM, Liotta JL, O'Neill EA, Roberts M, et al. Prolonged evaluation of patients

with corticosteroid-dependent asthma stage of allergic bronchopulmonary aspergillosis. J Allergy Clin Immunol. 1987;80(5):663-8.
21. Greenberger PA, Patterson R. Allergic bronchopulmonary aspergillosis and the evaluation of the patient with asthma. J Allergy Clin Immunol. 1988;81(4):646-50.
22. Greenberger PA, Miller TP, Roberts M, Smith LL. Allergic bronchopulmonary aspergillosis in patients with and without evidence of bronchiectasis. Ann Allergy. 1993;70(4):333-8.
23. Greenberger PA. Clinical aspects of allergic bronchopulmonary aspergillosis. Front Biosci. 2003;8:s119-27.
24. Bains SN, Judson MA. Allergic bronchopulmonary aspergillosis. Clin Chest Med. 2012;33(2):265-81.
25. Kirsten D, Nowak D, Rabe KF, Magnussen H. [Diagnosis of bronchopulmonary aspergillosis is often made too late]. Med Klin (Munich). 1993;88(6):353-6.
26. Behera D, Guleria R, Jindal SK, Chakrabarti A, Panigrahi D. Allergic bronchopulmonary aspergillosis: a retrospective study of 35 cases. Indian J Chest Dis Allied Sci. 1994;36(4):173-9.
27. Al-Mobeireek AF, El-Rab M, Al-Hedaithy SS, Alasali K, Al-Majed S, Joharjy I. Allergic bronchopulmonary mycosis in patients with asthma: period prevalence at a university hospital in Saudi Arabia. Respir Med. 2001;95(5):341-7.
28. Geiser DM, Klich MA, Frisvad JC, Peterson SW, Varga J, Samson RA. The current status of species recognition and identification in Aspergillus. Stud Mycol. 2007;59:1-10.
29. Walsh TJ, Anaissie EJ, Denning DW, Herbrecht R, Kontoyiannis DP, Marr KA, et al. Treatment of aspergillosis: clinical practice guidelines of the Infectious Diseases Society of America. Clin Infect Dis. 2008;46(3):327-60.
30. Bardana EJ Jr. The clinical spectrum of aspergillosis—part 1: epidemiology, pathogenicity, infection in animals and immunology of Aspergillus. Crit Rev Clin Lab Sci. 1981;13(1):21-83.
31. Franquet T, Muller NL, Gimenez A, Guembe P, de La Torre J, Bague S. Spectrum of pulmonary aspergillosis: histologic, clinical, and radiologic findings. Radiographics. 2001;21(4):825-37.
32. Soubani AO, Chandrasekar PH. The clinical spectrum of pulmonary aspergillosis. Chest. 2002;121(6):1988-99.
33. Shah A. Aspergillus-associated hypersensitivity respiratory disorders. Indian J Chest Dis Allied Sci. 2008;50(1):117-28.
34. Denning DW, O'Driscoll BR, Powell G, Chew F, Atherton GT, Vyas A, et al. Randomized controlled trial of oral antifungal treatment for severe asthma with fungal sensitization: The Fungal Asthma Sensitization Trial (FAST) study. Am J Respir Crit Care Med. 2009;179(1):11-8.
35. Sharma BB, Singh S, Singh V. Hypersensitivity pneumonitis: the dug-well lung. Allergy Asthma Proc. 2013;34(6):e59-64.
36. Chowdhary A, Agarwal K, Kathuria S, Gaur SN, Randhawa HS, Meis JF. Allergic bronchopulmonary mycosis due to fungi other than Aspergillus: a global overview. Crit Rev Microbiol. 2014;40(1):30-48.
37. Agarwal R, Chakrabarti A. Epidemiology of allergic bronchopulmonary aspergillosis. In: Pasqualotto AC (Ed). Aspergillosis from Diagnosis to Prevention. New York: Springer; 2010. pp. 671-88.
38. Agarwal R, Gupta D. Severe asthma and fungi: current evidence. Med Mycol. 2011;49(Suppl 1):S150-7.
39. Agarwal R. Severe asthma with fungal sensitization. Curr Allergy Asthma Rep. 2011;11(5):403-13.
40. Bateman ED. A new look at the natural history of Aspergillus hypersensitivity in asthmatics. Respir Med. 1994;88(5):325-7.
41. Agarwal R, Aggarwal AN, Gupta D, Jindal SK. Aspergillus hypersensitivity and allergic bronchopulmonary aspergillosis in patients with bronchial asthma: systematic review and meta-analysis. Int J Tuberc Lung Dis. 2009;13(8):936-44.
42. Gergen PJ, Arbes SJ Jr, Calatroni A, Mitchell HE, Zeldin DC. Total IgE levels and asthma prevalence in the US population: results from the National Health and Nutrition Examination Survey 2005-2006. J Allergy Clin Immunol. 2009;124(3):447-53.
43. Agarwal R, Noel V, Aggarwal AN, Gupta D, Chakrabarti A. Clinical significance of Aspergillus sensitisation in bronchial asthma. Mycoses. 2011;54(5):e531-8.
44. Malde B, Greenberger PA. Allergic bronchopulmonary aspergillosis. Allergy Asthma Proc. 2004;25(4 Suppl 1):S38-9.
45. Tillie-Leblond I, Tonnel AB. Allergic bronchopulmonary aspergillosis. Allergy. 2005;60(8):1004-13.
46. Donnelly SC, McLaughlin H, Bredin CP. Period prevalence of allergic bronchopulmonary mycosis in a regional hospital outpatient population in Ireland 1985-88. Ir J Med Sci. 1991;160(9):288-90.
47. Novey HS. Epidemiology of allergic bronchopulmonary aspergillosis. Immunol Allergy Clin North Am. 1998;18(3):641-53.
48. Denning DW, Pleuvry A, Cole DC. Global burden of allergic bronchopulmonary aspergillosis with asthma and its complication chronic pulmonary aspergillosis in adults. Med Mycol. 2013;51(4):361-70.
49. Eaton T, Garrett J, Milne D, Frankel A, Wells AU. Allergic bronchopulmonary aspergillosis in the asthma clinic. A prospective evaluation of CT in the diagnostic algorithm. Chest. 2000;118(1):66-72.
50. Kumar R, Gaur SN. Prevalence of allergic bronchopulmonary aspergillosis in patients with bronchial asthma. Asian Pac J Allergy Immunol. 2000;18(4):181-5.
51. Maurya V, Gugnani HC, Sarma PU, Madan T, Shah A. Sensitization to Aspergillus antigens and occurrence of allergic bronchopulmonary aspergillosis in patients with asthma. Chest. 2005;127(4):1252-9.
52. Prasad R, Garg R, Sanjay, Dixit RP. A study on prevalence of allergic bronchopulmonary aspergillosis in patients of bronchial asthma. Internet J Pulm Med. 2008;9(2).
53. Ghosh T, Dey A, Biswas D, Chatterjee S, Haldar N, Maiti PK. Aspergillus hypersensitivity and allergic bronchopulmonary aspergillosis among asthma patients in eastern India. J Indian Med Assoc. 2010;108(12):863-5.
54. Sarkar A, Mukherjee A, Ghoshal AG, Kundu S, Mitra S. Occurrence of allergic bronchopulmonary mycosis in patients with asthma: An Eastern India experience. Lung India. 2010;27(4):212-6.
55. Ma YL, Zhang WB, Yu B, Chen YW, Mu S, Cui YL. [Prevalence of allergic bronchopulmonary aspergillosis in Chinese patients with bronchial asthma]. Zhonghua Jie He He Hu Xi Za Zhi. 2011;34(12):909-13.
56. Agarwal R, Nath A, Aggarwal AN, Gupta D, Chakrabarti A. Aspergillus hypersensitivity and allergic bronchopulmonary aspergillosis in patients with acute severe asthma in a respiratory intensive care unit in North India. Mycoses. 2010;53(2):138-43.
57. Agarwal R, Denning DW, Chakrabarti A. Estimation of the burden of chronic and allergic pulmonary aspergillosis in India. PLoS One. 2014;9(12):e114745.

58. Henderson AH. Allergic aspergillosis; review of 32 cases. Thorax. 1968;23(5):513-23.
59. Kramer MN, Kurup VP, Fink JN. Allergic bronchopulmonary aspergillosis from a contaminated dump site. Am Rev Respir Dis. 1989;140(4):1086-8.
60. Kagen SL, Kurup VP, Sohnle PG, Fink JN. Marijuana smoking and fungal sensitization. J Allergy Clin Immunol. 1983;71(4):389-93.
61. Allmers H, Huber H, Baur X. Two year follow-up of a garbage collector with allergic bronchopulmonary aspergillosis (ABPA). Am J Ind Med. 2000;37(4):438-42.
62. Agarwal R, Devi D, Gupta D, Chakrabarti A. A questionnaire-based study on the role of environmental factors in allergic bronchopulmonary aspergillosis. Lung India. 2014;31(3):232-6.
63. Aimanianda V, Bayry J, Bozza S, Kniemeyer O, Perruccio K, Elluru SR, et al. Surface hydrophobin prevents immune recognition of airborne fungal spores. Nature. 2009;460(7259):1117-21.
64. Moss RB. Pathophysiology and immunology of allergic bronchopulmonary aspergillosis. Med Mycol. 2005;43(Suppl 1):S203-6.
65. Knutsen AP, Mueller KR, Levine AD, Chouhan B, Hutcheson PS, Slavin RG. Asp f I CD4+ TH2-like T-cell lines in allergic bronchopulmonary aspergillosis. J Allergy Clin Immunol. 1994;94(2 Pt 1):215-21.
66. Chauhan B, Knutsen A, Hutcheson PS, Slavin RG, Bellone CJ. T cell subsets, epitope mapping, and HLA-restriction in patients with allergic bronchopulmonary aspergillosis. J Clin Invest. 1996;97(10):2324-31.
67. Chauhan B, Santiago L, Kirschmann DA, Hauptfeld V, Knutsen AP, Hutcheson PS, et al. The association of HLA-DR alleles and T cell activation with allergic bronchopulmonary aspergillosis. J Immunol. 1997;159(8):4072-6.
68. Schuyler M. The Th1/Th2 paradigm in allergic bronchopulmonary aspergillosis. J Lab Clin Med. 1998;131(3):194-6.
69. Knutsen AP, Bellone C, Kauffman H. Immunopathogenesis of allergic bronchopulmonary aspergillosis in cystic fibrosis. Journal of cystic fibrosis : official journal of the European Cystic Fibrosis Society. 2002;1(2):76-89.
70. Murali PS, Kurup VP, Bansal NK, Fink JN, Greenberger PA. IgE down regulation and cytokine induction by Aspergillus antigens in human allergic bronchopulmonary aspergillosis. J Lab Clin Med. 1998;131(3):228-35.
71. Walker C, Bauer W, Braun RK, Menz G, Braun P, Schwarz F, et al. Activated T cells and cytokines in bronchoalveolar lavages from patients with various lung diseases associated with eosinophilia. Am J Respir Crit Care Med. 1994;150(4):1038-48.
72. Khan S, McClellan JS, Knutsen AP. Increased sensitivity to IL-4 in patients with allergic bronchopulmonary aspergillosis. Int Arch Allergy Immunol. 2000;123(4):319-26.
73. Agarwal R. Allergic bronchopulmonary aspergillosis: lessons learnt from genetics. Indian J Chest Dis Allied Sci. 2011;53(3):137-40.
74. Miller PW, Hamosh A, Macek M Jr, Greenberger PA, MacLean J, Walden SM, et al. Cystic fibrosis transmembrane conductance regulator (CFTR) gene mutations in allergic bronchopulmonary aspergillosis. Am J Hum Genet. 1996;59(1):45-51.
75. Aron Y, Bienvenu T, Hubert D, Dusser D, Dall'Ava J, Polla BS. HLA-DR polymorphism in allergic bronchopulmonary aspergillosis. J Allergy Clin Immunol. 1999;104(4 Pt 1):891-2.
76. Chauhan B, Santiago L, Hutcheson PS, Schwartz HJ, Spitznagel E, Castro M, et al. Evidence for the involvement of two different MHC class II regions in susceptibility or protection in allergic bronchopulmonary aspergillosis. J Allergy Clin Immunol. 2000;106(4):723-9.
77. Marchand E, Verellen-Dumoulin C, Mairesse M, Delaunois L, Brancaleone P, Rahier JF, et al. Frequency of cystic fibrosis transmembrane conductance regulator gene mutations and 5T allele in patients with allergic bronchopulmonary aspergillosis. Chest. 2001;119(3):762-7.
78. Eaton TE, Weiner Miller P, Garrett JE, Cutting GR. Cystic fibrosis transmembrane conductance regulator gene mutations: do they play a role in the aetiology of allergic bronchopulmonary aspergillosis? Clin Exp Allergy. 2002;32(5):756-61.
79. Saxena S, Madan T, Shah A, Muralidhar K, Sarma PU. Association of polymorphisms in the collagen region of SP-A2 with increased levels of total IgE antibodies and eosinophilia in patients with allergic bronchopulmonary aspergillosis. J Allergy Clin Immunol. 2003;111(5):1001-7.
80. Brouard J, Knauer N, Boelle PY, Corvol H, Henrion-Caude A, Flamant C, et al. Influence of interleukin-10 on Aspergillus fumigatus infection in patients with cystic fibrosis. J Infect Dis. 2005;191(11):1988-91.
81. Kaur S, Gupta VK, Shah A, Thiel S, Sarma PU, Madan T. Elevated levels of mannan-binding lectin [corrected] (MBL) and eosinophilia in patients of bronchial asthma with allergic rhinitis and allergic bronchopulmonary aspergillosis associate with a novel intronic polymorphism in MBL. Clin Exp Immunol. 2006;143(3):414-9.
82. Knutsen AP. Genetic and respiratory tract risk factors for aspergillosis: ABPA and asthma with fungal sensitization. Med Mycol. 2006;44(Suppl 1):61-70.
83. Knutsen AP, Kariuki B, Consolino JD, Warrier MR. IL-4 alpha chain receptor (IL-4 Ralpha) polymorphisms in allergic bronchopulmonary sspergillosis. Clin Mol Allergy. 2006;4:3.
84. Sambatakou H, Pravica V, Hutchinson IV, Denning DW. Cytokine profiling of pulmonary aspergillosis. Int J Immunogenet. 2006;33(4):297-302.
85. Vaid M, Kaur S, Sambatakou H, Madan T, Denning DW, Sarma PU. Distinct alleles of mannose-binding lectin (MBL) and surfactant proteins A (SP-A) in patients with chronic cavitary pulmonary aspergillosis and allergic bronchopulmonary aspergillosis. Clin Chem Lab Med. 2007;45(2):183-6.
86. Carvalho A, Pasqualotto AC, Pitzurra L, Romani L, Denning DW, Rodrigues F. Polymorphisms in toll-like receptor genes and susceptibility to pulmonary aspergillosis. J Infect Dis. 2008;197(4):618-21.
87. Vicencio AG, Chupp GL, Tsirilakis K, He X, Kessel A, Nandalike K, et al. CHIT1 mutations: genetic risk factor for severe asthma with fungal sensitization? Pediatrics. 2010;126(4):e982-5.
88. Lebecque P, Pepermans X, Marchand E, Leonard A, Leal T. ABPA in adulthood: a CFTR-related disorder. Thorax. 2011;66(6):540-1.
89. Agarwal R, Khan A, Aggarwal AN, Gupta D. Link between CFTR mutations and ABPA: a systematic review and meta-analysis. Mycoses. 2012;55(4):357-65.
90. Harrison E, Singh A, Morris J, Smith NL, Fraczek MG, Moore CB, et al. Mannose-binding lectin genotype and serum levels in patients with chronic and allergic pulmonary aspergillosis. Int J Immunogenet. 2012;39(3):224-32.
91. Muro M, Mondejar-Lopez P, Moya-Quiles MR, Salgado G, Pastor-Vivero MD, Lopez-Hernandez R, et al. HLA-DRB1 and

HLA-DQB1 genes on susceptibility to and protection from allergic bronchopulmonary aspergillosis in patients with cystic fibrosis. Microbiol Immunol. 2013;57(3):193-7.
92. Shah A, Kala J, Sahay S, Panjabi C. Frequency of familial occurrence in 164 patients with allergic bronchopulmonary aspergillosis. Ann Allergy Asthma Immunol. 2008;101(4):363-9.
93. Tomee JF, Wierenga AT, Hiemstra PS, Kauffman HK. Proteases from Aspergillus fumigatus induce release of proinflammatory cytokines and cell detachment in airway epithelial cell lines. J Infect Dis. 1997;176(1):300-3.
94. Tomee JF, Kauffman HF, Klimp AH, de Monchy JG, Koeter GH, Dubois AE. Immunologic significance of a collagen-derived culture filtrate containing proteolytic activity in Aspergillus-related diseases. J Allergy Clin Immunol. 1994;93(4):768-78.
95. Hogaboam CM, Blease K, Schuh JM. Cytokines and chemokines in allergic bronchopulmonary aspergillosis (ABPA) and experimental Aspergillus-induced allergic airway or asthmatic disease. Front Biosci. 2003;8:e147-56.
96. Kauffman HF. Immunopathogenesis of allergic bronchopulmonary aspergillosis and airway remodeling. Front Biosci. 2003;8:e190-6.
97. Kauffman HK, Tomee JFC. Inflammatory cells and airway defense against Aspergillus fumigatus. Immunol Allergy Clin North Am. 1998;18(3):619-40.
98. Kauffman HF, Tomee JF, van de Riet MA, Timmerman AJ, Borger P. Protease-dependent activation of epithelial cells by fungal allergens leads to morphologic changes and cytokine production. J Allergy Clin Immunol. 2000;105(6 Pt 1):1185-93.
99. Golbert TM, Patterson R. Pulmonary allergic aspergillosis. Ann Intern Med. 1970;72(3):395-403.
100. Slavin RG, Fischer VW, Levine EA, Tsai CC, Winzenburger P. A primate model of allergic bronchopulmonary aspergillosis. Int Arch Allergy Appl Immunol. 1978;56(4):325-33.
101. Slavin RG, Bedrossian CW, Hutcheson PS, Pittman S, Salinas-Madrigal L, Tsai CC, et al. A pathologic study of allergic bronchopulmonary aspergillosis. J Allergy Clin Immunol. 1988;81(4):718-25.
102. Chan-Yeung M, Chase WH, Trapp W, Grzybowski S. Allergic bronchopulmonary aspergillosis. Clinical and pathologic study of three cases. Chest. 1971;59(1):33-9.
103. Riley DJ, Mackenzie JW, Uhlman WE, Edelman NH. Allergic bronchopulmonary aspergillosis: evidence of limited tissue invasion. Am Rev Respir Dis. 1975;111(2):232-6.
104. Case records of the Massachusetts General Hospital. Weekly clinicopathological exercises. Case 24-2001. A 46-year-old woman with chronic sinsusitis, pulmonary nodules, and hemoptysis. N Engl J Med. 2001;345(6):443-9.
105. Hanson G, Flor N, Wells I, Novey H, Galant S. Bronchocentric granulomatosis: a complication of allergic bronchopulmonary aspergillosis. J Allergy Clin Immunol. 1977;59(1):83-90.
106. Kradin RL, Mark EJ. The pathology of pulmonary disorders due to Aspergillus spp. Arch Pathol Lab Med. 2008;132(4): 606-14.
107. Starke ID, Keal EE. Cerebral aspergilloma in a patient with allergic bronchopulmonary aspergillosis. Br J Dis Chest. 1980;74(3):301-5.
108. Bodey GP, Glann AS. Central nervous system aspergillosis following steroidal therapy for allergic bronchopulmonary aspergillosis. Chest. 1993;103(1):299-301.
109. Chung Y, Kraut JR, Stone AM, Valaitis J. Disseminated aspergillosis in a patient with cystic fibrosis and allergic bronchopulmonary aspergillosis. Pediatr Pulmonol. 1994;17(2):131-4.
110. Tsimikas S, Hollingsworth HM, Nash G. Aspergillus brain abscess complicating allergic Aspergillus sinusitis. J Allergy Clin Immunol. 1994;94(2 Pt 1):264-7.
111. Ganassini A, Cazzadori A. Invasive pulmonary aspergillosis complicating allergic bronchopulmonary aspergillosis. Respir Med. 1995;89(2):143-5.
112. Gupta K, Das A, Joshi K, Singh N, Aggarwal R, Prakash M. Aspergillus endocarditis in a known case of allergic bronchopulmonary aspergillosis: an autopsy report. Cardiovasc Pathol. 2010;19(4):e137-e9.
113. Agarwal R, Chakrabarti A. Clinical manifestations and natural history of allergic bronchopulmonary aspergillosis. In: Pasqualotto AC (Ed). Aspergillosis from Diagnosis to Prevention. New York: Springer; 2010. pp. 707-24.
114. Imbeau SA, Cohen M, Reed CE. Allergic bronchopulmonary aspergillosis in infants. Am J Dis Child. 1977;131(10):1127-30.
115. Shah A, Kala J, Sahay S. Allergic bronchopulmonary aspergillosis with hilar adenopathy in a 42-month-old boy. Pediatr Pulmonol. 2007;42(8):747-8.
116. McCarthy DS, Pepys S. Allergic broncho-pulmonary aspergillosis. Clinical immunology. Skin, nasal and bronchial tests. Clin Allergy. 1971;1(4):415-32.
117. Malo JL, Hawkins R, Pepys J. Studies in chronic allergic bronchopulmonary aspergillosis. Clinical and physiological findings. Thorax. 1977;32(3):254-61.
118. Agarwal R, Maskey D, Aggarwal AN, Saikia B, Garg M, Gupta D, et al. Diagnostic performance of various tests and criteria employed in allergic bronchopulmonary aspergillosis: a latent class analysis. PLoS One. 2013;8(4):e61105.
119. Agarwal AK, Bhagat R, Panchal N, Shah A. Allergic bronchopulmonary aspergillosis with aspergilloma mimicking fibrocavitary pulmonary tuberculosis. Asian Pac J Allergy Immunol. 1996;14(1):5-8.
120. Malo JL, Paquin R. Incidence of immediate sensitivity to Aspergillus fumigatus in a North American asthmatic population. Clin Allergy. 1979;9(4):377-84.
121. Ownby DR. Diagnostic tests in allergy. In: Lieberman P, Anderson JA (Eds). Allergic diseases diagnosis and treatment, 3rd edition. Totowa, NJ: Humana Press; 2007. pp. 27-38.
122. Agarwal R, Hazarika B, Gupta D, Aggarwal AN, Chakrabarti A, Jindal SK. Aspergillus hypersensitivity in patients with chronic obstructive pulmonary disease: COPD as a risk factor for ABPA? Med Mycol. 2010;48(7):988-94.
123. Rowe DS, Grab B, Anderson SG. An International Reference Preparation for human serum immunoglobulin E. Bull World Health Organ. 1973;49(3):320-1.
124. Bazaral M, Hamburger RN. Standardization and stability of immunoglobulin E (IgE). J Allergy Clin Immunol. 1972;49(3):189-91.
125. Heiner DC, Rose B. Elevated levels of gamma-E (IgE) in conditions other than classical allergy. J Allergy. 1970;45(1):30-42.
126. Wang JL, Patterson R, Rosenberg M, Roberts M, Cooper BJ. Serum IgE and IgG antibody activity against Aspergillus fumigatus as a diagnostic aid in allergic bronchopulmonary aspergillosis. Am Rev Respir Dis. 1978;117(5):917-27.
127. Greenberger PA, Patterson R. Diagnosis and management of allergic bronchopulmonary aspergillosis. Ann Allergy. 1986;56(6):444-8.

128. Vlahakis NE, Aksamit TR. Diagnosis and treatment of allergic bronchopulmonary aspergillosis. Mayo Clin Proc. 2001;76(9):930-8.
129. Wang JL, Patterson R, Roberts M, Ghory AC. The management of allergic bronchopulmonary aspergillosis. Am Rev Respir Dis. 1979;120(1):87-92.
130. Denning DW, O'Driscoll BR, Hogaboam CM, Bowyer P, Niven RM. The link between fungi and severe asthma: a summary of the evidence. Eur Respir J. 2006;27(3):615-26.
131. Wark PA, Hensley MJ, Saltos N, Boyle MJ, Toneguzzi RC, Epid GD, et al. Anti-inflammatory effect of itraconazole in stable allergic bronchopulmonary aspergillosis: a randomized controlled trial. J Allergy Clin Immunol. 2003;111(5):952-7.
132. Mahdavinia M, Grammer LC. Management of allergic bronchopulmonary aspergillosis: a review and update. Ther Adv Respir Dis. 2012;6(3):173-87.
133. Agarwal R, Aggarwal AN, Garg M, Saikia B, Chakrabarti A. Cut-off values of serum IgE (total and A. fumigatus-specific) and eosinophil count in differentiating allergic bronchopulmonary aspergillosis from asthma. Mycoses. 2014;57(11):659-63.
134. Ricketti AJ, Greenberger PA, Patterson R. Serum IgE as an important aid in management of allergic bronchopulmonary aspergillosis. J Allergy Clin Immunol. 1984;74(1):68-71.
135. Greenberger PA. When to suspect and work up allergic bronchopulmonary aspergillosis. Ann Allergy Asthma Immunol. 2013;111(1):1-4.
136. Mendelson EB, Fisher MR, Mintzer RA, Halwig JM, Greenberger PA. Roentgenographic and clinical staging of allergic bronchopulmonary aspergillosis. Chest. 1985;87(3):334-9.
137. Agarwal R. Allergic bronchopulmonary aspergillosis: Lessons for the busy radiologist. World journal of radiology. 2011;3(7):178-81.
138. McCarthy DS, Simon G, Hargreave FE. The radiological appearances in allergic broncho-pulmonary aspergillosis. Clin Radiol. 1970;21(4):366-75.
139. Mintzer RA, Rogers LF, Kruglik GD, Rosenberg M, Neiman HL, Patterson R. The spectrum of radiologic findings in allergic bronchopulmonary aspergillosis. Radiology. 1978;127(2):301-7.
140. Agarwal R, Khan A, Garg M, Aggarwal AN, Gupta D. Chest radiographic and computed tomographic manifestations in allergic bronchopulmonary aspergillosis. World J Radiol. 2012;4(4):141-50.
141. Shah A, Panchal N, Agarwal AK. Allergic bronchopulmonary aspergillosis: The spectrum of roentgenologic appearances. Indian J Radiol Imaging. 1999;9(3):107-12.
142. Shah A. Allergic bronchopulmonary and sinus aspergillosis: the roentgenologic spectrum. Front Biosci. 2003;8:e138-46.
143. Phelan MS, Kerr IH. Allergic bronchopulmonary aspergillosis: the radiological appearance during long-term follow-up. Clin Radiol. 1984;35(5):385-92.
144. Young K, Aspestrand F, Kolbenstvedt A. High resolution CT and bronchography in the assessment of bronchiectasis. Acta Radiol. 1991;32(6):439-41.
145. Grenier P, Maurice F, Musset D, Menu Y, Nahum H. Bronchiectasis: assessment by thin-section CT. Radiology. 1986;161(1):95-9.
146. Agarwal R, Khan A, Garg M, Aggarwal AN, Gupta D. Pictorial essay: Allergic bronchopulmonary aspergillosis. Indian J Radiol Imaging. 2011;21(4):242-52.
147. Panchal N, Pant C, Bhagat R, Shah A. Central bronchiectasis in allergic bronchopulmonary aspergillosis: comparative evaluation of computed tomography of the thorax with bronchography. Eur Respir J. 1994;7(7):1290-3.
148. Lynch DA. Imaging of asthma and allergic bronchopulmonary mycosis. Radiol Clin North Am. 1998;36(1):129-42.
149. Panchal N, Bhagat R, Pant C, Shah A. Allergic bronchopulmonary aspergillosis: the spectrum of computed tomography appearances. Respir Med. 1997;91(4):213-9.
150. Hansell DM, Strickland B. High-resolution computed tomography in pulmonary cystic fibrosis. Br J Radiol. 1989;62(733):1-5.
151. Scadding JG. The bronchi in allergic aspergillosis. Scand J Resp Dis. 1967;48:372-7.
152. Neeld DA, Goodman LR, Gurney JW, Greenberger PA, Fink JN. Computerized tomography in the evaluation of allergic bronchopulmonary aspergillosis. Am Rev Respir Dis. 1990;142(5):1200-5.
153. Angus RM, Davies ML, Cowan MD, McSharry C, Thomson NC. Computed tomographic scanning of the lung in patients with allergic bronchopulmonary aspergillosis and in asthmatic patients with a positive skin test to Aspergillus fumigatus. Thorax. 1994;49(6):586-9.
154. Ward S, Heyneman L, Lee MJ, Leung AN, Hansell DM, Muller NL. Accuracy of CT in the diagnosis of allergic bronchopulmonary aspergillosis in asthmatic patients. AJR Am J Roentgenol. 1999;173(4):937-42.
155. Menzies D, Holmes L, McCumesky G, Prys-Picard C, Niven R. Aspergillus sensitization is associated with airflow limitation and bronchiectasis in severe asthma. Allergy. 2011;66(5):679-85.
156. Mitchell TA, Hamilos DL, Lynch DA, Newell JD. Distribution and severity of bronchiectasis in allergic bronchopulmonary aspergillosis (ABPA). J Asthma. 2000;37(1):65-72.
157. Reiff DB, Wells AU, Carr DH, Cole PJ, Hansell DM. CT findings in bronchiectasis: limited value in distinguishing between idiopathic and specific types. AJR Am J Roentgenol. 1995;165(2):261-7.
158. Agarwal R, Khan A, Gupta D, Aggarwal AN, Saxena AK, Chakrabarti A. An alternate method of classifying allergic bronchopulmonary aspergillosis based on high-attenuation mucus. PLoS One. 2010;5(12):e15346.
159. Goyal R, White CS, Templeton PA, Britt EJ, Rubin LJ. High attenuation mucous plugs in allergic bronchopulmonary aspergillosis: CT appearance. J Comput Assist Tomogr. 1992;16(4):649-50.
160. Logan PM, Muller NL. High-attenuation mucous plugging in allergic bronchopulmonary aspergillosis. Can Assoc Radiol J. 1996;47(5):374-7.
161. Karunaratne N, Baraket M, Lim S, Ridley L. Case quiz. Thoracic CT illustrating hyperdense bronchial mucous plugging: allergic bronchopulmonary aspergillosis. Australas Radiol. 2003;47(3):336-8.
162. Molinari M, Ruiu A, Biondi M, Zompatori M. Hyperdense mucoid impaction in allergic bronchopulmonary aspergillosis: CT appearance. Monaldi Arch Chest Dis. 2004;61(1):62-4.
163. Agarwal R, Aggarwal AN, Gupta D. High-attenuation mucus in allergic bronchopulmonary aspergillosis: another cause of diffuse high-attenuation pulmonary abnormality. AJR Am J Roentgenol. 2006;186(3):904.
164. Morozov A, Applegate KE, Brown S, Howenstine M. High-attenuation mucus plugs on MDCT in a child with cystic fibrosis: potential cause and differential diagnosis. Pediatr Radiol. 2007;37(6):592-5.

165. Agarwal R. High attenuation mucoid impaction in allergic bronchopulmonary aspergillosis. World J Radiol. 2010;2(1): 41-3.
166. Agarwal R, Aggarwal AN, Gupta D, Bal A, Das A. Case report: A rare cause of miliary nodules–allergic bronchopulmonary aspergillosis. Br J Radiol. 2009;82(980):e151-4.
167. Aneja P, Singh UP, Kaur B, Patel K. Miliary nodules: An unusual presentation of allergic bronchopulmonary aspergillosis. Lung India. 2014;31(3):285-8.
168. Khan NA, Sumon SM, Rahman A, Hossain MA, Ferdous J, Bari MR. Miliary nodules in a patient of allergic bronchopulmonary aspergillosis. Mymensingh Med J. 2014;23(2):366-71.
169. Agarwal R, Reddy C, Gupta D. An unusual cause of hilar lymphadenopathy. Lung India. 2006;23(2):90-2.
170. Murphy D, Lane DJ. Pleural effusion in allergic bronchopulmonary aspergillosis: two case reports. Br J Dis Chest. 1981;75(1):91-5.
171. O'Connor TM, O'Donnell A, Hurley M, Bredin CP. Allergic bronchopulmonary aspergillosis: a rare cause of pleural effusion. Respirology. 2001;6(4):361-3.
172. Ogasawara T, Iesato K, Okabe H, Murata K, Kominami S, Tomita K, et al. [A case of pleural effusion associated with allergic bronchopulmonary aspergillosis during a relapse of the disease]. Nihon Kokyuki Gakkai Zasshi. 2003;41(12):905-10.
173. Madan K, Bal A, Agarwal R. Pleural effusion in a patient with allergic bronchopulmonary aspergillosis. Respir Care. 2012;57(9):1509-13.
174. Cote CG, Cicchelli R, Hassoun PM. Hemoptysis and a lung mass in a 51-year-old patient with asthma. Chest. 1998;114(5):1465-8.
175. Ko WK, Choi SW, Park JM, Ahn GH, Kim SK, Chang J, et al. A case of allergic bronchopulmonary aspergillosis shown as bilateral pulmonary masses. Tuberc Respir Dis. 1999;46(2):260-5.
176. Otero Gonzalez I, Montero Martinez C, Blanco Aparicio M, Valino Lopez P, Verea Hernando H. [Pseudotumoral allergic bronchopulmonary aspergillosis]. Arch Bronconeumol. 2000;36(6):351-3.
177. Sanchez-Alarcos JM, Martinez-Cruz R, Ortega L, Calle M, Rodriguez-Hermosa JL, Alvarez-Sala JL. ABPA mimicking bronchogenic cancer. Allergy. 2001;56(1):80-1.
178. Coop C, England RW, Quinn JM. Allergic bronchopulmonary aspergillosis masquerading as invasive pulmonary aspergillosis. Allergy Asthma Proc. 2004;25(4):263-6.
179. Agarwal R, Srinivas R, Agarwal AN, Saxena AK. Pulmonary masses in allergic bronchopulmonary aspergillosis: mechanistic explanations. Respir Care. 2008;53(12):1744-8.
180. Agarwal R, Aggarwal AN, Gupta N, Gupta D. A rare cause of acute respiratory failure-allergic bronchopulmonary aspergillosis. Mycoses. 2011;54(4):e223-7.
181. Garg M, Gupta P, Agarwal R, Khandelwal N. Magnetic resonance imaging (MRI): A new paradigm in imaging evaluation of allergic bronchopulmonary aspergillosis (ABPA)? Chest. 2015;147(2):e58-9.
182. Longbottom JL, Pepys J. Pulmonary aspergillosis: Diagnostic and immunological significance of antigens and C-Substance in Aspergillus Fumigatus. J Pathol Bacteriol. 1964;88:141-51.
183. Fairs A, Agbetile J, Hargadon B, Bourne M, Monteiro WR, Brightling CE, et al. IgE sensitisation to Aspergillus fumigatus is sssociated with reduced lung function in asthma. Am J Respir Crit Care Med. 2010;182(11):1362-8.
184. Baxter CG, Denning DW, Jones AM, Todd A, Moore CB, Richardson MD. Performance of two Aspergillus IgG EIA assays compared with the precipitin test in chronic and allergic aspergillosis. Clin Microbiol Infect. 2013;19(4):E197-204.
185. Campbell MJ, Clayton YM. Bronchopulmonary aspergillosis. A correlation of the clinical and laboratory findings in 272 patients investigated for bronchopulmonary aspergillosis. Am Rev Respir Dis. 1964;89:186-96.
186. McCarthy DS, Pepys J. Allergic bronchopulmonary aspergillosis. Clinical immunology. 2. Skin, nasal and bronchial tests. Clin Allergy. 1971;1(4):415-32.
187. Greenberger PA. Allergic bronchopulmonary aspergillosis. J Allergy Clin Immunol. 1984;74(5):645-53.
188. Denning DW. Chronic forms of pulmonary aspergillosis. Clin Microbiol Infect. 2001;7(Suppl 2):25-31.
189. Denning DW, Riniotis K, Dobrashian R, Sambatakou H. Chronic cavitary and fibrosing pulmonary and pleural aspergillosis: case series, proposed nomenclature change, and review. Clin Infect Dis. 2003;37 (Suppl 3):S265-80.
190. Guazzelli LS, Xavier MO, Oliveira FD, Severo LC. Chronic cavitary pulmonary aspergillosis and fungal balls. In: Pasqualotto AC (Ed). Aspergillosis from Diagnosis to Prevention. New York: Springer; 2009. pp. 585-620.
191. Murali PS, Dai G, Kumar A, Fink JN, Kurup VP. Aspergillus antigen-induced eosinophil differentiation in a murine model. Infect Immun. 1992;60(5):1952-6.
192. Wark PA, Saltos N, Simpson J, Slater S, Hensley MJ, Gibson PG. Induced sputum eosinophils and neutrophils and bronchiectasis severity in allergic bronchopulmonary aspergillosis. Eur Respir J. 2000;16(6):1095-101.
193. Agarwal R, Khan A, Aggarwal AN, Varma N, Garg M, Saikia B, et al. Clinical relevance of peripheral blood eosinophil count in allergic bronchopulmonary aspergillosis. J Infect Public Health. 2011;4(5-6):235-43.
194. Denning DW, Park S, Lass-Florl C, Fraczek MG, Kirwan M, Gore R, et al. High-frequency triazole resistance found in nonculturable Aspergillus fumigatus from lungs of patients with chronic fungal disease. Clin Infect Dis. 2011;52(9):1123-9.
195. Pashley CH, Fairs A, Morley JP, Tailor S, Agbetile J, Bafadhel M, et al. Routine processing procedures for isolating filamentous fungi from respiratory sputum samples may underestimate fungal prevalence. Med Mycol. 2012;50(4):433-8.
196. Klaassen CH, de Valk HA, Curfs-Breuker IM, Meis JF. Novel mixed-format real-time PCR assay to detect mutations conferring resistance to triazoles in Aspergillus fumigatus and prevalence of multi-triazole resistance among clinical isolates in the Netherlands. J Antimicrob Chemother. 2010;65(5): 901-5.
197. Nichols D, Dopico GA, Braun S, Imbeau S, Peters ME, Rankin J. Acute and chronic pulmonary function changes in allergic bronchopulmonary aspergillosis. Am J Med. 1979;67(4):631-7.
198. Kurup VP. Aspergillus antigens: which are important? Med Mycol. 2005;43 (Suppl 1):S189-96.
199. Crameri R, Lidholm J, Menz G, Gronlund H, Blaser K. Automated serology with recombinant allergens. A feasibility study. Adv Exp Med Biol. 1996;409:111-6.
200. Hemmann S, Nikolaizik WH, Schoni MH, Blaser K, Crameri R. Differential IgE recognition of recombinant Aspergillus fumigatus allergens by cystic fibrosis patients with allergic bronchopulmonary aspergillosis or Aspergillus allergy. Eur J Immunol. 1998;28(4):1155-60.

201. Kurup VP, Banerjee B, Hemmann S, Greenberger PA, Blaser K, Crameri R. Selected recombinant Aspergillus fumigatus allergens bind specifically to IgE in ABPA. Clin Exp Allergy. 2000;30(7):988-93.
202. Crameri R, Hemmann S, Ismail C, Menz G, Blaser K. Disease-specific recombinant allergens for the diagnosis of allergic bronchopulmonary aspergillosis. Int Immunol. 1998;10(8):1211-6.
203. Crameri R. Recombinant Aspergillus fumigatus allergens: from the nucleotide sequences to clinical applications. Int Arch Allergy Immunol. 1998;115(2):99-114.
204. Crameri R, Lidholm J, Gronlund H, Stuber D, Blaser K, Menz G. Automated specific IgE assay with recombinant allergens: evaluation of the recombinant Aspergillus fumigatus allergen I in the Pharmacia Cap System. Clin Exp Allergy. 1996;26(12):1411-9.
205. Nikolaizik WH, Moser M, Crameri R, Little S, Warner JO, Blaser K, et al. Identification of allergic bronchopulmonary aspergillosis in cystic fibrosis patients by recombinant Aspergillus fumigatus I/a-specific serology. Am J Respir Crit Care Med. 1995;152(2):634-9.
206. Nikolaizik WH, Weichel M, Blaser K, Crameri R. Intracutaneous tests with recombinant allergens in cystic fibrosis patients with allergic bronchopulmonary aspergillosis and Aspergillus allergy. Am J Respir Crit Care Med. 2002;165(7):916-21.
207. Arruda LK, Mann BJ, Chapman MD. Selective expression of a major allergen and cytotoxin, Asp f I, in Aspergillus fumigatus. Implications for the immunopathogenesis of Aspergillus-related diseases. J Immunol. 1992;149(10):3354-9.
208. Casaulta C, Fluckiger S, Crameri R, Blaser K, Schoeni MH. Time course of antibody response to recombinant Aspergillus fumigatus antigens in cystic fibrosis with and without ABPA. Pediatr Allergy Immunol. 2005;16(3):217-25.
209. Kurup VP, Knutsen AP, Moss RB, Bansal NK. Specific antibodies to recombinant allergens of Aspergillus fumigatus in cystic fibrosis patients with ABPA. Clin Mol Allergy. 2006;4:11.
210. Knutsen AP, Hutcheson PS, Slavin RG, Kurup VP. IgE antibody to Aspergillus fumigatus recombinant allergens in cystic fibrosis patients with allergic bronchopulmonary aspergillosis. Allergy. 2004;59(2):198-203.
211. Hemmann S, Ismail C, Blaser K, Menz G, Crameri R. Skin-test reactivity and isotype-specific immune responses to recombinant Asp f 3, a major allergen of Aspergillus fumigatus. Clin Exp Allergy. 1998;28(7):860-7.
212. de Oliveira E, Giavina-Bianchi P, Fonseca LA, Franca AT, Kalil J. Allergic bronchopulmonary aspergillosis' diagnosis remains a challenge. Respir Med. 2007;101(11):2352-7.
213. Denning DW, Pashley C, Hartl D, Wardlaw A, Godet C, Del Giacco S, et al. Fungal allergy in asthma-state of the art and research needs. Clinical and translational allergy. 2014; 4:14.
214. Agarwal R, Aggarwal AN, Sehgal IS, Dhooria S, Behera D, Chakrabarti A. Performance of serum galactomannan in patients with allergic bronchopulmonary aspergillosis. Mycoses. 2015;58(7):408-12.
215. Latzin P, Hartl D, Regamey N, Frey U, Schoeni MH, Casaulta C. Comparison of serum markers for allergic bronchopulmonary aspergillosis in cystic fibrosis. Eur Respir J. 2008;31(1):36-42.
216. Hartl D, Latzin P, Zissel G, Krane M, Krauss-Etschmann S, Griese M. Chemokines indicate allergic bronchopulmonary aspergillosis in patients with cystic fibrosis. Am J Respir Crit Care Med. 2006;173(12):1370-6.
217. Gernez Y, Dunn CE, Everson C, Mitsunaga E, Gudiputi L, Krasinska K, et al. Blood basophils from cystic fibrosis patients with allergic bronchopulmonary aspergillosis are primed and hyper-responsive to stimulation by aspergillus allergens. Journal of cystic fibrosis: official Journal of the European Cystic Fibrosis Society. 2012;11(6):502-10.
218. Schwartz HJ, Greenberger PA. The prevalence of allergic bronchopulmonary aspergillosis in patients with asthma, determined by serologic and radiologic criteria in patients at risk. J Lab Clin Med. 1991;117(2):138-42.
219. Imbeau SA, Nichols D, Flaherty D, Dickie H, Reed C. Relationships between prednisone therapy, disease activity, and the total serum IgE level in allergic bronchopulmonary aspergillosis. J Allergy Clin Immunol. 1978;62(2):91-5.
220. Leser C, Kauffman HF, Virchow C Sr, Menz G. Specific serum immunopatterns in clinical phases of allergic bronchopulmonary aspergillosis. J Allergy Clin Immunol. 1992;90(4 Pt 1):589-99.
221. Malo JL, Longbottom J, Mitchell J, Hawkins R, Pepys J. Studies in chronic allergic bronchopulmonary aspergillosis. 3. Immunological findings. Thorax. 1977;32(3):269-74.
222. Dhooria S, Agarwal R. Diagnosis of allergic bronchopulmonary aspergillosis: a case-based approach. Future Microbiol. 2014;9(10):1195-208.
223. Rosenberg M, Patterson R, Roberts M, Wang J. The assessment of immunologic and clinical changes occurring during corticosteroid therapy for allergic bronchopulmonary aspergillosis. Am J Med. 1978;64(4):599-606.
224. Ricketti AJ, Greenberger PA, Patterson R. Varying presentations of allergic bronchopulmonary aspergillosis. Int Arch Allergy Appl Immunol. 1984;73(3):283-5.
225. Halwig JM, Greenberger PA, Levine M, Patterson R. Recurrence of allergic bronchopulmonary aspergillosis after seven years of remission. J Allergy Clin Immunol. 1984;74(5):738-40.
226. Lee TM, Greenberger PA, Patterson R, Roberts M, Liotta JL. Stage V (fibrotic) allergic bronchopulmonary aspergillosis. A review of 17 cases followed from diagnosis. Arch Intern Med. 1987;147(2):319-23.
227. Skowronski E, Fitzgerald DA. Life-threatening allergic bronchopulmonary aspergillosis in a well child with cystic fibrosis. Med J Aust. 2005;182(9):482-3.
228. Thomas MF. Life-threatening allergic bronchopulomnary aspergillosis treated with methylprednisolone and anti-IgE monoclonal antibody. J R Soc Med. 2009;102 Suppl 1:49-53.
229. Patterson R. Allergic bronchopulmonary aspergillosis and hypersensitivity reactions to fungi. In: Fishman AP, Elias JA, Fishman JA, Grippi MA, Kaiser LR, Senior RM (Eds). Fishman's Pulmonary Diseases and Disorders, 3rd edition. New York: McGraw Hill; 1998. pp. 777-82.
230. Agarwal R, Aggarwal AN, Garg M, Saikia B, Gupta D, Chakrabarti A. Allergic bronchopulmonary aspergillosis with aspergilloma: an immunologically severe disease with poor outcome. Mycopathologia. 2012;174(3):193-201.
231. Agarwal R. What is the current place of azoles in allergic bronchopulmonary aspergillosis and severe asthma with fungal sensitization. Expert Rev Respir Med. 2012;6(4):363-71.
232. Sehgal IS, Agarwal R. Role of inhaled amphotericin in allergic bronchopulmonary aspergillosis. J Postgrad Med. 2014;60(1): 41-5.
233. Singh Sehgal I, Agarwal R. Pulse methylprednisolone in allergic bronchopulmonary aspergillosis exacerbations. Eur Respir Rev. 2014;23(131):149-52.

234. Baur X, Weiss W, Jarosch B, Menz G, Schoch C, Schmitz-Schumann M, et al. Immunoprint pattern in patients with allergic bronchopulmonary aspergillosis in different stages. J Allergy Clin Immunol. 1989;83(4):839-44.
235. Kumar R, Chopra D. Evaluation of allergic bronchopulmonary aspergillosis in patients with and without central bronchiectasis. J Asthma. 2002;39(6):473-7.
236. Kumar R. Mild, moderate, and severe forms of allergic bronchopulmonary aspergillosis: a clinical and serologic evaluation. Chest. 2003;124(3):890-2.
237. Agarwal R, Garg M, Aggarwal AN, Saikia B, Gupta D, Chakrabarti A. Serologic allergic bronchopulmonary aspergillosis (ABPA-S): Long-term outcomes. Respir Med. 2012;106(7):942-7.
238. Agarwal R, Chakrabarti A. Allergic bronchopulmonary aspergillosis. In: Chakrabarti A (Ed). Fungal Infections in Asia the Eastern frontier of Mycology. New Delhi: Elsevier; 2013. pp. 173-93.
239. Denning DW, Van Wye JE, Lewiston NJ, Stevens DA. Adjunctive therapy of allergic bronchopulmonary aspergillosis with itraconazole. Chest. 1991;100(3):813-9.
240. Hilton AM, Chatterjee SS. Bronchopulmonary aspergillosis-treatment with beclomethasone dipropionate. Postgrad Med J. 1975;51 (Suppl 4):98-103.
241. Inhaled beclomethasone dipropionate in allergic bronchopulmonary aspergillosis. Report to the Research Committee of the British Thoracic Association. Br J Dis Chest. 1979;73(4):349-56.
242. Heinig JH, Weeke ER, Groth S, Schwartz B. High-dose local steroid treatment in bronchopulmonary aspergillosis. A pilot study. Allergy. 1988;43(1):24-31.
243. Balter MS, Rebuck AS. Treatment of allergic bronchopulmonary aspergillosis with inhaled corticosteroids. Respir Med. 1992;86(5):441-2.
244. Imbeault B, Cormier Y. Usefulness of inhaled high-dose corticosteroids in allergic bronchopulmonary aspergillosis. Chest. 1993;103(5):1614-7.
245. Seaton A, Seaton RA, Wightman AJ. Management of allergic bronchopulmonary aspergillosis without maintenance oral corticosteroids: a fifteen-year follow-up. QJM. 1994;87(9): 529-37.
246. Agarwal R, Khan A, Aggarwal AN, Saikia B, Gupta D, Chakrabarti A. Role of inhaled corticosteroids in the management of serological allergic bronchopulmonary aspergillosis (ABPA). Intern Med. 2011;50(8):855-60.
247. Frauman AG. An overview of the adverse reactions to adrenal corticosteroids. Adverse Drug React Toxicol Rev. 1996;15(4):203-6.
248. Schacke H, Docke WD, Asadullah K. Mechanisms involved in the side effects of glucocorticoids. Pharmacol Ther. 2002;96(1):23-43.
249. Shale DJ, Faux JA, Lane DJ. Trial of ketoconazole in non-invasive pulmonary aspergillosis. Thorax. 1987;42(1):26-31.
250. De Beule K, De Doncker P, Cauwenbergh G, Koster M, Legendre R, Blatchford N, et al. The treatment of aspergillosis and aspergilloma with itraconazole, clinical results of an open international study (1982-1987). Mycoses. 1988;31(9):476-85.
251. Mannes GP, van der Heide S, van Aalderen WM, Gerritsen J. Itraconazole and allergic bronchopulmonary aspergillosis in twin brothers with cystic fibrosis. Lancet. 1993;341(8843):492.
252. Pacheco A, Martin JA, Cuevas M. Serologic response to itraconazole in allergic bronchopulmonary aspergillosis. Chest. 1993;103(3):980-1.
253. Germaud P, Tuchais E. Allergic bronchopulmonary aspergillosis treated with itraconazole. Chest. 1995;107(3):883.
254. Nikaido Y, Nagata N, Yamamoto T, Yoshii C, Ohmori H, Kido M. A case of allergic bronchopulmonary aspergillosis successfully treated with itraconazole. Respir Med. 1998;92(1):118-9.
255. Nepomuceno IB, Esrig S, Moss RB. Allergic bronchopulmonary aspergillosis in cystic fibrosis: role of atopy and response to itraconazole. Chest. 1999;115(2):364-70.
256. Salez F, Brichet A, Desurmont S, Grosbois JM, Wallaert B, Tonnel AB. Effects of itraconazole therapy in allergic bronchopulmonary aspergillosis. Chest. 1999;116(6):1665-8.
257. Suzuki M, Sugiyama Y, Kitamura S. A case of allergic bronchopulmonary aspergillosis refractory to the corticosteroid therapy and successfully treated by Itraconazole. Japanese J Chest Diseases. 1999;58(10):770-5.
258. Stevens DA, Schwartz HJ, Lee JY, Moskovitz BL, Jerome DC, Catanzaro A, et al. A randomized trial of itraconazole in allergic bronchopulmonary aspergillosis. N Engl J Med. 2000;342(11):756-62.
259. Skov M, Hoiby N, Koch C. Itraconazole treatment of allergic bronchopulmonary aspergillosis in patients with cystic fibrosis. Allergy. 2002;57(8):723-8.
260. Kumar R, Singh P, Arora R, Gaur SN. Effect of itraconazole therapy in allergic bronchopulmonary aspergillosis. Saudi Med J. 2003;24(5):546-7.
261. Morimoto T, Ohnishi H, Fujiyama R, Tomioka H, Sakurai T, Tada K, et al. Allergic bronchopulmonary aspergillosis successfully treated with itraconazole and fluticasone. Japanese Journal of Chest Diseases. 2003;62(1):55-60.
262. Ferrari M, Bodini I, Lo Cascio V. Rhabdomyolysis after the administration of itraconazole to an asthmatic patient with bronchopulmonary aspergillosis. Respiration. 2004;71(3):289-91.
263. Wark PA, Gibson PG, Wilson AJ. Azoles for allergic bronchopulmonary aspergillosis associated with asthma. The Cochrane database of systematic reviews. 2004(3):CD001108.
264. Pasqualotto AC, Denning DW. Generic substitution of itraconazole resulting in sub-therapeutic levels and resistance. Int J Antimicrob Agents. 2007;30(1):93-4.
265. Muthu V, Agarwal R. A report of a successfully treated case of ABPA in a HIV-infected individual. BMJ Case Rep. 2014;2014.
266. Howard SJ, Cerar D, Anderson MJ, Albarrag A, Fisher MC, Pasqualotto AC, et al. Frequency and evolution of azole resistance in Aspergillus fumigatus associated with treatment failure. Emerg Infect Dis. 2009;15(7):1068-76.
267. Lestner JM, Roberts SA, Moore CB, Howard SJ, Denning DW, Hope WW. Toxicodynamics of itraconazole: implications for therapeutic drug monitoring. Clin Infect Dis. 2009;49(6):928-30.
268. Hilliard T, Edwards S, Buchdahl R, Francis J, Rosenthal M, Balfour-Lynn I, et al. Voriconazole therapy in children with cystic fibrosis. JCyst Fibros. 2005;4(4):215-20.
269. McCallum BJ, Amrol D, Horvath J, Inayat N, Talwani R. A case of allergic bronchopulmonary aspergillosis leading to pneumonia with unusual organisms. South Med J. 2005;98(11):1135-8.
270. Mulliez P, Croxo C, Roy-Saint Georges F, Darras A. [Allergic broncho-pulmonary aspergillosis treated with voriconazole]. Rev Mal Respir. 2006;23(1 Pt 1):93-4.
271. Bandres Gimeno R, Munoz Martinez MJ. [Prolonged therapeutic response to voriconazole in a case of allergic bronchopulmonary aspergillosis]. Arch Bronconeumol. 2007;43(1):49-51.

272. Erwin GE, Fitzgerald JE. Case report: allergic bronchopulmonary aspergillosis and allergic fungal sinusitis successfully treated with voriconazole. J Asthma. 2007;44(10):891-5.
273. Glackin L, Leen G, Elnazir B, Greally P. Voriconazole in the treatment of allergic bronchopulmonary aspergillosis in cystic fibrosis. Ir Med J. 2009;102(1):29.
274. Gendrot A, de La Blanchardiere A, de La Gastine B, Fromager G, Massias L, Verdon R. [Painful peripheral neuropathy associated with voriconazole during the treatment of chronic cavitary pulmonary aspergillosis]. Rev Med Interne. 2010;31(2):163-6.
275. Mulliez P. [Treatment of ABPA: a place for voriconazole and omalizumab?]. Rev Mal Respir. 2010;27(7):670-2.
276. Mulliez P, Croxo C, Saint-Georges FR. [Rebound after ABPA treatment with voriconazole]. Rev Mal Respir. 2010;27(7): 786-7.
277. Skov M, Pressler T. High-dose IV-pulse methylprednisolone (HDIVPM) successful treatment of allergic bronchopulmonary aspergillosis (ABPA). Pediatr Pulmonol. 2010;45:365.
278. Chishimba L, Niven RM, Cooley J, Denning DW. Voriconazole and posaconazole improve asthma severity in allergic bronchopulmonary aspergillosis and severe asthma with fungal sensitization. J Asthma. 2012;49(4):423-33.
279. Kamei K, Kohno N, Tabeta H, Honda A, Unno H, Nagao K, et al. [The treatment of pulmonary aspergilloma with itraconazole]. Kansenshogaku Zasshi. 1991;65(7):808-12.
280. Tucker RM, Haq Y, Denning DW, Stevens DA. Adverse events associated with itraconazole in 189 patients on chronic therapy. J Antimicrob Chemother. 1990;26(4):561-6.
281. Lebrun-Vignes B, Archer VC, Diquet B, Levron JC, Chosidow O, Puech AJ, et al. Effect of itraconazole on the pharmacokinetics of prednisolone and methylprednisolone and cortisol secretion in healthy subjects. Br J Clin Pharmacol. 2001;51(5):443-50.
282. Main KM, Skov M, Sillesen IB, Dige-Petersen H, Muller J, Koch C, et al. Cushing's syndrome due to pharmacological interaction in a cystic fibrosis patient. Acta Paediatr. 2002;91(9):1008-11.
283. Skov M, Main KM, Sillesen IB, Muller J, Koch C, Lanng S. Iatrogenic adrenal insufficiency as a side-effect of combined treatment of itraconazole and budesonide. Eur Respir J. 2002;20(1):127-33.
284. Dupont B. Itraconazole therapy in aspergillosis: study in 49 patients. J Am Acad Dermatol. 1990;23(3 Pt 2):607-14.
285. Zwald FO, Spratt M, Lemos BD, Veledar E, Lawrence C, Marshall Lyon G, et al. Duration of voriconazole exposure: an independent risk factor for skin cancer after lung transplantation. Dermatol Surg. 2012;38(8):1369-74.
286. Lestner JM, Denning DW. Tremor: a newly described adverse event with long-term itraconazole therapy. J Neurol Neurosurg Psychiatry. 2010;81(3):327-9.
287. Laoudi Y, Paolini JB, Grimfed A, Just J. Nebulised corticosteroid and amphotericin B: an alternative treatment for ABPA? Eur Respir J. 2008;31(4):908-9.
288. Hayes D Jr, Murphy BS, Lynch JE, Feola DJ. Aerosolized amphotericin for the treatment of allergic bronchopulmonary aspergillosis. Pediatr Pulmonol. 2010;45(11):1145-8.
289. Proesmans M, Vermeulen F, Vreys M, De Boeck K. Use of nebulized amphotericin B in the treatment of allergic bronchopulmonary aspergillosis in cystic fibrosis. Int J Pediatr. 2010;2010:376287.
290. Godet C, Meurice JC, Roblot F, Kauffmann-Lacroix C, Verdaguer M, Frat JP, et al. Efficacy of nebulised liposomal amphotericin B in the attack and maintenance treatment of ABPA. Eur Respir J. 2012;39(5):1261-3.
291. van der Ent CK, Hoekstra H, Rijkers GT. Successful treatment of allergic bronchopulmonary aspergillosis with recombinant anti-IgE antibody. Thorax. 2007;62(3):276-7.
292. Kanu A, Patel K. Treatment of allergic bronchopulmonary aspergillosis (ABPA) in CF with anti-IgE antibody (omalizumab). Pediatr Pulmonol. 2008;43(12):1249-51.
293. Zirbes JM, Milla CE. Steroid-sparing effect of omalizumab for allergic bronchopulmonary aspergillosis and cystic fibrosis. Pediatr Pulmonol. 2008;43(6):607-10.
294. Alcorta A. Successful treatment of allergic bronchopulmonary aspergillosis with omalizumab. Allergy. 2009;64:477-8.
295. Gonzalez De Olano D, Gonzalez-Mancebo E, Gandolfo Cano M, Melendez Baltanas A, Valeri-Busto V, Racionero MA, et al. Successful treatment of allergic bronchopulmonary candidiasis with a recombinant anti-immunoglobulin E antibody. J Investig Allergol Clin Immunol. 2009;19(5):416-7.
296. Lebecque P, Leonard A, Argaz M, Godding V, Pilette C. Omalizumab for exacerbations of allergic bronchopulmonary aspergillosis in patients with cystic fibrosis. BMJ Case Rep. 2009;2009.
297. Quintas Vazquez LM, Ortiz Piquer M, Perez de Llano LA. [Effective anti-immunoglobulin-E antibody treatment of a patient with allergic bronchopulmonary aspergillosis]. Arch Bronconeumol. 2009;45(4):207.
298. Randhawa I, Chin T, Nussbaum E. Resolution of corticosteroid-induced diabetes in allergic bronchopulmonary aspergillosis with omalizumab therapy: a novel approach. J Asthma. 2009;46(5):445-7.
299. Schulze J, Christmann M, Rosewich M, Lieb A, Rose M, Posselt H, et al. Omalizumab for allergic bronchopulmonary aspergillosis. Allergy. 2009;64:97-8.
300. Brinkmann F, Schwerk N, Hansen G, Ballmann M. Steroid dependency despite omalizumab treatment of ABPA in cystic fibrosis. Allergy. 2010;65(1):134-5.
301. Gonzalez L, Aparicio M, Parra A. Asthma and allergic bronchopulmonary aspergillosis (ABPA). Response to omalizumab treatment. Allergy. 2010;65:531.
302. Lin RY, Sethi S, Bhargave GA. Measured immunoglobulin E in allergic bronchopulmonary aspergillosis treated with omalizumab. J Asthma. 2010;47(8):942-5.
303. Perez-de-Llano LA, Vennera MC, Parra A, Guallar J, Marin M, Asensio O, et al. Effects of omalizumab in Aspergillus-associated airway disease. Thorax. 2011;66(6):539-40.
304. Schulze J, Zissler U, Christmann M, Rosewich M, Zielen S. Allergic bronchopulmonary aspergillosis (ABPA) an IgE mediated disease? Respir Med CME. 2011;4(1):33-4.
305. Tillie-Leblond I, Germaud P, Leroyer C, Tetu L, Girard F, Devouassoux G, et al. Allergic bronchopulmonary aspergillosis and omalizumab. Allergy. 2011;66(9):1254-6.
306. Thomson JM, Wesley A, Byrnes CA, Nixon GM. Pulse intravenous methylprednisolone for resistant allergic bronchopulmonary aspergillosis in cystic fibrosis. Pediatr Pulmonol. 2006;41(2):164-70.
307. Cohen-Cymberknoh M, Blau H, Shoseyov D, Mei-Zahav M, Efrati O, Armoni S, et al. Intravenous monthly pulse methylprednisolone treatment for ABPA in patients with cystic fibrosis. J Cyst Fibros. 2009;8(4):253-7.
308. Ghdifan S, Couderc L, Michelet I, Leguillon C, Masseline B, Marguet C. Bolus methylprednisolone efficacy for uncontrolled

exacerbation of cystic fibrosis in children. Pediatrics. 2010;125(5):e1259-64.
309. Kreindler JL, Steele C, Nguyen N, Chan YR, Pilewski JM, Alcorn JF, et al. Vitamin D3 attenuates Th2 responses to Aspergillus fumigatus mounted by CD4+ T cells from cystic fibrosis patients with allergic bronchopulmonary aspergillosis. J Clin Invest. 2010;120(9):3242-54.
310. Nair P, Pizzichini MM, Kjarsgaard M, Inman MD, Efthimiadis A, Pizzichini E, et al. Mepolizumab for prednisone-dependent asthma with sputum eosinophilia. N Engl J Med. 2009;360(10):985-93.
311. Ortega HG, Liu MC, Pavord ID, Brusselle GG, FitzGerald JM, Chetta A, et al. Mepolizumab treatment in patients with severe eosinophilic asthma. N Engl J Med. 2014;371(13):1198-207.
312. Bel EH, Wenzel SE, Thompson PJ, Prazma CM, Keene ON, Yancey SW, et al. Oral glucocorticoid-sparing effect of mepolizumab in eosinophilic asthma. N Engl J Med. 2014;371(13):1189-97.
313. Corren J, Lemanske RF, Hanania NA, Korenblat PE, Parsey MV, Arron JR, et al. Lebrikizumab treatment in adults with asthma. N Engl J Med. 2011;365(12):1088-98.
314. Moss RB. The use of biological agents for the treatment of fungal asthma and allergic bronchopulmonary aspergillosis. Ann N Y Acad Sci. 2012;1272:49-57.
315. Moss RB. Treatment options in severe fungal asthma and allergic bronchopulmonary aspergillosis. Eur Respir J. 2014;43(5):1487-500.
316. Burgel PR, Baixench MT, Amsellem M, Audureau E, Chapron J, Kanaan R, et al. High prevalence of azole-resistant Aspergillus fumigatus in adults with cystic fibrosis exposed to itraconazole. Antimicrob Agents Chemother. 2012;56(2):869-74.
317. Agarwal R, Singh N, Gupta D. Pulmonary hypertension as a presenting manifestation of allergic bronchopulmonary aspergillosis. Indian J Chest Dis Allied Sci. 2009;51(1):37-40.
318. Agarwal R, Aggarwal AN, Gupta N, Gupta D. A rare cause of acute respiratory failure–allergic bronchopulmonary aspergillosis. Mycoses. 2011;54(4):e223-7.
319. Smith NL, Denning DW. Underlying conditions in chronic pulmonary aspergillosis including simple aspergilloma. Eur Respir J. 2011;37(4):865-72.
320. Gefter WB, Epstein DM, Miller WT. Allergic bronchopulmonary aspergillosis: Less common patterns. Radiology. 1981;140(2):307-12.
321. Menon MP, Das AK. Allergic bronchopulmonary aspergillosis (radiological aspects). Indian J Chest Dis Allied Sci. 1977;19(4): 157-69.
322. Felton TW, Baxter C, Moore CB, Roberts SA, Hope WW, Denning DW. Efficacy and safety of posaconazole for chronic pulmonary aspergillosis. Clin Infect Dis. 2010;51(12):1383-91.
323. Glancy JJ, Elder JL, McAleer R. Allergic bronchopulmonary fungal disease without clinical asthma. Thorax. 1981;36(5): 345-9.
324. Yoshida N, Suguro H, Kohara F, Akiyama Y, Katoh H, Hashimoto N, et al. [A case of allergic bronchopulmonary aspergillosis with no history of bronchial asthma]. Nihon Kyobu Shikkan Gakkai zasshi. 1992;30(12):2123-7.
325. Hoshino H, Tagaki S, Kon H, Shibusa T, Takabatake H, Fujita A, et al. Allergic bronchopulmonary aspergillosis due to Aspergillus niger without bronchial asthma. Respiration. 1999;66(4):369-72.
326. Shah A, Maurya V, Panjabi C, Khanna P. Allergic bronchopulmonary aspergillosis without clinical asthma caused by Aspergillus niger. Allergy. 2004;59(2):236-7.
327. Berkin KE, Vernon DR, Kerr JW. Lung collapse caused by allergic bronchopulmonary aspergillosis in non-asthmatic patients. Br Med J (Clin Res Ed). 1982;285(6341):552-3.
328. Bondue B, Remmelink M, Gevenois PA, Yernault JC, De Vuyst P. A pulmonary cavitated mass complicating long-standing allergic bronchopulmonary aspergillosis. Respir Med Extra. 2005;1(3):39-42.
329. Mearns M, Young W, Batten J. Transient pulmonary infiltrations in cystic fibrosis due to allergic aspergillosis. Thorax. 1965;20(9):385-92.
330. Stevens DA, Moss RB, Kurup VP, Knutsen AP, Greenberger P, Judson MA, et al. Allergic bronchopulmonary aspergillosis in cystic fibrosis–state of the art: Cystic Fibrosis Foundation Consensus Conference. Clin Infect Dis. 2003;37 (Suppl 3):S225-64.
331. de Almeida MB, Bussamra MH, Rodrigues JC. Allergic bronchopulmonary aspergillosis in paediatric cystic fibrosis patients. Paediatr Respir Rev. 2006;7(1):67-72.
332. Chen JH, Schulman H, Gardner P. A cAMP-regulated chloride channel in lymphocytes that is affected in cystic fibrosis. Science. 1989;243(4891):657-60.
333. Moss RB, Hsu YP, Olds L. Cytokine dysregulation in activated cystic fibrosis (CF) peripheral lymphocytes. Clin Exp Immunol. 2000;120(3):518-25.
334. Allard JB, Poynter ME, Marr KA, Cohn L, Rincon M, Whittaker LA. Aspergillus fumigatus generates an enhanced Th2-biased immune response in mice with defective cystic fibrosis transmembrane conductance regulator. J Immunol. 2006;177(8):5186-94.
335. Mueller C, Braag SA, Keeler A, Hodges C, Drumm M, Flotte TR. Lack of cystic fibrosis transmembrane conductance regulator in CD3+ lymphocytes leads to aberrant cytokine secretion and hyperinflammatory adaptive immune responses. Am J Respir Cell Mol Biol. 2011;44(6):922-9.
336. Chaudhary N, Datta K, Askin FB, Staab JF, Marr KA. Dysfunctional CFTR impacts pulmonary inflammatory responses to aspergillus fumigatus. Pediatr Pulmonol. 2011; 46:267.
337. Moss RB. Allergic bronchopulmonary aspergillosis and Aspergillus infection in cystic fibrosis. Curr Opin Pulm Med. 2010;16(6):598-603.
338. Mearns M, Longbottom J, Batten J. Precipitating antibodies to aspergillus fumigatus in cystic fibrosis. Lancet. 1967; 1(7489):538-9.
339. Allan JD, Moss AD, Wallwork JC, McFarlane H. Immediate hypersensitivity in patients with cystic fibrosis. Clin Allergy. 1975;5(3):255-61.
340. Silverman M, Hobbs FD, Gordon IR, Carswell F. Cystic fibrosis, atopy, and airways lability. Arch Dis Child. 1978;53(11):873-7.
341. Nelson LA, Callerame ML, Schwartz RH. Aspergillosis and atopy in cystic fibrosis. Am Rev Respir Dis. 1979;120(4):863-73.
342. Laufer P, Fink JN, Bruns WT, Unger GF, Kalbfleisch JH, Greenberger PA, et al. Allergic bronchopulmonary aspergillosis in cystic fibrosis. J Allergy Clin Immunol. 1984;73(1 Pt 1):44-8.
343. Feanny S, Forsyth S, Corey M, Levison H, Zimmerman B. Allergic bronchopulmonary aspergillosis in cystic fibrosis: a secretory immune response to a colonizing organism. Ann Allergy. 1988;60(1):64-8.
344. Schonheyder H, Jensen T, Hoiby N, Koch C. Clinical and serological survey of pulmonary aspergillosis in patients with cystic fibrosis. Int Arch Allergy Appl Immunol. 1988;85(4): 472-7.

345. Zeaske R, Bruns WT, Fink JN, Greenberger PA, Colby H, Liotta JL, et al. Immune responses to Aspergillus in cystic fibrosis. J Allergy Clin Immunol. 1988;82(1):73-7.
346. Knutsen AP, Hutcheson PS, Mueller KR, Slavin RG. Serum immunoglobulins E and G anti-Aspergillus fumigatus antibody in patients with cystic fibrosis who have allergic bronchopulmonary aspergillosis. J Lab Clin Med. 1990;116(5):724-7.
347. Nicolai T, Arleth S, Spaeth A, Bertele-Harms RM, Harms HK. Correlation of IgE antibody titer to Aspergillus fumigatus with decreased lung function in cystic fibrosis. Pediatr Pulmonol. 1990;8(1):12-5.
348. Simmonds EJ, Littlewood JM, Evans EG. Cystic fibrosis and allergic bronchopulmonary aspergillosis. Arch Dis Child. 1990;65(5):507-11.
349. Hutcheson PS, Rejent AJ, Slavin RG. Variability in parameters of allergic bronchopulmonary aspergillosis in patients with cystic fibrosis. J Allergy Clin Immunol. 1991;88(3 Pt 1):390-4.
350. el-Dahr JM, Fink R, Selden R, Arruda LK, Platts-Mills TA, Heymann PW. Development of immune responses to Aspergillus at an early age in children with cystic fibrosis. Am J Respir Crit Care Med. 1994;150(6 Pt 1):1513-8.
351. Marchant JL, Warner JO, Bush A. Rise in total IgE as an indicator of allergic bronchopulmonary aspergillosis in cystic fibrosis. Thorax. 1994;49(10):1002-5.
352. Mroueh S, Spock A. Allergic bronchopulmonary aspergillosis in patients with cystic fibrosis. Chest. 1994;105(1):32-6.
353. Becker JW, Burke W, McDonald G, Greenberger PA, Henderson WR, Aitken ML. Prevalence of allergic bronchopulmonary aspergillosis and atopy in adult patients with cystic fibrosis. Chest. 1996;109(6):1536-40.
354. Hutcheson PS, Knutsen AP, Rejent AJ, Slavin RG. A 12-year longitudinal study of Aspergillus sensitivity in patients with cystic fibrosis. Chest. 1996;110(2):363-6.
355. Geller DE, Kaplowitz H, Light MJ, Colin AA. Allergic bronchopulmonary aspergillosis in cystic fibrosis: reported prevalence, regional distribution, and patient characteristics. Scientific Advisory Group, Investigators, and Coordinators of the Epidemiologic Study of Cystic Fibrosis. Chest. 1999;116(3):639-46.
356. Cimon B, Carrere J, Chazalette JP, Ginies JL, Chabasse D, Bouchara JP. Bronchopulmonary mycoses in cystic fibrosis. Results of a five-year longitudinal study. J Mycol Med. 2000;10(3):128-35.
357. Mastella G, Rainisio M, Harms HK, Hodson ME, Koch C, Navarro J, et al. Allergic bronchopulmonary aspergillosis in cystic fibrosis. A European epidemiological study. Epidemiologic Registry of Cystic Fibrosis. Eur Respir J. 2000;16(3):464-71.
358. Taccetti G, Procopio E, Marianelli L, Campana S. Allergic bronchopulmonary aspergillosis in Italian cystic fibrosis patients: prevalence and percentage of positive tests in the employed diagnostic criteria. Eur J Epidemiol. 2000;16(9):837-42.
359. Ritz N, Ammann RA, Casaulta Aebischer C, Schoeni-Affolter F, Schoeni MH. Risk factors for allergic bronchopulmonary aspergillosis and sensitisation to Aspergillus fumigatus in patients with cystic fibrosis. Eur J Pediatr. 2005;164(9):577-82.
360. Skov M, McKay K, Koch C, Cooper PJ. Prevalence of allergic bronchopulmonary aspergillosis in cystic fibrosis in an area with a high frequency of atopy. Respir Med. 2005;99(7):887-93.
361. Almeida MB, Bussamra MH, Rodrigues JC. ABPA diagnosis in cystic fibrosis patients: the clinical utility of IgE specific to recombinant Aspergillus fumigatus allergens. J Pediatr (Rio J). 2006;82(3):215-20.
362. Kraemer R, Delosea N, Ballinari P, Gallati S, Crameri R. Effect of allergic bronchopulmonary aspergillosis on lung function in children with cystic fibrosis. Am J Respir Crit Care Med. 2006;174(11):1211-20.
363. Chotirmall SH, Branagan P, Gunaratnam C, McElvaney NG. Aspergillus/allergic bronchopulmonary aspergillosis in an Irish cystic fibrosis population: a diagnostically challenging entity. Respir Care. 2008;53(8):1035-41.
364. Rapaka RR, Kolls JK. Pathogenesis of allergic bronchopulmonary aspergillosis in cystic fibrosis: current understanding and future directions. Med Mycol. 2009;47 (Suppl 1):S331-7.
365. Cunningham S, Madge SL, Dinwiddie R. Survey of criteria used to diagnose allergic bronchopulmonary aspergillosis in cystic fibrosis. Arch Dis Child. 2001;84(1):89.
366. Amin R, Dupuis A, Aaron SD, Ratjen F. The effect of chronic infection with Aspergillus fumigatus on lung function and hospitalization in patients with cystic fibrosis. Chest. 2010;137(1):171-6.
367. Baxter CG, Dunn G, Jones AM, Webb K, Gore R, Richardson MD, et al. Novel immunologic classification of aspergillosis in adult cystic fibrosis. J Allergy Clin Immunol. 2013;132(3):560-6 e10.
368. Ein ME, Wallace RJ Jr, Williams TW Jr. Allergic bronchopulmonary aspergillosis-like syndrome consequent to aspergilloma. Am Rev Respir Dis. 1979;119(5):811-20.
369. Safirstein BH. Aspergilloma consequent to allergic bronchopulmonary aspergillosis. Am Rev Respir Dis. 1973;108(4):940-3.
370. Israel RH, Poe RH, Bomba PA, Gross RA. The rapid development of an aspergilloma secondary to allergic bronchopulmonary aspergillosis. Am J Med Sci. 1980;280(1):41-4.
371. Rosenberg IL, Greenberger PA. Allergic bronchopulmonary aspergillosis and aspergilloma. Long-term follow-up without enlargement of a large multiloculated cavity. Chest. 1984;85(1):123-5.
372. Sharma TN, Gupta PR, Mehrotra AK, Purohit SD, Mangal HN. Aspergilloma with ABPA due to Aspergillus niger. J Assoc Physicians India. 1985;33(11):748.
373. Shah A, Khan ZU, Chaturvedi S, Ramchandran S, Randhawa HS, Jaggi OP. Allergic bronchopulmonary aspergillosis with coexistent aspergilloma: a long-term follow-up. J Asthma. 1989;26(2):109-15.
374. Bhagat R, Shah A, Jaggi OP, Khan ZU. Concomitant allergic bronchopulmonary aspergillosis and allergic Aspergillus sinusitis with an operated aspergilloma. J Allergy Clin Immunol. 1993;91(5):1094-6.
375. Shah A, Bhagat R, Pant K, Jaggi OP, Khan ZU. Allergic bronchopulmonary aspergillosis with aspergilloma: Exacerbation after prolonged remission. Indian J Tuberc. 1993;40(1):39-41.
376. Jaques D, Bonzon M, Polla BS. Serological evidence of Aspergillus type I hypersensitivity in a subgroup of pulmonary aspergilloma patients. Int Arch Allergy Immunol. 1995;106(3):263-70.
377. Sharma P, Agarwal AK, Shah A. Formation of an aspergilloma in a patient with allergic bronchopulmonary aspergillosis on corticosteroid therapy. Indian J Chest Dis Allied Sci. 1998;40(4):269-73.

378. Shah A, Panjabi C. Contemporaneous occurrence of allergic bronchopulmonary aspergillosis, allergic Aspergillus sinusitis, and aspergilloma. Ann Allergy Asthma Immunol. 2006;96(6):874-8.
379. Dolan CT, Weed LA, Dines DE. Bronchopulmonary helminthosporiosis. Am J Clin Pathol. 1970;53(2):235-42.
380. Sahn SA, Lakshminarayan S. Allergic bronchopulmonary penicilliosis. Chest. 1973;63(2):286-8.
381. Novey HS, Wells ID. Allergic bronchopulmonary aspergillosis caused by Aspergillus ochraceus. Am J Clin Pathol. 1978;70(5):840-3.
382. Benatar SR, Allan B, Hewitson RP, Don PA. Allergic bronchopulmonary stemphyliosis. Thorax. 1980;35(7):515-8.
383. Laham MN, Allen RC, Greene JC. Allergic bronchopulmonary aspergillosis (ABPA) caused by Aspergillus terreus: specific lymphocyte sensitization and antigen-directed serum opsonic activity. Ann Allergy. 1981;46(2):74-80.
384. McAleer R, Kroenert DB, Elder JL, Froudist JH. Allergic bronchopulmonary disease caused by Curvularia lunata and Drechslera hawaiiensis. Thorax. 1981;36(5):338-44.
385. Patterson R, Samuels BS, Phair JJ, Roberts M. Bronchopulmonary torulopsosis. Int Arch Allergy Appl Immunol. 1982; 69(1):30-3.
386. Kino T, Yamada Y, Honda K, Fujimura N, Matsui Y, Izumi T, et al. [Diagnosis and treatment of a case of allergic bronchopulmonary mycosis caused by Mucor-like fungus]. Nihon Kyobu Shikkan Gakkai zasshi. 1983;21(9):896-903.
387. Akiyama K, Mathison DA, Riker JB, Greenberger PA, Patterson R. Allergic bronchopulmonary candidiasis. Chest. 1984;85(5): 699-701.
388. Lake FR, Tribe AE, McAleer R, Froudist J, Thompson PJ. Mixed allergic bronchopulmonary fungal disease due to Pseudallescheria boydii and Aspergillus. Thorax. 1990;45(6): 489-91.
389. Lake FR, Froudist JH, McAleer R, Gillon RL, Tribe AE, Thompson PJ. Allergic bronchopulmonary fungal disease caused by Bipolaris and Curvularia. Aust N Z J Med. 1991;21(6):871-4.
390. Kamei K, Unno H, Nagao K, Kuriyama T, Nishimura K, Miyaji M. Allergic bronchopulmonary mycosis caused by the basidiomycetous fungus Schizophyllum commune. Clin Infect Dis. 1994;18(3):305-9.
391. Backman KS, Roberts M, Patterson R. Allergic bronchopulmonary mycosis caused by Fusarium vasinfectum. Am J Respir Crit Care Med. 1995;152(4 Pt 1):1379-81.
392. Moreno-Ancillo A, Diaz-Pena JM, Ferrer A, Martin-Munoz F, Martin-Barroso JA, Martin-Esteban M, et al. Allergic bronchopulmonary cladosporiosis in a child. J Allergy Clin Immunol. 1996;97(2):714-5.
393. Ogawa H, Fujimura M, Tofuku Y. Allergic bronchopulmonary fungal disease caused by Saccharomyces cerevisiae. J Asthma. 2004;41(2):223-8.
394. Singh B, Denning DW. Allergic bronchopulmonary mycosis due to Alternaria: Case report and review. Med Mycol Case Rep. 2012;1(1):20-3.
395. Bahous J, Malo JL, Paquin R, Cartier A, Vyas P, Longbottom JL. Allergic bronchopulmonary aspergillosis and sensitization to Aspergillus fumigatus in chronic bronchiectasis in adults. Clin Allergy. 1985;15(6):571-9.
396. Agarwal R, Singh N, Aggarwal AN. An unusual association between Mycobacterium tuberculosis and Aspergillus fumigatus. Monaldi Arch Chest Dis. 2008;69(1):32-4.
397. Dhooria S, Kumar P, Saikia B, Aggarwal AN, Gupta D, Behera D, et al. Prevalence of Aspergillus sensitization in pulmonary tuberculosis-related fibrocavitary disease. Int J Tuberc Lung Dis. 2014;18(7)850-5.
398. Sharma B, Sharma M, Bondi E, Sharma M. Kartagener's syndrome associated with allergic bronchopulmonary aspergillosis. MedGenMed. 2005;7(2):25.
399. Agarwal R, Srinivas R, Jindal SK. Allergic bronchopulmonary aspergillosis complicating chronic obstructive pulmonary disease. Mycoses. 2008;51(1):83-5.
400. Pashley CH. Fungal culture and sensitisation in asthma, cystic fibrosis and chronic obstructive pulmonary disorder: what does it tell us? Mycopathologia. 2014;178(5-6):457-63.
401. Bafadhel M, McKenna S, Agbetile J, Fairs A, Desai D, Mistry V, et al. Aspergillus fumigatus during stable state and exacerbations of COPD. Eur Respir J. 2014;43(1):64-71.
402. Eppinger TM, Greenberger PA, White DA, Brown AE, Cunningham-Rundles C. Sensitization to Aspergillus species in the congenital neutrophil disorders chronic granulomatous disease and hyper-IgE syndrome. J Allergy Clin Immunol. 1999;104(6):1265-72.
403. Shah A, Panchal N, Agarwal AK. Concomitant allergic bronchopulmonary aspergillosis and allergic Aspergillus sinusitis: a review of an uncommon association. Clin Exp Allergy. 2001;31(12):1896-905.
404. Saravanan K, Panda NK, Chakrabarti A, Das A, Bapuraj RJ. Allergic fungal rhinosinusitis: an attempt to resolve the diagnostic dilemma. Arch Otolaryngol Head Neck Surg. 2006;132(2):173-8.
405. Chakrabarti A, Denning DW, Ferguson BJ, Ponikau J, Buzina W, Kita H, et al. Fungal rhinosinusitis: a categorization and definitional schema addressing current controversies. Laryngoscope. 2009;119(9):1809-18.
406. Shah TS, Sundaram P, Rege JD, Joshi JM. Proptosis in an asthmatic patient. Postgrad Med J. 2003;79(938):710.
407. Venarske DL, deShazo RD. Sinobronchial allergic mycosis: the SAM syndrome. Chest. 2002;121(5):1670-6.

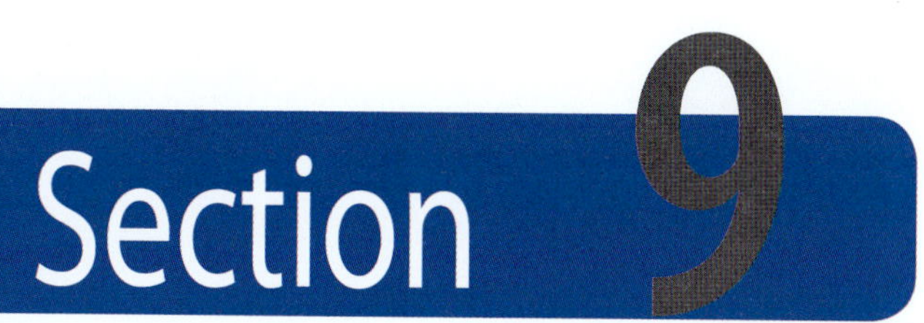

Chronic Obstructive Pulmonary Disease

Sundeep Salvi, Aditya Jindal

70 Chapter

Burden of Chronic Obstructive Pulmonary Disease

Monica Barne, Sundeep Salvi

INTRODUCTION

Chronic obstructive pulmonary disease (COPD) is one of the leading causes of morbidity and mortality and imposes major health and socioeconomic burden globally. The prevalence of COPD is substantial and increasing.[1] COPD prevalence, morbidity and mortality varies across countries and regions of the world and largely depends upon the exposure to various risk factors, mainly smoking, exposure to indoor air pollution, occupational exposure to particulate matter and other noxious agents and poor socioeconomic status. It also depends upon the existing health infrastructure and the primary preventive policies implemented in the country. With better focus on smoking cessation and antitobacco policies, the number of COPD cases in most of the developed countries has declined over the past 2 decades. But, the increasing use of tobacco amongst men and women of the developing countries is likely to reverse this trend soon.[2] The world needs to take cognizance of the impending epidemic of this major noncommunicable killer disease and take appropriate measures to curb this increasing burden.

MORTALITY DUE TO CHRONIC OBSTRUCTIVE PULMONARY DISEASE

Global Mortality

The World Health Organization (WHO) estimates about 3 million deaths due to COPD worldwide, which corresponds to almost 5% of all deaths globally. The publication of the global burden of disease (GBD) study 2010[3] gives us new insights into the number of deaths, and the ranking of diseases as major causes of mortality world over. The GBD report states that although the number of deaths dues to COPD has declined over the past 2 decades from 3.1 million to 2.9 million, COPD is still the third largest cause of mortality **(Fig. 1)**.

In 1990, COPD was the fourth leading cause of deaths worldwide. The WHO had ranked COPD as the fifth leading cause of deaths in 2002 and had predicted it would become the third leading cause of deaths by the year 2030.[4] However, COPD has managed to achieve this ranking 20 years before the estimated time[3] **(Fig. 2)** and this indeed is a matter of concern.

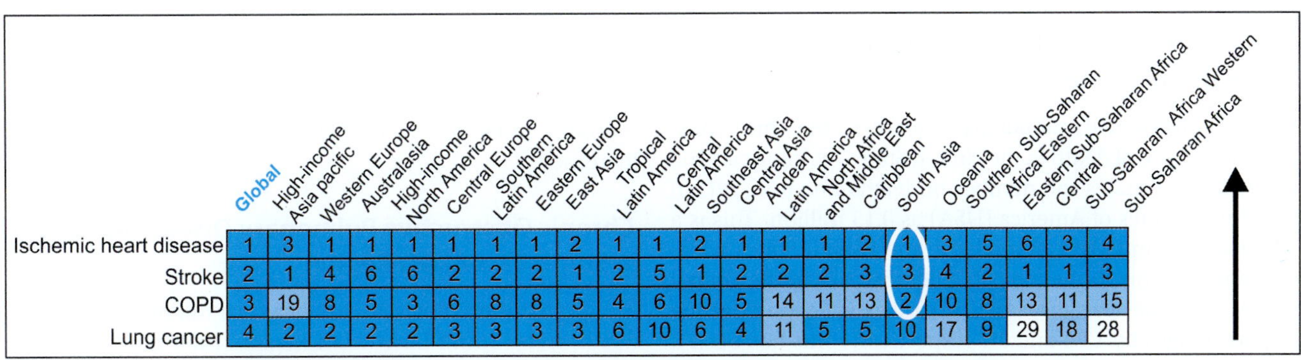

	Global	High-income Asia pacific	Western Europe	Australasia	High-income North America	Central Europe	Southern Latin America	Eastern Europe	East Asia	Tropical Latin America	Central Latin America	Southeast Asia	Central Asia	Andean Latin America	North Africa and Middle East	Caribbean	South Asia	Oceania	Southern Sub-Saharan Africa	Eastern Sub-Saharan Africa	Central Sub-Saharan Africa	Western Sub-Saharan Africa
Ischemic heart disease	1	3	1	1	1	1	1	1	2	1	1	2	1	1	1	2	1	3	5	6	3	4
Stroke	2	1	4	6	6	2	2	2	1	2	5	1	2	2	2	3	3	4	2	1	1	3
COPD	3	19	8	5	3	6	8	8	5	4	6	10	5	14	11	13	2	10	8	13	11	15
Lung cancer	4	2	2	2	2	3	3	3	3	6	10	6	4	11	5	5	10	17	9	29	18	28

Fig. 1 Rank of chronic obstructive pulmonary disease (COPD) as a cause of mortality globally

Reproduced with permission from the source: Institute for health metrics and evaluation (IHME). (2010). Global burden of disease (GBD). Health map. Seattle, WA: IHME, University of Washington; 2013. [online] Available from *http://vizhub.healthdata.org/irank/heat.php*. [Accessed 8 August, 2014].

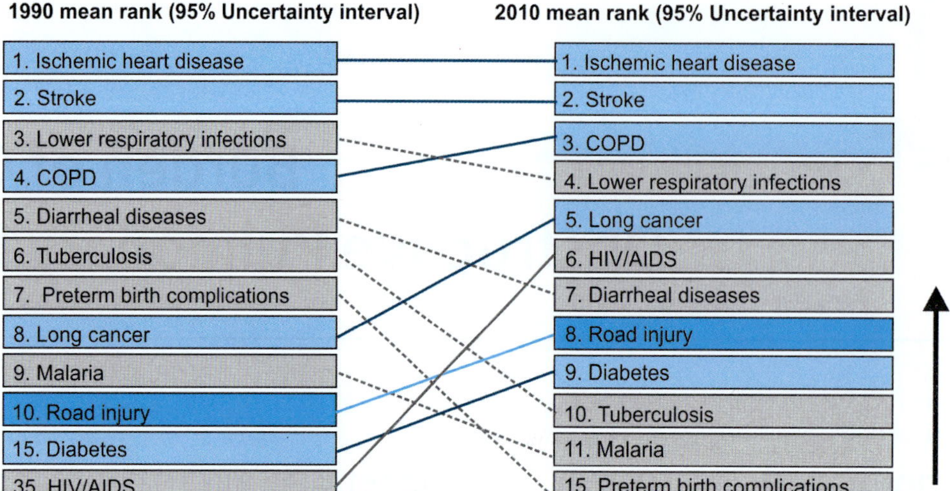

Fig. 2 Global rank of chronic obstructive pulmonary disease (COPD) as a cause of mortality in 1990 and 2010
Abbreviations: HIV/AIDS, human immunodeficiency virus/acquired immune deficiency syndrome; COPD, chronic obstructive pulmonary disease
Reproduced with permission from institute for health metrics and evaluation (IHME). (2010) Global burden of diseases (GBD) arrow diagram. Seattle, WA: IHME, University of Washington; 2013. [online] Available from *http://vizhub.healthdata.org/irank/arrow.php*. [Accessed 8 August, 2014].

India and China: Largest Contributors to the Global Chronic Obstructive Pulmonary Disease Mortality

Almost 90% of deaths from COPD occur in low- and middle-income countries.[5] India and China alone are responsible for 63% of deaths due to COPD.[3] The estimated deaths due to COPD in India in 2002, were over half a million, second only to China which was responsible for an estimated 1.3 million deaths.[6] The mortality rates were then projected to increase by over 30% every decade. But whereas the number of deaths in China has declined from 1.3 million to 0.93 million in 2010, India has overshot this 30% prediction and mortality due to COPD in India has increased from 0.59 million in 2002 to 0.91 million in 2010 making it the biggest contributor to the up scaled ranking of COPD.

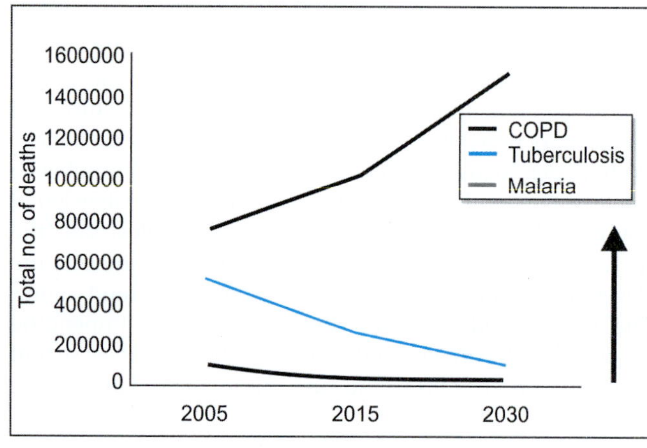

Fig. 3 Estimated mortality rate of COPD by 2030
Abbreviation: COPD, chronic obstructive pulmonary disease

Chronic Obstructive Pulmonary Disease Mortality in the United States of America

Chronic obstructive pulmonary disease is the third most common cause of death in the United States of America.[7] The GBD 2010 estimates the number of deaths due to COPD in the United States of America (USA) as 0.15 million. This is a 58% increase in COPD mortality in the United States while the mortality due to the top two killer diseases in the United States, ischemic heart diseases and stroke have seen a decline in percentages by 13% and 3% respectively. This has been a consistent trend in the United States since the past 4 decades which has shown that though coronary heart disease and stroke occupy the top two positions amongst all the causes of deaths, their mortality rates have steadily declined as against mortality rates due to COPD which have, in fact steadily increased.[8]

Chronic Obstructive Pulmonary Disease Mortality in South East Asian Region

Although, tuberculosis and malaria are still major causes of death in the South East Asian Region, their mortality rates are anticipated to reduce to almost half by the year 2030[9] **(Fig. 3)**. In contrast, mortality rates due to COPD which are over two-fold greater than those due to tuberculosis currently (900,000), are estimated to increase by over

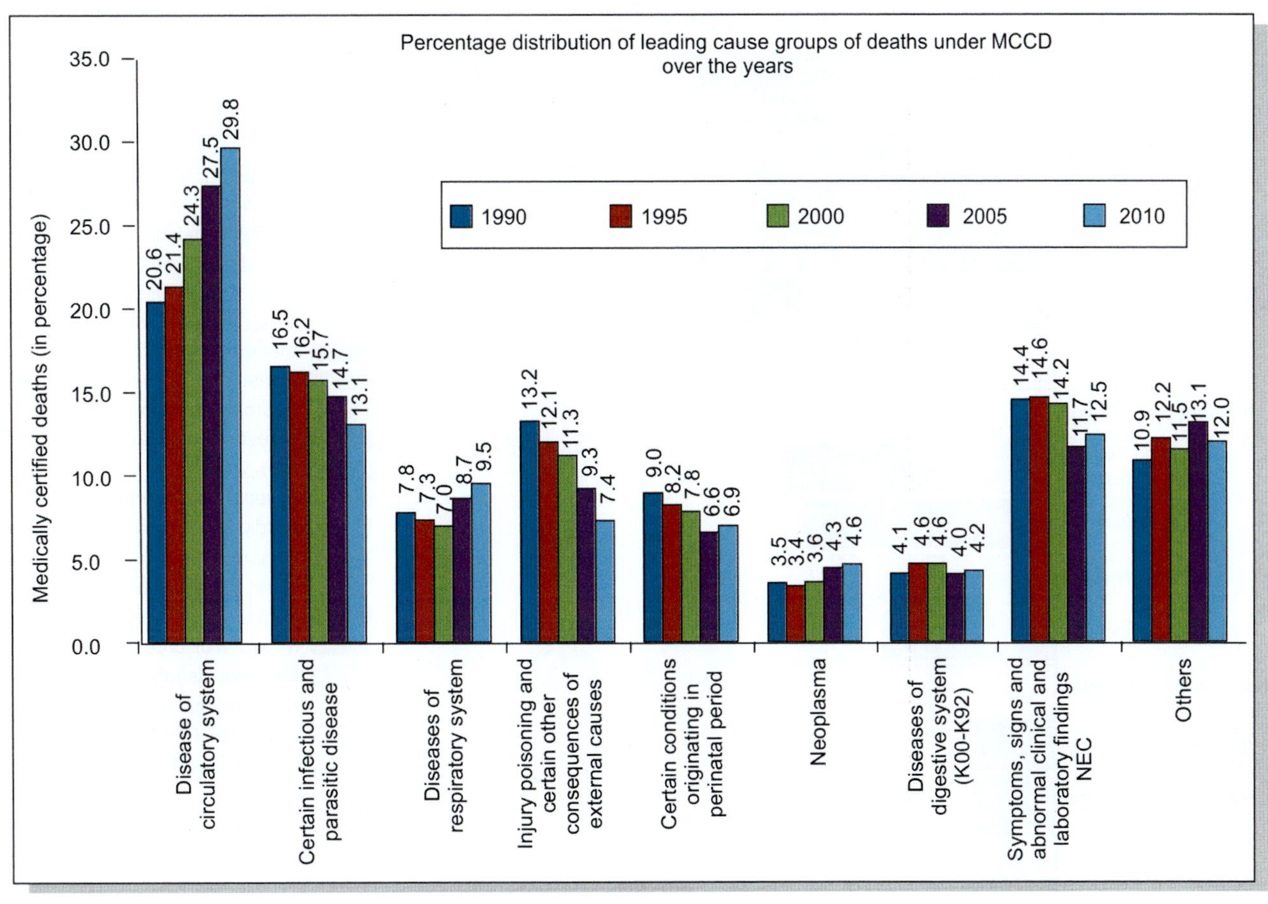

Fig. 4 Percentage distribution of leading cause groups of deaths under MCCD over the years

160% by the year 2030. These observations clearly highlight the fact that mortality rates due to COPD are increasing both in the developed as well as developing world.[9]

Chronic Obstructive Pulmonary Disease Mortality in India

As a result of industrialization, socioeconomic development, urbanization, changing age structure and changing lifestyles, India is facing a growing burden of noncommunicable diseases. Chronic respiratory diseases (namely COPD, asthma and other respiratory diseases) are the second leading cause of deaths among Indian adults between 25 years and 69 years of age and are responsible for about 10.2% of deaths in this age group.[10]

According to the government of India-medical certification of cause of death report for the year 2010, chronic respiratory diseases were the third largest cause of deaths and have shown a steadily increasing pattern over the past few decades whereas infectious disease which were the second largest cause of certified deaths, had shown a steady decline[11] **(Fig. 4)**.

As mentioned earlier in this chapter the death rate due to COPD in India has doubled in the past decade. With emergence of household air pollution and smoking as two of the top three risk factors[12] responsible for majority of disability adjusted life years (DALYs) lost due to respiratory diseases **(Fig. 5)**, unless an urgent action is taken to reduce the underlying risk factors, especially use of tobacco and exposure to biomass fuel smoke, the mortality will continue to rise over the next few decades.

PREVALENCE OF CHRONIC OBSTRUCTIVE PULMONARY DISEASE

Global Prevalence of Chronic Obstructive Pulmonary Disease

Two hundred ten million people, across the world are believed to suffer with COPD.[13] Prevalence of COPD varies from country-to-country and within the country from region to region not only due to the different levels of exposure to risk factors but also due to the remarkable variation in the survey methods, diagnostic criteria and analytical approaches. Several studies have estimated the prevalence of COPD

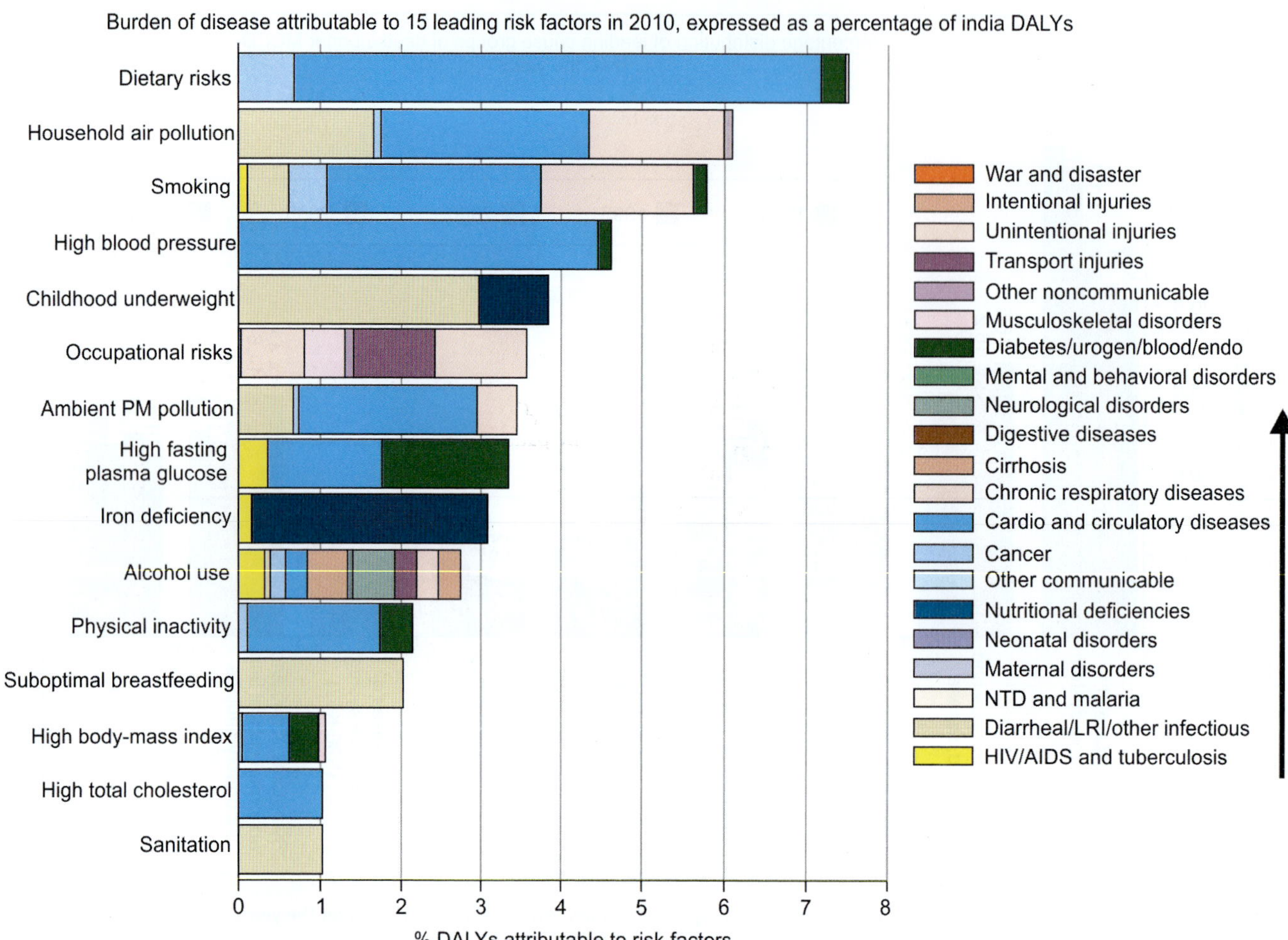

Fig. 5 The graph shows the top 15 risk factors for morbidity in India. The colored portion of each bar represents the specific disease attributable to that risk factor while bar size represents the percentage of disability-adjusted life years (DALYs) lost due to specific risk factors

Abbreviations: DALYs, disability-adjusted life years; NTD, neglected tropical diseases; HIV/AIDS, human immunodeficiency virus/acquired immune deficiency syndrome; PM, particulate matter

Reproduced with permission from the source: Institute for health metrics and evaluation (IHME). (2013) Global burden of disease (GBD) profile: India. Seattle, WA: IHME; [online] Available from *http://www.healthdata.org/sites/default/files/files/country_profiles/GBD/ihme_gbd_country_report_india.pdf.* [Accessed 8 August, 2014].

Table 1 Studies of chronic obstructive pulmonary disease (COPD) prevalence worldwide

	Study center	*Participants*	*Age (years)*	*Method of diagnosis*	*Prevalence of COPD*
Behrendt (2005)[17]	USA (nationwide NHANES III)	13,995	18–80	Prebronchodilator spirometry (FEV_1/FVC<0.70)	6.6%
Shahab et al. (2006)[18]	England (nationwide)	8,215	≥35	Prebronchodilator spirometry (FEV_1/FVC<0.70)	13.3%
Hardie et al. (2005)[19]	Bergen and Norway	1,649	≥70	Respiratory symptom questionnaire	4.0%
Lamprecht et al. (2008)[20]	Salzburg and Austria	1,258	≥40	Postbronchodilator spirometry (FEV_1/FVC <0.70)	26.1%
Lindström et al. (2001)[21]	Norrbotten, Sweden, Lapland and Finland	13,737	45–69	Symptoms; respiratory symptom questionnaire; self-reported physician	3.8% (Sweden) 3.2% (Finland)

Contd...

Contd...

Viegi et al. (2000)[22]	Po Delta and Italy	1,727	>25	*Spirometry:* ERS (prebronchodilator FEV_1/FVC <0.88 for men and <0.89 for women), BOLD (postbronchodilator FEV_1/FVC <0.70), ATS (prebronchodilator FEV_1/FVC <0.75); clinical examination	11.0% (ERS); 18.3% (BOLD); 40.4% (ATS)
De Marco et al. (2004)[23]	Multinational (16 countries;* ECRHS)	20,245	20–44	Prebronchodilator spirometry ($FEV_1/$ FVC,0.70)	2.5% (GOLD stage I); 1.1% (GOLD stage II/III)
Liu et al. (2007)[24]	Guangdong province and China	3,286	≥40	Postbronchodilator spirometry ($FEV_1/$ FVC <0.70); physician; respiratory symptoms questionnaire	9.4%; 12% (rural), 7.4% (urban)
Zhou et al. (2009)[25]	China (nationwide CESCOPD)	20,245	≥40	Postbronchodilator spirometry ($FEV_1/$ FVC <0.70)	5.2%
Ehrlich et al. (2004)[26]	South Africa	13,826	>18	Respiratory symptoms questionnaire	2.6%; 2.3% (men), 2.8% women
Brashier B et al. (2012)[27]	Pune, India (slum in city)	12,055	>45	Respiratory symptoms questionnaire	6.7%
Menzes et al. (2005)[28]	Brazil, Chile, Mexico, Uruguay and Venezuela (PLATINO)	5,571	≥40	Postbronchodilator spirometry ($FEV_1/$ FVC <0.70)	15.8% (Brazil), 16.9% (Chile), 7.8% (Mexico), 19.7% (Uruguay), 12.1% (Venezuela)
Caballero et al. (2008)[29]	Columbia (five cities;† PREPOCOL)	5,536	40	Postbronchodilator spirometry ($FEV_1/$ FVC <0.70); physician; respiratory symptoms questionnaire	8.9% (spirometry), 3.3% (physician), 2.7% (questionnaire)
Tan et al. (2003)[30]	Asia-pacific (12 countries‡)		≥30	Validate estimation model for prevalence of COPD	6.3% range from 3.5% (Hong Kong and Singapore) to 6.7% Vietnam
Kim et al. (2005)[31]	Korea (nationwide)	9,243	>18	Postbronchodilator spirometry ($FEV_1/$ FVC, 0.70)	7.8%
Lindberg et al. (2005)[32]	Norrbotten, Sweden	666	20–69	*Spirometry:* BTS (prebronchodilator FEV_1/FVC <0.70, FEV_1, 0.80), ERS (Prebronchodilator FEV_1/FVC <0.88 for men and <0.89 for women), GOLD (postbronchodilator FEV_1/FVC <0.70), ATS (Prebronchodilator FEV_1/FVC <0.75)	7.6% (BTS), 14.0% (ERS), 14.1% GOLD, 12.2% (ATS)
Fukuchi et al. (2004)[33]	Japan	2,343	≥40	Prebronchodilator spirometry (FEV_1/FVC <0.70)	10.9%
Cerveri et al. (2001)[34]	Multinational study (16 countries ECRHS)	17,966	20–44	British medical research council respiratory questionnaire; prebronchodilator spirometry (FEV_1/FVC, 0.70)	3.3%
von Hertzen et al. (2000)[35]	Finland (nationwide)	7,217	≥30	Respiratory symptoms questionnaire; clinical examination; Prebronchodilator spirometry (FEV_1/FVC <0.70); physician	14.1%

All studies were done in both men and women

Abbreviations: FEV_1/FVC, ratio of forced expiratory volume in 1 second/forced vital capacity; ERS, European Respiratory Society Guidelines; BOLD, burden of obstructive lung disease criteria; ATS, American Thoracic Society; GOLD, global initiative for chronic obstructive lung disease guidelines; BTS, British Thoracic Society; COPD, chronic obstructive pulmonary disease

*ECHRS, European community respiratory health survey; includes: Australia, Belgium, Denmark, France, Germany, Iceland, Ireland, Italy, Netherlands, New Zealand, Norway, Spain, Sweden, Switzerland, UK and USA

†Columbia 5 cities: Barranquilla, Bogota, Bucaramanga, Cali and Medellin

‡Asia Pacific (12 Countries): Australia, China, Hong Kong, Indonesia, Japan, Korea, Malaysia, Philippines, Singapore, Taiwan, Thailand and Vietnam

in the past, but the tools for diagnosis of COPD have been largely ill defined. On one hand, prevalence based on self-reported symptoms (chronic cough, sputum, etc.) most likely overestimated the true burden of COPD[14] while physician's diagnosis in absence of spirometry usually underestimates true COPD.[15]

Salvi and Barnes have summarized all the data available on prevalence of COPD from various countries[16] **(Table 1)**.

As is evident, there is considerable variation in the prevalence of COPD across the globe. The variations in prevalence rates may not necessarily be only due to the actual difference in prevalence in various countries but also likely depends upon the fact that the diagnostic and research tools vary from study to study. The tools used to define COPD have included respiratory symptoms, doctor diagnosed self-reported COPD and spirometry defined COPD [ratio between forced expiratory volume 1 (FEV_1) and forced vital capacity (FVC) measured either before bronchodilator or after bronchodilator]. Moreover, the cut-off value for the FEV_1/FVC ratio has also varied from study to study. There is considerable within study variation in the prevalence of COPD depending upon the criteria for defining COPD. For example, using the European Respiratory Society (ERS) definition of COPD (prebronchodilator FEV_1/FVC <0.88 for men and <0.89 for women) gives a prevalence of 11.0% which increases to 40% if the American Thoracic Society (ATS) criteria is used to define COPD in Po Delta, Italy.[22]

Considering this wide variation in the study methodology, and definitions of COPD, a worldwide study called burden of obstructive lung diseases (BOLD) was initiated in 2002[36] which has attempted to determine the prevalence of COPD using a standardized validated respiratory questionnaire and spirometry. A postbronchodilator FEV_1/FVC less than 70% on spirometry was used to define COPD which was the global initiative for chronic obstructive lung disease (GOLD) criteria for diagnosis of COPD. They published data of 9,425 participants from 12 sites in 2007 and reported a prevalence of stage II or higher COPD of 10·1% overall (11·8% for men and 8·5% for women).[37] The prevalence increased with age and pack years of smoking, but other less understood factors such as biomass heating and cooking exposures, occupational exposures and tuberculosis also contributed to the location specific variations in the disease.[38] With newer evidence suggesting that a fixed ratio of FEV_1/FVC for all ages is likely to under diagnose cases in the younger age group and over diagnose cases in the older age group. BOLD analyzed their existing data for prevalence using lower limit of normal (LLN) as the cut-off for defining COPD. The BOLD group stated that use of the FEV_1/FVC less than LLN criterion instead of the FEV_1/FVC less than 0.7 minimizes known age biases and is a better clinical parameter which reflects clinically significant irreversible airflow limitation.[39] Data from 22 of the BOLD completed sites with FEV_1/FVC less than LLN is now available and tabulated in **Table 2** with gender-specific prevalence rates. There are three sites from India which have been included in this report.[40]

In a multinational questionnaire based, patient reported survey of 12 countries (including Brazil, France, Germany, Italy, Japan, Mexico, Netherlands, Russia, South Korea, Spain, United Kingdom and United States of America) conducted between November 2012 and May 2013, which defined COPD as physician diagnosed COPD, or chronic obstructive pulmonary disease or emphysema or chronic bronchitis with reported use of regular medication for these symptoms or presence of symptoms of COPD on the basis of well-validated questionnaires showed that the overall COPD prevalence ranged from 7% to 12%, with the majority of individual country estimates ranging from 7% to 9%.[41]

Other studies done in 7,879 individuals in the United Kingdom[42] and 7,104 individuals in the United States,[43] National Health and Nutrition Examination Survey (NHANES) data (all age >40 years) showed a prevalence of 13.1–6.1% respectively, using the postbronchodilator LLN for FEV_1/FVC to define COPD. A Canadian study which identified prevalence of COPD on the basis of postbronchodilator FEV_1/FVC less than 0.70 and FEV_1 less than 80% reported a prevalence of 6.1–10.2% in Canada which reduced to 4.1–7.2% on applying the LLN for defining COPD.[44]

There is little existing research on COPD in sub-Saharan Africa.[45] A systematic review of articles published between 1990 and 2012 estimates the number of COPD cases to about 26.3 million (18.5–43.4 million) cases of COPD which is an estimated 31.5% increase as compared to the prevalence rates in 2000.[46] The only BOLD study conducted in South Africa which defined COPD by airflow obstruction on postbronchodilator FEV_1/FVC reported a prevalence of 22.2% in men and 16.7% in women aged more than equal 40 years.[37] This was by far the highest country rates reported within the global BOLD study till 2011.[47]

Chronic Obstructive Pulmonary Disease Prevalence in India

Jindal et al. performed an extensive review of all data published on COPD prevalence in India from 1964 to 1995.[48] This study has provided the backbone for the estimation of morbidity and mortality and projected economic burden of COPD in India. This review showed that there is a wide variation in the prevalence of COPD in different parts of India, the highest being reported from North Indian rural population (9.4%). This wide variation was explained by the wide variety in the exposure to risk factors like smoking, environmental tobacco smoke (ETS), biomass fuel, occupation and socioeconomic status.

Newer data from the BOLD study from three sites in India has been mentioned in **Table 2** earlier in this chapter. Latest Indian data from an extensive review of literature conducted by McKay[49] et al. is given in **Table 3**.

This review assimilated data from 16 studies on chronic bronchitis and COPD conducted after 1980 and presented the prevalence of COPD in different geographical, socioeconomic conditions in racially and culturally different populations in

Table 2 Prevalence of airflow obstruction defined by forced expiratory volume 1 (FEV_1)/forced vital capacity (FVC) less than lower limit of normal (LLN) in men and women separately from the burden of obstructive lung disease (BOLD) sites

		Prevalence of airflow obstruction (% FEV_1/FVC <LLN)	*Prevalence of airflow obstruction (%FEV_1/FVC <LLN)*
S. No.	Country	Men	Women
1.	China (Guangzhou) (2003)	9.3	6.3
2.	India (Mumbai) (2006/8)	6.0	7.6
3.	India (Pune) (2008/9)	5.7	6.8
4.	India (Srinagar) (2010/11)	17.3	14.8
5.	The Philippines (Manila) (2005/6)	15.1	4.2
6.	The Philippines (Nampicuan-Talugtug) (2008/9)	16.9	13.5
7.	Australia (Sydney) (2006/7)	7.6	14.1
8.	Poland (Krakow) (2005)	14.9	12.2
9.	Estonia (Tartu) (2008/10)	7.9	4.9
10.	Norway (Bergen) (2005-2006)	13.8	10.0
11.	Germany (Hannover) (2005)	9.9	6.8
12.	Portugal (Lisbon) (2008)	9.3	7.4
13.	United Kingdom (London) (2006/7)	19.5	16.0
14.	The Netherlands (Maastricht) (2007/9)	19.7	17.9
15.	Iceland (Reykjavik) (2004/5)	9.2	13.5
16.	Austria (Salzburg) (2004/5)	13.4	20.7
17.	Sweden (Uppsala) (2006/7)	10.5	8.7
18.	Turkey (Adana) (2003/4)	19.8	9.1
19.	United States of America (USA) (Lexington) (2005/6)	12.3	16.2
20.	Canada (Vancouver) (2005/6)	14.5	12.5
21.	South Africa (Cape Town) (2005)	23.0	16.9
22.	Tunisia (Sousse) (2010/12)	8.6	1.8

Adapted from "chronic obstructive pulmonary disease mortality and prevalence: the associations with smoking and poverty—a BOLD analysis. Burney P et al. Thorax 2014; 69:465-473" (PMC open source document)

India, which are exposed to different risk factors like tobacco smoke, indoor air pollution due to use of biomass fuel and outdoor air pollution. Despite the heterogeneity of these studies in their study population, methodology, study tools used, risk factors assessed and outcomes, the study concludes that the existing estimates of general prevalence of chronic bronchitis in rural areas was between 6.5% and 7.7%.

The study[51] which is probably the largest of its kind done in India and which deserves a special mention here is the large multicentric field survey that was conducted in both the urban as well as rural populations at Bangalore, Chandigarh, Delhi and Kanpur with the help of a structured and validated questionnaire. Prevalence of COPD amongst the 35,295 subjects investigated (age ≥35 years) was 4.1% with a male to female ratio of 1.6:1. Prevalence of COPD in smokers was 2.65 times higher than nonsmokers, and amongst the smokers, the prevalence was higher amongst *bidi* smokers as compared to cigarette smokers (8.2% and 5.9% respectively). Exposure to ETS was associated with a 40% increased odds of COPD which increased to 57% amongst those concomitantly exposed to biomass fuel. A questionnaire based study amongst 12,000 slum dwellers from Pune city in Maharashtra[27] is also notable for the fact that probably for the first time, this study showed that amongst those diagnosed with COPD, 69% were never smokers. The overall prevalence of questionnaire-diagnosed COPD amongst the never smoker males was 6.8% and females was 4.4%.

The national commission on macroeconomics and health in its background papers on the burden of diseases estimated that out of the 65 million cases of chronic respiratory diseases in India in 2005, about 17 million were due to COPD. The morbidity due to COPD was projected to increase to 22.2 million by the year 2016.[66] But, if we apply the current prevalence rate of about 7% to the population in India which

Table 3 Prevalence in India from various studies after 1980 Mc Kay et al.

Study date/location	*Population size*	*Age/gender*	*Risk factors*	*Study tools*	*Prevalence*
2010/Karnataka[50]	900	Males >40 years	Smokers males—71.9% Females—0% Biomass fuel exposure—80.9%	Questionnaire	7.1% (Males—11.1% Females—4.5%)
2006/Bengaluru, Chandigarh, Delhi and Kanpur[51]	35,295	Males >35 years	Smokers Male—43.8% Females—4% Biomass fuel Exposure—36%	Questionnaire	4.1% (Male—5% Female—3.2%)
2003–2005/ Unclear[52]	2,000–3,000	Males >65 years	Nil specified except old age	Questionnaire	Urban—1.8% Rural—7.6%
2002–2003 Dibrugarh/Assam[53]	293	>60 years	*Smokers*: Males—3.8% Females—1.8%	Questionnaire	Total—7.5% Males—8/8% Females—5.4%
2001–2/Shimla, Himachal Pradesh[54]	1,330	>18 years	Not specified	Questionnaire	Total—9.1% Males—11.1% Females—6.1%
2001/Delhi[55]	4,171	>18 years	Exposure to pollution	Questionnaire+ Spirometry	*Low pollution area*: Males—0.8–3.1% Females—0.3–2.1% *High pollution area*: Males–0.5–4.6% Females–1.1–5.9%
1999–2000 Haryana[56]	200	>60 years	Nil specified	COPD, clinical diagnosis, medical records and medication	Total—42% Urban Male—36.7% Female—31.4% *Rural* Male—57.1%, Female—43.1%
1994/Kashmir[57]	286–Gujjars 274– Nongujjars	>15 years	Low pollution smoking status and ventilation of homes	History+ Spirometry	Total—7.6% Gujjars—10.14% Nongujjars—5.11%
1982/Uttar Pradesh[58]	1,424	>20 years	Smoking status	Questionnaire	Total—6.5% Males—8.1% Females—4.5%
2010/West Bengal[59]	201	>35 years	Indoor stove usage	Questionnaire+ Spirometry	Airway obstruction in 58.5%
1999/Kashmir[60]	1,140	>30 years	Indoor room heating using biomass fuel smoking	History, clinical examination, spirometry	Chronic bronchitis—5.7% COPD—5.2%
1990/Chandigarh city and Mullanpur[61]	1,475	>15 years	Smoking	Questionnaire, examination and PEFR	Chronic bronchitis Total—3.6% Males—5% Females—2.7% COPD—1.8%
1987/Mumbai[62]	4,129	>45 years	Exposure to SO_2	Questionnaire, examination and spirometry	Chronic bronchitis: High SO_2—4.5% Medium SO_2—4.5% Low SO_2—2.3% Rural—5.0%

Contd...

Contd...

1981–86/Tamil Nadu[63]	9,946	>30 years	Low pollution atmosphere	Questionnaire and PEFR	*Chronic bronchitis*: Males—4.1 *COPD*: Total—2.5% Males—3.3% Females—1.8%
1986/Himachal Pradesh[64]	446	18–80 years	Smoking and poor ventilation	Questionnaire and spirometry	*Chronic bronchitis*: Total—20.9% Males—21.7% Females—19.0% *COPD*: Total—8.3% Males—7.2% Females—10.5%
1981 Chandigarh[65]	2,825	>16 years	Males—smoking Females—exposure to biomass fuel	Questionnaire and PEFR	*Chronic bronchitis*: Smoker males—9.9% Females—1.6% *COPD*: Smoker males—4.27% Females—1.02%
Abbreviations: COPD, chronic obstructive pulmonary disease; PEFR, peak expiratory flow rate					

is above 45 years, the estimated number of COPD patients in India would be about 25 million already **(Fig. 6)**.

DISABILITY ADJUSTED LIFE YEARS DUE TO CHRONIC OBSTRUCTIVE PULMONARY DISEASE

Mortality estimates give us the death rates due to a disease but the DALYs represent the morbidity that is caused by the illness with respect to the years lived with disability (YLD) which would otherwise have been years of good health and productivity for that individual and the years of life lost (YLL) (premature mortality) which the patient would have otherwise lived for, had the disease not occurred. According to the GBD study 2010[67] global all cause DALYs remained stable from 1990 (2·50 billion) to 2010 (2·49 billion). Crude DALYs per 1,000 have decreased by 23% (472 per 1,000 to 361 per 1,000). Chronic respiratory diseases as a group accounted for 4·7% of global DALYs, with COPD making up two-thirds of the total and asthma nearly a fifth of the total.

Globally, COPD is responsible for 76.8 million DALYs. 33% of these DALYs are contributed by India alone. COPD ranks third in DALYs globally due to the huge numbers contributed by China and India but though China leads in the number of deaths, the DALYs due to COPD are 16.7 million, much lesser than the 25.8 million DALYs from COPD in India. Though, COPD ranks second and third as a cause of DALYs in the United States and United Kingdom respectively, the DALYs lost are 3.6 million and 0.7 million in these developed countries, respectively.

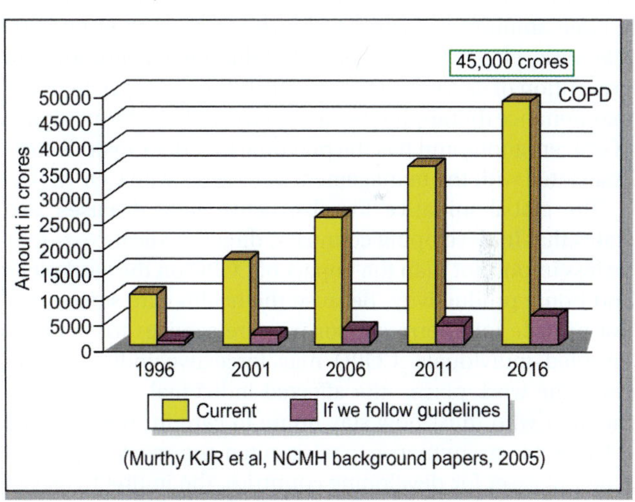

Fig. 6 Economic burden of COPD in India

ECONOMIC BURDEN OF CHRONIC OBSTRUCTIVE PULMONARY DISEASE

Global Economic Burden of Chronic Obstructive Pulmonary Disease

Chronic obstructive pulmonary disease is a costly disease with very high direct costs (value of health care resources devoted to diagnosis and medical management) as well as indirect costs[1] (monetary consequences of disability, missed work, premature mortality and cost of attendants or family costs resulting from the illness). In the European Union, the total direct costs of respiratory diseases is estimated to be about 6% of the total health care budget and COPD alone accounts for 56% of this budget amounting to about 38.6 billion Euro.[1] In the United States, the estimated direct costs of COPD are $29.5 billion and the indirect costs are $20.4 billion.[1]

The direct health-care costs for patients with COPD has increased by 38% between 1987 and 2007, and continued to increase by approximately 5% annually between 2006 and 2009.[68] The largest contributor to this increased expenditure was hospital admissions ($2,289 per admission in constant 2007 United States dollars).

The aggregate costs associated with the treatment of acute exacerbation of COPD for the United States are between $3.2 billion and $3.8 billion and an acute exacerbation imposes a 10-fold greater health-care cost as compared to stable COPD. Similar, data from another United States study suggest that 10% of persons with COPD account for more than 70% of all medical care costs.[69] Similar, data is available from several other countries including Poland,[70] Korea[71] and Singapore.[72] A systematic review of 259 articles[72] also showed a trend of direct cost growth in the elderly population, which was stated to be mainly due to more frequent use of acute health care services, especially for managing COPD exacerbations.[73] A large amount of this expenditure can be curbed by early diagnosis, effective management of the stable condition and prevention of exacerbations of COPD. The appropriate use of maintenance therapy has been shown to reduce the incidence of exacerbations and has the potential to reduce overall costs associated with the management of patients with COPD.

The global initiative for obstructive lung diseases also states that in developing countries, direct medical costs may be less important than the impact of COPD on the workplace and home productivity. Because the health care sector may not provide long-term supportive care services for severely disabled individuals, COPD may force two individuals to leave the work place—the affected individual and a family member who must now stay home to care for the disabled relative. Since, human capital is often the most important national asset for developing countries, the indirect costs of COPD may represent a serious threat to their economies.

Economic Burden of Chronic Obstructive Pulmonary Disease in India

There is no recent data on the economic burden from expenditures on management (both daily treatment and exacerbations (indoor/outdoor treatment) of COPD. Neither have the losses attributed to premature morbidity and mortality due to COPD been evaluated. COPD being a chronic, progressive disease poses a huge economic burden on the patient as well as the health-care systems. At individual level, it frequently proves to be financially ruin-some for families with average income. The cost-estimate assessed in an Indian Council of Medical Research (ICMR) sponsored project in 1998 showed about ₹ 2,440 as direct per capita expenditure, ₹ 1,340 on smoking products and ₹ 11,454 as indirect losses annually.[74] The assessment was an underestimation considering the facts that the State's expenditures on treatments and health-care related infrastructure were not accounted for. Importantly, however, the costs reflected an important financial burden of about 30% of the patient's income. According to national commission on macroeconomics and health published data[66] the per capita expenditure on COPD was ₹ 42,664 in 2006 and is expected to increase to ₹ 62,630 in 2016. India spent an estimated ₹ 25,209 crores for COPD (direct and indirect costs) in the year 2006 and this cost is expected to increase to about Rs. 45,000 crores in the year 2016 **(Fig. 6)**. A large part of this expenditure is because of delayed diagnosis and improper management and is preventable if we follow proper guidelines for diagnosis and management.

CONCLUSION

The incidence and prevalence of COPD is fast increasing not only in the industrialized countries but also in developing countries due to the ever increasing smoking epidemic compounded by poor socioeconomic status in countries like India and China. It has been estimated that almost 50% of smokers may develop COPD.[75] In addition; nonsmoking COPD caused mainly due to exposure to smoke from biomass fuel, occupational exposure to dust and gases, poor socioeconomic status, etc. is fast emerging as an entity that is causing considerable morbidity and mortality amongst nonsmokers too.[16]

The fact that the mortality rates due to COPD in India is second highest in the world and the huge economic burden of the disease on the country indicates that India needs to take aggressive measures to prevent the development of COPD and calls for major policy changes to equip the health care system with facilities for early diagnosis and appropriate management of COPD.

REFERENCES

1. Global Initiative for Chronic Lung Disease. GOLD 2014 update. Spain: GOLD Executive Committee; 2014.
2. Lozano R, Naghavi M, Foreman K, Lim S, Shibuya K, Aboyans V, et al. Global and regional mortality from 235 causes of death for 20 age groups in 1990 and 2010: a systematic analysis for the Global Burden of Disease Study 2010. Lancet. 2012;380(9859):2095-128.
3. Horton R. GBD 2010: understanding disease, injury, and risk. Lancet. 2012;380(9859):2053-4.
4. World Health Organization (WHO). (2014). Burden of COPD. [online] Available from *http://www.who.int/respiratory/copd/burden/en/*.[Accessed 29 July, 2014].
5. World Health Organization. (2010). Global status report on non-communicable diseases. [online] Available from *http://www.who.int/chp/ncd_global_status_report/en.* [Accessed April, 2016].
6. Lopez AD, Shibuya K, Rao C, Mathers CD, Hansell AL, Held LS, et al. Chronic obstructive pulmonary disease: current burden and future projections. Eur respir J. 2006;27(2):397-412.

7. Guarascio AJ, Ray SM, Finch CK, Self TH. The clinical and economic burden of chronic obstructive pulmonary disease in the USA. Clinicoecon Outcomes Res. 2013;5:235-45.
8. Jemal A, Ward E, Hao Y, Thun M. Trends in the leading causes of death in the United States, 1970-2002. JAMA. 2005;294(10):1255-9.
9. Mathers C, Loncar D. Updated projections of global mortality and burden of disease, 2002–2030: data sources, methods and results; evidence and information for policy working paper evidence and information for policy. World Health Organization. 2005.
10. Report on causes of death in India. (2001-03). [online] Available from *http://www. censusindia.gov.in/Vital_Statistics/Summary_Report_Death_01_03. Pdf.* [Accessed July, 2014].
11. Annual report on medical certification of cause of death. (2010). Available from *http://www.censusindia.gov.in/2011-Common/mccd.html.* [Accessed 30 July,2014].
12. Global burden of diseases, injuries, and risk factors study. (GBD). (2010). [online] Available from *http://www.healthdata.org/sites/default/files/files/country_profiles/GBD/ihme_gbd_country_report_india.pdf.* [Accessed 30 July, 2014].
13. World Health Organization. (2008) Global Alliance against Chronic Respiratory Diseases (GARD): general meeting report, Istanbul, Turkey. 2008.
14. Shibuya K, Mathers D, Lopez A. Chronic Obstructive Pulmonary Disease, consistent estimate of incidence, prevalence and mortality by WHO region, Global Programme on Evidence for Health Policy WHO. 2001.
15. Mannino D, Gagnon R, Petty T, et al. Obstructive lung disease and low lung function in adults in the United States: data from the National Health and Nutrition Examination Survey, 1988-1994. Arch Intern Med. 2000;160(11):1683-9.
16. Salvi SS, Barnes PJ. Chronic obstructive pulmonary disease in non-smokers. Lancet. 2009;374(9691):733-43.
17. Behrendt CE. Mild and moderate-to-severe COPD in nonsmokers: distinct demographic profiles. Chest. 2005;128(3): 1239-44.
18. Shahab L, Jarvis MJ, Britton J, West R. Prevalence, diagnosis and relation to tobacco dependence of chronic obstructive pulmonary disease in a nationally representative population sample. Thorax. 2006;61(12):1043-7.
19. Hardie JA, Vollmer WM, Buist AS, Bakke P, Mørkve O. Respiratory symptoms and obstructive pulmonary disease in a population aged over 70 years. Respir Med. 2005;99(2):186-95.
20. Lamprecht B, Schirnhofer L, Kaiser B, Buist S, Studnicka M. Non-reversible airway obstruction in never smokers: results from the Austrian BOLD study. Respir Med. 2008;102(12): 1833-8.
21. Lindström M, Kotaniemi J, Jönsson E, Lundbäck B. Smoking, respiratory symptoms, and diseases: a comparative study between northern Sweden and northern Finland: report from the FinEsS study. Chest. 2001;119(3):852-61.
22. Viegi G, Pedreschi M, Pistelli F, Di Pede F, Baldacci S, Carrozzi L, et al. Prevalence of airways obstruction in a general population: European Respiratory Society vs American Thoracic Society definition. Chest. 2000;117(5 Suppl 2): 339S-45S.
23. de Marco R, Accordini S, Cerveri I, Corsico A, Sunyer J, Neukirch F, et al. An international survey of chronic obstructive pulmonary disease in young adults according to GOLD stages. Thorax. 2004;59(2):120-5.
24. Liu S, Zhou Y, Wang X, Wang D, Lu J, Zheng J, et al. Biomass fuels are the probable risk factor for chronic obstructive pulmonary disease in rural South China. Thorax. 2007;62(10):889-97.
25. Zhou Y, Wang C, Yao W, Chen P, Kang J, Huang S, et al. COPD in Chinese nonsmokers. Eur Respir J. 2009;33(3):509-18.
26. Ehrlich RI, White N, Norman R, Laubscher R, Steyn K, Lombard C, et al. Predictors of chronic bronchitis in South African adults. Int J Tuberc Lung Dis. 2004;8(3):369-76.
27. Brashier B, Londhe J, Madas S, Vincent V, Salvi S. Prevalence of self-reported respiratory symptoms, asthma and chronic bronchitis in slum area of a rapidly developing Indian city. Open J Respir Dis. 2012;2:73-81.
28. Menzes AM, Perez Padilla R, Jardim JR, Muiño A, Lopez MV, Valdivia G, et al. Chronic obstructive pulmonary disease in five Latin American cities (the PLATINO study): a prevalence study. Lancet. 2005:366(9500):1875-81.
29. Caballero A, Torres-Duque CA, Jaramillo C, Bolívar F, Sanabria F, Osorio P, et al. Prevalence of COPD in five Colombian cities situated at low, medium, and high altitude (PREPOCOL study). Chest. 2008;133(2):343-9.
30. Regional COPD Working Group. COPD prevalence in 12 Asia-Pacific countries and regions: projections based on the COPD prevalence estimation model. Respirology. 2003;8(2):192-8.
31. Kim DS, Kim YS, Jung KS, Chang JH, Lim CM, Lee JH, et al. Prevalence of chronic obstructive pulmonary disease in Korea: a population-based spirometry survey. Am J Respir Crit Care Med. 2005;172(7):842-7.
32. Lindberg A, Jonsson AC, Rönmark E, Lundgren R, Larsson LG, Lundbäck B. Prevalence of chronic obstructive pulmonary disease according to BTS, ERS, GOLD and ATS criteria in relation to doctor's diagnosis, symptoms, age, gender, and smoking habits. Respiration. 2005;72(5):471-9.
33. Fukuchi Y, Nishimura M, Ichinose M, Adachi M, Nagai A, Kuriyama T, et al. COPD in Japan: the Nippon COPD Epidemiology study. Respir. 2004;9(4):458-65.
34. Cerveri I, Accordini S, Verlato G, Corsico A, Zoia MC, Casali L, et al. Variations in the prevalence across countries of chronic bronchitis and smoking habits in young adults. Eur Respir J. 2001;18(1): 85-92.
35. von Hertzen L, Reunanen A, Impivaara O, Mälkiä E, Aromaa A. Airway obstruction in relation to symptoms in chronic respiratory disease—a nationally representative population study. Respir Med. 2000;94(4):356-63.
36. Buist AS, Vollmer WM, Sullivan SD, Weiss KB, Lee TA, Menezes AM, et al. The Burden of Obstructive Lung Disease Initiative (BOLD):rationale and design. COPD. 2005;2(2):277-83.
37. Buist AS, McBurnie MA, Vollmer WM, Gillespie S, Burney P, Mannino DM, et al. International variation in the prevalence of COPD (the BOLD Study): a population-based prevalence study. Lancet. 2007;370(9589):741-50.
38. Buist AS, Vollmer WM, McBurnie MA. Worldwide burden of COPD in high- and low income countries. Part I. The burden of obstructive lung Diseases (BOLD) initiative. Int J Tuber Lung Dis. 2008;12(7):703-8.
39. Vollmer WM, Gíslason T, Burney P, Enright PL, Gulsvik A, Kocabas A, et al. Comparison of spirometry criteria for the diagnosis of COPD: results from the BOLD study. Eur Respir J. 2009;34(3):588-97.
40. Burney P, Jithoo A, Kato B, Janson C, Mannino D, Nizankowska-Mogilnicka E, et al. Chronic obstructive pulmonary disease mortality and prevalence: the associations with smoking and poverty—a BOLD analysis. Thorax. 2014;69(5):465-73.
41. Landis SH, Muellerova H, Mannino DM, Menezes AM, Han MK, van der Molen T, et al. Continuing to Confront COPD

International Patient Survey: methods, COPD prevalence, and disease burden in 2012-2013. Int J Chron Obstruct Pulmon Dis. 2014;9:597-611.

42. Scholes S, Moody A, Mindell JS. Estimating population prevalence of potential airflow obstruction using different spirometric criteria: a pooled cross-sectional analysis of persons aged 40-95 years in England and Wales. BMJ Open. 2014;4(7):e005685.
43. Tilert T, Dillon C, Paulose-Ram R, Hnizdo E, Doney B. Estimating the U.S. prevalence of chronic obstructive pulmonary disease using pre- and post-bronchodilator spirometry: the National Health and Nutrition Examination Survey (NHANES) 2007-2010. Respir Res. 2013;14:103.
44. Evans J, Chen Y, Camp PG, Bowie DM, McRae L, et al. Estimating the prevalence of COPD in Canada: Reported diagnosis versus measured airflow obstruction. Health Rep. 2014;25(3):3-11.
45. Finney LJ, Feary JR, Leonardi-Bee J, Gordon SB, Mortimer K. Chronic obstructive pulmonary disease in sub-Saharan Africa: a systematic review. Int J Tuberc Lung Dis. 2013;17(5):583-9.
46. Adeloye D, Basquill C, Papana A, Chan KY, Rudan I, Campbell H. An Estimate of the Prevalence of COPD in Africa: A Systematic Analysis. COPD. 2015;12(1):71-81.
47. van Germert F, van der Molen T, Jones R, Chavannes N. The impact of asthma and COPD in sub-Saharan Africa. Prim care respir j. 2011;20(3):240-8.
48. Jindal SK, Aggarwal AN, Gupta D. A review of population studies from India to estimate national burden of chronic obstructive pulmonary disease and its association with smoking. Indian J Chest Dis Allied Sci. 2001;43(3):139-47.
49. McKay AJ, Mahesh PA, Fordham JZ, Majeed A. Prevalence of COPD in India: a systematic review. Prim Care Respir J. 2012;21(3):313-21.
50. Mahesh PA, Jayaraj BS, Prahlad ST, Chaya SK, Prabhakar AK, Agarwal AN, et al. Validation of a structured questionnaire for COPD and prevalence of COPD in rural area of Mysore: a pilot study. Lung India. 2009;26(3):63-9.
51. Jindal S, Aggarwal A, Chaudhary K, Chhabra SK, D'Souza GA, Gupta D, et al. A multicentric study on epidemiology of chronic obstructive pulmonary disease and its relationship with tobacco smoking and environmental tobacco smoke exposure. Indian J Chest Dis Allied Sci. 2006;48(1):23-9.
52. Sousa R, Ferri C, Acosta D, Albanese E, Guerra M, Huang Y, et al. Contribution of chronic diseases to disability in elderly people in countries with low and middle incomes: a 10/66 Dementia Research Group population-based survey. Lancet. 2009;374(9704):1821-30.
53. Medhi GK, Hazarika NC, Borah PK, Mahanta J. Health problems and disability of elderly individuals in two population groups from same geographical location. J Assoc Physicians India. 2006;54:539-44.
54. Goel S, Gupta B, Kashyap S, Bhardwaj A. Epidemiological aspects of chronic bronchitis in Shimla hills. Indian J Chest Dis Allied Sci. 2007;49:144-7.
55. Chhabra SK, Chhabra P, Rajpal S, Gupta RK. Ambient air pollution and chronic respiratory morbidity in Delhi. Arch Environ Health. 2001;56(1):58-64.
56. Joshi K, Kumar R, Avasthi A. Morbidity profile and its relationship with disability and psychological distress among elderly people in Northern India. Int J Epidemiol. 2003;32(6): 978-87.
57. Qureshi KA. Domestic smoke pollution and prevalence of chronic bronchitis/asthma in a rural area of Kashmir. Indian J Chest Dis Allied Sci. 1994;36(2):61-72.
58. Nigam P, Verma BL, Srivastava RN. Chronic bronchitis in an Indian rural community. J Assoc Physicians India.1982;30(5): 277-80.
59. Mukherjee R, Moore V, Purkait S, Bhattacharya M, Warburton C, Calverley P, et al. Feasibility of performing valid spirometry in rural India: preliminary results from a population study assessing the prevalence of COPD. Conference Publication: British Thoracic Society Winter Meeting 2010, London, UK. Thorax. 2010;65: A129.
60. Akhtar MA, Latif PA. Prevalence of chronic bronchitis in urban population of Kashmir. J Indian Med Assoc. 1999;97(9):365-9.
61. Jindal S. A field study on follow up at 10 years of prevalence of chronic obstructive pulmonary disease and peak expiratory flow rate. Indian J Med Res. 1993;98:20-6.
62. Kamat SR, Doshi VB. Sequential health effect study in relation to air pollution in Bombay, India. Eur J Epidemiol. 1987;3(3):265-77.
63. Ray D, Abel R, Selvaraj K. A 5-yr prospective epidemiological study of chronic obstructive pulmonary disease in rural south India. Indian J Med Res. 1995;101:238-44.
64. Malik S, Kashyap S. Chronic bronchitis in rural hills of Himachal Pradesh, northern India. Indian J Chest Dis Allied Sci. 1986;28:70-5.
65. Malik S, Banga N, Qamra S. Chronic bronchitis in Chandigarh, North India. Bulletin Postgraduate Institute of Medical Education and Research. Chandigarh. 1981;15:161-3.
66. Murthy K, Sastry J. Economic burden of chronic obstructive pulmonary disease: NCMH Background Papers-Burden of Disease in India. 2005.
67. Murray C, Vos T, Lozano R, Naghavi M, Flaxman AD, Michaud C, et al. Disability-adjusted life years (DALYs) for 291 diseases and injuries in 21 regions, 1990-2010: a systematic analysis for the Global Burden of Disease Study 2010. Lancet. 2012;380(9859):2197–223.
68. Blanchette CM, Gross NJ, Altman P. Rising Costs of COPD and the potential for maintenance therapy to slow the trend. Am Health Drug Benefits. 2014;7(2):98-106.
69. Sullivan SD, Ramsey SD, Lee TA. The economic burden of COPD. Chest. 2000;117(2 Suppl):5S-9S.
70. Jahnz-Różyk K, Targowski T, From S, Faluta T, Borowiec L. [Costs of chronic obstructive pulmonary disease in patients treated in ambulatory care in Poland]. Pneumonol Alergol Pol. 2011;79(5):337-42.
71. Kim C, Yoo KH, Rhee CK, Yoon HK, Kim YS, Lee SW, et al. Health care use and economic burden of patients with diagnosed chronic obstructive pulmonary disease in Korea. Int J Tuberc Lung Dis. 2014;18(6):737-43.
72. Teo WS, Tan WS, Chong WF, Abisheganaden J, Lew YJ, Lim TK. (Abstract) Economic burden of chronic obstructive pulmonary disease. Respirology. 2012;17(1):120-6.
73. Bustacchini S, Chiatti C, Furneri G, Lattanzio F, Mantovani LG. The economic burden of chronic obstructive pulmonary disease in the elderly: results from a systematic review of the literature. Curr Opin Pulm Med. 2011;17(Suppl1):S35-41.
74. Jindal SK. Estimation of costs of management of smoking related COPD and CHD. Project Report Indian Council Med Res. 1998.
75. Lundbäck B, Lindberg A, Lindström M, Rönmark E, Jonsson AC, Jönsson E, et al. Not 15 but 50% of smokers develop COPD?—Report from the Obstructive Lung Disease in Northern Swedish Studies. Respir Med. 2003;97(2):115-22.

Risk Factors for Chronic Obstructive Pulmonary Disease

Sneha Limaye, Sundeep Salvi

INTRODUCTION

The risk of chronic obstructive pulmonary disease (COPD) is related to an interaction between genetic factors and many different environmental exposures, which could also be affected by the presence of comorbid diseases. Tobacco smoking is an established risk factor for COPD, but emerging evidence suggests that risk factors other than smoking are also associated with COPD.[1,2] These factors include exposure to indoor and outdoor air pollutants, workplace exposure to dust and fumes, history of repeated lower respiratory tract infections during childhood, history of pulmonary tuberculosis, chronic persistent, poorly treated asthma, intrauterine growth retardation, poor nourishment and poor socioeconomic status. The identification of risk factors is an important step towards not only developing strategies for prevention and treatment, but also to assist in the diagnosis of COPD.

TOBACCO SMOKING

Tobacco smoking was first shown to be associated with the risk of developing COPD during 1950s.[3,4] Later, Fletcher and Peto reported that lung function decreased markedly in those smokers who had symptoms of chronic cough and/or breathlessness.[5] A subsequent larger and longer Framingham cohort offspring study confirmed these results.[6] All subsequent research then focused on smoking as the most important risk factor for COPD and several prevalence as well as intervention studies, in fact, have been done only amongst smokers.

Tobacco smoking is more prevalent in the developed countries, although the number of smokers is now declining slowly. The prevalence is particularly high in Russia, China, Eastern Europe, Southeast Asia and South America **(Fig. 1)**. On the other hand, the number of smokers in the developing countries is increasing rapidly. There are an estimated 1.1 billion smokers worldwide and India's contribution is 110 million. Interestingly, India has the second largest number of female smokers in the world (12.1 million) after USA, although the prevalence is low, but rising in the cities. In India, an estimated 65% of all men and 33% of all women use some or other form of tobacco. According to 55th round (1999-2000) of NSS in India, 54% of tobacco consumers smoke *bidi*, 15% smoke cigarette and 30% consume different tobacco chewing products.

The prevalence of smoking in the Indian population is 28.5% in men and 2.1% in women.[7] It is estimated that by 2030, tobacco consumption in any form will account for 10 million deaths per year, half of them aged 35–69 years. Almost 82% of world's smokers reside in the developing countries, and nearly 17% of world's smoking population resides in India.[8] There is a wide range of the prevalence rate of smoking from the lowest of 13.9% in Punjab to the highest of 49.4% in Mizoram. *Bidi* is the most common form of smoking, more so in the rural areas. The different forms of tobacco smoking prevalent in India are cigarette, *bidi*, *hookah* and *chillum* smoking.

In India and other Southeast Asian countries, *bidi* smoking is more common than cigarette smoking. *Bidis* are made of tobacco wrapped in Tendu leaf **(Fig. 2)**. Although the amount of nicotine in a *bidi* is one-fourth that of a cigarette, the content of tar is roughly 5 times greater. From a COPD point of view, one *bidi* is as harmful as one cigarette. Because of low combustibility of the Tendu leaf wrapper, *bidi* smokers inhale more often and more deeply, thereby breathing greater amounts of tar.[9]

Cigarette smoke is a complex mixture of over 4,700 chemical compounds, generates high concentration of free radicals and oxidants like reactive oxygen species (ROS), epoxides, peroxides and nitric oxides (NO).[10] It contains two very different populations of free radicals, one in the tar and one in the gas phase. The tar phase contains several relatively stable free radicals, the principal radical being quinone/hydroquinone (Q/QH_2). The gas phase of cigarette smoke contains small oxygen- and carbon-centered radicals that are more reactive than are the tar phase radicals. One of the important mechanism through which tobacco smoke exerts its harmful effects on the lungs is the oxidative stress caused by release of ROS.

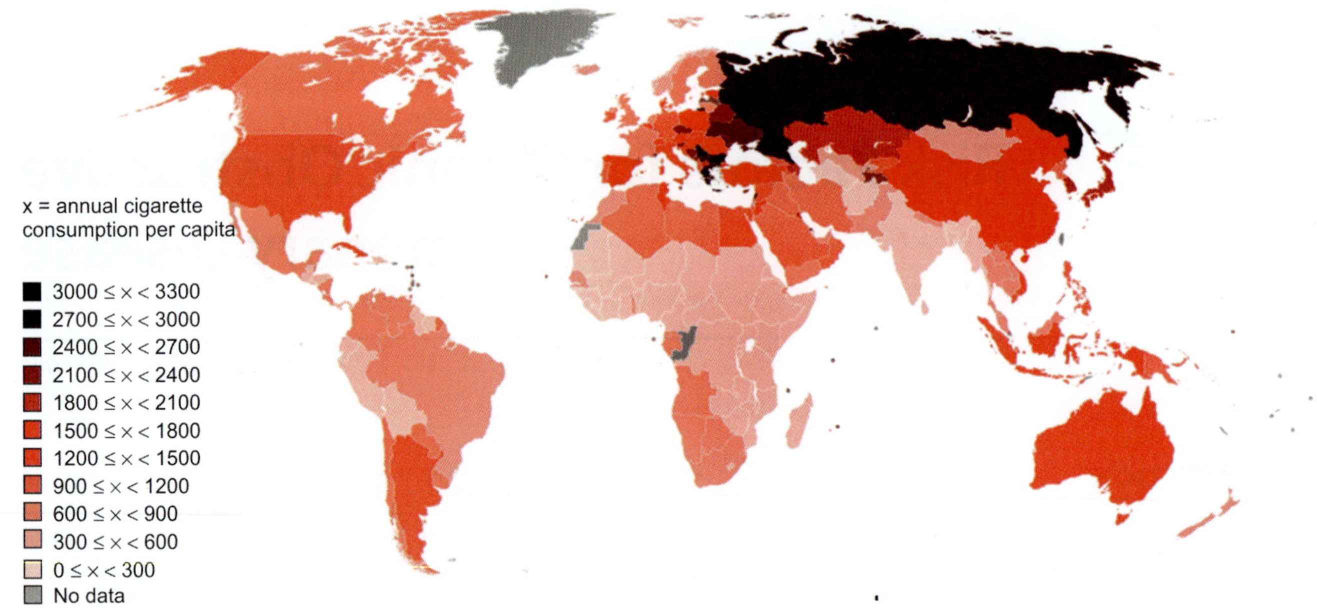

Fig. 1 Global smoking prevalence rates
Source: Jolly Janner. ERC. (2007). World Cigarettes 1: The 2007 Report. ERC Statistics Intl Plc. Population data is from Central Intelligence Agency. (2007). The World Factbook 2007. Washington: Government Printing Office.

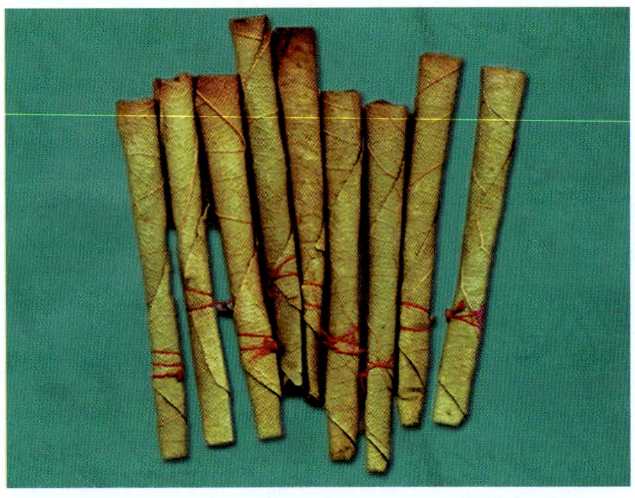

Fig. 2 *Bidis* are a more popular form of smoking than cigarette in India

Cigarette smoke contains 10^{17} oxidants per puff, of which 10^{14} are oxygen free radicals which have the potential to produce an enormous oxidant burden on the lungs.[11] All tissues are vulnerable to oxidant damage, but by virtue of its location, the airspace epithelium is particularly vulnerable. Tobacco smoking increases the risk of COPD by 2-3-fold, although not all smokers develop COPD. Some of the earlier reports estimated that only 15% of smokers develop COPD. New evidence suggests that up to 50% of smokers developed COPD.[12]

HOOKAH SMOKING AND RISK OF CHRONIC OBSTRUCTIVE PULMONARY DISEASE

Hookah, or water-pipe smoking (WPS), is a form of snuff smoking device used for tobacco smoking which has been used extensively in the Middle East. *Hookah* smoking has been practiced for hundreds of years, but has recently become a very popular form of social smoking as an emerging "trend" especially amongst the youth who believe *hookah* to be a less harmful than cigarettes and do not consider it as a health hazard or being addictive. Growing amount of evidences have associated *hookah* smoking as a risk factor for various diseases including COPD.[13]

The *hookah* smoke consists of 0.15–1 per puff, an average *hookah* session lasts 20–80 minutes which is equivalent of smoking 100 cigarettes or more.[14] The INSEARCH study reported *hookah* smoking was associated with higher odds of having chronic bronchitis in comparison to cigarette smoking.[15] These findings are consistent with studies from other parts of world, which showed that chronic bronchitis is most prevalent in *hookah* smokers than in cigarette smokers.[16,17]

ENVIRONMENTAL TOBACCO SMOKE AND THE RISK OF CHRONIC OBSTRUCTIVE PULMONARY DISEASE

Environmental tobacco smoke (ETS) is one of the most common and very harmful forms of indoor air pollutants. ETS is composed of midstream smoke (SS), emitted from the moldering tobacco between puffs and exhaled mainstream smoke (MS) from the smoker. When a cigarette is smoked, roughly half of the smoke generated is SS and the other half MS, while ETS is a diluted mixture of SS and exhaled MS. These smokes are a complex mixtures of over 4,000 chemicals, at least 50 of which are known to cause cancer, ischemic heart disease and respiratory diseases like asthma and COPD in humans. The particle sizes are smaller in ETS (0.01–1.0 μm) than in MS (0.1–1.0 μm), and are therefore more likely to penetrate deeper into the airways. Therefore, ETS seems to be more harmful in causing adverse respiratory health effects than MS.[18]

An increasing body of literature now supports an association between ETS exposure, passive smoke or second-hand smoke (SHS) and the development of COPD.[15,19-21] The risk of COPD also occurs amongst people who are exposed to SHS.[22,23] Interestingly, restaurant workers have been shown to experience a substantive decrement in spirometry after a single work shift in a smoky environment, suggesting that ETS has acute negative effects on pulmonary function. In addition, the cross-shift reduction of pulmonary function improved after a workplace smoking ban reduced SHS exposure.[23]

The association between ETS and COPD has been shown to be consistent across various cross-sectional and longitudinal cohort studies. The temporal relationship and a dose-response relationship have been established in studies that evaluated cumulative lifetime exposure.

HOUSEHOLD AIR POLLUTION AS A RISK FACTOR FOR CHRONIC OBSTRUCTIVE PULMONARY DISEASE

It is estimated that about half the global population (3 billion people) live in homes that use biomass fuel for cooking and heating purposes. Burning of biomass solid fuel (includes wood, twigs, crop residues, animal dung) **(Figs 3A to C)** emits very high levels of indoor air pollutants, both particulate matter as well as the gaseous pollutants. Many of these homes are poorly ventilated, exposing these individuals to very high levels of indoor air pollutants.

Women, young girls and small children are exposed for the longest duration because they spend more time in close vicinity to the biomass smoke. During their lifetime, women are exposed for around 30–40 years, equivalent to 60,000 hours of exposure to biomass smoke or inhaling a total volume of 25 million liters of highly polluted indoor air.[24] The levels of household air pollutants encountered in homes that use biomass fuel are several orders higher than the levels in the most polluted urban cities in the world. These pollutants have the potential to produce intense oxidative stress in the lungs, and the elastolytic effects of these pollutants have been found to be worse than those caused due to tobacco smoke.

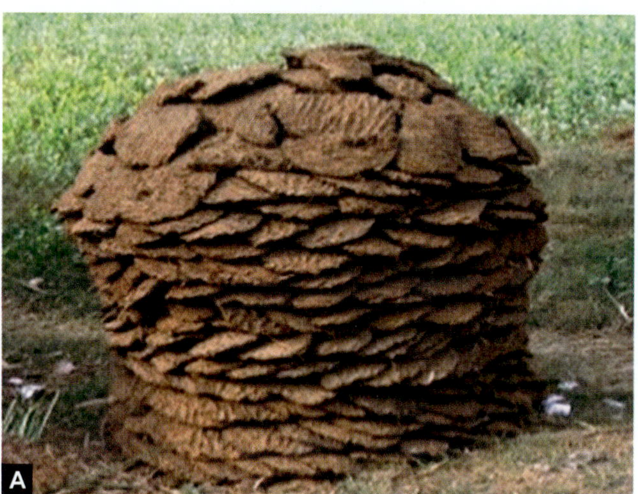

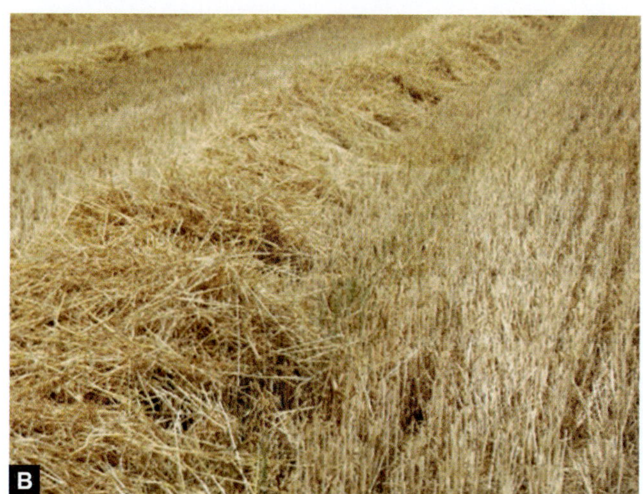

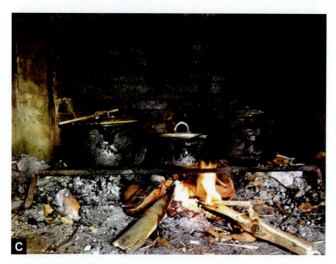

Figs 3A to C Sources of different biomass fuels. (A) Dung cake; (B) Crop residues; (C) Firewood

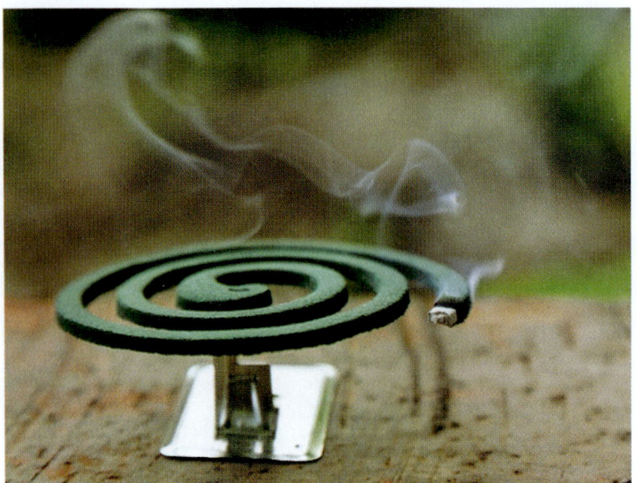

Fig. 4 Burning mosquito coil

The exposure to biomass smoke induces the same amount of risk of COPD as tobacco smoke.

MOSQUITO COIL SMOKE AND RISK OF CHRONIC OBSTRUCTIVE PULMONARY DISEASE

Mosquito bites transmit parasitic and viral infections, such as malaria, dengue, Japanese encephalitis, etc. which together affect 700 million people annually and cause several million deaths.[25]

Of the available forms of mosquito repellents, mosquito coils **(Fig. 4)** are the most widely used repellents in Asia, Africa and South America as they are cheap, easy to use and readily available. An estimated 29 billion mosquito coils are sold every year and are used by 2 billion people across the globe.[26] A recent study from South India reported that 73% of people living in rural areas and 42% of people living in urban areas burn mosquito coils at home.[27]

The main chemical repellent Pyrethrum present in the mosquito coils accounts for only 0.3–0.4% of the mosquito coil mass, while the bulk of the coil is made up of wood powder, coconut shell powder or joss powder, along with binders, dyes, oxidants and other additives which allow the coil to smolder for around 6–8 hours during the night. An earlier study from Malaysia reported that burning one mosquito coil over a period of 8 hours released the same amount of mass of particulate matter less than 2.5 microns ($PM_{2.5}$), that was equivalent to around 100 cigarettes, and formaldehyde that was equivalent to around 50 cigarettes.[28]

Both short-term and long-term animal exposure studies with mosquito coil smoke have shown significant adverse impacts on lung histology, including epithelial cell damage, interstitial cellular accumulation, pulmonary edema and emphysema.[29] Preliminary work from the author's laboratory indicates that the level of particulate matter emitted by different forms of mosquito repellents produced high indoor $PM_{2.5}$ and CO levels. Use of mosquito coils was associated with greater respiratory morbidity than liquid mosquito repellents.[30]

OUTDOOR AIR POLLUTION AND CHRONIC OBSTRUCTIVE PULMONARY DISEASE

Ambient air pollution is a growing problem in most urban cities of the world. Over the last few decades, air pollution in most cities in the developed countries has decreased appreciably due to the advent of strict legislation and improvements in engine technology, but it continues to increase markedly in most cities of the developing countries. Both the gaseous and particulate matter components of urban ambient air pollutants have been shown to be associated with increasing respiratory morbidity and cardiovascular mortality.

One of the earliest studies that investigated an association between ambient air pollution and COPD in 1958 reported that postmen from England and Wales who worked in areas with higher outdoor air pollution levels, had a greater prevalence of COPD than those who worked in areas with lower ambient air pollution levels.[31] A subsequent study from UK showed that postmen who worked in more polluted cities had lower lung function values than those who worked in less polluted areas.[32] Similar observations were later reported in the general population.[33] More recently, living in areas closer to roads with heavy motor vehicular traffic has been shown to be associated with significant decrements in lung function and increased prevalence of COPD in women.[34]

Adults exposed to high levels of ambient air pollutants have an increased risk of developing respiratory symptoms, asthma, COPD, allergic rhinitis, lower respiratory tract infections and lung cancers.[35] Apart from its impact on respiratory system, ambient air pollutants, and in particular, particulate matter also increase the risk of cardiovascular diseases and cardiovascular mortality. The harmful effects of ambient air pollutants are mediated by the formation of ROS, which in turn induce oxidative stress in the lung that incite a powerful cellular and mediator inflammatory response, which spills into the systemic circulation and causes harmful effects in other body organs. Exposure to high levels of respirable ambient air pollutants serves as an important risk factor for worsening or exacerbation of existing COPD.[36,37]

CHRONIC OBSTRUCTIVE PULMONARY DISEASE ASSOCIATED WITH OCCUPATIONAL EXPOSURES

The association between occupational exposures **(Figs 5A to C)** and COPD has been observed for at least four

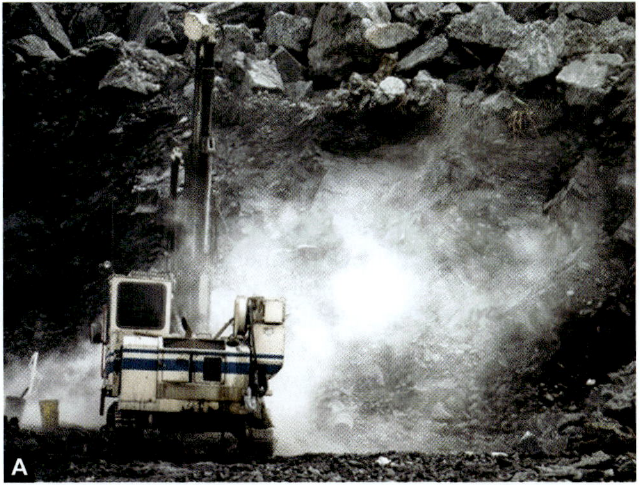

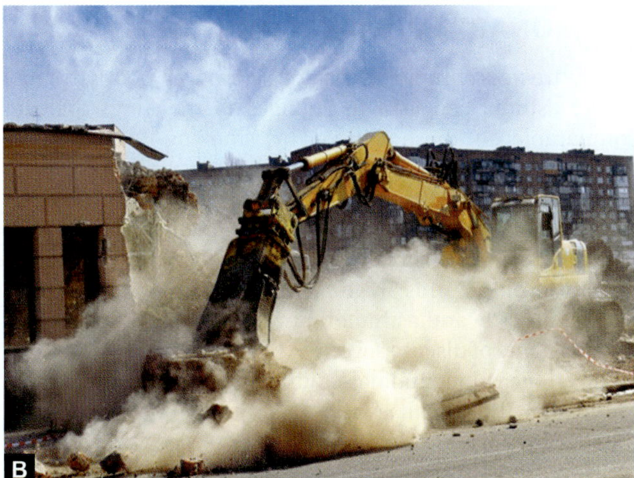

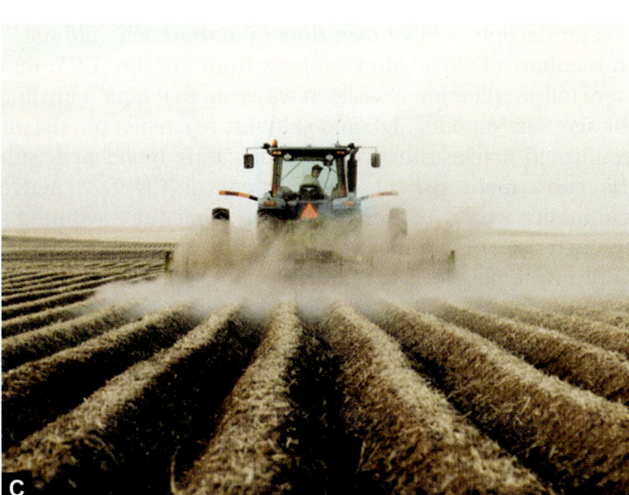

Figs 5A to C Dust exposures in different occupations. (A) Mining; (B) Construction; (C) Farming

Table 1 Occupations associated with risk of developing chronic obstructive pulmonary disease

Occupation	*Exposures causing COPD*
Crop farming	Inorganic and organic dust
Animal farming	Organic dust, bacteria, ammonia, hydrogen sulfide
Building and construction work	Dust exposures and fine particles, fumes
Mining, stone cutting and polishing	Fine dust exposure, fumes, mineral dust
Plastic, textile, rubber and leather industry	Chemical and dust exposures
Transportation industry and traffic duty	Vehicular emissions
Road sweeping	Road dust
Cooking and *dhaba*	Biomass smoke exposures

decades. Earlier studies revealed that exposure to toxic gases at workplace,[38] grain dust in farms,[39] and to dust and fumes in factories were strongly associated with the risk of development of COPD.

In 2003, the American Thoracic Society conducted a systematic epidemiological review of occupational factors associated with the development of COPD, and reported that approximately 15% of COPD may be attributable to workplace exposure.[40] A more recent follow-up of the review has provided similar estimates.[41] Several occupations are associated with an increased risk for COPD **(Table 1)**.

Farming as an occupation has been shown to be strongly associated with COPD. In a study of 1,258 adults of above the age of 40 years,[42] the association between farming and COPD prevalence (defined by a post-bronchodilator FEV1/FVC ratio less than 0.70 on spirometry), the risk of COPD, attributable to farming, was 7.7%, around 30% of the farmers had at least mild COPD. More recently, a study from Norway[43] demonstrated that livestock farmers compared to crop farmers, had a 40% greater risk of having COPD [95% confidence interval (CI): 10–70%], and that this correlated strongly with the levels of ammonia, hydrogen sulfide, inorganic dust and organic dusts measured by personal monitors at workplace.

Longitudinal studies have documented the association between COPD and occupational exposures in coal miners, hard rock miners, tunnel workers and concrete manufacturing workers. In heavily exposed workers, the effect of dust exposure may be even greater than that of cigarette smoking alone.[44] Construction workers exposed to fumes and mineral dust have been shown to have a significantly higher risk of death due to COPD.[45] Prolonged exposure to silica in occupations such as construction industry, brick manufacturing, gold mining and in iron and steel foundries (where average respirable dust levels reach up to 10,000 µg/m^3), is also strongly associated with the development of COPD.[46] The burden of occupational COPD is likely to be ever higher in countries of low and middle income, where occupational exposures to dust and fumes could be greater than in high income nations.

CHRONIC OBSTRUCTIVE PULMONARY DISEASE ASSOCIATED WITH PULMONARY TUBERCULOSIS

Pulmonary tuberculosis **(Fig. 6)** has been shown to be associated with chronic airflow obstruction, particularly of the COPD phenotype, at the time of diagnosis,[47-49] during treatment[50] and several years after the completion of treatment.[51] The amount of airflow obstruction is related to the extent of the disease determined radiologically, the amount of sputum produced, and the length of time after the diagnosis or completion of treatment.[51] Apart from the airway fibrosis that may follow tubercular infections, the immune response to mycobacteria may enhance the airway inflammation that is typical of COPD.

The prevalence of airflow obstruction in subjects with pulmonary tuberculosis has been shown to vary from 28% to 68% according to the study design, timing of assessment and medical or surgical treatment. In a nationwide household survey of 13,826 adults in South Africa, the strongest predictor of COPD, defined by self-reported symptoms of a chronic productive cough, was history of pulmonary tuberculosis. The odds ratios (OR) were 4.9 (95% CI 2.6–9.2) for men, and 6.6 (95% CI 3.7–11.9) for women.[52] More interestingly, this risk was stronger than the odds ratios associated with tobacco smoking or exposure to biomass fuel smoke.

More recently, a study from five cities in Colombia (PREPOCOL study)[53] that investigated the association between history of pulmonary tuberculosis and COPD (defined by post-bronchodilator FEV1/FVC ratio < 0.70), reported a strong association with an odds ratio of 2.9 (95% CI 1.6–5.5). Further, this association was even stronger than that noted with tobacco smoking [OR: 2.6, (95% CI 1.9–3.5)].

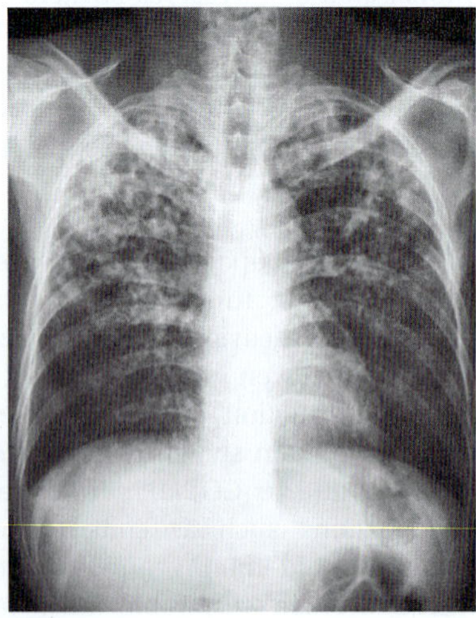

Fig. 6 Pulmonary TB: A risk factor for COPD

More than 2 billion people, equal to one-third of the world's population, are infected with tubercle bacilli, and an estimated 9.2 million new cases of tuberculosis are detected every year, 80% of them are present in 22 countries of the world.[54] Countries from Asia, Africa and Latin America have a particularly high burden of pulmonary tuberculosis. Studies from several different countries with high tuberculosis prevalence indicate that a history of pulmonary tuberculosis is a strong risk factor for COPD.[47-54] The cumulative burden of COPD associated with pulmonary tuberculosis is, therefore, likely to be much greater than previously believed, especially in the developing countries.[55]

CHRONIC ASTHMA AS A RISK FACTOR FOR CHRONIC OBSTRUCTIVE PULMONARY DISEASE

Poorly treated chronic persistent asthma or poorly treated severe asthma can lead to changes in the lungs that are comparable to those caused by smoking.[56] In patients with severe asthma, the inflammation in the airways becomes similar to those seen in COPD, with an increase in the number of neutrophils and IL-8, increased proteases, increased oxidative stress and a reduced responsiveness to corticosteroids.[57] This might reflect common mechanisms between COPD and asthma that are related to the intrinsic determinants of disease severity.

In a 5-year longitudinal study of 10,952 subjects, it was found that those with a new asthma diagnosis had lower initial values of lung function and an increased rate of decline in FEV1 compared to nonasthmatic subjects.[58] Subsequent analyses from the same study after 15-years of follow-up showed that subjects with self-reported asthma still had a greater decline in FEV1 over time than those who did not.[58] In a cohort of 3,099 adult subjects from Tucson, USA, that were followed up for 20 years, it was seen that after adjusting for age, sex, smoking, IgE and skin test reactivity, physician-confirmed active asthma was significantly associated with the subsequent risk of development of COPD.[59] Active asthmatics were 10 times more likely to acquire symptoms characteristic of chronic bronchitis and 17 times more likely to receive a diagnosis of emphysema by a physician. In this cohort, asthma was found to be the strongest risk factor for subsequent COPD [hazard ratio (HR)=12.5; attributable risk (AR)=18.5%], more than even tobacco smoking (HR=2.9; AR=6.7%). Primary care clinicians who practice long enough often report patients with acute bronchitis that morphs into chronic asthma that then develops into severe COPD.[60]

Poorly treated chronic persistent severe asthma may present with features of COPD in the subsequent years. In many regions of the developing world, as well as some parts of the developed world, asthma still remains poorly treated,

Table 2 Genes implicated in COPD

Genes for which association studies have shown a significant relationship between polymorphisms and COPD	*Candidate genes for which there are no significant associations at present*
Alpha 1-antitrypsin • Alpha 1-antichymotrypsin • Cystic fibrosis transmembrane regulator • Vitamin D-binding protein • Alpha 2-macroglobulin • Cytochrome P450A1 • ABH secretor, Lewis and ABO blood groups • HLA • Immunoglobulin deficiency • Haptoglobin	• Extracellular superoxide dismutase • Secretory leukocyte proteinase inhibitor • Cathepsin G

Abbreviations: COPD, chronic obstructive pulmonary disease; HLA, human leukocyte antigen

it is likely that this may contribute significantly to the global burden of COPD.

GENETIC FACTORS PREDISPOSING DEVELOPMENT OF CHRONIC OBSTRUCTIVE PULMONARY DISEASE

Although COPD is predominantly an environmental lung disease, it is clear that genetic susceptibility is also important. Recent studies have indicated that COPD can run in families, and several potential genes have been identified[61] **(Table 2)**. Though several genes have been implicated in COPD, work done to examine specific polymorphisms for the development of disease has been, at best, inconsistent. Functional genetic variants influencing the development of COPD have not been yet definitively identified.

The best known genetic factor linked to COPD is the deficiency of alpha 1-antitrypsin, a major circulating inhibitor of serine proteases, which arises in 1–3% of patients with COPD. Having low concentrations of this enzyme, particularly in combination with smoking or other pollutant exposures, increases the risk of developing panlobular emphysema. This rare recessive trait is most commonly seen in individuals of Northern European origin.

In addition to alpha 1-antitrypsin deficiency, various other genetic syndromes have been suggested to have a contributory role in development of COPD in nonsmokers. Of these, Cutis laxa, a rare inherited connective tissue disorder of elastic fibers, mostly caused by mutations in elastin genes has been clearly demonstrated to cause emphysema in adolescents and childhood even in some nonsmoker patients.[62]

FACIAL WRINKLING

Cigarette smoking is well-known to be associated with facial wrinkling that increases with the number of pack years smoked. Interestingly, COPD patients show exaggerated skin wrinkling compared to normal smokers, and this has been associated with increased MMP9 expression by keratinocytes. It has been suggested that there may be a common mechanism and a common genetic susceptibility.[63] Cigarette smoking (which is a proven risk factor for COPD) also results in cellular senescence. In vitro exposure of lung fibroblasts results in an increased expression of SA-β-gal (senescence-associated β-galactosidase), a marker of cellular senescence which is interestingly also shown to be expressed more in cultured lung fibroblasts from patients with emphysema,[64,65] hinting a common genetic linkage between facial wrinkling and COPD. These results suggest the importance of screening of wrinkled individuals for the presence of airflow obstruction.

More recently, work is underway to study the role of antioxidant genes as potential candidates for increasing genetic susceptibility. There are several antioxidant genes which play a major role in protecting the airways and lung parenchyma from environmental oxidative stress and a genetic defect in the production of these protective molecules may increase susceptibility to develop COPD.

SOCIOECONOMIC STATUS

Poor socioeconomic status is a risk factor independently associated with COPD, likely to be indicative of other factors such as intrauterine growth retardation, poor nutrition (low intake of antioxidants) housing conditions, childhood respiratory tract infections, exposure to tobacco smoke, biomass smoke and other indoor air pollutants, and occupational risks. These factors might collectively contribute to the risk of COPD. Socioeconomic status should therefore be treated as an independent risk factor for COPD.

In summary, there exist a host of risk factors important in the development of COPD. The environmental exposures such as the tobacco smoking and air pollution are most commonly identifiable. The genetic predisposition may play an equally important role, but remains an investigational issue at present.

REFERENCES

1. Celli BR, Halbert RJ, Nordyke RJ, Schau B. Airway obstruction in never smokers: results from the Third National Health and Nutrition Examination Survey. Am J Med. 2005;118:1364-72.
2. Behrendt CE. Mild and moderate-to-severe COPD in nonsmokers: distinct demographic profiles. Chest. 2005;128: 1239-44.
3. Oswald NC, Medvei VC. Chronic bronchitis: the effect of cigarette-smoking. Lancet. 1955;269:843-44.
4. Anderson D, Ferris BG. Role of tobacco smoking in the causation of chronic respiratory disease. N Engl J Med. 1962;267:787-94.
5. Fletcher C, Peto R. The natural history of chronic airflow obstruction. Br Med J. 1977;1:1645-48.
6. Kohansal R, Martinez-Camblor P, Agusti A, Buist AS, Mannino DM, Soriano JB. The natural history of chronic airflow obstruction revisited: an analysis of the Framingham offspring cohort. Am J Respir Crit Care Med. 2009;180:3-10.

7. Jindal SK, Aggarwal AN, Gupta D, Chhabra SK, D'Souza GA, Gupta D, et al. Tobacco smoking in India: prevalence, quit-rates and respiratory morbidity. Indian J Chest Dis Allied Sci. 2006;48:37-42.
8. John RM. Tobacco consumption patterns and its health implications in India. Health Policy. 2005;71:213-22.
9. Rickert WS. Determination of yields of "tar," nicotine and carbon monoxide from *bidi* cigarettes: Final report. Ontario: Lab Stat International Inc; 1999.
10. Rahman I, MacNee W. Role oxidants/antioxidants in smoking-induced lung diseases. Free Radic Biol Med. 1996;21:669-81.
11. Pryor W, Stone K. Oxidants in cigarette smoke. Radicals, hydrogen peroxide, peroxynitrate, and peroxynitrite. Ann N Y Acad Sci. 1993;686:12-28.
12. Lundbäck B, Lindberg A, Lindström M, Rönmark E, Jonsson AC, Jönsson E, et al. Not 15 but 50% of smokers develop COPD? Report from the Obstructive Lung Disease in Northern Sweden Studies. Respir Med. 2003;97(2):115-22.
13. Blachman-Braun R, Del Mazo-Rodríguez RL, López-Sámano G, Buendía-Roldán I. Hookah, is it really harmless? Respir Med. 2014;108(5):661-7.
14. WHO Study Group on Tobacoo Product Regulation. (2005) Tob Reg Advisory Note, waterpipe tobacoo smoking: health effects research needs and recommended actions by regulators. [online] Available from *http://www.who.int/tobacco/global_interaction/tobreg/Waterpipe%20recommendation_Final.pdf.* [Accessed March, 2016].
15. Jindal SK, Aggarwal AN, Gupta D, Agarwal R, Kumar R, Kaur T, et al. Indian study on epidemiology of asthma, respiratory symptoms and chronic bronchitis in adults (INSEARCH). Int J Tuberc Lung Dis. 2012;16:1270-77.
16. Mohammad Y, Kakah M, Mohammad Y. Chronic respiratory effect of narguileh smoking compared with cigarette smoking in women from the East Mediterranean region. Int J Chron Obstruct Pulmon Dis. 2008;3:405-14.
17. Al Mutairi S, Shihab-Eldeen A, Mojiminiyi O, Anwar AA. Comparative analysis of the effects of hubble-bubble (sheesha) and cigarette smoking on respiratory and metabolic parameters in hubble-bubble and cigarette smokers. Respirology. 2006;11:449-55.
18. Cheraghi M, Salvi S. Environmental tobacco smoke (ETS) and respiratory health in children. Eur J Pediatr. 2009;168(8):897-905.
19. Eisner M, Balmes J, Katz P, Trupin L, Yelin E, Blanc P. Lifetime environmental tobacco smoke exposure and the risk of chronic obstructive pulmonary disease. Environ Health. 2005;4:7.
20. Yin P, Jiang C, Cheng K, Lam T, Lam K, Miller M, et al. Passive smoking exposure and risk of COPD among adults in China: the Guangzhou Biobank Cohort Study. Lancet. 2007;370:751-7.
21. Sezer H, Akkurt I, Guler N, Marakoglu K, Berk S. A case-control study on the effect of exposure to different substances on the development of COPD. Ann Epidemiol. 2006;16:59-62.
22. Mark D. Indoor air, passive smoking, and COPD. Am J Respir Crit Care Med. 2007;176:426-7.
23. Eisner M, Anthonisen N, Coultas D, Kuenzli N, Perez-Padilla R, Postma D, et al. An official American Thoracic Society public policy statement: Novel risk factors and the global burden of chronic obstructive pulmonary disease. American journal of respiratory and critical care medicine. 2010;182(5):693-718.
24. Salvi S, Barnes PJ. Is exposure to biomass smoke the biggest risk factor for COPD globally? Chest. 2010;138(1):3-6.
25. Manimaran A, Cruz M, Muthu C, Vincent S, Ignacimuthu S. Larvicidal and knockdown effects of some essential oils against *Culex quinquefasciatus* Say, *Aedes aegypti* (L.) and *Anopheles stephensi* (Liston). Advances in Bioscience and Biotechnology. 2012;3:855-62.
26. Hill N, Zhou H, Wang P, Guo X, Carneiro I, Moore SJ. A household randomized, controlled trial of the efficacy of 0.03% transfluthrin coils alone and in combination with long-lasting insecticidal nets on the incidence of *Plasmodium falciparum* and *Plasmodium vivax* malaria in Western Yunnan Province, China. Malar. 2014;13(1):208.
27. Chitra GA, Kaur P, Bhatnagar T, Manickam P, Murhekar MV. High prevalence of household pesticides and their unsafe use in rural South India. Int J Occup Med Environ Health. 2013;26(2):275-82.
28. Liu W, Zhang J, Hashim J, Jalaludin J, Hashim Z, Goldstein B. Mosquito coil emissions and health implications. Environ Health Perspect. 2003;111(12):1454-60.
29. Idowu E, Aimufua O, Ejovwoke Y, Akinsanya B, Otubanjo O. Toxicological effects of prolonged and intense use of mosquito coil emission in rats and its implications on malaria control. Rev Biol Trop. 2013;61(3):1463-73.
30. Salvi D, Limaye S, Muralidharan V, et al. Indoor particulate matter < 2.5 μm in mean aerodynamic diameter and carbon monoxide levels during the burning of mosquito coils and their association with respiratory health. Chest. 2016;149: 459-66.
31. Fairbairn AS, Reid DD. Air pollution and other local factors in respiratory disease. Br J Prev Soc Med. 1958;12(2):94-103.
32. Holland WW, Reid DD. The urban factor in chronic bronchitis. Lancet. 1965;1(7383):445-8.
33. Burrows B, Kellogg A, Buskey J. Relationship of symptoms of chronic bronchitis and emphysema to weather and air pollution. Arch Environ Health. 1968;16(3):406-13.
34. Kan H, Heiss G, Rose KM, Whitsel E, Lurmann F, London SJ. Traffic exposure and lung function in adults: the Atherosclerosis Risk in Communities study. Thorax. 2007;62:873-9.
35. Sunyer J, Jarvis D, Gotschi T, Garcia-Esteban R, Jacquemin B, Aguilera I, et al. Chronic bronchitis and urban air pollution in an international study. Occup and Environ Med. 2006;63: 836-43.
36. Limaye S, Salvi S. Ambient air pollution and the lungs: what do clinicians need to know? Breathe. 2010;6(3):234-44.
37. Arbex M, de Souza C, Cendon S, Arbex FF, Lopes AC, Moyses EP, et al. Urban air pollution and COPD-related emergency visits. J Epidemiol Community Health. 2009;63(10):777-83.
38. Chester E, Gillespie D, Krause F. The prevalence of chronic obstructive pulmonary disease in chlorine gas workers. Am Rev Respir Dis. 1969;99(3):365-73.
39. Husman K, Koskenvuo M, Kaprio J, Terho EO, Vohlonen I. Role of environment in the development of chronic bronchitis. Eur J Respir Dis Suppl. 1987;152:57-63.
40. Balmes J, Becklake M, Blanc P, Henneberger P, Kreiss K, Mapp C, et al. American Thoracic Society statement: Occupational contribution to the burden of airway disease. Am J Respir Cit Care Med. 2003;167:787-97.
41. Blanc P, Toren K. Occupation in chronic obstructive pulmonary disease and chronic bronchitis: an update. Int J Tuberc Lung Dis. 2007;11(3):251-7.
42. Lamprecht B, Schirnhofer L, Kaiser B, Studnicka M, Buist A. Farming and the prevalence of non-reversible airways

obstruction: results from a population-based study. Am J Ind Med. 2007;50(6):421-6.
43. Eduard W, Pearce N, Douwes J. Chronic bronchitis, COPD, and lung function in farmers: the role of biological agents. Chest. 2009;136(3):716-25.
44. Ulvestad B, Bakke B, Eduard W, Kongerud J, Lund MB. Cumulative exposure to dust causes accelerated decline in lung function in tunnel workers. Occup Environ Med. 2001;58(10): 663-9.
45. Bergdahl I, Toren K, Eriksson K, Hedlund U, Nilsson T, Flodin R, et al. Increased mortality in COPD among construction workers exposed to inorganic dust. Eur Respir J. 2004;23(3):402-6.
46. Rushton L. Chronic obstructive pulmonary disease and occupational exposure to silica. Rev Environ Health. 2007;22(4): 255-72.
47. Birath G, Caro J, Malmberg R, Simonsson BG. Airways obstruction in pulmonary tuberculosis. Scand J Respir Dis. 1966;47(1):27-36.
48. Lancaster J, Tomashefski J. Tuberculosis: a cause of emphysema. Am Rev Respir Dis. 1963;87:435-57.
49. Snider G, Doctor L, Demas T, Shaw AR. Obstructive airway disease in patients with treated pulmonary tuberculosis. Am Rev Respir Dis. 1971;103(5):625-40.
50. Plit M, Anderson R, Van Rensburg C, Page-Shipp L, Blott JA, Fresen JL, et al. Influence of antimicrobial chemotherapy on spirometric parameters and pro-inflammatory indices in severe pulmonary tuberculosis. Eur Respir J. 1998;12(2):351-6.
51. Willcox P, Ferguson A. Chronic obstructive airways disease following treated pulmonary tuberculosis. Respir Med. 1989;83(3):195-8.
52. Ehrlich R, White N, Norman R, Laubscher R, Steyn K, Lombard C, et al. Predictors of chronic bronchitis in South African adults. Int J Tuberc Lung Dis. 2004;8(3):369-76.
53. Caballero A, Torres-Duque C, Jaramillo C, Bolívar F, Sanabria F, Osorio P, et al. Prevalence of COPD in five Colombian cities situated at low, medium, and high altitude (PREPOCOL study). Chest. 2008;133(2):343-9.
54. World Health Organisation. *www.who.int.org/healthtopics/tuberculosis*. [Accessed March, 2016].
55. Salvi S, Barnes P. Chronic obstructive pulmonary disease in non-smokers. Lancet. 2009;374:733-43.
56. Silva G, Sherrill D, Guerra S, Barbee R. Asthma as a risk factor for COPD in a longitudinal study. Chest. 2004;126(1):59-65.
57. Barnes PJ. Against the Dutch hypothesis: asthma and chronic obstructive pulmonary disease are distinct diseases. Am J Respir Crit Care Med. 2006;174(3):240-3.
58. Ulrik C, Lange P. Decline of lung function in adults with bronchial asthma. Am J Respir Crit Care Med. 1994;150(3):629-34.
59. Lange P, Parner J, Vestbo J, Schnohr P, Jensen G. A 15-year follow-up study of ventilatory function in adults with asthma. N Engl J Med. 1998;339(17):1194-200.
60. Hahn D. Evaluation and management of acute bronchitis. In: Hueston WJ (Ed). 20 common problems in respiratory disorders. New York: McGraw-Hill; 2002. pp. 141-53.
61. Sandford A, Weir T, Pare P. Genetic risk factors for chronic obstructive pulmonary disease. Eur Respir J. 1997;10(6): 1380-91.
62. Rodriguez-Revenga L, Iranzo P, Badenas C, Puig S, Carrio A, Mila M. A novel elastin gene mutation resulting in an auto-somal dominant form of cutis laxa. Arch Dermatol. 2004;140:1135-9.
63. Patel B, Loo W, Tasker A, Screaton N, Burrows N, Silverman E, et al. Smoking related COPD and facial wrinkling: is there a common susceptibility? Thorax. 2006;61:568-671.
64. MacNee W. Accelerated lung aging: a novel pathogenic mechanism of chronic obstructive pulmonary disease (COPD). Biochem Soc Trans. 2009;37(Pt 4):819-23.
65. Karrasch S, Holz O, Jörres RA. Aging and induced senescence as factors in the pathogenesis of lung emphysema. Resp Med. 2008;102: 1215-30.

Pathophysiology of Chronic Obstructive Pulmonary Disease

Bill Brashier, Baishakhi Ghosh, Sundeep Salvi

INTRODUCTION

Chronic obstructive pulmonary disease (COPD) is a disease syndrome characterized and defined by a single physiological parameter, limitation of expiratory airflow, which is accompanied by loss of lung elastic recoil, fibrosis, edema of the airways, intraluminal accumulation of secretions and bronchial smooth muscle contraction. Most often, these changes are slowly progressive over years. According to the current global initiative of obstructive lung disease (GOLD), COPD is defined as a "disease characterized by chronic airflow limitation and a range of pathological changes in the lungs, some significant extrapulmonary effects and important comorbidities which may contribute to severity of disease in individual patient",[1] and most interestingly with our improved understanding of pathogenic mechanisms, COPD now considered to be largely preventable, and to a certain extent treatable. All these changes in COPD are caused by a cascade of multiple complex inflammatory mechanisms occurring in the lung in response to chronic exposure to air pollutants, infections and various other risk factors.

The first evidence of COPD dates back to 1679 where COPD (defined as emphysema at that time) was first described as voluminous lung or turgid lung occurring as result of trumpet blowing.[2] In 1814, Badham described this disease as associated with chronic cough and mucus hypersecretion and called this disease "chronic bronchitis".[3] With the discovery of the stethoscope Laënnec gave a more vivid description of this disease as air entrapment in the lungs, which was caused not only by smoking, but also occurred in nonsmokers, especially those with familial predisposition, and suggested that this disease was very commonly prevalent in the general population.[2] Most of the earlier understanding of COPD was based on physiological and postmortem gross pathological observations. However, very little was known about the cellular and molecular changes of the disease, hence there was no optimal treatment available.

The first stride in our understanding of pathogenesis came in 1964 when Gross et al first demonstrated the protease-antiprotease animal model for emphysema. He suggested that emphysema was a disease caused by overproduction of proteases enzyme in the lung parenchyma accompanied by reduced antiprotease activity that caused alveolar wall destruction and development of emphysema.[4] Thereafter, over the next 50 years, understanding of the pathogenesis of COPD has advanced significantly, and new concepts still continue to emerge. Today it is clear that neutrophils, macrophages and T-lymphocytes along with various inflammatory mediators and proteases are the primary culprits in the pathogenesis of COPD. New concepts of protease/antiprotease imbalance, steroid tolerance, amplified oxidative stress, autoimmune character of COPD, disease of accelerated aging of the lung and more recently systemic inflammation have emerged, which are instrumental in altering the management in COPD patients and have given novel insights for new drug discoveries for this chronic disease.

The pathology of COPD is characterized by certain morphological and cellular changes occurring in the airways and lung parenchyma due to ongoing chronic inflammatory processes. Pathological changes such as subepithelial infiltration of mononuclear cells (macrophages, CD8+ T-lymphocytes), mucous gland hypertrophy and inflammation, subepithelial infiltration of eosinophils (during exacerbations of COPD), subepithelial infiltration of neutrophils, goblet cell hyperplasia, smooth muscle hypertrophy, wall fibrosis and destruction of the alveolar attachments, tend to occur in both proximal and peripheral airways of the lungs. Further, the inflammation of COPD also causes lung parenchymal changes such as, destruction and enlargement restricted to the respiratory bronchiole and the central portion of the acinus (centriacinar emphysema), destruction and enlargement uniformly involving the whole acinus (panacinar emphysema) and infiltration of CD8+ T-lymphocytes.

The basic pathophysiologic consequences of COPD inflammation consists of increased resistance to airflow, loss of elastic recoil and decreased expiratory flow rate. The alveolar walls frequently break because of the increased resistance of air flows and increased apoptosis of the alveolar epithelial cells. Consequently, more effort is required for the air to be exhaled, which happens mostly due to narrowed airway and pressure changes in the thorax. These physiological changes cause earlier closure of small airways resulting in more air trapped in the lungs. Further, hyperinflated lungs flatten the curvature of the diaphragm and enlarge the rib cage. The altered configuration of the chest cavity places the respiratory muscles, including the diaphragm, at a mechanical disadvantage and impairs their force-generating capacity. This results in increase the metabolic work of breathing, and the sensation of dyspnea heightens. All these changes occur due to inflammatory cells and mediators which are increased in COPD.

ROLE OF NEUTROPHILS IN CHRONIC OBSTRUCTIVE PULMONARY DISEASE

The neutrophil has been highly acclaimed as a key effector cell in the pathogenesis of COPD, to a degree that COPD has been characterized as neutrophil mediated disease. The presence of neutrophils has been inversely correlated with prebronchodilator and postbronchodilator forced expiratory volume in 1 second (FEV_1), with the strongest correlation in patients without bronchodilator reversibility.[5,6] Moreover, neutrophilic inflammation has been primarily implicated in steroid nonresponsiveness in COPD.[7,8] The respiratory symptoms in neutrophil directly correlate with neutrophils in COPD **(Fig. 1)**.

Normally there is sequestration of the neutrophils from the pulmonary vasculature into the lungs due to size dynamic interaction of pulmonary capillaries[9,10] and neutrophils which provides, along with resident macrophages, an enormous defense mechanism against invading microbes and environmental insults. However, in COPD there is a quantitative increase in lung neutrophils the reason for which is still elusive **(Figs 2A and B)**. However, in vitro experiment have shown that cigarette smoke has an ability to alter the kinetics of cytoskeletal-proteins such as filamentous actin (F-actin) which can impede contractile apparatus of neutrophils making them less plastic to negotiate a travel in very narrow pulmonary capillaries.[11-13] Further, in COPD there is also increased expression of adhesion molecules such as intercellular adhesion molecule-1 (ICAM-1) and endothelial adhesion molecules (E-selectin) in both the endothelium as well as neutrophils cell surface which can enhance neutrophil stickiness to the capillary endothelium and assist their migration into the lungs.[14-21] Also, inflammatory cells including neutrophils release various cytokines and chemoattractants such as interlukin-8 (IL-8),[22] leukotriene B4 (LTB4),[23] matrix metaloproteinase (MMP)-9[24] and neutrophil elastase, which provide a suitable milieu for the relentless migration of neutrophils and other inflammatory cells into the lungs even after the risk factors or triggers are removed **(Fig. 3)**.

Once the activated neutrophils enter the lung parenchyma, they start releasing battery of serine proteinase such as

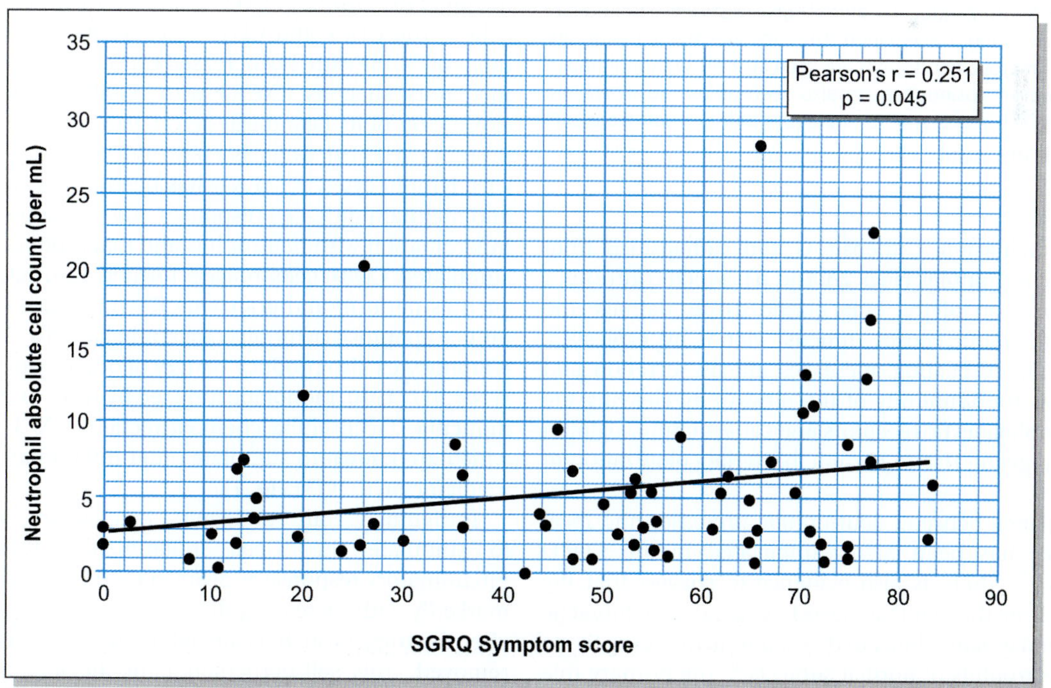

Fig. 1 Correlation association of neutrophil and chronic obstructive pulmonary disease symptoms. As symptoms increase neutrophils also increase

Source: Data derived from reference no. 89 smoking and nonsmoking COPD. This is unpublished of Chest Research Foundation

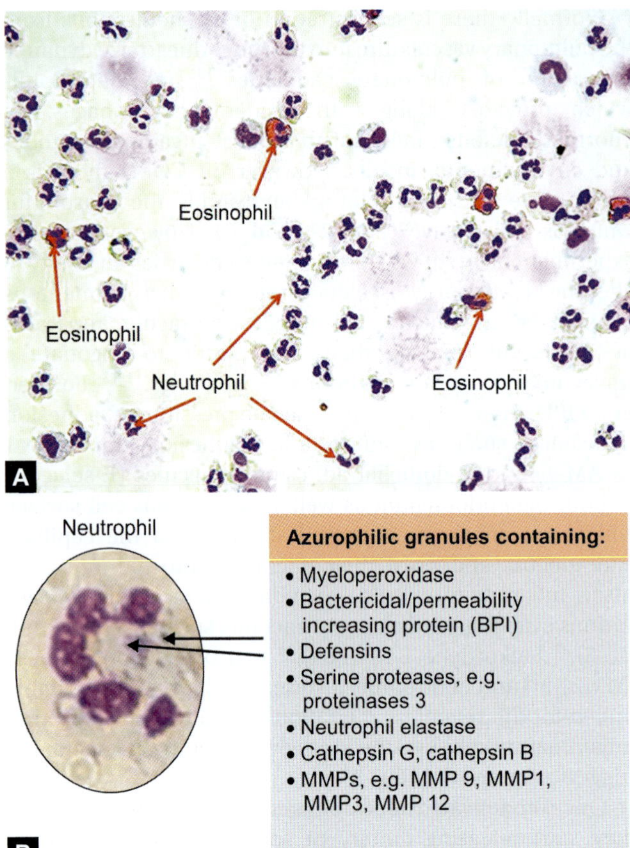

Figs 2A and B Sputum induction slide chronic obstructive pulmonary disease patient during exacerbation. The slide was stained with diff-quick stain. Numerous neutrophils are seen (as cells with multilobed nucleus). However, eosinophils are also seen as red eosin stained bilobed nuclear cell in exacerbation state (Unpublished data from CRF)

Abbreviation: MMPs, matrix metaloproteinases

elastase, proteinase-3, cathepsin-G and cathepsin-B from the azurophilic granules **(Figs 2A and B)**, which contributes to the destruction of the lung elastic tissue, damage the airway epithelium, causes mucus gland hyperplasia,[25] reduce the ciliary beating, increases mucus secretion and compromises the immunity of the airways by cleaving the C3Bi opsonophagocytic receptors and causes immunoglobin degradation, giving rise to chronic bacterial colonization of the airways.[26]

An imbalance between neutrophilic proteases and local antiproteases has been highly implicated in the COPD pathogenesis.[27] There is also evidence to suggest that the neutrophils from the COPD subjects have greater chemotactic responses and greater ability to digest the surrounding tissue than the neutrophils of normal subjects.[28] The primary role of these proteolytic enzymes is to generate a pathway for the movement of leukocytes into the tissue and in this process they unsparingly degenerate the elastic connective tissue of the lung parenchyma leading to emphysema. Restoring balance between proteases and antiproteases in the lungs of COPD seem to have promising prospects for future therapy in COPD management.[26]

ROLE OF T-LYMPHOCYTES IN CHRONIC OBSTRUCTIVE PULMONARY DISEASE

The first evidence of the role of T-lymphocytes in the pathogenesis COPD was demonstrated in 1995, wherein the correlation between the number of T-lymphocytes in the lung and extent of emphysema was first revealed. It was also realized that the inflammation of COPD was not only limited to the innate immune mechanisms but also involved adaptive immunity with the infiltration of CD8+ and CD4+ cells not only in the alveolar wall and small airways but also in the adventitia of pulmonary vasculature, indicating the importance of these cells in the development of pulmonary hypertension related to COPD. Subsequent studies have further shown that although both the CD4+ and CD8+ cells are increased in the airways and the lung parenchyma of the patients with COPD, it is the CD8+ cells which are more predominant and more likely involved in pathophysiology of COPD.[29,30]

The mucosal layers of the airways contains local lymphoid follicles that consists of a core B lymphocytes surrounded by T-cells and it has been suggested that the antigens are presented to the T-cells in these lymphoid nodes resulting in clonal expansion of CD4+ cells and to larger extent CD8+ cells.[31] The CD8+ and CD4+ cells are fully activated in the lungs of COPD with the increased expression of inflammatory mediators such as CXCR3 with parallel strong epithelial expression of its ligand interferon gamma (IFN-γ) inducible protein 10 (IP-10), which is a powerful chemoattractant of the CD8 lymphocytes.[32,33] IFN-γ has been implicated in driving and maintaining T-cell responses and promotes an immune inflammation with neutrophils and macrophages. The IFN-γ stimulated CD8+ cells release further destructive enzymes such as perforin and granzyme B which have the ability to induce apoptosis of the alveolar epithelial cells.[34-36] The CD8+ lymphocytes also produce battery of other cytokines such as IFN-γ, IL2, IP10, monokine induced by IFN-γ (CXCL9), IFN-γ inducible T-cell alpha chemoattractant (CXCL11) and IL4, which are known to stimulate other inflammatory cells and mediators in COPD **(Fig. 4)**.

Intriguingly, an antigenic mechanism is required to stimulate the T-cell inflammatory response. This inflammatory response appears in mild COPD and increases markedly with increasing disease severity and persists even after the triggers such as air-pollution or tobacco smoke are removed. This self-perpetuation of the adaptive immune system confers further understanding as it may explain the persistence of inflammation in the lungs of COPD patient. It is possible that the inflammatory and oxidative stress injury

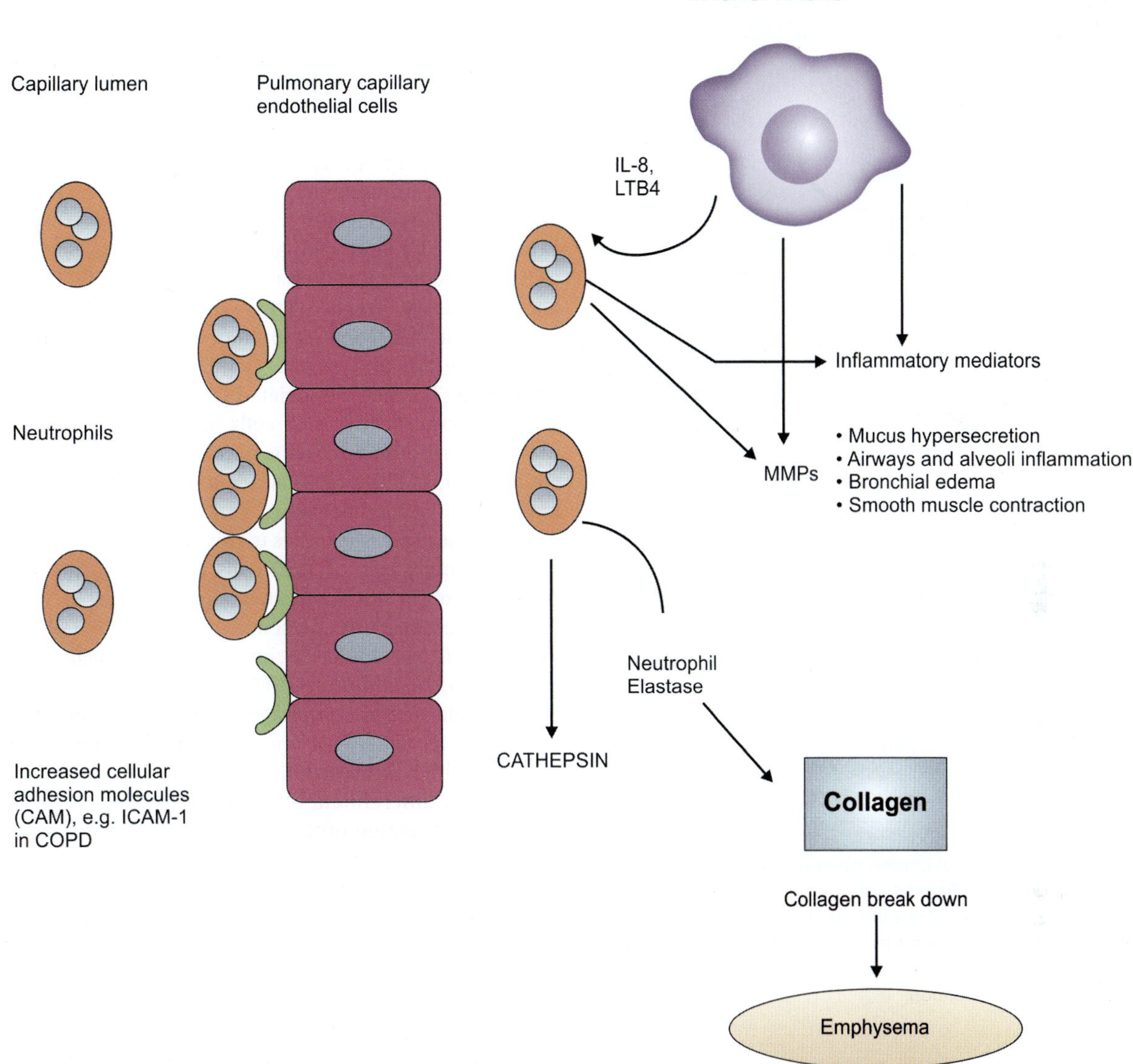

Fig. 3 Mechanisms of neutrophils migration from the pulmonary capillaries into the lungs. These mechanisms are amplified in chronic obstructive pulmonary disease (COPD)
Abbreviations: IL, interleukin; MMPs, matrix metalloproteinase; LTB, lymphotoxin beta

can create endogenous autoantigens in the lungs augmenting continued CD4/CD8 response in the lungs. There are also antigens in the tobacco smoke which may also induce the response.

Another possibility is that this chronic immune response is actuated, or at least continued, by chronic infectious processes of the respiratory tract often seen in the patients with severe disease, in which there is increased colonization of the lower airways. These infections could either co-stimulate or mimic as an antigen and provide a persisting antigenic stimulus that maintain the inflammatory processes.[25,37-39] The association between recurrent childhood viral infections and the development of COPD in adult life, indicate that viruses and bacteria recruit lymphocytes into the lungs as a part of the adaptive immunity.

Interestingly, in the chronic cigarette smokers who do not develop COPD the autoantigens generated by the oxidative stress and toxins may also induce the lymphocytic inflammation. But, this induction is controlled by subset of another CD4+ cells, collectively known as regulatory T-cells, which are capable of suppressing autoreactive lymphocytes through secretion of inhibitory mediators such as IL10

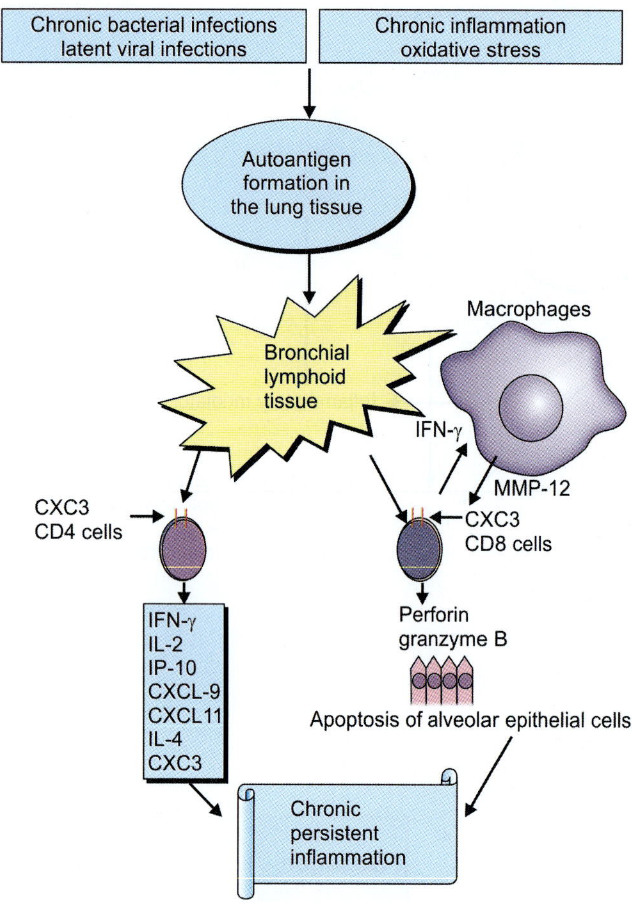

Fig. 4 Role of lymphocytes in chronic obstructive pulmonary disease inflammation—chronic inflammation and oxidative stress can modulate protein structures of the lung tissues to form autoantigens which can generate an autoimmune phenomenon attracting both CD4 and CD8 type lymphocytes. Lymphocytes can apoptosis and persistence of lung inflammation

or direct cell to cell contact.[40] In COPD there is a greater increase in CD8+ cells than the T regulatory cells and there is also evidence that the number of these cells may be reduced, thereby further enhancing the autoimmune processes.

Furthermore, inflammatory ligands of CXCR3 which have been shown to be increased in the lymphocytes of COPD lungs have also shown to increase the expression of MMP12 in the alveolar macrophages, thereby providing a direct link between T-cells and alveolar destruction.[41]

The mounting evidence implicating T-cells as important components of COPD inflammation is overwhelming. The understanding that the COPD inflammation is most likely driven by antigen has tremendous therapeutic interest. Currently, there is search of molecules that could inhibit receptors such as CXCR3 and block the trafficking of helper T1 (Th1) and cytotoxic T1 (Tc1) cells into the lungs.

HELPER T17 CELLS

Helper T17 and related cytokines such as IL17A, IL17F and IL22 and IL23 has been linked to various autoimmune diseases such as rheumatoid arthritis and psoriasis. The presence of Th17 cells in the inflammatory pool of COPD has also been implicated in association with autoimmune antielastin immunological response.[42,43] The Th-17 cells are known to correlate inversely with FEV1/forced vital capacity (FVC) and can also predict disease severity in COPD patients.[44] An imbalance of circulating Th17 cells and regulatory T-cells (Tregs) has shown to be linked with the deterioration of pulmonary function in patients with moderate and severe COPD.[45] Muscarinic receptor stimulation has been associated with pro-Th17 cytokine (IL-17) production[46] and Th17 cells have also been associated with autocrine acetylcholine production,[47] therefore there could be possibility of muscarinic receptor antagonists to have modulating effects in Th-17 related inflammation, however there are no studies in this context.

The primary role of Th17 cells is to rid-off bacteria and fungi which are not adequately eliminated by Th1 and Th2 cells.[48] Therefore the presence of microbial colonization in COPD lungs could be an important trigger for Th17 production. In addition, Th17 cells are known to regulate neutrophilic and macrophage inflammation in the lungs. Further, IL1β, IL23, IL6, and transforming growth factor-β (TGF-β) which are cardinal to COPD inflammation have potential to differentiate lymphocytes to Th17 cells.[49,50] The retinoic acid-related orphan receptor (ROR)-γt is one of the key transcription factors for the generation of Th17 cells.[51] ROR gene expression is induced by DNA damage caused by cigarette smoke and has been implicated in formation of emphysema and enhanced apoptosis **(Figs 5A and B)**.[52]

The bronchial epithelium and bronchial submucosa of COPD patients have shown to harbor higher numbers of Th17 cells compared to healthy control subjects **(Fig. 5)**.[53] FTh17 cells secrete unique set of cytokines including IL17, IL22 and IL23 which have important contribution in pathogenesis of COPD. IL17 family comprises of 6 members ranging from IL17A to IL17F[54] which function through five different receptors ranging from IL-17RA to IL17RE[55] respectively. IL17A and IL17F are the key IL17s in COPD inflammation.[56] IL17A has shown to be increased in the bronchial submucosa and subepithelium of COPD patients.[42,57] IL17 has been proposed to cause a crosstalk between the adaptive (TH17) and innate immune systems.[58] This begins with IL17 inducting pathogen clearance through IL17 receptors on epithelial cells, macrophages and dendritic cells to produce antimicrobial peptides including β-defensins, and chemokines, including tumor necrosis factor (TNF)-α, IL1b, IL6, granulocyte-macrophage colony-stimulating factor (GM-CSF), granulocyte colony-stimulating factor and IL8.[59] These chemokinesis are known to recruit neutrophils and macrophages at site of injury creating Th17 and cellular

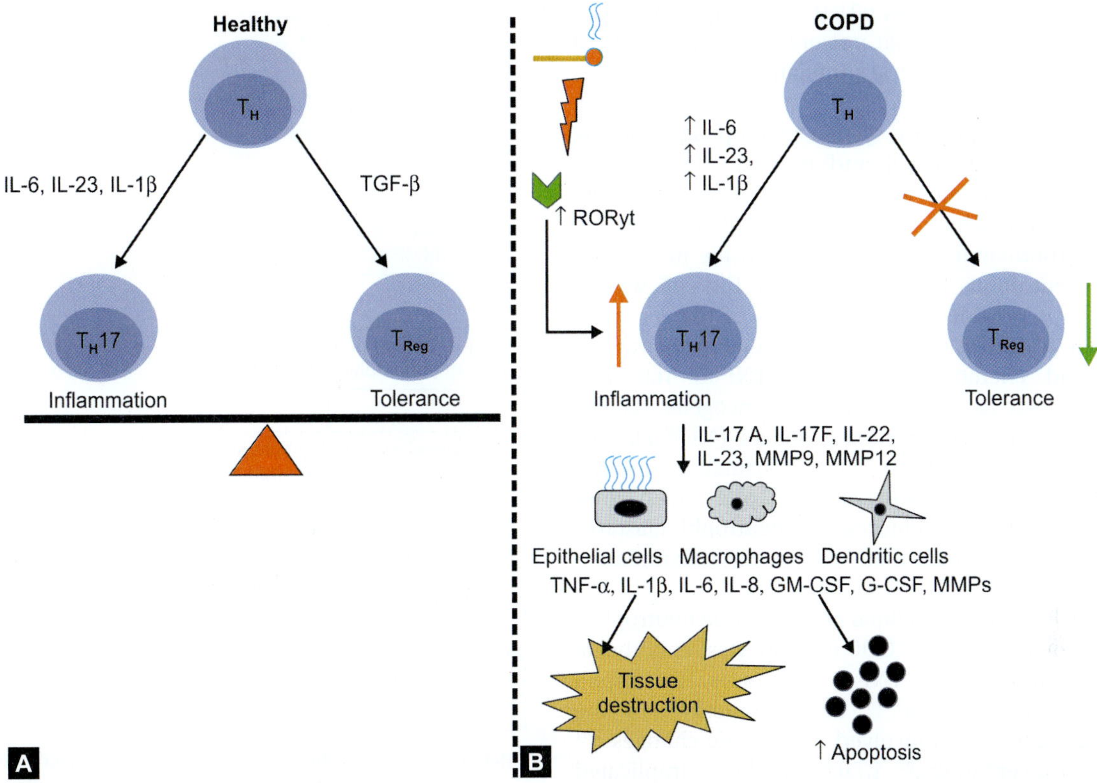

Figs 5A and B (A) Healthy subjects there is balance between Th17 and Treg cells. (B) In chronic obstructive pulmonary disease the environmental insults and inflammatory mediators skew the balance towards Th17 cell, which then secrete battery of cytokines [interleukin (IL)17A, IL17F, IL22, IL23 and matrix metalloproteinase (MMPs)] which can induce epithelial cells, macrophages and dendritic cells to release inflammatory mediators, which can also enhance cell apoptosis

Abbreviations: GM-CGF, granulocyte-macrophage colony-stimulating factor; G-CGF, gene-centric composite genomic factor

inflammation axis in COPD. Intriguingly, the Th17 cell-neutrophil axis demonstrates steroid resistance.[60] IL17 has also been involved in production of mucin which is important in bronchitis and regulates MMPs such as MMP9 and MMP12 involved in emphysema formation pathogenesis.[29]

Interlukin-17 is also known to damage structural cells such as epithelial cells, fibroblasts, and smooth muscle cells. Animal model studies have linked formation of emphysema with Th1 and Th17 cells, and IL17A in the development of elastase-induced pulmonary inflammation and emphysema.[61] Th17/Tc17 infiltration in lungs has also shown to play critical role in sustaining perpetuality in lung inflammation.[62] The patients with symptoms of chronic bronchitis, mucus production and frequent exacerbations have been proposed to be predominantly IL17 T-cell-mediated neutrophil phenotype.[63] IL6, IL8, granulocyte colony-stimulating factor, and monocyte chemotactic protein-1 which are the key mediators in COPD inflammation are IL17 gene dependent cytokines.[64]

Currently there is no evidence to show that Th17 cells modulation or treatment with anti-IL17 antibodies can cause any salutary benefits in COPD patients. The experience from rheumatoid arthritis and bronchiolitis obliterans clinical trials and animal model studies indicates that there could be a potential role of anti-IL17 antibody in COPD management in future.[65] However, mesenchymal stem cells have shown to inhibit Th17 and reduce tissue injury, and enhance tissue repair. Mesenchymal cells have been shown to reduce production of pro-TH17 cytokines such IL17, IL22, IFN-γ, TNF-α, and oncostatin M (OSM), and enhance the production of IL10 by the differentiating Th17, cells and induce regulatory transcription factors such as fork head box P3 protein (FOXP3) which are primarily involved in the development and function of regulatory T-cells.[66] Indeed, there could be potential role of stem cells in management of COPD in future.

MACROPHAGES

Prior understanding of COPD pathogenesis has largely been focused on potential role of neutrophils, however, it is now been realized that macrophages are perhaps the main culprits.[67] In COPD macrophage may increase by almost 20 times. The animal model studies have shown that the lung macrophages have potential to produce higher levels of antiapoptotic proteins such as p21 (CIP1/WAF1) and B cell lymphoma leukemia-x (L) that not only prolong the life of macrophages, but also causes accumulation of macrophages in COPD lung.[68]

In the human respiratory system macrophage line the whole of airway, the alveoli and even the interstitium, therefore they formulate a very strong innate immune system defense line which provides the first line protection from all environmental insults imposed on the lungs even before the neutrophils arrive at the site. The cell wall of macrophages is provided with wide array of CD receptors which when triggered can induce production of various cytokines and chemokines such as TNF-α, IL6, IL5, chemokines, such as growth-regulated oncogene (GRO)-alpha, monocyte chemoattractant protein-1 (MCP-1), MIG (IP10), lymphotoxin beta (LTB)-4 and IL8, oxidation products such as 8-isoprostane, hormones such as leptin and enzymes such as MMPs, serine proteinases, and neutrophil elastases and many more[69-75] which then triggers the inflammatory cascade of COPD.

Interlukin-8 can induce cellular chemotaxis in neutrophils and activate macrophages,[76] CD8 lymphocytes, endothelial cells[77] and mast cells. TNF-α enhances neutrophil chemotaxis and migration[78,79] and apoptosis[80] in the macrophages, and is also involved in cachexic changes[73,81] and COPD exacerbations.[82] LTB4 has been implicated as the major chemoattractant responsible for neutrophil and CD8 cell recruitment and activation in COPD.[70,83] IL6 is involved in causing symptoms of breathlessness, skeletal muscle weakness, insulin resistance, pulmonary hypertension, cardiovascular morbidity and most significantly exacerbations.[84,85] Further, in order to assist the inflammatory cell mobility in the nonfluidic environment of the lungs macrophage also secrete series of proteinases, particularly MMPs **(Fig. 6)**, and series of elastinolytic cysteine proteinases such as cathepsin-K, -L and -S which have potential elastolytic properties. MMPs degrade the connective tissue that has an important role in tissue development and remodeling of the damaged tissue. The MMP2 and MMP9 have very strong gelatin digesting and elastolytic properties respectively, while MMP12 is implicated in earlier stages of COPD.[67,86] Further the neutrophil elastase released by short lived neutrophil is also stored in the macrophages. There is a reasonable possibility that these inflammatory mechanisms are permanently switched on in COPD even in the absence of environmental trigger.

Second and one of the prime functions of COPD is phagocytosis which is a process of recognition and removal of foreign particles or microbes from the host and efferocytosis which is a process of engulfment of cellular debris of the local apoptotic bodies **(Fig. 7A)**. Phagocytosis process begin with coating of the foreign material with blood derived proteins such as complements (C3b or C3bi or C4b) or immunoglobulins (IgG or IgA), that are recognized by specific complement receptors (CRs such as CR1 or CR3), or immunoglobulin

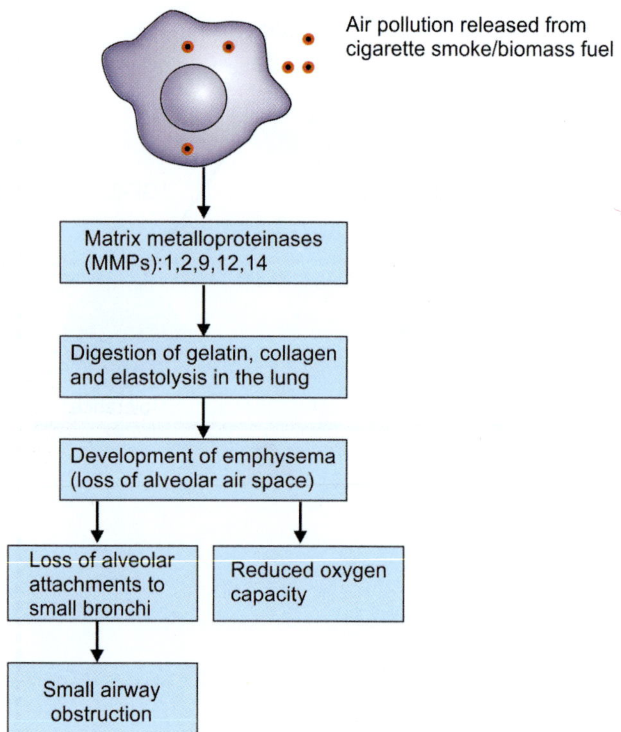

Fig. 6 Role of macrophages in tissue destruction seen in apoptosis through matrix metalloproteinase

receptors [such as FcγRI (CD64) or FcγRII (CD32) or FcγRIII (CD16)].[87,88] The process of coating the foreign material or microbe is called opsonization, and the particle is ready for the process of engulfment. The engulfment process initiates with cytoskeletal rearrangements of the macrophage leading to formation of phagolysosome (fusion of phagosome and lysosome) where the invading organisms are destroyed by the activity of proteolytic enzymes. Intriguingly, airways are the serum lacking regions; where nonopsonin phagocytosis occurs by recognition of invading particles by scavenger receptors (SRs) such as mannose receptors, macrophage receptor with collagenous structure (MARCO) and toll-like receptors (TLR).[87-89]

The TLRs expressed by macrophages are TLR2 and TLR4. The TLR2 receptor has the ability to bind to Gram-positive bacteria and its components (such as lipoteichoic acid, lipopeptides and peptidoglycan)[90] and mycobacterium,[91] whereas, TLR4 binds to lipopolysaccharide, a component of Gram-negative bacteria.[92] The expression of TLR2 is known to be reduced among COPD patients and smokers.[93] The TLR2 deficiency in the COPD pulmonary macrophage could also provide a link between recurrent exacerbations and tuberculosis amongst the COPD patients. However, there is still no data in this context. Further, there is also an evidence that there is a decline in lung function with the decrease in TLR4 expression in lung tissues among mice.[94] There is

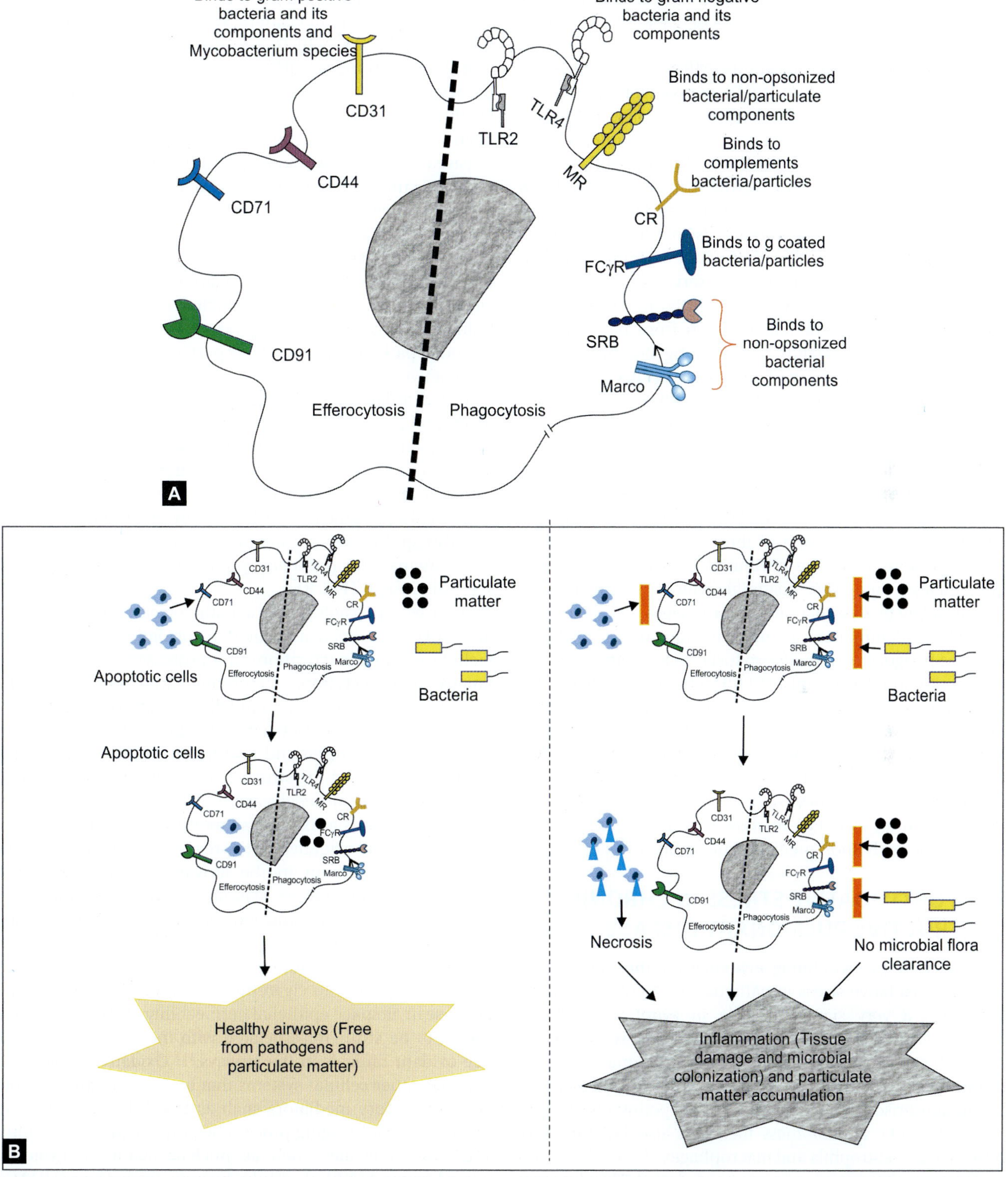

Figs 7A and B (A) The complex network of receptors involved in the phagocytosis and efferocytosis in macrophages. (B) Comparison of phagocytosis and efferocytosis of healthy and chronic obstructive pulmonary disease (COPD)—in healthy bacteria, remnant of dead cells and tissues are effectively phagocytized by resident macrophages to keep the lungs clean. In COPD compromised phagocytosis can cause bacterial colonization and perpetual presence of apoptotic and necrotic material contributing to perpetual inflammation

Source: Donnelly LE, Barnes PJ. Defective phagocytosis in airways disease. Chest. 2012;141(4):1055-62.

still lack of evidence on variability of expressions of these receptors in COPD. However, TLR4 deficiency is known to promote pulmonary emphysema.[95]

The other macrophage receptors (MRs) such as scavenger receptor A (SRAII and MARCO), Scavenger receptor B (CD36), and CD163 are also known to involve in binding of the unopsonized bacteria and inhaled particles such as dust.[96,97] It has been reported that upregulation of *Haemophilus influenzae* by MARCO receptors leads to enhanced phagocytosis.[98] However, there is lack of evidence to show whether these receptors are also modulated in COPD patients. MRs are another carbohydrate binding receptors involved in antigen presentation and serve as a link between innate and adaptive immunity.[87,99] MRs are found to be reduced among alveolar macrophages from patients with COPD compared to healthy,[100] indicating that nonopsonin phagocytosis is hindered in COPD subjects **(Figs 7A and B)**.

The lung macrophages from COPD patients also demonstrate decreased efferocytosis. The COPD macrophages have impaired effrocytic mechanism which can be attributed to alteration in its surface CD proteins such as CD31, CD91, CD44 and CD71, and antigen presenting proteins such as CD80 and CD86.[101-103] However, there is no alteration in expression of these proteins. The damage to CD proteins could be attributed to oxidative stress.[104] Nevertheless, apoptotic material which is not cleared appropriately by dysfunctional macrophages can be the situ for further inflammatory cascade. Therefore, drugs which can enhance phagocytosis or efferocytosis could be an important therapeutic strategy to control COPD inflammation **(Fig. 7B)**.

Counteracting oxidative stress with N-acetylcysteine has shown to improve phagocytosis in COPD macrophages in-vitro models.[105] Procysteine, improves efferocytosis in COPD macrophages.[106] Clinical trial with azithromycin has also shown to improve efferocytosis in the COPD macrophages.[100] There is also an evidence to show that statin can improve efferocytosis with RhoA mediated mechanism.[107]

ROLE OF OXIDATIVE STRESS IN CHRONIC OBSTRUCTIVE PULMONARY DISEASE

There is now overwhelming evidence for the presence of increased oxidative stress in patients with COPD. Oxidative stress has a very significant role in every stage of the pathogenesis in COPD. Increased oxidative stress in the airspaces can initiate a number of early inflammatory events in the lungs. The free oxidant radicals in the lungs and systemic circulation arise from the sources of air pollutants such as cigarette smoke and biomass fuel, and also inflammatory cells such as neutrophils and macrophages.[108]

Amongst the complex mixture of over 4,700 chemical compounds present in the cigarette smoke, free radicals and other oxidants account for the major deleterious effects on the respiratory system. It has been estimated that cigarette smoke contains approximately 10^{15} oxygen radicals per puff, primarily of the alkyl and peroxyl types. The other important compounds present in cigarette smoke include nitrous oxide and semiquinone, which are also capable of producing reactive oxygen species (ROS) such as superoxide anion (O_2^-), peroxynitrite, alkyl peroxynitrites and hydrogen peroxides.[109] On the other hand the oxidant burden of biomass fuel has not been yet demonstrated, but, considering inhaling the smoke released from burning biomass without intervention of filter could be a much higher source of reactive oxygen compounds than cigarette smoke.

The epithelial lining fluid and mucus are the first line of defence in the lungs against inhaled oxidants by quenching the short-lived radicals in the cigarette smoke.[110] However, cigarette smoke condensate, which forms in the epithelial lining fluid, may continue to produce ROS for a considerable period in patients with COPD, as part its pathogenesis.

Reactive oxygen species are also released from activated inflammatory leukocytes such as neutrophils and macrophages, which are known to present in increased numbers in the lungs of cigarette smokers. The inflammatory mediators released by these cells permanently switch on the oxidative stress mechanisms, providing a continuous source of free oxidant radicals which not only confine to the lungs but also spill into the systemic circulation and affect other body organs with particular predilection to the heart and skeletal muscles **(Fig. 8)**.

A series of physiological and pathological changes present in COPD have been attributed to oxidative stress, which include oxidative inactivation of antiproteases and surfactants, mucus hypersecretion, membrane lipid per oxidation, alveolar epithelial injury, remodeling of extracellular matrix, and apoptosis. ROS have been shown to reduce the synthesis of elastin and collagen and also fragmenting these skeletal proteins. ROS affect the structure of matrix proteins such as hyaluronate and proteoglycans and reduce the viscosity of the extracellular matrix for easy movement of inflammatory cells. Moreover, oxidative stress reacts with the membrane phospholipids present in the airway epithelial cells and activates the arachidonic acid in the cell membranes to release prostaglandins and leukotrienes, which are potent inflammatory agents.

Injury to the epithelium may be an important early event following exposure to cigarette smoke, and is shown by an increase in airspace epithelial permeability and this has been shown to be strongly associated with increased amount of free oxidant radicals in the airways.[111] Oxidative stress also activates other cellular systems that increase the production of inflammatory mediators such as IL8, IL1 and TNF-α. It also enhances the aging process by down regulating various antiaging molecules such as nuclear factor erythroid-2-related factor 2 (NRF2), sirtuin, histone deacetylase (HDAC) and oxidative protein, and also activates processes which are implicated in cell senescence and DNA damage. Furthermore steroid resistance of COPD inflammation has been implicated to be caused by increased oxidative stress.[112] Oxidative stress

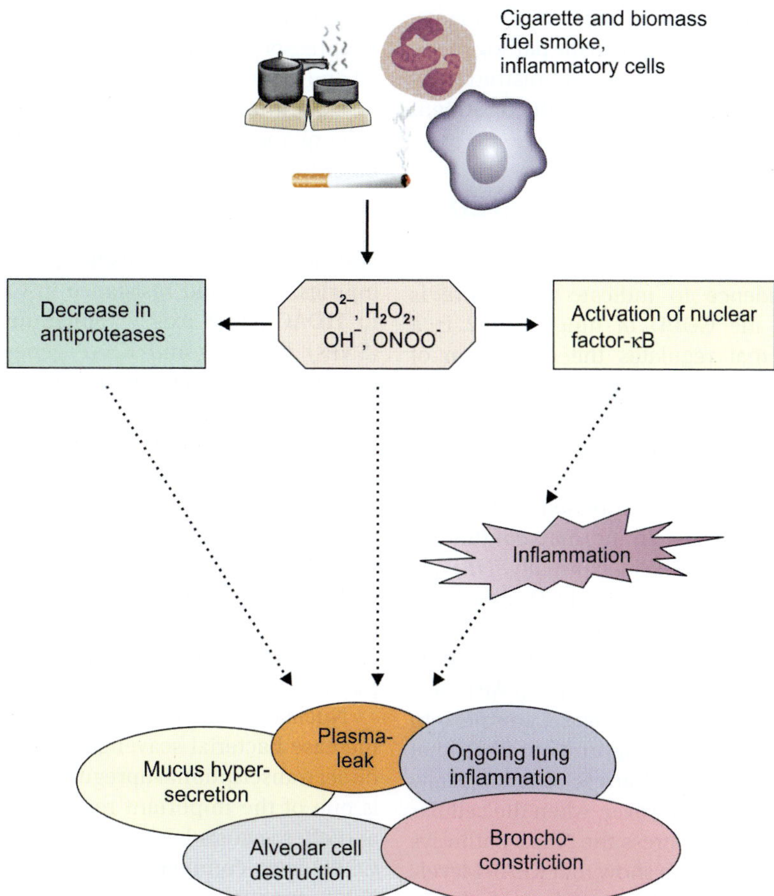

Fig. 8 Role of oxidative stress in pathogenesis of chronic obstructive pulmonary disease (COPD)—oxidant radicals from exogenous sources and from inflammatory cells such as neutrophils and macrophages can reduce the antiproteases and activate inflammatory transcription factors, and also directly damage the tissues, to cause emphysema, goblet cell hyperplasia, perpetuality of inflammation bronchoconstriction and plasma leaks to cause pathological changes of COPD. These changes also occur during normal aging process and therefore the COPD can be regarded as disease of accelerated aging of the lungs

reduces steroid responsiveness via a reduction in HDAC2 activity and expression.[113]

Airways are always exposed to various ambient pollutants, which are inhaled during respiration, that generate oxidative stress inside the airways. The airways are protected from this ongoing oxidative stress by a series of antioxidants which are found ubiquitously in the respiratory tract lining fluid throughout the respiratory tract. These antioxidants generally present in the fluid lining the airways are cysteine residues, such as mucin and glutathione, uric acid, albumin, vitamin E and vitamin C.

The reactive oxidant species enhance the secretions of mucin[114] and glutathione in the respiratory lining fluid to counteract the oxidant load, but in diseases like COPD this increase may not be sufficient to deal with excessive oxidant burden seen in this disease either due to is depletion of the antioxidants or reduced production. Therefore an improvement in the antioxidant capacity in COPD patients is an interesting therapeutic approach. Currently there is no effective antioxidant therapy which can effectively thwart the oxidative stress in the lungs of COPD patient. However, N-acetyl-cysteine (NAC), a precursor of glutathione, which is a very powerful and ubiquitously distributed antioxidant has met with varying success with more positive results in higher doses.[115]

Other interesting antioxidants such as dietary polyphenol [curcumin (diferuloylmethane), a principal component of turmeric], resveratrol (a flavonoid found in red wine), green tea (theophylline and epigallocatechin-3-gallate), ergothioneine (xanthine and peroxynitrite inhibitor), quercetin, erdosteine and carbocysteine lysine salt, spin traps such as α-phenyl-N-tert-butyl nitrone, a catalytic antioxidant (ECSOD mimetic), manganese(III) mesotetrakis (N,N'-diethyl-1,3-imidazolium-2-yl) porphyrin (AEOL 10150 and AEOL 10113), and a superoxide dismutase mimetic M40419 have also been reported to inhibit cigarette smoke-induced inflammatory responses in vivo.[112] Since a variety of oxidants, free radicals and aldehydes are implicated in the pathogenesis of COPD, it is possible that therapeutic administration of multiple antioxidants will likely be effective in the treatment of COPD.

NUCLEAR FACTOR ERYTHROID-2-RELATED FACTOR 2 IN COPD

There is burgeoning evidence to indicate that there is a depletion of NRF2 in the COPD of lungs. NRF2 is a key transcription factor that regulates the expression of antioxidant response element (ARE)-regulated antioxidant and cytoprotective genes.[116] NRF2 constitutes 605 amino acids which are spread into 6 domains called neutrophilic eccrine hidradenitis (NEH) (1-6).[117,118]

In the lungs, NRF2 is primarily expressed in alveolar macrophages and epithelial cells. In normal conditions, NRF2 is maintained at low basal levels. Normally, NRF2 is bound to a cytosolic inhibitor Kelch-like ECH-associated protein 1 (KEAP1) at its NEH2 regulatory domain.[119] KEAP1 ensures cytoplasmic sequestration of NRF2 and prevents its nuclear migration for functional activity. KEAP1 also initiates cullin-3 (CUL3) E3 ubiquitin ligase complex to initiate ubiquitination of NRF2 resulting in its proteasomal degradation, thus, keeping the NRF2 levels physiologically low in appropriate conditions.[116] However, when the cellular environment undergoes oxidative stress the NRF2 pathways get activated. There is an evidence to show that KEAP1 levels in COPD are increased,[120] indicating its possible reduction in NRF2 mechanism associated with disease. KEAP1 constitutes highly reactive sulfhydryl groups in its 27 cysteine residues. These sulfhydryl sites react with oxidant radicals inducing conformational changes in KEAP1, which then dissociate KEAP1 from NRF2. Hence, NRF2 becomes free for nuclear translocation. Further oxidation of cysteine residues and serine 40 phosphorylation of NRF2 molecule induced by oxidant-induced kinases can also trigger NRF2 nuclear translocation.

There is also evidence that activated phosphatidylinositol 3-kinase (PI3-kinase) in COPD, dysregulates KEAP1 function, depolymerizes and disrupts the cellular actin cytoskeleton which results in nuclear accumulation of NRF2.[121] In the nucleus NRF2 forms heterodimers with small MAF proteins, c-JUN, activating transcription factor-4, c-FOS and FRA-1 (FOS-related antigen-1). It also binds to cis-element of ARE in target gene promoters to enhance expression of ARE-dependent genes such as genes for glutathione S-transferases, nicotinamide adenine dinucleotide phosphate (NADPH), quinine oxidoreductase 1 (NQO1), heme oxygenase-1 (HO1) and UDP-glucuronosyltransferase 1A6. Also, NRF2 autoregulates its function by also regulating KEAP1 gene expression. Studies have also shown that NRF2 can exert its protective effect by upregulating transcriptional activation of antiproteinase as well.[122] NRF2 has also shown to induce peroxisome proliferator-activated receptor (gamma) which is a repressor of inflammatory transcription factor such as NF-kB and activator protein-1 (AP-1)[123] **(Figs 9A and B)**.

Experimental studies have shown that cigarette smoke can enhance expression and production of NRF2.[117] On the other hand, depletion of NRF2 can enhance susceptibility to develop emphysema, propagates inflammation, enhances neutrophil elastase activity, enhances oxidative stress and also increases the sensitivity to oxidative stress related injuries.[117] Steroid resistance in COPD has been attributed to HDAC-NRF2 axis.[124] Single-nucleotide polymorphisms (SNPs) in NRF2 and KEAP genes have been involved in modulation of lung volumes in population based studies.[125] The haplotype rs2001350T/rs6726395A/rs1962142A/rs2364722A/rs6721961T of NRF gene has been shown to be associated with lower annual decline in FEV_1. SNPs in the promoter region of human NRF2 have been associated with enhanced risk of acute lung injuries. The evidence indicates that there are marked decline NRF2-dependent antioxidants and NRF2 proteins in lungs of COPD patients.[126] Recently, role of azithromycin as anti-neutrophilic, anti-inflammatory agent has been attributed to induction of sestrin2 via NRF2 pathways.[127]

Nuclear factor erythroid-2-related factor 2 is known to increase bacterial scavenging capability of macrophages by direct transcriptional upregulation of MARCO receptor which is one of the important receptors involved in phagocytosis and efferocytosis in the lungs.[128] The association of NRF2 in COPD is so compelling that molecules which can enhance NRF2 functions such as curcumin, epicatechin, Ginkgo Biloba and sulforaphane could emerge as potential target for future COPD management.[117]

APOPTOSIS

Enhanced programmed cell death (apoptosis) of structural tissues is cardinal to various chronic inflammatory diseases. In COPD, apoptosis is independent of inflammation and has implicated the pathogenesis of emphysema.[129] In COPD endothelial cells, epithelial cells, interstitial tissue and inflammatory cells such as neutrophils and lymphocytes have shown to demonstrate enhanced apoptosis.[130] Usually apoptosis is compensated with cellular proliferation to replace the dying cells. However, evidence indicates that there is a presence of pertinent imbalance between cell death and cell proliferation as hallmark in COPD development.

Apoptosis is tightly regulated phenomenon of cell death, having a modulation potential. Normally, apoptosis is a part of cell regulation phenomenon, and cell apoptosis is usually accompanied by cell replenishment to maintain organ integrity and organ functionality. Apoptosis occurs primarily through five distinct, however, interlinked pathways.[131] In ligand death-receptor pathway apoptosis may get initiated through ligand such as TNF-α and FasL activation of death receptors such as TNF-α receptor1 (TNFR1) and Fas

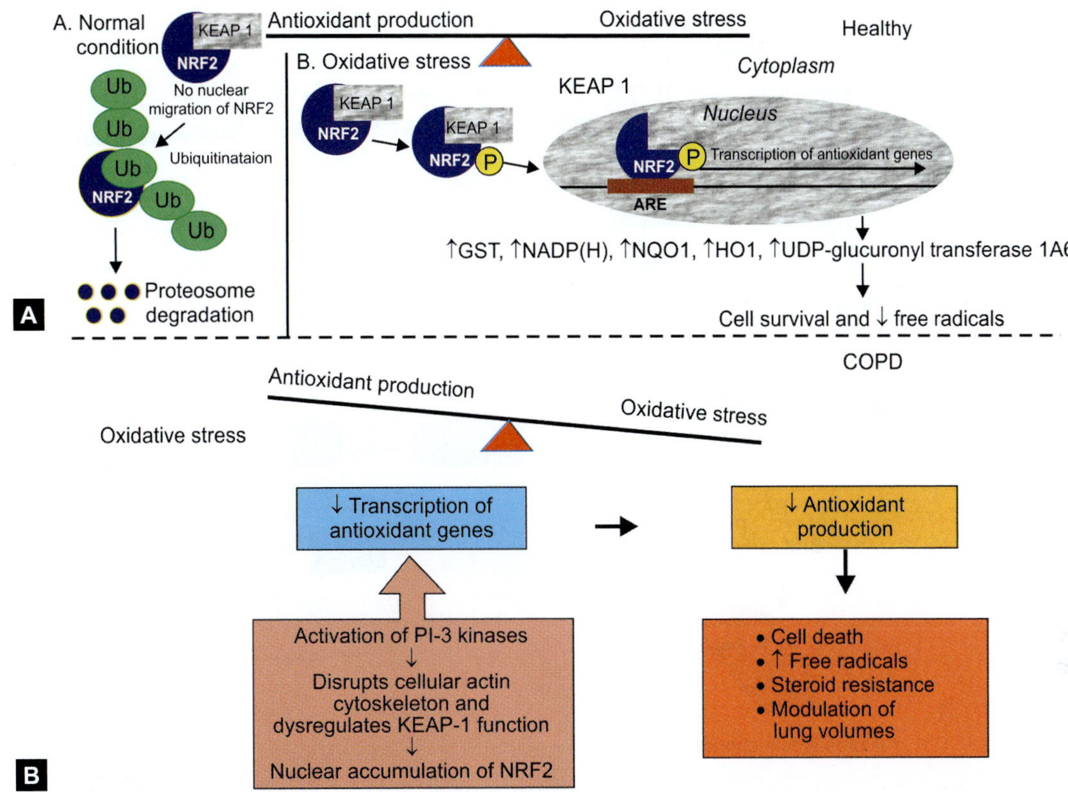

Figs 9A and B (A) NRF2-mediated antioxidant response. Under basal conditions, KEAP1, directly binds NRF2, thereby targeting it for destruction by the proteasome through ubiquitin (Ub) pathways, therefore at the basal levels of NRF2 is low. During oxidative stress, small amount of NRF2 dissociates from KEAP1 and translocates into the nucleus and heterodimerizes with other basic leucine zipper transcription factors such as small MAF proteins and the CBP/p300 coactivator, thereby increasing the transcription of ARE-driven genes (such as GST, NADPH, NQO1, UDP-glucuronyltransferase genes) protecting cell from oxidative stress. (B) In chronic obstructive pulmonary disease activation of PI3-kinase can disturb the activation and mobility of NRF2 which then fails to reach nucleus resulting in reduction in antioxidant production which induces unchecked oxidative stress related tissue damage and development of steroid resistance

respectively. This activation recruits procaspase-8 through an adaptor protein called Fas associated death domain protein (FADD) to form caspase-8. Caspase-8 then activates caspase-3 and cleaves proapoptotic BCL-2 family protein, BID to truncate BID. Caspase-3 is a key executioner of downstream events of all apoptotic pathways. Caspase-3 cleaves inhibitor of caspase-activated DNase (ICAD) to form caspase-activated DNase (CAD).

Caspase-activated DNase translocates from cytoplasm to nucleus, where it functions as endonuclease to fragment DNA to induce death. Further, the truncated BID interacts with other proapoptotic BCL-2 family proteins such as BAK and BAX to form pores in the mitochondria to release cytochrome C (Cyt C). The Cyt C together with apoptotic protease activating factor-1 (APAF-1) and procaspase-9 forms a complex to cleave procaspase-9 to caspase-9, which then switches caspase-3 to induce cell death as described above. Lack of survival factors and growth factors and stress on endoplasmic reticulum can also trigger BAX and BAK-mitochondrial cytochrome C-caspase-3 pathway. Endoplasmic reticulum stress can also directly target the nucleus to induce DNA fragmentation. The granzyme-B and perforin released by the T-cells can activate caspase-3 and caspase-8 pathways to induce DNA fragmentation **(Fig. 10)**.[129]

Studies have demonstrated increase in caspase-3 and proapoptotic proteins such as BAX and BAK in the lung tissue of COPD patients with emphysema.[132] Further, the emphysema was found to be associated with survival factor such as reduced vascular endothelial growth factor (VEGF) expression, which is a key molecule for endothelial survival.[133,134] Enhanced apoptosis was observed in the skeletal muscles of COPD patients that may cause skeletal muscles wasting in COPD patients.[135] The death cell-receptor ligand such as TNF-α and its receptors TNF-α-R55 was found to be increased in the serum of COPD patients.[136] Apoptosis has implicated in causing perpetuality of inflammation among COPD patients. The CD8 cells, the cardinal lymphocytes in COPD have propensity to induce apoptosis through perforin and granzyme B, the MMPs activate FasL and degrades the basement membrane to reduce survival signal to cause

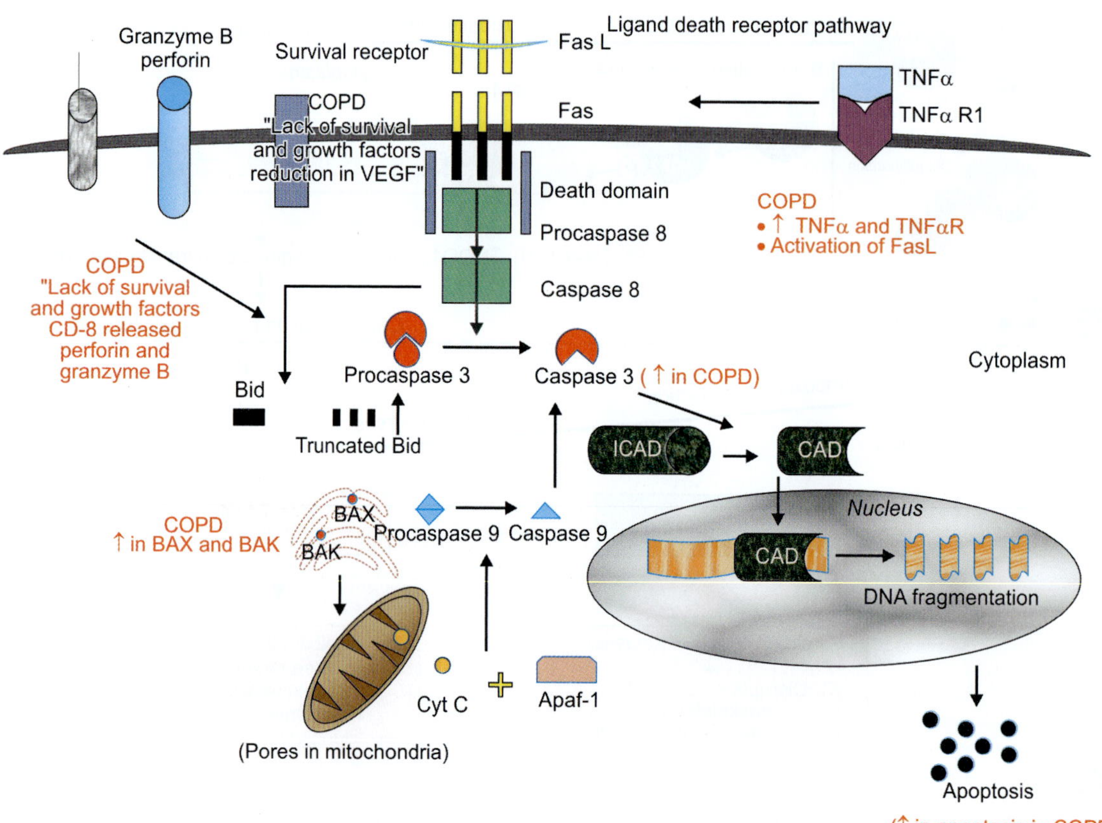

Fig. 10 Five complexly interlinked pathways of apoptosis. TNFα and FasL ligand activate death receptors [TNFα receptor1 (TNFR1) and Fas respectively] to recruit procaspase-8 through an adaptor protein [Fas associated death domain protein (FADD)] to form activated caspase-8. In chronic obstructive pulmonary disease (COPD) there is high TNFα and Fas and related receptors. Caspase-8 activates caspase-3 and cleaves BID to truncated BID. Caspase-3 is highly activated in COPD lungs. Caspase-3 cleaves inhibitor of caspase-activated DNase (ICAD) to form caspase activated Dnase (CAD). CAD translocates to nucleus to fragment DNA resulting in cell death. The truncated BID interacts with BAK and BAX to form pores in the mitochondria to release cytochrome C (Cyt C). The Cyt C together with apoptotic protease activating factor-1 (Apaf-1) converts procaspase-9 into caspase-9. Caspase-9 switches caspase-3. Lack of survival factors and growth factors and stress on endoplasmic reticulum can also trigger BAX and BAK-mitochondrial cytochrome C-caspase-3 pathway. Endoplasmic reticulum stress can also directly induce DNA fragmentation. There is lack of growth factors such as vascular endothelial growth factor (VEGF) in COPD. The T-cells associated granzyme-B and perforin can activate caspase-3 and caspase-8 pathways. In COPD CD8 cells enhance production of granzyme-3 and perforin

apoptosis and oxidative stress induces epithelial injury,[137,138] and reduce production of VEGF to induce apoptosis.[120]

Apoptotic by-product which is normally phagocytosized by macrophages fails to effectively clear the apoptotic material (efferocytosis) from the lungs. This could be because of the neutrophil elastase released by neutrophils to cleave the phosphatidyl serine receptors involved in efferocytosis rendering them nonfunctional in COPD.[136] The perpetual presence of apoptotic debris could be the trigger for an ongoing inflammation cascade. Currently, the pharmacological interventions that have the potential to reduce apoptosis and enhance apoptotic clearing mechanisms in the macrophage are being explored in new advancement of COPD treatments.

NEW INSIGHTS INTO SMALL AIRWAY OBSTRUCTION

Until now it has been largely believed that small airway obstruction in COPD is secondary consequence to destruction of alveoli and adjoining elastic tissue leading to kinking of small airways, in conjunction with small airway structural changes. However, microimaging computerized tomography (CT) studies indicate that terminal bronchioles undergo obliteration or apoptosis much before emphysema develops.[139] This has generated a possible hypothesis that loss of terminal bronchiole could precede emphysema in development stages of COPD pathologies.

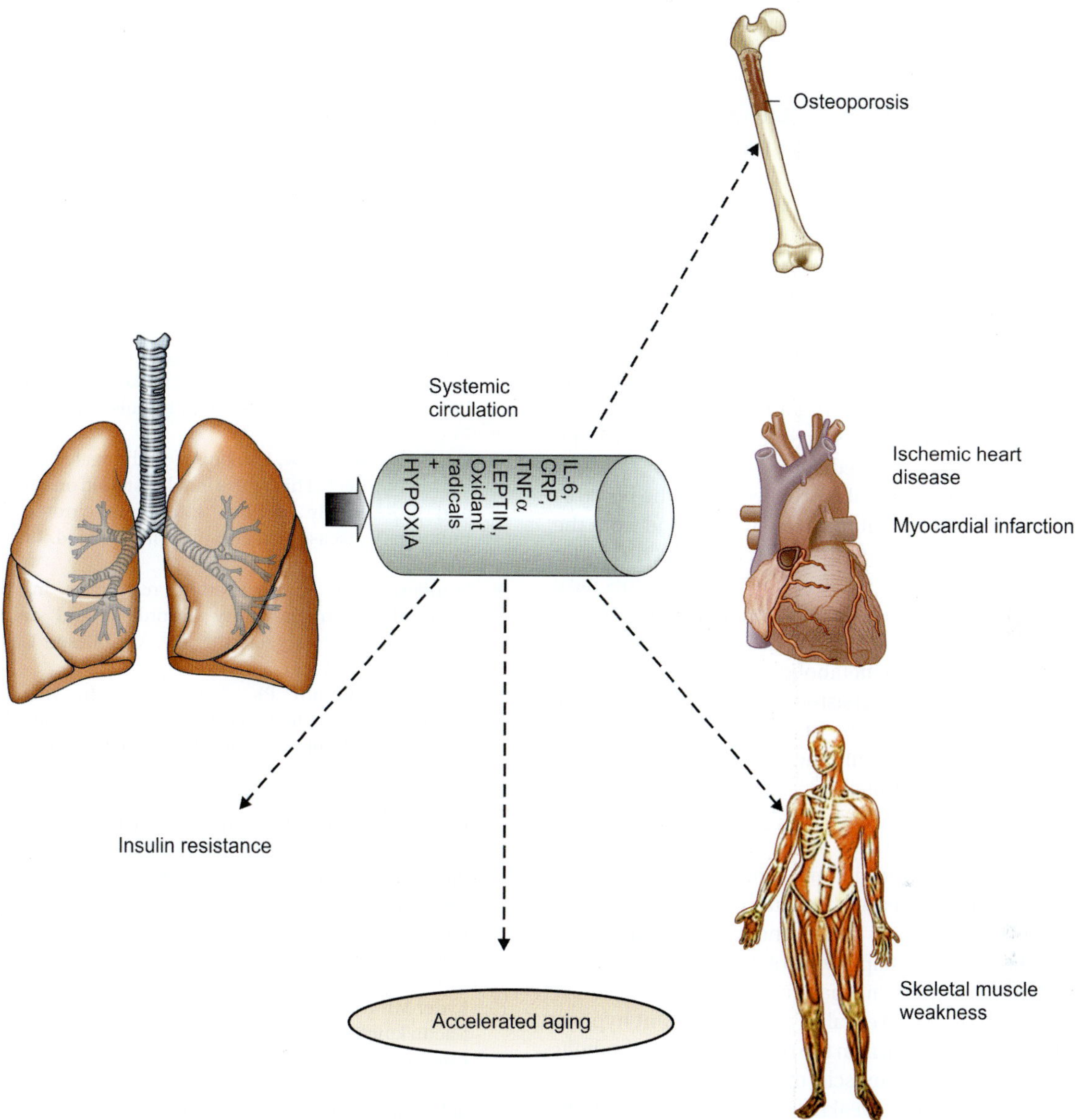

Fig. 11 Systemic effects of chronic obstructive pulmonary disease inflammation

There are approximately 44510 ± 15574 terminal bronchioles having a total cross-sectional area of 3,050.3 ± 576.6 mm.[2] Also, bronchioles less than 2 mm in diameter are spread across 4–14th generations indicating that terminal bronchi could be of varied luminal diameters.[140] The airflow in this area is slowest which physiologically allows adequate mixing of inspired and end-expiratory air for optimal gas diffusion. These physiological properties make the preterminal, terminal and first respiratory bronchiole domains an ideal situ for particulate matter impaction which are released from cigarette smoke or biomass fuel. Intriguingly, insults in less than 2 mm bronchiolar region do not manifest clinically and remains silent until appreciable damage to the bronchi-alveolar system occurs. This suggests that the pathologies of terminal bronchioles such as obliteration or apoptosis may occur much before COPD or emphysema is diagnosed clinically. The micro-CT imaging studies suggests that, number of the terminal bronchioles may reduce to 10% of normal in centrilobular emphysema and 25% in panlobular emphysema.[139] Also, evidence shows that there is reduction in number of terminal bronchiole in absence of histological emphysema.[139-141] There is a possibility that loss of terminal bronchioles compensates with dilatation of adjoining terminal bronchiole and respiratory bronchiole to reduce resistance in high resistance connecting bronchioles so that normal alveoli can receive proper ventilation. This dilatation could be harbinger of initial stages of centrilobular emphysema. However, there is still lot to be understood along with clinical implication of this hypothesis in understanding COPD pathogenesis.

CHRONIC OBSTRUCTIVE PULMONARY DISEASE: A DISEASE OF SYSTEMIC INFLAMMATION

Chronic obstructive pulmonary disease has classically been considered to be an intrathoracic condition characterized by poorly reversible airway obstruction. However, COPD has been recently recognized as a multicomponent disorder, associated with systemic inflammation and extrapulmonary manifestations. It has now been well documented that the inflammation that develops in the patient does not confine to the lungs but spills into the systemic circulation through the pulmonary vessels and predisposes almost every organ system in the body with particular predilection to the heart, as the heart is the first organ that receives all the blood from the pulmonary vasculature. More than 20% of cases of COPD suffer with chronic heart failure,[142] while up to 70% of patients have osteoporosis independent of steroid treatment or decreased physic activity.[143] Also almost 50% of COPD patients may have one or more components of metabolic syndrome.[144]

There is always a persistent low-grade systemic inflammatory response present in part of COPD patients. Various studies have shown enhanced levels of acute phase proteins like C-reactive protein[145,146] and proinflammatory cytokines such as TNF-α and IL6[147,148] in many COPD patients. Moreover, there has been a consistent strong association between reduced lung function and systemic inflammation. Even increased polymorphisms have been shown in the inflammatory genes and there is increasing interest in identifying a haplotype of inflammatory genes which predisposes to systemic manifestation of COPD.

These inflammatory makers along with persistent hypoxia increase the basal metabolism in the body leading to catabolic changes such as reduced muscle mass, wasting of skeletal muscles and diaphragmatic weakness. Notably, interventions such as regular exercise and physiotherapy have been shown to reduce systemic inflammation. There has also been a strong association between depression and COPD.[149] There is emerging evidence indicating insulin resistance in some COPD patients due to systemic inflammation and recently an association with diabetes and COPD has been demonstrated. COPD has also been related to metabolic syndrome as it predisposes patients to increased cardiovascular morbidity and diabetes mellitus **(Fig. 11)**.

REFERENCES

1. Vestbo J, Hurd SS, Agustí AG, Jones PW, Vogelmeier C, Anzueto A, et al. Global strategy for the diagnosis, management, and prevention of chronic obstructive pulmonary disease: GOLD executive summary. Am J Respir Crit Care Med. 2013;187(4):347-65.
2. Petty TL. The history of COPD. Int J Chron Obstruct Pulmon Dis. 2006;1(1):3-14.
3. Badham C. An Essay on Bronchitis: with Supplement Containing Remarks on Simple Pulmonary Abscess, 2nd edition. London: J Callow; 1814.
4. Gross P, Babyak MA, Tolker E, Kaschak M. Enzymatically produced pulmonary emphysema. A preliminary report. J. Occup Med. 1964;6:481-4.
5. O'Donnell RA, Peebles C, Ward JA, Daraker A, Angco G, Broberg P, et al. Relationship between peripheral airway dysfunction, airway obstruction, and neutrophilic inflammation in COPD. Thorax. 2004;59:837-42.
6. Stănescu D, Sanna A, Veriter C, Kostianev S, Calcagni PG, Fabbri LM, et al. Airways obstruction, chronic expectoration, and rapid decline of FEV1 in smokers are associated with increased levels of sputum neutrophils. Thorax. 1996;51:267-71.
7. Culpitt SV, Maziak W, Loukidis S, Nightingale JA, Matthews JL, Barnes PJ. Effect of high dose inhaled steroid on cells, cytokines, and proteases in induced sputum in chronic obstructive pulmonary disease. Am J Respir Crit Care Med. 1999;160:1635-39.
8. Wanderer AA. Corticosteroid resistance in pulmonary neutrophilic inflammatory disorders and rationale for adjunct IL-1beta targeted therapy. Am J Respir Cell Mol Biol. 2009;41(2):246-7.
9. Selby ED, Wraith PK, MacNee W. In vivo neutrophil sequestration within lungs of humans is determined by in vitro "filterability". J Appl Physiol. 1991;71:1996-2003.
10. Hogg JC. Neutrophil kinetics and lung injury. Physiological Reviews. 1987;67(4):1249-95.
11. Drost EM, Selby C, Lannan S, Lowe GD, MacNee W. Changes in neutrofil deformability following in vitro smoke exposure: mechanism and protection. Am J Resp Cell Mol Biol. 1992;6(3):287-95.
12. Rahman I, Morrison D, Donaldson K, MacNee W. Systemic oxidative stress in asthma, COPD, and smokers. Am. J Respir Crit Care Med. 1996;154(4 Pt 1):1055-60.
13. Ryder MI, Wu TC, Kallaos SS, Hyun W. Alterations of neutrophil f-actin kinetics by tobacco smoke: implications for periodontal diseases. J Periodontal Res. 2002;37(4):286-92.
14. Riise GC, Larsson S, Löfdahl CG, Andersson BA. Circulating cell adhesion molecules in bronchial lavage and serum in COPD patients with chronic bronchitis. Eur Respir J. 1994;7:1673-7.
15. Pilewski JM, Albelda SM. Adhesion molecules in the lung: an overview. Am Rev Respir Dis. 1993;148:S31-7.
16. Montefort S, Holgate ST, Howarth PH. Leucocyte-endothelial adhesion molecules and their role in bronchial asthma and allergic rhinitis. Eur Respir J. 1993;6:1044-54.
17. Lawrence MB, Springer TA. Leukocytes roll on a selectin at physiologic flow rates: distinction from and prerequisite for adhesion through integrins. Cell. 1991;65:859-73.
18. Wegner CD, Gundel RH, Reilly P, Haynes N, Gordon Letts L, Rothlein R. ICAM-1 in the pathogenesis of asthma. Science. 1990;247:416-8.
19. Montefort S, Feather IH, Wilson SJ, Haskard DO, Lee TH, Holgate ST, et al. The expression of leucocyte-endothelial adhesion molecules is increased in perennial allergic rhinitis. Am J Respir Cell Mol Biol. 1992;7:393-8.
20. Di Stefano A, Maestrelli P, Roggeri A, Turato G, Calabro S, Potena A, et al. Upregulation of adhesion molecules in the bronchial

mucosa of subjects with chronic obstructive bronchitis. Am J Respir Crit Care Med. 1994;149:803-10.

21. Seth R, Raymond FD, Makgoba MW. Circulating ICAM-1 isoforms: diagnostic prospects for inflammatory and immune disorders. Lancet. 1991;338:83-4.
22. Kaur M, Singh D. Neutrophil chemotaxis caused by chronic obstructive pulmonary disease alveolar macrophages: the role of CXCL8 and the receptors CXCR1/CXCR2. J Pharmacol Exp Ther. 2013;347(1):173-80.
23. Afonso PV, Janka-Junttila M, Lee YJ, McCann CP, Oliver CM, Aamer KA, et al. LTB4 is a signal-relay molecule during neutrophil chemotaxis. Dev Cell. 2012;22(5):1079-91.
24. Srivastava PK, Dastidar SG, Ray A. Chronic obstructive pulmonary disease: role of matrix metalloproteases and future challenges of drug therapy. Expert Opin Investig Drugs. 2007;16(7):1069-78.
25. Lee SH, Goswami S, Grudo A, Song LZ, Bandi V, Goodnight-White S, et al. Antielastin autoimmunity in tobacco smoking-induced emphysema. Nat Med. 2007;13:567-9.
26. Meijer M, Rijkers GT, van Overveld FJ. Neutrophils and emerging targets for treatment in chronic obstructive pulmonary disease. Expert Rev Clin Immunol. 2013;9(11):1055-68.
27. Fischer BM, Pavlisko E, Voynow JA. Pathogenic triad in COPD: oxidative stress, protease-antiprotease imbalance, and inflammation. Int J Chron Obstruct Pulmon Dis. 2011;6:413-21.
28. Stockley JA, Walton GM, Lord JM, Sapey E. Aberrant neutrophil functions in stable chronic obstructive pulmonary disease: the neutrophil as an immunotherapeutic target. Int Immunopharmacol. 2013;17(4):1211-7.
29. Saetta M, Baraldo S, Corbino L, Turato G, Braccioni F, Rea F, et al. CD8+ve cells in the lungs of smokers with chronic obstructive pulmonary disease. Am J Respir Crit Care Med. 1999;160:711-7.
30. O'Shaughnessy TC1, Ansari TW, Barnes NC, Jeffery PK. Inflammation in bronchial biopsies of subjects with chronic bronchitis: inverse relationship of CD8+ T lymphocytes with FEV1. Am J Respir Crit Care Med. 1997;155(3):852-7.
31. Hogg JC, Chu F, Utokaparch S, Woods R, Elliott WM, Buzatu L, et al. The nature of small airway obstruction in chronic obstructive pulmonary disease. N Engl J Med. 2004;350(26):2645-53.
32. Di Stefano A, Caramori G, Capelli A, Gnemmi I, Ricciardolo FL, Oates T, et al. STAT4 activation in smokers and patients with chronic obstructive pulmonary disease. Eur Resp J. 2004;24: 78-85.
33. Saetta M, Mariani M, Panina-Bordignon P, Turato G, Buonsanti C, Baraldo S, et al. Increased expression of the chemokine receptor CXCR3 and its ligand CXCL10 in peripheral airways of smokers with chronic obstructive pulmonary disease. Am J Respir Crit Care Med. 2002;165(10):1404-9.
34. Chrysofakis G, Tzanakis N, Kyriakoy D, Tsoumakidou M, Tsiligianni I, Klimathianaki M, et al. Perforin expression and cytotoxic activity of sputum CD8+ lymphocytes in patients with COPD. Chest. 2004;125:71-6.
35. Hodge S, Hodge G, Nairn J, Holmes M, Reynolds PN. Increased airway granzyme b and perforin in current and ex-smoking COPD subjects. COPD. 2006;3:179-87.
36. Majo J, Ghezzo H, Cosio MG. Lymphocyte population and apoptosis in the lungs of smokers and their relation to emphysema. Eur Respir J. 2001;17:946-53.
37. Taraseviciene-Stewart L, Scerbavicius R, Choe KH, Moore M, Sullivan A, Nicolls MR, et al. An animal model of autoimmune emphysema. Am J Respir Crit Care Med. 2005;171:734-42.
38. Sullivan AK, Simonian PL, Falta MT, Mitchell JD, Cosgrove GP, Brown KK, et al. Oligoclonal CD4+ T cells in the lungs of patients with severe emphysema. Am J Respir Crit Care Med. 2005;172:590-6.
39. Grumelli S, Corry DB, Song LZ, Song L, Green L, Huh J, et al. An immune basis for lung parenchymal destruction in chronic obstructive pulmonary disease. PLoS Med. 2004;1(1):e8.
40. Smyth LJ, Starkey C, Vestbo J, Singh D. CD4-regulatory cells in COPD patients. Chest. 2007;132:156-63.
41. Russell RE, Thorley A, Culpitt SV, Dodd S, Donnelly LE, Demattos C, et al. Alveolar macrophage mediated elastolysis: roles of matrix metalloproteinases, cysteine, and serine proteases. Am J Physiol Lung Cell Mol Physiol. 2002;283(4):L867-73.
42. Hong SC, Lee SH. Role of th17 cell and autoimmunity in chronic obstructive pulmonary disease. Immune Netw. 2010;10(4):109-14.
43. Kheradmand F, Shan M, Xu C, Corry DB. Autoimmunity in chronic obstructive pulmonary disease: clinical and experimental evidence. Expert Rev Clin Immunol. 2012;8(3):285-92.
44. Vargas-Rojas MI, Ramírez-Venegas A, Limón-Camacho L, Ochoa L, Hernández-Zenteno R, Sansores RH, et al. Increase of Th17 cells in peripheral blood of patients with chronic obstructive pulmonary disease. Respir Med. 2011;105:1648-54.
45. Wang H, Ying H, Wang S, Gu X, Weng Y, Peng W, et al. Imbalance of peripheral blood Th17 and Treg responses in patients with chronic obstructive pulmonary disease. Clin Respir J. 2015;9(3):330-41.
46. Qian J, Galitovskiy V, Chernyavsky AI, Marchenko S, Grando SA. Plasticity of the murine spleen T-cell cholinergic receptors and their role in in vitro differentiation of naïve CD4 T cells toward the Th1, Th2 and Th17 lineages. Genes Immun. 2011;12(3):222-30.
47. Profita M, Albano GD, Riccobono L, Di Sano C, Montalbano AM, Gagliardo R, et al. Increased levels of Th17 cells are associated with non-neuronal acetylcholine in COPD patients. Immunobiology. 2014;219(5):392-401.
48. Dubin PJ, Kolls JK. Th17 cytokines and mucosal immunity. Immunol Rev. 2008;226:160-71.
49. Jones CE, Chan K. Interleukin-17 stimulates the expression of interleukin-8, growth-related oncogene-alpha, and granulocyte-colony-stimulating factor by human airway epithelial cells. Am J Respir Cell Mol Biol. 2002;26:748-53.
50. Burgler S, Ouaked N, Bassin C, Basinski TM, Mantel PY, Siegmund K, et al. Differentiation and functional analysis of human TH17 cells. J Allergy Clin Immunol. 2009;123:588-95.
51. Chen Z, Lin F, Gao Y, Li Z, Zhang J, Xing Y, Deng Z, et al. FOXP3 and RORγt: transcriptional regulation of Treg and Th17. Int Immunopharmacol. 2011;11(5):536-42.
52. Steinman L. A brief history of T(H)17, the first major revision in the T(H)1/T(H)2 hypothesis of T cell-mediated tissue damage. Nat Med. 2007;13:139-45.
53. Di Stefano A, Caramori G, Gnemmi I, Contoli M, Vicari C, Capelli A, et al. T helper type 17-related cytokine expression is increased in the bronchial mucosa of stable chronic obstructive pulmonary disease patients. Clin Exp Immunol. 2009;157:316-24.
54. Kolls JK, Lindén A. Interleukin-17 family members and inflammation. Immunity. 2004;21:467-76.
55. Aggarwal S, Gurney AL. IL-17: prototype member of an emerging cytokine family. J Leukocyte Biol. 2002;71:1-8.

56. Eustace A, Smyth LJ, Mitchell L, Williamson K, Plumb J, Singh D. Identification of cells expressing IL-17A and IL-17F in the lungs of patients with COPD. Chest. 2011;139(5):1089-100.
57. Chang Y, Nadigel J, Boulais N, Bourbeau J, Maltais F, Eidelman DH, et al. CD8 positive T cells express IL-17 in patients with chronic obstructive pulmonary disease. Respir Res. 2011;12:43.
58. Miossec P, Korn T, Kuchroo VK. Interleukin-17 and type 17 helper T cells. N Engl J Med. 2009;361:888-98.
59. Lindén A, Laan M, Anderson GP. Neutrophils, interleukin-17A and lung disease. Eur Respir J. 2005;25:159-72.
60. McKinley L, Alcorn JF, Peterson A, Dupont RB, Kapadia S, Logar A, et al. TH17 cells mediate steroid-resistant airway inflammation and airway hyperresponsiveness in mice. J Immunol. 2008;181:4089-97.
61. Kurimoto E, Miyahara N, Kanehiro A, Waseda K, Taniguchi A, Ikeda G, et al. IL-17A is essential to the development of elastase-induced pulmonary inflammation and emphysema in mice. Respir Res. 2013;20:14:5.
62. Duan MC, Tang HJ, Zhong XN, Huang Y. Persistence of Th17/Tc17 cell expression upon smoking cessation in mice with cigarette smoke-induced emphysema. Clin Dev Immunol. 2013;2013:350727.
63. Vanaudenaerde BM, Verleden SE, Vos R, De Vleeschauwer SI, Willems-Widyastuti A, Geenens R, et al. Innate and adaptive interleukin-17-producing lymphocytes in chronic inflammatory lung disorders. Am J Respir Crit Care Med. 2011;183:977-86.
64. Halwani R, Al-Muhsen S, Hamid Q. T helper 17 cells in airway diseases: from laboratory bench to bedside. Chest. 2013;143(2):494-501.
65. Cazzola M, Matera MG. IL-17 in chronic obstructive pulmonary disease. Expert Rev Respir Med. 2012;6(2):135-38.
66. Ghannam S, Pène J, Moquet-Torcy G, Jorgensen C, Yssel H. Mesenchymal stem cells inhibit human Th17 cell differentiation and function and induce a T regulatory cell phenotype. J Immunol. 2010;185:302-12
67. Shapiro SD. The macrophage in chronic obstructive pulmonary disease. Am J Respir Crit Care Med. 1996;160(5 Pt 2):S29-32.
68. Kojima J, Araya J, Hara H, Ito S, Takasaka N, Kobayashi K, et al. Apoptosis inhibitor of macrophage (AIM) expression in alveolar macrophages in COPD. Respiratory Research. 2013;14(1):30.
69. Brozyna S, Ahern J, Hodge G, Nairn J, Holmes M, Reynolds PN, et al. Chemotactic Mediators of Th1 T-cell Trafficking in Smokers and COPD Patients. COPD. 2009;6(1):4-16.
70. Traves SL, Culpitt SV, Russell RE, Barnes PJ, Donnelly LE. Increased levels of the chemokines GROalpha and MCP-1 in sputum samples from patients with COPD. Thorax. 2002;57(7):590-5.
71. Hubbard RC, Fells G, Gadek J, Pacholok S, Humes J, Crystal RG. Neutrophil accumulation in the lung in alpha 1-antitrypsindeficiency: Spontaneous release of leukotriene B4 by alveolar macrophages. J Clin Invest. 1991;88(3):891-7.
72. Dentener MA, Louis R, Cloots RH, Henket M, Wouters EF. Differences in local versus systemic TNF alpha production in COPD: inhibitory effect of hyaluronan on LPS induced blood cell TNF alpha release. Thorax. 2006;61:478-84.
73. Sin DD, Man SF. Interleukin-6: a red herring or a real catch in COPD? Chest. 2008;133(1):4-6.
74. Montuschi P, Collins JV, Ciabattoni G, Lazzeri N, Corradi M, Kharitonov SA, et al. Exhaled 8-isoprostane as an in vivo biomarker of lung oxidative stress in patients with COPD and healthy smokers. Am J Respir Crit Care Med. 2000;162(3):1175-7.
75. Calikoglu M, Sahin G, Unlu A, Ozturk C, Tamer L, Ercan B, et al. Leptin and TNF-alpha levels in patients with chronic obstructive pulmonary disease and their relationship to nutritional parameters. Respiration. 2004;71(1):45-50.
76. Hata H, Yoshimoto T, Hayashi N, Hada T, Nakanishi K. IL-18 together with anti-CD3 antibody induces human Th1 cells to produce Th1- and Th2-cytokines and IL-8. Int Immunol. 2004;16(12):1733-9.
77. Solic N, Wilson J, Wilson SJ, Shute JK. Endothelial activation and increased heparan sulfate expression in cystic fibrosis. Am J Respir Crit Care Med. 2005;172:892-8.
78. Schulz C, Krätzel K, Wolf K, Schroll S, Köhler M, Pfeifer M. Activation of bronchial epithelial cells in smokers without airway obstruction and patients with COPD. Chest 2004;125:1706-13.
79. Schulz C, Wolf K, Harth M, Krätzel K, Kunz-Schughart L, Pfeifer M. Expression and release of interleukin-8 by human bronchial epithelial cells from patients with chronic obstructive pulmonary disease, smokers, and never-smokers. Respiration 2003;70(3):254-61.
80. Liu H, Ma Y, Pagliari LJ, Perlman H, Yu C, Lin A, et al. TNF-alpha-induced apoptosis of macrophages following inhibition of NF-kappa B: a central role for disruption of mitochondria. J Immunol. 2004;172(3):1907-15.
81. de Godoy I, Donahoe M, Calhoun WJ, Mancino J, Rogers RM. Elevated TNF-alpha production by peripheral blood monocytes of weight-losing COPD patients. Am J Respir Crit Care Med.1996;153(2):633-7.
82. Sethi S, Muscarella K, Evans N, Klingman KL, Grant BJ, Murphy TF. Airway inflammation and etiology of acute exacerbations of chronic bronchitis. Chest. 2000;118:1557-65.
83. Ott VL, Cambier JC, Kappler J, Marrack P, Swanson BJ. Mast cell-dependent migration of effector CD8+ T cells through production of leukotriene B4. Nat Immunol. 2003;4:974-81.
84. Bhowmik A, Seemungal TA, Sapsford RJ, Wedzicha JA. Relation of sputum inflammatory markers to symptoms and lung function changes in COPD exacerbations. Thorax. 2000;55:114-20.
85. Wedzicha JA, Seemungal TA, MacCallum PK, Paul EA, Donaldson GC, Bhowmik A, et al. Acute exacerbations of chronic obstructive pulmonary disease are accompanied by elevations of plasma fibrinogen and serum IL-6 levels. Thromb Haemost. 2000;84(2):210-5.
86. Finlay GA, O'Driscoll LR, Russell KJ, D'Arcy EM, Masterson JB, FitzGerald MX, et al. Matrix metalloproteinase expression and production by alveolar macrophages in emphysema. Am J Respir Crit Care Med. 1997;156(1):240-7.
87. Abbas AK, Lichtman AH, Shiv P. Cellular and Molecular Immunology. Philadelphia: Saunders Elsevier; 2012.
88. Janeway CA, Travers P, Walport M, Shlomchik MJ. Immunobiology: The Immune System in Health and Diseas, 5th edition. New York: Garland Science; 2001.
89. Linehan SA, Coulson PS, Wilson RA, Mountford AP, Brombacher F, Martínez-Pomares L, et al. IL-4 receptor signaling is required for mannose receptor expression by macrophages recruited to granulomata but not resident cells in mice infected with Schistosoma mansoni. Lab Invest. 2003;83(8):1223-31.
90. Lien E, Sellati TJ, Yoshimura A, Flo TH, Rawadi G, Finberg RW, et al. Toll-like receptor 2 functions as a pattern recognition

receptor for diverse bacterial products. J Biol Chem. 1999;274(47):33419-25.
91. Means TK, Wang S, Lien E, Yoshimura A, Golenbock DT, Fenton MJ. Human toll-like receptors mediate cellular activation by *Mycobacterium tuberculosis*. J Immunol. 1999;163(7):3920-7.
92. Lien E, Means TK, Heine H, Yoshimura A, Kusumoto S, Fukase K, et al. Toll-like receptor 4 imparts ligand-specific recognition of bacterial lipopolysaccharide. J Clin Invest. 2000;105(4):497-504.
93. Droemann D, Goldmann T, Tiedje T, Zabel P, Dalhoff K, Schaaf B. Toll-like receptor 2 expression is decreased on alveolar macrophages in cigarette smokers and COPD patients. Respir Res. 2005;6:68.
94. Lee SW, Kim DR, Kim TJ, Paik JH, Chung JH, Jheon S, et al. The association of down-regulated toll-like receptor 4 expression with airflow limitation and emphysema in smokers. Respir Res. 2012;13:106.
95. An CH, Wang XM, Lam HC, Ifedigbo E, Washko GR, Ryter SW, et al. TLR4 deficiency promotes autophagy during cigarette smoke-induced pulmonary emphysema. Am J Physiol Lung Cell Mol Physiol. 2012;303(9):L748-57.
96. Stuart LM, Ezekowitz RA. Phagocytosis: elegant complexity. Immunity. 2005;22(5):539-50.
97. Palecanda A, Kobzik L. Receptors for unopsonized particles: the role of alveolar macrophage scavenger receptors. Curr Mol Med. 2001;1(5):589-95.
98. Harvey CJ, Thimmulappa RK, Sethi S, Kong X, Yarmus L, Brown RH, et al. Targeting Nrf2 signaling improves bacterial clearance by alveolar macrophages in patients with COPD and in a mouse model. Sci Transl Med. 2011;3(78):78ra32.
99. Apostolopoulo V, McKenzie I. Role of mannose receptor in the immune response. Curr Mol Med. 2001;1(4):469-74.
100. Hodge S, Hodge G, Jersmann H, Matthews G, Ahern J, Holmes M, et al. Azithromycin improves macrophage phagocytic function and expression of mannose receptor in chronic obstructive pulmonary disease. Am J Respir Crit Care Med. 2008;178(2):139-48.
101. Löfdahl JM, Wahlström J, Sköld CM. Different inflammatory cell pattern and macrophage phenotype in chronic obstructive pulmonary disease patients, smokers and non-smokers. Clin Exp Immunol. 2006;145(3):428-37.
102. Hodge S, Hodge G, Ahern J, Jersmann H, Holmes M, Reynolds PN. Smoking alters alveolar macrophage recognition and phagocytic ability: implications in chronic obstructive pulmonary disease. Am J Respir Cell Mol Biol. 2007;37(6):748-55 .
103. Pons AR, Noguera A, Blanquer D, Sauleda J, Pons J, Agustí AG. Phenotypic characterisation of alveolar macrophages and peripheral blood monocytes in COPD. Eur Respir J. 2005;25(4):647-52.
104. Kirkham P. Oxidative stress and macrophage function: a failure to resolve the inflammatory response. Biochem Soc Trans. 2007;35(pt 2):284-7.
105. Vecchiarelli A, Dottorini M, Pietrella D, Cociani C, Eslami A, Todisco T, et al. Macrophage activation by N-acetyl-cysteine in COPD patients. Chest. 1994;105(3):806-11.
106. Brown LA, Ping XD, Harris FL, Gauthier TW. Glutathione availability modulates alveolar macrophage function in the chronic ethanol-fed rat. Am J Physiol Lung Cell Mol Physiol. 2007;292(4):L824-32.
107. Morimoto K, Janssen WJ, Fessler MB, McPhillips KA, Borges VM, Bowler RP, et al. Lovastatin enhances clearance of apoptotic cells (efferocytosis) with implications for chronic obstructive pulmonary disease. J Immunol. 2006;176(12):7657-65.
108. MacNee W. Oxidants/antioxidants and COPD. Chest. 2000;117(5 Suppl 1):303S-17S.
109. Pryor WA, Stone K. Oxidants in cigarette smoke: radicals hydrogen peroxides peroxynitrate and peroxynitrite. Ann N Y Acad Sci. 1993;686:12-27.
110. Bunnell E, Pacht ER. Oxidized glutathione is increased in the alveolar fluid of patients with the adult respiratory distress syndrome. Am Rev Respir Dis. 1993;148:1174-8.
111. Rahman I. Pharmacological antioxidant strategies as therapeutic interventions for COPD. Biochim Biophys Acta. 2012;1822(5):714-28.
112. Ito K, Barnes PJ. COPD as a disease of accelerated lung aging. Chest 2009;135:173-80.
113. Barnes PJ. Corticosteroid resistance in patients with asthma and chronic obstructive pulmonary disease. J Allergy Clin Immunol. 2013;131(3):636-45.
114. Fischer B, Voynow J. Neutrophil elastase induces MUC5AC messenger RNA expression by an oxidant-dependent mechanism. Chest. 2000;117(5 Suppl 1):317S-20S.
115. Tse HN, Raiteri L, Wong KY, Ng LY, Yee KS, Tseng CZ. Benefits of high-dose N-acetylcysteine to exacerbation-prone patients with COPD. Chest. 2014;146(3):611-23.
116. Kensler TW, Wakabayashi N, Biswal S. Cell survival responses to environmental stresses via the Keap1-Nrf2-ARE pathway. Annu Rev Pharmacol Toxicol. 2007;47:89-116.
117. Hybertson BM, Gao B. Role of the Nrf2 signaling system in health and disease. Clin Genet. 2014.
118. Boutten A, Goven D, Artaud-Macari E, Boczkowski J, Bonay M. NRF2 targeting: a promising therapeutic strategy in chronic obstructive pulmonary disease. Trends Mol Med. 2011;17(7):363-71.
119. Itoh K, Mimura J, Yamamoto M. Discovery of the negative regulator of Nrf2 Keap1: a historical overview. Antioxid Redox Signal. 2010;13:1665-78.
120. Goven D, Boutten A, Leçon-Malas V, Marchal-Sommé J, Amara N, Crestani B, et al. Altered Nrf2/Keap1-Bach1 equilibrium in pulmonary emphysema. Thorax. 2008;63(10):916-24.
121. Kang MI, Kobayashi A, Wakabayashi N, Kim SG, Yamamoto M. Scaffolding of Keap1 to the actin cytoskeleton controls the function of Nrf2 as key regulator of cytoprotective phase 2 genes. Proc Natl Acad Sci U S A. 2004;101(7):2046-51.
122. Ishii Y, Itoh K, Morishima Y, Kimura T, Kiwamoto T, Iizuka T, et al. Transcription factor Nrf2 plays a pivotal role in protection against elastase-induced pulmonary inflammation and emphysema. J Immunol. 2005;175(10):6968-75.
123. Cho HY, Gladwell W, Wang X, Chorley B, Bell D, Reddy SP, et al. Nrf2-regulated PPAR{gamma} expression is critical to protection against acute lung injury in mice. Am J Respir Crit Care Med. 210;182(2):170-82.
124. Adenuga D, Caito S, Yao H, Sundar IK, Hwang JW, Chung S, et al. Nrf2 deficiency influences susceptibility to steroid resistance via HDAC2 reduction. Biochem Biophys Res Commun. 2010;403(3-4):452-6.
125. Masuko H, Sakamoto T, Kaneko Y, Iijima H, Naito T, Noguchi E, et al. An interaction between Nrf2 polymorphisms and

smoking status affects annual decline in FEV1: a longitudinal retrospective cohort study. BMC Med Genet. 2011;12:97.

126. Malhotra D, Thimmulappa R, Navas-Acien A, Sandford A, Elliott M, Singh A, et al. Decline in NRF2-regulated antioxidants in chronic obstructive pulmonary disease lungs due to loss of its positive regulator, DJ-1. Am J Respir Crit Care Med. 2008;178(6):592-604.
127. Yu Yang Y, Cuevas S, Armando I, Jose P. Azithromycin induces sestrin2 expression through Nrf2 signaling pathway in lung epithelial cells stimulated with cigarette smoke extract (869.11). The FASEB Journal. 2014;28(1):869.11.
128. Harvey CJ, Thimmulappa RK, Sethi S, Kong X, Yarmus L, Brown RH, et al. Targeting Nrf2 signaling improves bacterial clearance by alveolar macrophages in patients with COPD and in a mouse model. Sci Transl Med. 2011;3(78).
129. Demedts IK, Demoor T, Bracke KR, Joos GF, Brusselle GG. Role of apoptosis in the pathogenesis of COPD and pulmonary emphysema. Respir Res. 2006;7:53.
130. Segura-Valdez L, Pardo A, Gaxiola M, Uhal BD, Becerril C, Selman M. Upregulation of gelatinases A and B, collagenases 1 and 2, and increased parenchymal cell death in COPD. Chest. 2000;117:684-94.
131. Degterev A, Boyce M, Yuan J. A decade of caspases. Oncogene. 2003;22:8543-67.
132. Imai K, Mercer BA, Schulman LL, Sonett JR, D'Armiento JM. Correlation of lung surface area to apoptosis and proliferation in human emphysema. Eur Respir J. 2005;25:250-8.
133. Kasahara Y, Tuder RM, Cool CD, Lynch DA, Flores SC, Voelkel NF. Endothelial cell death and decreased expression of vascular endothelial growth factor and vascular endothelial growth factor receptor 2 in emphysema. Am J Respir Crit Care Med. 2001;163:737-44.
134. Kanazawa H, Yoshikawa J. Elevated oxidative stress and reciprocal reduction of vascular endothelial growth factor levels with severity of COPD. Chest. 2005;128:3191-7.
135. Agusti AG, Sauleda J, Miralles C, Gomez C, Togores B, Sala E, et al. Skeletal muscle apoptosis and weight loss in chronic obstructive pulmonary disease. Am J Respir Crit Care Med. 2002;166(4):485-9.
136. Takabatake N, Nakamura H, Inoue S, Terashita K, Yuki H, Kato S, et al. Circulating levels of soluble Fas ligand and soluble Fas in patients with chronic obstructive pulmonary disease. Respir Med. 2000;94(12):1215-20.
137. Barry M, Bleackley RC. Cytotoxic T lymphocytes: all roads lead to death. Nat Rev Immunol. 2002;2:401-9.
138. Liu AN, Mohammed AZ, Rice WR, Fiedeldey DT, Liebermann JS, Whitsett JA, et al. Perforin-independent CD8(+) T-cell-mediated cytotoxicity of alveolar epithelial cells is preferentially mediated by tumor necrosis factor-alpha: relative insensitivity to Fas ligand. Am J Respir Cell Mol Biol. 1999;20(5):849-58.
139. McDonough JE, Yuan R, Suzuki M, Seyednejad N, Elliott WM, Sanchez PG, et al. Small-airway obstruction and emphysema in chronic obstructive pulmonary disease. N Engl J Med. 2011;365(17):1567-75.
140. Hogg JC, McDonough JE, Suzuki M. Small airway obstruction in COPD: new insights based on micro-CT imaging and MRI imaging. Chest. 2013;143(5):1436-43.
141. Burgel PR. The role of small airways in obstructive airway diseases. Eur Respir Rev. 2011;20(119):23-33.
142. Rutten FH, Cramer MJ, Lammers JW, Grobbee DE, Hoes AW. Heart failure and chronic obstructive pulmonary disease: An ignored combination? Eur J Heart Fail. 2006;8:706-11.
143. Jorgensen NR, Schwarz P, Holme I, Henriksen BM, Petersen LJ, Backer V. The prevalence of osteoporosis in patients with chronic obstructive pulmonary disease: a cross sectional study. Respir Med. 2007;101:177-85.
144. Marquis K, Maltais F, Duguay V, Bezeau AM, LeBlanc P, Jobin J, et al. The metabolic syndrome in patients with chronic obstructive pulmonary disease. J Cardiopulm Rehabil. 2005;25(4):226-32.
145. Gan WQ, Man SF, Senthilselvan A, Sin DD. Association between chronic obstructive pulmonary disease and systemic inflammation: a systematic review and a meta-analysis. Thorax. 2004;59:574-80.
146. Pinto-Plata VM, Müllerova H, Toso JF, Feudjo-Tepie M, Soriano JB, Vessey RS, et al. C-reactive protein in patients with COPD, control smokers and non-smokers. Thorax. 2006;61:23-8.
147. Wisniacki N, Taylor W, Lye M, Wilding JP. Insulin resistance and inflammatory activation in older patients with systolic and diastolic heart failure. Heart 2005;91:32-7.
148. McDermott MM, Guralnik JM, Corsi A, Albay M, Macchi C, Bandinelli S, et al. Patterns of inflammation associated with peripheral arterial disease: the InCHIANTI study. Am Heart J. 2005;150(2):276-81.
149. Janssen DJ, Müllerova H, Agusti A, Yates JC, Tal-Singer R, Rennard SI, et al. Persistent systemic inflammation and symptoms of depression among patients with COPD in the ECLIPSE cohort. Respir Med. 2014;108(11):1647-54.

Pulmonary Function Testing in Chronic Obstructive Pulmonary Disease

Tavpritesh Sethi, Anurag Agrawal

HISTORY AND EVOLUTION

The role of pulmonary function testing (PFT) in diagnosis and management of chronic obstructive pulmonary disease (COPD) has evolved over time. While accurate descriptions of the diseases grouped together under COPD predate any formal definitions,[1] the recognition of progressive respiratory symptoms and illnesses arising after exposure to noxious stimuli, especially cigarette smoke came much later in the mid-20th century. These illnesses were formerly known by multiple labels, of which two, namely chronic bronchitis and emphysema, were officially endorsed by the American Thoracic Society in 1962.

"Chronic bronchitis" was defined as a cough productive of sputum for at least 3 months of 2 consecutive years. Emphysema was defined in anatomic terms of enlarged alveolar spaces due to the destruction of alveolar walls. Neither definition encompassed any physiologic considerations. The term "COPD" encompassing both chronic bronchitis and emphysema is considered to have originated soon after.[1] In this era, the definition of COPD was mostly in clinical or structural terms and the disease was well-established by the time a diagnosis was made. While the scientific and technical basis of pulmonary function testings, including all current methods was already well-established by this time due to seminal work by stalwarts of the field, such as DuBois, Hyatt and Mead, the full recognition of the clinical utility of these tests in COPD came much later.

The 1959 Ciba symposium on "terminology, definitions and classification of chronic pulmonary emphysema and related conditions" presciently stated that the standardized collection of functional, clinical and pathological data may lead to the development of specific diagnostic criterion.[2] Forced expiratory tests of "ventilatory function", identical to modern spirometry and tests of "alveolar-capillary and circulatory function", such as arterial blood gases and cardiopulmonary exercise testing, were recommended as essential tests. Tests of lung compliance and resistance by the use of an esophageal balloon and a whole body plethysmograph (body box) were recommended as supplemental tests, amongst others such as gas diffusion and nitrogen washout. Over the next few decades, alterations in such measures of physiologic function were correlated to clinicopathological data and it became possible to reliably distinguish between the common lung diseases.

With the emergence of computed tomography as a preferred test to study structural lung diseases, such as emphysema, pulmonary fibrosis, etc. relatively simple and widely available tests like spirometry that primarily measure expiratory airflow limitation in obstructive airway disease (OAD), supplanted more complex methods. Over time, this has led to new definitions of COPD in which previous distinctions are done away with and the disease is simply defined in functional terms, as predicted in the 1959 Ciba symposium. The most recent guidelines from global obstructive lung disease (GOLD) initiative of the World Health Organization/National Heart Lung and Blood Institute state that COPD is a disease state characterized by airflow limitation that is not fully reversible.[3] The airflow limitation is usually both progressive and associated with an abnormal inflammatory response of the lungs to noxious particles and gases. The GOLD initiative revolutionized the definition of COPD by entirely basing the diagnosis of COPD upon the measurement of airflow limitation. It also emphasized the need to educate primary care and general practitioners, and to promote objective criterion.

Today, pulmonary function testing to evaluate airflow limitation is by definition necessary to diagnose COPD and also contributes immensely to its management. The various approaches and their relative merits are summarized in the following sections. To conform to the GOLD definition of COPD, pulmonary function testing needs to be done initially to look for airflow limitation, followed by the response to bronchodilators to look for reversibility and finally, multiple times thereafter to call the obstruction as persistent or progressive, these being key features of COPD. However, this does not mean that the GOLD definition is all inclusive and there is scope to incorporate factors such as dyspnea, which correlates well with subjective disability and quality of life (QoL); as well as other assessment of functional capacity like the 6-minute walk test.

CLINICAL NEED FOR PULMONARY FUNCTION TESTS

Early Diagnosis

The need for pulmonary function testing in diagnosing COPD is not just a question of semantics and academic distinctions. COPD has a relatively silent stage where measurable airflow limitation exists despite a paucity of symptoms. In this phase, smoking cessation, the most effective intervention, can arrest the progression of COPD. Therapeutic options in advanced stages are poor and cannot reverse the disease. In a large study conducted in the United States,[4] it was seen that most patients with spirometric abnormalities diagnostic of COPD or other obstructive disease never had their conditions diagnosed, nor were they receiving systematic therapy. Similar studies in the United Kingdom[5] and Canada[6] show strikingly similar figures with about 67% of patients who visited primary care for any reason having undiagnosed obstructive disease.[6] Importantly, poor lung function was strongly associated with adverse outcomes, which could have been avoided or delayed by early diagnosis and treatment. Thus, clinicians must become aware of the fact that OAD is no longer an exclusively clinical diagnosis and there is an unmet need for better detection early, because the true prevalence of COPD is much higher than it seems. It can be very conservatively estimated that in our own practices, in the absence of lung function testing, about half of the COPD cases might be missed.

Management

Optimal management of lung diseases, including COPD, requires objective assessment of lung function in addition to the subjective assessments of well-being. In addition to guide bronchodilator therapy, subsets of COPD patients identifiable by functional testing, may benefit from treatment with inhaled corticosteroids.[7] Some of these may have an asthmatic component characterized by partial reversibility to bronchodilators and increased exhaled nitric oxide. Other important uses for pulmonary function testing in routine practice include preoperative risk assessment and determination of suitability for pulmonary surgeries.[8,9]

PHYSIOLOGICAL PRINCIPLES

It may be pertinent to briefly review the physiology of the respiratory defect in COPD before discussing the findings and interpretation of the investigations. Airflow limitation, which defines COPD, refers to a reduced maximal expiratory flow of air despite normal respiratory effort. While a full review of the mechanical properties of the lung relating to the flow of air during breathing are beyond the scope of this chapter, a brief introduction is provided in a simple mechanical model of the lung.[10,11] It can be seen that expiratory flow of air can be diminished by increased resistance of the conducting airway, reduced driving pressure, or both **(Figs 1A and B)**. Key concepts of how these mechanisms relate to COPD are discussed further.

Airway Resistance in Chronic Obstructive Pulmonary Disease

The major mechanisms of increased resistance in COPD are narrowing, dynamic closure and occlusion of airways. Narrowing of airways is due to a multitude of causes such as thickened and inflamed mucosa, hypertrophied smooth muscle, and loss of expansile stretching effects of lung parenchyma. Airway closure is a physiological mechanism by which further exhalation at lower limits of lung volumes (residual volume, RV) is prevented by apposition of airway walls. This is exaggerated in narrowed and inflamed COPD airways, sometimes to the extent that it can be seen at tidal volumes of breathing. This pathological increase in RV is compensated by hyperinflation, which is the compensatory mechanism of the lung to "pull open" the airways. This has adverse mechanical consequences leading to increased work of breathing and ineffectiveness of respiratory muscles, as discussed in the next section.

The third mechanism of airflow limitation is the occlusion of the airways, most commonly by mucus plugs. This is distinct from the increased mucus production in the large airways,

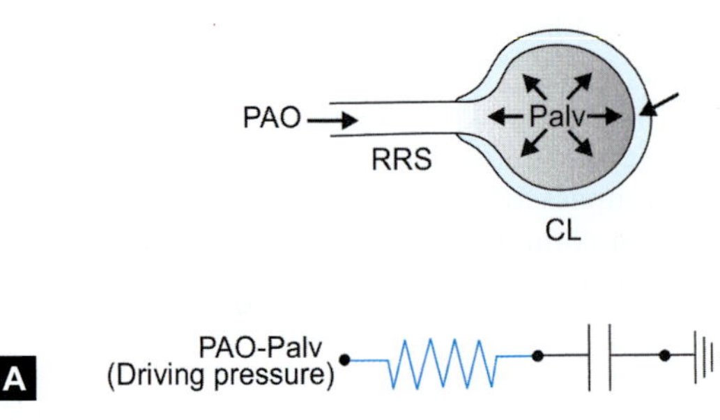

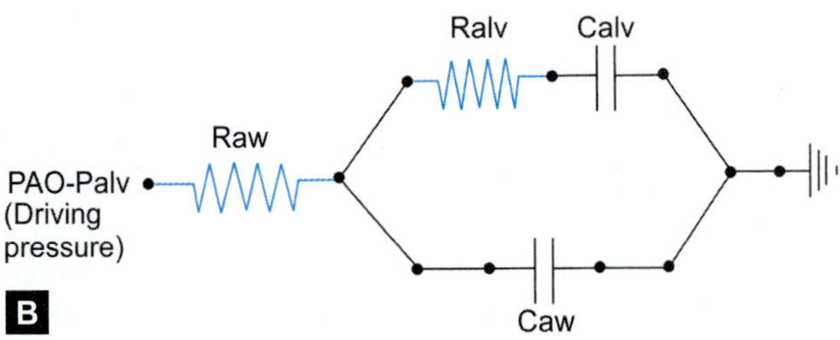

Figs 1A and B A simplified model of the lung showing airflow to the alveoli as a function of airway resistance, driving pressure and lung compliance

Abbreviations: PAO, pressure at the airway opening; Palv, alveolar pressure; PPL, pleural pressure

which while causing cough, does not cause airway occlusion. Here, it is important to realize that the bronchial tree is a parallel arrangement of resistances and hence, the increase in resistance is much greater with a homogeneous narrowing, even of a smaller degree than a localized complete obstruction. This is determined by the law of parallel resistances, $1/R = 1/R_1 + 1/R_2 + ... + 1/R_n$; such that homogeneous reduction of all airway diameters by half would lead to 16-fold increase in reductions (fourth power) while equivalent complete obstruction in terms of area, would lead to only fourfold increase in resistance. This translates conceptually to the fact that the total resistance in a parallel arrangement is lower than the lowest resistance, hence the lesser rise in resistance with a segmental collapse or a localized obstruction than with a total obstruction in a portion of the airways. Another fact to consider is that in normal lungs the cross-sectional area increases markedly while moving through the progressively higher generations of airways (Weibel's Trumpet Model).[12] Thus, the small airways with their maximal contribution to area contribute least to the resistance of the airways. Since, these are the initial sites of pathology, techniques that permit detection of small airway disease hold promise in COPD diagnosis.

Expiratory Driving Pressures in Chronic Obstructive Pulmonary Disease

In addition to obstruction, especially with emphysema as the predominant pathology, there is destruction of the lung tissue leading to a decrease in elasticity and loss of the supporting structures around airways and the alveolar walls. The loss of elastic recoil leads to reduced driving pressures for any given volume during expiratory flow, and higher volumes for a given transpulmonary pressure than the normal lung. The static expiratory pressure-volume curves **(Fig. 2)** show this as a marked deviation from the normal slope of the pressure volume relationship with a higher total lung capacity ratio (TLC), functional residual capacity (FRC) and RV. All the above changes in COPD are attended by mechanical consequences, such as flattening of the diaphragm and abnormal inspiratory muscle action angles on the ribcage. These are the primary causes for the feeling of breathlessness in COPD patients. The loss of parenchymal support also implies that airways are more prone to collapse.

The reduced driving pressures, hyperinflation and increased propensity to collapse are characteristic of COPD in contrast to increased airway resistance which is also seen in asthma. Together, these result in expiratory airflow limitation as discussed below.

Expiratory Airflow Limitation: Principles and Pitfalls

During forced exhalation, there is an effort-dependent phase, where the driving pressure is dependent upon the effort followed by an effort-independent phase where the elastic recoil of the lung determines the driving pressure. It is important to note that in the effort-independent phase, the resistive segment is not the entire airway but only the region proximal to the pressure equalization point. This point is referred to as the choke point, simplistically shown as collapse of the airway, but more accurately the point where local flow velocity reaches the local speed of wave propagation. **Figures 3A to D** show the common indices related to expiratory flow limitation during a forced exhalation maneuver. Notably, these correlate to the resistance of airways to airflow, but are only an indirect approximation since they are influenced by: Effort; lung recoil; location of choke point; and resistance of a variable segment defined by the location of choke point(s).

Other methods to indirectly assess airflow limitation include direct measurements of the resistance of the airways [whole body plethysmography (WBP), body box] or the respiratory system [impulse oscillometry system (IOS) or forced oscillation technique (FOT)].[13] These are substantially different from spirometry, which directly measures expiratory airflow limitation during a forced exhalation maneuver.

In WBP, the relationship of measured changes in airflow (dV') to calculated changes in alveolar pressure (dPalv) during breathing is used to estimate either airway resistance (Raw) or specific airway resistance [SRaw; SRaw = Thoracic gas volume (TGV) × Raw]. Since alveolar pressure changes cannot be directly measured, the patient breathes in a closed body box such that, using Boyle's law, they can be estimated (dPalv = PdV/V, where P is BTPS corrected atmospheric pressure and V is TGV). In contrast, impulse oscillometry

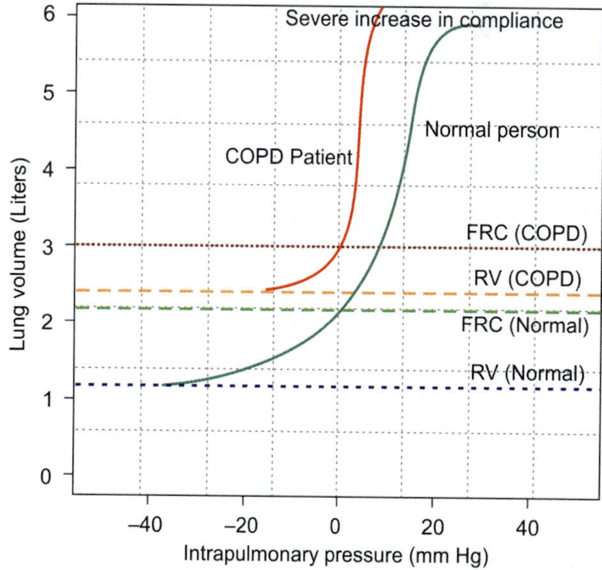

Fig. 2 Pressure-volume curve for the respiratory system of a healthy subject and a chronic obstructive pulmonary disease patient. The total lung capacity ratio (TLC), residual volume (RV) and functional residual capacity (FRC), all are increased in COPD

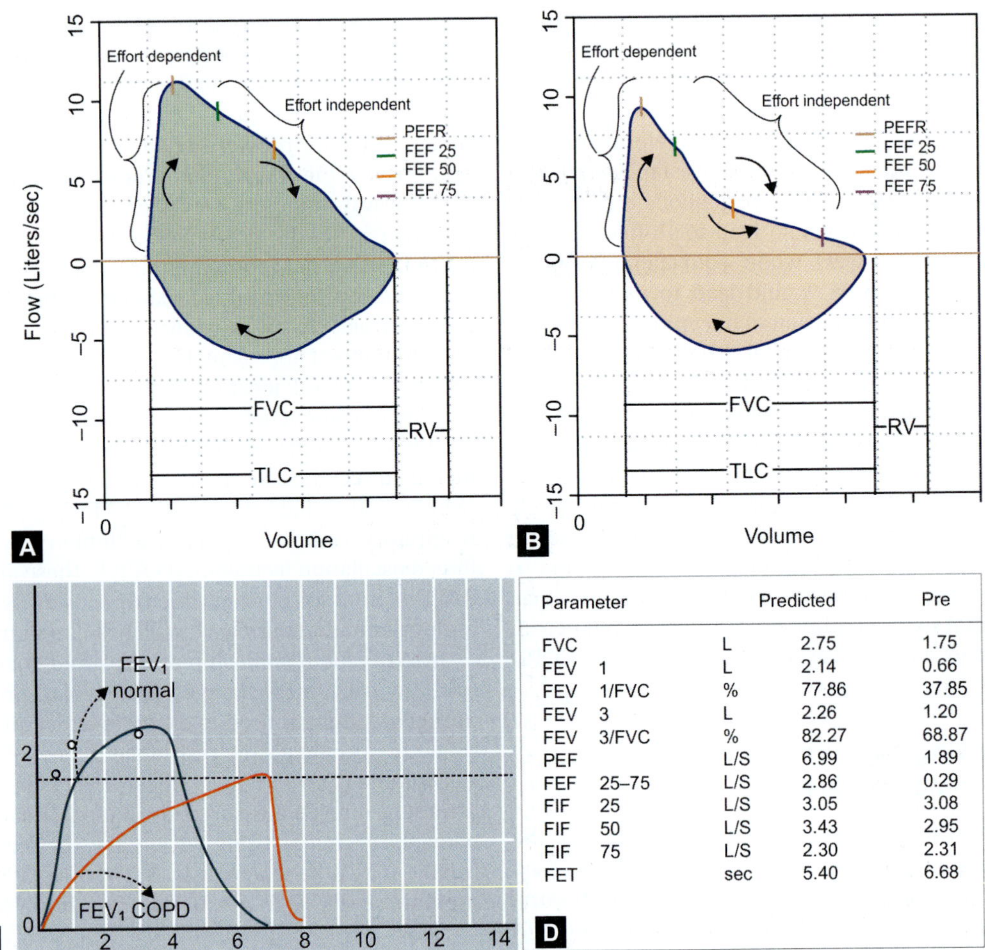

Parameter			Predicted	Pre
FVC		L	2.75	1.75
FEV	1	L	2.14	0.66
FEV	1/FVC	%	77.86	37.85
FEV	3	L	2.26	1.20
FEV	3/FVC	%	82.27	68.87
PEF		L/S	6.99	1.89
FEF	25–75	L/S	2.86	0.29
FIF	25	L/S	3.05	3.08
FIF	50	L/S	3.43	2.95
FIF	75	L/S	2.30	2.31
FET		sec	5.40	6.68

Figs 3A to D Common indices of expiratory airflow limitation (during a forced inhalation maneuver)

Abbreviations: PEFR, peak expiratory flow rate; FEF, forced expiratory flow; FVC, forced vital capacity; TLC, total lung capacity; RV, residual volume; FIF, forced inspiratory flow; FET, forced expiratory time; COPD, chronic obstructive pulmonary disease

system (IOS) or forced oscillation technique (FOT) rely upon the additional airflow (V') induced by applied pressure signal (P).

The use of suitable impulses (IOS) or pseudorandom noise (PRN-FOT), allows determination of respiratory system impedance [Zrs and its frequency dependence (Zrs{f} = P{f}/V'{f}/)]. Zrs being a complex parameter is further split into a resistive component (Rrs) and a reactive component (Xrs). The reactive component comprises of inertive behavior of air that resists acceleration and an opposing elastic behavior of lung (mostly parenchyma) that stores energy during volume expansion. Importantly, the elastic component is not the inverse of static compliance but reflects nondissipative energy storing properties of the lungs. Diseased stiff lungs that have a low compliance have reduced ability to store and return energy. In many ways, this is analogous to an electrical circuit. Advanced readers with interest in IOS can find more detailed information elsewhere.[14]

CLINICAL APPLICATIONS

Spirometry

Spirometry remains the cornerstone of diagnosis in COPD, but care must be exercised in following the procedure to the highest applicable standards.[15-19] Since, it measures flow limitation during a forced expiratory maneuver, the key aspects are adequacy of the maneuver, accurate measurement of flow, appropriate use of normal reference values, and last but not least—repetition. Quality assurance guidelines based on the standards defined by GOLD, are presented below, divided into test preparation, performance and evaluation.

Preparation

Spirometers should be calibrated on a regular basis, preferably weekly for machines that measure volume (bellows) and daily for machines that measure flow (differential pressure pneumotachograph, turbine, ultrasonic). Calibration is done by using a gas syringe that pushes known volume of air through the device at a representative flow rate. Some technologies, such as pneumotachographs, require more careful attention to calibration than others. Changes in ambient temperature may require recalibration.

The personnel conducting the test should be thoroughly trained for conducting spirometry. Since spirometers have individual quirks based on the technology used for volume/flow detection, the training must be relevant to the actual instrument in use. Except in rare circumstances, most modern spirometers provide equivalent data and are often precertified to comply with international guidelines. While a full discussion on choosing spirometers is beyond the scope of the current text, there is no such thing as "the best spirometer" and the choice depends upon the intended application.

Spirometers that provide visualization of the flow-volume loop should be used. Else, the equipment should have the capability to recognize a "bad-test", such as an inadequate expiration and prompt the possible reason for the error. It is preferable to use spirometers that conform to digital data standards that are portable across systems for easy collation of data.

Performance

Accurate and reproducible spirometry requires careful attention to the detail. The exhalation should be forceful, fast and complete. The posture of the individual should be straight to maximize the force developed by the chest and abdominal wall muscles.

At least three reproducible volume-time curves are necessary and at least two out of the three forced expiratory volume in 1 second (FEV_1) values should be within 5% or 100 mL of each other (whichever is greater). The best measurement is selected for comparison against the predicted values.

The expiratory volume-time curves should be smooth and free from irregularities. This is particularly troublesome in individuals with cough which creates irregular flows during the test. Ironically, the maneuver itself has a tendency to precipitate cough and airway closure in persons with airway disease.

The exhalation should begin from a full inspiration and should continue until it reaches a plateau. This might take anywhere between 6 and 15 seconds or even longer in severely diseased individuals.

Forced expiratory volume in 1 second (FEV_1)/forced vital capacity (FVC) ratio should be selected from the technically acceptable curve with the largest sum of FVC and FEV_1.

(*Note:* The above-mentioned procedure is repeated after a bronchodilator has been given to characterize the reversibility of the obstruction.)

Evaluation

The results are compared with the predicted normal values of FEV_1 and FVC for that particular age, sex, height and race. The ratio of FEV_1 to FVC is termed as forced expiratory ratio (FER). The postbronchodilator FER of less than 0.7, along with FEV_1 less than 80% predicted value confirms airflow limitation that is not fully reversible.

The predicted values should be appropriate for the population under study. In India, we should use local reference values rather than standard western standards that often come with the equipment.[19] However, the lack of such predictive values in the elderly creates a risk of overdiagnosing COPD due to the fall in normal lung function with age. GOLD mentions this as one of the urgent step to be taken for proper diagnosis.

The measurements should be serially repeated over time to assess the progression of airflow limitation. Typically COPD is defined as a progressive disorder without reversibility of airflow limitation. Typical shapes of flow volume loops from spirometry tests **(Fig. 4)** can help to identify the pattern and site of airway obstruction.

Spirometric Classification of Severity

In this chapter, we conform to the GOLD guidelines update 2009 for diagnosing and classifying COPD.[3] While these guidelines seem to result in the increased risk of false negatives in young and false positive in elderly subjects, compared to alternative recommendations from the American Thoracic Society (ATS) and the European Respiratory Societies (ERSs); they serve as important global standards. The spirometric classification stages the disease into four stages on the basis of severity. The initial diagnosis relies on the postbronchodilator spirometric cut-off of FEV_1/FVC as less than 0.7. These cut-off points are chosen for the sake of simplicity and have not been validated clinically, but support for taking FEV_1/FVC less than 0.7 as a diagnostic criterion comes from a study on a random sample which shows that in healthy people of all ages, the ratio was more than 0.7. This is the primary disagreement between GOLD criterion and the ATS/ERS recommendations that support use of population specific lower limit of normal (LLN) criterion that may vary with age, sex or even ethnicity. Consequently, the stages based upon these ratios are somewhat empirical **(Table 1)**. Nonetheless, for practical application, GOLD has made some effort to integrate spirometric classification with clinical picture although the synthesis is somewhat artificial because of imperfect relationship between the two.

Stage I

Mild COPD is characterized by mild airflow limitation (FEV_1/FVC <0.7; FEV_1 >80% predicted). Symptoms of chronic cough

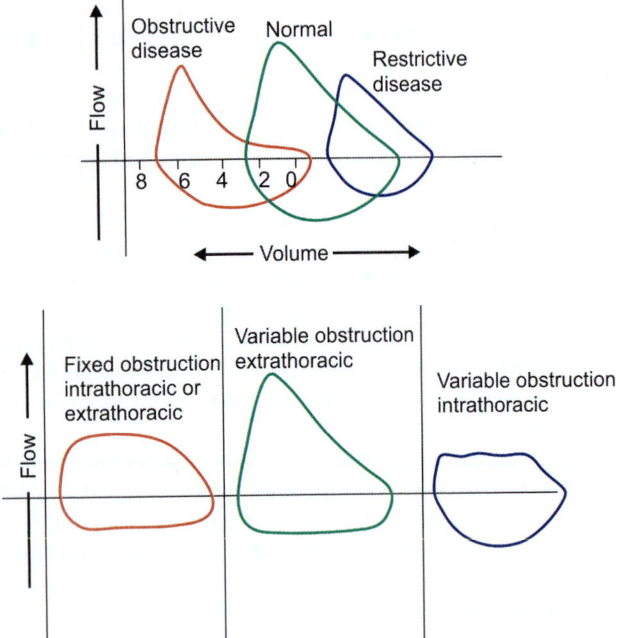

Fig. 4 Flow volume loops in some clinical situations as labeled. Extrathoracic obstructions affect inspiration, intrathoracic affect expiration and fixed such as tracheal stenosis affect both

Table 1 Summary of GOLD criterion for staging of severity of COPD

• *Stage I* – Mild FEV_1/FVC <0.7 – FEV_1 >80% predicted
• *Stage II* – Moderate FEV_1/FVC <0.7 – 50% <FEV_1 <80% predicted
• *Stage III* – Severe FEV_1/FVC <0.7 – 30% <FEV_1 <50% predicted
• *Stage IV* – Very Severe FEV_1/FVC <0.7 – FEV_1 <30% predicted or <50% predicted plus chronic respiratory failure
Respiratory failure: Arterial partial pressure of oxygen (PaO_2) <8 kPa (60 mm Hg) with or without arterial partial pressure of CO_2 ($PaCO^-_2$) greater than 6.7 kPa (50 mm Hg) while breathing at sea level
Abbreviations: FEV_1, forced expiratory volume in 1 second; FVC, forced vital capacity

and sputum may be present, but not always. The individual is usually unaware that his or her lung function is abnormal because of limitation starting with small airway involvement.

Stage II

Moderate is COPD characterized by worsening airflow limitation (FEV_1/FVC <0.7; 50%< FVC <80% predicted), with shortness of breath typically developing on exertion and cough and sputum sometimes also present. This is the stage at which patients typically seek medical attention because of chronic respiratory symptoms or an exacerbation of their disease.

Stage III

Severe COPD is characterized by further worsening of airflow limitation (FEV_1/FVC <0.7; 30% <FEV_1 <50% predicted), greater shortness of breath, reduced exercise capability, fatigue, repeated exacerbations that almost always affect the patients' quality of life.

Stage IV

Very severe COPD is characterized by severe airflow limitation (FEV_1/FVC <0.7; FEV_1 <30% predicted or <50% predicted plus chronic respiratory failure). Respiratory failure might lead to signs of right heart failure such as elevated jugular venous pressure (JVP), pitting edema at ankles and cor pulmonale due to effects on the right heart. Patients may also have stage IV (very severe COPD) even with FEV_1 more than 30% predicted if any of these complications are present. At this stage, the quality of life is appreciably impaired and exacerbations may be life threatening.

Since degree of airflow limitation correlates only modestly with the symptomatic disability, GOLD emphasizes that the spirometric classification is an educational tool and a pragmatic approach towards the initial management of the patient. It also suggests that the symptomatic impact of the disease should be taken into account because cough and sputum may precede the airflow limitation by years and hence may be important indicators for identifying the individuals at risk for developing COPD. Importantly, in the 2008 update, the previous category labeled as stage 0, aimed at identifying "at risk individuals" who were defined as "chronic cough and sputum without spirometric abnormality" has been dropped. This is because these individuals do not necessarily progress on to stage I. Nevertheless, the message that chronic cough and sputum are not normal is unchanged as before. Also, contrary to the earlier hopes of bronchodilator reversibility testing being a predictor of progression in COPD; unlike asthma, this test is now more or less abandoned except for a few indications. No clear relationship has been found between bronchodilator reversibility and disease progression. This was further complicated by increased probability of subjects with low initial FEV_1 being categorized as reversible, even with absolute increase in FEV_1 (200 mL) criterion being included. The test is presently indicated only for atypical COPD patients with history of childhood asthma or night-time awakening with cough and wheeze. The protocol for the same can be found in GOLD guidelines.

Limitations

There is a clear scope to improve upon the current spirometry based guidelines because of its limitations at the two ends of the disease spectrum, namely early disease and advanced disease. Small airway disease, which is an early marker of OADs such as COPD and asthma, is hard to detect by spirometry. This has been shown in clinical trials,[21,22] and is understandable in physiological terms because spirometry starts with a full inhalation to total lung capacity and operates over high lung volumes for most of the FEV_1 portion, thereby masking small airway disease. While indices related to the later part of the curve operating at low lung volumes, such as forced expiratory flow-25 (FEF25), are more sensitive to small airway disease, technical variability often precludes reliable use of these parameters. Very recent studies in COPD subjects report that more accurate quantification of small airway disease by impulse oscillometry correlates very well with the symptomatic disability and St George's Questionnaire measures.[23] This is discussed further in the next section.

Conventional spirometry also fails to live up to the expectations in severe disease. When a patient with severe COPD makes a maximal expiratory effort, he succeeds only in causing significant thoracic gas compression because the thoracic cage contracts, yet the gas cannot leave because of severely diminished airflow. This gas compression leads to distortion of the volume-flow relationship, inaccuracy of the FV loop and exaggerated estimates of flow limitation. In fact, if such patients were to make a submaximal effort, they would generate better airflow. This is a well-recognized problem that has been addressed by the late Joseph Rodarte's group.[24] Another important problem inherent to the current guidelines is that, they paradoxically use failure of therapeutic (bronchodilator) response for the diagnosis of COPD, yet propose to guide the therapy with the same test. However, in absence of other widely available alternatives, this represents a best possible solution focused at identifying declines in lung function and taking corrective measures.

MEASURING SMALL AIRWAY DISEASE: IMPULSE OSCILLOMETRY

As discussed in the above section on spirometry and in the introductory section in physiology, a major limitation of spirometry is that it neither truly measures resistance nor is sensitive to small airway disease which may identify early COPD. Early detection offers an opportunity for early intervention and perhaps delayed progression. Impulse oscillometry, a forced oscillation-based technique appears to be particularly promising in this regard[25,26] and is discussed in detail below.

Forced Oscillation Technique

Forced oscillation technique (FOT) is advancement in the direction of measuring pulmonary function by allowing measurements of central and peripheral respiratory resistance, without the need for performing any maneuvers. This allows the testing to be performed in subjects incapable of performing the maneuver and excludes the possibility of introducing changes in airway physiology that are attributable to the maneuver itself. As an example, investigators have observed that a forced expiration itself causes bronchoconstriction in individuals who have a tendency to develop bronchospasm. Therefore, the first measurement, which most often is not the best, affects the following measurements being performed in the same test. It has been noted previously that the deep inhalation that precedes the forced expiration, limits the ability to detect modest peripheral airway obstruction.[27]

The principle of the technique has been discussed in the section on physiology. Briefly, it uses superimposing or "forcing" external pressure signals upon the tidal volume breathing of the individual. The flow changes introduced by these small pressure changes are then utilized to calculate the "impedance of the respiratory system", as discussed earlier. The term resistance is replaced with impedance here because the pressure being applied is not constant but consists of mono- or multi-frequency sinusoidal pressure signals. In other words, it is analogous to an alternating current (AC) electrical circuit rather than a direct current (DC) one. An AC circuit has an "in phase" (real) component of impedance known as resistance and an "out of phase" (imaginary) component of impedance called reactance. Reactance can be further partitioned into the "energy storing and returning" component analogous to capacitance and an inertial component called inertance analogous to inductance in the electrical circuit theory. It is worth mentioning that the clinical use of the technique does not require much technical understanding, although an understanding of both is recommended for research related use.

A pure sinusoidal pressure wave is the basis for the mono-frequency forced oscillation technique, whereas pseudorandom noise (PRN-FOT) utilizes mathematical decomposition of a composite pressure signal generated through a computer algorithm to mimic random selection of frequencies (hence the name pseudorandom) into the component multiple frequencies.[20] Impulse oscillometry system (IOS) is a further advance that utilizes time-discrete pressure impulses (signals) rather than continuous signals, providing excellent temporal and spatial resolution. These signals are sufficiently different from the spontaneous respiratory patterns of people and do not require any special instructions to the patient in terms of breathing pattern. Impedance is a function of the forcing frequency and must be interpreted in this context. At low frequency (5 Hz), the pressure wave is able to influence flow in the entire lung, including the peripheral airways; while at higher frequencies (e.g. 20 Hz), it primarily influences the upper and central airways. Therefore, resistance at 5 Hz (R5), which is the real part of impedance, denotes the resistance of the total respiratory tree; while R20 corresponds to the upper and central airways. It can be seen that R5–R20 is a measure of peripheral airway resistance. Thus, IOS has a distinct advantage of giving differentiated spectral values of impedance at different frequencies. These parameters are quite well-studied and interpreted, although there is a much wider scope to the analysis of these measurements than is presently being employed.

Performance of the Test

The test is performed during normal tidal breathing. This makes it particularly attractive at extremes of age and in those where comprehension or circumstances, e.g. mental illness, postsurgical state, prevent performance of maneuvers. Specifically in IOS, a short reading of about 30 seconds with tidal volume breathing and impulses delivered at 0.02 second interval is recommended. Specific questions may be addressed by changing the impulse rate and the length of recording. The individual sits straight and relaxed while breathing in a relaxed manner. Swallowing movements or glottic closure is best avoided as they can cause artefacts in the reading. To avoid the dissipation of pressure at the cheeks, it is recommended to have hands kept on them, while the nose is closed off by using a nose clip.

Interpretation

A summary of the measured indices is shown in **Table 2**. Healthy lungs typically show R and Z values not more than 50% higher than the standard reference values calculated from age, sex, height and weight. Such equations are not yet published for India, but will be released soon. Our initial experience suggests that normal Indian values for these are somewhat higher than for western populations, especially in small-statured women, presumably due to smaller lungs. In health, R is minimally frequency dependent **(Fig. 5)** with R5–R20 being very low. Resonant frequency in adult subjects is typically less than 12 Hz. While a number of diseased patterns are described relating to peripheral airway obstruction, central airway obstruction and extrathoracic obstruction, a full discussion is beyond the scope of this chapter. In COPD, the pattern is typically of small airway obstruction, where R is increased beyond normal and R5 > R20. Almost invariably an increase in Fres and Ax is also seen. A volume dependence of R and Z can be seen such that they increase during expiration. IOS is extremely sensitive to small airway disease and correlates better with the symptomatic disability and St George's Questionnaire measures than spirometry.[22]

Table 2 Impulse oscillometry system parameters and typical reference values

IOS parameters	*Typical values**
Z5 (total impedance at 5 Hz)	0.33
R5 (resistance at 5 Hz)	0.31
R20 (resistance at 20 Hz)	0.30
X5 (reactance at 5 Hz)	–0.07
Fres (resonant frequency)	9.11
AX (area under the reactance curve)	1.4

* These values are for a normal Indian male, 165 cm tall, 65 kg weight. More than 50% elevation is considered abnormal.
Abbreviation: IOS, impulse oscillometry system

Impulse Oscillometry System in Diagnosis of Chronic Obstructive Pulmonary Disease

Impulse oscillometry system is a highly promising approach in COPD and was recently investigated in the ECLIPSE study (evaluation of COPD longitudinally for better definition of predictive surrogate endpoints). IOS was done in 2,054 subjects with COPD, 233 nonsmoking controls and 322 smoking

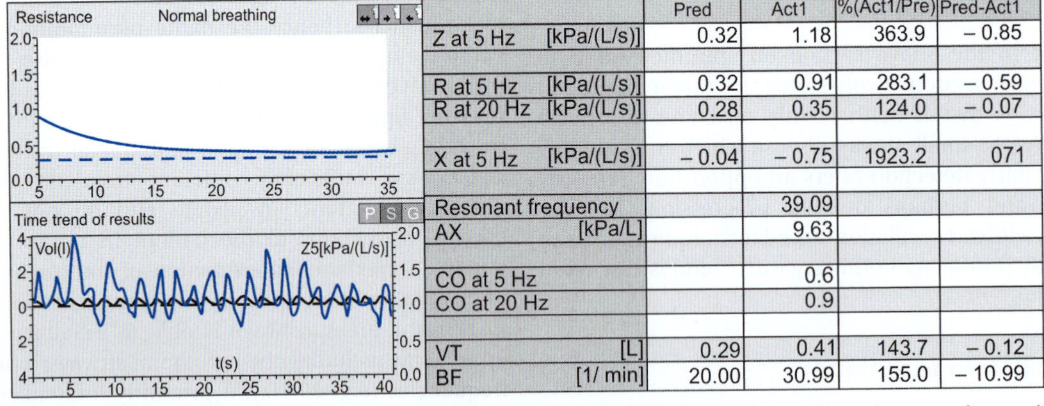

	Pred	Act1	%(Act1/Pre)	Pred-Act1
Z at 5 Hz [kPa/(L/s)]	0.32	1.18	363.9	– 0.85
R at 5 Hz [kPa/(L/s)]	0.32	0.91	283.1	– 0.59
R at 20 Hz [kPa/(L/s)]	0.28	0.35	124.0	– 0.07
X at 5 Hz [kPa/(L/s)]	– 0.04	– 0.75	1923.2	071
Resonant frequency		39.09		
AX [kPa/L]		9.63		
CO at 5 Hz		0.6		
CO at 20 Hz		0.9		
VT [L]	0.29	0.41	143.7	– 0.12
BF [1/ min]	20.00	30.99	155.0	– 10.99

Fig. 5 Representative impulse oscillometry system traces from normal (above) and chronic obstructive pulmonary disease (COPD) (below) subjects. Note the frequency dependence of R in COPD such that R5 > R20 as well as an absolute increase in R suggestive of peripheral and generalized airway obstruction respectively. Note the increase in R5 relative to R20 in COPD patient. Also note increase in total impedance at 5 Hz (Z5) during expiration in COPD

controls.[28] Computed tomography and plethysmography data were available along with spirometry. IOS measurements were only slightly more variable than spirometry and increased R5, R5–R20, and reactance were typical of COPD. While R5–R20 correlated modestly with FEF_{25-75}, the correlations were generally poor; plethysmography and reactance parameters of IOS were better correlated. Importantly, 5–10% of smokers with normal spirometry had "abnormal" IOS. These tended to be older and with a history of heavy smoking and therefore may represent small airway disease that was missed by spirometry. However, some nonsmoking controls were also found to have abnormal IOS and ranges derived from the nonsmoking controls overlapped with COPD. Further studies confirm the overlap between IOS values of patients with mild COPD and apparently healthy smokers[29] and abnormal IOS findings in apparently healthy smokers with normal spirometry,[30] suggesting that IOS provides different information than spirometry and may help in identifying early small airway disease that is missed by spirometry.

Limitations

Impulse oscillometry is not useful for the diagnosis of restrictive lung disease, since its emphasis is on resistances, not volumes. While Fres is increased in restrictive lung disease, that is a nonspecific sign. It should be noted that an IOS system is technically equipped for spirometry since it measures flow, which like spirometers is integrated to measure volumes.

OTHER TESTS

Body Plethysmography

Whole body plethysmography, more commonly known as body box because the patient sits inside a closed box, allows determination of airway resistances and TGV.[31] For any small instantaneous change in thoracic volume of the breathing subject, there is a corresponding opposite change in the box gas volume, which is detected as a box pressure change. Coupled with measurements of airflow at the mouth of the subject, this permits determination of specific airway resistance (SRaw). While techniques permitting measurements during natural breathing exist, commonly used commercial implementations require the patient to breathe in a fast and shallow pattern, similar to panting. This minimizes the glottic resistance and temperature artefacts, permitting estimation of SRaw from the slope of the trace between changes in box pressure versus airflow at the subject's mouth.

Specific airway resistance is an accurate and sensitive index of airway obstruction, being relatively independent of lung volumes and therefore insensitive to hyperinflation induced airway dilation. Interruption of airflow during panting by a shutter permits estimation of TGV from the trace between mouth pressure and box pressure. This can be readily understood as an application of Boyle's law to a closed (by shutter) thoracic gas compartment for which change in pressures during expansion and contraction is known, i.e. $PV = \text{constant} = (P + dp)\ (V + dV)$; $V = P\ (dV/dp)$ where P is atmospheric pressure and V is FRC, dP is pressure change at mouth during shutter occlusion, dV is change in thoracic volume obtained from box pressure signal. Knowledge of true FRC permits calculation of other lung volumes such as TLC, RV, etc. Lung volumes estimated by body plethysmography reflect the total compressible gas during breathing even if communication to airways is reduced or absent. Thus, volume measurements by plethysmography are superior to gas dilution methods in COPD, because of insensitivity to airway occlusion and closure that would otherwise cause systematic underestimates.

Spirometry can also be performed in the body box setup. Body box spirometry is free of compression artifacts mentioned previously and is more reliable than conventional spirometry in patients with severe COPD; however, it is technically more demanding. In addition to the regular calibration of airflow similar to spirometry, the equipment also needs to be calibrated daily for ambient conditions (room temperature, atmospheric pressure and humidity), box calibration (leak test result should typically be between 4s and 7s) and volume calibration. Regular calibration of volume and assessment of the dynamic responsiveness of the system to oscillating signals is particularly recommended. This is usually accomplished by alternately injecting and removing known volumes into the sealed body box by a piston or pump. Very importantly, the calibration factor requires adjustment for the air displaced when a subject is seated inside the box. This is a part of the standard analysis and the users only have to input correct values for the subject's weight. Importantly, patients must be adequately instructed for performance of suitable panting such that the traces obtained are reproducible and near-linear in the central regions of the trace. When used appropriately, the body box is a very sensitive pulmonary function test that can accurately measure the various components of COPD and distinguish between predominant emphysema and predominant bronchitis.

Peak Expiratory Flow Rate

Contrary to asthma, where peak expiratory flow has a distinct role in the management, it has a limited role in COPD management because the peak flow might be relatively well-preserved, despite the FEV_1/FVC ratio being low. Therefore, there is a weak correlation between the two, limiting its use in management of COPD.[32]

Helium Diffusion

Equilibration of known quantity of an inert gas that is neither consumed nor absorbed with the lungs followed by measurement of the concentration postequilibration permits determination of the unknown equilibration volume, i.e. lung volume. While this is a commonly used test in many conditions, it tends to systematically underestimate lung volume in COPD patients because equilibration can be slow and incomplete.[33]

Transfer Factor (Transfer Factor for Carbon Monoxide and Carbon Monoxide Transfer Coefficient)

This is a quantitative test for the quality of oxygen transfer across the lungs. It is based on measurement of the relative transfers of carbon monoxide (CO) and helium, when inhaled as a mixture. Helium is an inert gas and the concentration in the expired air is lesser than inspired air because of dilution with the resident gas in the lungs. On the other hand, CO is a surrogate for oxygen, since it additionally crosses the alveolar membrane and binds tightly to hemoglobin. Knowing the inhaled concentrations of these two gases, one can calculate the transfer factor expressed either as CO transfer factor (TLCO) or transfer factor per unit lung volume accessed (diffusion coefficient) to correct for nontransfer across the areas of lung which could not be accessed (e.g. pleural effusion). This is also known as carbon monoxide transfer coefficient (KCO). KCO tends to be high in airway disease, such as asthma, except when severe. Emphysema causes a fall in KCO because of loss in the area available for gas transfer by creating large airspaces and destruction of alveolar-capillary membrane. Hence, in an individual known to have COPD, KCO is a marker for the extent of emphysematous change in the lung. The utility of this test is limited by its nondiscriminatory power as KCO also decreases in conditions where restrictive or vascular changes are present in the lung.[32]

Fraction Exhaled Nitric Oxide

Although there is limited experience with this test in COPD patients, this might be useful in distinguishing cases where asthma seems to be a possible component of airflow limitation. This is because asthma, particularly of the "atopic" variety is characterized by higher levels of nitric oxide exhaled in the breath. This is correlated with the amount of eosinophilic inflammation in the airways and excellent reviews are available explaining the molecular mechanisms and the sites for generation of NO in airways.[34] The reader is encouraged to refer to these for further application.

THE FUTURE

Anticipated future trends in pulmonary function testing are described as follows:[35]

- Standardization with more physicians embracing the benefits of following common international guidelines; this seems inevitable
- *Focus on early detection:* It is increasingly recognized that onset of COPD predates onset of diagnostic changes in spirometry by many years. We hope that new guidelines will address this lacuna and move away from sole emphasis on airflow limitation.
- Convergence and portability of technology: Miniaturization of technology has already significantly reduced the size of pulmonary function testing equipment. This coupled with uniform standards, has permitted new generation devices with high user friendliness to penetrate the nonspecialist market.
- Innovative web-based applications, such as tele-pulmonary function testing, e-learning and internet-based distance education, are also likely to result in a paradigm shift in coming years.

REFERENCES

1. Petty TL. The history of COPD. Int J Chron Obstruct Pulmon Dis. 2006;1(1):3-14.
2. Ciba Guest Symposium. Terminology, definitions, and classification of chronic pulmonary emphysema and related conditions: a report of the conclusions of a Ciba guest symposium. Thorax. 1959;14:286-99.
3. Global Initiative for Chronic Obstructive Lung Disease. (2014). [online] Available from *http://www.goldcopd.org/uploads/users/files/GOLD_Report_2014_Jun11.pdf.* [Accessed in March 2016].
4. Mannino DM, Gagnon RC, Petty TL, Lydick E. Obstructive lung disease and low lung function in adults in the United States: data from the National Health and Nutrition Examination Survey, 1988-1994. Arch Intern Med. 2000;160(11):1683-9.
5. Bastin AJ, Starling L, Ahmed R, Dinham A, Hill N, Stern M, et al. High prevalence of undiagnosed and severe chronic obstructive pulmonary disease at first hospital admission with acute exacerbation. Chron Respir Disease. 2010;7(2):91-7.
6. Hill K, Goldstein RS, Guyatt GH, Blouin M, Tan WC, Davis LL, et al. Prevalence and underdiagnosis of chronic obstructive pulmonary disease among patients at risk in primary care. CMAJ. 2010;182(7):673-8.
7. Sin DD, Wu L, Anderson JA, Anthonisen NR, Buist AS, Burge PS, et al. Inhaled corticosteroids and mortality in chronic obstructive pulmonary disease. Thorax. 2005;60(12):992-7.
8. Fishman A, Martinez F, Naunheim K, Piantadosi S, Wise R, Ries A, et al. A randomized trial comparing lung-volume-reduction surgery with medical therapy for severe emphysema. N Engl J Med. 2003;348(21):2059-73.
9. Washko GR, Martinez FJ, Hoffman EA, Loring SH, Estépar RS, Diaz AA, et al. Physiological and computed tomographic predictors of outcome from lung volume reduction surgery. Am J Respir Critic Care Med. 2010;181(5):494-500.
10. Levitzky MG. Lange Physiology Series: Pulmonary Physiology, 6th edition. New York: McGraw Hill; 2003.
11. Lutchen KR, Primiano FP, Saidel GM. Nonlinear model combining pulmonary mechanics and gas concentration dynamics. IEEE Trans Biomed Eng. 1982;29(9):629-41.
12. Weibel ER. What makes a good lung? Swiss Med Wkly. 2009;139(27-28):375-86.
13. Borrill ZL, Houghton CM, Tal-Singer R, Vessey SR, Faiferman I, Langley SJ, et al. The use of plethysmography and oscillometry to compare long-acting bronchodilators in patients with COPD. Br J Clin Pharmacol. 2008;65(2):244-52.

14. Goldman MD, Saadeh C, Ross D. Clinical applications of forced oscillation to assess peripheral airway function. Respir Physiol Neurobiol. 2005;148(1-2):179-94.
15. Standardization of spirometry—1987 update. Statement of the American Thoracic Society. Am Rev Respir Dis. 1987;136(5):1285-98.
16. Standardized lung function testing. Report working party. Bull Eur Physiopathol Respir. 1983;19 (Suppl 5):1-95.
17. Derom E, van Weel C, Liistro G, Buffels J, Schermer T, Lammers E, et al. Primary care spirometry. Eur Respir J. 2008;31(1):197-203.
18. Global Initiative for Chronic Obstructive Lung Disease. (2010). _Spirometry. [online] *http://www.goldcopd.org/uploads/users/files/GOLD_Spirometry_2010.pdf.* [Accessed in April, 2016].
19. Global Initiative for Chronic Obstructive Lung Disease. (2010) [online] Available from *http://www.goldcopd.org/uploads/users/files/GOLD_SpirometryQuick_2010.pdf* [Accessed in March 2016].
20. Oostveen E, MacLeod D, Lorino H, Farré R, Hantos Z, Desager K, et al. The forced oscillation technique in clinical practice: methodology, recommendations and future developments. Eur Respir J. 2003;22(6):1026-41.
21. Verbanck S, Schuermans D, Paiva M, Vincken W. The functional benefit of anti-inflammatory aerosols in the lung periphery. J Allergy Clin Immunol. 2006;118(2):340-6.
22. Haruna A, Oga T, Muro S, Ohara T, Sato S, Marumo S, et al. Relationship between peripheral airway function and patient-reported outcomes in COPD: a cross-sectional study. BMC Pulm Med. 2010;10:10
23. Oppenheimer BW, Goldring RM, Herberg ME, Hofer IS, Reyfman PA, Liautaud S, et al. Distal airway function in symptomatic subjects with normal spirometry following World Trade Center dust exposure. Chest. 2007;132(4):1275-82.
24. Sharafkhaneh A, Goodnight-White S, Officer TM, Rodarte JR, Boriek AM. Altered thoracic gas compression contributes to improvement in spirometry with lung volume reduction surgery. Thorax. 2005;60(4):288-92.
25. Winkler J, Hagert-Winkler A, Wirtz H, Schauer J, Kahn T, Hoheisel G,.et al. Impulse oscillometry in the diagnosis of the severity of obstructive pulmonary disease. Pneumologie. 2009;63(5):266-75.
26. Winkler J, Hagert-Winkler A, Wirtz H, Hoheisel G. Modern impulse oscillometry in the spectrum of pulmonary function testing methods. Pneumologie. 2009;63(8):461-9.
27. Wang L, Paré PD. Deep inspiration and airway smooth muscle adaptation to length change. Respir Physiol Neurobiol. 2003;137(2-3):169-78.
28. Crim C, Celli B, Edwards LD, Wouters E, Coxson HO, Tal-Singer R, et al. Respiratory system impedance with impulse oscillometry in healthy and COPD subjects: ECLIPSE baseline results. Respir Med. 2011;105(7):1069-78.
29. Jarenbäck L, Ankerst J, Bjermer L, Tufvesson E. Flow-Volume Parameters in COPD Related to Extended Measurements of Lung Volume, Diffusion, and Resistance. Pulm Med. 2013.
30. Shinke H, Yamamoto M, Hazeki N, Kotani Y, Kobayashi K, Nishimura Y. Visualized changes in respiratory resistance and reactance along a time axis in smokers: a cross-sectional study. Respir Investig. 2013;51(3):166-74.
31. DuBois AB, Botelho SY, Comroe JH. A new method for measuring airway resistance in man using a body plethysmograph: values in normal subjects and in patients with respiratory disease. J Clin Invest. 1956;35(3):327-35.
32. Rees PJ, Calverley PM. Handbook of Chronic Obstructive Pulmonary Disease. London: Martin Dunitz; 2002. pp. 25-58.
33. O'Donnell CR, Bankier AA, Stiebellehner L, Reilly JJ, Brown R, Loring SH. Comparison of plethysmographic and helium dilution lung volumes: which is best in COPD? Chest. 2010;137(5):1108-15.
34. Stewart L, Katial R. Exhaled nitric oxide. Immunol Allergy Clin North Am. 2007;27(4):571-86.
35. Barnes PJ, Stockley RA. COPD: current therapeutic interventions and future approaches. Eur Respir J. 2005;25(6):1084-106.

74

Chapter

Systemic Manifestations and Comorbidities

SK Jindal, PS Shankar

INTRODUCTION

Chronic obstructive pulmonary disease (COPD), a syndrome of progressive airflow limitation caused by an abnormal inflammatory reaction of the airways and lung parenchyma, is now considered a systemic disease with widespread extrapulmonary manifestations.[1-6] There is a resultant increase in the overall morbidity, mortality, health care burden and costs. The systemic manifestations and comorbidities add to the total burden from disease morbidity and problems of management. While some of comorbidities are caused by COPD itself, the others result because of the common risk factors such as tobacco smoking or due to chronic systemic inflammation.[4] In view of the recognition of the multisystem involvement and manifestations, the disease in future may be well-classified and discussed as a disease with significant systemic component, if not a systemic disease per se.[5]

PATHOGENESIS

The mechanisms of systemic manifestations are not completely understood. The pathogenic process initiated in COPD is likely to have a variety of effects on target tissues. The pathologic changes in the lungs, such as peribronchial fibrosis, airway narrowing, destruction of alveolar walls and loss of elastic recoil lead to airflow limitation. An imbalance between oxidants and antioxidants plays an important role in the pathogenesis of COPD. Reactive oxygen species generated by neutrophils are removed by blood antioxidants and antioxidant enzymes. Thus, the ability to prevent the injurious effects of oxidative stress depends on the antioxidant capacity of the blood and the tissues. There is a marked oxidant-antioxidant imbalance in smokers and during acute exacerbations of COPD.[7] An increased oxidative burden is also likely to cause changes in fibrinolysis contributing to atherosclerosis.

Both systemic inflammation and oxidative stages are shown to play an important role in the association of COPD and atherosclerosis. A systematic search of studies had demonstrated that COPD patients had increased airway colonization presented with higher levels of both airway and systemic inflammation.[8]

The following mechanisms have been postulated to explain the pathogenesis of COPD:

Mediators and Cytokine Spillover from Lungs

There is an increase in the circulating levels of a variety of cytokine mediators such as interleukin (IL)-1 beta, IL6 and tumor necrosis factor (TNF)-alpha and interferon (IF)-gamma and leptin in patients with COPD.[9-18] Migration and activation of inflammatory cells are regulated by cytokines and chemokines, secreted by epithelial cells, endothelial cells, smooth muscle cells, fibroblasts and inflammatory cells. The systemic effects, however, are not directly attributed to the changes in the lungs. Possibly they are caused by low-grade systemic inflammation due to the presence of numerous inflammatory mediators and cytokines released from the lungs into the systemic circulation, i.e. lung to plasma spill-over.[2,11-13]

A large number of cytokines, chemoattractants and other mediators have been identified. Neutrophil granulocytes are the key players and the most important chemoattractants seem to be IL8 and leukotriene B4 (LTB4).[14]

Attempts have been made to study their role through analyses of exhaled air condensates. Inflammatory cytokines have been isolated from sputum exhaled breath condensate and bronchoalveolar lavage (BAL) fluid from COPD patients.[15] Unlike in asthma, the findings in COPD have not been very helpful. Inflammatory markers in the blood [e.g. IL6, C-reactive proteins (CRPs) and fibrinogen] have been also studied.[12]

Systemic inflammatory markers in COPD were assessed in the large Bergen COPD Cohort Study on 409 patients and 231 healthy subjects aged 40–75 years.[12] Plasma levels of CRP, soluble tumor necrosis factor receptor (sTNFR)-1, osteoprotegerin neutrophil activating peptide-2, CXCL16 and chemoattractant protein-4 were determined by enzyme-linked immunosorbent assay (ELISA) tests. COPD patients had significantly lower levels of osteoprotegerin and higher levels of CRP. sTNFR-1 was significantly associated with important comorbidities such as hypertension and depression. It was thus, concluded that the presence of these circulating inflammatory mediators was an important phenotypic feature of COPD.

Peripheral Blood Inflammatory and Other Cells

The evidence from other cross-sectional studies show no clear association between lung and systemic inflammation, which suggest that the systemic inflammatory response is not caused by the "spill-over" or overflow of inflammatory mediators from the pulmonary circulation, but by the systemic peripheral, inflammatory cells such as the neutrophils and lymphocytes.[18,19] There are several other cells including the macrophages and the mononuclear cells, which are attracted by mediators such as CCL2 and CCL3. Involvement of T-lymphocytes especially the cytotoxic $CD8^+$ cells has been also postulated.

The presence of hypoxia in severe COPD may also be responsible for an increased production of cytokines which activate TNF-alpha and soluble TNF-R.[20] It is also possible that the inflammatory mediators are produced by the muscle cells or other extrapulmonary cells located in the endothelium and fatty tissue.[21]

While it is likely that different systemic manifestations are explained by different mechanisms, the concept of inflammation as responsible for multisystem involvement has been established. The understanding of these pathogenic mechanisms is expected to change the clinical practice and pharmacotherapy of COPD.[22-26]

SYSTEMIC MANIFESTATIONS

There are a large number of systemic features and comorbidities seen in COPD **(Table 1)**. Interestingly some of the general clinical features, such as weakness, weight loss, anxiety, depression and others earlier considered as "vague" or nonspecific in nature, are now identified as more definitive and significant manifestations of nonpulmonary systemic involvement.

Table 1 Important systemic manifestations of chronic obstructive pulmonary disease

1.	General	Wasting and weight loss, nutritional anomalies, anemia
2.	Musculoskeletal	Skeletal muscle dysfunction, osteoporosis, reduction in exercise tolerance and performance
3.	Cardiovascular	Pulmonary vascular disease/chronic cor pulmonale, ischemic heart disease—acute cardiac events, cardiac failure, stroke
4.	Endocrinal	Diabetes, metabolic syndrome, dysfunction of pituitary, thyroid, gonads and adrenals
5.	Neuropsychiatric	Depression, disordered sleep, anxiety, cognitive function decline

Wasting and Weight Loss

Muscle wasting and weight loss are common manifestations of COPD. The body cell mass (BCM) is the actively metabolizing and contracting tissue. The alterations in BCM, recognized clinically by weight loss, essentially pertain to loss in fat-free mass (FFM) in COPD. Loss of FFM adversely affects muscle aerobic capacity and exercise capacity.[27,28] Weight loss appears to arise from an increased basal metabolic rate occurring due to an increased work of breathing. Inhaled salbutamol, altered amino acid composition and tissue hypoxia may result in an increased metabolic rate.[29-31]

Acidosis, infection, alteration in body composition and changes in intermediate metabolism or inadequate caloric intake, especially during acute exacerbations of the disease, are associated with an increased breakdown of cell proteins, especially in muscles. An important relationship is likely with acute exacerbations.[32] There is a preferential loss of skeletal muscles, especially in the lower extremities in patients with COPD. The muscle wasting is increasingly noticed in quadriceps muscles. Physical inactivity leads to quadriceps muscle weakness in patients with advanced COPD. Quadriceps muscle weakness is related to low circulating levels of testosterone in men with COPD.[33] Histologic study of biopsy specimens obtained from the quadriceps of patients with COPD has shown a loss of aerobic type I fibers and a reduction in oxidative enzymes.[34,35] It has been hypothesized that inflammatory cytokines may contribute to muscle wasting through the inhibition of myogenic differentiation.[36]

The mechanisms underlying weight loss and muscle wasting are incompletely understood, but likely to involve an imbalance in an ongoing process of protein degradation and replacement. It may include alteration in the relative levels or activities of endocrine hormones such as insulin, growth hormone, testosterone and glucocorticosteroids.[37]

Skeletal Muscle Dysfunction

The patients with COPD exhibit skeletal muscle dysfunction characterized by muscles atrophy and diminished strength.[38] It also results in marked reduction in exercise capacity.[39] Among the muscles, diaphragm is put into constant work and it has to work against an increased load. Other skeletal muscles are utilized less due to inactivity.[40]

Skeletal muscle dysfunction is likely to occur from sedentary lifestyle, tissue hypoxia and systemic inflammation.[39] Systemic inflammation, causing muscle dysfunction, is the result of the effects of cytokines such as TNF-alpha, IL6 and IL8, and oxidative and nitroactive stress.[41] They are likely to cause protein inactivation and degradation leading to dysfunction, atrophy and apoptosis.[42] It must be noted that an increased inflammation in the lung does not correlate with increased levels of circulating inflammatory markers.

The circulating neutrophils appear to be activated in patients with COPD and they show enhanced chemotaxis and extracellular proteolysis.[43] They produce greater amount of reactive oxygen species.[44] Besides low-grade systemic inflammation, nutritional depletion, corticosteroid medication, chronic inactivity, age, hypoxemia, smoking, oxidative and nitrosamine stresses, protein degradation and changes in vascular density are some other factors contributing to muscle dysfunction in COPD.[45]

Weight loss and skeletal muscle dysfunction cause limitation in the activities and the exercise capacity of the patient with COPD and indirectly on the quality of life. There is worsening of exercise tolerance and performance, increased healthcare utilization and increased mortality.[46,47] Muscle weakness is recognized to contribute independently to poor health status. Some of these manifestations, i.e. body mass index (B), degree of airflow obstruction (O), dyspnea (D) and exercise capacity (E) (the BODE index), have been used as measures of disease severity and mortality risk in COPD.[48-50]

Cardiovascular Problems

The link between COPD and cardiovascular disease (CVD) has been shown in a large number of epidemiological, clinical and pathogenetic studies. Cardiovascular system has a complex interaction with the respiratory system.[51] Pulmonary vascular abnormalities are common in the presence of a chronic lung disease such as the COPD. Pulmonary hypertension, right ventricular dysfunction and chronic cor pulmonale have been recognized since long.[52-53] It is now known that structural changes in pulmonary arteries can occur early in COPD before the onset of hypoxemia.[54] A review of the available evidence from recently published articles emphasize the role of chronic low-grade inflammation as a common mechanism for the presence of CVD in COPD.[55] Systemic inflammation, atherosclerotic coronary heart disease and cardiovascular deaths are known as important complications of COPD.

The burden of cardiovascular as well as the cerebrovascular disease is high in COPD patients. The prevalence was 20% in COPD, compared to 7.4% in non-COPD patients on an analysis of the pooled National Health And Nutritional Examination Survey (NHANES) 2007-2010 database.[56] Similarly, there was prevalence of airflow limitation compatible with COPD in 27% patients (995) of cardiovascular disease in a multicenter study from Japan.[57]

There is significant evidence to support the COPD-CVD association. There was a significant relationship of CVD with COPD associated with a marked impairment of functional capacity and quality of life (QoL) indices.[58] Presence of other comorbidities such as psychiatric problems, alcohol abuse and diabetes, along with cardiovascular disease, are important determinants for QoL impairment.[59] In another recent report, the cardiovascular disease in COPD was significantly more common in the presence of diabetes mellitus.[60]

Cardiac failure was seen in 10–46% of patients of COPD, while 40% of patients with cardiac failure showed some evidence of COPD, about half of whom were not earlier recognized.[61] It is also reported in a study from six European and three other countries that a large population of patients who present with acute heart failure and concomitant COPD had different clinical characteristics than those without the presence of COPD.[62] There is enough data from epidemiological and other studies to show that atherosclerosis and coronary artery disease are associated with decline in forced expiratory volume in one second (FEV1). The risk for cardiovascular death was 75% greater for patients who had a lower FEV1.[63] Cardiovascular death was also shown to increase by 28% and hospitalization for cardiovascular causes by 42% for every 10% decline in FEV1.[64]

Arrhythmias in COPD are common, but rarely fatal. The right ventricular arrhythmias are more often seen in the presence of chronic cor pulmonale. There is increased occurrence of arterial fibrillation, atrial flutter and no-sustained ventricular tachycardias.[65] The occurrence of both COPD and coronary artery disease is possibly due to the shared risk factors, such as tobacco smoking, as well as to the similar pathogenic mechanisms, i.e. systemic inflammation.[66]

There is clinical as well as pathological link between the chronic inflammation in the lungs and cardiovascular disease.[67] Systemic inflammation is also present in COPD patients who undergo percutaneous coronary intervention and elevated high-sensitivity C-reactive protein before the procedure is shown to relate to adverse outcomes in such patients.[68] Recently, the United Kingdom consortium has developed a longitudinal cohort, multicenter study, evaluating the role of inflammation chronic airway (ERICA) disease to assess the key parameters of inflammation as predictors for CVD and skeletal muscle dysfunction, etc.[69]

The COPD-CVD association raises several therapeutic issues for combined treatments of both the disorders. In particular, the use of statins has been advocated to reduce the morbidity and mortality. Several recent observational studies have suggested that statins may reduce all-cause CVD-related, cancer-related or respiratory-related mortality in COPD patients.[70] Statins are also reported to decrease the frequency and severity of COPD exacerbations, although the recent prospective randomized placebo-controlled trial of simvastatin in the prevention of COPD exacerbations (STATCOPE) has failed to show any effect in reducing acute exacerbation on the time to a first exacertation.[71]

There is new evidence to say that the use of inhaled bronchodilators and inhaled corticosteroids may affect the CVD management. A systemic review and meta-analysis of eight studies on tiotropium-use in COPD demonstrated reduced relative risk of myocardial infarction (MI).[72] It is also suggested that the MI-protective effect may in fact be attributed to an effective COPD treatment.

Arterial stiffness measured by aortic pulse wave velocity (aPWV) is an important determinant of cardiovascular events and mortality. Inhaled long-acting beta agonist (LABA) and inhaled corticosteroids (ICS) may lower the raised aPWV in COPD patients and thus reduce the CVD mortality. A multicenter study has however, failed to demonstrate any significant difference in aPWV in patients administered ICS plus LABA versus tiotropium at 12 weeks treatment.[73]

It is also hypothesized that the lower levels of vitamin D seen in COPD are associated with increased total and CVD mortality. Such an association was seen in 7,746 the United States' adults of age older than 40 years without any known CVD, though the authors pointed out that age and cardiovascular risk factors might explain the association to a large measure.[74]

Endocrinal Disorders

A number of endocrine functional disorders have been described in COPD.[75] Derangements of pituitary and thyroid function, gonads and adrenals have been seen in some studies. Hypogonadism in men has been reported in 22–69% of patients; testosterone replacement is associated with modest improvement in fat-free mass and limb muscle strength.[76] Diabetes along with other manifestations of metabolic syndrome has been described especially the presence of cardiovascular disease.[2,61,66,77] The presence of CVD disease in COPD is higher in the presence of type II diabetes mellitus.[78]

Several mechanisms have been proposed to cause endocrine dysfunction—hypoxemia, hypercapnia, systemic inflammation and glucocorticoid administration for airway obstruction. The presence of endocrine imbalance increases the overall morbidity and cardiovascular risks. The decreased protein anabolism and increased catabolism affect the body mass and also accounts for muscle dysfunction. Altered renin-angiotensin-aldosterone function affects the blood flow, fluid balance and the renal function. Other systemic effects of endocrinal disorders include the disturbances of control in breathing, worsening of respiratory mechanics and impairment of cardiac function.[75]

Neuropsychiatric Derangements

Depression and anxiety are more common in COPD than in healthy age-matched controls.[79,80] Psychiatric comorbidities and alcohol abuse were strong determinants of health-related QoL in COPD patients.[59] Disordered sleep is commonly ascribed to hypoxemia, hypercapnia and diminished ventilatory responses.[78,81] It is further aggravated by the concomitant presence of nocturnal respiratory symptoms, anxiety and depression. Obstructive sleep apnea is present in about 10–15% patients of COPD ("overlap syndrome").[81] Other sleep disturbances seen in more than half of the COPD patients include the diminished arousal responses, longer latency in falling asleep, more frequent awakenings or generalized insomnia.[82] The severity of sleep disturbances increase with the severity of disease.

Impairment of intellectual function is also common.[83] The cognitive decline, along with other neuropsychiatric problems, is attributed to the presence of hypoxemia and has shown to improve with long-term oxygen therapy in some small studies.[84] More work requires to be done on the subject.

Osteoporosis

Osteopenia and osteoporosis were reported in 68% of patients with COPD.[85] It is characterized by low bone mass and microarchitectural destruction of bones. Osteoporosis may lead to generalized bony pains, compression fracture of the spine and compromised lung function due to kyphosis and thoracic vertebral compression. Corticosteroid therapy, including inhaled steroids, is generally considered responsible for osteoporosis; although in one study, compression fractures were reported in 49% of patients who had COPD and had never received steroids.[86] Other common risk factors for COPD and osteoporosis include the older age, tobacco smoking, vitamin D deficiency and systemic inflammation.[87]

THERAPEUTIC CONSIDERATIONS

The recognition of systemic features has made the greatest impact on clinical course, complications and therapy of COPD. The variable host response and subsequent clinical phenotyping have made it possible to develop a targeted treatment with the help of a multisystem approach.[88] COPD treatment is no longer limited to inhalational and oral bronchodilators and ICS alone, but a multimodality treatment for multiple comorbidities.[89] Some of the treatment failures are possibly due to the phenotype heterogeneity of COPD and its different systemic manifestations. The future treatments with statins, angiotensin-converting enzyme inhibitors and anti-inflammatory drugs, targeting the comorbid conditions, may help to change the natural history of COPD and improve the mortality.[24-26,70,72] There are several novel anti-inflammatory agents such as the phosphodiesterase-4 inhibitor and other inhibitors of nuclear factor-κB and p38 mitogen-activated protein which may prove beneficial. Antioxidants may also help to control comorbidities.

Lastly, it is shown that the elderly patients, who are at an increased risk of almost all the comorbidities of COPD discussed earlier, may benefit from the treatment of concomitant comorbidities. Further, development of anti-aging molecules, such as sirtuin agonists, can be helpful and may also reduce the risk of lung cancer.[25] It should however, not be overlooked that aging alone is not an exclusion criterion for pulmonary rehabilitation and other treatment of COPD.[90] Assessment and appropriate treatments of COPD and the comorbid conditions have been shown to provide similar benefits of management.

Management of comorbidities has significantly added to medication burden and treatment costs as for most other chronic diseases. In a study from Australia, 57% patients were using 4–7 medications and 29% using 5 or more.[91] It is therefore, important to rationalize the treatment prescriptions.

REFERENCES

1. Evans RA, Morgan MD. The systemic nature of chronic lung disease. Clin Chest Med. 2014;35(2):283-93.
2. Barnes PJ, Celli BR. Systemic manifestations and comorbidities of COPD. Eur Respir J. 2009;33(5):1165-85.
3. Agusti A, Soriano JB. COPD as a systemic disease. COPD. 2008;5:133-8.
4. Cavailles A, Brinchault-Rabin G, Dixmier A, Goupil F, Gut-Gobert C, Marchand-Adam S, et al. Comorbidities of COPD. Eur Respir Rev. 2013;22(130):454-75.
5. Huertas A, Palange P. COPD: a multifactorial systemic disease. Ther Adv Respir Dis. 2011;5(3):217-24.
6. Stone AC, Nici L. Other systemic manifestations of chronic obstructive pulmonary disease. Clin Chest Med. 2007;28(3):553-7.
7. Rahman I, Morrison D, Donaldson K, MacNee W. Systemic oxidative stress in asthma, COPD and smokers. Am J Respir Crit Care Med. 1996;154(4 Pt 1):1055-60.
8. Fuschillo S, Martucci M, Donner CF, Balzano G. Airway bacterial colonization: the missing link between COPD and cardiovascular events? Respir Med. 2012;106:915-23.
9. Takabatake N, Nakamura H, Abe S, Hino T, Saito H, Yuki H, et al. Circulating leptin in patients with COPD. Am J Respir Crit Care Med. 1998;159(4 Pt 1):1215-9.
10. Majori M, Corradi M, Caminati A, Cacciani G, Bertacco S, Pesci A. Predominant TH1 cytokine pattern in peripheral blood from subjects with chronic obstructive pulmonary disease. J Allergy Clin Immunol. 1998;103(3 Pt 1):458-62.
11. Tkacova R. Systemic inflammation in chronic obstructive pulmonary disease: may adipose tissue play a role? Review of the literature and future perspectives. Mediators Inflamm. 2010;2010:585989.
12. Eagan TM, Ueland T, Wagner PD, Hardie JA, Mollnes TE, Damås JK, et al. Systemic inflammatory markers in COPD: results from the Bergen COPD Cohort Study. Eur Respir J. 2010;35(3):540-8.
13. Kardos P, Keenan J. Tackling COPD: a multicomponent disease driven by inflammation. Med Gen Med. 2006;8(3):54.
14. Larsson K. Inflammatory markers in COPD. Clin Respir J. 2008;2(Suppl)1:84-7.
15. Wouters EF. Local and systemic inflammation in chronic obstructive pulmonary disease. Proc Am Thorac Soc. 2005;2(1):26-33.
16. MacNee W. Pulmonary and systemic oxidant/antioxidant imbalance in chronic obstructive pulmonary disease. Proc Am Thorac Soc. 2005;2(1):50-60.
17. Oudijk EJ, Lammers JW, Koenderman L. Systemic inflammation in chronic obstructive pulmonary disease. Eur Respir J Suppl. 2003;46:5S-13S.
18. Vernooy JH, Küçükaycan M, Jacobs JA, Chavannes NH, Buurman WA, Dentener MA, et al. Local and systemic inflammation in patients with chronic obstructive pulmonary disease: soluble tumor necrosis factor receptors are increased in sputum. Am J Respir Crit Care Med. 2002;166(9):1218-24.
19. Noguera A, Busquets X, Sauleda J, Villaverde JM, MacNee W, Agustí AG. Expression of adhesion molecules and G proteins in circulating neutrophils in chronic obstructive pulmonary disease. Am J Respir Crit Care Med. 1998;158(5 Pt 1):1664-8.
20. Takabatake N, Nakamura H, Abe S, Inoue S, Hino T, Saito H, et al. The relationship between chronic hypoxemia and activation of the tumor necrosis factor-alpha system in patients with chronic obstructive pulmonary disease. Am J Respir Crit Care Med. 2000;161(4 Pt 1):1179-84.
21. Bartoccioni E, Michaelis D, Hohlfeld R. Constitutive and cytokine induced production of interleukin-6 by human myoblasts. Immunol Lett. 1994;42(3):135-8.
22. Couillard A, Muir JF, Veale D. COPD recent findings: impact on clinical practice. COPD. 2010;7(3):204-13.
23. Birrell MA, Patel HJ, McCluskie K, Wong S, Leonard T, Yacoub MH, et al. PPAR-gamma agonists as therapy for diseases involving airway neutrophilia. Eur Respir J. 2004;24(1):18-23.
24. Celli BR. Novel concepts in the pharmacotherapy of chronic obstructive pulmonary disease. Pneumonol Alergol Pol. 2009;77(1):82-90.
25. Barnes PJ. Future treatments for chronic obstructive pulmonary disease and its comorbidities. Proc Am Thorac Soc. 2008;5(8): 857-64.
26. Celli BR. Update on the management of COPD. Chest. 2008;133(6):1451-62.
27. Palange P, Forte S, Onorati P, Paravati V, Manfredi F, Serra P, et al. Effect of reduced body weight on muscle aerobic capacity in patients with COPD. Chest. 1998;114(1):12-8.
28. Palange P, Forte S, Felli A, Galassetti P, Serra P, Carlone S. Nutritional state and exercise tolerance in patients with chronic obstructive pulmonary disease. Chest. 1995;107(5):1206-12.
29. Amoroso P, Wilson SR, Moxham J, Ponte J. Acute effects of inhaled salbutamol on the metabolic rate of normal subjects. Thorax. 1993;48(9):882-5.
30. Pouw EM, Schols AM, Deutz NE, Wouters EF. Plasma and muscle amino acid levels in relation to resting energy expenditure and inflammation in stable chronic obstructive pulmonary disease. Am J Respir Crit Care Med. 1998;158(3):797-801.
31. Sridhar MK. Why do patients with emphysema lose weight? Lancet. 1995;345(8959):1190-1.
32. Wouters EF, Groenewegen KH, Dentener MA, Vernooy JH. Systemic inflammation in chronic obstructive pulmonary disease: the role of exacerbations. Proc Am Thorac Soc. 2007;4(8):626-34.
33. Van Vliet M, Spruit MA, Verleden G, Kasran A, Van Herck E, Pitta F, et al. Hypogonadism, quadriceps weakness, and exercise intolerance in chronic obstructive pulmonary disease. Am J Respir Crit Care Med. 2005;172(9):1105-11.
34. Jacobsson P, Jadeldt L, Brundin A. Skeletal muscle metabolites and five types in patients with advanced COPD with and without chronic respiratory failure. Eur Respir J. 1990;3:192-6.
35. Maltais F, Simard AA, Simard C, Jobin J, Desgagnés P, LeBlanc P. Oxidative capacity of the skeletal muscle and lactic acid kinetics during exercise in normal subjects and in patients with COPD. Am J Respir Crit Care Med. 1996;153(1):288-93.
36. Wouters EF, Creutzberg EC, Schols AM. Systemic effects in chronic obstructive pulmonary disease. Chest. 2002;121(5 Suppl):127S-30S.
37. Bernard S, LeBlanc P, Whittom F, Carrier G, Jobin J, Belleau R, et al. Peripheral muscle weakness in patients with chronic obstructive pulmonary disease. Am J Respir Crit Care Med. 1998;158(2):629-34.

38. Skeletal muscle dysfunction in chronic obstructive pulmonary disease. A statement of the American Thoracic Society and European Respiratory Society. Am J Respir Crit Care Med. 1999;159(4 Pt 2):S1-40.
39. Agustí AG. Systemic effects of chronic obstructive pulmonary disease. Proc Am Thorac Soc. 2005;2(4):367-70.
40. Agustí AG, Noguera A, Sauleda J, Sala E, Pons J, Busquets X. Systemic effects of chronic obstructive pulmonary disease. Eur Respir J. 2003;21(2):347-60.
41. Gan WQ, Man SF, Senthilselvan A, Sin DD. Association between chronic obstructive pulmonary disease and systemic inflammation: a systemic review and a meta-analysis. Thorax. 2004;59(7):574-80.
42. Li YP, Schwartz RJ, Waddell ID, Holloway BR, Reid MB. Skeletal muscle myocytes undergo protein loss and reactive oxygen-mediated NF-kappaB activation in response to tumor necrosis factor alpha. FASEB J. 1998;12(10):871-80.
43. Burnett D, Chamba A, Hill SL, Stockley RA. Neutrophils from subjects with chronic obstructive pulmonary disease show enhanced chemotaxis and extracellular proteolysis. Lancet. 1987;2(8567):1043-6.
44. Noguera A, Batle S, Miralles C, Iglesias J, Busquets X, MacNee W, et al. Enhanced neutrophil response in chronic obstructive pulmonary disease. Thorax. 2001;56(6):432-7.
45. Kim HC, Mofarrahi M, Hussain SN. Skeletal muscle dysfunction in patients with chronic obstructive pulmonary disease. Int J Chron Obstruct Pulmon Dis. 2008;3(4):637-58.
46. Dourado VZ, Tanni SE, Vale SA, Faganello MM, Sanchez FF, Godoy I. Systemic manifestations in chronic obstructive pulmonary disease. J Bras Pneumol. 2006;32(2):161-71.
47. Man WD, Kemp P, Moxham J, Polkey MI. Skeletal muscle dysfunction in COPD: clinical and laboratory observations. Clin Sci (Lond). 2009;117(7):251-64.
48. Cote CG. Surrogates of mortality in chronic obstructive pulmonary disease. Am J Med. 2006;119(10 Suppl 1):54-62.
49. Celli BR, Cote CG, Marin JM, Casanova C, Montes de Oca M, Mendez RA, et al. The body-mass index, airflow obstruction, dyspnea, and exercise capacity index in chronic obstructive pulmonary disease. N Engl J Med. 2004;350(10):1005-12.
50. Ramels AH, Gosker HR, van der Velden J, Langen RC, Schols AM. Systemic inflammation and skeletal muscle dysfunction in chronic obstructive pulmonary disease: state of the art and novel insights in regulation of muscle plasticity. Clin Chest Med. 2007;28(3):537-52.
51. Han MK, McLaughlin VV, Criner GJ, Martinez FJ. Pulmonary diseases and the heart. Circulation. 2007;116(25):2992-3005.
52. World Health Organization. Definition of chronic cor pulmonale. Circulation. 1963;27:594-615.
53. Voelkel NF, Tuder RM. Hypoxia-induced pulmonary vascular remodeling: a model for what human disease? J Clin Invest. 2000;106(6):733-8.
54. Wright JL, Levi RD, Churg A. Pulmonary hypertension in chronic obstructive pulmonary disease: current theories in pathogenesis and their implications for treatment. Thorax. 2005;60(7):605-11.
55. Roversi S, Roversi P, Spadafora G, Rossi R, Fabbri LM. Coronary artery disease concomitant with chronic obstructive pulmonary disease. Eur J Clin Invest. 2014;44:93-102.
56. Agarwal S, Rokadia H, Senn T, Menon V. Burden of cardiovascular disease in chronic obstructive pulmonary disease. Am J Prev Med. 2014;47(2):105-14.
57. Onishi K, Yoshimoto D, Hagan GW, Jones PW. Prevalence of airflow limitation in outpatients with cardiovascular diseases in Japan. Int J Chron Obstruct Pulmon Dis. 2014;9:563-8.
58. Black-Shinn JL, Kinney GL, Wise AL, Regan EA, Make B, Krantz MJ, et al. Cardiovascular disease is associated with COPD severity and reduced functional status and quality of life. COPD. 2014;11(5):546-51.
59. Koskela J, Kilpelainen M, Kupiainen H, Mazur W, Sintonen H, Boezen M, et al. Comorbidities are the key nominators of the health related quality of life in mild and moderate COPD. BMC Pulm Med. 2014;14(1):102.
60. Rogliani P, Calzetta L, Segreti A, Barrile A, Cazzola M. Diabetes mellitus among outpatients with COPD attending a university hospital. Acta Diabetol. 2014;51(6):933-40.
61. Löfdahl CG. COPD and co-morbidities, with special emphasis on cardiovascular conditions. Clin Respir J. 2008;2 (Suppl)1:59-63.
62. Parissis JT, Andreoli C, Kadoglou N, Ikonomidis I, Farmakis D, Dimopoulou I, et al. Differences in clinical characteristics, management and short-term outcome between acute heart failure patients, chronic obstructive pulmonary disease and those without this co-morbidity. Clin Res Cardiol. 2014;103(9):733-41.
63. Sin DD, Man SF. Chronic obstructive pulmonary disease as a risk factor for cardiovascular morbidity and mortality. Proc Am Thorac Soc. 2005;2(1):8-11.
64. Anthonisen NR, Connett JE, Enright PL, Manfreda J. Lung Health Study Research Group. Hospitalization and mortality in the Lung Health Study. Am J Respir Crit Care Med. 2002;166(3): 333-9.
65. Konecny T, Park JY, Somers KR, Konecny D, Orban M, Soucek F, et al. Relation of chronic obstructive pulmonary disease to atrial and ventricular arrhythmias. Am J Cardiol. 2014;114(2):272-7.
66. Falk JA, Kadiev S, Criner GJ, Scharf SM, Minai OA, Diaz P. Cardiac disease in chronic obstructive pulmonary disease. Proc Am Thorac Soc. 2008;5(4):543-8.
67. Laratta CR, van Eeden S. Acute exacerbation of chronic obstructive pulmonary disease: cardiovascular links. Biomed Res Int. 2014;2014:528789.
68. Zhang XL, Chi YN, Wang le F, Wang HS, Lin XM. Systemic inflammation in patients with chronic obstructive pulmonary disease undergoing percutaneous coronary intervention. Respirology. 2014;19(5):723-9.
69. Mohan D, Gale NS, McEniery CM, Bolton CE, Cockcroft JR, MacNee W, et al. Evaluating the role of inflammation in chronic airways disease: the ERICA study. COPD. 2015;1(5):552-9.
70. Horita N, Miyazawa N, Kojima R, Inoue M, Ishigatsubo Y, Ueda A, et al. Statins reduce all-cause mortality in chronic obstructive pulmonary disease: a systematic review and meta-analysis of observational studies. Respir Res. 2014;15:80.
71. Criner GJ, Connett JE, Aaron SD, Albert RK, Bailey WC, Casaburi R, et al. Simvastatin for the prevention of exacerbations in moderate to severe COPD. N Engl J Med. 2014;370:2201-10.
72. Rottenkolber M, Rottenkolber D, Fischer R, Ibáñez L, Fortuny J, Ballarin E, et al. Inhaled beta-2-agonists/muscarinic antagonists and acute myocardial infarction in COPD patients. Respir Med. 2014;108(8):1075-90.
73. Pepin JL, Cockcroft JR, Midwinter D, Sharma S, Rubin DB, Andreas S. Long-acting bronchodilators and arterial stiffness in patients with COPD: a comparison of fluticasone furoate/ vilanterol with tiotropium. Chest. 2014;146(6):1521-30.

74. Lee HM, Liu M, Lee K, Luo Y, Wong ND. Does low vitamin D amplify the association of COPD with total and cardiovascular disease mortality? Clin Cardiol. 2014;37(8):473-8.
75. Laghi F, Adiguzel N, Tobin MJ. Endocrinological derangements in COPD. Eur Respir J. 2009;34(4):975-96.
76. Balasubramanian V, Naing S. Hypogonadism in chronic obstructive pulmonary disease: incidence and effects. Curr Opin Pulm Med. 2012;18(2):112-7.
77. Fabbri LM, Luppi F, Beghé B, Rabe KF. Complex chronic comorbidities of COPD. Eur Respir J. 2008;31(1): 204-12.
78. Mohsenin V. Sleep in chronic obstructive pulmonary disease. Semin Respir Crit Care Med. 2005;26(1):109-16.
79. Ferguson DM, Lynskey MT, Horwood LJ. Comorbidity between depressive disorders and nicotine dependence in a cohort of 16-year-olds. Arch Gen Psychiatry. 1996;53(11):1043-7.
80. Norwood R. Prevalence and impact of depression in chronic obstructive pulmonary disease patients. Curr Opin Pulm Med. 2006;12(2):113-7.
81. Bhullar S, Phillips B. Sleep in COPD patients. COPD. 2005;2(3): 355-61.
82. George CF, Bayliff CD. Management of insomnia in patients with chronic obstructive pulmonary disease. Drugs. 2003;63(4): 379-87.
83. Liesker JJ, Postma DS, Beukema RJ, ten Hacken NH, van der Molen T, Riemersma RA, et al. Cognitive performance in patients with COPD. Respir Med. 2004;98(4):351-6.
84. Hjalmarsen A, Waterloo K, Dahl A, Jorde R, Viitanen M. Effect of long-term oxygen therapy on cognitive and neurological dysfunction in chronic obstructive pulmonary disease. Eur Neurol. 1999;42(1):27-35.
85. Jørgensen NR, Schwarz P, Holme I, Henriksen BM, Petersen LJ, Backer V. The prevalence of osteoporosis in patients with chronic obstructive pulmonary disease: a cross sectional study. Respir Med. 2007;101(1):177-85.
86. McEvoy CE, Ensrud KE, Bender E, Genant HK, Yu W, Griffith JM, et al. Association between corticosteroid use and vertebral fractures in older men with chronic obstructive pulmonary disease. Am J Respir Crit Care Med. 1998;157(3 Pt 1):704-9.
87. Romme EA, Smeenk FW, Rutten EP, Wouters EF. Osteoporosis in chronic obstructive pulmonary disease. Expert Rev Respir Med. 2013;7(4):397-410.
88. Anderson D, Macnee W. Targeted treatment in COPD: a multi-system approach for a multi-system disease. Int J Chron Obstruct Pulmon Dis. 2009;4:321-35.
89. Nussbaumer-Ochsner Y, Rabe KF. Systemic manifestations of COPD. Chest 2011;139(1):165-73.
90. Gelberg J, Mclvor RA. Overcoming gaps in the management of chronic obstructive pulmonary disease in older patients: new insights. Drugs Aging. 2010;27(5):367-75.
91. Noteboom B, Jenkins S, Maiorana A, Cecins N, Ng C, Hill K. Comorbidities and medication burden in patients with chronic obstructive pulmonary disease attending chronic obstructive pulmonary disease pulmonary rehabilitation. J Cardiopulm Rehabil Prev. 2014;34(1):75-9.

Role of Infections in Chronic Obstructive Pulmonary Disease

Kamlesh Pandey, Suruchi Mandrekar, Sundeep Salvi

INTRODUCTION

Chronic obstructive pulmonary disease (COPD) is a leading cause of morbidity and mortality worldwide and results in an economic and social burden that is both substantial and increasing.[1] The role of infections in the pathogenesis of COPD has been the focus of interest in recent years with the introduction of new research techniques which have provided interesting information on this topic. Infections play a larger role than currently recognized in the pathogenesis of COPD, and the relationship between the two is a complicated comorbid one, which may affect both the direction and course of each problem. Historically, bacteria have been considered the main infectious cause of COPD exacerbations.[2] However, a growing body of evidence, has implicated viral respiratory infections as playing an important role in the exacerbations of COPD.[3,4] The role of chronic infection in the pathogenesis of COPD has been an active area of research with several types of pathogens potentially implicated. COPD patients have an increased risk of developing active tuberculosis (TB) compared to the general population.[5] Pulmonary TB is associated with chronic airflow obstruction, especially of the COPD phenotype, at diagnosis, during treatment, and even several years after the treatment has ended.[6] Several studies have shown that human immunodeficiency virus (HIV) infection is an independent risk factor for the development of COPD.[7] A complex picture is emerging as the epidemics of HIV, tobacco smoking and biomass fuel exposure, pulmonary TB and COPD are interacting on a global scale.[8]

INFECTION CYCLES IN CHRONIC OBSTRUCTIVE PULMONARY DISEASE

In a normal healthy subject, the respiratory tract has a remarkable ability to maintain sterility, despite having repetitive exposures to microbial inocula from micro-aspiration as well as the inhalational route. In patients of COPD the innate lung defences are impaired as a result of exposure to smoke and other toxic environmental irritants. This impairment in lung defence results in two distinct infection cycles in COPD that could contribute to progressive loss of lung function.[9]

Acute Cycle

Recurrent acute exacerbations are commonly seen in patients with COPD due to secondary bacterial or viral pathogens. Infection with these pathogens may lead to episodes of increased inflammation and worsened symptoms, which are clinically diagnosed as exacerbations of COPD. Evidence suggests that these exacerbations contribute to poor quality of life, increased mortality and further progression of the disease in COPD. Acute exacerbations are also associated with increased health-care costs for the COPD patients.

Chronic Cycle

Patients with COPD have microbial colonization in the lower airways of lung even when they are stable. This microbial colonization leads to chronic airway mucosal inflammation and lung parenchymal destruction, conceptualized as the "vicious circle hypothesis" **(Fig. 1)**.[9] This hypothesis suggests that in the presence of an impaired innate lung defence due

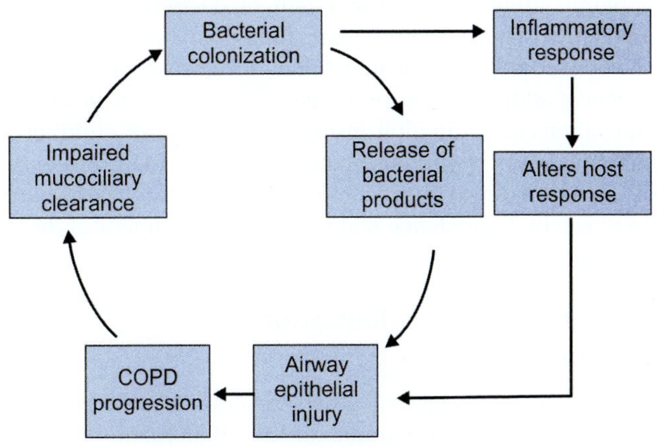

Fig. 1 The vicious circle hypothesis
Abbreviation: COPD, chronic obstructive pulmonary disease

BOX 1 Role of bacterial infection in the etiology, pathogenesis, and the clinical course of chronic obstructive pulmonary disease

- Chronic childhood lower respiratory tract infection impairs lung growth as reflected by a lower FEV_1 during adulthood
- Chronic colonization of the lower respiratory tract by bacterial pathogens induces a chronic inflammatory response with subsequent lung damage (the vicious circle hypothesis)
- Chronic infection of respiratory tissues by bacterial pathogens contributes to the pathogenesis of COPD by altering the host response to cigarette smoke or by inducing a chronic inflammatory response
- Bacteria cause acute exacerbations of chronic bronchitis, which contribute significantly to the morbidity and mortality of COPD
- Bacterial antigens in the lower airway induce hypersensitivity that enhances bronchial hyperreactivity.

Abbreviations: FEV_1, forced expiratory volume in one second; COPD, chronic obstructive pulmonary disease

BOX 2 Bacterial pathogens isolated from respiratory secretions

Potentially pathogenic microorganism PPM (infectious)	Nonpathogenic microorganism PPM (normal flora)
Haemophilus spp.—[nontypeable *Haemophilus* influenzae (NTHi)]	*Corynebacterium* spp.
Streptococcus pneumoniae	Neisseria spp.
Moraxella catarrhalis	*Enterococcus* spp.
Staphylococcus aureus	Coagulase-negative *Staphylococcus* spp.
Pseudomonas aeruginosa	*Streptococcus viridans* group
Enterobacteriaceae family (some members)	Candida spp.

Abbreviation: PPM, potentially pathogenic microorganism

to tobacco smoking or other causes, microbial pathogens become established in the lower respiratory tract, which causes further impairment of mucociliary clearance and lung defence. The chronic presence of microorganisms induces persistent airway inflammation and thus lung damage and progressive airflow obstruction.

Several putative roles of bacterial infection in the etiology, pathogenesis, and the clinical course of COPD have been identified and are described in **Box 1**.[10,11]

RECURRENT RESPIRATORY TRACT INFECTIONS IN CHILDHOOD AND ADULT LUNG FUNCTION[11,12]

Several studies have shown a lower FEV_1 and often a lower FVC among adults who experienced recurrent lower respiratory tract infection during childhood. This association has been observed even after controlling for confounding factors such as tobacco exposure and other exposures. The defect in lung function is consistent with "smaller lungs", suggesting impaired lung growth. The extent of decrease in FEV_1 is unlikely to cause symptomatic pulmonary disease on its own, but could make the individual further susceptible to the effects of additional injurious agents such as tobacco smoke and other environmental insults. The impact of childhood bacterial lower respiratory tract infection on the prevalence of COPD is likely to be greater in developing countries where there is a high incidence and inadequate treatment of these infections.[12]

Chronic Microbial Colonization or Chronic Infection

Studies have suggested that several microorganisms actively contribute to chronic airway inflammation leading to progression of COPD. In recent years, new research techniques, including molecular typing, sophisticated diagnostic tools and application of molecular technologies have been used to explore the causal relationship between chronic respiratory tract infection and exacerbation. Bacterial pathogens isolated from respiratory secretions can be divided into two groups: potentially pathogenic microorganisms (PPMs) and nonpotentially pathogenic microorganisms (non-PPMs) **(Boxes 2 and 3)**.[13]

BOX 3 Risk factors for colonization with potentially pathogenic microorganisms

- Current or previous smoking
- Impaired lung function
- Recurrent exacerbations
- Bronchiectasis

Potentially pathogenic microorganisms commonly cause respiratory infections.[14] Non-PPMs belong to the normal oropharyngeal or gastrointestinal flora and they are usually not involved in respiratory infections in immunocompetent individuals.[15] The most frequently isolated organisms (PPMs) in stable COPD are nontypeable *Haemophilus influenzae (NTHi), Streptococcus pneumoniae, Moraxella catarrhalis* and *Haemophilus parainfluenzae* patients while *Pseudomonas* spp. predominantly appear in more advanced disease.[16] Sometimes more than one pathogen can be isolated simultaneously in the same patient.

Pathogenesis

For the establishment and proliferation of microorganisms in the lower airways the host-pathogen interaction is very important. Impaired lung defense can manifest as defective phagocytosis and hyporesponsiveness of alveolar macrophages to bacterial antigens, leading to reduced clearance of bacterial pathogens and subsequent predisposition to colonization and infection.[17] It is not clear whether reduced mucociliary clearance and increased mucus hypersecretion are the

BOX 4 Important host factors

- Impaired innate immunity
- Reduced mucociliary clearance
- Mucus hypersecretion
- Bronchiectasis

causes or results of bacterial presence in the lower airways.[18] Important host factors are described in **Box 4**.

Bacteria release molecules with potent proinflammatory effects such as endotoxins (e.g. lipopolysaccharide of nontypeable *H. influenzae*), outer membrane lipoproteins (e.g. outer membrane protein (OMP) P2 and OMP P6 of nontypeable *H. influenzae*), peptydoglycan fragments, lipoteichoic acid and toxins such as pneumolysin from *S. pneumoniae*.[19] As a response to these bacterial molecules, airway epithelial cells and macrophages produce a variety of different inflammatory mediators, e.g. interleukin (IL)-6, IL8, IL10, tumor necrosis factor (TNF-α), macrophage chemotactic protein (MCP)-1, macrophage inflammatory protein (MIP)-1α, which further leads to recruitment and activation of neutrophils, macrophages and other inflammatory cells.[20-23]

Different bacterial species and even different strains of the same species differ in virulence and inflammatory potential. There is an interspecies diversity in the duration of colonization. Bacterial colonization is a dynamic process with changes in pathogens, their strains and loads occurring over time. A change in bacterial strain and/or a rise in bacterial load can increase the degree of airway and systemic inflammation and trigger the onset of an exacerbation.[24]

Nontypeable *H. influenzae* involves adherence to mucous membranes and extracellular matrix, damages epithelial cells, has ciliotoxic activity, leads to increase in mucin production as well as has complex mechanisms of evading host immune defences such as invasion into the epithelial cells, production of IgA proteases and antigenic heterogeneity.[25,26]

Chronic obstructive pulmonary disease patients who have chronic microbial colonization have higher concentrations of inflammatory cytokines, greater neutrophils number and their proinflammatory products in respiratory secretions in comparison with noncolonized patients with a similar degree of airflow obstruction. Chronic colonizers have worse health status, increased frequency of exacerbation, are more symptomatic, and have an accelerated decline in lung function. Bacteria accelerate decline in FEV_1 by increasing the number of exacerbations and increasing the basal chronic inflammation in the lungs of stable state.[27-29] Recently it was suggested that the term chronic bronchial infection would be more appropriate for the presence of significant concentrations of PPMs in the lower airways of stable COPD patients.[17] The presence of PPM is associated with inflammatory response in the lungs and also causes damage to the lungs and hence does not fit with the definition of colonization. Such patients have chronic production of purulent sputum.

Respiratory viruses and atypical bacteria may also be present in the form of chronic infection. A study on stable COPD patients that analyzed the nasal aspirates and blood samples by polymerase chain reaction (PCR) methods detected presence of low grade viral infection with the respiratory syncitial virus (RSV) in 24% patients and other viruses in 16% patients.[4] These patients had higher concentrations of IL6 and plasma fibrinogen and had increased exacerbation frequency. Latent adenoviral infection has been shown to amplifiy the effect of cigarette smoke-induced lung inflammation in patients with emphysema.[30] These viruses and atypical bacteria promote inflammation and also increase the susceptibility of the airways to other pathogens.

Acute Exacerbation of Chronic Obstructive Pulmonary Disease

The American Thoracic Society/European Respiratory Society (ATS/ERS) Task Force on COPD defines acute exacerbation of chronic obstructive pulmonary disease (AECOPD) as an increase in respiratory symptoms over baseline that usually requires a change in therapy. The most widely used clinical criteria for AECOPD are increased dyspnea, sputum volume and sputum purulence.[31] The estimated annual cost of COPD is $32.1 billion in the United States and 70% of this cost is related to acute exacerbations that require hospitalization.[32,33] Acute exacerbations are the most important cause of mortality and morbidity in patients with COPD. A recent study demonstrated an in-hospital mortality rate of 8% and a 1-year mortality rate of 23%.[34] Patients with frequent exacerbations of COPD have a more rapid decline in lung function and report worse health-related quality of life than those who do not have frequent exacerbations.

During an acute exacerbation of COPD there is increased airway inflammation as well as systemic inflammation when compared to the stable state. The number of inflammatory cells like neutrophils, eosinophils and lymphocytes increase along with an increase in inflammatory mediators, including IL6, IL8, leukotriene B4 (LTB4), TNF-α, neutrophil proteases, myeloperoxidase, eosinophil cationic protein (ECP) and regulated upon activation, normal T-cell expressed and secreted (RANTES).[35] Increased inflammation induces airway mucosal edema, bronchospasm and mucus hypersecretion, which leads to increased respiratory symptoms.[36] Sputum neutrophilia is associated with airways inflammation, sputum purulence, bacterial exacerbations and also correlates with the severity of exacerbation.[35] Data suggest that up to 70% of exacerbations are caused by respiratory infections including aerobic bacteria (40–60%), respiratory viruses (about 30%) and atypical bacteria (5–10%).[37] Some authors have demonstrated polymicrobial etiology in as much as 33% of exacerbations, being particularly important in the most severe cases.[38] Environmental factors including low temperature and air pollution, noncompliance with therapy and/or abrupt withdrawal of therapy are provocation factors in some exacerbations. In certain proportion of exacerbation of chronic obstructive pulmonary disease (ECOPD) the etiology remains unknown.

The earlier pathogenesis of acute exacerbations was based on bacterial load model in which increased bacterial concentration in the lower airways was attributed as the cause of exacerbation.[39] Recent findings suggest that acquisition of new strains of bacteria or antigenic change in pre-existing strains are crucial in the pathogenesis of bacterial exacerbations, and that the change in the bacterial load with subsequent enhancement of inflammation are a secondary phenomena.[24] For example acquisition of a new strain of nontypeable *H. influenzae, S. pneumoniae* and *M. catarrhalis* was associated with a more than a twofold greater risk for an exacerbation in a cohort of stable COPD patients. Similar associations were shown by another study between change in the bacterial strain and the occurrence of exacerbations with *Pseudomonas aeruginosa.*[40]

Role of Viruses and Atypical Bacteria in Exacerbations of Chronic Obstructive Pulmonary Disease

The prevalence of viral infection in patients with AECOPD using PCR in sputum and nasal lavage was shown to be 34%.[41] The most commonly detected viruses are Picornavirus (rhinovirus), followed by influenza and RSV. Coronavirus, parainfluenza, adenovirus and human metapneumovirus are detected in significantly smaller percentages.[42] An earlier study[43] found that experimental rhinovirus infection in subjects with COPD-induced inflammatory changes similar to those are seen in naturally occurring exacerbations. Those infected COPD patients developed more severe and prolonged respiratory symptoms, greater lung function impairment and increased airway inflammation in comparison with healthy controls. The role of atypical bacteria in acute exacerbation is not completely clear. They are involved in 5–10% of exacerbations either as an independent factor or as a co-pathogen. Some exacerbations may have polymicrobial etiology with multiple interacting pathogens that can be simultaneous coinfection, secondary bacterial after a viral infection or vice versa.[44] The patients with such exacerbations are more symptomatic. The proposed mechanism is that one microorganism leads to increased susceptibility of airways to other microorganism.

Diagnosis and Management of Acute Exacerbation of Chronic Obstructive Pulmonary Disease

The clinical diagnosis of AECOPD traditionally uses some combination of the original three Anthonisen criteria: (1) increased cough, (2) dyspnea, or (3) increased sputum purulence from baseline. There are no characteristic laboratory or radiographic tests that can confirm the diagnosis of AECOPD. There are no characteristic physical findings in AECOPD. The severity of exacerbation should be assessed based on the patient's medical history and clinical signs of severity and some laboratory test. Chest radiographs are useful in excluding alternative diagnosis. Pulse oximetry is useful for adjusting supplemental oxygen levels. Arterial blood gas measurement is useful for understanding acid-base balance and presence of chronic respiratory failure and also provides vital information before initiating mechanical ventilation. Sputum gram stain and culture have a limited role in diagnosing AECOPD due to frequent colonization of airways in chronic bronchitis patients. Sputum analysis should be reserved only for patients with frequent exacerbations or in patients with purulent sputum in whom there is a suspicion of more virulent or resistant bacteria. Other tests like routine electrocardiogram (ECG), biochemical tests and whole blood counts can give vital information. Spirometry is not recommended during an acute exacerbation as it becomes difficult to perform and gives inaccurate results.

An exacerbation can be managed in an outpatient or inpatient setting depending upon the severity. The goals of treatment of COPD exacerbations are to minimize the impact of current exacerbation and to prevent development of subsequent exacerbations. The most commonly used medications in COPD exacerbations are bronchodilators, corticosteroids and antibiotics.

Short acting bronchodilators with or without short-acting anticholinergics are the preferred bronchodilators for treatment of COPD exacerbation. It can be given by metered dose inhalers or nebulizers, although nebulizers are more convenient to use in sicker patients. Sometimes intravenous methylxanthines may be used as a second-line bronchodilator in selected cases with inadequate response to short-acting bronchodilators. Systemic corticosteroids have been shown to decrease time to recovery, decrease hypoxemia, and improve FEV_1. Previous global initiative for obstructive lung disease (GOLD) guidelines recommended 30–40 mg of oral prednisolone daily for 10–14 days. The most recent iteration of the guidelines recommend a shorter duration of 5 days based on the findings from the recently published REduction by DUtasteride of prostate Cancer Events (REDUCE) trial.[45]

Role of Antibiotics in the Treatment of Exacerbations of Chronic Obstructive Pulmonary Disease

As per the GOLD guidelines antibiotics should be given to only those COPD patients:[1]

- Who have all three cardinal symptoms—(1) increase in dyspnea, (2) sputum volume, and (3) sputum purulence
- Who have two of the three cardinal symptoms, if increased purulence is one of the two symptoms
- COPD patients who are on mechanical ventilator.

The recommended duration of therapy is 5–10 days. The antibiotic choice should be based on the local bacterial resistance pattern. The initial empirical antibiotic can be an aminopenicillin with or without clavulanic acid, or a macrolide. In high risk patients culture of the respiratory secretions should guide the further antibiotic choice. The route of administration depends upon the patients ability to take oral antibiotics. The use of antibiotics in acute exacerbation is associated with reduction in short-term mortality. Patients with high risk of poor outcome are the ones who can derive the greatest benefit from early treatment with the most potent antibiotic therapy. The use of efficacious antibiotics is crucial in such patients may help prevent relapses and delay subsequent exacerbations.

Smoking Cessation for Prevention of Exacerbation of Chronic Obstructive Pulmonary Disease

Smoking cessation is the most crucial intervention that is known to reduce mortality in patients with COPD. In the lung health study,[46] there was no significant difference in the risk of hospital admission between current smokers and ex-smokers. In a large prospective population study in Denmark,[47] previous smokers had a lower risk of hospitalization for COPD [relative hazard (HR) 0.57, 95% CI 0.73 to 1.18] compared to current smokers. Another population study[48] showed a reduced risk of COPD exacerbations in ex-smokers compared with current smokers when adjusted for comorbidity, markers of COPD severity, and socioeconomic status (adjusted HR 0.78, 95% CI 0.75 to 0.87). Smoking cessation is associated with a reduced risk of COPD exacerbations, and the reduction is dependent upon the duration of abstinence.

Pulmonary Rehabilitation for Prevention of Acute Exacerbation of Chronic Obstructive Pulmonary Disease

Pulmonary rehabilitation (PR) is "an evidence-based, multidisciplinary and comprehensive intervention" for patients with COPD that is designed to reduce symptoms, optimize functional status, increase patient participation and reduce health-care costs through stabilizing or reversing systemic manifestations of the disease. Exercise training, nutrition, education and psychosocial support are important components of pulmonary rehabilitation.[49] Recently there is increasing evidence of utility of PR in early recovery period following an exacerbation. Data supports the role of PR in preventing exacerbations and in reducing acute health-care utilization. A recent Cochrane systematic review[50] of five randomized controlled trials (RCTs) of early PR postacute exacerbation concluded that there was a significant reduction in hospital admissions in patients enrolled in PR programs following an exacerbation (odds ratio 0.22, 95% confidence interval 0.08 to 0.58). More importantly, these data showed that only four patients need to receive PR in the postacute phase in order to prevent one readmission, with an overall reduction in mortality observed also (OR 0.28; CI 0.10 to 0.84). There were no serious adverse events in any of the five studies reviewed.

Role of Immunomodulators in the Prevention of Acute Exacerbation of Chronic Obstructive Pulmonary Disease

Immunity against bacteria can be achieved as a result of natural infection and an immune response following it, or due to vaccination. Bacterial immunomodulators contain killed bacteria, their lysate or components of bacterial cells. Immunomodulators are known to increase the efficiency of immune system response via both cellular and humoral mechanisms.[51] OM-85 (Broncho-Vaxom) is a preparation that contains lysates of eight bacterial pathogens, most commonly involved in respiratory tract infections viz *H. influenzae, S. pneumoniae, Klebsiella pneumoniae, Klebsiella ozaenae, Staphylococcus aureus, Streptococcus pyogenes,* the viridans group streptococci, *Neisseria catarrhalis.*

Immunoprotector effects of OM-85 are mediated by stimulation of Th1 cellular response and by inducing immunoglobulin synthesis [secretory IgA (sIgA) by B-cells].[52] The mechanism of action of OM-85 bacterial lysate is illustrated in **Figure 2**. Clinical studies have confirmed the efficacy and safety of OM-85 bacterial lysate to prevent and treat recurrent respiratory infections in children. A study evaluating the effect of OM-85,[53] in 290 elderly population found that it was associated with significant decrease in number of patients with respiratory tract infections ($p < 0.05$) and an overall reduction in antibiotic prescriptions. Another study[54] of 191 elderly patients with chronic bronchitis and COPD, found a 55% reduction in the number of days of

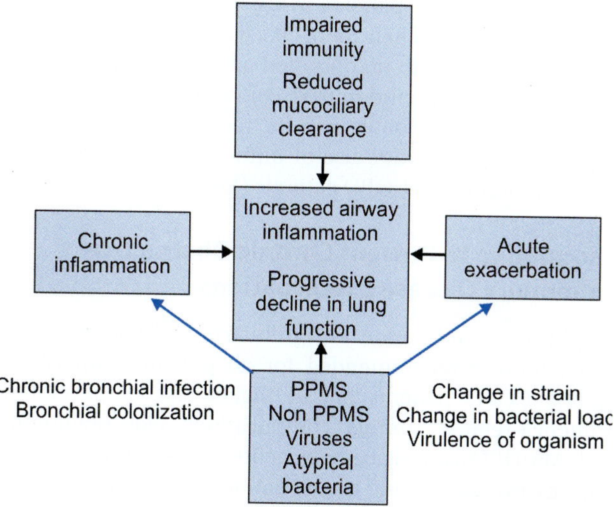

Fig. 2 Role of infections in pathogenesis of chronic obstructive pulmonary disease in stable state and in acute exacerbations
Abbreviations: PPMs, potentially pathogenic microorganisms; non-PPMs, non-potentially pathogenic microorganisms

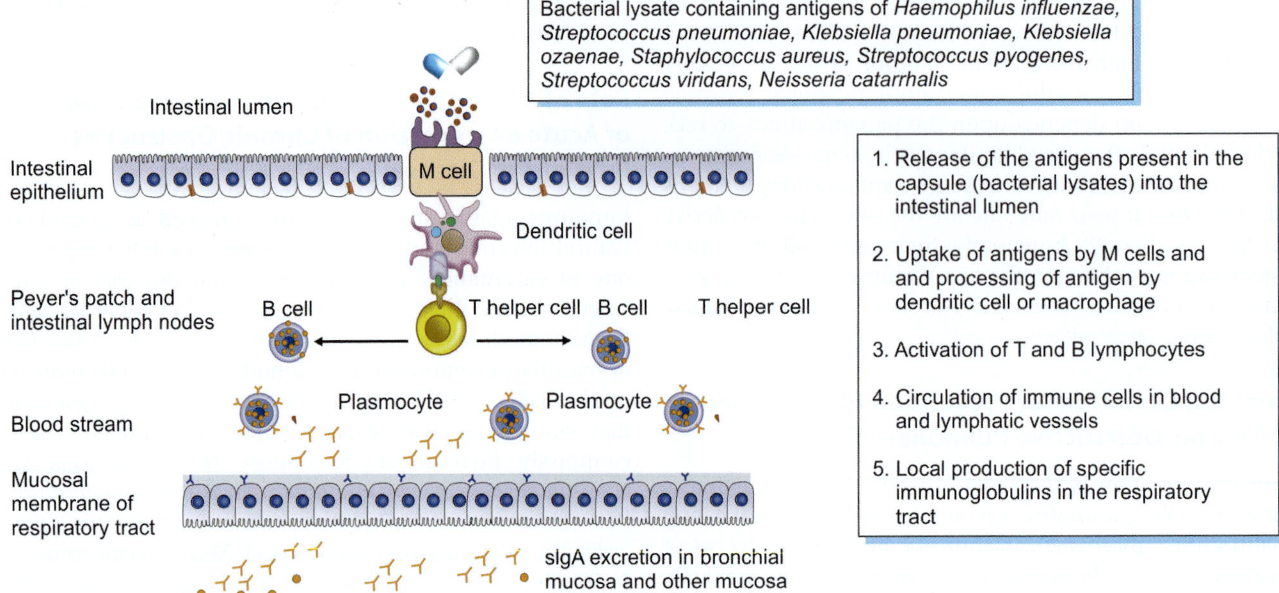

Bacterial lysate containing antigens of Haemophilus influenzae, Streptococcus pneumoniae, Klebsiella pneumoniae, Klebsiella ozaenae, Staphylococcus aureus, Streptococcus pyogenes, Streptococcus viridans, Neisseria catarrhalis
Intestinal lumen
Intestinal epithelium
M cell
Dendritic cell
Peyer's patch and intestinal lymph nodes
B cell
T helper cell
B cell
T helper cell
Blood stream
Plasmocyte
Plasmocyte
Mucosal membrane of respiratory tract
sIgA excretion in bronchial mucosa and other mucosa
1. Release of the antigens present in the capsule (bacterial lysates) into the intestinal lumen
2. Uptake of antigens by M cells and and processing of antigen by dendritic cell or macrophage
3. Activation of T and B lymphocytes
4. Circulation of immune cells in blood and lymphatic vessels
5. Local production of specific immunoglobulins in the respiratory tract

Fig. 3 Mechanism of action of immunomodulators

hospitalization and in duration of stay in the active group compared to placebo (p = 0.037). In a systematic analysis of 13 trials[55] encompassing 1,971 patients treated with bacterial extracts or placebo, sufficient evidence was not found to suggest that treatment could prevent exacerbations. However, treatment with OM-85 BV resulted in improvements of symptoms as assessed by both observers and patients, and shortening of the average duration of exacerbation. Another systematic review[56] evaluated the effect and safety of OM-85 on COPD patients in 2,066 patients and found a nonsignificant trend in favor of OM-85 in reducing frequency of exacerbations with no observed adverse effects. However more high quality randomized controlled trials with well-defined COPD outcomes will be required before we can recommend the routine use of immunomodulators for the regular treatment in COPD patients **(Fig. 3)**.

Vaccination to Prevent Chronic Obstructive Pulmonary Disease Exacerbations

Prophylactic vaccination with influenza and pneumococcal vaccination is recommended for all patients with COPD. Elderly COPD patients are at higher risk of developing influenza-related serious complications like pneumonia and AECOPD can exacerbate acute cardiovascular events such as myocardial infarction. Influenza vaccine has been shown to reduce the number of acute exacerbations and mortality in patients with COPD. A study[57] confirmed that there is increased risk of myocardial infarction after an acute lower respiratory tract infection by about five times during the first 3 days. A recent study[58] found that elderly COPD patients who had received annual influenza vaccine, had a lower risk of hospitalization for acute coronary syndrome. The antigenic content of influenza virus vaccines is changed annually due to antigenic changes in influenza viruses. The influenza vaccine is an injectable trivalent inactivated influenza vaccine (TIV) composed of seasonal H3N2, H1N1, and influenza B. The recommended regimen is influenza vaccine once a year before winter every year. The Japanese government amended preventive vaccination law to give influenza vaccine to all the elderly people who are greater than 65 years of age in November 2001. A study evaluating the effect of this amendment on nationwide mortality rate of COPD found that there was a significant reduction on the COPD mortality.[59]

Pneumococcal vaccine reduces the incidence of invasive pneumococcal disease. There are two types of pneumococcal vaccine currently available, pneumococcal capsular polysaccharide vaccine contains capsular polysaccharides from twenty-three common serotypes of *S. pneumoniae (PPSV23)* and the protein-conjugate pneumococcal vaccine that contains capsular material from thirteen pneumococcal serotypes (PCV13). All COPD patients should receive a single dose of PCV13, which should be followed by a dose of PPSV23 at least 8 weeks later. The next dose of PPSV23 is recommended at the age of 65 years or 5 years from the last dose whichever is later. Patients who are previously vaccinated with PPSV23 should receive a dose of PCV13 at least 1 year after the last PPSV23 dose and the next dose of PPSV23 should be at the age of 65 years or 5 years from the last dose,

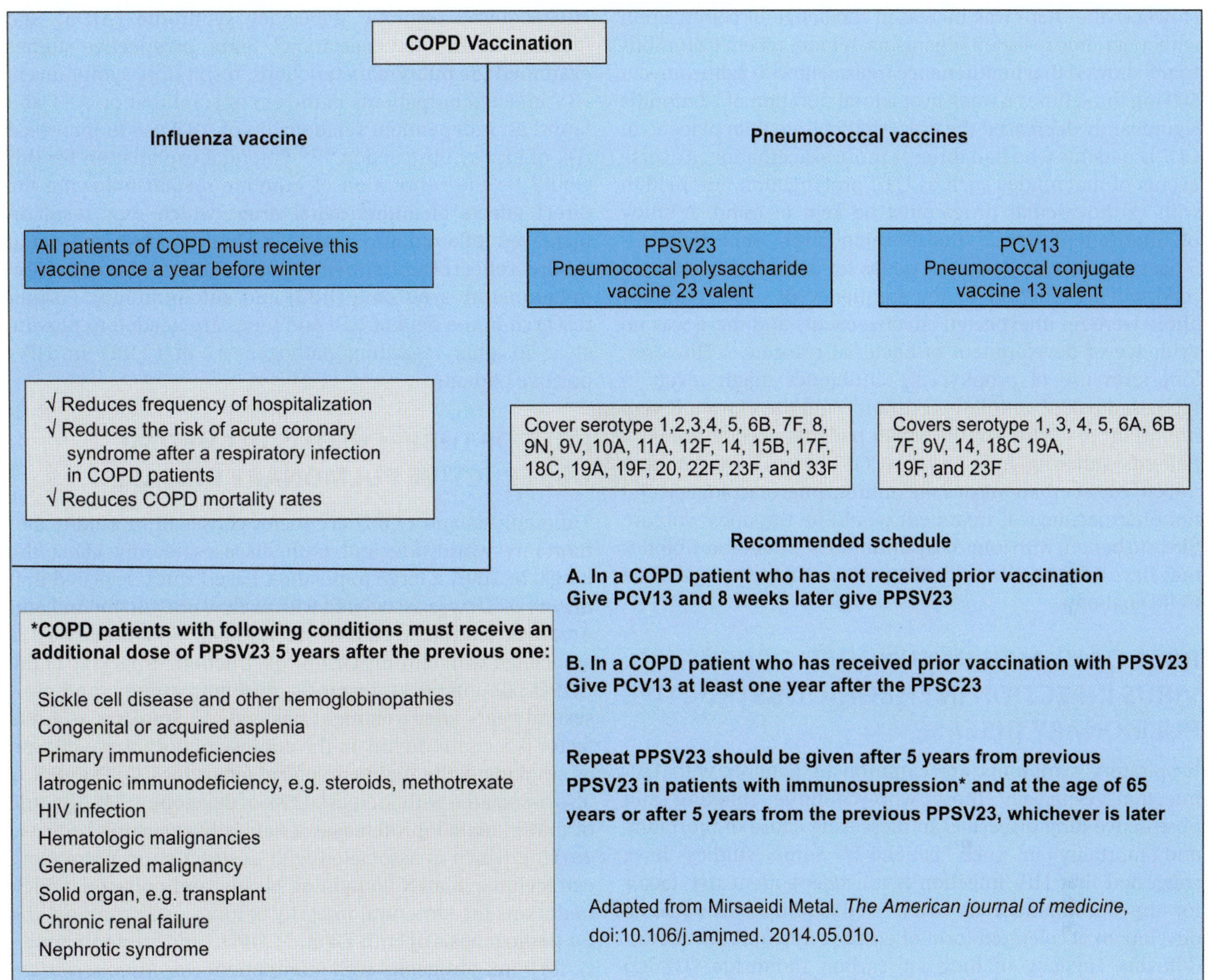

Fig. 4 Summary of recommendations for chronic obstructive pulmonary disease vaccination
Abbreviation: COPD, chronic obstructive pulmonary disease

whichever is later.[60] COPD patients with conditions causing immunosuppression must be revaccinated with additional dose of PPSV23 5 years after the previous dose. PCV13 must not be administered at the same time with influenza vaccine because it might diminish the antibody response to PCV13. Vaccination with both influenza and pneumococcal vaccine may produce an additive effect that reduces exacerbations more effectively than either vaccine alone. Future research is needed to develop newer vaccines against pathogens that are known to cause exacerbations of COPD **(Fig. 4)**.

Role of Prophylactic Antibiotics in Preventing Acute Bacterial Exacerbations of COPD

Patients with COPD may present as different clinical phenotypes. Chronic infective phenotype is one such subgroup of patients who are characterized to have frequent bacterial exacerbations, chronic dark/purulent sputum and may have underlying bronchiectasis.[17] Such patients continue to have frequent bacterial exacerbations despite optimal medications. In stable COPD patients there is presence of PPM which contribute to chronic airway inflammation and further progression of COPD. With the use of prophylactic antibiotics it may be possible to reduce the bacterial load and prevent acquisition of new strain, which may reduce frequency and severity of COPD exacerbation in these chronically infected patients. Macrolides are known to have immunomodulatory, anti-inflammatory and antibacterial effects. Recently, a large randomized controlled trial showed that in COPD patients, azithromycin taken daily for 1 year, when added to usual COPD treatment, decreased the frequency of exacerbations and improved quality of life.[61]

However the there was increased incidence of colonization with macrolide resistant organisms. A more recent Columbus trial[62] showed that maintenance treatment with azithromycin 500 mg three times a week over a total duration of 12 months significantly decreased the exacerbation rate than placebo in COPD patients who had three or more exacerbation. Adverse events of macrolides such as QTc prolongation, interaction with cardiovascular drugs must be kept in mind. A study of intermittent pulsed moxifloxacin given once daily for 5 days and repeated every 8 weeks for a total of six courses reported a reduction in the frequency of exacerbation.[63] There were no unexpected adverse events and there was no evidence of development of bacterial resistance. However, long-term use of prophylactic antibiotics might result in increased risk of antibiotic resistance and therefore it is very important to clearly stratify which patients need antibiotics. Patients suffering from severe COPD who have frequent infective exacerbations despite optimal pharmacological and nonpharmacological treatment would be the ones who are likely to benefit with long-term antibiotics. Inhaled antibiotics may have a future role in the long-term management of these COPD patients.

ROLE OF HUMAN IMMUNODEFICIENCY VIRUS INFECTION IN CHRONIC OBSTRUCTIVE PULMONARY DISEASE

Respiratory symptoms are common in patients with HIV infection, especially those who continue smoking and obstructive lung disease is an increasing cause of morbidity and mortality in such patients.[64] Some studies have suggested that HIV infection is an independent risk factor for the development of COPD.[7] HIV seropositive people develop an accelerated form of emphysema and have lower diffusing capacity of lung for carbon monoxide (DLCO) values as compared to HIV negative patients.[65,66] There have been reports of emphysema in a HIV seropositive who are nonsmoker. The potential mechanisms involved in HIV-associated COPD are listed in the **Box 5**. With the development and use of combination antiretroviral therapy (ART) there has been decline in morbidity and mortality from HIV/acquired immune deficiency syndrome (AIDS) and increase in the life expectancy.[67] Some prospective studies examined the pulmonary functions, respiratory symptoms in HIV infected outpatients in the era of combination ART and found an independent relationship of ART use to increased risk of airway obstruction.[68,69] Potential explanation for this would be the restoration of immune system following the direct effects of antiretroviral drugs which may result in increased inflammatory response. Other mechanisms could be direct effect of antiretroviral agents, immune reconstitution inflammatory syndrome (IRIS) and autoimmunity. Further research in the field of HIV and lungs are needed to provide clear insights regarding pathogenesis of COPD in HIV-positive patients.

BOX 5 Potential mechanisms involved in human immunodeficiency virus-associated chronic obstructive pulmonary disease

- Excess risk behaviors (e.g. cigarette smoking)
- Increased susceptibility to pulmonary infections and colonization
- Aberrant inflammatory responses
- Altered oxidant/antioxidant balance
- Increased apoptosis
- Effects of antiretroviral therapy:
  - Direct effects of antiretroviral drugs
  - Modified immune inflammatory response to colonizing pathogens
  - Autoimmunity.

ROLE OF TUBERCULOSIS IN CHRONIC OBSTRUCTIVE PULMONARY DISEASE

Tuberculosis and COPD are major causes of morbidity and mortality worldwide and both diseases mainly affect the lungs. In 2007, a large population based study revealed that history of TB was associated with airflow obstruction in Latin American middle-aged and older adults.[70] Pulmonary TB is associated with chronic airflow obstruction, especially of the COPD phenotype, at diagnosis, during treatment, and even several years after treatment has ended.[6] Smoking as a risk factor is a common link in the etiology of both these disease as smoking is the main etiological factor for COPD and it is also associated with increased risk of developing TB. The role of matrix metalloproteinases a naturally occurring protease enzyme which is associated with destruction of pulmonary extracellular matrix containing elastin and collagen, which maintains the structural integrity of lungs, is a common link for pathogenesis of both TB and COPD. Lipoarabinomannan (LAM) an antigenic wall component of *Mycobacterium tuberculosis* stimulates release of MMP9 and upregulates genetic expression of MMP1 and MMP9, resulting in damage to lungs and further activation of inflammatory mediators. MMPs are associated with remodeling of the pulmonary extracellular matrix (ECM) and structural changes seen in lung that is seen in both TB and COPD.[71] Recent studies suggest that COPD patients are at high risk of developing active pulmonary TB, particularly the ones who receive frequent course of oral steroids and have other comorbidities.[5,72] In developing countries, high prevalence of infectious diseases like HIV, TB and high number of smoking population and high incidence of indoor biomass fuel exposure interact together and result in a very complex lung disease. Understanding of these interactions will help in formulating policy recommendation and health planning in these countries.

In conclusion, respiratory infections play a crucial role in acute exacerbations of COPD and also during stable state in the form of chronic infection and colonization which is associated with chronic airway inflammation and progressive loss of lung function. Better understanding of the host pathogen interaction will provide us with new strategies for prevention of exacerbations and prevention of progression of disease. The interaction of HIV and TB in COPD needs attention and further research.

REFERENCES

1. Global initiative for chronic obstructive lung disease. (2014). Global strategy for the diagnosis, management, and prevention of chronic obstructive pulmonary disease. [online] Available from *http://www.goldcopd.org/uploads/users/files/GOLD_Report_2014_Jan23.pdf.* Updated January 23, 2014. [Accessed March 2016].
2. Mallia P, Johnston SL. How viral infections cause exacerbations of airway diseases. Chest. 2006;130:1203-10.
3. Role of viral infections in asthma and chronic obstructive pulmonary disease. Am J Respir Cell Mol Biol. 2006;35:513-8.
4. Seemungal T, Harper-Own R, Bhowmik A, Moric I, Sanderson G, Message S, et al. Respiratory viruses, symptoms, and inflammatory markers in acute exacerbations and stable chronic obstructive pulmonary disease. Am J Respir Crit Care Med. 2001;164(9):1618-23.
5. Inghammar M, Ekbom A, Engström G, Ljungberg B, Romanus V, Löfdahl CG, et al. COPD and the risk of tuberculosis--a population-based cohort study. PLoS One. 2010;5(4):e10138.
6. Salvi SS, Barnes PJ. Chronic obstructive pulmonary disease in non-smokers. Lancet. 2009;374(9691):733-43.
7. Crothers K. Chronic obstructive pulmonary disease in patients who have HIV infection. Clin Chest Med. 2007;28(3):575-87.
8. van Zyl Smit RN, Pai M, Yew WW, Leung CC, Zumla A, Bateman ED, et al. Global lung health: the colliding epidemics of tuberculosis, tobacco smoking, HIV and COPD. Eur Respir J. 2010;35(1):27-33.
9. Sethi S, Murphy TF. Bacterial infection in chronic obstructive pulmonary disease in 2000: a state-of-the-art review. Clin Microbiol Rev. 2001;14(2):336-63.
10. Murphy TF, Sethi S. Bacterial infection in chronic obstructive pulmonary disease. Am Rev Respir Dis. 1992;146(4):1067-83.
11. Tager I, Speizer FE. Role of infection in chronic bronchitis. N Engl J Med. 1975;292(11):563-71.
12. Shaheen SO, Sterne JA, Tucker JS, Florey CD. Birth weight, childhood lower respiratory tract infection, and adult lung function. Thorax. 1998;53:549-53.
13. Sethi S, Maloney J, Grove L, Wrona C, Berenson CS. Airway inflammation and bronchial bacterial colonization in chronic obstructive pulmonary disease. Am J Respir Crit Care Med. 2006;173(9):991-8.
14. Cabello H, Torres A, Celis R, El-Ebiary M, Puig de la Bellacasa J, Xaubet A, et al. Bacterial colonization of distal airways in healthy subjects and chronic lung disease: a bronchoscopic study. Eur Respir J. 1997;10(5):1137-44.
15. Weinreich UM, Korsgaard J. Bacterial colonisation of lower airways in health and chronic lung disease. Clin Respir J. 2008;2(2):116-22.
16. Monsó E, Rosell A, Bonet G, Manterola J, Cardona PJ, Ruiz J, et al. Risk factors for lower airway bacterial colonization in chronic bronchitis. Eur Respir J. 1999;13(2):338-42.
17. Matkovic Z, Miravitlles M. Chronic bronchial infection in COPD. Is there an infective phenotype? Respir Med. 2013;107(1):10-22.
18. Berenson CS, Wrona CT, Grove LJ, Maloney J, Garlipp MA, Wallace PK, et al. Impaired alveolar macrophage response to Haemophilus antigens in chronic obstructive lung disease. Am J Respir Crit Care Med. 2006;174(1):31-40.
19. Murphy TF. The role of bacteria in airway inflammation in exacerbations of chronic obstructive pulmonary disease. Curr Opin Infect Dis. 2006;19(3):225-30.
20. Clemans DL, Bauer RJ, Hanson JA, Hobbs MV, St Geme JW, Marrs CF, et al. Induction of proinflammatory cytokines from human respiratory epithelial cells after stimulation by nontypeable *Haemophilus influenza*. Infect Immun. 2000;68(8):4430-40.
21. Berenson CS, Murphy TF, Wrona CT, Sethi S. Outer membrane protein P6 of nontypeable Haemophilus influenzae is a potent and selective inducer of human macrophage proinflammatory cytokines. Infect Immun. 2005;73(5):2728-35.
22. Hill A, Gompertz S, Stockley R. Factors influencing airway inflammation in chronic obstructive pulmonary disease. Thorax. 2000;55(11):970-7.
23. Fuke S, Betsuyaku T, Nasuhara Y, Morikawa T, Katoh H, Nishimura M. Chemokines in bronchiolar epithelium in the development of chronic obstructive pulmonary disease. Am J Respir Cell Mol Biol. 2004;31(4):405-12.
24. Sethi S, Evans N, Grant BJ, Murphy TF. New strains of bacteria and exacerbations of chronic obstructive pulmonary disease. N Engl J Med. 2002;347(7):465-71.
25. Foxwell AR, Kyd JM, Cripps AW. Nontypeable *Haemophilus influenzae:* pathogenesis and prevention. Microbiol Mol Biol Rev. 1998;62(2):294-308.
26. van Alphen L, Jansen HM, Dankert J. Virulence factors in the colonization and persistence of bacteria in the airways. Am J Respir Crit Care Med. 1995;151(6):2094-9.
27. Patel IS, Seemungal TA, Wilks M, Lloyd-Owen SJ, Donaldson GC, Wedzicha JA. Relationship between bacterial colonisation and the frequency, character, and severity of COPD exacerbations. Thorax. 2002;57(9):759-64.
28. Banerjee D, Khair OA, Honeybourne D. Impact of sputum bacteria on airway inflammation and health status in clinical stable COPD. Eur Respir J. 2004;23(5):685-91.
29. Marin A, Monsó E, Garcia-Nuñez M, Sauleda J, Noguera A, Pons J, et al. Variability and effects of bronchial colonisation in patients with moderate COPD. Eur Respir J. 2010;35(2):295-302.
30. Retamales I, Elliott WM, Meshi B, Coxson HO, Pare PD, Sciurba FC, et al. Amplification of inflammation in emphysema and its association with latent adenoviral infection. Am J Respir Crit Care Med. 2001;164(3):469-73.
31. Anthonisen NR, Manfreda J, Warren CP, Hershfield ES, Harding GK, Nelson NA. Antibiotic therapy in exacerbations of chronic obstructive pulmonary disease. Ann Intern Med. 1987;106(2):196-204.
32. Sullivan SD, Ramsey SD, Lee TA. The economic burden of COPD. Chest. 2000;117:5-9S.
33. Ruckdeschel EA, Kirkham C, Lesse AJ, Hu Z, Murphy TF. Mining the Moraxella catarrhalis genome: identification of potential vaccine antigens expressed during human infection. Infect Immun. 2008;76(4):1599-607.
34. Groenewegen KH, Schols AM, Wouters EF. Mortality and mortality-related factors after hospitalization for acute exacerbation of COPD. Chest. 2003;124(2):459-67.

35. Sethi S, Muscarella K, Evans N, Klingman KL, Grant BJ, Murphy TF. Airway inflammation and etiology of acute exacerbations of chronic bronchitis. Chest. 2000;118(6):1557-65.
36. Veeramachaneni SB, Sethi S. Pathogenesis of bacterial exacerbations of COPD. COPD. 2006;3(2):109-15.
37. Sethi S. Infectious etiology of acute exacerbations of chronic bronchitis. Chest. 2000;117(5 Suppl 2):380S-5S.
38. Papi A, Bellettato CM, Braccioni F, Romagnoli M, Casolari P, Caramori G, et al. Infections and airway inflammation in chronic obstructive pulmonary disease severe exacerbations. Am J Respir Crit Care Med. 2006;173(10):1114-21.
39. Gompertz S, O'Brien C, Bayley DL, Hill SL, Stockley RA. Changes in bronchial inflammation during acute exacerbations of chronic bronchitis. Eur Respir J. 2001;17(6):1112-9.
40. Murphy TF, Brauer AL, Eschberger K, Lobbins P, Grove L, Cai X, et al. Pseudomonas aeruginosa in chronic obstructive pulmonary disease. Am J Respir Crit Care Med. 2008;177(8): 853-60.
41. Rohde G, Wiethege A, Borg I, Kauth M, Bauer TT, Gillissen A, et al. Respiratory viruses in exacerbations of chronic obstructive pulmonary disease requiring hospitalisation: a case-control study. Thorax. 2003;58(1):37-42.
42. Mohan A, Chandra S, Agarwal D, Guleria R, Broor S, Gaur B, et al. Prevalence of viral infection detected by PCR and RT-PCR in patients with acute exacerbation of COPD: A systematic review. Respirology. 2010;15(3):536-42.
43. Mallia P, Message SD, Gielen V, Contoli M, Gray K, Kebadze T, et al. Experimental rhinovirus infection as a human model of chronic obstructive pulmonary disease exacerbation. Am J Respir Crit Care Med. 2011;183(6):734-42.
44. Bandi V, Jakubowycz M, Kinyon C, Mason EO, Atmar RL, Greenberg SB, et al. Infectious exacerbations of chronic obstructive pulmonary disease associated with respiratory viruses and non-typeable Haemophilus influenzae. FEMS Immunol Med Microbiol. 2003;37(1):69-75.
45. Leuppi JD, Schuetz P, Bingisser R, Bodmer M, Briel M, Drescher T, et al. Short-term vs conventional glucocorticoid therapy in acute exacerbations of chronic obstructive pulmonary disease: the REDUCE randomized clinical trial. JAMA. 2013;309(21):2223-31.
46. Anthonisen NR, Connett JE, Murray RP. Smoking and lung function of Lung Health Study participants after 11 years. Am J Respir Crit Care Med. 2002;166(5):675-9.
47. Godtfredsen NS, Vestbo J, Osler M, Prescott E. Risk of hospital admission for COPD following smoking cessation and reduction: a Danish population study. Thorax. 2002;57(11): 967-72.
48. Au DH, Bryson CL, Chien JW, Sun H, Udris EM, Evans LE, et al. The effects of smoking cessation on the risk of chronic obstructive pulmonary disease exacerbations. J Gen Intern Med. 2009;24(4):457-63.
49. Nici L, ZuWallack R, Wouters E, Donner CF. On pulmonary rehabilitation and the flight of the bumblebee: the ATS/ERS Statement on Pulmonary Rehabilitation. Eur Respir J. 2006;28(3):461-2.
50. Puhan MA, Gimeno-Santos E, Scharplatz M, Troosters T, Walters EH, Steurer J. Pulmonary rehabilitation following exacerbations of chronic obstructive pulmonary disease. Cochrane Database Syst Rev. 2011.
51. De Benedetto F, Sevieri G. Prevention of respiratory tract infections with bacterial lysate OM-85 bronchomunal in children and adults: a state of the art. Multidiscip Respir Med. 2013;8(1):33.
52. Huber M, Mossmann H, Bessler WG. Th1-orientated immunological properties of the bacterial extract OM-85-BV. Eur J Med Res. 2005;10(5):209-17.
53. Orcel B, Delclaux B, Baud M, Derenne JP. Oral immunization with bacterial extracts for protection against acute bronchitis in elderly institutionalized patients with chronic bronchitis. Eur Respir J. 1994;7(3):446-52.
54. Collet JP, Shapiro P, Ernst P, Renzi T, Ducruet T, Robinson A. Effects of an immunostimulating agent on acute exacerbations and hospitalizations in patients with chronic obstructive pulmonary disease. The PARI-IS Study Steering Committee and Research Group. Prevention of Acute Respiratory Infection by an Immunostimulant. Am J Respir Crit Care Med. 1997;156(6):1719-24.
55. Steurer-Stey C, Bachmann LM, Steurer J, Tramèr MR. Oral purified bacterial extracts in chronic bronchitis and COPD: systematic review. Chest. 2004;126(5):1645-55.
56. Sprenkle MD, Niewoehner DE, MacDonald R, Rutks I, Wilt TJ. Clinical efficacy of OM-85 BV in COPD and chronic bronchitis: a systematic review. COPD. 2005;2(1):167-75.
57. Smeeth L, Thomas SL, Hall AJ, Hubbard R, Farrington P, Vallance P. Risk of myocardial infarction and stroke after acute infection or vaccination. N Engl J Med. 2004;351(25):2611-8.
58. Sung LC, Chen CI, Fang YA, Lai CH, Hsu YP, Cheng TH, et al. Influenza vaccination reduces hospitalization for acute coronary syndrome in elderly patients with chronic obstructive pulmonary disease: a population-based cohort study. Vaccine. 2014;32(30):3843-9.
59. Kiyohara K, Kojimahara N, Sato Y, Yamaguchi N. Changes in COPD mortality rate after amendments to the Preventive Vaccination Law in Japan. Eur J Public Health. 2013;23(1): 133-9.
60. Mirsaeidi M, Ebrahimi G, Allen MB, Aliberti S. Pneumococcal vaccine and patients with pulmonary diseases. Am J Med. 2014;127(9):886.
61. Albert RK, Connett J, Bailey WC, Casaburi R, Cooper JA, Criner GJ, et al. Azithromycin for prevention of exacerbations of COPD. N Engl J Med. 2011;365(8):689-98.
62. Uzun S, Djamin RS, Kluytmans JA, Mulder PG, van't Veer NE, Ermens AA, et al. Azithromycin maintenance treatment in patients with frequent exacerbations of chronic obstructive pulmonary disease (COLUMBUS): a randomised, double-blind, placebo-controlled trial. Lancet Respir Med. 2014;2(5):361-8.
63. Sethi S, Jones PW, Theron MS, Miravitlles M, Rubinstein E, Wedzicha JA, et al. Pulsed moxifloxacin for the prevention of exacerbations of chronic obstructive pulmonary disease: a randomized controlled trial. Respir Res. 2010;11:10.
64. Morris A, George MP, Crothers K, Huang L, Lucht L, Kessinger C, et al. HIV and chronic obstructive pulmonary disease: is it worse and why? Proc Am Thoracic Soc. 2011;8(3):320-5.
65. Diaz PT, King MA, Pacht ER, Wewers MD, Gadek JE, Nagaraja HN, et al. Increased susceptibility to pulmonary emphysema among HIV-seropositive smokers. Ann Intern Med. 2000;132(5):369-72.
66. Diaz PT, Clanton TL, Pacht ER. Emphysema-like pulmonary disease associated with human immunodeficiency virus infection. Ann Intern Med. 1992;116(2):124-8.
67. Palella FJ, Delaney KM, Moorman AC, Loveless MO, Fuhrer J, Satten GA, et al. Declining morbidity and mortality among patients with advanced human immunodeficiency virus

infection. HIV Outpatient Study Investigators. N Engl J Med. 1998;338(13):853-60.

68. George MP, Kannass M, Huang L, Sciurba FC, Morris A. Respiratory symptoms and airway obstruction in HIV-infected subjects in the HAART era. PLoS One. 2009.
69. Gingo M, George MP, Kessinger C, Lucht L, Rissler B, Weinmann R, et al. Pulmonary function abnormalities in HIV-infected patients during the current antiretroviral therapy era. Am J Respir Crit Care Med. 2010;182:790-6.
70. Menezes AM, Hallal PC, Perez-Padilla R, Jardim JR, Muiño A, Lopez MV, et al. Tuberculosis and airflow obstruction: evidence from the PLATINO study in Latin America. Eur Respir J. 2007;30(6):1180-5.
71. Chakrabarti B, Calverley PM, Davies PD. Tuberculosis and its incidence, special nature, and relationship with chronic obstructive pulmonary disease. Int J Chron Obstruct Pulmon Dis. 2007;2(3):263-72.
72. Lee CH, Lee MC, Shu CC, Lim CS, Wang JY, Lee LN, et al. Risk factors for pulmonary tuberculosis in patients with chronic obstructive airway disease in Taiwan: a nationwide cohort study. BMC Infect Dis. 2013;13:194.

Treatment of Chronic Obstructive Pulmonary Disease

Peter J Barnes

INTRODUCTION

Chronic obstructive pulmonary disease (COPD) is characterized in most patients by slowly progressive development of airflow limitation that is not fully reversible.[1-3] COPD encompasses chronic obstructive bronchiolitis with obstruction of small airways and emphysema with enlargement of airspaces and destruction of lung parenchyma, loss of lung elasticity and closure of small airways.[4] Chronic bronchitis, by contrast, is defined by a productive cough of more than 3 months duration for more than two successive years; this reflects mucous hypersecretion and is not necessarily associated with airflow limitation. Most patients with COPD have all three pathological mechanisms (chronic obstructive bronchitis, emphysema and mucus plugging), but may differ in the proportion of emphysema and obstructive bronchitis. At present, these different phenotypes of COPD do not appear to affect the choice of therapy. However, in the future as more specific therapies are developed, careful phenotyping may be important in selecting optimal therapy.

Chronic obstructive pulmonary disease is one of the common chronic diseases in elderly people and one of the most frequent causes of hospital admission. Globally, COPD is now the fourth most common cause of death and the only one that is increasing.[5] It is one of the most common causes of death in India.[6] Despite the enormous advances in asthma management that have taken place over the last 10 years, there have been relatively few new developments in the management of COPD. None of the existing drug therapies are able to significantly slow the relentless progression of airway obstruction, so treatment is based largely on improving lung function with bronchodilators, together with changes in lifestyle. Since, the airflow obstruction in COPD is largely irreversible and current therapies do not alter the course of the disease, existing drug treatments provide only limited benefit to the patients. There is now an urgent search for new classes of treatment that might alter the course of disease in the future.

The management of COPD has now been formalized in guidelines produced in several countries and all-propose escalating treatment, depending on the severity of airflow obstruction, symptoms and the risk of exacerbations.[7,8]

RISK FACTORS AND THEIR PREVENTION

It is likely that there are important interactions between environmental factors and a genetic predisposition to develop the disease.

Environmental Risk Factors

In industrialized countries, cigarette smoking accounts for most cases of COPD, but in developing countries, other environmental pollutants, such as particulates associated with cooking with biomass fuels in confined spaces, are important causes.[9] Even in developed countries, nonsmoking COPD may account for over 20% of COPD patients.[10] Much less is known about nonsmoking forms of COPD. Some cases are due to progression of asthma which loses its reversibility, but these are usually identified by early onset and a typical history of variable symptoms at least in the early history of the disease. In developing and emerging countries such as India, exposure to biomass fuels is an important cause of COPD, especially in women, and accounts for over 50% of cases.[11]

Air pollution (particularly sulfur dioxide and particulates), exposure to certain occupational chemicals such as cadmium and passive smoking may all be additional risk factors. The role of airway hyper-responsiveness and allergy as risk factors for COPD is still uncertain. Atopy, serum IgE and blood eosinophilia are not important risk factors. However, this is not necessarily the same type of abnormal airway responsiveness that is seen in asthma. Low birth weight is also a risk factor for COPD, probably because poor nutrition in fetal life results in small lungs, so that decline in lung function with age starts from a lower peak value. Poor nutrition may contribute to COPD and a lack of antioxidants may be particularly important.

Chest infections during the first year of life are associated with COPD in later life. There is some evidence that certain latent virus infections (such as adenovirus) may predispose

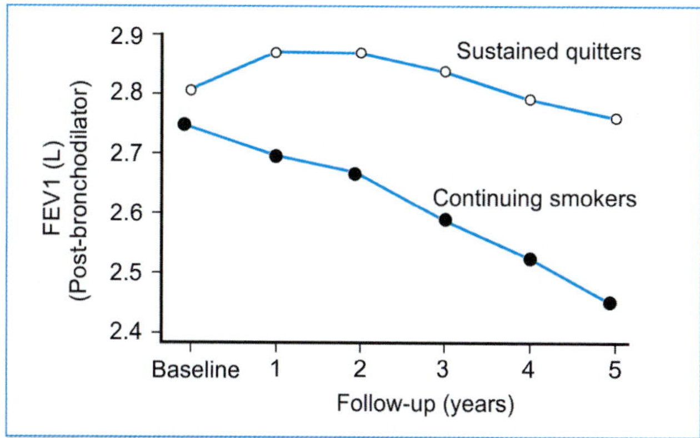

Fig. 1 Smoking cessation reduces the rate of decline of lung function in patients with COPD, if instituted early in the course of the disease[13]

to the development of COPD, but this is controversial. Many patients with COPD have a history of previous tuberculosis, whereas patients with COPD have an increased risk of developing tuberculosis, although the relationship between COPD and tuberculosis is not clear.[12]

The most important treatment strategy is avoidance of environmental risk factors wherever possible to prevent disease progression. Most attention has focused on smoking cessation strategies.

Stopping Smoking

Stopping smoking is the single most beneficial management strategy and the only intervention that reduces the accelerated decline in lung function and the number of exacerbations, and is important even in elderly patients **(Fig. 1)**. Stopping smoking also reduces the mucus hypersecretion of chronic bronchitis and markedly reduces the risks of associated cardiovascular disease.[13] Smoking cessation is more effective early in the course of disease, becomes less effective as the disease progresses to severe and very severe stage.[14]

Nicotine is addictive and stopping smoking should be viewed as the treatment of drug addiction. Abrupt quitting is more successful than gradual reduction, but even after an intensive smoking cessation program, 75% of smokers are still smoking 1 year later. There are several ways to encourage smoking cessation. Psychological counseling, group therapy and smoking reduction measures may be useful in some patients. Nicotine replacement therapy available as chewing-gum, skin patches, nasal spray and inhaler doubles long-term (6–12 months) abstinence rates.[15] Bupropion is an atypical antidepressant that acts through stimulating noradrenergic activity and has double the quit rate of nicotine replacement therapies.[16] More recently varenicline, which is a partial nicotinic agonist, has been introduced and shown to be the most effective way of quitting smoking.[17] Varenicline is usually given for 12 weeks and is well-tolerated, but some patients develop nausea, insomnia and depression.

Avoiding Biomass Fuel Exposure

It is exposure to biomass fuels (wood, charcoal, animal dung) in unventilated houses which is a major risk factor for COPD in developing countries.[18] This may be addressed by using alternative fuels, such as liquefied petroleum gas or natural gas, ethanol or biogas, although this may not be available or affordable in poor rural communities. Improving ventilation of the cooking area, reducing cooking time or cooking outdoors may also help. Substitution of traditional open fires with locally produced improved stoves has been shown to improve respiratory health in women and to improve lung function and disease progression.[19]

Genetic Factors

Longitudinal monitoring of lung function in cigarette smokers reveals that only a minority (15–40% depending on definition) develop significant airflow obstruction due to an accelerated decline in lung function (2–5-fold higher than the normal decline of 15–30 mL FEV1/year compared to the normal population and the remainder of smokers who have consumed an equivalent number of cigarettes.[20] This strongly suggests that genetic factors may determine which smokers are susceptible and develop airflow limitation. Further evidence that genetic factors are important is the familial clustering of patients with early onset COPD and the differences in COPD prevalence between different ethnic groups.[21] Patients with α_1-antitrypsin deficiency [proteinase inhibitor (Pi)ZZ phenotype with α_1-antitrypsin levels <10% of normal values] develop early emphysema which is exacerbated by smoking, indicating a clear genetic predisposition to COPD. However, α_1-antitrypsin deficiency accounts for less than 1% of patients with COPD and many other genetic variants of α_1-antitrypsin that are associated with lower than normal serum levels of this proteinase inhibitor have not been clearly associated with an increased risk of COPD. This has led to a search for associations between COPD and polymorphisms of other genes that may be involved in its pathophysiology.

So far, few significant associations have been detected and even those reported have not been replicated in other studies. A 10-fold increased risk of COPD in individuals who have a polymorphism in the promoter region of the gene for tumor necrosis factor-α (TNF-α) that is associated with increased TNF-α production has been reported in a Chinese population, but not confirmed in Caucasian populations. Several other genes have been implicated in COPD, but few have been replicated in different populations. Genome-wide association studies in COPD have found susceptibility related to two polymorphisms of the nicotinic receptor, which probably reflect propensity to nicotine addiction.[22] It is unlikely that molecular genetics will identify new therapeutic targets. Even in patients with α_1-antitrypsin deficiency, replacement therapy has been poorly effective as well as very expensive.[23] Techniques such as DNA microarray (gene chips) to detect single nucleotide polymorphisms, proteomics to detect novel proteins and gene expression profiling to measure which known and novel genes are expressed are now being employed in cigarette smokers who develop COPD compared with matched smokers who do not. This may identify markers of risk, but may also reveal novel molecular targets for the development of treatments of the future.

PHARMACOTHERAPY

Bronchodilators

Bronchodilators are the mainstay of current drug therapy for COPD, although the degree of bronchodilation is less than seen in asthma (typically about 5% improvement in FEV1, although some patients show greater responses). Bronchodilators may improve dyspnea and exercise tolerance, despite little or no effect on spirometry, by reducing lung volumes and therefore hyperinflation (air trapping). In addition, bronchodilators may reduce respiratory muscle fatigue (controversial) and improve mucociliary clearance. The choice of bronchodilator includes short- and long-acting β_2-agonists, anticholinergics (muscarinic receptor antagonists) and high doses of theophylline, will partly be determined by patient preference and cost. The preferred bronchodilators are long-acting inhaled drugs such as long-acting β_2-agonists (LABA: formoterol, salmeterol, indacaterol) or long-acting muscarinic antagonist (LAMA: tiotropium bromide, glycopyrronium, aclidinium). Several bronchodilators are available for COPD **(Table 1)**.[24]

Anticholinergics

Atropine is a naturally occurring compound that was introduced for the treatment of asthma, but because of side effects (particularly drying of secretions), less soluble quaternary compounds (e.g. ipratropium bromide) were developed. Anticholinergics are probably the most effective bronchodilators in the treatment of COPD and vagal cholinergic tone appears to be the only reversible element in the airflow obstruction of COPD.

Mode of action: Anticholinergics are specific antagonists of muscarinic receptors and inhibit cholinergic nerve-induced bronchoconstriction. A small degree of resting bronchomotor tone is present because of tonic cholinergic nerve impulses, which release acetylcholine in the vicinity of airway smooth muscle, and cholinergic reflex bronchoconstriction may be initiated by irritants, cold air and stress **(Fig. 2)**. Anticholinergics reduce air trapping by acting on small airways and thereby improve dyspnea and symptoms.

Clinical use: Ipratropium bromide and oxitropium bromide are administered three or four times daily via inhalation, whereas tiotropium bromide is given once daily by inhalation. Tiotropium is very effective in improving lung function and quality of life at all stages of disease even when added to other therapies, as shown in the large UPLIFT study[25] **(Fig. 3)**. Tiotropium also reduces severe exacerbations and hospital admissions, as well as mortality from COPD and cardiovascular disease. In addition to tiotropium, there are other long-acting muscarinic antagonists (LAMA) now

Table 1 Bronchodilators for COPD

Drug	*MDI (μg)*	*Nebulizer (mg)*	*Oral (mg)*	*Duration (hr)*
β_2-agonists				
Salbutamol	100–200	2.5–5.0	4	4–6
Terbutaline	250–500	5–10	-	4–6
Indacaterol	150–300	-	-	24
Formoterol	12–24	-	-	12
Salmeterol	50–100	-	-	12
Bambuterol	-	-	10–20	12
Anticholinergics				
Ipratropium	40–80	0.25–0.5	-	6–8
Oxitropium	200	-	-	7–8
Tiotropium	18	-	-	>24
Glycopyrronium	50	-	-	24
Aclidinium	400	-	-	12
Theophyllines				
Theophylline SR	-	-	200–400	12–24
Aminophylline SR			200–400	12–24

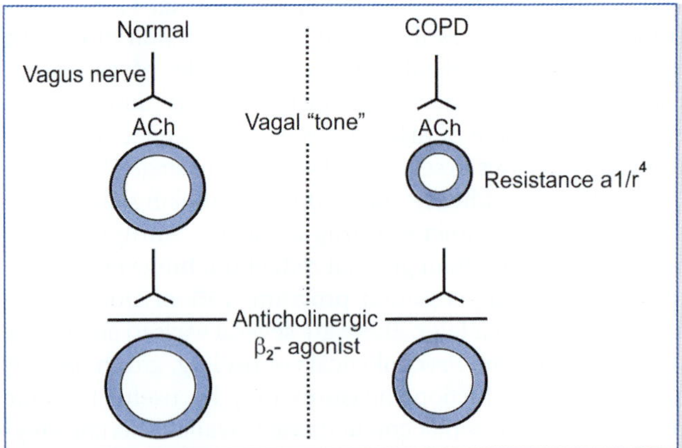

Fig. 2 Cholinergic control of airways in COPD. Normally there is a certain amount of cholinergic tone. This is exaggerated in COPD because of geometric factors related to the fixed narrowing of the airways (airway resistance R is proportional to $1/r^4$, where r is airway radius), so that airway resistance improves to a greater extent than in normal airways with an anticholinergic drug, which blocks the effect of acetylcholine (ACh) on muscarinic receptors in airway smooth muscle. Beta-agonists, which block all known bronchoconstrictor mechanisms, have a similar effect to anticholinergics suggesting that vagal tone is the only reversible component in COPD

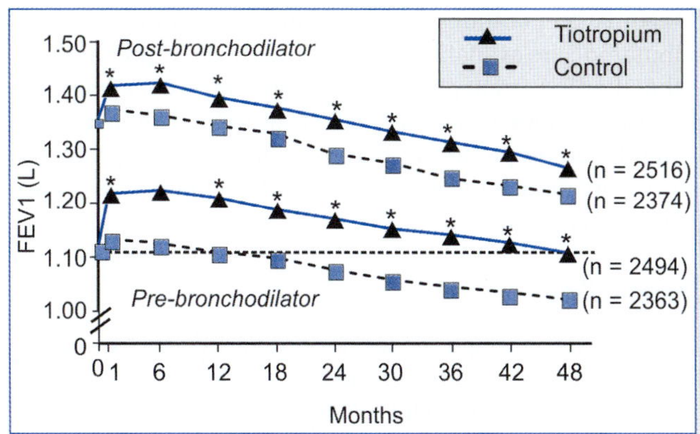

Fig. 3 The UPLIFT study. This large study of approximately 6,000 COPD patients compared tiotropium bromide (18 μg once daily) with placebo when added to current therapy. Tiotropium resulted in a greater increase in FEV1 pre- and post-bronchodilator, which was sustained throughout the 4 years of the study[25]

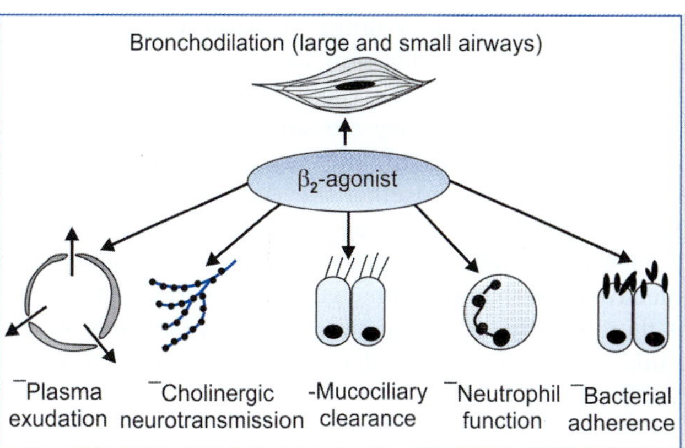

Fig. 4 Mechanism of action of β_2 agonists in COPD. Although their primary action is likely to be on airway smooth muscle, there are additional effects of β_2 agonists that may be beneficial

available, including glycopyrronium and umeclidinium, which are once daily and aclidinium, which is twice daily.[26,27]

Anticholinergic drugs may have additive bronchodilator effects with β_2-agonists so may be given together. For short-acting drugs, ipratropium-salbutamol inhalers are popular, whereas once daily combination inhalers containing tiotropium with formoterol are also available.[28] Several LABA-LAMA fixed combination inhalers are now available and in the development (discussed later).

Side effects: Inhaled anticholinergic drugs are well-tolerated, and systemic side effects are uncommon because almost no systemic absorption occurs. Ipratropium bromide, even in high doses, has no detectable effect on airway secretions. Nebulized ipratropium bromide may precipitate glaucoma in elderly patients as a result of a direct effect of the nebulized drug on the eye; this is avoided by use of a mouthpiece rather than a face mask. Dry mouth occurs in about 5–10% of patients on LAMA, but rarely requires discontinuation of treatment.

β_2-Agonists

Short-acting β_2-agonists are used mainly as required for symptom relief, but may be used four times a day on a regular basis. LABA are preferred therapy for COPD as they give better control of symptoms and are used as a maintenance therapy.[29]

Mode of action: β_2-agonists have several beneficial effects on the airways in COPD **(Fig. 4)**. These drugs act on airway smooth muscle causing a relaxation in large and small airways. They act as functional antagonists and reverse bronchoconstriction irrespective of the cause. Experimentally, they reduce plasma exudation and cholinergic reflexes. They also increase mucociliary clearance (when it is reduced), have no effect on chronic inflammation. Evidence suggests that β_2-agonists may reduce adherence of bacteria to airway epithelial cells and this may reduce infective exacerbations.[28] There is some evidence that β_2-agonists may increase the ventilatory drive to hypercapnia (but not to hypoxia).

Side effects: Side effects are not usually a problem; excessive use does not appear to be dangerous, even in patients with hypoxia and with cardiovascular disease.

- Muscle tremor (direct effect on skeletal muscle β_2-receptors)—more common in elderly patients
- Tachycardia (direct effect on atrial β_2-receptors, reflex effect from increased peripheral vasodilatation via β_2-receptors)
- Hypokalemia (direct effect on skeletal muscle uptake of potassium ions via β_2-receptors)—usually a small effect
- Restlessness
- Hypoxemia (increased V/Q mismatch due to pulmonary vasodilatation).

Short-acting β_2 Agonists

Short-acting inhaled β_2 agonists, such as salbutamol and terbutaline, are recommended for the immediate relief of symptoms. Ideally, they should not be used regularly (as tolerance to their protective effects occurs), although in patients with severe COPD regular nebulized β_2 agonists may be indicated.

Long-acting Inhaled β_2 Agonists

Salmeterol and formoterol give bronchodilation and protection against bronchoconstriction for over 12 hours. Indacaterol is a once daily LABA that is approved for use in COPD. Other once daily LABAs, including vilanterol and olodaterol are also becoming available. There is compelling evidence that these LABAs are useful as bronchodilators in patients with COPD and that once daily drugs are more effective than twice daily drugs. These drugs may improve symptoms, quality of life and exercise performance and reduce air trapping through relaxant effects on small airways. In long-term studies, they are safe, reduce exacerbations and mortality[30,31] **(Fig. 5)**. They have a similar efficacy to anticholinergics, but together they have additive effects. If the inhibitory effect of β_2-agonists on bacterial adhesion is relevant *in vivo,* they may also reduce the frequency of infective exacerbations, although this is yet to be determined as there is little difference between LABA (salmeterol) and LAMA (tiotropium) in reducing severe exacerbations of COPD **(Fig. 6)**.[32]

Oral β_2 Agonists

Although inhaled β_2-agonists are preferred, some elderly patients have problems with using inhalers. Slow-release oral β_2-agonist preparations, such as bambuterol and slow-release salbutamol, are available. An advantage of these preparations is that they may treat peripheral airways more effectively, but the disadvantage is that side effects are more frequent than with inhaled preparations. Bambuterol is a prodrug which is slowly metabolized to terbutaline and is effective as a once daily preparation.[33]

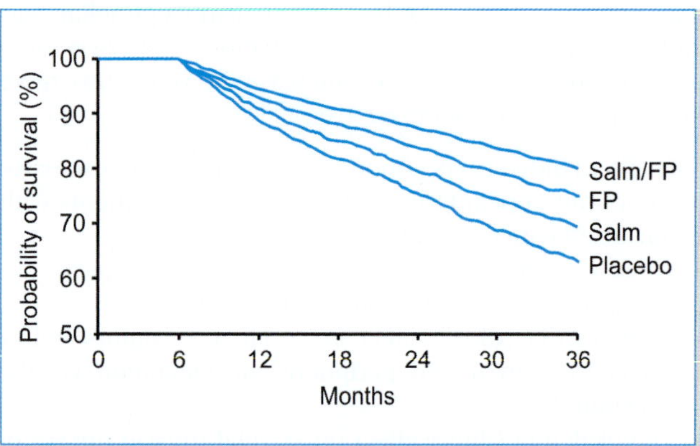

Fig. 5 TORCH study. This large study of approximately 6,000 COPD patients showed that fluticasone propionate/salmeterol reduced all cause mortality over 3 years, although this did not quite reach statistical significance ($p = 0.052$), whereas salmeterol and fluticasone alone had less effect[30]

Theophylline

Theophylline in high doses (with plasma concentration 10–20 mg/L) is a useful additional bronchodilator in patients with severe COPD,[34] oral administration has the advantage of treating small airways. It may have additional properties such as effects on mucociliary clearance and on respiratory muscles that are useful **(Fig. 7)**. The major limitation to the use of theophylline is its side effects, when high doses are used. Lower doses of theophylline (plasma concentration 5–10 mg/L) have anti-inflammatory effects in COPD patients and specifically reduce neutrophilic inflammation.[35,36]

Mode of action: Theophylline acts through nonselective inhibition of phosphodiesterases (PDEs), resulting in increased intracellular concentrations of cyclic AMP and cyclic GMP.[37] This effect is important for bronchodilator action, and might also be important in reducing neutrophilic inflammation. The drug also has some adenosine receptor antagonism, which accounts for some of the side effects, but there is little evidence that this is relevant for bronchodilator effects. Theophylline increases adrenaline secretion, but this is unlikely to account for the effects of the drug in COPD. Theophylline inhibits calcium entry and release and phosphoinositide hydrolysis. It is difficult to explain all of the beneficial effects of theophylline through these mechanisms alone, as many only occur at concentrations higher than those used therapeutically. More recently, it

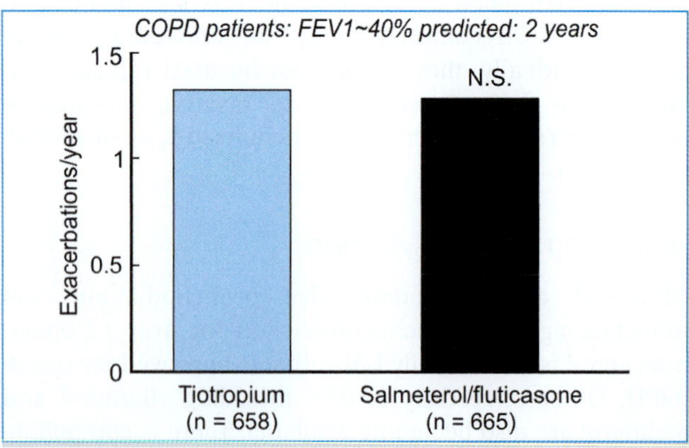

Fig. 6 Comparison between tiotropium and fluticasone/salmeterol in reducing acute exacerbations of COPD, showing no difference between these therapies[59]

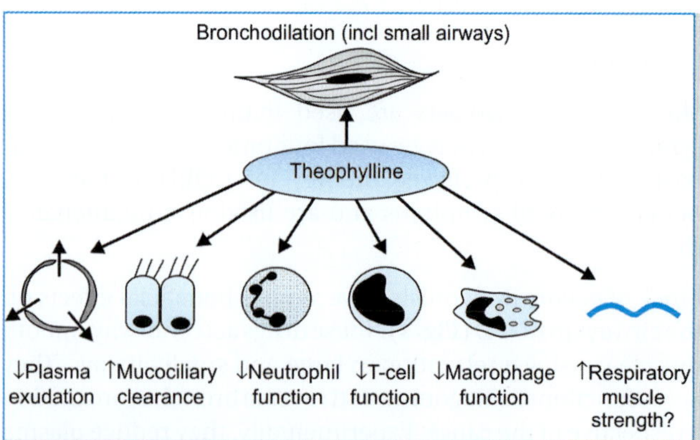

Fig. 7 Mechanism of action of theophylline in COPD. There may be several mechanisms of action of this drug, apart from bronchodilation. At subbronchodilator doses theophylline reduces neutrophilic inflammation in COPD

has been shown that low concentrations of theophylline are able to reverse corticosteroid resistance in COPD cells *in vitro* and preliminary studies have confirmed this in COPD patients.[37-39] This effect of theophylline is through direct inhibition of oxidative stress-activated phosphoinositide-3-kinase-δ, which results in increased histone deacetylase-2 activity.[40]

Recommended Use in COPD

Theophylline is recommended as an additional bronchodilator in patients not controlled on regular inhaled LAMA and LABA. A slow-release preparation should be given twice daily to achieve plasma concentrations of 10–20 mg/L. The recent demonstration that theophylline has anti-inflammatory effects and reverses corticosteroid resistance in COPD may lead to the use of low doses (plasma concentration 1–5 mg/L) as a maintenance treatment combined with low doses of inhaled corticosteroids (ICS).[37] Low dose theophylline reduces exacerbations of COPD[41] and large trials studying the effects of low dose theophylline and inhaled or oral corticosteroids are needed.

Side effects: Side effects are related to plasma concentration, although some patients may be particularly susceptible to side effects. They may be reduced by slowly increasing the dose when the drug is introduced. Side effects are mainly due to PDE inhibition and include:

- Nausea and vomiting
- Headache
- Restlessness
- Gastroesophageal reflux
- Diuresis
- Cardiac arrhythmias (usually plasma concentration >20 mg/L and due to adenosine receptor antagonism)
- Epileptic seizures (usually plasma concentration >30 mg/L and due to adenosine receptor antagonism).

Clearance of theophylline: The therapeutic effect is related to plasma concentration, which is affected by several factors that alter clearance. If in doubt, plasma concentrations should be measured.

Increased clearance (increase dose)

- Enzyme induction (rifampicin, phenobarbitone, ethanol)
- Smoking (tobacco, marijuana)
- Childhood
- High-protein, low-carbohydrate diet
- Barbecued meat.

Decreased clearance (decrease dose)

- Enzyme inhibition (cimetidine, erythromycin, ciprofloxacin, allopurinol, ketoconazole)
- Congestive heart failure
- Liver disease
- Pneumonia
- Viral infection and vaccination
- High carbohydrate diet.

Doxofylline

Doxofylline is a methylxanthine with similar bronchodilator properties to theophylline.[42] It is not an adenosine receptor antagonist, so there is reduced risk of cardiac arrhythmias or seizures. It does not significantly inhibit PDE isoenzymes which may also contribute to its better safety profile.[43] In addition, there are fewer drug interactions.[44]

Corticosteroids

The role of corticosteroids in the management of COPD remains controversial.[45] Maintenance treatment with oral corticosteroids should be avoided as there is no evidence of benefit and a high-risk of side effects in COPD populations. ICSs are commonly prescribed in high doses on the basis that COPD is like poorly responsive asthma, but there is little evidence that they are beneficial in patients with pure COPD. Approximately, 10% of patients with COPD have a positive response to oral corticosteroids and it is likely that these patients have coexisting asthma (asthma-COPD overlap syndrome, ACOS) and should therefore be treated as if they are asthmatic with regular ICSs. These patients may be recognized by increased eosinophils in the sputum and nitric oxide in the breath.[46]

Patients with COPD have a poor response to corticosteroids in comparison to asthma with little improvement in lung function. High doses of ICSs have consistently been shown a reduction (20–25%) in exacerbations in patients with severe disease and this is the main clinical indication for their use.[8] Several large studies have shown that corticosteroids fail to reduce the progression in COPD (measured by annual fall in FEV1)[47] and they have not been found to reduce mortality in a large study.[30] These results are likely to reflect the resistance of pulmonary inflammation to corticosteroids in COPD patients as a result of the reduction in HDAC2.[48]

Side effects: The reduction in the frequency of exacerbations, may be offset by systemic side effects such as osteoporosis, particularly in an elderly population that may be poorly nourished with reduced mobility. There is evidence that high dose ICSs are associated with increased cataracts in COPD patients[49] and that there is an increased risk of diabetes.[50] Several large trials of high dose ICSs have shown an increase in pneumonia amongst COPD patients.[51,52] The role of ICSs in nonreversible COPD is, therefore, currently uncertain. Lower doses of ICSs will have less risk of side effects, budesonide may be less likely to have adverse effects than fluticasone propionate.[51] Slow withdrawal of inhaled steroids in COPD patients, even with severe disease and a history of exacerbations is not associated with increased exacerbations and a small fall in FEV1.[53]

Phosphodiesterase Inhibitors

Theophylline is a weak nonselective inhibitor of PDEs, which breakdown cyclic nucleotides and may result in bronchodilation and anti-inflammatory effects. PDE4 inhibitors have a broad spectrum of anti-inflammatory effects, in vitro and animal models of COPD show good anti-inflammatory effects.[54] Several selective PDE4 inhibits have been tested in COPD and most failed because of insufficient clinical efficacy or unacceptable side effects (most commonly nausea, vomiting, diarrhea, headaches). Roflumilast is the only PDE4 inhibitor approved for COPD which provides only modest clinical benefit in COPD patients with severe disease, and frequent exacerbations. There is a small improvement in lung function, but no significant improvement in symptoms or quality of life and a small (~20%) reduction in exacerbation frequency.[55,56] However, many patients develop side effects and discontinue therapy. It may be indicated for patients with frequent exacerbations instead of high dose ICS.

Combination Inhalers

Several fixed combination inhalers are now available and several more in development for COPD patients. These combinations are more convenient and may improve adherence. Several studies have demonstrated a benefit of combination inhalers containing a corticosteroids and an LABA. Most of the benefit is provided by the LABA component.[31] Any superiority of combination inhalers over LABA alone in reducing exacerbations may be counteracted by the higher risk of side effects due to the corticosteroids component.[57] ICS-LABA combination inhalers improve symptoms and reduce exacerbations with a reduction in all cause mortality, although this does not quite reach statistical significance **(Fig. 6)**.[58] The reduction in exacerbation between twice daily fluticasone/salmeterol is similar to that seen with tiotropium **(Fig. 7)**.[59] ICS-LABA combination inhalers may be useful when patients with FEV1 less than 50% predicted and with frequent exacerbations (≥ 2/year) who are already on tiotropium and need further treatment. Recently, a once daily ICS-LABA combination inhaler (fluticasone furoate/vilanterol–Relvar) has been approved for use in COPD, although there is little difference in comparison with vilanterol alone.[60]

Several LABA-LAMA combination inhalers have been developed and some have reached the clinic.[61] These are based on the additive bronchodilator effects of LABA and LAMA that have been demonstrated in several studies. In one study, a maximally effective dose of indacaterol was given and since LABA inhibit all bronchoconstrictor mechanisms, including choliner tone, no further bronchodilation should be possible.[62] Addition of glycopyrronium in combination with indacaterol (QVA149, Ultibro) doubled the bronchodilator response. This may be explained by cross-talk between the cholinergic and β_2-agonist signaling pathways in airway smooth muscle cells. This additive bronchodilator effect is seen after chronic dosing, with reduction in symptoms and exacerbations.[63,64] Other LABA-LAMA combination inhalers include vilanterol/umeclidinium (Anoro) and olodaterol/tiotropium (once daily), formoterol/glycopyrronium and formoterol/aclidinium (twice daily).[65] It is likely that these will become first-line therapy, especially as they are more effective than an ICS-LABA combination.[66]

SUPPLEMENTARY OXYGEN

Poor oxygenation is one of the fundamental problem of severe COPD, and therefore supplementary oxygen is an important part of therapy in patients with severe disease.[67] Controlled oxygen (24%) is used acutely in the treatment of acute exacerbations in all patients who are hospitalized. Long-term oxygen therapy (LTOT, domiciliary oxygen) is indicated in selected patients with COPD. Two large multicenter trials demonstrated that long-term oxygen administration (>15 hours daily) prolongs survival (by about 30%) in patients with COPD. The goal of oxygen therapy is to increase PaO_2 to around 60 mm Hg or oxygen saturation of more than 90%; increasing PaO_2 above 60 mm Hg has little further benefit and increases the risk of CO_2 retention.[68,69] There is a danger of inducing respiratory failure if supplementary oxygen is used in patients with CO_2 retention, so careful assessment is required before oxygen is prescribed.

Long-term oxygen therapy may have several beneficial effects:
- Improvement in exercise capacity (increased endurance)
- Reduction in dyspnea
- Reduction in pulmonary hypertension, by reducing hypoxic pulmonary vasoconstriction
- Reduction in hematocrit by reducing erythropoietin levels
- Improved quality of life and neuropsychiatric function
- Reduction in severe desaturation episodes during sleep.

There are three methods of providing domiciliary oxygen therapy:
1. Long-term, low-dose oxygen for patients with chronic respiratory failure.
2. Portable oxygen therapy for exercise-related hypoxia and dyspnea.
3. Short-burst oxygen therapy for temporary relief of symptoms.

Selection of Patients for Long-term Oxygen Therapy

In some countries, guidelines (Department of Health) have been drawn up for the provision of Long-term oxygen therapy (LTOT). LTOT should not be considered in patients who continue to smoke. All patients should be assessed by a pulmonary specialist.

Absolute indications are:
- Stable COPD with hypoxemia and edema
- FEV1 <1.5L, FVC <2.0 L, and
- PaO_2 < 55 mm Hg (<7.3 kPa), $Paco_2$ >45 mm Hg (>6 kPa) and
- Stability demonstrated over 3 weeks on optimal therapy.

Relative indications are:

- As above, but without edema or $PaCO_2$ > 45 mm Hg
- Palliative (symptom relief).

Portable oxygen is indicated in patients who desaturate during exercise and its efficacy needs to be assessed during a treadmill or 6-minute walk test with patients wearing the portable oxygen cylinder. Portable oxygen may also be indicated in patients with severe exercise limitation irrespective of oxygen desaturation. Portable oxygen may also be needed in such patients during commercial airline flights (provided by airline).

ANTIBIOTICS

Infection is often the cause of progression or acute deterioration in patients with COPD, the combating of infection by the appropriate use of antibiotics is an important part of therapy.[70] In fact, the organisms causing pulmonary infections are often the same as those found normally in the upper respiratory tract. It may be difficult to know if a pathogen isolated from the sputum is responsible for the exacerbation. For most of the time, the sputum in COPD is mucoid, but becomes yellow or green with exacerbations of infection and when this occurs, it is usual to begin empirical antibiotic therapy. Purulence of sputum is due to an increase in degranulating neutrophils and may not necessarily imply bacterial infection. Indeed, many exacerbations of COPD are likely to be due to upper respiratory tract virus infections, such as *Rhinovirus, Corona* virus and *Parainfluenza* virus.[71] This means that antibiotics are often used inappropriately, but it is difficult to tell clinically whether an infection is viral or bacterial in origin. In a meta-analysis of placebo controlled trials of antibiotics for COPD, there was a small, but significant difference in peak expiratory flow (PEF) between patients treated with antibiotics and placebo.[72,73]

The common bacterial organisms responsible for exacerbations of COPD include *Streptococcus pneumoniae, Hemophilus influenzae, Moraxella catarrhalis* and *Mycoplasma pneumoniae* (less common). The choice of antibiotic depends upon the likely organisms, the likely sensitivity of the organisms in the community, the tolerance of the patient for the drug and the response to treatment. The treatment of choice in the community will often be either amoxicillin or co-trimoxazole (Septrin). Co-trimoxazole is not recommended as development of resistance and side effects due to the sulfonamide component are relatively common. Since, many strains of *H. influenzae* are now β-lactamase producers and hence resistant to ampicillin/amoxicillin, the choice for initial therapy commonly lies between–

- Amoxicillin/clavulanic acid (Augmentin)
- Erythromycin or other macrolides (clarithromycin, azithromycin)
- A cephalosporin, e.g. cefaclor
- A tetracycline, e.g. doxycycline.

There are advantages and disadvantages of each drug and the choice may finally be based on finding out which drug works for a given patient. Cost is also a factor and there is no justification for using an expensive drug when a cheaper one works just as well. In most cases, the choice usually falls between amoxicillin, amoxicillin/clavulanic acid or doxycycline for the typical ambulatory patient.

The antibiotic should be given in full therapeutic doses for a course lasting about 10–14 days except for clarithromycin and azithromycin which are given for shorter periods (3 days). Treatment is then stopped provided the patient has responded. If there has been a poor response, a change of antibiotic may be indicated, usually to one of the newer broad spectrum agents such as clarithromycin if this has not already been tried. Continuous antibiotic administration is not recommended as this has not been shown to alter the course of the disease and is likely to lead to an increase in resistant organisms. Macrolide antibiotics (erythromycin and azithromycin) reduce exacerbations of COPD, but it is not certain whether this is an antibiotic or an anti-inflammatory effect of the macrolide.[74,75] Since, long-term antibiotic treatment may have adverse effects (cardiovascular risk, deafness) and increase bacterial resistance, they may be only indicated in selected patients, such as those with coexistent bronchiectasis who have persistently purulent sputum.

OTHER DRUG THERAPIES

Mucolytics

Because mucus hypersecretion is a prominent feature of chronic bronchitis, various mucolytic therapies have been used to increase the ease of mucus expectoration, in the belief that this will improve lung function.[76]

- Stopping smoking is the most effective way to reduce mucus hypersecretion
- Anticholinergics may decrease mucus hypersecretion
- β_2-agonists and theophylline may improve mucus clearance
- Steam inhalation (with or without aromatics) may provide symptomatic relief, but there is no evidence that it improves lung function or long-term symptom control
- Several drugs, such as bromhexine and ambroxol, reduce mucus viscosity *in vitro*, but there is little evidence from controlled trials that they improve lung function in patients with COPD, and cannot be recommended as routine therapy
- Expectorants, such as guaifenesin and potassium iodide, similarly have no proven beneficial effects
- Recombinant human DNAse (alfadornase, pulmozyme) has beneficial effects in some patients with cystic fibrosis, but its role in COPD is not yet clear. Until there is clear evidence of benefit, it should not be used in view of its high cost.

Antioxidants

Since, oxidant damage may be critical in the pathophysiology of COPD, antioxidant therapy is logical. N-acetylcysteine (NAC) and carbocisteine were originally developed as mucolytics, but have well-documented antioxidant effects.[77] Several small studies demonstrated a beneficial effect of NAC in reducing exacerbations of COPD by approximately 25%, meta-analysis has shown little effect and no effect on the quality of life.[78] In a large prospective controlled trial NAC failed to reduce exacerbations, improve health status or reduce disease progression.[79] Large studies from China showed that carbocisteine and NAC significantly reduced exacerbations, especially is less in severe patients.[80,81] At present, these therapies are not recommended for routine use.

Vaccines

- Influenza vaccine is recommended as patients with COPD are subject to severe exacerbations with this infection and there is evidence for a reduction in acute exacerbations and hospital admissions. Influenza vaccination is cost-effective in elderly people and should be more so in patients with COPD. Influenza vaccination reduces all-cause mortality.[82] It should be given prior to the winter season
- Polyvalent pneumococcal vaccine is used in many countries to protect against the development of pneumococcal lung infections. Pneumococcal vaccination does not reduce mortality[82] and there are no convincing large trials to show a reduction in exacerbations.[83] Improved vaccines are now in development
- OM85-BV (Broncho-vaxom) is a mixture of bacterial products that activate macrophage function (the advantage of which is obscure!). There is some evidence that it may reduce the severity of acute exacerbations, but there are no consistent clinical benefits, so it cannot be recommended as a routine treatment.[84]

Neuraminidase Inhibitors

Inhibitors of neuraminidase, such as zanamivir (inhaled) and oseltamivir (oral) speed the recovery from influenza. However, there are no specific trials in patients with COPD and it is not yet certain whether this treatment is cost-effective.[85]

Treatment of Dyspnea

Breathlessness is a problem in many patients, particularly in those with severe emphysema. Several drugs, including nebulized opiates, slow-release morphine, dihydrocodeine and benzodiazepines, may reduce the sensation of dyspnea, but the reduction in ventilatory drive is potentially dangerous and these drugs should be avoided, particularly during exacerbations.[86]

Respiratory Stimulants

There is no role for respiratory stimulants, such as doxapram or almitrine, in the long-term management of COPD, since there is no evidence that central ventilatory drive is impaired. Ventilation is limited by mechanical rather than neurophysiological factors. However, doxapram may be indicated in the management of an acute exacerbation of COPD, if there is hypercapnia and hypoventilation in order to tide the patient over 24–36 hours until the underlying cause (e.g. infection) is controlled. It is likely that the use of doxapram in this situation will decline as nasal intermittent positive pressure ventilation (NIPPV) becomes more widely available.

Antitussives

Cough is often a troublesome symptom of COPD, but may have a protective effect in clearing secretions. The regular use of antitussives is therefore not recommended in COPD.[87]

NONPHARMACOLOGICAL TREATMENTS

Several nonpharmacological approaches have also been used in the management of COPD and may form part of a comprehensive rehabilitation program in elderly patients.

Exercise

Exercise training to improve cardiorespiratory function is helpful; the type of exercise does not appear to be important and aerobic exercise or upper limb exercises are equally effective. Respiratory muscle training using resistive inspiratory loading may reduce breathlessness, but an analysis of several controlled studies of respiratory muscle training alone has provided no evidence of clear overall benefit.[88] Controlled breathing techniques, such as pursed lip breathing and diaphragmatic breathing, result in reduced dyspnea, particularly in patients with hyperventilation.

Nutrition

Nutrition is important in patients with COPD, many patients are malnourished and underweight, although marked cachexia is uncommon. Many COPD patients are obese because of reduced physical activity who should lose weight, particularly if there are sleep disturbances or they have metabolic syndrome or Frank type II diabetes. Antioxidant vitamin supplements may also be used. There is no convincing evidence that improved nutrition is beneficial in COPD patients and there is no evidence that nutritional supplements with a high fat content that are marketed for use in COPD have any special value.[89] The place of androgens and anabolic steroids to build muscle bulk in COPD has not been established.[90]

Pulmonary Rehabilitation

Rehabilitation concerns prevention of deconditioning and allowing the patient to cope with his/her disease. Rehabilitation programs are successful in prospective randomized trials in terms of increased performance and quality of life and reduce exacerbations, even though they may not improve lung function.[91,92] Patients with moderate to severe COPD should be considered for pulmonary rehabilitation programs, which include educational advise and physiotherapy. There is evidence that pulmonary rehabilitation also increases the efficacy of bronchodilator therapy.[93]

Artificial Ventilation

Artificial ventilation devices have improved enormously. Noninvasive ventilation using NIPPV has been an important advance in the management of acute exacerbations of COPD in hospital and more recently in the control of hypercapnic respiratory failure at home, thus reducing the need for hospitalization. There is no good evidence for the use of nocturnal NIPPV in stable COPD[94] NIPPV corrects hypercapnia and respiratory acidosis. Good results in management of acute exacerbations have been reported, with significant reduction in mortality and time spent in hospital.[95]

Surgery

Several surgical techniques have been successfully applied to more severe emphysema. These include heart-lung transplantation, now largely replaced by single lung transplantation in carefully selected patients.[96] Lung volume reduction surgery by excision of badly affected emphysematous lung is effective in highly selected patients with bilateral, predominantly upper lobe emphysema and evidence of air trapping. There is sustained improvement in lung function, reduction in symptoms and exacerbations.[97] Patients with a very poor diffusing capacity had an increased mortality. More recently, bronchoscopic lung volume reduction surgery has been developed to avoid the surgical morbidity and mortality of lung volume reduction surgery (LVRS). Several devices, including one way valves, coils, sealants, airway bypass stents and bronchoscopic thermal vapor ablation, designed to collapse and remodel hyperinflated lung are currently being tried in clinical trials.[98]

MANAGING CHRONIC DISEASE

It is important that an accurate diagnosis is made and COPD differentiated from asthma, which is usually possible from the history. Spirometry is important to diagnose airway obstruction objectively and to stage the disease in order to decide on the most appropriate therapy. In the GOLD strategy for COPD, treatment of chronic disease follows a stepwise escalation based on disease severity, symptoms and risk of exacerbations.[8] At all stages, smoking cessation is important, particularly in the early stages of disease and patients should routinely receive immunization against seasonal influenza. In GOLD 1 patients, there is usually little functional impairment, the only treatment needed is "as required", inhaled short-acting bronchodilator such as salbutamol, ipratropium or a combination of the two. In patients with GOLD 2, the preferred therapy is a long-acting bronchodilator—either LAMA once daily (tiotropium, glycopyrronium) or LABA once (indacaterol) or twice (salmeterol, formoterol) daily. Patients often prefer the once daily regime.

There are additive effects between LABA and LAMA; fixed dose LABA-LAMA inhalers are now available. If long-acting bronchodilators are too expensive, it may be necessary to use a short-acting bronchodilator, such as salbutamol or ipratropium bromide, regularly four times daily or an oral bronchodilator, such as slow-release theophylline twice daily, or bambuterol once daily. For GOLD 3 patients, an inhaled corticosteroid may be added, this is often done by using a combination inhaler with a steroid and LABA. Oral theophylline may also be added at this stage as it may have an anti-inflammatory effect.

Pulmonary rehabilitation is also useful in some patients, if it is available. In GOLD 4 patients, it is necessary to consider the use of supplementary oxygen, and for very selected patients lung surgery.

Referral to Hospital

Referral to a respiratory physician is useful to:

- Establish the diagnosis and differentiate from asthma
- Exclude other pathology, including malignancy
- Reinforce the need to stop smoking
- Optimize therapy.

Referral is indicated particularly in following conditions:

- Early onset of disease or family history of α_1-antitrypsin deficiency
- Signs of *cor pulmonale*
- Assessment of LTOT or nebulizer therapy
- Those with a rapid decline in lung function (>100 mL/year)
- Those with frequent infections to exclude bronchiectasis.

TREATMENT OF ACUTE EXACERBATIONS

An important aim of treatment is to prevent exacerbations. Several of the treatments for chronic disease including long-acting bronchodilators (both β_2-agonists and anticholinergic), low dose theophylline, high dose ICSs, pulmonary rehabilitation and smoking cessation have been shown to reduce exacerbation rates and hospitalization.[99]

Chronic obstructive pulmonary disease exacerbations are one of the most common causes of hospital admission. Apart from the treatment of underlying bacterial infection with antibiotics (as discussed above), exacerbations are treated symptomatically by increasing the dose of short-acting β_2-agonist and anticholinergic bronchodilators delivered by nebulizer. The place of antibiotics is not certain as controlled trials show little clinical benefit; this may reflect the fact that over half of the exacerbations are due to viral or noninfective causes. Oxygen (24 or 28% via Venturi mask) should be given to achieve a PaO_2 of at least 60 mm Hg without a fall in pH to less than 7.26 (indicating an acute change). Blood gases should be checked within 1 hour of starting oxygen therapy.

Oxygen saturation by pulse oximetry may be used to monitor response provided $PaCO_2$ and pH are normal. A course of oral corticosteroids is usually indicated, but only reduces in-patient stay by about 1 day. Very high doses of oral corticosteroids, or intravenous steroids, such as hydrocortisone or methylprednisolone, are no better than low oral doses, and there is a greater risk of side effects.[100] Diuretics are indicated, if there is peripheral edema. Chest physiotherapy may be useful, although there is no evidence from controlled studies that it improves recovery. Development of respiratory failure with a rising $PaCO_2$ may necessitate NPPV or intubation.

TREATMENT OF COR PULMONALE

Cor pulmonale (right heart failure) is due to the effect of chronic hypoxia on pulmonary vasculature resulting in pulmonary hypertension. It is usual to treat with LTOT. Diuretics are used to reduce fluid retention. Digoxin is only indicated if there is coexistent atrial fibrillation. Vasodilators may be hazardous as they lower systemic as well as pulmonary blood pressure.

FUTURE THERAPIES

There is a pressing need to develop new therapies, as existing treatments do not alter the progressive course of the disease or reduce mortality. There have been relatively few advances in the therapeutic options for the treatment of COPD, but better understanding of the molecular mechanisms involved in the pathogenesis of COPD will undoubtedly lead to improved therapies in the future.[101]

Several inhaled long-acting bronchodilators and combinations are currently in development. There are currently no treatments, apart from theophylline, that reduce inflammation in COPD and there is an intense search for drugs that are effective against steroid-resistant inflammation. Drugs that block specific mediators, such as leukotriene B_4 and TNF, have not been shown to have any benefit. Because of the problem with side effects of oral PDE4 inhibitors, there are now attempts to develop inhaled PDE4 inhibitors to avoid these side effects, so far most inhaled PDE4 inhalers have lacked clinical efficacy. Several other anti-inflammatory drugs including p38 MAP kinase, JAK and NF-κB inhibitors are also in clinical development stage, but these drugs also have side effect issues and may need to be given by the inhaled route.

REFERENCES

1. Barnes PJ. Chronic obstructive pulmonary disease. N Engl J Med. 2000;343:269-80.
2. Decramer M, Janssens W, Miravitlles M. Chronic obstructive pulmonary disease. Lancet. 2012;379(9823):1341-51.
3. Barnes PJ. Chronic obstructive pulmonary disease. Clin Chest Med. 2014;35(1):xiii.
4. Hogg JC, Timens W. The pathology of chronic obstructive pulmonary disease. Annu Rev Pathol. 2009;4:435-59.
5. Lozano, R, Naghavi M, Foreman K, Lim S, Shibuya K, Aboyans V, et al. Global and regional mortality from 235 causes of death for 20 age groups in 1990 and 2010: a systematic analysis for the Global Burden of Disease Study 2010. Lancet. 2012;380(9859):2095-128.
6. Salvi S, Agrawal A. India needs a national COPD prevention and control programme. J Assoc Physicians India. 2012;(Suppl 60): 5-7.
7. Gupta D, Agarwal R, Aggarwal AN, Maturu VN, Dhooria S, Prasad KT, et al. Guidelines for diagnosis and management of chronic obstructive pulmonary disease: joint recommendations of Indian Chest Society and National College of Chest Physicians (India). Indian J Chest Dis Allied Sci. 2014;56 Spec No:5-54.
8. Vestbo J, Hurd SS, Agustí AG, Jones PW, Vogelmeier C, Anzueto A, et al. Global strategy for the diagnosis, management and prevention of chronic obstructive pulmonary disease, GOLD executive summary. Am J Respir Crit Care Med. 2013;187:347-65.
9. Salvi SS, Barnes PJ. Chronic obstructive pulmonary disease in non-smokers. Lancet. 2009;374(9691):733-43.
10. García Rodríguez LA, Wallander MA, Tolosa LB, Johansson S. Chronic obstructive pulmonary disease in UK primary care: incidence and risk factors. COPD. 2009;6(5):369-79.
11. Salvi S. Tobacco smoking and environmental risk factors for chronic obstructive pulmonary disease. Clin Chest Med. 2014;35(1):17-27.
12. Allwood BW, Myer L, Bateman ED. A systematic review of the association between pulmonary tuberculosis and the development of chronic airflow obstruction in adults. Respiration. 2013;86(1):76-85.
13. Anthonisen NR, Skeans MA, Wise RA, Manfreda J, Kanner RE, Connett JE, et al. The effects of a smoking cessation intervention on 14.5-year mortality: a randomized clinical trial. Ann Intern Med. 2005;142(4):233-9.
14. Vestbo J, Edwards LD, Scanlon PD, Yates JC, Agusti A, Bakke P, et al. Changes in forced expiratory volume in 1 second over time in COPD. N Engl J Med. 2011;365(13):1184-92.
15. Tashkin DP, Murray RP. Smoking cessation in chronic obstructive pulmonary disease. Respir Med. 2009;103(7):963-74.
16. Rennard SI, Daughton DM. Smoking cessation. Clin Chest Med. 2014;35(1):165-76.
17. Cahill K, Stevens S, Lancaster T. Pharmacological treatments for smoking cessation. JAMA. 2014;311(2):193-4.
18. Fullerton DG, Bruce N, Gordon SB. Indoor air pollution from biomass fuel smoke is a major health concern in the developing world. Trans R Soc Trop Med Hyg. 2008;102(9):843-51.

19. Zhou Y, Zou Y, Li X, Chen S, Zhao Z, He F, et al. Lung function and incidence of chronic obstructive pulmonary disease after improved cooking fuels and kitchen ventilation: a 9-year prospective cohort study. PLoS Med. 2014;11(3):e1001621.
20. Lokke A, Lange P, Scharling H, Fabricius P, Vestbo J. Developing COPD: a 25-year follow up study of the general population. Thorax. 2006;61(11):935-9.
21. Wan ES, Silverman EK. Genetics of COPD and emphysema. Chest. 2009;136(3):859-66.
22. Pillai SG, Ge D, Zhu G, Kong X, Shianna KV, Need AC, et al. A genome-wide association study in chronic obstructive pulmonary disease (COPD): identification of two major susceptibility loci. PLoS Genet. 2009;5(3):e1000421.
23. Campos MA, Lascano J. α1 Antitrypsin deficiency: current best practice in testing and augmentation therapy. Ther Adv Respir Dis. 2014;8(5):150-61.
24. Cazzola M, Page CP, Calzetta L, Matera MG. Pharmacology and therapeutics of bronchodilators. Pharmacol Rev. 2012;64(3):450-504.
25. Tashkin DP, Celli B, Senn S, Burkhart D, Kesten S, Menjoge S, et al. A 4-year trial of tiotropium in chronic obstructive pulmonary disease. N Engl J Med. 2008;359(15):1543-54.
26. Carter NJ. Inhaled glycopyrronium bromide: a review of its use in patients with moderate to severe chronic obstructive pulmonary disease. Drugs. 2013;73(7):741-53.
27. Ni H, Soe Z, Moe S. Aclidinium bromide for stable chronic obstructive pulmonary disease. Cochrane Database Syst Rev. 2014;9:CD010509.
28. Tashkin DP, Pearle J, Iezzoni D, Varghese ST. Formoterol and tiotropium compared with tiotropium alone for treatment of COPD. COPD. 2009;6(1):17-25.
29. Kew KM, Mavergames C, Walters JA. Long-acting beta2-agonists for chronic obstructive pulmonary disease. Cochrane Database Syst Rev. 2013;10:CD010177.
30. Calverley PM, Anderson JA, Celli B, Ferguson GT, Jenkins C, Jones PW, et al. Salmeterol and fluticasone propionate and survival in chronic obstructive pulmonary disease. N Engl J Med. 2007;356(8):775-89.
31. Suissa S, Ernst P, Vandemheen KL, Aaron SD. Methodological issues in therapeutic trials of COPD. Eur Respir J. 2008;31(5):927-33.
32. Vogelmeier C, Hederer B, Glaab T, Schmidt H, Rutten-van Mölken MP, Beeh KM, et al. Tiotropium versus salmeterol for the prevention of exacerbations of COPD. N Engl J Med. 2011;364(12):1093-103.
33. Cazzola M, Calderaro F, Califano C, Di Pema F, Vinciguerra A, Donner CF, et al. Oral bambuterol compared to inhaled salmeterol in patients with partially reversible chronic obstructive pulmonary disease. Eur J Clin.Pharmacol. 1999;54(11):829-33.
34. ZuWallack RL, Mahler DA, Reilly D, Church N, Emmett A, Rickard K, et al. Salmeterol plus theophylline combination therapy in the treatment of COPD. Chest. 2001;119(6):1661-70.
35. Culpitt SV, de Matos C, Russell RE, Donnelly LE, Rogers DF, Barnes PJ. Effect of theophylline on induced sputum inflammatory indices and neutrophil chemotaxis in COPD. Am J Respir Crit Care Med. 2002;165:1371-6.
36. Kanehara M, Yokoyama A, Tomoda Y, Shiota N, Iwamoto H, Ishikawa N, et al. Anti-inflammatory effects and clinical efficacy of theophylline and tulobuterol in mild-to-moderate chronic obstructive pulmonary disease. Pulm Pharmacol Ther. 2008;21(6):874-8.
37. Barnes PJ. Theophylline. Am J Respir Crit Care Med. 2013;188:901-6.
38. Cosio BG, Tsaprouni L, Ito K, Jazrawi E, Adcock IM, Barnes PJ. Theophylline restores histone deacetylase activity and steroid responses in COPD macrophages. J Exp Med. 2004;200:689-95.
39. Ford PA, Durham AL, Russell RE, Gordon F, Adcock IM, Barnes PJ. Treatment effects of low dose theophylline combined with an inhaled corticosteroid in COPD. Chest. 2010;137:1338-44.
40. To Y, Ito K, Kizawa Y, Failla M, Ito M, Kusama T, et al. Targeting phosphoinositide-3-kinase-δ with theophylline reverses corticosteroid insensitivity in COPD. Am J Resp Crit Care Med. 2010;182:897-904.
41. Zhou Y, Wang X, Zeng X, Qiu R, Xie J, Liu S, et al. Positive benefits of theophylline in a randomized, double-blind, parallel-group, placebo-controlled study of low-dose, slow-release theophylline in the treatment of COPD for 1 year. Respirology. 2006;11(5):603-10.
42. Dini FL, Cogo R. Doxofylline: a new generation xanthine bronchodilator devoid of major cardiovascular adverse effects. Curr Med Res Opin. 2001;16(4):258-68.
43. van Mastbergen J, Jolas T, Allegra L, Page CP. The mechanism of action of doxofylline is unrelated to HDAC inhibition, PDE inhibition or adenosine receptor antagonism. Pulm Pharmacol Ther. 2012;25(1):55-61.
44. Shukla D, Chakraborty S, Singh S, Mishra B. Doxofylline: a promising methylxanthine derivative for the treatment of asthma and chronic obstructive pulmonary disease. Expert Opin Pharmacother. 2009;10(14):2343-56.
45. Barnes PJ. Inhaled corticosteroids in COPD: a controversy. Respiration. 2010;80(2):89-95.
46. Brightling CE, McKenna S, Hargadon B, Birring S, Green R, Siva R, et al. Sputum eosinophilia and the short-term response to inhaled mometasone in chronic obstructive pulmonary disease. Thorax. 2005;60(3):193-8.
47. Yang IA, Clarke MS, Sim EH, Fong KM. Inhaled corticosteroids for stable chronic obstructive pulmonary disease. Cochrane Database Syst Rev. 2012;7:CD002991.
48. Barnes PJ. Role of HDAC2 in the pathophysiology of COPD. Annu Rev Physiol. 2009;71:451-64.
49. Ernst P, Baltzan M, Deschênes J, Suissa S. Low-dose inhaled and nasal corticosteroid use and the risk of cataracts. Eur Respir J. 2006;27(6):1168-74.
50. Suissa S, Kezouh A, Ernst P. Inhaled corticosteroids and the risks of diabetes onset and progression. Am J Med. 2010;123(11):1001-6.
51. Suissa S, Patenaude V, Lapi F, Ernst P. Inhaled corticosteroids in COPD and the risk of serious pneumonia. Thorax. 2013; 68(11):1029-36.
52. Finney L, Berry M, Singanayagam A, Elkin SL, Johnston SL, Mallia P. Inhaled corticosteroids and pneumonia in chronic obstructive pulmonary disease. Lancet Respir Med. 2014;2(11):919-32.
53. Magnussen H, Disse B, Rodriguez-Roisin R, Kirsten A, Watz H, Tetzlaff K, et al. Withdrawal of Inhaled Glucocorticoids and Exacerbations of COPD. N Engl J Med. 2014;371(14):1285-94.
54. Hatzelmann A, Morcillo EJ, Lungarella G, Adnot S, Sanjar S, et al. The preclinical pharmacology of roflumilast--a selective, oral phosphodiesterase 4 inhibitor in development for chronic obstructive pulmonary disease. Pulm Pharmacol Ther. 2010;23(4):235-56.
55. Calverley PM, Rabe KF, Goehring UM, Kristiansen S, Fabbri LM, Martinez FJ, et al. Roflumilast in symptomatic chronic

obstructive pulmonary disease: two randomised clinical trials. Lancet. 2009;374(9691):685-94.
56. Fabbri LM, Calverley PM, Izquierdo-Alonso JL, Bundschuh DS, Brose M, Martinez FJ, et al. Roflumilast in moderate-to-severe chronic obstructive pulmonary disease treated with long-acting bronchodilators: two randomised clinical trials. Lancet. 2009;374(9691):695-703.
57. Suissa S, Barnes PJ. Inhaled corticosteroids in COPD: the case against. Eur Respir J. 2009;34(1):13-6.
58. Nannini LJ, Poole P, Milan SJ, Kesterton A. Combined corticosteroid and long-acting beta(2)-agonist in one inhaler versus inhaled corticosteroids alone for chronic obstructive pulmonary disease. Cochrane Database Syst Rev. 2013;8:CD006826.
59. Wedzicha JA, Calverley PM, Seemungal TA, Hagan G, Ansari Z, Stockley RA, et al. The prevention of chronic obstructive pulmonary disease exacerbations by salmeterol/fluticasone propionate or tiotropium bromide. Am J Respir Crit Care Med. 2008;177(1):19-26.
60. Dransfield, MT, Bourbeau J, Jones PW, Hanania NA, Mahler AD, Vestbo J, Wachtel A, et al. Once-daily inhaled fluticasone furoate and vilanterol versus vilanterol only for prevention of exacerbations of COPD: two replicate double-blind, parallel-group, randomised controlled trials. Lancet Respir Med. 2013;1(3):210-23.
61. de Miguel-Díez, J, Jiménez-García G. Considerations for new dual-acting bronchodilator treatments for chronic obstructive pulmonary disease. Expert Opin Investig Drugs. 2014;23(4):453-6.
62. van Noord JA, Buhl R, Laforce C, Martin C, Jones F, Dolker M, et al. QVA149 demonstrates superior bronchodilation compared with indacaterol or placebo in patients with chronic obstructive pulmonary disease. Thorax. 2010;65(12):1086-91.
63. Bateman ED, Ferguson GT, Barnes N, Gallagher N, Green Y, Henley M, et al. Dual bronchodilation with QVA149 versus single bronchodilator therapy: the SHINE study. Eur Respir J. 2013;42(6):1484-94.
64. Wedzicha JA, Decramer M, Ficker JH, Niewoehner DE, Sandström T, Taylor AF, et al. Analysis of chronic obstructive pulmonary disease exacerbations with the dual bronchodilator QVA149 compared with glycopyrronium and tiotropium (SPARK): a randomised, double-blind, parallel-group study. Lancet Respir Med. 2013;1(3):199-209.
65. Bateman ED, Mahler DA, Vogelmeier CF, Wedzicha JA, Patalano F, Banerji D. Recent advances in COPD disease management with fixed-dose long-acting combination therapies. Expert Rev Respir Med. 2014;8(3):357-79.
66. Vogelmeier CF, Bateman ED, Pallante J, Alagappan VK, D'Andrea P, Chen H, et al. Efficacy and safety of once-daily QVA149 compared with twice-daily salmeterol-fluticasone in patients with chronic obstructive pulmonary disease (ILLUMINATE): a randomised, double-blind, parallel group study. Lancet Respir Med. 2013;1(1):51-60.
67. Tarpy SP, Celli B. Long-term oxygen therapy. New Engl J Med. 1995;333:710-4.
68. Cranston JM, Crockett AJ, Moss JR, Alpers JH. Domiciliary oxygen for chronic obstructive pulmonary disease. Cochrane Database Syst Rev. 2005;19(4):CD001744.
69. Moore RP, Berlowitz DJ, Denehy L, Pretto JJ, Brazzale DJ, Sharpe K, et al. A randomised trial of domiciliary, ambulatory oxygen in patients with COPD and dyspnoea but without resting hypoxaemia. Thorax. 2011;66(1):32-7.
70. Sethi S, Murphy TF. Infection in the pathogenesis and course of chronic obstructive pulmonary disease. N Engl J Med. 2008;359(22):2355-65.
71. Papi A, Bellettato CM, Braccioni F, Romagnoli M, Casolari P, Caramori G, et al. Infections and airway inflammation in chronic obstructive pulmonary disease severe exacerbations. Am J Respir Crit Care Med. 2006;173(10):1114-21.
72. Saint S, Bent S, Vittinghoff E, Grady D. Antibiotics in chronic obstructive pulmonary disease exacerbations. A meta-analysis. JAMA. 1995;273(12):957-60.
73. Vollenweider DJ, Jarrett H, Steurer-Stey CA, Garcia-Aymerich J, Puhan MA. Antibiotics for exacerbations of chronic obstructive pulmonary disease. Cochrane Database Syst Rev. 2012;12:CD010257.
74. Seemungal TA, Wilkinson TM, Hurst JR, Perera WR, Sapsford RJ, Wedzicha JA. Long-term erythromycin therapy is associated with decreased chronic obstructive pulmonary disease exacerbations. Am J Respir Crit Care Med. 2008;178(11):1139-47.
75. Albert RK, Connett J, Bailey WC, Casaburi R, Cooper JA, Criner GJ, et al. Azithromycin for prevention of exacerbations of COPD. N Engl J Med. 2011;365(8):689-98.
76. Fahy JV, Dickey BF. Airway mucus function and dysfunction. N Engl J Med. 2010;363(23):2233-47.
77. Kirkham PA, Barnes PJ. Oxidative stress in COPD. Chest. 2013;144:266-73.
78. Poole P, Black PN, Cates CJ. Mucolytic agents for chronic bronchitis or chronic obstructive pulmonary disease. Cochrane Database Syst Rev. 2012;8:CD001287.
79. Decramer M, Rutten-van Mölken M, Dekhuijzen PN, Troosters T, van Herwaarden C, Pellegrino R, et al. Effects of N-acetylcysteine on outcomes in chronic obstructive pulmonary disease (Bronchitis Randomized on NAC Cost-Utility Study, BRONCUS): a randomised placebo-controlled trial. Lancet. 2005;365(9470):1552-60.
80. Zheng JP, Kang J, Huang SG, Chen P, Yao WZ, Yang L, et al. Effect of carbocisteine on acute exacerbation of chronic obstructive pulmonary disease (PEACE Study): a randomised placebo-controlled study. Lancet. 2008;371(9629):2013-8.
81. Zheng JP, Wen FQ, Bai CX, Wan HY, Kang J, Chen P, et al. Twice daily N-acetylcysteine 600 mg for exacerbations of chronic obstructive pulmonary disease (PANTHEON): a randomised, double-blind placebo-controlled trial. Lancet Respir Med. 2014;2(3):187-94.
82. Schembri S, Morant S, Winter JH, MacDonald TM. Influenza but not pneumococcal vaccination protects against all-cause mortality in patients with COPD. Thorax. 2009;64(7):567-72.
83. Schenkein JG, Nahm MH, Dransfield MT. Pneumococcal vaccination for patients with COPD: current practice and future directions. Chest. 2008;133(3):767-74.
84. Sprenkle MD, Niewoehner DE, MacDonald R, Rutks I, Wilt TJ. Clinical efficacy of OM-85 BV in COPD and chronic bronchitis: a systematic review. COPD. 2005;2(1):167-75.
85. Williamson JC, Pegram PS. Neuraminidase inhibitors in patients with underlying airways disease. Am J Respir Med. 2002;1(2):85-90.
86. Currow DC, Abernethy AP. Pharmacological management of dyspnoea. Curr Opin Support Palliat Care. 2007;1(2):96-101.
87. Molassiotis A. Bryan G, Caress A, Bailey C, Smith J. Pharmacological and non-pharmacological interventions for cough in adults with respiratory and non-respiratory diseases: A systematic review of the literature. Respir Med. 2010;104(7):934-44.

88. Holland AE, Hill CJ, Jones AY, McDonald CF. Breathing exercises for chronic obstructive pulmonary disease. Cochrane Database Syst Rev. 2012;10:CD008250.
89. Collins PF, Elia M, Stratton RJ. Nutritional support and functional capacity in chronic obstructive pulmonary disease: a systematic review and meta-analysis. Respirology. 2013;18(4): 616-29.
90. Collins A, Koppen G, Valdiglesias V, Dusinska M, Kruszewski M, Møller P, et al. The comet assay as a tool for human biomonitoring studies: The ComNet Project. Mutat Res. 2014;759c:27-39.
91. Casaburi R, ZuWallack R. Pulmonary rehabilitation for management of chronic obstructive pulmonary disease. N Engl J Med. 2009;360(13):1329-35.
92. Troosters T, Hornikx M, Demeyer H, Camillo CA, Janssens W. Pulmonary rehabilitation: timing, location, and duration. Clin Chest Med. 2014;35(2):303-11.
93. Casaburi R, Kukafka D, Cooper CB, Witek TJ, Kesten S. Improvement in exercise tolerance with the combination of tiotropium and pulmonary rehabilitation in patients with COPD. Chest. 2005;127(3):809-17.
94. Struik FM, Lacasse Y, Goldstein RS, Kerstjens HA, Wijkstra PJ. Nocturnal noninvasive positive pressure ventilation in stable COPD: a systematic review and individual patient data meta-analysis. Respir Med. 2014;108(2):329-37.
95. Plant PK, Owen JL, Parrott S, Elliott MW. Cost-effectiveness of ward based non-invasive ventilation for acute exacerbations of chronic obstructive pulmonary disease: economic analysis of randomised controlled trial. BMJ. 2003;326(7396): 956.
96. Patel N, M DeCamp, Criner GJ. Lung transplantation and lung volume reduction surgery versus transplantation in chronic obstructive pulmonary disease. Proc Am Thorac Soc. 2008;5(4):447-53.
97. Criner GJ, Cordova F, Sternberg AL, Martinez FJ. The National Emphysema Treatment Trial (NETT) Part II: Lessons learned about lung volume reduction surgery. Am J Respir Crit Care Med. 2011;184(8):881-93.
98. Iftikhar IH, McGuire FR, Musani AI. Efficacy of bronchoscopic lung volume reduction: a meta-analysis. Int J Chron Obstruct Pulmon Dis. 2014;9:481-91.
99. Wedzicha JA, Singh R, Mackay AJ. Acute COPD exacerbations. Clin Chest Med. 2014;35(1):157-63.
100. Woods JA, Wheeler JS, Finch CK, Pinner NA. Corticosteroids in the treatment of acute exacerbations of chronic obstructive pulmonary disease. Int J Chron Obstruct Pulmon Dis. 2014;9:421-30.
101. Barnes PJ. New anti-inflammatory treatments for chronic obstructive pulmonary disease. Nat Rev Drug Discov. 2013;12:543-59.

Acute Exacerbations of Chronic Obstructive Pulmonary Disease

Raja Dhar, AG Ghoshal

INTRODUCTION

Chronic obstructive pulmonary disease (COPD) exacerbation occurs despite adequate control. Most patients experience episodes of exacerbations at least one or more times during their lifetime and many suffer with these episodes at least 1-3 times a year. These episodes may vary immensely in terms of frequency and severity. COPD exacerbations have a huge impact on the overall health condition of the patient, both physically as well as emotionally. Moreover, exacerbation costs a huge amount of money to the patient and the family. It must be remembered that even in patients with stable COPD, a severe exacerbation episode can cause a significant dent in pulmonary function and adversely affect the quality of his or her life. It is therefore, extremely important for practicing physicians to learn the early identification of crisis, perform optimal management under appropriate settings, escalate and de-escalate the therapy based on patient's response, bring back the patient to the initial baseline status, help the patient and family to cope up with the situation with adequate support, discharge the patient in a stable clinical conditions, give necessary instruction about the proper follow-up.

Thankfully, with modern evidence-based treatment modalities, successful management of COPD exacerbation can be done in the majority of patients.

CHRONIC OBSTRUCTIVE PULMONARY DISEASE EXACERBATION

An acute exacerbation of COPD (AECOPD) is an event in the natural course of COPD characterized by an acute change in the patient's baseline dyspnea or breathing difficulty, cough and/or sputum production beyond day-to-day variability sufficient to warrant a change in management.

It can be infective or noninfective in nature. In the absence of a universal agreed criterion, the following operational classification can help to rank the clinical severity of the episode and its outcome:

- *Level I:* Treated at home
- *Level II:* Requires hospitalization
- *Level III:* Leads to respiratory failure.

CAUSES OF CHRONIC OBSTRUCTIVE PULMONARY DISEASE EXACERBATIONS

About 50% of COPD exacerbations are caused by lower respiratory tract infections, while the remaining are caused by exposure to indoor or outdoor air pollutants, changes in weather and several host factors including peer compliance to therapy **(Box 1)**.[1,2]

A recent study has tried to identify the "exacerbation phenotype" in COPD. Following literature review, the established etiologies of AECOPD have been précised in the acronym—ABCDEFGX;[3]

Airway viral infection
Bacterial infection
Coinfection
Depression or Anxiety
Embolism (pulmonary)
Failure (cardiac, or failure of lung integrity—pneumothorax)
General environment
X (unknown).

Each patient in this study underwent nasopharyngeal sampling for respiratory virus multiplex polymerase chain reaction in addition to sputum culture and a host of other basic investigations. It showed coinfection (simultaneous bacterial and viral infection) resulted in a statistically longer length of hospital stay. This pilot study emphasizes the

BOX 1 Causes of chronic obstructive pulmonary disease exacerbations

Infectious process: Viral (Rhinovirus spp., influenza); Bacterial (*Haemophilus influenzae*, *Streptococcus pneumoniae*, *Moraxella catarrhalis*, *Enterobacteriaceae* species, *Pseudomonas* spp.)

Environmental conditions: Sudden change in temperature, humidity, etc. air pollution exposure, exposure to tobacco smoke, noxious gases or irritating chemicals

Host factors: Patients with poor general health condition, poor nutritional status, immunocompromised status, lack of compliance with prescribed medical therapy, adoption of unhealthy lifestyle modes like lack of continuing with advised exercises, improper diet, poor level of personal hygiene, lack of compliance with long-term oxygen therapy, failure to participate in pulmonary rehabilitation.

heterogeneity of AECOPD and demonstrates that refining the term "COPD exacerbation" to reflect underlying exacerbation etiology may be feasible and clinically relevant.[4]

SYMPTOMS OF CHRONIC OBSTRUCTIVE PULMONARY DISEASE EXACERBATION

Usually, patients present with one or more symptoms of acute exacerbation **(Box 2)**. During clinical assessment, further objective evaluation is necessary. Several clinical elements must be considered when evaluating patients with exacerbations. These include the assessment of the severity of the underlying COPD, the presence of comorbidities and the history of previous exacerbation. The physical examination should evaluate the effects of the episode on hemodynamic and respiratory systems. The diagnostic procedures such as chest radiography, sputum and blood examination and spirometry to be performed depend on the setting of the evaluation.[5,6]

MANAGEMENT OF CHRONIC OBSTRUCTIVE PULMONARY DISEASE EXACERBATION

The decision to treat a patient at home or in the hospital is based both on subjective evaluation as well as objective criteria **(Table 1)**. The choice of the patient or patients' family should also be taken into account. However, it must be noted that there may be a sudden deterioration of condition and the decision to treat at home or at hospital can change rapidly **(Box 3)**. Development of new situations may warrant further evaluation and subsequent hospitalization. Diagnosis of an exacerbation is primarily clinical and dependent on investigation though they are useful in assessing the severity and planning the optimum treatment **(Table 2)**.

Primary Care

In patients with an exacerbation managed in primary care:

- Sending sputum samples for culture is not recommended in routine practice
- Pulse oximetry may be useful if there are clinical features of a severe exacerbation.

BOX 2 Symptoms of chronic obstructive pulmonary disease exacerbation

- Increase in cough
- Chest pain
- Increase in breathlessness
- Increase in sputum volume and change in its color (white to green, yellow or blood streaked)
- Fever
- Increased tiredness
- Increase in oxygen requirement (for those on long-term oxygen therapy)

Prognostication

The CRB65 score, a risk stratification method validated for use in community-acquired pneumonia, has recently been shown to have utility in AECOPD. In-hospital and 30-day mortality increased progressively with increasing CRB65 score

Table 1 Clinical factors that determine whether the patient should be treated at home or hospital

Factor	*Indication to treat at home*	*Indication to treat at hospital*
Able to cope at home	Yes	No
Severity of breathlessness	Mild	Severe
General health condition	Good/ Satisfactory	Poor/ deteriorating
Level of activity	Good	Poor/confined to bed
Cyanosis	No	Yes
Worsening peripheral edema	No	Yes
Level of consciousness	Normal	Impaired
Already receiving LTOT	No	Yes
Social circumstances	Good/adequate support	Living alone/ not coping
Acute confusion/altered mental status	No	Yes
Rapid rate of onset	No	Yes
Significant comorbidity (particularly heart disease and insulin-dependent diabetes)	No	Yes
$SaO_2 < 90\%$	No	Yes
Changes on the chest radiograph	No	Present
Arterial pH level	>7.35	< 7.35
Arterial PaO_2	>7 kPa	< 7 kPa

Abbreviations: LTOT, long-term oxygen therapy; SaO_2, arterial oxygen saturation; PaO_2, partial pressure of O_2 in arterial blood

BOX 3 The situations for immediate reassessment of the patient condition

- Marked increase in dyspnea
- Inability to eat or sleep due to respiratory symptoms
- Inadequate response to the outpatient management
- Worsening of hypoxemia
- Worsening of hypercarbia
- Change in mental status
- Poor perception of severity
- Inability of the patient to take care of himself/herself/lack of home support
- Documented noncompliance to prescribed therapy
- Development of new symptoms
- Uncertain diagnosis

Table 2 Elements of the clinical evaluation and diagnostic procedures that are usually informative in patients with exacerbations according to the severity of the episode

	Level I (Treated at home)	*Level II (Requires hospitalization)*	*Level III (Leads to respiratory failure)*
Clinical history:			
Comorbid conditions*	+	+++	+++
Frequent exacerbations	+	+++	+++
Severity of COPD	Mild/Moderate	Moderate/Severe	Severe
Physical findings:			
Hemodynamics	Stable	Stable	Stable/unstable
Use of accessory muscles while breathing/tachypnea	Not present	++	+++
Persistent symptoms after initial therapy	No	++	+++
Diagnostic procedures:			
Oxygen saturation	Yes	Yes	Yes
Arterial blood gases	No	Yes	Yes
Chest radiograph	No	Yes	Yes
Blood tests†	No	Yes	Yes
Serum drug concentration‡	If applicable	If applicable	If applicable
Sputum Gram stain and culture	No¶	Yes	Yes
Electrocardiogram	No	Yes	Yes

Abbreviation: COPD, chronic obstructive pulmonary disease
Keys:
*The more common comorbid conditions associated with poor prognosis in exacerbations are congestive heart failure, coronary artery disease, diabetes mellitus, renal and liver failure
†Blood tests include cell blood count, serum electrolytes, renal and liver function
‡Consider if patients are using theophylline, warfarin, carbamazepine, digoxin
¶Consider if patient has been recently on antibiotics
+unlikely to be present ++likely to be present +++very likely to be present

and was markedly higher in the CRB 3–4 group. Differences in 1-year mortality were less apparent. We recommend its use in clinical practice, particularly in patients with a score 3, which is associated with a high risk of early mortality, and need for intensive hospital management.[7]

A study at Oslo University Hospital looked to establish a prediction model for length of stay (LOS) in hospital in patients with AECOPD. Admission between Thursday and Saturday, heart failure, diabetes, stroke, high arterial partial pressure of carbon dioxide (PCO_2), and low serum albumin level were associated with a prolonged LOS.[8] A Spanish study had also predicted a poorer outcome in patients admitted on a weekend. These findings may help physicians to identify patients that will need a prolonged LOS in the early stages of admission. However, these are only clinical pointers and will need to be studied further before we can use them in clinical practice.[9]

Serum procalcitonin has recently been advocated for use in deciding regarding antibiotic treatment in patients with AECOPD. However, recent studies show that procalcitonin is useful in COPD patients for alerting clinicians to invasive bacterial infections such as pneumonia but it does not distinguish bacterial from viral and noninfectious causes of AECOPD.[10]

Serum uric acid is increased in respiratory disease, especially in the presence of hypoxia and systemic inflammation. High uric acid levels (>6.9 mg/dL) in AECOPD were an independent predictor of 30-day mortality, but not of 1-year mortality. Patients with high serum uric acid required more prolonged hospitalization, and more often needed noninvasive ventilation (NIV) and admission to the intensive care unit (ICU) within 30 days.[11]

During AECOPD, poor outcome is predicted from elevated cardiac biomarkers such as brain natriuretic peptide (BNP) or troponin.[1,2] There is strong recent evidence which shows that higher levels of NT-Pro BNP is associated with increased long-term mortality in patients with AECOPD. It appears that AECOPD may have an impact on plasma BNP levels that is not attributable to heart failure.[12]

In another study, subtle subclinical left ventricular performance impairment detected by transthoracic echocardiogram was associated with poor prognosis in acutely decompensated COPD patients. Early detection of left ventricular (LV) function impairment during exacerbation could lead to the optimization of pharmacotherapy strategies. The early use of diuretics could lower filling pressures for symptom improvement. After exacerbation, patients could benefit from the use of cardioselective beta-blockers, while betamimetics are known to potentially worsen myocardial dysfunction.[13]

PATIENTS REFERRED TO HOSPITAL

In all patients with an exacerbation referred to hospital:

- A chest radiograph should be obtained
- Arterial blood gas tensions should be measured and the inspired oxygen concentration recorded
- An electrocardiogram (ECG) should be recorded to exclude cardiac comorbidities
- A full blood count should be performed; urea and electrolyte concentrations should be measured
- A theophylline level should be measured in patients who are on theophylline therapy at admission
- If sputum is purulent, a sample should be sent for microscopy and culture
- Blood cultures should be taken if the patient has fever.

OUTPATIENT MANAGEMENT FOR CHRONIC OBSTRUCTIVE PULMONARY DISEASE EXACERBATION (LEVEL I)

The treatment of exacerbation has to be based on the clinical presentation of the patient.

The essential components of treatment are shown in **Box 4**.

BOX 4 The essential components of treatment of chronic obstructive pulmonary disease exacerbation

Bronchodilators:
- Short-acting beta 2-agonist* and/or ipratropium by metered dose inhaler with spacer or hand-held nebulizer as needed[14-16]
- Consider adding long-acting bronchodilator, e.g. formoterol [by metered-dose inhaler (MDI) plus spacer or nebulized route] if patient is not using it.

Corticosteroids (the actual dose may vary):
- Oral prednisone 30–40 mg per os q.d. for 10 days[17-19]
- Consider using an inhaled corticosteroid[20]

Antibiotics:[1,21-26]
- May be initiated in patients with altered sputum characteristics
- Choice should be based on local bacteria resistance patterns
- Amoxicillin/ampicillin†, cephalosporins§
- Doxycycline
- Macrolides¶[27-29]
- If the patient has failed prior antibiotic therapy consider:
  - Amoxicillin/clavulanate[28]
  - Respiratory fluoroquinolones**[22,30,31]
- Cefdinir, cefprozil, cefuroxime

Patient education:
- Check inhalation technique
- Consider use of spacer devices.

Keys:
*Metered-dose inhaler: salbutamol/levosalbutamol
†Terbutaline: depending on local prevalence of bacterial beta-lactamases
§Cefpodoxime, cefprozil, cefuroxime, cefdinir
¶Azithromycin, clarithromycin, dirithromycin, roxithromycin
**Gatifloxacin, levofloxacin and moxifloxacin

INPATIENT MANAGEMENT OF CHRONIC OBSTRUCTIVE PULMONARY DISEASE EXACERBATION (LEVELS II AND III)

As mentioned earlier, the decision to admit a patient is derived from the subjective interpretation of clinical features, such as the severity of dyspnea, determination of respiratory failure, short-term response to emergency room therapy, degree of cor pulmonale and the presence of complicating features such as severe bronchitis, pneumonia or other comorbid conditions.

Very few clinical studies have investigated patient-specific objective clinical and laboratory features that identify patients with COPD who require hospitalization. General consensus supports the need for hospitalization in patients with severe acute hypoxemia or acute hypercarbia. Less extreme arterial blood gas abnormalities, however, do not assist decision analysis. Other factors that identify "high-risk" patients include a previous emergency room visit within 7 days, the number of doses of nebulized bronchodilators, use of home oxygen, previous relapse rate, administration of aminophylline and the use of corticosteroids and antibiotics at the time of previous emergency room discharge.[32-35]

Pharmacologic management remains the mainstay of COPD exacerbation along with other supportive measures.

INHALED BRONCHODILATORS

- Short-acting beta 2-agonist (salbutamol 100–200 mcg inhaler/levosalbutamol) and/or
- Ipratropium MDI (20, 40 mcg) with spacer or hand-held nebulizer as needed.[14-16]

Delivery systems for inhaled therapy during exacerbations:

- Both nebulizers and hand-held inhalers can be used to administer inhaled therapy during exacerbations of COPD
- The choice of delivery system should reflect the dose of drug required, the ability of the patient to use the device and the resources available to supervise the administration of the therapy
- If a patient is hypercapnic or acidotic, the nebulizer should be driven by compressed air, not oxygen (to avoid worsening hypercapnia). If oxygen therapy is needed, it should be administered simultaneously by nasal cannulae
- The driving gas for nebulized therapy should always be specified in the prescription.

SYSTEMIC CORTICOSTEROIDS

- Inhaled corticosteroids by MDI or hand-held nebulizer should be considered.[20] For example, beclomethasone 50–400 mcg; budesonide 100, 200, 400 mcg; fluticasone 50–500 mcg inhaler
- In the absence of significant contraindications, oral corticosteroids should be used in conjunction with other therapies in all patients admitted to hospital with an exacerbation of COPD
- In the absence of significant contraindications, oral corticosteroids should be considered in patients managed in the community who have an exacerbation with a significant increase in breathlessness which interferes with daily activities
- Patients requiring corticosteroid therapy should be encouraged to present early to get maximum benefits
- Prednisolone 30 mg orally should be prescribed for 7–14 days
- If patient tolerates, prednisone 30–40 mg/day should be prescribed for 10 days[17-19]
- If patient cannot tolerate oral intake, consider equivalent dose intravenous (IV) for up to 14 days (20 mg hydrocortisone is equivalent to 5 mg prednisolone, 4 mg methylprednisolone and 0.75 mg dexamethasone)
- It is recommended that a course of corticosteroid treatment should not be longer than 14 days as there is no advantage in prolonged therapy
- Osteoporosis prophylaxis should be considered in patients requiring frequent courses of oral corticosteroids
- Patients should be made aware of the optimum duration of treatment and the adverse effects of prolonged therapy
- Patients, particularly those discharged from hospital, should be given clear instructions about why, when and how to stop their corticosteroid treatment.

ANTIBIOTICS[1,2,18-28,32,36]

- Antibiotics based on local bacteria resistance patterns should be started for patients with the history of producing purulent sputum. Any change in sputum characteristics like color, consistency and volume should also prompt the initiation
- Antibiotics need not be started for patients having exacerbations without increase in sputum purulence, unless there are signs of consolidation on chest radiograph or clinical symptoms of pneumonia
- Antibiotic choice should be based on local bacteria resistance patterns, if available. However, when this information is not available, macrolides or second-generation cephalosporins can be used
- Initial empirical treatment should consist of an aminopenicillin, a macrolide or a tetracycline. When initiating empirical antibiotic treatment, one should always take account of any guidance issued by the local microbiologists
- When sputum has been sent for culture, the sensitivity to antibiotics should be checked to ensure appropriate therapy:
- Amoxicillin/clavulanate[28] and respiratory fluoroquinolones (levofloxacin, moxifloxacin)[22,30,31] are commonly used
- If *Pseudomonas* spp. and/or other enterobacteriaceae spp. are suspected, consider combination therapy [e.g. piperacillin/tazobactam (3.375 g q 4 hours IV) or imipenem (500 mg q 6 hours IV) or meropenem (1 g q 8 hours IV) plus amikacin (7.5 mg/kg q 12 hours or 15 mg/kg q 24 hours IV) or levofloxacin (500 mg daily) for 10–14 days].

THEOPHYLLINE AND OTHER METHYLXANTHINES

- Intravenous theophylline should only be used as an adjunct to the management of exacerbations of COPD, if there is an inadequate response to nebulized bronchodilators
- Care should be taken when using intravenous theophylline because of its interactions with other drugs (e.g. ciprofloxacin, clarithromycin, allopurinol, phenytoin, etc.) and potential toxicity if the patient has been on oral theophylline
- Within 24 hours of starting the treatment, the theophylline levels should be monitored to maintain within therapeutic range (10–20 mcg/mL). Thereafter, monitoring should be done as frequently as indicated by clinical circumstances.

RESPIRATORY STIMULANTS

It is recommended that doxapram is used only when NIV is either unavailable or considered inappropriate (e.g. hypersensitivity, pulmonary embolism, severe hypertension, cerebral edema, epilepsy, hyperthyroidism, etc.).

OXYGEN THERAPY

Oxygen therapy is recommended to relieve severe respiratory distress and prevent tissue hypoxia.

- The goal is to prevent tissue hypoxia by maintaining arterial oxygen saturation (SaO_2) at more than 90%
- All patients with COPD exacerbation should have their arterial oxygen tension (PaO_2), arterial carbon dioxide tension ($PaCO_2$) and pH measured upon admission, during the course of treatment and whenever there is any change in patient's clinical condition
- In case of unavailability of arterial blood gas measurement facility, oxygen saturation should be measured. Pulse oximeters should be available to all healthcare professionals managing patients with exacerbations of COPD and they should be trained in their use. Clinicians should be aware that pulse oximetry gives no information about the PCO_2 or pH
- Even if oximeter is not available for any reason, oxygen should be given to all patients with an exacerbation of

COPD who are breathless, even if the oxygen saturations are not known, but careful monitoring of the patient condition is essential to prevent excessive CO_2 washout and cause respiratory depression since CO_2 acts as the respiratory drive for many COPD patients
- The principal delivery device for oxygen comprises of nasal cannula and venturi mask. Alternative delivery devices include nonrebreather mask, reservoir cannula or transtracheal catheter
- During the transfer to hospital, the following points should be considered:
  - It is not desirable to exceed an oxygen saturation of 93%. Oxygen therapy should be commenced at approximately 40% and titrated upward if saturation falls below 90% and downward if the patient becomes drowsy or if the saturation exceeds 93–94%
  - Patients with known type II respiratory failure need special care, especially if they require a long ambulance journey or if they are given oxygen at home for a prolonged period before the ambulance arrives. It is important to remember that the prevention of tissue hypoxia supercedes CO_2 retention issue
- The aim of oxygen therapy during exacerbation of COPD is to maintain adequate level of oxygen (SaO_2 > 90%) without worsening or precipitating respiratory acidosis or worsening hypercapnia. If pH falls below 7.35 (acidemia), consider mechanical ventilation.

ADMISSION TO INTENSIVE CARE UNIT OR CRITICAL CARE UNIT

The decision to shift or admit a patient to the critical care unit largely depends on subjective assessment and clinician's judgment, although various diagnostic parameters help in decision making. Presence of the following features merit consideration for shifting to intermediate respiratory care unit (IRCU):
- Persistent respiratory distress despite standard management
- Inability to maintain oxygen level above 90% despite oxygen therapy by high-flow mask
- Persistent hypercapnia
- Abnormal blood gas parameters (PaO_2 < 60 mm Hg and/or $PaCO_2$ > 60 mm Hg)
- Alteration of mental status, acute confusion, drowsiness
- Increased signs of infection (pyrexia, increased sputum purulence/volume, etc.)
- Significant abnormal changes in chest radiograph
- Clinical deterioration.

An integrative review of prognostic variables predictive of intermediate-term mortality in AECOPD were low Glasgow coma scale (GCS) on admission to ICU, cardiorespiratory arrest prior to ICU admission, cardiac dysrhythmia prior to ICU admission, length of hospital stay prior to ICU admission and higher values of acute physiology scoring systems. Premorbid variables such as age, functional capacity, pulmonary function tests, prior hospital or ICU admissions, body mass index and long-term oxygen therapy were not found to be associated with intermediate-term mortality, nor were the diagnosis attributed to the cause of the AECOPD.[37]

ASSISTED VENTILATION

Despite optimal pharmacologic management, severe cases of exacerbation necessitates ventilatory support, when the patient is unable to maintain the breathing function and/or unable to maintain sufficient gaseous exchange for normal physiologic function.

Ventilatory support, either "invasive" or "noninvasive", is not a therapy but a form of life support until the cause of underlying acute respiratory failure is reversed with medical therapy.[38-40]

Noninvasive ventilation (NIV) is an alternative for patients who have respiratory failure and can no longer breathe on their own. It enhances the breathing process by giving the patient a mixture of air and oxygen from a flow generator through a tightly fitted facial or nasal mask. NIV assists the patient in taking a full breath and helps to maintain an adequate oxygen supply to the body.[41]

Noninvasive positive pressure ventilation (NIPPV) is by far the most popular mode of providing NIV[40,42] in combination with some continuous positive airway pressure (CPAP) plus pressure support ventilation (PSV).[38,43] It improves the gas exchange by improving the alveolar ventilation, without causing significant modifications in the alveolar ventilation or perfusion mismatching and gas exchange in the lungs.[44] The application of the combination of CPAP and PSV offers a better outcome than either alone because the CPAP counterbalances the intrinsic positive end expiratory pressure.[45]

Noninvasive ventilation should be used as the treatment of choice for persistent hypercapnic ventilatory failure during exacerbations despite optimal medical therapy. Noninvasive positive pressure ventilation should be offered to patients with exacerbations when, after optimal medical therapy and oxygenation, respiratory acidosis (pH < 7.36) and or excessive breathlessness persist. All patients considered for mechanical ventilation should have arterial blood gases measured.
- If pH < 7.30, NIPPV should be delivered under controlled environments such as intermediate ICUs and/or high-dependency units. If pH < 7.25, NIPPV should be administered in the ICU and intubation should be readily available
- It is important to ensure that the NIV be administered by a dedicated team by its staff, with necessary training for the same, well conversant with its application as well as the limitations
- The combination of some CPAP (e.g. 4–8 cm H_2O) and PSV (e.g. 10–15 cm H_2O) provides the most effective mode of NIPPV

- NIV should also be a consideration for patients who are slow from weaning from ventilator (factors influencing slow weaning are not provided in guideline)
- The combination of some CPAP (e.g. 4–8 cm H_2O) and PSV (e.g. 10–15 cm H_2O) provides the most effective mode of NIPPV
- In the first few hours, the level of assistance and monitoring of NIPPV is same as mechanical ventilation
- When put on NIV, there should be a well-defined plan for every patient on course of action on deterioration as well clear indicators of the limits of such deterioration, when the next action is to be taken.

CLINICAL SETTINGS

Noninvasive positive pressure ventilation can be delivered in different clinical settings which are as follows.

- *Medical ward:* Patients with moderate acidosis (pH 7.30–7.35) and hypercapnia (6–8 kPa ($PaCO_2$ 45–60 mm Hg)[46,47]
- Intermediate or high-dependency respiratory unit[48,49] patients who present moderate-to-severe acidosis (pH < 7.30); the facilities for rapid endotracheal intubation and institution of conventional mechanical ventilation should be promptly available
- *ICU:*[50] Patients with severe respiratory acidosis (pH < 7.25); in this particular setting, NIPPV may be as effective as conventional mechanical ventilation to reverse acute respiratory failure due to COPD[51]
- It is important to note that the 1-year mortality was reported to be lower in patients receiving NIPPV for exacerbations of COPD, compared to both optimal medical therapy alone[52] and conventional mechanical ventilation.[51]

MECHANICAL VENTILATION

Mechanical ventilation is a mode of assisted or controlled ventilation using mechanical devices that cycle automatically to generate airway pressure.[53] *Intubation should be considered in patients with the following:*

- *NIPPV failure:* Worsening of arterial blood gases and or pH in 1–2 hours; lack of improvement in arterial blood gases and or pH after 4 hours
- *Severe acidosis* (pH < 7.25) and hypercapnia [$PaCO_2$ > 8 kPa (60 mm Hg)]
- *Tachypnea* > 35 breaths/minute
- *Other complications:* Metabolic abnormalities, sepsis, pneumonia, pulmonary embolism, barotrauma, massive pleural effusion[50]
- During exacerbations of COPD, functional status, body mass index, requirement for oxygen when stable, comorbidities and previous admissions to ICUs should be considered, in addition to age and forced expiratory volume in 1 second (FEV1), when assessing suitability for intubation and ventilation. Neither age nor FEV1 should be used in isolation when assessing suitability
- Noninvasive positive pressure ventilation should be considered as the first-line intervention, in addition to optimal mechanical therapy, for the management of patients with respiratory failure due to exacerbation of COPD.[42] In the first few hours, NIPPV requires the same level of assistance as conventional mechanical ventilation[54]
- The fact that NIPPV is cost-effective is clearly demonstrated by a study[30,55] and it can also be used as a potential successful strategy of weaning[31,56] the patients from mechanical ventilation, in cases where the patients need an intermediate care between complete machine-dependent and totally independent for breathing
- The NIPPV may also be considered for those with history of previous persistent weaning failure.[57]

DE-ESCALATION OF THERAPY

- Patients' recovery should be monitored by regular clinical assessment of their symptoms and observation of their functional capacity
- For patients with nonhypercapnic failure, nonacidotic failure can be monitored with pulse oximetry
- For hypercapnic or acidotic patients, intermittent blood gas monitoring should be done to evaluate the situation. The frequency of such tests largely depends on the clinical judgment of the treating physician
- During recovery from an exacerbation from COPD, daily performance of FEV1 or peak expiratory flow is not advised since the magnitude of change is small as compared to the variability of measurement.

Discharge should be planned when:

- There is significant improvement in the clinical status of the patient
- Significant improvement of symptoms like breathlessness, cough, remission or steady improvement in infection symptoms (reduction in sputum volume, nonpyrexial status, nonpurulence of sputum as confirmed by culture)
- Ability to maintain blood gas at acceptable range
- Ability and inclination to perform day to day activities, even with some degree of assistance.

On the other hand of the spectrum, discharge or hospice care needs to be planned when the patient has already reached the end-stage and no significant improvement in clinical and cognitive status is unlikely.

- Spirometry measurement is a must for all patients before discharge. This helps in assessing the impact of the exacerbation episode on the pulmonary function and reassign the baseline values, in case of any alteration
- Patients should be re-established on their optimal maintenance bronchodilators
- Patients and/or home carers must be given the necessary information so that they fully understand the correct usage of medication including oxygen (if applicable)

- Follow-up visits must be scheduled and communicated to the patient/family
- Follow-up care like refilling of medication, visiting nurse, oxygen delivery and referral for other support must be made before discharge
- Before the patient is discharged, the patient, family members and the treating physician must be confident that the patient will be able to manage successfully. In case of doubts, formal assessments can be initiated
- All aspects of the routine care that patients receive (including appropriateness and risk of side effects) should be assessed before discharge
- An early rehabilitation program following AECOPD (2–3 weeks after discharge) led to improvement in quality of life up to 6 months. This needs to be investigated further[58]
- It is useful to hand over a written plan on daily self care, medication management, emergency action plan during exacerbation to all patients/carers before discharge, with adequate explanation.

REFERENCES

1. Adams SG, Anzueto A. Treatment of acute exacerbations of chronic bronchitis. Seminar Respir Infect. 2000;15:234-47.
2. Fagon JY, Chastre J. Severe exacerbations of COPD patients: the role of pulmonary infections. Semin Respir Infect. 1996;11(2): 109-18.
3. MacDonald M, Bardin P, Beasley R, Irving L. A hypothesis to phenotype COPD exacerbations by aetiology. Respirology. 2011;16:264-8.
4. MacDonald M, Korman T, King P, Hamza K, Bardin P. Exacerbation phenotyping in chronic obstructive pulmonary disease. Respirology. 2013;18:1280-1.
5. Emerman CL, Cydulka RA. Evaluation of high-yield criteria for chest radiography in acute exacerbation of chronic obstructive pulmonary disease. Ann Emerg Med. 1993;22(4);680-4.
6. O'Brien C, Guest PJ, Hill SL. Physiological and radiological characterization of patients diagnosed with chronic obstructive pulmonary disease in primary care. Thorax. 2000;55(8):635-42.
7. Edwards L, Perrin K, Wijesinghe M, Weatherall M, Beasley R, Travers J. The value of the CRB65 score to predict mortality in exacerbations of COPD requiring hospital admission. Respirology. 2011;16(4):625-9.
8. Wang Y, Stavem K, Dahl FA, Humerfelt S, Haugen T. Factors associated with a prolonged length of stay after acute exacerbation of chronic obstructive pulmonary disease (AECOPD). Int J Chron Obstruct Pulmon Dis. 2014;9:99-105.
9. Barba R, Zapatero A, Losa JE, Marco J, Plaza S, Rosado C, et al. The impact of weekends on outcome for acute exacerbations of COPD. Eur Respir J. 2012;39(1):46-50.
10. Falsey AR, Becker KL, Swinburne AJ, Nylen ES, Snider RH, Formica MA, et al. Utility of serum procalcitonin values in patients with acute exacerbations of chronic obstructive pulmonary disease: a cautionary note. Int J Chron Obstruct Pulmon Dis. 2012;7:127-35.
11. Bartziokas K, Papaioannou A, Loukides S, Papadopoulos A, Haniotou A, Papiris S, et al. Serum uric acid as a predictor of mortality and future exacerbations of COPD. Eur Respir J. 2014;43(1):43-53.
12. Nishimura K, Nishimura T, Onishi K, Oga T, Hasegawa Y, Jones PW, et al. Changes in plasma levels of B-type natriuretic peptide with acute exacerbations of chronic obstructive pulmonary disease. Int J Chron Obstruct Pulmon Dis. 2014;9:155-62.
13. Escande W, Duva Pentiah A, Coisne A, Mouton S, Richardson M, Polge AS, et al. Left ventricular myocardial performance index predicts poor outcome during COPD exacerbation. International Journal of Cardiology. 2014;173(3):575-9.
14. Karpel JP, Pesin J, Greenberg D, Gentry E. A comparison of the effects of ipratropium bromide and metaproterenol sulfate in acute exacerbation of COPD. Chest. 1990;98(4):835-9.
15. Emerman CL, Cydulka RK. Effect of different albuterol dosing regimens in the treatment of acute exacerbation of chronic obstructive disease. Ann Emerg Med. 1997;29(4):474-8.
16. Turner MO, Patel A, Ginsburg S, FitzGerald JM. Bronchodilator delivery in acute airflow obstruction. A meta-analysis. Arch Intern Med. 1997;157(15):1736-44.
17. Hudson LD, Monti M. Rationale and use of corticosteroids in chronic obstructive pulmonary disease. Med Clin N Am. 1990;74(3):661-90.
18. Davies L, Angus RM, Calverley PM. Oral corticosteroids in patients admitted to hospital with exacerbations of chronic obstructive pulmonary disease: a prospective randomized controlled trial. Lancet. 1999;345(9177):456-60.
19. Thompson WH, Nielson CP, Carvalho P, Charan NB, Crowley JJ. Controlled trial of oral prednisone in outpatients with acute COPD exacerbation. Am J Respir Crit Care Med. 1996;154(2 Pt 1):407-12.
20. Maltais F, Ostinelli J, Bourbeau J, Tonnel AB, Jacquemet N, Haddon J, et al. Comparison of nebulized budesonide and oral prednisolone with placebo in the treatment of acute exacerbations of chronic obstructive pulmonary disease: a randomized controlled trial. Am J Respir Crit Care Med. 2002;165(5):698-703.
21. Miravitlles M, Guerrero T, Mayordomo C, Sánchez-Agudo L, Nicolau F, Segú JL. Factors associated with increased risk of exacerbation and hospital admission in a cohort of ambulatory COPD patients: a multiple logistic regression analysis. The EOLO Study Group. Respiration. 2000;67(5):495-501.
22. Wilson R, Schentag JJ, Ball P, Mandell L, 068 Study Group. A comparison of gemifloxacin and clarithromycin in acute exacerbations of chronic bronchitis and long-term clinical outcomes. Clin Ther. 2002;24(4):639-52.
23. Anthonisen NR, Manfreda J, Warren CP, Hershfield ES, Harding GK, Nelson NA. Antibiotic therapy in exacerbations of chronic obstructive pulmonary disease. Ann Intern Med. 1987;106(2):196-204.
24. Saint SK, Bent S, Vittinghoff E, Grady D. Antibiotics in chronic obstructive pulmonary disease exacerbations. A meta-analysis. JAMA. 1995;273(12):957-60.
25. Wilson R, Tillotson G, Ball P. Clinical studies in chronic bronchitis: a need for better definition and classification of severity. J Antimicrob Chemother. 1996;37(2):205-8.
26. Nouira S, Marghli S, Belghith M, Besbes L, Elatrous S, Abroug F. Once daily oral ofloxacin in chronic obstructive pulmonary disease exacerbation requiring mechanical ventilation: a randomized placebo-controlled trial. Lancet. 2001;358(9298):2020-35.
27. Swanson RN, Lainez-Ventosilla A, De Salvo MC, Dunne MW, Amsden GW. Once-daily azithromycin for 3 days compared with clarithromycin for 10 days for acute exacerbation of

chronic bronchitis: a multicenter, double-blind, randomized study. Treat Respir Med. 2005;4(1):31-9.

28. Anzueto A, Fisher CL, Busman T, Olson CA. Comparison of the efficacy of extended-release clarithromycin tablets and amoxicillin/clavulanate tablets in the treatment of acute exacerbations of chronic bronchitis. Clin Ther. 2001;23(1):72-86.
29. Cazzola M, Vinciguerra A, Di Perna F, Califano C, Calderaro F, Salzillo A, et al. Comparative study of dirithromycin and azithromycin in the treatment of acute bacterial exacerbation of chronic bronchitis. J Chemother. 1999;11(2):119-25.
30. Gotfried MH, DeAbate A, Fogarty C, Mathew CP, Sokol WN. Comparison of 5-day, short course gatifloxacin therapy with 7-day gatifloxacin therapy and 10-day clarithromycin therapy for acute exacerbation of chronic bronchitis. Clin Ther. 2001;23(1):97-107.
31. Wilson R, Kubin R, Ballin I, Deppermann KM, Bassaris HP, Leophonte P, et al. Five day moxifloxacin therapy compared with 7 day clarithromycin therapy for the treatment of acute exacerbations of chronic bronchitis. J Antimicrobial Chemother. 1999;44(4):501-13.
32. Emerman CL, Effron D, Lukens TW. Spirometric criteria for hospital admission of patients with acute exacerbations of COPD. Chest. 1991;99(3):595-9.
33. Grossman R, Mukherjee J, Vaughan D, Eastwood C, Cook R, LaForge J, et al. A 1-year community-based health economic study of ciprofloxacin vs usual antibiotic treatment in acute exacerbations of chronic bronchitis: the Canadian Ciprofloxacin Health Economic Study Group. Chest. 1998;113(1): 131-41.
34. Kessler R, Faller M, Fourgaut G, Mennecier B, Weitzenblum E. Predictive factors of hospitalization for acute exacerbation in a series of 64 patients with chronic obstructive pulmonary disease. Am J Crit Care Med. 1999;159(1):158-64.
35. Garcia-Aymerich J, Monsó E, Marrades RM, Escarrabill J, Félez MA, Sunyer J, et al. Risk factors for a chronic obstructive pulmonary disease exacerbation. EFRAM study. Am J Respir Crit Care Med. 2001;164(6):1002-7.
36. Wedzicha JA. The heterogeneity of chronic obstructive pulmonary disease. Thorax. 2000;55(8):631-2.
37. Messer B, Griffiths J, Baudouin SV. The prognostic variables predictive of mortality in patients with an exacerbation of COPD admitted to the ICU: an integrative review. QJM. 2012;105(2):115-26.
38. International Consensus Conferences in Intensive Care Medicine: noninvasive positive pressure ventilation in acute Respiratory failure. Am J Respir Crit Care Med. 2001;163(1):283-91.
39. British Thoracic Society Standards of Care Committee. Non-invasive ventilation in acute respiratory failure. Thorax. 2002;57(3):192-211.
40. Mehta S, Hill NS. Noninvasive ventilation. Am J Respir Crit Care Med. 2001;163(2):540-77.
41. Ram FS, Picot J, Lightowler J, Wedzicha JA. Non-invasive positive pressure ventilation for treatment of respiratory failure due to exacerbations of chronic obstructive pulmonary disease. Cochrane Database Sys Rev. 2004;3:CD004104.
42. Lightowler JV, Wedzicha JA, Elliot MW, Ram FS. Non-invasive positive pressure ventilation to treat respiratory failure resulting from exacerbations of chronic obstructive pulmonary disease: Cochrane systematic review and meta-analysis. BMJ. 2003;326(7382):185.
43. Rossi A, Appendini L, Roca J. Physiological aspects of noninvasive positive pressure ventilation. Eur Respir Mon. 2001;16:1-10.
44. Diaz O, Iglesia R, Ferrer M, Zavala E, Santos C, Wagner PD, et al. Effects of noninvasive ventilation on pulmonary gas exchange and hemodynamics during acute hypercapnic exacerbations of chronic obstructive pulmonary disease. Am J Respir Crit Care Med. 1997;156(6):1840-5.
45. Appendini L, Patessio A, Zanaboni S, Carone M, Gukov B, Donner CF, et al. Physiologic effects of positive end expiratory pressure and mask pressure support during exacerbation of chronic obstructive pulmonary disease. Am J Respir Crit Care Med. 1994;149(5):1069-76.
46. Bott J, Carroll MP, Conway JH, Keilty SE, Ward EM, Brown AM, et al. Randomised controlled trial of nasal ventilation in acute ventilatory failure due to chronic obstructive airways disease. Lancet. 1993;341(8860):1555-7.
47. Plant PK, Owen JL, Elliott MW. Early use of non-invasive ventilation for acute exacerbations of chronic obstructive pulmonary disease on general respiratory wards: a multicentre randomised controlled trial. Lancet. 2000;355(9219):1931-5.
48. Kramer N, Meyer TJ, Meharg J, Cece RD, Hill NS. Randomized, preospective trial of non invasive positive pressure ventilation in acute respiratory failure. Am J Respir Crit Care Med. 1995;151(6):1799-806.
49. Celikel T, Sungur M, Ceyhan B, Karakurt S. Comparison of noninvasive positive pressure ventilation with standard medical therapy in hypercapnic acute respiratory failure. Chest. 1998;114(6):1636-42.
50. Brochard L, Mancebo J, Wysocki M, Lofaso F, Conti G, Rauss A, et al. Noninvasive ventilation for acute exacerbations of chronic obstructive pulmonary disease. N Eng J Med. 1995;333(13):817-22.
51. Conti G, Antonelli M, Navalesi P, Rocco M, Bufi M, Spadetta G, et al. Noninvaisve vs conventional mechanical ventilation in patients with chronic obstructive pulmonary disease after failure of medical treatment in the ward: a randomized trial. Intensive Care Med. 2002;28(12):1701-7.
52. Plant PK, Owen JL, Elliott MW. Non-invasive ventilation in acute exacerbations of chronic obstructive pulmonary disease: long term survival and predictors of in-hospital outcome. Thorax. 2001;56(9):708 12.
53. Slutsky AS. Mechanical ventilation. American College of Chest Physicians Consensus Conference. Chest. 1993;194:1833-59.
54. Nava S, Evangelisti I, Rampulla C, Ompagnoni ML, Fracchia C, Rubini F. Human and financial costs of non invasive mechanical ventilation in patients affected by COPD and acute respiratory failure. Chest. 1997;111(6):1631-8.
55. Plant PK, Owen JL, Parrott S, Elliott MW. Cost-effectiveness of ward based non-invasive ventilation for acute exacerbations of chronic obstructive pulmonary disease: economic analysis of randomised controlled trial. BMJ. 2003;326(7396):956.
56. Nava S, Ambrosino N, Clini E, Prato M, Orlando G, Vitacca M, et al. Noninvasive mechanical ventilation in the weaning of patients with respiratory failure due to chronic obstructive pulmonary disease. A randomized, controlled trial. Ann Intern Med. 1998;128(9):721-8.
57. Ferrer M, Esquinas A, Arancibia F, Bauer TT, Gonzalez G, Carrillo A, et al. Noninvasive ventilation during persitent weaning failure: a randomized controlled trial. Am J Respir Crit Care Med. 2003;168(1):70-6.
58. Ko FW, Dai DL, Ngai J, Tung A, Ng S, Lai K, et al. Effect of early pulmonary rehabilitation on health care utilization and health status in patients hospitalized with acute exacerbations of COPD. Respirology. 2011;16(4):617-24.

78
Chapter

End-of-life Communication and Palliative Care in Advanced Chronic Obstructive Pulmonary Disease

Sujeet Rajan

INTRODUCTION

This is by far the most challenging part of managing advanced chronic obstructive pulmonary disease (COPD) for respiratory physicians. Physicians managing COPD must be both confident and competent in caring for their patients in the final phase of their illness. Both the patient and his family must be assisted to face inevitable death. It is not surprising that in a study of 100 patients with COPD, 58% preferred a plan of comfort care over a plan to extend life and 78% did not want ventilation in intensive care.[1] Decisions to limit support in terminal illness have become routine in Europe and the United States. In India, however, these decisions are far more difficult due to the lack of palliative care orientation, unawareness of ethical issues, culture of "fighting till the end" and legal and administrative prejudices.[2]

DEFINITIONS

At the end-of-life, potentially important decisions are needed. The correct definition of each possible intervention is extremely important. The definitions below are from the International Consensus Conference on end-of-life care in the intensive care unit (ICU) published in 2004.[3,4]

Withholding: A planned decision not to introduce therapies that are otherwise warranted (i.e. intubation, renal replacement therapy, increased doses of vasopressor infusions, surgery, transfusion, nutrition and hydration).

Withdrawal: Discontinuation of treatments that have been started (i.e. decreasing inspiratory oxygen fraction to 21%, extubation, turning off the ventilator and suspending the vasopressors).

Terminal sedation: Pain and symptom treatment with the possible side effect of shortening life.

Euthanasia: From the Greek words *eu* and *thanatos* meaning "good death". It means that a doctor is intentionally killing a person who is suffering unbearably and hopelessly at the latter's voluntary, explicit, repeated, well-considered and informed request.

Physician-assisted suicide: It means that a doctor is intentionally helping or assisting or co-operating in the suicide of a person who is suffering unbearably and hopelessly at the latter's voluntary, explicit, repeated, well-considered and informed request. These acts do not include withholding or withdrawing treatments although these may occur prior to physician-assisted suicide.

Cardiopulmonary resuscitation failure: Defined as death despite the use of a ventilator or cardiac massage.

Brain death: Documented cessation of cerebral function and meeting the criteria for brain death.

Palliative care: Any interventions aimed to prevent and relieve suffering by controlling symptoms and providing other support to patients and families in order to maintain and improve their quality of living during all stages of chronic life-threatening (or terminal) illness.

End-of-life care: It is the care (comfort, supportive or symptom care) provided to a person in their final stages of life.

ADVANCED TERMINAL CHRONIC OBSTRUCTIVE PULMONARY DISEASE

Advanced terminal chronic obstructive pulmonary disease (COPD) comes under the spectrum of "end-stage lung disease" which basically implies that the patient now has very severe airflow obstruction, often with a forced expiratory volume in one second (FEV_1) of 0.5 L. There is chronic hypoxemia with or without hypercapnia. The terminal phase of COPD is difficult to define, it can vary from one patient to another based on the actual lung function, presence of pulmonary hypertension, personality and attitude toward illness, and of course, the social status of the patient. At one spectrum, one could get a patient with an FEV_1 of 45% of predicted, from lower socioeconomic strata who has almost permanently confined himself to his home, to another from higher socioeconomic strata with an FEV_1 of 34% who is raring to play golf.

A good way to define terminal disease is when survival is expected to be less than 2 years. This allows the primary care physician with help from the specialist to guide the patient and the family on how the future is likely to evolve. Though 2 years sound a realistic end-point before which to start communicating, it is not so easy in COPD, which reflects certain death at an uncertain time. Many, in fact most patients with COPD, do not die of progressive respiratory failure, but of cardiac disease or cancers. This was clearly evident from the review of the mortality data from the toward a revolution in COPD Health (TORCH) Study.[5] Therefore, a reasonably healthy COPD patient may actually and very often die suddenly of myocardial infarction. This may not be easily predictable. However, that needs to be a factored point when discussing end-of-life issues with the patient.

PROGNOSIS OF ADVANCED CHRONIC OBSTRUCTIVE PULMONARY DISEASE

Equally important is to realize the prognosis of patients with COPD. **Table 1** lists a good guide in deciding when to bring up the topic for discussion with patients discharged after an acute exacerbation of chronic bronchitis (AECB).

A Canadian study suggested that after 6 months of discharge from a hospital following AECB, only 25% of patients were well and with a good quality of life; 44% of them had been re-admitted by then.[8] This illustrates how important it is to bring up this issue at the stage of hospital discharge from an AECB. The author will discuss other situations to define advanced terminal COPD, but equally important is the presence of pulmonary hypertension and right ventricle (RV) dysfunction, the presence of which itself, is indicative of a 4-year mortality of 73%.[7] The timing of death, however, remains almost impossible to predict. As mentioned in the example earlier of myocardial infarction as a cause of death, the timing of death is poorly estimated even within a week of death.[9]

Issues Involved in Treating Advanced Terminal Chronic Obstructive Pulmonary Disease

When the disease gets worse, and as the pharmacological options become limited, the care gets harder and more challenging. *Some of the questions to handle at this stage are as follows:*

- Handling the fear of a dying patient. The fear of suffocation or choking to death is real; watching someone going through this stage can be equally devastating for the family

Table 1 Postdischarge mortality in two studies

Ai Ping et al.[6]	*Breen et al.[7]*
• *6 months*: 39%	*6 months*: 41%
• *1 year*: 43%	*1 year*: 49%
• *3 years*: 61%	*2 years*: 58%
• *5 years*: 76%	*3 years*: 64%

- When the next exacerbation occurs, should the patient be *actively* treated to prolong life, or treated so as to allow smooth transition from life to death?
- How *much* active treatment is appropriate? Should the next exacerbation be treated at home (especially in a financially drained patient) or at a hospital?
- If treated at home, should noninvasive ventilation (NIV) be used (machines can now be rented or bought by patients)?
- If treated in the hospital, should the patient be treated in the room/ward or ICU (distanced from relatives and loved ones)?
- If a decision has been taken that patient is not to be transferred to ICU, what is the maximum time for the patient to remain in the ward/room setting?
- If a decision to transfer to ICU is taken, is the patient agreeable to be *invasively* ventilated?
- If *no* to the above question, what will be the maximum care offered to the patient in the ICU, which cannot be given in a room/ward?
- If the patient has said no to any of the above "active treatment" options, has an "advance directive" been obtained from the patient?
- Are the relatives taking most of the decisions for the patient (common in Indian scenario, where shielding the patient from an adverse diagnosis or prognosis is common)? Is the patient educated enough to take a better decision himself? If so, is the "relatives" opinion/decision final?
- If the patient is unconscious (with no advance directives), how does the discussion with family ensue?

GOOD DEATH IN CHRONIC OBSTRUCTIVE PULMONARY DISEASE: IMPLICATIONS

An excellent study identified five issues that a patient may wish to see addressed before he dies.[10] *As a physician, it is important to be very sensitive to these issues:*

1. Adequate relief of symptoms, especially pain and dyspnea
2. No inappropriate prolongation of life
3. Sense of control of their own person
4. Relief of the burden to their family
5. Strengthening of family relationships.

Patients with COPD are not always able to die quietly, peacefully, or in their own homes. The patient and the families' descriptions of breathlessness challenge the definitions of a "good death". Patients often die in the ICU or hospital, and it could be argued that dying in an environment away from the home setting has meant that we have lost our ability to communicate with the dying patient.[11]

For the COPD patient, this is a constant dilemma. By suffering at home all the time, he has already experienced a "social" death for years. He is often "dying and living" at the same time. At the end, when brought to a hospital, he is additionally subjected to the regular procedures of a "hospital management", which could range from simple intravenous lines to endotracheal intubation and invasive ventilation.

Having undergone a prolonged period of reduced physical and social functioning, they are actually hardly "living" in the true sense much before they die. The COPD patient, therefore, challenges the concept of a "good death." This remains one of the most difficult situations in dealing with patients with any kind of advanced lung disease.[12]

Appropriate Time to Begin Discussions on End-of-Life Issues with Chronic Obstructive Pulmonary Disease Patients

As mentioned earlier, when survival is expected to be below 2 years, the time has come to start a discussion with the patient. Studies have shown that patients appreciate physicians who discuss these issues with them, in contrast to many physicians believing that patients may not be ready for the same.[13] Patients appreciated physicians who are honest and straightforward, are willing to talk about dying, are good at listening, give bad news in a sensitive way and most importantly, are sensitive to the timing of such discussions. By avoiding the topic, patients are less satisfied. Introduction of the topic actually allows patients to engage in a good discussion and maintain a sense of hope with less depression, even when the prognosis is poor.

Patients perceive their physicians based on *what* (the content) they communicate and *how* (the process) they do it largely. Unfortunately, most of these discussions take place outside the ICU, and often when the patient himself is unable to take a decision on his own. This delay in communication must be avoided and every attempt should be made at the out-patient level to start such discussions where appropriate and of course after a full review of diagnostic tests and ongoing treatments. Sometimes, even a second opinion helps before deciding that the patient and the family needs such a discussion. End-of-life discussions in COPD can be started in the presence of different disease criteria **(Box 1)**.

Appropriate Time to Begin Discussions on End-of-Life Issues

Despite these criteria, less than 15% of ICU patients retain decision making capacity so it is impossible to discuss the decision with them in ICU.[14] Also, though the patient's family is often involved in decision-making in India (largely shielding the patient), studies have shown that relatives rate the communication with hospital staff as poor.

Additionally, many of these discussions occur outside an ICU and during an exacerbation[14] hardly the appropriate place to start of such discussions, but sadly this is where most such discussions occur.

BOX 1 Different criteria in chronic obstructive pulmonary disease when end-of-life discussion can happen

- FEV1 < 30% (during the stable period)
- Oxygen dependence
- One or more hospitalizations in the past 1 year with AECB
- Left heart failure
- Weight loss/cachexia and increasing dependence on others
- Age more than 70 years.

Abbreviations: AECB, acute exacerbation of chronic bronchitis; FEV1, forced expiratory volume in 1 second.

Identifying the High-risk Patient

More recently, a decision tree (CART) has been proposed and validated. It can identify patients at a high risk of mortality in the next 5 years, and takes into account five easily available parameters in clinical practice:[15]

1. Age
2. FEV1
3. Dyspnea
4. Physical activity
5. Number of hospital admissions in the previous 2 years.

It would be worth using such decision trees in prognosticating severe COPD in clinical practice.

PRINCIPLES OF END-OF-LIFE COMMUNICATION IN CHRONIC OBSTRUCTIVE PULMONARY DISEASE

- *Ethical principles:* The basic ethical principles consist of beneficence; nonmaleficence; autonomy and justice, i.e. fairness in the physician's approach.[16] Physician should not provide investigation or treatment that will harm or serve no purpose. Avoid imposing futile treatments on the patient. Treatment aimed at a specific symptom may have adverse effects that may shorten life, e.g. morphine. When the benefits of alleviating the patient's suffering outweigh the risks, then such therapy is acceptable, and is not considered euthanasia.
- *Cultural principles:* Surprisingly, there is very little information on how the influence of culture affects the patient and family. Culture encompasses the patient's beliefs, life's experiences, values, attitudes and assumptions. This is not necessarily related to the ethnicity of the patient. Culture can affect the entire way in which a patient approaches his life, disease and death. This culture needs to be respected by the physician. Eye contact with the patient, physical touch and privacy often varies between cultures. The entire communication process of "breaking bad news" can vary between cultures, and understandably, this can have profound effects on management planning. Respect given to the patient's cultural preferences has a tremendous positive impact on the patient and the family. Trust is immensely improved and strengthened when this aspect of the patient's whole is also respected.
- *Incompetent patient:* Depression can often affect the decision-making process of COPD patients. This must be carefully looked for before labeling the patient as poorly

responsive to suggestions *or* incompetent in making a decision. For the actual incompetent patient, one has to often ask the family for end-of-life directives. Ideally, this should be the spouse or children. It is important here to understand, if the patient had ever expressed any desires about the way he should be managed toward the end of his life. Often, the patient has expressed such views to the family, such as not being ventilated or brought to ICU at all. Our culture often shields the patient from bad news, despite the patient realizing, long before the family, that he is headed in a downward trajectory.

Sadly, even in competent patients, the family often incorrectly states a patient's wishes.[17] When life and death decisions are at play, the family must be told that the decision is not their responsibility, but that they are simply guiding the physicians in their decisions.

Place where End-of-Life Communication should be Done

Communication is most often done outside an ICU cubicle. This should be avoided as far as possible. A large quiet room with privacy and confidentiality is the best. Emotional outbursts are not uncommon by family members. In some cultures, the patient is asked as to whom he would like to have present in the room. In others, the patient is often left out of the discussion, leaving this to responsible family members whom he entrusts with all decisions pertaining to his life and death. It is important to counsel these members extensively.

When such discussions occur, ensure that everyone's opinion in the room is heard out and try to end it on a final collective decision that everyone is agreeable to.

How and What Needs to be Done?[18]

- After listening well to the patient and the family, you will be able to understand their expectations and come to a consensus on what needs to be done. The levels at which things for advanced COPD can be planned are outlined here:
  - *Level 4:* All conditions investigated and treated, including cardiopulmonary resuscitation (CPR)
  - *Level 3:* Above, except CPR (the patient can still be intubated and ventilated)
  - *Level 2:* Potentially reversible conditions are investigated and treated (can be done at home or hospital)
  - *Level 1:* Main focus is on palliative care—symptom relief is the focus of all treatment (intravenous feeds and Ryle tube feeds are avoided).
- As mentioned earlier, when planning the foreseeable level of care, always use words like "if" rather than "when". "When" seems to be a prediction of doom, but "if" is more often seen as uncertainty and allows patients to balance hope and acceptance
- Discuss the implications and consequences of treatments, in the light of the disease prognosis. It is imperative that patients' and their families' understand the "misery of doing everything". Often patients with unlimited financial resources believe that "everything" must be done for a dying patient. "Everything" includes more drugs with adverse effects; mechanical ventilation; more procedures on an ill patient; and not to forget the ongoing mental stress to the patient and the family members, many of whom have not been actively involved in this decision to do "everything"
- *Do not forget about depression and COPD*: Depression often affects decision-making by the COPD patient and this should not preclude the introduction of an intervention when it can actually help to improve the patient's quality of life
- Manage symptoms as possible in the following ways:

Dyspnea: Over 50% patients suffer from dyspnea, 90% by the end of their life. Dyspnea is often aggravated by anxiety, low-dose anxiolytics like alprazolam can often help, especially if back-up NIV is available. Pharmacologic therapy is often limited after nebulized bronchodilators and systemic steroid have been used. Though oxygen and NIV help, morphine may need to be used when dyspnea worsens. The only drugs with a proven effect on dyspnea are opioids. An excellent recent randomized, placebo-controlled trial was performed on patients with refractory dyspnea, the large majority having COPD.[19] Not only did the dyspnea scores improve significantly with morphine, the patients reported much better sleep too. The only concern was distressing constipation despite laxatives. Though the global initiative for chronic obstructive lung disease (GOLD) guidelines state that opioids are contraindicated in COPD management, physicians should refer to the American Thoracic Society (ATS) clinical policy statement on palliative care where the principle holds that relief of suffering is adequate justification of the use of opioids to control dyspnea or pain.[20] Sadly, in many countries, "morphine-phobia" among clinicians and the general population leads to inappropriate management of terminal pain and dyspnea.

The benefits are largely related to reduced ventilation and the sensation of dyspnea. Unlike pain management, the long-term effects are not so beneficial and side effects are common. Relaxation breathing, upright posture and sometimes music therapy can also help in palliative care. Slow-paced music is usually preferred over fast pace. Music therapy is shown to be superior to progressive muscle relaxation in acute exacerbations.[21]

Cough: Often, suppressive therapy works for cough. Sometimes systemic steroids are needed. Inhaled local anesthetics can help at times. Physiotherapy may help to control secretions, but adequate hydration goes a long way in ensuring that thick secretions do not impair the ability of the patient to protect his airway.

Insomnia: Not uncommon in advanced COPD, usually due to orthopnea. Anxiety, depression and theophylline can also contribute. Oxygen to relieve nocturnal desaturation often helps. Non-benzodiazepine sedatives such as zolpidem and amitriptyline may help. Benzodiazepines should be avoided as far as possible.

Fatigue: Lack of exercise, low body mass index and insomnia all contribute to fatigue. Never miss out treatable causes like anemia (iron or B_{12} deficiency) or thyroid disease. Sleep disturbance is often a cause of fatigue and must be addressed.

Delirium: Confusion occurs in a large number of patients as they approach death. Medications, especially opioids and metabolic disturbances can contribute. After correction of hypoxia and hyponatremia, haloperidol can be tried as a good first-line choice for this symptom. As the need for haloperidol increases, more aggressive sedation may be required and the family should be informed about this requirement.

Cachexia and weight loss: A poor prognostic sign, this catabolic state often is a result of increased minute ventilation. Mouth breathing and aerophagy aggravate anorexia. High calorie supplements can help. Sometimes, prokinetics help by improving gastric emptying. Foods liked by patient should be provided, including alcohol. Though weight loss can be explained to families as a body's way of shutting down, it is often followed by desperate attempts to feed (and often overfeed) the patient. This must be avoided as metabolism will increase further, putting further load on the respiratory system.

Judicious use of NIV: NIV has significantly helped many COPD patients die a more comfortable death. Just the ability to speak and eat a bit too makes NIV so much less intrusive than an endotracheal tube or a tracheostomy. NIV at home has also reduced the number of terminally ill COPD patients reaching the hospital for the inevitable. Though the machines are expensive to purchase, rentals on a daily or monthly basis are now available in several cities.

In the era before NIV, COPD patients admitted to an ICU for an acute exacerbation aged more than 65 years had a mortality rate of 30%, which doubled after 1 year to 60%. A more recent retrospective study aimed at looking at long-term survival of patients treated with NIV for the first time. Survival here was 72%, 52% and 26% at 1, 2 and 5 years, respectively.[22] The survival rate was also influenced by the need for readmission. Those who needed readmission had a 20% survival chance at 5 years.

Though we are aware that numerous studies have shown improved survival with invasive and non-invasive ventilation, these patients require physiotherapy and intensive nursing for weeks after recovery. In the rare situations where even tracheostomies have been done, and the patient sent home, the quality of life can really take a huge dip, despite improved "survival". Many of these patients live the last phase of their lives in a hospital or protected environment, with reduced privacy and restricted policies to meet their relatives.[23]

In the final analysis, NIV has improved survival, but the quality of life of COPD patients on long-term NIV needs to be seriously examined in the Indian setting. It is always helpful to proceed according to the decision-tree to appropriate the management of COPD.[15]

CONCLUSION

To conclude, end-of-life communication and palliative care is cardinal in the overall management of severe, advanced COPD. As the disease gets more and more severe, less and less specific therapies are likely to benefit the patient and more supportive and palliative care becomes the order of the day. It is imperative that not just respiratory physicians, but primary care physicians too, better understand the process of dying in these patients. It will help them deal with death much better.

REFERENCES

1. Claessens MT, Lynn J, Zhong Z, Desbiens NA, Phillips RS, Wu AW, et al. Dying with lung cancer or chronic obstructive pulmonary disease: Insights from SUPPORT. Study to Understand Prognoses and Preferences for Outcomes and Risks of Treatments. J Am Geriatr Soc. 2000;48(5 Suppl):S146-53.
2. Mani RK. End-of-life care in India. Intensive Care Med. 2006;32(7):1066-8.
3. Carlet J, Thiijs LG, Antonelli M, Cassell J, Cox P, Hill N, et al. Challenges in end-of-life care in the ICU. Statement of the 5th International Consensus Conference. Intensive Care Med. 2004;30:770-84.
4. Carlucci A, Guerrieri A, Nava Stefano. Eur Respir Rev. 2012 ;21: 26:347-54.
5. Calverley PM, Anderson JA, Celli B, Ferguson GT, Jenkins C, Jones PW, et al. Salmeterol and fluticasone propionate and survival in chronic obstructive pulmonary disease. N Engl J Med. 2007;356(8):775-89.
6. Ai-Ping C, Lee KH, Lim TK. In-hospital and 5-year mortality of patients treated in the ICU for acute exacerbation of COPD: a retrospective study. Chest. 2005;128(2):518-24.
7. Breen D, Churches T, Hawker F, Torzillo PJ. Acute respiratory failure secondary to chronic obstructive pulmonary disease treated in the intensive care unit: a long term follow up study. Thorax. 2002;57(1):29-33.
8. Connors AF, Dawson NV, Thomas C, Harrell FE, Desbiens N, Fulkerson WJ, et al. Outcomes following acute exacerbation of severe chronic obstructive lung disease. The SUPPORT investigators (Study to Understand Prognoses and Preferences for Outcomes and Risks of Treatments). Am J Respir Crit Care Med. 1996;154(4 Pt 1):959-67.
9. Budev MM, Arroliga AC, Wiedemann HP, Matthay RA. Cor pulmonale: an overview. Semin Respir Crit Care Med. 2003;24(3):233-44.
10. Singer PA, Martin DK, Kelner M. Quality end-of-life care: patients' perspectives. JAMA. 1999;281(2):163-8.
11. Costello J. Dying well: nurses' experiences of 'good and bad' deaths in hospital. J Adv Nurs. 2006;54(5):594-601.
12. Russel SJ, Russel RE. Challenges in end-of-life communication in COPD. Breathe. 2007;4(2):133-9.

13. Wenrich MD, Curtis JR, Shannon SE, Carline JD, Ambrozy DM, Ramsey PG, et al. Communicating with dying patients within the spectrum of medical care from terminal diagnosis to death. Arch Intern Med. 2001;161(6):868-74.
14. Curtis JR, Engelberg RA, Nielsen EL, Au DH, Patrick DL. Patient-physician communication about end-of-life care for patients with severe COPD. Eur Respir J. 2004;24:200-5.
15. Esteban C, Arostegui I, Moraza J, Aburto M, Quintana JM, Pérez-Izquierdo J, et al. Development of a decision tree to assess the severity and progress of stable COPD. Eur Respir J. 2011;38:1294-300.
16. Selecky PA, Eliasson CA, Hall RI, et al. American College of Chest Physicians. Palliative and end-of-life care for patients with cardiopulmonary diseases: American College of Chest Physicians position statement. Chest. 2005;128:3599-610.
17. Layde PM, Beam CA, Broste SK, Connors AF, Desbiens N, Lynn J, et al. Surrogates' predictions of seriously ill patients' resuscitation preferences. Arch Farm Med. 1995;4(6):518-23.
18. Bourbeau J, Nault D, Borycki E. The Final illness: Palliative Care in Terminal COPD. In: BC Decker, Warren P, Barnett B, Cathcart A, et al (Eds.). Comprehensive Management of Chronic Pulmonary Disease, 1st edition. Hamilton; 2002. pp. 319-38.
19. Abernethy AP, Currow DC, Frith P, Fazekas BS, McHugh A, Bui C, et al. Randomised double-blind, placebo-controlled crossover trial of sustained-release morphine for the management of refractory dyspnoea. BMJ. 2003;327:523-28.
20. Lanken PN, Terry PB, Delisser HM, Fahy BF, Hansen-Flaschen J, Heffner JE, et al. An official American Thoracic Society clinical policy statement: palliative care for patients with respiratory diseases and critical illnesses. Am J Respir Crit care Med. 2008;177:912-27.
21. Seneff MG, Wagner DP, Wagner RP, Zimmerman JE, Knaus WA. Hospital and 1-year survival of patients admitted to intensive care units with acute exacerbation of chronic obstructive pulmonary disease. JAMA. 1995;274:1852-7.
22. Chung LP, Winship P, Phung S, Lake F, Waterer G. Five year outcome in COPD patients after their first episode of acute exacerbation treated with non-invasive ventilation. Respirology. 2010;15:1084-91.
23. Soler-Cataluna JJ, Martinez Garcia MA, Roman Sanchez P, Salcedo E, Navarro M, Ochando R. Severe acute exacerbations and mortality in patients with chronic obstructive pulmonary disease. Thorax. 2005;60:925-31.

79

Chapter

Smoking/Tobacco Control

Virendra Singh, Bharat Bhushan Sharma

INTRODUCTION

Tobacco smoking is one of the most important factors in the occurrence and progression of chronic respiratory illnesses. It is also considered the most preventable factor leading to morbidity and mortality.[1] Tobacco cessation confers health benefits, which are evident in former smokers who have lower relative risk of death in all disease categories.[2] Quitting smoking slows down the accelerated rate of lung function decline that occurs in susceptible smokers.[3] Despite the knowledge of beneficial effects of cessation of tobacco, a large number of users fail to stop smoking. Although, 70% of the smokers think of quitting and approximately 40% try to quit each year, hardly 5% remain abstinent.[4] In addition, tobacco contributes to the generation of revenue and employment for people of many developing countries. Tobacco product manufacturing companies have exploited all these factors nicely to their advantage.

Recent scientific advancements have led to the development of effective treatment modalities for tobacco addiction. However, overall emphasis on smoking cessation activities is poor, at the same time there is a growing number of new smokers, especially in developing countries. Thus, tobacco smoking continues to remain a big public health problem. The present chapter is divided into two parts. First part gives a brief description of magnitude of problem related to tobacco use and smoking. The second part deals with evidence-based recommendations for smoking control methods.

TOBACCO SMOKING

Historical Aspects

Tobacco cultivation was started around 8,000 years back in the American continent. Nevertheless, it was introduced to the rest of the world only about 500 years back. In later part of 15th century, Christopher Columbus while discovering America, found that native people cultivated and used tobacco.[5] Columbus brought tobacco to his country, Spain.[6] Within a few decades, tobacco use spread to the rest of the world from Europe. Portuguese merchants brought tobacco to India. Harmful effects of tobacco use were identified quite early and many European countries started imposing bans on smoking in the 17th century.[7]

However, smoking bans were lifted subsequently because medicinal properties of tobacco were highlighted and tobacco trade became an important source of income for governments. Around middle of the 20th century, tobacco use was linked to development of lung cancer.[8] Subsequently, it was linked to many other diseases. Environmental tobacco smoke (ETS) exposure (passive or secondhand smoking) was also linked to a variety of health problems. Despite of all these, tobacco use continued to increase, especially in the developing countries.

Epidemiology

Prevalence of Use

India is the second largest producer and consumer of tobacco products worldwide.[5] According to a national survey on adults in India, 47% of males and 14% of females are current tobacco users. Among male tobacco users, 30% are smokers while the rest use chewing tobacco.[9] Though in adults, tobacco use among males is 10–15 times higher in comparison to females, in adolescents this gap is reducing fast. Global youth tobacco survey (GYTS) has shown that in 8th–10th grade school-going adolescents, in 13–15 year age group, male users were only about one and a half times the female counterparts.[10]

In developed countries, tobacco use is showing a decreasing trend. Among adults in USA, 27% males and 19% of females are current tobacco users. More than 75% of them are smokers and the rest use smokeless tobacco.[4]

Types of Smoking

Cigarettes are the most common mode of tobacco use globally. Smoking pattern in India shows that around 70–80% of people use *bidis*, 15–25% cigarettes and about 4% smoke *hookah*.[11]

Mortality Attributed to Tobacco Use

Almost half of people who use tobacco are killed by tobacco-related diseases. World Health Organization estimated that 100 million deaths were caused by tobacco in the 20th century. If current trends remain unaltered, there will be up to one billion deaths due to tobacco use in the 21st century. There are around one billion smokers in the world today and 500 million are expected to die due to tobacco-induced diseases. Approximately, one million people are killed by tobacco-related diseases each year in India, where 10% of the world's smokers live.[12] Tobacco-related diseases are important cause of death among middle-aged men in India; almost 25% deaths in this group are due to tobacco-related diseases.[13]

Factors Responsible for Smoking

It is still quite intriguing why some people are able to quit smoking quickly and easily while others smoke right up to their untimely death. Apart from strong addiction power of tobacco, the answer to this question lies in variable nature of tobacco smoking behavior. Tobacco habit may be considered as a complex chronic disease just like diabetes or chronic obstructive pulmonary disease (COPD). Early life exposures, environmental factors like living in an area that restricts smoking and genetic factors play important role in the continuation of smoking **(Fig. 1)**.[14] A study among school children in Rajasthan showed that children were more likely to smoke when they were exposed to smoking advertisement or to other smokers in the family.[15] Therefore, strategies to persuade a person to stop smoking must address all of these issues.

Neuronal Pathophysiology

Various neural pathways and transmitter systems have emerged to explain the psychoactive and addictive properties of nicotine. Nicotinic acetylcholine neurons located in the ventral tegmental area show increased activity with nicotine administration. They concomitantly trigger the increased release of dopamine into the nucleus accumbens **(Fig. 2)**. Addiction to nicotine is believed to result from increased release of dopamine in the region of nucleus acumbens.[16,17] The evidence suggests that excitatory amino acid systems, in particular, N-methyl D-aspartate (NMDA) receptors are implicated in the behavioral changes that occur following long-term nicotine use, including tolerance, sensitization and physical dependence.[18]

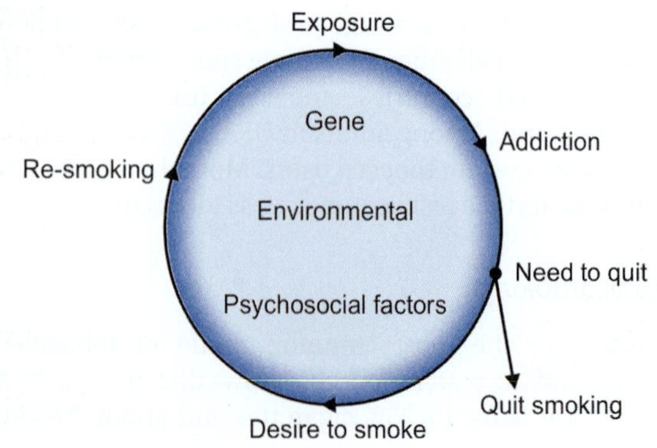

Fig. 1 Origin and perpetuation of addiction[5,14]

Withdrawal Symptoms

Similar to addiction with other drugs, nicotine withdrawal leads to a number of clinical manifestations **(Fig. 2)**. Nicotine withdrawal symptoms are time-dependent, at times lasting for many weeks. These include symptoms like irritability, anxiety, depression, difficulty in concentrating, weight gain, restlessness and many more.[19,20] The level of nicotine dependence is the most important factor that determines the intensity of withdrawal symptoms. We can assess the level of nicotine dependence by objective measures such as Fagerström's test for nicotine dependence, which measures addiction on a 0–10 scale. The two most important parameters of the test are the length of time after waking before the first cigarette is taken by individual and the number of cigarettes smoked per day.[21]

Harmful Effects of Smoking

Toxins of Smoke

Cigarette smokes contain a significant concentration of oxidants, which are responsible for damage and causation of respiratory and other illnesses. Approximately, 4,000 chemicals have been identified in tobacco smoke of which at least 250 are known to be harmful **(Fig. 3)**. These substances generated by smoking stimulate inflammation in the lung and its airways.[22] Cigarette smoking leads to inflammatory changes in the central and peripheral airways as well as the lung parenchyma. These changes finally lead to structural remodeling because of repeated injury and repair.[23] Respiratory morbidity due to tobacco smoking is varied and vast in nature, includes obstructive as well as restrictive lung diseases and lung cancer.[24]

Types of Smoking and Harm

Bidis produce three times more carbon monoxide and nicotine and five times more tar than regular cigarettes.[25] *Bidi* smokers have a three-fold higher risk of oral cancer compared with nonsmokers and are also at increased risk of lung cancer. *Hookahs*, a popular form of smoking in rural areas of India, are also linked to lung disease and cancer.[26]

Sidestream or Secondhand Smoke

Smoke emitted from the burning end of a cigarette or *bidi* while not being smoked, is called sidestream tobacco smoke.

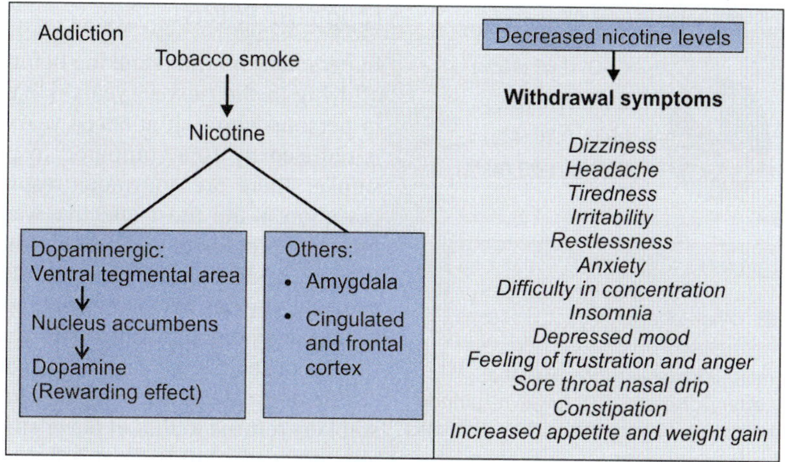

Fig. 2 Nicotine addiction and withdrawal symptoms[16,17]

Both the mainstream and the sidestream smoke contain similar components, but the sidestream smoke is three to four times more toxic per gram of particulate matter than the mainstream tobacco smoke **(Fig. 3)**.[27] Toxic chemicals from secondhand tobacco smoke stick to rugs, curtains, clothes, food or furniture and can remain in a room even for weeks and months after someone has smoked there.[28] Tobacco toxins that build up over time, coat the surfaces of room and materials are sometimes referred to as thirdhand smoke, approximately 50 of which are known to cause cancer.[29]

Passive smoking during childhood is considered as a risk factor for the development of asthma. Uncontrolled asthma is associated with parental smoking. Furthermore, asthmatic symptoms decline sharply after the ETS exposure is controlled.[30]

Tobacco-related Diseases

Smoking causes cancers of many organs. Cancer of lungs, tracheobronchial tree, mouth, esophagus, stomach and urinary bladder are mainly linked to tobacco use. Tobacco use is associated with higher rates of coronary artery disease, stroke and atherosclerosis.[31] Respiratory diseases caused by smoking include COPD, tuberculosis and lower respiratory tract infection[31] **(Fig. 4)**. Globally, COPD is the most common cause of death among smokers. Likewise, smoking is responsible for half of all male deaths from tuberculosis in India.[13]

Loss of Revenue Due to Tobacco

In India, the cost of treating tobacco-related disease is more than double than the revenue the government gets from the tobacco industry.[32] Besides this, there is an uncountable fiscal and personal loss to the families and society due to early deaths of the smokers.[33]

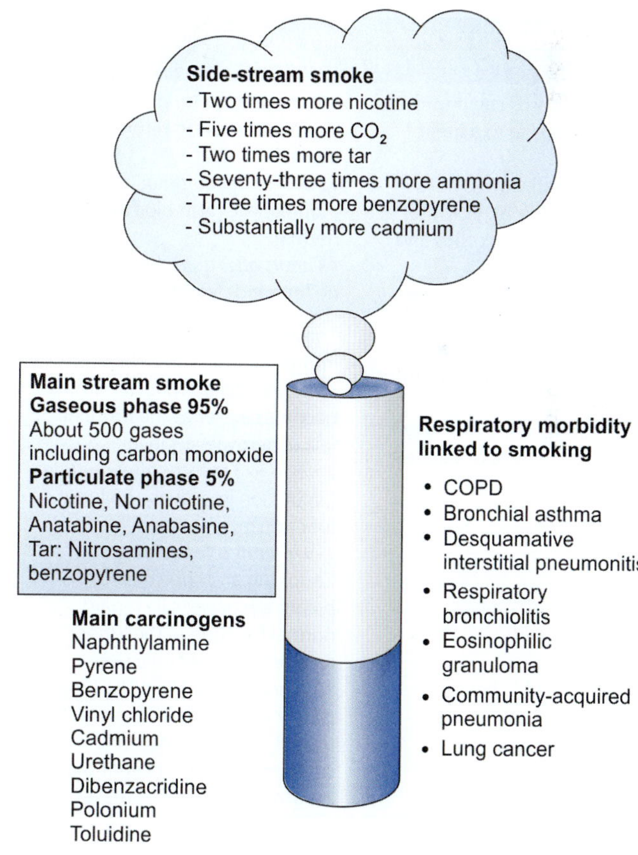

Fig. 3 Tobacco toxins and respiratory ailments
Abbreviation: COPD, chronic obstructive pulmonary disease

Benefits of Smoking Cessation

Smoking cessation has definite personal and health benefits that may be divided into short-term and long-term benefits **(Table 1)**.[20,34]

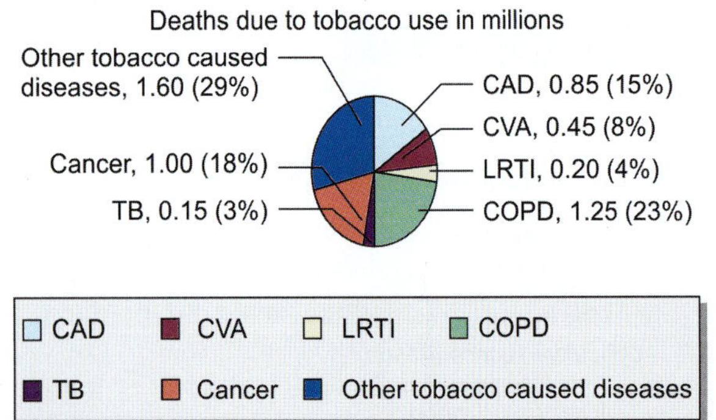

Fig. 4 Leading causes of mortality due to tobacco: Globally[31]
Abbreviations: CAD, coronary artery disease; LRTI, lower respiratory tract infection; CVA, cerebrovascular accidents; COPD, chronic obstructive pulmonary disease; TB, tuberculosis

Table 1 Beneficial effects of smoking cessation[20,34]

Immediate rewards of quitting	*Respiratory benefits of quitting over time*
These rewards can improve day-to-day life to a great extent: • The breath smells better • Stained teeth get whiter • Bad smelling clothes and hair disappear • Yellow fingers and finger nails disappear • The food tastes better • The sense of smell returns to normal • Breathlessness on everyday relax activities is reduced	*8 hours after quitting*: Oxygen levels in the blood return to normal. *12 hours after quitting*: The carbon monoxide level in blood drops to normal *48 hours after quitting*: Nicotine is no longer detectable in body.
	The ability to taste and smell improves *72 hours after quitting*: Breathing becomes easier as the bronchi relax Energy levels increase. *2 weeks to 3 months after quitting*: Circulation improves and lung function increases. *1–9 months after quitting*: Coughing and shortness of breath decrease; cilia regain normal function in the lungs, reduce the risk of infection. *10 years after quitting*: The lung cancer death rate is about half that of a person who continues smoking. Risk of cancer of the mouth/throat also decreases.

Short-term Benefits

Immediate benefits of smoking cessation include a decline in carbon monoxide levels in the blood, return of pulse rate and blood pressure to normal levels. Personal benefits include improvements in breath smells, stained teeth, bad smelling clothes or hair, colored fingers and fingernails, taste of food, sense of smell and breathlessness on everyday activities.

Long-term Effects

In persons who quit smoking before 50 years of age, the risk of dying in the next 15 years is half that of a smoker. Even in persons who quit at 60–64 years of age, the risk of dying is reduced by 10% compared to persons who continue to smoke. There are enormous respiratory benefits. Smoking cessation is the most effective way to reduce the risk and improve prognosis of COPD.[1] Smoking cessation reduces the risk of developing cancer. Ten years after cessation of smoking, the risk of dying from lung cancer is about one-half to that of smoking persons. Smoking cessation also reduces the risk of acquiring a second primary cancer.[35]

The rate of decline in lung function in COPD among former smokers returns to that of never smokers. Smoking cessation also decreases the risk of influenza and pneumonia. If a mother stops smoking before becoming pregnant or within 3–4 months of pregnancy, the birth weight of the infant will be the same as that of infants of nonsmokers. Even cessation at later stage of pregnancy will lead to higher birth weight than those of babies of regular smokers. Smoking cessation also eliminates the risk of passive smoking-induced diseases, including pneumonias and exacerbations of bronchial asthma in relatives.[36]

SMOKING CONTROL INTERVENTIONS

Controlling smoking addiction is quite demanding and also unpredictable. A multitude of interventions have been tried with variable rates of success. Smoking cessation is defined as validated sustained abstinence from cigarettes and/or other tobacco products for at least 6 months, preferably for a year.[37] The available smoking cessation interventions can be classified into behavioral, pharmacologic, combined and alternative methods. Behavioral interventions are physician guidance, individual counseling and group counseling, or counseling by telephone. Pharmacologic interventions include nicotine replacement therapy (NRT), sustained-release bupropion, varenicline as first-line agents and clonidine and nortriptyline as second-line agents. The alternative, less evidence-based interventions are hypnosis, acupuncture, aversive therapy, exercise, lobeline, anxiolytics, mecamylamine and silver acetate. Nicotine vaccine is among some of more promising agents for future therapy of tobacco dependence. Above all, it is most important to prevent the initiation of smoking in unexposed individuals.

How to Restrict Tobacco use in the Society?

First Level Prevention

The target population may be divided in two categories nonsmokers and smokers. They may be further classified as nonsmoking children and adolescents, grown-up adults; sick and healthy smokers.

Nonsmoking children and adolescents: They belong to the age group when a smoker learns smoking. Efforts should be made to make these children aware of harmful effects of smoking. It is easy not to start than to quit smoking. Pamphlets, stickers, articles in newspapers, television serials and a chapter in curriculum books may play an important role in dissuading adolescents from initiating smoking. In a study, use of posters; curriculum changes; parental involvement and peer-led activism reduced self-reported tobacco use, as well as future intentions to start tobacco chewing or smoking.[38]

Nonsmoking grown-up adults: Usually grown-up nonsmoker adults are unlikely to initiate smoking in later years of life. They are probably most receptive in accepting dangers of passive smoking and therefore must be motivated to resist anyone else smoking in their presence. Efforts should be made to make these people aware that breathing clean air is very important for health. It will ensure the compliance of ban on smoking at public places.[39]

Sick smokers: Sick smokers can be motivated more readily. Appropriate advice by healthcare workers can motivate a sick smoker for cessation of smoking. Timely advice by doctors, nurses, pharmacists and other healthcare personnel is crucial for a smoker who is interacting with them during his illness. Current evidence-based opinion regarding smoking cessation is that it should be done for every smoker during every healthcare visit.[40,41] Even a short period of counseling at the clinician's office, to ask a smoker to quit, results in cessation rates of up to 10%.[42,43] All smokers including those at risk for COPD already having disease should be offered the most possible and rigorous cessation intervention. The rate of successful smoking cessation at 1 year is 7–16%, if the smoker undergoes behavioral intervention alone and up to 24% when receiving pharmacological treatment plus behavioral support.[44]

Healthy Smokers

Healthy smokers are least receptive to no-smoking advice. However, their tobacco use can be restricted by means such as making cigarettes more expensive, ban on public smoking and ban on sale to minors. Sometimes, peer pressure, family persuasion and religious appeal may motivate smokers in this category.

Efforts must be made to register the smokers for subsequent detailed interventional plans. This form of counseling takes less than 10-minute of clinicians. For such brief intervention used to initiate smoking cessation, a mnemonic five "A's" is commonly used. All patients should be *asked* about tobacco use and their smoking status is recorded. A strong *advice* is given to all tobacco users to quit. Their willingness to make a quit attempt is assessed. The smokers are assisted with a quit plan, practical counseling, social support and medications. Finally, follow-up visits are arranged for the smokers willing to quit. For those smokers not willing to undergo cessation, five "R's" are used to enhance motivation and decrease mental inertia to quit: relevance, risks, rewards, roadblocks and repetition **(Fig. 5)**.[45]

Behavioral Interventions

Initial approaches to smoking cessation during mid-20th century were based on the behavioral therapy alone. For next few decades, cognitive therapy gained momentum but finally pharmacotherapy started emerging around 1990s. Behavioral interventions are effective in smoking cessation, although there is insufficient information to know which elements of behavioral support or type of approach (like motivational interviewing or cognitive behavioral therapy) is more effective.[40]

Basically, three behavioral interventions approaches are utilized: (1) practical counseling-problem solving or skill training, (2) giving intratreatment support, (3) provision of extratreatment support. The physician, nurse or telephone counselor may assist in the process or it is performed as self-help by the patient himself.

Among the simplest of behavioral interventions, even brief, but direct physician advice to quit smoking is effective. Furthermore, the rate of smoking abstinence increases when the intensity of advice is increased and when follow-up visits are included.

Types of Behavioral Interventions

- *Individual counseling:* A review of studies about individual behavioral counseling by trained therapists with a follow-

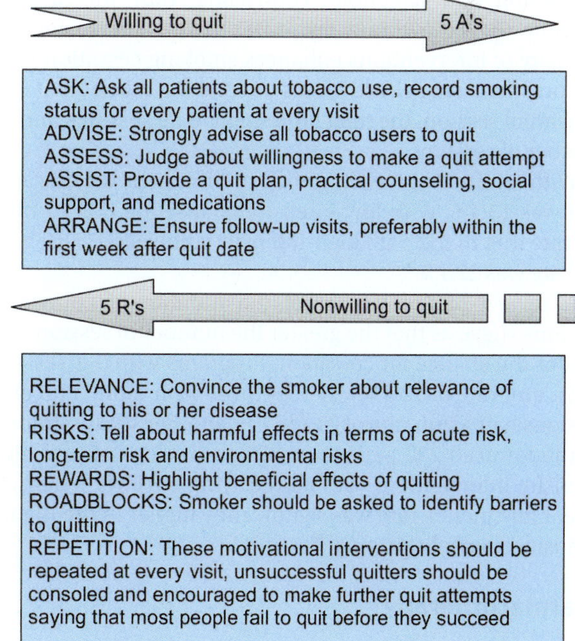

Fig. 5 Initiation of smoking cessation effort[43,45]

up of at least 6 months indicated benefits of counseling as compared to no intervention. Individual counseling usually consists of one or more direct interview sessions, often followed by telephone contact for the support.[19]

- *Group counseling:* Available studies also suggest that group counseling is effective in promoting smoking cessation.[19,46] Overall, the evidence supporting the efficacy of group counseling satisfies level A.[46]
- *Telephone counseling:* It is simple, can reach a large number of people at a time. Proactive telephone counseling, which the counselor initiates, is more effective than reactive counseling, which is client initiated.[19]
- *Self-help information:* It is marginally beneficial for increasing smoking cessation.[19,46] Examples of self-help materials include booklets, leaflets, brochures, videotapes, compact discs, help lines, and various other computer and Internet interventions. Enhanced or tailored self-help material was associated with better cessation rate than standard self-help material.[47] Though the effectiveness is nominal, self-help also achieves evidence level A.[46] Other reasons that self-help, despite its small impact, should be included in smoking programs are increased population awareness, low expense and the opportunity to customize the message. Cessation programs available on the Internet are also found to be effective in smoking cessation.[48,49]

Increasing Effectiveness of Interventions

Another lesson from available meta-analyses of behavioral interventions is that adding cessation formats confers incremental effectiveness. Combining up to 3–4 formats, e.g. self-help with individual counseling or individual counseling and telephone counseling, may increase the absolute cessation rate by 12%.[46] Also, increasing the intensity of interventions enhances smoking cessation rates. Factors increasing effectiveness include the duration of each individual session, the total time spent in all sessions and the number of sessions.

With minimal counseling of up to 3 minutes, the cessation rate was 13.4%; with low-intensity counseling (32–10 min), the rate was 16.0%; with high-intensity counseling (> 10 min), the rate was 22.1%.[46]

A review of the impact of the number of counseling sessions suggests that the greater the number of sessions, the greater the chance for cessation. Programs with 0–1 sessions had a quit rate of 12.4%, whereas those with more than eight sessions had a quit rate of 24.7%.[40] In another study, Simon et al. randomized 228 patients to either low-intensity or high-intensity intervention, with all receiving NRT via patch; the 1-year abstinence rate was significantly higher in the higher-intensity counseling group.[50]

Pharmacotherapy

Pharmacotherapy aimed to quit smoking is very different from that used for the treatment of a disease. Success of pharmacotherapy of quit smoking depends substantially on the desire or motivation of a patient. Pharmacotherapy fails to produce effect if the patient does not have a desire or motivation to quit. Unfortunately, we do not have any medicine to induce a desire to quit smoking. Personalized counseling to induce motivation for quitting smoking should be a prerequisite for the use of pharmacotherapy.

A number of meta-analyses have revealed that all current medications for smoking cessation are twice more efficacious than placebo.[15] However, there is limited data to guide clinicians to advocate one type of medication over another or the use of combinations. Lately, a Delphi method was used by a group of international experts for clinicians to guide the tailoring of medication for individual smoking cessation.[19] Levels of scientific evidence, patient preference, previous experience and failed attempts with monotherapy are some of the factors which should determine the prescription. Other important factors include the presence of comorbidities and contraindications to the medications.[1]

Current Medications for Smoking Cessation

All smokers who have previously relapsed when attempting to quit are questioned about their prior use of pharmacotherapy and their perceptions of the treatment options. Even light smokers or those who have failed in earlier attempts to give up, can benefit from pharmacotherapy.[52]

Beside decreasing the withdrawal symptoms and craving, pharmacotherapy decreases the short-term reinforcing effects of tobacco. This form of relief can help to ease the process of a patient learning new coping skills. The addition of a pharmacologic agent to a quit plan can have a positive psychological impact on those making quit attempts, especially if previous quit attempts had fared poorly.[53,54] All first-line medications appear to similar effectiveness, but there have been few direct comparisons **(Table 2)**.[51,52]

The medication is selected on the basis of medical conditions, potential adverse effects, individual preference, previous smoking cessation, level of dependence and any apprehension of weight gain. Current medications may be grossly divided into NRT and non-nicotine pharmacotherapy.

Nicotine Replacement Therapy

Nicotine replacement therapy is the most common medication to assist smoking cessation, probably because there are more data available on its effectiveness and safety.[53] It is important to explain to the patient that NRT will help diminish nicotine craving, will make it controllable but will not completely eradicate.

Rationale: Nicotine is the substance to which a smoker is addicted. In smokers, when the blood level of nicotine decreases, withdrawal symptoms begin within a few hours after having the last puff of smoke. Smoking relieves these symptoms immediately. If smoking is not done, withdrawal

Table 2 Various medications for smoking cessation[51,52]

Type		*Requirements*	*Dose*	*Duration*	*Drawbacks*
NRT	Gum	Start on quit date	2 mg up to 24 cigarettes/d 4 mg > 25 cigarettes/d	Up to 12 weeks	Mouth soreness, dyspepsia
	Patch	Start on quit date Worn 24 hours	21 mg, 14 mg, 7 mg depending on level of addiction	8 weeks	Insomnia, local skin reaction
	Inhaler	Start on quit date, inhaled into mouth, not lungs	6–16 cartridges/d	Up to 6 months	Local irritation of mouth and throat
	Lozenge	Start on quit date	2 mg: 1st cigarette >30 min, postawakening 4 mg: 1st cigarette < 30 min, post-awakening	8 weeks	Mouth soreness, dyspepsia
Bupropion SR			150 mg OD for 3 days then 150 mg BID for rest of treatment	Up to 6 months	Insomnia, dry mouth, contraindicated in seizures
Varenicline		Quit date two weeks after initiation. Taken after meals with a full glass of water	0.5 mg OD for 3 days, 0.5 mg BID for next 4 days then 1 mg BID for rest of treatment	12 weeks treatment and 1 week maintenance	
Clonidine		Quit date 1 week after initiation. Taken after meals with a full glass of water	0.15–0.75 mg/d	3–10 weeks	Dry mouth, dizziness, drowsiness, sedation, rebound hypertension
Nortriptyline		Quit date 2–3 weeks after initiation. Taken after meals with a full glass of water	75–100 mg/d	12 weeks	Dry mouth, sedation, risk.of arrhythmia

Abbreviation: NRT, nicotine replacement therapy.

symptoms will continue to manifest with increasing severity. NRT will maintain a stable nicotine level in the bloodstream of the smoker, who is trying to quit, avoiding withdrawal symptoms.[55] When NRT via transdermal patch is used, more constant delivery of nicotine helps to desensitize nicotine receptors and therefore further inhibit withdrawal symptoms. NRT is available in form of nicotine gum, patches, lozenges and inhalers. In tobacco chewers, nicotine gum may be more effective since it provides the physical sensation of manipulating tobacco in the mouth.

A systematic review of randomized clinical trials including smokers not ready to stop, reveals that with NRT, twice as many quitters achieve 6 months of sustained abstinence.[56] It is also shown that the nicotine patch used along with another NRT is more effective than any of the single NRT.[57] It is customary to equate 1 mg of NRT to each cigarette smoked and start 2 weeks prior to the quit date while the patient goes on smoking on NRT. However, both these practices are not based on sound scientific evidence. Ideally, smoking should be stopped before starting NRT.

- *Transdermal nicotine patch:* It is the most common form of NRT, which has been available for more than two decades. It is available in different strengths but 21 mg patch over a 24-hour period is commonly used. Current trend involves increasing the NRT patch dosage and duration for heavy tobacco users. The final goal is to supply the dosage necessary to equate the nicotine level to body's accustomed state. Side effect may consist of local irritation, headache, dizziness, nausea and sleep disturbances.
- *Nicotine gum or lozenge:* They contain polacrilex compounds that are resin carriers. Both forms (gums and lozenge) of polacrilex are sugarless and available in different flavors. One should not eat or drink just before and during the use of these compounds. Acidic food and drinks like coffee or carbonated beverages interfere with drug delivery by these compounds, hence best avoided. Side effects of nicotine gum include dyspepsia, hiccups and mandible pain.
- *The nicotine inhaler:* Unlike the usual pressurized metered-dose inhaler, nicotine inhaler is a cartridge, from which, on suction a nicotine vapor is released in mouth and throat. For heavy tobacco users, it is not a good option as a monotherapy because of its poorer dose delivery. To deliver high doses, nicotine nasal spray can be used, but it is not popular as it is costly and can cause substantial nasal and eye irritation. NRT is usually considered safe for most patients.[53,58]

Contraindications to Nicotine Replacement Therapy's

Nicotine replacement therapy should not be started if within the past 6 weeks there is a history of myocardial infarction, unstable angina, uncontrolled hypertension, hypertension during treatment and severe rhythm disturbance. Relative contraindications include severe COPD, uncontrolled diabetes mellitus, and some cardiovascular disorders like coronary artery disease. Vivid dreams or insomnia may indicate a high NRT dose. NRT may interact with other drugs; it can lead to an increase in blood pressure when used along with bupropion. Drugs taken concomitantly, like insulin, benzodiazepines, caffeine and ergot may need dose adjustment. Irritation at application-site may suggest a need for a change in type of NRT. Insomnia with NRT is dealt by removing patch 1-hour prior to bedtime or by reducing the dose. Sublingual tablet is a new form of NRT, but the superiority of this formulation over NRT lozenge has not been proved.[56]

Non-nicotine Pharmacotherapy

Bupropion: Bupropion can reduce the severity of nicotine cravings and withdrawal symptoms. It was originally introduced in 1997 as a smoking cessation aid. Now, it has been approved in more than 50 countries across the globe.[56] The proposed mechanism of the effectiveness of bupropion in smoking cessation is blockade of the reuptake of dopamine and norepinephrine.

For tobacco-dependence treatment, sustained release variety of bupropion is preferred over the instant release. Bupropion SR needs to be taken twice daily and bupropion XL only once daily.

Side effects: Most common adverse effects of bupropion are dry mouth and insomnia. Agitation is an adverse effect that can be mostly avoided by the gradual escalation of dose from 150–300 mg daily by 1 week rather than just 3 days. Duration of treatment is typically 7–12 weeks with no tapering. The risk of seizures (one-in-a-thousand) is more common in epilepsy and some eating disorders. In a dose of 450 mg in treating depression, bupropion increases the risk of seizures, but the 300 mg dose used for tobacco cessation has very little risk of seizure. Bupropion should not be used by people with active use of alcohol who takes more than three drinks per day or by people with sudden alcohol withdrawal. It should also not be used by pregnant women. One significant advantage of bupropion is that it typically does not cause weight gain, may rather suppress it.

- *Varenicline:* Varenicline is an effective oral smoking cessation product to be approved by the US Food and Drug Administration. It was launched in mid-2006 in some parts of the world and was launched in India in 2008. Several trials have shown the benefits of varenicline in cessation rates. Bupropion was compared with varenicline in recent randomized controlled trials. In a meta-analysis it was found that rates of smoking cessation associated with varenicline were superior to those of bupropion and NRT.[60-63] Varenicline acts as a partial agonist of the a4b2 nicotinic acetylcholine receptor through which nicotine dependence is mediated. It also stimulates the dopaminergic system, which results in reduced withdrawal symptoms. The drug also blocks nicotinic receptors, which prevents the dopamine release in response to nicotine. Additionally, reinforcing effects of nicotine exposure is blocked because varenicline is expected to occupy this receptor.[64] The current recommendation state that the drug should be started 1 week prior to quit date, the full therapeutic effect may not occur until following a few weeks.

Side effects: The most common side effect of varenicline is nausea occurring in about 30% of patients. The nausea is generally short-lived, taking varenicline with a full glass of water and after eating helps to reduce this unfavorable effect. Less common side effects are insomnia, abnormal vivid dreams, constipation and flatulence.[53]

Varenicline has been associated with some psychiatric adverse effects. These include erratic behavior, new appearance of depressed mood, agitation, suicidal ideation, suicidal attempts and completed suicides within days to weeks after initiating varenicline.

Patients should be asked about any prior history of mental illness before starting varenicline and monitoring for changes in mood and behavior. It is important to note that in clinical trials, prevalence of behavioral changes with varenicline were similar to those with placebo. Varenicline poses a low burden on the kidney and liver, therefore may be used in end-stage renal disease with a reduced dosage.

Second-line Drugs

- *Nortriptyline:* It is a second-generation tricyclic antidepressant used in the treatment of major depression. It is recommended as a second-line medication in recent guidelines for the treatment of tobacco dependence.[53,59,65] Nortriptyline can have a sedating effect, it is more practical to take it in the evening. There are a number of other potential adverse effects including dizziness, blurring of vision, tinnitus, tremor, weakness, insomnia, nausea, constipation and rash. In patients with cardiovascular disease, it can increase the risk of serious dysrhythmia.[59] Nortriptyline can interact with a variety of medications. It is usually started earlier than other tobacco cessation medications, i.e. up to three weeks prior to quit date, to allow for a gradual build of dosage.
- *Clonidine:* It is also a second-line tobacco-cessation drug, is effective in reducing symptoms of opioid and alcohol withdrawal.[59] It can be taken orally in tablet form or via transdermal patch, and is started a week prior to quit date. Possible adverse effects include drowsiness, dizziness, fatigue, agitation, depression, constipation, nausea, weight gain and rebound hypertension.[53] A specific dosing regimen for tobacco cessation has not been established and there are several important drug interactions.

Combination Treatments

Nicotine patch can be combined with other formulations of NRTs in the cases of heavy addiction. Bupropion or varenicline should not be combined together or theoretically, with any of NRTs, no sound evidence is available for such an approach. They also should not be given to children, pregnant or lactating mothers. However, both of these can be used safely for people with stable cardiovascular disease.

Any of above pharmacological therapy may be advantageously combined with all types of behavioral interventions.[66]

Novel Therapies: Hope for the Future

We have seen that drug therapy for smoking is effective, but a significant number of patients fail to gain significant advantage on a long-term basis. Therefore, there is a continuous need for search of an agent, which would be ideal to tackle this problem more effectively. Agents which are of some hope include new non-nicotine replacement medications such as selegiline, fluoxetine and naltrexone.[19,67]

Newest strategies are related to search for a vaccine against nicotine addiction and application of pharmacogenetic principles to smoking cessation. A safe and effective vaccine would lead to better compliance than the existing pharmacotherapy. Such a proposed vaccine is based on stimulation of immune system to form specific antibodies (Nic-IgG) to nicotine to make the molecule too large to cross the blood-brain barrier and act on its central receptors.[68-70]

Nicotine is principally metabolized by cytochrome 450 enzyme coded by *CYP2A6* gene. Fast metabolizers need high amount of nicotine to maintain the addiction, and hence chance of high level addiction. Various other genes related to signaling molecules and *CYP2B7P1* or *CYP2B6* gene responsible for bupropion metabolism, are under evaluation. With better knowledge of pharmacogenomics, we will be able to design the medication for individual patients better.

CONCLUSION

Tobacco smoking is responsible for enormous adverse respiratory health consequences. Smoking cessation interventions are rewarding and should be attempted for all patients and at every healthcare visit. Effective and relatively safe pharmacotherapy in the form of first-line drugs like NRT, bupropion and varenicline are now available all over the world. India and other developing countries have started developing an antismoking momentum that needs to be build up with greater force by healthcare providers, supported by better responsiveness of smoking individuals. Tobacco cessation clinics and self-help material, including the information books on the subject are now widely available.[71] World Health Organization with its resolve to create smoke free and tobacco-free world has taken several steps toward accomplishing the ultimate goal of a smoking-free society.

REFERENCES

1. Global Strategy for the Diagnosis, Management and Prevention of COPD. Global Initiative for Chronic Obstructive Lung Disease (GOLD). 2014. [online] Available from *http:// www.goldcopd.com* [Accessed January 2015].
2. Centers for Disease Control and Prevention. Smoking attributable mortality, morbidity, and economic costs (SAMMEC): Adult SAMMEC and Maternal and Child Health (MCH) SAMMEC software, 2002c. [online] Available from *http://www.cdc.gov/tobacco/sammec* [Accessed May 2010].
3. Anthonisen NR, Connett JE, Murray RP. Smoking and lung function of Lung Health Study participants after 11 years. Am J Respir Crit Care Med. 2002;166(5):675-9.
4. Centers for Disease Control and Prevention (CDC). Cigarette smoking among adults—United States, 2000. MMWR Morb Mortal Wkly Rep. 2002;51(29):642-5.
5. Reddy KS, Gupta PC. Tobacco control in India. New Delhi: Ministry of Health and Family Welfare, Government of India; 2004.
6. Musk AW, de Klerk NH. History of tobacco and health. Respirology. 2003;8(3):286-90.
7. Borio G. The Tobacco Timeline: The Seventeenth Century—"The Great Age of the Pipe." [online] Available from *http:// wwww.tobacco.org/resources /history/tobacco_History 17th.* html [Accessed in May 2010].
8. Proctor RN, The anti-tobacco campaign of the Nazis: a little known aspect of public health in Germany, 1933-1945. BMJ. 1996;313(7070):1450-3.
9. Rani M, Bonu S, Jha P, Nguyen SN, Jamjoum L. Tobacco use in India: prevalence and predictors of smoking and chewing in a national cross sectional household survey. Tobacco Control. 2003;12(4):e4.
10. CDC Fact Sheet: South-East Asia Region Region. Global Youth Tobacco Survey (GYTS) India. [online] Available from *http:// www.cdc.gov/tobacco/global/gyts/factsheets/sear/2006/ India_factsheet. htm.* [Accessedin May 2010].
11. Jindal SK, Aggarwal AN, Chaudhry K. Tobacco smoking in India: prevalence, quit-rates and respiratory morbidity. Indian J Chest Dis Allied Sci. 2006;48(1):37-42.
12. WHO report on the global tobacco epidemic, 2009. MPOWER. [online] Available from *www.who.int/tobacco/mpower/en* [Accessed May 2010).
13. Gajalakshmi V, Peto R, Kanaka TS, Jha P. Smoking and mortality from tuberculosis and other diseases in India: Retrospective study of 43000 adult male deaths and 35000 controls. Lancet. 2003;362(9383):507-15.
14. Mannino DM. Why won't our patients stop smoking? The power of nicotine addiction. Diabetes Care. 2009;32 Suppl 2:S426-8.
15. Singh V, Gupta R. Prevalence of tobacco use and awareness of risks among school children in Jaipur. J Assoc Phys India. 2006;54:609-12.
16. Pidoplichko VI, DeBiasi M, Williams JT, Dani JA. Nicotine activates and desensitizes midbrain dopamine neurons. Nature. 1997;390(6658):401-4.
17. Corrigal WA, Coen KM, Adamson KL. Self-administered nicotine activates the mesolimbic dopamine system through the ventral tegmental area. Brain Res. 1994;653(1-2):278-84.
18. Jain R, Mukherjee K, Balhara YP. The role of NMDA receptor antagonists in nicotine tolerance, sensitization, and physical dependence: a preclinical review. Yonsei Med J. 2008;49(2): 175-88.

19. Laniado-Laborín R. Smoking and chronic obstructive pulmonary disease (COPD). Parallel epidemics of the 21st century. Int J Environ Res Public Health. 2009;6(1):209-24.
20. American Cancer Society: guide to quitting. [online] Available from *http://www.cancer.org/docroot/PED/content/PED_10_13X_Guide_for_Quitting_Smoking.asp.* [Accessed May 2010].
21. Heatherton TF, Kozlowski LT, Frecker RC, Fagerström KO. The Fagerström Test for Nicotine Dependence: a revision of the Fagerström Tolerance Questionnaire. Br J Addict. 1991;86(9):1119-27.
22. Saetta M. Airway inflammation in chronic obstructive pulmonary disease. Am J Respir Crit Care Med. 1999;160(5 Pt 2):S17-20.
23. Saetta M, Di Stefano A, Maestrelli P, et al. Activated T-lymphocytes and macrophages in bronchial mucosa of subjects with chronic bronchitis. Am Rev Respir Dis. 1993;147(2): 301-6.
24. Brody JS, Spira A. Chronic obstructive pulmonary disease, inflammation, and lung cancer. Proc Am Thorac Soc. 2006;3:535-8.
25. World Health Organization. Tobacco: deadly in any form or disguise. Geneva, World Health Organization, 2006. [online] Available from *http://www.who.int/tobacco/communications/events/wntd/2006/Tfi.* [Accessed May 2010).
26. Tobacco smoke and involuntary smoking: summary of data reported and evaluation. Geneva, World Health Organization, International Agency for Research on Cancer, 2002 (IARC Monographs on the Evaluation of Carcinogenic Risks to Humans, Vol. 83. [online] Available from *http://monographs.iarc.fr/ENG/Monographs/vol83/ volume83.pdf.* [Accessed May 2010].
27. Singer BC, Hodgson AT, Guevarra KS, Hawley EL, Nazaroff WW. Gas-phase organics in environmental tobacco smoke. 1. Effects of smoking rate, ventilation, and furnishing level on emission factors. Environ Sci Technol. 2002;36(5):846-53.
28. Winickoff JP, Friebely J, Tanski SE, Sherrod C, Matt GE, Hovell MF, et al. Beliefs about the health effects of "thirdhand" smoke and home smoking bans. Pediatrics. 2009;123(1):e74-9.
29. Invernizzi G, Ruprecht A, Mazza R, Rossetti E, Sasco A, Nardini S, et al. Particulate matter from tobacco versus diesel car exhaust: an educational perspective. Tob Control. 2004;13(3):219-21.
30. Jindal SK, Gupta D. The relationship between tobacco smoke and bronchial asthma. Indian J Med Res. 2004;120(5):443-53.
31. WHO report on the global tobacco epidemic, 2008 MPOWER. [online] Available from *www.who.int/tobacco/mpower* [Accessed May 2010].
32. India's new smoking laws--progress or politics? Lancet Oncol. 2001;2(3):123.
33. Thankappan KR, Thresia CU. Tobacco use and social status in Kerala. Indian J Med Res. 2007;126(4):300-8.
34. American Cancer Society. Guidelines for quitting tobacco. [online] Available from *www.quittobacco.org/whyquit/physicalbenefits.html.* [Accessed May 2010).
35. Sarnet JM. The health benefits of smoking cessation. Med Clin North Am. 1992;76(2):399-414.
36. Vijayan VK, Kumar R. Tobacco cessation in India. Indian J Chest Dis Allied Sci. 2005;47(1):5-8.
37. Campbell I. Nicotine replacement therapy in smoking cessation. Thorax. 2003;58(6):464-5.
38. Perry CL, Stigler MH, Arora M, Reddy KS. Preventing tobacco use among young people in India: Project MYTRI. Am J Public Health. 2009;99(5):899-906.
39. Public Health Service (PHS) Clinical Practice Guideline: Treating Tobacco Use and Dependence—2008 Update. Agency for Healthcare Research and Quality, Rockville, MD. [online] Available from *http://www.ahrq.gov/path/tobacco.htm#Clinic.* [Accessed May 2010].
40. The World Bank South Asia Human Development, Health, Nutrition, and Population Unit. Tobacco in South Asia. [online] Available from http://*go.worldbank.org/*. [Accessed September 2010].
41. Fiore MC, Bailey WC, Cohen SJ, et al. A clinical practice guideline for treating tobacco use and dependence: A US Public Health Service report. The Tobacco Use and Dependence Clinical Practice Guideline Panel, Staff, and Consortium Representatives. JAMA. 2000;283:3244-54.
42. Morgan MD, Britton JR. Chronic obstructive pulmonary disease 8: Non-pharmacological management of COPD. Thorax. 2003;58(5):453-7.
43. Wu P, Wilson K, Dimoulas P, Mills EJ. Effectiveness of smoking cessation therapies: a systematic review and meta-analysis. BMC Public Health. 2006;6:300.
44. van Schayck CP, Kaper J. Smoking and COPD: will they ever vanish into smoke? Prim Care Respir J. 2006;15(2):81-3.
45. Pohlig C. Smoking cessation counseling. A Practice Management Perspective. Chest. 2006;130(4):1231-33.
46. Marlow SP, Stoller JK. Smoking Cessation. Respir Care. 2003;48(12):1238-54.
47. Anderson JE, Jorenby DE, Scott WJ, Fiore MC. Treating tobacco use and dependence: an evidence-based clinical practice guideline for tobacco cessation. Chest. 2002;121(3):932-41.
48. Swartz LH, Noell JW, Schroeder SW, Ary DV. A randomised control study of a fully automated internet based smoking cessation programme. Tob Control. 2006;15(1):7-12.
49. Strecher VJ, Shiffman S, West R. Randomized controlled trial of a web-based computer-tailored smoking cessation program as a supplement to nicotine patch therapy. Addiction. 2005;100(5):682-8.
50. Simon JA, Carmody TP, Hudes ES, Snyder E, Murray J. Intensive smoking cessation counseling versus minimal counseling among hospitalized smokers treated with transdermal nicotine replacement: a randomized trial. Am J Med. 2003;114(7): 555-62.
51. Ranney L, Melvin C, Lux L, McClain EMA, Lohr KN. Systematic Review: Smoking Cessation Intervention Strategies for Adults and Adults in Special Populations. Ann Intern Med. 2006;145:845-56.
52. Talwar A, Jain M, Vijayan VK. Pharmacotherapy of tobacco dependence. Med Clin N Am. 2004;88(6):1517-34.
53. Hughes JR. Motivating and helping smokers to stop smoking. J Gen Intern Med. 2003;18(12):1053-7.
54. American College of Physicians. In the clinic. Smoking cessation. Ann Intern Med. 2007(online) ITC2-1 to ICT2-16.
55. Galanti LM. Tobacco smoking cessation management: integrating varenicline in current practice. Vasc Health Risk Manag. 2008;4(4):837-45.
56. Moore D, Aveyard P, Connock M. Effectiveness and safety of nicotine replacement therapy assisted reduction to stop smoking: systematic review and meta-analysis. BMJ. 2009;338:b1024.

57. Jorenby DE, Leischow SJ, Nides MA, Rennard SI, Johnston JA, Hughes AR, et al. A controlled trial of sustained-release bupropion, a nicotine patch, or both for smoking cessation. N Engl J Med. 1999;340(9):685-91.
58. Bohadana A, Nilsson F, Rasmussen T, Martinet Y. Nicotine inhaler and nicotine patch as a combination therapy for smoking cessation: a randomized, double-blind, placebo-controlled trial. Arch Intern Med. 2000;160(20):3128-34.
59. Goodfellow LT, Waugh JB. Tobacco treatment and prevention: what works and why. Respir Care. 2009;54(8):1082-90.
60. Aubin HJ. Tolerability and safety of sustained-release bupropion in the management of smoking cessation. Drugs. 2002;62:45-52.
61. Oncken C, Gonzales D, Nides M, Rennard S, Watsky E, Billing CB, et al. Efficacy and safety of the novel selective nicotinic acetylcholine receptor partial agonist, varenicline, for smoking cessation. Arch Intern Med. 2006;166(15):1571-7.
62. Tonstad S, Tønnesen P, Hajek P, Williams KE, Billing CB, Reeves KR, et al. Effect of maintenance therapy with varenicline on smoking cessation: a randomized controlled trial. JAMA. 2006;296(1):64-71.
63. Hind D, Tappenden P, Peters J, Kenjegalieva K. Varenicline in the management of smoking cessation: a single technology appraisal. Health Technol Assess. 2009;13 Suppl 2:9-13.
64. Jorenby DE, Hays JT, Rigotti NA, Azoulay S, Watsky EJ, Williams KE, et al. Efficacy of varenicline, an á4b2 nicotinic acetylcholine receptor partial agonist, vs. placebo or sustained-release bupropion for smoking cessation: a randomized controlled trial. JAMA. 2006;296(1):56-63.
65. 2008 PHS Panel, liaisons, and staff. Treating tobacco use and dependence: 2008 update. US Public Health Service clinical practice guideline: executive summary. Respir Care. 2008;53(9):1217-22.66.
66. NICE public health guidelines 10. [online] Available from *www.nice.org.uk/PH010.* [Accessed May 2010].
67. Maseeh A, Kwatra G. A review of smoking cessation interventions. Med Gen Med. 2005;7(2):24.
68. Lindblom N, de Villiers SH, Kalayanov G, Gordon S, Johansson AM, Svensson TH. Active immunization against nicotine prevents reinstatement of nicotine-seeking behavior in rats. Respiration. 2002;69(3):254-60.
69. De Villiers SH, Lindblom N, Kalayanov G, Gordon S, Malmerfelt A, Johansson AM, et al. Active immunization against nicotine suppresses nicotine-induced dopamine release in the rat nucleus accumbens shell. Respiration. 2002;69(3):247-53.
70. Hall W. The prospects for immunotherapy in smoking cessation. Lancet. 2002;360(9339):1089-91.
71. Jindal SK. Quit Smoking-Why and How? New Delhi: Vitasta Publications; 2008.

Pulmonary Rehabilitation

Rachael A Evans, Roger S Goldstein

INTRODUCTION

Pulmonary rehabilitation is an important component of management of chronic obstructive pulmonary disease (COPD).

The term "rehabilitation" refers to the process of restoration of function despite physical or psychological disability. Pulmonary rehabilitation (PR) programs have developed over the last few decades as a therapy targeted at the secondary alterations of COPD, aiming at improving both the functional and psychosocial aspects of an individual.

SYMPTOMS AND DISABILITY ASSOCIATED WITH COPD

Patients with chronic obstructive pulmonary disease (COPD) commonly present with exertional breathlessness and fatigue[1] and typically they become less active to avoid these symptoms. This reduction in activity can lead to loss of confidence, depression, loss of work or inability to perform hobbies and social isolation, resulting in substantial disability. Although the primary pathological process of COPD results in a progressive reduction in airflow, the correlation between the degree of lung function impairment and the severity of symptoms is weak. Abnormalities in gas exchange as well as the restrictive ventilatory limitation associated with hyperinflation contribute to the symptoms of exertional breathlessness and diminished exercise capacity.

Systemic Consequences of Chronic Obstructive Pulmonary Disease

In addition to the primary pulmonary pathology, there are secondary alterations in skeletal muscle function, nutrition, bone density, gonadal hormones, hemoglobin and mood,[2-4] many of which influence exercise tolerance and health-related quality of life (HRQL). The skeletal muscles of locomotion are altered on multiple levels. Morphologically, there is a reduction in muscle mass and strength of the quadriceps compared to age-matched healthy controls.[5] The muscle fiber types are altered with an increase in proportion of the type II, fast twitch, glycolytic fibers (more fatigable) compared to the type I, slow twitch, oxidative fibers.[6] Muscle metabolism is altered, with a reduction in oxidative enzymes and a reduction in mitochondrial density. Energy metabolism during exercise is altered with a more rapid loss of phosphocreatine at lower workloads than age-matched healthy controls and a failure of adenosine triphosphate (ATP) replenishment to meet the demand.[7]

Skeletal muscle dysfunction contributes to reduced exercise tolerance by promoting an earlier rise in the level of lactic acid, which when buffered, increases CO_2 production which, in turn, increases the ventilatory load applied to a system which already has an impaired ventilatory capacity. Whether the skeletal muscle dysfunction relates to deconditioning or whether it relates to an underlying inflammatory myopathy, remains an area of interest. Although people with COPD do enter a vicious cycle of inactivity **(Fig. 1)** which does influence the function of their leg muscles, muscles not involved in ambulation such as the adductor pollicis retains normal function. Moreover, much of the reduced ambulatory muscle function can be reversed with exercise training. In favor of an underlying systemic inflammatory process are the increased levels of systemic markers of inflammation as well as oxidative stress and nutritional depletion. Hypoxia and medications such as corticosteroids also contribute toward the skeletal muscle alteration.

The spiral of inactivity is also affected by symptoms of anxiety and depression experienced by many patients with COPD. The sensation of dyspnea generates feelings of anxiety, but anxiety itself can manifest as dyspnea. Low mood is frequently reported by patients with COPD-related to their disability and loss of function, but may also be a pre-existing phenomenon predisposing to smoking. Unfortunately, the effect of low mood on motivation and self-esteem further impacts on the inactivity.

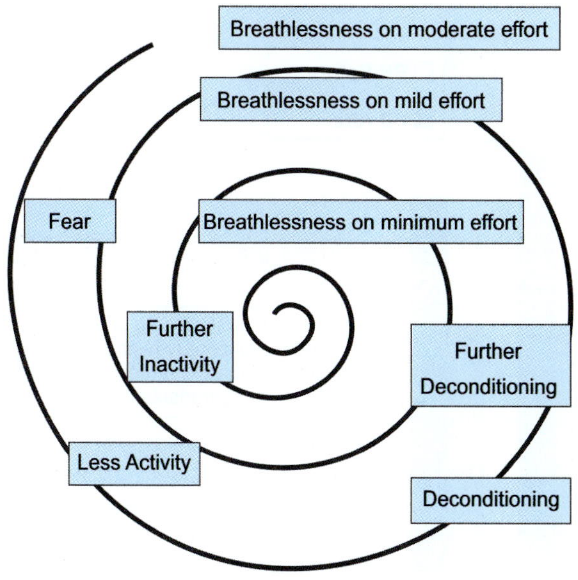

Fig. 1 Spiral of inactivity
Note: The diminishing cycle of dyspnea and reduced exercise tolerance

ROLE AND DEFINITION OF PULMONARY REHABILITATION

Pulmonary rehabilitation is now recommended as an integral part of the clinical management of patients with COPD and has a strong, supportive evidence base demonstrating a reduction in dyspnea, and improvements in both exercise tolerance and HRQL.[8] There is also the evidence to support a reduction in health care costs following a rehabilitation program.[9] It has yet to be established whether pulmonary rehabilitation impacts directly on mortality, although it clearly impacts on many of the factors that affect mortality, such as dyspnea, exercise tolerance and HRQL.[10,11]

The international guidelines of the American Thoracic Society (ATS) and the European Respiratory Society (ERS) adopted the following definition for pulmonary rehabilitation. "Pulmonary rehabilitation is a comprehensive intervention based on a thorough patient assessment followed by patient tailored therapies that include, but are not limited to, exercise training, education, and behavior change, designed to improve the physical and psychological condition of people with chronic respiratory disease and to promote the long-term adherence to health-enhancing behaviors."

Pulmonary rehabilitation programs include several evidence-based components and should not be mistaken for more general programs of activity promotion, convalescence or pure self-management programs.

CHANGING PULMONARY REHABILITATION POPULATION: WHOM TO REFER?

Patients with COPD are the traditional target population for pulmonary rehabilitation. However, the spiral of inactivity also applies to other chronic respiratory diseases, providing a rationale for rehabilitation which has been reported to be beneficial in other conditions including pulmonary fibrosis, post-tuberculosis lung disease, thoracic restriction, bronchiectasis, cystic fibrosis, asthma, pulmonary hypertension, preoperatively and postoperatively for lung resection, volume reduction or transplantation **(Fig. 2)**. Certain program adaptations for non-COPD patients are required, such as the exclusion of exercise induced arrhythmias in pulmonary hypertension and education about chest clearance for patients with chronic suppurative lung diseases.

The predominant clinical inclusion criterion, for referral for pulmonary rehabilitation, is exertional dyspnea that interferes with function as assessed by the Medical Research Council (MRC) dyspnea scale **(Table 1)**. This is a simple, self-scale and can easily be used to screen those who may benefit from rehabilitation. International guidelines suggest referral for pulmonary rehabilitation for Grades III–V. There is evidence to suggest that patients with milder levels of breathlessness may also benefit.[12] The World Health Organization [global initiative for obstructive lung disease, (GOLD)] recommends rehabilitation for any symptomatic patients with GOLD stage II and above [forced expiratory volume in one second (FEV_1) < 80% predicted].

Both the primary respiratory disease and existing co-morbid conditions should be optimally managed prior to enrolment. Patients with obstructive disease should receive optimal airway care. Any pre-existing depression should be addressed as it is known to be associated with poor compliance and response to rehabilitation. Diagnostic assessment and optimizing management should occur prior to commencing pulmonary rehabilitation.

Table 1 The Medical Research Council (MRC) dyspnea scale[7]

Grade	*Description of limitation*
I	I get breathless only with strenuous exercise
II	I get breathless when hurrying or walking or walking uphill
III	I walk slower than people of the same age on the level or I have to stop because of breathlessness on the level
IV	I can only walk 100 yards before stopping because of breathlessness or after a few minutes on the level
V	I am breathless when dressing or undressing or I am too breathless to leave the house

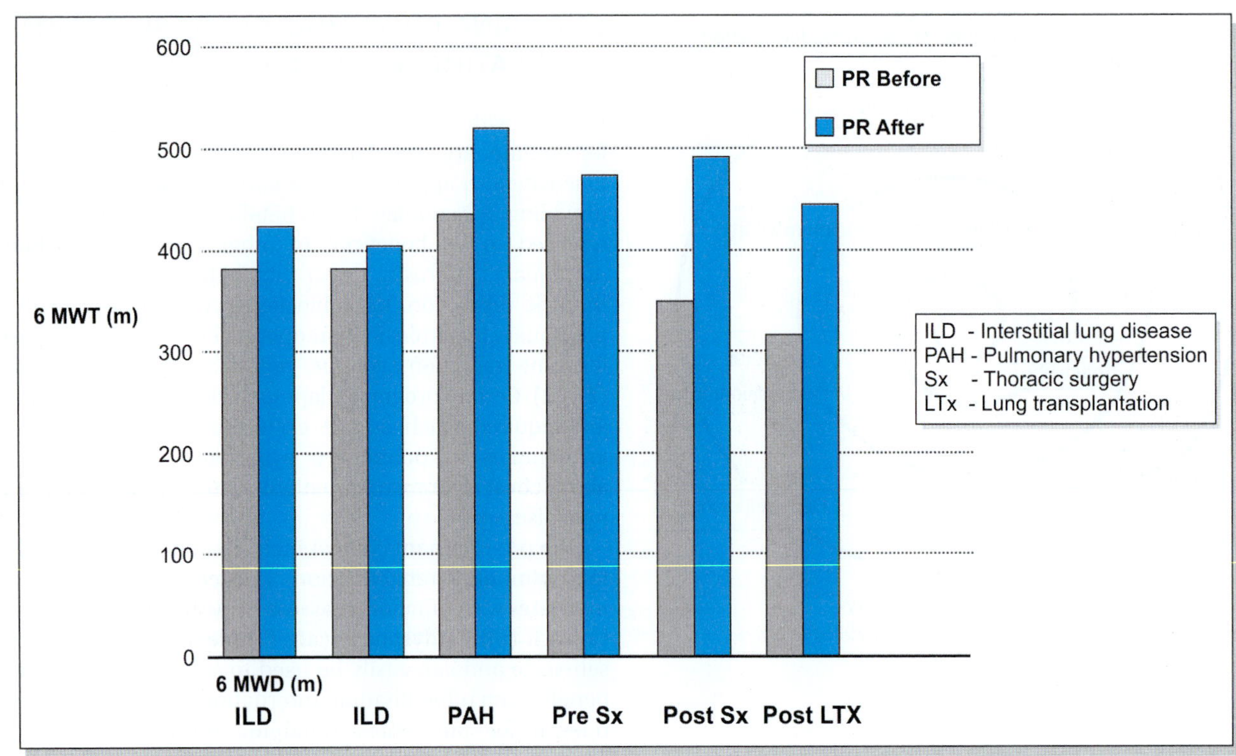

Fig. 2 Six-minute walk test distance before and after pulmonary rehabilitation in different populations
Note: Similar increments in 6MW test can be achieved among a variety of respiratory populations[9]

Patients need to be able to participate in endurance exercises and those with a predominantly orthopedic, neurological or peripheral vascular limitation to exercise, are commonly excluded. Safety criteria should be adhered to, for example a myocardial infarction sustained within three months, unstable angina, moderate to severe aortic stenosis or uncontrolled blood pressure will all exclude patients from being enrolled. Patients with unstable cardiovascular disease must be assessed and treated appropriately prior to inclusion to a program. Nonclinical factors may be pivotal. These include a reasonable level of comprehension, realistic expectations of the program, motivation to improve, an ability to follow instructions, acceptable health literacy and a supportive home and family.

COMPONENTS OF A PULMONARY REHABILITATION PROGRAM ASSESSMENT

The assessment should systematically address the inclusion and exclusion criteria and further inform the patients about the process of pulmonary rehabilitation. An assessment of dyspnea, exercise performance and health status is standard and can inform both individual progress and program quality.[13] An exercise assessment for the program exercise prescription, requirements for safety and as a baseline for the exercise outcome, is increasingly performed using simple, inexpensive field tests rather than expensive laboratory-based exercise equipment. Patients with resting hypoxia should exercise with supplemental oxygen. The criterion for ambulatory oxygen varies among jurisdictions. Those who desaturate markedly on exercise less than 85% are often offered supplementary oxygen during training. In many countries, the expense of oxygen makes it prohibitive except in patients with profound hypoxemia.

OUTCOME MEASURES

Full Cardiopulmonary Exercise Tests

The gold standard measurement of exercise capacity is peak oxygen consumption. A maximal, incremental, symptom limited cardiopulmonary test with expiratory gas analysis can provide this as well as comprehensive information about the precise limitation to exercise. However, it involves expensive equipment and expertise. Typically tests are performed on a cycle ergometer providing a stable platform, but a treadmill can also be used particularly, if cycling is not familiar. Endurance tests can be performed using the same equipment

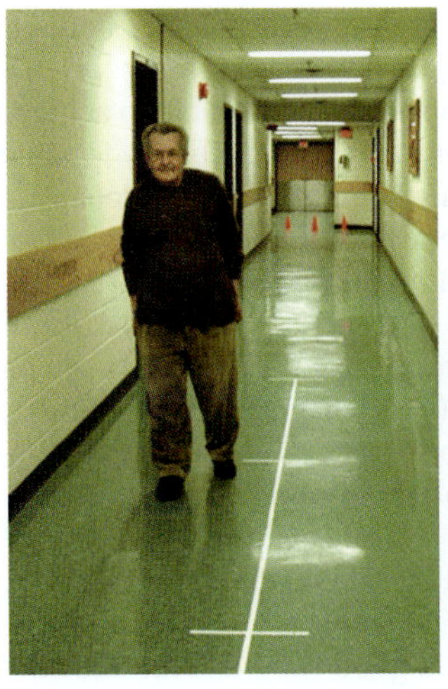
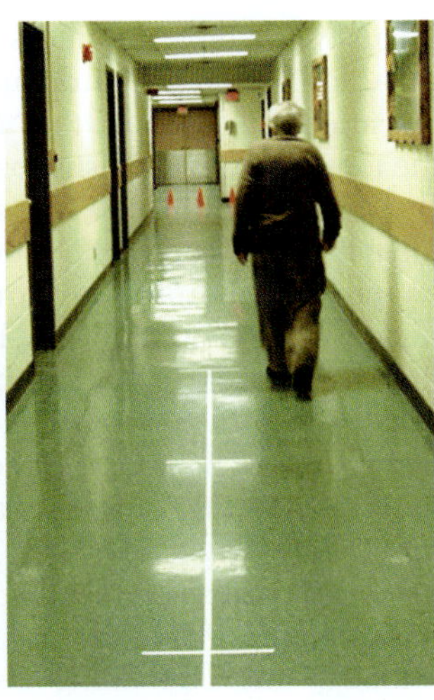

Fig. 3 Six-minute walk test
Note: This is carried out on a flat surface in a temperature and humidity controlled environment.

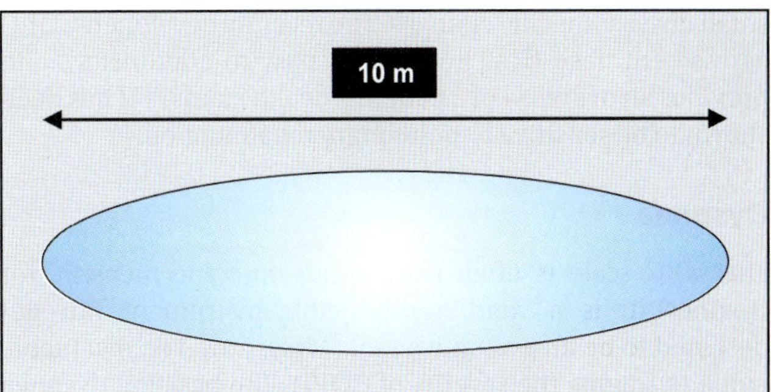

Fig. 4 Diagram of the shuttle walking course

set at an intensity relative to the peak performance. Although the variability of endurance testing is greater than for maximal testing, endurance tests are often a more sensitive outcome measure for pulmonary rehabilitation.

Six-minute Walk Test

The most commonly used field test is the six-minute walk test (6MWT).[14] The test is completed over a 30 meter flat course. It is self-paced and standardized instructions are given. Patients are asked to walk as far as they can for 6 minutes and the result is usually presented as the distance walked, although the speed can be calculated. The test is reproducible after two practice tests and is responsive. Unlike other field tests, normal reference values are available. The 6MWT can be influenced by encouragement, which is, therefore, standardized. It is likely closer to peak exercise capacity although the distance walked is referred to as a measure of functional capacity. The 6MWT distance is highly co-related with other outcomes of COPD such as mortality and is featured in the multidimensional severity index; the body-mass index, airflow obstruction, dyspnea and exercise (BODE) index.[15] It has been used to set exercise prescription (usually as a percentage of the overall speed), but the intensity will vary between individuals. It is reliable, valid and interpretable, all important qualities for its use in clinical research **(Fig. 3)**.[14]

Incremental Shuttle Walk Test

The incremental shuttle walk test (ISWT) is a symptom limited, externally paced test, conducted along a 10 meter course **(Fig. 4)** and reflects maximal exercise capacity.[16] The walking speed increases every minute until the patient is too breathless or fatigued to continue or can no longer maintain the required speed. The result is presented as the total distance achieved. It is reproducible after a single practice test. In contrast to the 6MWT the ISWT has a graded physiological response. However, normal reference values are not currently available. The test is also reliable, valid and interpretable,[16,17] making it an excellent evaluative test just like the 6MWT.

Endurance Shuttle Walk Test

The endurance shuttle walk test (ESWT) was developed as a test of submaximal exercise capacity. It is similarly symptom limited, externally paced and uses the same 10 meter course as the ISWT.[18] After a 2-minute warm up, the patients walk at the set speed until they can no longer maintain the required speed or are too breathless or fatigued to continue. The result is presented as the time walked after the warm up and is reproducible after a familiarization test. The ISWT and ESWT can be used to develop individualized exercise prescriptions for pulmonary rehabilitation. The speed of the walk can be set at a high intensity (85% of the predicted peak oxygen consumption) derived from the ISWT distance. The duration of the walk can then be progressed throughout the program. Both the ISWT and ESWT are responsive outcome measures.

Health Status

Health-related quality of life has become an important outcome for assessing chronic disease interventions. Most disease-specific questionnaires have components that assess dyspnea, and activity limitation. The two most commonly used and therefore, the best understood are the chronic respiratory questionnaire (CRQ)[19] and St. George's respiratory questionnaire (SGRQ).[20] They are both reproducible and evaluative, but the SGRQ has the advantage of also being discriminative. Generic questionnaires such as the Medical Outcomes Short Form-36 Questionnaire (SF-36) can also be used. This has the advantage of being able to compare across different disease populations and has normative values, but it is more discriminative than evaluative and may not identify small disease specific changes. The recently developed COPD assessment test (CAT) is short, easy-to-administer, and provides an overview of a patient's health status.[21] It has been shown to be sensitive to pulmonary rehabilitation.[22]

Dyspnea

The MRC scale is often used as an outcome measure for dyspnea. It is a valid, reproducible instrument but not designed to be an evaluative tool.[23] It is, however, a valuable guide to staging the severity of COPD. The baseline dyspnea index and the transition dyspnea index (BDI/TDI) are disease specific valid, reproducible and interpretable. Together with the SGRQ and the CRQ, the BDI-TDI is among the most frequently employed measure of outcome in pulmonary rehabilitation.[24]

Clinical Important Difference

For many of the outcome measures described a "clinically meaningful" change has been evaluated. This adds to clinical interpretation of results from an intervention. A minimum clinically important difference exists for the 6MWT, ISWT, ESWT, CRQ, SGRQ and the BDI or TDI. If achieved, it provides a rationale for introducing or withdrawing a management intervention.

CORE COMPONENTS OF A PULMONARY REHABILITATION PROGRAM

The core components of a program are summarized in **Box 1**.

Exercise Training

Exercise training is an essential component to pulmonary rehabilitation and has the largest supporting evidence base of all the other components.

Lower Limb Endurance Training

Lower limb endurance training is mandatory for the individuals who wish to improve exercise tolerance and reduce dyspnea on exertion. It is individually prescribed, based on an assessment exercise test and progressed throughout the program. High intensity training is recommended in the healthy population for achieving cardio-respiratory fitness. Similar principles apply to patients with COPD and high intensity training produces greater physiologic benefits than lower intensity training.[25] However, many are so constrained by dyspnea that they are often unable to achieve the ideal training intensity, but the highest intensity feasible should be the aim. The training schedule should detail the intensity, duration and frequency of training. Intensity can be prescribed from the cardiopulmonary exercise (CPX) test performed on a treadmill or a cycle ergometer, or from the various field tests. The training speed or load can be calculated from the measured (CPX) or predicted (field tests) percentage of peak oxygen consumption (typically 60–80% for high intensity) or from peak heart rate (similarly 60–80% predicted for high intensity).

An exercise session should last between 20–30 minutes. Walking and cycling are both effective training modalities. Although interval training has a good rationale for allowing the muscles to recover during the lower intensity periods, studies have not identified interval training as being more effective than constant load training for those with COPD.[26]

BOX 1 Core components of a pulmonary rehabilitation program

- Exercise training
  - Lower limb endurance training
  - Lower and upper limb resistance training
- Multidisciplinary education
- Psychological support
- Self-management

Resistance Training

Resistance (strength) training has received much attention over the last two decades and is recommended by international guidelines. Although muscle strength is improved compared to endurance training alone, this has not translated to additional improvements in exercise tolerance or health status. The effect of strength training on daily physically activity has yet to be thoroughly investigated. Ideally, resistance training should be individually prescribed, for example, at 40–60% of the one repetition maximum, and progressed through the program. The studies advocating resistance training were performed on gym equipment **(Fig. 5)**. Lower limb exercise often consists of sit to stand, step ups, leg raises, which can be progressed throughout the program, but these exercises have not been thoroughly evaluated. Ankle weights can also be employed to add resistance.

Upper limb resistance training is commonly performed using free weights and currently unsupported endurance

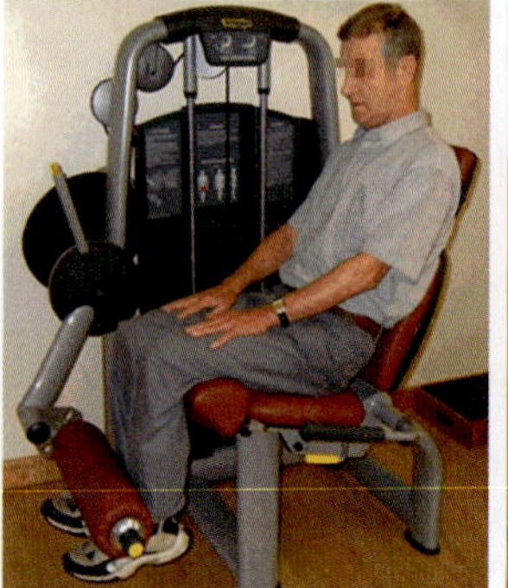
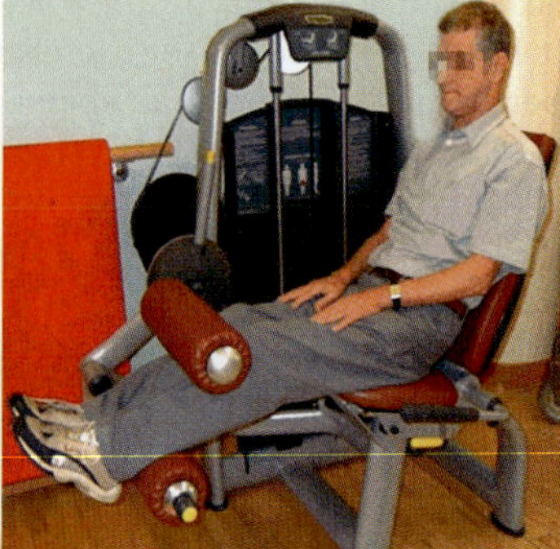

Fig. 5 Lower limb resistance training

BOX 2 Example of topics for the education component

Multidisciplinary education:
- Exercise
- Nutritional advice
- Relaxation
- Devices and oxygen therapy
- Benefits advice
- Energy conservation
- Travel
- Sexual intercourse advice
- Disease education
- Pharmacology

exercises are recommended in the guidelines. There are theoretical reasons why improving upper limb strength may help dyspnea and activities of daily living, but the results of small studies so far are varied.[27] Nevertheless most pulmonary rehabilitation programs include upper limb exercise.

Multidisciplinary Education

It is widely accepted that education is a logical and necessary component of pulmonary rehabilitation, but less is known about which topics are essential. Examples of typical education topics are shown in **Box 2**. Education is commonly delivered in a group setting, but should be supplemented with individual support and other ongoing educational materials such as computer-based and on-line learning modules. Psychological support is a core component of pulmonary rehabilitation as many patients experience symptoms of anxiety or depression. Psychological status should be first assessed using a standardized measuring tool such as the hospital anxiety and depression scale (HADS).[28] Support is usually delivered by the rehabilitation team, but for some patients with more severe symptoms a psychologist is consulted. The process of pulmonary rehabilitation has been shown to improve low mood and reduce anxiety.[29]

EDUCATION SELF-MANAGEMENT

Self-management can be taught within or outside of pulmonary rehabilitation.[30] It increases patients' involvement and control of their disease and improves their sense of well-being. It has been shown to reduce resource utilization especially that attributable to unscheduled visits to the hospital. Patients learn to cope and react to their disease. With new skills of decision making, early symptom recognition and action plans patients are able to recognize and respond to respiratory exacerbations and avoid hospital admissions. Exercise, nutritional management and the correct administration of medications are all assisted by self-management education.

INTENSITY AND DURATION OF A PROGRAM

Intensity can refer to the intensity of the exercise prescription or the number of sessions per week. A minimum of three supervised sessions per week for 6 weeks is recommended, but due to recognized financial and time constraints, two supervised sessions with at least one other home session is acceptable. Additional home training alongside the supervised sessions should be commenced from the outset. There is ongoing debate about the optimum length of a program. Even very short programs (4 weeks) can significantly improve exercise performance and HRQL, but longer programs (>12 weeks) may help sustain the benefits. A minimum length of 6 weeks is recommended for the supervised program. As with many approaches to chronic conditions, the initial improvements will diminish in time in the absence of good adherence to the program guidelines.[9]

MAINTENANCE

Follow up and maintenance are required to sustain the benefits of pulmonary rehabilitation in keeping with the principles of long-term chronic disease management. A close relationship between primary and specialist care is also important as the majority of patients with COPD will be managed by their primary care physician or nurse practitioner.

As adherence to the exercise protocol decreases, the level of exercise achieved is often reduced. This is especially the case following a respiratory exacerbation.[31] There are many approaches to the frequency and location of the maintenance process including whether it is necessary for this to be institutionally based or whether effective programs can be accessed through community centers. Repeat modified (short-term) programs result in similar short-term gains in exercise tolerance, but without an overall long-term benefit.[32]

Maintenance programs are modest in their effects[33,34] in part because they rely on behavioral changes to impact on lifestyle. In many healthcare systems, cost is an obstacle, which makes any out-of-hospital solutions more attractive. Nevertheless, patients do discontinue pulmonary rehabilitation for a variety of social, motivational or medical reasons, including an acute exacerbation of COPD and intercurrent illnesses. Prediction of adherence is difficult, but it is likely that those who benefitted little from the program will not subsequently maintain their exercise habits. Rolling programs have the advantage over fixed entry programs in that patients may enter or re-enter at any time.

OXYGEN

Supplemental oxygen during exercise may be required for safety reasons in those who exhibit profound desaturation. Under laboratory and field exercise conditions, oxygen can improve exercise performance by reducing the ventilatory

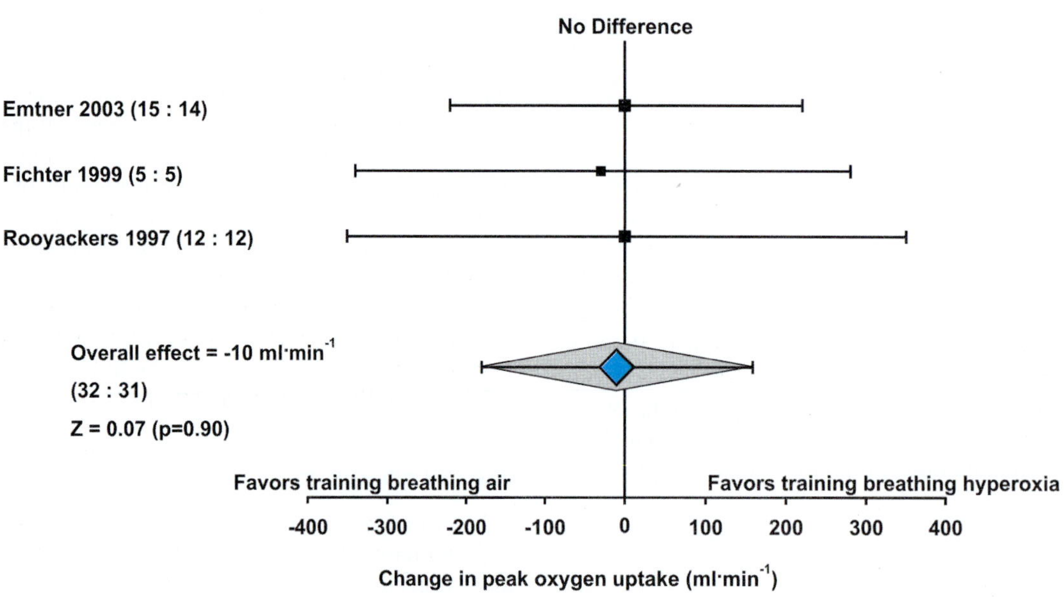

Fig. 6 Effect of training with supplemental oxygen
Note: The three studies included do not show evidence of change in peak oxygen uptake[25,26]

requirements. However, the effects of training with supplemental oxygen have been variable **(Fig. 6)**.[35,36] Carrying the weight of the cylinder may negate any additional benefits. Although liquid oxygen is lighter to carry, it is expensive and not widely available.

MOBILITY AIDS

Although walking sticks can improve balance and posture, rollators **(Fig. 7)** provide more stable support, improve balance and enable the user to sit comfortably on the seat provided. Rollators have been shown to improve walking distance especially among the more limited patients unassisted 6MWD less than 375 m.[37] These benefits are sustained, if the patients continue to use the rollator at home.[38] Rollators also have the advantage of being able to carry oxygen or other small items such as groceries.

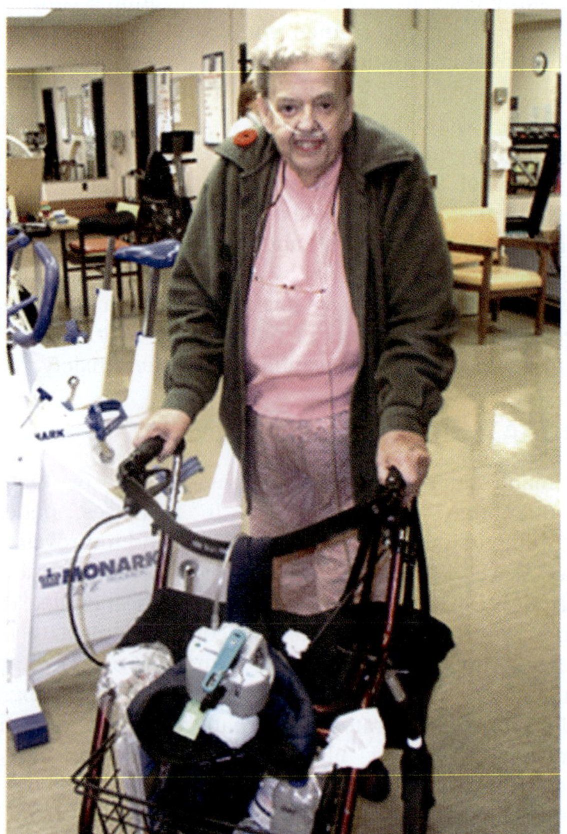

Fig. 7 Patient with rollator and oxygen

REHABILITATION TEAM

The multidisciplinary team should encompass the skills of respiratory physiotherapists, occupational therapists, nurses, assistants and physicians. It is often not possible to have the complete range of disciplines in person, but the skill set should be available. Team members should all have basic and intermediate life-support skills and at least one member in the exercise sessions should have advanced life support. A minimum of one professional to eight patients is recommended. Experienced patients are a useful addition to the team, usually on a voluntary basis, and can provide further support to the patient group.

QUALITY ASSURANCE AND AUDIT

Programs should set up a regular audit to ensure that the results are in keeping with acceptable standards. Group aggregate data on walking distance and health status are frequently used. Feedback from patients can be collected by anonymous satisfaction questionnaire and data on compliance and dropout rates should also be recorded.

SETTING

Pulmonary rehabilitation programs have been hospital-based for stable disease both as in-patient and out-patient settings. There are limitations with this approach namely transport and accessibility. As in most countries, the provision of pulmonary rehabilitation does not reach the demand, and community and home-based programs are sometimes available.[39,40] These alternate settings may be advantageous for patients still at work or wishing to avoid the difficulties of travel to a central site.

EXACERBATIONS

Exacerbations are the real enemy of pulmonary rehabilitation as all the components that improve with pulmonary rehabilitation dyspnea, exercise tolerance, muscle strength and HRQL are all reduced following an acute exacerbation.[41-43] Many patients do not reach their pre-exacerbation level of functioning and clinical practice is of repeat referral for a shorter (booster) program. There is the evidence that undergoing pulmonary rehabilitation immediately post-exacerbation is beneficial and not associated with adverse effects.[44] Targeting exercise therapy immediately post-exacerbation has a strong rationale, but there are significant challenges in engaging patients immediately post-exacerbation,[45] and whether morbidity can be improved long term needs to be investigated. Although there is evidence supporting early mobilization strategies within the intensive care setting, a recently published randomized controlled trial showed no benefit of a similar strategy during hospitalization for an exacerbation of COPD.[46] How to manage patients post-exacerbation remains an area for further research.

PERFORMANCE ENHANCEMENT

Several approaches to enhancement have been evaluated. Calorie supplementation appears to help normal weight patients, but not those with cachexia.[47] Creatine supplementation has not been demonstrated to impact on exercise performance.[48] Anabolic agents are not currently recommended. Patients should be optimally pharmacologically managed prior to entry into pulmonary rehabilitation and the addition of a long-acting anticholinergic has been shown to improve pulmonary rehabilitation compared to placebo.[49]

Training Adjuncts or Strategies

These experimental strategies are included out of interest and to reflect the exciting ways in which exercise rehabilitation is challenging, healthcare professionals need to be creative. As ventilatory limitation is a major barrier to exercise training the use of proportional assist ventilation (noninvasive ventilation), by means of a tight-fitting mask, will improve endurance under laboratory conditions.[50] The use of a helium-hyperoxic mixture improves endurance time and enables a faster progression of training intensity, resulting in greater improvements in HRQL.[51] As helium is less dense, turbulence is reduced and laminar flow is improved thereby reducing the work of breathing.

An approach that reduces the ventilatory load by limiting the muscle mass being exercised has generated considerable interest.[52] The reduced muscle mass reduces the amount of lactic acid. As the latter is buffered to release carbon dioxide, this reduction enables a lower ventilatory drive and, therefore increases endurance. A training study has demonstrated that this is one of the few approaches to exercise training in COPD that will improve the peak oxygen consumption **(Fig. 8)**.[53]

SUMMARY

Key features of a pulmonary rehabilitation program:

- Assessment for suitability and safety
- Provision by a multidisciplinary team
- Individually prescribed exercise training combined with education and self-management advice
- Minimum of two supervised and one unsupervised sessions per week
- Exercise sessions each of 20–30 minutes duration
- Minimum of 6 weeks duration
- Individual progress assessed by appropriate outcome measures usually exercise performance and health status
- Audit for quality control
- Ideally to have a subsequent maintenance program or potentially further programs after an exacerbation.

Future Work

Although much is known about the efficacy of short-term pulmonary rehabilitation, healthcare strategies are needed to ensure adequate access for the large population who stand to benefit from it. Pulmonary rehabilitation skills workshops, especially when augmented by distance learning, can assist with dissemination of information required to develop small local programs. A clearer understanding of adherence requires an understanding of self-efficacy, behavioral adaptations and other determinant factors. Maintenance programs are necessary for comprehensive long-term

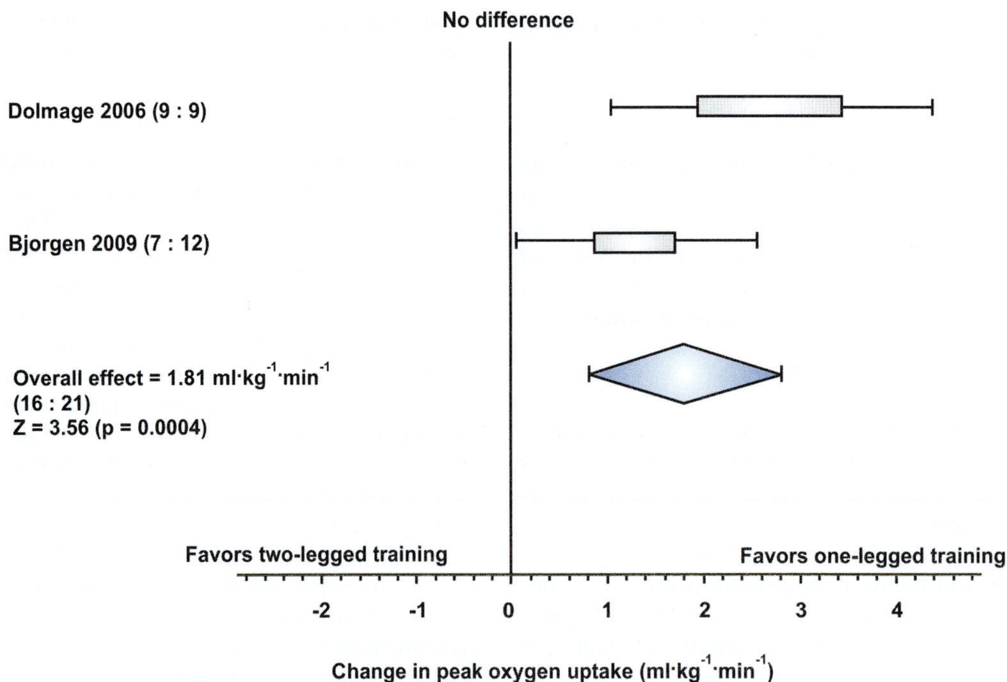

Fig. 8 Effect of one-legged training on peak oxygen uptake
Note: Improvement in peak oxygen uptake favors one-legged training[53]

management of chronic respiratory diseases, just as they are for nonrespiratory conditions. The frequency, content and duration of maintenance programs need to be better defined. Frequent exacerbations are likely to remain a large healthcare burden for patients with COPD and particular attention should be given to integrating exercise therapy early in the recovery period.

Pulmonary rehabilitation is an exciting field that has accomplished much over the last 25 years. Its growth and acceptance as mainstream management opens the way for further innovations.

REFERENCES

1. Pauwels RA, Buist AS, Calverley PM, Jenkins CR, Hurd SS. Global strategy for the diagnosis, management, and prevention of chronic obstructive pulmonary disease. NHLBI/WHO Global Initiative for Chronic Obstructive Lung Disease (GOLD) Workshop summary. Am J Respir Crit Care Med. 2001;163(5):1256-76.
2. Agusti A, Soriano JB. COPD as a systemic disease. COPD. 2008;5(2):133-8.
3. Agusti AG, Noguera A, Sauleda J, Sala E, Pons J, Busquets X. Systemic effects of chronic obstructive pulmonary disease. Eur Respir J. 2003;21(2):347-60.
4. Similowski T, Agusti A, MacNee W, Schonhofer B. The potential impact of anaemia of chronic disease in COPD. Eur Respir J. 2006;27(2):390-6.
5. Gosselink R, Troosters T, Decramer M. Peripheral muscle weakness contributes to exercise limitation in COPD. Am J Respir Crit Care Med. 1996;153(3):976-80.
6. Maltais F, Sullivan MJ, LeBlanc P, Duscha BD, Schachat FH, Simard C, et al. Altered expression of myosin heavy chain in the vastus lateralis muscle in patients with COPD. Eur Respir J. 1999;13(4):850-4.
7. Steiner MC, Evans R, Deacon SJ, Singh SJ, Patel P, Fox J, et al. Adenine nucleotide loss in the skeletal muscles during exercise in chronic obstructive pulmonary disease. Thorax. 2005;60(11):932-6.
8. Spruit MA, Singh SJ, Garvey C, Zuwallack R, Nici L, Rochester C, et al. An official American Thoracic Society/European Respiratory Society statement: key concepts and advances in pulmonary rehabilitation. Am J Respir Crit Care Med. 2013;188(8):e13-64.
9. Griffiths TL, Burr ML, Campbell IA, Lewis-Jenkins V, Mullins J, Shiels K, et al. Results at 1 year of outpatient multidisciplinary pulmonary rehabilitation: a randomised controlled trial. Lancet. 2000;355(9201):362-8.
10. Nishimura K, Izumi T, Tsukino M, Oga T. Dyspnea is a better predictor of 5-year survival than airway obstruction in patients with COPD. Chest. 2002;121(5):1434-40.
11. Oga T, Nishimura K, Tsukino M, Sato S, Hajiro T. Analysis of the factors related to mortality in chronic obstructive pulmonary disease: role of exercise capacity and health status. Am J Respir Crit Care Med. 2003;167(4):544-9.
12. Evans RA, Singh SJ, Collier R, Williams JE, Morgan MD. Pulmonary rehabilitation is successful for COPD irrespective of MRC dyspnoea grade. Respir Med. 2009;103(7):1070-5.
13. Brooks D, Sottana R, Bell B, Hanna M, Laframboise L, Selvanayagarajah S, et al. Characterization of pulmonary rehabilitation programs in Canada in 2005. Can Respir J. 2007;14(2):87-92.
14. ATS statement: guidelines for the six-minute walk test. Am J Respir Crit Care Med. 2002;166(1):111-7.

15. Celli BR, Cote CG, Marin JM, Casanova C, Montes dO, Mendez RA, et al. The body-mass index, airflow obstruction, dyspnea, and exercise capacity index in chronic obstructive pulmonary disease. N Engl J Med. 2004;350(10):1005-12.
16. Singh SJ, Morgan MD, Hardman AE, Rowe C, Bardsley PA. Comparison of oxygen uptake during a conventional treadmill test and the shuttle walking test in chronic airflow limitation. Eur Respir J. 1994;7(11):2016-20.
17. Singh SJ, Morgan MD, Scott S, Walters D, Hardman AE. Development of a shuttle walking test of disability in patients with chronic airways obstruction. Thorax. 1992;47(12):1019-24.
18. Revill SM, Morgan MD, Singh SJ, Williams J, Hardman AE. The endurance shuttle walk: a new field test for the assessment of endurance capacity in chronic obstructive pulmonary disease. Thorax. 1999;54(3):213-22.
19. Schunemann HJ, Goldstein R, Mador MJ, McKim D, Stahl E, Puhan M, et al. A randomised trial to evaluate the self-administered standardised chronic respiratory questionnaire. Eur Respir J. 2005;25(1):31-40.
20. Jones PW, Quirk FH, Baveystock CM, Littlejohns P. A self-complete measure of health status for chronic airflow limitation. The St. George's Respiratory Questionnaire. Am Rev Respir Dis. 1992;145(6):1321-7.
21. Jones PW, Harding G, Berry P, Wiklund I, Chen WH, Kline LN. Development and first validation of the COPD Assessment Test. Eur Respir J. 2009;34(3):648-54.
22. Dodd JW, Hogg L, Nolan J, Jefford H, Grant A, Lord VM, et al. The COPD assessment test (CAT): response to pulmonary rehabilitation. A multicentre, prospective study. Thorax. 2011;66(5):425-9.
23. Bestall JC, Paul EA, Garrod R, Garnham R, Jones PW, Wedzicha JA. Usefulness of the Medical Research Council (MRC) dyspnoea scale as a measure of disability in patients with chronic obstructive pulmonary disease. Thorax. 1999;54(7):581-6.
24. Mahler DA, Waterman LA, Ward J, McCusker C, Zuwallack R, Baird JC. Validity and responsiveness of the self-administered computerized versions of the baseline and transition dyspnea indexes. Chest. 2007;132(4):1283-90.
25. Vallet G, Ahmaidi S, Serres I, Fabre C, Bourgouin D, Desplan J, et al. Comparison of two training programmes in chronic airway limitation patients: standardized versus individualized protocols. Eur Respir J. 1997;10(1):114-22.
26. Beauchamp MK, Nonoyama M, Goldstein RS, Hill K, Dolmage TE, Mathur S, et al. Interval versus continuous training in individuals with chronic obstructive pulmonary disease--a systematic review. Thorax. 2010;65(2):157-64.
27. Janaudis-Ferreira T, Hill K, Goldstein R, Wadell K, Brooks D. Arm exercise training in patients with chronic obstructive pulmonary disease: a systematic review. J Cardiopulm Rehabil Prev. 2009;29(5):277-83.
28. Bjelland I, Dahl AA, Haug TT, Neckelmann D. The validity of the Hospital Anxiety and Depression Scale. An updated literature review. J Psychosom Res. 2002;52(2):69-77.
29. Paz-Diaz H, Montes dO, Lopez JM, Celli BR. Pulmonary rehabilitation improves depression, anxiety, dyspnea and health status in patients with COPD. Am J Phys Med Rehabil. 2007;86(1):30-6.
30. Bourbeau J, Julien M, Maltais F, Rouleau M, Beaupre A, Begin R, et al. Reduction of hospital utilization in patients with chronic obstructive pulmonary disease: a disease-specific self-management intervention. Arch Intern Med. 2003;163(5):585-91.
31. Cote CG, Dordelly LJ, Celli BR. Impact of COPD exacerbations on patient-centered outcomes. Chest. 2007;131(3):696-704.
32. Foglio K, Bianchi L, Ambrosino N. Is it really useful to repeat outpatient pulmonary rehabilitation programs in patients with chronic airway obstruction? A 2-year controlled study. Chest. 2001;119(6):1696-704.
33. Ries AL, Bauldoff GS, Carlin BW, Casaburi R, Emery CF, Mahler DA, et al. Pulmonary Rehabilitation: Joint ACCP/AACVPR Evidence-based Clinical Practice Guidelines. Chest. 2007;131(5 Suppl):4S-42S.
34. Beauchamp MK, Evans R, Janaudis-Ferreira T, Goldstein RS, Brooks D. Systematic review of supervised exercise programs after pulmonary rehabilitation in individuals with COPD. Chest. 2013;144(4):1124-33.
35. Garrod R, Paul EA, Wedzicha JA. Supplemental oxygen during pulmonary rehabilitation in patients with COPD with exercise hypoxaemia. Thorax. 2000;55(7):539-43.
36. Nonoyama ML, Brooks D, Lacasse Y, Guyatt GH, Goldstein RS. Oxygen therapy during exercise training in chronic obstructive pulmonary disease. Cochrane Database Syst Rev. 2007;(2):CD005372.
37. Probst VS, Troosters T, Coosemans I, Spruit MA, Pitta FO, Decramer M, et al. Mechanisms of improvement in exercise capacity using a rollator in patients with COPD. Chest. 2004;126(4):1102-7.
38. Gupta R, Goldstein R, Brooks D. The acute effects of a rollator in individuals with COPD. J Cardiopulm Rehabil. 2006;26(2):107-11.
39. van Wetering CR, Hoogendoorn M, Mol SJ, Rutten-van Molken MP, Schols AM. Short- and long-term efficacy of a community-based COPD management programme in less advanced COPD: a randomised controlled trial. Thorax. 2010;65(1):7-13.
40. Maltais F, Bourbeau J, Shapiro S, Lacasse Y, Perrault H, Baltzan M, et al. Effects of home-based pulmonary rehabilitation in patients with chronic obstructive pulmonary disease: a randomized trial. Ann Intern Med. 2008;149(12):869-78.
41. Cote CG, Dordelly LJ, Celli BR. Impact of COPD exacerbations on patient-centered outcomes. Chest. 2007;131(3):696-704.
42. Spruit MA, Gosselink R, Troosters T, Kasran A, Gayan-Ramirez G, Bogaerts P, et al. Muscle force during an acute exacerbation in hospitalised patients with COPD and its relationship with CXCL8 and IGF-I. Thorax. 2003;58(9):752-6.
43. Pitta F, Troosters T, Probst VS, Spruit MA, Decramer M, Gosselink R. Physical activity and hospitalization for exacerbation of COPD. Chest. 2006;129(3):536-44.
44. Puhan M, Scharplatz M, Troosters T, Walters EH, Steurer J. Pulmonary rehabilitation following exacerbations of chronic obstructive pulmonary disease. Cochrane Database Syst Rev. 2009;(1):CD005305.
45. Jones SE, Green SA, Clark AL, Dickson MJ, Nolan AM, Moloney C, et al. Pulmonary rehabilitation following hospitalisation for acute exacerbation of COPD: referrals, uptake and adherence. Thorax. 2014;69(2):181-2.
46. Greening NJ, Williams JE, Hussain SF, Harvey-Dunstan TC, Bankart MJ, Chaplin EJ, et al. An early rehabilitation intervention to enhance recovery during hospital admission for an exacerbation of chronic respiratory disease: randomised controlled trial. BMJ. 2014;349:g4315.

47. Steiner MC, Barton RL, Singh SJ, Morgan MD. Nutritional enhancement of exercise performance in chronic obstructive pulmonary disease: a randomised controlled trial. Thorax. 2003;58(9):745-51.
48. Deacon SJ, Vincent EE, Greenhaff PL, Fox J, Steiner MC, Singh SJ, et al. Randomized controlled trial of dietary creatine as an adjunct therapy to physical training in chronic obstructive pulmonary disease. Am J Respir Crit Care Med. 2008;178(3):233-9.
49. Casaburi R, Kukafka D, Cooper CB, Witek TJ, Kesten S. Improvement in exercise tolerance with the combination of tiotropium and pulmonary rehabilitation in patients with COPD. Chest. 2005;127(3):809-17.
50. Hawkins P, Johnson LC, Nikoletou D, Hamnegard CH, Sherwood R, Polkey MI, et al. Proportional assist ventilation as an aid to exercise training in severe chronic obstructive pulmonary disease. Thorax. 2002;57(10):853-9.
51. Eves ND, Sandmeyer LC, Wong EY, Jones LW, MacDonald GF, Ford GT, et al. Helium-hyperoxia: a novel intervention to improve the benefits of pulmonary rehabilitation for patients with COPD. Chest. 2009;135(3):609-18.
52. Dolmage TE, Goldstein RS. Response to one-legged cycling in patients with COPD. Chest 2006;129(2):325-32.
53. Dolmage TE, Goldstein RS. Effects of one-legged exercise training of patients with COPD. Chest. 2008;133(2):370-6.

81

Chapter

Bullous Lung Diseases

Aditya Jindal, Gyanendra Agrawal

INTRODUCTION

A "bulla" is an air-containing emphysematous space within the lungs that has a diameter of more than 1 cm in the distended state and causes a local protrusion from the surface of the removed lung. The terminology "bullous lung disease" is reserved for an entity characterized by the presence of bullae in one or both the lung fields, with normal intervening lung.[1] This entity is different in etiology and pathogenesis from "bullous emphysema", a condition in which bullae occur in conjunction with the emphysematous changes in the nonbullous lung.[2-4] "Giant bullous lung disease" is said to be present if the bullae occupy at least one-third of the hemithorax and compress the surrounding lung parenchyma.[2] It is a rare form of bullous lung disease which may frequently need differential diagnosis from pneumothorax.[5]

It is important to differentiate between the terms bulla, bleb and cyst. "Bleb" is an accumulation of air between the two layers of visceral pleura and lined by the elastic lamina. Whereas, "bulla" is present deep to the internal elastic layer of the visceral pleura and is confined by connective tissue septa of the lung. In contrast, "cyst" is lined by epithelium and can be present in the lung parenchyma or mediastinum. Pathologically, three types of bullae are recognized which differ in location, size of neck, and amount of contained residual lung tissue; the clinical significance of which is unclear.

PATHOGENESIS

The pathogenesis of bullae formation is complex and poorly understood. Bulla arises from destruction, dilatation and confluence of airspaces distal to terminal bronchioles, the walls of which are composed of attenuated and compressed parenchyma. Of all the hypotheses, that of an underlying paraseptal emphysema is the most popular. The structural weakness of the interalveolar septa caused by elastolysis, which itself may be secondary either to a constitutional disorder or to enhanced proteolysis, is the predominant mechanism for the development of paraseptal emphysema. Airspaces in paraseptal emphysema may become confluent and develop into bullae, which may be large. Airway obstruction caused either by loss of airway support or by inflammatory changes in the walls of small airways also contributes to progressive enlargement of these airspaces; ultimately resulting in the formation of bullous emphysema.

In patients of "bullous lung disease" with normal intervening lung, a mechanism different from that of bullae occurring in conjunction with emphysema is more likely. Several hypotheses have been proposed over the years, but none has been proved. Two hypotheses which have attracted most of the attention are "paper bag hypothesis" and a "ball valve mechanism" for bulla formation. Chronic inflammation of the airways especially terminal bronchioles causes airway obstruction, which acts as ball valve allowing air to enter during inspiration, leading to progressive air trapping and tension airspaces. However, this theory of bulla formation by positive pressure within the airspace has been refuted by the studies of dynamic computerized tomography and intrabulla pressure measurements. Moreover, in studies performed in subjects with bullae who were taken to altitudes of 18,500 feet (at an ascent rate of 1,000 feet per minute), little increase in bulla volume was noted, probably reflecting good communication between bullae and airways and adequate pressure equalization.

The pressure in bullae is normally negative and same as that of pleural pressure.[6] The lung surrounding the bulla is less compliant than the bulla itself. Therefore, the pressure required to inflate the surrounding lung is greater than that necessary to inflate the bulla. During inspiration, when bullae and the adjacent lung parenchyma are subjected to same negative pleural pressure, bulla fills preferentially than the surrounding lung like a "paper bag". This "paper bag compliance" is seen up to a critical lung volume, after which they become stiff and much less compliant than lung.[7] Bullae communicate with the rest of the bronchial tree, but air enters or leaves the bullae quite slowly. So, bullae generally do not act as clinically important dead space. During tidal breathing, PO_2 in bullae is higher than arterial PO_2.

Chronic marijuana smoking is also believed to cause bullae formation through microscopic injury to the airways or other unknown mechanisms.[8,9]

ETIOLOGY

Bullae may originate in a variety of clinical and pathogenetic settings **(Table 1)**. Smoking and alpha 1-antitrypsin deficiency are the two most important risk factors for bullous emphysema.[10-12] A hereditary predisposition to bullous emphysema is also suggested by its association with a variety of rare familial disorders, including Fabry's disease, cutis laxa, Ehlers-Danlos syndrome and Marfan's syndrome.[13-17] In a cohort of 166 patients of Marfan syndrome, 16 (9.6%) had apical blebs or bullae.[17] Marijuana smoking has been implicated as the cause of large upper zone bullae in some individuals.[8,9,18] Concomitant use of marijuana and tobacco frequently makes it difficult to isolate the damaging effects of marijuana on lung micro-structure and function.[19]

Upper zone "fibrobullous disease" is also reported in ankylosing spondylitis, usually seen in patients of long-standing disease of 15–20 years duration with marked spinal involvement.[20] It is possible that some patients labeled as having giant bullous disease harbor an unusual condition like pulmonary sarcoidosis, Langerhans cell histiocytosis, idiopathic pulmonary fibrosis or progressive massive fibrosis.[21-23] Post-tubercular fibrosis may sometimes present as bullous disease.[24] Bullae are occasionally described in association with other rare conditions such as neurofibromatosis, Proteus syndrome and absent unilateral pulmonary artery.[25-27]

The cause cannot be ascertained in a subset of patients with bullous disease; they are labeled as idiopathic bullous disease. Pleural blebs or bullae were seen in 6% of 250 young healthy adults on thoracoscopic examination performed for thoracic sympathectomy for essential hyperhidrosis.[28] Transport and retail trade industrial workers exposed to exhaust gas had significant increased risk for bullae on chest radiographs performed on 27,361 men in their 50s in Japan.[29]

Table 1 Causes of bullae in the lungs

Causes
I. Extraneous/environmental
• Tobacco smoking
• Marijuana smoking
• HIV infection
• Post-tubercular fibrosis
II. Rare familial disorders
• Alpha-1 antitrypsin deficiency
• Fabry's disease
• Cutis laxa
• Ehlers-Danlos syndrome
• Marfan's syndrome
• Neurofibromatosis
III. Miscellaneous
• Ankylosing spondylitis
• Sarcoidosis
• Langerhans cell histiocytosis
• Idiopathic pulmonary fibrosis
IV. Idiopathic bullous disease

CLINICAL PRESENTATION

As a rule, small bullae usually produce no symptoms, signs or discernible alterations in pulmonary function, and are detected during routine chest radiography. Rupture of one or more bullae may lead to spontaneous pneumothorax.[30] Most of the causes of bullae formation are therefore responsible for recurrent pneumothraces.[17,20,30]

The most common presenting symptom in bullous lung disease is of gradually progressive exertional dyspnea. Occasionally they may develop sudden severe increase in breathlessness either due to pneumothorax or overdistension due to air-trapping. Chest pain may occur in a patient with bullous lung disease.[5] This is also due to overdistension of the large bullae or development of pneumothorax. Overdistension causes a diffuse dull aching type of chest pain, usually located retrosternally. Hemoptysis is an uncommon presentation, and usually indicates hemorrhage inside the bullae. Increase in cough and sputum production, in patients with known bullous disease, usually heralds the presence of infection in a bulla.

The findings on physical examination are usually dominated by the presence of associated disease. Occasionally, giant bullae may cause localized hyperresonant note and decreased breath sounds. Giant bullae may commonly present with vanishing lung syndrome.[31,32]

RADIOLOGIC FEATURES

Small bullae rarely become visible on the chest radiograph, but they are easily visible by computed tomography (CT). Apical bullae may sometimes be misinterpreted as cavitation on plain radiographs. They can be differentiated if it is remembered that cavities are centered within areas of consolidation and they do not merely overlap them.

High resolution computed tomography is an important tool as it can locate the bullae with considerable accuracy, even when their presence is not suspected on the basis of clinical and radiographic data.[31] It also helps in assessing the extent and localization of bullae and associated diffuse nonbullous emphysema. It also allows assessment of associated diseases such as bronchiectasis, infected cysts, pleural disease and pulmonary hypertension.[1] CT scans can help in differentiating bullous lung disease from bullous emphysema. The intervening lung parenchyma is normal in bullous lung disease as opposed to changes of emphysema seem in emphysematous bullae **(Figs 1A and B)**.

A bulla is seen as an avascular transradiant area separated from the rest of lung parenchyma by a thin curvilinear wall. The wall is usually of hairline thickness. They are of variable

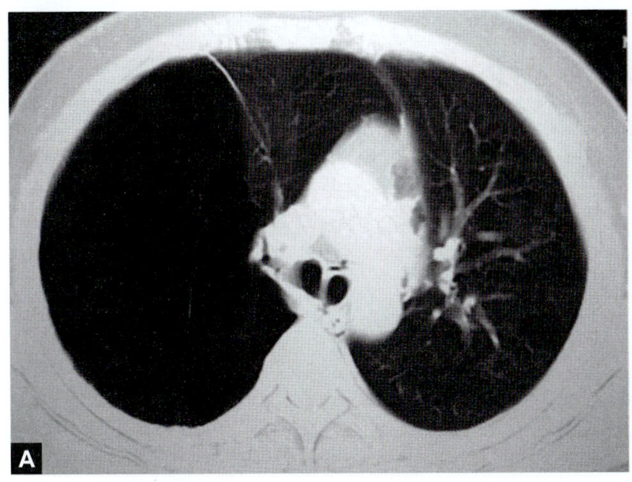

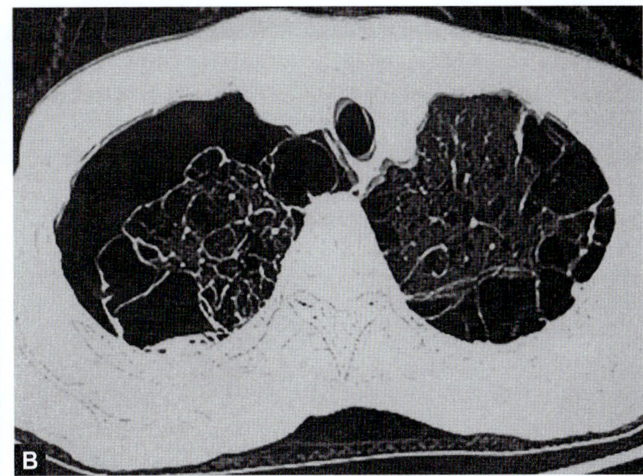

Figs 1A and B (A) High-resolution computed tomography (HRCT) scan in bullous lung disease; (B) Bullous emphysema

sizes ranging from 1 cm to almost half of the hemithorax. Bullae are more common in the upper zones, especially those associated with paraseptal emphysema. The difficult distinction between bullous disease and pneumothorax can be made with CT through the "double-wall sign" (i.e. air visible on either side of the wall of bulla). CT has also been used to create 3-D reconstructions of bullae, which can then be used to calculate bullae volumes.

PULMONARY FUNCTION TESTS

Detailed pulmonary function tests (PFTs) have an important place in the assessment of these conditions and to differentiate bullous disease from bullous emphysema. This distinction is important since patients with bullous emphysema are poor surgical candidates as compared to patients with bullous lung disease. Pulmonary function tests can also help to make an objective assessment of the severity of underlying disease, quantifying the size of bulla and monitor the response to treatment.

Spirometry in patients with bullous lung disease usually shows restrictive defect, presumably as a result of the bulla compressing intervening normal lung; whereas a predominant obstructive defect is seen in patients having bullous emphysema. The diffusing capacity is reduced to a greater extent in bullous emphysema as compared to bullous lung disease; this test correlates better with morphologic estimates of emphysema than do most other tests. The diffusing capacity fails to increase normally during exercise. With exercise, the arterial oxygenation, ratio of dead space to tidal volume and the alveolar-arterial difference in PaO_2 tend to remain normal or near normal in patients with a few circumscribed bullae and otherwise normal lungs, as compared to patients with bullous emphysema where they uniformly decrease, indicating progressive alveolar hypoventilation.

In patients with bullous lung disease, the lung volumes should be assessed by both the helium dilution technique and body plethysmography. A known volume of gas and a trace amount of helium (an inert gas, very little of which absorbs into the pulmonary circulation) is breathed in and out of a reservoir in the helium dilution technique. The helium is diluted by the gas that was previously present in the lung. With the knowledge of the gas in the reservoir and the initial and final helium concentrations, the functional residual capacity and the total lung capacity (TLC) can be calculated. However, because of inadequate time to equilibrate with slowly communicating and noncommunicating air spaces such as bullae, this technique may underestimate the TLC. So, lung volumes should also be measured with body plethysmography, which measures the total volume of the thorax. The difference in TLC measured by body plethysmography and that by the helium dilution technique approximates the volume of the bullae.[1]

Bullae volume = TLC by body plethysmography – TLC by helium dilution

In some patients with bullous emphysema, respiratory muscle strength improves after bullectomy, as assessed by the measurements of maximal inspiratory and transdiaphragmatic pressures.[33] In patients with bullous emphysema, due to reduction in the pulmonary vascular bed, the resting pulmonary artery pressures are increased which further exaggerate during exercise. However, isolated bullae act like amputated segments of the lung, and resting pulmonary arterial pressure and blood flow are within normal limits.

NATURAL HISTORY

Systematic long-term studies on the natural history of bullous lung disease are lacking. Patients with bullous disease should be monitored by chest radiography at regular intervals to

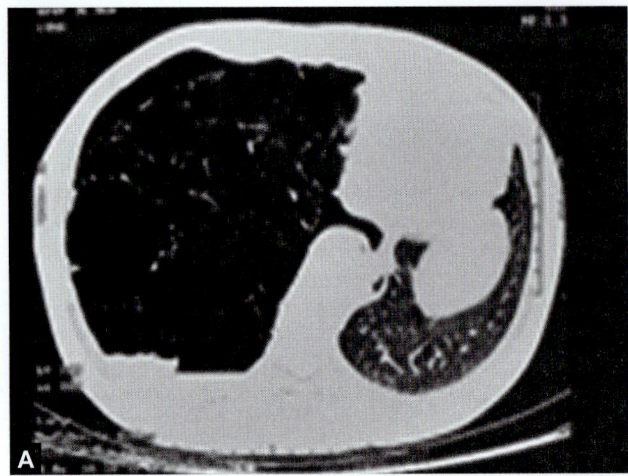

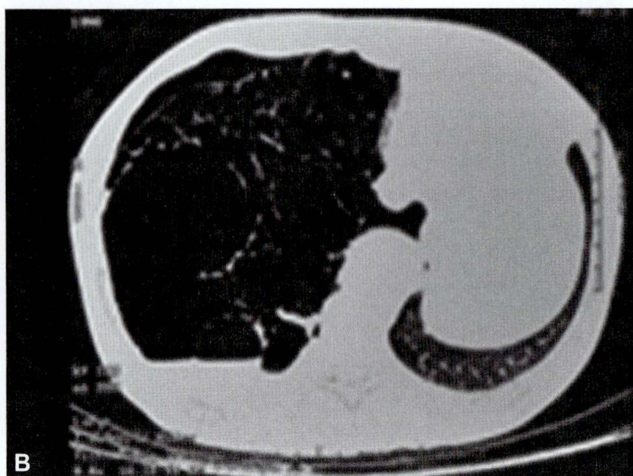

Figs 2A and B Giant bullae with fluid levels
Abbreviation: HRCT, high-resolution computed tomography.

ensure that the disease is stable. Bullae usually enlarge over months and years at a variable rate, the period of stability may be followed by a sudden expansion. In some patients, often young men, there may be the inexorable progression of idiopathic giant bullous disease. The alternative name given for the devastating nature of this condition is "vanishing lung syndrome." In some patients bulla may disappear either spontaneously[34] or following infection and hemorrhage,[35] or with medical therapy alone.[36]

COMPLICATIONS

The main complications of bullae are pneumothorax, infection or hemorrhage. When infected, bullae usually contain fluid and develop an air-fluid level. Air fluid levels within the bullae **(Figs 2A and B)** are relatively uncommon.[37] Fluid may be frequently resorbed, and cause complete resolution of the bulla. The hair-line wall often becomes thickened, and indeed this may be the only sign of infection. An infected bulla differs from an abscess in that the patient is less ill, the wall of the ring shadow is thinner and has a sharp margin, and there is less adjacent pneumonitis. Sometimes, a fungus colonizes a bulla and may form a mycetoma or fungal ball. Hemorrhage inside the bulla is a less common complication and it manifests as hemoptysis or decrease in hemoglobin level.[36] As with infection, bulla may disappear after bleeding occurs. Pneumothorax may occur due to the rupture of the bulla in pleural cavity or as a complication of paraseptal emphysema. Patients tend to have a prolonged air-leak in such cases.[38]

Isolated cases of carcinomas arising in bullous lung diseases have been reported during the past 40 years. The majority of lung cancers associated with bullous disease are non-small-cell tumors. The frequency of lung cancer in subjects with bullous disease is approximately 32 times higher than in those without these abnormalities.[39] High resolution computed tomography signs which could suggest the presence of carcinoma include mural nodule, mural thickening, fluid within bulla and change in bulla diameter.[40,41] The possible carcinogenic mechanism of bullous disease remains uncertain. The proposed mechanisms are: (1) carcinogens may inhibit antielastase enzymes, resulting in interalveolar-septal destruction with subsequent bulla formation; (2) constitutional or congenital factors may cause bullous disease and simultaneously may also predispose to lung cancer; and (3) impaired ventilation of bullae may facilitate the deposition of carcinogens.

TREATMENT

An asymptomatic patient diagnosed to have bullous lung disease should be reassured and educated about the disease. All attempts should be made to quit smoking. The patients should be asked to avoid activities that promote rupture of bulla like "scuba-diving." Appropriate treatment for the associated disease like asthma or chronic obstructive pulmonary disease (COPD) should be given. There are case reports of spontaneous resolution of progressively enlarging giant bullous emphysema after medical therapy for COPD was instituted.[35] Appropriate antibiotics and chest physiotherapy should be started as soon as the diagnosis of infected bullae is established.

Because of the impairment of respiratory function, and the higher incidence of coexisting infection and cancer, the giant bulla should be resected in all patients, even if they are asymptomatic. Enlarging bullae causing incapacitating dyspnea or chest pain or impending respiratory insufficiency also need to be resected. Any lung mass associated with bullae should be considered as an indication for surgery. Other indications of bullectomy include infected bullae and that causing recurrent pneumothorax **(Table 2)**.

Even in bullectomy cases without the evidence of parenchymal lesions, the surgical resection should be as

Table 2 Indications of bullectomy

- Giant bullae
- Symptomatic bullous lung disease
  - Incapacitating dyspnea
  - Chest pain
- Complications
  - Infection
  - Recurrent pneumothorax
  - Cancer

complete as possible. Pathological examination of the resected specimen should be performed because of the suspected existing occult or small sized lung cancer. Bullectomy can be done either via video-thoracoscopy (using a stapling device) or conventional thoracotomy. Giant bullae in vanishing lung syndrome have also been removed by video-assisted thoracoscopic surgery.[42] Thoracoscopic bullapasty performed in fully awake patients is reported to be well tolerated and effective.[43] Antilogous pleural reinforcement of staple line in surgery is another safe and cost effective measure.[44] Mortality and complication rates are usually lower with thoracoscopy than with other surgical approaches.

Lung volume reduction surgery (LVRS) is the surgical removal of 20–30% of nonbullous emphysematous lung from each side. The greatest benefit from surgery is seen in a patient with a large bulla (occupying 50% or more of hemithorax), a moderate reduction in forced expiratory volume in 1 second (FEV_1), a rapid onset of dyspnea and no evidence of generalized emphysema.[45,46] The physiologic basis of functional improvement after bullectomy is similar to that following LVRS.[47]

Other treatment approaches for giant bullae include reduction pneumoplasty and Brompton's procedure (endocavitary aspiration with sclerosis and pleurodesis); the latter is preferred in patients with poor pulmonary function.[48]

Distinction between widespread obstructive airways disease with concomitant bullae and bullous lung disease has practical significance, since surgical lung resection in generalized emphysema offers a less certain therapeutic response than does resection of giant bullae in the absence of widespread obstructive lung disease. As a rule, surgical intervention is avoided in bullae associated with either obstructive or fibrotic lung disease, unless life-threatening complication arises.

REFERENCES

1. Agarwal R, Aggarwal AN. Bullous lung disease or bullous emphysema? Respir Care. 2006;51(5):532-4.
2. Stern EJ, Webb WR, Weinacker A, Müller NL. Idiopathic giant bullous emphysema (vanishing lung syndrome): imaging findings in nine patients. AJR Am J Roentgenol. 1994;162(2):279-82.
3. Carr DH, Pride NB. Computed tomography in preoperative assessment of bullous emphysema. Clin Radiol. 1984;35(1):43-5.
4. Morgan MD, Strickland B. Computed tomography in the assessment of bullous lung disease. Br J Dis Chest. 1984;78(1):10-25.
5. Ghattas C, Barreiro TJ, Gemmel DJ. Giant bullae emphysema. Lung. 2013;191:573-4.
6. Morgan MD, Edwards CW, Morris J, Matthews HR. Origin and behaviour of emphysematous bullae. Thorax. 1989;44(7):533-8.
7. Ting EY, Klopstock R, Lyons HA. Mechanical properties of pulmonary cysts and bullae. Am Rev Respir Dis. 1963;87:538-44.
8. Tashkin DP. Effects of marijuana smoking on the lung. Ann Am Thorac Soc. 2013;10(3):239-47.
9. Lee MH, Hancox RJ. Effects of smoking cannabis on lung function. Expert Rev Respir Med. 2011;5(4):537-46.
10. Paulose-Ram R, Tilert T, Dillon CF, Brody DJ. Cigarette smoking and lung obstruction among adults aged 40-79: United States, 2007-2012. NCHS Data Brief. 2015;(181):1-8.
11. Doney B, Hnizdo E, Syamlal G, Kullman G, Burchfiel C, Martin CJ, et al. Prevalence of chronic obstructive pulmonary disease among US working adults aged 40-70 years. National Health Interview Survey data 2004-2011. J Occup Environ Med. 2014;56:1088-93.
12. Stockley RA. Aphal-antitrypsin review. Clin Chest Med. 2014;35:39-50.
13. Brown LK, Miller A, Bhuptani A, Sloane MF, Zimmerman MI, Schilero G, et al. Pulmonary involvement in Fabry disease. Am J Respir Crit Care Med. 1997;155:1004-10.
14. Franzen D, Krayenbuehl PA, Lidove O, Aubert JD, Barbey F. Pulmonary involvement in Fabry disease: overview and perspectives. Eur J Intern Med. 2013;24:707-13.
15. Ayres JG, Pope FM, Reidy JF, Clark TJ. Abnormalities of the lungs and thoracic cage in the Ehlers-Danlos syndrome. Thorax. 1985;40(4):300-5.
16. Dyhdalo K, Farver C. Pulmonary histologic changes in Marfan syndrome: a case series and literature review. Am J Clin Pathol. 2011;136:857-63.
17. Karpman C, Aughenbaugh GL, Ryu JH. Pneumothorax and bullae in Marfan syndrome. Respiration. 2011;82:219-24.
18. Tan C, Hatam N, Treasure T. Bullous disease of the lung and cannabis smoking: insufficient evidence for a causative link. J R Soc Med. 2006;99(2):77-80.
19. Howden ML, Naughton MT. Pulmonary effects of marijuana inhalation. Expert Rev Respir Med. 2011;5:87-92.
20. Rumancik WM, Firooznia H, Davis MS Jr, Leitman BS, Golimbu C, Rafi M, et al. Fibrobullous disease of the upper lobes: an extra-skeletal manifestation of ankylosing spondylitis. J Comput Tomogr. 1984;8(3):225-9.
21. Jeebun V, Forrest IA. Sarcoidosis: an underrecognized cause for bullous lung disease? Eur Respir J. 2009;34:999-1001.
22. Braier J, Chantada G, Resso D, Bernaldez P, Amaral D, Latella A, et al. Langerhans cell histiocytosis: retrospective evaluation of 123 patients a single institution. Pediatr Hemat Oncol. 1999;16:377-85.
23. Ryu JH, Tian X, Baqir M, Xu K. Diffuse cystic lung diseases. Front Med. 2013;7:316-27.
24. Yen YT, Wu MH, Cheng L, Liu YS, Lin SH, Wang JD, et al. Image characteristics as predictors for thoracoscopic anatomic lung resection in patients with pulmonary tuberculosis. Ann Thorac Surg. 2011;92(1):290-5.
25. Nardecchia E, Perfetti L, Castiglioni M, Di Natale D, Imperatori A, Rotolo N. Bullous lung disease and neurofibromatosis type-1. Monaldi Arch Chest Dis. 2012;77(2):105-7.

26. Lim GY, Kim OH, Kim HW, Lee KS, Kang KH, Song HR, et al. Pulmonary manifestations in Proteus syndrome: pulmonary varicosities and bullous lung disease. Am J Med Genet A. 2011;155A(4):865-9.
27. Betigeri VM, Betigery AV, Saichandran BV, Subbarao. Bullous lung disease and bronchiectasis in unilateral absent right pulmonary artery. Gen Thorac Cardiovasc Surg. 2013;61:100-3.
28. Amjadi K, Alvarez GG, Vanderhelst E, Velkeniers B, Lam M, Noppen M. The prevalence of blebs or bullae among young healthy adults: a thoracoscopic investigation. Chest. 2007;132: 1140-5.
29. Mitsumune T, Senoh E, Kayashima E. Occupations associated with bullae on chest radiographs in Japanese middle-aged men. Int Arch Occup Environ Health. 2005;78:185-8.
30. Van Berkel V, Kuo E, Meyers BF. Pneumothorax, bullous disease and emphysema. Surg Clin North Am. 2010;90:935-53.
31. Sharma N, Justaniah AM, Kanne JP, Gurney JW, Mohammed TL. Vanishing lung syndrome (giant bullous emphysema): CT findings in 7 patients and a literature review. J Thorac Imaging. 2009;24(3):227-30.
32. Mani D, Guinee DG Jr, Aboulafia DM. Vanishing lung syndrome and HIV infection: an uncommon yet potentially fatal sequel of cigarette smoking. J Int Assoc Physicians AIDS Care (Chic). 2012;11(4):230-3.
33. Travaline JM, Addonizio VP, Criner GJ. Effect of bullectomy on diaphragm strength. Am J RespirCrit Care Med. 1995; 152(5 Pt 1):1697-701.
34. Satoh H, Suyama T, Yamashita YT, Ohtsuka M, Sekizawa K. Spontaneous regression of multiple emphysematous bullae. Can Respir J. 1999;6(5):458-60.
35. Park HY, Lim SY, Park HK, Park SY, Kim TS, Suh GY. Regression of giant bullous emphysema. Intern Med. 2010;49(1):55-7.
36. Jay SJ, Johanson WG. Massive intrapulmonary hemorrhage: an uncommon complication of bullous emphysema. Am Rev Respir Dis. 1974;110(4):497-501.
37. Henao-Martinez AF, Fernandez JF, Adams SG, Restrepo C. Lung bullae with air-fluid levels: what is the appropriate therapeutic approach? Respir Care. 2012;57(4):642-5.
38. Smit HJ, Wienk MA, Schreurs AJ, Schramel FM, Postmus PE. Do bullae indicate a predisposition to recurrent pneumothorax? Br J Radiol. 2000;73(868):356-9.
39. Ogawa D, Shiota Y, Marukawa M, Hiyama J, Mashiba H, Yunoki K, et al. Lung cancer associated with pulmonary bulla. case report and review of literature. Respiration. 1999;66(6):555-8.
40. Tsutsui M, Araki Y, Shirakusa T, Inutsuka S. Characteristic radiographic features of pulmonary carcinoma associated with large bulla. Ann Thorac Surg. 1988;46(6):679-83.
41. Richardson MS, Reddy VD, Read CA. New air-fluid levels in bullous lung disease: a reevaluation. J Natl Med Assoc. 1996;88(3):185-7.
42. Van Bael K, La Meir M, Vanoverbeke H. Video-assisted thoracoscopic resection of a giant bulla in vanishing lung syndrome: case report and a short literature review. J Cardiothorac Surg. 2014;9:4.
43. Pompeo E, Tacconi F, Frasca L, Mineo TC. Awake thoracoscopic bullaplasty. Eur J Cardiothorac Surg. 2011;39(6):1012-7.
44. Baysungur V, Tezel C, Ergene G, Sevilgen G, Okur E, Uskul B, et al. The autologous pleural buttressing of staple lines in surgery for bullous lung disease. Eur J Cardiothorac Surg. 2010;38(6):679-82.
45. Gaensler EA, Cugell DW, Knudson RJ, FitzGerald MX. Surgical management of emphysema. Clin Chest Med. 1983;4(3): 443-63.
46. Sardenberg RA, Younes RN, Deheizelin D. Lung volume reduction surgery: an overview. Rev Assoc Med Bras. 2010;56(6): 719-23.
47. De Giacomo T, Rendina EA, Venuta F, Moretti M, Mercadante E, Mohsen I, et al. Bullectomy is comparable to lung volume reduction in patients with end-stage emphysema. Eur J Cardiothorac Surg. 2002;22(3):357-62.
48. Shah SS, Goldstraw P. Surgical treatment of bullous emphysema: experience with the Brompton technique. Ann Thorac Surg. 1994;58(5):1452-6.

82

Chapter

Upper and Central Airway Obstruction

VR Pattabhi Raman

INTRODUCTION

Upper airway obstruction (UAO) can be classified as acute and chronic; the causes for both are quite different. Chronic UAO poses a diagnostic dilemma, and is frequently misdiagnosed and managed as bronchial asthma. On the other hand, acute UAO poses a therapeutic challenge and is best managed in a well-equipped setting that has physicians trained in difficult airway management.

ANATOMICAL CONSIDERATIONS

Upper airways obstruction is defined as the obstruction of the airways at or proximal to carina, including the nose, mouth, pharynx and larynx.[1] The problems relevant to these areas are usually dealt by the otorhinolaryngologists, therefore readers interested in details are advised to refer to otorhinolaryngology textbooks. Also, obstructive sleep apnea, an important disorder causing UAO is dealt separately in this textbook. This chapter essentially focuses on disorders that cause obstruction between the vocal cords and the carina. Tracheal obstruction at the level of thoracic inlet, including in the vocal cords and the cervical portion of trachea is called extrathoracic UAO whereas the obstruction in the thoracic portion of trachea till the carina is called intrathoracic UAO. This distinction is helpful as the changes in the airway dynamics that happen during respiratory cycle are different in the two segments. The intrathoracic segment of trachea increases in dimension during inspiration and decreases during expiration whereas it is the opposite in the cervical trachea and the airways above. The pressure that affects the caliber of upper airways in the extrathoracic region is atmospheric pressure **(Fig. 1)** and the intrathoracic pressure is the pleural pressure.[2] It is therefore easy to imagine how narrowed (extrathoracic) upper airways cause snoring, which is typically associated with inspiratory collapse of the airways.

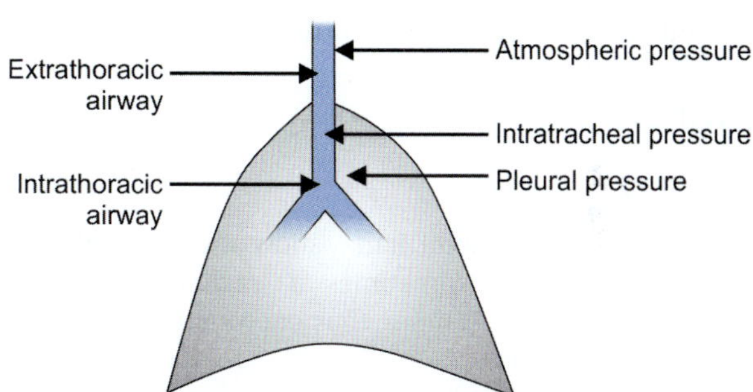

Fig. 1 Pressure affecting upper airways
Source: Acres JC, Kryger MH. Clinical significance of pulmonary function tests: upper airway obstruction. Chest. 1981;80(2):207-11.

PHYSIOLOGICAL CONSIDERATIONS

The classification of UAO on the basis of the anatomical landmark, i.e. the thoracic inlet has also got physiological significance and helps in the understanding of the differences that one sees when one assesses the flow-volume loops of extrathoracic and intrathoracic obstruction. Also, the nature of obstruction, whether it is stiff or pliable, determines whether there will be changes in severity in relation to changes in the transmural pressure. A stiff lesion as in some cases of postintubation tracheal stenosis (PITS) does not allow dynamic differences in the diameter of the stenosis and in the airflow between inspiration and expiration.[2] This is called fixed airway obstruction. In cases of bilateral abductor palsy of vocal cords, there are differences in the caliber and the airflow during the respiratory cycle. Because of the extrathoracic nature of the obstruction, inspiration worsens and expiration lessens the obstruction. This is an example of variable airway obstruction. Based on these parameters, UAO can be divided into fixed obstruction, variable extrathoracic obstruction and variable intrathoracic obstruction.

CLINICAL FEATURES

Acute airway obstruction usually has a dramatic presentation and seldom poses a diagnostic challenge. It usually presents as severe breathlessness and agitation. Stridor is the usual diagnostic sign. Stridor is frequently audible unaided and stethoscope is seldom required.

Chronic obstruction is frequently misdiagnosed and managed as asthma and/or chronic obstructive pulmonary disease (COPD) for a variable period of time before the recognition of upper airway problem. The patient may also present very late in the course of the disease. The presence of stridor in UAO means a fairly severe narrowing. It has been known for almost four decades that tracheal lumen of less than 8 mm produces symptoms after exercise[3] and of less than 5 mm produces stridor.[4] High index of suspicion is usually required in chronic UAO. Diligent history-taking including the history of intubation and of thyroid surgery could serve as a clue. Many cases of chronic UAO have periods of worsening, which get better with antibiotics and steroids, further delaying the diagnosis. Certain features, such as hemoptysis, and relative refractoriness to asthma treatment should alert the physicians about the possibility of UAO and the need for further investigations.

DIAGNOSIS

Radiology

Plain X-ray is seldom useful. It may show obvious mediastinal lymphadenopathy or sometimes a tracheal tumor with extramural extension. At times, the penetrated film may show the site of obstruction.

Computed tomography (CT) is very valuable to diagnose airway obstruction. In particular, the reconstructed images **(Fig. 2)** provide relevant details about the site, the extent and the nature of obstruction. The diameter at the most narrow portion and the length of the stenosis are critical details that are required to plan treatment. The present generation multiplanar CT provides this information in a very short time. Some patients with very severe stenosis may not be able to lie down flat and hold their breath for the study. Magnetic resonance imaging (MRI) is not very commonly sought. It may give valuable information by its superior contrast resolution.

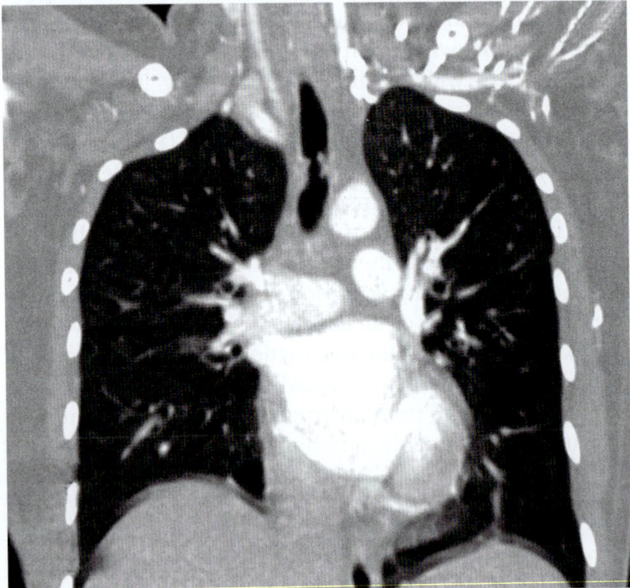

Fig. 2 Reconstructed computed tomography (CT) image of a patient with tracheal stenosis

Spirometry

In normal subjects, during a forced expiration from total lung capacity (TLC), the maximum airflow is achieved during the first 25% of the vital capacity (VC), which is directly dependent on effort and inversely to the resistance. In the remaining 75%, the flow is limited in such a way that an increase in effort (and the associated increase of pleural pressure) does not result in increased flows.[3] With UAO, flow at higher lung volume may be limited by obstruction. UAO causes more pronounced decrease in peak expiratory flow (PEF) than in the forced expiratory volume in one second (FEV_1).[5] Therefore, an increased ratio of FEV_1 (mL) divided by PEF (L/mL) can alert the clinician to the need for an inspiratory and expiratory flow-volume loop.[6] This ratio is called as Empey's index, the value of more than eight suggests the presence of central or UAO.[7] Poor initial effort by the patient can also increase the index. Hence, it is very important that the patient's inspiratory and expiratory efforts are maximal and the technician should confirm this in the quality pattern of repeatable plateau of forced inspiratory flow, notes.[5] Miller and Hyatt[8] did elegant experiments by simulating UAO in normal subjects and found that flow-volume loop would be particularly useful in diagnosing and categorizing UAO[8]. When patient effort is good, the pattern of repeatable plateau of forced inspiratory flow along with a preserved expiratory flow loop indicates variable extrathoracic UAO **(Fig. 3A)** while the pattern of repeatable plateau of forced expiratory flow with a preserved inspiratory loop indicates variable intrathoracic UAO **(Fig. 3B)**. The pattern of repeatable plateau of a similar flow in both inspiratory and expiratory flows suggests a fixed UAO **(Fig. 3C)**. When patient's effort is good, the absence of classic patterns does not rule out UAO. The presence of specific UAO patterns would also warrant confirmation of the presence of UAO, hence, bronchoscopy is required as the next important step.

Bronchoscopy

Bronchoscopy, which provides the most useful information in UAO, is the procedure of choice. It is useful to have an idea about the lesion with a CT done before bronchoscopy so that planning could be better. The cause of the anatomical obstruction can be diagnosed in the case of an intramural pathology like a tumor. Care, however, has to be taken while passing a flexible bronchoscope through a very narrow lumen, since even a minor hemorrhage can become catastrophic by causing critical airway narrowing. It is wise to employ

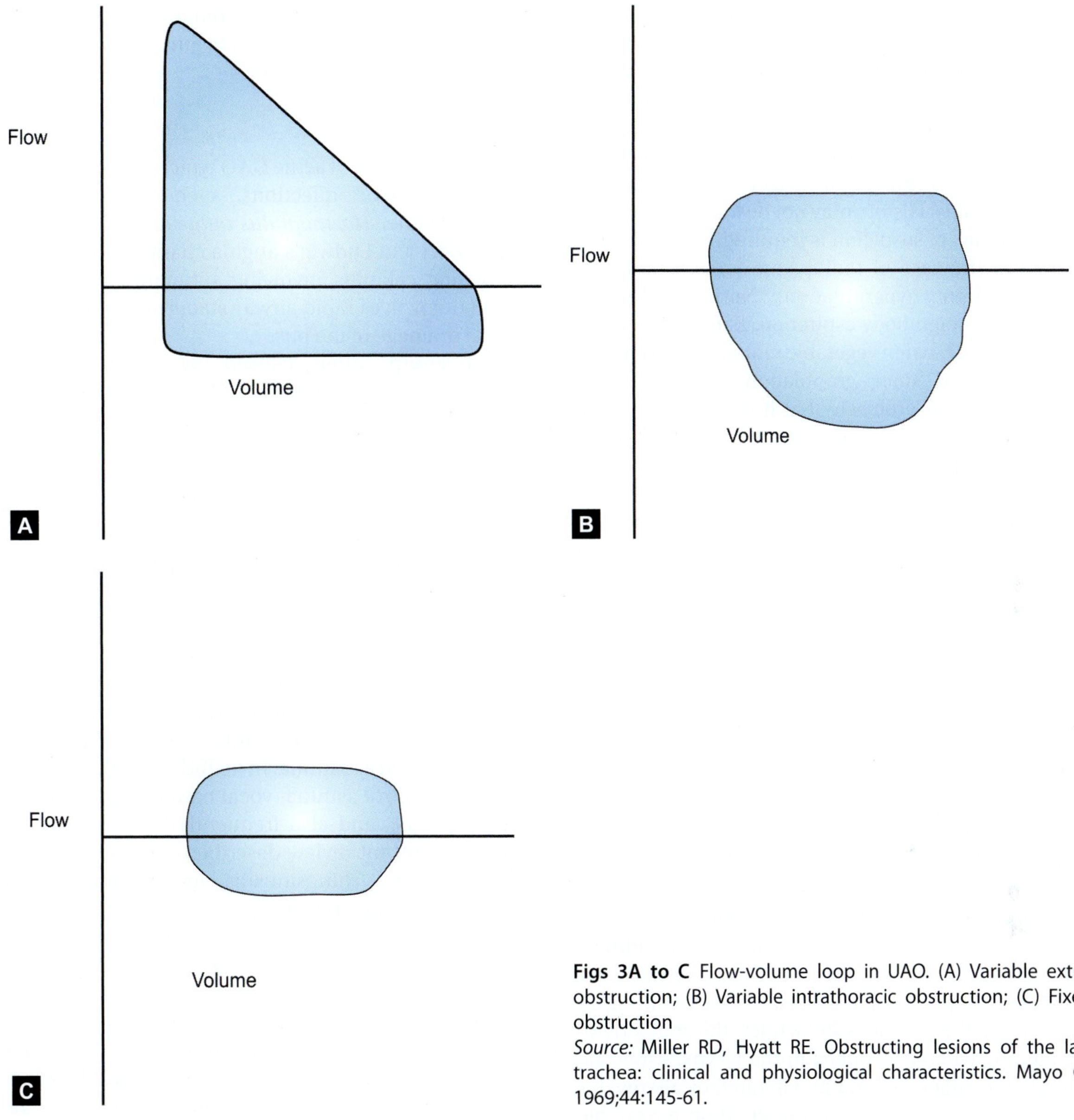

Figs 3A to C Flow-volume loop in UAO. (A) Variable extrathoracic obstruction; (B) Variable intrathoracic obstruction; (C) Fixed airway obstruction

Source: Miller RD, Hyatt RE. Obstructing lesions of the larynx and trachea: clinical and physiological characteristics. Mayo Clin Proc. 1969;44:145-61.

rigid bronchoscopy in such a case of severe obstruction. During rigid bronchoscopy, ventilation can be done during the procedure and therefore, oxygenation is easy. Moreover, the larger bore of the rigid barrel allows the passage of instruments simultaneously, and procedures like biopsy can be safely done. Also, the barrel of the bronchoscope could be used to tamponade bleeding points and to mechanically dilate the tracheal stenosis. Another significant advantage of rigid bronchoscopy is the deployment of silicone stents, making it the investigation of choice in severe UAO.

In cases of extrinsic obstruction, bronchoscopy could be valuable in assessing the mucosa, if there is a transmural invasion. It also helps in assessing the extent of involvement to guide a definitive therapy. In the cases of functional obstruction, such as in tracheomalacia (TM), bronchoscopy is mandatory. Here, flexible bronchoscopy scores over the rigid bronchoscopy to identify abnormal airway dynamics during respiration would mandate an awake and cooperative patient on the table, which is not possible in an anesthetized patient undergoing rigid bronchoscopy.

ACUTE UPPER AIRWAY OBSTRUCTION

Foreign Body

Typically seen in children aged between 2 years and 4 years, aspiration of foreign bodies can also be seen in older children and the elderly individuals. In the elderly patients, it commonly occurs in the presence of comorbidities with depressed consciousness and poor swallowing reflex.[9] In pediatric population, choking is the most common symptom followed by a protracted cough.[10] There is a male preponderance and more often when there is an elderly sibling. No predilection between right and left bronchial tree is seen, at that age the bronchial division makes a similar angle on both the sides. History may not be forthcoming in all cases and high index of suspicion is required.[11] Radiography is useful only in the case of radiopaque foreign bodies or when there is expiratory hyperinflation.[10] Normal chest X-ray does not exclude foreign body aspiration. Early intervention is important especially when vegetable matter like groundnut or bean is aspirated since granulation happens rather rapidly and at times so profusely that it may not be visible in bronchoscopy.[12] Also, delayed removal may not result in complete healing of the granulation tissue. Groundnut is probably the most common foreign body among children in India.[11] Though rigid bronchoscopy is considered the gold standard for the retrieval of an aspirated foreign body, there is a definite role for flexible pediatric bronchoscopes for both diagnosis and retrieval of pediatric foreign bodies.[13-15]

Acute Laryngeal Edema

Acute laryngeal edema may happen following anaphylactic reactions causing life-threatening angioedema, prototype being the penicillin allergy or nonsteroidal anti-inflammatory drugs (NSAID) allergy in aspirin-sensitive asthma. The deterioration is rapid and early intervention is crucial. Parenteral administration of adrenaline can be life saving.

This has to be distinguished from a rare autosomal dominant condition called hereditary angioedema. This condition happens secondary to deficiency of C1 inhibitor enzyme due to mutations of its gene.[16] Localized swelling that is self-limiting can happen at any site of the body including the skin, genitalia, and the gastrointestinal tract. The angioedema is life-threatening when it happens in the larynx, especially if untreated.[17] The attacks are not precipitated by allergy, but by trauma and stress.[17] The age of presentation is variable. Prophylaxis is useful if started early (with tranexamic acid) or attenuated with androgens like danazol.[18] In patients refractory to prophylaxis of danazol, pasteurized plasma-derived C1 inhibitor (pC1-INH) concentrate has been found to be useful in reducing the recurrence.[19] In acute attacks, pC1-INH concentrate (intravenous dose of 20 U/kg) and newer drugs like icatibant, bradykinin receptor-2 antagonist (30 mg subcutaneous injection) have been shown to provide rapid relief.[20,21]

Another important cause for nonallergic laryngeal edema is the administration of angiotensin-converting enzyme inhibitors (ACEIs) which, like hereditary angioedema, is not associated with itching or urticaria.

Prompt recognition and stopping the drug will stop the recurrence. Recent studies have described the increased incidence of angioedema in renal transplant recipients receiving a combination of ACEIs and mammalian target of rapamycin (mTOR) inhibitors.[22]

Infection

Infection as a cause of acute UAO typically occurs in children. This may include infections, such as acute epiglottitis caused by either *Haemophilus influenzae* or beta-hemolytic streptococci and Ludwig's angina characterized by a rapidly progressing cellulitis involving submandibular space. The treatment involves rapid airway stabilization, antibiotics and surgical drainage of the pus.

Viral croup, often caused by parainfluenza virus, is managed by nebulized adrenaline and parenteral corticosteroids. Bacterial tracheitis is usually caused by *Staphylococcus aureus* infection. Bronchoscopic appearance shows the presence of erythema, edema, thick secretions and at times, plaques in the trachea.

CHRONIC UPPER AIRWAY OBSTRUCTION

Vocal Cord Dysfunction

This is a syndrome in which the vocal cords adduct during inspiration producing UAO like features. Patients are usually females in the age group of 20–40 years.[23-25] It masquerades the diagnosis of refractory asthma with multiple attacks, is usually managed as asthma. In an Indian study that evaluated difficult to control asthma, vocal cord dysfunction was seen in about 23.5%, and also frequently found to coexist with asthma.[26] A recent review described exercise, psychological stress, irritants, rhinosinusitis, gastroesophageal reflux disease as the usual triggers.[27]

The "wheeze" typically appears at lower lung volumes since the obstruction happens during the inspiration and for the same reason, the chest X-ray does not show hyperinflation. Spirometry done during the episode may show the classical loop of extrathoracic UAO. Flexible laryngoscopy is considered the gold standard for diagnosis, especially when done during the episode. The classical description during the inspiration consists of adduction of the vocal cords, with a small diamond-shaped chink in the posterior region of the vocal cords. Reassurance and breathing exercises may reduce the intensity during the acute episode and interestingly, rapid shallow breathing (like panting) has been found to be useful.[28] Speech therapy, psychological counseling and avoidance of triggers would help in long-term management.

Tracheobronchomalacia

Tracheomalacia (TM) refers to the weakness of tracheal walls, frequently due to reduction and/or atrophy of the longitudinal elastic fibers of the pars membrane; or cartilage integrity, such that the airway is softer and more susceptible to collapse.[29] TM may be localized or diffuse and usually affects intrathoracic portion of trachea. If main bronchi are also involved, it is called tracheobronchomalacia (TBM).

Pediatric TM

Tracheomalacia is the most common congenital abnormality of trachea.[30] There is a strong association with prematurity,[31] mucopolysaccharidosis and tracheoesophageal fistula,[29] and some congenital heart diseases.[29] There is a male preponderance. Acquired causes include long-standing tracheostomy, and pressure from vascular slings. Congenital TM is usually self-limiting and the children outgrow the disease by the age of 2–3 years. Severe cases are managed by the use of continuous positive airway pressure (CPAP), or by surgical procedures like aortopexy.[32] Aortopexy which is a procedure where the aortic arch is stiched to the sternum and thus relieving the pressure on the trachea is gaining popularity in surgical approach to pediatric TM especially if they become life-threatening, and some authors report the success of thoracoscopic aortopexy with its attendant advantages including shorter hospital stay and no additional complications.[33]

Adult TM and TBM

There is an increased awareness in recognizing and implicating TM as an important cause for pulmonary symptoms. This can be attributed to the advances in CT technology and virtual bronchoscopy, increasing availability of bronchoscopes and of better therapeutic options.

Tracheomalacia in adults is predominantly seen in the middle-aged male individuals who are also smokers. Adult cases most commonly happen following the trauma, including after intubation, tracheostomy, external chest trauma, and after lung transplantation. Emphysema, chronic bronchitis, chronic inflammation like relapsing polychondritis (RP), and chronic extrinsic compression of the trachea are the other important reasons.

Acquired TM is commonly seen in association with long-term intubation and tracheostomy. It is usually a short segment stenosis. A comprehensive in depth review on TM describes that the length of malacic segment secondary to postintubation is usually less than 3 cm.[29] More than 50% decrease in airway caliber occurring during expiration is diagnostic of TM. *Three types are described*:[29]

1. Saber-sheath type (Ω)—lateral wall narrowing
2. Scabbard type (⌓)—anteroposterior (AP) narrowing-crescentic type
3. Circumferential type (O)—all round narrowing.

The TM secondary to COPD is usually diffuse, and also, difficult to treat. The patient presents with symptoms such as cough, dyspnea and wheeze. Dynamic CT, which is noninvasive, is useful for diagnosis. The multidetector CT technology shows very good promise.[34]

Symptomatic cases need to be treated depending on the etiology. Focal TM in postintubation or post-traumatic cases should be respected, if possible. Alternatively, it can be managed with tracheostomy, if the segment can be byepassed. The advantages of tracheostomy in such a situation are that the tube acts like a stent. Long flange tracheostomy tubes are available for the purpose. The tracheostomy can also be an interface for CPAP application. However, tracheostomy can also predispose to TM of a different segment of trachea.

In TM secondary to COPD, the optimization of medications for COPD can help reduce symptoms. Severe cases can be managed with silicone stents. However, it is not effective in all patients and there is a high chance of migration of these stents. Metallic stents should be avoided because of the difficulty of removal and replacement. Different surgical means have been tried. Strengthening the posterior membranous portion using various prostheses like crystalline polypropylene mesh has been tried with variable success.[35]

Polychondritis

Relapsing polychondritis (RP) is a rare and interesting disease. It is a multisystem disorder with unknown etiology, characterized by recurrent progressive inflammation and degeneration of the cartilage and the connective tissue.[34] RP affects people between 2 years and 80 years of age and has equal gender distribution. The airway complications in about 50% of the cases are seen more often in females than in males, and carry a poorer prognosis.[36-38]

Diagnostic Criteria

Criteria for the diagnosis of RP were described initially by McAdam and associates.[37]

Presence of three or more of the following criteria is employed for diagnosis:

- Chondritis of larynx, trachea or bronchitis
- Chondritis of nasal cartilages
- Chondritis of both auricles
- Audiovestibular damage (sensory-neural hearing loss, tinnitus and vertigo)
- Ocular inflammation
- Nonerosive seronegative inflammatory polyarthritis.

The criteria were modified by Damiani and Levine[39] to include histological features and therapeutic responses. *The modified criteria include the presence of any one of the following combinations:*

- Three or more of McAdam's criteria (no tissue confirmation needed)
- One or more of McAdam's criteria with positive histological confirmation by biopsy of the cartilage
- Involvement of two or more separate anatomic locations with response to steroids and/or dapsone.

Clinical Features

Clinical features depend on the cartilage that is involved. It is important to understand that apart from cartilaginous structure of the external ear, nose, peripheral joints, larynx and tracheobronchial tree, other proteoglycan-rich structures can become involved, including the heart, blood vessels and inner ear.[40]

Airway Complications

The prevalence of symptomatic airway involvement was reported in 21% with female preponderance in about 70% patients.[38] The usual symptoms were progressive dyspnea, cough, stridor, hoarseness, chest discomfort and features of respiratory failure. The presence of airway symptoms was the first manifestation of RP is about 50% of patients with airway manifestation. *Airway obstruction in RP can occur due to any of the following:*[41]

- Acute airway inflammatory swelling and airway narrowing.
- TBM—due to progressive destructions of the cartilage.
- Formation of fibrous tissue and cicatricial contraction at a later stage.

Investigations

Pulmonary function tests show mixed pattern.[38] Dynamic CT scan and bronchoscopy **(Fig. 4)** provide the vital details in RP regarding the extent and severity of the airway problem. Typical CT findings include the presence of diffuse tracheobronchial stenosis (better seen with reconstructed CT images), dynamic expiratory collapse or anterior bronchial wall thickening with posterior sparing. Recently PET CT is being used to diagnose and even identify site for TBNA.[42] Typical bronchoscopic findings include supraglottic and false vocal cord edema, subglottic stenosis or TM.[38]

Treatment

Many medications such as the steroids, mycophenolate mofetil, methotrexate and dapsone have been tried, but the response to treatment is variable. Newer biological agents like rituximab, etanercept and abatacept show some promise. Bronchoscopic techniques, such as balloon dilatation and tracheobronchial stenting used alone or in combination, might give some respite from symptoms for patients with airway complications.[43] Interventional procedures provide a good short-term relief. However, long-term outcome is quite variable.

Tracheopathia Osteochondroplastica

It is a rare, slowly progressive disorder of unknown etiology. Endoluminal projections of bony and cartilaginous nodules arise from the submucosa of the trachea. There appears to be a male predominance and usually presents in the sixth or seventh decades of life.[44] The nodules characteristically spare the posterior membrane **(Fig. 5)**, but may be present in the proximal, main bronchi also. The presentation is usually with chronic cough, dyspnea in advanced cases and minimal hemoptysis due to the ulceration of the overlying mucosa.[45] Diagnosis is based on typical bronchoscopic appearances, biopsy is not generally needed. There is no definitive treatment. Severe obstruction may warrant therapeutic interventions.

Tracheobronchial Amyloidosis

Tracheobronchial amyloidosis (TBA) is very rare, characterized by endoluminal accumulation of abnormal proteins in the form of fibrils, which cause obstructive symptoms. In a retrospective review of 17 biopsy proven TBA over a 26-year

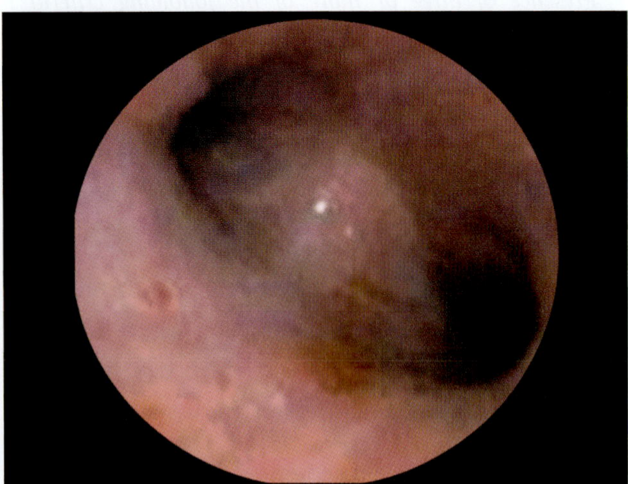

Fig. 4 Relapsing polychondritis. A 50-year-old lady: Biopsy proven relapsing polychondritis. Note the absence of cartilage prominence at the level of distal trachea

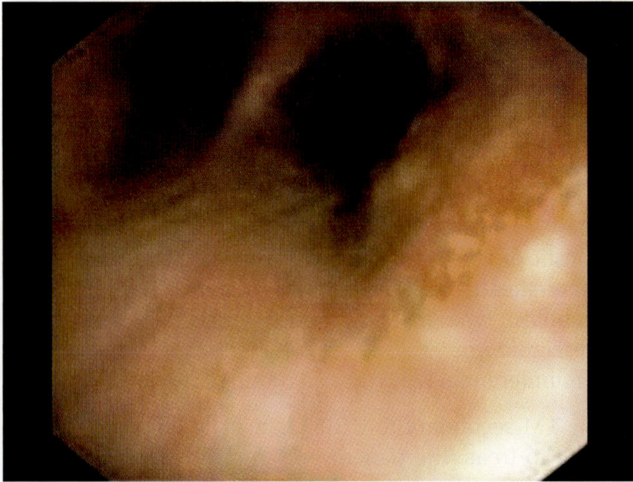

Fig. 5 Case of tracheopathia osteochondroplastica. Note the nodules seen only on the cartilaginous portion of trachea and sparing of membranous portion

period, Capizzi and colleagues from Mayo Clinic described dyspnea, cough, hemoptysis and hoarseness as presenting symptoms.[46] Diagnosis is made by bronchoscopy and biopsy with specific Congo red staining. Response to medications like steroids and Melphalan is suboptimal, severe obstruction warrant debulking.

Tuberculosis

Endobronchial tuberculosis (TB) is not an uncommon problem in the developing world. The true incidence in patients with sputum-positive pulmonary TB is difficult to estimate because bronchoscopy is usually avoided. Endobronchial TB is seen more commonly in females, perhaps because they tend to retain the infected secretions in the bronchial tree and avoid expectoration. It is also more common in the left than the right-side bronchi probably because the left main bronchus is narrow and lengthy and hence the infected sputum may remain in contact with the bronchi for a longer time. Endotracheal TB **(Fig. 6)** is very rare, but presents a formidable challenge to the treating clinician. The disease is quite refractory to chemotherapy alone. *Chung and Lee classified endobronchial TB into seven types based on the bronchoscopic appearance*:[47,48]

1. Active caseating
2. Edematous-hyperemic
3. Fibrostenotic
4. Tumorous
5. Granular
6. Ulcerative
7. Nonspecific bronchitic

Once the lesion becomes fibrostenotic, which is a final path for all the types, it becomes resistant to therapy.

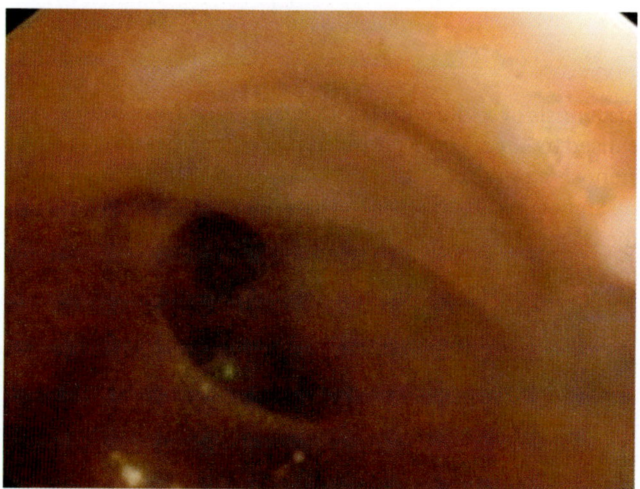

Fig. 6 A 21-year-old lady known case of sputum-positive pulmonary Kochs developed severe respiratory distress despite therapy. She had endotracheal fibrostenosis in distal trachea, which was dilated

Hence, early identification by bronchoscopy is encouraged in a suspected patient. Suspicion arises if a patient with TB develops wheeze or breathlessness. Surgery is ideal if the involved segment is small. If the disease is extensive, balloon dilatation or thermal desobstruction followed by silicone stenting can be tried.[49]

Sarcoidosis

As in TB, an airway abnormality in sarcoidosis is often overlooked. Endobronchial involvement is usually seen in the elderly age groups, smokers during advanced stages of parenchymal involvement and with thickening of bronchovascular bundles on high resolution computed tomography. It carries a relatively poorer prognosis.[50] Flow limitation is seen in about 9% of patients with sarcoidosis.[48] Sarcoidosis can affect every part of upper airway. Sarcoid involvement of the supraglottic airways, larynx, and central and peripheral airways is also described.[51] Obstructive sleep apnea syndrome is seen more often in patients with sarcoidosis, especially lupus pernio.[52]

Tracheal obstruction secondary to sarcoidosis is very rare. After an early case in 1981, not many reports of tracheal obstruction have appeared.[53] The classic endobronchial sarcoidosis is characterized by mucosal islands of waxy yellow mucosal nodules, measuring 2–4 mm in diameter.[51] The nodules are sparse in the trachea, but abundant in the main, lobar and segmental bronchi. Other changes are mucosal erythema, granular mucosa, cobblestone mucosa, mucosal plaques, bronchial stenosis, airway distortion due to cicatricial changes in parenchyma, bronchiectasis, extrinsic compression due to mediastinal lymphadenopathy or airway hyper-responsiveness.[51]

Tracheal Stenosis

Tracheal stenosis is an important cause of UAO. It may happen secondary to trauma to trachea, following prolonged intubation, i.e. PITS and after tracheostomy, i.e. post-tracheostomy tracheal stenosis (PTTS). Idiopathic stenosis is rare.

Mechanical ventilation has made a great difference in the outcome of many sick patients with respiratory failure, but the use of endotracheal tube has resulted in a group of diseases that have become more common than before. Despite the use of low pressure cuffs, which have reduced the incidence of tracheal stenosis significantly, the incidence of PITS and PTTS is high, i.e. 0.6–21%.[54-59] It is seen predominantly in females, presumably because of smaller tracheal lumen and hence, prone to injury.[54,55,60,61]

Classification

Brichet and colleagues[62] classified the PITS based on bronchoscopic appearance into three types.

1. *Web-like membranous stenosis:* A short segment (<1 cm) concentric stenosis with no cartilage damage **(Fig. 7A)**.

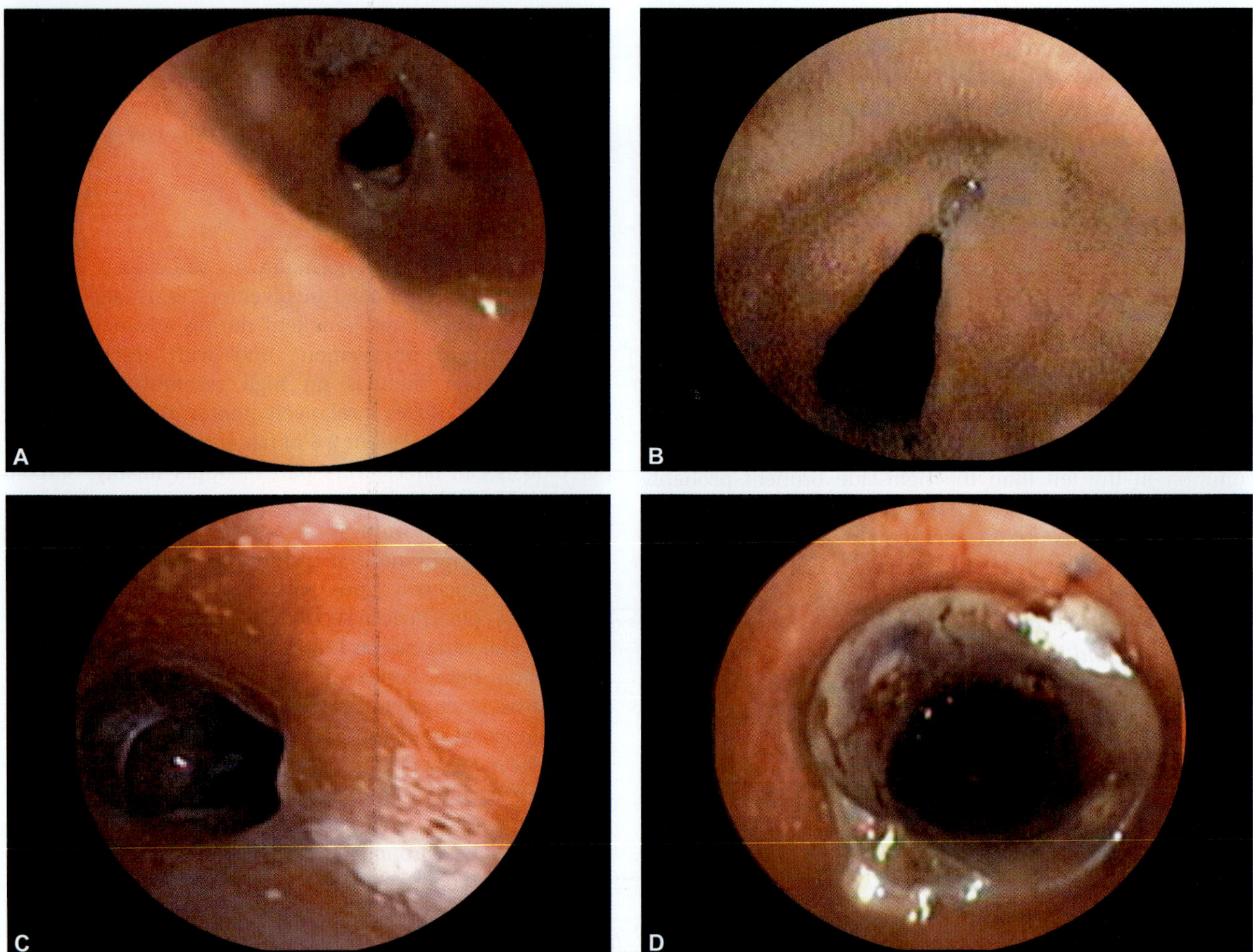

Figs 7A to D (A) A 24-year-old lady, postintubation; (B) Example of pseudoglottis stenosis. There is with membranous stenosis a remarkable resemblance to vocal cords; (C and D) Complex stenosis. A complex stenosis involving more than one cartilage, managed. These patients are typically managed by dilatation followed by silicone stenting
Courtesy: Dr Ravindra Mehta, Bengaluru

2. *Pseudoglottic stenosis:* "A" shaped stenosis secondary to lateral impacted fracture of cartilage in patients following tracheostomy. Since the stenosis resembles a vocal cord, it is called pseudoglottic stenosis **(Fig. 7B)**.
3. *Complex stenosis:* It includes all other varieties, including extensive (>1 cm), circumferential hourglass-like contraction scarring or malacia. Basically, there is cartilage damage along with the narrow lumen **(Figs 7C and D)**. The membranous and complex types are most common.

Pathogenesis

Usage of high cuff pressure in an intubated patient predisposes to mucosal ischemia, which also worsens in the presence of hypotension when the capillary pressure is lower. Pressure necrosis and chondritis result, which lead to either the development of cicatricial tissue and membranous type of stenosis or to the cartilage damage when compared to that caused by surgical tracheo and weakening causing a complex stenosis stomy.[58]

Stenosis usually develops at the site of the cuff, though the distal end of the tube, because of the repetitive *Management* injury, may also be involved. In post-tracheostomy management of tracheal stenosis depends on the type of stenosis, stoma of the tracheostomy is an additional site stenosis, presence of comorbidities, functional status of stenosis. Stenosis caused by percutaneous the patient, and the length of the stenosis. While surgical tracheostomy occurs earlier and subglottic in nature tracheal sleeve resection is a permanent solution considered the gold standard, it carries 3% mortality in trained hands. A multidisciplinary approach incorporating both surgical and bronchoscopic techniques is preferably employed.[62]

Bronchoscopic Management

Bronchoscopic management is sufficient in a majority of cases of membranous stenosis and can be very useful as either a stand-alone therapy or as a bridge to surgery in very sick patients. Bronchoscopy is used both for achieving and maintaining an effective lumen. Some of procedures to tackle membranous stenosis can be done with a flexible bronchoscope, but it is important that the bronchoscopist is trained in rigid bronchoscopy as well. Better ventilation, better control of secretions and of bleeding during the procedure and more importantly, the option of deploying silicone stents makes rigid bronchoscopy the procedure of choice.

The general recommendation by the FDA is to avoid metallic stents for such benign causes of tracheal obstruction.[63] Since the stent placement for benign lesions (PITS being the prototype) is usually temporary, it is customary to remove the stent and assess after 12–18 months of deployment to see the tracheal function effectively without the stent. Deploying metal stents is easy, can be done through flexible scope and can be done with little training, hence very popular. However, removal of stent after it is deployed is a messy affair. It cannot be removed in toto, needs trained physician with rigid bronchoscopy skills. Hence, a silicone stent is the standard choice for supporting stenosis secondary to cartilage weakness.

In membranous stenosis, stent is not required after dilatation since the cartilage is not involved, and the stability of airway is not affected. In complex stenosis, however, the underlying cartilage is damaged and collapsible. Therefore, despite achieving a good lumen by bronchoscopic means, it has to be followed by leaving a stent at the end of procedure.

Managing patients with tracheal stenosis is all about two important components: (1) to achieve an effective lumen, and (2) to maintain the lumen.

1. *Achieving effective lumen:* Many techniques are described, which are broadly classified as mechanical or thermal. Dilatation using rigid bronchoscope-barrels of increasing diameters, dilators, balloon dilatation and making nicks in the membrane using rigid scissors are some of the techniques. Laser and electrocautery can be used to cut the membranes with Mercedes Benz incisions which are mucosa sparing. They prove to be curative in about 65% cases when repeated up to three times.[64]
2. *Maintaining the lumen:* For membranous stenosis, achieving an effective lumen would suffice. However, in complex stenosis, because of cartilaginous weakness, achieving effective lumen shall usually be followed by silicone stenting.

It is important to realize the importance of being gentle with the airways since the best approach to tracheal stenosis is to prevent its occurrence. Using appropriate cuff pressures and using noninvasive ventilation when indicated are important considerations. Newer endotracheal tubes that do not have cuffs and have ability to mold to the shape of the intratracheal airways have been tested in animals and show good promise in reducing tracheal injury.[65]

Idiopathic Tracheal Stenosis

Idiopathic tracheal stenosis is a rare condition. It is seen almost exclusively in females, involves the upper trachea, predominantly, the immediate subglottic portion.[66] Many causes have been proposed, it may represent some form of fibromatosis.[66] Immunohistochemical staining for estrogen receptors is usually positive. Gastroesophageal reflux disease is seen in about a third of cases. Usual treatment consists of dilatation, tracheostomy or if feasible, resection of the involved cartilage.

Extrinsic Compression

Extrinsic compression of trachea occurs from the enlargement of structures nearby such as the malignant lymph nodes, thyroid enlargement (both benign and malignant), esophageal tumors and occasionally vascular problems. Vascular problems may more often cause TM secondary to a long-standing pressure effect than anatomical obstruction. In a patient with esophageal malignancy for whom surgery is not done due to any reason, stenting the esophagus is a popular intervention. However, in the presence of partial tracheal obstruction, stenting the esophagus may precipitate severe airway obstruction. In such a situation, trachea is stented first, followed by esophageal stenting **(Fig. 8)**.

Both benign and malignant disorders of thyroid can cause UAO. Airway obstruction is an indication for surgery in both benign and malignant thyroid problems. Mechanisms of airway obstruction include extrinsic tracheal compression (e.g. benign intrathoracic or substernal goiter), tracheal invasion by a growth, vocal cord paralysis (e.g. recurrent nerve paralysis after thyroidectomy) or a combination of the above **(Fig. 9)**.[67] In a series of 30 patients with thyroid disorders causing UAO who were also not candidates for surgery due to various reasons, there is a great utility of rigid bronchoscopy and laser application in providing both immediate and long-term benefits.

Wegener's Granulomatosis

Upper airways are commonly involved in Wegener's granulomatosis most of the times. Nasal and oral ulcerations, granulomatous inflammation, epistaxis, sinusitis and otitis are common manifestations.[68,69] Usual features are ulceration of larynx and trachea. However, a rare but a significant airway problem is subglottis stenosis. This has been reported to develop during treatment with steroid and cyclophosphamide.[70] It is typically dealt by interventional techniques like laser application[68] or dilatation.[71] Recently, intralesional long-acting corticosteroids have found to be effective.[72]

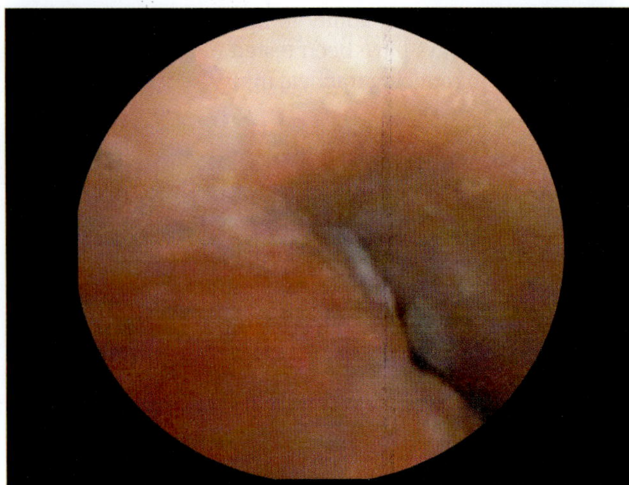

Fig. 8 A 60-year-old lady with esophageal malignancy causing near total occlusion at subglottic region

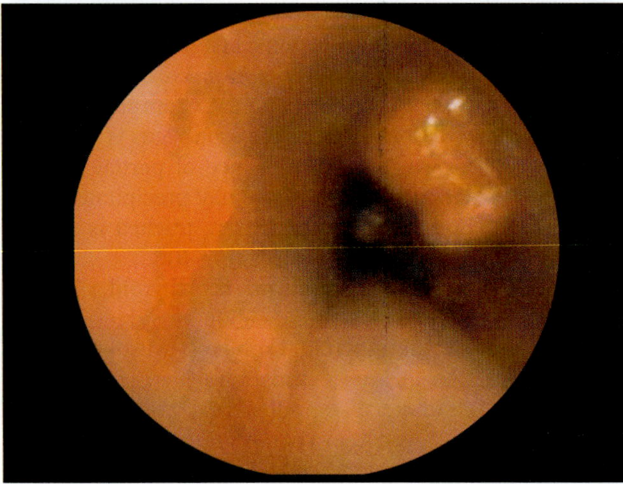

Fig. 9 Elderly lady with thyroid malignancy causing both extrinsic compression and tumor infiltration of upper trachea

Tumors

Primary tracheal tumors are very rare, seen in about 0.2 per 100,000 persons[73] of whom about 80% are malignant. Primary tracheal tumors can arise from the respiratory epithelium, salivary glands, and mesenchymal structures of the trachea.[74] Squamous and adenoid cystic carcinoma account for about two-thirds of tumors from trachea. The other malignant tumors are mucoepidermoid carcinoma, arising from the submucosal glands. Neuroendocrine neoplasms are seen more in bronchi than in trachea and include typical and atypical carcinoids, large cell neuroendocrine tumors and small cell carcinoma. The difference between the primary tracheal tumors and the bronchogenic malignancies is that the tracheal tumors have a better long-term prognosis and need more aggressive approach in providing good palliation or a cure.[75] Benign tumors of the trachea include tumors from surface epithelium like papilloma, papillomatosis, tumors from glands (like pleomorphic adenoma, mucous gland adenoma, myoepithelioma and oncocytoma) and tumors from mesenchymal structures (like fibroma, benign fibrous histiocytoma, hemangioma, paraganglioma (chemodectoma), hemangiopericytoma, glomus tumor, chondroma, lipoma and leiomyoma granular cell tumors.[74]

Endotracheal metastases are much less common than endobronchial metastasis. Endobronchial metastasis commonly arises from renal, colon, or bronchogenic malignancy, melanoma and osteosarcoma. Presentation of metastases as UAO is very rare.

Other Causes

Bilateral vocal cord palsy can happen secondary to thyroid malignancy or thyroid surgery. Others include the neurological diseases or idiopathic causes. Cases of bilateral vocal cord palsy have been reported following nasogastric tube, systemic lupus erythematosus (SLE) and esophageal surgeries.[76-78] Other rare and diverse causes of UAO have been described as anecdotal case reports.[79-85]

THERAPEUTIC CONSIDERATIONS

As is true with many other conditions in medicine, treating the primary cause of the UAO is important. However, it is also important to manage the obstruction. Obstruction can occur due to intrinsic pathology as in the case of tumors or tracheal stenosis, extrinsic compression as in compression from thyroid swelling or esophageal cancer. Functional obstruction without significant anatomic narrowing can happen secondary to TM. In cases where surgery is feasible, especially in short segment complex stenosis or tracheal tumors, it should be offered. Several other interventional approaches provide a good quality of life in most of the conditions.

In the cases of intramural pathology, achieving a patent lumen is accomplished by techniques like rigid bronchoscopy, laser, electrocautery, and argon plasma coagulation, while airway stenting is necessary for extramural compression or TM where maintaining lumen is the key issue. Silicone stents are preferred over metallic stents because the latter are difficult to remove after deployment. A recent study shows that most of the cases of UAO secondary to tracheal stenosis could be managed using flexible bronchoscopy, for balloon dilatation, laser application, stent placement and brachytherapy.[86] But rigid bronchoscopy is generally preferred because of a better control of airway, ventilation and for deployment of silicone stents.

REFERENCES

1. Rotman HH, Liss HP, Weg JG. Diagnosis of upper airway obstruction by pulmonary function testing. Chest. 1975;68(6):796-9.
2. Acres JC, Kryger MH. Clinical significance of pulmonary function tests: upper airway obstruction. Chest. 1981;80(2):207-11.
3. Al-Bazzaz F, Grillo H, Kazemi H. Response to exercise in upper airway obstruction. Am Rev Respir Dis. 1975;111(5):631-40.
4. Geffin B, Grillo HC, Cooper JD, Pontoppidan H. Stenosis following tracheostomy for respiratory care. JAMA. 1971; 216(12):1984-8.
5. Pellegrino R, Viegi G, Brusasco V, Crapo RO, Burgos F, Casaburi R, et al. Interpretative strategies for lung function tests. Eur Repir J. 2005:26(5):948-68.
6. Empey DW. Assessment of upper airways obstruction. Br Med J. 1972;3(5825):503-5.
7. Miller MR, Pincock AC, Oates GD, Wilkinson R, Skene-Smith H. Upper airway obstruction due to goiter: detection, prevalence and results of surgical management. Q J Med. 1990;74(274): 177-88.
8. Miller RD, Hyatt RE. Obstructing lesions of the larynx and trachea: clinical and physiologic characteristics. Mayo Clin Proc. 1969;44(3):145-61.
9. Boyd M, Chatterjee A, Chiles C, Chin R Jr. Tracheobronchial foreign body aspiration in adults. South Med J. 2009;102(2): 171-4.
10. Swanson KL, Edell ES. Tracheobronchial foreign bodies. Chest Surg Clin N Am. 2001;11(4):861-72.
11. Gulati SP, Kumar A, Sachdeva A, Arora S. Groundnut as the commonest foreign body of tracheobronchial tree in winter in Northern India. An analysis of fourteen cases. Indian J Med Sci. 2003;57(6):244-8.
12. Moura e Sá J, Oliveira A, Caiado A, Neves S, Barroso A, Almeida J, et al. Tracheobronchial foreign bodies in adults—experience of the Bronchology Unit of Centro Hospitalar de Vila Nova de Gaia. Rev Port Pneumol. 2006;12(1):31-43.
13. Tang LF, Xu YC, Wang YS, Wang CF, Zhu GH, Bao XE, et al. Airway foreign body removal by flexible bronchoscopy: experience with 1027 children during 2000-2008. World J Pediatr. 2009;5(3):191-5.
14. Castro M, Midthun DE, Edell ES, Stelck MJ, Prakash,UBS. Flexible bronchoscopic removal of foreign bodies from pediatric airways. J Bronchol. 1994;1(2):92-8.
15. Swanson KL, Prakash UB, Midthun DE, Edell ES, Utz JP, McDougall JC, et al. Flexible bronchoscopic management of airway foreign bodies in children. Chest. 2002;121(5):1695-700.
16. Papadopoulou-Alataki E. Upper airway considerations in hereditary angioedema. Curr Opin Allergy Clin Immunol. 2010;10(1):20-5.
17. Weis M. Clinical review of hereditary angioedema: diagnosis and management. Postgrad Med. 2009;121(6):113-20.
18. Gompels MM, Lock RJ, Abinun M, Bethune CA, Davies G, Grattan C, et al. C1 inhibitor deficiency: consensus document. Clin Exp Immunol. 2005;139(3):379-94.
19. Kreuz W, Martinez-Saguer I, Aygören-Pürsün E, Rusicke E, Heller C, Klingebiel T. C1 inhibitor concentrate for individual replacement therapy in patients with severe hereditary angioedema refractory to danazol prophylaxis. Transfusion. 2009;49(9):1987-95.
20. Craig TJ, Levy RJ, Wasserman RL, Bewtra AK, Hurewitz D, Obtułowicz K, et al. Efficacy of human C1 esterase inhibitor concentrate compared with placebo in acute hereditary angioedema attacks. J Allergy Clin Immunol. 2009;124(4): 801-8.
21. Gras J. Icatibant for hereditary angioedema. Drugs Today (Barc). 2009;45(12):855-64.
22. Duerr M, Glander P, Diekmann F, Dragun D, Neumayer HH, Budde K. Increased Incidence of angioedema with ACE Inhibitors in combination with mTOR inhibitors in kidney transplant recipients. Clin J Am Soc Nephrol. 2010;5(4):703-8.
23. Newman KB, Mason UG, Schmaling KB. Clinical features of vocal cord dysfunction. Am J Respir Crit Care Med. 1995; 152(4 Pt 1):1382-6.
24. Morris MJ, Allan PF, Perkins PJ. Vocal cord dysfunction: etiologies and treatment. Clin Pulmonary Med. 2006;13(2): 73-86.
25. Morris MJ, Deal LE, Bean DR, Grbach VX, Morgan JA. Vocal cord dysfunction in patients with exertional dyspnea. Chest. 1999;116(6):1676-82.
26. Hira HS, Singh A. Significance of upper airway influence among patients of vocal cord dysfunction for its diagnosis: Role of impulse oscillometry. Lung India. 2009;26(1):5-8.
27. Deckert J, Deckert L. Vocal cord dysfunction. Am Fam Physician. 2010;81(2):156-9.
28. Pitchenik AE. Functional laryngeal obstruction relieved by panting. Chest. 1991;100(5):1465-7.
29. Carden KA, Boiselle PM, Waltz DA, Ernst A. Tracheomalacia and tracheobronchomalacia in children and adults: an in depth review. Chest. 2005;127(3):984-1005.
30. Holinger LD. Etiology of stridor in the neonate, infant and child. Ann Otol Rhinol Laryngol. 1980;89(5 Pt 1):397-400.
31. Jacobs IN, Wetmore RF, Tom LW, Handler SD, Potsic WP. Tracheobronchomalacia in children. Arch Otolaryngol Head Neck Surg. 1994;120(2):154-8.
32. Blair GK, Cohen R, Filler RM. Treatment of tracheomalacia: eight years' experience. J Pediatr Surg. 1986;21(9):781-5.
33. van der Zee DC, Straver M. Thoracoscopic aortopexy for tracheomalacia. World J Surg. 2014;39(1):158-64.
34. Wagnetz U, Roberts HC, Chung T, Patsios D, Chapman KR, Paul NS. Dynamic airway evaluation with volume CT: initial experience. Can Assoc Radiol J. 2010;61(2)90-7.
35. Hanawa T, Ikeda S, Funatsu T, Matsubara Y, Hatakenaka R, Mitsuoka A, et al. Development of a new surgical procedure for repairing tracheobronchomalacia. J Thorac Cardiovasc Surg. 1990;100(4):587-94.
36. Michet CJ, Mckenna CH, Luthra HS, O'Fallon WM. Relapsing polychondritis survival and predictive role of early disease manifestations. Ann Intern Med. 1986;104(1):74-8.
37. McAdam LP, O'Hanlan MA, Bluestone R, Pearson CM. Relapsing polychondritis: prospective study of 23 patients and a review of the literature. Medicine (Baltimore). 1976;55(3): 193-215.
38. Ernst A, Rafeq S, Boiselle P, Sung A, Reddy C, Michaud G, et al. Relapsing polychondritis and airway involvement. Chest. 2009;135(4):1024-30.
39. Damiani JM, Levine HL. Relapsing polychondritis—report of ten cases. Laryngoscope. 1979;89(6 Pt 1):929-46.
40. Trentham DE, Le CH. Relapsing polychontritis. Ann Intern Med. 1998;129(2):114-22.
41. Mohsenifar Z, Tashleus DP, Careson SA, Bellamy PE. Pulmonary function in patients with relapsing polychondritis. Chest. 1982;81(6):711-7.

42. Lei W, Zeng DX, Chen T, Jiang JH, Wang CG, Zhu YH, et al. FDG PET-CT combined with TBNA for the diagnosis of atypical relapsing polychondritis: report of 2 cases and a literature review. J Thorac Dis. 2014;6(9):1285-92.
43. Sarodia BD, Dasgupta A, Mehta AC. Management of airway manifestations of relapsing polychondritis: case reports and review of literature. Chest. 1999;116(6):1669-75.
44. Lundgren R, Stjernberg NL. Tracheobronchopathia osteochondroplastica. A clinical bronchoscopic and spirometric study. Chest. 1981;80(6):706-9.
45. Decalmer S, Woodcock A, Greaves M, Howe M, Smith J. Airway abnormalities at flexible bronchoscopy in patients with chronic cough. Eur Respir J. 2007;30(6):1138-42.
46. Capizzi SA, Betancourt EM, Prakash UB. Tracheobronchial amyloidosis. Mayo Clin Proc. 2000;75(11):1148-52.
47. Chung HS, Lee JH, Han SK, et al. Classification of endobronchial tuberculosis by the bronchoscopic features. Tuberc Respir Dis. 1991;38:108-15.
48. Chung HS, Lee JH. Bronchoscopic assessment of the evolution of endobronchial tuberculosis. Chest. 2000;117(2):385-92.
49. Low SY, Hsu A, Eng P. Interventional bronchoscopy for tuberculous tracheobronchial stenosis. Eur Respir J. 2004;24(3):345-7.
50. Handa T, Nagai S, Fushimi Y, Miki S, Ohta K, Niimi A, et al. Clinical and radiographic indices associated with airflow limitation in patients with sarcoidosis. Chest. 2006;130(6): 1851-6.
51. Polychronopoulos VS, Prakash UB. Airway involvement in sarcoidosis. Chest. 2009;136(5):1371-80.
52. Turner GA, Lower EE, Corser BC, Gunther KL, Baughman RP. Sleep apnea in sarcoidosis. Sarcoidosis Vasc Diffuse Lung Dis. 1997;14(1):61-4.
53. Brandstetter RD, Messina MS, Sprince NL, Sprince NL, Grillo HC. Tracheal stenosis due to sarcoidosis. Chest. 1981;80(5):656.
54. Rumbak MJ, Graves AE, Scott MP, Sporn GK, Walsh FW, Anderson WM, et al. Tracheostomy tube occlusion protocol predicts significant tracheal obstruction to air flow in patients requiring prolonged mechanical ventilation. Crit Care Med. 1997;25(3):413-7.
55. Law JH, Barnhart K, Rowlett W, de la Rocha O, Lowenberg S. Increased frequency of obstructive airway abnormalities with long-term tracheostomy. Chest. 1993;104(1):136-8.
56. Pearson FG, Andrews MJ. Detection and management of tracheal stenosis following cuffed tube tracheostomy. Ann Thorac Surg. 1971;12(4):359-74.
57. Grillo HC, Donahue DM, Mathisen DJ, Wain JC, Wright CD. Postintubation tracheal stenosis. Treatment and results. J Thorac Cardiovasc Surg. 1995;109(3):486-92.
58. Raghuraman G, Rajan S, Marzouk JK, Mullhi D, Smith FG. Is tracheal stenosis caused by percutaneous tracheostomy different from that by surgical tracheostomy? Chest. 2005;127(3):879-85.
59. Stauffer JL, Olson DE, Petty TL. Complications and consequences of endotracheal intubation and tracheostomy. A prospective study of 150 critically ill adult patients. Am J Med. 1981;70(1):65-76.
60. Ferris MC, Rumbak MJ. Life-threatening tracheal obstruction due to tracheomalacia and granulation tissue in a long-term acute-care ventilator patient. J Bronchol. 1994; 1:223-5.
61. Rumbak MJ, Walsh FW, Anderson WM, Rolfe MW, Solomon DA. Significant tracheal obstruction causing failure to wean in patients requiring prolonged mechanical ventilation: a forgotten complication of long-term mechanical ventilation. Chest. 1999;115(4):1092-5.
62. Brichet A, Verkindre C, Dupont J, Carlier ML, Darras J, Wurtz A, et al. Multidisciplinary approach to management of post-intubation tracheal stenoses. Eur Respir J. 1999;13(4):888-93.
63. FDA (Food and Drug Association). (2005). Recommendations to avoid metallic stents in benign stenosis. [online] Available from *http://www.fda.gov/cdrh/safety/072905-tracheal.html*. [Accessed June 2016].
64. Mehta AC, Lee FY, Cordasco EM, Kirby T, Eliachar I, De Boer G. Concentric tracheal and subglottic stenosis. Management using the Nd-YAG laser for mucosal sparing followed by gentle dilatation. Chest. 1993;104(3):673-7.
65. Gordin A, Chadha NK, Campisi P, Luginbuehl I, Taylor G, Forte V. Effect of a novel anatomically shaped endotracheal tube on intubation-related injury. Arch Otolaryngol Head Neck Surg. 2010;136(1):54-9.
66. Mark EJ, Meng F, Kradin RL, Mathisen DJ, Matsubara O. Idiopathic tracheal stenosis: a clinicopathologic study of 63 cases and comparison of the pathology with chondromalacia. Am J Surg Pathol. 2008;32(8):1138-43.
67. Noppen M, Poppe K, D'Haese J, Meysman M, Velkeniers B, Vincken W. Interventional bronchoscopy for treatment of tracheal obstruction secondary to benign or malignant thyroid disease. Chest. 2004;125(2):723-30.
68. Fauci AS, Haynes BF, Katz P, Wolff SM. Wegener's granulomatosis: prospective clinical and therapeuticexperience with 85 patients for 21 years. Ann Intern Med. 1983;98(1):76-85.
69. Fahey JL, Leonard E, Churg J, Godman G. Wegener's granulomatosis. Am J Med. 1954;17(2):168-79.
70. Strange C, Halstead L, Baumann M, Sahn SA. Subglottic stenosis in Wegener's granulomatosis: development during cyclophosphamide treatment with response to carbon dioxide laser therapy. Thorax. 1990;45(4):300-1.
71. Schokkenbroek AA, Franssen CF, Dikkers FG. Dilatation tracheoscopy for laryngeal and tracheal stenosis in patients with Wegener's granulomatosis. Eur Arch Otorhinolaryngol. 2008;265(5):549-55.
72. Solans-Laqué R, Bosch-Gil J, Canela M, Lorente J, Pallisa E, Vilardell-Tarrés M. Clinical features and therapeutic management of subglottic stenosis in patients with Wegener's granulomatosis. Lupus. 2008;17(9):832-6.
73. Pearson FG, Cardoso P, Keshavjee S. Primary tumours of the upper airway. In: Pearson FG (Ed). Thoracic Surgery, 1st edition. New York: Churchill Livingstone; 1995. pp. 285-99.
74. Macchiarini P. Primary tracheal tumours. Lancet Oncol. 2006;7(1):83-91.
75. Maziak DE, Todd TR, Keshavjee SH, et al. Adenoid cystic carcinoma of the airway: thirty-two-year experience. J Thorac Cardiovasc Surg. 1996; 112(6):1522-31.
76. Brousseau VJ, Kost KM. A rare but serious entity: nasogastric tube syndrome. Otolaryngol Head Neck Surg. 2006; 135(5): 677-9.
77. Jayachandran NV, Agrawal S, Rajasekhar L, et al. Bilateral vocal cord palsy as a manifestation of systemic lupus erythematosus. Lupus. 2010; 19(1):109-10.
78. Hamer PW, Thompson SK, Rees GL, et al. Bilateral recurrent laryngeal nerve palsy after Ivor Lewis oesophagectomy. ANZ J Surg. 2009; 79(12):959-60.

79. Lippmann M, Solit R, Goldberg SK, Najjar D. Mediastinal bronchogenic cyst. A cause of upper airway obstruction. Chest. 1992;102(6):1901-3.
80. Schwartz JR, Nagle MG, Elkins RC, Mohr JA. Mucormycosis of the trachea: an unusual cause of acute upper airway obstruction. Chest. 1982;81(5):653-4.
81. Karim A, Ahmed S, Siddiqui R, Marder GS, Mattana J. Severe upper airway obstruction from cricoarytenoiditis as the sole presenting manifestation of a systemic lupus erythematosus flare. Chest. 2002;121(3):990-3.
82. Alday LE, Vega PJ, Heller A. Congenital ankylosis of the temporomandibular joint: resultant upper airway obstruction and corpulmonale. Chest. 1979;75(3):384-6.
83. Demuynck K, Van Calenbergh F, Goffin J, Verschakelen J, Demedts M, Van de Woestijne K. Upper airway obstruction caused by a cervical osteophyte. Chest. 1995;108(1):283-4.
84. Theaker NJ, Brady PW, Fisher MM. Postesophagectomy mediastinal chylothorax causing upperairway obstruction misdiagnosed as asthma: a report of two cases. Chest. 1997;111(4):1126-8.
85. Almarri M. A case of intratracheal schwannoma presenting to the emergency department with a diagnosis of asthmatic attack: a clue to suspect the cause of upper airway obstruction to be other than asthma. J Emerg Med. 2010;38(2):245-6.
86. Rahman NA, Fruchter O, Shitrit D, Fox BD, Kramer MR. Flexible bronchoscopic management of benign tracheal stenosis: long term follow-up of 115 patients. J Cardiothorac Surg. 2010;5(1):2.

Section 10

Interstitial Lung Diseases

Aditya Jindal, Sahajal Dhooria

An Introduction to Interstitial Lung Diseases

Venkata Nagarjuna Maturu, Dheeraj Gupta

INTRODUCTION

Diffuse interstitial lung disease (ILD) encompasses a group of disorders of diverse etiologies with common feature of generalized involvement of lung interstitium. ILD encompasses a heterogeneous group of diseases, includes over 200 different diseases, which, in spite of their heterogeneous nature have several common clinical, radiological and histological manifestations. The presenting symptoms such as dry cough and dyspnea, are nonspecific, the diagnosis is often delayed unless the examining physician has a high level of suspicion. Diagnosis comes from a thoughtful history/physical examination, specific laboratory tests and X-rays. The etiology may be further clarified by lung biopsy; however, it is not essential in all patients. Depending on the etiology, therapy may include immunosuppression, trigger avoidance or observation alone. The prognosis is closely tied to the etiology. Overall, early diagnosis is critical for best patient outcomes and is dependent on physician awareness of this often deadly disease.

ETIOLOGY AND CLASSIFICATION

The classification of ILD is confusing and evolving. Several terminologies and classifications have been used to describe the same clinicopathological disease. ILD is broadly grouped as (a) primary, when the cause is unknown, and (b) secondary when there is an identifiable disease responsible for the interstitial involvement **(Table 1)**.

Primary ILD

Primary interstitial lung disease (ILD) is idiopathic in origin. No secondary cause or association is identifiable. The latest ATS/ERS update (2013) classified idiopathic interstitial pneumonias (IIP) based on clinicoradiological, pathological features, the incidence and natural course of the disease.[1] They classified IIPs into major IIPs, rare IIPs and unclassifiable IIPs (those in which the diagnosis remained inconclusive even after a multidisciplinary meet). The major IIPs include

Table 1 Important causes of interstitial lung diseases

I. *Primary or idiopathic interstitial pneumonias*
• Major idiopathic interstitial pneumonias
– Idiopathic pulmonary fibrosis
– Idiopathic nonspecific interstitial pneumonia
– Respiratory bronchiolitis–interstitial lung disease
– Desquamative interstitial pneumonia
– Cryptogenic organizing pneumonia
– Acute interstitial pneumonia
• Rare idiopathic interstitial pneumonias
– Idiopathic lymphoid interstitial pneumonia
– Idiopathic pleuroparenchymal fibroelastosis
• Unclassifiable idiopathic interstitial pneumonias
II. *Secondary*
A. Known causes
1. *Infections*
• Tuberculosis (Miliary)
• Bacterial (Atypical pneumonias)
• Fungal
• Parasitic
• Viral
2. *Noninfectious causes*
• Hypersensitivity pneumonitis
• Pneumoconioses
• Drug-induced
• Radiation-induced
• Malignancies
• Systemic vasculitides
B. Association with diseases of unknown etiology
1. *Sarcoidosis*
2. *Connective tissue disorders*
• Systemic sclerosis
• Rheumatoid arthritis
• Polymyositis, dermatomyositis
• Systemic lupus erythematosus
• Sjögren syndrome
3. *Chronic eosinophilic pneumonia*
4. *Miscellaneous*
• Histiocytosis
• Eosinophilic granuloma
• Lymphangioleiomyomatosis
• Tuberous sclerosis

chronic fibrosing IIPs [idiopathic pulmonary fibrosis (IPF) and idiopathic nonspecific interstitial pneumonia (NSIP)], acute/subacute IIPs [acute interstitial pneumonia (AIP) and cryptogenic organizing pneumonia (COP)] and smoking-related IIPs [desquamative interstitial pneumonia (DIP) and respiratory bronchiolitis-related ILD (RB-ILD)]. Lymphocytic interstitial pneumonia (LIP) is usually secondary to infections/autoimmune diseases and hence idiopathic LIP has been classified as a rare IIP. An ILD is considered to be idiopathic only after a carefully history and focused investigations have ruled out secondary causes of the same.

Secondary ILDs

Most forms of secondary ILDs have either a known etiological cause or an association with another disease of known (or unknown) etiology **(Table 1)**. An ILD secondary to another illness factually represents the pulmonary involvement of the primary disease than a separate entity. There are more than 200 conditions/exposures known to be associated with ILD. American Thoracic Society (ATS) and the European Respiratory Society (ERS) international consensus statement on ILD categorized ILDs into three broad groups:[2] (1) Diffuse parenchymal lung disease (DPLD) with known cause [e.g. connective tissue disease (CTD), hypersensitivity pneumonia, toxins, infections, inherited, malignancy, pneumoconiosis]; (2) Granulomatous DPLD (e.g. sarcoidosis) and (3) Other DPLDS [e.g. lymphangioleiomyomatosis (LAM), histiocytosis, eosinophilic lung diseases, etc.]. Even in cases of ILD with a defined etiology, the mechanisms of lung injury and fibrosis are largely undefined.

It is important to understand that the clinicoradiologic and pathologic features of primary and secondary ILDs may be similar **(Tables 2 and 3)**. It is only the identification of an antecedent cause, which shall differentiate secondary from primary ILDs. For example, NSIP pattern can occur secondary to drugs, and several CTDs. When no cause is identified, it is labeled as idiopathic NSIP. Similarly, the usual interstitial pneumonia (UIP) pattern can either be idiopathic

Table 2 Patterns of interstitial lung disease and their causes

S. no.	*Histologic/ Radiologic pattern*	*Idiopathic interstitial pneumonia*	*Secondary ILDs*
1	Usual interstitial pneumonia (UIP)	Idiopathic pulmonary fibrosis (IPF)	• Chronic hypersensitivity pneumonitis • Asbestosis • CTD (RA, PSS) • Drugs (Amiodarone)
2	Nonspecific interstitial pneumonia (NSIP)	Idiopathic NSIP	• CTD • HIV • Drugs • Hypersensitivity pneumonias
3	Organizing pneumonia	Cryptogenic organizing pneumonia (COP)	• Postinfectious • CTD (RA, PM, DM) • Drugs (Methotrexate) • Inhalational toxicity • Postobstruction
4	Diffuse alveolar damage (DAD)	Acute interstitial pneumonia (AIP)	• Infections • Trauma • CTD (SLE, PM, DM) • TRALI • Drugs • Inhalational agents
5	Desquamative interstitial pneumonia (DIP)	Idiopathic DIP	• CTD (RA) • Infections (HCV) • Drugs (Sirolimus)
6	Respiratory bronchiolitis ILD	RB-ILD	None
7	Lymphocytic interstitial pneumonia (LIP)	Idiopathic LIP	• HIV • Immunodeficiency disorders (SCID, CVID) • CTD (Sjögrens, RA) • Autoimmune diseases • Drugs

Abbreviations: CTD, connective tissue disease; CVID, common variable immunodeficiency; DM, dermatomyositis; HCV, hepatitis C virus; HIV, human immunodeficiency virus; RA, rheumatoid arthritis; PM, polymyositis; PSS, progressive systemic sclerosis; SCID, severe combined immunodeficiency; SLE, systematic lupus erythematosis; TRALI, transfusion-related acute lung injury.

Table 3 Radiologic and pathologic characteristics of the patterns of interstitial lung disease

ILD pattern	*High resolution CT features*	*Histopathology features*
Usual interstitial pneumonia (UIP)	• Subpleural basal predominance • Intralobular septal thickening • Honeycombing • Absence of mosaic, ground glass opacities, pleural abnormalities, nodules and cysts.	• Temporal and spatial heterogeneity • Fibroblastic foci • Marked fibrosis/honeycombing in a subpleural distribution • Absence of hyaline membranes, inflammatory infiltrate, organizing pneumonia and airway centered changes
Nonspecific interstitial pneumonia (NSIP)	• Bilateral symmetrical changes • Ground glass opacities • Inter- and intralobular septal thickening ± traction bronchiectasis • Subpleural sparing (only in 30%) • Lack of an apicobasal gradient and predominant honeycombing	• Uniform involvement of the interstitium • Spectrum of findings from a predominantly inflammatory infiltrate (Cellular NSIP) to a predominantly fibrotic process (Fibrotic NSIP)
Organizing pneumonia (OP)	• Patchy and often migratory airspace consolidation in subpleural or peribronchial distribution • Reversed halo sign (Atoll sign)	• Intraluminal organizing fibrosis in distal airspaces (bronchioles, alveolar ducts and alveoli)—Massons bodies • Preservation of lung architecture
Diffuse alveolar damage (DAD)	• Bilateral diffuse ground glass opacities, more in the bases	• Presence of edema, hyaline membranes and acute interstitial inflammatory infiltrate
Desquamative interstitial pneumonia (DIP)	• Bilateral ground glass opacities • Diffuse or patchy distribution	• Diffuse intra-alveolar macrophage accumulation
Respiratory bronchiolitis ILD	• Centrilobular nodules and patchy ground glass opacities • Predominant upper lobe distribution	• Bronchiolocentric distribution • Intra-alveolar pigmented macrophage accumulation
Lymphocytic interstitial pneumonia (LIP)	• Presence of cysts, nodules, ground glass opacities and septal thickening in varying proportions	• Diffuse interstitial polyclonal lymphocytic infiltration • Lymphoid follicles may be present

or secondary to CTDs like rheumatoid arthritis (RA) or chronic hypersensitivity pneumonitis. When idiopathic, it is called as IPF.

Connective Tissue Diseases

The most important association of ILD is with different connective tissue diseases (CTDs). Pulmonary fibrosis is most prevalent in systemic sclerosis (SSc)—SSc-PF, forming part of the American Rheumatism Association minor diagnostic criteria for SSc.[3] Clinically, significant pulmonary fibrosis occurs in approximately 30% of patients with systemic sclerosis and polymyositis/dermatomyositis (PM/DM), 10% with Sjögren's syndrome (SS), and in less than 5% with systemic lupus erythematosus (SLE) or rheumatoid arthritis (RA).[4] Studies of lung function and high resolution CT scan (HRCT) suggest a much higher prevalence of subclinical disease in all of these disorders.[5-8] Ankylosing spondylitis (AS) is frequently associated with limited nonspecific HRCT abnormalities, but clinically significant upper zone fibrobullous disease is relatively uncommon.[9] The most common pattern seen with CTDs is the NSIP pattern. Virtually any pattern including the UIP pattern (commoner in RA/SSc), organizing pneumonia pattern (RA/PM/DM), AIP pattern (SLE/PM/DM) and the LIP pattern (Sjögren) may be seen secondary to CTDs.

Occupational and Environmental Exposures

Occupational exposure to different inorganic and metal dusts is another important cause. Silica dust causes progressive fibrosis (Silicosis). Massive progressive fibrosis can occur in a much shorter period of a few weeks to a few months in case of a heavy exposure. Asbestosis and anthracosis are also associated with pulmonary fibrosis. Inhalation of toxic gases and fumes, such as methyl isocyanate and nitrogen dioxide can cause interstitial involvement. In view of a shorter exposure, it is generally self-limiting, but chronic pulmonary involvement from inhalational exposure is also possible.

Drugs

Several drugs are known to cause ILD. Pneumotox® *(www.pneumotox.com)* provides free and updated information on drug-induced respiratory disease. Drugs and drug classes, which more often cause ILD, include amiodarone, cancer chemotherapy agents [bleomycin, busulfan, chlorambucil, cyclophosphamide, gemcitabine, imatinib, methotrexate, mitomycin C, nitrosoureas (BCNU, CCNU and newer nitrosoureas), rituximab, trastuzumab and taxanes], disease-modifying antirheumatic drugs (methotrexate, anti-TNF-alpha antibody therapy), interferon, minocycline, nitrofurantoin, nonsteroidal anti-inflammatory drugs (NSAIDs) and rapamycin.[10] Drugs given by almost any route of administration [oral, parenteral, inhaled, topical (ophthalmic, dermal, intranasal), intrathecal, intracavitary and intra-arterial] can cause ILD, but the vast majority of cases result from oral or parenteral administration. The incidence rate of drug-induced ILD varies with different drug in different studies from 1/100,000 and 1/5,000 treatment courses for nitrofurantoin to 1–5% of patients exposed to regular doses of long-term amiodarone, 17–36% of patients treated with rapamycin and congeners[11] and more than 30% in patients exposed to high-dose amiodarone (>1,200 mg/day).[12]

Radiation

Radiation administered for thoracic malignancies, especially when used in a higher dose, is another iatrogenic cause of ILD.[13] Radiation can induce both pulmonary and mediastinal fibrosis. Radiation lung injury can manifest during or weeks to years after radiation therapy for lung cancer, breast carcinoma, Hodgkin's and non-Hodgkin's lymphomas, or following total body irradiation in recipients of bone marrow or stem cell transplant. Radiation-induced changes may involve the pleura, heart, pulmonary veins, mediastinum, lymphatic vessels and nerves in addition to the lung, creating manifold possibilities and patterns of involvement.

Hypersensitivity Pneumonias

Hypersensitivity pneumonias (extrinsic allergic alveolitis) of acute, subacute or chronic onset, which occur on exposure to known environmental or occupational antigens, include farmer's lung, byssinosis, air-conditioner's lung, bird-fancier's disease and mushroom picker's disease. They may also occur in individuals working with different chemicals, drugs, pharmaceutical agents and laboratory animals. This is especially so in the industrial workers engaged in the manufacturing/processing of rubber foam, azo-dyes, tetracyclines, ampicillin, antihypertensive drugs and others.[14]

EPIDEMIOLOGY

Although the exact incidence and prevalence of ILD are not known, patients with this disease comprise about 15% of a pulmonary physician's practice.[15,16] Mortality from cryptogenic fibrosing alveolitis continues to increase in many countries.[17] In India, this was earlier considered to be a rare disease until 1979, when Jindal, et al. published their data on 61 cases of DPLD seen over a period of 5 years.[18] The scenario is different now and the disease is no longer rare or uncommon. Recently the same center published data on 76 patients with IPF diagnosed over a 16-month period showing a definite increase in the frequency of diagnosis.[19] A number of other publications from India have described various aspects of the disease.[20-32] The increase in the number of studies from India may be a true reflection of the increase in incidence or may be apparent because of increased awareness or due to better availability of diagnostic facilities (like high-resolution CT and fiberoptic bronchoscopy).

Globally also, the incidence and prevalence of ILD are unclear. IPF is the most common and best studied ILD. The prevalence of this disease was studied in Bernalillo County, New Mexico, estimated to be 13.2–20.2 per 100,000, with an annual incidence of 7.4–10.7 per 100,000 cases/year.[16] Since IPF accounts for 60% of the ILD cases, one can anticipate the true incidence of ILD in the general population as much greater.[16] Furthermore, the prevalence of IPF in individuals older than 75 years of age has been estimated to be as high as 175 per 100,000.[16] Given that two-thirds of patients with IPF are over 60 years of age at diagnosis and the population is ageing globally, ILDs are likely to be encountered with increasing frequency.[33] In a recent population-based study from Olmsted County, Minnesota, from 1997 to 2005, the age- and sex-adjusted incidence was 8.8/100,000 and 17.4/100,000 person-years, using narrow or broad criteria, respectively. The age-adjusted incidence was higher in men than in women, and among patients aged 70–79 years, had shown a significant decline during the study period.[34]

PATHOLOGY

As is implied in the name, the primary site of pathology lies in the pulmonary interstitium. The diverse etiologies cause pulmonary inflammation and/or fibrosis as the final common pathways to lung damage. Hence, the ILDs are often referred to collectively as "pulmonary fibrosis." The normal pulmonary interstitium comprises of the anatomical space between the alveolar and the capillary basement membranes. In a normal lung, this space is occupied by a single cell layer, only 10 microns in width, allowing passive diffusion of oxygen between the alveolus and blood in the capillaries. It also contains mesenchymal and connective tissue cells and extracellular matrix composed of collagen, elastin and proteoglycans. Characteristically, there is cellular infiltration and thickening of pulmonary interstitium and of alveolar walls, as well as the presence of mononuclear cells in the alveolar lumen. The cellular exudate comprises primarily of alveolar macrophages, but lymphocytes, neutrophils, eosinophils and plasma cells are also present. Although the total collagen component of lungs remains normal, the ratio of type I to type III collagen is increased. The interstitial involvement progressively encroaches the alveolar spaces, the terminal bronchioles and also the overlying pleura. It is for this reason that the ILDs are also referred to as DPLDs. The advanced-stage disease is characterized by extensive fibrosis, obliteration of the lumen of alveoli and formation of multiple cysts, also called as the honeycomb lung. The ILDs are distinguished from diseases predominantly affecting the airways and blood vessels.

PATHOGENESIS

There is no clear understanding of disease-pathogenesis. Chronic inflammation, recurrent epithelial injury and impaired wound repair are some of the possible reasons of pulmonary fibrosis.[35] Several new mechanisms of pulmonary fibrosis have evolved in the last decade. Pulmonary fibrosis is considered to result from an aberrant defense reaction with failure of mechanisms, which are normally responsible for repair. It is now recognized that there is persistent and/or repetitive injury responsible for inflammation followed by recruitment of a host of inflammatory cells.[36]

An interesting perspective has been recently proposed that ILD (IPF) should be considered as a neoproliferative disorder of the lung. Genetic alterations, response to growth and inhibitory signals, resistance to apoptosis, myofibroblast origin and behavior, altered cellular communications, and intracellular signaling pathways are all fundamental pathogenic hallmarks of both IPF and cancer and IPF is associated with a poor prognosis, like the cancers.[37]

Several pathobiological processes have been identified or proposed, some of which have been outlined below **(Fig. 1)**.

Inflammatory Hypothesis

Inflammation as the central mechanism causing IPF was largely derived from the observation that bronchoalveolar lavage (BAL) fluid from patients with IPF had increased numbers of inflammatory cells (mostly neutrophils and eosinophils) relative to normal individuals. Therapies were therefore directed at abrogating inflammation with corticosteroids. However, lack of response to corticosteroids leads to the belief that inflammation may be a result, rather than a cause of fibrosis. This was supported by studies showing increased levels of inflammatory mediators such as CXC chemokine IL-8/CXCL8, a potent chemotactic cytokine for neutrophils in lung tissue.[38]

Vascular Hypothesis

Increased angiogenesis has been suggested to play an important role in the progression of pulmonary fibrosis in both animal models and clinical specimens.[39,40] This increased angiogenic activity has been attributed to an imbalance of proangiogenic chemokines (IL-8, ENA-78) and anti-angiogenic CXC chemokines (IP-10/CXCL10).[41,42] In contrast, recent reports have shown decreased expression of VEGF and endothelial cell proliferation in IPF.[41,43] It is likely that angiogenesis may be enhanced in the earlier stages of the development of UIP, while there is a loss of blood vessels in the more advanced stages. Pulmonary hypertension is becoming recognized as an important clinical component of progressive IPF in some patients.[22,44]

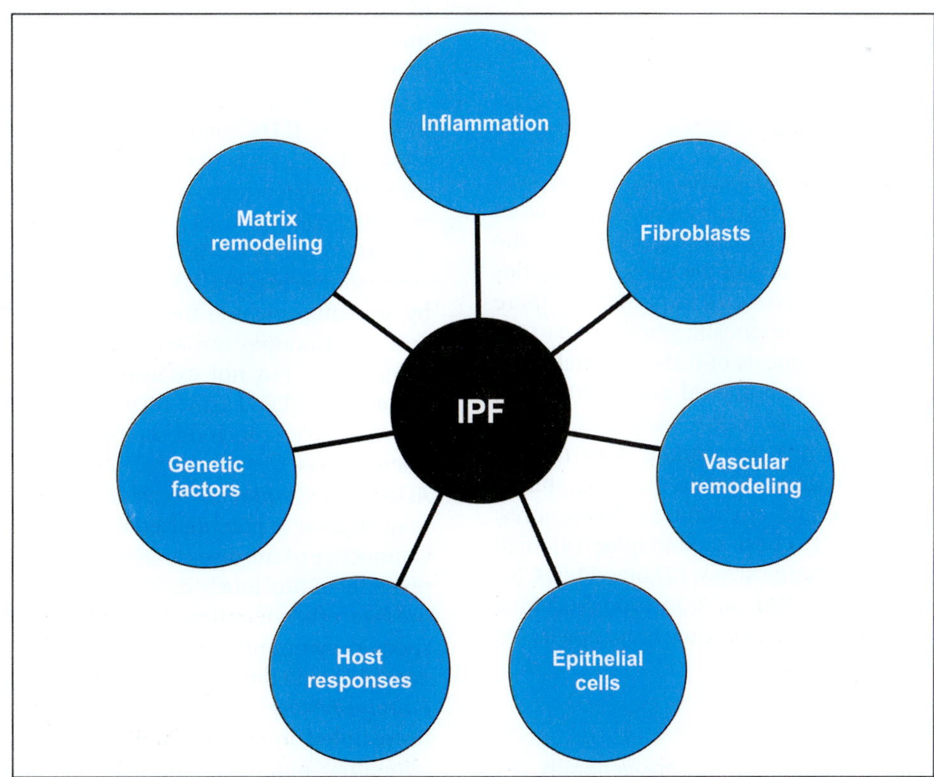

Fig. 1 Proposed mechanisms for development of pulmonary fibrosis

Alveolar Epithelial Cells

Abnormalities in alveolar type II cell injury and repair may be a critical feature in the pathogenesis of pulmonary fibrosis. Ultrastructural studies have demonstrated alveolar type II cell injury and apoptosis in lung biopsies from IPF patients. Studies have demonstrated increased expression of proapoptotic proteins in alveolar epithelial cells and in BAL from IPF patients. More recent data have suggested that there is increased oxidative stress in alveolar epithelium in IPF patients.[45-50]

Matrix Remodeling

There is an imbalance between the production and degrada tion of extracellular matrix, which leads to excessive production of extracellular matrix molecules including collagens, tenascin, and proteoglycans and glycosamino-glycans.[51] TGF-β promotes matrix production and inhibits inhibitors of matrix degradation (TIMPs), and thus could be a key mediator in this process.[52,53]

Fibroblast Activation and Dysfunction

A variety of growth factors that influence fibroblast and myofibroblast functions have been shown to be produced in the lung tissue of IPF patients. These include Th2 cytokines (IL-4, IL-5 and IL-13), growth factors such as TGF-β, IGF-1,[54] PDGF A or B and CTGF.[55] Also, the fibroblasts in IPF may have unique phenotype that can have different growth rates.[56,57] Recent studies suggest that myofibroblasts may also have an important role in mediating lung fibrosis.[47,58,59]

DIAGNOSTIC APPROACH

Diagnosis of ILD is generally suspected on history and clinical examination. A comprehensive evaluation is required to narrow down the possible predisposing factors in the secondary ILD or to assign it to one of the known categories of idiopathic varieties. This exercise is important as there are important treatment and prognostic implications to a proper diagnosis. The final diagnosis of ILDs essentially rest on the evaluation of *c*linical, *r*adiological and *p*athological data in unison, referred to as *C-R-P diagnosis*. While approaching a patient with ILD the various steps needed include: (1) a methodical history to include demographics, family history, occupational and environmental exposures; (2) physical examination; (3) chest radiographs; (4) high resolution computed tomographic scans; (5) blood tests; (6) fiberoptic bronchoscopy with BAL or transbronchial lung biopsies (selected patients); (7) surgical lung biopsy (selected patients).

Clinical History

The clinical signs and symptoms of ILD are generally not specific to a diagnosis of ILD. Individuals present with progressive dyspnea on exertion and dry cough. Symptoms are usually progressive. This combination of dry cough and dyspnea can also be due to various other diseases including cardiac failure, airway diseases (bronchiolitis, asthma), mediastinal pathologies, pleural diseases and pulmonary vascular causes. Careful history and examination can often exclude these differentials and help in coming to a clinical diagnosis of an ILD. The initial symptoms may be attributed to cardiac disease, deconditioning or advancing age, thus delaying the ultimate diagnosis and treatment.[27] The various factors in history, which need to be taken into consideration while framing a differential diagnosis, include:

a. *Age at diagnosis*: Most ILDs, including IPF present in the fifth to seventh decade of life. Earlier presentation is common with familial ILDs, CTD, occupation and exposure-related ILDs (pneumoconiosis, hypersensitivity pneumonias). Similarly, sarcoidosis most often occurs in the third to fifth decade of the life.
b. *Progression of the disease*: A thoughtful assessment of the course and progression of the illness (weeks, months, years) provides some suggestions regarding etiology. Gradual progression over months to years suggests chronic fibrosing ILDs like IPF and NSIP. If the disease is indolent to run over decades, it is unlikely to be IPF; the median survival of IPF is only 3–5 years.[60] A more acute/subacute presentation is suggestive of COP or AIP. An acute exacerbation of an underlying ILD also may be the initial presentation of an underlying chronic ILD. Other causes of an acute presentation include acute hypersensitivity pneumonias, acute eosinophilic pneumonia and CTD-related ILDs.
c. *Sex of the patient*: Most ILDs are common in men compared to women. ILDs, which occur only in women, include LAM, others which, occur more commonly in women, are the CTD-related ILDs.
d. *Smoking status*: ILDs, which are causally related to smoking, include RB-ILD, DIP and pulmonary Langerhans cell histiocytosis (PLCH). The ILDs, which are precipitated by smoking, include the acute eosinophilic pneumonia and the Goodpasture syndrome. ILDs which are more common in but not exclusively limited to smokers are IPF and RA-ILD. Lastly, ILDs, which are less common in active smokers, include sarcoidosis and hypersensitivity pneumonias.[61]
e. *Associated symptoms*: Occasionally, additional symptoms, may suggest a potential etiology for the ILD **(Table 4)**. Connective tissue disease-associated ILD (CTD-ILD) often presents in previously diagnosed CTD, although ILD may predate other manifestations of CTD. In these patients, specific symptoms related to various CTDs provide a critical clue to the etiology of lung disease.
f. *Family history*: An increased incidence of ILD has been noted in certain families. These cases of "familial idiopathic pulmonary fibrosis" are thought to account for less than 3% of all cases and may be associated with a

defect in surfactant protein C.[62] Careful history of drug and tobacco use is also important.[63,64]

g. *Occupational history*: A detailed occupational history is an essential component in the assessment of patients with ILD. It is important to enquire not only the current occupation but also the past occupations as many a times the onset of symptoms may occur with a lag period.
h. *History of drug intake*: An often forgotten part of history is the past/ongoing exposure to drugs. A careful history may identify the culprit drug. All medications, which the patient is currently taking or has taken in the recent past have to be identified and screened for their potential to cause ILD.

Physical Examination

Physical examination is helpful to suggest interstitial involvement, but rarely does it lead to a specific diagnosis **(Table 4)**. The bibasal dry, end-inspiratory "velcro" crackles are quite characteristically heard in most patients of IPF. These crackles are attributed to the opening up of collapsed alveoli when equalization of pressure occurs between the alveolar spaces and the proximal bronchiole during inspiration.[2,65] Finger-clubbing is present in about one-third of patients. Hypertrophic osteoarthropathy is rarely seen. Physical examination of chest may reveal tachypnea, reduced chest expansion and intercostal retractions. Breath sounds are vesicular and quite distinct. Bronchovesicular or bronchial breathing is heard in the presence of a consolidation, a cavity or an advanced disease. Cyanosis is generally absent at rest but desaturation occurs and cyanosis appears after even mild exercise. Cyanosis may be present even at rest in an advanced disease. Similarly, pulmonary hypertension and chronic cor pulmonale, and chronic congestive failure develop in a long-standing disease.[66,67]

Patients with secondary ILD may also have signs of the underlying disease. Patients with CREST syndrome (calcinosis, Raynaud's phenomenon, esophageal dysfunction, sclerodactyly and telangiectasia) or mixed connective tissue disease (MCTD) may present with pulmonary hypertension as the primary manifestation.

Chest Radiography

A diffusely abnormal chest radiograph often is the first leading clue to a diagnosis of ILD; however, a normal chest X-ray does not exclude ILD.[2] The interstitial infiltrates are seen as discrete linear, nodular or reticulonodular shadows diffusely distributed in both the lungs. The individual nodular shadows are usually of less than 2 mm in diameter. They may also

Table 4 Clinical clues to specific diagnosis of interstitial lung disease

Clinical clue	*Diagnostic possibilities*
A. History	
• Age	
60 years	IPF
Younger (20–40 years)	CTD
• Gender	LAM exclusively in women
• Acute onset, fever	Infections, AIP, CTD (acute lupus), AEP, COP, HP, drugs
• History of smoking	RB-ILD, DIP, UIP, PLCH, Goodpasture syndrome, less in HP
• Specific exposures	Occupational ILD, pneumoconioses, HP
• Hemoptysis	Alveolar hemorrhage syndromes, LAM,
• Arthralgia	IPF, CTD (arthritis with morning stiffness)
• Skin rash, dysphagia, Raynaud's, skin tightness, dryness	CTD
B. Physical examination	
• Typical 'velcro' crepts	IPF, crepts frequently absent in sarcoidosis
• Inspiratory squeaks	COP
• Clubbing	IPF, DIP, IBD
• Skin involvement	Sarcoidosis, CTD, vasculitis, tuberous sclerosis
• Arthritis	CTD, sarcoidosis
• Eye changes (uveitis, conjunctivitis)	Sarcoidosis, CTD
• Muscle weakness	Polymyositis, dermatomyositis
• Neuropathy	Sarcoidosis, CTD
• Lymphadenopathy	Sarcoidosis, CTD

Source: Adapted from Raghu G, Brown KK. Interstitial lung disease: clinical evaluation and keys to an accurate diagnosis. Clin Chest Med. 2004;25:409-19, v.

Abbreviations: IPF, idiopathic pulmonary fibrosis; CTD, connective tissue diseases; LAM, lymphangioleiomyomatosis; AIP, acute interstitial pneumonia; AEP, acute eosinophilic pneumonia; COP, cryptogenic organizing pneumonia; HP, hypersensitivity pneumonitis; RB-ILD, respiratory bronchiolitis-associated ILD; DIP, desquamative interstitial pneumonia; UIP, usual interstitial pneumonia; PLCH, pulmonary Langerhans cell histiocytosis; IBD, inflammatory bowel disease.

coalesce and form larger nodules. The shadows are generally bibasilar in distribution in early stages. In later stages, diffuse involvement occurs all over the lungs. Upper lobe involvement suggests diseases such as pneumoconiosis, sarcoidosis and hypersensitivity pneumonias. The abnormalities on chest radiograph often provide useful clues, are a good starting point in narrowing the differential diagnoses **(Table 3)**.

Presence of diffuse mottling or ground-glass appearances may suggest an active stage of diffuse alveolitis. Miliary distribution throughout the lung fields is characteristically seen in tuberculosis, pneumoconiosis and sometimes in sarcoidosis. Occasionally, fluffy alveolar shadows may be present due to the coalescence of interstitial shadows or a complicating infection. In advanced disease when fibrosis is extensive, the lungs get shrunken and reduced in volume. Small, uniform sized, quadrangular cystic spaces, representing patent bronchioles, give the typical appearances of a honeycomb lung.

High-resolution CT of the Chest

High-resolution computed tomographic (CT) scanning offers a much better view of lung parenchymal/interstitial involvement and has become an integral part of diagnostic algorithm in all suspect patients of ILDs.[68] Recognition of the pattern on HRCT is of utmost importance while approaching patients with ILD **(Table 3)**. The presence of symmetrical, bibasal (apicobasal gradient), subpleural intralobular septal thickening with or without honeycombing is considered characteristic of UIP pattern on HRCT chest.[69,70] In the absence of secondary causes, this pattern is considered diagnostic of IPF. The positive predictive value of HRCT findings in the diagnosis of IPF is as high as 90–100% and typical HRCT findings can even negate a surgical biopsy.[70-72] Diseases such as sarcoidosis, histiocytosis and lymphangitis have more characteristic patterns. HRCT is also of some help in making a quantitative assessment of pulmonary fibrosis.[73] Spiral CT scan gives an even better resolution, especially in a patient with tachypnea who cannot hold his breath.

Pulmonary Function Tests

Most ILDs demonstrate a restrictive defect on spirometry and pulmonary function tests (PFT) cannot help in differential diagnosis. They are important however for functional assessment and to monitor therapy. Tidal volumes are generally small and both the vital capacity and the total lung capacity are reduced.[74,75] Expiratory flows are normal or even "supranormal". Airway obstruction, characterized by reduced forced vital capacity (FVC) and forced expiratory flows, can occur in certain ILDs which can have concomitant small airway involvement like hypersensitivity pneumonias, sarcoidosis, PLCH and LAM. Reduced diffusing capacity (DLCO) and arterial hypoxemia (reduced PaO_2) may not be present in the early stages. Some degree of arterial hypoxemia on exercise is almost always demonstrable. Measurements of pulmonary compliance can pick up early lung involvement in CT-ILDs.[7,8]

Bronchoalveolar Lavage

Assessment of cellular response in the BAL fluid, although nonconclusive, may help in the differential diagnosis.[76] BAL is more often used to rule out the differentials to ILD-like infections and malignancy. BAL may be adequate to diagnose infections (e.g. tuberculosis, histoplasmosis, coccidioidomycosis, endemic fungal infections) and selected noninfectious diseases (e.g. PLCH[77], LAM[78], DAH). Increases in BAL lymphocytes suggest sarcoidosis, hypersensitivity pneumonitis, or other granulomatous processes. When BAL lymphocytes exceed 50%, hypersensitivity pneumonitis is likely.[76] Similarly high CD4/CD8 ratio (>3.5) of BAL lymphocytes favors sarcoidosis and a low value (<1) favors hypersensitivity pneumonitis. Presence of eosinophils (>25%) may suggest acute or chronic eosinophilic pneumonia.[79] Mild increases in lymphocytes or eosinophils have no diagnostic value.[80] Increases in neutrophils can be seen in a wide array of fibrotic disorders.[81] The interstitial lung diseases differ in the pattern of cytokines expressed in BAL and thus the measurement of cytokine levels could be diagnostically useful.[82] Infective microorganisms such as the mycobacteria, fungi or *Pneumocystis jerovecii* can be isolated from BAL fluid. Presence of lymphocytosis in the BAL fluid is shown to predict a better response to corticosteroid therapy. An increase in the alkaline phosphatase/albumin ratio in BAL fluid on a repeat study reflects progression of fibrosis.[83] The role of BAL differential cell count in predicting response to therapy or prognostication is not established.

Other Investigations

Although nonspecific, hematological investigations provide useful information **(Table 5)**. A high erythrocyte sedimentation rate (ESR) of more than 50 mm in first hour occurs in connective tissue disorders, malignancies, infections and systemic vasculitides. Unexplained anemia is seen in diffuse alveolar hemorrhage and connective tissue diseases. Mild-to-moderate leukocytosis is common in both primary and secondary ILDs. Eosinophilia is more characteristically seen in eosinophilic pneumonias, vasculitides, sarcoidosis and drug-induced lung disease. Occasionally, there is leukopenia and/or thrombocytopenia.

Abnormal liver or renal function tests suggest the involvement of these organs. Elevated calcium may be seen in sarcoidosis and malignancies. Increased enzymes such as creatinine phosphokinase and aldolase are present in polymyositis and dermatomyositis. Increased serum angiotensin converting enzyme (SACE) in sarcoidosis is quite characteristic but may be seen in silicosis, hypersensitivity pneumonias and other diseases like tuberculosis.

Table 5 Some important clues to specific diagnoses in ILD on investigations

Investigation	*Diagnostic possibilities*
A. Chest radiographs	
• Normal	Sarcoidosis, CTD, RB-ILD
• Increased or preserved lung volumes	RB-ILD, CPFE, LAM, AHP
• Upper lobe predominance	Sarcoidosis, HP, pneumoconioses, AS
• Lower lobe predominance	IPF, CTD
• Peripheral (Reverse pulmonary edema)	CEP
• Honeycombing	IPF, CTD, chronic HP
• Spontaneous pneumothorax	LAM, PLCH,
• Pleural effusions	CTD, asbestosis, sarcoidosis
• Fleeting infiltrates	COP, HP
• Miliary pattern	Infections, HP, sarcoidosis
B. High resolution CT scans	
• Interlobular and intralobular septal thickening, honeycombing, traction bronchiectasis	CTD, IPF, asbestosis
• Alveolar shadows, ground glassing	COP, AIP, PAP, AEP
• Nodules	Sarcoidosis, pneumoconioses, RA
• Cystic ILD	LAM, PLCH, LIP
C. Laboratory investigations	
• Eosinophilia	AEP, CEP
• Iron deficiency anemia	DAH
• Leukopenia/thrombocytopenia	CTD
• Creatinine kinase, Jo-1 antibody	Polymyositis
• ANA, RF	
• Serum precipitins to specific	CTD, IPF (low titers)
antigens	HP
• ANCA, Anti-GBM antibodies	Vasculitides, Goodpasture syndrome

Source: Adapted from Raghu G, Brown KK. Interstitial lung disease: clinical evaluation and keys to an accurate diagnosis. Clin Chest Med. 2004;25:409-19, v.
Abbreviations: CTD, connective tissue diseases; RB-ILD, respiratory bronchiolitis-associated ILD; CPFE, combine pulmonary fibrosis and emphysema; LAM, lymphangioleiomyomatosis; AHP, acute hypersensitivity pneumonitis; AS, ankylosing spondylitis; IPF, idiopathic pulmonary fibrosis; AIP, acute interstitial pneumonia; AEP, acute eosinophilic pneumonia; COP, cryptogenic organizing pneumonia; HP, hypersensitivity pneumonitis; PLCH, pulmonary Langerhans cell histiocytosis.

A number of immunological parameters are described in connective tissue disorders and other ILDs. Hypergammaglobulinemia, positive serum autoantibodies (e.g. the antinuclear factor) and circulating immune complexes may be seen. Antibasement membrane antibodies in Goodpasture syndrome, antineutrophil cytoplasmic antibody (C-ANCA) in Wegener's granulomatosis, Churg-Strauss syndrome and systemic necrotizing vasculitis, and anti-Jo-1 antibody in polymyositis-dermatomyositis are generally considered characteristic.

Radionuclide scanning using Gallium[67,84,85] and position emission tomography (PET) scans[86,87] with 18F-FDG glucose isotope have a place to identify disease-activity and to predict response to therapy. Similarly, the clearance of aerosolized technetium-99m diethylenetriamine penta-acetic acid (DTPA) is markedly increased in patients with inflammatory lung diseases including sarcoidosis.[88]

Lung Biopsy

Diagnosis of IIPs is fairly specific on clinical features and roentgenographic characteristics seen on HRCT scanning. Lung biopsy is required only when the clinicoradiologic findings are atypical, to exclude an infection, vasculitides or malignancy. It may also help to predict the response to treatment and prognosis of a patient.[89] Transbronchial lung biopsy (TBLB) with the help of fiberoptic bronchoscopy is less rewarding especially in patients with IPF. In diseases like sarcoidosis, the positivity rates of endobronchial biopsies (EBB) and TBLB may be as high as 70–80%. Many a patient of IPF cannot be subjected to TBLB in view of an inadequate biopsy size and risks involved with fiberoptic bronchoscopy. Transthoracic or open surgical approach provides a better option to obtain lung tissue.[90,91] Surgical lung biopsy achieves three purposes: (1) establishes a precise diagnosis; (2) assesses the extent of inflammation and fibrosis; (3) identifies a histopathological pattern for IIPs.[92,93] Surgical lung biopsy is also not without risks; there is an increased risk of death in the month following surgery, especially in patients with IPF, as surgery itself can trigger an acute exacerbation. Hence, a decision for surgical lung biopsy has to be taken after carefully considering the risk benefit ratio and only when the pathologic diagnosis is likely to alter the management approach to the patient.[94]

TREATMENT

Treatment options for ILD are limited, especially for chronic fibrosing ILDs like IPF. Establishing a clear diagnosis of ILD and identifying a potential etiology are critical in determining appropriate therapeutic interventions.[95] In the absence of a satisfactory, definitive treatment for IPF, most objectives **(Box 1)** are achieved with supportive and symptomatic therapy.[65] Several different groups of drugs have been tried in its treatment **(Table 6)**. Supportive treatment is provided for respiratory failure, pulmonary hypertension, cor pulmonale and congestive cardiac failure, wherever indicated. Long-term pulmonary vasodilators have not shown to prevent the development of pulmonary hypertension.

An acute increase in symptoms and presence of fever with or without mucopurulent expectoration raise the suspicion of a respiratory infection necessitating treatment with antibiotics. To assess the response to therapy and monitor its

BOX 1 Treatment objectives in interstitial lung disease

- Provide symptom-relief
- Slow down disease—progression
- Prevent complications
- Improve quality of life
- Prolong survival
- Prevent treatment-complications
- End-of-life care—palliation treatment

Table 6 List of drugs used in the treatment of interstitial lung disease

Treatment of primary ILD 1. Anti-inflammatory drugs • Corticosteroids • Azathioprine • Cyclophosphamide • Mycophenolate mofetil • Methotrexate 2. Antifibrotic agents • Pirfenidone • Nintedanib (BIBF 1120) • Colchicine • Pentoxifylline • D-penicillamine • TGF beta antagonist • Interferon-gamma 3. Antioxidant agents • N-acetyl cysteine • Nitric oxide synthase inhibition 4. Receptor antagonists 5. Antiapoptosis agents 6. Antiangiogenesis agents
Supportive and symptomatic drugs 1. Oxygen 2. Pulmonary vasodilators 3. Diuretics 4. Antibiotics (if infection)
Rehabilitation 1. Nutrition and dietary supplements 2. Graded, regulated exercises

progress a clinical, roentgenological and physiological (CRP) score has been used in the past. It is difficult to frequently repeat invasive investigations such as the BAL or lung biopsy. It is generally adequate to rely on clinical picture, simple spirometry and a plain chest roentgenogram. The American Thoracic Society/European Respiratory Society has published therapeutic guidelines for specific subtypes of ILD.[70] Broad approaches are discussed below.

Anti-inflammatory Therapy

Anti-inflammatory therapy has remained the mainstay of treatment for several different groups of ILDs. The IIPs, which respond to corticosteroids/immunosuppressants, include the NSIP (the cellular variant), COP, DIP and LIP. Acute interstitial pneumonia also responds to steroids in up to 50% of the patients. Corticosteroids also form the initial line of management for connective tissue disease ILDs, eosinophilic pneumonias, hypersensitivity pneumonias (along with trigger avoidance) and sarcoidosis. Many a times, corticosteroid-sparing agents may be needed especially when the treatment is needed for a prolonged duration. Severe forms of ILDs may need concomitant agents like cyclophosphamide.

The role of corticosteroids in fibrotic ILDs like IPF and the fibrotic NSIP is limited. Corticosteroids had been used in the management of IPF in the past either as monotherapy[96] or in combination with azathioprine and N-acetylcysteine (NAC) (triple therapy).[97] The PANTHER-IPF study had shown that the triple therapy increases the mortality; treatment-related side effects and the hospitalizations does not have any clinical benefit.[98] Another study suggested that combined corticosteroid and cyclophosphamide therapy has no impact on survival in patients with IPF.[99] The recent guidelines on IPF recommend not using any of these drugs for managing patients with IPF. The only indication for the use of corticosteroids in patients with IPF is an acute exacerbation of the underlying disease.

Antifibrotic Agents

There is a greater trend to rely on antifibrotic drugs for the treatment of fibrosing ILDs. Of the several antifibrotic agents, which had been tried, pirfenidone, an orally administered pyridine, is the only drug, which has shown clinical promise.[100] It has antifibrotic, antioxidant and anti-inflammatory properties. It has been used in doses ranging from 1200 mg/day to 2400 mg/day. Pirfenidone has so far been tested in five randomized controlled studies (two CAPACITY trials,[101] two Japanese trials[102,103] and the ASCEND trial[104]). All the trials have consistently shown that this drug slows the disease progression (rate of decline in FVC), improves the progression free survival and is well-tolerated. Some of the trials have also shown reduced rate of acute exacerbations and reduced IPF-related mortality. The common side effects of pirfenidone are gastrointestinal intolerance, skin rash and hepatotoxicity. This drug is currently approved for clinical use in India.

Nintedanib (BIBF 1120), a multiple tyrosine kinase inhibitor (VEGF, FGF and PDGF), also has antifibrotic properties and is the other drug to have shown some clinical promise. The recent phase three trials (INPULSIS 1 and 2) have shown that when used at a dose of 150 mg twice a day, this drug slows the decline in FVC and decreases the acute exacerbations,[105] but the patients included in these trials had milder IPF with mean FVC of 70–80% predicted. These results have to be replicated in other trials before this drug can be routinely used in clinical practice.

The other drugs, which have been tried, include colchicine, D-penicillamine, interferon gamma and others. Colchicine inhibits collagen formation, modulates the extracellular milieu and suppresses the release of alveolar macrophage-derived growth factor and fibronectin.[106] Initial studies were encouraging with trend towards improved outcome.[107] Subsequent studies have failed to demonstrate any benefit of treatment with colchicine over no treatment at all.[108,109] D-penicillamine and other drugs, which have been tried with variable results.[109,110] Interferon (IF)-γ inhibits the proliferation of lung fibroblasts in a dose-dependent manner and reduces the synthesis of protein in fibroblasts. It had generated great interest in IF as the magic cure for IPF but subsequent studies dampened the hopes.[111] In a large double-blinded trial with 330 patients with IPF who did not respond to corticosteroid therapy, it was found that IF γ-1b did not affect progression-free survival, pulmonary function, or the quality of life over 58 weeks.[112] None of these agents are currently recommended for clinical use.

Other Treatments

Antioxidants, such as NAC to reduce oxidative stress, are shown to offer some clinical advantage when used along with antifibrotic agents. A double-blind, randomized, placebo-controlled multicenter study (the IFIGENIA trial) assessed the effectiveness over one year of a high oral dose of acetylcysteine (600 mg three times daily) added to standard therapy with prednisone plus azathioprine.[113] This landmark trial showed that acetylcysteine slowed the deterioration of vital capacity and DLCO at 12 months without significant differences in the type or severity of adverse events. The results of the subsequent PANTHER-IPF study were contradicting to these results. The triple therapy arm was shown to have a higher mortality and the triple therapy arm was prematurely stopped after an interim analysis.[98] The results of the NAC monotherapy arm have also been recently published. The NAC monotherapy (600 mg thrice a day) also did not confer any clinical benefit.[114] Thus, the role of NAC in managing patients with IPF is debatable.

Drugs targeted to prevent or reduce apoptosis, angiogenesis and coagulant activity may find some use in the future. Presently, no drug from these groups is available for clinical use. It is a better option to resort to symptomatic palliative therapy and withdraw immunosuppressive drugs in case there is no response in the initial 3–6 months of use and for end-stage disease.

Transplantation

Lung transplantation is the only hope for the advanced, end-stage disease.[115] Single lung transplantation is recommended in most patients. Five years survival is reported in up to 40–60% of patients. The common post-transplant complications include the risk of resection, multiple opportunistic infections in an immunosuppressed host and organizing pneumonias. The lack of availability of organ for transplantation and very high costs involved in the procedure are the limited factors. Living-donor lobar lung transplantation (LDLLT) is a new and evolving option for patients with end-stage lung disease.[116]

Other Supportive Measures

The primary goal in managing a patient with IPF is to restore them to the highest possible functional state. Patients should be encouraged to enroll in a pulmonary physical rehabilitation program. Daily walks or use of a stationary bicycle is useful. Those with hypoxemia at rest or during exercise should be managed by supplemental oxygen. Higher flow rates than those needed in COPD may be frequently required. Dry cough may be controlled with antitussives. Low-dose opioids are effective and safe in the palliative management of dyspnea in terminally-ill IPF patients.[117]

Pulmonary hypertension, cor pulmonale and right heart failure, which complicate late stages of IPF, should be appropriately managed. In randomized controlled, open-label trials, the phosphodiesterase type 5-inhibitor sildenafil causes preferential pulmonary vasodilatation and improves gas exchange in patients with severe lung fibrosis and secondary pulmonary hypertension.[118,119] There was no improvement in the primary end point, exercise tolerance. Other vasodilator agents, which have been tried in managing patients, include bosentan, ambrisentan and macitentan. The results of all these trials have been negative.[120-124]

ACUTE EXACERBATION OF INTERSTITIAL LUNG DISEASES

Acute exacerbation of idiopathic pulmonary fibrosis (AE-IPF) is a clinical entity characterized by rapid deterioration of IPF during the course of disease that is not due to infections, pulmonary embolism or heart failure. The simplified 2007 consensus criteria for the diagnosis of AE-IPF include: (a) Previous or concurrent diagnosis of IPF; (b) worsening of dyspnea over the last 30 days; (c) new onset infiltrates (ground glass opacities or consolidation) on CT chest and (d) absence of infection and other causes of deterioration including pulmonary edema and pulmonary thromboembolism.[125] This condition needs to be differentiated from acute interstitial pneumonia (or Hamman-Rich syndrome), which occurs in patients with no underlying lung disease.

The exact etiology and pathogenesis remain unknown, but the condition is characterized by diffuse alveolar damage (on a background of IPF) that probably occurs as a result of a massive lung injury due to some unknown etiologic agent. HRCT can help in prognostication and management of this condition. Once infections and other causes of worsening have been excluded, treatment involves enhanced immunosuppression with pulse doses of methyl prednisolone and cytotoxic agents. Our systematic review shows that the outcome is poor with 1-month and 3-month mortality around 60% and 67%, respectively.[126] Few studies have shown beneficial effects of cyclosporine, pirfenidone, and anticoagulants in the management and prevention of AE-IPF.[126] Acute exacerbation of the underlying ILD can also occur in fibrotic NSIP and CTD-related ILDs. The approach and the management are the same as that of AE-IPF.

PROGNOSIS

Prognosis of ILDs, secondary to systemic diseases or other causes is determined by the natural course of the underlying disease. Prognosis of primary IIPs is variable. While NSIP, COP, DIP and RB-ILD respond better, the IPF is progressive and fatal. The survival has not significantly improved in the last 50 years or so from that reported in the 1960s. The median survival of IPF is about 4 years. Acute interstitial pneumonia and acute exacerbation of IPF are rapidly fatal, sometimes in a course of a few weeks or months.[127]

It is unclear how many ILD patients actually die of their lung disease.[128,129]

Given the age of many with ILD, patients are at risk for other age-related diseases and need close follow-up with their internists. Survival for ILD is worse if at time of diagnosis there is advanced age (>50), male gender, moderate/severe dyspnea on exertion, history of tobacco use, moderate loss of lung function (TLC <45%, DLCO <40%), neutrophilia/eosinophilia on BAL, honeycombing on HRCT, lack of a response to corticosteroids, or moderate/severe fibrosis and fibroblastic foci on histology.[129,130]

REFERENCES

1. Travis WD, Costabel U, Hansell DM, King TE Jr, Lynch DA, Nicholson AG, et al. An official American Thoracic Society/European Respiratory Society statement: Update of the international multidisciplinary classification of the idiopathic interstitial pneumonias. Am J Respir Crit Care Med. 2013;188:733-48.
2. American Thoracic Society. Idiopathic pulmonary fibrosis: diagnosis and treatment. International consensus statement. American Thoracic Society (ATS), and the European Respiratory Society (ERS). Am J Respir Crit Care Med. 2000;161:646-64.
3. Masi AT. Classification of systemic sclerosis (scleroderma): relationship of cutaneous subgroups in early disease to outcome and serologic reactivity. J Rheumatol. 1988;15:894-8.
4. Tansey D, Wells AU, Colby TV, Ip S, Nikolakoupolou A, du Bois RM, et al. Variations in histological patterns of interstitial pneumonia between connective tissue disorders and their relationship to prognosis. Histopathology. 2004;44:585-96.
5. Dawson JK, Fewins HE, Desmond J, Lynch MP, Graham DR. Fibrosing alveolitis in patients with rheumatoid arthritis as assessed by high-resolution computed tomography, chest radiography, and pulmonary function tests. Thorax. 2001;56:622-7.
6. Harrison NK, Glanville AR, Strickland B, Haslam PL, Corrin B, Addis BJ, et al. Pulmonary involvement in systemic sclerosis: the detection of early changes by thin section CT scan, bronchoalveolar lavage and 99mTc-DTPA clearance. Respir Med. 1989;83:403-14.
7. Aggarwal AN, Gupta D, Wanchu A, Jindal SK. Use of static lung mechanics to identify early pulmonary involvement in patients with ankylosing spondylitis. J Postgrad Med. 2001;47:89-94.
8. Gupta D, Aggarwal AN, Sud A, Jindal SK. Static lung mechanics in patients of progressive systemic sclerosis without obvious pulmonary involvement. Indian J Chest Dis Allied Sci. 2001;43:97-101.
9. Casserly IP, Fenlon HM, Breatnach E, Sant SM. Lung findings on high-resolution computed tomography in idiopathic ankylosing spondylitis—correlation with clinical findings, pulmonary function testing and plain radiography. Br J Rheumatol. 1997;36:677-82.
10. Foucher P, Camus P. (2010). Pneumotox[(r)] Dijon. [online] Available from *http://www.pneumotox.com. online database.* [Accessed March, 2016].
11. Duran I, Siu LL, Oza AM, Chung TB, Sturgeon J, Townsley CA, et al. Characterisation of the lung toxicity of the cell cycle inhibitor temsirolimus. Eur J Cancer. 2006;42:1875-80.
12. Camus P, Martin WJ 2nd, Rosenow EC 3rd. Amiodarone pulmonary toxicity. Clin Chest Med. 2004;25:65-75.
13. Abratt RP, Morgan GW, Silvestri G, Willcox P. Pulmonary complications of radiation therapy. Clin Chest Med. 2004;25:167-77.
14. Bertorelli G, Bocchino V, Oliveri D. Hypersensitivity pneumonitis. Interstitial lung diseases. Eur Respir Monograph. 2000;14:120-36.
15. Coultas DB, Hughes MP. Accuracy of mortality data for interstitial lung diseases in New Mexico, USA. Thorax. 1996;51:717-20.
16. Coultas DB, Zumwalt RE, Black WC, Sobonya RE. The epidemiology of interstitial lung diseases. Am J Respir Crit Care Med. 1994;150:967-72.
17. Hubbard R, Johnston I, Coultas DB, Britton J. Mortality rates from cryptogenic fibrosing alveolitis in seven countries. Thorax. 1996;51:711-6.
18. Jindal SK, Malik SK, Deodhar SD, Sharma BK. Fibrosing alveolitis: a report of 61 cases seen over the past five years. Indian J Chest Dis Allied Sci. 1979;21:174-9.
19. Maheshwari U, Gupta D, Aggarwal AN, Jindal SK. Spectrum and diagnosis of idiopathic pulmonary fibrosis. Indian J Chest Dis Allied Sci. 2004;46:23-6.
20. Ghanem MK, Makhlouf HA, Agmy GR, Imam HM, Fouad DA. Evaluation of recently validated non-invasive formula using basic lung functions as new screening tool for pulmonary hypertension in idiopathic pulmonary fibrosis patients. Ann Thorac Med. 2009;4:187-96.
21. Balamugesh T, Behera D. Idiopathic pulmonary fibrosis. J Assoc Physicians India. 2007;55:363-70.
22. Agarwal R, Gupta D, Verma JS, Aggarwal AN, Jindal SK. Noninvasive estimation of clinically asymptomatic pulmonary hypertension in idiopathic pulmonary fibrosis. Indian J Chest Dis Allied Sci. 2005;47:267-71.
23. Subhash HS, Ashwin I, Solomon SK, David T, Cherian AM, Thomas K. A comparative study on idiopathic pulmonary fibrosis and secondary diffuse parenchymal lung disease. Indian J Med Sci. 2004;58:185-90.

24. Sharma R, Guleria R, Pande JN. Idiopathic pulmonary fibrosis: newer concepts and management strategies. Indian J Chest Dis Allied Sci. 2003;45:31-49.
25. Behera D, Kaur S, Sathyanarayana G, Majumdar S. Surfactant protein-A in lung lavage fluid obtained from patients with idiopathic pulmonary fibrosis. J Assoc Physicians India. 2002; 50:1409-12.
26. Behera D, Kaur S, Sathyanarayana G, Bhatnagar A, Majumdar S. Nitric oxide derivative in bronchoalveolar lavage fluid from patients with idiopathic pulmonary fibrosis. Indian J Chest Dis Allied Sci. 2002;44:21-4.
27. Jindal SK, Gupta D. Algorithm for diagnosing pulmonary fibrosis in tropical countries. Curr Opin Pulm Med. 1998;4: 294-9.
28. Chhabra SK. Idiopathic pulmonary fibrosis: prognostic indicators. Indian J Chest Dis Allied Sci. 1998;40:159-61.
29. Jindal SK, Gupta D. Incidence and recognition of interstitial pulmonary fibrosis in developing countries. Curr Opin Pulm Med. 1997;3:378-83.
30. Behera D, D'Souza G, Rajwanshi A, Jindal SK. Bronchoalveolar lavage—cellular characteristics in patients with idiopathic pulmonary fibrosis and sarcoidosis. Indian J Chest Dis Allied Sci. 1990;32:107-10.
31. Sharma SK, Pande JN, Verma K, Guleria JS. Bronchoalveolar lavage fluid (BALF) analysis in interstitial lung diseases—a 7-year experience. Indian J Chest Dis Allied Sci. 1989;31:187-96.
32. Sharma SK, Pande JN, Guleria JS. Diffuse interstitial pulmonary fibrosis. Indian J Chest Dis Allied Sci. 1984;26:214-9.
33. Johnston ID, Prescott RJ, Chalmers JC, Rudd RM. British Thoracic Society study of cryptogenic fibrosing alveolitis: current presentation and initial management. Fibrosing Alveolitis Subcommittee of the Research Committee of the British Thoracic Society. Thorax. 1997;52:38-44.
34. Fernandez Perez ER, Daniels CE, Schroeder DR, St Sauver J, Hartman TE, Bartholmai BJ, et al. Incidence, prevalence, and clinical course of idiopathic pulmonary fibrosis: a population-based study. Chest. 2010;137:129-37.
35. Kuhn C. The pathogenesis of pulmonary fibrosis. Monogr Pathol; 1993.pp.78-92.
36. Martinez FJ, Keane MP. Update in diffuse parenchymal lung diseases 2005. Am J Respir Crit Care Med. 2006;173:1066-71.
37. Vancheri C, Failla M, Crimi N, Raghu G. Idiopathic pulmonary fibrosis: a disease with similarities and links to cancer biology. Eur Respir J. 2010;35:496-504.
38. Carre PC, Mortenson RL, King TE, Noble PW, Sable CL, Riches DW Jr. Increased expression of the interleukin-8 gene by alveolar macrophages in idiopathic pulmonary fibrosis. A potential mechanism for the recruitment and activation of neutrophils in lung fibrosis. J Clin Invest. 1991;88:1802-10.
39. Keane MP. Angiogenesis and pulmonary fibrosis: feast or famine? Am J Respir Crit Care Med. 2004;170:207-9.
40. Keane MP, Arenberg DA, Lynch JP 3rd, Whyte RI, Iannettoni MD, Burdick MD, et al. The CXC chemokines, IL-8 and IP-10, regulate angiogenic activity in idiopathic pulmonary fibrosis. J Immunol. 1997;159:1437-43.
41. Antoniou KM, Soufla G, Lymbouridou R, Economidou F, Lasithiotaki I, Manousakis M, et al. Expression analysis of angiogenic growth factors and biological axis CXCL12/CXCR4 axis in idiopathic pulmonary fibrosis. Connect Tissue Res. 2010;51:71-80.
42. Cui A, Anhenn O, Theegarten D, Ohshimo S, Bonella F, Sixt SU, et al. Angiogenic and angiostatic chemokines in idiopathic pulmonary fibrosis and granulomatous lung disease. Respiration. 2010;80(5):372-8.
43. Tzouvelekis A, Aidinis V, Harokopos V, Karameris A, Zacharis G, Mikroulis D, et al. Down-regulation of the inhibitor of growth family member 4 (ING4) in different forms of pulmonary fibrosis. Respir Res. 2009;10:14.
44. Nadrous HF, Pellikka PA, Krowka MJ, Swanson KL, Chaowalit N, Decker PA, et al. The impact of pulmonary hypertension on survival in patients with idiopathic pulmonary fibrosis. Chest. 2005;128:616S-7S.
45. Waisberg DR, Barbas-Filho JV, Parra ER, Fernezlian S, de Carvalho CR, Kairalla RA, et al. Abnormal expression of telomerase/apoptosis limits type II alveolar epithelial cell replication in the early remodeling of usual interstitial pneumonia/idiopathic pulmonary fibrosis. Hum Pathol. 2010;41:385-91.
46. Kliment CR, Englert JM, Gochuico BR, Yu G, Kaminski N, Rosas I, et al. Oxidative stress alters syndecan-1 distribution in lungs with pulmonary fibrosis. J Biol Chem. 2009;284:3537-45.
47. Gharaee-Kermani M, Hu B, Phan SH, Gyetko MR. Recent advances in molecular targets and treatment of idiopathic pulmonary fibrosis: focus on TGFbeta signaling and the myofibroblast. Curr Med Chem. 2009;16:1400-17.
48. Selman M, Pardo A. Role of epithelial cells in idiopathic pulmonary fibrosis: from innocent targets to serial killers. Proc Am Thorac Soc. 2006;3:364-72.
49. Selman M, Thannickal VJ, Pardo A, Zisman DA, Martinez FJ, Lynch JP 3rd. Idiopathic pulmonary fibrosis: pathogenesis and therapeutic approaches. Drugs. 2004;64:405-30.
50. Pan LH, Yamauchi K, Uzuki M, Nakanishi T, Takigawa M, Inoue H, et al. Type II alveolar epithelial cells and interstitial fibroblasts express connective tissue growth factor in IPF. Eur Respir J. 2001;17:1220-7.
51. Ramos C, Montano M, Garcia-Alvarez J, Ruiz V, Uhal BD, Selman M, et al. Fibroblasts from idiopathic pulmonary fibrosis and normal lungs differ in growth rate, apoptosis, and tissue inhibitor of metalloproteinases expression. Am J Respir Cell Mol Biol. 2001;24:591-8.
52. Ask K, Bonniaud P, Maass K, Eickelberg O, Margetts PJ, Warburton D, et al. Progressive pulmonary fibrosis is mediated by TGF-beta isoform 1 but not TGF-beta3. Int J Biochem Cell Biol. 2008;40:484-95.
53. Kang HR, Cho SJ, Lee CG, Homer RJ, Elias JA. Transforming growth factor (TGF)-beta1 stimulates pulmonary fibrosis and inflammation via a Bax-dependent, bid-activated pathway that involves matrix metalloproteinase-12. J Biol Chem. 2007;282:7723-32.
54. Ruan W, Ying K. Abnormal expression of IGF-binding proteins, an initiating event in idiopathic pulmonary fibrosis? Pathol Res Pract. 2010;206:537-43.
55. Cao B, Guo Z, Zhu Y, Xu W. The potential role of PDGF, IGF-1, TGF-beta expression in idiopathic pulmonary fibrosis. Chin Med J (Engl). 2000; 113:776-82.
56. Zhao HW, Lu CJ, Yu RJ, Hou XM. An increase in hyaluronan by lung fibroblasts: a biomarker for intensity and activity of interstitial pulmonary fibrosis? Respirology. 1999;4:131-8.
57. Raghu G, Chen YY, Rusch V, Rabinovitch PS. Differential proliferation of fibroblasts cultured from normal and fibrotic human lungs. Am Rev Respir Dis. 1988;138:703-8.

58. Strieter RM, Keeley EC, Hughes MA, Burdick MD, Mehrad B. The role of circulating mesenchymal progenitor cells (fibrocytes) in the pathogenesis of pulmonary fibrosis. J Leukoc Biol. 2009;86:1111-8.
59. Schissel SL, Layne MD. Telomerase, myofibroblasts, and pulmonary fibrosis. Am J Respir Cell Mol Biol. 2006;34:520-2.
60. Fell CD, Martinez FJ, Liu LX, Murray S, Han MK, Kazerooni EA, et al. Clinical predictors of a diagnosis of idiopathic pulmonary fibrosis. Am J Respir Crit Care Med. 2010;181:832-7.
61. Vassallo R, Ryu JH. Smoking-related interstitial lung diseases. Clin Chest Med. 2012;33:165-78.
62. Loyd JE. Pulmonary fibrosis in families. Am J Respir Cell Mol Biol. 2003;29:S47-50.
63. Chung JH, Kanne JP. Smoking-related interstitial lung diseases. Semin Roentgenol. 2010;45:29-35.
64. Hubbard R, Venn A, Smith C, Cooper M, Johnston I, Britton J. Exposure to commonly prescribed drugs and the etiology of cryptogenic fibrosing alveolitis: a case-control study. Am J Respir Crit Care Med. 1998;157:743-7.
65. King TE Jr. Clinical advances in the diagnosis and therapy of the interstitial lung diseases. Am J Respir Crit Care Med. 2005;172:268-79.
66. Tonelli AR, Fernandez-Bussy S, Lodhi S, Akindipe OA, Carrie RD, Hamilton K, et al. Prevalence of pulmonary hypertension in end-stage cystic fibrosis and correlation with survival. J Heart Lung Transplant. 2010;29:865-72.
67. Glaser S, Noga O, Koch B, Opitz CF, Schmidt B, Temmesfeld B, et al. Impact of pulmonary hypertension on gas exchange and exercise capacity in patients with pulmonary fibrosis. Respir Med. 2009;103:317-24.
68. Raghu G, Mageto YN, Lockhart D, Schmidt RA, Wood DE, Godwin JD. The accuracy of the clinical diagnosis of new-onset idiopathic pulmonary fibrosis and other interstitial lung disease: A prospective study. Chest. 1999;116:1168-74.
69. Sverzellati N, Wells AU, Tomassetti S, Desai SR, Copley SJ, Aziz ZA, et al. Biopsy-proved idiopathic pulmonary fibrosis: spectrum of nondiagnostic thin-section CT diagnoses. Radiology. 2010;254:957-64.
70. Raghu G, Collard HR, Egan JJ, Martinez FJ, Behr J, Brown KK, et al. An official ATS/ERS/JRS/ALAT statement: idiopathic pulmonary fibrosis: evidence-based guidelines for diagnosis and management. Am J Respir Crit Care Med. 2011;183:788-824.
71. MacDonald SL, Rubens MB, Hansell DM, Copley SJ, Desai SR, du Bois RM, et al. Nonspecific interstitial pneumonia and usual interstitial pneumonia: comparative appearances at and diagnostic accuracy of thin-section CT. Radiology. 2001;221:600-5.
72. Elliot TL, Lynch DA, Newell JD J., Cool C, Tuder R, Markopoulou K, et al. High-resolution computed tomography features of nonspecific interstitial pneumonia and usual interstitial pneumonia. J Comput Assist Tomogr. 2005;29:339-45.
73. Lynch DA, Godwin JD, Safrin S, Starko KM, Hormel P, Brown KK, et al. High-resolution computed tomography in idiopathic pulmonary fibrosis: diagnosis and prognosis. Am J Respir Crit Care Med. 2005;172:488-93.
74. Wanchu A, Gupta D, Deodhar SD. Pulmonary function abnormalities in rheumatoid arthritis subjects with no cardio-respiratory symptoms: DLCO does not add to the diagnosis. J Assoc Physician India. 1997;45:91-3. (Editorial comment by Chowgle AR, pp. 87-9).
75. Wanchu A, Gupta D, Deodhar SD, Jindal SK. Cross-sectional analysis of pulmonary function abnormalities among patients with systemic lupus erythematosus. J Assoc Physicians India. 1998;46:998-1000.
76. Welker L, Jorres RA, Costabel U, Magnussen H. Predictive value of BAL cell differentials in the diagnosis of interstitial lung diseases. Eur Respir J. 2004;24:1000-6.
77. Vassallo R, Ryu JH, Colby TV, et al. Pulmonary Langerhans'-cell histiocytosis. N Engl J Med. 2000;342:1969-78.
78. Johnson SR, Tattersfield AE. Clinical experience of lymphangioleiomyomatosis in the UK. Thorax. 2000;55:1052-7.
79. Marchand E, Cordier JF. Idiopathic chronic eosinophilic pneumonia. Semin Respir Crit Care Med. 2006;27:134-41.
80. Veeraraghavan S, Latsi PI, Wells AU, Pantelidis P, Nicholson AG, Colby TV, et al. BAL findings in idiopathic nonspecific interstitial pneumonia and usual interstitial pneumonia. Eur Respir J. 2003;22:239-44.
81. Bronchoalveolar lavage constituents in healthy individuals, idiopathic pulmonary fibrosis, and selected comparison groups. The BAL Cooperative Group Steering Committee. Am Rev Respir Dis. 1990;141:S169-202.
82. Wolff H, Teppo AM, Mutanen P, Sutinen S, Backman R, Sutinen S, et al. Studies of cytokine levels in bronchoalveolar fluid lavage from patients with interstitial lung diseases. Scand J Clin Lab Invest. 2003;63:27-36.
83. Capelli A, Lusuardi M, Cerutti CG, Donner CF. Lung alkaline phosphatase as a marker of fibrosis in chronic interstitial disorders. Am J Respir Crit Care Med. 1997;155:249-53.
84. Teirstein AT, Morgenthau AS. "End-stage" pulmonary fibrosis in sarcoidosis. Mt Sinai J Med. 2009;76:30-6.
85. Jin S, Wang G, He B, Zhu M. Gallium-67 scanning for detection of alveolitis in idiopathic pulmonary fibrosis and sarcoidosis. Chin Med J (Engl). 1996;109:519-21.
86. Eastwood PR, Maher TM, Wells AU, Lam B. Year in review 2009: Interstitial lung diseases, acute injury, sleep, physiology, imaging and bronchoscopic intervention. Respirology. 2010;15:172-81.
87. Inoue K, Okada K, Taki Y, Goto R, Kinomura S, Fukuda H. 18FDG uptake associated with CT density on PET/CT in lungs with and without chronic interstitial lung diseases. Ann Nucl Med. 2009;23:277-81.
88. Antoniou KM, Malagari K, Tzanakis N, Perisinakis K, Symvoulakis EK, Karkavitsas N, et al. Clearance of technetium-99m-DTPA and HRCT findings in the evaluation of patients with Idiopathic Pulmonary Fibrosis. BMC Pulm Med. 2006;6:4.
89. Nicholson AG, Fulford LG, Colby TV, du Bois RM, Hansell DM, Wells AU. The relationship between individual histologic features and disease progression in idiopathic pulmonary fibrosis. Am J Respir Crit Care Med. 2002;166:173-7.
90. Lettieri CJ, Veerappan GR, Helman DL, Mulligan CR, Shorr AF. Outcomes and safety of surgical lung biopsy for interstitial lung disease. Chest. 2005;127:1600-5.
91. Tiitto L, Heiskanen U, Bloigu R, Pääkkö P, Kinnula V, Kaarteenaho-Wiik R. Thoracoscopic lung biopsy is a safe procedure in diagnosing usual interstitial pneumonia. Chest. 2005;128:2375-80.
92. American Thoracic Society; European Respiratory Society. American Thoracic Society/European Respiratory Society International Multidisciplinary Consensus Classification of the Idiopathic Interstitial Pneumonias. This joint statement of the American Thoracic Society (ATS), and the European

Respiratory Society (ERS) was adopted by the ATS board of directors, June 2001 and by the ERS Executive Committee, June 2001. Am J Respir Crit Care Med. 2002;165:277-304.
93. Katzenstein AL, Myers JL. Idiopathic pulmonary fibrosis: clinical relevance of pathologic classification. Am J Respir Crit Care Med. 1998;157:1301-15.
94. Kaarteenaho R. The current position of surgical lung biopsy in the diagnosis of idiopathic pulmonary fibrosis. Respir Res. 2013;14:43.
95. Raghu G, Brown KK. Interstitial lung disease: clinical evaluation and keys to an accurate diagnosis. Clin Chest Med. 2004;25:409-19, v.
96. Mapel DW, Samet JM, Coultas DB. Corticosteroids and the treatment of idiopathic pulmonary fibrosis. Past, present, and future. Chest. 1996;110:1058-67.
97. Raghu G, Depaso WJ, Cain K, Hammar SP, Wetzel CE, Dreis DF, et al. Azathioprine combined with prednisone in the treatment of idiopathic pulmonary fibrosis: a prospective double-blind, randomized, placebo-controlled clinical trial. Am Rev Respir Dis. 1991;144:291-6.
98. Raghu G, Anstrom KJ, King TE Jr, Lasky JA, Martinez FJ, Idiopathic Pulmonary Fibrosis Clinical Research Network. Prednisone, azathioprine, and N-acetylcysteine for pulmonary fibrosis. N Engl J Med. 2012;366:1968-77.
99. Collard HR, Ryu JH, Douglas WW, Schwarz MI, Curran-Everett D, King TE Jr, et al. Combined corticosteroid and cyclophosphamide therapy does not alter survival in idiopathic pulmonary fibrosis. Chest. 2004;125:2169-74.
100. Kreuter M. Pirfenidone: an update on clinical trial data and insights from everyday practice. Eur Respir Rev. 2014;23:111-7.
101. Noble PW, Albera C, Bradford WZ, Costabel U, Glassberg MK, Kardatzke D, et al. Pirfenidone in patients with idiopathic pulmonary fibrosis (CAPACITY): two randomised trials. Lancet. 2011;377:1760-9.
102. Azuma A, Nukiwa T, Tsuboi E, Suga M, Abe S, Nakata K, et al. Double-blind, placebo-controlled trial of pirfenidone in patients with idiopathic pulmonary fibrosis. Am J Respir Crit Care Med. 2005;171:1040-7.
103. Taniguchi H, Ebina M, Kondoh Y, Ogura T, Azuma A, Suga M, et al. Pirfenidone in idiopathic pulmonary fibrosis. Eur Respir J. 2010;35:821-9.
104. King TE Jr, Bradford WZ, Castro-Bernardini S, Fagan EA, Glaspole I, Glassberg MK, et al. A phase 3 trial of pirfenidone in patients with idiopathic pulmonary fibrosis. N Engl J Med. 2014;370:2083-92.
105. Richeldi L, du Bois RM, Raghu G, Azuma A, Brown KK, Costabel U, et al. Efficacy and safety of nintedanib in idiopathic pulmonary fibrosis. N Engl J Med. 2014;370:2071-82.
106. Rennard SI, Bitterman PB, Ozaki T, Rom WN, Crystal RG. Colchicine suppresses the release of fibroblast growth factors from alveolar macrophages in vitro. The basis of a possible therapeutic approach to the fibrotic disorders. Am Rev Respir Dis. 1988;137:181-5.
107. Douglas WW, Ryu JH, Swensen SJ, Offord KP, Schroeder DR, Caron GM, et al. Colchicine versus prednisone in the treatment of idiopathic pulmonary fibrosis. A randomized prospective study. Members of the Lung Study Group. Am J Respir Crit Care Med. 1998;158:220-5.
108. Douglas WW, Ryu JH, Schroeder DR. Idiopathic pulmonary fibrosis: Impact of oxygen and colchicine, prednisone, or no therapy on survival. Am J Respir Crit Care Med. 2000;161:1172-8.
109. Selman M, Carrillo G, Salas J, Padilla RP, Pérez-Chavira R, Sansores R, et al. Colchicine, D-penicillamine, and prednisone in the treatment of idiopathic pulmonary fibrosis: a controlled clinical trial. Chest. 1998;114:507-12.
110. Raghu G, Johnson WC, Lockhart D, Mageto Y. Treatment of idiopathic pulmonary fibrosis with a new antifibrotic agent, pirfenidone: results of a prospective, open-label Phase II study. Am J Respir Crit Care Med. 1999;159:1061-9.
111. Ziesche R, Hofbauer E, Wittmann K, Petkov V, Block LH. A preliminary study of long-term treatment with interferon gamma-1b and low-dose prednisolone in patients with idiopathic pulmonary fibrosis. N Engl J Med. 1999;341:1264-9.
112. Raghu G, Brown KK, Bradford WZ, Starko K, Noble PW, Schwartz DA, et al. A placebo-controlled trial of interferon gamma-1b in patients with idiopathic pulmonary fibrosis. N Engl J Med. 2004;350:125-33.
113. Demedts M, Behr J, Buhl R, Costabel U, Dekhuijzen R, Jansen HM, et al. High-dose acetylcysteine in idiopathic pulmonary fibrosis. N Engl J Med. 2005;353:2229-42.
114. Idiopathic Pulmonary Fibrosis Clinical Research Network, Martinez FJ, de Andrade JA, Anstrom KJ, King TE Jr, Raghu G. Randomized trial of acetylcysteine in idiopathic pulmonary fibrosis. N Engl J Med. 2014;370:2093-101.
115. Sulica R, Teirstein A, Padilla ML. Lung transplantation in interstitial lung disease. Curr Opin Pulm Med. 2001;7:314-22.
116. Date H, Tanimoto Y, Goto K, Yamadori I, Aoe M, Sano Y, et al. A new treatment strategy for advanced idiopathic interstitial pneumonia: living-donor lobar lung transplantation. Chest. 2005;128:1364-70.
117. Allen S, Raut S, Woollard J, Vassallo M. Low dose diamorphine reduces breathlessness without causing a fall in oxygen saturation in elderly patients with end-stage idiopathic pulmonary fibrosis. Palliat Med. 2005;19:128-30.
118. Ghofrani HA, Wiedemann R, Rose F, Schermuly RT, Olschewski H, Weissmann N, et al. Sildenafil for treatment of lung fibrosis and pulmonary hypertension: a randomised controlled trial. Lancet. 2002;360:895-900.
119. Zisman DA, Schwarz M, Anstrom KJ, Collard HR, Flaherty KR, Hunninghake GW, et al. A controlled trial of sildenafil in advanced idiopathic pulmonary fibrosis. N Engl J Med. 2010;363:620-8.
120. King TE Jr, Behr J, Brown KK, du Bois RM, Lancaster L, de Andrade JA, et al. BUILD-1: a randomized placebo-controlled trial of bosentan in idiopathic pulmonary fibrosis. Am J Respir Crit Care Med. 2008;177:75-81.
121. King TE Jr, Brown KK, Raghu G, du Bois RM, Lynch DA, Martinez F, et al. BUILD-3: a randomized, controlled trial of bosentan in idiopathic pulmonary fibrosis. Am J Respir Crit Care Med. 2011;184:92-9.
122. Raghu G, Behr J, Brown KK, Egan JJ, Kawut SM, Flaherty KR, et al. Treatment of idiopathic pulmonary fibrosis with ambrisentan: a parallel, randomized trial. Ann Intern Med. 2013;158:641-9.
123. Raghu G, Million-Rousseau R, Morganti A, Perchenet L, Behr J; MUSIC Study Group. Macitentan for the treatment of idiopathic pulmonary fibrosis: the randomised controlled MUSIC trial. Eur Respir J. 2013;42:1622-32.

124. Corte TJ, Keir GJ, Dimopoulos K, Howard L, Corris PA, Parfitt L, et al. Bosentan in pulmonary hypertension associated with fibrotic idiopathic interstitial pneumonia. Am J Respir Crit Care Med. 2014;190:208-17.
125. Collard HR, Moore BB, Flaherty KR, Brown KK, Kaner RJ, King TE Jr, et al. Acute exacerbations of idiopathic pulmo-nary fibrosis. Am J Respir Crit Care Med. 2007;176: 636-43.
126. Agarwal R, Jindal SK. Acute exacerbation of idiopathic pulmonary fibrosis: a systematic review. Eur J Intern Med. 2008;19:227-35.
127. Saydain G, Islam A, Afessa B, Ryu JH, Scott JP, Peters SG. Outcome of patients with idiopathic pulmonary fibrosis admitted to the intensive care unit. Am J Respir Crit Care Med. 2002;166:839-42.
128. Martinez FJ, Safrin S, Weycker D, Starko KM, Bradford WZ, King TE Jr, et al. The clinical course of patients with idiopathic pulmonary fibrosis. Ann Intern Med. 2005;142:963-7.
129. Schwartz DA, Helmers RA, Galvin JR, Van Fossen DS, Frees KL, Dayton CS, et al. Determinants of survival in idiopathic pulmonary fibrosis. Am J Respir Crit Care Med. 1994;149: 450-4.
130. King TE Jr, Tooze JA, Schwarz MI, Brown KR, Cherniack RM. Predicting survival in idiopathic pulmonary fibrosis: scoring system and survival model. Am J Respir Crit Care Med. 2001;164:1171-81.

84

Chapter

Pathology of Interstitial Lung Diseases

Amanjit Bal, Kusum Joshi

INTRODUCTION

Interstitial lung disease (ILD) is a heterogeneous group and refers to a diverse range of acute, subacute and chronic diseases that produce inflammation and fibrosis of the alveoli, distal airways and septal interstitium of the lungs. The "interstitium" is a connective tissue framework, which is abundant around the airways and arteries in the center of the lobules and around the veins at the periphery. At the alveolar level, it includes the space between the epithelial and endothelial basement membranes. Its matrix consists of collagen and elastin fibers; and the cellular components include fibroblasts, myofibroblasts, histiocytes, lymphocytes, dendritic cells, Langerhans cells and mast cells. Though ILD involves the interstitium dominantly, these disorders may affect the airspaces, peripheral airways and blood vessels along with their respective epithelial and endothelial linings. Hence, an alternative term of "diffuse parenchymal lung disease" has been used to define the same group of disorders **(Box 1)**.

IDIOPATHIC INTERSTITIAL PNEUMONIA

The idiopathic interstitial pneumonias (IIPs) are a group of diffuse parenchymal diseases of unknown etiology. The American Thoracic Society or European Respiratory Society (ATS/ERS) sponsored committee comprising of the clinicians, radiologists and pathologists developed a consensus classification system in 2002 for IIPs.[1] This classification was based on the seven histopathologic patterns seen on surgical lung biopsies. The ATS or ERS 2011 classification updated the 2002 classification and grouped IIPs into two categories; major IIPs and rare IIPs. The usual interstitial pneumonia (UIP), nonspecific interstitial pneumonia (NSIP), cryptogenic organizing pneumonia (COP), acute interstitial pneumonia (AIP), respiratory bronchiolitis-associated interstitial lung disease (RB-ILD) and desquamative interstitial pneumonia (DIP) are categorized under major IIPs and the lymphoid interstitial pneumonia (LIP) which is mostly seen in association with other conditions and is rarely seen as idiopathic form has been shifted to rare IIPs. Also in the rare group a new entity pleuroparenchymal fibroelastosis (PPFE) has been added. In addition, the two rare histologic patterns of ILD have been described which includes acute fibrinous and organizing pneumonia (AFOP) and bronchiolocentric ILD (BrILD), though these are not included in the classification of IIPs.[2,3]

Pathogenesis of Idiopathic Interstitial Pneumonias

Despite intensive research, the etiology and pathogenesis of IIPs remain poorly understood. Increased number of inflammatory cells in bronchoalveolar lavage (BAL) in

BOX 1 Classification of interstitial (diffuse parenchymal) lung disease

Idiopathic interstitial pneumonias (IIPs) (ATS/ERS 2011)
- Major idiopathic interstitial pneumonias
  - Chronic fibrosing IIPs:
    - Usual interstitial pneumonia/idiopathic pulmonary fibrosis (UIP/IPF)
    - Nonspecific interstitial pneumonia (NSIP)
  - *Smoking-related IIPs:*
    - Desquamative interstitial pneumonia (DIP)
    - Respiratory bronchiolitis-associated interstitial lung disease (RB-ILD)
  - *Acute/subacute IIPs:*
    - Acute interstitial pneumonia (AIP)
    - Cryptogenic organizing pneumonia (COP)
- *Rare idiopathic interstitial pneumonias:*
  - Lymphoid interstitial pneumonia (LIP)
  - Pleuroparenchymal fibroelastosis (PPFE)

Multisystem diseases:
- Sarcoidosis
- Connective tissue disorders
- Drug reactions

Environmental and occupational diseases
- Pneumoconiosis
- Hypersensitivity pneumonitis/extrinsic allergic alveolitis

Rare lung diseases
- Lymphangioleiomyomatosis
- Pulmonary alveolar proteinosis
- Pulmonary Langerhans cell histiocytosis
- Pulmonary eosinophilia
- Idiopathic pulmonary hemosiderosis.

patients with IIPs, led to the prevailing hypothesis that the disease process begins as an "alveolitis" and progresses to interstitial fibrosis. It is speculated that chronic inflammatory process injures the lung and modulates fibrogenesis, leading to the end-stage fibrotic scar. Tansforming growth factor (TGF)-β activation which is responsible for maintaining the mesenchymal cells and regulating extracellular matrix (ECM) synthesis and degradation is a proposed key element in promoting the progression of pulmonary fibrosis.[4] Though, at present, the inflammatory cells are the principle source for fibrogenic mediators, but there is evidence that supports the essential role of activation of alveolar epithelial cells after injury. Alveolar epithelial cells are being considered as the main source of platelet-derived growth factor (PDGF), TGF-β1, tumor necrosis factor (TNF)-α, endothelin (ET)-1 and connective tissue growth factor (CTGF); the mediators implicated in pathogenesis of pulmonary fibrosis. Recently, polymorphism in the promoter region of the MUC5B gene has been shown to be associated with increase in risk of idiopathic pulmonary fibrosis (IPF) in both heterozygotes and homozygotes.[5]

Utility of Bronchoalveolar Lavage and Lung Biopsy

Bronchoalveolar lavage is useful for detecting infections as a cause of diffuse lung infiltrates. In RB-ILD, BAL demonstrates smokers' macrophages and the absence of lymphocytosis. An excess of lymphocytes can be indicative of sarcoidosis; whereas, an increase in neutrophils and eosinophils is typically found in IPF. Rarely, Langerhans cells can be identified in a case of Langerhans cell histiocytosis (LCH). Presence of hemosiderin laden macrophages indicates old hemorrhage in pulmonary hemosiderosis, vasculitis or other causes.

Lung biopsy is often required to clinch the diagnosis. Although, lung biopsy is said to be the gold standard, it is limited by the fact that only a small tissue is being sampled in a disease which is heterogeneous from area to area. Transbronchial lung biopsy is usually inadequate for the diagnosis as it samples only centrilobular areas; however, it may be of value to diagnose organizing pneumonia (OP), and RB-ILD and to exclude granulomatous lesions, neoplasms as well as infectious etiologies. Thus, surgical lung biopsy is almost always required to determine the histological pattern in IIPs. It is important to avoid areas of end-stage disease and biopsies from multiple sites provide diagnostic tissue and reduce sampling errors.

Chronic Fibrosing Idiopathic Interstitial Pneumonias

Usual Interstitial Pneumonia

Usual interstitial pneumonia is the most common of IIPs. IPF and UIP are interchangeable terms; IPF being a chronic fibrosing interstitial pneumonia of unknown cause with a surgical lung biopsy showing a histologic pattern of UIP.[6] Patients with UIP usually present with slowly progressive dyspnea and restrictive abnormalities on pulmonary function studies. High-resolution computed tomography (HRCT) shows a characteristic combination of peripheral (subpleural), irregular, linear "reticular" opacities involving predominantly the lower lung zones with associated architectural distortion in the form of traction bronchiectasis and honeycomb change. The 2011 update emphasizes the importance of a multidisciplinary approach to diagnose UIP and has introduced three levels of certainty for interpretation of HRCT; UIP, possible UIP and inconsistent with UIP. Similarly, the histologic levels of certainty were also introduced which included; UIP, "probable UIP", "possible UIP", and "not UIP".[3]

Histopathological features: Histologically UIP is a specific morphological entity defined by a combination of (i) fibrosis distributed in a heterogeneous fashion, (ii) fibroblastic foci, and (iii) honeycomb change and scars **(Figs 1A and B)**.[7] On examination at low magnification, UIP is characterized by "spatial heterogeneity" and nonuniform distribution of the inflammatory and fibrosing process **(Fig. 1C)**. These morphological changes are sharply demarcated from the adjacent normal areas. The fibrosis is more marked at the periphery and paraseptal region in the lower lobes. The other cardinal feature of UIP is the presence of active fibroblastic foci which comprises plump spindle cells with little intervening collagen. The other areas of fibrosis show poorly cellular foci with deeply eosinophilic hyalinized collagen **(Fig. 1D)**. This variation in age of fibrosis is termed as "temporal heterogeneity". The inflammatory component in UIP is usually mild-to-moderate and is composed of lymphocytes and plasma cells with occasional aggregate formation. In advanced stages, fibrosis leads to distortion of the lung parenchyma and cystic dilatation of air spaces resulting in end-stage lung or honeycomb change. The end-stage lung shows bronchiolar metaplasia of alveoli, prominence of type II pneumocytes and smooth muscle hyperplasia. These end-stage changes when florid have been termed as "muscular cirrhosis" of the lungs. Vascular changes in the scarred areas show intimal proliferation and medial hypertrophy resulting in endarteritis obliterans.

Treatment and prognosis: There is no optimal treatment for UIP. Low dose prednisolone along with immunosupression is the first-line treatment. The patients with UIP have chronically progressive disease with mean survival of 2–3 years. BAL fluid with an overall increase in cell count and excess of neutrophils has been associated with worse prognosis; however, it has no role in the management. Death is usually due to acute exacerbation, cardiac failure or lung cancer.

Nonspecific Interstitial Pneumonia

Nonspecific interstitial pneumonia which was regarded as a provisional entity in ATS or ERS 2002, has now been accepted

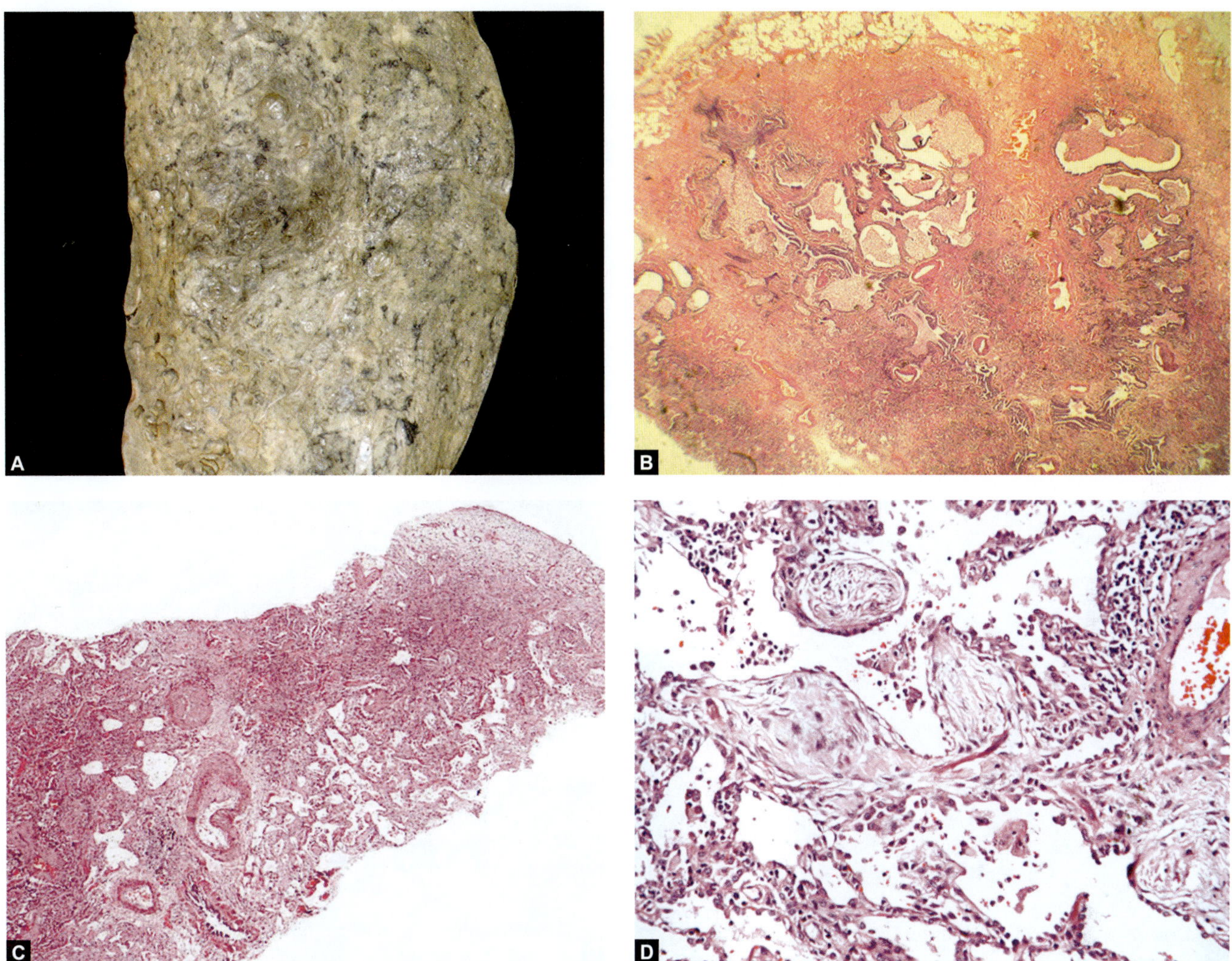

Figs 1A to D (A) Gross photograph of cut surface of the lung in usual interstitial pneumonia showing extensive peripheral honeycombing; (B) Honeycomb change in usual interstitial pneumonia characterized by enlarged airspaces lined by bronchiolar type of epithelium, surrounded by dense fibrosis and lumen filled with mucin and inflammatory cells; (C) Patchy heterogeneous inflammation and fibrosis with subpleural localization, and alternating with normal lung parenchyma in a case of usual interstitial pneumonia; (D) Fibroblastic foci composed of plump spindle-shaped fibroblasts in the interstitium and lifting the alveolar lining epithelial cells in usual interstitial pneumonia

as a specific clinicopathologic entity in the 2011 update. Nonspecific interstitial pneumonia is currently the second most common (after UIP) histopathological pattern of the IIPs and is characterized by a temporally and spatially uniform pattern that suggests that the lesions are of the same age.

Histopathological features: Nonspecific interstitial pneumonia is characterized by "temporal homogeneity". The NSIP has three major subgroups based on the amount of inflammation and/or fibrosis in the lung biopsies: *Group I (cellular NSIP):* primarily with interstitial inflammation, *Group II:* with both inflammation and fibrosis, and *Group III (fibrotic NSIP):* primarily with fibrosis.[4] The cellular end of the spectrum has mild-to-moderate interstitial inflammation comprising lymphocytes and plasma cells with minimal or no fibrosis **(Figs 2A and B)**. The fibrotic end of spectrum shows interstitial fibrosis composed of mature collagen and only a few fibroblasts **(Figs 2C and D)**. Intermediate stage of cellular and fibrotic NSIP shows mixture of inflammatory cells and collagen type fibrosis **(Fig. 2E)**. The lung architecture may appear to be lost on examination of routine hematoxylin and eosin-stained sections, but is relatively preserved with elastic stains. The NSIP lacks alveolar remodeling with honeycomb cyst formation and active fibroblastic foci distinguishing it from UIP.[8]

Treatment and prognosis: Cellular phase of NSIP is responsive to steroids and the 5-year survival is almost 100%. Survival in fibrotic phase of NSIP is variable, however, is significantly better than UIP.

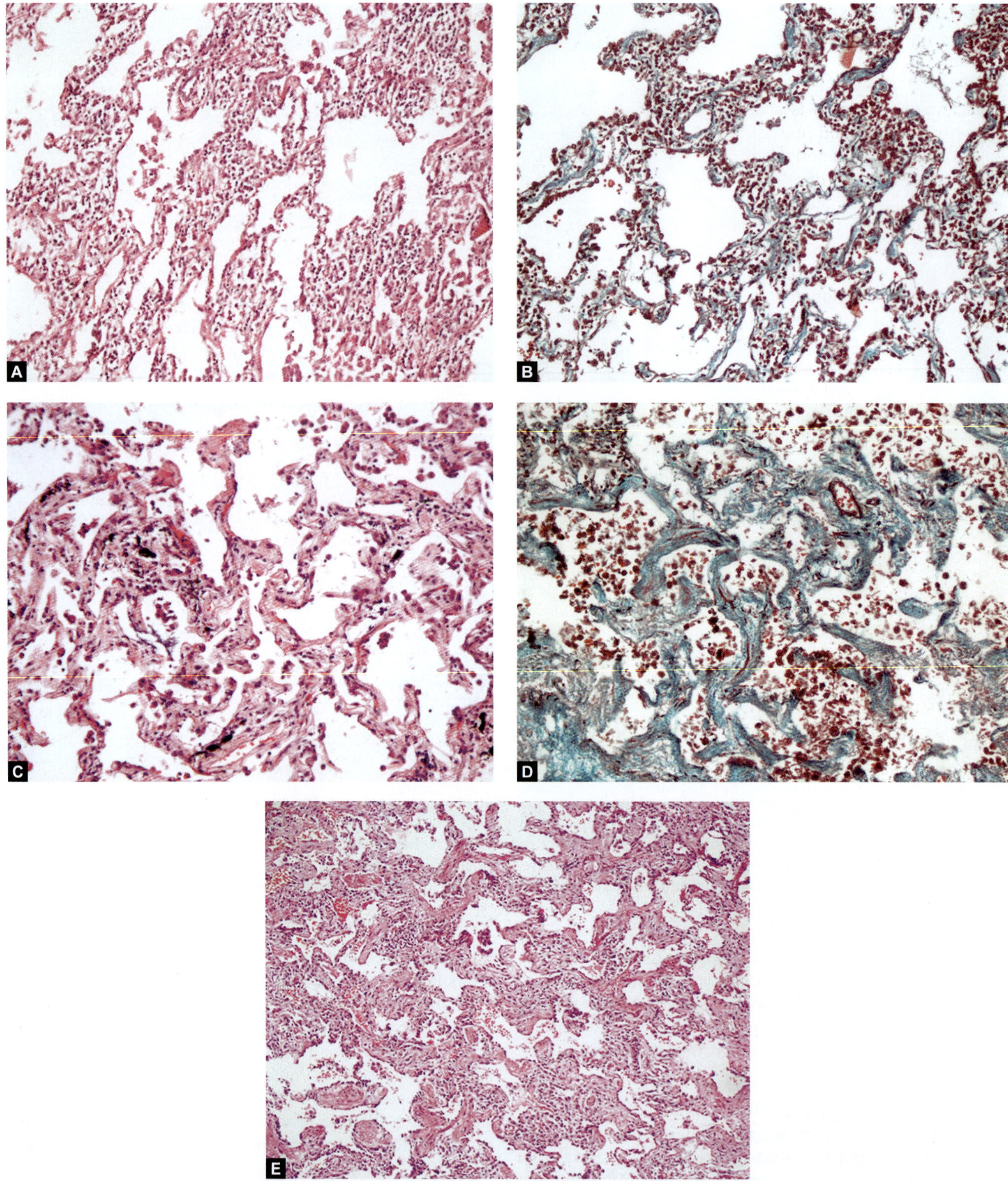

Figs 2A to E (A) Cellular nonspecific interstitial pneumonia showing diffuse interstitial infiltrate of chronic inflammatory cells with no interstitial fibrosis along with mild prominence of type II pneumocytes; (B) Masson's trichrome stain in cellular nonspecific interstitial pneumonia showing lack of interstitial fibrosis; (C) Fibrotic nonspecific interstitial pneumonia showing diffuse collagen-rich interstitial fibrosis; (D) Masson's trichrome in fibrotic nonspecific interstitial pneumonia showing interstitial fibrosis of same age without active fibroblastic foci; (E) Nonspecific interstitial pneumonia where interalveolar interstitium is thickened by the mixture of inflammatory cells and collagen type fibrosis

Subacute or Acute Idiopathic Interstitial Pneumonias

Cryptogenic Organizing Pneumonia

Organizing pneumonia is a histologic pattern of repair in response to injury and presents as subacute illness of short duration. It is characterized by air space filling fibrosing process that involves distal bronchioles, alveolar ducts and peribronchiolar alveolar spaces. Different terminologies have been used for this lesion which includes; *bronchiolitis obliterans-organizing pneumonia (BOOP)* in cases where luminal fibrosis is seen in the bronchioles as well; *COP*, a preferred term for idiopathic disease. ATS or ERS consensus classification has proposed the term *organizing pneumonia* for the histologic pattern on biopsy. Organizing pattern of ILD is also seen secondary to various underlying etiologies like infections; bacterial, viral and fungal, collagen vascular diseases (CVD) and drugs.

Histopathological features: Organizing pneumonia is characterized by patchy areas of loose fibroblastic intraluminal plugs involving alveolar ducts and alveolar spaces.[9] This process is centered on bronchioles and obliterative bronchiolitis may be seen in many cases. These intraluminal fibroblastic plugs called "Masson's bodies" are rich in mucopolysaccharides and assume the oval, elongated or serpiginous shapes of air spaces in which they are formed **(Figs 3A and B)**. The adjoining interalveolar interstitium shows varying degrees of inflammatory infiltrate. In addition there is accumulation of foamy, lipid-containing macrophages in the air spaces that represent postobstructive or endogenous lipoid pneumonia due to bronchiolar obstruction.

Treatment and prognosis: Steroid therapy is the treatment of choice for complete resolution of idiopathic organizing pneumonia. A small number of cases resolve spontaneously.

Acute Interstitial Pneumonia

Acute interstitial pneumonia is a diffuse alveolar damage (DAD) occurring in an idiopathic setting. It is a very aggressive form of ILD that may occur as an acute phase of acceleration of UIP and is also termed as Hamman-Rich disease. The AIP is the least common, rapidly progressive and histologically distinct form of interstitial pneumonia analogous to acute respiratory distress syndrome (ARDS) caused by sepsis and shock.[10] Patients with the AIP present with rapidly evolving shortness of breath and nonproductive cough of 1–3 weeks duration preceded by a flu-like illness. Most patients are severely hypoxemic at the time of diagnosis and require hospitalization and mechanical ventilation. The HRCT shows ground glass attenuation and consolidation in a bilateral and symmetrical distribution.

Histopathological features: Biopsy specimens from patients with AIP demonstrate DAD, usually in the late or organizing stage. The lung biopsy typically shows diffuse involvement, although there may be variation in the severity of the changes among different histologic fields. Alveolar septa are thickened and distorted by proliferating spindle cells (fibroblasts and myofibroblasts) within a pale-staining basophilic matrix **(Fig. 4A)**. The uniformity of the findings contrasts sharply with the heterogeneous distribution of varying abnormalities in the UIP. Fibroblast proliferation is accompanied by marked hyperplasia of type II pneumocytes which may show cytological atypia characterized by nuclear enlargement and prominent nucleoli **(Fig. 4B)**. Remnants of hyaline membranes may be present in some cases, but are often inconspicuous. Hyaline membranes are a histologic hallmark of DAD in early exudative phase and their presence is helpful in the distinction from the UIP, NSIP or organizing pneumonia patterns **(Fig. 4C)**. Thrombi in small to medium-sized pulmonary arterioles and squamous metaplasia of

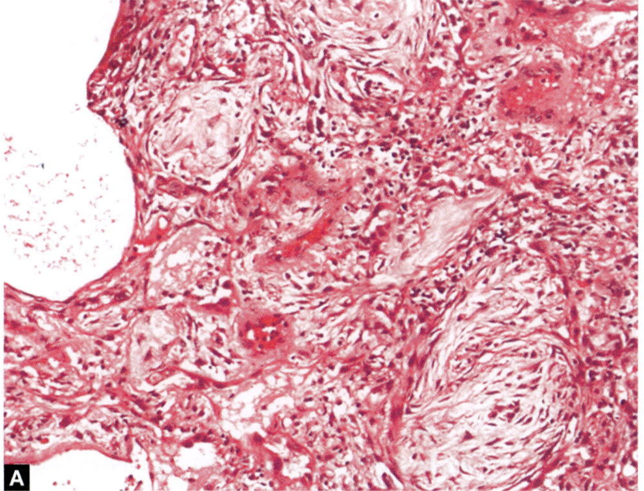

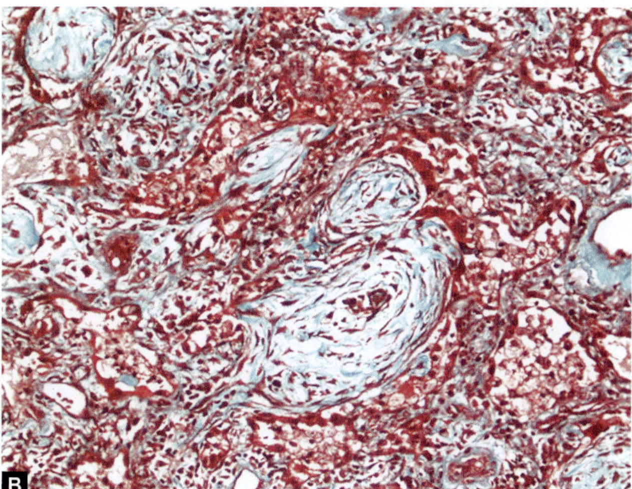

Figs 3A and B (A) Loose plugs of fibroblastic tissue, "Masson's bodies" filling the alveolar spaces in organizing pneumonia; (B) Masson's trichrome highlighting the inluminal fibroblastic plugs in organizing pneumonia

bronchiolar epithelium, which are features of acute lung injury, can provide an important clue to the diagnosis **(Fig. 4D)**.

No histological features can reliably distinguish DAD in the setting of AIP from DAD of other known causes. Therefore, before making a diagnosis of AIP, all potential causes of DAD should be excluded. The presence of granulomas, viral inclusions, foci of necrosis or neutrophilic abscesses suggest infection.

Treatment and prognosis: The AIP is associated with a poor prognosis with a mortality rate of about 70%. If the patient survives, the lungs may resolve to normal. Some cases may have repeated episodes and the lungs may progress to end-stage honeycomb fibrosis.

Smoking-related Idiopathic Interstitial Pneumonias

In spite of the strong association with smoking, RB-ILD and DIP were retained in the updated classification of IIP's.

Respiratory Bronchiolitis-associated Interstitial Lung Disease

Respiratory bronchiolitis-associated ILD is the clinical manifestation of ILD associated with the pathologic lesion of respiratory bronchiolitis. Nearly, all patients have strong history of cigarette smoking, thus RB-ILD is being considered as a smoking-related ILD. It is rarely symptomatic and is usually associated with no more than minor small airway

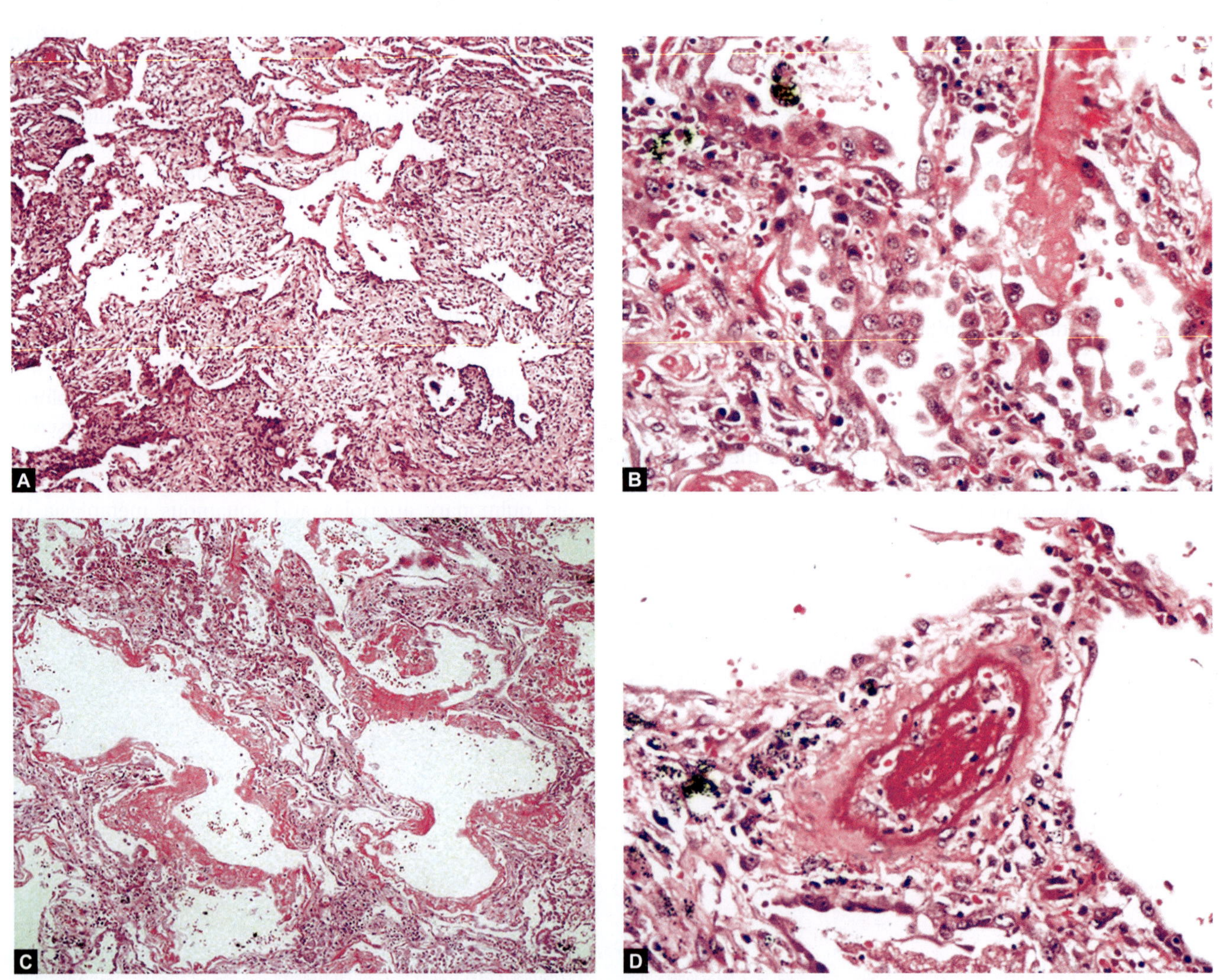

Figs 4A to D (A) Organizing phase of acute interstitial pneumonia-marked interstitial thickening by prominent fibroblast proliferation and scanty inflammatory infiltrate; (B) Proliferation and prominence of type 2 pneumocytes in acute interstitial pneumonia. The lining cells are hobnail shaped and have prominent nucleoli; (C) Exudative phase of acute interstitial pneumonia showing hyaline membranes lining alveolar ducts and alveolar spaces. The alveolar septa are thickened by interstitial edema; (D) Fibrin thrombi in small vessels in acute interstitial pneumonia

dysfunction. In rare cases, the condition presents as a form of ILD with significant pulmonary symptoms, abnormal pulmonary function, and imaging abnormalities; it is then described as RB-ILD.[11] The HRCT shows patchy ground glass opacities and centrilobular nodules often with a lower lung zone distribution, without fibrotic scars and honeycomb change.

Histopathological features: In respiratory bronchiolitis the changes are patchy at low magnification and have a bronchiolocentric distribution. Respiratory bronchioles, alveolar ducts, and peribronchiolar alveolar spaces contain clusters of pigmented (smoker's) macrophages **(Fig. 5)**. The macrophages have abundant cytoplasm containing finely granular dusty brown pigment that stains faintly with Perl's stain. Mild peribronchiolar fibrosis is also seen that radiates to and expands contiguous alveolar septa, which are lined by hyperplastic type II pneumocytes. It is also frequently associated with the presence of centrilobular emphysema and this pattern is termed as combined pulmonary fibrosis and emphysema (CPFE).

Desquamative Interstitial Pneumonia

Desquamative interstitial pneumonia is a rare form of ILD that affects smokers and is characterized by desquamation of alveolar macrophages with minimal fibrosis. Previously the intra-alveolar cells were thought to represent alveolar epithelial cells that had desquamated from alveolar septa. This condition is considered by many to represent the end of a spectrum of RB-ILD in view of its similar pathology and almost invariable association with cigarette smoke.[12]

Histopathological features: The DIP pattern is characterized by diffuse involvement of the lungs by numerous macrophage accumulations within most of the distal airspaces **(Fig. 6)**. The alveolar macrophages form loose clusters and have round nuclei with abundant eosinophilic cytoplasm containing golden brown pigment that stains weakly with Perl's stain. The alveolar septa are thickened by a sparse inflammatory infiltrate that often includes plasma cells and occasional eosinophils, and they are lined by plump type II pneumocytes. The main feature that distinguishes DIP from RB-ILD is that the former affects the lung in a uniform diffuse manner and lacks the bronchiolocentric distribution seen in RB-ILD.

DIP-like reactions: Areas resembling RB-ILD and DIP are commonly seen as incidental findings in cigarette smokers with other lung diseases. No histological changes can reliably separate patients with RB-ILD or DIP from those with other lung diseases in whom RB and "DIP-like reactions" represent incidental findings. Thus, RB-ILD or DIP should be diagnosed only when other forms of ILD have been excluded by careful examination of the surgical lung biopsy, clinical features and radiological findings.

Rare Idiopathic Interstitial Pneumonias

Lymphoid Interstitial Pneumonia

Lymphoid interstitial pneumonia usually occurs in association with connective tissue diseases, autoimmune diseases, or HIV infection and is rarely idiopathic, thus it has been shifted to the category of rare IIPs.[2] It is characterized by the expansion of the interstitium by sheets of lymphoid cells that are histologically benign and immunophenotypically polyclonal. Most of the cases previously diagnosed as LIP are now considered as cellular NSIP.

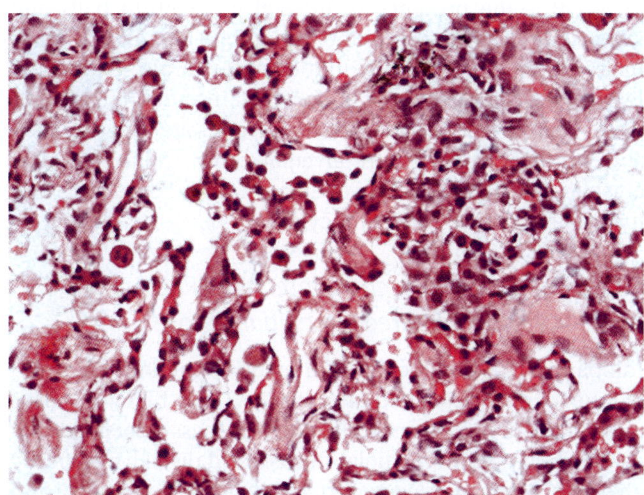

Fig. 5 Respiratory bronchiolitis associated interstitial lung disease showing collection of smoker's macrophages in respiratory bronchiole and adjoining alveolar spaces

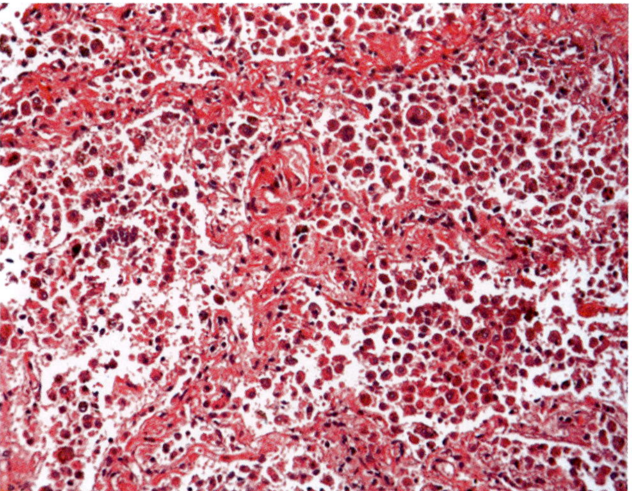

Fig. 6 Desquamative interstitial pneumonia showing diffuse distribution of macrophages in alveolar spaces. Macrophages have abundant eosinophilic cytoplasm with granular brown pigment

Histopathological features: LIP is defined as a dense and diffuse interstitial lymphoid infiltrate, comprising lymphocytes, plasma cells, and histiocytes **(Fig. 7)**. The alveolar septa should be extensively infiltrated and lymphoid follicles including follicles with germinal centers are often present. Some architectural derangement (including honeycombing) and non-necrotizing granulomas may be seen. The pertinent negative findings are lack of tracking along lymphatic routes (bronchovascular bundles, pleura, and interlobular septa) which are characteristic of lymphomas, inconspicuous or absent organizing pneumonia, lack of Dutcher bodies, lack of monoclonality on immunohistochemistry for light chains, lack of extensive pleural involvement or lymph node involvement and lack of necrotizing granuloma.[1,13]

The differential diagnosis for LIP includes diffuse lymphoid hyperplasia [hyperplasia of bronchial mucosa-associated lymphoid tissue (BALT))] nodular lymphoid hyperplasia, lymphoma (of mucosa-associated lymphoid tissue or small lymphocytic types), and the patterns of OP, NSIP, hypersensitivity pneumonitis (HP) and UIP.[1] The hypersensitivity pneumonitis tends to have lesser inflammation, a peribronchiolar distribution, poorly formed granulomas and intraluminal organizing fibrosis. The bronchus-associated lymphoid tissue differs from LIP in that it lacks extensive alveolar septal infiltration. Malignant lymphomas show a monomorphic population of lymphoid cells with destruction of alveolar architecture, pleural infiltration, and tracking along lymphatic routes.

Pleuroparenchymal Fibroelastosis

Pleuroparenchymal fibroelastosis is a rare and recently described entity characterized by fibrotic thickening of the pleura and subpleural parenchyma dominantly involving the upper lobes.[14] The upper lobes are always more severely involved, whereas the involvement of the lower lobes is absent or show less severe fibrosis. These patients are prone to the development of secondary spontaneous pneumothoraces and persistent postoperative bronchopleural fistulae. The etiology and pathogenesis of this entity remains unknown.

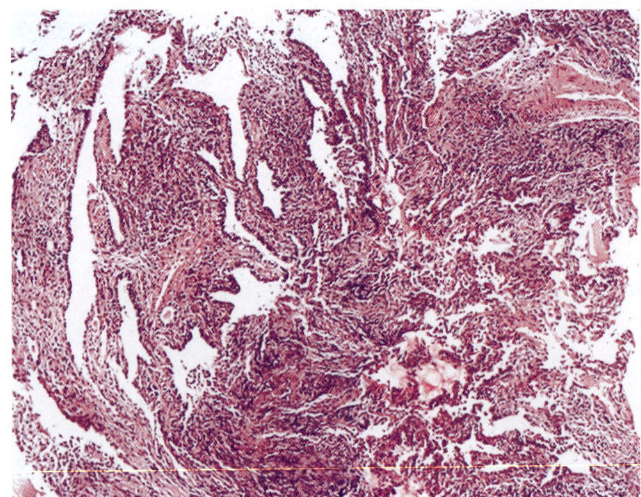

Fig. 7 Lymphocytic interstitial pneumonia showing diffuse dense lymphomononuclear cell infiltrate in the interstitium

Histopathological features: It is characterized by markedly thickened visceral pleura and prominent subpleural fibrosis which is composed of both elastic tissue and dense collagen. This differs from the usual forms of fibrosis, which almost invariably shows predominance of collagen. This lesion is rich in randomly oriented elastic fibers which can be demonstrated with the help of special stains like elastic Van Gieson (EVG) stain and can be differentiated from UIP which has collagenous fibrosis. The demarcation between fibrotic areas and adjacent lung parenchyma is abrupt. Mostly the distant lung parenchyma is spared of fibrotic process.

Treatment: Currently, there is no effective treatment and the only available option for these patients is the lung transplantation.

Rare Histologic Patterns

Acute Fibrinous and Organizing Pneumonia

Acute fibrinous and organizing pneumonia is a pattern of acute lung injury used for cases which do not meet the criteria for classical patterns of acute lung injury, i.e. DAD or organizing pneumonia.[15] The potential underlying etiologies for AFOP are many and range from drugs, infection, connective tissue disorders (CTDs) to idiopathic. Patients present with acute and subacute respiratory symptoms. The mortality rate is similar to that of DAD, therefore, AFOP is thought to represent its poorly described histologic variant.

Histopathological features: The dominant histological feature of AFOP is the presence of intra-alveolar fibrin balls and absence of hyaline membrane formation **(Fig. 8)**. The fibrin balls can be patchy in distribution but can also be diffuse. Evidence of organization in form of intraluminal fibrous plugs composed of loose connective tissue can be seen surrounding cores of intra-alveolar fibrin. Adjacent inter-alveolar interstitum shows edema, mild inflammation and hyperplasia of type II pneumocytes.

Idiopathic Bronchiolocentric Interstitial Pneumonia (BrIP) or Airway-centered Interstitial Fibrosis

Idiopathic bronchiolocentric interstitial pneumonia (BrIP) is a new entity described after 2002 ATS or ERS consensus classification. It is a bronchiolocentric process associated with centrilobular peribronchiolar fibrosis and distal lymphocytic alveolitis.[16] Studies have reported female predominance and history of inhalational exposure to smoke, birds, cotton and agrochemicals. Chest radiographs and HRCT show bilateral dominant lower lobe reticular and reticulonodular infiltrates.

Histopathological features: The most striking finding is the centrilobular and bronchiolocentric nature of inflammatory infiltrate with relative sparing of the subpleural and peripheral lung parenchyma.[17,18] The inflammation extends into the peribronchiolar alveolar septa and distal interstitium of the acinus and is accompanied by peribronchiolar fibrosis and bronchiolar metaplasia **(Figs 9A and B)**. There is ingrowth of bronchiolar epithelium along the alveolar ducts to alveoli through canal of Lambert. This process of bronchiolar metaplasia of alveolar lining is termed as "lambertosis' or "microscopic honeycomb change". BrIP has histologic similarity to hypersensitivity pneumonia with a higher degree of centrilobular fibrosis and absent granulomas. It can hypothesized that BrIP represents chronic hypersensitivity pneumonia.

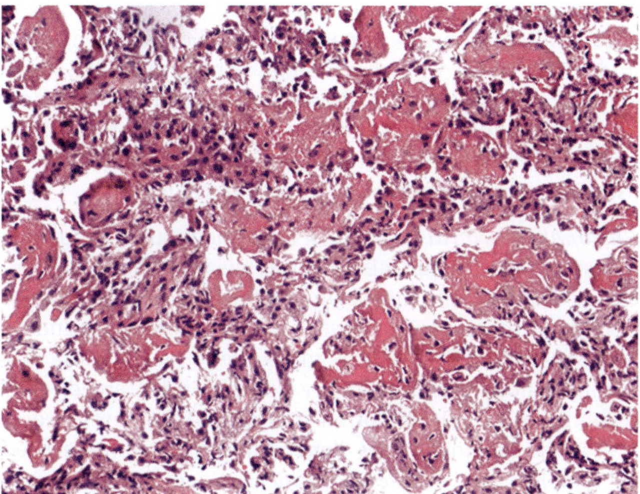

Fig. 8 Acute fibrinous and organizing pneumonia showing presence of intra-alveolar fibrin balls and absence of hyaline membrane formation

Treatment and prognosis: Bronchiolocentric interstitial pneumonia in contrast to other centrilobular ILD, i.e. RB-ILD and hypersensitivity pneumonia has significantly poor prognosis with persistent or progressive disease. On a 4-year follow up 33% patients died of the disease and 56% patients had a persistent or progressive disease.[18]

DRUG-INDUCED INTERSTITIAL LUNG DISEASE

An increasing number of drugs are recognized to induce distinctive patterns of ILD, ranging from benign infiltrates to life-threatening adult respiratory distress syndromes. In addition to drugs, biomolecules such as proteins and cytokines, and medicinal plants are also capable of inducing respiratory disease. A list of drugs having the potential to cause pulmonary disease continues to grow and now at least 350 agents are recognized **(Table 1)**.[19]

A carefully obtained history that includes medications is essential to suspecting a drug-induced reaction. A major, but largely unresolved question is why, out of the treated population of patients, only some individuals will develop drug-induced interstitial lung disease (DI-ILD). Explanations for the unequal risks among patients include the following (i) prior respiratory reactions to the drug, or to unrelated compounds, (ii) type of underlying disease for which the drug is being given. Diseases such as rheumatoid arthritis (RA) or ulcerative colitis may increase the relative risk of developing respiratory disease from disease modifying drugs, (iii) occupational factors, such as exposure to asbestos, may potentiate the noxious respiratory effects of ergot drugs, and (iv) activation and detoxication pathways of drugs and chemicals, which differ quantitatively and qualitatively among individuals.

Drug-induced pulmonary diseases can present in a variety of syndromes, clinical presentations, and radiographic

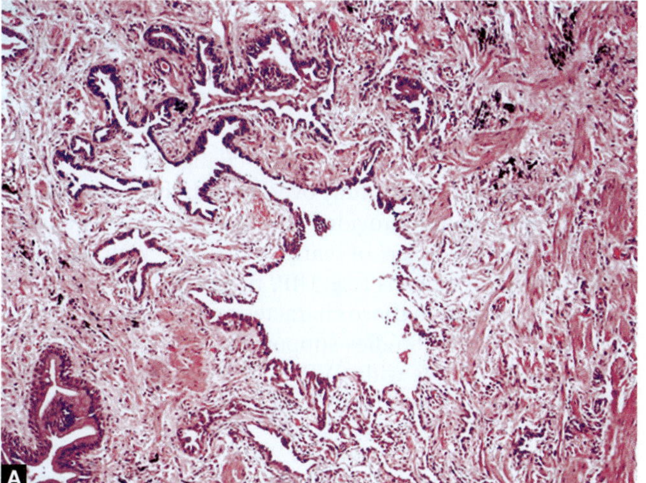

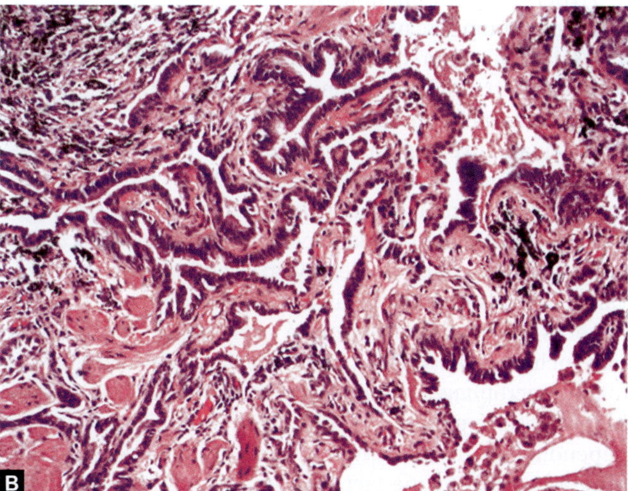

Figs 9A and B (A) Bronchiolocentric interstitial pneumonia showing interstitial fibrosis and bronchiolar metaplasia of the adjoining alveolar spaces termed as lambertosis; (B) Higher power showing metaplastic bronchiolar epithelium in bronchiolocentric interstitial pneumonia

Table 1 Drugs known to cause interstitial lung disease

Action	Drugs
Anticonvulsant, antipsychotic, antidepressant	Carbamazepine, chlordiazepoxide, fluoxetine Phenothiazines, phenytoin
Anti-inflammatory	Aspirin, gold, methotrexate, penicillamine
Antimetabolic	Azathioprine, cytarabine, fludarabine Gemcitabine, 6-mercaptopurine
Antimicrobial	Amphotericin B, ethambutol, isoniazid Minocycline, nitrofurantoin
Biologic response modifiers	Granulocyte-macrophage colony-stimulating factor, interferon, interleukin-2, tumor necrosis factor
Cardiovascular	Amiodarone, angiotensin-converting enzyme inhibitors, anticoagulants
Chemotherapeutic and immunosuppressive	Bleomycin, busulfan, chlorambucil cyclophosphamide, cyclosporin A
Illicit drugs	Cocaine, heroin, methadone, methylphenidate narcotic and sedative drugs

patterns. The most common presentations of drug-induced pulmonary disease are an abnormality on a chest radiograph or a symptom complex.

Clinicoradiological patterns: The clinicoradiological correlates of DI-ILD range from subclinical opacities to a picture of white lungs with the criteria of ARDS. In the patient with migratory opacities with or without chest pain that could be suggestive of organizing pneumonia, a careful drug history should be taken, as this clinical pattern may relate to exposure to drugs, or radiation. Transient infiltrates have been described in mild form of DI-ILD.

Pathology: Reports of DI-ILD in which histological data were obtained indicate that drugs can induce many distinctive histopathological patterns of ILD.[20] Drugs can trigger the development of such conventional patterns of ILD as:

- Hypersensitivity pneumonia
- Mild eosinophilic pneumonia
- Nonspecific interstitial pneumonia (cellular or fibrotic)
- Usual interstitial pneumonia
- Organizing pneumonia (or BOOP)
- Desquamative interstitial pneumonia.

While some drugs (e.g. minocycline, nitrofurantoin) induce quite stereotyped reactions in the lung (eosinophilic pneumonia and the cellular type of NSIP, respectively) other drugs (e.g. amiodarone, bleomycin), can induce a palette of variegated histopathological patterns in different patients. Patterns described under the term "amiodarone pneumonitis" may include NSIP (cellular or fibrotic type), alveolar filling by foamy macrophages, organizing pneumonia, DAD, interstitial lung fibrosis, a pattern of "UIP", or any combination thereof depending on the patient. A notable clue that suggests the drug as a cause is the fact that the ILD will demonstrate a relative refractoriness to steroids, or will recur while the patient is still receiving relatively high dosages of steroids. Early diagnosis is important, because stopping the drug usually reverses toxicity, whereas unrecognized toxicity can be progressive and even fatal.

CONNECTIVE TISSUE DISORDERS-ASSOCIATED INTERSTITIAL LUNG DISEASE

The connective tissue disorders (CTDs) comprise a heterogeneous group of diseases including rheumatoid arthritis, systemic sclerosis, polymyositis or dermatomyositis (PM/DM), systemic lupus erythematosus (SLE), Sjogren's syndrome and mixed connective tissue disorders. Pulmonary complications are commonly associated with CTDs and can affect various anatomical compartments of the lung (airways, vasculature, interstitium, pleura, etc.) either individually or in combination. The reported prevalence of clinically overt pulmonary parenchymal disease ranges from 30% in patients with PM or DM to 10% in patients with Sjogren's syndrome and 5% in those with rheumatoid arthritis and SLE.[21] On some occasions, the lung disease precedes the more typical systemic manifestations and the evolution of the pulmonary disease is independent from the systemic disease and is associated with greater mortality and morbidity.

Rheumatoid arthritis-associated ILD: Rheumatoid arthritis is a destructive systemic inflammatory disorder that is defined by its characteristic attack on diarthroidal joints. A major portion of rheumatoid arthritis's disease burden, including the excess mortality, appears to be due to its extra-articular manifestations and pulmonary complications are directly responsible for 10–20% of all mortality. The prevalence of ILD in rheumatoid varies depending on the criteria used to establish the diagnosis. Clinically significant ILD has been described in approximately 7% of subjects, whereas autopsy studies have described a prevalence of up to 35%.[22] Histopathological patterns of ILD associated with RA include: UIP, followed by NSIP (cellular and fibrotic), and rarely DAD, OP and LIP. Other respiratory manifestations of RA include; rheumatoid nodules, follicular bronchiolitis and pulmonary arterial hypertension.

In rheumatoid arthritis, UIP pattern is more commonly seen on surgical lung biopsy than NSIP.[23] In RA-ILD, cellular inflammatory, fibrosing, and mixed changes are seen, and these pathologic patterns fully overlap with those seen in the IIPs. The information provided by these pathologic patterns is important predictor of early mortality, with patterns characterized by fibrosis (e.g. UIP, fibrosing NSIP) having a worse prognosis than those characterized by cellular disease (e.g. cellular NSIP). Studies support the hypothesis that the prognosis of subjects with CVD-ILD, and particularly those with CVD-UIP, is better than that of patients with idiopathic UIP.

Systemic lupus erythematosis: Parenchymal lung lesions especially NSIP and LIP are more common in SLE as compared to extensive fibrotic lesions seen in other CVDs.

Less commonly, the pathological changes include alveolar hemorrhages with associated expansion and destruction of alveolar septa by capillaritis. In addition, variety of pulmonary vascular changes like intimal thickening, medial hypertrophy and periadventitial fibrosis have been reported.

Polymyositis or dermatomyositis: NSIP and OP are the most common patterns of ILD associated with PM or DM. Antibodies against aminoacyl-tRNA synthetases (anti-synthetases) have been linked to ILD. The presence of one of the anti-synthetases, in association with PM, arthritis and ILD, is the hallmark of the anti-synthetase syndrome, in which ILD is responsible for a 40% excess mortality.[24]

Sjogren's syndrome: Lymphocytic interstitial pneumonia and amyloidosis are the most common pattern of ILD associated with Sjogren's syndrome.

HYPERSENSITIVITY PNEUMONITIS

Hypersensitivity pneumonitis (HP) also known as extrinsic allergic alveolitis is an ILD caused by immunological response to inhalation of organic substances and certain inorganic chemicals. Chronic hypersensitivity pneumonitis is considered as the most important differential diagnosis of IIPs. It is thought to result from combination of type III (immune complex) and type IV (cell-mediated) immune reactions.[25] The main etiological agents include thermophilic bacteria, fungi and animal proteins. The most common occupation related hypersensitivity pneumonitis is farmer's lung followed by air conditioner lung, humidifier lung and pigeon breeder's lung. Hypersensitivity pneumonitis may present in three forms: acute, subacute, and chronic depending upon the intensity and frequency of exposure. HRCT findings include centrilobular nodular opacities and areas of ground glass attenuation.

Histopathological features: The diagnostic features of hypersensitivity pneumonitis include triad of patchy nonspecific interstitial pneumonia with peribronchiolar attenuation, nonnecrotizing granulomas and foci of bronchiolitis obliterans **(Fig. 10)**. The inflammatory infiltrate is composed of lymphocytes and plasma cells present around bronchioles and extending into alveolar septa. The granulomas are interstitial, poorly formed and composed of epithelioid histiocytes and Langhans' giant cells. In absence of granulomas, the morphological changes can resemble cellular NSIP, thus requiring careful identification of specific antigen.

Treatment and prognosis: The therapeutic strategy for hypersensitivity pneumonitis is avoidance of offending agent. The prognosis depends upon the amount and reversibility of damage.

LYMPHANGIOLEIOMYOMATOSIS

Pulmonary lymphangioleiomyomatosis is a rare disease characterized by haphazard proliferation of immature myoid cells throughout the interstitium of the lung. Lymphangioleiomyomatosis is currently classified by the WHO under the broad group of tumors known as perivascular epithelioid cell tumors (PEComas), derived from perivascular epithelioid cells (PECs).[26] The PEC cells are perivascular cells with myoid features characterized by positivity for smooth muscle actin, HMB45 and Melan A immunostains. It occurs exclusively in women during reproductive years of life, either sporadically or in association with tuberous sclerosis. Patients present with progressive dyspnea, chylous pleural effusions and recurrent pneumothoraces. Radiological examination shows diffuse reticular or reticulonodular shadows. Thin walled cystic spaces seen on HRCT are highly suggestive of LAM.

Histopathological features: Gross appearance of lungs in LAM is characteristic and shows multiple air filled cysts **(Fig. 11A)**. Microscopically, cystic change is the striking feature. There is randomly distributed proliferation of immature smooth muscle cells in the interstitium **(Fig. 11B)**, around bronchioles, blood vessels, lymphatics, alveolar septa and walls of cystic spaces. These myoid cells are positive for smooth muscle actin **(Fig. 11C)**, HMB45 and Melan A **(Fig. 11D)**.

Treatment and prognosis: Since estrogen and progesterone receptor antigens have been identified in some cases of LAM, hormonal treatment has been advocated. Lymphangioleiomyomatosis is a slowly progressive disease with 5-year survival ranging from 50–80%.

PULMONARY LANGERHANS CELL HISTIOCYTOSIS

Pulmonary LCH, also known as pulmonary eosinophilic granuloma and pulmonary histiocytosis X is characterized

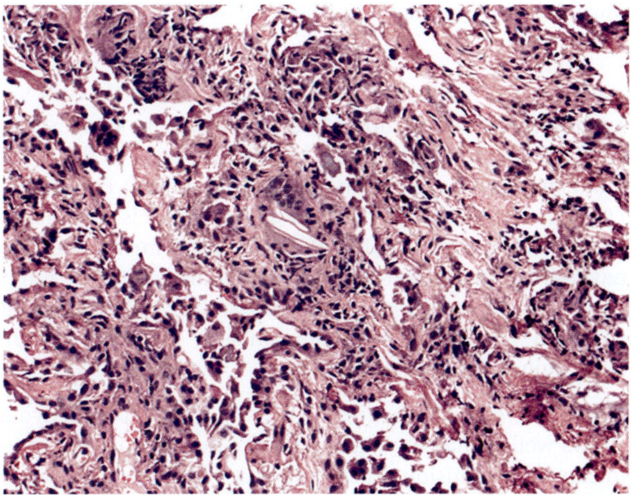

Fig. 10 Hypersensitivity pneumonia showing patchy nonspecific interstitial inflammation with peribronchiolar attenuation, and ill-formed non-necrotizing granuloma

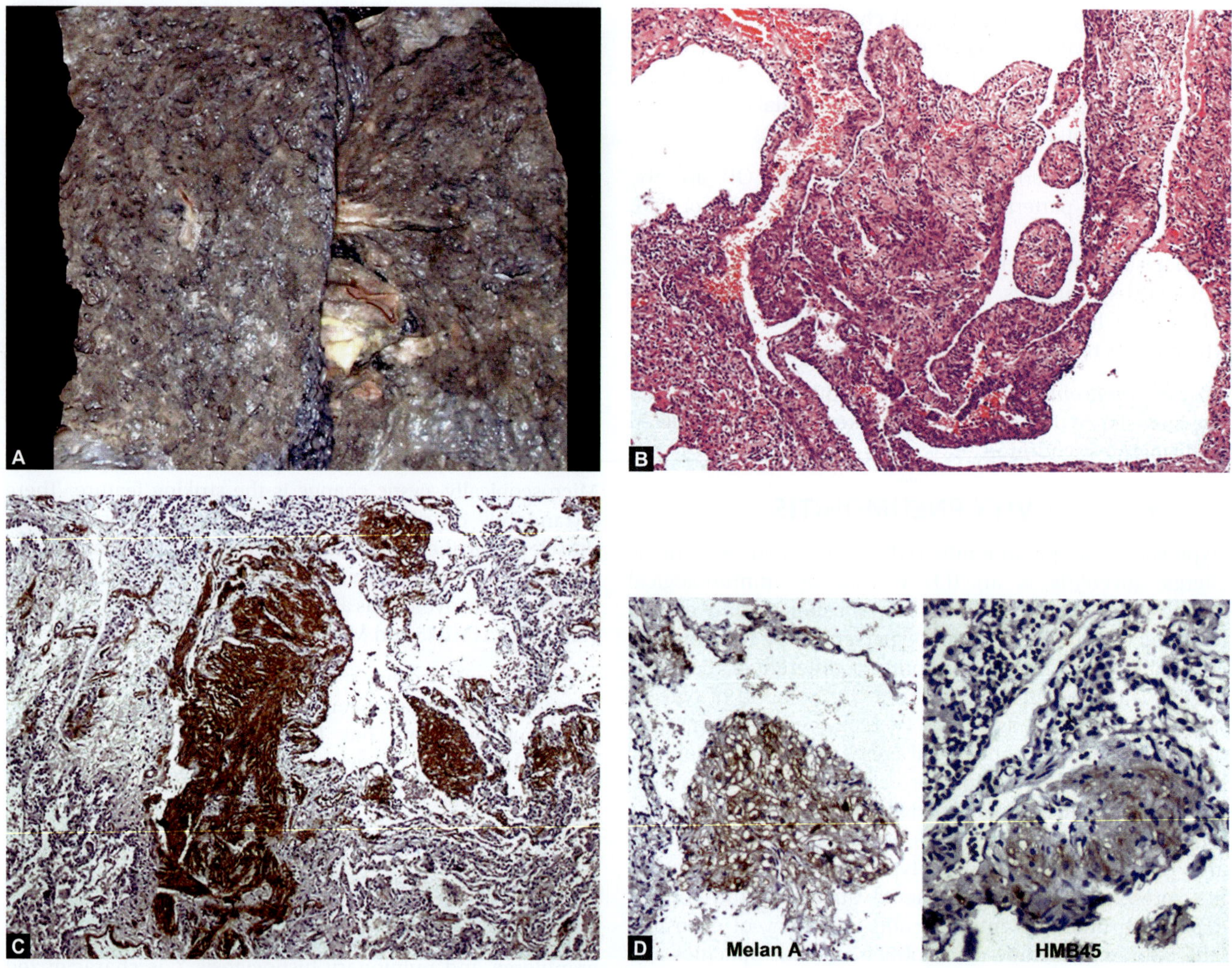

Figs11A to D (A) Lymphangioleiomyomatosis; gross showing innumerable cysts throughout the lung; (B) Varying smooth muscle cell proliferation in the wall of cystic spaces in lymphangioleiomyomatosis; (C) Smooth muscle cells positive for smooth muscle actin in lymphangioleiomyomatosis; (D) Smooth muscle cells positive for Melan A and HMB45 in lymphangioleiomyomatosis

by abnormal proliferation of Langerhans cells. Langerhans cells are dendritic or antigen presenting cells of the body that express CD1a, langerin and S-100 protein.[27] Pulmonary LCH has been linked to cigarette smoking and is considered as smoking-associated ILD of adults. Experimental studies have shown increased number of dendritic cells in lungs chronically exposed to cigarette smoke.[28,29] The most common presenting symptoms include dyspnea, cough, chest pain, fever and hemoptysis.

Histopathological features: Grossly lung parenchyma shows well-demarcated grayish white nodules of 1–2 cm in maximum dimension. In chronic phases there is pulmonary fibrosis, cystic change and honeycombing. The characteristic microscopic feature is nodular aggregates of Langerhans cells in the interstitium **(Fig.12A)**. These cells have pale convoluted nuclei with small nucleoli, pale eosinophilic cytoplasm and ill-defined cell borders **(Fig. 12B)**. These cells are associated with other inflammatory cells like lymphocytes, plasma cells and eosinophils. These Langerhans cells are positive for S-100 **(Fig. 12C)** and CD1a immunostains. The adjacent lung parenchyma shows interstitial fibrosis and alveolar cell hyperplasia. With the evolution of the disease, fibrosis evolves and cellular nodules are replaced by stellate fibrous nodules.

Treatment and prognosis: Cessation of smoking and prednisone is effective in controlling the signs and symptoms of LCH.

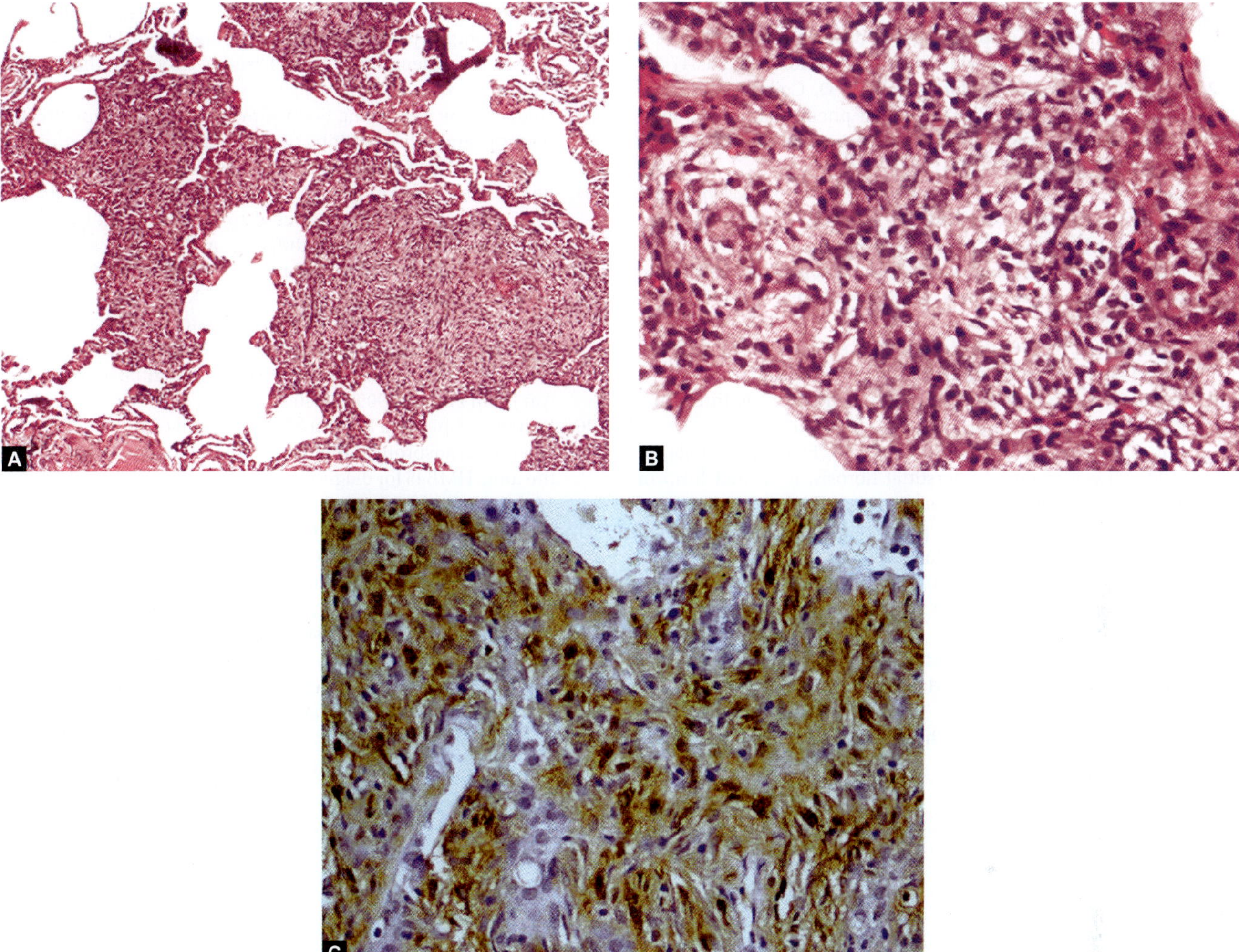

Figs 12A to C (A) Nodules of Langerhans cell histiocytosis admixed with other inflammatory cells; (B) High-power showing Langerhans cells pale nuclear chromatin and convoluted nuclear membranes, admixed with lymphocytes and plasma cells; (C) S-100 immunostain highlighting Langerhans histiocytosis cells

REFERENCES

1. American Thoracic Society, European Respiratory Society. International Multidisciplinary Consensus Classification of the Idiopathic Interstitial Pneumonias. Am J Respir Crit Care Med. 2002;165:277-304.
2. Antoniou KM, Margaritopoulos GA, Tomassetti S, Bonella F, Costabe U, Poletti V. Interstitial lung disease. Eur Respir Rev. 2014;23:40-54.
3. Travis WD, Costabe U, Hansell DM, King TE, Lynch DA, Nicholson AG, et al. An official American Thoracic Society/ European Respiratory Society Statement: Update of the International Multidisciplinary Classification of the Idiopathic Interstitial Pneumonias. Am J Respir Crit Care. Med. 2013;188(6):733-48.
4. WANG Zeng-li. Advances in understanding of idiopathic pulmonary fibrosis. Chin Med J. 2009;122(7):844-57.
5. Seibold MA, Wise AL, Speer MC, Steele MP, Brown KK, Loyd JE, et al. A common MUC5B promoter polymorphism and pulmonary fibrosis. N Engl J Med. 2011;364:1503-12.
6. Myers JL, Katzenstein Ala. Beyond a consensus classification for idiopathic interstitial pneumonias: progress and controversies. Histopathology. 2009;54:90-103.
7. Bourke SJ. Interstitial lung disease: progress and problems. Postgrad Med J. 2006;82:494-9.
8. Martinez FJ. Idiopathic Interstitial Pneumonias; Usual interstitial pneumonia versus nonspecific interstitial pneumonia. Proc Am Thorac Soc. 2006;3(1):81-95.
9. Visscher DW, Myers JL. Histologic spectrum of idiopathic interstitial pneumonias. Proc Am Thorac Soc. 2006;3:322-9.
10. Avnon LS, Pikovsky O, Sion-Vardy N, Almog Y. Acute interstitial pneumonia–Hamman-Rich syndrome: clinical characteristics and diagnostic and therapeutic considerations. Anesth Analg. 2009;108:232-7.

11. Fraig M, Shreesha U, Savici D, Katzenstein AL. Respiratory bronchiolitis: a clinicopathologic study in current smokers, ex-smokers, and never smokers. Am J Surg Pathol. 2002;26:647-53.
12. Craig PJ, Wells AU, Doffman S, Rassl D, Colby TV, Hansell DM, et al. Desquamative interstitial pneumonia, respiratory bronchiolitis and their relationship to smoking. Histopathology. 2004;45:275-82.
13. Cha SI, Fessler MB, Cool CD, Schwarz MI, Brown KK. Lymphoid interstitial pneumonia: clinical features, associations and prognosis. Eur Respir J. 2006;28:364-9.
14. Beasley MB. Classification of idiopathic interstitial pneumonias: what is new since 2002? Diagn Histopathol. 2013;19:8;267-72.
15. Hernandez-Prera JC, Beasley MB. Novel patterns of interstitial lung disease. Diagn Histopathol. 2013;19:8;276-81.
16. Yousem SA, Dacic S. Idiopathic Bronchiolocentric Interstitial Pneumonia. Mod Pathol. 2002;15(11):1148-53.
17. Churg A, Myers J, Suarez T, Gaxiola M, Estrada A, Mejia M, et al. Airway-centered interstitial fibrosis; a distinct form of aggressive diffuse lung disease. Am J Surg Pathol. 2004;28:62-8.
18. Rice A, Nicholson AG. The pathologist's approach to small airways disease. Histopathology. 2009;54:117-33.
19. Camus P, Foucher P, Bonniaud P, Ask K. Drug-induced infiltrative lung disease. Eur Respir J Suppl. 2001;18 (Suppl. 32):93s-100s.
20. Özkan M, Dweik RA, Ahmad M. Drug-induced lung disease. Cleveland Clinic Journal of Medicine. 2001;68:762-95.
21. Tansey D, Wells AU, Colby TV, Ip S, Nikolakoupolou A, du Bois RM, et al. Variations in histological patterns of interstitial pneumonia between connective tissue disorders and their relationship to prognosis. Histopathology. 2004;44:585-96.
22. Brown KK. Rheumatoid Lung Disease. Proc Am Thorac Soc. 2007;4:443-8.
23. Hyun-Kyung Lee, Dong Soon Kim, Bin Yoo. Histopathologic pattern and clinical interstitial lung disease features of rheumatoid arthritis-associated. Chest. 2005;127;2019-27.
24. de Lauretis A, Veeraraghavan S, Renzoni E. Aspects of interstitial lung disease: connective tissue disease-associated interstitial lung disease: how does it differ from IPF? How should the clinical approach differ? Chron Respir Dis. 2011;8:53-82.
25. Akashi T, Takemura T, Ando N, Eishi Y, Kitagawa M, Takizawa T, et al. Histopathologic analysis of sixteen autopsy cases of chronic hypersensitivity pneumonitis and comparison with idiopathic pulmonary fibrosis/usual interstitial pneumonia. Am J Clin Pathol. 2009;131:405-15.
26. Bonetti F, Chiodera PL, Pea M, Martignoni G, Bosi F, Zamboni G, et al. Transbronchial biopsy in lymphangiomyomatosis of the lung. HMB45 for diagnosis. Am J Surg Pathol. 1993;17:1092-102.
27. Yousem SA, Colby TV, Chen YY, Chen WG, Weiss LM. Pulmonary Langerhans' cell histiocytosis: molecular analysis of clonality. Am J Surg Pathol. 2001;25:630-6.
28. Vassalo R, Ryu JH, Colby TV, Hartman T, Limper AH. Pulmonary Langerhans cell histiocytosis. N Engl J Med. 2000;342:1969-78.
29. Sundar KM, Gosselin MV, Chung HL, Cahill BC. Pulmonary Langerhans cell histiocytosis: emerging concepts in pathobiology, radiology, and clinical evolution of disease. Chest. 2003;123:1673-83.

Idiopathic Interstitial Pneumonias

Hidenobu Shigemitsu, Ngozi Orjioke, Carmen Luraschi-Monjagatta

INTRODUCTION

Pulmonary interstitium is defined as the loose connective tissue surrounding the alveolar spaces. It consists of alveolar epithelium, pulmonary capillary endothelium, basement membrane, and perivascular and perilymphatic tissues. Idiopathic interstitial pneumonias (IIPs) is a condition in which the interstitium is replaced with extracellular matrix and inflammatory cells resulting in impaired gas exchange. As the name suggests, the IIPs are a heterogeneous group of diseases of unknown etiology that share some common clinical features and are distinguished primarily by radiography and histopathology. This distinction is important as it impacts therapeutic options and prognosis.

EPIDEMIOLOGY

Among the IIPs, idiopathic pulmonary fibrosis (IPF) is the most commonly described with annual incidence in the US estimated at 6.8–16.3 per 1,00,000 and a prevalence of 14.0–42.7 per 1,00,000.[1] Nearly two-third of patients are men above 60 years of age. Reports from India suggests that there is a trend towards higher incidence of IPF with advancing age; however, age at presentation is almost a decade earlier.[2]

CLASSIFICATION

Although, the initial classification in 2002 American Thoracic Society (ATS)/European Respiratory Society (ERS) statement is mainly based on the histologic patterns, the new classification was based on a *"dynamic integrated approach"* including histological, clinical and radiological features in a multidisciplinary discussion.[3,4]

The major and rare idiopathic interstitial pneumonia are further classified into following disorders: idiopathic pulmonary fibrosis (IPF), idiopathic nonspecific interstitial pneumonia (NSIP), respiratory bronchiolitis-interstitial lung disease (RB-ILD), desquamative interstitial pneumonia (DIP), cryptogenic organizing pneumonia (COP) and acute interstitial pneumonia (AIP), meanwhile the rare idiopathic pneumonias include lymphoid interstitial pneumonia (LIP) and idiopathic pleuroparenchymal fibroelastosis (PPFE) and as a last group, the unclassifiable IIP.[4]

CLINICAL FEATURES

It has been recognized and emphasized that the diagnosis of IIPs requires an interdisciplinary approach between the clinicians, radiologists and the pathologists. The signs and symptoms are usually nonspecific, but referable to the pulmonary system **(Table 1)**.[1-6] Nonproductive cough and progressive dyspnea with exertion usually prompt the patient to seek medical attention. The onset and progression can be variable, thus a detailed history of onset and duration of symptoms, and associated features must be obtained. Furthermore, particular attention should be paid to obtain detailed history of tobacco use; family history of lung disease especially with pulmonary fibrosis and to the current and prior drug use to rule out medication induced lung fibrosis. Occupational exposure history with attention to duration, degree and latency of exposure must also be carefully elucidated.[3] In the developing countries where expensive diagnostic equipment and surgical personnel may not be readily available, such detailed history in combination with the clinical features and radiographic features **(Table 2)**, may help the diagnostic approach and rule out other diseases in the differential diagnosis.[4,5]

When the clinico-radiological features are atypical of IPF, lung tissue obtained by surgical biopsy or bronchoalveolar lavage (BAL) with transbronchial biopsy (TBBx), based on available modalities to evaluate the histopathology may be helpful to rule out other possible etiologies as infections or diffuse alveolar hemorrhage **(Flow chart 1)**.[4,5] Laboratory tests for autoimmune disease, vasculitides and immunological response to organic inhalational exposure may assist in directing the clinician to various etiologies that are known to cause IIPs. Routine laboratory investigations usually play no significant role in the diagnostic process.[4]

Table 1 Summary of clinical features of idiopathic interstitial pneumonias

Diagnosis	*Features*	*PFTS*	*BAL*	*Histological pattern*	*Treatment*	*Prognosis*
Major idiopathic interstitial pneumonias						
IPF	Gradual onset, > men >50 years. Constitutional symptoms are usual. Associated to smoking	Restrictive pattern, ↓ DLCO, low resting PaO_2	Ne predominant, mild-to-moderate ↑ in eosinophilia usually < 20%	UIP	Generally ineffective, Pirfenidone, lung transplantation	50–70% mortality in 5 years
NSIP	Gradual onset, mean age 40–50, M = W, constitutional symptoms may be present	Restrictive pattern, ↓ DLCO, Mild airflow limitation in minority, hypoxemia on exercise	Lymphocytic predominant	NSIP: Cellular and fibrosing pattern	Immunosuppression	<10% mortality in 5 years
RB-ILD	Smokers, 40–60 years/ old	Obstructive/restrictive patterns, ↓ DLCO, isolated increase in RV	Alveolar macrophages with black pigmented inclusions	RB	Smoking cessation	Mortality rare
DIP	Insidious onset, smokers, 40–50 years, M:F 2:1	Normal or restrictive pattern, ↓ DLCO	Alveolar macrophages with black pigmented inclusions, modest increase in neutrophils, eosinophils and lymphocytes	DIP	Smoking cessation	5% mortality in 5 years
COP	Mean age 55 years, M = F, nonsmokers > smokers, neutrophilia with ↑ ESR/CRP	Restrictive, mild airflow limitation, ↓ DLCO, mild resting hypoxemia	Lymphocytic predominant with ↑ CD4 + /CD8 +	OP	Corticosteroids	Mortality rare
AIP	Acute and rapidly progressive. Prior illness suggestive of viral URI.	Restrictive pattern, hypoxemia, ↓ DLCO	Increase total cells, hemorrhage, atypical pneumocytes and fragments of hyaline membrane, modest ↑ in neutrophils	DAD	No proven treatment	>50% mortality in 1–2 months
Rare idiopathic interstitial pneumonias						
LIP	F > M, 50 years, insidious constitutional symptoms +/- adenopathy, mild anemia		Lymphocytes without clonality on immunophenotyping	LIP	Corticosteroids	Unknown
PPFE	F = M, 30–40 years, tall individuals	Restrictive, ↓ DLCO, increase RV/TLC			No proven treatment	
Unclassifiable IIP						

Abbreviations: AIP, acute interstitial pneumonia; BAL, bronchoalveolar lavage; COP, cryptogenic fibrosing alveolitis; DAD, diffuse alveolar damage; DIP, desquamative interstitial pneumonia; IPF, idiopathic pulmonary fibrosis; LIP, lymphoid interstitial pneumonia; NSIP, nonspecific interstitial pneumonia; OP, organizing pneumonia; PFTS, pulmonary function tests; RB-ILD, respiratory bronchiolitis-associated interstitial lung disease; UIP, usual interstitial pneumonia; PPFE, pleuroparechymal fibroelastosis, ↓ decrease, ↑ increase; DLCO, diffusing capacity of the lung for carbon monoxide; PaO2, partial pressure of arterial oxygen; ESR, erythrocyte sedimentation rate; URI, upper respiratory infection; RV, residual volume; TLC, total lung capacity; CRP, C-reactive protein; RV, residual volume.
Source: Adapted from reference 4.

HISTOLOGICAL FEATURES

Histopathological examination of lung is helpful in the diagnosis of IIPs. The patterns have been shown to correlate with the clinical course and response to treatment. In IPF, the characteristic injury pattern is usual interstitial pneumonia (UIP). The hallmark of UIP is fibroblastic foci which consist of dense eosinophilic fibrosis with scattered foci of young myxoid fibrosis and fibroblasts. These foci represent the advancing or progressive edge of disease and are required

Table 2 Radiographic features of idiopathic interstitial pneumonias

Clinical diagnosis	*Radiographic features*	*CT distribution*	*CT findings*
Major idiopathic interstitial pneumonias			
IPF	Reticular, basilar, low lung volumes	Peripheral, subpleural/basal	Architectural distortion, honeycombing, traction bronchiectasis
NSIP	Reticular	Peripheral, subpleural/basal, symmetric	Ground glass opacification (GGO) intermixed with reticular lines
RB-ILD	Ground glass, bronchial thickening	Diffuse	Patchy GGO, bronchial thickening, centrilobular nodules
DIP	Ground glass	Peripheral, lower lobes	Reticular lines, nodular to GGO
COP	Patchy bilateral consolidations	Subpleural, peribronchial, lower lobes	Patchy consolidation, nodules
AIP	Progressive diffuse consolidation	Diffuse	Consolidation, GGO with lobar sparing, traction bronchiectasis
Rare idiopathic interstitial pneumonias			
LIP	Reticulonodular	Diffuse	GGO, septal/ bronchovascular thickening, centrilobular nodules, thin-wall cyst
PPFE	Reticular and nodular in upper lobes	Subpleural, upper lobes	Reticular, nodular opacities, interlobular septal thickening
Unclassifiable IIP			

Abbreviations: AIP, acute interstitial pneumonia; COP, cryptogenic fibrosing alveolitis; DIP, desquamative interstitial pneumonia; IPF, idiopathic pulmonary fibrosis; LIP, lymphoid interstitial pneumonia; NSIP, nonspecific interstitial pneumonia; RB-ILD, respiratory bronchiolitis-associated interstitial lung disease; PPFE, pleuroparechymal fibroelastosis, GGO, ground glass opacity; CT, computed tomography

Source: Adapted from reference 4.

Flow chart 1: Simplified algorithm for diagnosis of idiopathic interstitial pneumonias

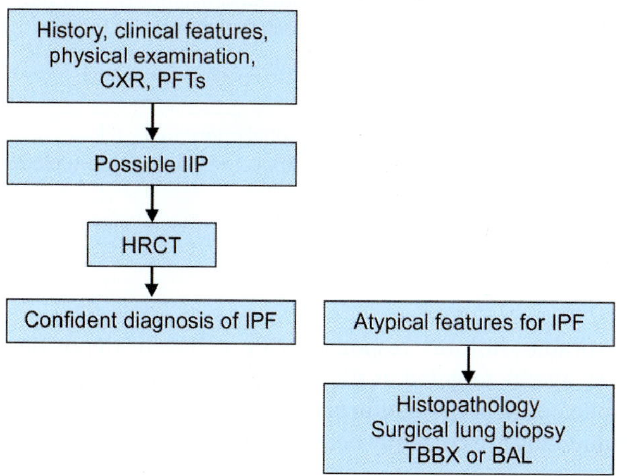

Abbreviations: CXR, chest X-ray; PFTs, pulmonary function tests; IIP, idiopathic interstitial pneumonias; HRCT, high-resolution computed tomography; IPF, idiopathic pulmonary fibrosis; TBBX, transbronchial biopsy; BAL, bronchoalveolar lavage

to be a major component of the histological pattern for a confident diagnosis. The injury is predominantly seen in the subpleural region, consists of a pattern of temporal heterogeneity.[2-8] In other words, the areas of injury with fibroblastic foci and honeycomb changes are seen adjacent to relatively unaffected tissue. Other histological patterns of IIPs are summarized in **Table 3**.[4]

TREATMENT

Management usually involves supportive therapy with oxygen supplementation, immunizations, treatment of intercurrent infections and management of complications that may arise from treatment.[6,7] For some of the IIPs, the mainstay of treatment is corticosteroids. Other treatments options, including immunosuppressive therapies and antifibrotic agents, are discussed individually.

Idiopathic Pulmonary Fibrosis

Epidemiology

Idiopathic pulmonary fibrosis, also known as cryptogenic fibrosing alveolitis, is a distinctive type of chronic fibrosing interstitial pneumonitis of unknown etiology accounting for over 50% of all IIPs.[9] It is associated with surgical lung biopsy showing a UIP pattern. It is predominantly seen in middle-aged men with a median age of 66 years at time of diagnosis.[7,8] In a series from India, the age of presentation was a decade earlier.[6] The incidence is higher with the increasing age.[7]

Table 3 Histological patterns in the idiopathic interstitial pneumonias

Diagnosis	*Histological pattern*	*Description*
Major idiopathic interstitial pneumonias		
IPF	Usual interstitial pneumonia	Patchy/focal involvement of the lung: dense fibrosis and honeycombing with areas of "normal lung" adjacent to heavily involved areas. Subpleural distribution, paraseptal and peribronchiolar. Fibrosis, temporal heterogeneity. Alveolar component reduced or completely lost in affected areas. Bronchiolar component damage and abnormal regeneration
NSIP	Nonspecific interstitial pneumonitis	*Cellular pattern*: Homogenous interstitial chronic inflammatory infiltrate focal alveolar collections of macrophages. Focal alveolar damage with pneumocyte type II hyperplasia and organizing pneumonia *Fibrosing pattern*: Dense or loose interstitial fibrosis with homogeneous involvement of the lung. Mild inflammatory infiltrate. No evidence of fibroblast foci or honeycombing
RB-ILD	Respiratory bronchiolitis	Bronchiolocentric alveolar macrophage accumulation. Mild bronchiolar fibrosis and chronic inflammation. Macrophages have dusty brown cytoplasm (may be positive for iron stains)
DIP	Desquamative interstitial pneumonia	Chronic interstitial inflammation and numerous intra-alveolar mononuclear cells, macrophages. Diffuse alveolar mononuclear cell (macrophage) accumulation. Cuboidal epithelial cells (type 2 cells) line alveoli. Mild diffuse interstitial fibrosis and chronic inflammation. Occasional lymphoid follicles. No dense scarring or revamping of architecture
COP	Organizing pneumonia	Organizing tissue (polyps) within alveolar ducts and alveoli. Mild interstitial inflammatory infiltrate/intra-alveolar foamy macrophages. Focal alveolar damage with pneumocyte type II hyperplasia. Preservation of lung structure, the process appears mainly centered in small airways
AIP	Diffuse alveolar damage	Diffuse involvement of the lung parenchyma. Fibrosis of uniform temporal appearance with myofibroblast accumulation within alveolar interstitial spaces. Diffuse features of acute alveolar damage with pneumocyte type II hyperplasia, atypia and hyaline membranes.
Rare idiopathic interstitial pneumonias		
LIP	Lymphoid interstitial pneumonia	Intense and diffuse chronic accumulation of lymphocytes occurs in alveolar interstitial spaces. Follicular reaction may occur along lymphatic routes.
PPFE	Pleuroparenchimal fibroelastosis	Upper lobe predominant fibrosis of the visceral pleura, with intra-alveolar fibrosis and septal elastosis. Variable lymphocytic inflammation, rare fibroblast foci, demarcation of the healthy lung parenchyma.
Unclassifiable IIP		

Abbreviations: AIP, acute interstitial pneumonia; COP, cryptogenic fibrosing alveolitis; DIP, desquamative interstitial pneumonia; IPF, idiopathic pulmonary fibrosis; LIP, lymphoid interstitial pneumonia; NSIP, nonspecific interstitial pneumonia; RB-ILD, respiratory bronchiolitis-associated interstitial lung disease; PPFE, pleuroparechymal fibroelastosis

Source: Adapted from reference 4.

Etiology

The cause of IPF is unclear, but it is increasingly becoming clear that it represents in part a response to injurious agent(s) in genetically predisposed individuals, followed by deregulated inflammation, repair of the interstitium and alveolar epithelium. The possible risk factors for alveolar injury include but are not limited to cigarette smoking, environmental exposures (metal and wood dust, farming, other inorganic particles), infections (viral) and gastroesophageal reflux disease (GERD) with microaspiration.[8] Eventually chronic inflammation and an imbalance in the production of various cytokines, growth factors and profibrotic agents result in inexorable fibrotic response with collagen deposition.[10] Thus, agents targeted at the cytokine release and processes implicated in perpetuation of pulmonary fibrosis and vascular remodeling are currently being investigated for treatment.

Signs and Symptoms

Paroxysmal nonproductive cough associated with progressively worsening of shortness of breath are the most common symptoms. These symptoms have an insidious onset and are often present for months prior to the diagnosis.[7,8] End inspiratory crackles are present on lung examination, with finger clubbing in 25–50% of patients. In late stages of disease,

Table 4 Diagnosis of idiopathic pulmonary fibrosis based in high-resolution computed tomography and surgical lung biopsy

HRCT pattern	*Histopathological pattern*	
UIP	UIP, probable UIP, possible UIP and nonclassifiable fibrosis	IPF diagnosis
	Not UIP	Other IIP
Possible UIP	UIP, probable UIP	IPF diagnosis
	Possible UIP, nonclassifiable fibrosis	Probable IPF diagnosis
	Not UIP	Other IIP
Inconsistent with UIP	UIP	Probable IPF diagnosis
	Probable UIP, possible UIP, nonclassifiable fibrosis, not UIP	Other IIP

Abbreviations: HRCT, high-resolution computed tomography; UIP, usual interstitial pneumonia; IIP, idiopathic interstitial pneumonias; IPF, idiopathic pulmonary fibrosis

Source: Adapted from reference 11.

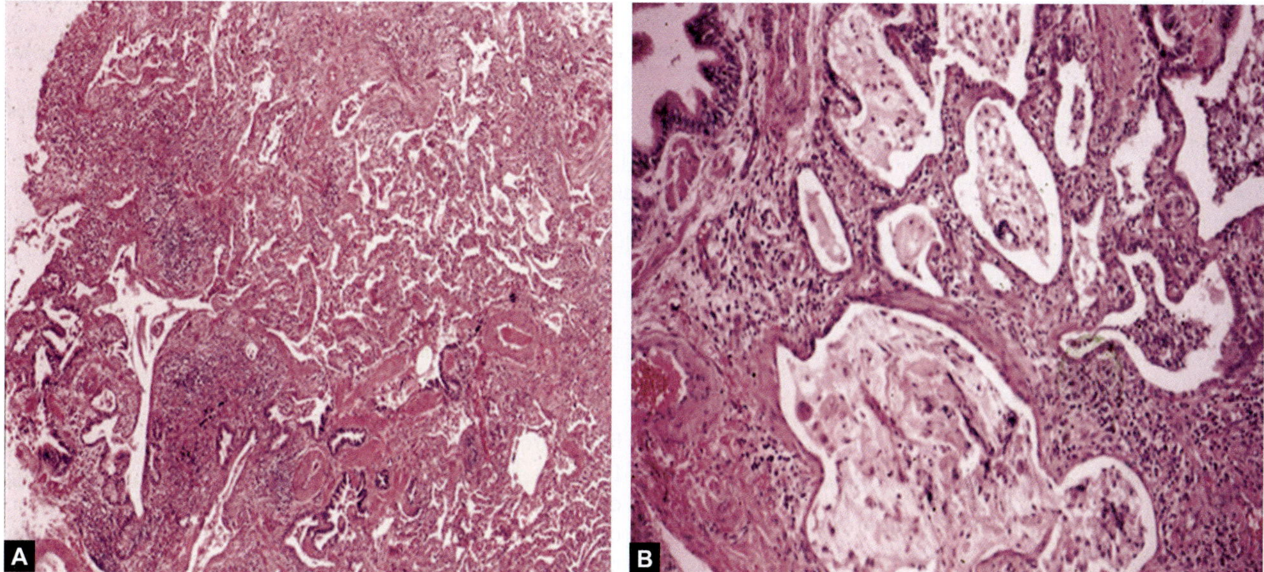

Figs 1A and B: UIP pattern on histopathology. Temporal heterogeneity and geographic heterogeneity. Patchy involvement of the lung with variation in the age of the fibrosis. Interstitial and alveolar inflammation, cellular proliferation and honeycombing cysts

signs attributable to pulmonary hypertension or right heart failure may be present.

Diagnosis

The diagnosis of IPF in the new ATS/ERS statement requires a multidisciplinary approach based on clinical, radiological and if a lung biopsy has been performed, pathological patterns that correlate with the radiological patterns **(Table 4)**.[11] Other causes of ILD must be excluded before diagnosing IPF.[8]

The pulmonary function test usually reveal a restrictive physiology with abnormal gas exchange.[3] The typical chest radiographic features include diffuse peripheral reticular opacities with basilar predilection.[3,7]

The high specificity of the high-resolution computed tomography (HRCT) of chest in many instances allow a reasonably confident diagnosis without a lung biopsy.[8] The typical findings on HRCT scan consist of predominantly peripheral, subpleural, bibasilar reticular abnormalities; traction bronchiectasis and subpleural honeycombing. If ground-glass opacities appear to be the predominant radiographic finding, an alternate diagnosis other than IPF must be strongly considered. IPF is characterized morphologically with a UIP pattern on pathology **(Figs 1A and B)**. HRCT and histopathological criteria for UIP pattern are described in **Tables 4 to 6**.[11] The findings on chest radiography, CT and gross pathological examination of lung with IPF/UIP are demonstrated in **Figures 2A to C**.

Table 5 High-resolution computed tomography criteria for usual interstitial pneumonia pattern

UIP pattern: Needs all four features	*Possible UIP: Needs all three features*	*Inconsistent with UIP if any of the seven features*
Subpleural, basal predominance reticular abnormality	Subpleural, basal predominance reticular abnormality	Upper or mid-lung predominance peribronchovascular predominance
Honeycombing with or without traction bronchiectasis absence of features listed as inconsistent with UIP	Absence of features listed as inconsistent with UIP	Extensive GGO or > reticular abnormality profuse micronodules Discrete cyst diffuse mosaic attenuation/air trapping consolidations

Abbreviations: HRCT, high resolution computed tomography; UIP, usual interstitial pneumonia; GGO, ground glass opacity.
Source: Adapted from reference 11.

Table 6 Histopathological criteria

UIP pattern: Needs all four	*Probable*	*Possible: Needs all three*	*Not UIP*
1. Evidence of marked fibrosis/architectural distortion, ± predominant subpleural/paraseptal honeycombing 2. Patchy lung involvement 3. Fibroblast foci 4. Absence of features against a diagnosis of UIP suggesting an alternate diagnosis	1. Evidence of marked fibrosis/ architectural distortion, ± honeycombing 2. Absence of patchy lung involvement or fibroblast foci 3. Absence of features against a diagnosis of UIP suggesting an alternate diagnosis or 4. Honeycoomb changes only	1. Patchy or diffuse lung fibrosis with or without interstitial inflammation 2. Absence of other criteria for UIP 3. Absence of features against a diagnosis of UIP suggesting an alternate diagnosis	1. Hyaline membranes 2. Organizing pneumonia 3. Granulomas 4. Marked interstitial 5. Inflammatory cell infiltrate away from honeycombing 6. Predominant airway centered changes 7. Other features suggestive of an alternate diagnosis

Abbreviation: UIP, usual interstitial pneumonia
Source: Adapted from reference 11.

Treatment

Treatment is targeted at resolution and slowing down the progression of disease.[6-8] There is no treatment that improves survival in IPF. The new ATS/ERS/JRS/ALAT guidelines of 2011 make emphasis against treatment with monotherapy with steroids, colchicine, cyclosporine a, interferon gamma, bosentan and etanercept since none those medication improve survival nor slow the progression of the disease.[8] The guidelines actually recommend the use of combined corticosteroid with azathioprine and acetylcysteine or acetylcysteine alone in selected patients, but recent data show no significant benefit in the use of this medication rather a trend toward increased mortality with the combination of azathioprine and steroids.[12,13]

A trial with pirfenidone was found to be effective in stabilizing lung function and reducing the frequency of acute exacerbations in Japanese patients.[14] Recently, a phase 3 trial of pirfenidone for 52 weeks and a randomized trial of nintedanib (intracellular inhibitor of tyrosine kinase), at several centres including the United States, showed slow decline in forced vital capacity (FVC) and progression-free survival providing hope for better treatment options.[15,16]

Supportive care with supplemental oxygen, immunizations, prompt treatment of infections and pulmonary rehabilitation help to improve the quality of life.[6,8] In spite of these therapies, IPF portends a poor prognosis with a median 5 year survival of less than 50%.[2,4-6] Lung transplantation becomes the only option for treatment for eligible patients, although this is not readily available in many developing countries.

Prognosis

The general clinical course is variable, some patients stay with stable lung function for many years, while others show slow progression of impairment and some may report even accelerated progression. Acute worsening of function due to acute IPF exacerbations, infections or other comorbidities can be part of this disease behavior.[8]

Factors associated with increased risk of mortality include level of dyspnea, severity on baseline DLCO or % of worsening, extension of honeycombing, worsening of fibrosis on HRCT, desaturation less than 88% on 6-minute walk test (6MWT) as well pulmonary hypertension.[8]

Nonspecific Interstitial Pneumonia

Idiopathic nonspecific interstitial pneumonia is defined now as a distinct clinical entity, although it is most frequently associated with other pathologic conditions such as

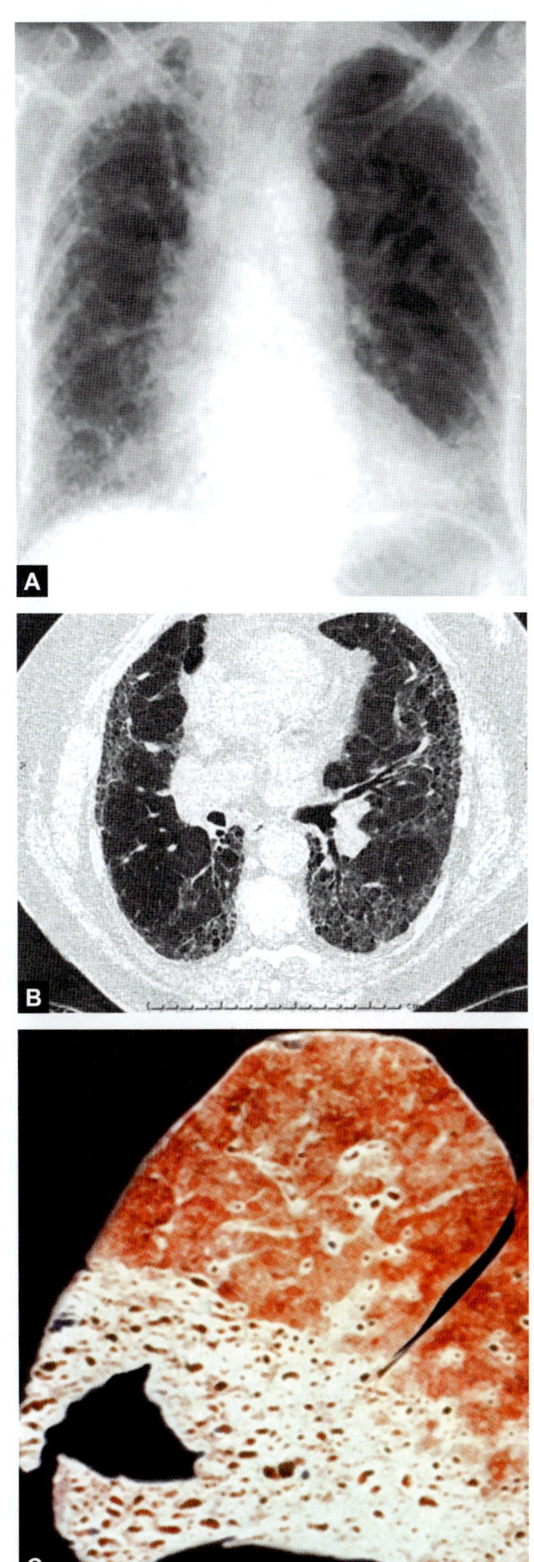

Figs 2A to C: Chest radiograph, computed tomography chest, and gross pathology of the explanted lung with idiopathic pulmonary fibrosis/usual interstitial pneumonia. Note that the distribution is predominantly at the bases and subpleural region

connective tissue disorders, drug toxicity, hypersensitivity pneumonitis, and human immunodeficiency virus (HIV) infection.[4,17]

Epidemiology

The mean age of onset is 40–50 years of age, which is about a decade earlier than in IPF. It has been also reported in the pediatric population.[18] It occurs equally in both men and women, has no known association with cigarette smoking.[4,17]

Etiology

Unlike IPF, the etiology of NSIP may be more evident with autoimmune diseases, hypersensitivity pneumonitis and certain inhalational exposure. Therefore, a diagnosis of NSIP should prompt clinical evaluation for an underlying etiology. The etiology in a significant number of patients with NSIP, remains elusive and coined as idiopathic NSIP which has unique features than other forms of NSIP.

Signs and Symptoms

Onset is gradual and some patients have associated constitutional symptoms such as fever and weight loss in addition to respiratory symptoms such as chronic cough and dyspnea.[3,17,19] Finger clubbing is less common than in IPF, can occur in 8% of patients.[17] Inspiratory crackles are usually present on lung examination.

Diagnosis

Clinical features in the presence of a restrictive pattern and a reduction in DLCO suggest the diagnosis of an interstitial pulmonary disease. Histologically, NSIP consist of varying degree of inflammation and involvement; it can be further separated into cellular and fibrotic NSIP.[17] In cellular NSIP, mild-to-moderate homogenous interstitial chronic inflammation is the predominant feature, unlike fibrosing NSIP where uniformly dense fibrosis is the prominent feature.[18] Temporal uniformity, the paucity of fibroblastic foci and honeycomb lesions are the features that histologically differentiate NSIP from UIP.[3,4,17,19]

Radiographically, cellular NSIP in contrary to IPF, show diffuse symmetric interstitial infiltrates and ground-glass opacities, with subpleural sparing.[4,17,19] In fibrotic NSIP, the radiographic signs of fibrotic disease are similar to those of IPF.

Treatment/Prognosis

Treatment for NSIP is based mostly on expert opinion, since randomized trials are not available. Katzenstein classified NSIP into three subgroups based on the degree of inflammation and fibrosis on histopathology: Group 1 primarily has interstitial fibrosis; group 2 inflammation and fibrosis; and group 3 primarily fibrosis.[18] Patients with

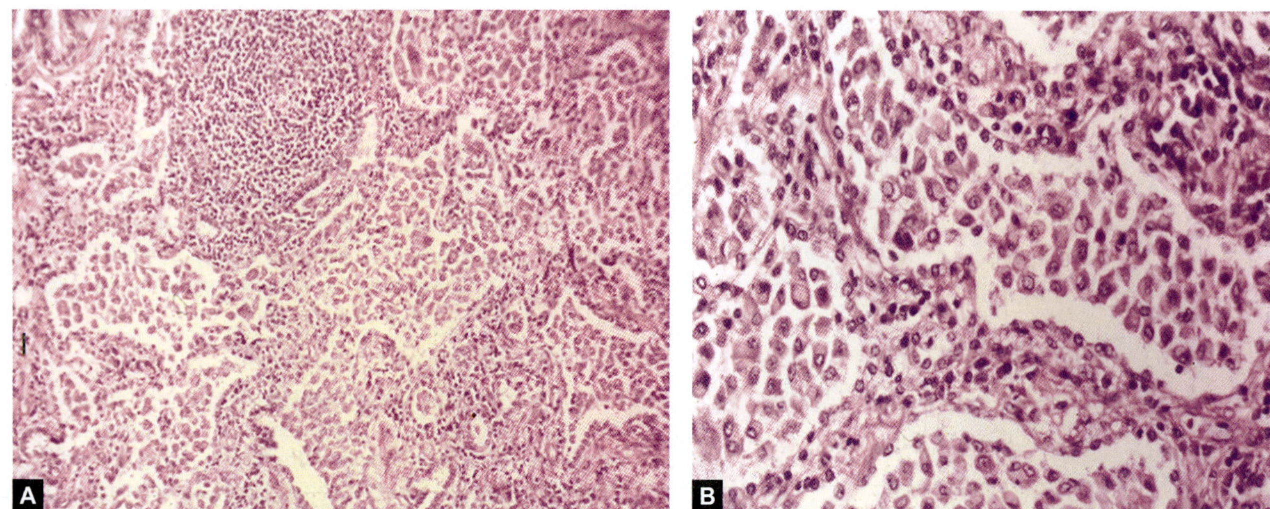

Figs 3A and B: Desquamative interstitial pneumonia pattern on histopathology. Diffuse macrophage accumulation with type 2 cells lining alveoli. Mild interstitial fibrosis, chronic inflammation and no dense scarring or architectural distortion is seen

cellular NSIP usually respond well to corticosteroids unlike fibrotic NSIP.[3] Thus the prognosis is good in cellular NSIP, as opposed to fibrotic NSIP, which has been shown to mirror that of IPF, given the similarities in histology and clinical features.

Desquamative Interstitial Pneumonia

Epidemiology

Desquamative interstitial pneumonia is a rare IIP primarily seen in smokers in the 4–5 decades of life.[3,20] The term DIP was coined by Myers et al. based on findings in six patients who had interstitial pattern on chest radiograph with restrictive pulmonary function test and respiratory bronchiolitis (RB) on histopathology.[21]

Etiology

In at-risk patients, tobacco induces injury to the bronchiolar and alveolar epithelium. The pathobiology is not completely understood as to why and how this occurs.[22] As in patients with pulmonary Langerhans cell histiocytosis, abnormal T-cell proliferation and increased secretion of peptides has been described.[22] It is likely that this disorder, like other cigarette smoking related lung diseases, occurs in susceptible individuals following initial injury to the pulmonary epithelium.

Signs and Symptoms

Dyspnea at rest or on exertion is the most common presenting symptom. Onset is insidious, cough may be dry or productive of nonpurulent sputum.[20] Systemic symptoms are usually absent, digital clubbing is seen in some patients.[3] Physical examination shows crackles in less than 50% of patients.[3,20]

Diagnosis

The diagnosis should be suspected when these clinical and epidemiological features are seen in combination with radiographic findings. Typical radiographic findings include patchy ground glass opacification with a predilection for the lower zones, in rare cases it can even be normal. The PFTs can show a combined obstructive and restrictive defect, often with a decrease in DLCO.[3,21]

The histological pattern is characterized by chronic interstitial inflammation and numerous intra-alveolar mononuclear cells, thought to be desquamated epithelial cells (hence the name) which subsequently proved to be macrophages. It is common to find multinucleated giants cells **(Figs 3A and B)**.[23,24]

Treatment

There is clinical response to smoking cessation alone or in combination with corticosteroid therapy, as well as some possible spontaneous resolution.[3,25,26] In some cases, in spite of clinical stability, abnormal radiographic features may persist.[26]

Respiratory Bronchiolitis-associated Interstitial Lung Disease

Epidemiology

Recent studies have linked idiopathic DIP to RB and RB-ILD in a spectrum of smoking related lung injury.[23] It is considered

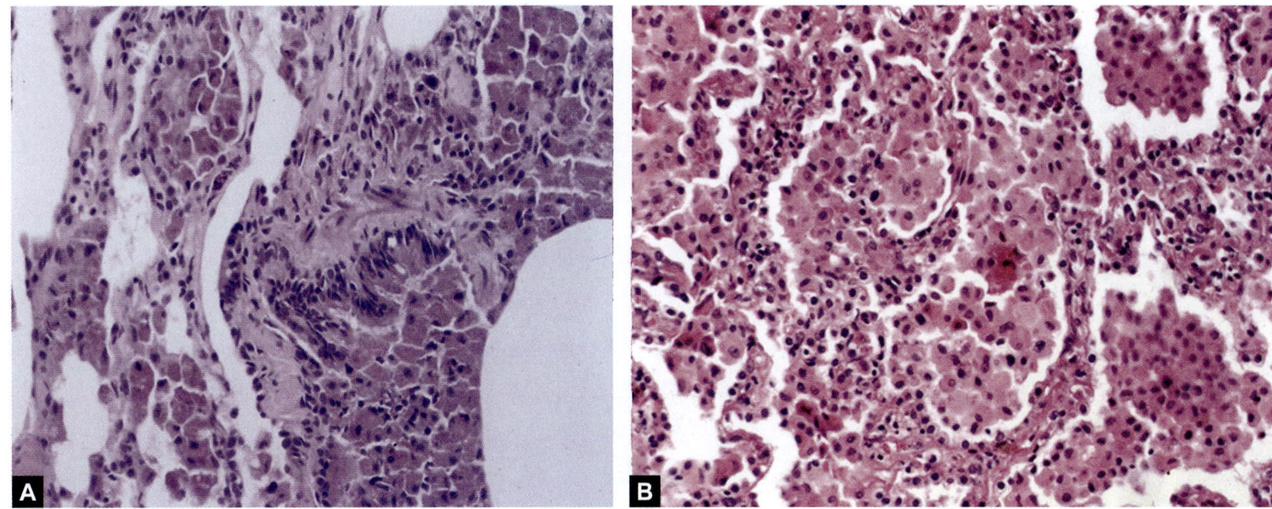

Figs 4A and B: Respiratory bronchiolitis-associated interstitial lung disease pattern on histopathology. Clusters of dusty brown macrophages in respiratory bronchioles, alveolar ducts and peribronchiolar alveolar spaces are seen in respiratory bronchiolitis-associated interstitial lung disease

a variant of DIP and has a patchy distribution rather than a diffuse process. Smokers in the 3–4 decade of life are usually affected.[27]

Signs and Symptoms

Most patients are asymptomatic or have mild symptoms of dyspnea and cough of insidious onset.[3,4,20,26] Inspiratory crackles are present on lung examination, digital clubbing in up to 25% in one series.[26]

Diagnosis

On spirometry, a combined defect with abnormalities of gas exchange is often seen.[3,20] Ground glass opacities and attenuation may be seen on chest imaging, associated with thickening of walls of central and peripheral airways. These findings are ultimately associated with the pathological lesions of RB consistent with macrophages infiltration with more peribronchiolar distribution than intra-alveolar as in DIP[28] **(Figs 4A and B)**.

Treatment

The only proven therapy for RB-ILD is smoking cessation. Only those who continue to be symptomatic in spite of smoking cessation should be considered for corticosteroid therapy.[3,22]

Prognosis

Prognosis is good and patients usually improve with smoking cessation. To date, there are no documented cases of respiratory failure or death directly attributable to RB-ILD.[3,22]

Cryptogenic Organizing Pneumonia

Epidemiology

Cryptogenic organizing pneumonia, previously known as bronchiolitis obliterans with organizing pneumonia (BOOP), often presents clinically as a flu-like illness of subacute onset (weeks to a few months). The disease process was initially described by Grinblat and colleagues in two patients.[25] Organizing pneumonia is often a nonspecific response to lung injury, classified as cryptogenic when an underlying disease cannot be identified.

Cryptogenic organizing pneumonia is commonly diagnosed during the fifth decade of life; there have been case reports in adolescence.[29] In most series from developing countries including from the Middle East and Southeast Asia, no correlation was seen between smoking status and the disease.[30-32] Men and women are equally affected.

Etiology

Organizing pneumonia is a nonspecific response of the lung to injury. It is termed cryptogenic when an inciting agent or disease process is absent. Increased expression of interleukin-8 and fibronectin genes by alveolar macrophages has been described in COP.[33] This suggests that the lung injury and inflammation may be initiated and perpetuated by inflammatory cytokines produced in situ by alveolar macrophages. In mice models, there is a suggestion that genetic host factors play an important role in the development of lung fibrosis in COP.[33]

Signs and Symptoms

Cryptogenic organizing pneumonia often presents clinically as a flu-like illness of subacute onset (weeks to a few months).[3]

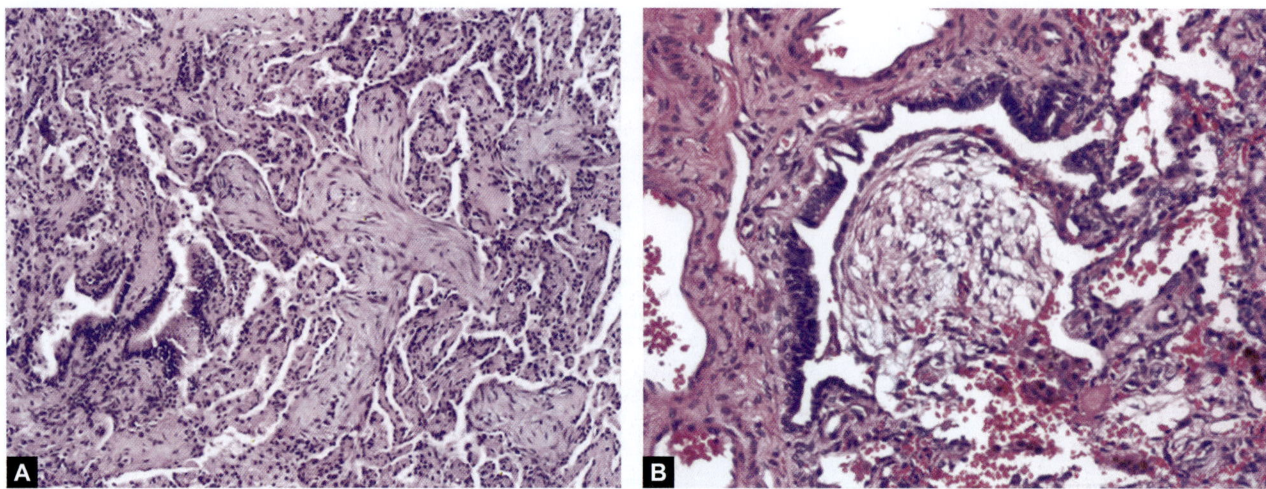

Figs 5A and B: Cryptogenic organizing pneumonia pattern on histopathology

Fever, dry cough with malaise, anorexia and weight loss are often present with mild dyspnea, especially on exertion.[3] Physical findings are sparse, inspiratory crackles are present on lung examination.[3]

Diagnosis

The diagnosis should be considered in patients with features of nonresolving pneumonia. Chest X-ray shows patchy migratory, unilateral or bilateral airspace disease with predominantly peripheral distribution.[3] On CT scan, the opacities range from ground glass to dense peribronchial consolidation, with multifocal and subpleural involvement.[4] These radiographic findings can also be seen in other conditions.[33] Less commonly, radiographic features of diffuse interstitial opacities and solitary focal lesions may be seen.[33] Spirometry may be normal; it typically reveals a restrictive pattern with some gas exchange abnormalities. BAL may reveal an increase in all cell lines, with occasional foamy macrophages. Lymphocytosis with CD4/CD8 ratio less than 0.9 has been described in COP.[34] In smokers, there may be an obstructive component to pulmonary function tests (PFTs). Buds of granulation tissue are found within the lumen of the distal airways (alveolar ducts and alveoli) on histology (Masson bodies).[35] This pattern is nonspecific and reflects an inflammatory response to lung injury. There is a preservation of lung architecture with the absence of scarring or honeycombing on histopathology **(Figs 5A and B)**.

Polypoid plugs of fibrous tissue (Masson bodies) within bronchiolar lumens, alveolar ducts and alveoli. Clusters of alveolar foamy macrophages are also present.

Treatment/Prognosis

Most patients respond well to corticosteroids, but relapses can occur requiring chronic steroid therapy.[3] Cytotoxic drugs and steroid sparing agents are used in addition to corticosteroid where there is slow response to steroids alone.[33] A small group (10–15%) may progress to pulmonary fibrosis and one third of patient can relapse.[3] Factors that may predict poor outcomes include the lack of lymphocytosis on BAL, predominantly interstitial pattern on imaging and histological features of scarring and remodeling of lung parenchyma.[33]

Acute Interstitial Pneumonia

Epidemiology

Hamman-Rich described a series of four patients who died from rapidly progressive lung disease, associated with respiratory failure and death within a few months of onset. Autopsy was characterized by a diffuse interstitial pneumonia and fibrosis.[36] Acute interstitial pneumonia is a rare and often fatal disease encountered in apparently healthy individuals after an acute respiratory illness characterized by diffuse alveolar damage (DAD).[36] The syndrome mimics acute respiratory distress syndrome (ARDS).

Etiology

The exact mechanisms responsible for AIP are poorly understood; however, there is diffuse acute lung injury resulting in acute respiratory failure.[37] Several mediators have been described and implicated in this process. Proinflammatory, anti-inflammatory, metalloproteinases and proteins regulating apoptosis have all been implicated.[38-40]

Signs and Symptoms

The presentation is similar to that of ARDS. There is no predilection for age and sex, but are mostly seen in adults.[41]

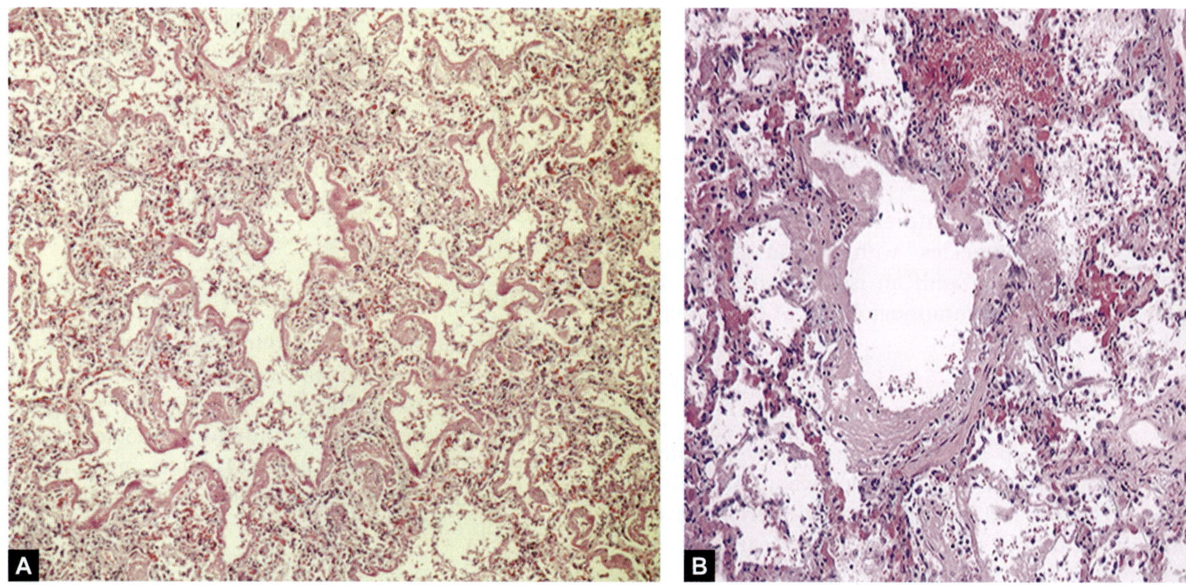

Figs 6A and B: Acute interstitial pneumonia pattern on histopathology. Hyaline membranes with eosinophilic material lining alveolar spaces consistent with diffuse alveolar damage are present with areas of progressive fibrosis

The onset is acute and often preceded by symptoms suggestive of viral upper respiratory tract infection followed by widespread pneumonia. Hypoxemia develops early followed by respiratory failure requiring mechanical ventilatory support. There is no association with smoking.

Diagnosis

Based on the ATS/ETS guidelines[3] the criteria include rapidly progressive clinical course (less than 2 months) leading to respiratory failure; exclusion of infectious, toxic, autoimmune or any other cause of ARDS; DAD with hyalines membranes in early or exudative stages,[41,42] observed on biopsy specimens; radiological findings consistent with ILD as bilateral ground glass opacity (GGO) with consolidation;[4,41] and absence of chronic lung disease.[2] Bilateral airspace disease seen radiographically correlates with DAD seen on histology **(Figs 6A and B)**. BAL is not helpful in diagnosis, but it is useful to rule out other possible etiologies such as infections, acute eosinophilic pneumonia and diffuse alveolar hemorrhage.[42]

Treatment

Since there is no proven treatment, supportive care with oxygen supplementation and mechanical ventilation is indicated.[41] Early corticosteroid therapy and combination therapy with intravenous cyclophosphamide and vincristine have been reported.[43] Newer agents, such as inhaled nitric oxide, anticytokine antibodies and surfactant, may be useful.[44,45] There is a report of single lung transplantation as therapy for AIP.[46]

Prognosis

Mortality is greater than 60%.[3,37] Based on the morphology of lung parenchyma on CT, some authors report that this may help to differentiate fulminant forms of AIP.[41,42,47,48] Those who survive may have no residual lung damage, residual pulmonary fibrosis or recurrent disease.[42]

Lymphoid Interstitial Pneumonia

Epidemiology

Lymphoid interstitial pneumonia (LIP) is considered as a rare IIP in the 2013 ATS/ERS statement, it mostly affects women in the fifth decade of life but can occur at any age.[3,4,36] Although, a part of IIPs, there is a thought that LIP possibly represents a lymphoproliferative disorder confined to the lungs that was initially described by Liebow and Carrington.[49] Lymphoid interstitial pneumonia has also been described in developing countries such as Africa and the Caribbean, but all in association with systemic diseases, most notably HIV infection [or acquired immunodeficiency syndrome (AIDS)] although some cases remain idiopathic. It has also been described in post bone marrow transplantation.[50]

Etiology

There is some evidence that this is a lymphoproliferative disorder rather than a primary interstitial pulmonary process.[51] It may result from a lymphoproliferative response to chronically presented viral antigens or cytokines with or without recruitment of circulating lymphocytes. Mutations of the B-cell CLL/lymphoma 6 gene have been associated with LIP.[51]

Signs and Symptoms

It is slow in onset with increasing cough and breathlessness. Constitutional symptoms, such as fever, weight loss, arthralgias, may be prominent features.[3] Chest examination often reveals bibasilar crackles with digital clubbing being rare.[51] Dysproteinemia with an isolated increase in immunoglobulin G (IgG) or immunoglobulin M (IgM) may be present in 75% of cases.[3,49]

Diagnosis

Chest X-ray may show an alveolar pattern predominantly at the bases or a diffuse disease with honeycombing. The predominant cell type on BAL is lymphocyte, with a restrictive pattern on lung function tests. Histology reveals dense interstitial lymphoid infiltrate. This pathological finding has been described in other connective tissue disorders, such that the diagnosis can only be made once underlying connective tissue or systemic diseases have been excluded.[3]

Treatment

Some patients improve spontaneously without any treatment. Clinical improvement to corticosteroid therapy has been reported. In some cases, cytotoxic agents including cyclophosphamide, azathioprine and cyclosporine have been used.[51,52] Supplemental oxygen therapy and treatment of pulmonary infections may be necessary.

Prognosis

Survival is impaired; but mortality data are sparse because of the rarity of the condition.[3,51]

Idiopathic Pleuroparenchymal Fibroelastosis

Idiopathic pleuroparenchymal fibroelastosis is a new and rare IIP described for the first time in 1992 as idiopathic upper lobe fibrosis by Amitani et al. and later further described in 2004 by Frankel et al.[53,54] It is characterized by predominant pleural and subpleural upper lobe fibrosis.[4,52,53]

Diagnosis and Treatment

Pleuroparenchymal fibroelastosis is a disease of adults, more frequent in their fourth and fifth decades of life, with a median of 57 years of age.[4,55] Progressive dyspnea on exertion and nonproductive cough are the main symptoms. Pneumothorax is frequent. It is associated with decrease anterior-posterior diameter of the thoracic cage know as *"flattened thoracic cage"*.[55] HRCT chest shows pleural thickening along with nodular and reticular opacities in bilateral upper lobes. Restrictive physiology with increased residual volume (RV)/ total lung capacity (TLC) can be found on PFTs.[54] Intra-alveolar fibrosis, septal fibroelastosis of the visceral pleural with lymphoplasmocytic infiltrates and fibroblast foci can be observed in the histology.[56] PPFE appears to be resistant to any kind of immunosuppressive therapy. The disease is progressive with a poor prognosis close to 50% survival at 10 years.[55]

Unclassifiable Idiopathic Interstitial Pneumonia

Unclassifiable category is applied to those cases where there is discrepancy in the clinical, radiological or histological characteristics, or where previous treatment of the patient modified the primary findings or the new histological patterns are found. Multidisciplinary discussion is essential in these cases to determine the best course of further diagnostic and treatment approaches.[4]

REFERENCES

1. Wyngarden JB, Smith LH. Cecil Textbook of Medicine, 19th edition. Philadelphia: WB Saunders; 1992.
2. Maheshwari U, Gupta D, Aggarwal AN, Jindal SK. Spectrum and diagnosis of idiopathic pulmonary fibrosis. Indian J Chest Dis Allied Sci. 2004;46(1):23-6.
3. American Thoracic Society/European Respiratory Society international multidisciplinary consensus classification of idiopathic interstitial pneumonias. This joint statement of the American Thoracic Society (ATS), and the European Respiratory Society (ERS) was adopted by the ATS board of directors, June 2001 and by the ERS Executive Committee, June 2001. Am J Respir Crit Care Med. 2002;165(2):277-304.
4. American Thoracic Society/European Respiratory Society statement: update in the international multidisciplinary classification of the idiopathic interstitial pneumonias. Am J Respir Crit Care Med. 2013;188(6):733-48.
5. Jindal SK, Gupta D. Algorithm for diagnosing pulmonary fibrosis in tropical countries. Curr Opin Pulm Med. 1998;4(5):294-9.
6. Jindal SK, Gupta D, Aggarwal AN. Treatment issues in interstitial lung disease in tropical countries. Curr Opin Pulm Med. 1999;5(5):287-92.
7. American Thoracic Society. Idiopathic Pulmonary Fibrosis: diagnosis and treatment International Consensus Statement. Am J Respir Crit Care Med. 2000;161(2 Pt 1):646-64.
8. Raghu G, Collard HR, Egan JJ, Martinez FJ, Behr J, Brown KK, et al. An official ATS/ERS/JRS/ALAT statement: idiopathic pulmonary fibrosis-evidence-based guidelines for diagnosis and management. Am J Respir Crit Care Med. 2011;183:788-824.
9. Rudd RM, Haslam PL, Turner-Warwick M. Cryptogenic fibrosing alveolitis. Relationships of pulmonary physiology and bronchoalveolar lavage to treatment and prognosis. Am Rev Respir Dis. 1981;124(1):1-8.
10. Wilson MS, Wynn TA. Pulmonary fibrosis: pathogenesis, etiology and regulation. Mucosal Immunol. 2009;2(2):103-21.
11. ATS/ERS/JRT/ALAT Statement: Idiopathic pulmonary fibrosis: evidence based guidelines for diagnosis and management. Am J Respir Crit Care. 2011.

12. Demedts M, Behr J, Buhl R, Costabel U, Dekhuijzen R, Jansen HM, et al. High dose acetylcysteine in idiopathic pulmonary fibrosis. N Engl J Med. 2005;353(21):2229-42.
13. Martinez FJ, de Andrade JA, Anstrom KJ, King TE, Raghu G. Idiopathic Pulmonary Fibrosis Clinical Research Network. Randomized trial of acetylcysteine in idiopathic pulmonary fibrosis. N Engl J Med. 2014;370:2093-101.
14. Azuma A, Tsuboi E, Abe S. A Placebo Control and Double Blind Phase 2 Clinical Study of Pirfenidone in Patients with Idiopathic Pulmonary Fibrosis in Japan. Am J Respir Crit Care Med. 2002;165:A728.
15. King TE, Bradford WZ, Castro-Bernardini S, Fagan EA, Glaspole I, Glassberg MK, et al. A phase 3 trial of pirfenidone in patients with idiopathic pulmonary fibrosis. N Engl J Med. 2014;370:2083-92.
16. Richeldi L, M du Bois R, Raghu G, Azuma A, Brown KK, Costabel U, et al. Efficacy and safety of nintedanib in idiophatic pulmonary fibrosis. N Engl J Med. 2014;370:2071-82.
17. Travis WD, Hunninghake G, King TE, Lynch DA, Colby TV, Galvin JR, et al. Idiopathic nonspecific interstitial pneumonia. Report of the American Thoracic Society Project. Am J Respir Crit Care Med. 2008;177:1338-47.
18. Katzenstein AL, Fiorelli RF. Nonspecific interstitial pneumonia/fibrosis: histologic features and clinical significance. Am J Surg Pathol. 1994;18(2):136-47.
19. Cottin V, Donsbeck AV, Revel D, Loire R, Cordier JF. Nonspecific interstitial pneumonia. Individualization of a clinicopathologic entity in a series of 12 patients. Am J Respir Crit Care Med. 1998;158(4):1286-93.
20. Yousem SA, Colby TV, Gaensler EA. Respiratory bronchiolitis-associated interstitial lung disease and its relationship to desquamative interstitial pneumonia. Mayo Clin Proc. 1989;64(11):1373-80.
21. Myers JL, Veal CF, Shin MS, Katzenstein AL. Respiratory bronchiolitis causing interstitial lung disease. A clinicopathologic study of six cases. Am Rev Respir Dis. 1987;135(4):880-4.
22. Caminati A, Harari S. Smoking-related interstitial pneumonias and pulmonary Langerhans cell histiocytosis. Proc Am Thorac Soc. 2006;3(4):299-306.
23. Liebow AA, Steer A, Billingsley JG. Desquamative interstitial pneumonia. Am J Med. 1965;39:369-404.
24. Godbert B, Wissler MP, Vignaud JM. Desquamative interstitial pneumonia. An analytic review with emphasis on etiology. Eur Respir Rev. 2013;22(128):117-123.
25. Grinblat J, Mechlis S, Lewitus Z. Organizing pneumonia-like process: an unusual observation in steroid responsive cases with features of chronic interstitial pneumonia. Chest. 1981;80(3):259-63.
26. Ryu JH, Myers JL, Capizzi SA, Douglas WW, Vassallo R, Decker PA. Desquamative interstitial pneumonia and respiratory bronchiolitis-associated interstitial lung disease. Chest. 2005;127(1):178-84.
27. Moon J, du Bois RM, Colby TV, Hansell DM, Nicholson AG. Clinical significance of respiratory bronchiolitis on open biopsy and its relationship to smoking related interstitial lung diseases. Thorax. 1999;54(11):1009-14.
28. Hidalgo A, Franquet T, Gimenez A, Bordes R, Pineda R, Madrid M. Smoking-related interstitial lung disease: radiologic-pathologic correlation. Eur Radiol. 2006;16:2463-70.
29. Inoue T, Toyoshima K, Kikui M. Idiopathic broncholitis obliterans organizing pneumonia (idiopathic BOOP) in childhood. Pediatr Pulmonol. 1996;22(1):67-72.
30. Oymak FS, Demirbaş HM, Mavili E, Akgun H, Gulmez I, Demir R, et al. Bronchiolitis obliterans organizing pneumonia. Clinical and roentgenological features in 26 cases. Respiration. 2005;72(3):254-62.
31. Alsaghir AH, Al-Mobeireek AF, Al-Jahdali H, Al-Eithan A, Al-Otair H, Al-Dayel F. Bronchiolitis obliterans organizing pneumonia: experience at three hospitals in Riyadh. Ann Saudi Med. 2007;27(1):32-5.
32. Chang J, Han J, Kim DW, Lee I, Lee KY, Jung S, et al. Bronchiolitis obliterans organizing pneumonia: clinicopathologic review of a series of 45 Korean patients including rapidly progressive form. J Korean Med Sci. 2002;17(2):179-86.
33. Cordier JF. Organising pneumonia. Thorax. 2000;55(4):318-28.
34. Drakopanagiotakis F, Paschalaki K, Abu-Hijleh M, Aswad B, Karagianidis N, Kastanakis E, et al. Cryptogenic and secondary organizing pneumonia: clinical presentation, radiographic findings, treatment response and prognosis. Chest. 2011;139(4):893-900.
35. Robertson BJ, Hansell DM. Organizing pneumonia: a kaleidoscope of concepts and morphology. Eur Radiol. 2011;21:2244-54.
36. Hamman L, Rich AR. Acute diffuse interstitial fibrosis of the lungs. Bull Johns Hopkins Hosp. 1944;74:177-212.
37. Bouros D, Nicholson AC, Polychronopoulos V, du Bois RM. Acute interstitial pneumonia. Eur Respir J. 2000;15(2):412-8.
38. Bitterman PB. Pathogenesis of fibrosis in acute lung injury. Am J Med. 1992;92(6A):39S-43S.
39. Downey GP, Granton JT. Mechanisms of acute lung injury. Curr Opin Pulm Med. 1997;3(3):234-41.
40. Hayashi T, Stetler-Stevenson WG, Fleming MV, Fishback N, Koss MN, Liotta LA, et al. Immunohistochemical study of metalloproteinases and their tissue inhibitors in the lungs of patients with diffuse alveolar damage and idiopathic pulmonary fibrosis. Am J Pathol. 1996;149(4):1241-56.
41. Mukhopadhyay S, Parambil JG. Acute interstitial pneumonia (AIP): relationship to Hamman-Rich syndrome, diffuse alveolar damage (DAD), and acute respiratory distress syndrome (ARDS). Semin Respir Crit Care Med. 2012;33:476-85.
42. Vourlekis JS. Acute interstitial pneumonia. Clin Chest Med. 2004;25:739-47.
43. Peabody JW, Buechner HA, Anderson AE. Hamman-Rich syndrome; analysis of current concepts and report of three precipitous deaths following cortisone and corticotropin (ACTH) withdrawal. AMA Arch Intern Med. 1953;92(6):806-24.
44. Luce JM. Acute lung injury and the acute respiratory distress syndrome. Crit Care Med. 1998;26(2):369-76.
45. Primack SL, Hartman TE, Ikezoe J, Akira M, Sakatani M, Müller NL. Acute interstitial pneumonia: radiographic and CT findings in nine patients. Radiology. 1993;188(3):817-20.
46. Robinson DS, Geddes DM, Hansell DM, Shee CD, Corbishley C, Murday A, et al. Partial resolution of acute interstitial pneumonia in native lung after single lung transplantation. Thorax. 1996;51(11):1158-9.
47. Ichikado K, Suga M, Müller NL, Taniguchi H, Kondoh Y, Akira M, et al. Acute interstitial pneumonia: comparison of high-resolution computed tomography findings between

survivors and nonsurvivors. Am J Respir Crit Care Med. 2002;165(11):1551-6.
48. Akira M. Computed tomography and pathologic findings in fulminant forms of idiopathic interstitial pneumonia. J Thorac Imaging. 1999;14(2):76-84.
49. Liebow AA, Carrington CB. Diffuse pulmonary lymphoreticular infiltrations associated with dysproteinemia. Med Clin North Am. 1973;57(3):809-43.
50. Rio B, Louvet C, Gessain A, Dormont D, Gisselbrecht C, Martoia R, et al. Adult T-cell leukemia and non-malignant adenopathies associated with HTLV I virus. Apropos of 17 patients born in the Caribbean region and Africa. Presse Med. 1990;21(16):746-51.
51. Kurosu K, Weiden MD, Takiguchi Y, Rom WN, Yumoto N, Jaishree J, et al. BCL-6 mutations in pulmonary lymphoproliferative disorders: demonstration of an aberrant immunological reaction in HIV-related lymphoid interstitial pneumonia. J Immunol. 2004;172(11):7116-22.
52. Cha SI, Fessler MB, Cool CD, Schwarz MI, Brown KK. Lymphoid interstitial pneumonia: clinical features, associations and prognosis. Eur Respir J. 2006;28(2):364-9.
53. Amitani R, Niimi A, Kuse F. Idiopathic pulmonary upper lobe fibrosis (IPUF). Kokyu. 1992;11:693-9.
54. Frankel SK, Cool CD, Lynch DA, Brown KK. Idiopathic pleuroparenchymal fibroelastosis: description of a novel clinicopathologic entity. Chest. 2004;126(6):2007-13.
55. Watanabe K. Pleuroparenchymal fibroelastosis: its clinical characteristics. Current Respiratory Medicine Review. 2013;9:229-37.
56. Von Der Thusen JH. Pleuroparenchymal fibroelastosis: its pathological characteristics. Current Respiratory Medicine Review. 2013;9:238-47.

Sarcoidosis

Dheeraj Gupta, Sahajal Dhooria, Om P Sharma

INTRODUCTION

Sarcoidosis is a multisystem granulomatous disorder of unknown etiology. The disease occurs worldwide and affects young and middle-aged adults of both sexes. The lungs are the most frequently involved organs, but its chameleon-like presentation can involve any organ including the eyes, skin, bones, heart, liver and the brain. Despite extensive research carried out over a century, the cause of sarcoidosis remains unknown. The most accepted hypothesis favors an environmental or infectious agent in a genetically susceptible host. In the past, sarcoidosis was considered rare in India and other developing countries. However, due to increasing awareness and the availability of better diagnostic modalities, sarcoidosis is now more readily diagnosed by clinicians in this country as compared to the situation two decades ago. Still the differential diagnosis from tuberculosis, which is far more prevalent in developing countries and is a close clinical mimic of sarcoidosis, remains a challenge.

HISTORY

The early descriptions of sarcoidosis were limited only to its skin manifestations. In 1877, Jonathan Hutchinson, a general practitioner in London described a patient with chronic multiple, raised, purplish cutaneous patches over hands and feet. This was probably the first reported case of sarcoidosis.[1] The term "sarcoidosis" is credited to Caesar Boeck, who described histological findings of epithelioid cells and giant cells in a skin biopsy specimen and termed it "multiple benign sarcoid of the skin", implying that the histology resembled "sarcoma" but was benign.[2] The major landmarks in the description and understanding of the disease are summarized in **Table 1**. Detailed accounts of the history of sarcoidosis have appeared elsewhere.[3,4]

Table 1 Some important historical landmarks in sarcoidosis

Year(s)	*Landmark*
1869	Hutchinson describes skin lesions
1889	Besnier describes "Lupus pernio"[5]
1904	Kreibich describes sarcoid bone cysts[6]
1909	Heerfordt describes uveoparotid fever[7]
1916–17	Schaumann recognizes multiple organ involvement and separates sarcoidosis from lymphoma[8]
1939	Association of hypercalcemia or hypercalciuria with sarcoidosis is described[9]
1941	Kveim describes a test to help diagnose sarcoidosis,[10] Siltzbach later refines and popularizes the test,[11] James christens the test as Kveim-Siltzbach test
1946	Löfgren links erythema nodosum, bilateral hilar lymphadenopathy, fever and polyarthritis[12]
1951	Corticosteroids are first used to treat sarcoidosis[13]
1958	Wurm and colleagues proposed radiographic staging[14] First International Conference held in London, UK
1975	Serum angiotensin-converting enzyme (ACE) is first recognized as a possible biochemical marker by Lieberman[15]
1984	Rizzato starts the journal sarcoidosis (now called sarcoidosis, vasculitis and diffuse lung diseases)
1987	Rizzato and James form the World Association of Sarcoidosis and Other Granulomatous Disorders (WASOG)

EPIDEMIOLOGY

Sarcoidosis has evolved from a dermatological curiosity in the 19th century to a common multisystem disorder in the 21st century. The epidemiology of sarcoidosis has been a confusing field because of the varied clinical presentation of the disease in different parts of the world, despite the fact that there is a vast body of evidence worldwide on the prevalence, racial predilection, and the familial, geographic, climatic and occupational clustering of sarcoidosis.[16-20] There are significant differences in disease prevalence between countries, e.g. compared to a high prevalence rate of 28.2/100,000 in Finland, it is as low as 3.7/100,000 population in Japan.[16] The definite prevalence figures are not available from India, but the disorder has moved from the position of a disease of relative obscurity to that of increasing recognition.[17-23] At our hospital, which is a tertiary care referral center for the region in Northern India, North of Delhi, we have been diagnosing over 100 new cases every year since 2001.

The ACCESS (A Case Control Etiologic Study of Sarcoidosis) study conducted across 10 centers in the United States has clarified and confirmed some epidemiological and etiologic aspects of the disease.[24,25] In addition to investigating the possible etiology of the disease, this study examined the psychosocial characteristics[26] and clinical course of 736 patients enrolled in the first 6 months after histological diagnosis of sarcoidosis and compared them with control subjects paired by age, sex and race. A follow-up study of the first 215 cases was undertaken 2 years after enrollment.[27] Women were somewhat more likely to be affected, and there were sex differences in clinical manifestations; women tended to have more ocular and neurological involvement, whereas men had a higher risk of hypercalcemia. African-Americans were more likely to have uveitis, skin and liver disease. In the United States, the lifetime risk of sarcoidosis for those of Afro-Caribbean origin is nearly three times that for Caucasians (2.4 vs 0.85%, respectively).[28]

RISK FACTORS

Genetic Predisposition

Clustering of sarcoidosis occurs in families. Nearly 6% of patients in the United Kingdom have an affected relative[29] and the relative risk (RR) of sarcoidosis for family members in the United States is 4.7, siblings have the highest (RR = 5.8) risk.[30] The familial clustering is higher for White than Black families. The majority of familial "clusters" involve only parent–child pairs or sibling pairs, more complex pedigrees are rare. This suggests a summation of more than one minor genetic influences rather than a single causative gene mutation.

Blau syndrome, an autosomal dominant chronic granulomatous disease clinically identical to sporadic infantile-onset sarcoidosis, had its gene locus mapped 16–16p12-q21 and subsequently both diseases were found to be associated with mutations in the *CARD15* gene.[31] However, no association is found with adult sarcoidosis.[32] In recent years, many of class II major histocompatibility complex (MHC) alleles have been implicated in certain aspects of sarcoidosis. HLA-DR5, HLA-DR6, HLA-DR8 and HLA-DR9 seem to confer risk of having disease in Japanese patients, although HLA-DR9 is protective in the Scandinavian population. In German patients, HLA-DR5 is associated with chronic disease and HLA-DR3 with acute forms. Likewise, in Scandinavians, HLA-DR14 and HLA-DR15 are associated with chronic forms and HLA-DR17 with self-limiting ones.[33] The ACCESS study identified a significant association between HLA-DRB1 alleles (specifically HLA-DRB1*1101) and the development of the disease, both in Blacks and Caucasians.[24] The only class II allele that was distributed differently among different races with respect to the disease was HLA-DRB1*1501, which was associated with controls in blacks and with cases in whites. This would indicate that, in general, alleles similar to class II HLA may be associated with sarcoidosis in both populations. Similarly, other studies have identified specific alleles of HLA-DQB1 as determining susceptibility to sarcoidosis in the African-American population.[25,34,35] In a study from India presence of DRB1*11 and DRB1*14, and absence of DRB1*07 and DQB1*0201 alleles, were found to be independent predictors of sarcoidosis.[36] Recently, genome-wide association studies (GWAS) have identified new predisposing genes. Advances in molecular techniques like large-scale and systematic genetic sequencing will help in discovering further risk loci.

Environmental and Occupational Risk Factors

Many studies support the possibility that environmental and occupational exposures to inflammation-evoking stimuli may trigger sarcoidosis-like illness.[37] Barnard et al.[38] based on data from the ACCESS study, observed a greater risk among workers with industrial exposure to organic powders, particularly in those who worked for suppliers of building materials, hardware and gardening material. The jobs associated with childcare and occupational exposure to metal vapors or dusts were not associated with sarcoidosis. These associations were seen particularly among Caucasians.

Occupational exposures identified in the case-control studies among Afro-American patients of sarcoidosis were of wood-burning stoves, fireplaces, consumption of water from wells (not from the public mains supply), living or working on a farm,[39] exposed to metals at work, and working in humid places with musty smells.[40]

The data on the seasonality in the occurrence of this disease is conflicting.[41,42] In a study, we have found seasonal clustering of sarcoidosis during summer months.[43] This is depicted in **Figure 1**.

Tobacco smoking is considered protective for sarcoidosis. In 1961, Comstock et al., in their study of possible risk factors for sarcoidosis, observed that patients with sarcoidosis smoked less than matched controls. This inverse association was however noted only among white subjects.[44] Similar findings were subsequently reported in several studies with a reduction in prevalence of smokers among sarcoidosis patients varying between 21% and 79%.[45-52] The large multicentric ACCESS study demonstrated lesser odds for ever-smoking among patients (OR 0.65, CI 0.51–0.82).[53] Fewer alveolar macrophages are recovered by lavage from smokers with sarcoidosis than from normal subjects with a similar smoking history. This supports the possibility that smokers, particularly those with a lower accumulation of

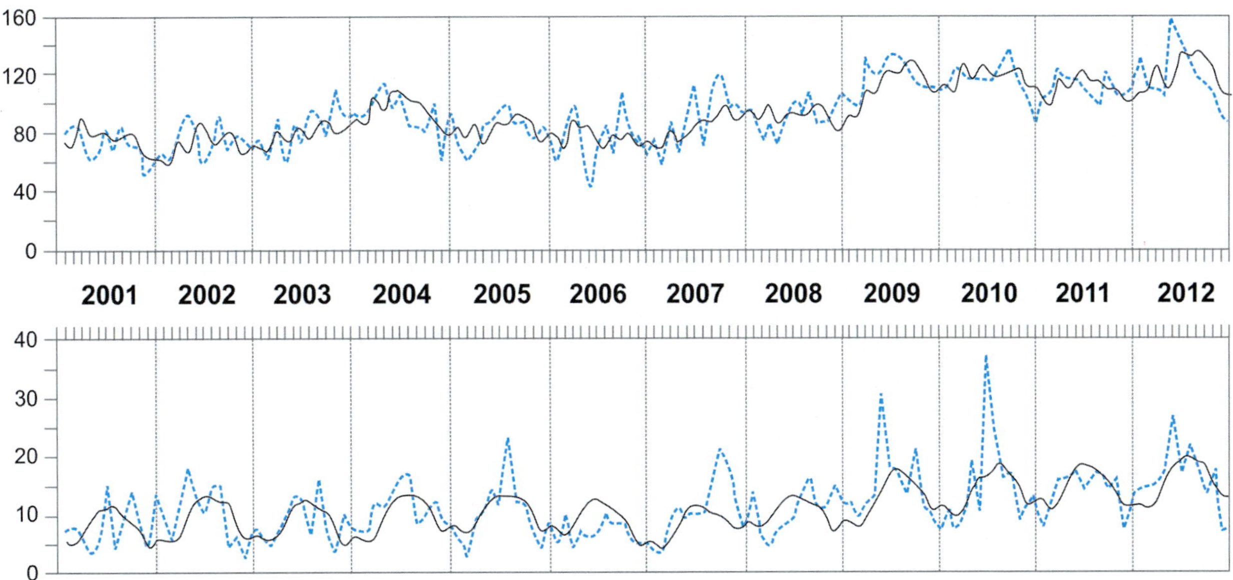

Fig. 1 Chart depicting month-wise distribution of total number of flexible bronchoscopies (upper panel) and number of patients with sarcoidosis (bottom panel) in the years 2001–2012 at our center

alveolar macrophages in the lower respiratory tract, may be less prone to develop sarcoidosis.[45,51] This was further supported by Blanchet and coworkers, who demonstrated in animal models and cell lines that concomitant exposure to nicotine with agents known to induce granulomatous inflammation, had a protective effect.[54] Contrary to above data, many studies have reported insignificant association or even increased prevalence of smoking among sarcoidosis patients.[55,56] A recent study has reported impact of active smoking and environmental tobacco smoke (ETS) exposure on disease severity in newly diagnosed cases of sarcoidosis from India. In this study smoking or ETS exposure did not have any significant negative association with sarcoidosis.[57] Also, tobacco smoke did not have any effect on the clinical behavior or disease severity in sarcoidosis.

Infectious Agents as Risk Factors

Granulomatous diseases are the result of continued presentation of a poorly degradable antigen.[58] In the case of sarcoidosis, numerous etiologic agents have been incriminated, both infective and noninfective.[59] Noninfective agents have been implicated because of their epidemiologic association,[60] but have not stood the test of time.[61] Examination of the sarcoid granuloma with an electron microscope and immunohistochemical techniques has identified structures similar to organisms such as *Leptospira* species, *Mycoplasma* species and *Propionibacterium* species.[59] Other microbiological agents that have been implicated from time to time include herpes virus, retrovirus, *Chlamydia pneumoniae, Borrelia burgdorferi, Rickettsia helvetica,* and finally *Pneumocystis jiroveci.*[59,62] The two strongest contenders are the *Propionibacterium* and the *Mycobacterium.*[63-65]

From the time sarcoidosis has been described, there has always been a belief that the disease is in some way related to tuberculosis.[66] However, the inability to identify mycobacteria by histologic staining or culture from pathologic tissues continues to be one of the strongest arguments against a potential role for mycobacteria. A recent meta-analysis suggested a 30% prevalence rate of mycobacterial DNA in sarcoid samples but the individual studies reported detection rates from 0% to 50%.[67] Moreover, most of these studies were published from countries with low prevalence for tuberculosis. If indeed mycobacteria are etiologically linked to sarcoidosis then the detection rates for mycobacterial DNA in sarcoid samples would be higher in countries with high prevalence of tuberculosis. In a recent prospective case-control study aimed at detection of mycobacterial DNA in patients with sarcoidosis from India, reinforced the hypothesis by showing mycobacterial DNA with polymerase chain reaction (PCR) for 65 kDa protein gene in 48% of samples [bronchoalveolar lavage (BAL or biopsy)] from freshly diagnosed patients of sarcoidosis.[68]

The factors that favor mycobacteria being a trigger for sarcoidosis include histopathologic appearances of the granulomas,[58] reports of mycobacterial disease either existing before, during or after sarcoidosis,[69,70] and the finding of mycobacteria in occasional granulomas of sarcoidosis.[71-73] Passage experiments have also suggested that mycobacteria with characteristics of *Mycobacterium tuberculosis* may be the incriminating agent.[74-77] Recent studies on humoral immunity to mycobacterial antigens from sarcoidosis patients have renewed interest in a potential role of mycobacteria in sarcoidosis.[78] It has been shown that mycobacterial early secreted antigenic target 6 (ESAT-6) and katG are recognized by sarcoidosis CD4+ T-cells when presented by known sarcoidosis susceptibility allele, DRB1*1101.[79] Interestingly, we have also found similar frequency of circulating antibodies to the RD1 antigens used in interferon gamma release assays (IGRAs) [ESAT-6 and culture filtrate protein (CFP-10)] in patients with pulmonary tuberculosis and sarcoidosis, indicating a possible pathogenic role of mycobacterial antigens in sarcoidosis.[80] However, the antibody response to a combination of epitopes from the RD-1 and RD-2 antigens is significantly different between tuberculosis and sarcoidosis.[81]

It is possible that the presence of mycobacterial infection or Bacille-Calmette Guerin (BCG) vaccination in genetically predisposed host may be involved in the development of autoimmunity.[82] It has also been suggested that the organism might exist in a cell wall deficient L-form and may be difficult to isolate.[83] Nevertheless, the jury is still out on the issue whether the tubercle bacillus causes sarcoidosis.

PATHOGENESIS AND IMMUNOLOGY

Granulomatous inflammation is the central feature in the pathogenesis of sarcoidosis. The granulomatous reaction is a protective response to an inciting agent. It limits inflammation and protects the tissue. Though the exact antigen inciting this response in sarcoidosis is yet unclear and it may, in fact be different in different patients and different demographic areas **(Fig. 2)**. Essentially there are four stages involved. First is the presence of the inciting antigen and its contact with antigen processing cells (APC), which are mostly the alveolar macrophages. The second stage is the interaction between APCs and CD4+ T lymphocytes to initiate the formation of a simple granuloma. The third stage includes further recruitment of CD4+ T-lymphocytes and elicitation of type 1 and type 2 helper responses, which lead to the final or fourth stage of formation and maintenance of complex granulomas. Macrophages differentiate to form epithelioid cells under the influence of cytokine production. These epithelioid cells fuse to form multinucleated giant cells (MNGC) and gain secretory properties. Granulomas secrete many chemicals including calcitriol and angiotensin-converting enzyme. These events, however, are dependent on a susceptible genetic background described by a variety of functional polymorphisms.[84,85]

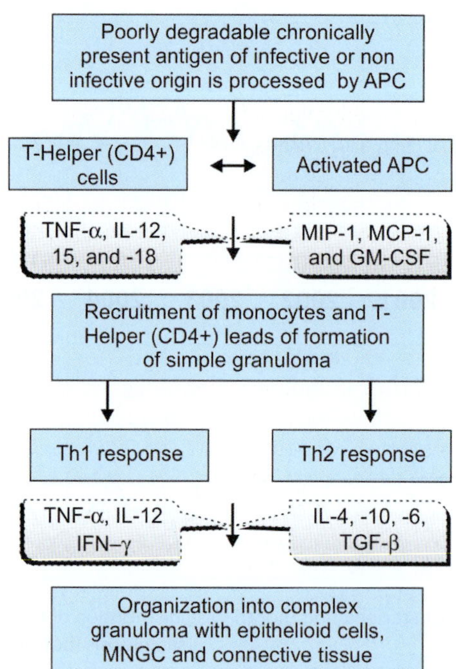

Fig. 2 A possible sequence of development of granulomatous inflammation in sarcoidosis

Abbreviations: APC, antigen processing cells; TNF-α, tumor necrosis factor-α; IL-12; interleukin-12; MIP-1, macrophage inflammatory protein; MCP-1, monocyte chemoattractant protein-1; GM-CSF, granulocyte macrophage colony-stimulating factor; IFN-γ, interferon-γ; MNGC, multinucleated giant cells.

What Controls the Course of Granulomas?

Extensive research over the past two decades has helped to delineate the sequence of events in the immunopathogenesis of sarcoidosis. The sarcoid granulomatous inflammation is characterized by an altered balance of Th1 or Th2 responses with a dominant expression of Th1 cytokines [interferon-γ (IFN-γ) and interleukin-2 (IL-2)] with low levels of expression of T helper 2 (Th2) cytokines (IL-4 and IL-5).[86,87] The earliest event is accumulation CD4+ helper T-cells and release of IL-2 in the alveoli and interstitium.[86,88,89] This is followed by a progressive and selective oligoclonal expansion of αβ T-cell.[90] There is increased in situ production of Th1 cell-derived cytokines (IL-2 and IFN-γ) during granuloma formation.[91,92] The alveolar macrophages in sarcoidosis have immense secretory properties and there is an increased release of macrophage-derived cytokines [IL-1, IL-6, IL-8, IL-15, tumor necrosis factor-α (TNF-α), IFN-γ, granulocyte-macrophage colony-stimulating factor (GM-CSF)] and chemokines [regulated on activation, normal T-cell expressed and secreted (RANTES), macrophage inflammatory protein-1α (MIP-1α), IL-16]. Most of these cytokines favor granuloma formation and lung damage.[93-96] IL-12 contributes to proliferation of activated T-cells in early disease. Elevated levels of IL-6 and IL-8 are reported in the BAL fluid of active sarcoidosis, and these may modify the disease process. IL-15 may aid in the proliferation of T- and B-cells.[97] IL-12 and IL-18 are also increased in the lungs of sarcoidosis and they stimulate IFN-production.[86,98] The chemoattractant cytokines like IL-8, IL-15, IL-16 and RANTES recruit the CD4+ T-cells from the peripheral blood to the site of inflammation,[85-87] while IL-2 induces an in situ proliferation of these cells.[99,100]

The progression and maintenance of granulomatous reaction is also helped by accumulation of these monocyte-macrophages with antigen-presenting cell capacity and expressing increased levels of activation markers (HLA-DR, HLA-DQ, CD71) and adhesion molecules (CD49a, CD54, CD102). The mechanism(s) that result in spontaneous resolution or progression to chronic disease and fibrosis are unclear but may be linked to host susceptibility and genetic factors. Transforming growth factor-beta (TGF-β) is an inhibitor of IL-12 and IFN-production. Its production is increased in those patients undergoing remission of sarcoidosis, suggesting a key role for TGF-β in the downregulation of granulomatous inflammation of sarcoidosis.[101] Oxidative stress may also have a role to play in the pathogenesis of sarcoidosis. A detailed discussion of this aspect of pathogenesis can be found elsewhere.[102]

Another clinically important phenomenon that occurs in sarcoidosis is the depression of delayed type hypersensitivity. Commonly utilized as a diagnostic tool, this is often impaired in active sarcoidosis and not seen when sarcoidosis resolves. A subgroup of CD4 T-cells may account for this anergy by abolishing IL-2 production and inhibiting T-cell proliferation.[103,104] It is also suggested that anergy state may be related to diminished dendritic cell function.[105]

PATHOLOGY

The most common organs of involvement are lymph nodes, lungs, liver, spleen and skin. In the lungs, the common site of involvement is along the bronchovascular spaces (lymphangitic pattern), that makes the transbronchial biopsy a preferred choice for obtaining histological diagnosis. Pulmonary vascular involvement has also been reported quite frequently.[106] Nevertheless, any organ can be involved and the histological features are similar in all the organs.[13,107,108] Many a times the pathological involvement of organs may remain clinically silent, making sarcoidosis an iceberg syndrome **(Fig. 3)**.

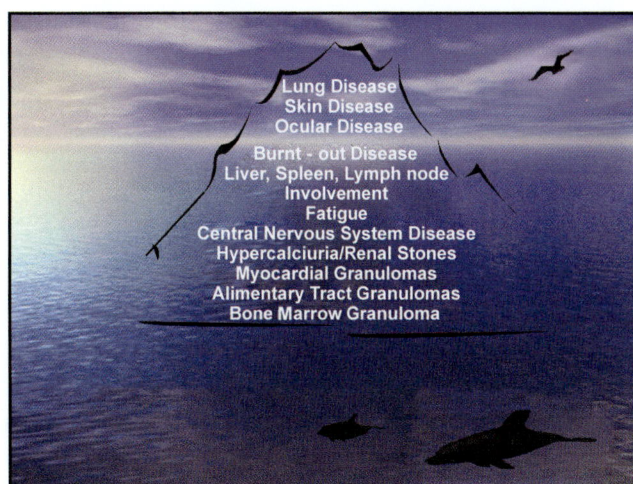

Fig. 3 Sarcoidosis: An Iceberg syndrome. Pathological involvement of various organs may not be clinically apparent

The hallmark of sarcoidosis is the presence of noncaseating, compact, "naked" granulomas. On histology, a sarcoid granuloma is comprised of lymphocytes, macrophages, well-differentiated epithelioid cells, MNGC, fibroblasts and mast cells. The sarcoid granulomas have CD4 T-cells in the center and CD8 T-cells and B lymphocytes in the periphery.[13,109-111] Histologic findings differ based on the stage of the disease. In early stages of disease, the sarcoid granuloma is a compact structure consisting of radially arranged pale, pink epithelioid cells seen most often in the center of the granulomas. Lymphocytes and fibroblasts form a surrounding rim. Multinucleated Langerhans' type giant cells, usually only a few, are often seen in the granuloma. Caseation is absent. However, focal coagulative necrosis may be seen.[110] In rare cases, fibrinoid necrosis is seen in nodular and necrotizing sarcoid granulomatosis.[112,113] Nonspecific cytoplasmic inclusions can be seen in sarcoidosis, such as asteroid bodies, Schaumann's bodies, Hamazaki-Wesenberg bodies and calcium oxalate crystals. Granulomatous inflammation may resolve totally with or without therapy. It may also persist and show hyalinization. In chronic sarcoidosis, fibrosis and scarring occur.[110,112]

CLINICAL FEATURES

Though the lung is the most common organ affected with sarcoidosis, the disease may involve any part of the body.[27] A systematic review and cumulative analysis of all the major studies from India that have reported on clinical features show almost similar figures as reported from other countries while extrapulmonary lymphadenopathy is distinctly more frequent **(Table 2)**.[114]

Pulmonary Involvement

Clinical Findings

The symptoms of sarcoidosis are often nonspecific and 20–50% of patients with sarcoidosis are asymptomatic. The diagnosis is pursued after an abnormality is detected on a chest X-ray film obtained for an unrelated reason.[125] Dry cough and dyspnea are the most common clinical signs and symptoms attributable to the intrathoracic manifestations of sarcoidosis. Chest pain may be present and is often vague and nonspecific; however, it may be severe and suggestive of cardiac pain.[126,127] Chest pain may also indicate an unusual complication such as pleuritis or pneumothorax, or even pulmonary embolism, as antiphospholipid antibody syndrome has been associated with sarcoidosis on rare occasions.[125] Wheezing suggests airway obstruction secondary to endobronchial granulomatous disease, extrinsic compression by mediastinal adenopathy, or bronchial

Table 2 Summary of clinical findings as computed from major studies published from India

	Center (reference)					Total n/N	%
	AIIMS, Delhi		Eastern India[115]	South India[19]	PGI, Chandigarh [19,57,116-122]		
	Sharma[123]	Tahir[124]					
Total patients	106	72	200	22	492	892	-
Gender (Females)	38	36	89	13	203	379/892	42.48%
Constitutional Symptoms:							
Arthralgia	47	27	122	6	124	326/892	36.54%
Malaise	NA	NA	26	NA	73	99/692	13.29%
Fever	60	NA	140	9	224	433/820	52.8%
Pulmonary symptoms:							
Cough/dyspnea	88	NA	186	17	338	629/820	76.7%
Extrapulmonary symptoms:							
Eye	19	17	NA	2	54	92/692	13.29%
Lymph nodes	48	NA	44	NA	21	113/698	16.18%
Liver	48	9	87	NA	41	185/870	21.26%
Spleen	NA	6	65	NA	17	88/764	11.5%
Skin	45	22	NA	7	43	117/692	16.9%
Parotidomegaly	13	6	NA	NA	12	31/670	4.62%
Neurological	9	3	NA	1	7	20/692	2.89%
Chest radiograph:							
Stage I	25	1	NA	8	216	250/692	36.12%
Stage II	67	35	NA	10	244	356/692	51.44%
Stage III	14	35	NA	3	24	76/692	10.98%
Stage IV	NA	1	NA	1	8	10/692	1.44%

distortion secondary to fibrotic lung disease. Wheezing may also be contributed by bronchial hyperreactivity.[128,129] A productive cough may indicate traction bronchiectasis due to parenchymal fibrosis. Hemoptysis suggests bronchiectasis or the presence of an aspergilloma.

Radiographic Findings

The chest radiograph is abnormal in more than 90% of sarcoidosis patients and diagnosis of sarcoidosis is first suspected on routine chest roentgenography in most patients. Bilateral hilar lymphadenopathy is noted in 50–85% of cases. The presence of symmetrical bihilar and mediastinal lymphadenopathy is almost characteristic in sarcoidosis. Lymph nodes are generally big and sharply defined, with a clear line of translucency between the mediastinal shadow and the nodes classically described as "potato nodes". Unilateral hilar adenopathy is rare. Pulmonary parenchymal infiltrates are seen in 25–60%. Typically, the infiltrates are bilateral and symmetrical and are most common in the upper and mid-lung fields.[130,131]

A chest radiographic staging system[132] for sarcoidosis is as follows **(Table 3 and Figs 4A to D)**:

Higher radiographic stages have been associated with poorer prognosis.[133,134] However, there is significant overlap between the groups and prognosticating individual patients based on radiographic stage alone is unreliable. Nevertheless, once patients develop stage IV disease spontaneous remission is rare. In Stage IV pulmonary sarcoidosis, the lung parenchyma is destroyed with upward traction of the hila, lung distortion, upper lobe volume loss, fibrocystic disease, honeycombed cysts, and reduced lung volumes. Large bullae may house one or more fungus balls (aspergillomas) **(Figs 5A and B)**.[135] Cystic or traction bronchiectasis may develop.

Chest computed tomography (CT) though is more sensitive in revealing the extent of involvement than the chest radiograph, there is no evidence that CT has a superior prognostic or therapeutic value compared with the chest

Table 3 Chest radiographic staging of sarcoidosis

Stage	*Features*
Stage 0	No involvement
Stage 1	Bilateral hilar adenopathy, often with right paratracheal adenopathy
Stage 2	Stage 1 + Pulmonary infiltrates
Stage 3	Pulmonary infiltrates without adenopathy as described in stage 1
Stage 4	Advanced parenchymal lung disease, including fibrosis, honeycomb lung, traction bronchiectasis, cysts, bullae and emphysema, with or without adenopathy

radiograph in the management of pulmonary sarcoidosis. CT scans can have several typical and atypical findings.[130,136] Typically the high-resolution CT (HRCT) reveals nodules along the bronchovascular bundle and subpleural regions.[136,137] Coalescence of these granulomata may result in mass-like lesions with or without air bronchograms. Occasionally, these conglomerate nodules are surrounded by small nodules giving an appearance that is known as "sarcoid galaxy sign" **(Figs 6A to D)**.[138] More extensive lymphadenopathy is also more commonly seen on CT than the typical hilar and paratracheal nodes seen on chest radiograph. Ground glass attenuation, often thought to represent acute alveolitis, has been shown to represent granulomatous inflammation.[139]

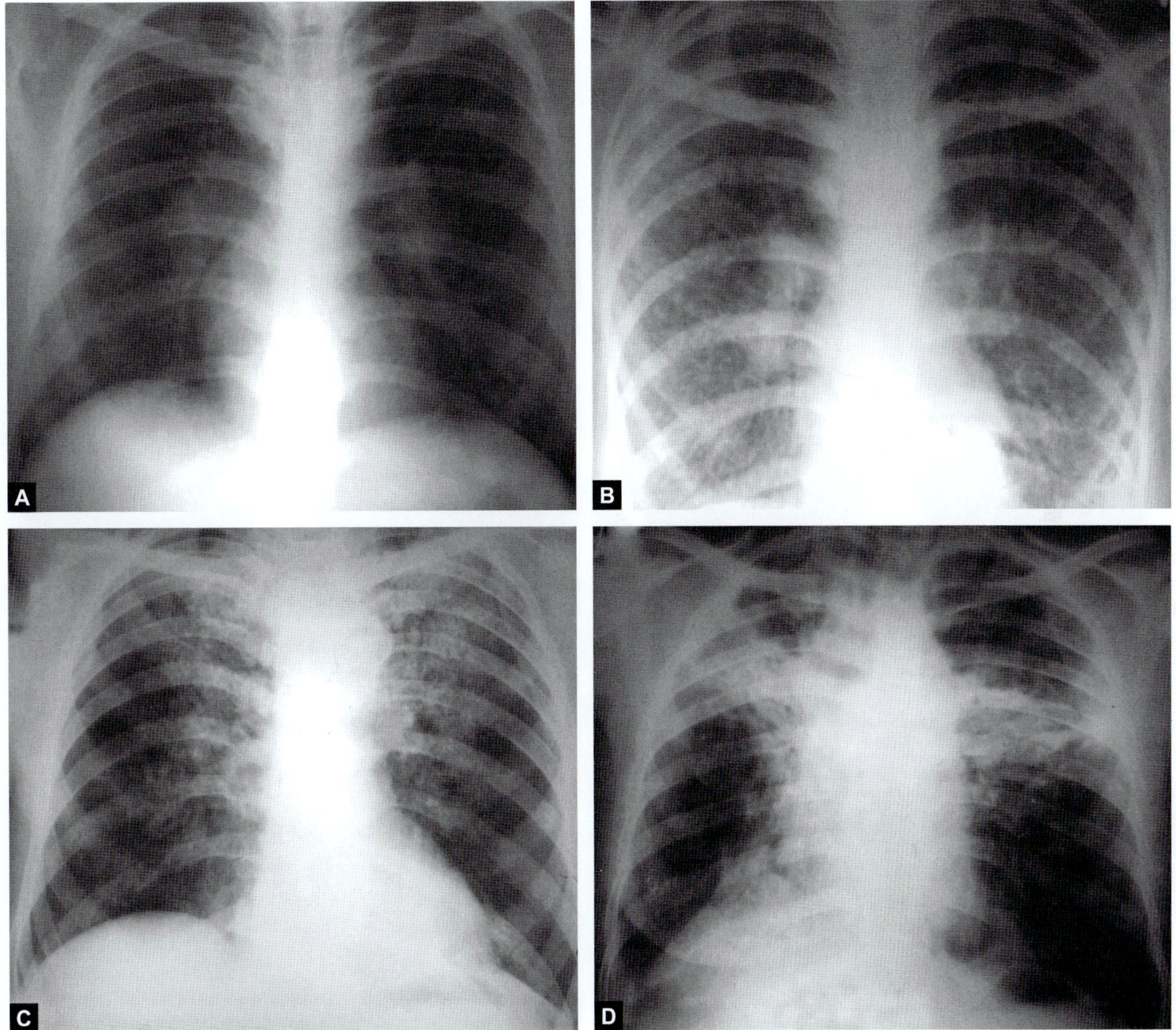

Figs 4A to D Typical chest radiographs in sarcoidosis. (A) Stage 1, showing bilateral hilar and paratracheal lymphadenopathy; (B) Stage 2, hilar and paratracheal lymphadenopathy with pulmonary infiltrates; (C) Stage 3, pulmonary infiltrates with no lymphadenopathy; (D) Stage 4, pulmonary fibrosis with architectural distortion

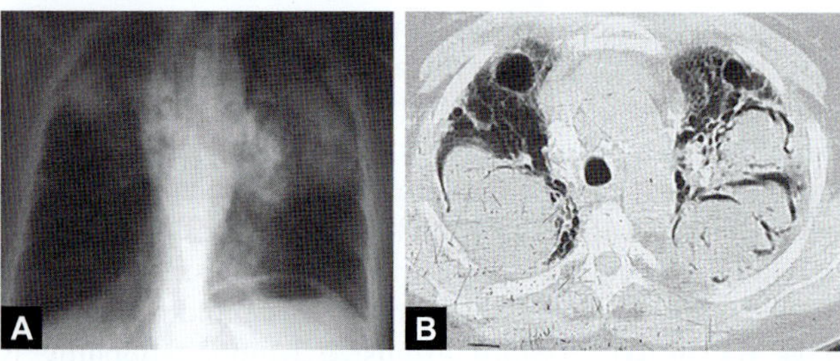

Figs 5A and B Bilateral upper lobe aspergillomas in sarcoidosis

"Reverse halo" sign typically described with invasive fungal infections has also been reported in sarcoidosis.[140] Typical findings, if found, may be useful in suggesting sarcoidosis in the evaluation of an undiagnosed interstitial lung disease.

Functional Abnormalities

Pulmonary function abnormalities can be seen in 20–40% sarcoidosis patients with a normal lung parenchyma on a chest radiograph and 50–70% of cases when the lung parenchyma is visibly abnormal.[141] These include abnormalities in the vital capacity, diffusing capacity, partial pressure of oxygen (PAO_2) at rest, PAO_2 with exercise, and lung compliance.[141] Lung function testing with the help of spirometry is a simple procedure to grade the disease extent. Lung function changes have been shown to bear a clinical correlation with overall histopathological scoring assessed from the granuloma load and interstitial inflammation.[120,142] Lung functions have also been correlated with radiological extent of the parenchymal disease; patients with stage IV fibrocystic disease have the most severe pulmonary function impairment.[143] Being an interstitial lung disease, a restrictive ventilatory defect is to be expected. However, as mentioned previously, endobronchial involvement may result in airflow obstruction being the major abnormality on pulmonary function testing. Airflow obstruction in chronic sarcoidosis may possibly be due to airway distortion from lung fibrosis. Granulomatous involvement of skeletal muscle occurs in 50–80% of patients with sarcoidosis and

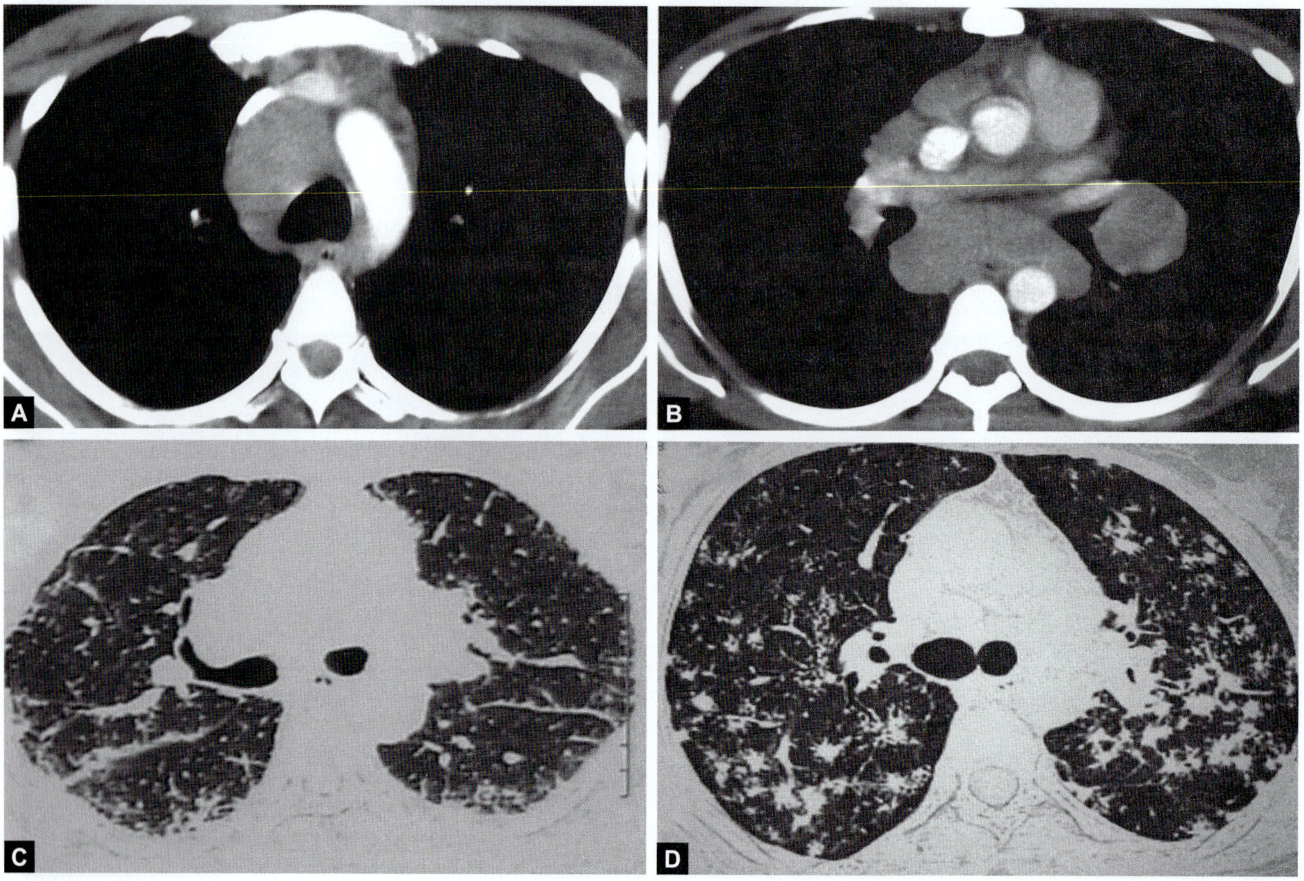

Figs 6A to D Some representative computed tomography pictures in sarcoidosis. (A) Paratracheal lymphadenopathy; (B) Hilar and subcarinal lymphadenopathy. Lymph nodes are typically homogenous with no central necrosis; (C) Pulmonary nodular infiltrates with typical lymphangitic distribution; panel; (D) "S arcoid galaxy" sign: large conglomerate nodules surrounded by small nodules

this may affect respiratory muscle function in sarcoidosis.[144] Measurements of respiratory pressures has been used as an index of functional work capacity and reflection of activities of daily living.[145] Pulmonary hypertension is a serious complication of pulmonary sarcoidosis and is a risk factor for death.[146] Pulmonary hypertension may occur via a number of mechanisms including parenchymal fibrosis distorting the pulmonary vasculature (pulmonary arterial or venous system), granulomatous inflammation of the pulmonary vasculature, hypoxic pulmonary arterial vasoconstriction from parenchymal sarcoidosis pulmonary disease, and from elevated left ventricular end diastolic pressure because of cardiac involvement with sarcoidosis.[146,147]

Other Intrathoracic Manifestations

Pleural involvement (including effusions and thickening) may be detected in 5–10% of patients with sarcoidosis **(Fig. 7)**. Pleural effusions are estimated to occur in 1–3% of patients with sarcoidosis and are more likely to be seen in patients with stages 2 and 3 disease.[148,149] These effusions are more often right-sided (45% vs 33% left-sided and 22% bilateral), have relatively few cells (mostly lymphocytes), and are often discordant with respect to Light's criteria in that the effusions are characteristically exudative by protein criteria and transudative by lactate dehydrogenase (LDH) criteria.[148] Chylothorax, hemothorax, and pneumothorax have also been reported rarely.[150-152] Contrary to the infrequency with which the above pleural diseases affect the patients with sarcoidosis, pleural thickening on CT scan may be seen in up to one-third of patients, the clinical significance of which remains unclear.[153]

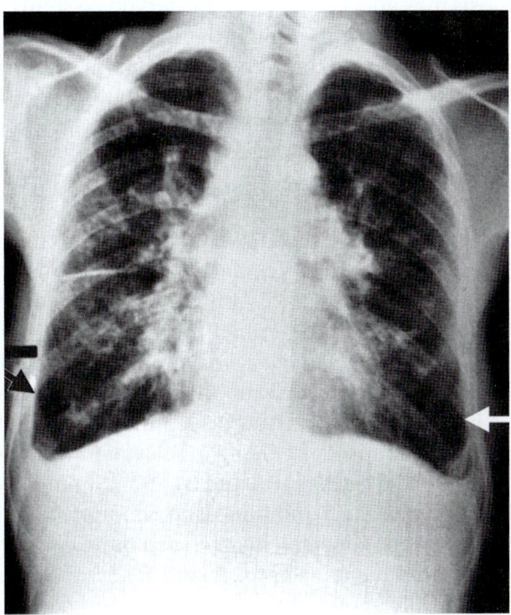

Fig. 7 Bilateral pleural thickening in sarcoidosis

Hemoptysis, at times, serious, can occur due to variety of reasons such as formation of a fungal ball (aspergilloma) in a preexisting cyst or cavity, bronchiectasis (most often due to traction in association with parenchymal fibrosis) and necrotizing sarcoid angiitis.[154,155] Rare consequences of mediastinal lymphadenopathy include superior vena cava syndrome,[156] mediastinal lymph node calcification and mediastinal fibrosis.[157] Rarely giant bullae resulting from sarcoidosis may lead to the "vanishing lung syndrome".[158] Several of these rare manifestations have also been documented from India.[159]

Extrapulmonary Involvement

Involvement of extrapulmonary sites is fairly common and often of major clinical importance. When carefully looked for, one or more of the other extrapulmonary organs were involved in about two-thirds of patients at our center.[21] Constitutional symptoms of fever, night sweats, weight loss, fatigue, myalgia and arthralgia occur very frequently with extrathoracic sarcoidosis. Fatigue, in particular, is an important symptom.[160] Although any organ can be involved, skin and eye are the most common, whereas cardiac and neurological involvement are most serious. Major extra-pulmonary manifestations of sarcoidosis are outlined below, detailed descriptions can be found elsewhere.[161,162]

Skin

Erythema nodosum (EN), subcutaneous nodules and plaques, lupus pernio and maculopapular eruptions are the important manifestations of sarcoidosis.[163] Skin lesions are divided into two categories: (1) specific and (2) nonspecific. Specific lesions demonstrate granulomatous inflammation on biopsy. Nonspecific skin lesions are inflammatory skin reactions with no evidence of granulomatous inflammation. EN is the most common nonspecific skin lesion of sarcoidosis. It presents as tender nodules on the extremities. EN with hilar lymphadenopathy (Löfgren's syndrome, also often with polyarthropathy and nongranulomatous uveitis) is a typical subset of sarcoidosis with particular characteristics **(Figs 8A and B)**. Known to carry a very favorable prognosis for resolution, it has been described with a spring seasonal peak in both the Northern and Southern hemisphere.[140,141] Specific skin lesions are usually asymptomatic. Disfigurement is the most common complaint. The most common lesions are firm, 2 to 5 mm papules that often have a translucent red-brown or yellow-brown appearance. Lupus pernio is the most severe form of dermatological manifestation that usually affects the nose, cheeks, lips, and ears in form of indolent, red-purple or violaceous skin lesions. These lesions can erode into cartilage and bone, especially around the nose.[164-166] Lupus pernio is associated with poor prognosis of sarcoidosis and is associated with more severe pulmonary disease.[167,168]

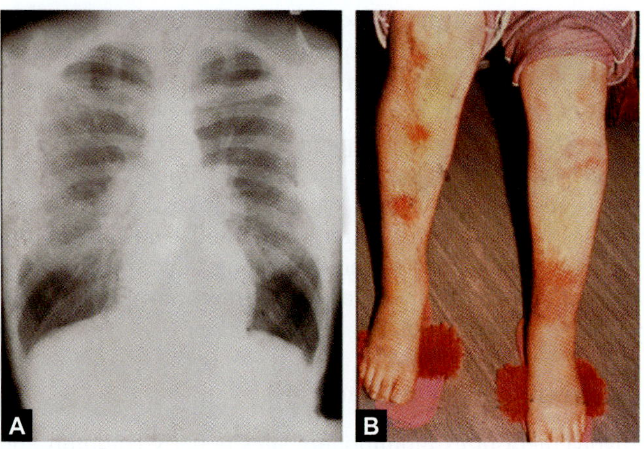

Figs 8A and B Lofgren syndrome: Bilateral hilar adenopathy with erythema nodosum

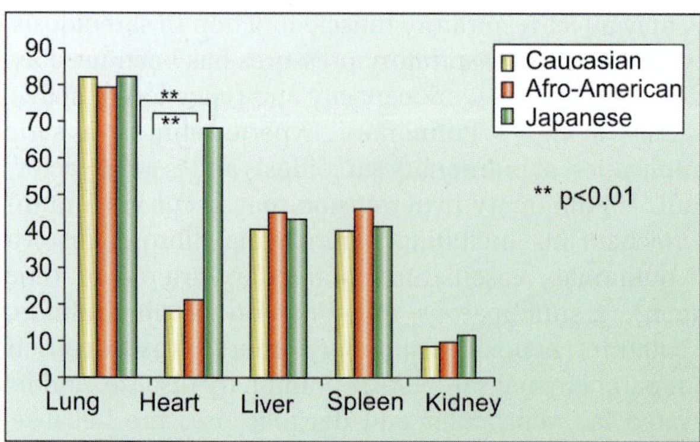

Fig. 9 Frequency of organ involvement in sarcoidosis. Cardiac involvement is much higher in Japanese patients than other groups

Eye

Eyes are involved in sarcoidosis in up to 25% patients and it can affect any part of the eye and may be the major manifestation of the disease.[169,170] Ocular involvement is present in more than 70% Japanese patients.[171] A careful eye check-up should be a part of routine clinical work-up of sarcoidosis. Uveitis is the most common ocular manifestation of sarcoidosis.[172] Depending upon the site of involvement, the symptoms vary from blurred vision, red eye, painful eye or photophobia in anterior uveitis to vision loss in posterior uveitis. Retinal perivasculitis, retinal scarring, and glaucoma can occur. One-third of the patients with anterior uveitis have no symptoms (a "quiet eye").[170,173] Besides uveitis, involvement of lacrimal glands is also common, which may occasionally cause dry eyes. Optic neuropathy is rare but can result in rapid, permanent vision loss.[170,173,174] Funduscopic examination shows papillitis, papilledema, and neovascularization with optic atrophy ultimately. This condition is an ophthalmologic emergency and mandates immediate systemic therapy.

Cardiac

Though rare, both cardiac and neurologic sarcoidosis may be life-threatening and are, therefore, important to recognize. Though clinically detectable in only 5% of sarcoidosis patients, cardiac involvement may be picked up in 25% patients at autopsy.[175,176] Japanese show a markedly higher rate of cardiac involvement compared to Caucasians and African-Americans **(Fig. 9)**. Cardiac sarcoidosis may cause left ventricular dysfunction, heart block and cardiac arrhythmias that can result in sudden death.[177-180] Endomyocardial biopsy is the gold standard diagnostic test which is very specific, however, it has a poor sensitivity of less than 25% because of sampling error.[181] For the noninvasive diagnosis of cardiac involvement in sarcoidosis, various investigations such as echocardiography, thallium scanning, gallium scanning, magnetic resonance imaging (MRI), or positron emission tomography (PET) scanning can be used coupled with a typical clinical presentation.[180,182-188]

Neurosarcoidosis

Overall, central nervous system (CNS) involvement may be seen in about 10% patients of sarcoidosis.[189] Neurosarcoidosis can mimic diverse neurological conditions. Diagnosis of neurosarcoidosis is based on a confirmation of systemic sarcoidosis since pathologic confirmation is rarely available from the central nervous system. CNS infection and malignancy should be reasonably excluded before making a diagnosis of CNS sarcoidosis.[190] The most common manifestation of neurosarcoidosis is seventh cranial nerve palsy and it may precede the diagnosis of the disease. Sarcoidosis may affect any part of the nervous system causing a cranial nerve palsy, mononeuropathy or polyneuropathy, aseptic meningitis, seizures, mass lesions in the brain or spinal cord, and encephalopathy.[191,192] Rarely, it may also mimic multiple sclerosis.[193]

Other Extrapulmonary Organ Involvement

Sarcoidosis may affect the upper airways, and the gastrointestinal, hematological, endocrine, genitourinary and musculoskeletal systems.[194] Almost all types of organs involvement have been described from India and the other developing countries as well. Asymptomatic histological involvement of liver may be seen in 50–65% patients. Abnormalities in liver function tests are seen in less than 35%, the most common abnormality being an elevation in the serum alkaline phosphatase **(Figs 10A and B)**.[195-199] Similarly, spleen may also be involved with minimal or no symptoms. Significant splenomegaly with hypersplenism is seen more commonly in Afro-American patients **(Figs 11A and B)**.[200-203] Sarcoidosis causes clinically apparent peripheral lymphadenopathy in more than 10% of patients.[204] Sarcoidosis of the upper

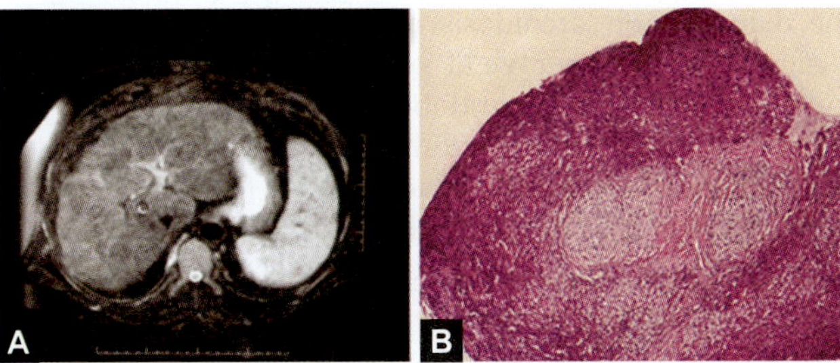

Figs 10A and B Hepatic sarcoidosis

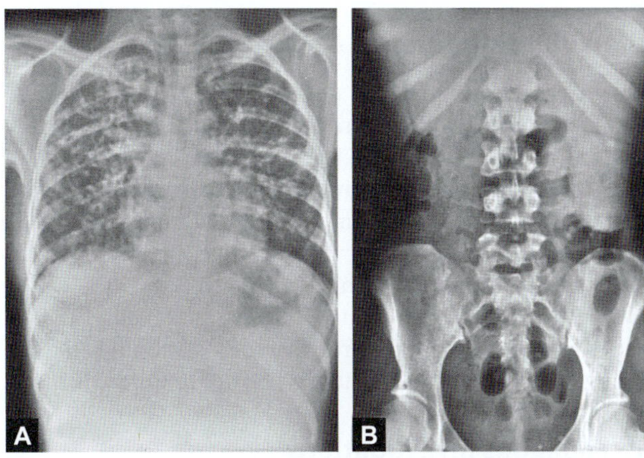

Figs 11A and B A patient with sarcoidosis and massive splenomegaly. Enlarged spleen and hypersplenism is common in African-American patients

respiratory tract is underappreciated. It may occur in the nasopharynx, hypopharynx, larynx, or sinuses and rarely vocal cord palsy may be a feature.[205,206]

Typical bone lesions of sarcoidosis are small cysts or cortical defects in the small bones of the hands or feet, which occur occasionally (about 4% in one series) and are possibly more frequent in females and in patients with lupus pernio.[207] Joints if involved acutely, as is often seen in patients with Lofgren's syndrome, carry a good prognosis.[208] Chronic sarcoid arthritis is rare but can progress to cause joint deformities.[209,210]

Abnormalities of Calcium Metabolism

In any general medical ward, there are three common causes of hypercalcemia: hyperparathyroidism, lymphoma or malignancy, and sarcoidosis. In sarcoidosis, hyperkalemia has been reported to occur in 2–63% of patients; hypercalciuria is three times more common than hypercalcemia.[211] Therefore, serum and urine calcium levels should be measured regularly over the whole course of the illness. The mechanism of hypercalcemia in sarcoidosis is due to excess extrarenal calcitriol production.[212] The alveolar macrophages present within the granulomas contain the enzyme 1-α hydroxylase which converts precursor vitamin D to active calcitriol.[213] Normally, high levels of calcitriol cause feedback inhibition of 1-α hydroxylase; calcitriol also causes upregulation of 25 $(OH)D_3$ 24 hydroxylase, the enzyme which converts 25 $(OH)D_3$ to 24, 25 $(OH)_2D_3$, the metabolically inactive form of vitamin D. Both the feedback mechanisms are lost in alveolar macrophages which lead to continuous production of calcitriol.[214] Another recently described mechanism is excess production of parathyroid-hormone related peptide (PTHrp), which like parathyroid hormone, causes upregulation of 1-α hydroxylase.[215] Unlike parathyroid hormone, PTHrp is not regulated by calcium but by IL-2 and TNF-α both of which are increased in sarcoidosis.[216] It is possible that these cytokines released by the alveolar macrophages act in a paracrine fashion to upregulate PTHrp production by the macrophages.[214] Hypercalciuria or hypercalcemia can lead to nephrolithiasis and renal failure. Rarely hypercalcemia may cause acute pancreatitis.[217]

DIAGNOSIS

The diagnosis of sarcoidosis rests on a triad of clinical, radiologic and histological criteria. Although the diagnosis of sarcoidosis can be reached with a high level of confidence in up to 80% of patients using clinical data and HRCT imaging, it is imperative that a histological diagnosis be obtained in all patients as far as circumstances permit (except in those with the classic Löfgren's syndrome). This is especially so in tuberculosis-endemic areas, because the clinical and radiologic picture of the two diseases may be overlapping. The other diagnostic possibilities in patients with hilar and mediastinal lymphadenopathy are enumerated in **Box 1** (marked with an asterisk). Another point worth mentioning is that sarcoidosis may come to clinical attention due to any of its pulmonary or extrapulmonary features. However, as the lungs and mediastinum are involved in most cases, even in extrapulmonary disease; these are usually the most appropriate sites to access (barring the case in cutaneous sarcoidosis) for establishing a histologic diagnosis.

Histological Diagnosis

In general, the least invasive method of obtaining a histological diagnosis should be selected.[218] Biopsy of the skin or peripheral lymph nodes, if enlarged, may yield the diagnosis in a few cases. However, most patients having thoracic or internal organ involvement would require a sampling of the mediastinal lymph nodes, the airway mucosa, and/or the lung parenchyma. Transbronchial lung biopsy obtained with the help of fiberoptic bronchoscopy has traditionally been the most commonly used procedure in the diagnosis of pulmonary sarcoidosis and has made a major difference in diagnosis of sarcoidosis in India.[17,219,220] Its yield varies from 40% to over 80% depending on operator experience.[221-224]

BOX 1 Common pathological differential diagnosis of sarcoidosis

Mycobacterial:*
- Tuberculosis
- Atypical mycobacteria

Fungal infections:*
- Cryptococcosis
- Aspergillosis
- Histoplasmosis
- Coccidioidomycosis
- Blastomycosis
- Pneumocystis

Bacterial:
- Mycoplasma
- Brucella

Hypersenstivity pneumonias

Drug Reactions*

Pneumoconiosis:
- Beryllium (chronic beryllium disease)*
- Titanium
- Aluminum

Malignancy:
- Lymphoma*

Others:
- Wegener's granulomatosis (sarcoid-type granulomas are rare)
- Chronic interstitial pneumonia (UIP, LIP)
- Necrotizing sarcoid granulomatosis (NSG)
- Granulomatous lesions of unknown significance (GLUS syndrome)

Source: Statement on Sarcoidosis. Joint Statement of the American Thoracic Society (ATS), the European Respiratory Society (ERS) and the World Association of Sarcoidosis and Other Granulomatous Disorders (WASOG) adopted by the ATS Board of Directors and by the ERS Executive Committee, February 1999. Am J Respir Crit Care Med. 1999;160(2):736-55. Conditions marked with (*) can also present with hilar and mediastinal lymphadenopathy

Abbreviations: LIP, lymphocytic interstitial pneumonia; UIP, usual interstitial pneumonitis.

Granulomatous inflammation may be encountered in lung biopsies even in stage I sarcoidosis. Combining endobronchial with transbronchial biopsy improves the diagnostic yield by about 10%.[223,225] Endobronchial abnormalities are more commonly seen in patients with respiratory symptoms.[225] In stages I and II disease, in which mediastinal lymph nodes are involved, transbronchial needle aspiration (TBNA) during flexible bronchoscopy is very useful.[226] "Blind" or "conventional" TBNA (i.e. TBNA performed without ultrasound image guidance) has an average yield of around 60% (varies from 6% to 90% in different studies).[227] Adding transbronchial lung biopsy (TBLB) to TBNA increases the yield by 20%.[227]

Endobronchial ultrasound (EBUS) is a novel bronchoscopic modality, which helps to improve the yield of TBNA. Endobronchial ultrasound-guided TBNA (EBUS-TBNA) has an average yield of around 80% (range, 54–93%) in the diagnosis of sarcoidosis. A recent large trial reported a significantly higher yield of EBUS-TBNA as compared to a combination of endobronchial biopsy (EBB) and TBLB.[228] However, a later study has reaffirmed the utility of conventional bronchoscopic techniques (TBNA plus TBLB plus EBB) by demonstrating their equivalence to a combination of EBUS-TBNA and TBLB.[224]

The characteristic findings on biopsy is the presence of compact noncaseating epithelioid cell granulomas, however, an alternative diagnosis has to be excluded. A general differential diagnosis of granulomatous inflammation is given **(Box 1)**.

Tuberculin Skin Test

The tuberculin sensitivity is depressed in sarcoidosis even in the background of high prevalence of tuberculosis and a cut-off of 10 mm reaction to 5 tuberculin unit (TU) tuberculin test has virtually 100% sensitivity for sarcoidosis, however, it is not specific.[117] The problem is further confounded by the coexistence of two diseases.[229] A negative tuberculin test is heavily relied upon for diagnosis of sarcoidosis. It is cheap and simple to perform. A positive tuberculin skin test (TST) in a patient suspected to suffer from sarcoidosis should alert the treating physician for a thorough work-up for tuberculosis.

Miscellaneous Investigations

Bronchoalveolar lavage: Bronchoalveolar lavage has a high positive predictive value for the diagnosis of sarcoidosis with an elevated ratio of CD4 or CD8 in BAL fluid. However, the samples require more than 15% lymphocytes on cell count to be useful.[230] A CD4:CD8 ratio greater than 3.5 shows a high specificity of 93–96% for sarcoidosis, but the sensitivity is low (53–59%).[228,231]

Kveim test: The Kveim-Siltzbach test is performed using intradermal injections of human sarcoid tissue. Four weeks later the papule that forms at the site of the injection is biopsied. Though the mechanism of the Kveim test vis-à-vis sarcoidosis is still not clearly understood,[232] it has been traditionally considered a reliable test for diagnosis of sarcoidosis with positivity of even up to 98%.[11,233] However, it has some limitations. A validated good quality antigen is not available.[234] The frequency of positivity depends upon the duration of disease. The test requires a long period of 4–6 weeks following intradermal injection of the antigen before a positive reaction is obtained. Further, there is a risk of transmission of the etiological agent by the Kveim test. Therefore, the clinical application of this test remains limited.

Serum angiotensin-converting enzyme (SACE): Angiotensin-converting enzyme is produced by the epithelioid cells of sarcoid granulomas. SACE estimation was introduced as a promising test of diagnosis in the mid-seventies.[15] A rise in SACE activity in active sarcoidosis has been shown in a few reports from this country as well.[235,236] However, the test is neither sensitive nor specific to be useful as a diagnostic tool.[237,238] It may be normal in patients with sarcoidosis and other disorders such as diabetes mellitus, cirrhosis, acute hepatitis, chronic renal disease, silicosis, Gaucher's disease, leprosy, asbestosis, and berylliosis may demonstrate elevated SACE levels. Overall, the sensitivity and specificity of elevated SACE levels are 55% and 90%, respectively.[239] Also, there is no apparent association between serum ACE level and radiographic staging.[237] In spite of lack of specificity as a test for sarcoidosis, SACE provides a fairly good monitor of disease activity. It is to be borne in mind that the presence of inhibitors may interfere with SACE levels unless sensitive radioimmunoassay techniques are used for assessment.[240] Some studies have suggested that SACE levels may vary with genetic factors and the use of genotype corrected ACE levels may make it a more useful diagnostic tool.[241-243]

Gallium scanning: It demonstrates inflammation throughout the body and is associated with specific findings in sarcoidosis. Uptake in the hilar lymph nodes and right paratracheal nodes results in the "lambda sign", whereas lacrimal and salivary gland uptake results in the "panda sign".[244] Its use has largely fallen out of favor due to the advances in bronchoscopic techniques and availability of a better radionuclide study, 18-fluorodeoxyglucose-PET (^{18}FDG-PET) scanning.

18-Fluorodeoxyglucose-positron emission tomography (^{18}FDG-PET) scanning: ^{18} FDG-PET plays an important role in the diagnosis and management of sarcoidosis, although it is not indispensable. It acts as an adjunct to the routine investigations in assessing disease activity especially in extrapulmonary sites, and monitoring treatment response and also helps to identify occult sites for biopsy.[245,246] It is especially useful in cardiac sarcoidosis, where it can help in identifying potentially life-threatening disease in an asymptomatic patient.[247] However, it is not useful for differentiating sarcoidosis from other inflammatory diseases, especially tuberculosis.[248] F-methyltyrosine-PET (FMT-PET) uses an amino acid that is preferentially taken up and expressed on the surface of tumor cells, and is negative in patients with sarcoidosis.[249]

Assessment of Activity

Assessing activity and/or severity of disease in sarcoidosis is a tough task as no single variable in isolation is accurate.[250] Imaging with 18-FDG PET scanning and several laboratory and cell biological markers in serum [e.g. SACE, lysozyme, neopterin, soluble IL-2-receptor, soluble intracellular adhesion molecule (ICAM)-1, IFN-c] or in BAL fluid (e.g. high lymphocytes, activation marker expression on T-cells, CD4/C8 ratio, macrophage TNF-α release, collagenase, procollagen-III-peptide, vitronectin, fibronectin and hyaluronan) have been studied as potential indices of active disease.[251-253] Out of these, only SACE has found some clinical utility, while PET is emerging as a useful tool.[254,255] The magnitude of the initial SACE levels has no prognostic significance as the levels are no different between patients who deteriorate and those who improve. After initiation of treatment, serum ACE levels might be helpful in monitoring the treatment effect, since an initially elevated serum ACE activity will usually come down within a few weeks of the start of corticosteroid treatment. Initial evaluation suggests that 18-FDG PET might help in assessing the total burden of disease activity in systemic sarcoidosis, and can prove particularly useful in cardiac and stage IV pulmonary sarcoidosis.[255] Yet, as of now, the best way to assess the activity of sarcoidosis is still through clinical assessment. This is based on the mode of onset, the worsening or persistence of symptoms, and the presence of skin lesions, in combination with changes in chest radiography and lung function tests, with or without treatment. Pulmonary function studies have shown rough correlation with histological severity and may be used as a surrogate.[120]

SARCOIDOSIS-TUBERCULOSIS ENIGMA

The relationship between sarcoidosis and tuberculosis remains a riddle. The remarkable similarity of sarcoidosis to tuberculosis in both the clinical and histological features has perplexed investigators for decades and a possible link between the two conditions has been debated.[66,256-259] The possible relationship has implications in pathogenesis, diagnosis as well as treatment.

Almost a quarter of a century ago, in a cooperative study of sarcoidosis in several countries of Asia, the authors commented that the chronological increase in sarcoidosis was related to the decrease in infectious diseases represented by tuberculosis.[260] This proposed relationship of tuberculosis to sarcoidosis is weak and needs to be reanalyzed as the situation in India contradicts this hypothesis. The prevalence of sarcoidosis has increased in this country despite the continued high prevalence of tuberculosis.

There are many similarities between these two granulomatous diseases, however, certain features can help in distinguishing between the two. Certain demographic factors may be different between patients with sarcoidosis and those with tuberculosis. In a study, we found that compared to tuberculosis, patients with sarcoidosis were older, had a higher body mass index, residence in urban areas, were better educated, had higher per capita income and belonged to better socioeconomic status.[261] All these differences were also significant when sarcoidosis patients were compared to healthy controls albeit to a lesser degree. Tobacco smoking, ETS exposure and use of fossil or biomass fuels for cooking were more commonly seen in tuberculosis patients.

Both tuberculosis and sarcoidosis can present with similar constitutional symptoms (fever, easy fatigability, anorexia and weight loss) and respiratory symptoms (cough and breathlessness), although expectoration and hemoptysis are distinctly more frequent in fibro-cavitary tuberculosis.

In general, patients with untreated tuberculosis have more signs and symptoms compared to sarcoidosis. But the severity and magnitude may not always help in the differential diagnosis.

Hilar lymphadenopathy, the most common clinical presentation of sarcoidosis, is also a manifestation of tuberculosis.[262] However, the nodes in sarcoidosis only rarely show a central hypodensity on CT scan, which is frequently observed in tuberculosis.[136] Further, the characteristics of mediastinal lymph nodes on EBUS can help in differentiating sarcoidosis from tuberculosis.[263] The presence of heterogeneous echotexture or coagulation necrosis sign in lymph nodes on EBUS imaging has good specificity and positive predictive value for the diagnosis of tuberculosis.[263] Fibrosis, especially in the apical regions, can occur in both conditions although cavitation is rarer in sarcoidosis.[264] Similarly, miliary distribution of lesions, characteristically described in tuberculosis, can also occur in sarcoidosis.[265,266] Miliary disease in particular poses a great difficulty in differential diagnosis particularly in India where it is considered a sine quo non for tuberculosis.[267] In fact, most patients of miliary sarcoidosis, described from India, had received antituberculosis therapy before the diagnosis of sarcoidosis was established.[265,266]

The tuberculin sensitivity is depressed in sarcoidosis even in the background of high prevalence of tuberculosis and a less than 10 mm reaction to 5TU tuberculin test has virtually 100% sensitivity for sarcoidosis.[117] A negative tuberculin test excludes tuberculosis except in seriously sick or otherwise immunosuppressed individuals. Diagnosis of tuberculosis in tuberculin negative individuals is required to be supported by strong bacteriological evidence.[268] A positive tuberculin test in sarcoidosis should also be looked with high suspicion as discussed above. In India, tuberculin test is positive in about 30–50% of general population and in 64–85% in the 25–45 years age groups.[269,270] A higher cut-off point of tuberculin test is, therefore, suggested to diagnose tuberculosis.[271]

Interferon gamma release assays have a higher sensitivity and specificity for detecting *Mycobacterium tuberculosis* (MTB) infection than the conventional TST, as they utilize antigens specific for MTB complex.[272] Clinicians in high prevalence countries erroneously make a diagnosis of tuberculosis based on a positive IGRA test. We have observed that IGRA (Quantiferon in tube[r]) being more sensitive test than TST continues to remain positive in many patients with sarcoidosis and in high prevalence countries it should not be a deterrent for making a diagnosis of sarcoidosis, since it merely represents an underlying tubercular infection.[273,274]

Although nonnecrotizing granulomas are the usual findings in sarcoidosis, necrosis can occur. Prior to the widespread use of transbronchial biopsy necrosis was reported in up to 30% of large biopsy specimens (open lung, lymph node). The incidence of necrosis is far lower in small specimens such as transbronchial biopsies because of the small number of granulomas usually sampled. Compared with the "caseous" necrosis seen in tuberculosis granulomas, the necrosis in the granulomas of sarcoidosis is most often focal, involving small areas and very few of the granulomas and is not discernible on gross examination of the specimen. The foci of necrosis are acidophilic with a fibrinoid, granular appearance and usually located within the centers of granulomas. Rarely, biopsy material from patients with well-documented sarcoidosis will exhibit extensive necrosis.[110,275]

The site and type of organ involvement may help in making a distinction. For example, lacrimal and parotid glands and myocardium are rarely involved in tuberculosis. Labial biopsy has also been shown to have a high discriminatory value in differentiation of sarcoidosis from tuberculosis.[276] Subtle differences which may help in differential diagnosis from tuberculosis are summarized in **Table 4**. However, in some situations the differential diagnosis may become impossible, particularly when the two diseases can even coexist, albeit rarely.[229]

Finally, there are treatment issues to be considered in the relationship of sarcoidosis and tuberculosis. Reactivation of tuberculosis after corticosteroid treatment is instituted for sarcoidosis is a genuine concern, given the high prevalence of latent infection in our country.[278] If indeed tuberculosis is a causal factor in sarcoidosis, then the hypothesis can be further reinforced, if antitubercular therapy (ATT) is useful in treatment of sarcoidosis. Very few trials have been conducted in the past but the results of these trials have been discouraging. These trials were generally small studies and limited by time bias and used older regimens based on isoniazid, amino-salicylic acid and streptomycin.[279,280] In our experience, nearly one third of patients who are finally diagnosed to have sarcoidosis, have received ATT for variable length of time, but its impact of final outcome of sarcoidosis has not been studied. Role of antimicrobial therapy in sarcoidosis has recently been reviewed and it gives us a definite thought for the future.[281]

TREATMENT

The treatment of sarcoidosis is even more challenging than its diagnosis. This is especially so in developing countries, where the availability of medical expertise is limited, the referral system insufficient, and facilities to monitor efficacy and complications of treatment inadequate. In tuberculosis-endemic areas, the problem is twofold. Patients with sarcoidosis may be treated inappropriately with anti-tuberculosis drugs for long periods and may be correctly diagnosed only after they have already developed end-stage fibrosis making treatment difficult. Conversely, corticosteroids prescribed to patients harboring mycobacteria in quiescent lesions may lead to reactivation of tuberculosis.

Not all patients diagnosed with sarcoidosis need pharmacological therapy, as the disease is often self-limiting. Moreover, most therapeutic options are not without significant adverse effects. Even in case of multisystem involvement, the decision to treat depends on the nature and severity of individual organ involvement.[282]

Table 4 Differentiating sarcoidosis form tuberculosis in high tuberculosis prevalence countries, some useful "INDICATORS"*

Indicator	*Sarcoidosis*	*Tuberculosis*
Demographic:		
Age	Generally older (third to fourth decade)	Younger
Body mass index	Higher	Lower
Socioeconomic status	Higher	Lower
Clinical:		
History of close contact with patient having tuberculosis infection	Not present	May be present
Constitutional symptoms	Asymptomatic or with mild fever, anorexia and loss of weight	More prominent fever, anorexia, and weight loss
Cough	Mainly dry, hemoptysis is rare	Usually productive, hemoptysis is common
Peripheral lymph node involvement	Seen in about 10% patients only	Cervical and axillary lymph node involvement is common
Lacrimal, parotid and myocardial involvement	May be seen	Rare
Pleural, peritoneal, meningeal and adrenal involvement	Rarely, if ever **(Fig. 12)**	May be seen
Radiology:		
Intrathoracic lymph node involvement	Typically symmetrical bi-hilar and paratracheal; smooth, discrete, and solid-looking nodes	Asymmetrical, large, may be conglomerate, usually with central areas of hypodensity
Radiology: Necrotizing pneumonia, cavitation and pleural involvement with effusion	Rare	Common
HRCT scan of lungs **(Figs 13A to D)**	Micronodules and macronodules which have characteristic distribution in peribronchovascular region, subpleural interstitium and interlobular septa	Micronodules, randomly distributed with tree-in-bud appearance
Clinicoradiological dissociation i.e. patient relatively asymptomatic despite extensive pulmonary involvement	Even with advanced radiological abnormalities, usually the "patients walk-in"	Rare: usually the patients are "brought-in"
Other investigations:		
Tuberculin test	Nearly always negative	Nearly always positive
Increased SACE level	More common	Less common
Increased serum calcium or hypercalciuria	May be seen	Not seen
Sputum: Positive for *M. tuberculosis* on smear or culture	False-positive acid fast bacilli or rarely coexisting TB with sarcoidosis. Patient should never receive glucocorticoids alone	Confirmatory for TB
PCR of biopsy tissues is positive for *M. tuberculosis* DNA	Quantitative tests can be positive in up to half of the patients in high TB prevalence countries Qualitative test shows low copy numbers[277]	Positive with high copy numbers if quantitative tests are done
Biopsy of involved site **(Figs 13A to D)**	Noncaseating, compact granulomas, sparse lymphocytic cuffing around granuloma (naked) with inclusion bodies at times	Caseating necrosis, ill-formed granuloma with intense inflammatory reaction and may be positive for acid-fast bacilli
Response to treatment:		
No expected response to anti-tubercular therapy	Very common, however, spontaneous resolution in sarcoidosis is known	Very rare, only in case of primary multi-drug resistance
Dramatic clinic-radiological response to steroids	Usual	No response or may worsen

*These indicators are only based on common clinical observations with unknown sensitivity and specificity for most of them

Abbreviations: TB, tuberculosis; PCR, polymerase chain recation; DNA, deoxyribonucleic acid; SACE, serum angiotensin-converting enzyme; HRCT, high-resolution computed tomography.

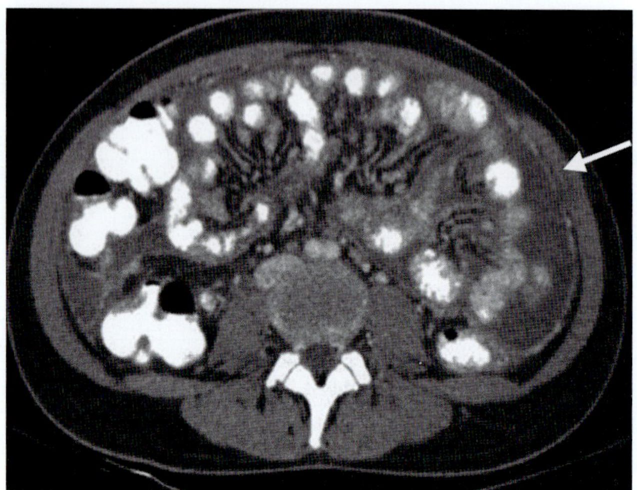

Fig. 12 Peritoneal sarcoidosis is rare and it resembles tuberculous peritonitis

When to Treat?

Pulmonary Sarcoidosis

Unless there is extrapulmonary involvement requiring treatment, the general rule of managing pulmonary sarcoidosis is not to treat asymptomatic disease. Patients having moderate-to-severe symptoms, a decrement in the quality of life, or significant physiological impairment should be treated.[282] It should be confirmed that the symptoms are attributable to pulmonary sarcoidosis and not to any alternate cause. There remains a paucity of high quality evidence from large randomized controlled trials on steroid treatment of pulmonary sarcoidosis regarding the timing, dose, and duration of treatment. However, the following may serve as guiding principles of treatment of pulmonary sarcoidosis according to the radiological stage:

Stage 0, I: Asymptomatic patients with stage 0 or stage I disease nearly always remain free of symptoms without treatment,

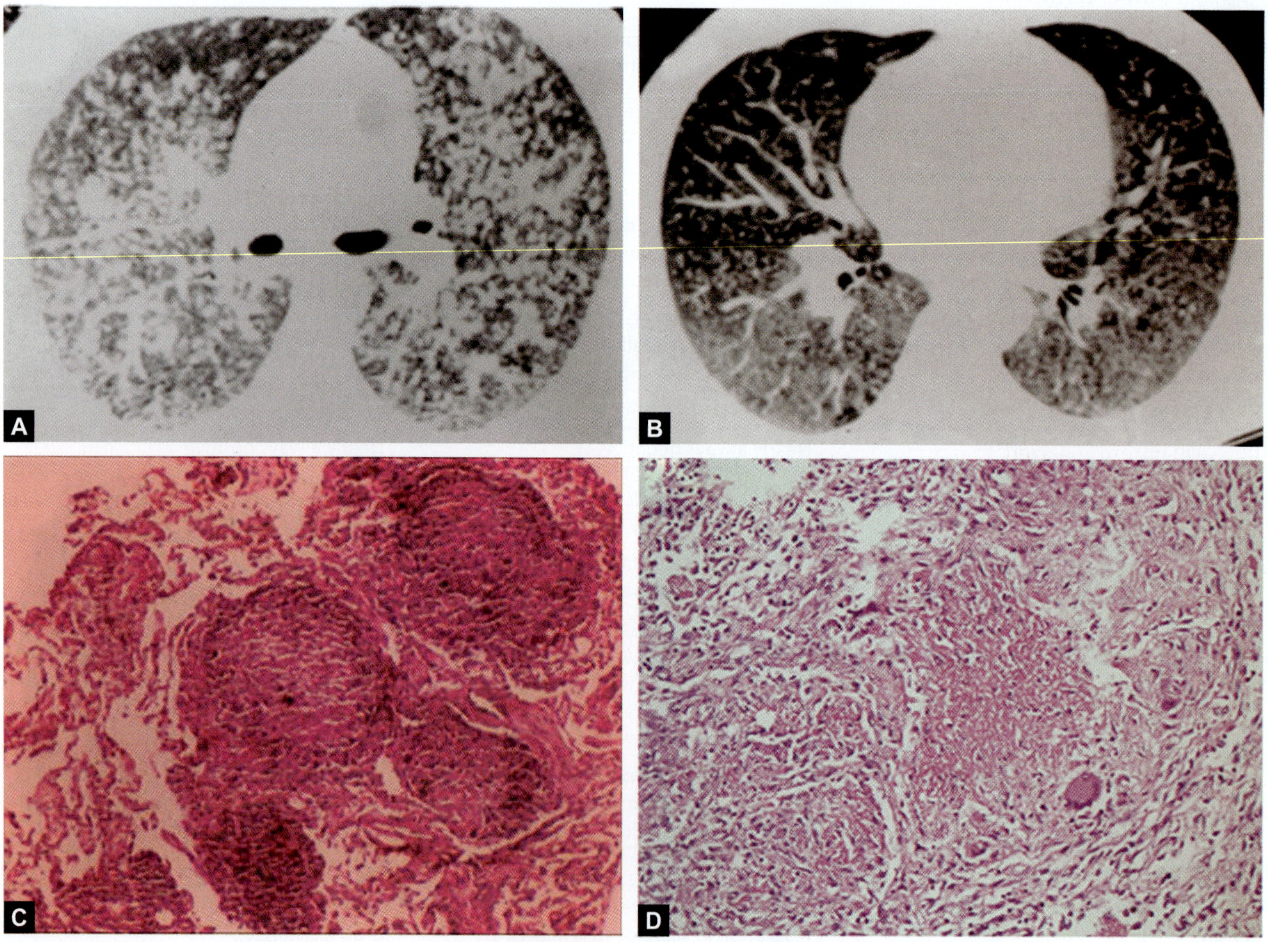

Figs 13A to D Miliary sarcoidosis (A, C) versus miliary tuberculosis (B, D). On computed tomography, the nodules in sarcoidosis are larger than tuberculosis with typical lymphangitic distribution. On histopathology, the granulomas in sarcoidosis are typically compact, with no necrosis and minimal lymphocytic cuffing (C) compared to large areas of necrosis and intense lymphomononuclear cell infiltrates in tuberculosis (D)

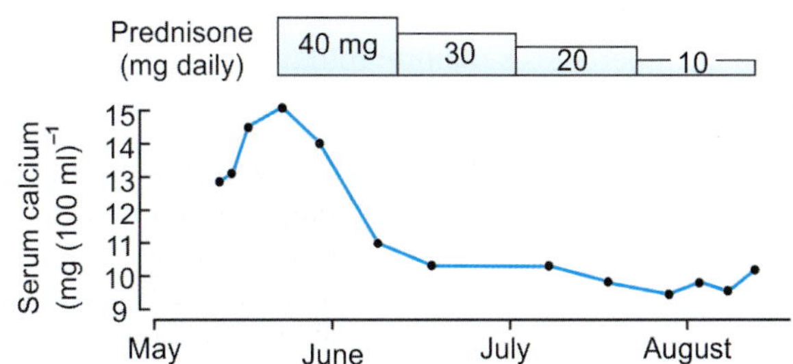

Fig. 14 Response of serum calcium level to steroid treatment over a period of several months

hence do not require treatment.[133,283] Patients having fever and joint pains may be observed or treated with nonsteroidal anti-inflammatory drugs (NSAIDs). Occasionally, a short-term course of prednisone 15–20 mg/day may be needed to control symptoms that do not respond to NSAIDs.

Stage II: Patients who are asymptomatic and have only mild lung function impairment can be followed without any specific treatment. However, if deterioration of lung function [10% decrease in forced vital capacity (FVC) or 20% decrease in diffusing capacity of carbon monoxide] should occur over a period of 3–6 months, immunosuppressive treatment should be instituted.[284,285] Those with symptoms (cough, dyspnea, chest pain, and effort intolerance) or significant lung function impairment should be treated.[286]

Stage III: These patients usually have symptoms along with lung function abnormalities and almost always need treatment. Asymptomatic stage III patients with progressive pulmonary function impairment should also be treated.

Stage IV: These patients, especially those with extensive fibrosis and bullae formation respond poorly or not at all to corticosteroids and immunosuppressive therapy. It should however, be emphasized that some stage IV patients with irreversible fibrosis may have coexisting active inflammation and the treatment should be strongly considered in order to control symptoms and progression of functional impairment.[287] Patients with stage 4 sarcoidosis frequently develop complications and should be managed for the same as detailed later in the chapter.

Extrapulmonary Sarcoidosis

Patients with certain extrapulmonary manifestations of sarcoidosis need to be treated right away with immunosuppressive therapy. These include symptomatic patients with ocular, neurologic, cardiac, upper airway involvement, lupus pernio and those with hypercalcemia. Ocular involvement in the form of mild anterior uveitis may be treated with topical steroids only. For more severe or unresponsive disease, intravitreal steroid injections and/or systemic steroids may be indicated.[171] In both neurosarcoidosis and cardiac sarcoidosis, higher initial doses of steroids (1 mg/kg/day) might be required.[288-290] In severe cases, initial treatment with high dose methylprednisolone pulses may be required.[288-290] Atrioventricular conduction blocks and left ventricular function generally show recovery, while the data on ventricular tachycardia, and mortality are sparse.[291] It should be remembered that therapy in these scenario needs experience and individualization as there are no evidence-based guidelines on these entities.[290] A Delphi study failed to reach any consensus on the appropriate doses and duration of steroid treatment in cardiac sarcoidosis.[292] Asymptomatic hypercalciuria and hypercalcemia can cause nephrocalcinosis and renal failure.[282] Hypercalcemia should be treated with steroids **(Fig. 14)** apart from hydration, diuretics and low calcium diet.

Patients with sarcoidosis frequently have asymptomatic elevations in liver transaminases, which should not be treated. In those with elevation of enzymes more than twice the upper limit of normal, liver functions must be monitored.[293] Any patient with symptoms (jaundice or pruritus), worsening of liver function test abnormalities, cholestasis or abnormal synthetic liver function should be treated.[293] Mild and cosmetically unimportant skin lesions do not require any treatment.[294] Others may be treated with topical and intralesional steroid treatment. Lupus pernio and other disfiguring lesions require systemic corticosteroids, which should be started early.[294] Initial observation is suggested in asymptomatic patients with lymph node involvement, splenic enlargement, and parotid swelling. If symptomatic, they generally respond to modest doses of prednisolone (20–30 mg daily).

Drugs Used to Treat Sarcoidosis

Corticosteroids

Corticosteroids have been used for the treatment of sarcoidosis for the past six decades.[295] They suppress inflammation by deactivating several proinflammatory genes (by repressing nuclear factor kappa B) and activation of multiple anti-inflammatory genes. In stages II to IV, in a Cochrane database, systematic review of available trials on the efficacy of corticosteroids in pulmonary sarcoidosis, it was concluded that treatment with oral corticosteroids led to improvements in chest radiography, although there was no evidence for improvement in lung function.[296] According to expert consensus reached by a Delphi method, corticosteroids are the initial therapy of choice and 40 mg of daily prednisone equivalent is the maximum dose recommended for the treatment of pulmonary sarcoidosis.[297]

A six-phase treatment is suggested.[298] Treatment is started at a dose of 20–40 mg/day of prednisolone administered for around 4–6 weeks (phase 1).[3] This is followed by tapering (phase 2) to a daily dose of 5–10 mg over a period of 1–6 months. The maintenance (phase 3) dosing is continued for 3–9 months followed by tapering off (phase 4) and stoppage of steroids after a total duration of 12 months. The patient should then be observed (phase 5) and treated for a relapse if it occurs (phase 6). Administration of steroids every other day is equally effective as daily dosing and may be used for patients developing significant adverse effects.[299-301]

There is insufficient data to recommend routine use of inhaled corticosteroids for treatment of pulmonary disease.[297,302] A meta-analysis found inconclusive evidence to support the use of inhaled corticosteroids.[296] Isolated studies have demonstrated a slight improvement in diffusing capacity or improved symptoms.[303,304] A study indicates that inhaled budesonide administered after a course of oral steroids may lead to improved pulmonary function over a long term.[305] We suggest the use of inhaled steroids after the completion of oral steroid treatment in patients having an obstructive defect on spirometry.

Corticosteroid therapy is associated with significant adverse effects. The important adverse effects of the drugs used in treatment of sarcoidosis are listed in **Table 5**. Clinicians should consider calcium and vitamin D supplementation, after excluding hypercalcemia and hypercalciuria and monitoring for the same thereafter. Use of bisphosphonate has been recommended by the American College of Rheumatology in patients receiving more than 5 mg of prednisone per day or its equivalent for greater than 3 months.[306] Gastrointestinal bleeding risk is low in ambulatory patients treated with steroids.[307] Proton pump inhibitors or histamine H2 receptor antagonists should be considered if patients have significant dyspepsia due to steroids.

Reactivation of latent tuberculosis is an important concern with steroid therapy. However, the usual recommendation by the American Thoracic Society to undertake skin testing for latent tuberculosis before initiation of corticosteroid therapy[308] is not practical for India for two reasons. One, there is high prevalence of tuberculosis infection in population and a vast majority of our patients with sarcoidosis would be infected and two, as already discussed, tuberculin test is likely to be negative in active sarcoidosis. Another major complication of chronic glucocorticoid therapy is osteoporosis.

Alternatives to Corticosteroids

Alternatives to steroids are required due to the following reasons: (1) steroid treatment causes side effects which may be unacceptable; (2) the disease may relapse after stopping or tapering of steroids;[3] as a maintenance dose of prednisolone above 10 mg/day is unacceptable for long-term use,[297] an alternate medication may be required; (3) occasionally extrapulmonary disease may be refractory to corticosteroids.[309] The options for nonsteroidal treatment [also called disease modifying antisarcoid drugs (DMASDs)] are cytotoxic drugs, antimalarials, biologics and other agents.[310] Barring the anti-TNF-α drugs, most of these agents take a few weeks to months to be effective. Therefore, steroid treatment should not be tapered for at least a month after the addition of an alternative agent, unless the steroid adverse effects are major.[282]

Cytotoxic drugs: These include methotrexate (MTX), azathioprine, leflunomide, mycophenolate mofetil, cyclophosphamide and chlorambucil and constitute the most promising alternative to corticosteroids.[311-314] Methotrexate is the preferred second-line drug for steroid refractory

Table 5 Important adverse effects of drugs used in the management of sarcoidosis

Drug	*Adverse effects*
Corticosteroids	Weight gain, skin thinning, acne, mood changes, increased risk of infection, hypertension, diabetes, cataracts and osteoporosis
Methotrexate	Hepatitis, hepatic fibrosis, interstitial pneumonia, pulmonary fibrosis, leucopenia, gastrointestinal intolerance, teratogenicity
Azathioprine	Myelosuppression, opportunistic infections, hepatitis, teratogenicity
Leflunomide	Rash, alopecia, peripheral neuropathy, interstitial pneumonia, gastrointestinal intolerance, teratogenicity
Mycophenolate mofetil	Hyperglycemia, hypercholesterolemia, gastrointestinal intolerance, bone marrow suppression, hepatitis, teratogenicity
Cyclophosphamide	Myelosuppression, opportunistic infections, hemorrhagic cystitis, bladder malignancy, cardiomyopathy, infertility, teratogenicity
Chloroquine, hydroxychloroquine	Retinopathy, corneal changes, muscle weakness, gastrointestinal intolerance
TNF-antagonists	Infections (especially reactivation of tuberculosis), infusion reactions, gastrointestinal intolerance, headache
Rituximab	Infusion reactions, lymphopenia, opportunistic infections, asthenia

Abbreviation: TNF, tumor necrosis factor

cases and can be used as a steroid sparing drug as well.[297,315-317] Occasionally, it may be used as a first-line agent in combination with steroids.[317] The recommended initial dose is 10–15 mg once a week along with folic acid 5 mg weekly or 1 mg daily. If gastrointestinal effects occur, splitting the dose may be useful. Response is relatively slower in onset. Methotrexate may take up to 6 months to be effective.[317] Azathioprine (2 mg/kg/day) may also be used as a steroid-sparing agent.[318,319] It is equally efficacious as methotrexate, but results in a higher risk of infections.[320] Leflunomide (20 mg/day) is also effective as a steroid sparing agent. Though it has been touted as a less toxic alternative to methotrexate although similar to methotrexate, it may also occasionally cause interstitial pneumonitis as an adverse effect.[321,322] The data mycophenolate mofetil are limited, but it may also be considered as a steroid sparing option in pulmonary and extrapulmonary sarcoidosis.[323-325] Cyclophosphamide is mostly reserved for use in steroid refractory cases of severe cardiac or neurosarcoidosis, while chlorambucil is practically no longer in use.[326,327] Careful monitoring is required for toxicity of cytotoxic drugs with the help of repeated liver and renal function tests and hematological assessment.

Antimalarial drugs: Antimalarials such as chloroquine and hydroxychloroquine act as immunomodulators and have been successfully used for cutaneous sarcoidosis involving the paranasal sinuses, sarcoid-related hypercalcemia and neurosarcoidosis.[328-331] Hydroxychloroquine has also been found to be effective in treating chronic pulmonary sarcoidosis.[332] The usual dose of hydroxychloroquine is 200–400 mg daily. The risk of irreversible retinopathy and blindness greatly restricts its use for longer periods. This is significantly more likely with chloroquine than hydroxychloroquine, so hydroxychloroquine is the preferred agent. Rare side effects include agranulocytosis and myopathy, so periodic monitoring of the complete blood count and neuromuscular strength are recommended.

Biologic therapy: TNF-α antagonists (infliximab, adalimumab, etanercept) are the major biologic agents used for the treatment of sarcoidosis. TNF-α is believed to play a central role in granuloma formation thus its inhibition might effectively control the disease.[333-341] A systematic review and Delphi study reported recently found that most of the published data on these agents is observational with few randomized trials.[342] They are recommended as the third-line agents for the treatment of sarcoidosis.[282]

Of all the agents in this class infliximab is the most studied. It is typically administered as an intravenous infusion of 3–5 mg/kg on weeks 0 and 2, with repeat dosing every 4–8 weeks thereafter.[335,342] In one of the trials of infliximab in pulmonary sarcoidosis there was an improvement in lung function while the other study did not find any significant improvement.[339,340] For extrapulmonary sarcoidosis although there was improvement after 24 weeks of therapy, but this benefit was not sustained after a 24-week washout.[334] More than half of the patients relapse after discontinuation of treatment.[343] Trials demonstrating long-term safety and efficacy of infliximab therapy are lacking. Adalimumab can be given subcutaneously and being a fully humanized antibody has lower allergic reaction rate than infliximab.[344] It has been shown to be efficacious in a few small studies.[345-347] Eternacept has been found to be associated with treatment failure and is not recommended for treatment of sarcoidosis.[348,349]

One of the major concerns for use of TNF-α inhibitors is the increased risk of reactivation of latent tuberculosis and other opportunistic infections. In fact, in the United States, careful screening for latent tuberculosis and isoniazid (INH) prophylaxis for all those found positive is recommended for all patients planning to start therapy with a TNF-α inhibitor,[350] a recommendation that is not possible to implement in countries with high burden of tuberculosis. Therefore, the role of these therapies for treatment of sarcoidosis in India would remain limited to a few carefully selected patients, where other therapies fail. Other known side effects include a possible increase in malignancy, such as lymphoma, new onset and worsening of congestive heart failure, and demyelinating diseases. Surprisingly, there are also several reports of development of sarcoidosis during treatment with TNF-α antagonists, which represents a rare and paradoxical adverse event. The occurrence of sarcoidosis has been reported with all the three available agents and is probably linked to a cytokine disequilibrium.[351]

Rituximab, an antibody directed against CD20+ cells has been reported to be efficacious in a few case reports, although a recent small study has found its effect to be inconsistent.[352-355] Ustekinumab and golimumab are other biologics studied in sarcoidosis but not found to be effective.[356]

Other agents: Several other drugs which have been employed in sporadic cases or short trials include thalidomide, colchicine, pentoxifylline and cyclosporin A. None has found an established role as yet.[343]

How Long to Continue?

The duration in each patient is individualized on the basis of symptoms, organ involvement and response to therapy. There is frequent relapse of symptoms when the treatment is tapered off.[357-360] Prolonged treatment is recommended for the continued suppression of disease-activity. Most clinicians continue treatment for about 1 year.[3,335] Significantly better results were observed in patients who had received prolonged treatment for 4 years or more in the British Thoracic Society (BTS) study.[286]

There is a small group of patients with limited but symptomatic disease in whom the treatment is discontinued after a period of 3–6 months. On the other hand, some of the patients may require low dose prednisolone treatment for much longer periods of 10 years or more. Alternate-day treatment is preferred if required for longer periods. It is considered safer than the daily dose regimen, even when the total dose is similar.[301]

Acute pulmonary exacerbation of sarcoidosis (APES): It may be defined as worsening of pulmonary symptoms (present for at least 1 month) in a patient with sarcoidosis that are not explained by another cause, along with a decline in spirometry [≥10% decrease from previous baseline FVC and/or forced expiratory volume (FEV_1)].[361] They usually occur after tapering or stoppage of steroids. These exacerbations can be treated with 20 mg prednisone for a median of 21 days followed by tapering to a level at which the patient remains free of symptoms.[362]

The status of long-term treatment in developing countries is somewhat depressing.[122] There is a general trend to taper treatment earlier than required, largely for the fear of steroid-induced complications and poor patient compliance. Patients often stop treatment on their own and report back only when symptoms relapse. It is not infrequent to encounter patients who have received multiple courses of steroid treatment for short periods.

Treatment of Complications

Management of complications of disease, adverse events due to different treatments and of comorbid conditions is also important. Sarcoidosis patients should be screened for depression and, if present, should be treated appropriately. Systemic, constitutional symptoms of sarcoidosis are treated with analgesics and nonsteroidal anti-inflammatory drugs. An often overlooked aspect of sarcoidosis is fatigue. Regardless of disease activity, patients often report fatigue, sleep disturbance, and impaired general quality of life (QOL).[363] One study had shown good results with use of dexmethylphenidate hydrochloride for the treatment of sarcoidosis-associated fatigue.[364]

Bronchiectasis requires treatment like any other bronchiectasis patient, with anti-inflammatory therapy, mucociliary clearance, and appropriate antibiotic therapy for exacerbations.[365] Patients with aspergilloma, if symptomatic, may be treated conservatively with appropriate antifungal agents. An occasional patient with aspergilloma causing hemoptysis may benefit from intracavitary instillation of antifungal agents or arterial embolization. Resection may be necessary for severe hemoptysis if lung function is not severely impaired. Bronchoscopic balloon dilation with adjunctive topical mitomycin C has been tried in bronchostenosis following sarcoidosis.[366] Extensive fibrosis causing hypoxemia requires supplemental long-term oxygen therapy. With severe functional impairment and patient disability, pulmonary hypertension and right heart failure may supervene for which the patient will require oxygen and diuretics. Sildenafil and bosentan may be used with caution for pulmonary hypertension.[367] These patients are candidates for lung transplantation. Survival rates following lung transplantation for sarcoidosis are generally comparable to other indications. Sarcoidosis can recur in lung allografts but does not affect survival or risk for complications.

Additional treatments for complications due to extra-pulmonary organ involvement are needed as appropriate. Decongestive therapy is required for heart failure due to sarcoid cardiomyopathy. A pacemaker or implantable cardioverter defibrillator (ICD) may also be indicated.[288] Radiation therapy has been successfully used for refractory neurosarcoidosis.[368] Elderly sarcoidosis patients often present with unusual clinical features of sarcoidosis. Occasionally, these features resemble malignancy; rarely sarcoidosis and malignancy may coexist.[369]

PROGNOSIS AND MORTALITY

Sarcoidosis is a benign process. Many patients remain asymptomatic and spontaneous remission is common. The disease, however, follows a chronic course in 10–30% of the cases, sometimes leading to significant deterioration in lung function. Mortality rates of 1–6% have been reported.[370] Fibrosis in the chest radiograph and an FVC below 1.5 L are predictive of death due to respiratory failure caused by sarcoidosis.[371] When fibrosis and pulmonary hypertension are present at the same time, there is a sharp drop in respiratory functions and such findings should alert the clinician to this serious complication.[372] In the survival analysis, sarcoidosis has a better prognosis at 5 years (91.6% survival) compared to other diffuse interstitial lung diseases such as nonspecific or desquamative interstitial pneumonia (85.5%), hypersensitivity pneumonitis (84.1%), collagen-related diffuse interstitial lung disease (69.7%), undefined forms of pulmonary fibrosis (69.5%), and idiopathic pulmonary fibrosis (35.4%).[371] One case-control study points to a possible increased risk for developing neoplastic processes such as lymphomas, lung cancer, or cancer of other organs affected by the disease, but these findings have not been confirmed in other studies with long-term follow-up.[373,374] In short, the prognosis of sarcoidosis is linked to the severity of the disease.

FUTURE DIRECTIONS

Despite extensive research, sarcoidosis remains an enigmatic disease. A working group of the National Heart, Lung and Blood Institute identified several future research directions and opportunities for sarcoidosis. These include developing a tissue bank, using novel methods to identify genetic factors, studying the immunopathogenesis with human tissue and animal models, exploring new approaches to diagnose and manage disease and finally conducting randomized controlled trials to assess new therapies.[375] The remarkable similarity of sarcoidosis to tuberculosis and the continued interrelationship of the two conditions is of special interest to clinicians and researchers from countries with ongoing tuberculosis epidemic. The wish list for sarcoidosis research in these countries would, therefore, include development of definitive test/s for differentiating the two conditions and also looking for newer therapies or standardizing the existing treatments in a fashion that would reduce the risk of common complications such as reactivation of latent tuberculosis.

REFERENCES

1. Hutchinson J. Case of livid papillary psoriasis. Illustrations of Clinical Surgery. Vol 1. London: J and A Churchill; 1877. pp. 42-3.
2. Boeck C. Multiple benign sarcoid of the skin. J Cutan Genitourinary Dis. 1899;17:543-50.
3. Statement on sarcoidosis. Joint Statement of the American Thoracic Society (ATS), the European Respiratory Society (ERS) and the World Association of Sarcoidosis and Other Granulomatous Disorders (WASOG) adopted by the ATS Board of Directors and by the ERS Executive Committee, February 1999. Am J Respir Crit Care Med. 1999;160(2):736-55.
4. James DG. Descriptive definition and historic aspects of sarcoidosis. Clin Chest Med. 1997;18(4):663-79.
5. Besnier M. Lupus pernio de la face: synovites funguesues (scrofulo-tuberculeuses) symetriques des extremities superieures. Ann Dermatol Syphiligr. 1899;10:33-6.
6. Kreibich K. Ueber lupus pernio. Arch Derm Syph (Wien). 1904;71:417-9.
7. Heerfordt C. Uber eine Febris uveo-parotidea subchronica. Von Graefe's Arch Opthalmol. 1909;70:254-73.
8. Schaumann J. Etude sur le lupus pernio et ses rapports avec les sarcoides et la tuberculose. Ann Dermatol Syphiligr. 1916-1917:357-63.
9. Harrell GT, Fisher S. Blood Chemical Changes in Boeck's Sarcoid with Particular Reference to Protein, Calcium and Phosphatase Values. J Clin Invest. 1939;18(6):687-93.
10. Kveim A. En ny og spesifikk kutan-reaksjon ved Boecks sarcoid. Nord Med. 1941;9:169-72.
11. Siltzbach LE. The Kveim test in sarcoidosis. A study of 750 patients. JAMA: the Journal of the American Medical Association. 1961;178:476-82.
12. Löfgren S. Erythema nodosum: studies on etiology and pathogenesis in 185 adult cases. Acta Med Scand. 1946;124:1-197.
13. Longcope WT, Freiman DG. A study of sarcoidosis; based on a combined investigation of 160 cases including 30 autopsies from the Johns Hopkins Hospital and Massachusetts General Hospital. Medicine (Baltimore). 1952;31(1):1-132.
14. Wurm K, Reindell H, Heilmeyer. L. Der Lungenboeck *Röntgenbild.* Stuttgart, Germany: Thieme; 1958.
15. Lieberman J. Elevation of serum angiotensin-converting-enzyme (ACE) level in sarcoidosis. Am J Med. 1975;59(3):365-72.
16. Pietinalho A, Hiraga Y, Hosoda Y, Lofroos AB, Yamaguchi M, Selroos O. The frequency of sarcoidosis in Finland and Hokkaido, Japan. A comparative epidemiological study. Sarcoidosis. 1995;12(1):61-7.
17. Jindal SK, Gupta D, Aggarwal AN. Sarcoidosis in developing countries. Curr Opin Pulm Med. 2000;6(5):448-54.
18. Gupta SK. Clinical profile of sarcoidosis in Eastern India. Indian J Chest Dis Allied Sci. 1981;23(4):173-8.
19. Singh RB, Babu KS. Pulmonary sarcoidosis in a south Indian hospital: clinical and lung function profile. Indian J Chest Dis Allied Sci. 1999;41(3):145-51.
20. Kim DS. Sarcoidosis in Korea: report of the Second Nationwide Survey. Sarcoidosis Vasc Diffuse Lung Dis. 2001;18(2):176-80.
21. Bambery P, Behera D, Gupta AK, Kaur U, Jindal SK, Deodhar SD, et al. Sarcoidosis in North India: the clinical profile of 40 patients. Sarcoidosis. 1987;4(2):155-8.
22. Samman Y, Ibrahim M, Wali S. Sarcoidosis in the western region of Saudi Arabia. Sarcoidosis Vasc Diffuse Lung Dis. 1999;16(2):215-8.
23. Liam CK, Menon A. Sarcoidosis: a review of cases seen at the University Hospital, Kuala Lumpur. Singapore Med J. 1993;34(2):153-6.
24. Rossman MD, Thompson B, Frederick M, Maliarik M, Iannuzzi MC, Rybicki BA, et al. HLA-DRB1*1101: a significant risk factor for sarcoidosis in blacks and whites. Am J Hum Genet. 2003;73(4):720-35.
25. Iannuzzi MC, Maliarik MJ, Poisson LM, Rybicki BA. Sarcoidosis susceptibility and resistance HLA-DQB1 alleles in African Americans. Am J Respir Crit Care Med. 2003;167(9):1225-31.
26. Yeager H, Rossman MD, Baughman RP, Teirstein AS, Judson MA, Rabin DL, et al. Pulmonary and psychosocial findings at enrollment in the ACCESS study. Sarcoidosis Vasc Diffuse Lung Dis. 2005;22(2):147-53.
27. Baughman RP, Teirstein AS, Judson MA, Rossman MD, Yeager H Jr, Bresnitz EA, et al. Clinical characteristics of patients in a case control study of sarcoidosis. Am J Respir Crit Care Med. 2001;164(10 Pt 1):1885-9.
28. Rybicki BA, Major M, Popovich J, Maliarik MJ, Iannuzzi MC. Racial differences in sarcoidosis incidence: a 5-year study in a health maintenance organization. Am J Epidemiol. 1997;145(3):234-41.
29. McGrath DS, Daniil Z, Foley P, du Bois JL, Lympany PA, Cullinan P, et al. Epidemiology of familial sarcoidosis in the UK. Thorax. 2000;55(9):751-4.
30. Rybicki BA, Iannuzzi MC, Frederick MM, Thompson BW, Rossman MD, Bresnitz EA, et al. Familial aggregation of sarcoidosis. A case-control etiologic study of sarcoidosis (ACCESS). Am J Respir Crit Care Med. 2001;164(11):2085-91.
31. Becker ML, Martin TM, Doyle TM, Rose CD. Interstitial pneumonitis in Blau syndrome with documented mutation in CARD15. Arthritis Rheum. 2007;56(4):1292-4.
32. Schurmann M, Valentonyte R, Hampe J, Muller-Quernheim J, Schwinger E, Schreiber S. CARD15 gene mutations in sarcoidosis. Eur Respir J. 2003;22(5):748-54.
33. du Bois RM, Beirne PA, Anevlavis SE. Genetics of sarcoidosis. Eur Resp Mon. 2005;32:64-81.
34. Schurmann M, Reichel P, Muller-Myhsok B, Schlaak M, Muller-Quernheim J, Schwinger E. Results from a genome-wide search for predisposing genes in sarcoidosis. Am J Respir Crit Care Med. 2001;164(5):840-6.
35. Rybicki BA, Maliarik MJ, Poisson LM, Sheffer R, Chen KM, Major M, et al. The major histocompatibility complex gene region and sarcoidosis susceptibility in African Americans. Am J Respir Crit Care Med. 2003;167(3):444-9.
36. Sharma SK, Balamurugan A, Pandey RM, Saha PK, Mehra NK. Human leukocyte antigen-DR alleles influence the clinical course of pulmonary sarcoidosis in Asian Indians. Am J Respir Cell Mol Biol. 2003;29(2):225-31.

37. Newman KL, Newman LS. Occupational causes of sarcoidosis. Current opinion in allergy and clinical immunology. 2012;12(2):145-50.
38. Barnard J, Rose C, Newman L, Canner M, Martyny J, McCammon C, et al. Job and industry classifications associated with sarcoidosis in A Case-Control Etiologic Study of Sarcoidosis (ACCESS). J Occup Environ Med. 2005;47(3):226-34.
39. Kajdasz DK, Judson MA, Mohr LC, Lackland DT. Geographic variation in sarcoidosis in South Carolina: its relation to socioeconomic status and health care indicators. American Journal of Epidemiology. 1999;150(3):271-8.
40. Kucera GP, Rybicki BA, Kirkey KL, Coon SW, Major ML, Maliarik MJ, et al. Occupational risk factors for sarcoidosis in African-American siblings. Chest. 2003;123(5):1527-35.
41. Gerke AK, Tangh F, Yang M, Cavanaugh JE, Polgreen PM. An analysis of seasonality of sarcoidosis in the United States veteran population: 2000-2007. Sarcoidosis Vasc Diffuse Lung Dis. 2012;29(2):155-8.
42. Demirkok SS, Basaranoglu M, Coker E, Karayel T. Seasonality of the onset of symptoms, tuberculin test anergy and Kveim positive reaction in a large cohort of patients with sarcoidosis. Respirology. 2007;12(4):591-3.
43. Gupta D. Seasonality of Sarcoidosis: the 'heat' is on. Sarcoidosis Vasc Diffuse Lung Dis. 2013;30(3):241-3.
44. Comstock GW, Keltz H, Sencer DJ. Clay eating and sarcoidosis: a controlled study in the State of Georgia. Am Rev Respir Dis. 1961;76 (Suppl):130-4.
45. Hance AJ, Basset F, Saumon G, Danel C, Valeyre D, Battesti JP, et al. Smoking and interstitial lung disease. The effect of cigarette smoking on the incidence of pulmonary histiocytosis X and sarcoidosis. Ann NY Acad Sci. 1986;465:643-56.
46. Harf RA, Ethevenaux C, Gleize J, Perrin-Fayolle M, Guerin JC, Ollagnier C. Reduced prevalence of smokers in sarcoidosis. Results of a case-control study. Ann N Y Acad Sci. 1986;465: 625-31.
47. Hinman LM, Stevens C, Matthay RA, Bernard J, Gee L. Angiotensin convertase activities in human alveolar macrophages: effects of cigarette smoking and sarcoidosis. Science. 1979;205(4402):202-3.
48. Lawrence EC, Fox TB, Teague RB, Bloom K, Wilson RK. Cigarette smoking and bronchoalveolar T cell populations in sarcoidosis. Ann NY Acad Sci. 1986;465:657-64.
49. Peros-Golubicic T, Ljubic S. Cigarette smoking and sarcoidosis. Acta medica Croatica: casopis Hravatske akademije medicinskih znanosti. 1995;49(4-5):187-93.
50. Revsbech P. Is sarcoidosis related to exposure to pets or the housing conditions? A case-referent study. Sarcoidosis. 1992;9(2):101-3.
51. Valeyre D, Soler P, Clerici C, Pré J, Battesti JP, Georges R, et al. Smoking and pulmonary sarcoidosis: effect of cigarette smoking on prevalence, clinical manifestations, alveolitis, and evolution of the disease. Thorax. 1988;43(7):516-24.
52. Visser H, Vos K, Zanelli E, Verduyn W, Schreuder GM, Speyer I, et al. Sarcoid arthritis: clinical characteristics, diagnostic aspects, and risk factors. Annals of the rheumatic diseases. 2002;61(6):499-504.
53. Newman LS, Rose CS, Bresnitz EA, Rossman MD, Barnard J, Frederick M, et al. A case control etiologic study of sarcoidosis: environmental and occupational risk factors. Am J Respir Crit Care Med. 2004;170(12):1324-30.
54. Blanchet MR, Israel-Assayag E, Cormier Y. Inhibitory effect of nicotine on experimental hypersensitivity pneumonitis in vivo and in vitro. Am J Respir Crit Care Med. 2004;169(8):903-9.
55. Terris M, Chaves AD. An epidemiologic study of sarcoidosis. Am Rev Respir Dis. 1966;94(1):50-5.
56. Warren CP. Extrinsic allergic alveolitis: a disease commoner in non-smokers. Thorax. 1977;32(5):567-9.
57. Gupta D, Singh AD, Agarwal R, Aggarwal AN, Joshi K, Jindal SK. Is tobacco smoking protective for sarcoidosis? A case-control study from North India. Sarcoidosis Vasc Diffuse Lung Dis. 2010;27(1):19-26.
58. Perez RL, Rivera-Marrero CA, Roman J. Pulmonary granulomatous inflammation: From sarcoidosis to tuberculosis. Semin Respir Infect. 2003;18(1):23-32.
59. Newman LS. Aetiologies of sarcoidosis. Eur Resp Mon. 2005;32:23-48.
60. Thomeer M, Demedts M, Wuyts W. Epidemiology of sarcoidosis. Eur Respir Mon. 2005;32:13-22.
61. du Bois RM, Goh N, McGrath D, Cullinan P. Is there a role for microorganisms in the pathogenesis of sarcoidosis? J Intern Med. 2003;253(1):4-17.
62. Vidal S, de la Horra C, Martin J, Montes-Cano MA, Rodríguez E, Respaldiza N, et al. *Pneumocystis jirovecii* colonisation in patients with interstitial lung disease. Clin Microbiol Infect. 2006;12(3):231-5.
63. Drake WP, Newman LS. Mycobacterial antigens may be important in sarcoidosis pathogenesis. Curr Opin Pulm Med. 2006;12(5):359-63.
64. Ishige I, Eishi Y, Takemura T, Kobayashi I, Nakata K, Tanaka I, et al. Propionibacterium acnes is the most common bacterium commensal in peripheral lung tissue and mediastinal lymph nodes from subjects without sarcoidosis. Sarcoidosis Vasc Diffuse Lung Dis. 2005;22(1):33-42.
65. Oswald-Richter KA, Drake WP. The etiologic role of infectious antigens in sarcoidosis pathogenesis. Seminars in respiratory and critical care medicine. 2010;31(4):375-9.
66. Sharma OP. Murray Kornfeld, American College of Chest Physician, and sarcoidosis: a historical footnote: 2004 Murray Kornfeld Memorial Founders Lecture. Chest. 2005;128(3): 1830-5.
67. Gupta D, Agarwal R, Aggarwal AN, Jindal SK. Molecular evidence for the role of mycobacteria in sarcoidosis: a meta-analysis. Eur Respir J. 2007;30(3):508-16.
68. Mootha VK, Agarwal R, Aggarwal AN, Gupta D, Ahmed J, Verma I, et al. The Sarcoid-Tuberculosis link: evidence from a high TB prevalence country. J Infect. 2010;60(6):501-3.
69. Kent DC, Houk VN, Elliott RC, Sokolowski JW, Baker JH, Sorensen K. The definitive evaluation of sarcoidosis. Am Rev Respir Dis. 1970;101(5):721-7.
70. Hatzakis K, Siafakas NM, Bouros D. Miliary sarcoidosis following miliary tuberculosis. Respiration. 2000;67(2):219-22.
71. Vanek J, Schwarz J. Demonstration of acid-fast rods in sarcoidosis. Am Rev Respir Dis. 1970;101(3):395-400.
72. Cantwell AR. Variably acid-fast bacteria in a case of systemic sarcoidosis and hypodermitis sclerodermiformis. Dermatologica. 1981;163(3):239-48.
73. Cantwell AR. Histologic observations of variably acid-fast pleomorphic bacteria in systemic sarcoidosis: a report of 3 cases. Growth. 1982;46(2):113-25.
74. Mitchell DN, Rees RJ. A transmissible agent from sarcoid tissue. Lancet. 1969;2(7611):81-4.

75. Mitchell DN, Rees RJ. An attempt to demonstrate a transmissible agent from sarcoid material. Postgrad Med J. 1970;46(538):510-4.
76. Mitchell DN, Rees RJ, Goswami KK. Transmissible agents from human sarcoid and Crohn's disease tissues. Lancet. 1976;2(7989):761-5.
77. Mitchell DN. The nature and physical characteristics of a transmissible agent from human sarcoid tissue. Ann NY Acad Sci. 1976;278:233-48.
78. Song Z, Marzilli L, Greenlee BM, Chen ES, Silver RF, Askin FB, et al. Mycobacterial catalase-peroxidase is a tissue antigen and target of the adaptive immune response in systemic sarcoidosis. J Exp Med. 2005;201(5):755-67.
79. Oswald-Richter K, Sato H, Hajizadeh R, Shepherd BE, Sidney J, Sette A, et al. Mycobacterial ESAT-6 and katG are recognized by sarcoidosis CD4+ T cells when presented by the American sarcoidosis susceptibility allele, DRB1*1101. J Clin Immunol. 2010;30(1):157-66.
80. Agarwal R, Gupta D, Srinivas R, Verma I, Aggarwal AN, Laal S. Analysis of humoral responses to proteins encoded by region of difference 1 of Mycobacterium tuberculosis in sarcoidosis in a high tuberculosis prevalence country. Indian J Med Res. 2012;135(6):920-3.
81. Goyal B, Kumar K, Gupta D, Agarwal R, Latawa R, Sheikh JA, et al. Utility of B-cell epitopes based peptides of RD1 and RD2 antigens for immunodiagnosis of pulmonary tuberculosis. Diagn Microbiol Infect Dis. 2014;78(4):391-7.
82. Dubaniewicz A. *Mycobacterium tuberculosis* heat shock proteins and autoimmunity in sarcoidosis. Autoimmun Rev. 2010;9(6):419-24.
83. Almenoff PL, Johnson A, Lesser M, Mattman LH. Growth of acid fast L forms from the blood of patients with sarcoidosis. Thorax. 1996;51(5):530-3.
84. Rybicki BA, Hirst K, Iyengar SK, Barnard JG, Judson MA, Rose CS, et al. A sarcoidosis genetic linkage consortium: the sarcoidosis genetic analysis (SAGA) study. Sarcoidosis Vasc Diffuse Lung Dis. 2005;22(2):115-22.
85. Schurmann M. Genetics of sarcoidosis. Seminars in respiratory and critical care medicine. 2003;24(2):213-22.
86. Grunewald J, Eklund A. Role of CD4+ T cells in sarcoidosis. Proc Am Thorac Soc. 2007;4(5):461-4.
87. Agostini C, Adami F, Semenzato G. New pathogenetic insights into the sarcoid granuloma. Current opinion in rheumatology. 2000;12(1):71-6.
88. Hunninghake GW, Crystal RG. Pulmonary sarcoidosis: a disorder mediated by excess helper T-lymphocyte activity at sites of disease activity. N Engl J Med. 1981;305(8):429-34.
89. Semenzato G, Pezzutto A, Chilosi M, Pizzolo G. Redistribution of T lymphocytes in the lymph nodes of patients with sarcoidosis. N Engl J Med. 1982;306(1):48-9.
90. Silver RF, Crystal RG, Moller DR. Limited heterogeneity of biased T-cell receptor V beta gene usage in lung but not blood T cells in active pulmonary sarcoidosis. Immunology. 1996;88(4):516-23.
91. Konishi K, Moller DR, Saltini C, Kirby M, Crystal RG. Spontaneous expression of the interleukin 2 receptor gene and presence of functional interleukin 2 receptors on T lymphocytes in the blood of individuals with active pulmonary sarcoidosis. J Clin Invest. 1988;82(3):775-81.
92. Robinson BW, McLemore TL, Crystal RG. Gamma interferon is spontaneously released by alveolar macrophages and lung T lymphocytes in patients with pulmonary sarcoidosis. J Clin Invest. 1985;75(5):1488-95.
93. Baughman RP, Strohofer SA, Buchsbaum J, Lower EE. Release of tumor necrosis factor by alveolar macrophages of patients with sarcoidosis. J Lab Clin Med. 1990;115(1):36-42.
94. Moller DR, Forman JD, Liu MC, Noble PW, Greenlee BM, Vyas P, et al. Enhanced expression of IL-12 associated with Th1 cytokine profiles in active pulmonary sarcoidosis. J Immunol. 1996;156(12):4952-60.
95. Agostini C, Trentin L, Facco M, Sancetta R, Cerutti A, Tassinari C, et al. Role of IL-15, IL-2, and their receptors in the development of T cell alveolitis in pulmonary sarcoidosis. J Immunol. 1996;157(2):910-8.
96. Kreipe H, Radzun HJ, Heidorn K, Barth J, Kiemle-Kallee J, Petermann W, et al. Proliferation, macrophage colony-stimulating factor, and macrophage colony-stimulating factor-receptor expression of alveolar macrophages in active sarcoidosis. Lab Invest. 1990;62(6):697-703.
97. Girgis RE, Basha MA, Maliarik M, Popovich J, Iannuzzi MC. Cytokines in the bronchoalveolar lavage fluid of patients with active pulmonary sarcoidosis. Am J Respir Crit Care Med. 1995;152(1):71-5.
98. Shigehara K, Shijubo N, Ohmichi M, Takahashi R, Kon S, Okamura H, et al. IL-12 and IL-18 are increased and stimulate IFN-gamma production in sarcoid lungs. J Immunol. 2001;166(1):642-9.
99. Pinkston P, Bitterman PB, Crystal RG. Spontaneous release of interleukin-2 by lung T lymphocytes in active pulmonary sarcoidosis. N Engl J Med. 1983;308(14):793-800.
100. Hunninghake GW, Bedell GN, Zavala DC, Monick M, Brady M. Role of interleukin-2 release by lung T-cells in active pulmonary sarcoidosis. Am Rev Respir Dis. 1983;128(4):634-8.
101. Bingisser R, Speich R, Zollinger A, Russi E, Frei K. Interleukin-10 secretion by alveolar macrophages and monocytes in sarcoidosis. Respiration. 2000;67(3):280-6.
102. Dhooria S, Gupta D. Oxidative Stress in Sarcoidosis. In: Ganguly NK (Ed) Studies on Respiratory Disorders. New York: Springer; 2014. pp. 191-201.
103. Miyara M, Amoura Z, Parizot C, Badoual C, Dorgham K, Trad S, et al. The immune paradox of sarcoidosis and regulatory T cells. J Exp Med. 2006;203(2):359-70.
104. Hudspith BN, Flint KC, Geraint-James D, Brostoff J, Johnson NM. Lack of immune deficiency in sarcoidosis: compartmentalisation of the immune response. Thorax. 1987;42(4):250-5.
105. Mathew S, Bauer KL, Fischoeder A, Bhardwaj N, Oliver SJ. The anergic state in sarcoidosis is associated with diminished dendritic cell function. J Immunol. 2008;181(1):746-55.
106. Takemura T, Matsui Y, Saiki S, Mikami R. Pulmonary vascular involvement in sarcoidosis: a report of 40 autopsy cases. Human pathology. 1992;23(11):1216-23.
107. Perry A, Vuitch F. Causes of death in patients with sarcoidosis. A morphologic study of 38 autopsies with clinicopathologic correlations. Arch Pathol Lab Med. 1995;119(2):167-72.
108. Iwai K, Takemura T, Kitaichi M, Kawabata Y, Matsui Y. Pathological studies on sarcoidosis autopsy. II. Early change, mode of progression and death pattern. Acta Pathol Jpn. 1993;43(7-8):377-85.
109. Kitaichi M. Pathology of pulmonary sarcoidosis. Clin Dermatol. 1986;4(4):108-15.

110. Rosen Y. Pathology of sarcoidosis. Seminars in respiratory and critical care medicine. 2007;28(1):36-52.
111. Sheffield EA. Pathology of sarcoidosis. Clin Chest Med. 1997;18(4):741-54.
112. Ma Y, Gal A, Koss MN. The pathology of pulmonary sarcoidosis: update. Seminars in diagnostic pathology. 2007;24(3):150-61.
113. Churg A, Carrington CB, Gupta R. Necrotizing sarcoid granulomatosis. Chest. 1979;76(4):406-13.
114. Lynch JP, Sharma OP, Baughman RP. Extrapulmonary sarcoidosis. Semin Respir Infect. 1998;13(3):229-54.
115. Gupta SK. Sarcoidosis: a journey through 50 years. Indian J Chest Dis Allied Sci. 2002;44(4):247-53.
116. Balamugesh T, Behera D, Bhatnagar A, Majumdar S. Inflammatory cytokine levels in induced sputum and bronchoalveolar lavage fluid in pulmonary sarcoidosis. Indian J Chest Dis Allied Sci. 2006;48(3):177-81.
117. Gupta D, Chetty M, Kumar N, Aggarwal AN, Jindal SK. Anergy to tuberculin in sarcoidosis is not influenced by high prevalence of tuberculin sensitivity in the population. Sarcoidosis Vasc Diffuse Lung Dis. 2003;20(1):40-5.
118. Gupta D, Gupta S, Balamugesh T, Aggarwal AN, Das R. Circulating D-dimers as a marker of disease activity in pulmonary sarcoidosis. Indian J Chest Dis Allied Sci. 2005;47(3):175-9.
119. Gupta D, Jain P, Wanchu A, Arora S. Serum interleukin-2 and interleukin-4 levels in patients with sarcoidosis: influence of corticosteroid therapy. Lung India. 2005;22(1):12-5.
120. Gupta D, Jorapur V, Bambery P, Joshi K, Jindal SK. Pulmonary sarcoidosis: spirometric correlation with transbronchial biopsy. Sarcoidosis Vasc Diffuse Lung Dis. 1997;14(1):77-80.
121. Gupta D, Rao VM, Aggarwal AN, Garewal G, Jindal SK. Haematological abnormalities in patients of sarcoidosis. Indian J Chest Dis Allied Sci. 2002;44(4):233-6.
122. Jindal SK, Gupta D, Aggarwal AN. Sarcoidosis in India: practical issues and difficulties in diagnosis and management. Sarcoidosis Vasc Diffuse Lung Dis. 2002;19(3):176-84.
123. Sharma SK, Mohan A, Guleria JS. Clinical characteristics, pulmonary function abnormalities and outcome of prednisolone treatment in 106 patients with sarcoidosis. J Assoc Physicians India. 2001;49:697-704.
124. Tahir M, Sharma SK, Ashraf S, Mishra HK. Angiotensin-converting enzyme genotype affects development and course of sarcoidosis in Asian Indians. Sarcoidosis Vasc Diffuse Lung Dis. 2007;24(2):106-12.
125. Lynch JP, Kazerooni EA, Gay SE. Pulmonary sarcoidosis. Clin Chest Med. 1997;18(4):755-85.
126. Highland KB, Retalis P, Coppage L, Schabel SI, Judson MA. Is there an anatomic explanation for chest pain in patients with pulmonary sarcoidosis? Southern Medical Journal. 1997;90(9):911-4.
127. Hendrick DJ, Blackwood RA, Black JM. Chest pain in the presentation of sarcoidosis. Br J Dis Chest. 1976;70(3):206-10.
128. Bechtel JJ, Starr T, Dantzker DR, Bower JS. Airway hyper-reactivity in patients with sarcoidosis. Am Rev Respir Dis. 1981;124(6):759-61.
129. Aggarwal AN, Gupta D, Chandrasekhar G, Jindal SK. Bronchial hyperresponsiveness in patients with sarcoidosis. J Assoc Physicians India. 2004;52:21-3.
130. Hoang DQ, Nguyen ET. Sarcoidosis. Semin Roentgenol. 2010;45(1):36-42.
131. Sones M, Israel HL. Course and prognosis of sarcoidosis. Am J Med. 1960;29:84-93.
132. Wurm K. [The significance of stage classification of sarcoidosis (Boeck's disease.]. Deutsche medizinische Wochenschrift (1946). 1960;85:1541-8.
133. Mana J, Salazar A, Manresa F. Clinical factors predicting persistence of activity in sarcoidosis: a multivariate analysis of 193 cases. Respiration. 1994;61(4):219-25.
134. Winterbauer RH, Belic N, Moores KD. Clinical interpretation of bilateral hilar adenopathy. Ann Intern Med. 1973;78(1):65-71.
135. Judson MA. Sarcoidosis: clinical presentation, diagnosis, and approach to treatment. Am J Med Sci. 2008;335(1):26-33.
136. Nishino M, Lee KS, Itoh H, Hatabu H. The spectrum of pulmonary sarcoidosis: variations of high-resolution CT findings and clues for specific diagnosis. Eur J Radiol. 2010;73(1):66-73.
137. Dawson WB, Muller NL. High-resolution computed tomography in pulmonary sarcoidosis. Seminars in ultrasound, CT and MR. 1990;11(5):423-9.
138. Nakatsu M, Hatabu H, Morikawa K, Uematsu H, Ohno Y, Nishimura K, et al. Large coalescent parenchymal nodules in pulmonary sarcoidosis: "sarcoid galaxy" sign. AJR Am J Roentgenol. 2002;178(6):1389-93.
139. Nishimura K, Itoh H, Kitaichi M, Nagai S, Izumi T. Pulmonary sarcoidosis: correlation of CT and histopathologic findings. Radiology. 1993;189(1):105-9.
140. Marchiori E, Zanetti G, Hochhegger B, Carvalho JF. Sarcoid cluster sign and the reversed halo sign: Extending the spectrum of radiographic manifestations in sarcoidosis. Eur J Radiol. 2010;80(2):567-8.
141. Winterbauer RH, Hutchinson JF. Use of pulmonary function tests in the management of sarcoidosis. Chest. 1980;78(4):640-7.
142. Huang CT, Heurich AE, Rosen Y, Moon S, Lyons HA. Pulmonary sarcoidosis: Roentgenographic, functional, and pathologic correlations. Respiration. 1979;37(6):337-45.
143. Bergin CJ, Bell DY, Coblentz CL, Chiles C, Gamsu G, MacIntyre NR, et al. Sarcoidosis: correlation of pulmonary parenchymal pattern at CT with results of pulmonary function tests. Radiology. 1989;171(3):619-24.
144. Baydur A, Pandya K, Sharma OP, Kanel GC, Carlson M. Control of ventilation, respiratory muscle strength, and granulomatous involvement of skeletal muscle in patients with sarcoidosis. Chest. 1993;103(2):396-402.
145. Baydur A, Alsalek M, Louie SG, Sharma OP. Respiratory muscle strength, lung function, and dyspnea in patients with sarcoidosis. Chest. 2001;120(1):102-8.
146. Shorr AF, Helman DL, Davies DB, Nathan SD. Pulmonary hypertension in advanced sarcoidosis: epidemiology and clinical characteristics. Eur Respir J. 2005;25(5):783-8.
147. Handa T, Nagai S, Miki S, Fushimi Y, Ohta K, Mishima M, et al. Incidence of pulmonary hypertension and its clinical relevance in patients with sarcoidosis. Chest. 2006;129(5):1246-52.
148. Huggins JT, Doelken P, Sahn SA, King L, Judson MA. Pleural effusions in a series of 181 outpatients with sarcoidosis. Chest. 2006;129(6):1599-604.
149. Salerno D. Sarcoidosis pleural effusion: a not so common feature of a well-known pulmonary disease. Respir Care. 2010;55(4):478-80.
150. Soskel NT, Sharma OP. Pleural involvement in sarcoidosis. Curr Opin Pulm Med. 2000;6(5):455-68.
151. Jarman PR, Whyte MK, Sabroe I, Hughes JM. Sarcoidosis presenting with chylothorax. Thorax. 1995;50(12):1324-5.
152. Rockoff SD, Rohatgi PK. Unusual manifestations of thoracic sarcoidosis. Am J Roentgenol. 1985;144(3):513-28.

153. Szwarcberg JB, Glajchen N, Teirstein AS. Pleural involvement in chronic sarcoidosis detected by thoracic CT scanning. Sarcoidosis Vasc Diffuse Lung Dis. 2005;22(1):58-62.
154. Lemay V, Carette MF, Parrot A, Bazelly B, Grivaux M, Milleron B. [Hemoptysis in sarcoidosis. Apropos of 6 cases including 4 with fatal outcome]. Revue de pneumologie clinique. 1995;51(2): 61-70.
155. Koss MN, Hochholzer L, Feigin DS, Garancis JC, Ward PA. Necrotizing sarcoid-like granulomatosis: clinical, pathologic, and immunopathologic findings. Human pathology. 1980;11(5 Suppl):510-9.
156. Gordonson J, Trachtenberg S, Sargent EN. Superior vena cava obstruction due to sarcoidosis. Chest. 1973;63(2):292-3.
157. Hietala SO, Stinnett RG, Faunce HF, Sharpe AR, Scoggins WG, Smith RH. Pulmonary artery narrowing in sarcoidosis. JAMA: the Journal of the American Medical Association. 1977;237(6):572-3.
158. Miller A. The vanishing lung syndrome associated with pulmonary sarcoidosis. Br J Dis Chest. 1981;75(2):209-14.
159. Sharma SK, Mohan A. Uncommon manifestations of sarcoidosis. J Assoc Physicians India. 2004;52:210-4.
160. Sharma OP. Fatigue and sarcoidosis. Eur Respir J. 1999;13(4):713-4.
161. Judson MA. Extrapulmonary sarcoidosis. Seminars in respiratory and critical care medicine. 2007;28(1):83-101.
162. Holmes J, Lazarus A. Sarcoidosis: extrathoracic manifestations. Dis Mon. 2009;55(11):675-92.
163. Sharma OP. Cutaneous sarcoidosis: clinical features and management. Chest. 1972;61(4):320-5.
164. Collin B, Rajaratnam R, Lim R, Lewis H. A retrospective analysis of 34 patients with cutaneous sarcoidosis assessed in a dermatology department. Clin Exp Dermatol. 2009;35(2):131-4.
165. Fernandez-Faith E, McDonnell J. Cutaneous sarcoidosis: differential diagnosis. Clin Dermatol. 2007;25(3):276-87.
166. Yanardag H, Pamuk ON, Pamuk GE. Lupus pernio in sarcoidosis: clinical features and treatment outcomes of 14 patients. Journal of clinical rheumatology : practical reports on rheumatic and musculoskeletal diseases. 2003;9(2):72-6.
167. Yanardag H, Pamuk ON, Karayel T. Cutaneous involvement in sarcoidosis: analysis of the features in 170 patients. Respir Med. 2003;97(8):978-82.
168. Mana J, Marcoval J, Graells J, Salazar A, Peyri J, Pujol R. Cutaneous involvement in sarcoidosis. Relationship to systemic disease. Archives of dermatology. 1997;133(7):882-8.
169. James DG. Ocular sarcoidosis. Ann NY Acad Sci. 1986;465:551-63.
170. Mayers M. Ocular sarcoidosis. International ophthalmology clinics. 1990;30(4):257-63.
171. Baughman RP, Lower EE, Kaufman AH. Ocular sarcoidosis. Seminars in respiratory and critical care medicine. 2010;31(4):452-62.
172. Bradley D, Baughman RP, Raymond L, Kaufman AH. Ocular manifestations of sarcoidosis. Seminars in respiratory and critical care medicine. 2002;23(6):543-8.
173. Jabs DA, Johns CJ. Ocular involvement in chronic sarcoidosis. American Journal of Ophthalmology. 1986;102(3):297-301.
174. Ohara K, Okubo A, Sasaki H, Kamata K. Intraocular manifestations of systemic sarcoidosis. Jpn J Ophthalmol. 1992;36(4):452-7.
175. Silverman KJ, Hutchins GM, Bulkley BH. Cardiac sarcoid: a clinicopathologic study of 84 unselected patients with systemic sarcoidosis. Circulation. 1978;58(6):1204-11.
176. Sharma OP, Maheshwari A, Thaker K. Myocardial sarcoidosis. Chest. 1993;103(1):253-8.
177. Dubrey SW, Falk RH. Diagnosis and management of cardiac sarcoidosis. Prog Cardiovas Dis. 2010;52(4):336-46.
178. Pierre-Louis B, Prasad A, Frishman WH. Cardiac manifestations of sarcoidosis and therapeutic options. Cardiol Rev. 2009;17(4):153-8.
179. Boglioli LR, Taff ML, Funke S, Mihalakis I. Sudden death due to sarcoid heart disease. J Forensic Sci. 1998;43(5):1072-3.
180. Suranagi VV, Malur PR, Bannur HB. Cardiac sarcoidosis causing sudden death. Indian Journal of Pathology and Microbiology. 2009;52(4):566-7.
181. Uemura A, Morimoto S, Hiramitsu S, Kato Y, Ito T, Hishida H. Histologic diagnostic rate of cardiac sarcoidosis: evaluation of endomyocardial biopsies. Am Heart J. 1999;138(2 Pt 1):299-302.
182. Chandra M, Silverman ME, Oshinski J, Pettigrew R. Diagnosis of cardiac sarcoidosis aided by MRI. Chest. 1996;110(2):562-5.
183. Chapelon-Abric C, de Zuttere D, Duhaut P, Veyssier P, Wechsler B, Huong DL, et al. Cardiac sarcoidosis: a retrospective study of 41 cases. Medicine (Baltimore). 2004;83(6):315-34.
184. Cheong BY, Muthupillai R, Nemeth M, Lambert B, Dees D, Huber S, et al. The utility of delayed-enhancement magnetic resonance imaging for identifying nonischemic myocardial fibrosis in asymptomatic patients with biopsy-proven systemic sarcoidosis. Sarcoidosis Vasc Diffuse Lung Dis. 2009;26(1): 39-46.
185. Nomura S, Funabashi N, Tsubura M, Uehara M, Shiina Y, Daimon M, et al. Cardiac sarcoidosis evaluated by multimodality imaging. Int J Cardiol. 2011;150(2):e81-4.
186. Kudoh H, Fujiwara S, Shiotani H, Kawai H, Hirata K. Myocardial washout of (99m)Tc-tetrofosmin and response to steroid therapy in patients with cardiac sarcoidosis. Ann Nucl Med. 2010;24(5):379-85.
187. Sharma S. Cardiac imaging in myocardial sarcoidosis and other cardiomyopathies. Curr Opin Pulm Med. 2009;15(5):507-12.
188. Sharma PS, Lubahn JG, Donsky AS, Yoon AD, Carry MM, Grayburn PA, et al. Diagnosing cardiac sarcoidosis clinically without tissue confirmation. Proceedings (Baylor University. Medical Center). 2009;22(3):236-8.
189. Sharma OP, Sharma AM. Sarcoidosis of the nervous system. A clinical approach. Arch Intern Med. 1991;151(7):1317-21.
190. Stern BJ, Aksamit A, Clifford D, Scott TF. Neurologic presentations of sarcoidosis. Neurologic clinics. 2010;28(1):185-98.
191. Chen RC, McLeod JG. Neurological complications of sarcoidosis. Clin Exp Neurol. 1989;26:99-112.
192. Stern BJ. Neurological complications of sarcoidosis. Current opinion in neurology. 2004;17(3):311-6.
193. Gupta D, Gupta ML, Ghosh D, Parihar PS, Behera D. Sarcoidosis presenting as multifocal remitting and relapsing neurological illness: A diagnostic dilemma. Neurol India. 1995;43:219-21.
194. Giovinale M, Fonnesu C, Soriano A, Cerquaglia C, Curigliano V, Verrecchia E, et al. Atypical sarcoidosis: case reports and review of the literature. European review for medical and pharmacological sciences. 2009;13 Suppl 1:37-44.
195. Vatti R, Sharma OP. Course of asymptomatic liver involvement in sarcoidosis: role of therapy in selected cases. Sarcoidosis Vasc Diffuse Lung Dis. 1997;14(1):73-6.

196. James DG, Sherlock S. Sarcoidosis of the liver. Sarcoidosis. 1994;11(1):2-6.
197. Ebert EC, Kierson M, Hagspiel KD. Gastrointestinal and hepatic manifestations of sarcoidosis. Am J Gastroenterol. 2008;103(12):3184-92.
198. Karagiannidis A, Karavalaki M, Koulaouzidis A. Hepatic sarcoidosis. Annals of hepatology. 2006;5(4):251-6.
199. Kahi CJ, Saxena R, Temkit M, Canlas K, Roberts S, Knox K, et al. Hepatobiliary disease in sarcoidosis. Sarcoidosis Vasc Diffuse Lung Dis. 2006;23(2):117-23.
200. Warshauer DM. Splenic sarcoidosis. Seminars in ultrasound, CT, and MR. 2007;28(1):21-7.
201. Perez-Grueso MJ, Repiso A, Gomez R, Gonzalez C, de Artaza T, Valle J, et al. Splenic focal lesions as manifestation of sarcoidosis: Characterization with contrast-enhanced sonography. Journal of clinical ultrasound: JCU. 2007;35(7):405-8.
202. Kessler A, Mitchell DG, Israel HL, Goldberg BB. Hepatic and splenic sarcoidosis: ultrasound and MR imaging. Abdom Imaging. 1993;18(2):159-63.
203. Kataria YP, Whitcomb ME. Splenomegaly in sarcoidosis. Arch Intern Med. 1980;140(1):35-7.
204. Rizzato G, Montemurro L. The clinical spectrum of the sarcoid peripheral lymph node. Sarcoidosis Vasc Diffuse Lung Dis. 2000;17(1):71-80.
205. Sharma OP. Sarcoidosis of the upper respiratory tract. Selected cases emphasizing diagnostic and therapeutic difficulties. Sarcoidosis Vasc Diffuse Lung Dis. 2002;19(3):227-33.
206. Sarnaik RM, Nair N, Guleria R, Jindal SK. Sarcoidosis in two brothers, manifesting in one with vocal cord palsy. Lung India. 1992;11(4):147-8.
207. Yanardag H, Pamuk ON. Bone cysts in sarcoidosis: what is their clinical significance? Rheumatol Int. 2004;24(5):294-6.
208. Mana J, Gomez-Vaquero C, Montero A, et al. Lofgren's syndrome revisited: a study of 186 patients. Am J Med. 1999;107(3):240-5.
209. Grigor RR, Hughes GR. Chronic sarcoid arthritis. Br Med J. 1976;2(6043):1044.
210. Torralba KD, Quismorio FP. Sarcoid arthritis: a review of clinical features, pathology and therapy. Sarcoidosis Vasc Diffuse Lung Dis. 2003;20(2):95-103.
211. Sharma OP. Hypercalcemia in granulomatous disorders: a clinical review. Curr Opin Pulm Med. 2000;6(5):442-7.
212. Burke RR, Rybicki BA, Rao DS. Calcium and vitamin D in sarcoidosis: how to assess and manage. Seminars in respiratory and critical care medicine. 2010;31(4):474-84.
213. Bell NH, Stern PH, Pantzer E, Sinha TK, DeLuca HF. Evidence that increased circulating 1 alpha, 25-dihydroxyvitamin D is the probable cause for abnormal calcium metabolism in sarcoidosis. J Clin Invest. 1979;64(1):218-25.
214. Conron M, Young C, Beynon HL. Calcium metabolism in sarcoidosis and its clinical implications. Rheumatology (Oxford). 2000;39(7):707-13.
215. Zeimer HJ, Greenaway TM, Slavin J, Hards DK, Zhou H, Doery JC, et al. Parathyroid-hormone-related protein in sarcoidosis. Am J Pathol. 1998;152(1):17-21.
216. Muller-Quernheim J. Sarcoidosis: immunopathogenetic concepts and their clinical application. Eur Respir J. 1998;12(3):716-38.
217. Gupta D, Agarwal R, Singh A, Joshi K. A "respiratory" cause of abdominal pain. Eur Respir J. 2006;27(2):430-3.
218. Teirstein AS, Judson MA, Baughman RP, Rossman MD, Yeager H Jr., Moller DR. The spectrum of biopsy sites for the diagnosis of sarcoidosis. Sarcoidosis Vasc Diffuse Lung Dis. 2005;22(2):139-46.
219. Jindal SK, Gupta D. Incidence and recognition of interstitial pulmonary fibrosis in developing countries. Curr Opin Pulm Med. 1997;3(5):378-83.
220. Gupta D, Behera D, Joshi K, Jindal SK. Role of fiberoptic bronchoscopy (transbronchial lung biopsy) in diagnosis of parenchymatous lung diseases. J Assoc Physicians India. 1997;45:371-3.
221. Gilman MJ. Transbronchial biopsy in sarcoidosis. Chest. 1983;83(1):159.
222. Oki M, Saka H, Kitagawa C, Kogure Y, Murata N, Ichihara S, et al. Prospective study of endobronchial ultrasound-guided transbronchial needle aspiration of lymph nodes versus transbronchial lung biopsy of lung tissue for diagnosis of sarcoidosis. J Thorac Cardiovas Surg. 2012;143(6):1324-9.
223. Goyal A, Gupta D, Agarwal R, Bal A, Nijhawan R, Aggarwal AN. Value of different bronchoscopic sampling techniques in diagnosis of sarcoidosis: a prospective study of 151 patients. J Bronchology Interv Pulmonol. 2014;21(3):220-6.
224. Gupta D, Dadhwal DS, Agarwal R, Gupta N, Bal A, Aggarwal AN. Endobronchial Ultrasound Guided TBNA vs. Conventional TBNA in the diagnosis of sarcoidosis. Chest. 2014;146(3):547-56.
225. Gupta D, Mahendran C, Aggarwal AN, Joshi K, Jindal SK. Endobronchial vis a vis transbronchial involvement on fiberoptic bronchoscopy in sarcoidosis. Sarcoidosis Vasc Diffuse Lung Dis. 2001;18(1):91-2.
226. Khan A, Agarwal R, Aggarwal AN, Gupta N, Bal A, Singh N, et al. Blind transbronchial needle aspiration without an on-site cytopathologist: experience of 473 procedures. Natl Med J India. 2011;24(3):136-9.
227. Agarwal R, Aggarwal AN, Gupta D. Efficacy and safety of conventional transbronchial needle aspiration in sarcoidosis: a systematic review and meta-analysis. Respir Care. 2013;58(4):683-93.
228. von Bartheld MB, Dekkers OM, Szlubowski A, Eberhardt R, Herth FJ, in 't Veen JC, et al. Endosonography vs conventional bronchoscopy for the diagnosis of sarcoidosis: the GRANULOMA randomized clinical trial. JAMA: the journal of the American Medical Association. 2013;309(23):2457-64.
229. Smith-Rohrberg D, Sharma SK. Tuberculin skin test among pulmonary sarcoidosis patients with and without tuberculosis: its utility for the screening of the two conditions in tuberculosis-endemic regions. Sarcoidosis Vasc Diffuse Lung Dis. 2006;23(2):130-4.
230. Winterbauer RH, Lammert J, Selland M, Wu R, Corley D, Springmeyer SC. Bronchoalveolar lavage cell populations in the diagnosis of sarcoidosis. Chest. 1993;104(2):352-61.
231. Costabel U, Bonella F, Ohshimo S, Guzman J. Diagnostic modalities in sarcoidosis: BAL, EBUS, and PET. Seminars in respiratory and critical care medicine. 2010;31(4):404-8.
232. Munro CS, Mitchell DN. The Kveim response: still useful, still a puzzle. Thorax. 1987;42(5):321-31.
233. Siltzbach LE, Ehrlich JC. The Nickerson-Kveim reaction in sarcoidosis. Am J Med. 1954;16(6):790-803.
234. Siltzbach LE. Qualities and behavior of satisfactory Kveim suspensions. Ann N Y Acad Sci. 1976;278:665-9.
235. Gupta SK. Markers of activity in sarcoidosis with a special reference to serum angiotensin converting enzyme (SACE). Indian J Chest Dis Allied Sci. 1993;35(3):117-27.

236. Sainani GS, Mahbubani V, Trikannad V. Serum angiotensin converting enzyme activity in sarcoidosis and pulmonary tuberculosis. J Assoc Physicians India. 1996;44(1):29-30.
237. Shorr AF, Torrington KG, Parker JM. Serum angiotensin converting enzyme does not correlate with radiographic stage at initial diagnosis of sarcoidosis. Respir Med. 1997;91(7): 399-401.
238. Silverstein E, Brunswick J, Rao TK, Friedland J. Increased serum angiotensin-converting enzyme in chronic renal disease. Nephron. 1984;37(3):206-10.
239. Studdy PR, Bird R. Serum angiotensin converting enzyme in sarcoidosis--its value in present clinical practice. Annals of clinical biochemistry. 1989;26 (Pt 1):13-8.
240. Brice EA, Friedlander W, Bateman ED, Kirsch RE. Serum angiotensin-converting enzyme activity, concentration, and specific activity in granulomatous interstitial lung disease, tuberculosis, and COPD. Chest. 1995;107(3):706-10.
241. Kruit A, Ruven HJ, Grutters JC, van den Bosch JM. Angiotensin-converting enzyme 2 (ACE2) haplotypes are associated with pulmonary disease phenotypes in sarcoidosis patients. Sarcoidosis Vasc Diffuse Lung Dis. 2005;22(3):195-203.
242. Kruit A, Grutters JC, Gerritsen WB, Kos S, Wodzig WK, van den Bosch JM, et al. ACE I/D-corrected Z-scores to identify normal and elevated ACE activity in sarcoidosis. Respir Med. 2007;101(3):510-5.
243. Floe A, Hoffmann HJ, Nissen PH, Moller HJ, Hilberg O. Genotyping increases the yield of angiotensin-converting enzyme in sarcoidosis--a systematic review. Danish Medical Journal. 2014;61(5):A4815.
244. Costabel U, Ohshimo S, Guzman J. Diagnosis of sarcoidosis. Curr Opin Pulm Med. 2008;14(5):455-61.
245. Treglia G, Taralli S, Giordano A. Emerging role of whole-body 18F-fluorodeoxyglucose positron emission tomography as a marker of disease activity in patients with sarcoidosis: a systematic review. Sarcoidosis Vasc Diffuse Lung Dis. 2011;28(2):87-94.
246. Jung RS, Mittal BR, Maturu NV, Kumar R, Bhattacharya A, Gupta D. Ocular sarcoidosis: does (18)F-FDG PET/CT have any role? Clin Nucl Med. 2014;39(5):464-6.
247. Sobic-Saranovic D, Artiko V, Obradovic V. FDG PET imaging in sarcoidosis. Seminars in nuclear medicine. 2013;43(6):404-11.
248. Maturu VN, Agarwal R, Aggarwal AN, Mittal BR, Bal A, Gupta N, et al. Dual time point whole body 18F-fluorodeoxyglucose PET/ CT imaging in undiagnosed mediastinal lymphadenopathy: a prospective study of 117 patients with sarcoidosis and TB. Chest. 2014;146(6):e216-20.
249. Kaira K, Oriuchi N, Otani Y, Yanagitani N, Sunaga N, Hisada T, et al. Diagnostic usefulness of fluorine-18-alpha-methyltyrosine positron emission tomography in combination with 18F-fluorodeoxyglucose in sarcoidosis patients. Chest. 2007;131(4):1019-27.
250. Keir G, Wells AU. Assessing pulmonary disease and response to therapy: which test? Semin Respir Critical Care Med. 2010;31(4):409-18.
251. Costabel U, Du Bois RD, Eklund A. Consensus conference: activity of sarcoidosis. Sarcoidosis. 1994;11(1):27-33.
252. Muller-Quernheim J. Serum markers for the staging of disease activity of sarcoidosis and other interstitial lung diseases of unknown etiology. Sarcoidosis Vasc Diffuse Lung Dis. 1998;15(1):22-37.
253. Drent M, Jacobs JA, de Vries J, Lamers RJ, Liem IH, Wouters EF. Does the cellular bronchoalveolar lavage fluid profile reflect the severity of sarcoidosis? Eur Respir J. 1999;13(6):1338-44.
254. Costabel U, Teschler H. Biochemical changes in sarcoidosis. Clin Chest Med. 1997;18(4):827-42.
255. Keijsers RG, van den Heuvel DA, Grutters JC. Imaging the inflammatory activity of sarcoidosis. Eur Respir J. 2013;41(3):743-51.
256. Hadley GD, Emanuel RW. Diagnostic problems. No. 3. Tuberculosis and sarcoidosis? Arch Middx Hosp. 1951;1(4):288-91.
257. Lees AW. Tuberculin-negative tuberculosis presenting as sarcoidosis. Lancet. 1956;271(6944):656-8.
258. Editorial: Sarcoidosis and tuberculosis. Br Med J. 1974;4(5937): 124-5.
259. Gupta D, Agarwal R, Aggarwal AN, Jindal SK. Sarcoidosis and tuberculosis: the same disease with different manifestations or similar manifestations of different disorders. Curr Opin Pulm Med. 2012;18(5):506-16.
260. Hosoda Y, Hiraga Y, Odaka M, Yangawa H, Ito Y, Shiegematsu I, et al. A cooperative study of sarcoidosis in Asia and Africa: analytic epidemiology. Ann NY Acad Sci. 1976;278:355-67.
261. Gupta D, Vinay N, Agarwal R, Agarwal AN. Socio-demographic profile of patients with sarcoidosis vis-a-vis tuberculosis. Sarcoidosis Vasc Diffuse Lung Dis. 2013;30(3):186-93.
262. Woodring JH, Vandiviere HM, Fried AM, Dillon ML, Williams TD, Melvin IG. Update: the radiographic features of pulmonary tuberculosis. AJR Am J Roentgenol. 1986;146(3):497-506.
263. Dhooria S, Agarwal R, Aggarwal AN, Bal A, Gupta N, Gupta D. Differentiating tuberculosis from sarcoidosis by sonographic characteristics of lymph nodes on endobronchial ultrasonography: A study of 165 patients. J Thorac Cardiovasc Surg. 2014;148(2):662-7.
264. DeRemee RA. The roentgenographic staging of sarcoidosis. Historic and contemporary perspectives. Chest. 1983;83(1):128-33.
265. Chugh IM, Agarwal AK, Arora VK, Shah A. Bilateral miliary pattern in sarcoidosis. Indian J Chest Dis Allied Sci. 1997;39(4):245-9.
266. Gupta D, Kumar S, Jindal SK. Bilateral miliary mottling without hilar lymphadenopathy: a rare presentation of sarcoidosis. Lung India. 1996;14:87-8.
267. Sharma SK, Mohan A, Pande JN, Prasad KL, Gupta AK, Khilnani GC. Clinical profile, laboratory characteristics and outcome in miliary tuberculosis. QJM. 1995;88(1):29-37.
268. Israel HL, Sones M. Sarcoidosis, tuberculosis, and tuberculin anergy. A prospective study. Am Rev Respir Dis. 1966;94(6):887-95.
269. Trial of BCG vaccines in south India for tuberculosis prevention. Indian J Med Res. 1979;70:349-63.
270. Trial of BCG vaccines in south India for tuberculosis prevention: first report--Tuberculosis Prevention Trial. Bull World Health Organ. 1979;57(5):819-27.
271. Gupta D, Saiprakash BV, Aggarwal AN, Muralidhar S, Kumar B, Jindal SK. Value of different cut-off points of tuberculin skin test to diagnose tuberculosis among patients with respiratory symptoms in a chest clinic. J Assoc Physicians India. 2001;49:332-5.
272. Lee SS, Liu YC, Huang TS, Chen YS, Tsai HC, Wann SR, et al. Comparison of the interferon gamma release assay and the tuberculin skin test for contact investigation of tuberculosis

in BCG-vaccinated health care workers. Scand J Infect Dis. 2008;40(5):373-80.
273. Gupta D, Kumar S, Aggarwal AN, Verma I, Agarwal R. Interferon gamma release assay (QuantiFERON-TB Gold In Tube) in patients of sarcoidosis from a population with high prevalence of tuberculosis infection. Sarcoidosis Vasc Diffuse Lung Dis. 2011;28(2):95-101.
274. Gupta D, Kumar S, Verma I, Agarwal R. Interferon Gamma Release Assay (IGRA) in Sarcoidosis Patients from A High Tuberculosis (TB) Prevalence Country. Am J Respir Crit Care Med. 2010;181:A2366.
275. Reid L, Lorriman G. Lung biopsy in sarcoidosis, with special reference to bacteriological and microscopic features. Br J Dis Chest. 1960;54:321-34.
276. Tabak L, Agirbas E, Yilmazbayhan D, Tanyeri H, Guc U. The value of labial biopsy in the differentiation of sarcoidosis from tuberculosis. Sarcoidosis Vasc Diffuse Lung Dis. 2001;18(2): 191-5.
277. Zhou Y, Li HP, Li QH, Zheng H, Zhang RX, Chen G, et al. Differentiation of sarcoidosis from tuberculosis using real-time PCR assay for the detection and quantification of *Mycobacterium tuberculosis*. Sarcoidosis Vasc Diffuse Lung Dis. 2008;25(2):93-9.
278. Pal D, Behera D, Gupta D, Aggarwal AN. Tuberculosis in patients receiving prolonged treatment with oral corticosteroids for respiratory disorders. Indian J Tuberc. 2002;49:83-6.
279. Hoyle C, Dawson J, Mather G. Treatment of pulmonary sarcoidosis with streptomycin and cortisone. Lancet. 1955;268(6865):638-43.
280. James DG, Thomson AD. The course of sarcoidosis and its modification by treatment. Lancet. 1959;1(7082):1057-61.
281. Tercelj M, Salobir B, Rylander R. Microbial antigen treatment in sarcoidosis--a new paradigm? Medical hypotheses. 2008;70(4):831-4.
282. Beegle SH, Barba K, Gobunsuy R, Judson MA. Current and emerging pharmacological treatments for sarcoidosis: a review. Drug Des Develop Ther. 2013;7:325-38.
283. Scadding JG. Prognosis of intrathoracic sarcoidosis in England. A review of 136 cases after five years' observation. Br Med J. 1961;2(5261):1165-72.
284. Lazar CA, Culver DA. Treatment of sarcoidosis. Semin Respir Crit Care Med. 2010;31(4):501-18.
285. Lynch JP 3rd, Ma YL, Koss MN, White ES. Pulmonary sarcoidosis. Semin Respir Crit Care Med. 2007;28(1):53-74.
286. Gibson GJ, Prescott RJ, Muers MF, Middleton WG, Mitchell DN, Connolly CK, et al. British Thoracic Society Sarcoidosis study: effects of long-term corticosteroid treatment. Thorax. 1996;51(3):238-47.
287. Teirstein AT, Morgenthau AS. "End-stage" pulmonary fibrosis in sarcoidosis. Mt Sinai J Med. 2009;76(1):30-6.
288. Chapelon-Abric C. Cardiac sarcoidosis. Curr Opin Pulm Med. 2013;19(5):493-502.
289. Hoitsma E, Drent M, Sharma OP. A pragmatic approach to diagnosing and treating neurosarcoidosis in the 21st century. Curr Opin Pulm Med. 2010;16(5):472-9.
290. Segal BM. Neurosarcoidosis: diagnostic approaches and therapeutic strategies. Curr Opin Neurol. 2013;26(3):307-13.
291. Sadek MM, Yung D, Birnie DH, Beanlands RS, Nery PB. Corticosteroid therapy for cardiac sarcoidosis: a systematic review. Can J Cardiol. 2013;29(9):1034-41.
292. Hamzeh NY, Wamboldt FS, Weinberger HD. Management of cardiac sarcoidosis in the United States: a Delphi study. Chest. 2012;141(1):154-62.
293. Cremers JP, Drent M, Baughman RP, Wijnen PA, Koek GH. Therapeutic approach of hepatic sarcoidosis. Curr Opin Pulm Med. 2012;18(5):472-82.
294. Marchell RM, Judson MA. Cutaneous sarcoidosis. Semin Respir Crit Care Med. 2010;31(4):442-51.
295. Israel HL, Sones M, Harrell D. Cortisone treatment of sarcoidosis: experience with thirty-six cases. J Am Med Assoc. 1954;156(5):461-6.
296. Paramothayan NS, Lasserson TJ, Jones PW. Corticosteroids for pulmonary sarcoidosis. Cochrane Database Syst Rev. 2005(2):CD001114.
297. Schutt AC, Bullington WM, Judson MA. Pharmacotherapy for pulmonary sarcoidosis: A Delphi consensus study. Respir Med. 2010.
298. Judson MA. An approach to the treatment of pulmonary sarcoidosis with corticosteroids: the six phases of treatment. Chest. 1999;115(4):1158-65.
299. Block AJ, Light RW. Alternate-day steroid therapy in diffuse pulmonary sarcoidosis. Chest. 1973;63(4):495-504.
300. Selroos O, Sellergren TL. Corticosteroid therapy of pulmonary sarcoidosis. A prospective evaluation of alternate-day and daily dosage in stage II disease. Scand J Respir Dis. 1979;60(4): 215-21.
301. Spratling L, Tenholder MF, Underwood GH, Feaster BL, Requa RK. Daily vs alternate-day prednisone therapy for stage II sarcoidosis. Chest. 1985;88(5):687-90.
302. Gupta SK. Treatment of sarcoidosis patients by steroid aerosol: a ten-year prospective study from Eastern India. Sarcoidosis. 1989;6(1):51-4.
303. Erkkila S, Froseth B, Hellstrom PE, Kaltiokallio K, Taskinen E, Viljanen A, et al. Inhaled budesonide influences cellular and biochemical abnormalities in pulmonary sarcoidosis. Sarcoidosis. 1988;5(2):106-10.
304. Alberts C, van der Mark TW, Jansen HM. Inhaled budesonide in pulmonary sarcoidosis: a double-blind, placebo-controlled study. Dutch Study Group on Pulmonary Sarcoidosis. Eur Respir J. 1995;8(5):682-8.
305. Pietinalho A, Tukiainen P, Haahtela T, Persson T, Selroos O. Early treatment of stage II sarcoidosis improves 5-year pulmonary function. Chest. 2002;121(1):24-31.
306. Recommendations for the prevention and treatment of glucocorticoid-induced osteoporosis: 2001 update. American College of Rheumatology Ad Hoc Committee on Glucocorticoid-induced Osteoporosis. Arthritis Rheum. 2001;44(7):1496-503.
307. Narum S, Westergren T, Klemp M. Corticosteroids and risk of gastrointestinal bleeding: a systematic review and meta-analysis. BMJ Open. 2014;4(5):e004587.
308. Targeted tuberculin testing and treatment of latent tuberculosis infection. American Thoracic Society. MMWR Recomm Rep. 2000;49(RR-6):1-51.
309. Lower EE, Broderick JP, Brott TG, Baughman RP. Diagnosis and management of neurological sarcoidosis. Arch Intern Med. 1997;157(16):1864-8.
310. Korsten P, Mirsaeidi M, Sweiss NJ. Nonsteroidal therapy of sarcoidosis. Curr Opin Pulm Med. 2013;19(5):516-23.
311. Gibson GJ. Sarcoidosis: old and new treatments. Thorax. 2001;56(5):336-9.

312. Baughman RP, Lower EE. Alternatives to corticosteroids in the treatment of sarcoidosis. Sarcoidosis Vasc Diffuse Lung Dis. 1997;14(2):121-30.
313. Kataria YP. Chlorambucil in sarcoidosis. Chest. 1980;78(1): 36-43.
314. Pacheco Y, Marechal C, Marechal F, Biot N, Perrin Fayolle M. Azathioprine treatment of chronic pulmonary sarcoidosis. Sarcoidosis. 1985;2(2):107-13.
315. Lynch JP, 3rd, McCune WJ. Immunosuppressive and cytotoxic pharmacotherapy for pulmonary disorders. Am J Respir Crit Care Med. 1997;155(2):395-420.
316. Baughman RP, Winget DB, Lower EE. Methotrexate is steroid sparing in acute sarcoidosis: results of a double blind, randomized trial. Sarcoidosis Vasc Diffuse Lung Dis. 2000; 17(1):60-6.
317. Cremers JP, Drent M, Bast A, Shigemitsu H, Baughman RP, Valeyre D, et al. Multinational evidence-based World Association of Sarcoidosis and Other Granulomatous Disorders recommendations for the use of methotrexate in sarcoidosis: integrating systematic literature research and expert opinion of sarcoidologists worldwide. Curr Opin Pulm Med. 2013;19(5):545-61.
318. Muller-Quernheim J, Kienast K, Held M, Pfeifer S, Costabel U. Treatment of chronic sarcoidosis with an azathioprine/ prednisolone regimen. Eur Respir J. 1999;14(5):1117-22.
319. Lewis SJ, Ainslie GM, Bateman ED. Efficacy of azathioprine as second-line treatment in pulmonary sarcoidosis. Sarcoidosis Vasc Diffuse Lung Dis. 1999;16(1):87-92.
320. Vorselaars AD, Wuyts WA, Vorselaars VM, Zanen P, Deneer VH, Veltkamp M, et al. Methotrexate vs azathioprine in second-line therapy of sarcoidosis. Chest. 2013;144(3):805-12.
321. Baughman RP, Lower EE. Leflunomide for chronic sarcoidosis. Sarcoidosis Vasc Diffuse Lung Dis. 2004;21(1):43-8.
322. Raj R, Nugent K. Leflunomide-induced interstitial lung disease (a systematic review). Sarcoidosis Vasc Diffuse Lung Dis. 2013;30(3):167-76.
323. Androdias G, Maillet D, Marignier R, Pinède L, Confavreux C, Broussolle C, et al. Mycophenolate mofetil may be effective in CNS sarcoidosis but not in sarcoid myopathy. Neurology. 2011;76(13):1168-72.
324. Brill AK, Ott SR, Geiser T. Effect and safety of mycophenolate mofetil in chronic pulmonary sarcoidosis: a retrospective study. Respiration. 2013;86(5):376-83.
325. Zaidi AA, Devita MV, Michelis MF, Rosenstock JL. Mycophenolate mofetil as a steroid-sparing agent in sarcoid-associated renal disease. Clinical nephrology. 2015;83(1):41-4.
326. Demeter SL. Myocardial sarcoidosis unresponsive to steroids. Treatment with cyclophosphamide. Chest. 1988;94(1):202-3.
327. Doty JD, Mazur JE, Judson MA. Treatment of corticosteroid-resistant neurosarcoidosis with a short-course cyclophosphamide regimen. Chest. 2003;124(5):2023-6.
328. Siltzbach LE, Teirstein AS. Chloroquine therapy in 43 patients with intrathoracic and cutaneous sarcoidosis. Acta Med Scand Suppl. 1964;425:302-8.
329. Hassid S, Choufani G, Saussez S, Dubois M, Salmon I, Soupart A. Sarcoidosis of the paranasal sinuses treated with hydroxychloroquine. Postgrad Med J. 1998;74(869):172-4.
330. Barre PE, Gascon-Barre M, Meakins JL, Goltzman D. Hydroxychloroquine treatment of hypercalcemia in a patient with sarcoidosis undergoing hemodialysis. Am J Med. 1987;82(6):1259-62.
331. Sharma OP. Effectiveness of chloroquine and hydroxychloroquine in treating selected patients with sarcoidosis with neurological involvement. Arch Neurol. 1998;55(9):1248-54.
332. Baltzan M, Mehta S, Kirkham TH, Cosio MG. Randomized trial of prolonged chloroquine therapy in advanced pulmonary sarcoidosis. Am J Respir Crit Care Med. 1999;160(1):192-7.
333. Zissel G, Muller-Quernheim J. Sarcoidosis: historical perspective and immunopathogenesis (Part I). Respir Med. 1998;92(2):126-39.
334. Judson MA, Baughman RP, Costabel U, Flavin S, Lo KH, Kavuru MS, et al. Efficacy of infliximab in extrapulmonary sarcoidosis: results from a randomised trial. Eur Respir J. 2008;31(6): 1189-96.
335. Baughman RP, Costabel U, du Bois RM. Treatment of sarcoidosis. Clin Chest Med. 2008;29(3):533-48, ix-x.
336. Rosen T, Doherty C. Successful long-term management of refractory cutaneous and upper airway sarcoidosis with periodic infliximab infusion. Dermatol Online J. 2007;13(3):14.
337. Kahler CM, Heininger P, Loeffler-Ragg J, Vogelsinger H. Infliximab therapy in pulmonary sarcoidosis. Am J Respir Crit Care Med. 2007;176(4):417-8.
338. Denys BG, Bogaerts Y, Coenegrachts KL, De Vriese AS. Steroid-resistant sarcoidosis: is antagonism of TNF-alpha the answer? Clin Sci (Lond). 2007;112(5):281-9.
339. Rossman MD, Newman LS, Baughman RP, Teirstein A, Weinberger SE, Miller W, et al. A double-blinded, randomized, placebo-controlled trial of infliximab in subjects with active pulmonary sarcoidosis. Sarcoidosis Vasc Diffuse Lung Dis. 2006;23(3):201-8.
340. Baughman RP, Drent M, Kavuru M, et al. Infliximab therapy in patients with chronic sarcoidosis and pulmonary involvement. Am J Respir Crit Care Med. 2006;174(7):795-802.
341. Doty JD, Mazur JE, Judson MA. Treatment of sarcoidosis with infliximab. Chest. 2005;127(3):1064-71.
342. Drent M, Cremers JP, Jansen TL, Baughman RP. Practical eminence and experience-based recommendations for use of TNF-alpha inhibitors in sarcoidosis. Sarcoidosis Vasc Diffuse Lung Dis. 2014;31(2):91-107.
343. Vorselaars AD, Verwoerd A, van Moorsel CH, Keijsers RG, Rijkers GT, Grutters JC. Prediction of relapse after discontinuation of infliximab therapy in severe sarcoidosis. Eur Respir J. 2014;43(2):602-9.
344. Baughman RP, Nunes H, Sweiss NJ, Lower EE. Established and experimental medical therapy of pulmonary sarcoidosis. Eur Respir J. 2013;41(6):1424-38.
345. Sweiss NJ, Noth I, Mirsaeidi M, Zhang W, Naureckas ET, Hogarth DK, et al. Efficacy Results of a 52-week Trial of Adalimumab in the Treatment of Refractory Sarcoidosis. Sarcoidosis Vasc Diffuse Lung Dis. 2014;31(1):46-54.
346. Pariser RJ, Paul J, Hirano S, Torosky C, Smith M. A double-blind, randomized, placebo-controlled trial of adalimumab in the treatment of cutaneous sarcoidosis. J Am Acad Dermatol. 2013;68(5):765-73.
347. Milman N, Graudal N, Loft A, Mortensen J, Larsen J, Baslund B. Effect of the TNF-alpha inhibitor adalimumab in patients with recalcitrant sarcoidosis: a prospective observational study using FDG-PET. Clin Resp J. 2012;6(4):238-47.
348. Field S, Regan AO, Sheahan K, Collins P. Recalcitrant cutaneous sarcoidosis responding to adalimumab but not to etanercept. Clin Exp Dermatol. 2010;35(7):795-6.

349. Utz JP, Limper AH, Kalra S, Specks U, Scott JP, Vuk-Pavlovic Z, et al. Etanercept for the treatment of stage II and III progressive pulmonary sarcoidosis. Chest. 2003;124(1):177-85.
350. Tuberculosis associated with blocking agents against tumor necrosis factor-alpha. California, 2002-2003. MMWR Morb Mortal Wkly Rep. 2004;53(30):683-6.
351. Massara A, Cavazzini L, La Corte R, Trotta F. Sarcoidosis appearing during anti-tumor necrosis factor alpha therapy: a new "class effect" paradoxical phenomenon. Two case reports and literature review. Semin Arthritis Rheum. 2010;39(4):313-9.
352. Sweiss NJ, Lower EE, Mirsaeidi M, Dudek S, Garcia JG, Perkins D, et al. Rituximab in the treatment of refractory pulmonary sarcoidosis. Eur Respir J. 2014;43(5):1525-8.
353. Lower EE, Baughman RP, Kaufman AH. Rituximab for refractory granulomatous eye disease. Clinical ophthalmology (Auckland, N.Z.). 2012;6:1613-8.
354. Bomprezzi R, Pati S, Chansakul C, Vollmer T. A case of neurosarcoidosis successfully treated with rituximab. Neurology. 2010;75(6):568-70.
355. Belkhou A, Younsi R, El Bouchti I, El Hassani S. Rituximab as a treatment alternative in sarcoidosis. Joint, bone, spine: revue du rhumatisme. 2008;75(4):511-2.
356. Judson MA, Baughman RP, Costabel U, Drent M4, Gibson KF5, Raghu G, et al. Safety and efficacy of ustekinumab or golimumab in patients with chronic sarcoidosis. Eur Respir J. 2014;44(5):1296-307.
357. Johns CJ, Michele TM. The clinical management of sarcoidosis. A 50-year experience at the Johns Hopkins Hospital. Medicine (Baltimore). 1999;78(2):65-111.
358. Hoyle C, Smyllie H, Leak D. Prolonged treatment of pulmonary sarcoidosis with corticosteroids. Thorax. 1967;22(6):519-24.
359. Johns CJ, Macgregor MI, Zachary JB, Ball WC. Extended experience in the long-term corticosteroid treatment of pulmonary sarcoidosis. Ann NY Acad Sci. 1976;278:722-31.
360. Rizzato G, Montemurro L, Colombo P. The late follow-up of chronic sarcoid patients previously treated with corticosteroids. Sarcoidosis Vasc Diffuse Lung Dis. 1998;15(1):52-8.
361. Panselinas E, Judson MA. Acute pulmonary exacerbations of sarcoidosis. Chest. 2012;142(4):827-36.
362. McKinzie BP, Bullington WM, Mazur JE, Judson MA. Efficacy of short-course, low-dose corticosteroid therapy for acute pulmonary sarcoidosis exacerbations. Am J Med Sci. 2010;339(1):1-4.
363. Wirnsberger RM, de Vries J, Breteler MH, van Heck GL, Wouters EF, Drent M. Evaluation of quality of life in sarcoidosis patients. Respir Med. 1998;92(5):750-6.
364. Lower EE, Harman S, Baughman RP. Double-blind, randomized trial of dexmethylphenidate hydrochloride for the treatment of sarcoidosis-associated fatigue. Chest. 2008;133(5):1189-95.
365. O'Donnell AE. Bronchiectasis. Chest. 2008;134(4):815-23.
366. Teo F, Anantham D, Feller-Kopman D, Ernst A. Bronchoscopic management of sarcoidosis related bronchial stenosis with adjunctive topical mitomycin C. Ann Thorac Surg. 2010;89(6):2005-7.
367. Palmero V, Sulica R. Sarcoidosis-associated pulmonary hypertension: assessment and management. Semin Respir Crit Care Med. 2010;31(4):494-500.
368. Agbogu BN, Stern BJ, Sewell C, Yang G. Therapeutic considerations in patients with refractory neurosarcoidosis. Arch Neurol. 1995;52(9):875-9.
369. Tachibana T, Iwai K, Takemura T. Sarcoidosis in the aged: review and management. Curr Opin Pulm Med. 2010;16(5):465-71.
370. Chappell AG, Cheung WY, Hutchings HA. Sarcoidosis: a long-term follow up study. Sarcoidosis Vasc Diffuse Lung Dis. 2000;17(2):167-73.
371. Thomeer MJ, Vansteenkiste J, Verbeken EK, Demedts M. Interstitial lung diseases: characteristics at diagnosis and mortality risk assessment. Respir Med. 2004;98(6):567-73.
372. Sulica R, Teirstein AS, Kakarla S, Nemani N, Behnegar A, Padilla ML. Distinctive clinical, radiographic, and functional characteristics of patients with sarcoidosis-related pulmonary hypertension. Chest. 2005;128(3):1483-9.
373. Askling J, Grunewald J, Eklund A, Hillerdal G, Ekbom A. Increased risk for cancer following sarcoidosis. Am J Respir Crit Care Med. 1999;160(5 Pt 1):1668-72.
374. Romer FK, Hommelgaard P, Schou G. Sarcoidosis and cancer revisited: a long-term follow-up study of 555 Danish sarcoidosis patients. Eur Respir J. 1998;12(4):906-12.
375. Martin WJ, Iannuzzi MC, Gail DB, Peavy HH. Future directions in sarcoidosis research: summary of an NHLBI working group. Am J Respir Crit Care Med. 2004;170(5):567-71.

Pulmonary Eosinophilic Disorders

Subhash Varma, Aditya Jindal

INTRODUCTION

Though eosinophils were first described by Paul Ehrlich in 1879,[1] the association between pulmonary infiltrates and eosinophilia was described by Löeffler in 1932[2] and the term "pulmonary infiltrates with eosinophilia" (PIE) was coined by Reeder and Goodrich in 1952.[3] It has been just over 30 years that the role of these cells in the etiopathogenesis of systemic disease, including that of the lungs, has been better understood and defined.

Eosinophilia and lung disease is currently recognized to be either secondary to known causes or a primary involvement. Eosinophilic lung disease, therefore, includes conditions known to involve the lung that are associated with peripheral and/or pulmonary eosinophilia.

EOSINOPHILS

Eosinophils originate from CD34+ myeloid progenitor cells; they share a common immediate precursor with basophils that differentiates toward the eosinophilic lineage under the influence of various cytokines, mainly interleukin-5 (IL-5), granulocyte-macrophage colony-stimulating factor (GM-CSF) and IL3.[4] Expression of high-affinity IL-5 receptors is a prerequisite and an early lineage specific event in this process. IL-5 gene knockout mice produce basal levels of eosinophils but fail to mount expected blood and/or tissue eosinophilia in response to various stimuli. IL-5 is produced by T cells and endothelial cells in the bone marrow, and T cells and parenchymal cells in the lung. Along with the differentiation of eosinophils, it also promotes the release of eosinophils into the bloodstream.

The mature eosinophil varies from 12–17 μm in diameter and has a bilobed nucleus in an eosinophilic cytoplasm.[5] It is characterized by the presence of primary and secondary granules in the cytoplasm, which are clearly visible on electron microscopy. Primary granules are rounded, membrane limited structures and contain Charcot Leyden crystal protein. The secondary granules are somewhat oval and consist of a dense core clearly visible in a less dense matrix. The core of these granules is formed by major basic protein (MBP) while the matrix contains various other enzymes such as eosinophil-derived neurotoxin (EDN), eosinophil cationic protein (ECP) and eosinophil peroxidase. Additionally, dense lipid bodies that are not membrane bound and contain enzymes for metabolizing arachidonic acid, are present. These serve as sites of eicosanoid synthesis.

After a brief intravascular stay of 3–8 hours following its release, the mature eosinophil enters various tissues—predominantly those having an epithelial-environment interface such as the respiratory, gastrointestinal and genitourinary tracts. Once in tissues, survival depends upon the local production of cytokines regulating eosinophil apoptosis. It is eventually phagocytosed by tissue macrophages after a few days.[5] Eosinophils have a diurnal variation in response to the level of endogenous steroids with higher levels in the morning.[6] Pyogenic infections lead to eosinopenia, while parasitic infestations and drugs cause eosinophilia. Eosinopenia can also occur in response to exogenous steroids, estrogens and epinephrine.[7,8]

Circulating eosinophils, like other leukocytes, first move to the margins of the bloodstream where, by the process of rolling, they adhere to the vascular endothelium. They enter the interstitium by passing in between the endothelial cells by diapedesis and then migrate to the site of inflammation under the influence of various cytokines and chemokines. After their arrival, they are primed by cytokines, especially IL-5, platelet activating factor and complement fragment of C5a that through piecemeal degranulation results in the release of various mediators by piecemeal degranulation like MBP, ECP, EDN, erythropoietin (EPO), substance P and also oxygen radicals, lipid mediators and cytokines like IL1, IL3, IL5, IL6, IL8, GM-CSF, transforming growth factor-α (TGF)-α and β, eotaxin, the prostaglandins, leukotrienes and platelet-activating factor. These contribute to the inflammatory actions of the eosinophils.

As a part of the human leukocyte system, eosinophils have a variety of functions to perform. They are especially important in the defense against helminthic infestations—eosinophilic products are lethal to the larval stages of these

BOX 1 Defining limits of eosinophilia

- *Normal counts:* Differential ≤ 5%
- *AEC:* ≤ 0.5×10^9/l
- *Eosinophilia*
- *Mild:* AEC 0.5–1.5×10^9/l
- *Moderate:* AEC 1.5–5.0×10^9/l
- Severe: AEC > 5.0×10^9/l HES
- *AEC:* > 1.5×10^9/l lasting for 6 months
- Lack of evidence for known causes of eosinophilia
- Signs and symptoms of organ involvement/dysfunction

Abbreviations: AEC, absolute eosinophil count; HES, hypereosinophilic syndrome.
Source: Reference 9.

parasites. The role of eosinophils in allergic disorders, parasitic and neoplastic diseases, tissue inflammation or idiopathic eosinophilia as a result of their proinflammatory and cytotoxic effects is also now better understood. As discussed, these effects are related to the release of preformed granule constituents and inducible lipid mediators, cytokines and oxidative products. The role of eosinophils in tissue injury has been elucidated by the demonstration of protein constituents of primary and secondary granules in the tissues involved in eosinophilia related disorders.

A large number of conditions are associated with the development of eosinophilia **(Box 1)** with manifestations in different organ systems necessitating a careful search for the cause. Though secondary causes of eosinophilia are more likely (allergic disorders in the west and parasitic infections in rest of the world), in many cases an underlying myeloid malignancy may be detected (clonal eosinophilia); the search may be inconclusive in several instances and lead to a diagnosis of idiopathic hypereosinophilic syndrome (HES).

PULMONARY EOSINOPHILIC DISORDERS

A holistic approach to pulmonary eosinophilic disorders involves understanding the place of lung diseases associated with eosinophilia in the overall gamut of eosinophilic disorders. In recent years, a significant evolution in classification and differentiation has taken place. *Broadly, eosinophilic disorders are divided into the following categories:*[4]

- Hypereosinophilic syndromes previously considered idiopathic for which the causes are now known. These include PDGFRA-associated myeloproliferative neoplasms and lymphocytic variants of HESs. The eosinophilia here is driven by eosinophilopoietic cytokines produced by T cells that are clonal and/or express aberrant surface phenotypes, most commonly cluster of differentiation 3 $(CD3)^-$ $CD4^+$[22]
- Organ restricted eosinophilic syndromes; pulmonary eosinophilic disorders and eosinophilic gastrointestinal disorders

BOX 2 Pulmonary eosinophilic disorders

Primary pulmonary eosinophilia
- Predominant involving lung
  - Acute eosinophilic pneumonia
  - Chronic eosinophilic pneumonia
- Systemic disease with lung disease
  - Churg-Strauss syndrome
  - Idiopathic hypereosinophilic syndrome

Secondary pulmonary eosinophilia
- Infections
  - Parasitic infestations
    - Transient passage (Löffler's syndrome):
      - Ancylostoma, ascaris, strongyloides
    - *Tissue resident:* Paragonimiasis, echinococcosis
    - Heavy hematogenous seeding
      - Trichinella
      - Visceral larva migrans
      - Disseminated strongyloidiasis
      - Schistosomiasis
    - *Fungal infections:* Coccidioimycosis, histoplasmosis
    - *Other infections:* Tuberculosis, brucellosis
- Tropical pulmonary eosinophilia
- Allergic bronchopulmonary aspergillosis
- Hypersensitivity pneumonia
- Drugs, toxins and radiation

Lung disorders with associated eosinophilia
- Interstitial lung disease, sarcoidosis idiopathic pulmonary fibrosis, Langerhans cell histiocytosis connective tissue disease
- Asthma
- Bronchiolitis obliterans-organizing pneumonia
- Neoplastic disorders, hematological malignancies solid organ tumors
- Postlung transplant.

- Syndromes in which eosinophilia and eosinophil-associated pathogenesis are central to the diagnosis; Churg-Strauss syndrome
- Hereditary disorders characterized by eosinophilia.

Pulmonary eosinophilic disorders may occur with or without a known cause or as an association of known lung disease **(Box 2)**. Since many of these disorders have been dealt with in detail elsewhere discussion will be restricted to that of primary pulmonary eosinophilic disorders [acute eosinophilic pneumonia (AEP), idiopathic chronic eosinophilic pneumonia (ICEP), Churg-Strauss syndrome (CSS) and HES] and those related to drugs and toxins. AEP and ICEP are only occasionally associated with extrapulmonary involvement and predominant systemic symptoms suggest the possibility of systemic vasculitis, idiopathic HES or other causes.

LÖFFLER'S SYNDROME

This syndrome was first described by Löffler in 1932. The original description was of a syndrome consisting of no to minimal respiratory symptoms along with fleeting pulmonary opacities and peripheral eosinophilia. A similar syndrome may be seen secondary to drug reactions. There is no age or sex predilection and the patients typically present with an acute, self-limiting disease comprising of low-grade fever, dry cough, dyspnea and rarely, hemoptysis. Blood examination shows moderate to marked eosinophilia; respiratory secretions may also show eosinophilia. The chest X-ray will show transient, migratory, nonsegmental interstitial or alveolar infiltrates. The symptoms typically resolve within 1-2 weeks.[2,5]

ACUTE EOSINOPHILIC PNEUMONIA

Acute eosinophilic pneumonia is an acute onset rapidly progressive disorder that occurs in the previously normal young adult population and causes acute onset, severe respiratory failure.[10,11] The median age at onset is approximately 30 years and has a slight male preponderance.[12,13] The exact cause in the majority of individuals is not known though it has been associated with unusual activities such as cave exploring and wood working.[14] This has led to a hypothesis that AEP is due to a hypersensitivity reaction to fungal antigens; though nothing has been proven as yet. Also, cases have been reported in individuals who have recently taken up smoking; interestingly, cases have been reported recently after exposure to e-cigarettes and to second hand smoke.[15-18]

The clinical presentation is that of acute onset disease with rapid progression to acute respiratory distress syndrome (ARDS) over 2-3 days. Patients may present with fever, cough, myalgias, dyspnea, pleuritic chest pain that progresses to frank respiratory failure.[19] A somewhat characteristic feature is the absence of any multisystem involvement despite severe respiratory failure.[12] A possibility of AEP should always be kept in mind during the evaluation of any ARDS patient.

Investigations typically show leukocytosis with initial absence of peripheral blood eosinophilia, though the immunoglobulin E (IgE) levels may be moderately increased. However, a recent study demonstrated that up to 28% of patients may have peripheral blood eosinophilia at presentation; also it may be associated with a better prognosis as compared to patients without initial eosinophilia.[20] The chest X-ray shows bilateral patchy reticular infiltrates that progress rapidly to an ARDS like picture with diffuse alveolar or interstitial infiltrates. The computed tomography (CT) scan shows ground glass opacities and/or consolidation which may patchy or diffuse in nature and smooth interlobular septal thickening distributed in a random manner without any zonal predominance.[21,22] Bilateral pleural effusions may also be seen while pleural fluid analysis shows marked eosinophilia and high pH. Bronchoalveolar lavage (BAL) shows marked eosinophilia along with variably elevated levels of beta-D-glucan and many cytokines such as IL-5 and IL-18. Pulmonary function tests (PFTs) during the acute phase show a restrictive defect with reduced diffusing capacity of lung for carbon monoxide (DLCO).

Pathologically, the main finding is that of a diffuse alveolar damage syndrome, with marked eosinophilic infiltration in the interstitium and in the alveolar spaces. Fibrinous membranes are commonly seen; airway involvement with mucus plugs has also been described. AEP is not characterized by either formation of granulomas or by alveolar hemorrhage. Pleural eosinophilic infiltration has been noted in 10% of cases.[19]

Despite its severe clinical presentation, AEP is highly responsive to corticosteroids. Mechanical ventilation may be required for severe cases, with ventilation strategies as for ARDS. The mortality rate is low with prompt treatment that results in a rapid and sustained response and infrequent relapses. The diagnosis requires a high index of suspicion and is made only after exclusion of all other causes.

IDIOPATHIC CHRONIC EOSINOPHILIC PNEUMONIA

Idiopathic chronic eosinophilic pneumonia was first described by Carrington in 1969.[23] Though it may occur at any age, the peak incidence of the disease is seen between the ages of 30-40 years[24] with a female preponderance. Patients with CEP are generally nonsmokers. A history of antecedent atopy, allergic rhinitis or nasal polyps is present in one-third to half of the patients and that of asthma in about two-third of the patients. The asthma is adult onset and may arise spontaneously or precede ICEP by some time.

The disease generally has an insidious onset and indolent course.[25] Predominant symptoms are low-grade fever, drenching night sweats and weight loss. Associated productive or nonproductive cough, dyspnea and wheezing are the other presenting features. Dyspnea is generally mild, but at times may progress to a point that mechanical ventilation may be required.[25] Extrapulmonary manifestations other than fever, asthenia and weight loss occur rarely; they include arthralgias, joint pains and heart failure. In fact, presence of significant extrapulmonary symptoms should necessitate a search for other systemic disorders such as vasculitis or hypereosinophilic syndrome.

Diagnosis

The peripheral blood examination shows normocytic-normochromic anemia with a mild to moderately elevated erythrocyte sedimentaion rate (ESR). There is usually a moderate leukocytosis with an elevated eosinophil count; the platelet count may also be elevated.[26] However, the absence of peripheral eosinophilia should not preclude the diagnosis. BAL fluid also shows marked eosinophilia ranging from 12–95% of the total. Serum IgE levels are moderately elevated in about half of the cases. Pulmonary function testing may either be normal or show an obstructive or restrictive defect. The obstructive defect may occur in patients with asthma though patients without asthma may also develop the same. The restrictive pattern occurs due to eosinophil infiltration into the interstitium. The DLCO is mildly reduced.

The radiographic features of CEP are quite variable. Characteristically, infiltrates are dense, patchy, bilateral, peripheral and symmetrical, involve the upper and mid zones and are progressive in nature.[27] They may be subpleural in location. The characteristic "photographic negative of pulmonary edema" that occurs following involvement of extensive areas or whole lung is seen in less than 25% of cases.[24] Pleural effusions are uncommon though reported.[28] High-resolution computed tomography (HRCT) shows bilateral involvement with areas of ill-defined consolidation and ground glass opacification, areas of patchy consolidation with atelectasis and septal thickening. There may be mediastinal lymphadenopathy and nodular infiltrates.[26,29]

Histopathologic examination reveals infiltration of the interstitium and alveoli by eosinophils, lymphocytes, macrophages and plasma cells with disruption of the local architecture. Evidence of proliferative bronchiolitis obliterans, microangiitis and microabscesses may also be seen. The diagnosis is suggested by appropriate investigations in the presence of a suitable clinical background. The differential diagnosis includes tuberculosis, fungal infections (like cryptococcosis), sarcoidosis, Löffler's syndrome, desquamative interstitial pneumonia (DIP) and bronchiolitis obliterans with organizing pneumonia (BOOP), among others.

Management

There is a dramatic response to corticosteroids in CEP with symptoms decreasing within 6–48 hours and radiological clearing within two months. Oral steroids with dose ranging from 0.5–1 mg/kg/day can be used and treatment in low doses is maintained for at least 6 months to one year or longer. Relapse occurs in half to two-thirds of treated patients after discontinuation of steroids.[24,25,30] However, currently no risk factors indicative of relapse are recognized. The relapse can usually be controlled by reinstitution of steroids which may need to be given for prolonged periods of time.[24,26,29-31] The dose of oral steroids can be brought down by the addition of inhaled corticosteroids.[5,29] The use of Omalizumab, an anti IgE antibody, has been described recently as a steroid sparing agent in CEP with good results.[32,33]

CHURG-STRAUSS SYNDROME (EOSINOPHILIC GRANULOMATOSIS WITH POLYANGIITIS)

Churg-Strauss syndrome was first described as a separate entity in the early 1950s.[34,35] The nomenclature was recently revised and it has now been renamed as eosinophilic granulomatosis with polyangiitis (EGPA).[36-39] It has now been defined as an eosinophil-rich and necrotizing granulomatous inflammation often involving the respiratory tract, and necrotizing vasculitis predominantly affecting small to medium vessels, and associated with asthma and eosinophilia.[36] The diverse clinical presentation and the difficulty in differentiating the disease often lead to a delay in the diagnosis. It is 2–10 times less common than the other antinuclear cytotoxic antibodies (ANCA) associated vasculitis with an incidence of 0.5–3.7 per million and a prevalence of 2–22 per million population.[38] It can affect any age group with peak incidence between 30 years and 50 years, without any sex predilection.[40]

The underlying pathology is believed to be an immune hypersensitivity, accounting for the presence of ANCA and nearly universal finding of an atopic state in these individuals. The presence or absence of ANCA allows the differentiation of these patients into two subgroups. The group with ANCA positivity has more frequent mononeuritis multiplex, glomerulonephritis, purpura and alveolar hemorrhage while the ANCA negative group has more frequent cardiomyopathic features and lung infiltrates.[37-39,41]

Eosinophilic granulomatosis with polyangiitis has been associated with the use of leukotriene inhibitors, montelukast more than zafirlukast.[42] The onset of the disease is variable from 2 days to 12 months after the initiation of therapy and it occurs almost exclusively as corticosteroids are being tapered off. This is considered to be an unmasking of the underlying disease rather than the result of drug use. There have also been reports of EGPA occurring after the use of omalizumab.[39]

Clinical Features

Eosinophilic granulomatosis with polyangiitis is commonly diagnosed when a patient with long standing asthma develops symptoms suggestive of vasculitis, i.e. mononeuritis multiplex, purpura, etc. along with peripheral eosinophilia and lung infiltrates. Three stages have been described clinically:

Prodromal stage: This can last for months to years. The patient usually presents with late onset atopic states such as allergic rhinitis, nasal polyposis and asthma in the absence of any family history.

Eosinophilic stage: This stage is characterized by the infiltration of various tissues by eosinophils, especially the skin, gastrointestinal tract (GIT) and lungs.

Vasculitic stage: Characterized clinically by the onset of constitutional symptoms and microscopically by eosinophilic infiltration, vasculitis and granulomatous infiltration.

The clinical course can be variable and may not strictly adhere to the mentioned stages. The respiratory manifestations of EGPA include upper respiratory tract disease, asthma, pleural effusions and Löffler's like syndrome. The upper respiratory tract is involved in approximately 75–85% of cases and manifests as allergic rhinitis, sinusitis and nasal polyposis. No necrosis is seen unlike in Wegener's granulomatosis.[43]

Asthma is the predominant feature of EGPA. It may be present for many years before the diagnosis of EGPA is made.[44] It is usually predominant in the prodromal and eosinophilic stages of the disease and may subside with the onset of the vasculitic phases. A short interval between the onset of asthma and that of vasculitis is considered a sign of increased severity.[45]

Other pulmonary manifestations include a Löffler's like syndrome (40%) and unilateral or bilateral pleural effusions or pleurisy without effusions in up to one-third of patients.

The cardiovascular system is commonly involved and is the leading cause of mortality.[40] Patients may develop coronary vasculitis leading to myocardial infarction and ischemic cardiomyopathy or congestive cardiac failure secondary to eosinophilic myocardial infiltration. Acute and chronic constrictive pericarditis and pericardial tamponade may also occur. The development of coronary vasculitis is associated with high risk of mortality of around 60%.[46]

Systemic manifestations may be prominent, include fever, weight loss, arthralgias and arthritis, lymphadenopathy, splenomegaly, urological and ocular disease. These generally herald the onset of extrapulmonary disease. Neurological manifestations are seen in up to two-thirds of patients, include mononeuropathy and polyneuropathy, cranial neuropathy especially optic neuritis, mononeuritis multiplex, seizures, cerebrovascular accidents and subarachnoid hemorrhage.[44]

Gastrointestinal tract manifestations generally consist of eosinophilic gastroenteritis or vasculitis causing abdominal pain, bleeding, diarrhea, intestinal obstruction, bowel perforation, gastric ulcers and liver function test abnormalities.[47] Dermatologic manifestations like palpable purpura, nodules, ulcers, maculopapular rashes and livedo reticularis may occur. Renal involvement consists of interstitial nephritis, focal segmental glomerulosclerosis, hematuria and hypertension following renal infarction. However, chronic renal failure is unusual in EGPA as compared to other forms of vasculitis.

Diagnosis

Laboratory examination shows normocytic-normochromic anemia, normal platelet counts and a high ESR. Leukocytosis with variable eosinophilia is commonly noted. IgE and IgG levels are elevated and there is hypergammaglobulinemia with rheumatoid factor seropositivity. IgE levels may parallel the disease activity. Overall, about 40% of patients have ANCA positivity; this is generally perinuclear (pANCA) with specificity against myeloperoxidase. However, only 25% of patients with EGPA who have no renal disease are ANCA positive, while ANCA is positive in 75% of patients with any renal disease and in 100% with documented necrotizing glomerulonephritis.[36] The titers of ANCA do not have utility as a marker of disease activity on follow-up examinations.[37-39]

The chest X-ray may be normal or nonspecific. Löffler's syndrome like infiltrates may be present in up to 40% of individuals **(Figs 1A and B)** and pleural effusions may be seen in one-third of cases. Other findings on radiology include noncavitatory nodules, patchy areas of consolidation or ground glass opacification, septal thickening, pulmonary artery enlargement and peribronchial thickening. Pleural fluid is acidic with high eosinophil count and low glucose levels. The imaging findings are not specific to EGPA and should be interpreted in the overall clinical context.

Pulmonary function tests show an obstructive physiology while BAL shows variable eosinophilia. Positron emission tomography (PET) may show cardiac involvement. Histopathological examination of various tissues, including the lungs, pleura, skin, GIT and nervous tissue reveals both intravascular and extravascular noncaseating granulomas with eosinophilic infiltration accompanied by vasculitis of the small and medium-sized arteries, veins, venules and capillaries.[40] Peripheral nerves are more commonly involved in EGPA as compared to other ANCA associated

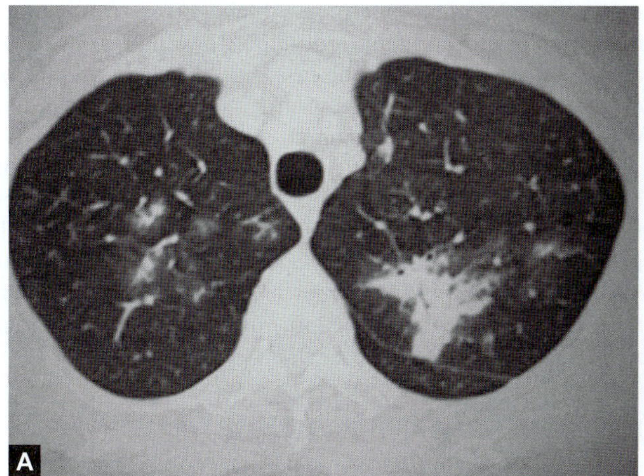

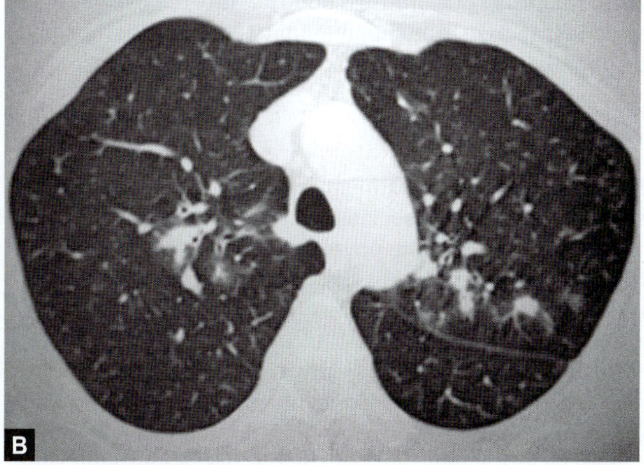

Figs 1A and B High-resolution computed tomography of a patient with eosinophilic granulomatosis with polyangiitis with pulmonary infiltrates

Table 1 Classification and diagnostic criteria for eosinophilic granulomatosis with polyangiitis

Lanham et al[40]	*ACR 1990*[48]	*CHCC 1994*[49]	*CHCC 2012*[36]
Asthma	Asthma	Eosinophil-rich and granulomatous inflammation involving the respiratory tract, necrotizing vasculitis affecting small to medium-sized vessels, and associated with asthma and eosinophilia	Eosinophil-rich and necrotizing granulomatous inflammation often involving the respiratory tract, and necrotizing vasculitis predominantly affecting small to medium vessels, and associated with asthma and eosinophilia
Eosinophilia >1.5 × 10^9/l	Eosinophilia >10%		
Clinical or pathological evidence of vasculitis involving at least two organs	Neuropathy (mono- or poly-neuropathy) Nonfixed pulmonary infiltrates Paranasal sinus abnormalities Extravascular eosinophil infiltration on biopsy		
Abbreviations: ACR, American College of Rheumatolology; CHCC, Chapel Hill Consensus Conference ACR criteria require 4 out of 6 to be present.			

vasculitides.[38] The inflammation may resolve with time and treatment, or lead further to fibrous scarring.

In the absence of universally accepted diagnostic criteria, the diagnosis of EGPA is challenging. There are several diagnostic criteria that rely on symptoms of asthma, eosinophilia and evidence of organ involvement secondary to medium and small vessel vasculitis. The American College of Rheumatology criteria published in 1990 **(Table 1)** require the presence of at least four out of the six given criteria, which give a sensitivity and specificity of 85% and 99.7%, respectively.[48] These include (i) asthma, (ii) paranasal sinusitis, (iii) monoarthropathy or polyarthropathy, (iv) migratory or transient pulmonary infiltrates, (v) peripheral blood eosinophilia greater than 10%, and (vi) extravascular eosinophils in a blood vessel on a biopsy specimen.

The differential diagnosis includes other ANCA associated vasculitis like granulomatosis with polyangiitis or Wegener's granulomatosis, polyarteritis nodosa, tuberculosis, fungal infections, allergic bronchopulmonary aspergillosis, chronic eosinophilic pneumonia, asthma and Hodgkin's disease.

Treatment

There is no stratified treatment schedule available in EGPA as in other ANCA associated vasculitis.[50] The choice of treatment is based on the presence of systemic involvement. The five factor score (FFS) is the most commonly used guide for treatment initiation. The five factors are; (1) proteinuria more than 1 g/24 h; (2) serum creatinine level more than 140 mmol/L; (3) myocardial involvement; (4) severe gastrointestinal involvement; and (5) central nervous system involvement.[39] Presence of more than or equal to 1 of these factors is indicative of a higher risk of morbidity and mortality; if the FFS is more than or equal to 1 treatment is started with both steroids and immunosuppressive agents while steroids alone would suffice with a FFS of 0.[44,46] Oral prednisolone may be started at a dose of 1 mg/kg/day and continued for 6–12 weeks followed by a gradual taper to a maintenance dose, which might be continued for a year or more. Disease activity may be followed by the disappearance of constitutional symptoms, hypertension, cardiac, renal, neurological and vasculitic disease. Laboratory markers of disease activity include ESR, IgE levels and leukocyte counts; pANCA is not useful for follow-up.

Indications for the use of cytotoxic chemotherapy include nonresponsiveness to steroids and severe systemic disease including cardiac, GIT and renal disease (proteinuria > 1 g/day or renal insufficiency). Pulse cyclophosphamide is probably the immunosuppressive treatment of choice in an acute phase, whereas azathioprine may be useful for maintenance. Pulse steroids may also be used in acute settings. Other immunomodulators such as high dose intravenous immunoglobulin and interferon-alpha in standard dose have also been used in severe disease and so has been plasma exchange.[44] There have been recent case reports of treatment with rituximab and mepolizumab. [51-58]

The prognosis of EGPA is very poor without treatment. However, the use of corticosteroids has dramatically reduced the mortality rate.[44] Long-term remissions are usually achieved, though relapses may occur. The use of steroids and immunosuppressive agents may cause significant morbidity though, in the form of infections, osteoporosis, solid organ malignancies, etc.

HYPEREOSINOPHILIC SYNDROME

Also known as Löffler's endocarditis and eosinophilic leukemia, HES is a disorder characterized by multisystem involvement and a variable presentation.[9,59-61] It predominantly affects males and is more common from ages 20–50 years, though it can occur at any age.[59] The diagnostic criteria, initially proposed by Chusid have been subsequently expanded to include the World Health Organization (WHO) criteria for diagnosis **(Table 1 and Box 3)**.[9,62] There has been a significant confusion in the past over the terminology and at times it was thought that HES constitutes a spectrum of illness with minimal involvement on one hand and eosinophilic leukemia on the other extreme. Recent WHO classification suggests that clonal disorders that show chromosomal or molecular clonality should be classified as neoplastic and HES should include the rest of the disorders without any clear cause for eosinophilia.

The cause of this disorder is unknown and the various hypotheses propose it as a disorder ranging from a primary disturbance of myelopoiesis to a monoclonal expansion of T lymphocytes producing cytokines to an immune hypersensitivity reaction. The organ damage is the result of eosinophilic infiltration and/or thromboembolic phenomena.

Clinical Features

Three major clinical variants of HES are recognized,[63] i.e. myeloproliferative variant, lymphoproliferative and familial HES. The myeloproliferative variant has been shown to be associated with FIP1LI-PDGFR α fusion gene. Since these patients have a clonal abnormality, these may also be classified by some as CEL. The lymphoproliferative variant is associated with monoclonal expansion of T cells that result in increased IL-5 secretion and hypereosinophilia. Familial HES is secondary to a genetic defect that results in increased IL-5 and eosinophilia. Currently, even after detailed investigations, a subset of patients may not reveal any cause, termed as true idiopathic HES.

BOX 3 WHO criteria for diagnosis of chronic eosinophilic leukemia and hypereosinophilic syndrome[62]

Persistent eosinophilia > 1.5×10^9/l
Increased number of eosinophils in the bone marrow
Myeloblasts < 20% in both blood and bone marrow

- Exclude all causes of reactive eosinophilia (secondary to allergy, parasitic diseases, infectious diseases, pulmonary diseases, collagen vascular diseases, etc.)
- Exclude all neoplastic disorders with reactive eosinophilia (T-cell lymphomas, Hodgkin's lymphoma, ALL, B-cell lymphomas, mastocytosis)
- Exclude other neoplastic disorders in which eosinophils are part of neoplastic clone [Philadelphia (Ph) chromosome &/and/or BCRABL positive chronic myelogenous leukemia; acute myeloid leukemia, including those with inv(16), t(16;16)(p13;q22); other myeloproliferative diseases like polycythemia vera (PV), essential thrombocythemia (ET), idiopathic myelofibrosis (IMF)]
- Exclude T cell populations with aberrant phenotype and abnormal cytokine production
- Diagnose HES, if there is no demonstrable disease that can cause eosinophilia, no evidence of abnormal T cell population and no evidence of clonal myeloid disorder
- Diagnose chronic eosinophilic leukemia (CEL) if all of the requirements (including conditions 1–4) have been met, and if the myeloid cells demonstrate a clonal cytogenetic abnormality or are shown to be clonal by other means, or if blast cells are present in peripheral blood (< 2%) or bone marrow (5–19%).

Hypereosinophilic syndrome is a heterogeneous disease. Its clinical manifestations are highly variable in the terms of duration, severity and organ involvement. The symptoms most often are indolent; include fever, weight loss, fatigue, anorexia, night sweats, skin rash, hepatosplenomegaly, angioedema and other system involvement.

The respiratory system is involved in approximately 40% of cases, manifested predominantly by nocturnal cough, which is usually nonproductive.[9,61,63] Wheezing and dyspnea also occur and occasionally the disease can progress to ARDS. Pleural effusion, pulmonary hypertension and thromboembolism may develop over a period of time.

The cardiovascular system is most common involved.[59,64] There is an eosinophilic infiltration of the endocardium and myocardium leading to restrictive cardiomyopathy,[65,66] endocardial fibrosis and mitral regurgitation. Intracardiac thrombus formation occurs, leading to pulmonary thromboembolism. Associated peripheral arterial or venous thrombosis has also been reported.[67]

Neurological manifestations include encephalopathy, neuropsychiatric disturbances, memory loss, visual changes and cerebrovascular accidents secondary to thromboembolism.[68] Other systems are involved less frequently; the symptomatology varies according to the system involved **(Table 2)**.

Diagnosis

Blood examination shows anemia, leukocytosis (10,000–50,000/mm^3) with 30–70% eosinophils; associated may be blood and or bone marrow neutrophilia, basophilia and eosinophilic dysplasia[69] ESR, serum IgE and gamma globulins are elevated. Also noted are elevated levels of serum B_{12} and leukocyte alkaline phosphatase. Circulating immune complexes are occasionally found. Bone marrow shows an increase in eosinophils and eosinophil precursors **(Fig. 2)**. Eosinophilic blast transformation has been noted in 28–51% of patients. Eosinophilic infiltration of other organs is also demonstrable on histopathological examination **(Fig. 3)**.

Chest X-ray shows focal or diffuse nonspecific infiltrates and pleural effusions. PFTs demonstrate an obstructive physiology. Echocardiography may show evidence of intracardiac thrombi; should be done 6-monthly in follow-up as cardiovascular disease is the major cause of mortality and morbidity in this disease.[67]

The differential diagnosis includes the different eosinophilic disorders like CEP, CSS, AEP, tropical pulmonary eosinophilia, fungal infections and parasitic infestations,

Table 2 End-organ damage in hypereosinophilic syndrome and hypereosinophilic disorders

System	*Clinical manifestations*
Cardiac	Pericarditis, EMF, cardiomyopathy, myocarditis, intramural thrombi, regurgitation
Neurologic	Thromboemboli, peripheral neuropathy, dementia/psychosis, meningitis, epilepsy
Dermatologic	Angioedema, urticaria, papulonodular lesions, mucosal ulcers, vesiculobullous, microthrombi, Raynaud's phenomenon, digital necrosis
Pulmonary	Infiltrates, fibrosis, effusion, emboli
Ocular	Microthrombi, vasculitis, retinal arteritis
Joints	Arthralgia, effusions, polyarthritis
Gastrointestinal	Ascites, diarrhea, gastritis, colitis, pancreatitis, cholangitis, Budd-Chiari syndrome
Abbreviation: EMF, endomyocardial fibrosis	

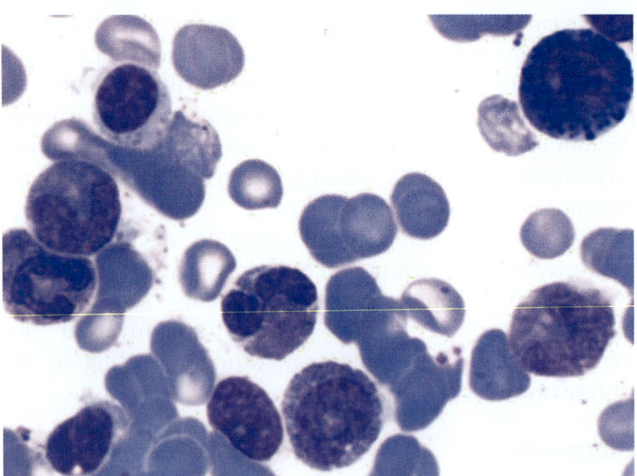

Fig. 2 Bone marrow smear in hypereosinophilic syndrome patient showing two metamyelocytes, one basophil and two eosinophils (one has a ring nucleus)

etc. Different laboratory criteria are used for the differential diagnosis of lymphoproliferative and myeloproliferative variants **(Box 4)**.

Treatment

Treatment depends upon the presence of end-organ dysfunction. In clonal and idiopathic hypereosinophilia, the aim of the treatment is to limit or reverse end-organ damage and provide symptomatic improvement. In asymptomatic patients without any evidence of end-organ damage, a careful follow-up and assessment of any end-organ damage may be a prudent policy.

Asymptomatic peripheral eosinophilia can be followed up every 3–6 months without any treatment. The first line of therapy consists of steroids, which are given orally. Prednisone, in a dose of 1 mg/kg/day for 1–2 months is followed by a slow taper to a maintenance dose, which can be continued for 1 year or longer as required. In refractory cases, treatment with hydroxyurea, vincristine, chlorambucil, cyclosporine or interferon-α, can be tried.[59,70] The anti-IL5

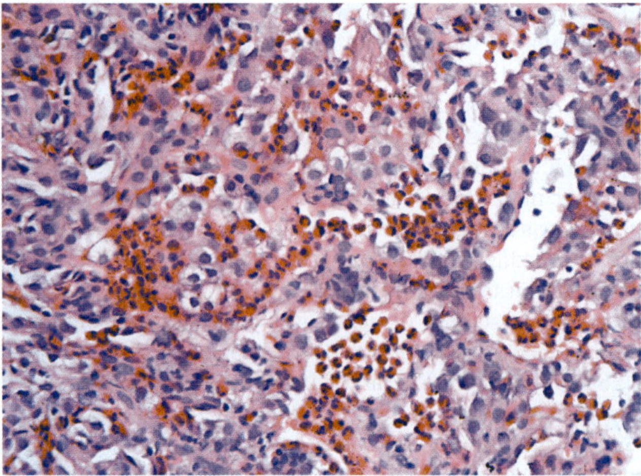

Fig. 3 Extensive eosinophilic infiltration of tissues on histopathological examination

BOX 4 Laboratory diagnosis of myeloproliferative and lymphoproliferative variants of hypereosinophilic syndrome

Myeloproliferative variant

Definitive evidence:
- FIP1L1-PDGFRA fusion
- Eosinophil clonality.

Supportive evidence:
≥ 4 of
- Increased serum tryptase
- Increased serum B12
- Splenomegaly
- Anemia, thrombocytopenia
- Increased circulating myeloid precursors
- Dysplastic eosinophils
- Myelofibrosis
- Increased spindle shaped mast cells in bone marrow

Lymphoproliferative variant

Definitive evidence:
- Phenotypically aberrant T Cells
- TCR rearrangement
- Increased eosinophilopoietic cytokines.

Supportive evidence:
- Increased serum thymus and activation-regulated chemokine (TARC)
- Increased serum IgE
- Predominantly cutaneous manifestations
- H/O atopy
- Steroid responsive.

antibody, mepolizumab has also been used in patients with high IL5 levels.[71,72]

Even though steroids had been the mainstay of treatment in the past, it is now realized that patients with myeloproliferative variant do not respond well to steroids and in case of FIP1L1-PDGFRA positive patients, use of tyrosine-kinase inhibitors such as imatinib[73,74] and dasatinib results in a gratifying response. Initial dose for a rapid cytogenetic response should be 400 mg/day with a lower maintenance dose. Whereas, this variant is associated with exquisite sensitivity to imatinib even at a dose of 100 mg/day, other variants may require higher dosage and have variable response. Steroids should be added to imatinib in patients with evidence of myocarditis on echocardiography, electrocardiography or biochemical parameters (elevated serum troponin). The anti-CD 52 antibody, alemtuzumab has been tried in refractory cases especially those of lymphoproliferative variant.[75,76] There are several reports of successful treatment using hematopoietic stem cell transplant in refractory cases.[77-83]

The causes of mortality in HES include refractory congestive cardiac failure, renal failure, hepatic failure, venous thromboembolism, gut perforation and infections. However, proper treatment leads to a mean survival of greater than 10 years. In a recent study, 23 of 247 patients died over a 19-year follow-up, with the cause of death identified as cardiac dysfunction in 5 patients (33%), infection in 3 (20%), unrelated malignancy in 3 (20%), thromboembolic phenomena in 2 (13%), and vascular disease in 2 (13%) patients.[84]

Other Eosinophilic Lung Diseases

Langerhans Cell Granulomatosis

Histiocytosis X consists of three closely-related disorders, occurring at different ages: Langerhans cell histiocytosis, Letterer-Siwe disease and Hand-Schüller-Christian disease.[85] Primary pulmonary histiocytosis X, earlier known as eosinophilic granuloma of the lung, is almost exclusively found in smokers. The male to female ratio is 1:1; patients in the third and fourth decades of life are commonly affected.

It presents with cough, dyspnea, hemoptysis, chest pain, fever, wheezing, weight loss and recurrent, often bilateral pneumothorax. Patients also develop diabetes insipidus and bony disease. Chest X-ray shows involvement of the upper and middle zones with sparing of the costophrenic angles, reticulonodular changes, cystic lesions and bullae that may rupture to cause recurrent pneumothorax. PFTs may show either a restrictive or an obstructive defect.

Histopathologically, a granulomatous infiltrate of histiocytes, eosinophils and other cells can be seen. The histiocyte is a large cell with an indented nucleus that has Birbeck granules on electron microscopy. S-100 antibody can also be found **(Figs 2 and 3)**.

Treatment is based on the severity of the disease. Smoking should be stopped and patient treated with corticosteroids. Vincristine, cyclophosphamide and fludarabine have also been used. The mortality rate is less than 5% in adults.

Sarcoidosis

It is a multisystem disorder with pulmonary involvement in the majority of cases. Patients may present with fever, weight loss, mediastinal lymphadenopathy and lung infiltrates.

Histopathological examination reveals noncaseating epithelioid granulomas. Tuberculosis is a close differential diagnosis, especially in the Indian subcontinent. The incidence of eosinophilia in sarcoidosis ranges from 10% to 67%.[86]

Neoplastic Disorders

Eosinophilia may occur in association with several neoplastic conditions, both with hematological malignancies and solid organ tumors. The presence of eosinophilia may or may not be an adverse prognostic sign, depending upon the underlying disorder.

Hematological disorders associated with eosinophilia include systemic mastocytosis (in approximately 20%),[87,88] nodular sclerosing Hodgkin's disease (15%),[89] B-cell non-Hodgkin's disease,[89] T-cell leukemia and Sézary syndrome.[90] Of course, eosinophilic leukemia is a well-known variant of acute myelomonocytic leukemia (M4).[91]

Solid organ malignancies include large cell cancer of the lung, squamous cell carcinomas of cervix, skin, nasopharynx, bladder transitional cell carcinoma, etc.[92-96]

Tropical Pulmonary Eosinophilia

It is an important cause of marked eosinophilia, hence an important differential diagnosis.

Infections

Eosinophilia occurs with a variety of infectious agents, which include bacterial, fungal and parasitic diseases. An undulating pattern of eosinophilia that corresponds to disease activity has been noted in tuberculosis.[97] It has been shown that eosinophilia correlates with a good prognosis while eosinopenia was noted in fulminant or miliary disease.

Chronic brucellosis is also known to be associated with eosinophilia.[98] The fungal infection most commonly associated with eosinophilia is coccidioidomycosis in which it occurs as a hypersensitivity phenomenon.[99,100] Other fungal infections include rare case reports of eosinophilia associated with *Histoplasma capsulatum* and cryptococcosis.

Drug-induced and Toxin-induced Pulmonary Eosinophilia

A variety of drugs and toxins are associated with eosinophilic lung disease **(Box 5)**.[101] The signs and symptoms of disease may manifest anywhere from a few minutes after exposure to weeks afterwards. One of the more common drugs to be

BOX 5 Drugs causing eosinophilic lung disease

- Antimicrobials
  - Para-amino salicylic acid
  - Nitrofurantoin
  - Penicillin
  - Tetracycline
  - Streptomycin
  - Isoniazid
  - Sulfonamides
  - Tetracycline
  - Minocycline
  - Dapsone + pyrimethamine
- Antineoplastic and immunosuppressives
  - Bleomycin
  - Methotrexate
  - Melphalan
  - Gold salts
  - Azathioprine
  - Penicillamine
  - Beclomethasone
- Nonsteroidal anti-inflammatory drugs (NSAIDs):
  - Aspirin
  - Naproxen
  - Piroxicam
  - Nimesulide
  - Phenylbutazone
- Cardiovascular and antidiabetics:
  - Amiodarone
  - Hydralazine
  - Thiazides
  - Clofibrate
  - Sulfonylureas
- Miscellaneous
  - Carbamazepine
  - Phenytoin
  - Dantrolene
  - Methylphenidate
  - Imipramine
  - Cocaine or heroin exposure
  - Iodinated contrast media
  - L-tryptophan.

implicated is nitrofurantoin, which causes acute, subacute and chronic reactions.[102]

Symptoms, as already detailed, occur variably after exposure to the drug. These include low-grade fever, cough and dyspnea with or without wheezing. Examination might show wheezing and crackles and the peripheral blood will show eosinophilia. Chest X-ray may reveal diffuse or patchy pulmonary infiltrates; CT scans show bilateral consolidation and ground-glass opacification, both of which may be peripheral. PFTs may either be absolutely normal, or show a reduced DLCO or a mild restrictive defect.

The syndrome usually disappears after discontinuation of the responsible drug. Corticosteroids are not universally beneficial, though their use may hasten recovery, especially in sick patients.

Flow chart 1 Proposed diagnostic algorithm for pulmonary eosinophilic disorders

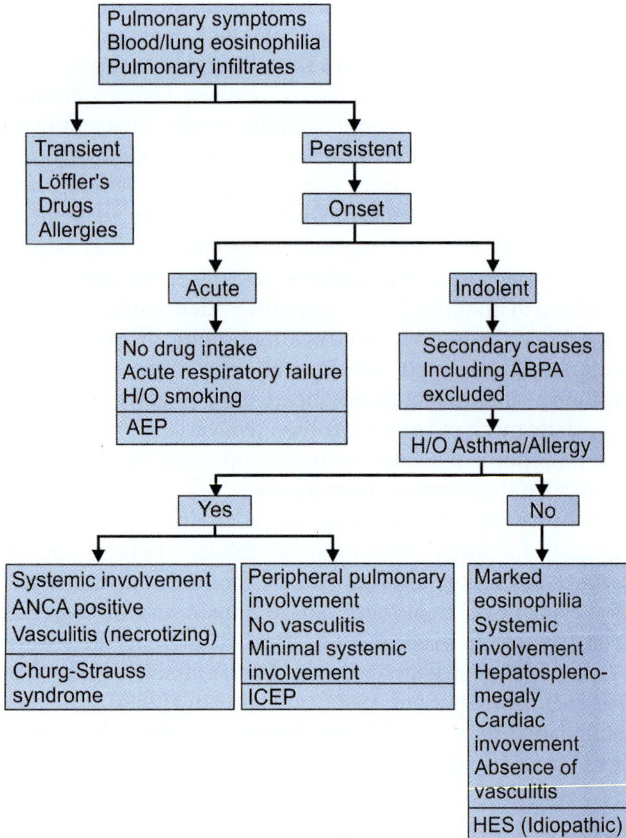

Abbreviations: AEP, acute eosinophilic pneumonia; HES, hypereosinophilic syndrome; ICEP, idiopathic chronic eosinophilic pneumonia; ABPA, allergic bronchopulmonary aspergillosis

APPROACH TO DIAGNOSIS AND CONCLUSION

It is apparent that eosinophilic lung diseases are heterogeneous disorders that require a meticulous history taking, painstaking examination and judicious use of investigations to reach a definite diagnosis (**Flow chart 1**). It is important to reach a diagnosis because these illnesses have different course and complications and thus involve important treatment decisions.

REFERENCES

1. Hirsch JG, Hirsch BI. Paul Ehrlich and the discovery of the eosinophil. In: Mahmoud AAF, Austen KF (Eds). The Eosinophil in Health and Disease. New York: Grune and Stratton; 1980. pp. 3-13.
2. LofflerW.Zurdifferential-diagnosederlungeninfiltrierungen:II. Uber fluchtige succedan-infiltrate (mit eosinopile). Beitr Klin Tuberk. 1932;79:368-82.

3. Reeder WH, Goodrich BE. Pulmonary infiltration with eosinophilia (PIE syndrome). Annals of Internal Medicine. 1952;36(5):1217-40.
4. Wechsler ME, Fulkerson PC, Bochner BS, Gauvreau GM, Gleich GJ, Henkel T, et al. Novel targeted therapies for eosinophilic disorders. The Journal of Allergy and Clinical Immunology. 2012;130(3):563-71.
5. Savani DM, Sharma OP. Eosinophilic lung disease in the tropics. Clinics in Chest Medicine. 2002;23(2):377-96, ix.
6. Uhrbrand H. The number of circulating eosinophils; normal figures and spontaneous variations. Acta Medica Scandinavica. 1958;160(2):99-104.
7. Bass DA. Behavior of eosinophil leukocytes in acute inflammation. I. Lack of dependence on adrenal function. The Journal of Clinical Investigation. 1975;55(6):1229-36.
8. Beeson PB, Bass DA. The eosinophil. Major Problems in Internal Medicine. 1977;14:1-269.
9. Chusid MJ, Dale DC, West BC, Wolff SM. The hypereosinophilic syndrome: analysis of fourteen cases with review of the literature. Medicine. 1975;54(1):1-27.
10. Badesch DB, King TE, Schwarz MI. Acute eosinophilic pneumonia: a hypersensitivity phenomenon? The American Review of Respiratory Disease. 1989;139(1):249-52.
11. Allen JN, Pacht ER, Gadek JE, Davis WB. Acute eosinophilic pneumonia as a reversible cause of noninfectious respiratory failure. The New England Journal of Medicine. 1989;321(9): 569-74.
12. Wechsler ME. Pulmonary eosinophilic syndromes. Immunology and Allergy Clinics of North America. 2007;27(3):477-92.
13. Al-Jahdali H, Waness A, Al-Jawder S, Baharoon SA, Al-Muhsen S, Al-Mobeireek A, et al. Eosinophilic pneumonia: experience at two tertiary care referral hospitals in Saudi Arabia. Annals of Saudi Medicine. 2012;32(1):32-6.
14. Allen J. Acute eosinophilic pneumonia. Seminars in respiratory and critical care medicine. 2006;27(2):142-7.
15. Abe K, Yanagi S, Imadsu Y, Sano A, Iiboshi H, Mukae H, et al. Acute eosinophilic pneumonia with fine nodular shadows. Internal Medicine (Tokyo, Japan). 2003;42(1):88-91.
16. Thota D, Latham E. Case report of electronic cigarettes possibly associated with eosinophilic pneumonitis in a previously healthy active-duty sailor. The Journal of Emergency Medicine. 2014;47(1):15-7.
17. Chung MK, Lee SJ, Kim MY, Lee JH, Chang JH, Sim SS, et al. Acute eosinophilic pneumonia following secondhand cigarette smoke exposure. Tuberculosis and Respiratory Diseases. 2014;76(4): 188-91.
18. Natarajan A, Shah P, Mirrakhimov AE, Hussain N. Eosinophilic pneumonia associated with concomitant cigarette and marijuana smoking. BMJ Case Rep. 2013;2013.
19. Vahid B, Marik PE. An 18-year-old woman with fever, diffuse pulmonary opacities, and rapid onset of respiratory failure: idiopathic acute eosinophilic pneumonia. Chest. 2006;130(6): 1938-41.
20. Jhun BW, Kim SJ, Kim K, Lee JE. Clinical implications of initial peripheral eosinophilia in acute eosinophilic pneumonia. Respirology (Carlton, Vic). 2014.
21. Cheon JE, Lee KS, Jung GS, Chung MH, Cho YD. Acute eosinophilic pneumonia: radiographic and CT findings in six patients. AJR American Journal of Roentgenology. 1996;167(5):1195-9.
22. Daimon T, Johkoh T, Sumikawa H, Honda O, Fujimoto K, Koga T, et al. Acute eosinophilic pneumonia: Thin-section CT findings in 29 patients. European Journal of Radiology. 2008;65(3):462-7.
23. Carrington CB, Addington WW, Goff AM, Madoff IM, Marks A, Schwaber JR, et al. Chronic eosinophilic pneumonia. The New England Journal of Medicine. 1969;280(15):787-98.
24. Jederlinic PJ, Sicilian L, Gaensler EA. Chronic eosinophilic pneumonia. A report of 19 cases and a review of the literature. Medicine. 1988;67(3):154-62.
25. Allen JN, Davis WB. Eosinophilic lung diseases. American Journal of Respiratory and Critical Care Medicine. 1994; 150(5 Pt 1):1423-38.
26. Marchand E, Reynaud-Gaubert M, Lauque D, Durieu J, Tonnel AB, Cordier JF. Idiopathic chronic eosinophilic pneumonia. A clinical and follow-up study of 62 cases. The Groupe d'Etudes et de Recherche sur les Maladies "Orphelines" Pulmonaires (GERM"O"P). Medicine. 1998;77(5):299-312.
27. Gaensler EA, Carrington CB. Peripheral opacities in chronic eosinophilic pneumonia: the photographic negative of pulmonary edema. AJR American Journal of Roentgenology. 1977;128(1):1-13.
28. Samman YS, Wali SO, Abdelaal MA, Gangi MT, Krayem AB. Chronic eosinophilic pneumonia presenting with recurrent massive bilateral pleural effusion: case report. Chest. 2001;119(3):968-70.
29. Marchand E, Cordier JF. Idiopathic chronic eosinophilic pneumonia. Orphanet Journal of Rare Diseases. 2006;1:11.
30. Naughton M, Fahy J, FitzGerald MX. Chronic eosinophilic pneumonia. A long-term follow-up of 12 patients. Chest. 1993;103(1):162-5.
31. Fox B, Seed WA. Chronic eosinophilic pneumonia. Thorax. 1980;35(8):570-80.
32. Kaya H, Gumus S, Ucar E, Aydogan M, Musabak U, Tozkoparan E, et al. Omalizumab as a steroid-sparing agent in chronic eosinophilic pneumonia. Chest. 2012;142(2):513-6.
33. Shin YS, Jin HJ, Yoo HS, Hwang EK, Nam YH, Ye YM, et al. Successful treatment of chronic eosinophilic pneumonia with anti-IgE therapy. Journal of Korean Medical Science. 2012;27(10):1261-4.
34. Keogh KA, Specks U. Churg-Strauss syndrome. Seminars in respiratory and critical care medicine. 2006;27(2):148-57.
35. Barros JM, Antunes T, Barbas CS. Churg-Strauss syndrome. J Bras Pneumol. 2005;31(Suppl 1):S27-31.
36. Jennette JC, Falk RJ, Bacon PA, Basu N, Cid MC, Ferrario F, et al. 2012 revised International Chapel Hill Consensus Conference Nomenclature of Vasculitides. Arthritis and Rheumatism. 2013;65(1):1-11.
37. Vaglio A, Buzio C, Zwerina J. Eosinophilic granulomatosis with polyangiitis (Churg-Strauss): state of the art. Allergy. 2013;68(3):261-73.
38. Mahr A, Moosig F, Neumann T, Szczeklik W, Taille C, Vaglio A, et al. Eosinophilic granulomatosis with polyangiitis (Churg-Strauss): evolutions in classification, etiopathogenesis, assessment and management. Current Opinion in Rheumatology. 2014;26(1):16-23.
39. Mouthon L, Dunogue B, Guillevin L. Diagnosis and classification of eosinophilic granulomatosis with polyangiitis (formerly named Churg-Strauss syndrome). Journal of Autoimmunity. 2014;48-49:99-103.
40. Lanham JG, Elkon KB, Pusey CD, Hughes GR. Systemic vasculitis with asthma and eosinophilia: a clinical approach to the Churg-Strauss syndrome. Medicine. 1984;63(2):65-81.

41. Vaglio A, Moosig F, Zwerina J. Churg-Strauss syndrome: update on pathophysiology and treatment. Current Opinion in Rheumatology. 2012;24(1):24-30.
42. Wechsler ME, Pauwels R, Drazen JM. Leukotriene modifiers and Churg-Strauss syndrome: adverse effect or response to corticosteroid withdrawal? Drug safety: an International Journal of Medical Toxicology and Drug Experience. 1999;21(4):241-51.
43. Antunes T, Barbas CS. Wegener's granulomatosis. J Bras Pneumol. 2005; 31(Suppl 1):S21-6.
44. Guillevin L, Cohen P, Gayraud M, Lhote F, Jarrousse B, Casassus P. Churg-Strauss syndrome. Clinical study and long-term follow-up of 96 patients. Medicine. 1999;78(1):26-37.
45. Chumbley LC, Harrison EG, DeRemee RA. Allergic granulomatosis and angiitis (Churg-Strauss syndrome). Report and analysis of 30 cases. Mayo Clinic proceedings. 1977;52(8):477-84.
46. Conron M, Beynon HL. Churg-Strauss syndrome. Thorax. 2000;55(10):870-7.
47. Hagen EC, Daha MR, Hermans J, Andrassy K, Csernok E, Gaskin G, et al. Diagnostic value of standardized assays for anti-neutrophil cytoplasmic antibodies in idiopathic systemic vasculitis. EC/BCR Project for ANCA Assay Standardization. Kidney international. 1998;53(3):743-53.
48. Masi AT, Hunder GG, Lie JT, Michel BA, Bloch DA, Arend WP, et al. The American College of Rheumatology 1990 criteria for the classification of Churg-Strauss syndrome (allergic granulomatosis and angiitis). Arthritis and rheumatism. 1990;33(8):1094-100.
49. Jennette JC, Falk RJ, Andrassy K, Bacon PA, Churg J, Gross WL, et al. Nomenclature of systemic vasculitides. Proposal of an international consensus conference. Arthritis and rheumatism. 1994;37:187-92.
50. Mukhtyar C, Guillevin L, Cid MC, Dasgupta B, de Groot K, Gross W, et al. EULAR recommendations for the management of primary small and medium vessel vasculitis. Annals of the Rheumatic Diseases. 2009;68(3):310-7.
51. Koukoulaki M, Smith KG, Jayne DR. Rituximab in Churg-Strauss syndrome. Annals of the rheumatic diseases. 2006;65(4):557-9.
52. Taniguchi M, Tsurikisawa N, Higashi N, Saito H, Mita H, Mori A, et al. Treatment for Churg-Strauss syndrome: induction of remission and efficacy of intravenous immunoglobulin therapy. Allergology international: Official Journal of the Japanese Society of Allergology. 2007;56(2):97-103.
53. Pepper RJ, Fabre MA, Pavesio C, Gaskin G, Jones RB, Jayne D, et al. Rituximab is effective in the treatment of refractory Churg-Strauss syndrome and is associated with diminished T-cell interleukin-5 production. Rheumatology (Oxford, England). 2008;47(7):1104-5.
54. Kim S, Marigowda G, Oren E, Israel E, Wechsler ME. Mepolizumab as a steroid-sparing treatment option in patients with Churg-Strauss syndrome. The Journal of Allergy and Clinical Immunology. 2010;125(6):1336-43.
55. Moosig F, Gross WL, Herrmann K, Bremer JP, Hellmich B. Targeting interleukin-5 in refractory and relapsing Churg-Strauss syndrome. Annals of Internal Medicine. 2011;155(5):341-3.
56. Herrmann K, Gross WL, Moosig F. Extended follow-up after stopping mepolizumab in relapsing/refractory Churg-Strauss syndrome. Clinical and experimental rheumatology. 2012;30(1 Suppl 70):S62-5.
57. Thiel J, Hassler F, Salzer U, Voll RE, Venhoff N. Rituximab in the treatment of refractory or relapsing eosinophilic granulomatosis with polyangiitis (Churg-Strauss syndrome). Arthritis Research and Therapy. 2013;15(5):R133.
58. Umezawa N, Kohsaka H, Nanki T, Watanabe K, Tanaka M, Shane PY, et al. Successful treatment of eosinophilic granulomatosis with polyangiitis (EGPA; formerly Churg-Strauss syndrome) with rituximab in a case refractory to glucocorticoids, cyclophosphamide, and IVIG. Modern rheumatology/the Japan Rheumatism Association. 2014;24(4):685-7.
59. Weller PF, Bubley GJ. The idiopathic hypereosinophilic syndrome. Blood. 1994;83(10):2759-79.
60. Spry CJ, Kumaraswami V. Tropical eosinophilia. Seminars in hematology. 1982;19(2):107-15.
61. Hardy WR, Anderson RE. The hypereosinophilic syndromes. Annals of Internal Medicine. 1968;68(6):1220-9.
62. Jaffe ES, Harris NL, Stein H, et al. WHO classification of tumours. Pathology and genetics of tumours of the hematopoietic and lymphoid tissues: In: Press I, (Ed). Lyon. 2001. pp. 29-31.
63. Klion AD, Bochner BS, Gleich GJ, Nutman TB, Rothenberg ME, Simon HU, et al. Approaches to the treatment of hypereosinophilic syndromes: a workshop summary report. The Journal of Allergy and Clinical Immunology. 2006;117(6):1292-302.
64. Cottin V, Cordier JF. Eosinophilic pneumonias. Allergy. 2005;60(7):841-57.
65. Klion AD. Recent advances in the diagnosis and treatment of hypereosinophilic syndromes. Hematology/the Education Program of the American Society of Hematology American Society of Hematology Education Program. 2005:209-14.
66. Ogbogu PU, Rosing DR, Horne MK. Cardiovascular manifestations of hypereosinophilic syndromes. Immunology and allergy clinics of North America. 2007;27(3):457-75.
67. Varma N, Varma S, Marwaha N, Dash S. Hypereosinophilic syndrome: the spectrum of clinical, haematological and morphological features. The Journal of the Association of Physicians of India. 1994;42(3):242-4.
68. Fauci AS, Harley JB, Roberts WC, Ferrans VJ, Gralnick HR, Bjornson BH. NIH conference. The idiopathic hypereosinophilic syndrome. Clinical, pathophysiologic, and therapeutic considerations. Annals of Internal Medicine. 1982;97(1):78-92.
69. Gotlib J. World Health Organization-defined eosinophilic disorders: 2014 update on diagnosis, risk stratification, and management. American Journal of Hematology. 2014;89(3):325-37.
70. Parrillo JE, Fauci AS, Wolff SM. Therapy of the hypereosinophilic syndrome. Annals of Internal Medicine. 1978;89(2):167-72.
71. Rothenberg ME, Klion AD, Roufosse FE, Kahn JE, Weller PF, Simon HU, et al. Treatment of patients with the hypereosinophilic syndrome with mepolizumab. The New England Journal of Medicine. 2008;358(12):1215-28.
72. Rosenwasser LJ, Schwartz LB, Sheikh J, et al. Corticosteroid-sparing effects of mepolizumab, an anti-interleukin-5 monoclonal antibody, in patients with hypereosinophilic syndrome. J Allergy Clin Immunol. 2007;119:S160.
73. Cools J, DeAngelo DJ, Gotlib J, Stover EH, Legare RD, Cortes J, et al. A tyrosine kinase created by fusion of the PDGFRA and FIP1L1 genes as a therapeutic target of imatinib in idiopathic hypereosinophilic syndrome. The New England Journal of Medicine. 2003;348(13):1201-14.

74. Klion AD. How I treat hypereosinophilic syndromes. Blood. 2009;114(18):3736-41.
75. Sefcick A, Sowter D, DasGupta E, Russell NH, Byrne JL. Alemtuzumab therapy for refractory idiopathic hypereosinophilic syndrome. British Journal of Haematology. 2004;124(4):558-9.
76. Pitini V, Teti D, Arrigo C, Righi M. Alemtuzumab therapy for refractory idiopathic hypereosinophilic syndrome with abnormal T cells: a case report. British Journal of Haematology. 2004;127(5):477.
77. Esteva-Lorenzo FJ, Meehan KR, Spitzer TR, Mazumder A. Allogeneic bone marrow transplantation in a patient with hypereosinophilic syndrome. American Journal of Hematology. 1996;51(2):164-5.
78. Sadoun A, Lacotte L, Delwail V, Randriamalala E, Patri S, Babin P, et al. Allogeneic bone marrow transplantation for hypereosinophilic syndrome with advanced myelofibrosis. Bone marrow transplantation. 1997;19(7):741-3.
79. Basara N, Markova J, Schmetzer B, Blau IW, Kiehl MG, Bischoff M, et al. Chronic eosinophilic leukemia: successful treatment with an unrelated bone marrow transplantation. Leukemia and Lymphoma. 1998;32(1-2):189-93.
80. Vazquez L, Caballero D, Canizo CD, Lopez C, Hernandez R, Gonzalez I, et al. Allogeneic peripheral blood cell transplantation for hypereosinophilic syndrome with myelofibrosis. Bone Marrow Transplantation. 2000;25(2):217-8.
81. Ueno NT, Anagnostopoulos A, Rondon G, Champlin RE, Mikhailova N, Pankratova OS, et al. Successful non-myeloablative allogeneic transplantation for treatment of idiopathic hypereosinophilic syndrome. British Journal of Haematology. 2002;119(1):131-4.
82. Cooper MA, Akard LP, Thompson JM, Dugan MJ, Jansen J. Hypereosinophilic syndrome: long-term remission following allogeneic stem cell transplant in spite of transient eosinophilia post-transplant. American Journal of Hematology. 2005;78(1):33-6.
83. Halaburda K, Prejzner W, Szatkowski D, Limon J, Hellmann A. Allogeneic bone marrow transplantation for hypereosinophilic syndrome: long-term follow-up with eradication of FIP1L1-PDGFRA fusion transcript. Bone Marrow Transplantation. 2006;38(4):319-20.
84. Podjasek JC, Butterfield JH. Mortality in hypereosinophilic syndrome: 19 years of experience at Mayo Clinic with a review of the literature. Leukemia Research. 2013;37(4):392-5.
85. Lichtenstein L. Histiocytosis X; integration of eosinophilic granuloma of bone, Letterer-Siwe disease, and Schuller-Christian disease as related manifestations of a single nosologic entity. AMA Archives of Pathology. 1953;56(1):84-102.
86. Renston JP, Goldman ES, Hsu RM, Tomashefski JF. Peripheral blood eosinophilia in association with sarcoidosis. Mayo Clinic Proceedings. 2000;75(6):586-90.
87. Golkar L, Bernhard JD. Mastocytosis. Lancet. 1997;349(9062):1379-85.
88. Miranda RN, Esparza AR, Sambandam S, Medeiros LJ. Systemic mast cell disease presenting with peripheral blood eosinophilia. Human Pathology. 1994;25(7):727-30.
89. Navarro-Roman L, Medeiros LJ, Kingma DW, Zarate-Osorno A, Nguyen V, Samoszuk M, et al. Malignant lymphomas of B-cell lineage with marked tissue eosinophilia. A report of five cases. The American Journal of Surgical Pathology. 1994;18(4):347-56.
90. Borish L, Dishuck J, Cox L, Mascali JJ, Williams J, Rosenwasser LJ. Sezary syndrome with elevated serum IgE and hypereosinophilia: role of dysregulated cytokine production. The Journal of Allergy and Clinical Immunology. 1993;92(1 Pt 1):123-31.
91. Bain BJ. Eosinophilic leukaemias and the idiopathic hypereosinophilic syndrome. British Journal of Haematology. 1996;95(1):2-9.
92. Berkompas RJ. Isolated eosinophilia associated with a squamous cell lung cancer. Journal of the Tennessee Medical Association. 1989;82(5):241-2.
93. Knox AJ, Johnson CE, Page RL. Eosinophilia associated with thoracic malignancy. British Journal of Diseases of the Chest. 1986;80(1):92-5.
94. Lowe D, Fletcher CD. Eosinophilia in squamous cell carcinoma of the oral cavity, external genitalia and anus—clinical correlations. Histopathology. 1984;8(4):627-32.
95. Lowe D, Fletcher CD, Gower RL. Tumour-associated eosinophilia in the bladder. Journal of Clinical Pathology. 1984;37(5):500-2.
96. Lowe D, Jorizzo J, Hutt MS. Tumour-associated eosinophilia: a review. Journal of Clinical Pathology. 1981;34(12):1343-8.
97. Muller GL. Clinical significance of the blood in tuberculosis. Commonwealth Fund. New York; 1943. pp. 95-121.
98. Elsom KA, Ingelfinger FJ. Eosinophilia and pneumonitis in chronic brucellosis: report of 2 cases. Ann Intern Med. 1942;16:995-1002.
99. Lombard CM, Tazelaar HD, Krasne DL. Pulmonary eosinophilia in coccidioidal infections. Chest. 1987;91(5):734-6.
100. Drutz DJ, Catanzaro A. Coccidioidomycosis. Part II. The American review of respiratory disease. 1978;117(4):727-71.
101. Rosenow EC, Limper AH. Drug-induced pulmonary disease. Seminars in respiratory infections. 1995;10(2):86-95.
102. Sovijarvi AR, Lemola M, Stenius B, Idanpaan-Heikkila J. Nitrofurantoin-induced acute, subacute and chronic pulmonary reactions. Scandinavian Journal of Respiratory Diseases. 1977;58(1):41-50.

Infiltrative and Deposition Diseases

Pralay Sarkar, Arunabh Talwar

INTRODUCTION

There are several different diseases characterized by the deposition of abnormal materials, either endogenous or exogenous, in the pulmonary parenchyma or in other areas of the respiratory system. Although rare, they frequently pose problems in the differential diagnosis of common clinical conditions, which present with similar respiratory or other clinical manifestations. Not infrequently, they are responsible for long delays in establishing the diagnoses.

PULMONARY AMYLOIDOSIS

Amyloidosis is a group of disorders characterized by the extracellular tissue deposition of fibrils as beta-pleated sheets and disruption of organ function. These deposits are composed of low molecular weight subunits (most in the molecular weight range of 5–25 kD) of a variety of proteins, which circulate as the constituents of plasma. Current nomenclature of amyloid is based on the precursor proteins.[1] The pattern of organ involvement often depends on the nature of the precursor protein, many of which are associated with specific disease entities[1] **(Table 1)**. Most common types of amyloidosis associated with pulmonary involvement are either amyloid light chain type (AL) or amyloid A (AA) amyloidosis (see below). Amyloidosis has association with a wide range of systemic diseases, most commonly plasma cell dyscrasias, chronic infections or inflammatory conditions **(Table 2)**.

Pulmonary Involvement in Amyloidosis

The first case of amyloidosis confined to the lower respiratory tract was described by Lesser in 1857, based on an autopsy. Pulmonary involvement with amyloidosis can occur in one of the three circumstances **(Table 3)**. The Mayo clinic experience, based on retrospective review of pathological specimens, remains one of the best descriptions of pulmonary involvement with amyloidosis.[2] In their 55 patients recorded over a period of 13 years, 35 patients (66%) had primary systemic amyloidosis (including 3 of 35 patients with multiple myeloma), while 30% patients had localized (primary) pulmonary involvement. In systemic amyloidosis, lung is rarely the predominant organ involved

Table 1 Major types of amyloidosis

Protein class	*Protein name*	*Amyloid type*	*Clinical presentation*	*Pulmonary involvement*
Immunoglobulin gene superfamily	Ig light chain/Ig heavy chain (IgL/IgH)	AL/AH	• Primary systemic amyloidosis • Amyloidosis associated with multiple myeloma and other monoclonal gammopathies	Yes, almost universal in autopsy studies
	Beta-2 microglobulin	Aβ2m	Dialysis amyloidosis	Yes
High-density apolipoproteins	(Apo) serum AA	AA	Amyloid complicating chronic infections or inflammatory diseases; some heredofamilial periodic fever syndromes, such as familial mediterranean fever (FMF)	Less frequent, usually not significant clinically
Transport protein	Transthyretin (TTR; prealbumin)	ATTR	Hereditary neuropathic and/or cardiopathic amyloids; senile systemic amyloidosis	

Abbreviations: AL, amyloid light; AH, amyloid heavy; AA, amyloid A; ATTR, amyloidosis transthyretin.

Table 2 Different diseases and other conditions associated with (pulmonary) amyloidosis

• Blood dyscrasias/hematologic malignancies/lymphoproliferative disorders – Multiple myeloma – Waldenstrom's macroglobulinemia – Non-Hodgkin's lymphoma (NHL) – Mucosa-associated lymphoid tissue (MALT) lymphoma of the lung
• Connective tissue disorders – Rheumatoid arthritis – Systemic lupus erythematosus – Mixed connective tissue disorder – Primary Sjögren's syndrome
• Other conditions – End-stage renal disease on hemodialysis – Asbestos inhalation – Liver transplantation – Bone marrow transplant – Sarcoidosis – Familial mediterranean fever – Dystrophic epidermolysis bullosa

Table 3 Pulmonary amyloidosis

1. *Pulmonary involvement in systemic amyloidosis*: Lung involvement as part of multisystem involvement • *Primary systemic amyloidosis*: Pulmonary involvement is almost universal • *Secondary systemic amyloidosis*: Pulmonary involvement is infrequent and mild
2. *Organ specific involvement of lung without any evidence of systemic amyloidosis*: Primary (localized) pulmonary amyloidosis
3. Organ specific pulmonary amyloidosis in association with other pulmonary disorders • Sarcoidosis • Sjögren's syndrome with multiple pulmonary cysts • *Pulmonary neoplasms*: Anaplastic tumor or carcinoid • Lymphocytic interstitial pneumonia • Pulmonary mucosa-associated lymphoid tissue (MALT) lymphoma

clinically.[3] Pathological involvement of lung, however, has been described as a rule in primary systemic amyloidosis with amyloid deposition noted at autopsy in over 90% of patients.[2,4,5] In secondary systemic amyloidosis, pulmonary involvement is reported to be low, is usually mild and takes a different pattern of deposition with prominent perivascular component; most of these patients have no respiratory symptoms attributable to amyloid deposition and have normal chest radiograph.[4-6] Amyloid deposition limited only to lungs, called primary (localized) pulmonary amyloidosis, is diagnosed on the basis of following criteria:[7] (a) positive immunohistochemical staining for k and λ light chains (AL amyloid) in a respiratory tract biopsy or negative staining

Table 4 Clinicopathological patterns of respiratory system involvement in amyloidosis

• Tracheobronchial amyloidosis • Solitary pulmonary nodule • Nodular amyloidosis • Alveolar septal amyloidosis • Pulmonary vascular amyloidosis • *Pleural amyloidosis*: Pleural effusion and spontaneous hemothorax • Other thoracic or respiratory tract amyloidosis – Laryngeal – Intrathoracic lymphadenopathy – Mediastinal mass – Mediastinal hemorrhage – Pulmonary hypertension – Diaphragmatic paralysis

for serum AA protein, hereditary amyloid of transthyretin-type (TTR); (b) no evidence of plasma cell dyscrasias on bone marrow biopsy; (c) negative urine or serum studies for paraproteins; (d) characteristic distribution and pattern of localized respiratory tract disease on computed tomography (CT) scan; (e) no extrapulmonary involvement on serum amyloid P component (SAP) scan; and (f) negative echocardiogram. Amyloid can involve both the upper and the lower respiratory tracts in a variety of pathological patterns **(Table 4)**.

Pathogenesis

The pathogenesis of localized pulmonary amyloidosis remains obscure. In case of immunoglobulin light-chain (AL) amyloid, deposition is postulated to occur following a localized monoclonal proliferation of lymphoplasmacytic cells in pulmonary parenchyma; however, monoclonal plasma cell proliferation is not found in many such cases. Another theory postulates that the circulating amyloid precursor molecule is deposited in the lung as a result of increased regional vascular permeability, possibly due to local inflammation. Polyclonal plasma cell infiltrates, often found in association with the amyloid deposits in the lung, are considered to reflect residual inflammation or a reactive inflammatory reaction to amyloid deposition. It is also possible that lung being in direct contact with environmental antigens, an abnormality of the local secretory immune system may contribute to amyloid deposition. Low pH and interaction with glycosaminoglycan help in deposition of amyloid.[8]

Clinical Types, Presentation and Diagnosis

Tracheobronchial Amyloidosis

Tracheobronchial amyloidosis is a rare disease. Here amyloid deposition typically occurs in the submucosa of trachea and main bronchi, sometimes extending to the level of segmental bronchi. Tracheobronchial amyloidosis usually occurs as an isolated airway involvement without that of lung parenchyma or other organs. Tracheobronchial involvement may be focal or diffuse, the latter being more common.[9,10] Tracheobronchial amyloidosis has been associated with tracheobronchopathia osteochondroplastica though the causative relationship of these two rare conditions remains debatable.

Clinical presentation: Most cases have been reported in the 5th and 6th decades of life.[9] The presentation is predictable from the site of involvement: cough, dyspnea, recurrent hemoptysis and wheezing are common symptoms. Significant narrowing of airway can happen, leading to consequences like atelectasis and recurrent pneumonia.[11] Rarely, tracheobronchomalacia due to amyloidosis of the trachea has been reported.[12]

Diagnosis: The nonspecific clinical presentation of tracheobronchial amyloidosis can lead to delay in diagnosis. Often the disease is misdiagnosed as (refractory) asthma or chronic bronchitis for a long period of time.[11] Lung function tests may show evidence of large airway obstruction. Chest X-ray (CXR) and CT may show focal or diffuse thickening of the airway wall **(Figs 1A and B)**, nodular and irregular narrowing of airway lumen **(Fig. 1C)** and localized nodule in the airway lumen **(Fig. 1D)**. CXR can also show the consequences of airway obstruction like pneumonia, distal atelectasis or hyperinflation of lung distal to the obstruction.[10,13] CXR sometimes may be normal adding initial difficulty to the diagnosis.[14] Bronchoscopy shows different endoscopic patterns: submucosal plaques, pseudotumor appearance and circumferential wall thickening; these are believed to represent different stages of the same process of amyloid deposition.[15] The deposits on bronchoscopy typically appear yellowish, often shiny and pale, with indistinct outline of cartilaginous rings and intact overlying mucosa **(Fig. 2)**.[14] On macroscopic examination of the affected tissue, the amyloid deposits appear as irregular nodular masses or as diffuse sheets. Microscopically, the nodular masses or diffuse sheets are made of pink, amorphous, acellular material on hematoxylin and eosin (H and E) stain (hyaline deposits) **(Fig. 3)**. Congo red staining shows apple-green birefringence under polarized light. Macrophages, foreign-body giant cells, microscopic calcifications, osseous metaplasia can be seen.[9] Submucosal blood vessels may also show amyloid deposition. Localized tracheobronchial amyloidosis is usually AL type, but AA type amyloid has been found in rare cases.[16]

Nodular Pulmonary Amyloidosis

In this type of pulmonary amyloidosis, nodular deposits of amyloid occur in pulmonary parenchyma, usually bilaterally at multiple sites. Nodular pulmonary amyloidosis is usually not associated with systemic amyloidosis. Presentation as a single nodular lesion/mass (amyloidoma) may also occur.[17]

Diagnosis: Average age of presentation is in the 6th decade of life. Nodular amyloid is commonly asymptomatic, often found incidentally on CXR or at autopsy.[9] Symptoms arise when a large mass produces its mechanical effects: patients present with cough and progressive dyspnea. Significant weight loss has also been reported.[18] CXR and CT of the thorax show single or multiple pulmonary nodular opacities/masses of soft tissue density. These masses have irregular contour and are distributed diffusely, bilaterally and often asymmetrically.[18] Distribution of nodules may show lower lobe and subpleural preponderance. The size of most nodules ranges from 0.4 cm to 5 cm; an average nodule is approximately 3 cm in size and size up to 15 cm has been reported.[9,19] A solitary amyloidoma can grow unusually big with extension into the surrounding tissues **(Fig. 4)**.[20] The nodular deposits may contain areas of calcification, may rarely cavitate.[21,22] Calcification is often subtle, apparent only on CT scan and can be the only clue to the diagnosis. Nodular pulmonary amyloidosis has close radiological resemblance with primary/metastatic lung cancer. Therefore, biopsy is required to reach a diagnosis. Image-guided transthoracic fine needle aspiration (FNA) biopsy can be attempted, but the firm-to-hard consistency of deposits may cause difficulty in obtaining an adequate sample.[23] Bronchoscopic tissue sampling, including transbronchial lung biopsy, can give diagnosis in some cases.[2] Occasional report of accurate diagnosis with CT-guided bronchoscopic sampling can also be found.[24] However, serious adverse consequences have been reported in some cases following transbronchial biopsy, including reports of fatal pulmonary hemorrhage and arterial air embolism.[2,25] Open lung biopsy by thoracotomy or video-assisted thoracoscopy should often be the preferred approach for safe and adequate tissue sampling. In pathological specimens, nodular amyloid deposits appear as irregular masses of eosinophilic amorphous material. Some nodules can have areas of ossification and/or calcification. Small arteries or veins adjacent to or within the lesions may contain amyloid. Clusters of plasma cells and giant cells are seen adjacent to or within the amyloid deposits (more frequently in the nodular parenchymal than in the tracheobronchial variant). A histological picture consistent with interstitial pneumonitis or granulomatous pneumonitis can be found in a small number of cases.[9] Immunohistochemistry usually reveals AL amyloid; amyloid composed predominantly of beta-2-microglobulin has also been described.[23] Differential diagnoses include primary and secondary neoplasms and granulomatous disorders.[26] In cases of solitary nodule/mass, careful sectioning of pathological specimen is necessary to rule out any neoplastic process as amyloid deposition has been described in association with primary lung tumor.[27,28] Amyloid deposits are usually fluorodeoxyglucose positron emission tomography (FDG-PET) negative, a point which may be useful in diagnosis; false positive results are, however, known adding difficulty to the diagnosis.[29]

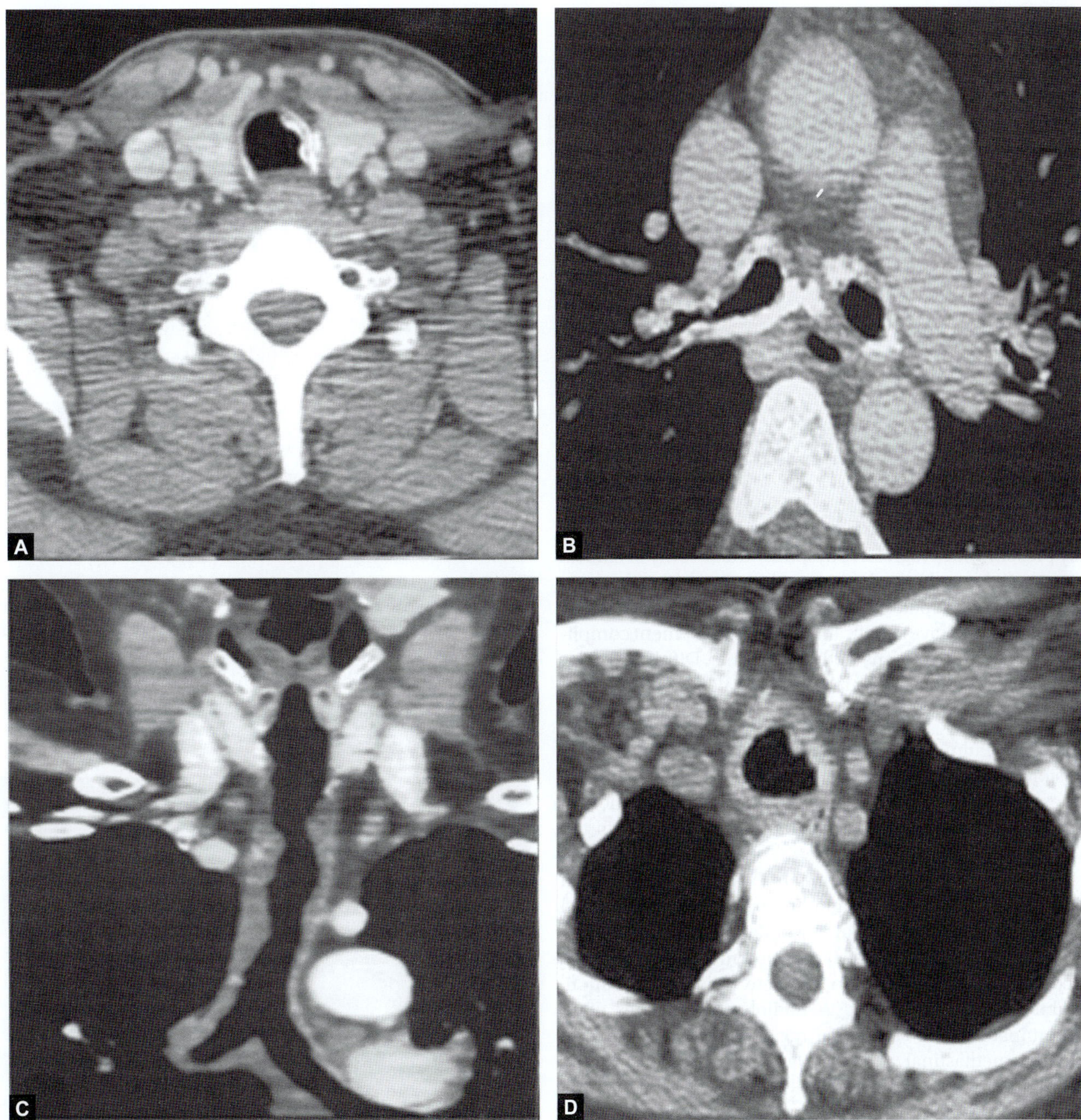

Figs 1A to D Tracheobronchial amyloidosis: (A) Localized thickening of upper trachea; (B) Diffuse thickening of tracheal wall at the level of carina; (C) Sagittal section of trachea showing and irregular narrowing of airway; (D) Localized amyloid nodule in the airway lumen
Courtesy: Dr Rakesh Shah, Consultant Radiologist, North Shore University Hospital, Manhasset, New York, USA (Figs A, B and C)
Dr Subha Ghosh, Consultant Radiologist, Ohio State University, Columbus, Ohio, USA (Fig. D)

Diffuse Alveolar Septal Amyloidosis

In this pathological pattern of pulmonary involvement, the microscopic deposits of amyloid occur diffusely within the alveolar septae and the interstitial tissue. Interstitial/alveolar septal pulmonary amyloidosis is usually seen as a part of the systemic amyloidosis.[2] It is rare for primary/localized pulmonary amyloidosis to show a diffuse interstitial pattern and only a handful of well-documented cases have been reported in the literature.[30]

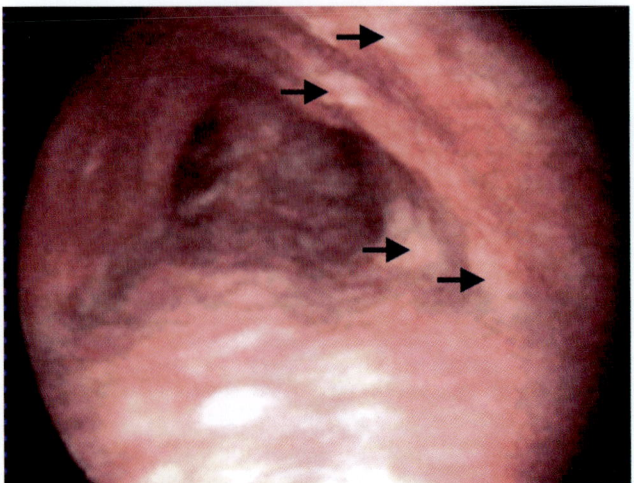

Fig. 2 Bronchoscopic view of tracheobronchial amyloidosis showing multiple yellowish, shiny submucosal deposits (marked with arrow)

Clinical presentation: The patient may be asymptomatic or may present with progressive dyspnea. The severity of clinical symptoms depends on the extent the gas exchange zones, namely alveolar septae and capillaries are involved. Majority of these patients have significant cardiac involvement complicating the picture in many of these patients. Diffuse alveolar hemorrhage (DAH) leading to fatality has been reported with this form of amyloidosis.[31]

Diagnosis: Pulmonary function tests reveal a restrictive physiology with impaired gas exchange that parallels with the extent and pattern of interstitial amyloid deposition. A high-resolution computed tomography (HRCT) scan of the thorax reveals interlobular septal thickening or irregular lines that frequently have a predominant basilar and peripheral distribution.[32] Small (2–4 mm in diameter) well-defined nodules and confluent areas of consolidations can also be seen. Some nodules may show calcifications and some of the areas of consolidation may contain punctate foci of calcification, a subtle clue to the diagnosis. Radiological changes often predominate in the subpleural regions. Associated pleural effusion, mediastinal and hilar lymphadenopathy may be seen. Rarely, CT scan might reveal multiple cysts of variable size with surrounding high-density areas.[21,33-35]

Histopathologically, variable amount of amyloid deposition is found in the pulmonary interstitium: alveolar septa, capillaries, as well as in the wall of bronchioles, arterioles, venules and in lymphatic vessels.[36,37] Interstitial/septal amyloid deposit may be present as diffuse and uniform or as multiple small interstitial nodules.[9] Correlating with radiological findings, thickening of interlobular septa with amyloid deposition can be shown in histological specimens. Extensive deposits are also found beneath the visceral pleura. Areas of calcification and ossification are found within the affected areas.[34]

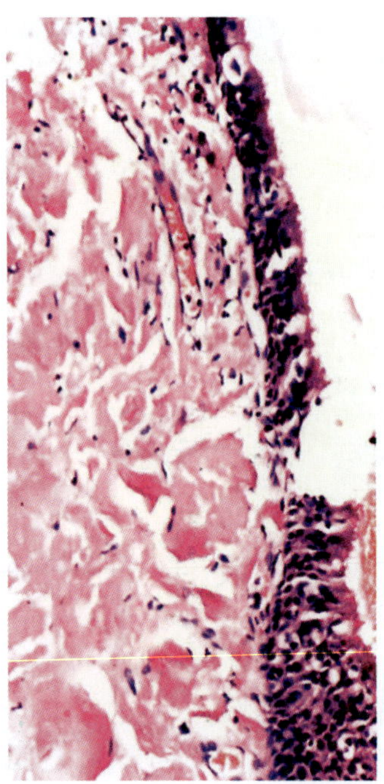

Fig. 3 Light microscopic appearance of a bronchoscopic biopsy specimen in a case of tracheobronchial amyloidosis. Diffuse sheets of pink, amorphous, acellular material are seen [hematoxylin and eosin (H and E) stain, 100x]

Courtesy: Dr Ritesh Aggarwal, Associate Professor, Department of Pulmonary Medicine, Postgraduate Institute of Medical Education and Research, Chandigarh, India

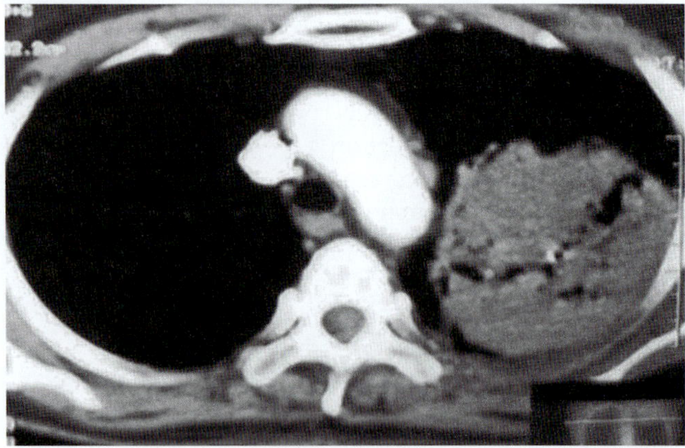

Fig. 4 Large solitary mass of amyloid deposit in the pulmonary parenchyma

Courtesy: Dr Ritesh Aggarwal, Associate Professor, Department of Pulmonary Medicine, Postgraduate Institute of Medical Education and Research, Chandigarh, India

Pleural Disease

Pleural effusion is a rare manifestation of systemic amyloidosis. Significantly large, persistent pleural effusions have been reported in 6% cases in a large series of AL amyloidosis; less significant effusions are seen in approximately 10–15% cases. Pleural effusions are not usually seen in secondary (AA) amyloidosis.[4,5] Cardiac involvement and congestive heart failure are common in AL amyloidosis. Pleural effusions may result from congestive heart failure; the pleural fluid in these cases is expected to be transudative in character. However, one-third of the persistent pleural effusions in primary amyloidosis are exudative, which cannot be explained by cardiac involvement alone.[38] Large persistent effusions are the result of direct involvement of the parietal pleura.[39] Apart from being exudative, cellular characteristics of the effusions do not have any distinctive feature to point to the diagnosis. Pleural infiltration by amyloid can be demonstrated by thoracoscopy and can be proven by pleural biopsy.[40-42] AL amyloidosis patients sometimes develop nephrotic syndrome and hypothyroidism, secondary to infiltration of the kidney and the thyroid gland respectively. Both nephrotic syndrome and hypothyroidism may contribute to pleural effusions in these patients, though their contribution remains debated.[38] Lymphatic infiltration with amyloid can lead to chylous effusion.[43]

Other Manifestations of Respiratory System Amyloidosis

Pulmonary arterial hypertension (PAH) has been known to develop in systemic amyloidosis with or without the presence of parenchymal lung involvement.[44,45] Deposition of amyloid in the pulmonary vasculature is responsible for this uncommon development.[46] PAH has been described in primary systemic AL amyloidosis, as well as in AA amyloidosis related to familial mediterranean fever (FMF). "Diffuse pulmonary hemorrhage" has been described as a first manifestation of pulmonary amyloidosis. Amyloid angiopathy, involving small- and medium-sized pulmonary arteries, may cause "pulmonary arterial dissection", presenting with recurrent hemoptysis.[47] Rupture of an amyloid-involved vessel may cause "pulmonary hematoma".[48] Amyloid deposition in vessel wall may cause fragility and lead to the formation of "arteriovenous fistula".[49]

Involvement of nasopharynx and paranasal sinuses: Leads to chronic infections and contribute to obstructive sleep apnea.

Laryngeal amyloidosis: Laryngeal involvement causes long-standing hoarseness of voice. It may also cause airway obstruction. Amyloidosis localized to the larynx has been rarely reported to cause fatal upper respiratory tract hemorrhage.[50]

Mediastinal lymphadenopathy: Mediastinal as well as unilateral or bilateral hilar lymphadenopathy can be seen in amyloidosis. Lymph node involvement is usually a part of systemic amyloidosis.[21] It is an unusual manifestation in localized pulmonary amyloidosis though hilar or mediastinal lymphadenopathy has been described in conjunction with tracheobronchial amyloidosis. Very rarely, mediastinal or hilar lymphadenopathy in the absence of pulmonary involvement has been reported as the only manifestation of localized amyloidosis.[51] Lymph nodes involved in amyloidosis present homogeneous low attenuation and faint or stippled calcification.

Diaphragmatic paralysis: Diaphragm dysfunction has been reported in systemic amyloidosis as a result of infiltrative myopathy.[52,53] Alternatively, diaphragm paralysis may result from amyloid-induced mononeuritis multiplex.[54]

Treatment

A variety of management strategies, such as observation in selected cases, intermittent bronchoscopic intervention, surgical resection and external beam radiation are used in laryngotracheobronchial amyloidosis.[15] In a given case, the choice of treatment strategy depends on the extent of involvement, the size, location and appearance of the lesions, the functional consequences of amyloid deposition and the availability of expertise in a particular institution. Bronchoscopic procedures include the mechanical debulking/resection with/without dilatation, transmucosal neodymium-doped: yttrium aluminum garnet (Nd:YAG) laser treatment (for pseudotumoral mass or circumferential thickening), carbon dioxide laser ablation (for submucosal lesions) and stent placement (after establishing patency of airway lumen).[15,55,56] Majority of the cases can be managed by bronchoscopic procedures. Open neck surgical approach for the management of laryngotracheal amyloidosis is rarely necessary.[57] External beam radiation has been successfully used in the treatment with functional improvement as well as the regression of lesions.[58] Bronchoscopic debulking and external beam radiation have been used in combination.[59] In patients with secondary systemic amyloidosis, treatment of the underlying inflammatory or chronic condition is recommended. The response to tumor necrosis factor-α blockade has been described in patients with rheumatic diseases who developed systemic AA amyloidosis.[60-62] Sustained improvement in proteinuria and renal function has been consistently reported though no information is available about the efficacy of these agents for the pulmonary involvement. Patients with systemic amyloidosis, who have an underlying hematological condition like multiple myeloma, Waldenström's macroglobulinemia or other monoclonal gammopathies need treatment for the underlying condition. Various treatment options are available for primary systemic amyloidosis (AL amyloidosis) **(Table 5)**. For decades, alkylating agents have been the mainstay of treatment, often in combination with high-dose dexamethasone **(Table 5)**. Intermediate dose chemotherapy regimens, adopted from chemotherapy of multiple myeloma, have also been used with success. As the general prognosis of primary systemic amyloidosis remains poor, hematopoietic stem-cell transplantation (HSCT) has been advocated as one

Table 5 Treatment of primary systemic amyloidosis

• Standard dose alkylating agents with dexamethasone – Monthly courses of oral melphalan (10 mg per square meter of body-surface area on days 1–4) plus high-dose oral dexamethasone (40 mg per day on days 1–4): for up to 18 treatment courses (12 courses if complete remission has been achieved)
• High dose melphalan with autologous hematopoietic stem cell transplantation (HSCT) – Melphalan, 200 mg per square meter given intravenously on day 0, and stem cells were infused on day 2 – Risk adapted HSCT with post-transplant adjuvant chemotherapy with thalidomide/bortezomib and dexamethasone
• Intermediate dose chemotherapy regimens (regimens adapted from multiple myeloma treatment) – Vincristine, adriamycin and dexamethasone (VAD) – Cyclophosphamide, vincristine, adriamycin and methylprednisolone (C-VAMP) – Intermediate-dose melphalan (IDM)
• Newer regimens – Cyclophosphamide, thalidomide, dexamethasone – Lenalidomide, dexamethasone – Melphalan, lenalidomide, dexamethasone – Bortezomib with/without dexamethasone – Bortezomib, melphalan, dexamethasone

approach to achieve survival better than chemotherapy.[63,64] Caution should be exercised while interpreting the available data, particularly while choosing HSCT over chemotherapy. Patients who are considered eligible for HSCT comprise a good-risk population. This group of patients do relatively well with chemotherapy (median survival 42 months), substantially better than the expected median survival of 18 months for all patients with AL amyloidosis on chemotherapy.[65] Using a variety of chemotherapy or cytotoxic regimens, (adopted from multiple myeloma therapy) **(Table 5)**, result comparable to HSCT (survival of ~60% after a median follow-up of >20 months) were found.[66-68] Chemotherapy remains the first-line management for primary systemic amyloidosis. In selected patients or in patients who fail to respond to chemotherapy, HSCT is a choice. Various other newer regimens have been tried in recent years with success, often in relapsed disease[69] **(Table 5)**. Specific clinical or radiological response of pulmonary lesions to any form of treatment has scarcely been reported.[70] The optimal approach for treating isolated pulmonary interstitial amyloidosis is undefined. Colchicine has been tried. Symptomatic improvement with prednisone and azathioprine has been reported.[30] Management of heart failure is the mainstay of treatment in the cases where the effusions result from heart failure. Refractory pleural effusions, secondary to direct amyloid involvement of pleura, pose a difficult therapeutic challenge. These patients should be managed with diuretic therapy and intermittent thoracentesis. When thoracentesis is required weekly or more frequently, measures of a more sustained nature should be adopted to prevent accumulation of pleural fluid. These measures include one of the following: tube thoracostomy and pleurodesis, video-assisted thoracoscopy with talc insufflations for pleurodesis, or placement of a drainage system that can be kept in place for long time and be intermittently drained at home (e.g. PleurX tube). Recently, four patients reported with AL amyloidosis who presented with bilateral pleural effusions, refractory to diuretic therapy were treated with bevacizumab, an antivascular endothelial growth factor (VEGF) antibody.[71] Three of the four patients had improvement in their pleural effusions. Further studies are required to define the role of this novel agent in the management of amyloidosis-related pleural effusion.

Prognosis

The prognosis of pulmonary amyloidosis depends on the type and extent of lung involvement, as well as on the involvement of other major organs. In tracheobronchial amyloidosis, the prognosis is not always benign. Some patients die of respiratory failure or recurrent pneumonia secondary to bronchial obstruction.[9] Severe hemoptysis also remains an important complication. Recurrence of isolated endobronchial masses after resection is rare. Nodular pulmonary amyloidosis typically runs a benign course, generally has an excellent prognosis. Nodules grow slowly over years without any regression. Follow-up of cases over 6–20 years has been reported.[72-74] Occasionally, patients may develop large lesions producing space-occupying effects. Long-term prognosis of patients with primary systemic amyloidosis remains poor. A median survival of 16 months was reported in the Mayo clinic series.[2] Pulmonary involvement in itself contributes to death in a small proportion of cases.[4,36] Many of the patients with primary amyloidosis have other major organ involvement, notably cardiac and renal involvement, causing death. Overall, the presence of pulmonary amyloidosis in patients with primary systemic amyloidosis portends a poor outcome, whether the pulmonary component of the disease is directly related to death or is simply a marker of an otherwise advanced disease.[2] In the rare presentation of alveolo-septal form of localized pulmonary amyloidosis, the prognosis is generally poor with death occurring from progressive respiratory failure within 2 years.

LYSOSOMAL STORAGE DISORDERS

Lysosomal storage disorders (LSDs) are a diverse group of hereditary metabolic disorders caused by defects in lysosomal function. Most commonly, these disorders result from mutations in genes that encode catabolic enzymes (e.g. lysosomal hydrolases) involved in the degradation of macromolecules. Failure to degrade macromolecules causes accumulation of the same in the cells leading to cellular dysfunction and progressive clinical manifestations. More

Table 6 Classification of lysosomal storage disorders (by affected lysosomal function)

Nature of defective lysosomal function	*Prototype disorder*
Defective metabolism of glycosaminoglycans	Mucopolysaccharidoses (MPS) I–IX
Defective degradation of glycan portion of glycoproteins	Aspartylglucosaminuria, fucosidosis, mannosidosis, Schindler disease, sialidosis type I
Defective degradation of sphingolipid components	Fabry disease, Farber disease, Gaucher disease (types I–III), GM1-gangliosidosis, GM2-gangliosidoses (Tay-Sachs disease, Sandhoff disease, GM2 activator disease), Krabbe disease, metachromatic leukodystrophy, Niemann-Pick disease (type A or B).
Defective degradation of glycogen	Pompe disease
Defective degradation of polypeptides	Pycnodysostosis
Defective degradation or transport of cholesterol, cholesterol esters or other complex lipids	Ceroid lipofuscinosis, cholesterol ester storage disease, Niemann-Pick disease type C, Wolman disease
Multiple deficiencies of lysosomal enzymes multiple sulfatase	Galactosialidosis
Transport and trafficking defects	Cystinosis, mucolipidosis IV, sialic acid storage disorder, chylomicron retention disease, Hermansky-Pudlak syndrome (several forms), Chediak-Higashi syndrome
Unknown defects	Geleophysic dysplasia, Marinesco–Sjögren syndrome

than 45 diseases have been described till date, most being inherited in an autosomal recessive manner **(Table 6)**.[75] The clinical expression of LSDs is variable. The age of onset, the severity of symptoms and the pattern of organ involvement can vary markedly within a single disorder type or subtype. Clinical manifestations differ according to the residual enzyme function, genetic and environmental factors. Many of these disorders, e.g. Gaucher, Tay-Sachs, Pompe, metachromatic leukodystrophy, and GM1 gangliosidosis have infantile, juvenile and adult forms. Many LSDs have upper and/or lower respiratory tract involvement. A detailed description of all the entities is beyond the scope of this chapter. Respiratory involvement can occur in various LSDs **(Table 7)**, some of which have also been reported in adult patients.

Anderson-Fabry Disease

Fabry disease is an X-linked recessive disease as a result of the deficiency of the lysosomal enzyme alpha-galactosidase A (α-gal A). It has no ethnic predilection and occurs in about 1:117,000 live births. Anderson-Fabry disease (AFD) leads to progressive accumulation of glycosphingolipids, predominantly globotriaosylceramide (GL-3), in many body tissues over a period of years or decades. Clinical manifestations include renal failure in about 30% of patients and cerebrovascular accidents in about 25% of patients. A 15-year follow-up of patients from AFD clinical and genetic register (UK) reported the median age of 21.9 years at diagnosis and median cumulative survival of 50 years.[76] Obligate carrier females have also been reported to have clinical manifestations with a high frequency.[77]

Pulmonary Manifestations

The extent of pulmonary involvement and the significance of the same in AFD are still debated. In one report, investigators found mild reduction in forced expiratory volume (FEV_1) and forced vital capacity (FVC) with normal diffusing capacity of lung for carbon monoxide (DLCO) in a cohort of 13 patients.[78] In other reports, respiratory symptoms, consistent with airway involvement, are common in AFD patients.[79] In a cohort of 25 consecutive male patients with AFD, 36% complained of dyspnea and 24% had cough and/or wheezing.[80] Hemoptysis has also been reported. Interstitial involvement can also occur in AFD.[81] In line with symptoms of airway disease, chronic airflow obstruction is commonly reported on spirometry in AFD patients and is said to be more common in those who smoke.[80,82] An accelerated decline in FEV_1 is also a known feature.[83] Other investigators have reported features consistent with small airway disease, in more than half of both men and women with AFD.[79] A reduced diffusion capacity (DLCO) is also a common finding. The disease manifestations can be explained by the deposition of GL-3 within various compartments of the lower respiratory tract. The airflow obstruction is thought to be due to fixed airway narrowing secondary to deposition of GL-3 in airway epithelial cells as has been demonstrated by presence of inclusion bodies in bronchoscopic biopsy specimens.[82] Pathologic evidence for pulmonary parenchymal and vascular involvement has also been reported; hemoptysis may result from such direct vascular involvement or from angiectatic lesions in bronchi.

Table 7 Respiratory manifestations of lysosomal storage disorders

Disease	*Upper respiratory tract involvement*	*Lower respiratory tract involvement*
(MPS I) disease* (Hurler, Hurler-Scheie, Scheie syndromes)	• Chronic rhinitis and rhinorrhea • Enlarged tongue, tonsils, adenoids • Obstructive sleep apnea	• Narrowing of trachea • Thickened vocal cords • Reduced lung volumes • Recurrent respiratory infections • Respiratory failure common cause of death
(MPS II) disease* (Hunter syndrome)	• Recurrent ear infections • Upper airway obstruction • Progressive hearing loss	Pulmonary hypertension
(MPS III) disease* (Sanfilippo syndrome)	Airway obstruction common cause of death	
(MPS IV) disease* (Morquio syndrome)	Upper airway obstruction	Restricted chest wall movement leads to restrictive ventilator defect
(MPS VI) disease* (Maroteaux-Lamy syndrome)	Enlarged tongue	
(MPS VII) disease* (Sly syndrome)		• Chronic inflammatory lung disease • Recurrent respiratory infections
Aspartylglycosaminuria*		• Kyphoscoliosis • Recurrent respiratory infections
Fucosidosis type I	Macroglossia	Recurrent lung infections
Mannosidosis*		Recurrent respiratory infections
Pompe disease*	• Macroglossia • Sleep apnea	Recurrent lung infections
Acid sphingomyelinase deficiency (Niemann-Pick disease types A and B*)		Alveolar proteinosis
Fabry disease*		Chronic airflow obstruction
Farber disease	• Vocal cord infiltration • Hoarseness of voice	Recurrent respiratory infections
Gaucher disease—type I* (non-neuronopathic)		• Pulmonary infiltration • Kyphoscoliosis • Pulmonary hypertension • Restrictive lung disease • Hypoxia secondary to liver disease
Gaucher disease—type II (acute infantile neuronopathic)	• Laryngospasm • Apneic episodes	
Gaucher disease—type III (chronic neuronopathic)*		• Pulmonary infiltration • Kyphoscoliosis • Pulmonary hypertension • Restrictive lung disease
GM1 gangliosidosis—type I (infantile form)		• Dorsolumbar kyphoscoliosis • Recurrent pneumonia
GM1 gangliosidosis—type II (infantile form)		Recurrent pneumonia
Sandhoff disease—type I Mucolipidosis II (I-cell disease)	• Loss of swallowing • Recurrent and persistent upper respiratory tract infections	Recurrent aspiration and pneumonia

Abbreviations: MPS, mucopolysaccharidoses; I-cell, inclusion-cell.
*Survival into adulthood known
Note: Disease entities marked in bold are discussed in detail in the text.

Diagnosis

Chest X-ray can be normal in many patients. In keeping with the occurrence of airway disease, some of the patients have CXR changes suggestive of emphysema with or without bulla.[82] Pneumothorax can also occur. HRCT findings of lung involvement in AFD have been infrequently reported. In a recent report, HRCT demonstrated bilateral mosaic attenuation pattern. Regions of both abnormally lucent and dense lung parenchyma were present, reflecting a combination of ground-glass opacity and air trapping.[84] In a patient known to have AFD, characteristic manifestations point to pulmonary involvement and a tissue diagnosis may not be warranted. Where needed, diagnosis can be confirmed by demonstrating typical lamellar inclusion bodies in bronchial biopsy or brushings.[80,82] Cells present in induced sputum may also show inclusion bodies clinching the diagnosis.[85] Whether similar inclusion bodies are present in AFD patients without clinical lung involvement is not known. In a patient with the evidence of interstitial lung disease (ILD), lung biopsy may be indicated to rule out other diagnoses.

Management

Enzyme replacement therapy (ERT) for AFD has been available since 2003. Agalsidase-β (Fabrazyme®, Genzyme Corporation) and agalsidase-α (Replagal®, Shire) are approved in the United States of America, Europe and some other countries for treatment of AFD. ERT has been shown to improve symptoms, as well as renal and cardiac function.[86,87] ERT with agalsidase-α 0.2 mg/kg every other week (EOW) or agalsidase-β 1.0 mg/kg EOW is the standard of treatment for this disease. Controlled data about the effect of ERT on progression of pulmonary function abnormalities are either scant or absent. Isolated case reports have shown significant improvement or stabilization in radiological abnormalities and spirometry on ERT.[81,88] Renal involvement and neuropathy usually dominate the clinical picture in AFD; it can be anticipated that pulmonary involvement alone will rarely be the sole indication for ERT.

Gaucher Disease

Gaucher disease is an autosomal recessive disorder as a result of the deficiency of the lysosomal enzyme glucocerebrosidase. It is the most prevalent LSD. Gaucher disease leads to the accumulation of the lipid glucocerebroside within the lysosomes of the monocyte-macrophage system. Lipid engorged cells (Gaucher cells) accumulate and cause organ dysfunction. Age of the onset of symptoms and their severity is variable. At an incidence of 1 in 40-60,000 live births, type I is the most common type. Type 1 is pan-ethnic, but has higher frequency among Ashkenazi Jews. Type 1 Gaucher disease patients have normal life-expectancy and may present for the first time in adult life. Type III presents in late childhood/early adolescence and has more severe and rapidly progressive visceral disease. Type II disease rarely survives beyond the age of 2 years.

Pulmonary Manifestations

Pulmonary involvement has been reported in both type I and type III Gaucher disease, is more rare in type I and more severe in type III.[89] The frequency of symptomatic pulmonary involvement varies in literature from uncommon to common presentation.[90,91] Clinical picture is characterized by gradual onset and progression of dyspnea that in some cases culminates to respiratory failure and death. (Lung involvement is the second most common cause of death in type III Gaucher disease). Pulmonary involvement occurs due to infiltration by the Gaucher cells giving a pattern of ILD. PAH has been reported in a significant proportion of adult patients and may be particularly severe, life-threatening in those who have had splenectomy for the management of the disease.[92] PAH in Gaucher disease can result from chronic hypoxemia secondary to interstitial disease, secondary to liver disease or due to long bone infarction and fracture with pulmonary emboli. Severe PAH can also occur in these patients primarily due to pulmonary capillary blockage by Gaucher cells, in absence of significant parenchymal involvement.[93] Other intrathoracic manifestations of Gaucher disease include: enlarged hilar and mediastinal lymph nodes that can sometimes lead to bronchial obstruction; increased incidence of pulmonary infections and hypoxemia due to intrapulmonary arterial-venous shunts in patients with severe hepatic disease. Large hepatosplenomegaly can cause the elevation of diaphragm and contribute to dyspnea.

Diagnosis

Clinical examination may show clubbing as a result of hepatopulmonary syndrome. Additional clue may be an expansion of the proximal digit due to deposition of lipid laden cells **(Fig. 5)**. The chest radiograph may be abnormal with or without symptoms and show bilateral diffuse reticulonodular or miliary opacities. HRCT shows bilateral irregular interlobular, as well as intralobular septal thickening. The interstitial changes are more common in lower lung zones. Irregular costal margin and fissures indicate subpleural interstitial thickening. Additional ground-glass opacities reflect interstitial and alveolar space disease.[94,95] Other reported HRCT findings include consolidation, alveolar opacities and bronchial wall thickening.[96] Additional findings also may include prominent pulmonary arteries as a result of the PAH. The diagnosis of PAH should be actively looked for in these patients with echocardiographic screening. Osteopenia, cortical thinning and the widening of medullary spaces of clavicles and ribs can also be evident on the CXR. Diagnosis is established by showing deficient glucocerebrosidase

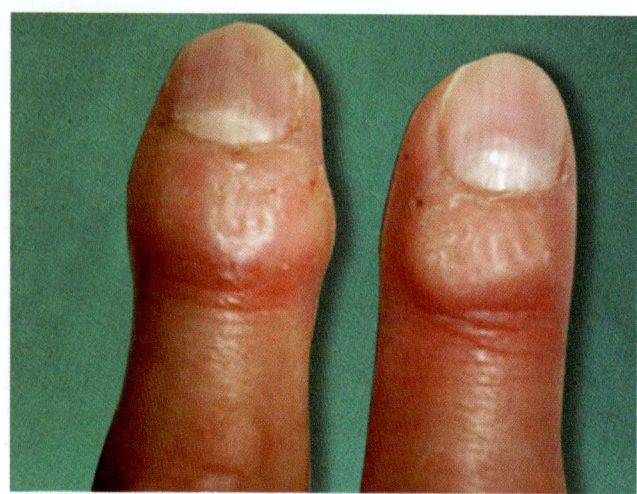

Fig. 5 Expansion of the proximal digit due to deposition of lipid laden cells

activity in peripheral blood leukocytes. In patients with respiratory involvement, bronchoalveolar lavage (BAL) reveals Gaucher cells;[97] these cells resemble macrophages with eccentric, small, oval nuclei and abundant cytoplasm with the characteristic "crumpled tissue paper" appearance. Gaucher cells stain strongly positive with periodic acid-Schiff (PAS) stain. Electron microscopy reveals lysosomes containing the characteristic twisted tubular structures. Lung biopsy specimens also reveal similar cells. Lung biopsy may not be needed in known patients of Gaucher disease with typical respiratory manifestations. Pathologic examination of the lungs reveals massive infiltration of alveolar septal walls, interstitial spaces in a lymphatic distribution, perivascular septal regions by Gaucher cells. Clumps of these cells also fill alveolar spaces and obliterate functional air exchanging tissue. In some cases, interstitial fibrosis may result. Alveolar hemorrhage and multiple pulmonary emboli are also seen in some cases.[98] In patients with PAH, apart from the characteristic arterial/arteriolar changes associated with PAH, the histological sections of lung disclose widespread plugging of the lumina of precapillary arterioles and alveolar capillaries by Gaucher cells.[93,99]

Management

Gaucher disease is the first LSD for which macrophage targeted ERT was introduced in clinical practice (in 1991): the placental-derived macrophage-targeted glucocerebrosidase, alglucerase. (Ceredase®, Genzyme Corporation, Cambridge, Massachusetts). Currently, three analogs of glucocerebrosidase developed by recombinant DNA technology are in use: (1) imiglucerase (Cerezyme®, Genzyme Corporation), (2) velaglucerase alfa (VPRIV®, Shire Human Genetics Therapies Inc) and (3) taliglucerase alfa (ELELYSO®, Pfizer Inc, or, outside the United States, Protalix BioTherapeutics). With imiglucerase, majority of the patients initiate therapy with doses ranging from 30 units/kg to 60 units/kg body weight given every fortnight. Taliglucerase alfa is a plant derived product with possibility of being cheaper with large scale production. Dose ranges from 11 units/kg to 73 units/kg once every 2 weeks as intravenous infusion.[100] ERT is started in early childhood and has been found to be safe and effective in reducing organomegaly, skeletal complications and in improving hematological parameters.[101-103] Improvement in clinical signs of pulmonary disease, increased sense of well-being, stabilization of lung function, stabilization or improvement in chest radiological changes and improvement in lung pathology have been reported on ERT.[91,104] Lungs may be slow to respond to ERT in some patients and in some cases, pulmonary changes may be irreversible. ERT has been reported to improve outcome in hepatopulmonary syndrome and pulmonary arterial hypertension in Gaucher disease.[105] In recent years, substrate reduction therapy (SRT) has come in practice in type I Gaucher disease; these medications (e.g. miglustat, a small iminosugar), given orally, act to reduce substrate load either by inhibiting its synthesis or enhancing the residual activity of the endogenous mutant enzyme. The effect of SRT on lung disease is unknown.[106]

Niemann-Pick Disease

Niemann-Pick disease (type A and B) is due to the deficiency of the enzyme acid sphingomyelinase (ASM). When ASM is deficient, sphingomyelin and cholesterol accumulate in lysosomes. Clinical manifestations are due to fat deposition in one or more organs. ASM deficiency can present along a continuum of severity. Severe ASM deficiency is associated with the type A phenotype (neuronopathic form presenting in infancy, death before 5 years of age). Non-neuronopathic ASM deficiency can present at any age and historically has been classified as Niemann-Pick disease type B phenotype. Niemann-Pick type C is a genetically distinct disorder resulting from defective intracellular trafficking of cholesterol and secondary accumulation of glycosphingolipids. Niemann-Pick disease is pan-ethnic though type A has higher frequency among Ashkenazi Jews; the incidence is 1 in 248,000 live births.

Pulmonary Manifestations

Pulmonary involvement has been reported in all types of Niemann-Pick disease.[107-109] Pulmonary symptoms result from alveolar lipoproteinosis. Pulmonary disease has been best described in type B disease. Respiratory manifestations may present at a variable age and rarely may be the initial presentation of this disease.[110,111] In the largest reported cohort of patients with type B disease, (59 patients, >6 years of age; 50% >18 years of age), shortness of breath and respiratory infections were common symptoms.[107] Various bleeding manifestations are common in this disease and hemoptysis and hemothorax have been reported. Cyanosis, clubbing, rales and wheezing may be present on physical examination. Pulmonary function tests are abnormal in vast majority of patients with type B disease, including those who have no symptoms.

Diagnosis

Chest X-ray shows reticulonodular opacities with the areas of ground glass haziness, often out of proportion to clinical manifestations.[110] HRCT shows variable combination of septal thickening and ground glass, diffuse and homogeneous.[108,111,112] The radiological evidence of ILD has been reported to be present in nearly all patients with type B Niemann-Pick disease.[113] Diagnosis of Niemann-Pick disease is based on the deficiency of ASM activity in peripheral leukocytes or in cultured skin fibroblasts/lymphocytes in the presence of characteristic clinical features. BAL shows numerous foamy macrophages (Niemann-Pick cells), helps to establish diagnosis and avoid lung biopsy in many patients.[108] On lung biopsy, finely vacuolated foamy macrophages are seen to fill the alveolar space along with the thickening of alveolar septa. Foamy macrophages also fill the lymphatic space around peripheral bronchioles, pulmonary artery branches and the interstitial tissues in subpleural area and interlobular septa. Pneumocytes and clara cells remain unaffected.[108] Foamy changes have also been seen in ciliated epithelial cells. Inflammation and fibrosis are minimal and pulmonary architecture is usually preserved. In short, the histological picture can be described as diffuse endogenous lipoid pneumonia or alveolar proteinosis.[111]

Management

No specific therapy is available for ASM deficiency. Both ERT and gene therapy have shown promising results in the mouse model. Slow and inexorable progress is the natural history of respiratory disease. Treatment with whole lung lavage has been described with clinical improvement in isolated case reports.[111,114]

Hermansky-Pudlak Syndrome

Hermansky-Pudlak syndrome (HPS) is an autosomal recessive disorder characterized by the triad of oculocutaneous albinism, bleeding diathesis (secondary to defect in platelet function) and (in some cases) lysosomal accumulation of ceroid lipofuscin. Eight human subtypes have been described, each one resulting from mutation in one of eight different human genes. HPS has been described in many different ethnic groups; HPS1 is the most frequently described subtype; it is particularly common in individuals from North West Puerto Rico and accounts for approximately 50% of non-Puerto Rican cases. Mutations in both HPS1 and HPS4 genes have been described in Indian patients.[115,116]

Pathogenesis

The function of HPS genes is thought to involve intracellular vesicle formation and trafficking. The mutations of HPS genes cause defective formation, trafficking or function of intracellular lysosome-related organelles, e.g. melanosomes, platelet dense granules and lamellar bodies in alveolar type II pneumocytes.[117] A suggested mechanism for lung disease is that intracellular disruption of type II pneumocytes by ceroid deposition triggers a cascade of inflammation, cytokine production and fibroblast proliferation, leading to fibrosis. Interaction with external/environmental noxious stimuli has also been postulated to contribute to the development of fibrosis.

Pulmonary Manifestations

Hermansky-Pudlak syndrome causes ILD. Pulmonary involvement has been described in HPS1 and HPS4.[115,118] Studies exploring pulmonary involvement in other subtypes of HPS are lacking. Lung fibrosis typically develops in the 2nd or 3rd decade of life in HPS1. In a series of 38 patients with HPS1, 61% had the onset of pulmonary symptoms at the mean age of 35 years.[119] However, a wide individual variability in clinical presentation and pulmonary function is known. Clinical presentation is akin to usual interstitial pneumonia (UIP): exertional dyspnea and dry cough are the usual presenting symptoms; physical examination is conspicuous for clubbing and velcro crepitations.[120] Pulmonary function tests reveal restrictive physiology with reduced DLCO. CXR shows bilateral reticulonodular opacities. HRCT scan shows septal thickening, ground glass pattern and mild reticulation in early cases; in the more advanced stages of disease, moderate to severe reticulation, traction bronchiectasis, subpleural cysts, and peribronchovascular thickening are seen. The changes have fairly even distribution within the lung zones with peripheral predominance.[121]

Diagnosis

This diagnosis can be suspected when a young patient presents with pulmonary fibrosis and shows typical ocular features, albinism and platelet dysfunction. Absence of platelet dense bodies on electron microscopy has been described as a rapid and reliable method of diagnosing HPS.[122] The diagnosis can also be established by the genotyping of DNA samples or the demonstration of ceroid accumulation in pathological specimens. Pathological examination of the lungs shows a picture of pulmonary fibrosis, architectural distortion and diffuse lymphocytic infiltration. Pathological pattern may resemble UIP or nonspecific interstitial pneumonitis (NSIP).[123] In addition, a distinctive feature is the presence of large vacuolated histiocytes and pneumocytes containing PAS positive fine and coarse brown pigment within areas of interstitial fibrosis.[124] Numerous giant lamellar bodies can be seen in the macrophages and type II pneumocytes by ultrastructural examination. The fibrosis is also unevenly distributed without any subpleural or peribronchial predilection.

Management

Antifibrotic agent, pirfenidone, has been tried in pulmonary fibrosis of HPS. In an earlier study pirfenidone appeared to slow progression of the disease when started at a stage when good residual function is still left.[125] However, a more recent double blind placebo controlled trial did not show any therapeutic benefit in patients with mild to moderate disease.[126] As it is true in many other chronic lung diseases, measures like the avoidance of smoking and environmental tobacco smoke, prompt treatment of respiratory infections, and administration of influenza and pneumococcal vaccines are recommended to preserve residual lung function.[119] In HPS patients with end-stage lung fibrosis, lung transplantation has been used successfully.[127] Pulmonary fibrosis in HPS is usually fatal in 4th or 5th decade and accounts for death in approximately 50% of HPS patients.

Lipoid Pneumonia

Lipoid pneumonia is a pattern of pathological involvement of lungs characterized by prominent deposition/filling of alveolar spaces with lipoid material. It can be called exogenous when the source of the aspirated lipoid material is from external sources and endogenous when the lipid deposition occurs without an exogenous source. Also called "cholesterol pneumonia", endogenous lipoid pneumonia typically occurs from accumulation of lipid-filled macrophages, surfactant and eosinophilic proteinaceous material derived from degenerating cells, in the alveoli distal to the bronchial obstruction. Diffuse intra-alveolar deposition of lipoprotein material, either as an idiopathic process or in the association of systemic diseases, e.g. chronic myeloid leukemia, is better termed pulmonary alveolar proteinosis (PAP). In this section, we will limit our discussion to exogenous lipoid pneumonia.

Pathogenesis

Exogenous lipoid pneumonia is an uncommon condition that occurs as a result of aspiration or inhalation of lipids: mineral oils (hydrocarbons obtained from petroleum), vegetable-based oils or animal fats. Mineral oils and vegetable-based oils cause milder inflammatory reactions with local encapsulation and fibrosis; animal fats, on the other hand, are hydrolyzed by lung lipases and the resultant free fatty acids trigger a severe inflammatory reaction, both in the alveolar space and the interlobular septa. Progression to fibrosis and end-stage lung disease may occur.

Risk Factors

Exogenous lipoid pneumonia has been reported in two familiar settings: (1) ingestion of paraffin for chronic constipation, and (2) the use of oily nasal preparations for rhinopharyngeal obstruction (often as a part of folk remedies).[128] In both scenarios, it involves aspiration of mineral oil that cannot be cleared by the lungs. Patients with the high risk of aspiration, due to anatomic or functional alterations of swallowing, such as patients with achalasia, gastroesophageal reflux, scleroderma, Zenker's diverticulum, and neurological and psychiatric disorders, etc. are at the increased risk of exogenous lipoid pneumonia.[129] Accidental aspiration of isoparaffin and the development of exogenous lipoid pneumonia have also been reported as a peril of fire eating as a recreational activity.[130,131] Exogenous lipoid pneumonia, usually in the chronic form, has been described in a variety of industrial occupations involving the lubrication and cleaning of machinery and the spraying of pesticides or paints. It has been described as a result of "diesel siphoning", a common practice in many developing countries.[132] It has also been reported as a result of embolization following rectal or subcutaneous administration of mineral oils. Rarely, it has been reported as a consequence of substance abuse, e.g. the inhalation of crack cocaine mixed with petroleum jelly or smoking of weed oil.[133,134]

Clinical Presentation

The clinical presentation depends on the volume and acuity of the aspiration episode(s). Acute exogenous lipoid pneumonia results as a consequence of aspiration of large amount of oil/hydrocarbons, e.g. accidental poisoning in children. Here the presentation is with acute respiratory symptoms: cough, respiratory distress and low-grade fever. Repeated aspirations of small amounts of lipids result in the chronic form of exogenous lipoid pneumonia. Here the onset of symptoms is insidious with chronic cough and/or dyspnea; fever, weight loss, chest pain and hemoptysis are less common at presentation.[128,135] Often the presentation is that of nonresolving pneumonia. Sometimes, the patient may present with chronic fibrosis. Auscultation of lungs may be normal or may reveal crepitations or wheezes. Lung function can be normal or may show a restrictive pattern, with reduced DLCO.

Imaging Features

Different radiological patterns can be seen in the cases of lipoid pneumonia. In acute cases, radiological changes develop within the first few hours and usually within 24 hours. CXR and CT scan show: (a) focal or multifocal consolidation with air bronchogram; (b) areas of ground glass haziness; (c) CT lesions typically with negative attenuation values (HU < 0); (d) pneumatoceles (as a late complication);

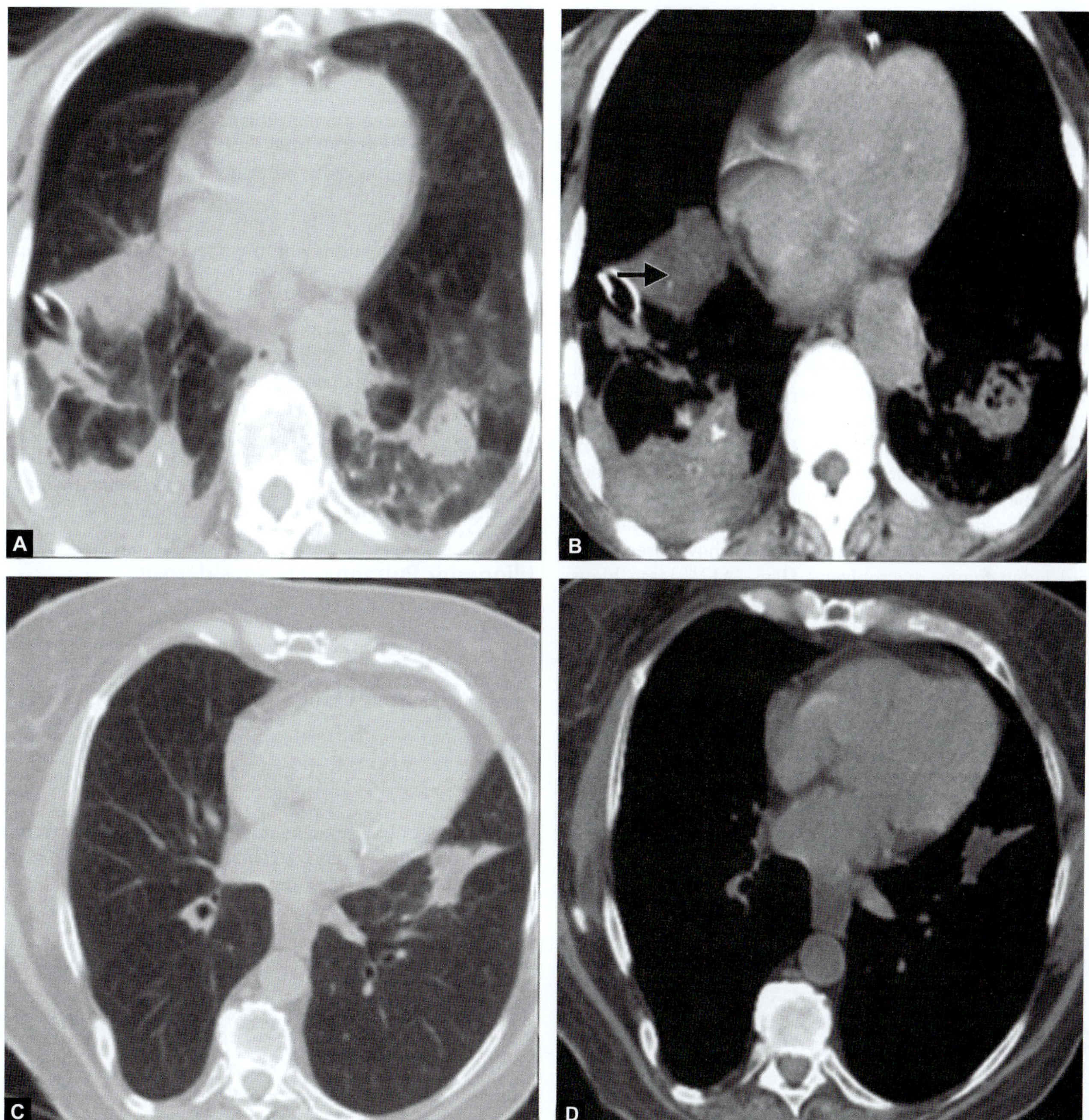

Figs 6A to D CT scan appearance of lipoid pneumonia: (A) Lung window showing multiple bilateral areas of alveolar consolidation/nodule. (*Note*: right pneumothorax following CT-guided lung biopsy); (B) Mediastinal window showing an area of low attenuation within the consolidation (arrow); (C) Small area of consolidation in left upper lobe; (D) Mediastinal window from the same case showing an area of low attenuation
Courtesy: Dr Linda Haramati, Professor of Radiology, Albert Einstein College of Medicine, Bronx, New York, USA (Figs A and B).
Dr Rakesh Shah, Consultant Radiologist, North Shore University Hospital, Manhasset, New York, USA (Figs C and D).

(e) pneumomediastinum, pneumothorax and pleural effusions (rarely). The changes predominate in lower and middle lobes and are segmental or lobar in distribution. The radiologic manifestations of acute exogenous lipoid pneumonia improve or resolve over a variable period of time. Chronic lipoid pneumonia may show: (a) multiple areas of low-attenuation consolidation **(Figs 6A to D)**; (b) areas of ground glass with septal thickening giving rise to a "crazy pavement" pattern; (c) single or multiple nodules or masses resembling primary or metastatic lung cancer; (d) multilobar centrilobular nodularity, tree-in-bud; (e) predominant peri-bronchovascular and lower lobe distribution; (f) architectural distortion and fibrosis in late cases.[129,136-139] False positive result with 18F fluorodeoxy-D-glucose (FDG) positron emission tomography (PET) scan has been reported and may raise the suspicion of lung cancer.[139] The radiological manifestations of chronic lipoid pneumonia remain stable or slowly improve over time if exposure can be halted.

Diagnosis

Making a diagnosis of lipoid pneumonia requires a high degree of clinical suspicion and meticulous history taking. Diagnosis is difficult as the aspiration episodes are often unrecognized and clinical and radiological features mimic many other pulmonary diseases. On CT scan, the demonstration of fat-density areas within the lesions is considered diagnostic of lipoid pneumonia. Diagnosis can be confirmed by BAL. Fat globules are found in the bronchoalveolar fluid; cytological examination of the BAL fluid shows presence of lipid laden foamy macrophages **(Fig. 7A)**.[140] Lung biopsy specimens show alveoli filled with macrophages containing lipid vacuoles **(Fig. 7B)**. Advanced lesions show larger lipid vacuoles surrounded by inflammatory infiltrates. Formation of giant cells and fibrosis are also seen.[141]

Management

Prompt identification and prevention of further aspiration prevent the progression of the disease, and in some cases allow resolution.[128,142] Anecdotal case reports of improvement with steroids are there; the beneficial effects in these cases may be attributed to the effect of steroids on the inflammatory process in lipoid pneumonia.[143,144] Similar results, however, have not been supported in data from large series.[128] Bronchoscopy with therapeutic BAL for the clearance of mineral oil from the lung parenchyma has been reported as the treatment for this condition. This strategy can lead to improvement in lung function, can prevent fibrosis and reduce the morbidity from lipoid pneumonia. Use of a fat emulsifier (sorbitan mono-oleate) during the lung lavage has also been reported.[145-147.] BAL may not be effective in all cases, particularly in the chronic ones; each individual case should be carefully reviewed to decide whether therapeutic lavage will be effective.[128] The prognosis is generally good in most of the cases. However, complications like fibrosis, lung abscess formation, pleural effusion, bronchopulmonary fistula and bacterial/mycobacterial/fungal superinfection may occur. Infections with mycobacterial species like *Mycobacterium chelonae* and *Mycobacterium fortuitum* and fungal pathogens like *Aspergillus fumigatus*, *Nocardia* species have been reported.[148,149] These infections should be looked for when appropriate and treated.

Idiopathic Pulmonary Hemosiderosis

Idiopathic pulmonary hemosiderosis (IPH) is an uncommon disease of unknown etiology characterized by the repetitive episodes of DAH. The causes of DAH are diverse and other causes need to be excluded before a diagnosis of IPH can be reached.

Pathogenesis

The etiology of IPH remains unknown. Several theories have been proposed.[150] Familial clustering has been reported, which may suggest the inheritance of a rare genetic defect,

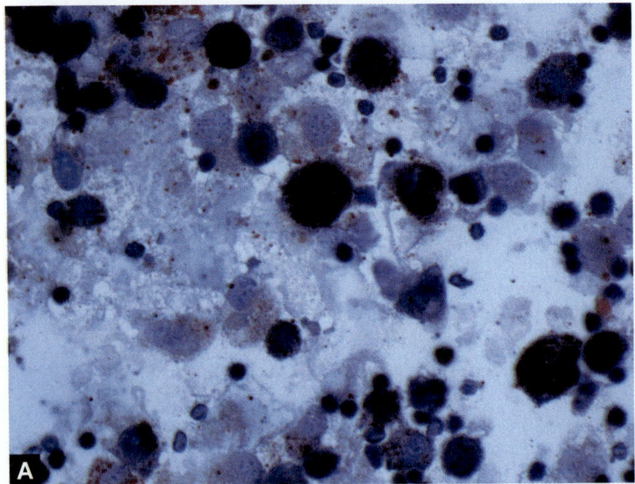

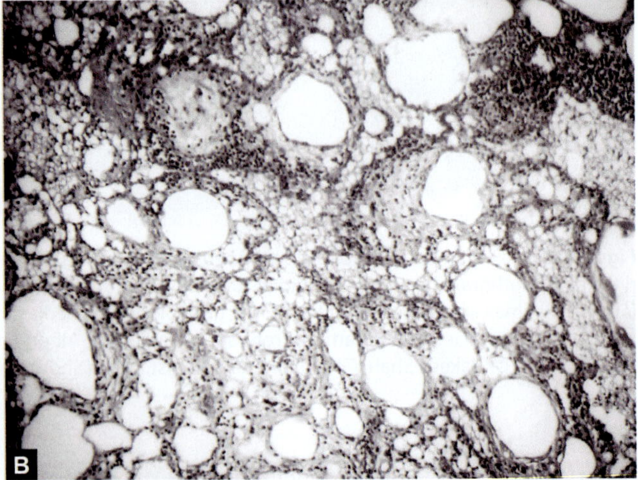

Figures 7A and B (A) Bronchoalveolar lavage in a patient with aspiration, showing multiple lipid laden macrophages. (Sudan Red/Oil Red stain; magnification 400X); (B) Lung biopsy showing an area of lipoid pneumonia with large vacuoles surrounded by histiocytes in the interstitium (From Reference 139 with permission) [hematoxylin and eosin stain; magnification: 100X]

predisposition and common exposure to environmental antigens. Suggestions of an autoimmune pathogenesis are based on indirect evidences like the presence of circulating immune complexes and the development of other autoimmune diseases in many patients of IPH who survive for more than a decade. An allergic theory has been proposed based on the presence of antibodies against cow milk and coexistence with celiac disease.[151-153] Reports of the potential association of IPH and exposure to insecticides or fungal toxins have never been conclusively proven. A metabolic role of toxic oxidative radicals is likely to perpetuate lung pathology in IPH. Alveolar macrophages have only a limited capacity for iron metabolism. After an episode of DAH, alveolar macrophage apparatus becomes exhausted and excess free iron can be present in the alveoli; within the alveoli, the free iron leads to the formation of highly reactive hydroxyl radicals, eventually leading to damage to alveolar structure and fibrosis.[154,155]

Clinical Presentation

About 80% of all cases of IPH occur in children, most of them being diagnosed in the 1st decade of life.[156] The rest of the cases are diagnosed in young adults, some of which may have remained undiagnosed till the adulthood.[150] Among adult patients, slight male preponderance is found. The clinical presentation widely varies. Some patients have a fulminant presentation with catastrophic DAH and respiratory failure. Some patients are present with the nonspecific symptoms of chronic cough and dyspnea. Recurrent hemoptysis is yet another presentation.[157] Patients may present with symptomatic or asymptomatic anemia without any respiratory symptoms.[158] All adult patients report hemoptysis at some point in time. As the alveolar hemorrhage is intermittent, waxing and waning of symptoms are usual in the clinical course. Exacerbations can occur during the tapering of steroids/immunosuppressive therapy. Other factors causing exacerbations are not clearly known. Fulminant DAH has been reported in the peripartum period.[159] Pulmonary function tests reveal a pattern of restrictive ventilatory defect. Increased DLCO is the hallmark abnormality in pulmonary function tests during an acute episode of DAH. When chronic changes of the disease such as fibrosis set in, DLCO is either low or normal.[160]

Laboratory and Radiological Features

Investigations often reveal hypochromic microcytic anemia, a reflection of repeated DAH, binding of iron with pulmonary hemosiderin (an unusable form) and iron loss in the sputum. Plasma ferritin level does not reflect the iron deficiency state; it is normal or elevated as a result of alveolar synthesis and subsequent release into the circulation of ferritin.[161] Bone marrow examination is consistent with an iron deficiency state. During or few days before an episode of bleeding, peripheral blood neutrophilia and eosinophilia may be seen.[162] During an acute phase of IPH, CXR reveals diffuse alveolar opacities and HRCT reveals bilateral ground-glass opacities. After multiple episodes of bleeding, chronic changes, evident as reticulonodular interstitial shadows, are seen on HRCT **(Figs 8A and B)**. Variable amount of fibrosis eventually develops.[163,164]

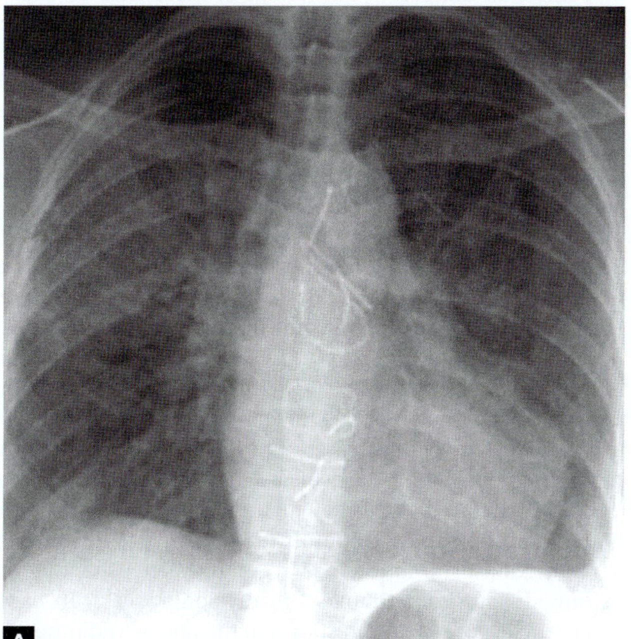

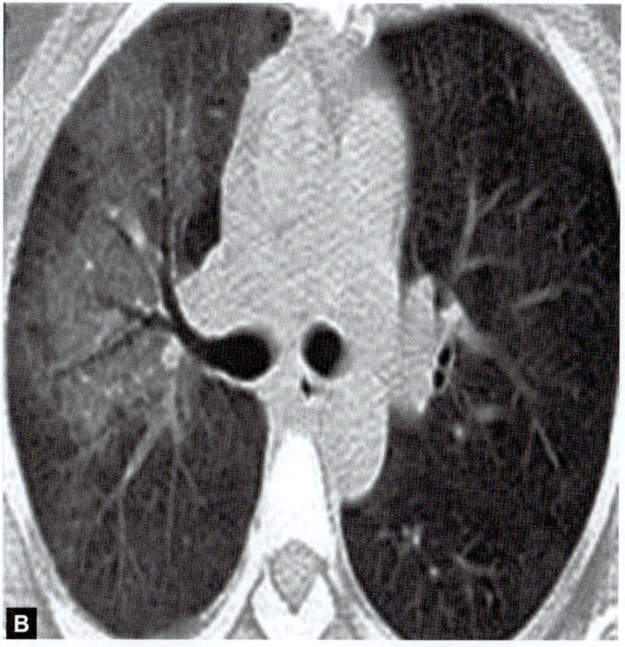

Figs 8A and B Idiopathic pulmonary hemosiderosis: (A) CXR during an acute phase of bleeding showing the alveolar opacities in left middle and lower lung zones. Note the underlying mild reticulonodular opacities that represent the fibrosis from multiple previous episodes of alveolar hemorrhage; (B) CT scan delineates the bilateral fibrotic changes better

Diagnosis

Proof of intrapulmonary hemorrhage is an essential part of diagnosis of IPH. History of repeated episodes of cough, dyspnea and hemoptysis along with a consistent picture on CXR and HRCT, point towards the diagnosis. The demonstration of hemosiderin-laden macrophages in the sputum or in the BAL fluid confirms alveolar hemorrhage. Sometimes, the pulmonary hemorrhage is occult and the patient presents with iron deficiency anemia only; a comprehensive investigation of the cause is required before a diagnosis of IPH is suspected and established.[158,162] Serological studies for the markers of autoimmune diseases, e.g. antinuclear factor (ANF), anti-double-stranded DNA, antineutrophilic cytoplasmic antibody (ANCA, both perinuclear and cytoplasmic variants), antiglomerular basement membrane (GBM) antibody, antiphospholipid antibodies, IgG and IgE cow's milk antibodies and rheumatoid factor (RF) are negative in IPH. A lung biopsy is required to rule out other causes of DAH. Transbronchial lung biopsy may be tried initially; if inadequate, video-assisted thoracoscopic biopsy or open lung biopsy can be obtained to get adequate tissue for study. Characteristic light microscopic features of IPH include: (1) the presence of intact or minimally fragmented erythrocytes in the distal airways and alveoli, an indication of recent alveolar hemorrhage; (2) hemosiderin-laden macrophages as an evidence of recurrent alveolar hemorrhage; (3) absence of vasculitis, granuloma, vascular malformation, neoplasm, infections, pulmonary infarct or evidence of any other lung disease. Thickening of the alveolar septae with the evidence of interstitial fibrosis is seen in the long-standing cases. Immunofluorescence and immunohistochemistry studies do not show any immunoglobulin or immune complex deposition, an important step to rule out autoimmune diseases causing DAH.[165,166] Some authors suggest that celiac disease should be routinely looked for in patients with IPH.[152]

Management

Systemic glucocorticoids remain the mainstay of treatment. Occasional reports of the successful use of inhaled corticosteroids are there, but the strength of evidence is not sufficient to support their use as a routine therapy.[150,167] Treatment, when started during an acute phase, helps to control symptoms and reduce mortality. Once started during the acute phase, steroids are continued till the new pulmonary infiltrates have resolved.

A slow taper-off over a few months follows, if symptoms do not recur. Corticosteroids, when chronically administered, reduce the number of acute episodes and the occurrence of pulmonary fibrosis.[168,169] The indefinite administration of glucocorticoids, however, may lead to troublesome adverse effects; also in some cases, symptoms may not be adequately controlled by corticosteroids. As maintenance therapy, various immunosuppressive agents, e.g. azathioprine, cyclophosphamide and chloroquine have been tried with or without corticosteroids, with variable success.[157,165,170-174] Cyclophosphamide infusion has been tried with success as a salvage therapy in IPH exacerbation with life-threatening DAH.[175] Gluten-free diet should be instituted in patients who have coexistent celiac disease and IPH (Lane-Hamilton syndrome).[176] IPH patients, who had advanced chronic lung diseases requiring lung transplantation, had recurrence of disease in the transplanted lung.[177]

Prognosis

Idiopathic pulmonary hemosiderosis patients have substantial mortality from acute, severe DAH and significant morbidity from the recurrent episodes of bleeding and chronic lung disease. Prognosis and mortality vary in the reported literature.[169,178,179] In general, better outcome has been reported when prolonged immunosuppressive therapy has been used. Prognosis is better in adult patients than in children and adolescents. No other clinical or biological parameter predicts prognosis in IPH.[180]

Intrathoracic Extramedullary Hematopoiesis

In many hematological disorders, such as thalassemia, sickle-cell anemia, hereditary spherocytosis, polycythemia vera and myelofibrosis, intense compensatory hematopoiesis lead to the formation of foci of extramedullary hematopoiesis. Extramedullary hematopoiesis can be present within the thoracic cavity, described most frequently in patients with sickle-cell anemia and thalassemia.[181,182] Intrathoracic extramedullary hematopoiesis appears as paravertebral and/or paracostal masses.[183] Formation of these masses occurs from the extrusion from the bone marrow through the cortex. A common site in the thorax is the costovertebral junction leading to a paraspinal mass. These masses have smooth, sharply defined margins, may be unilateral or bilateral in distribution **(Figs 9A to C)**. No erosion of the adjacent bone is seen. The masses may show initial rapid growth and subsequently remain stable in size. The patients usually do not have any symptoms attributable to the masses. Occasional cases with symptoms due to mass effect from the large foci of extramedullary hematopoiesis and other complications, e.g. exudative pleural effusion, hemothorax have been described.[184-186] In the case of presentation as intrathoracic masses, classic location and clinical setting make the diagnosis obvious; invasive diagnostic studies should be avoided. In symptomatic cases, a variety of treatment options may be tried. Blood transfusion (hypertransfusion) and hydroxyurea have been used with improvement in symptoms and should be the first line of treatment.[181,187] Ruxolitinib, a Janus kinase inhibitor, has recently been used to treat extramedullary hematopoiesis in myelofibrosis.[188] In cases where the lesions do not respond to the above, radiotherapy and surgical resection remain other treatment options. Pleural effusion and hemothorax are managed with pleural drainage and pleurodesis.[189]

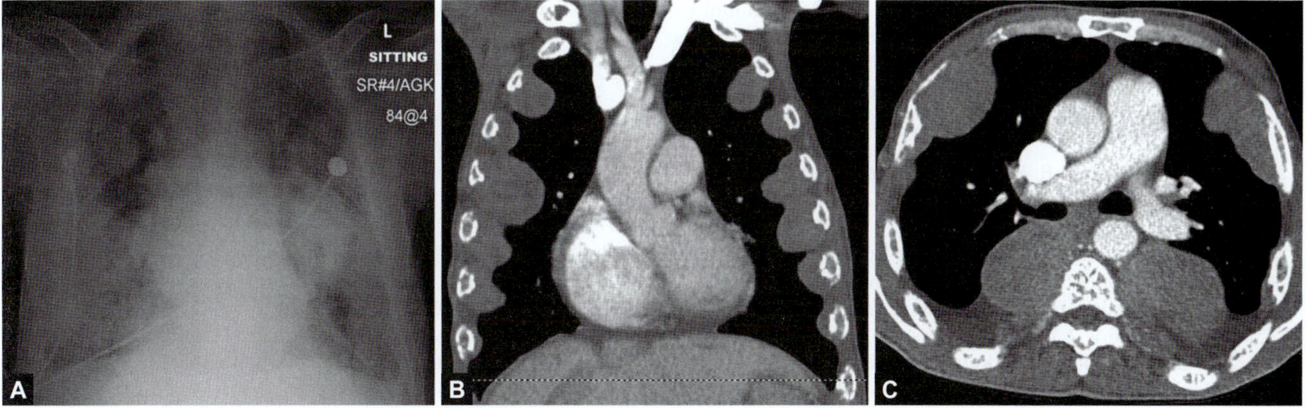

Figs 9A to C Extramedullary intrathoracic hematopoiesis. CXR (A) and CT scan [(B) coronal section and (C), axial section] showing bilateral multiple soft tissue density opacities in paraspinal location and in relation to multiple ribs

Neurofibromatosis

Von Recklinghausen's disease or neurofibromatosis (NF) type 1 is an autosomal dominant disorder with characteristic neurocutaneous manifestations. NF causes ILD. In an analysis of 64 cases of ILD in NF patients, the mean age of presentation of 50 years and a male preponderance was reported.[190] Most NF patients with lung involvement by ILD report dyspnea. Pulmonary function tests show an obstructive pattern with reduced DLCO. CXR and HRCT show bilateral cystic lesions with upper lobe predominance.[191] Other radiological findings include ground-glass opacities, bibasilar subpleural reticular opacities and bullae. On pathological specimens, the involvement is patchy; areas of normal lung alternate with the areas of interstitial involvement. In the involved areas, the alveolar septae demonstrate lymphoplasmacytic inflammation and fibrosis consistent with nonspecific idiopathic pneumonia (NSIP) pattern. The etiological role of smoking in NF related ILD is debated; it has been suggested that smoking is the actual risk factor for the development and severity of ILD in NF patients.[192,193]

REFERENCES

1. Westermark P, Benson MD, Buxbaum JN, Cohen AS, Frangione B, Ikeda S, et al. Amyloid: toward terminology clarification. Report from the Nomenclature Committee of the International Society of Amyloidosis. Amyloid. 2005;12(1):1-4.
2. Utz JP, Swensen SJ, Gertz MA. Pulmonary amyloidosis. The Mayo Clinic experience from 1980 to 1993. Ann Intern Med. 1996;124(4):407-13.
3. Howard ME, Ireton J, Daniels F, Langton D, Manolitsas ND, Fogarty P, et al. Pulmonary presentations of amyloidosis. Respirology. 2001;6(1):61-4.
4. Celli BR, Rubinow A, Cohen AS, Brody JS. Patterns of pulmonary involvement in systemic amyloidosis. Chest. 1978;74(5):543-7.
5. Smith RR, Hutchins GM, Moore GW, Humphrey RL. Type and distribution of pulmonary parenchymal and vascular amyloid. Correlation with cardiac amyloid. Am J Med. 1979;66(1): 96-104.
6. Thompson PJ, Citron KM. Amyloid and the lower respiratory tract. Thorax. 1983;38(2):84-7.
7. Shah PL, Gillmore JD, Copley SJ, Collins JV, Wells AU, du Bois RM, et al. The importance of complete screening for amyloid fibril type and systemic disease in patients with amyloidosis in the respiratory tract. Sarcoidosis Vasc Diffuse Lung Dis. 2002;19(2):134-42.
8. Merlini G, Bellotti V. Molecular mechanisms of amyloidosis. N Engl J Med. 2003;349(6):583-96.
9. Hui AN, Koss MN, Hochholzer L, Wehunt WD. Amyloidosis presenting in the lower respiratory tract. Clinicopathologic, radiologic, immunohistochemical, and histochemical studies on 48 cases. Arch Pathol Lab Med. 1986;110(3):212-8.
10. Tariq SM, Morrison D, McConnochie K. Solitary bronchial amyloid presenting with haemoptysis. Eur Respir J. 1990;3(10): 1230-1.
11. Antunes ML, Vieira da Luz JM. Primary diffuse tracheobronchial amyloidosis. Thorax. 1969;24(3):307-11.
12. Turkstra F, Rinkel RN, Biermann H, van der Valk P, Voskuyl AE. Tracheobronchomalacia due to amyloidosis in a patient with rheumatoid arthritis. Clin Rheumatol. 2008;27(6):807-8.
13. Kirchner J, Jacobi V, Kardos P, Kollath J. CT findings in extensive tracheobronchial amyloidosis. Eur Radiol. 1998; 8(3):352-4.
14. Xu L, Cai BQ, Zhong X, Zhu YJ. Respiratory manifestations in amyloidosis. Chin Med J (Engl). 2005;118(24):2027-33.
15. Piazza C, Cavaliere S, Foccoli P, Toninelli C, Bolzoni A, Peretti G. Endoscopic management of laryngo-tracheobronchial amyloidosis: a series of 32 patients. Eur Arch Otorhinolaryngol. 2003;260(7):349-4.
16. Dzingozovova M, Skrickova J, Macak J, Múcková K, Adam Z. Localized tracheobronchial amyloidosis, type AA, and its differentiation from the systemic form of amyloidosis in clinical practice. Vnitr Lek. 2009;55(6):593-8.
17. Singh J, Rana SS. Solitary intrapulmonary nodular amyloidoma. Asian Cardiovasc Thorac Ann. 2009;17(3):329-31.
18. Vieira IG, Marchiori E, Zanetti G, Cabral RF, Takayassu TC, Spilberg G, et al. Pulmonary amyloidosis with calcified nodules and masses–a six-year computed tomography follow-up: a case report. Cases J. 2009;2:6540.
19. Gillmore JD, Hawkins PN. Amyloidosis and the respiratory tract. Thorax. 1999;54(5):444-51.

20. Rosen DJ, Stavropoulos C, Travis WD, Ashton RC, Bhora FY, Connery CP. Transdiaphragmatic amyloidoma. Ann Thorac Surg. 2008;86(1):310-2.
21. Pickford HA, Swensen SJ, Utz JP. Thoracic cross-sectional imaging of amyloidosis. Am J Roentgenol. 1997;168(2): 351-5.
22. Ayuso MC, Gilabert R, Bombi JA, Salvador A. CT appearance of localized pulmonary amyloidosis. J Comput Assist Tomogr. 1987;11(1):197-9.
23. Yang MC, Blutreich A, Das K. Nodular pulmonary amyloidosis with an unusual protein composition diagnosed by fine-needle aspiration biopsy: a case report. Diagn Cytopathol. 2009;37(4):286-9.
24. Kitamura H, Kobayashi T, Kaneko M, Kusumoto M, Kodama T, Matsuno Y, et al. Pulmonary amyloidosis diagnosed by CT-guided transbronchial biopsy: a case report. Jpn J Clin Oncol. 2001;31(5):209-11.
25. Strange C, Heffner JE, Collins BS, Brown FM, Sahn SA. Pulmonary hemorrhage and air embolism complicating transbronchial biopsy in pulmonary amyloidosis. Chest. 1987;92(2): 367-9.
26. Pusztaszeri M, Kamel EM, Artemisia S, Genevay M, McKee T. Nodular pseudotumoral pulmonary amyloidosis mimicking pulmonary carcinoma. Thorax. 2005;60(5):440.
27. Hacihanefioglu U, Uzgoren E. Amyloid producing tumour of the lung. Thorax. 1981;36(5):395-6.
28. Gordon HW, Miller R Jr, Mittman C. Medullary carcinoma of the lung with amyloid stroma: a counterpart of medullary carcinoma of the thyroid. Hum Pathol. 1973;4(3):431-6.
29. Ollenberger GP, Knight S, Tauro AJ. False-positive FDG positron emission tomography in pulmonary amyloidosis. Clin Nucl Med. 2004;29(10):657-8.
30. BoydKing A, Sharma O, Stevenson K. Localized interstitial pulmonary amyloid: a case report and review of the literature. Curr Opin Pulm Med. 2009;15(5):517-20.
31. Sterlacci W, Veits L, Moser P, Steiner HJ, Rüscher S, Jamnig H, et al. Idiopathic systemic amyloidosis primarily affecting the lungs with fatal pulmonary haemorrhage due to vascular involvement. Pathol Oncol Res. 2009;15(1):133-6.
32. Cottin V, Cordier JF. Interstitial pulmonary amyloidosis. Respiration. 2008;75(2):210.
33. Ohdama S, Akagawa S, Matsubara O, Yoshizawa Y. Primary diffuse alveolar septal amyloidosis with multiple cysts and calcification. Eur Respir J. 1996;9(7):1569-71.
34. Graham CM, Stern EJ, Finkbeiner WE, Webb WR. High-resolution CT appearance of diffuse alveolar septal amyloidosis. Am J Roentgenol. 1992;158(2):265-7.
35. Geusens EA, Verschakelen JA, Bogaert JG. Primary pulmonary amyloidosis as a cause of interlobular septal thickening. AJR Am J Roentgenol. 1997;168(4):1116-7.
36. Cordier JF, Loire R, Brune J. Amyloidosis of the lower respiratory tract. Clinical and pathologic features in a series of 21 patients. Chest. 1986;90(6):827-31.
37. Kaiserling E, Krober S. Lymphatic amyloidosis, a previously unrecognized form of amyloid deposition in generalized amyloidosis. Histopathology. 1994;24(3):215-21.
38. Berk JL. Pleural effusions in systemic amyloidosis. Curr Opin Pulm Med. 2005;11(4):324-8.
39. Berk JL, Keane J, Seldin DC, Sanchorawala V, Koyama J, Dember LM, et al. Persistent pleural effusions in primary systemic amyloidosis: etiology and prognosis. Chest. 2003;124(3): 969-77.
40. Mansalis KA, Klein DA, Demartini SD, Powers JF, Danielson DS. Pleural findings in a patient with persistent pulmonary effusions from systemic amyloidosis. Amyloid. 2011;18(1):29-31.
41. Maeno T, Sando Y, Tsukagoshi M, Suga T, Endo M, Seki R, et al. Pleural amyloidosis in a patient with intractable pleural effusion and multiple myeloma. Respirology. 2000;5(1):79-80.
42. Bontemps F, Tillie-Leblond I, Coppin MC, Frehart P, Wallaert B, Ramon P, et al. Pleural amyloidosis: thoracoscopic aspects. Eur Respir J. 1995;8(6):1025-7.
43. Davis SN, Clark F. Multiple myeloma as a cause of chylothorax. JR Soc Med. 1986;79(1):49.
44. Eder L, Zisman D, Wolf R, Bitterman H. Pulmonary hypertension and amyloidosis—an uncommon association: a case report and review of the literature. J Gen Intern Med. 2007;22(3):416-9.
45. Dingli D, Utz JP, Gertz MA. Pulmonary hypertension in patients with amyloidosis. Chest. 2001;120(5):1735-8.
46. Shiue ST, McNally DP. Pulmonary hypertension from prominent vascular involvement in diffuse amyloidosis. Arch Intern Med. 1988;148(3):687-9.
47. Road JD, Jacques J, Sparling JR. Diffuse alveolar septal amyloidosis presenting with recurrent hemoptysis and medial dissection of pulmonary arteries. Am Rev Respir Dis. 1985;132(6):1368-70.
48. Case records of the Massachusetts General Hospital. Weekly clinicopathological exercises. Case 20-1998. A 53-year-old man with cardiac amyloidosis and a left pulmonary mass. N Engl J Med. 1998;338(26):1905-13.
49. Kamei K, Kusumoto K, Suzuki T. Pulmonary amyloidosis with pulmonary arteriovenous fistula. Chest. 1989;96(6):1435-6.
50. Chow LT, Chow WH, Shum BS. Fatal massive upper respiratory tract haemorrhage: an unusual complication of localized amyloidosis of the larynx. J Laryngol Otol. 1993;107(1):51-3.
51. Yong HS, Woo OH, Lee JW, Suh SI, Oh YW, Kang EY. Primary localized amyloidosis manifested as supraclavicular and mediastinal lymphadenopathy. Br J Radiol. 2007;80(955): e131-3.
52. Ashe J, Borel CO, Hart G, Humphrey RL, Derrick DA, Kuncl RW. Amyloid myopathy presenting with respiratory failure. J Neurol Neurosurg Psychiatry. 1992;55(2):162-5.
53. Streeten EA, de la Monte SM, Kennedy TP. Amyloid infiltration of the diaphragm as a cause of respiratory failure. Chest. 1986;89(5):760-2.
54. Berk JL, Wiesman JF, Skinner M, Sanchorawala V. Diaphragm paralysis in primary systemic amyloidosis. Amyloid. 2005;12(3):193-6.
55. Hanon S, De Keukeleire T, Dieriks B, Bultynck W, Vanmaele L, Meysman M, et al. Primary tracheobronchial amyloidosis: a series of 3 cases. Acta Clin Belg. 2007;62(1):56-60.
56. Alloubi I, Thumerel M, Begueret H, Baste JM, Velly JF, Jougon J. Outcomes after bronchoscopic procedures for primary tracheobronchial amyloidosis: retrospective study of 6 cases. Pulm Med. 2012;2012:352719.
57. Kennedy TL, Patel NM. Surgical management of localized amyloidosis. Laryngoscope. 2000;110(6):918-23.
58. Monroe AT, Walia R, Zlotecki RA, Jantz MA. Tracheobronchial amyloidosis: a case report of successful treatment with external beam radiation therapy. Chest. 2004;125(2):784-9.
59. Firlinger I, Setinek U, Koller H, Feurstein P, Prosch H, Burghuber OC, et al. A case of tracheobronchial amyloidosis treated with endoscopic debulking and external beam radiation therapy. Pneumologie. 2013;67(7):398-400.

60. Fernandez-Nebro A, Olive A, Castro MC, Varela AH, Riera E, Irigoyen MV, et al. Long-term TNF-alpha blockade in patients with amyloid A amyloidosis complicating rheumatic diseases. Am J Med. 2010;123(5):454-61.
61. Nakamura T, Higashi S, Tomoda K, Tsukano M, Baba S. Efficacy of etanercept in patients with AA amyloidosis secondary to rheumatoid arthritis. Clin Exp Rheumatol. 2007;25(4): 518-22.
62. Gottenberg JE, Merle-Vincent F, Bentaberry F, Allanore Y, Berenbaum F, Fautrel B, et al. Anti-tumor necrosis factor alpha therapy in fifteen patients with AA amyloidosis secondary to inflammatory arthritides: a followup report of tolerability and efficacy. Arthritis Rheum. 2003;48(7):2019-24.
63. Gertz MA, Lacy MQ, Dispenzieri A. Myeloablative chemotherapy with stem cell rescue for the treatment of primary systemic amyloidosis: a status report. Bone Marrow Transplant. 2000;25(5):465-70.
64. Sanchorawala V, Wright DG, Seldin DC, Dember LM, Finn K, Falk RH, et al. An overview of the use of high-dose melphalan with autologous stem cell transplantation for the treatment of AL amyloidosis. Bone Marrow Transplant. 2001;28(7):637-42.
65. Dispenzieri A, Lacy MQ, Kyle RA, Therneau TM, Larson DR, Rajkumar SV, et al. Eligibility for hematopoietic stem-cell transplantation for primary systemic amyloidosis is a favorable prognostic factor for survival. J Clin Oncol. 2001;19(14):3350-6.
66. Jaccard A, Moreau P, Leblond V, Leleu X, Benboubker L, Hermine O, et al. High-dose melphalan versus melphalan plus dexamethasone for AL amyloidosis. N Engl J Med. 2007; 357(11):1083-93.
67. Palladini G, Perfetti V, Obici L, Caccialanza R, Semino A, Adami F, et al. Association of melphalan and high-dose dexamethasone is effective and well tolerated in patients with AL (primary) amyloidosis who are ineligible for stem cell transplantation. Blood. 2004;103(8):2936-8.
68. Lachmann HJ, Gallimore R, Gillmore JD, Carr-Smith HD, Bradwell AR, Pepys MB, et al. Outcome in systemic AL amyloidosis in relation to changes in concentration of circulating free immunoglobulin light chains following chemotherapy. Br J Haematol. 2003;122(1):78-84.
69. Cohen AD, Comenzo RL. Systemic light-chain amyloidosis: advances in diagnosis, prognosis, and therapy. Hematology Am Soc Hematol Educ Program. 2010;2010:287-94.
70. Horger M, Lengerke C, Pfannenberg C, Wehrmann M, Einsele H, Knop S, et al. Significance of the "halo" sign for progression and regression of nodular pulmonary amyloidosis: radiographic-pathological correlation (2005:6b). Eur Radiol. 2005;15(9):2037-40.
71. Hoyer RJ, Leung N, Witzig TE, Lacy MQ. Treatment of diuretic refractory pleural effusions with bevacizumab in four patients with primary systemic amyloidosis. Am J Hematol. 2007;82(5):409-13.
72. Suzuki H, Matsui K, Hirashima T, Kobayashi M, Sasada S, Okamato N, et al. Three cases of the nodular pulmonary amyloidosis with a long-term observation. Intern Med. 2006;45(5):283-6.
73. Eisenberg R, Sharma OP. Primary pulmonary amyloidosis. An unusual case with 14 years' survival. Chest. 1986;89(6):889-91.
74. Young WA. Bronchopulmonary amyloidosis-multiple tissue involvement and long follow-up. Aust NZJ Med. 1989;19(5): 463-5.
75. Wilcox WR. Lysosomal storage disorders: the need for better pediatric recognition and comprehensive care. J Pediatr. 2004;144(5 Suppl):S3-14.
76. MacDermot KD, Holmes A, Miners AH. Anderson-Fabry disease: clinical manifestations and impact of disease in a cohort of 98 hemizygous males. J Med Genet. 2001;38(11): 750-60.
77. MacDermot KD, Holmes A, Miners AH. Anderson-Fabry disease: clinical manifestations and impact of disease in a cohort of 60 obligate carrier females. J Med Genet. 2001;38(11): 769-75.
78. Koskenvuo JW, Kantola IM, Nuutila P, Knuuti J, Parkkola R, Mononen I, et al. Cardiopulmonary involvement in Fabry's disease. Acta Cardiol. 2010;65(2):185-92.
79. Bierer G, Kamangar N, Balfe D, Wilcox WR, Mosenifar Z. Cardiopulmonary exercise testing in Fabry disease. Respiration. 2005;72(5):504-11.
80. Brown LK, Miller A, Bhuptani A, Sloane MF, Zimmerman MI, Schilero G, et al. Pulmonary involvement in Fabry disease. Am J Respir Crit Care Med. 1997;155(3):1004-10.
81. Kim W, Pyeritz RE, Bernhardt BA, Casey M, Litt HI. Pulmonary manifestations of Fabry disease and positive response to enzyme replacement therapy. Am J Med Genet A. 2007;143(4):377-81.
82. Rosenberg DM, Ferrans VJ, Fulmer JD, Line BR, Barranger JA, Brady RO, et al. Chronic airflow obstruction in Fabry's disease. Am J Med. 1980;68(6):898-905.
83. Franzen D, Krayenbuehl PA, Lidove O, Aubert JD, Barbey F. Pulmonary involvement in Fabry disease: overview and perspectives. Eur J Intern Med. 2013;24(8):707-13.
84. Bartimmo EE Jr, Guisan M, Moser KM. Pulmonary involvement in Fabry's disease: a reappraisal follow-up of a San Diego kindred and review of literature. Am J Med. 1972;53(6):755-64.
85. Kelly MM, Leigh R, McKenzie R, Kamada D, Ramsdale EH, Hargreave FE. Induced sputum examination: diagnosis of pulmonary involvement in Fabry's disease. Thorax. 2000;55(8):720-1.
86. Beck M, Ricci R, Widmer U, Dehout F, de Lorenzo AG, Kampmann C, et al. Fabry disease: overall effects of agalsidase alfa treatment. Eur J Clin Invest. 2004;34(12):838-44.
87. Kampmann C, Linhart A, Devereux RB, Schiffmann R. Effect of agalsidase alfa replacement therapy on Fabry disease-related hypertrophic cardiomyopathy: a 12-to 36-month, retrospective, blinded echocardiographic pooled analysis. Clin Ther. 2009;31(9):1966-76.
88. Wang RY, Abe JT, Cohen AH, Wilcox WR. Enzyme replacement therapy stabilizes obstructive pulmonary Fabry disease associated with respiratory globotriaosylceramide storage. J Inherit Metab Dis. 2008;31(Suppl 2):S369-74.
89. Hill SC, Damaska BM, Tsokos M, Kreps C, Brady RO, Barton NW. Radiographic findings in type 3b Gaucher disease. Pediatr Radiol. 1996;26(12):852-60.
90. Yassa NA, Wilcox AG. High-resolution CT pulmonary findings in adults with Gaucher's disease. Clin Imaging. 1998;22(5):339-42.
91. Banjar H. Pulmonary involvement of Gaucher's disease in children: a common presentation in Saudi Arabia. Ann Trop Paediatr. 1998;18(1):55-9.
92. Roberts WC, Fredrickson DS. Gaucher's disease of the lung causing severe pulmonary hypertension with associated acute recurrent pericarditis. Circulation. 1967;35(4):783-9.

93. Wolson AH. Pulmonary findings in Gaucher's disease. Am J Roentgenol Radium Ther Nucl Med. 1975;123(4):712-15.
94. Tunaci A, Berkmen YM, Gokmen E. Pulmonary Gaucher's disease: high-resolution computed tomographic features. Pediatr Radiol. 1995;25(3):237-8.
95. Aydin K, Karabulut N, Demirkazik F, Arat A. Pulmonary involvement in adult Gaucher's disease: high resolution CT appearance. Br J Radiol. 1997;70:93-5.
96. McHugh K, Olsen E ØE, Vellodi A. Gaucher disease in children: radiology of non-central nervous system manifestations. Clin Radiol. 2004;59(2):117-23.
97. Carson KF, Williams CA, Rosenthal DL, Bhuta S, Kleerup E, Diaz RP, et al. Bronchoalveolar lavage in a girl with Gaucher's disease. A case report. Acta Cytol. 1994;38(4):597-600.
98. Gribetz AR, Kasen L, Teirstein AS. Respiratory distress, pericarditis and inappropriate antidiuretic hormone secretion in a patient with infectious mononucleosis and Gaucher's disease. Mt Sinai J Med. 1980;47(6):589-91.
99. Smith RL, Hutchins GM, Sack GH Jr, Ridolfi RL. Unusual cardiac, renal and pulmonary involvement in Gaucher's disease. Intersitial glucocerebroside accumulation, pulmonary hypertension and fatal bone marrow embolization. Am J Med. 1978;65(2):352-60.
100. Bennett LL, Mohan D. Gaucher disease and its treatment options. Ann Pharmacother. 2013;47(9):1182-93.
101. Barton NW, Brady RO, Dambrosia JM, Di Bisceglie AM, Doppelt SH, Hill SC, et al. Replacement therapy for inherited enzyme deficiency–macrophage-targeted glucocerebrosidase for Gaucher's disease. N Engl J Med. 1991;324(21): 1464-70.
102. Weinreb NJ, Charrow J, Andersson HC, Kaplan P, Kolodny EH, Mistry P, et al. Effectiveness of enzyme replacement therapy in 1028 patients with type 1 Gaucher disease after 2 to 5 years of treatment: a report from the Gaucher Registry. Am J Med. 2002;113(2):112-9.
103. Rohrbach M, Clarke JT. Treatment of lysosomal storage disorders: progress with enzyme replacement therapy. Drugs. 2007;67(18):2697-716.
104. Goitein O, Elstein D, Abrahamov A, Hadas-Halpern I, Melzer E, Kerem E, et al. Lung involvement and enzyme replacement therapy in Gaucher's disease. QJM. 2001;94(8):407-15.
105. Lo SM, Liu J, Chen F, Pastores GM, Knowles J, Boxer M, et al. Pulmonary vascular disease in Gaucher disease: clinical spectrum, determinants of phenotype and long-term outcomes of therapy. J Inherit Metab Dis. 2011;34(3):643-50.
106. Pastores GM, Giraldo P, Cherin P, Mehta A. Goal-oriented therapy with miglustat in Gaucher disease. Curr Med Res Opin. 2009;25(1):23-37.
107. McGovern MM, Wasserstein MP, Giugliani R, Bembi B, Vanier MT, Mengel E, et al. A prospective, cross-sectional survey study of the natural history of Niemann-Pick disease type B. Pediatrics. 2008;122(2):e341-9.
108. Guillemot N, Troadec C, de Villemeur TB, Clément A, Fauroux B. Lung disease in Niemann-Pick disease. Pediatr Pulmonol. 2007;42(12):1207-14.
109. McGovern MM, Aron A, Brodie SE, Desnick RJ, Wasserstein MP. Natural history of Type A Niemann-Pick disease: possible endpoints for therapeutic trials. Neurology. 2006;66(2):228-32.
110. Niggemann B, Rebien W, Rahn W, Wahn U. Asymptomatic pulmonary involvement in 2 children with Niemann-Pick disease type B. Respiration. 1994;61(1):55-7.
111. Nicholson AG, Florio R, Hansell DM, Bois RM, Wells AU, Hughes P, et al. Pulmonary involvement by Niemann-Pick disease. A report of six cases. Histopathology. 2006;48(5):596-603.
112. Rodrigues R, Marchiori E, Muller NL. Niemann-Pick disease: high-resolution CT findings in two siblings. J Comput Assist Tomogr. 2004;28(1):52-4.
113. Mendelson DS, Wasserstein MP, Desnick RJ, Glass R, Simpson W, Skloot G, et al. Type B Niemann-Pick disease: findings at chest radiography, thin-section CT, and pulmonary function testing. Radiology. 2006;238(1):339-45.
114. Nicholson AG, Wells AU, Hooper J, Hansell DM, Kelleher A, Morgan C. Successful treatment of endogenous lipoid pneumonia due to Niemann-Pick Type B disease with whole-lung lavage. Am J Respir Crit Care Med. 2002;165(1):128-31.
115. Anderson PD, Huizing M, Claassen DA, White J, Gahl WA. Hermansky-Pudlak syndrome type 4 (HPS-4): clinical and molecular characteristics. Hum Genet. 2003;113(1):10-7.
116. Vincent LM, Adams D, Hess RA, Ziegler SG, Tsilou E, Golas G, et al. Hermansky-Pudlak syndrome type 1 in patients of Indian descent. Mol Genet Metab. 2009;97(3):227-33.
117. Wei ML. Hermansky-Pudlak syndrome: a disease of protein trafficking and organelle function. Pigment Cell Res. 2006;19(1): 19-42.
118. Gahl WA, Brantly M, Kaiser-Kupfer MI, Iwata F, Hazelwood S, Shotelersuk V, et al. Genetic defects and clinical characteristics of patients with a form of oculocutaneous albinism (Hermansky-Pudlak syndrome). N Engl J Med. 1998;338(18):1258-64.
119. Brantly M, Avila NA, Shotelersuk V, Lucero C, Huizing M, Gahl WA. Pulmonary function and high-resolution CT findings in patients with an inherited form of pulmonary fibrosis, Hermansky-Pudlak syndrome, due to mutations in HPS-1. Chest. 2000;117(1):129-36.
120. Sen T, Mullerpattan J, Agarwal D, Naphde D, Deshpande R, Mahashur AA. Hermansky-Pudlak syndrome. J Assoc Physicians India. 2009;57:660-2.
121. Avila NA, Brantly M, Premkumar A, Huizing M, Dwyer A, Gahl WA. Hermansky-Pudlak syndrome: radiography and CT of the chest compared with pulmonary function tests and genetic studies. Am J Roentgenol. 2002;179(4):887-92.
122. Witkop CJ, Krumwiede M, Sedano H, White JG. Reliability of absent platelet dense bodies as a diagnostic criterion for Hermansky-Pudlak syndrome. Am J Hematol. 1987;26(4):305-11.
123. Furuhashi K, Enomoto N, Fujisawa T, Hashimoto D, Inui N, Nakamura Y, et al. Hermansky-Pudlak syndrome with non-specific interstitial pneumonia. Intern Med. 2014;53(5):449-53.
124. Tager AM, Sharma A, Mark EJ. Case records of the Massachusetts General Hospital. Case 32-2009. A 27-year-old man with progressive dyspnea. N Engl J Med. 2009;361(16):1585-93.
125. Gahl WA, Brantly M, Troendle J, Avila NA, Padua A, Montalvo C, et al. Effect of pirfenidone on the pulmonary fibrosis of Hermansky-Pudlak syndrome. Mol Genet Metab. 2002;76(3):234-42.
126. O'Brien K, Troendle J, Gochuico BR, Markello TC, Salas J, Cardona H, et al. Pirfenidone for the treatment of Hermansky-Pudlak syndrome pulmonary fibrosis. Mol Genet Metab. 2011;103(2):128-34.
127. Lederer DJ, Kawut SM, Sonett JR, Vakiani E, Seward SL Jr, White JG, et al. Successful bilateral lung transplantation for pulmonary fibrosis associated with the Hermansky-Pudlak syndrome. J Heart Lung Transplant. 2005;24(10):1697-9.

128. Gondouin A, Manzoni P, Ranfaing E, Brun J, Cadranel J, Sadoun D, et al. Exogenous lipid pneumonia: a retrospective multicentre study of 44 cases in France. Eur Respir J. 1996;9(7):1463-9.
129. Cardasis JJ, MacMahon H, Husain AN. The spectrum of lung disease due to chronic occult aspiration. Ann Am Thorac Soc. 2014;11(6):865-73.
130. Kitchen JM, O'Brien DE, McLaughlin AM. Perils of fire eating. An acute form of lipoid pneumonia or fire eater's lung. Thorax. 2008;63(5):401, 439.
131. Shaikh AY, Oliveira PJ. Exogenous lipoid pneumonia (fire-eater's lung). Am J Med. 2014;127(2):e3-4.
132. Venkatnarayan K, Madan K, Walia R, Kumar J, Jain D, Guleria R. "Diesel siphoner's lung": Exogenous lipoid pneumonia following hydrocarbon aspiration. Lung India. 2014;31(1):63-6.
133. Gurell MN, Kottmann RM, Xu H, Sime PJ. Exogenous lipoid pneumonia: an unexpected complication of substance abuse. Ann Intern Med. 2008;149(5):364-5.
134. Vethanayagam D, Pugsley S, Dunn EJ, Russell D, Kay JM, Allen C. Exogenous lipid pneumonia related to smoking weed oil following cadaveric renal transplantation. Can Respir J. 2000;7(4):338-42.
135. Baron SE, Haramati LB, Rivera VT. Radiological and clinical findings in acute and chronic exogenous lipoid pneumonia. J Thorac Imaging. 2003;18(4):217-24.
136. Agarwal R. Low-attenuation consolidation—the most characteristic finding in lipoid pneumonia. Eur J Intern Med. 2006;17(4):307.
137. Franquet T, Gimenez A, Bordes R, Rodríguez-Arias JM, Castella J. The crazy-paving pattern in exogenous lipoid pneumonia: CT-pathologic correlation. Am J Roentgenol. 1998;170(2): 315-7.
138. Laurent F, Philippe JC, Vergier B, Granger-Veron B, Darpeix B, Vergeret J, et al. Exogenous lipoid pneumonia: HRCT, MR, and pathologic findings. Eur Radiol. 1999;9(6):1190-6.
139. Talwar A, Mayerhoff R, London D, Shah R, Stanek A, Epstein M. False-positive PET scan in a patient with lipoid pneumonia simulating lung cancer. Clin Nucl Med. 2004;29(7):426-8.
140. Kameswaran M, Annobil SH, Benjamin B, Salim M. Bronchoscopy in lipoid pneumonia. Arch Dis Child. 1992;67(11): 1376-7.
141. Spickard A 3rd, Hirschmann JV. Exogenous lipoid pneumonia. Arch Intern Med. 1994;154(6):686-92.
142. Chiang IC, Lin YT, Liu GC, Chiu CC, Tsai MS, Kao EL. Exogenous lipoid pneumonia: serial chest plain roentgenography and high-resolution computerized tomography findings. Kaohsiung J Med Sci. 2003;19(12):593-8.
143. Segev D, Szold O, Fireman E, Kluger Y, Sorkine P. Kerosene-induced severe acute respiratory failure in near drowning: reports on four cases and review of the literature. Crit Care Med. 1999;27(8):1437-40.
144. Indumathi CK, Vikram KS, Paul P, Lewin S. Severe lipoid pneumonia following aspiration of machine oil: successful treatment with steroids. Indian J Chest Dis Allied Sci. 2012; 54(3):197-9.
145. Chang HY, Chen CW, Chen CY, Hsuie TR, Chen CR, Lei WW, et al. Successful treatment of diffuse lipoid pneumonitis with whole lung lavage. Thorax. 1993;48(9):947-8.
146. Russo R, Chiumello D, Cassani G, Maiocchi G, Gattinoni L. Case of exogenous lipoid pneumonia: steroid therapy and lung lavage with an emulsifier. Anesthesiology. 2006;104(1): 197-8.
147. Sias SM, Daltro PA, Marchiori E, Ferreira AS, Caetano RL, Silva CS, et al. Clinic and radiological improvement of lipoid pneumonia with multiple bronchoalveolar lavages. Pediatr Pulmonol. 2009;44(4):309-15.
148. Jouannic I, Desrues B, Lena H, Quinquenel ML, Donnio PY, Delaval P. Exogenous lipoid pneumonia complicated by *Mycobacterium fortuitum* and *Aspergillus fumigatus* infections. Eur Respir J. 1996;9(1):172-4.
149. Abe M, Kondo K, Fujino S, Hirasawa Y, Yokoyama A, Kohno N, et al. [Lipoid pneumonia combined with pulmonary nocardiosis caused by inhalation of amphotericin-B after renal transplantation]. Nihon Kyobu Shikkan Gakkai Zasshi. 1996;34(6):737-40.
150. Ioachimescu OC, Sieber S, Kotch A. Idiopathic pulmonary haemosiderosis revisited. Eur Respir J. 2004;24(1):162-70.
151. Ertekin V, Selimoglu MA, Gursan N, Ozkan B. Idiopathic pulmonary hemosiderosis in children with celiac disease. Respir Med. 2006;100(3):568-9.
152. Khemiri M, Ouederni M, Khaldi F, Barsaoui S. Screening for celiac disease in idiopathic pulmonary hemosiderosis. Gastroenterol Clin Biol 2008; 32(8-9):745-8.
153. Bhattacharya M, Kapoor S, Dubey AP. Celiac disease presentation in a tertiary referral centre in India: current scenario. Indian J Gastroenterol. 2013;32(2):98-102.
154. Castranova V, Bowman L, Miles PR, Reasor MJ. Toxicity of metal ions to alveolar macrophages. Am J Ind Med. 1980;1(3-4):349-57.
155. Mateos F, Brock JH, Perez-Arellano JL. Iron metabolism in the lower respiratory tract. Thorax. 1998;53(7):594-600.
156. Morgan PG, Turner-Warwick M. Pulmonary haemosiderosis and pulmonary haemorrhage. Br J Dis Chest. 1981;75(3): 225-42.
157. Kabra SK, Bhargava S, Lodha R, Satyavani A, Walia M. Idiopathic pulmonary hemosiderosis: clinical profile and follow up of 26 children. Indian Pediatr. 2007;44(5):333-8.
158. Minkov M, Kovacs J, Wiesbauer P, Dekan G, Gadner H. Severe anemia owing to occult pulmonary hemorrhage: a diagnostic pitfall. J Pediatr Hematol Oncol. 2006;28(7):467-70.
159. Foglia LM, Deering SH. Post-partum exacerbation of idiopathic pulmonary hemosiderosis. J Matern Fetal Neonatal Med. 2008;21(12):895-7.
160. Allue X, Wise MB, Beaudry PH. Pulmonary function studies in idiopathic pulmonary hemosiderosis in children. Am Rev Respir Dis. 1973;107(3):410-5.
161. Milman N, Pedersen FM. Idiopathic pulmonary haemosiderosis. Epidemiology, pathogenic aspects and diagnosis. Respir Med. 1998;92(7):902-7.
162. Chen RL, Chuang SS. Silent idiopathic pulmonary hemosiderosis with iron-deficiency anemia but normal serum ferritin. J Pediatr Hematol Oncol. 2007;29(7):509-11.
163. Akyar S, Ozbek SS. Computed tomography findings in idiopathic pulmonary hemosiderosis. Respiration. 1993;60(1):63-4.
164. Buschman DL, Ballard R. Progressive massive fibrosis associated with idiopathic pulmonary hemosiderosis. Chest. 1993;104(1):293-5.
165. Yeager H Jr, Powell D, Weinberg RM, Bauer H, Bellanti JA, Katz S. Idiopathic pulmonary hemosiderosis: ultrastructural studies and responses to azathioprine. Arch Intern Med. 1976;136(10):1145-9.
166. Corrin B, Jagusch M, Dewar A, Tungekar MF, Davies DR, Warner JO, et al. Fine structural changes in idiopathic pulmonary haemosiderosis. J Pathol, 1987;153(3):249-56.

167. Tutor JD, Eid NS. Treatment of idiopathic pulmonary hemosiderosis with inhaled flunisolide. South Med J. 1995;88(9): 984-6.
168. Kiper N, Gocmen A, Ozcelik U, Dilber E, Anadol D. Long-term clinical course of patients with idiopathic pulmonary hemosiderosis (1979-1994): prolonged survival with low-dose corticosteroid therapy. Pediatr Pulmonol. 1999;27(3):180-4.
169. Saeed MM, Woo MS, MacLaughlin EF, Margetis MF,Keens TG. Prognosis in pediatric idiopathic pulmonary hemosiderosis. Chest. 1999;116(3):721-5.
170. Rossi GA, Balzano E, Battistini E, Oddera S, Marchese P, Acquila M, et al. Long-term prednisone and azathioprine treatment of a patient with idiopathic pulmonary hemosiderosis. Pediatr Pulmonol. 1992;13(3):176-80.
171. Airaghi L, Ciceri L, Giannini S, Ferrero S, Meroni PL, Tedeschi A. Idiopathic pulmonary hemosiderosis in an adult. Favourable response to azathioprine. Monaldi Arch Chest Dis. 2001;56(3):211-3.
172. Bagnato L, Grilli C, Portioli P, Biella C, Carnelli V. [Long-term evaluation of immunosuppressive therapy in childhood idiopathic pulmonary hemosiderosis]. Pediatr Med Chir. 1986;8(5):671-4.
173. Huang SH, Lee PY, Niu CK. Treatment of pediatric idiopathic pulmonary hemosiderosis with low-dose cyclophosphamide. Ann Pharmacother. 2003;37(11):1618-21.
174. Taytard J, Nathan N, de Blic J, Fayon M, Epaud R, Deschildre A, et al. New insights into pediatric idiopathic pulmonary hemosiderosis: the French RespiRare(®) cohort. Orphanet J Rare Dis. 2013;8:161.
175. Naithani R, Chandra J, Singh V, Kumar V, Dubey NK. Life-threatening exacerbation in idiopathic pulmonary hemosiderosis salvaged by cyclophosphamide infusion. Indian J Chest Dis Allied Sci. 2006;48(4):287-9.
176. Sethi GR, Singhal KK, Puri AS, Mantan M. Benefit of gluten-free diet in idiopathic pulmonary hemosiderosis in association with celiac disease. Pediatr Pulmonol. 2011;46(3):302-5.
177. Calabrese F, Giacometti C, Rea F, Loy M, Sartori F, Di Vittorio G, et al. Recurrence of idiopathic pulmonary hemosiderosis in a young adult patient after bilateral single-lung transplantation. Transplantation. 2002;74(11):1643-5.
178. Chryssanthopoulos C, Cassimos C, Panagiotidou C. Prognostic criteria in idiopathic pulmonary hemosiderosis in children. Eur J Pediatr. 1983;140(2):123-5.
179. Le Clainche L, Le Bourgeois M, Fauroux B, Forenza N, Dommergues JP, Desbois JC, et al. Long-term outcome of idiopathic pulmonary hemosiderosis in children. Medicine (Baltimore). 2000;79(5):318-26.
180. Miwa S, Imokawa S, Kato M, Ide K, Uchiyama H, Yokomura K, et al. Prognosis in adult patients with idiopathic pulmonary hemosiderosis. Intern Med. 2011;50(17):1803-8.
181. Meo A, Cassinerio E, Castelli R, Bignamini D, Perego L, Cappellini MD. Effect of hydroxyurea on extramedullary haematopoiesis in thalassaemia intermedia: case reports and literature review. Int J Lab Hematol. 2008;30(5):425-31.
182. Verani R, Olson J, Moake JL. Intrathoracic extramedullary hematopoiesis: report of a case in a patient with sickle-cell disease-beta-thalassemia. Am J Clin Pathol. 1980;73(1):133-7.
183. Delavaud C, Lincot J, Debray MP, Schouman-Claeys E, Dallaudière B. Paravertebral extramedullary hematopoiesis. Diagn Interv Imaging. 2014;95(4):457-60.
184. Aessopos A, Tassiopoulos S, Farmakis D, Moyssakis I, Kati M, Polonifi K, et al. Extramedullary hematopoiesis-related pleural effusion: the case of beta-thalassemia. Ann Thorac Surg. 2006;81(6):2037-43.
185. Tassiopoulos S, Konstantopoulos K, Rombos Y, Aessopos A. Hemothorax due to extramedullary erythropoietic masses. Ann Thorac Surg. 2004;77(1):323-4.
186. Luo Y, Zhang Y, Lou SF. Bilateral pleural effusion in a patient with an extensive extramedullary hematopoietic mass. Case Rep Hematol. 2013;2013:857610.
187. Karimi M, Cohan N, Pishdad P. Hydroxyurea as a first-line treatment of extramedullary hematopoiesis in patients with beta thalassemia: Four case reports. Hematology. 2015;20(1): 53-7.
188. Maccaferri M, Leonardi G, Marasca R, Colaci E, Paolini A, Soci F, et al. Ruxolitinib for pulmonary extramedullary hematopoiesis in myelofibrosis. Leuk Lymphoma. 2014;55(9):2207-8.
189. Peng MJ, Kuo HT, Chang MC. A case of intrathoracic extramedullary hematopoiesis with massive pleural effusion: successful pleurodesis with intrapleural minocycline. J Formos Med Assoc. 1994;93(5):445-7.
190. Zamora AC, Collard HR, Wolters PJ, Webb WR, King TE. Neurofibromatosis-associated lung disease: a case series and literature review. Eur Respir J. 2007;29(1):210-4.
191. Chang ET, Hu Wang A, Lin CB, Lee JJ, Yang GG. Pulmonary manifestation in neurofibromatosis type 1. Intern Med. 2007;46(8):527-8.
192. Ryu JH, Parambil JG, McGrann PS, Aughenbaugh GL. Lack of evidence for an association between neurofibromatosis and pulmonary fibrosis. Chest. 2005;128(4):2381-6.
193. Yokoyama A, Kohno N, Sakai K, Kondo K, Hirasawa Y, Hiwada K. Distal acinar emphysema and interstitial pneumonia in a patient with von Recklinghausen's disease: five-year observation following quitting smoking. Intern Med. 1997; 36(6):413-6.

Bronchiolitis

Gyanendra Agrawal, Dheeraj Gupta

INTRODUCTION

The term "small airways" refers to airways of less than 3 mm in diameter.[1,2] This definition includes small bronchi, bronchioles and respiratory bronchioles. Bronchioles are small airways of less than 2 mm in diameter without cartilage or submucosal glands. This includes terminal bronchioles, whose principal role is to conduct air to the respiratory bronchioles. The latter contain alveoli, which are the site of air conduction and gas exchange. Although not strictly synonymous, the terms "bronchioles" and "small airways" are used interchangeably.

Bronchiolitis is nonspecific inflammation of the respiratory bronchioles and peribronchiolar alveolar sacs of variable causes, clinical manifestations and evolution. Bronchiolitis is traditionally classified as one of the interstitial lung disease (ILD). The diseases affecting bronchioles can be classified into primary bronchiolar disorders—those diseases in which the pathologic process is centered in the bronchioles—and those disorders in which the bronchioles are secondarily involved by a pathologic process that is centered in the lung parenchyma or proximal large airways **(Box 1)**.[3]

No single classification for bronchiolar disorders is widely accepted. Classification schemes have been proposed based on causes and underlying diseases, radiologic features, histopathologic findings, or some combination of these parameters. Unavoidable overlaps exist, no matter which classification is chosen.

The clinical classification is primarily based on the proved or presumed etiology, related systemic diseases or other associations **(Box 2)**.[4] An etiologic classification is useful to remind the physician when to suspect the presence of bronchiolitis.

BOX 1 Classification of bronchiolar disorders*

- Primary bronchiolar disorders:
  - Constrictive bronchiolitis (bronchiolitis obliterans)
  - Diffuse panbronchiolitis
  - Respiratory bronchiolitis
  - Acute bronchiolitis
  - Mineral dust airway disease
  - Follicular bronchiolitis
  - Others (diffuse aspiration bronchiolitis, lymphocytic bronchiolitis)
- Parenchymal disorders with prominent bronchiolar involvement
  - RB-ILD and DIP
  - Hypersensitivity pneumonitis (HP)
  - Cryptogenic organizing pneumonia (idiopathic BOOP)
  - Others (PLCH, sarcoidosis)
- Large airway diseases with bronchiolar involvement
  - Bronchiectasis
  - Chronic bronchitis
  - Asthma

Abbreviations: RB-ILD, respiratory bronchiolitis-associated interstitial lung disease; DIP, desquamative interstitial pneumonia; BOOP, bronchiolitis obliterans organizing pneumonia; PLCH, pulmonary Langerhans cell histiocytosis.
Source: *Modified from Ryu JH, Myers JL, Swensen SJ. Bronchiolar disorders. Am J Respir Crit Care Med. 2003;168(11):1277-92.

GENERAL FEATURES OF BRONCHIOLAR DISORDERS

Bronchiolitis, a cellular and mesenchymal inflammatory reaction that follows damage to the bronchiolar epithelium of small conducting airways, is the most common form of disease affecting small airways. This entity is relatively uncommon in adults. Neutrophils which accumulate at the site of injury causes further damage to the airway epithelium and matrix by the release of inflammatory mediators. Depending on the disease stage, the repair process may cause narrowing and distortion of small airways (constrictive bronchiolitis) or complete obliteration (bronchiolitis obliterans).

CLINICAL PRESENTATIONS

Most commonly, the patients present with slowly progressive exertional dyspnea and dry cough. Onset of symptoms is relatively acute in bronchiolitis from infections, inhalational injury or drugs; subacute in organizing pneumonia; and indolent and chronic in patients with post-transplant

BOX 2 Clinical classification of bronchiolitis

- *Infectious bronchiolitis:* Respiratory syncytial virus, *Mycoplasma pneumoniae*, parainfluenza, adenovirus, measles, rubella, rubeola
- *Drug-induced bronchiolitis:* D-penicillamine, gold, sulfasalazine, amiodarone, interferon, phenytoin, cocaine, minocycline, nitrofurantoin, carmustine, bleomycin, busulfan, *Sauropus androgynus*, paraquat
- *Inhalational injury:* Toxic fumes and gases, mineral dusts, organic dusts, volatile flavoring agents, flock worker's lung (fine nylon fiber), grain dusts, fire smoke (World Trade Center lung)
- *Post-transplant:* Bone marrow, heart-lung, lung
- *Connective tissue diseases:* Rheumatoid arthritis, Sjögren's syndrome, systemic lupus erythematosus, polymyositis, dermatomyositis
- *Idiopathic:* Cryptogenic adult bronchiolitis, respiratory bronchiolitis, diffuse panbronchiolitis, cryptogenic organizing pneumonia, diffuse aspiration bronchiolitis
- *Systemic diseases:* Ulcerative colitis, chronic eosinophilic pneumonia, Wegener's granulomatosis, chronic thyroiditis, ataxia-telangiectasia, immunoglobulin A (IgA) nephropathy
- *Other rare:* Eosinophilic bronchiolitis, lymphocytic bronchiolitis, radiation pneumonitis, primary diffuse hyperplasia of pulmonary neuroendocrine cells

bronchiolitis. Cough with copious expectoration may be seen in infectious bronchiolitis and diffuse panbronchiolitis (DPB). Fever and constitutional symptoms are mainly seen in infectious bronchiolitis and collagen vascular diseases. Some patients may even present with pulmonary hypertension and respiratory failure in advanced stages. Due to extensive air trapping, the physiologic dead space gradually increases to the extent insufficient to washout normal carbon dioxide from the lungs, ultimately leading to hypercapnic respiratory failure.

Pulmonary Function Tests

Depending on the predominant physiology, pulmonary function tests (PFTs) may yield variable results. Most of the primary bronchiolar disorders and large airway diseases are associated with obstructive physiologic defects. In contrast, most of the distal acinar interstitial diseases with secondary bronchiolar involvement show restrictive or mixed pattern. Abnormal values for forced expiratory flow (FEF) 25–75%, in conjunction with normal values for forced vital capacity (FVC) and forced expiratory volume in one second (FEV_1), are often useful in identifying small airway disease. Primary bronchiolar disorders show nonreversibility with inhaled bronchodilators. In addition, these patients also demonstrate reduced diffusion capacity. The obstruction of small airways results in abnormal distribution of ventilation to peripheral lung units. This principle forms the basis of two tests: Frequency dependence of dynamic compliance and closing volumes. The tests of small airway function **(Box 3)**, however, are rarely performed in clinical practice.

BOX 3 Tests of small airway function

- Increase in mid-expiratory flow rate
- Frequency dependence of dynamic compliance
- Increase in closing volume
- Increased volume of isoflow

Chest X-ray Findings

Chest radiography in bronchiolar disorders may be normal or demonstrate nonspecific findings like hyperinflation and peripheral attenuation of vascular markings in purely obstructive bronchiolar lesions such as constrictive bronchiolitis. In other primary bronchiolar disorders, small nodules or reticulonodular infiltrates may be observed. Increased bronchial wall thickening may also be seen. In distal acinar interstitial diseases with secondary bronchiolar involvement, chest radiography usually demonstrates features of the underlying parenchymal disease such as cryptogenic organizing pneumonia (COP) or hypersensitivity pneumonitis.

High-resolution Computed Tomography Findings

High-resolution computed tomography (HRCT) is perhaps the most important tool for the diagnostic evaluation of bronchiolitis.[5] Normal bronchioles cannot be seen on computed tomography (CT) scans, since airways less than 2 mm in diameter are not visible on CT; however, diseased bronchioles with dilated lumen (>2 mm in diameter) or thickened walls can be visualized. HRCT scan abnormalities that reflect bronchiolar diseases can be categorized into direct and indirect signs **(Table 1)**.

Bronchiolar wall thickening may occur due to inflammation and fibrosis, with or without dilatation (bronchiolectasis). Bronchiolar luminal impaction manifests as 2–4 mm nodular and linear branching centrilobular opacities on CT. The "tree-in-bud" pattern represents a form of bronchiolar impaction in which branching linear structures have more than one contiguous branching site. Apart from direct signs, the most important indirect finding consists of mosaic attenuation, which occurs due to air trapping. This sign is not specific for bronchiolitis. In bronchiolar diseases, the mosaic pattern is caused by hypoventilation of alveoli distal to bronchiolar obstruction, which leads to secondary vasoconstriction is seen on CT scans as areas of decreased attenuation. Paired CT scans performed in both inspiration and expiration are useful for distinguishing bronchiolar from pulmonary vascular disease and some diffuse infiltrative diseases that may also cause a mosaic pattern.

Based on the radiologic features, bronchiolar diseases have been classified into four dominant CT patterns **(Box 4)**.[2] "Centrilobular opacities with tree-in-bud" pattern is seen in infectious bronchiolitis, DPB **(Figs 1A and B)**, diffuse aspiration bronchiolitis (DAB) and immunodeficiency

BOX 4 Radiologic classification of bronchiolar diseases

- Centrilobular nodules with/without tree-in-bud
- Ground-glass attenuation and alveolar consolidation
- Mosaic perfusion
- Mixed or different pictures

Table 1 High-resolution computed tomography signs of bronchiolar disorders

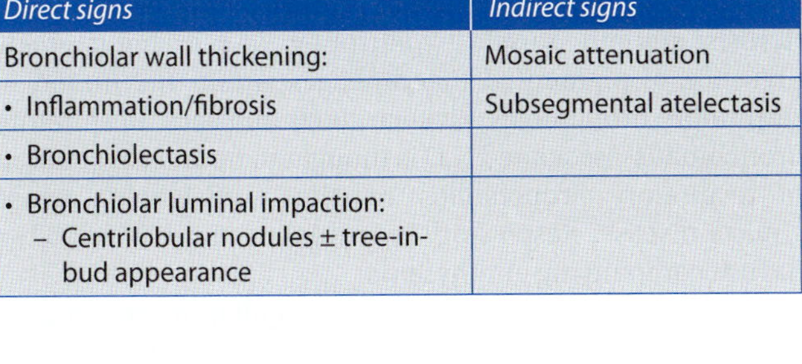

Direct signs	*Indirect signs*
Bronchiolar wall thickening:	Mosaic attenuation
• Inflammation/fibrosis	Subsegmental atelectasis
• Bronchiolectasis	
• Bronchiolar luminal impaction: – Centrilobular nodules ± tree-in-bud appearance	

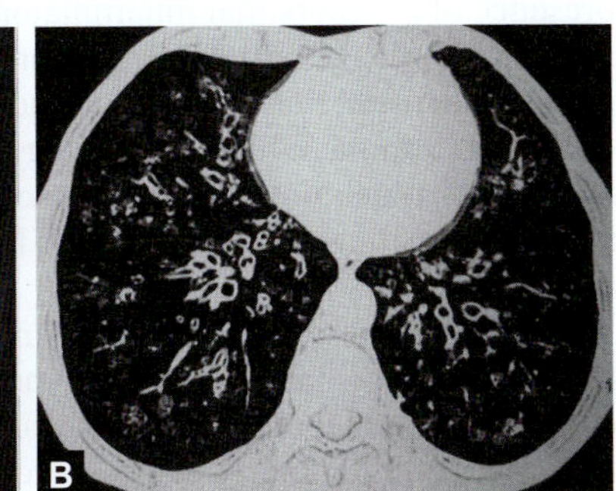

Figs 1A and B A case of diffuse panbronchiolitis. (A) X-ray paranasal sinuses shows sinusitis and (B) the HRCT scan shows centrilobular nodules with bronchiectasis

syndromes. Centrilobular opacities appearing as ill-defined ground-glass nodules in the absence of a tree-in-bud pattern are associated with respiratory bronchiolitis, hypersensitivity pneumonitis and follicular bronchiolitis. "Ground-glass attenuation" or consolidation is due mainly to alveolar filling that occurs in bronchiolitis obliterans organizing pneumonia (BOOP) **(Fig. 2)** or in respiratory bronchiolitis-interstitial lung disease (RB-ILD). The prototype of the third type of CT pattern, "mosaic lung attenuation," is constrictive bronchiolitis **(Figs 3A and B)**.

Other conditions resulting in a pattern of mosaic attenuation include connective tissue disorders, bone marrow and lung transplantation, toxic fume inhalation and drugs. Quite often many diseases will have a "mixed pattern"

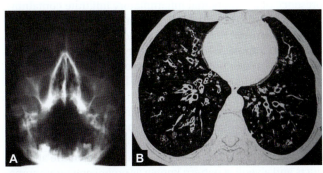

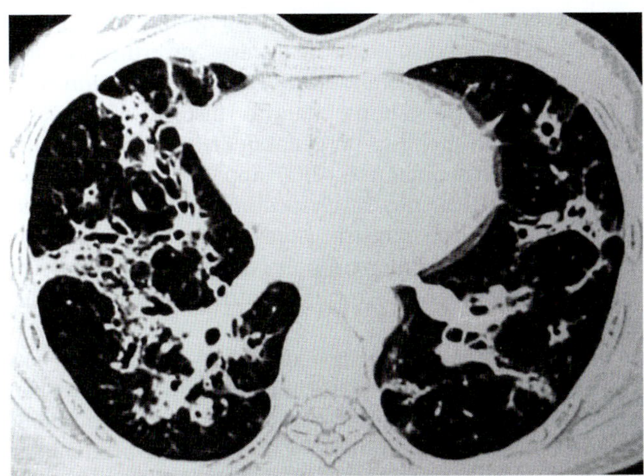

Fig. 2 A case of biopsy proven bronchiolitis obliterans organizing pneumonia showing diffuse patchy consolidations and ground-glass opacities

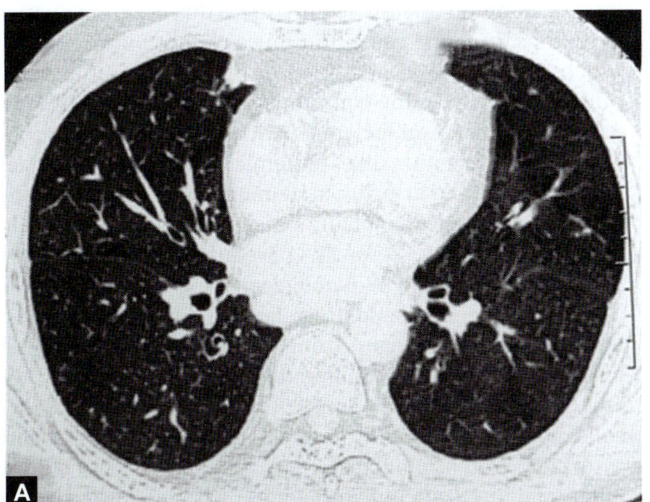

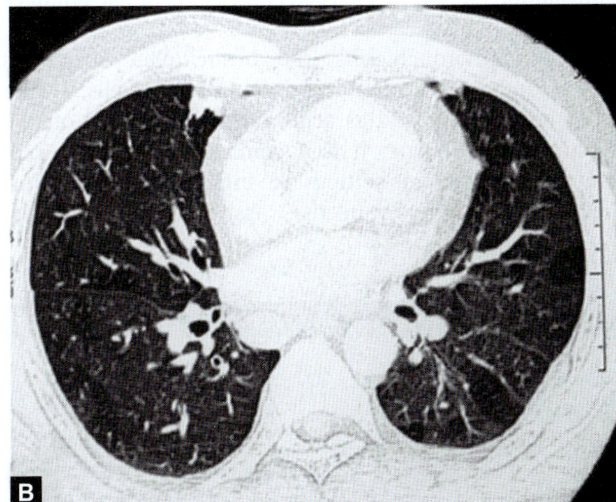

Figs 3A and B (A) Paired inspiratory and (B) expiratory HRCT scans in bronchiolitis, mosaic attenuation and air trapping becomes more apparent on expiratory scans

on HRCT. Association of tree-in-bud with mosaic perfusion can be seen in different entities, such as bronchiectasis and acute bronchopulmonary infections. The combination of mosaic perfusion and ground-glass opacities in the same patient, referred to as the "headcheese sign" is very suggestive of HP.[5] HRCT findings in chemical-induced lung injuries are variable and nonspecific but may help to distinguish from other forms of injuries.[6]

Histologic Findings

Histologically, bronchiolitis can have a wide variety of patterns **(Box 5)**. Most morphological abnormalities of the bronchioles are not specific, since bronchiolitis arises from a variety of sources of injury that result in the diversity of clinical, radiological and functional patterns. Bronchiolar changes should not be ascribed an etiology or pathogenesis based solely on histologic features. Nevertheless, the histologic patterns generally show a better correlation with radiological manifestations, natural history of disease, and response to therapy.[7] In general, cellular bronchiolitis and bronchiolitis obliterans (BO) appear to be common "early" lesions that may resolve completely or partly, and are corticosteroid-responsive. Constrictive bronchiolitis is relatively corticosteroid unresponsive, usually progressive with the development of irreversible airflow obstruction and air trapping.

It is difficult to recognize and classify bronchiolitis in transbronchial biopsies because of the limited sampling size, hence surgical biopsy is preferred. It is important to obtain wedge biopsies from multiple lobes because the bronchiolar pathology is often patchy. Transbronchial biopsies may be sufficient for diagnosis in certain clinical settings, such as those in post-transplant settings. It is recommended to obtain at least five pieces of well-expanded alveolar parenchyma with transbronchial biopsies.[8] The severity of clinical manifestations frequently exceeds that of histologic changes seen on lung biopsy.

In cellular bronchiolitis, the bronchioles' structures show an increased number of inflammatory cells. It can further be characterized as acute or chronic based on the inflammatory cell type. It is a common pattern seen in many clinicopathologic settings like infectious bronchiolitis, inhalational injury, connective tissue diseases (CTDs) and aspiration. "Follicular bronchiolitis" represents hyperplasia of the mucosa-associated lymphatic tissue (MALT) and chronic peribronchiolar infiltrate along with secondary germinal centers. This pattern is associated with congenital or acquired immunodeficiency syndromes (AIDS), including human immunodeficiency virus (HIV) infection; collagen vascular diseases, especially rheumatoid arthritis and Sjögren's syndrome; and lymphoproliferative diseases. Respiratory bronchiolitis is a mild inflammatory reaction to cigarette smoke[9] which consists of slight fibrosis, smooth muscle hypertrophy, and a characteristic presence of pigmented macrophages within the lumen of respiratory bronchioles, alveolar ducts and sacs. Respiratory bronchiolitis-associated ILD is thought to be an exaggeration of respiratory bronchiolitis reaction sufficient to cause clinical disease. Respiratory bronchiolitis and RB-ILD often have accompanying emphysema.

BOX 5 Histologic patterns of bronchiolitis

- Cellular bronchiolitis
  - Follicular bronchiolitis
  - Respiratory bronchiolitis
  - Diffuse panbronchiolitis
- Organizing pneumonia/bronchiolitis obliterans with intraluminal polyps
- Constrictive bronchiolitis
- Peribronchiolar metaplasia and fibrosis

"Diffuse panbronchiolitis" is a peculiar morphological form of cellular bronchiolitis largely restricted to the adult individuals of Japanese heritage. Its histologic hallmark is the presence of an interstitial inflammatory infiltrate containing foamy macrophages around respiratory bronchioles. Polyps of granulation tissue may partially occlude adjacent bronchiolar or alveolar lumina. When the histology of DPB is encountered in an individual not of Asian descent, the possibility of inflammatory bowel disease-related bronchiolitis should be considered.

Bronchiolitis obliterans with intraluminal polyps is characterized by intrabronchiolar polypoid protrusions of connective tissue that partially fill bronchiolar lumens. These polypoid proliferations usually extend distally in the alveolar ducts and alveoli, a pattern known as organizing pneumonia. This combination of changes is referred to as BOOP pattern. The airway lumen appears to be occluded from within, as opposed to the concentric narrowing seen in constrictive bronchiolitis. Bronchiolitis obliterans organizing pneumonia is a very common tissue reaction pattern that occurs in a variety of settings. In many cases, the cause cannot be ascertained, which is referred as cryptogenic organizing pneumonia (idiopathic BOOP). The common secondary causes of BOOP pattern are those associated with a variety of infections; CTDs and vasculitis like systemic lupus erythematosus (SLE), rheumatoid arthritis, systemic sclerosis, inflammatory myopathies; post-transplant; inhalational injury like silo-filler's lung, paint aerosols, paraquat poisoning; drugs, radiation therapy and hematological malignancies.

Constrictive bronchiolitis refers to luminal narrowing by scarring that ranges from very subtle abnormalities to complete luminal obliteration. The hallmark of this type of bronchiolitis is mural thickening by submucosal collagenous fibrosis with progressive concentric narrowing associated with luminal distortion, mucus stasis and chronic inflammation. Bronchiolar dilatation with mucus impaction and smooth muscle hypertrophy may also be seen. There are many conditions and disorders which are associated with

BOX 6 Disorders associated with constrictive bronchiolitis

Postinfectious:
- *Viruses:* Respiratory syncytial virus, influenza, parainfluenza, adenovirus, HIV
- *Bacteria:* Mycoplasma, Chlamydia
- *Parasites: Plasmodium vivax*
- *Fungi: Pneumocystis jirovecii, Cryptococcus*

Connective tissue diseases:
- Rheumatoid arthritis, SLE
- Inhalational injury (toxic fumes or smoke) phosgene, hot gases, nitrogen dioxide, sulfur dioxide, ammonia, chlorine

Drugs:
Penicillamine, lomustine, gold, amiodarone, interferon, nitrofurantoin, etc.

Post-transplant: Bone marrow, heart-lung or lung, graft-versus-host-disease

Idiopathic

Others:
Radiation, cocaine abuse, inflammatory bowel disease

Abbreviations: HIV, human immunodeficiency virus; SLE, systemic lupus erythematosus.

this type of bronchiolitis **(Box 6)**; some specific ones are post-transplant bronchiolitis, bronchiolitis associated with rheumatoid arthritis and World Trade Center lung.[10-12]

Peribronchiolar fibrosis and bronchiolar metaplasia is a rare condition characterized by the growth of bronchiolar epithelium into the adjacent fibrotic alveolar walls (so-called lambertosis).[13] Inflammatory cells are scanty and usually present in the bronchiolar lumen. It represents a manifestation of previous bronchiolar injury/scarring such as viral bronchiolitis or extrinsic allergic alveolitis.

PRACTICAL APPROACH FOR DIAGNOSIS OF BRONCHIOLAR DISORDERS

The broad clinical spectrum of bronchiolar inflammatory disorders in adults can be diagnosed with the help of a practical algorithmic approach **(Flow chart 1)**.

A detailed history of symptoms suggestive of CTD, as well as exposure to inhalational irritants and radiation, should be elicited in order to identify a possible cause. A potential relationship with drug intake should be investigated in depth and taken into account in combination with the underlying disease. On auscultation, the presence of wheezing, inspiratory squeaks, or crackles should point to the bronchioles as the likely anatomic site involved. After history and physical examination, posteroanterior and lateral chest radiographs (CXRs) and PFTs are typically obtained. These tests are of limited value in directing the diagnostic workup of primary bronchiolar disorders as they rarely establish specific diagnoses. However, they are important to exclude large airway diseases in which secondary bronchiolar changes may be seen.

Flow chart 1 Algorithm for practical approach to patients with supposed bronchiolitis

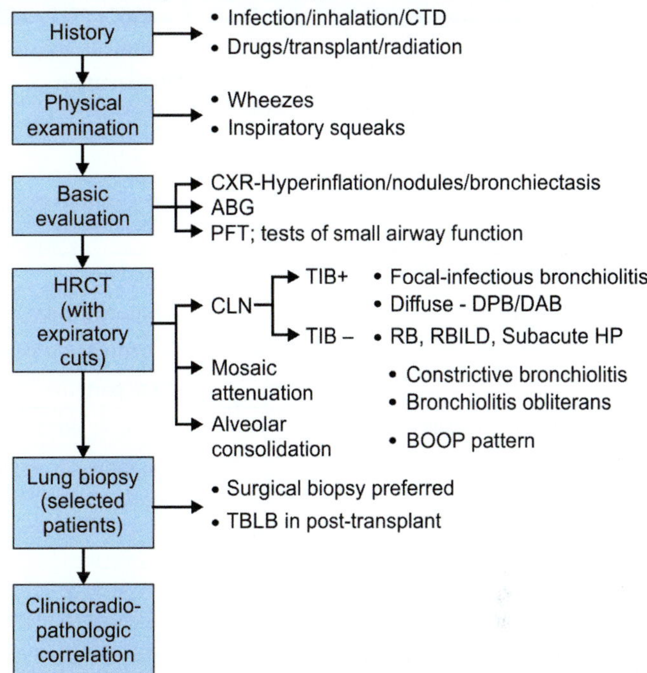

Abbreviations: ABG, arterial blood gases; BOOP, bronchiolitis obliterans with organizing pneumonia; CLN, centrilobular nodules; CTD, connective tissue diseases; CXR, chest X-ray; DAB, diffuse aspiration bronchiolitis; DPB, diffuse panbronchiolitis; HP, hypersensitivity pneumonitis; PFT, pulmonary function tests; RB, respiratory bronchiolitis; RB-ILD, respiratory bronchiolitis interstitial lung disease; TBLB, transbronchial lung biopsy; TIB, tree-in-bud.

As both CXR and PFT findings are frequently nonspecific, a high index of clinical suspicion should be maintained in order to diagnose and/or exclude bronchiolar disease. HRCT scanning (inspiratory and expiratory) may play a critical role in both suggesting the specific causes of bronchiolar disease and directing optimal management. In select cases, the diagnosis may be made solely using HRCT scans in combination with the history and clinical presentation, thus obviating more invasive diagnostic testing. In patients where the diagnosis of bronchiolitis and its cause is not clear, the clinical relevance of a bronchiolar lesion is best determined by identifying the underlying histopathologic pattern and assessing the correlative clinico-physiologic-radiologic context. The interdependence of clinical, radiological and pathologic findings in assessing the significance of bronchiolar lesions and the necessity of a multidisciplinary (clinical-radiological-pathologic)[4] approach cannot be overemphasized **(Table 2)**.

SPECIFIC FORMS OF BRONCHIOLITIS

Infectious Causes of Bronchiolitis

Infection is the most common cause of acute bronchiolitis, mostly seen in children of less than 1 year of age, especially

Table 2 Clinicoradiological-pathological correlation of bronchiolitis*

Histopathologic findings	*Radiological findings*	*Common clinical conditions*
Cellular bronchiolitis	CL nodules, TIB Mixed pattern	Respiratory bronchiolitis Infectious bronchiolitis DPB, DAB Collagen vascular diseases Post-transplant Immunodeficiency
Bronchiolitis with intraluminal polyps	CL nodules Mosaic oligemia Air trapping on expiratory CT Mixed pattern	COP Drug-induced bronchiolitis Collagen vascular diseases Post-transplant
Constrictive bronchiolitis	Mosaic oligemia Air trapping on expiratory CT	Postinfectious (MacLeod's syndrome) Inhalational injury Collagen vascular diseases Idiopathic
Peribronchiolar metaplasia and fibrosis	CL areas of increased attenuation	Chronic hypersensitivity pneumonitis

Source: *Modified from Poletti V, Costabel U. Bronchiolar disorders: classification and diagnostic approach. Semin Respir Crit Care Med. 2003;24(5):457-64.
Abbreviations: CL, centrilobular; TIB, tree-in-bud; CT, computed tomography scan; DPB, diffuse panbronchiolitis; DAB, diffuse aspiration bronchiolitis; COP, cryptogenic organizing pneumonia.

during the winter season. Respiratory syncytial virus (RSV) is the etiologic agent in the majority of these patients, but other viruses (adenovirus, influenza, parainfluenza) and nonviral pathogens (mycoplasma, chlamydia) can cause a similar syndrome.[3,14] Symptomatic acute bronchiolitis in adults is relatively rare, but can be caused by infectious agents such as *Mycoplasma pneumoniae* and RSV.[14] No systematic study has been reported; therefore, the clinical presentation of infectious bronchiolitis in adults is ill defined.[15]

Most patients with acute viral bronchiolitis can be managed at home with supportive care since respiratory symptoms are generally mild. Although bronchodilators, epinephrine and corticosteroids have been commonly used in more severe cases of acute viral bronchiolitis, there is considerable disagreement regarding optimal treatment strategies. Beyond the use of supportive care and supplemental oxygen, there is little evidence to support a routine role for any of these drugs.[16,17]

One of the long-term complications of postinfectious constrictive bronchiolitis occurring in childhood is the development of the Swyer-James (or MacLeod's) syndrome, that is, unilateral hyperlucent lung with the evidence of air trapping and decreased vascularity especially after adenoviral infection occurring in infancy.

Inhalational Lung Injury

Several irritant gases like sulfur dioxide, chlorine gas, ammonia, nitrogen dioxide (NO_2), phosgene, photochemical air pollutants, and ozone have been occasionally associated with bronchitis or bronchiolitis. Two distinct and uncommon types of airway processes can follow exposure to noxious fumes, gases or mists: Reactive airway dysfunction syndrome (RADS) and constrictive bronchiolitis. Reactive airway dysfunction syndrome is defined as the development of respiratory symptoms in minutes or hours after a single accidental inhalation of high concentrations of irritant gas and aerosol. These symptoms are followed by asthma-like symptoms and airway hyperresponsiveness.

Mineral dust airways disease occurs because of the inhalation of a number of inorganic dusts, including asbestos, iron oxide, aluminum oxide, talc, mica, silica and coal. Inflammatory response induced by the dust likely leads to the local production of fibrogenic factors and morphogenesis of the bronchiolar lesion. Poorly defined centrilobular opacities can be seen on HRCT scans early in the course of the disease; these predominate posteriorly and at the lung bases owing to the gravitational effects of fiber deposition. Peribronchial infiltration of dust-laden macrophages is often noted on microscopy. Inhalations of "organic dusts" are associated with the development of hypersensitivity pneumonitis. Interstitial pneumonitis with granulomas is seen in most of the patients on lung biopsy.

Volatile flavoring agents used in the microwave popcorn industry can cause a respiratory illness resembling bronchiolitis obliterans, especially in workers who work nearest to the mixing tank. Lung function testing shows severe airflow obstruction, which does not recover after removal from exposure. There does not appear to be any risk to the general population who use microwave popcorn products.

Bronchiolitis Associated with Connective Tissue Diseases

A wide spectrum of inflammatory and fibrotic disorders involving the small airways may complicate CTDs which include COP; constrictive (obliterative) bronchiolitis; small airways disease; cellular or follicular bronchiolitis; and bronchiectasis (most often seen in late rheumatoid arthritis). In addition, medications used to treat CTDs, penicillamine, methotrexate and gold can cause histologic abnormalities similar to those seen in the primary disease. Small airway diseases are most commonly seen in the following CTDs: Rheumatoid arthritis, Sjögren's syndrome, SLE, systemic sclerosis and polymyositis-dermatomyositis.[18] Corticosteroids are highly efficacious for COP, but therapeutic options for constrictive bronchiolitis are disappointing. Prophylactic antibiotics and good pulmonary hygiene remains the mainstay of therapy for patients with bronchiectasis.

Idiopathic Cryptogenic Adult Bronchiolitis

It is a rare entity, the diagnosis of which is made on exclusion of other causes. Most patients are middle-aged women with symptoms usually of 6–24 months' duration. Lung biopsies show cellular constrictive bronchiolitis, often quite subtle. Early treatment with corticosteroids might be of benefit in some patients.[19-22]

Respiratory bronchiolitis is a specific form of smoking-related small airway disease.[23] Respiratory bronchiolitis usually occurs without symptoms or physiologic evidence of lung disease.[9] In some patients, respiratory bronchiolitis can cause symptomatic diffuse parenchymal lung infiltrates, a syndrome referred to as RB-ILD. Respiratory bronchiolitis per say does not require any treatment other than smoking cessation. Most studies suggest a favorable response to steroids in RB-ILD.

Diffuse aspiration bronchiolitis is a term used to define a clinical entity characterized by the chronic inflammation of bronchioles caused by recurrent aspiration of foreign particles.[24] Most previously described patients with this disorder have been elderly and bedridden.[24] This disorder can be seen in the adults of varying ages with gastroesophageal reflux disease that may be clinically occult.[25]

Drug-induced Bronchiolitis

Several drugs are reported to have an association with the development of bronchiolitis, usually with organizing pneumonia. A definite "cause and effect" relationship between these drugs and the development of BO is uncertain, because most reports are of single cases or small case series. Pure bronchiolitis obliterans, with airflow obstruction, has been associated with gold therapy.[26] It is difficult to state that these cases resulted from gold-induced airway injury, because patients with rheumatoid arthritis also are prone to develop pure bronchiolitis obliterans. Pulmonary complications of penicillamine therapy are uncommon, but may include BO and diffuse interstitial infiltrates.[27,28] This form of BO may be characterized by a rapidly deteriorating course and pulmonary insufficiency. Up to 25% cases of amiodarone lung disease may develop organizing pneumonia (BOOP pattern), which mimic an infectious pneumonitis. Treatment primarily consists of stopping the offending drug. Corticosteroid therapy (prednisone 40–60 mg a day, tapering over 2–6 months) can be life-saving in severe cases.

In Taiwan, an outbreak of rapidly progressive respiratory distress associated with consumption of uncooked *Sauropus androgynus,* a vegetable, claimed to be effective in weight control, has been reported. No effective treatment has been reported and the clinical response to prednisolone was limited.[29]

Bronchiolitis Associated with Organ Transplantation

Patients with bone marrow transplantation, heart-lung transplantation, or lung transplantation may develop BO as a chronic rejection phenomenon. This type of bronchiolitis remains the most common form of chronic rejection in patients with lung transplants, occurring in up to 50% of patients.[30] Constrictive bronchiolitis is also seen as a manifestation of graft-versus-host-disease in 10% of people who have received allogeneic bone marrow transplants.[31] This problem is a major threat to long-term survival in these transplant recipients and is the leading cause of late death after lung transplantation.[32]

Three major kinds of airway injury may be seen in allograft recipients: Acute (cellular) rejection, bronchiolitis obliterans and lymphocytic bronchitis. The lesions of BO are characterized by the features of constrictive bronchiolitis. Ultimately, smooth muscle cells, myofibroblasts and mature collagen obliterate the airways ("vanishing airways disease").[33,34] Occasionally, classic BOOP, with patchy organizing pneumonia and granulation tissue plugs extending into the alveolar ducts, is observed as the predominant lesion.

The pathogenesis of post-transplant bronchiolitis is a finely orchestrated process involving multiple events. Alloreactive injury to the bronchial epithelium is considered as the key pathogenetic mechanism. Other possible mechanisms like recurrent, persistent bacterial or viral infections; graft-versus-host disease or transplant rejection; impaired repair of injured airways due to bronchial artery ligation; altered mucociliary clearance; and recurrent aspiration also contribute to the development of BO.

Because of the patchy distribution of lesions and difficulties in obtaining adequate samples of bronchioles, confirming the diagnosis of constrictive bronchiolitis in transplant recipients by transbronchial lung biopsies is problematic. Thus, the phenomenon of progressive airway obstruction in lung transplant recipients is termed bronchiolitis obliterans syndrome (BOS), a clinical diagnosis, and is defined physiologically by a decrement in FEV_1 of 20% or more below a stable baseline.[32,35]

Most patients with BO progress to respiratory failure, and some patients develop bronchiectasis with frequent bacterial exacerbations. Aggressive therapy results in improvement of lung function in only 8–20% of patients.[36] Intensification of immunosuppressive therapy is the mainstay of therapy. The maintenance therapy with macrolides has demonstrated significant functional improvement in BOS,[37] which is used as an adjunct to immunosuppressive regimen.

Diffuse Panbronchiolitis

Diffuse panbronchiolitis is a progressive inflammatory disease characterized by chronic sinusitis, bronchiolitis and progressive obstructive airway disease that rapidly progresses to bronchiectasis, respiratory failure and death. While DPB is prevalent in Asian countries especially Japan, it has been rarely described among non-Asian patients.[38,39] It has a strong genetic predisposition with HLA-B54 common among the Japanese.[38] The precise etiology is unknown.

It usually affects people in the second to fifth decade of life. If DPB is left untreated, only 12–25% of patients survive for up to 10 years.

The plain CXR film reveals bilateral, diffuse, small nodular shadows predominantly in the lower field of the lung with hyperinflation. In advanced cases, ring shaped or tram-line shadows indicating bronchiectasis appear. HRCT is extremely useful for the detection of characteristic pulmonary lesions of DPB **(Figs 1A and B)**. In fact a system for grading these HRCT scan changes has been described.[40] Stage I is characterized by multiple centrilobular nodules usually of less than 5 mm in diameter, which are present at the end of bronchovascular branching structures. In stage II, these centrilobular nodules are seen connected to distal branching bronchovascular structures in a Y-shaped configuration, which provide the tree-in-bud appearance. Early-stage bronchiectasis is seen in stage III, while the presence of large cysts makes it stage IV. The diagnosis of DPB is often made on clinicoradiologic grounds by demonstrating its distinctive features and excluding other sinobronchial disorders. Lung biopsy shows transmural and peribronchiolar infiltration with lymphocytes and plasma cells. It is usually not necessary in countries where the disease is of high prevalence **(Box 7)**.

BOX 7 Diagnostic criteria for diffuse panbronchiolitis*

Major:
- Persistent cough, sputum and exertional dyspnea
- History suggestive of chronic paranasal sinusitis
- Bilateral small nodular shadows on plain chest radiograph or centrilobular nodules on high-resolution computed tomography (HRCT)

Minor:
- Coarse crackles
- FEV_1/FVC <70% and PaO_2 <80 mm Hg
- Cold hemagglutinin titer ≥64

Abbreviations: FEV1, forced expiratory volume in 1 second; FVC forced vital capacity; PaO_2, arterial oxygen tension
Definite diagnosis made if all three major and two out of three minor criteria present.
Source: *Modified from Kelly K, Hertz MI. Obliterative bronchiolitis. Clin Chest Med. 1997;18(2):319-38.

Erythromycin therapy has been shown to improve symptoms, lung functions, CT scan changes and survival rates in patients of DPB. Most patients are treated for more than 2 years until the resolution of symptoms and disappearance of centrilobular nodules. Treatment should be resumed if symptoms reappear after the cessation. Other members of the macrolide family are also efficacious in treating patients with DPB. An immune system modulating effect is more likely than antibacterial activity, as the mechanism of erythromycin therapy. It has been demonstrated by the ability of erythromycin to reduce neutrophil influx by decreasing levels of interleukins that are chemoattractants.[41]

Other Rare Forms of Primary Bronchiolar Disorders

A relatively new entity termed eosinophilic bronchiolitis has been described wherein the lung biopsy specimen demonstrated peri- and transmural bronchiolar infiltration by massive numbers of eosinophils along with plasma cells and degenerating eosinophils with Charcot-Leyden crystals within bronchiolar lumina, with minimal alveolar involvement.[42] Most cases of eosinophilic were earlier reported from Japan, but a few cases from the Western hemisphere have now been recognized.[42,43] Diagnosis is based on high blood and/or bronchoalveolar lavage eosinophil count; persistent airflow obstruction despite treatment with corticosteroids; and eosinophilic bronchiolitis at lung biopsy and/or computed tomography.[43] This disease responds fairly well to oral steroid therapy.

REFERENCES

1. Hansell DM. Small airways diseases: detection and insights with computed tomography. Eur Respir J. 2001;17(6):1294-313.
2. Müller NL, Miller RR. Diseases of the bronchioles: CT and histopathologic findings. Radiology. 1995;196(1):3-12.

3. Ryu JH, Myers JL, Swensen SJ. Bronchiolar disorders. Am J Respir Crit Care Med. 2003;168(11):1277-92.
4. Poletti V, Costabel U. Bronchiolar disorders: classification and diagnostic approach. Semin Respir Crit Care Med. 2003;24(5):457-64.
5. Devakonda A, Raoof S, Sung A, Travis WD, Naidich D. Bronchiolar disorders: a clinical-radiological diagnostic algorithm. Chest. 2010;137(4):938-51.
6. Akira M, Suganuma N. Acute and subacute chemical-induced lung injuries: HRCT findings. Eur J Radiol. 2014;83:1461-9.
7. Poletti V, Zompatori M, Cancellieri A. Clinical spectrum of adult chronic bronchiolitis. Sarcoidosis Vasc Diffuse Lung Dis. 1999;16(2):183-96.
8. Stewart S, Fishbein MC, Snell GI, Berry GJ, Boehler A, Burke MM, et al. Revision of the 1996 working formulation for the standardization of nomenclature in the diagnosis of lung rejection. J Heart Lung Transplant. 2007;26(12):1229-42.
9. Niewoehner DE, Kleinerman J, Rice DB. Pathologic changes in the peripheral airways of young cigarette smokers. N Engl J Med. 1974;291(15):755-8.
10. Prezant DJ, Weiden M, Banauch GI, McGuinness G, Rom WN, Aldrich TK, et al. Cough and bronchial responsiveness in firefighters at the World Trade Center site. N Engl J Med. 2002;347(11):806-15.
11. Sieminska A, Kuziemski K. Respiratory bronchiolitis-interstitial lung disease. Orphanet J Rare Dis. 2014;11:106.
12. Thompson BR, Hodgson YM, Kotsimbos T, Liakakos P, Enjis MJ, Snell GI, et al. Bronchiolitis obliterans syndrome leads to a functional deterioration of the acinus post lung transplant. Thorax. 2014;69:487-8.
13. Colby TV. Bronchiolitis. Pathologic considerations. Am J Clin Pathol. 1998;109(1):101-9.
14. Pickles RJ, Devincenzo JP. Respiratory syncytial virus (RSV) and its protensity causing bronchiolitis. J Pathol. 2015;235:288-76.
15. Marinopoulos GC, Huddle KR, Wainwright H. Obliterative bronchiolitis: virus induced? Chest. 1991;99(1):243-5.
16. Davison C, Ventre KM, Luchetti M, Randolph AG. Efficacy of interventions for bronchiolitis in critically ill infants: a systematic review and meta-analysis. Pediatr Crit Care Med. 2004;5(5):482-9.
17. King VJ, Viswanathan M, Bordley WC, Jackman AM, Sutton SF, Lohr KN, et al. Pharmacologic treatment of bronchiolitis in infants and children: a systematic review. Arch Pediatr Adolesc Med. 2004;158(2):127-37.
18. White ES, Tazelaar HD, Lynch JP. Bronchiolar complications of connective tissue diseases. Semin Respir Crit Care Med. 2003;24(5):543-66.
19. Turton CW, Williams G, Green M. Cryptogenic obliterative bronchiolitis in adults. Thorax. 1981;36(11):805-10.
20. Dorinsky PM, Davis WB, Lucas JG, Weiland JE, Gadek JE, et al. Adult bronchiolitis. Evaluation by bronchoalveolar lavage and response to prednisone therapy. Chest. 1985;88(1):58-63.
21. Kindt GC, Weiland JE, Davis WB, Gadek JE, Dorinsky PM. Bronchiolitis in adults. A reversible cause of airway obstruction associated with airway neutrophils and neutrophil products. Am Rev Respir Dis. 1989;140(2):483-92.
22. Kraft M, Mortenson RL, Colby TV, Newman L, Waldron JA Jr, King TE Jr. Cryptogenic constrictive bronchiolitis. A clinicopathologic study. Am Rev Respir Dis. 1993;148(4 Pt 1):1093-101.
23. Vassallo R. Diffuse lung diseases in cigarette smokers. Semin Respir Crit Care Med. 2012;33(5):533-42.
24. Matsuse T, Oka T, Kida K, Fukuchi Y. Importance of diffuse aspiration bronchiolitis caused by chronic occult aspiration in the elderly. Chest. 1996;110(5):1289-93.
25. Ryu JH. Classification and approach to bronchiolar diseases. Curr Opin Pulm Med. 2006;12(2):145-51.
26. Holness L, Tenenbaum J, Cooter NB, Grossman RF. Fatal bronchiolitis obliterans associated with chrysotherapy. Ann Rheum Dis. 1983;42(5):593-6.
27. Yam LY, Wong R. Bronchiolitis obliterans and rheumatoid arthritis. Report of a case in a Chinese patient on d-penicillamine and review of the literature. Ann Acad Med Singapore. 1993;22(3):365-8.
28. Turner-Warwick M. Adverse reactions affecting the lung: possible association with D-penicillamine. J Rheumatol Suppl. 1981;7:166-8.
29. Lai RS, Chiang AA, Wu MT, Wang JS, Lai NS, Lu JY, et al. Outbreak of bronchiolitis obliterans associated with consumption of Sauropus androgynus in Taiwan. Lancet. 1996;348(9020):83-5.
30. Burke CM, Theodore J, Dawkins KD, Yousem SA, Blank N, Billingham ME, et al. Post-transplant obliterative bronchiolitis and other late lung sequelae in human heart-lung transplantation. Chest. 1984;86(6):824-9.
31. Estenne M, Hertz MI. Bronchiolitis obliterans after human lung transplantation. Am J Respir Crit Care Med. 2002;166(4):440-4.
32. Estenne M, Maurer JR, Boehler A, Egan JJ, Frost A, Hertz M, et al. Bronchiolitis obliterans syndrome 2001: an update of the diagnostic criteria. J Heart Lung Transplant. 2002;21(3):297-310.
33. Paradis I, Yousem S, Griffith B. Airway obstruction and bronchiolitis obliterans after lung transplantation. Clin Chest Med. 1993;14(4):751-63.
34. Kelly K, Hertz MI. Obliterative bronchiolitis. Clin Chest Med. 1997;18(2):319-38.
35. Cooper JD, Billingham M, Egan T, Hertz MI, Higenbottam T, Lynch J, et al. A working formulation for the standardization of nomenclature and for clinical staging of chronic dysfunction in lung allografts. International Society for Heart and Lung Transplantation. J Heart Lung Transplant. 1993;12(5):713-6.
36. Soubani AO, Uberti JP. Bronchiolitis obliterans following haematopoietic stem cell transplantation. Eur Respir J. 2007;29(5):1007-19.
37. Gerhardt SG, McDyer JF, Girgis RE, Conte JV, Yang SC, Orens JB, et al. Maintenance azithromycin therapy for bronchiolitis obliterans syndrome: results of a pilot study. Am J Respir Crit Care Med. 2003;168(1):121-5.
38. Tsang KW, Lam W, Ip M, Tanaka E. Diffuse panbronchiolitis in the United States. Am J Respir Crit Care Med. 1997;155(6):2114.
39. Tsang KW, Ooi CG, Ip MS, Lam WK, Ngan H, Chan EY, et al. Clinical profiles of Chinese patients with diffuse panbronchiolitis. Thorax. 1998;53(4):274-80.
40. Akira M, Kitatani F, Lee YS, Kita N, Yamamoto S, Higashihara T, et al. Diffuse panbronchiolitis: evaluation with high-resolution CT. Radiology. 1988;168(2):433-8.
41. Nagai H, Shishido H, Yoneda R, Yamaguchi E, Tamura A, Kurashima A, et al. Long-term low-dose administration of erythromycin to patients with diffuse panbronchiolitis. Respiration. 1991;58(3-4):145-9.
42. Takayanagi N, Kanazawa M, Kawabata Y, Colby TV. Chronic bronchiolitis with associated eosinophilic lung disease (eosinophilic bronchiolitis). Respiration. 2001;68(3):319-22.
43. Cordier JF, Cottin V, Khouatra C, Revel D, Proust C, Freymond N, et al. Hypereosinophilic obliterative bronchiolitis: a distinct, unrecognized syndrome. Eur Respir J. 2013;41(5):1126-34.